CAMPBELL'S
UROLOGY

Edited by

Patrick C. Walsh, M.D.

David Hall McConnell Professor and Director
The Johns Hopkins University School of Medicine
Urologist-in-Chief
Brady Urological Institute
The Johns Hopkins Hospital
Baltimore, Maryland

Alan B. Retik, M.D.

Professor of Surgery (Urology)
Harvard Medical School
Chief, Department of Urology
Children's Hospital
Boston, Massachusetts

E. Darracott Vaughan, Jr., M.D.

James J. Colt Professor of Urology
Cornell University Medical College
Urologist-in-Chief
The New York Hospital–Cornell Medical Center
New York, New York

Alan J. Wein, M.D.

Professor and Chair, Division of Urology
University of Pennsylvania School of Medicine
Chief of Urology
University of Pennsylvania Medical Center
Philadelphia, Pennsylvania

CAMPBELL'S UROLOGY

Seventh Edition

VOLUME

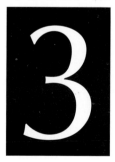

3

W.B. SAUNDERS COMPANY
A Division of Harcourt Brace & Company
Philadelphia   London   Toronto   Montreal   Sydney   Tokyo

W.B. SAUNDERS COMPANY
A Division of Harcourt Brace & Company

The Curtis Center
Independence Square West
Philadelphia, Pennsylvania 19106

Library of Congress Cataloging-in-Publication Data

Campbell's Urology / [edited by] Patrick C. Walsh [et al.].—7th ed.

    p.   cm.

Includes bibliographical references and index.

ISBN 0–7216–4461–9

1. Urology.   I. Campbell, Meredith F. (Meredith Fairfax).   II. Walsh, Patrick C.
  [DNLM: 1. Urogenital Diseases.   2. Urology—methods.
  WJ 100 C192 1997]

RC871.C33 1998 616.6—dc21

DNLM/DLC   96–40836

Volume 1 ISBN 0–7216–4462–7
Volume 2 ISBN 0–7216–4463–5
Volume 3 ISBN 0–7216–4464–3
Set   ISBN 0–7216–4461–9

Campbell's Urology

Copyright © 1998, 1992, 1986, 1978, 1970, 1963 by W.B. Saunders Company

Copyright © 1954 by W.B. Saunders Company

Copyright renewed 1982 by Evelyn S. Campbell

All rights reserved. No part of this publication may be reproduced or transmitted in any form or by any means, electronic or mechanical, including photocopy, recording, or any information storage and retrieval system, without permission in writing from the publisher.

Printed in the United States of America

Last digit is the print number: 9   8   7   6   5   4   3   2   1

CONTRIBUTORS

Mark C. Adams, M.D.
Associate Professor of Urology and Pediatrics, Vanderbilt University School of Medicine, Vanderbilt University and The Vanderbilt University Children's Hospital, Nashville, Tennessee
AUGMENTATION CYSTOPLASTY

Ahmed Alkhunaizi, M.D.
Renal Fellow, University of Colorado School of Medicine, Denver, Colorado
ETIOLOGY, PATHOGENESIS, AND MANAGEMENT OF RENAL FAILURE

Rodney A. Appell, M.D.
Head, Section of Voiding Dysfunction and Female Urology, Department of Urology, The Cleveland Clinic Foundation, Cleveland, Ohio
PERIURETHRAL INJECTION THERAPY

Anthony Atala, M.D.
Assistant Professor, Harvard Medical School; Assistant in Surgery, Children's Hospital, Boston, Massachusetts
VESICOURETERAL REFLUX AND MEGAURETER

David M. Barrett, M.D.
Professor and Chair, Department of Urology, Mayo Clinic, Rochester, Minnesota
IMPLANTATION OF THE ARTIFICIAL GENITOURINARY SPHINCTER IN MEN AND WOMEN

John M. Barry, M.D.
Professor of Surgery and Chairman, Division of Urology and Renal Transplantation, The Oregon Health Sciences University; Staff Surgeon, University Hospital, Portland, Oregon
RENAL TRANSPLANTATION

Stuart B. Bauer, M.D.
Associate Professor of Urology, Harvard Medical School; Senior Associate in Surgery (Urology), The Children's Hospital, Boston, Massachusetts
ANOMALIES OF THE KIDNEY AND URETEROPELVIC JUNCTION
NEUROGENIC DYSFUNCTION OF THE LOWER URINARY TRACT IN CHILDREN

Arie Belldegrun, M.D.
Professor of Urology, Chief, Division of Urologic Oncology, and Director of Urological Research, Department of Urology, University of California, Los Angeles, School of Medicine, Los Angeles, California
RENAL TUMORS

Mitchell C. Benson, M.D.
Professor of Urology, Columbia University College of Physicians and Surgeons; Director, Urologic Oncology, Columbia-Presbyterian Medical Center, New York, New York
CONTINENT URINARY DIVERSION

Richard E. Berger, M.D.
Professor of Urology, University of Washington, Seattle, Washington
SEXUALLY TRANSMITTED DISEASES: THE CLASSIC DISEASES

Jerry G. Blaivas, M.D., FACS
Clinical Professor of Urology, Cornell University Medical College, The New York Hospital–Cornell Medical Center, New York, New York
URINARY INCONTINENCE: PATHOPHYSIOLOGY, EVALUATION, TREATMENT OVERVIEW, AND NONSURGICAL MANAGEMENT

David A. Bloom, M.D.
Professor of Surgery and Chief of Pediatric
Urology, University of Michigan Medical
School; Chief of Pediatric Urology, Mott
Children's Hospital, Ann Arbor, Michigan
SURGERY OF THE SCROTUM AND TESTIS IN
CHILDREN

Jon D. Blumenfeld, M.D.
Associate Professor of Medicine, Cornell
University Medical College, New York, New
York; Associate Attending in Medicine,
Department of Medicine, The New York
Hospital–Cornell Medical Center, New York,
New York
RENAL PHYSIOLOGY
THE ADRENALS

Michael K. Brawer, M.D.
Professor, University of Washington; Chief,
Urology Section, Seattle Veterans
Administration Medical Center, Seattle,
Washington
ULTRASONOGRAPHY OF THE PROSTATE AND
BIOPSY

Charles B. Brendler, M.D.
Professor and Chief, Section of Urology,
University of Chicago Hospitals and Pritzker
School of Medicine, Chicago, Illinois
EVALUATION OF THE UROLOGIC PATIENT:
HISTORY, PHYSICAL EXAMINATION, AND
URINALYSIS

Gregory Broderick, M.D., FACS
Associate Professor of Surgery in Urology,
University of Pennsylvania School of
Medicine; Director of the Center for the Study
of Male Sexual Dysfunction, University of
Pennsylvania Health Systems, Philadelphia,
Pennsylvania
EVALUATION AND NONSURGICAL
MANAGEMENT OF ERECTILE DYSFUNCTION
AND PRIAPISM

James D. Brooks, M.D.
Instructor of Urology, Department of Urology,
Johns Hopkins Medical Institute, Baltimore,
Maryland
ANATOMY OF THE LOWER URINARY TRACT
AND MALE GENITALIA

H. Ballentine Carter, M.D.
Associate Professor of Urology and Oncology,
The Johns Hopkins University School of
Medicine; Department of Urology, The Johns
Hopkins Hospital and Bayview Medical
Center, Baltimore, Maryland
INSTRUMENTATION AND ENDOSCOPY
DIAGNOSIS AND STAGING OF PROSTATE
CANCER

William Catalona, M.D.
Professor and Director, Division of Urology,
Washington University School of Medicine, St.
Louis, Missouri
UROTHELIAL TUMORS OF THE URINARY TRACT

Thomas S.K. Chang, Ph.D.
Associate Professor of Urology, Johns Hopkins
School of Medicine, Baltimore, Maryland
PHYSIOLOGY OF MALE REPRODUCTION: THE
TESTIS, EPIDIDYMIS, AND DUCTUS DEFERENS

Michael P. Chetner, M.D.
Associate Clinical Professor of Surgery and
Oncology, University of Alberta; Director,
Division of Urology, University of Alberta
Hospital, Edmonton, Alberta, Canada
ULTRASONOGRAPHY OF THE PROSTATE AND
BIOPSY

Robert L. Chevalier, M.D.
Genentech Professor of Pediatrics, University of
Virginia School of Medicine; Director of
Research, Children's Medical Center,
University of Virginia, Health Sciences Center,
Charlottesville, Virginia
RENAL FUNCTION IN THE FETUS, NEONATE,
AND CHILD

Ashok Chopra, M.D.
Fellow of Reconstruction, Neurourology and
Female Urology, Center for Health Sciences,
University of California School of Medicine,
Los Angeles, California
VAGINAL RECONSTRUCTIVE SURGERY FOR
INCONTINENCE AND PROLAPSE

Ralph V. Clayman, M.D.
Professor of Urologic Surgery and Radiology,
Washington University School of Medicine, St.
Louis, Missouri
ENDOUROLOGY OF THE UPPER URINARY
TRACT: PERCUTANEOUS RENAL AND
URETERAL PROCEDURES

Donald S. Coffey, Ph.D.
Professor of Urology, Oncology, Pharmacology, and Experimental Therapeutics, Department of Urology, The Johns Hopkins Medical Institute, Baltimore, Maryland
THE MOLECULAR BIOLOGY, ENDOCRINOLOGY, AND PHYSIOLOGY OF THE PROSTATE AND SEMINAL VESICLES

Arnold Colodny, M.D.
Clinical Professor of Surgery, Harvard Medical School; Senior Surgeon and Associate Director of Urology, Boston Children's Hospital, Boston, Massachusetts
SURGERY OF THE SCROTUM AND TESTIS IN CHILDREN

Carlos Cordon-Cardo, M.D., Ph.D.
Associate Professor, Cornell University Medical Center; Director, Division of Molecular Pathology, Memorial Sloan-Kettering Cancer Center, New York, New York
AN OVERVIEW OF CANCER BIOLOGY

Jean B. deKernion, M.D.
Professor of Surgery/Urology, University of California, Los Angeles, School of Medicine; The Fran and Ray Stark Professor of Urology and Chairman, Department of Urology, UCLA Medical Center, Los Angeles, California
RENAL TUMORS

Charles J. Devine, M.D.
Professor of Urology, Eastern Virginia Medical School, Norfolk, Virginia
SURGERY OF THE PENIS AND URETHRA

William C. De Wolf, M.D.
Professor of Surgery, Harvard Medical School; Urologist-in-Chief, Division of Urology, Beth Israel Deaconess Medical Center, Boston, Massachusetts
PRINCIPLES OF MOLECULAR GENETICS

David A. Diamond, M.D.
Associate Professor of Surgery (Urology), Harvard Medical School; Associate in Surgery (Urology), Children's Hospital, Boston, Massachusetts
NEONATAL UROLOGIC EMERGENCIES

Giulio J. D'Angio, M.D.
Professor of Radiation Oncology Emeritus, University of Pennsylvania School of Medicine, Philadelphia, Pennsylvania
PEDIATRIC ONCOLOGY

George W. Drach, M.D.
Professor of Urology, University of Texas, Southwestern School of Medicine, Dallas, Texas
URINARY LITHIASIS: ETIOLOGY, DIAGNOSIS, AND MEDICAL MANAGEMENT

John W. Duckett, M.D.
Professor of Urology, University of Pennsylvania; Director of Pediatric Urology, Children's Hospital of Philadelphia, Philadelphia, Pennsylvania
HYPOSPADIAS

James A. Eastham, M.D.
Assistant Professor of Urology and Director of Urologic Oncology, Louisiana State University School of Medicine–Shreveport, Shreveport, Louisiana
RADICAL PROSTATECTOMY

Charles L. Edelstein, M.B., Ch.B., M.Med.
Renal Fellow, University of Colorado School of Medicine, Denver, Colorado; Senior Consultant Physician, Renal Unit, Department of Internal Medicine, University of Stellenbosch and The Tygerberg Hospital, Tygerberg, South Africa
ETIOLOGY, PATHOGENESIS, AND MANAGEMENT OF RENAL FAILURE

Mario A. Eisenberger, M.D.
Associate Professor of Oncology and Urology, Johns Hopkins Medical Institute, Baltimore, Maryland
CHEMOTHERAPY FOR HORMONE-RESISTANT PROSTATE CANCER

Jack S. Elder, M.D.
Professor of Urology and Pediatrics, Case Western Reserve University School of Medicine; Director of Pediatric Urology, Rainbow Babies and Children's Hospital, Cleveland, Ohio
CONGENITAL ANOMALIES OF THE GENITALIA

Jonathan I. Epstein, M.D.
Professor of Pathology, Urology, and Oncology, Johns Hopkins University School of Medicine; Associate Director of Surgical Pathology, The Johns Hopkins Hospital, Baltimore, Maryland
PATHOLOGY OF ADENOCARCINOMA OF THE PROSTATE

Audrey E. Evans, M.D.
Professor of Pediatrics, University of
   Pennsylvania School of Medicine,
   Philadelphia, Pennsylvania
   PEDIATRIC ONCOLOGY

William R. Fair, M.D.
Professor of Urology, Cornell University Medical
   College; Chief of Urology and Vice-Chairman,
   Department of Surgery, Memorial Sloan-
   Kettering Cancer Center, New York, New York
   AN OVERVIEW OF CANCER BIOLOGY

Diane Felsen, Ph.D.
Associate Research Professor of Pharmacology in
   Urology, Cornell University Medical College,
   The New York Hospital–Cornell Medical
   Center, New York, New York
   PATHOPHYSIOLOGY OF URINARY TRACT
      OBSTRUCTION

Jeffrey Forman, M.D.
Professor of Radiation Oncology, Wayne State
   University School of Medicine, Detroit,
   Michigan
   RADIOTHERAPY AND CRYOTHERAPY FOR
      PROSTATE CANCER

Jenny J. Franke, M.D.
Assistant Professor, Department of Urologic
   Surgery, Vanderbilt University, Nashville,
   Tennessee
   SURGERY OF THE URETER

John P. Gearhart, M.D.
Professor of Pediatric Urology and Pediatrics,
   The Johns Hopkins University School of
   Medicine; Director of Pediatric Urology, The
   Johns Hopkins Hospital and Johns Hopkins
   Children's Center, Baltimore, Maryland
   EXSTROPHY-EPISPADIAS COMPLEX AND
      BLADDER ANOMALIES

Robert P. Gibbons, M.D.
Chief of Staff, Section of Urology and Renal
   Transplantation, Virginia Mason Medical
   Center; Clinical Professor of Urology,
   University of Washington, Seattle, Washington
   RADICAL PERINEAL PROSTATECTOMY

Kenneth I. Glassberg, M.D.
Professor of Urology, State University of New
   York, Health Science Center at Brooklyn;
   Director, Divisions of Pediatric Urology at

University Hospital of Brooklyn, Kings County
   Hospital Center, Long Island College Hospital,
   Brooklyn; and Staten Island University
   Hospital, Staten Island, New York
   RENAL DYSPLASIA AND CYSTIC DISEASE OF
      THE KIDNEY

Marc Goldstein, M.D.
Professor of Urology, Cornell University Medical
   College; Staff Scientist, Center for Biomedical
   Research, The Population Council; Attending
   Urologist and Director, Center for Male
   Reproductive Medicine and Microsurgery,
   Department of Urology, The New York
   Hospital–Cornell Medical Center, New York,
   New York
   SURGICAL MANAGEMENT OF MALE
      INFERTILITY AND OTHER SCROTAL
      DISORDERS

Edmond T. Gonzales, Jr., M.D.
Professor of Urology, Scott Department of
   Urology, Baylor College of Medicine; Head,
   Department of Surgery, and Chief, Urology
   Service, Texas Children's Hospital, Houston,
   Texas
   POSTERIOR URETHRAL VALVES AND OTHER
      URETHRAL ANOMALIES

Rafael Gosalbez, M.D.
Assistant Professor of Urology and Pediatrics and
   Chief of Pediatric Urology, Jackson Memorial
   Hospital, University of Miami, Miami, Florida
   NEONATAL UROLOGIC EMERGENCIES

James E. Gow, M.D., Ch.M., FRCS
Late Clinical Lecturer, University of Liverpool,
   Liverpool, United Kingdom
   GENITOURINARY TUBERCULOSIS

David Grignon, M.D.
Director of Anatomic Pathology, Harper Hospital;
   Associate Professor of Pathology, Detroit,
   Michigan
   RADIOTHERAPY AND CRYOTHERAPY FOR
      PROSTATE CANCER

Frederick A. Gulmi, M.D.
Clinical Assistant Professor of Urology, State
   University of New York Health Sciences
   Center at Brooklyn; Associate Attending,
   Brookdale University Hospital and Medical
   Center, Brooklyn, New York
   PATHOPHYSIOLOGY OF URINARY TRACT
      OBSTRUCTION

Philip Hanno, M.D.
Professor and Chairman, Department of Urology,
Temple University School of Medicine,
Philadelphia, Pennsylvania
INTERSTITIAL CYSTITIS AND RELATED
DISEASES

W. Hardy Hendren, M.D., FACS, FAAP, FRCS(I)Hon.
Robert E. Gross Professor of Surgery, Harvard
Medical School; Chief of Surgery,
Massachusetts General Hospital; Visiting
Surgeon, Children's Hospital, Boston,
Massachusetts
CLOACAL MALFORMATIONS
URINARY UNDIVERSION:
REFUNCTIONALIZATION OF THE PREVIOUSLY
DIVERTED URINARY TRACT

Terry W. Hensle, M.D.
Professor of Urology, Columbia University,
College of Physicians and Surgeons; Director
of Pediatric Urology, Babies and Children's
Hospital of New York, New York, New York
SURGICAL MANAGEMENT OF INTERSEXUALITY

Dianne M. Heritz, M.D., FRCSC
Lecturer, University of Toronto, Women's
College Hospital, Toronto, Ontario, Canada
URINARY INCONTINENCE: PATHOPHYSIOLOGY,
EVALUATION, TREATMENT OVERVIEW, AND
NONSURGICAL MANAGEMENT

Harry W. Herr, M.D.
Associate Professor, Department of Urology,
Cornell University Medical College; Associate
Attending Surgeon, Urology Service,
Department of Surgery, Memorial Sloan-
Kettering Cancer Center, New York, New York
SURGERY OF PENILE AND URETHRAL
CARCINOMA

Warren D. W. Heston, Ph.D.
Director, George M. O'Brien Urology Research
for Prostate Cancer, Memorial Sloan-Kettering
Cancer Center, New York, New York
AN OVERVIEW OF CANCER BIOLOGY

Stuart S. Howards, M.D.
Professor of Urology and Physiology, University
of Virginia, Charlottesville, Virginia
MALE INFERTILITY
RENAL FUNCTION IN THE FETUS, NEONATE,
AND CHILD

Jeffrey L. Huffman, M.D., M.H.A.
Professor of Urology, School of Medicine, and
Associate Vice President for Health Affairs,
University of Southern California, Los
Angeles, California
URETEROSCOPY

Robert D. Jeffs, M.D.
Professor of Pediatric Urology and Pediatrics,
The Johns Hopkins University School of
Medicine, The Johns Hopkins Hospital, and
Johns Hopkins Children's Center, Baltimore,
Maryland
EXSTROPHY-EPISPADIAS COMPLEX AND
BLADDER ANOMALIES

Gerald H. Jordan, M.D.
Professor of Urology, Eastern Virginia Medical
School, Norfolk, Virginia
SURGERY OF THE PENIS AND URETHRA

John N. Kabalin, M.D.
Assistant Professor of Urology, Stanford
University School of Medicine, Stanford,
California
SURGICAL ANATOMY OF THE
RETROPERITONEUM, KIDNEYS, AND URETERS

Louis R. Kavoussi, M.D.
Associate Professor and Director, Division of
Endourology, Brady Urological Institute, The
Johns Hopkins School of Medicine; Chief of
Urology, Johns Hopkins Bayview Medical
Center, Baltimore, Maryland
LAPAROSCOPY IN CHILDREN AND ADULTS

Michael A. Keating, M.D.
Private Practice, Orlando, Florida
VESICOURETERAL REFLUX AND MEGAURETER

William A. Kennedy II, M.D.
Fellow in Pediatric Urology, Children's Hospital
of Philadelphia, Philadelphia, Pennsylvania
SURGICAL MANAGEMENT OF INTERSEXUALITY

Joseph M. Khoury, M.D.
Associate Professor of Surgery and Director,
Urophysiology Division of Urology,
Department of Surgery, University of North
Carolina School of Medicine, Chapel Hill,
North Carolina
RETROPUBIC SUSPENSION SURGERY FOR
FEMALE SPHINCTERIC INCONTINENCE

Stephen A. Koff, M.D.
Professor of Surgery, The Ohio State University
Medical Center; Chief, Section of Urology,
Children's Hospital, Columbus, Ohio
ENURESIS

Karl J. Kreder, M.D.
Associate Professor of Urology, Department of
Urology, University of Iowa Hospital and
Clinics, Iowa City, Iowa
THE NEUROUROLOGIC EVALUATION

John N. Krieger, M.D.
Professor, Department of Urology, University of
Washington School of Medicine; Attending
Surgeon, University of Washington Medical
Center, Seattle Veterans Administration
Medical Center, Harborview Medical Center,
and Children's Orthopedic Hospital, Seattle,
Washington
ACQUIRED IMMUNODEFICIENCY SYNDROME
AND RELATED CONDITIONS

Elroy D. Kursh, M.D.
Department of Urology, Cleveland Clinic,
Cleveland, Ohio
EXTRINSIC OBSTRUCTION OF THE URETER

Gary E. Leach, M.D.
Associate Clinical Professor of Urology,
University of California, Los Angeles; Chief of
Urology, Kaiser-Permanente Medical Center,
Los Angeles, California
SURGERY FOR CERVICOVAGINAL AND
URETHROVAGINAL FISTULA AND URETHRAL
DIVERTICULUM

Herbert Lepor, M.D.
Professor and Chairman, Department of Urology,
and Professor, Department of Pharmacology,
New York University School of Medicine;
Urologist-in-Chief, New York University
Medical Center, New York, New York
NATURAL HISTORY, EVALUATION, AND
NONSURGICAL MANAGEMENT OF BENIGN
PROSTATIC HYPERPLASIA

Ronald Lewis, M.D.
Professor of Surgery (Urology), Medical College
of Georgia; Chief, Section of Urology, Medical
College of Georgia Hospital, Augusta, Georgia
SURGERY FOR ERECTILE DYSFUNCTION

John A. Libertino, M.D.
Clinical Assistant Professor, Harvard Medical
School, Boston; Chairman of Urology, Lahey
Hitchcock Medical Center, Burlington,
Massachusetts
RENOVASCULAR SURGERY

Mark R. Licht, M.D.
Head, Section of Sexual Dysfunction, and Staff,
Department of Urology, Cleveland Clinic
Florida, Ft. Lauderdale, Florida
IMPLANTATION OF THE ARTIFICIAL
GENITOURINARY SPHINCTER IN MEN AND
WOMEN

Peter Littrup, M.D.
Associate Professor of Radiology, Urology, and
Radiation Oncology, Wayne State University
School of Medicine, Detroit, Michigan
RADIOTHERAPY AND CRYOTHERAPY FOR
PROSTATE CANCER

Tom F. Lue, M.D.
Professor of Urology, University of California
School of Medicine, San Francisco, California
PHYSIOLOGY OF PENILE ERECTION AND
PATHOPHYSIOLOGY OF ERECTILE
DYSFUNCTION AND PRIAPISM
EVALUATION AND NONSURGICAL
MANAGEMENT OF ERECTILE DYSFUNCTION
AND PRIAPISM

Donald F. Lynch, Jr., M.D.
Associate Professor, Department of Urology,
Eastern Virginia Medical School, Norfolk,
Virginia
TUMORS OF THE PENIS

Max Maizels, M.D.
Professor of Urology, Northwestern University
School of Medicine; Attending Pediatric
Urologist, The Children's Memorial Hospital,
Chicago, Illinois
NORMAL AND ANOMALOUS DEVELOPMENT OF
THE URINARY TRACT

James Mandell, M.D.
Professor of Surgery and Pediatrics and Chief,
Division of Urology, Albany Medical College,
Albany, New York
PERINATAL UROLOGY
SEXUAL DIFFERENTIATION: NORMAL AND
ABNORMAL

David J. Margolis, M.D.
Assistant Professor of Dermatology, University of
Pennsylvania School of Medicine,
Philadelphia, Pennsylvania
COLOR ATLAS OF GENITAL DERMATOLOGY
CUTANEOUS DISEASES OF THE MALE
EXTERNAL GENITALIA

Fray F. Marshall, M.D.
Professor of Urology and Professor of Oncology,
The Johns Hopkins University School of
Medicine; Director, Division of Adult Urology,
James Buchanan Brady Urological Institute,
The Johns Hopkins Medical Institute,
Baltimore, Maryland
SURGERY OF THE BLADDER

Thomas V. Martin, M.D.
Yale–New Haven Medical Center, New Haven,
Connecticut
SHOCK-WAVE LITHOTRIPSY

John D. McConnell, M.D.
Professor and Chairman, Department of Urology,
University of Texas Southwestern Medical
Center, Dallas, Texas
EPIDEMIOLOGY, ETIOLOGY, PATHOPHYSIOLOGY,
AND DIAGNOSIS OF BENIGN PROSTATIC
HYPERPLASIA

David L. McCullough, M.D.
William H. Boyce Professor and Chairman of
Department of Urology, Bowman Gray School
of Medicine of Wake Forest University; Chief
of Urology, North Carolina Baptist/Wake
Forest University Medical Center, Winston-
Salem, North Carolina
MINIMALLY INVASIVE TREATMENT OF BENIGN
PROSTATIC HYPERPLASIA

W. Scott McDougal, M.D.
Walter S. Kerr, Jr., Professor of Urology, Harvard
Medical School; Chief of Urology,
Massachusetts General Hospital, Boston,
Massachusetts
USE OF INTESTINAL SEGMENTS AND URINARY
DIVERSION

Elspeth M. McDougall, M.D., FRCSC
Associate Professor of Urologic Surgery,
Washington University School of Medicine, St.
Louis, Missouri
ENDOUROLOGY OF THE UPPER URINARY
TRACT: PERCUTANEOUS RENAL AND
URETERAL PROCEDURES

Edward J. McGuire, M.D.
Professor and Director, Division of Urology, The
University of Texas Health Science Center,
Houston, Texas
PUBOVAGINAL SLINGS

Mani Menon, M.D.
Professor and Director, Division of Urology,
University of Massachusetts, Worcester,
Massachusetts
URINARY LITHIASIS: ETIOLOGY, DIAGNOSIS,
AND MEDICAL MANAGEMENT

Edwin M. Meares, Jr., M.D.
Professor of Urology, Emeritus, Tufts University
School of Medicine; Chairman, Department of
Urology (Retired), New England Medical
Center, Boston, Massachusetts
PROSTATITIS AND RELATED DISORDERS

Winston K. Mebust, M.D.
Valk Professor of Surgery/Urology and
Chairman, Section of Urologic Surgery,
University of Kansas Medical Center, Kansas
City, Kansas
TRANSURETHRAL SURGERY

Edward M. Messing, M.D.
Winfield W. Scott Professor of Urology and
Chairman, Department of Urology, University
of Rochester Medical Center, Rochester, New
York
UROTHELIAL TUMORS OF THE URINARY TRACT

James E. Montie, M.D.
Professor of Urology, University of Michigan,
Ann Arbor, Michigan
RADIOTHERAPY AND CRYOTHERAPY FOR
PROSTATE CANCER

Randall E. Morris, M.D.
Research Professor of Cardiothoracic Surgery and
Director of Transplantation Immunology in the
Department of Cardiothoracic Surgery,
Stanford University School of Medicine,
Stanford, California
TRANSPLANTATION IMMUNOBIOLOGY

Stephen Y. Nakada, M.D.
Assistant Professor of Surgery (Urology) and
Head, Section of Endourology and Stone
Disease, University of Wisconsin Medical
School and University of Wisconsin Hospital
and Clinics, Madison, Wisconsin

ENDOUROLOGY OF THE UPPER URINARY
TRACT: PERCUTANEOUS RENAL AND
URETERAL PROCEDURES

H. Norman Noe, M.D.
Professor of Urology and Chief of Pediatric
Urology, University of Tennessee, Memphis;
Chief of Pediatric Urology, LeBonheur
Children's Medical Center, Memphis,
Tennessee
RENAL DISEASE IN CHILDHOOD

Andrew C. Novick, M.D.
Professor of Surgery (Urology) Ohio State
University School of Medicine; Chairman,
Department of Urology, Cleveland Clinic
Foundation, Cleveland, Ohio
SURGERY OF THE KIDNEY

Helen E. O'Connell, M.D.
Senior Lecturer, University of Melbourne,
Department of Surgery; Attending Urologist,
Royal Melbourne Hospital, Melbourne,
Australia
PUBOVAGINAL SLINGS

Joseph E. Oesterling, M.D.
Professor and Urologist-in-Chief and Director,
The Michigan Prostate Institute, University of
Michigan, Ann Arbor, Michigan
RETROPUBIC AND SUPRAPUBIC
PROSTATECTOMY

Carl A. Olsson, M.D.
John K. Lattimer Professor and Chairman,
Department of Urology, College of Physicians
and Surgeons of Columbia University;
Director, Squier Urologic Clinic at The
Columbia Presbyterian Hospital, New York,
New York
CONTINENT URINARY DIVERSION

Nicholas Papanicolaou, M.D.
Professor of Clinical Radiology, Cornell
University College of Medicine; Chief,
Division of Abdominal Imaging, The New
York Hospital–Cornell Medical Center, New
York, New York
URINARY TRACT IMAGING AND INTERVENTION:
BASIC PRINCIPLES

Alan W. Partin, M.D., Ph.D.
Associate Professor of Urology, Department of
Urology, The Johns Hopkins Medical Institute,
Baltimore, Maryland
THE MOLECULAR BIOLOGY, ENDOCRINOLOGY,
AND PHYSIOLOGY OF THE PROSTATE AND
SEMINAL VESICLES
DIAGNOSIS AND STAGING OF PROSTATE
CANCER

Bhalchondra G. Parulkar, M.D.
Chief Resident, Division of Urological and
Transplant Surgery, University of
Massachusetts Medical Center, Worcester,
Massachusetts
URINARY LITHIASIS: ETIOLOGY, DIAGNOSIS,
AND MEDICAL MANAGEMENT

Craig A. Peters, M.D.
Assistant Professor of Surgery, Harvard Medical
School; Assistant in Surgery, Children's
Hospital, Boston, Massachusetts
PERINATAL UROLOGY
LAPAROSCOPY IN CHILDREN AND ADULTS

Paul C. Peters, M.D.
Professor Emeritus, University of Texas
Southwestern Medical Center, Dallas, Texas
GENITOURINARY TRAUMA

Kenneth J. Pienta, M.D.
Associate Professor, University of Michigan
School of Medicine, Ann Arbor, Michigan
ETIOLOGY, EPIDEMIOLOGY, AND PREVENTION
OF CARCINOMA OF THE PROSTATE

Arthur T. Porter, M.D., FRCPC
Professor and Chairman, Wayne State University;
Director of Clinical Care, Barbara Ann
Karmanos Cancer Institute, Detroit, Michigan
RADIOTHERAPY AND CRYOTHERAPY FOR
PROSTATE CANCER

Jacob Rajfer, M.D.
Professor of Surgery/Urology, University of
California, Los Angeles, School of Medicine,
Los Angeles; Chief, Division of Urology,
Harbor–UCLA Medical Center, Torrance,
California
CONGENITAL ANOMALIES OF THE TESTIS AND
SCROTUM

R. Beverly Raney, M.D.
Professor of Pediatrics, University of Texas,
M.D. Anderson Cancer Center, Houston, Texas
PEDIATRIC ONCOLOGY

Shlomo Raz, M.D.
Professor of Surgery/Urology, Center for Health
Sciences, University of California School of
Medicine, Los Angeles, Los Angeles,
California
VAGINAL RECONSTRUCTIVE SURGERY FOR
INCONTINENCE AND PROLAPSE

Martin I. Resnick, M.D.
Lester Persky Professor and Chairman,
Department of Urology, Case Western Reserve
University School of Medicine; Director,
Department of Urology, University Hospitals
of Cleveland, Cleveland, Ohio
EXTRINSIC OBSTRUCTION OF THE URETER

Neil M. Resnick, M.D.
Assistant Professor of Medicine, Harvard
Medical School; Chief of Gerontology,
Brigham and Women's Hospital, Boston,
Massachusetts
GERIATRIC INCONTINENCE AND VOIDING
DYSFUNCTION

Alan B. Retik, M.D.
Professor of Surgery/Urology, Harvard Medical
School; Chief, Department of Urology,
Children's Hospital, Boston, Massachusetts
PERINATAL UROLOGY
ANOMALIES OF THE URETER

Jerome P. Richie, M.D.
Elliott C. Cutler Professor of Surgery, Harvard
Medical School; Chief of Urology, Brigham
and Women's Hospital, and Chairman, Harvard
Program in Urology (Longwood Area), Boston,
Massachusetts
NEOPLASMS OF THE TESTIS

Richard C. Rink, M.D.
Associate Professor of Urology and Chief,
Pediatric Urology, James Whitcomb Riley
Hospital for Children, Indiana University
School of Medicine, Indianapolis, Indiana
AUGMENTATION CYSTOPLASTY

Lauri J. Romanzi, M.D., FACOG
Assistant Professor, Cornell University Medical
College; Director of Urogynecology, The New
York Hospital–Cornell Medical Center, New
York, New York
URINARY INCONTINENCE: PATHOPHYSIOLOGY,
EVALUATION, TREATMENT OVERVIEW, AND
NONSURGICAL MANAGEMENT

Shane Roy III, M.D.
Professor of Pediatrics, Section of Pediatric
Nephrology, University of Tennessee,
Memphis; Chief, Pediatric Nephrology,
LeBonheur Children's Medical Center,
Memphis, Tennessee
RENAL DISEASE IN CHILDHOOD

Thomas Rozanski, M.D.
Chief of Urology and Chief of Pediatric Urology,
Brooke Army Medical Center, Ft. Sam
Houston, Texas
SURGERY OF THE SCROTUM AND TESTIS IN
CHILDREN

Daniel B. Rukstalis, M.D.
Chief of Urology, Allegheny University Hospital/
Hahnemann, Philadelphia, Pennsylvania
PRINCIPLES OF MOLECULAR GENETICS

Arthur I. Sagalowsky, M.D.
Professor and Chief, Urologic Oncology,
Department of Urology, The University of
Texas Southwestern Medical Center;
Attending, Zale Lipshy University Hospital,
Dallas, Texas
GENITOURINARY TRAUMA

Jay I. Sandlow, M.D.
Assistant Professor, Department of Urology, The
University of Iowa, Iowa City, Iowa
SURGERY OF THE SEMINAL VESICLES

Peter T. Scardino, M.D.
Russell and Mary Hugh Scott Professor and
Chairman, Scott Department of Urology,
Baylor College of Medicine; Chief, Urology
Service, The Methodist Hospital, Houston,
Texas
RADICAL PROSTATECTOMY

Anthony J. Schaeffer, M.D.
Professor and Chairman, Department of Urology,
Northwestern University Medical School,
Chicago, Illinois
INFECTIONS OF THE URINARY TRACT

Paul F. Schellhammer, M.D.
Professor and Chairman, Eastern Virginia
Medical School, Norfolk; Active Staff, Sentara
Health System: Norfolk General Hospital,
Leigh Memorial Hospital, and Bayside,
Norfolk and Virginia Beach, Virginia
TUMORS OF THE PENIS

Peter N. Schlegel, M.D.
Associate Professor of Urology, Cornell
University Medical College; Staff Scientist,
The Population Council; Associate Attending
Urologist, The New York Hospital; Associate
Visiting Physician, The Rockefeller University
Hospital, New York, New York
PHYSIOLOGY OF MALE REPRODUCTION: THE
TESTIS, EPIDIDYMIS, AND DUCTUS DEFERENS

Steven M. Schlossberg, M.D.
Professor of Urology, Eastern Virginia School of
Medicine, Norfolk, Virginia
SURGERY OF THE PENIS AND URETHRA

Richard N. Schlussel, M.D.
Assistant Professor of Urology, Mount Sinai
School of Medicine; Chief, Pediatric Urology,
Mount Sinai Medical Center, New York, New
York
ANOMALIES OF THE URETER

Robert W. Schrier, M.D.
Professor and Chairman, Department of
Medicine, University of Colorado School of
Medicine, Denver, Colorado
ETIOLOGY, PATHOGENESIS, AND MANAGEMENT
OF RENAL FAILURE

Fritz H. Schröder, M.D.
Professor and Chairman, Department of Urology,
Erasmus University, Rotterdam, The
Netherlands
ENDOCRINE TREATMENT OF PROSTATE CANCER

Joseph I. Shapiro, M.D.
Associate Professor of Medicine and Radiology,
University of Colorado School of Medicine,
Denver, Colorado
ETIOLOGY, PATHOGENESIS, AND MANAGEMENT
OF RENAL FAILURE

Linda M. Dairiki Shortliffe, M.D.
Professor and Chair of Urology, Stanford
University School of Medicine; Chief of
Pediatric Urology, Lucile Salter Packard
Children's Hospital, Stanford, California
URINARY TRACT INFECTIONS IN INFANTS AND
CHILDREN

Mark Sigman, M.D.
Assistant Professor of Urology, Brown
University; Staff, Rhode Island Hospital,
Veterans Administration Hospital, Providence,
Rhode Island
MALE INFERTILITY

Donald G. Skinner, M.D.
Professor and Chairman, Department of Urology,
University of Southern California School of
Medicine, Los Angeles, California
SURGERY OF TESTICULAR NEOPLASMS

Eila C. Skinner, M.D.
Associate Professor of Clinical Urology,
University of Southern California, Department
of Urology, School of Medicine, Los Angeles,
California
SURGERY OF TESTICULAR NEOPLASMS

Edwin A. Smith, M.D.
Assistant Clinical Professor of Surgery
(Urology), Emory University School of
Medicine; Attending, Egleston Children's
Hospital and Scottish Rite Children's Medical
Center, Atlanta, Georgia
PRUNE-BELLY SYNDROME

Jerome Hazen Smith, M.S.(Anat), M.Sc.Hyg., M.D.
Professor in Pathology, University of Texas
Medical Branch; Pathologist, University of
Texas Medical Branch Hospitals, Galveston,
Texas
PARASITIC DISEASES OF THE GENITOURINARY
SYSTEM

Joseph A. Smith, Jr., M.D.
William L. Bray Professor and Chairman,
Department of Urologic Surgery, Vanderbilt
University, Nashville, Tennessee
SURGERY OF THE URETER

Howard M. Snyder III, M.D.
Professor of Surgery in Urology, University of
Pennsylvania School of Medicine,
Philadelphia, Pennsylvania
PEDIATRIC ONCOLOGY
PRINCIPLES OF CONTINENT RECONSTRUCTION

R. Ernest Sosa, M.D.
Associate Professor of Urology, Cornell
University Medical College; Associate
Attending Urologist, The New York
Hospital–Cornell Medical Center, New York,
New York
RENOVASCULAR HYPERTENSION AND OTHER
RENAL VASCULAR DISEASES
SHOCK-WAVE LITHOTRIPSY

William D. Steers, M.D.
Chairman and J.Y. Gillenwater Professor of
  Urology, University of Virginia School of
  Medicine, Charlottesville, Virginia
  PHYSIOLOGY AND PHARMACOLOGY OF THE
    BLADDER AND URETHRA

Lynn Stothers, M.D., M.H.Sc.
Fellow of Reconstruction, Neurology, and Female
  Urology, Center for Health Sciences,
  University of California, Los Angeles, School
  of Medicine, Los Angeles, California
  VAGINAL RECONSTRUCTIVE SURGERY FOR
    INCONTINENCE AND PROLAPSE

Stevan B. Streem, M.D.
Head, Section of Stone Disease and Endourology,
  Department of Urology, Cleveland Clinic
  Foundation, Cleveland, Ohio
  SURGERY OF THE KIDNEY

Terry B. Strom, M.D.
Professor of Medicine, Harvard Medical School;
  Medical Director, Renal Transplant Service,
  and Director, Division of Immunology, Beth
  Israel Hospital; Physician, Brigham and
  Women's Hospital, Boston, Massachusetts
  TRANSPLANTATION IMMUNOBIOLOGY

Manikkam Suthanthiran, M.D.
Professor of Medicine, Biochemistry, and
  Surgery, Cornell University Medical College;
  Chief, Division of Transplantation Medicine
  and Extracorporeal Therapy, and Chief,
  Division of Nephrology, Department of
  Medicine, The New York Hospital–Cornell
  Medical Center; Director, Immunogenetics and
  Transplantation Center, The Rogosin Institute,
  New York, New York
  TRANSPLANTATION IMMUNOBIOLOGY

Ronald S. Swerdloff, M.D.
Professor of Medicine, University of California,
  Los Angeles, School of Medicine, Los
  Angeles; Chief, Division of Endocrinology,
  Harbor–UCLA Medical Center; Director,
  World Health Organization Collaborating
  Center of Reproduction, Torrance, California
  PHYSIOLOGY OF HYPOTHALAMIC-PITUITARY
    FUNCTION

Brett A. Trockman, M.D.
Clinical Instructor, Department of Urology,
  Loyola University Medical Center, Maywood,
  Illinois
  SURGERY FOR CERVICOVAGINAL AND
    URETHROVAGINAL FISTULA AND URETHRAL
    DIVERTICULUM

E. Darracott Vaughan, Jr., M.D.
James J. Colt Professor of Urology, Cornell
  University Medical College; Chairman,
  Department of Urology, and Attending
  Urologist-in-Chief, The New York
  Hospital–Cornell University Medical Center,
  New York, New York
  RENAL PHYSIOLOGY
  PATHOPHYSIOLOGY OF URINARY TRACT
    OBSTRUCTION
  RENOVASCULAR HYPERTENSION AND OTHER
    RENAL VASCULAR DISEASES
  THE ADRENALS

Franz von Lichtenberg, M.D.
Professor Emeritus of Pathology, Harvard
  Medical School; Senior Pathologist, Brigham
  and Women's Hospital, Boston, Massachusetts
  PARASITIC DISEASES OF THE GENITOURINARY
    SYSTEM

R. Dixon Walker III, M.D.
Professor of Surgery and Pediatrics, University of
  Florida College of Medicine; Chief of Pediatric
  Urology, Shands Children's Hospital,
  Gainesville, Florida
  EVALUATION OF THE PEDIATRIC UROLOGIC
    PATIENT

Patrick C. Walsh, M.D.
David Hall McConnell Professor and Director,
  Department of Urology, Johns Hopkins
  University School of Medicine; Urologist in
  Chief, James Buchanan Brady Urological
  Institute, Johns Hopkins Hospital, Baltimore,
  Maryland
  THE NATURAL HISTORY OF LOCALIZED
    PROSTATE CANCER: A GUIDE TO THERAPY
  ANATOMIC RADICAL RETROPUBIC
    PROSTATECTOMY

Christina Wang, M.D., FRACP, FRCP(Glas.)
Professor of Medicine, University of California,
  Los Angeles, School of Medicine, Los
  Angeles; Director, Clinical Study Center,
  Harbor–UCLA Medical Center, Torrance,
  California
  PHYSIOLOGY OF HYPOTHALAMIC-PITUITARY
    FUNCTION

George D. Webster, M.B., Ch.B., FRCS
Professor of Surgery, Department of Surgery, Division of Urology, Duke University School of Medicine, Durham, North Carolina
THE NEUROUROLOGIC EVALUATION
RETROPUBIC SUSPENSION SURGERY FOR FEMALE SPHINCTERIC INCONTINENCE

Alan J. Wein, M.D.
Professor and Chair, Division of Urology, University of Pennsylvania School of Medicine; Chief of Urology, University of Pennsylvania Medical Center, Philadelphia, Pennsylvania
COLOR ATLAS OF GENITAL DERMATOLOGY
PATHOPHYSIOLOGY AND CHARACTERIZATION OF VOIDING DYSFUNCTION
NEUROMUSCULAR DYSFUNCTION OF THE LOWER URINARY TRACT AND ITS TREATMENT

Robert M. Weiss, M.D.
Professor and Chief, Section of Urology, Yale University School of Medicine, New Haven, Connecticut
PHYSIOLOGY AND PHARMACOLOGY OF THE RENAL PELVIS AND URETER

Richard D. Williams, M.D.
Professor and Head, Rubin H. Flocks Chair, Department of Urology, The University of Iowa, Iowa City, Iowa
SURGERY OF THE SEMINAL VESICLES

Gilbert J. Wise, M.D.
Professor of Urology, Health Science Center, State University of New York; Director of Urology, Maimonides Medical Center, Brooklyn, New York
FUNGAL INFECTIONS OF THE URINARY TRACT

John R. Woodard, M.D.
Clinical Professor of Surgery (Urology) and Director of Pediatric Urology, Emory University School of Medicine; Chief of Urology, Egleston Hospital for Children at Emory University, Atlanta, Georgia
PRUNE-BELLY SYNDROME

Subbarao V. Yalla, M.D.
Associate Professor of Surgery (Urology), Harvard Medical School, Boston, Massachusetts
GERIATRIC INCONTINENCE AND VOIDING DYSFUNCTION

Muhammad M. Yaqoob, M.D., Ph.D., MRCP
Consultant Nephrologist, The Royal London and St. Bartholomew's Hospitals, London, United Kingdom
ETIOLOGY, PATHOGENESIS, AND MANAGEMENT OF RENAL FAILURE

PREFACE
Seventh Edition of Campbell's Urology

The seventh edition of *Campbell's Urology* perpetuates over 70 years of association between the W.B. Saunders Company and the field of urology. In 1926, the classic textbook by Hugh Hampton Young, *Young's Practice of Urology* was first published. This was followed in 1935 by Frank Hinman Sr.'s *Textbook of Urology*. The first edition of *Campbell's Urology*, which was published in 1954, was edited by Meredith Campbell, Professor and Chairman of Urology at New York University. After his first and second editions he invited J. Hartwell Harrison to join him as a co-editor of the third edition. When Dr. Harrison expanded the editorial board for the fourth edition, the editors believed that Dr. Campbell's contribution to urology should be recognized in perpetuity by officially naming the textbook in his honor. This tradition continues today with the publication of the seventh edition.

With the field of urology undergoing rapid transformation, the editors believed that a major complete revision of *Campbell's Urology* was necessary within 5 years of publishing the last edition. This edition has been greatly expanded with the addition of 22 new chapters and 32 new authors. Dr. Alan Wein, Professor and Chairman of Urology at the University of Pennsylvania, has joined as a new editor and has added immeasurably to the sections on neuromuscular dysfunction of the urinary tract and incontinence.

In this edition we have used an organ systems orientation attempting wherever possible to aggregate physiology, pathophysiology, and medical and surgical management into individual sections, thereby providing a "mini" textbook for each subspecialty. We also believed that multidisciplinary authorship of some areas was very important, especially oncology. For this reason, you will note that prostate cancer is now subdivided into multiple chapters written by basic scientists, surgeons, medical oncologists, and radiation therapists. We have maintained an encyclopedic approach to each topic, but have encouraged the authors to use bold type to emphasize important concepts, thus making it easier to glean the essence from each chapter. Also, to make this edition more user friendly we have expanded the use of algorithms and decision trees wherever possible. Finally, this book will be accompanied by a study guide, which we have created to provide a structured approach to urologic education for residents, program directors, and certified urologists. At present, there is no structured curriculum for this purpose and it

is the hope of the editors that this study guide will provide a systematic way to review many of the important areas in each field.

As we enter the 21st century it seemed appropriate to begin the book with the principles of molecular genetics, followed by the more traditional basic sciences such as anatomy. We have grouped renal physiology and pathophysiology together so that the reader can review the entire spectrum from normal physiology to the management of end-stage renal disease and hypertension. By building on a firm base of renal physiology, the reader can better understand the current thinking on acute renal failure, urinary tract obstruction, and renovascular disease.

Section V deals with the transport of urine to the lower urinary tract, normal and abnormal lower urinary tract storage and emptying, and the treatment of voiding dysfunction. Urinary incontinence is such an important topic that it and its treatment are considered in separate chapters in this section even though some overlap with other material is inevitable. Reconstructive and prosthetic surgery for sphincter incontinence are also considered separately here as well as other topics specifically related to female urology. Geriatric voiding dysfunction is likewise important enough to be accorded a separate chapter.

Sexual function and dysfunction, as well as reproductive function and dysfunction, follow in separate sections combining physiology, pathophysiology, and surgery. Benign prostatic hyperplasia represents one of the most common disorders managed by urologists. For this reason, it is now represented as a separate section with six chapters.

The entire section on pediatric urology has been reorganized, with new chapters "Evaluation of the Pediatric Urologic Patient" and "Renal Disease in Childhood." The chapter on "Normal and Anomalous Development of the Urinary Tract" has been expanded to include a section on molecular biology, and the chapter "Neonatal Urologic Emergencies" has been totally reorganized and stresses the most common conditions. In the chapter "Urinary Tract Infections in Infants and Children," there are now new sections discussing the management of girls with recurrent urinary tract infections without anatomic abnormalities and the incidence and detection of pyelonephritis in the absence of vesicoureteral reflux. Congenital disorders of the urinary tract have been subdivided into anomalies of the kidney and ureter, and the chapter "Vesicoureteral Reflux and Megaureter" has been totally rewritten with new authorship. Long-term results are now emphasized in the chapters on prune-belly syndrome, exstrophy of the bladder, cloacal malformations, and urinary undiversion.

The current approach to urinary stone disease as well as the use of emerging techniques in endourology and laparoscopy is now condensed. The chapter on the pathogenesis of urinary stone disease is immediately followed by alternatives for therapy including ESWL, ureteroscopy, and percutaneous approaches. These sections conclude with the chapter on percutaneous approaches for indications other than stone

disease and an updated overview of the role of laparoscopy in both adults and children with urological problems. These chapters interface well with the following section, which is a compendium of the current status of urologic surgery, and includes open approaches to stone disease.

The editors are grateful for the support of the W.B. Saunders Company and especially to Richard Zorab, the editorial manager, who has facilitated our interactions. We also wish to express our thanks to Faith Voit, Hazel Hacker, Linda R. Garber, and the staff of the W.B. Saunders Company for their patience and help in bringing this ambitious undertaking to publication.

PATRICK C. WALSH, M.D.
For the Editors

CONTENTS

VIII
BENIGN PROSTATIC HYPERPLASIA

45
The Molecular Biology, Endocrinology, and Physiology of the Prostate and Seminal Vesicles

Alan W. Partin, M.D., Ph.D. and
Donald S. Coffey, Ph.D.

46
Epidemiology, Etiology, Pathophysiology, and Diagnosis of Benign Prostatic Hyperplasia

John D. McConnell, M.D.

47
Natural History, Evaluation, and Nonsurgical Management of Benign Prostatic Hyperplasia

Herbert Lepor, M.D.

48
Minimally Invasive Treatment of Benign Prostatic Hyperplasia

David L. McCullough, M.D.

Urothelial Tumors of the Renal Pelvis and Ureter 2383

78
Neoplasms of the Testis 2411
Jerome P. Richie, M.D.

79
Tumors of the Penis 2453
Donald F. Lynch, Jr., M.D. and
Paul F. Schellhammer, M.D.

XI
CARCINOMA OF THE PROSTATE

80
Etiology, Epidemiology, and Prevention of Carcinoma of the Prostate

Kenneth J. Pienta, M.D.

81
Pathology of Adenocarcinoma of the Prostate

Jonathan I. Epstein, M.D.

82
Ultrasonography of the Prostate and Biopsy

Michael K. Brawer, M.D. and
Michael P. Chetner, M.D.

83
Diagnosis and Staging of Prostate Cancer

H. Ballentine Carter, M.D. and
Alan W. Partin, M.D., Ph.D.

94
Endourology of the Upper Urinary Tract: Percutaneous Renal and Ureteral Procedures

Ralph V. Clayman, M.D.,
Elspeth M. McDougall, M.D., and
Stephen Y. Nakada, M.D.

95
Laparoscopy in Children and Adults

Craig A. Peters, M.D. and
Louis R. Kavoussi, M.D.

XIV
UROLOGIC SURGERY

96
The Adrenals

E. Darracott Vaughan, Jr., M.D. and
Jon D. Blumenfeld, M.D.

108
Surgery of Penile and Urethral Carcinoma 3395
Harry W. Herr, M.D.

109
Surgery of Testicular Neoplasms 3410
Eila C. Skinner, M.D. and
Donald G. Skinner, M.D.

Index i

DRUG NOTICE

Medicine is an ever-changing field. Standard safety precautions must be followed, but as new research and clinical experience broaden our knowledge, changes in treatment and drug therapy become necessary or appropriate. Readers are advised to check the product information currently provided by the manufacturer of each drug to be administered to verify the recommended dose, the method and duration of administration, and contraindications. It is the responsibility of the treating physician, relying on experience and knowledge of the patient, to determine dosages and the best treatment for the patient. Neither the Publisher nor the editor assumes any responsibility for any injury and/or damage to persons or property.

The Publisher

X
ONCOLOGY

75
AN OVERVIEW OF CANCER BIOLOGY

William R. Fair, M.D.
Warren D. W. Heston, Ph.D.
Carlos Cordon-Cardo, M.D., Ph.D.

Cancerous cells reflect a broad spectrum of altered biologic behavior relative to their cell of origin. In the minimum, this alteration is barely discernable, and in the extreme, the anaplastic cell no longer possesses distinguishing features to characterize its tissue of origin. In the steady-state maintenance of normal adult tissue, there is an invariant routine of stem cell division, differentiation, and cell death maintaining the tissue at a fairly constant mass and configuration. This steady state results from complex, tightly controlled interplay of extracellular signals, intracellular signal transduction, and the response of the genomic DNA to these signals. The final arbiter of interpretation and response to these signals is the information of the genomic DNA itself. In normal somatic cells, this is a constant. The DNA of cancer cells is unstable, and any chromosomal alterations that have occurred tend to accumulate and become more frequent with time, resulting in abnormal responses to intracellular and extracellular signals and to tumor progression

from a well-differentiated to an anaplastic state (Heim et al, 1988; Pierce and Speers, 1988; Pienta et al, 1989). **Thus, cancer is a disease of damaged DNA and altered genetic code. The four hallmarks of cancerous cells are**

1. **Loss of growth regulation.**
2. **Immortalization.**
3. **Induction of angiogenesis.**
4. **Capability to metastasize.**

It is appreciated that there needs to be more than one DNA-damaging hit for a cell to become cancerous. Often the genetic changes occurring in tumors are so numerous that it is difficult to tell what the important genetic lesions critical for the cancer are. **Minimal requirements for malignant transformation often involve at least two interactive changes.** One is a positive growth regulator, often a cell surface–associated protein, which becomes abnormally activated, such as the mutated Ras protein or an abnormal growth factor/receptor combination. Second is the loss of a growth suppressor function or nuclear regulator, such as retinoblastoma gene Rb or P53, or activation of a suppressor of apoptotic cell death, such as bcl-2.

For example, in bladder cancer, using the sensitive technique of polymerase chain reaction, 40% of bladder neoplasms were found to harbor H-*ras* 12-point mutations (Czerniak et al, 1990; Ooi et al, 1994). High-stage and high-grade bladder tumors have been reported to overexpress epidermal growth factor receptor. Deletions in Rb and P53 genes and increases in MDM2, which inactivates both Rb and P53, have been documented. Indeed, many chromosomal alterations have been observed to occur in bladder cancer, but those at 9p and 9q, 5q, 3p, 17p, 11p, 6q, 13q, and 18q appear to be most associated with malignant progression of bladder cancer (Fig. 75–1).

Normal cell fibroblasts can be grown and repeatedly passaged, but after a defined number of passages the cells reach a stage at which they do not grow further. This time period is called the **"crisis period."** Certain cells mutate, however, becoming immortal and passaged forever. In becoming immortalized and able to replicate indefinitely, cells, whether normal or malignant, **activate the enzyme telomerase.** Telomerase is involved in the lengthening of the ends of the chromosomes, which would otherwise shorten with each cell division. With continued shortening, the cell is eventually unable to divide and dies. Telomerase was discussed in Chapter 1 and is not discussed further except to emphasize that for unlimited tumor growth, the tumor must express this enzyme.

Further changes occur that allow the growing tumor to develop a blood supply to grow bigger than just a few millimeters in diameter. Aggressive tumors are angiogenic, that is, active in their ability to recruit a vascular supply. A count of the vessels in a tumor may predict its biologic behavior. Tumor progression includes the ability to gain access to the vasculature and to disseminate, followed by implantation and growth at other distant sites. Many of these processes are now being elucidated at the molecular level. It is always the hope that this knowledge will enable the development of rational therapeutic approaches to eliminate

the malignant cell specifically, avoiding the use of toxic therapies that are intensely harmful to the patient.

LOSS OF GROWTH REGULATION

Cell Clock and Its Dysregulation in Cancer

Neoplastic diseases are proliferative disorders characterized by an uncoordinated cell growth (Willis, 1952). To reach a better understanding of cancer, it is important to have an in-depth knowledge of the mechanisms that control cell division. This process is the basis for the continuity of life and underlies the complexity of growth, renewal, and repair active in all multicellular organisms. **Historically, cell division was morphologically separated into two events: karyokinesis (nuclear division) and cytokinesis (cytoplasmic division).** Two major prototypic mechanisms prevail in either somatic cells (mitosis) or gametes (meiosis). This section concentrates on the events that occur during cell division of somatic cells and the alterations they undergo in human cancer.

Somatic cell division may be conceptualized as a linear model composed of two major stages: interphase and mitosis. The latter can be compartmentalized into four phases: prophase, metaphase, anaphase, and telophase. Completion of the process includes chromosome replication and segregation into two daughter cells. A clinical application derived from these initial observations was the morphologic assessment of tumor cell proliferation, based on counting mitotic figures detectable in tissue sections. This method, however, measures only the shortest period of the proliferating tumor cell population, as discussed later, and has major drawbacks, such as lack of standardization and reproducibility (Hall et al, 1992; Linden et al, 1992). Nevertheless, it is still employed as a marker of cell proliferation in many morphologic studies, and it is a component of some tumor grading systems (Coindre et al, 1986).

The linear model was subsequently revised to formulate the current cell cycle theory (Murray and Hunt, 1993). The

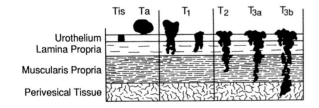

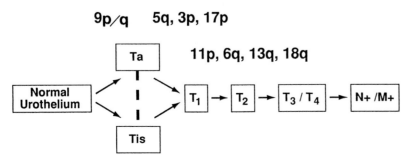

Figure 75–1. Proposed model of bladder cancer progression as it may relate to the pathology staging of these cancers.

Table 75–1. RELATIONSHIP OF HISTOLOGIC PATTERN AND MITOTIC INDEX IN PROSTATIC CANCER

Histologic Pattern	Mitotic Index*
Well differentiated (N = 10)	0.9 + 0.3
Moderately differentiated (N = 16)	2.3 + 1.3
Poorly differentiated (N = 28)	3.6 + 0.8
Anaplastic (N = 4)	12.1 + 5.5

*Determined by counting 6000 cells of similar histologic type within each tumor. Values represent mean ± SEM.
Adapted from Alison MR, Wright NA: Rec Results Cancer Res 1981; 41:29–43.

typical cycle of cultured cells lasts about 24 hours, although it can vary widely, and comprises two readily detectable phases: **S-phase** (DNA synthesis—6 hours—(^{3}H)thymidine incorporation and autoradiography) and **M-phase** (mitosis—approximately 30 minutes—chromosomal condensation), **separated from each other by two gap phases (G1 and G2**—12 hours and 6 hours).

Examples of Predicted Tumor Cell Growth Based on Mitotic Index

The **mitotic index** is the number of mitoses as a percentage of the cells counted. It is a direct measure and a reliable indication of proliferation rate. Alison and Wright (1981) reported the relationship of increasing mitotic index and decreased differentiation as seen in Table 75–1.

If there is no cell loss, the cell production rate remains constant in relation to population size, and growth is exponential; the potential doubling time (T_{pot}) is a fraction of the turnover time [turnover time (T_t) = t_M/MI] in the population, which is equal to the time required to replace all of the cells (double), where t_m is the duration of mitosis and MI is the mitotic index [$T_{pot} = 0.693\ t_m/MI$]. Usually the time cells spend in mitosis is 30 minutes to 2 hours. If one assumes exponential growth, the poorly differentiated cells would have a potential population doubling time of 1.6 days if there was no cell loss fraction (Steel, 1977; Alison and Wright, 1981). Obviously, even poorly differentiated prostatic cancer does not grow with such a rapid doubling time. These and other data suggest **a high rate of cell loss** from these tumors, an observation common to most adenocarcinomas. Although metaphase and anaphase are easily recognized, prophase and telophase are not. Agents such as colchicine cause metaphase arrest. Metaphase-arresting agents can be used to determine the rate at which cells accumulate in metaphase as an index of the rate of entry into mitosis, provided that they have no effect on other phases of the cell cycle. This procedure is referred to as the stathmokinetic method (Steel, 1977; Alison and Wright, 1981). Fulker and co-workers used the stathmokinetic method to determine potential growth rates of bladder cancer (Fulker et al, 1971). They obtained mitotic indices of 1.3, 4.8, and 13.1 and potential doubling times of 22, 6, and 2.2 days for well-differentiated, poorly differentiated, and undifferentiated tumors. The authors also point out that the true doubling times observed clinically are much longer, again suggesting a substantial **cell loss fraction.** Cell loss is only recently being appreciated by using methods to measure the process of

active cell death, apoptosis. Apoptosis can be measured using the so-called TUNEL (terminal uridine deoxynucleotide nick end labeling) technique, and similar to mitosis, apoptosis occurs quickly. Thus, the rate of cell loss can negate the growth activity of a rapidly proliferating tumor, whereas a slowly proliferating tumor with no cell loss can double in tumor volume faster.

Cells not only change their DNA content as they progress through the cell cycle, but also, as the damaged DNA accumulates, the chromosomal DNA content becomes abnormal. This **aneuploid** DNA population can be followed in proliferation by measuring chromosomal abnormalities in cancer cells with the aid of cell sorters and flow cytometry instruments (Melamed et al, 1990). DNA histograms display defined G_1, S, and G_2/M phases, and a large series of clinically relevant reports dealing with proliferative activity and abnormal DNA content (aneuploidy) have been documented (Barlogie, 1984; Badalament et al, 1987; Koss et al, 1989; Melamed et al, 1990). The prognostic value of flow cytometry parameters for certain tumor types, including bladder and breast carcinomas as well as non-Hodgkin's lymphoma, has been established (Macartney and Camplejohn, 1990; Merkel and McGuire, 1990; Wheeless et al, 1993). The implementation of multiparameter flow cytometry enhances the quality of tumor DNA profiles and allows combined measurements of DNA and RNA.

Examples of Aneuploidy and Cell Proliferation Measured by Flow Cytometry

The technique of flow cytometry quantitating the amount of fluorescent dye bound to a single cell's DNA can be used to determine cell cycle parameters as the cell goes through S and G_2/M phases, returning to baseline following cell division (Melamed et al, 1990; Raber and Barlogie, 1990). S phase has been examined in a number of urologic tumors by Frankfurt and co-workers, and they found the characteristics listed in Table 75–2 (Frankfurt et al, 1984).

In these studies, it is not always possible to correlate the apparent degree of differentiation and the proliferation index, so that some well-differentiated tumors can have high prolif-

Table 75–2. S-INDEX IN PRIMARY AND METASTATIC UROLOGIC SOLID TUMORS

Diagnosis	Site	DNA Ploidy	Median S-Index (%)
Renal carcinoma	Primary	Diploid	5.7
Renal carcinoma	Metastasis	Diploid	18.9
Renal carcinoma	Primary	Aneuploid	13.4
Renal carcinoma	Metastasis	Aneuploid	19.6
Bladder carcinoma	Primary	Diploid	6.9
Bladder carcinoma	Metastasis	Diploid	9.3
Bladder carcinoma	Primary	Aneuploid	22.6
Bladder carcinoma	Metastasis	Aneuploid	26.5
Prostate cancer	Primary	Diploid	6.3
Prostate cancer	Primary	Aneuploid	11.9

Data adapted from Frankfurt OS, Greco WR, Slocum HK, et al: Cytometry 1984; 5:629–635.

eration rates, and some poorly differentiated tumors can have low proliferation rates (Frankfurt et al, 1984). In studies involving prostatic cancer patients with microscopic lymph node metastases, those with aneuploid metastatic lesions survived only half as long as individuals with diploid or tetraploid tumors (Stephenson et al, 1987). Even though aneuploidy is associated with a higher proliferative rate, however, it does not always correlate with survival (Raber and Barlogie, 1990). More recently, the development of immunoflow cytometry methods has added the capabilities of retrieving kinetic information and phenotype characterization.

There are, however, several limitations in these assays, including the need to disaggregate tissue samples into suspensions of single cells or nuclei and the loss of tissue morphology (Melamed et al, 1990; Hall et al, 1992). Indeed, the use of modern **molecular histologic techniques** allows for multiple correlations to be performed from limited patient specimens, and they can be performed in a quantitative manner with the use of a cell analysis system (CAS) machine. These measures can then be correlated with patient response to therapy (Fig. 75–2).

Molecular Determinants of the Cell Cycle

Since 1991, mainly because of the advent of genetic engineering and powerful technical tools, there has been a tremendous amount of information generated dealing with the principles that govern the cell cycle of eukaryotes or nucleated cells. Moreover, clinical and basic research findings have linked mutations of otherwise orphan genes, now known to be involved in cell cycle control, with underlying processes of tumorigenesis and tumor progression (Freeman and Donoghue, 1991; Hartwell and Kastan, 1994; Hunter and Pines, 1994). In the following sections, the structure and functions of key cell cycle regulatory elements, their reported mutations, and altered patterns of expression in human neoplasms are reviewed. The potential implications of

detecting such alterations in distinctive clinical settings and tumor types are discussed.

Cyclins and Cyclin-Dependent Kinases Are Positive Control Complexes

Cellular proliferation follows an orderly progression through the cell cycle, which is controlled by protein complexes composed of cyclins and cyclin-dependent kinases (Cdk) (Nurse, 1990; Reed, 1992; Murray and Hunt, 1993). Studies using cytoplasmic transfer experiments revealed the existence of the so-called **maturation promoting factor,** found to be a heterodimer with kinase activity that controlled the balance of phosphorylation/dephosphorylation events observed during the cycle (Masui and Markert, 1971; Lohka et al, 1988). These findings were followed by the characterization of a family of genes in yeast known as **cell division control (cdc) genes,** some of which also encoded protein kinases and were later termed **cyclin-dependent kinase (cdk) genes** (Draetta and Beach, 1988; Gould and Nurse, 1989). The p34[cdc2] was identified as the kinase component of the maturation promoting factor (Dunphy et al, 1988). Concomitant biochemical and genetic analyses led to the discovery of a set of periodic proteins that were synthesized at determined phases of the cell cycle and suddenly degraded, therefore being referred to as **cyclins** (Evans et al, 1983). Further studies revealed cyclin B as the regulatory subunit of the maturation promoting factor (Richardson et al, 1989; Gautier et al, 1990).

The current model for the **enzymatically active complexes** consists of **a cyclin as a regulatory molecule and a Cdk as a catalytic subunit** (Fig. 75–3A). Their regulatory function is achieved by **phosphorylation** of fundamental elements involved in cell cycle transitions, such as the retinoblastoma protein (pRB) (see later). An analogy may be drawn between these cyclin-Cdk complexes and those formed by growth factor receptors with kinase activity. Binding to their corresponding physiologic ligands results in the phosphorylation of particular substrates.

Multiple cyclins have been isolated and characterized and a temporal map of their expression during cell cycle progres-

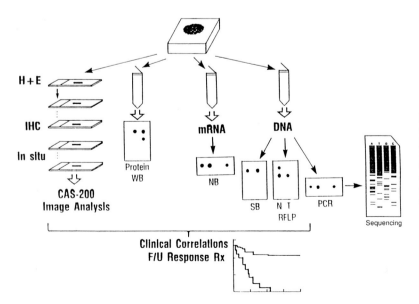

Figure 75–2. The multiple potential determinations that can be made on sequential sections of material from a patient. This includes ploidy and cell cycle determinations, immunohistochemical determination of cell cycle regulatory genes, mRNA expression and determination by Northern blot, DNA determinations by Southern blot, polymerase chain reaction for genetic alterations, and the outcome correlated with patient response to therapy and survival.

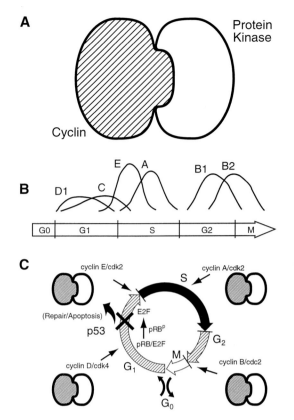

Figure 75–3. *A,* Cell cycle progression is controlled by protein complexes composed of cyclins and cyclin-dependent kinases (Cdk), in which the cyclin acts as a regulatory molecule and the Cdk as a catalytic subunit. *B,* Multiple cyclins have been isolated and characterized, and a temporal map of their expression during cell cycle progression is shown. Cyclins C, D1-3, and E reach their maximum synthesis and peak of activity during G1 phase. Cyclins A and B1-2 achieve their maximum levels during S and G2 phases. Specific heterodimers composed of a cyclin and a Cdk are regarded as regulators of cell cycle transitions. It is postulated that the complexes formed by cyclin D1 and Cdk4 govern G1 progression, whereas cyclin E-Cdk2 controls entry into S phase. *C,* Cyclin A-Cdk2 units produce their regulation through S phase and cyclin B-cdc2 control entry into mitosis. The so-called P53 G1-checkpoint is illustrated. Increases in cellular levels of wild-type P53 occur in response to DNA damage, which may result in either G1 arrest or activation of apoptosis, depending on the cell type in which damage develops. Also depicted in *C* is the proposed function of pRB, forming complexes while underphosphorylated with DNA-binding proteins such as E2F. On pRB phosphorylation, unbound E2F transcription factors appear to stimulate transcription of cellular genes implicated in induction of S phase.

sion delineated (Fig. 75–3*B*). Briefly, five major classes of mammalian cyclins (termed A–E) have been described. **Cyclins C, D1–3, and E reach their peak of synthesis and activity during the G$_1$ phase and apparently regulate the transition of G$_1$ to S phase. Cyclins A and B1–2 achieve their maximal levels later in the cycle, during S and G$_2$ phases, and are regarded as regulators of the transition to mitosis.** Similarly, multiple Cdk molecules are being identified and their cyclin partners and patterns of cell cycle specificity distinguished. It is postulated that the complexes formed by cyclin D1 and Cdk4 govern G$_1$ progression, whereas cyclin E-Cdk2 controls entry into S phase. Cyclin A-Cdk2 units effect their regulation through S phase, and cyclin B-cdc2 units (also known as Cdk1) control entry into mitosis (Fig. 75–3*C*) (Lewin, 1990; Nurse, 1990).

As a corollary to these findings, it has been proposed that **two major checkpoints exist during cell cycle progression and have been established at the mid-end of G$_1$ and G$_2$.** These, in turn, ensure fidelity of genetic information before DNA replication as well as structural accuracy before chromosome segregation and cell division (King et al, 1994; Nurse, 1994; Sherr, 1994).

Mutations of Cyclins and Cyclin-Dependent Kinases Convert Them into Activated Oncogenes

The search for molecular alterations modifying crucial cell cycle regulators in human tumors revealed that the cyclin D1/CCND1 gene, located at chromosome 11q13, is amplified in a subset of cancers, mainly breast and non–small cell lung carcinomas (Lammie and Peters, 1991; Keyomarsi and Pardee, 1993; Schauer et al, 1994). In addition, overexpression of cyclin D1 was found to be a common feature in the tumors harboring this specific 11q13 amplicon. CDK4 is amplified as part of an amplicon on 12q13, where it is encoded, in a series of tumor types. Similar stories are developing for the other cyclins, and more information is required to determine their role in the progression of urologic tumors.

P53 and pRB Are Cell Cycle Regulators

Findings from several lines of investigation suggest that **P53 controls a cell cycle checkpoint responsible for maintaining the integrity of the genome** (see Fig. 75–3*C*). Wild-type P53 (wt P53) mediates arrest of the cell cycle in the G$_1$ phase after sublethal DNA damage (Kastan et al, 1991); P53 also appears to be involved in transcriptional control (Kern et al, 1992; Zambetti et al, 1992). Similar to most well-characterized transcription factors, P53 proteins possess a nuclear localization signal and a sequence-specific DNA-binding domain (Fields and Jang, 1990). An oligomerization domain at the C-terminus has been characterized, suggesting that P53 proteins form tetrameric complexes in solution, yielding the active units that interact with putative P53-binding sites (Stenger et al, 1992). The crystal structure of the P53 fragment that extends from amino acid residue 94 to 312, containing the critical site-specific DNA-binding core domain (residues 102–292), has been resolved (Cho et al, 1994). Analysis of the structure demonstrated that the conserved regions of the core domain are the site of the majority of TP53 mutations identified in human primary tumors, further supporting the hypothesis that DNA binding is critical for the biologic activity of P53. These studies provide a framework for understanding how mutations inactivate P53 functions.

The retinoblastoma gene encodes an approximately 105-kDa nuclear phosphoprotein (Friend et al, 1987; Fung et al, 1987; Lee et al, 1987). **Although the amount of pRB does not change during progression of the cell cycle, the phosphorylation state of pRB is cell cycle dependent and is a target for the enzymatic activity of cyclin-Cdk complexes** (DeCaprio et al, 1988; Buchkovich et al, 1989; Chen et al, 1989). pRB is in the **underphosphorylated form in G$_1$,** and as **cells progress into late G$_1$ and early S phase, pRB becomes highly phosphorylated and remains**

phosphorylated in G_2 (see Fig. 75–3C). The underphosphorylated form of pRB is believed to be the functionally active form of pRB in G_0/middle G_1 (Mittnacht and Weinberg, 1991). pRB does not appear to possess sequence-specific DNA-binding activity, and the underphosphorylated form of pRB most likely exerts its negative regulatory effect on gene expression through complex formation with DNA-binding proteins. A colinear segment comprising more than 350 amino acids, located within the carboxyl two thirds of pRB, has been identified as a functional internal protein receptor and is designated **the "pocket" domain** (Kaelin et al, 1991). **pRB can complex stably** by the interaction of this region with cellular proteins, including members of the **E2F** family (Chellappan et al, 1991; DeFeo-Jones et al, 1991). E2F is a 60-kDa transcription factor originally identified through its role in transcriptional activation of the adenovirus E2 promoter (Kovesdi et al, 1986). **Unbound E2F transcription factors could stimulate transcription of cellular genes.** E2F sites are present in genes implicated in induction of S phase, such as thymidine kinase, *myc*, *myb*, dihydrofolate reductase, and DNA polymerase (Johnson et al, 1993). This suggests that **E2F family members may be responsible for transversing the G_1/S restriction point of the cell cycle** (Weintraub et al, 1992) (see Fig. 75–3C). It may then be concluded that **pRB functions by sequestering other cellular proteins with growth-promoting activities.** The fact that the operative "pocket" region is the target for viral oncoproteins that inhibit pRB as well as a common site for RB mutations provides insight into how specific alterations inactivate pRB (see later).

A relationship between P53 and pRB in cell cycle regulation is suggested based on the action of two novel genes that are regulated by P53: **the MDM2 and the P21** (also known as WAF1, Cip1 and Sdi1) genes (Fig. 75–4). The MDM2 gene maps to the long arm of chromosome 12 and is under transcriptional control by wt P53 (Fakharzadeh et al, 1991; Momand et al, 1992; Oliner et al, 1992). The product encoded by MDM2 is a 90-kDa zinc-finger protein (mdm2), which also contains a P53-binding site (Oliner et al, 1992). It has been shown that mdm2 proteins bind to P53 and act as a negative regulator, inhibiting wt P53 transcriptional regulatory activity and creating an autoregulatory feedback loop. A pRB-binding site has also been identified at the carboxy-terminal domain of mdm2 that interacts with pRB and restrains its functions by altering the conformation of the "pocket" region (Xiao et al, 1995). It is postulated that overexpression of mdm2 inactivates both P53 and pRB in a fashion similar to some viral oncoprotein products, as discussed later. An alternative pathway of P53-pRB interaction is mediated by P21. The P21 gene belongs to a new family of negative cell cycle regulators, functioning as cyclin-dependent kinase inhibitory molecules (discussed later). P21 inactivates cyclin-Cdk complexes that, as described, target pRB phosphorylation (El-Deiry et al, 1993; Harper et al, 1993; Xiong et al, 1993a). In that context, P21 serves as an effector of cell cycle arrest in response to activation of the P53 G_1 phase checkpoint pathway. Figure 75–4 schematically illustrates the previous summary and delineates a model of molecular networking and cross-talk. **These findings imply a potential link between P53 and pRB in cell cycle regulation, apoptosis, and tumor progression.**

Inhibition of P53 and pRB Functions Deregulate Cell Growth and Apoptotic Cell Death

Several viral and cellular proteins have been shown to interact with P53, pRB or both, altering their functions. The SV40 large **T antigen,** the adenovirus **E1B** 55-kDa protein, and the human papillomavirus **E6** protein **each bind to P53 and inactivate its transcriptional activity** (Linzer and Levine, 1979; Sarnow et al, 1982; Werness et al, 1990). Similarly, **underphosphorylated pRB** molecules may form **complexes** with viral transforming proteins, including the SV40 large **T antigen,** the adenovirus **E1A** protein, and the papillomavirus **E7** protein (DeCaprio et al, 1988; Whyte et al, 1988; Dyson et al, 1989). **Complex formation with these proteins inactivates pRB function and leads to cellular immortalization.** It is believed that the growth deregulation produced by pRB inhibition is counteracted by apoptotic cell death orchestrated by normal P53 function. Therefore, the loss of one tumor suppressor gene is compensated by the activity of the other, serving as a safeguard mechanism to protect against the emergence of neoplastic cell growth. Without both pRB and P53, it appears that E2F activation stimulates cell proliferation permitting tumor formation (Morgenbesser et al, 1994). High transformation strains of tumor viruses encode proteins that bind and inactivate both P53 and pRB, revealing the crucial role of these molecules and their close interaction (Fig. 75–4).

In an effort to establish biologic systems to study P53 and pRB, targeted gene expression and knockout murine models for these genes have been developed and characterized. **Germ line mutations in P53 and Rb each predispose mice to cancer.** Animals homozygous for an Rb mutation die in utero with defects in fetal hematopoiesis and widespread neuronal cell death (Jacks et al, 1992; Lee et al, 1992). P53 homozygous mice as well as Rb heterozygous and P53 heterozygous mice, however, are viable but develop a variety

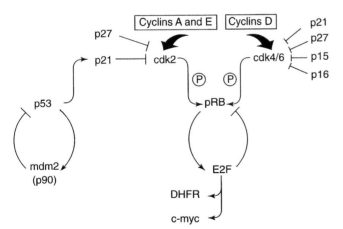

Figure 75–4. Molecular networking model for P53 and pRB. pRB is one of the targets for the enzymatic activity of cyclin-Cdk complexes. P21 is transcriptionally regulated by P53 and inactivates cyclin E-Cdk2; cyclin A-Cdk2; and cyclins D1-, D2-, and D3-Cdk4 complexes; by doing so, P21 also inhibits pRB phosphorylation. P27 inactivates the same complexes that P21 inactivates. P16 and P15, however, have a more restricted activity and form binary complexes only with Cdk4 and Cdk6.

of tumors. The most common neoplasms after P53 disruption are sarcomas and lymphomas (Donehower et al, 1992; Williams et al, 1994), whereas pinealoblastomas and medullary thyroid carcinomas are usually found in heterozygous Rb mice (Williams et al, 1994). **It should be emphasized that germ line homozygosity for P53 mutation causes a pronounced cancer susceptibility, as 90% of the P53-deficient animals develop one or more tumors by 6 months of age.** In one study, the cooperative tumorigenic effects of germ line mutations in P53 and Rb have been established. Heterozygous mice mutant for both genes have reduced viability and exhibit novel pathology, including retinal dysplasia as well as increased tumor burden and metastatic spread (Williams et al, 1994). Taken together, these observations parallel observations in the clinical setting, as is discussed subsequently.

Germline Mutations of TP53 and RB Genes Predispose Individuals to Cancer

The concept of the existence of **tumor suppressor genes** was formulated by Knudson (1971). He postulated that **two independent events** were needed to inactivate a given gene, resulting in malignant transformation. **This hypothesis was based on the model of retinoblastoma, in which susceptible individuals with a germ line RB mutation required inactivation of the remaining allele to develop the malignant tumor.** Children affected with the hereditary form of retinoblastoma often develop a second malignancy several years after successful treatment of the primary tumor (Abramson et al, 1984). In contrast, secondary tumors are uncommon in patients with the sporadic form of the disease (Hansen et al, 1985).

Similar to the RB gene, germ line mutations of the TP53 gene are detected in patients with the **Li-Fraumeni syndrome,** a rare autosomal dominant trait (Li and Fraumeni, 1969; Malkin et al, 1990). These patients are susceptible to a variety of cancers, such as sarcomas, leukemias, and breast carcinomas. TP53 germ line mutations were also detected in patients with no apparent family history (Toguchida et al, 1992) as well as in a subset of patients presenting with a second primary neoplasm (Malkin et al, 1992).

Mutations of TP53 and RB Are Frequent Somatic Events in Primary Tumors

Loss of heterozygosity of chromosome 17 at the TP53 locus (17p13.1) and somatic mutations of TP53 are the most common genetic alterations reported to date in human cancer. These molecular aberrations have been associated with the development and progression of a large number of human tumors (Thor et al, 1992; Allred et al, 1993; Mitsudomi et al, 1993; Sarkis et al, 1993; Drobnjak et al, 1994; Esrig et al, 1994; Greenblatt et al, 1994; Zeng et al, 1994). Striking significant correlations between TP53 mutations or altered patterns of P53 expression and poor survival of cancer patients have been independently documented by different groups studying common human neoplasms (Thor et al, 1992; Allred et al, 1993; Mitsudomi et

al, 1993; Sarkis et al, 1993; Drobnjak et al, 1994; Esrig et al, 1994; Zeng et al, 1994). Moreover, the majority of the tumor-associated mutations are found at or near the DNA binding domain at the so-called hot spots (Cho et al, 1994; Greenblatt et al, 1994). Two classes of mutations have been characterized: mutations that involve residues that contact the DNA (functional mutants) and mutations altering residues important for the structural integrity of the core domain, in particular, the DNA-binding surface of the wt P53 protein (structural mutants) (Cho et al, 1994). The resolution of the crystal structure of P53 solidified the hypothesis that **DNA-binding and transactivation** are the critical activities of P53 required for tumor suppression and confirms the relationship between basic and clinical findings. On the basis of these observations, it has been postulated that detection of these abnormalities may become important adjuncts to the main factors associated with outcome in patients with particular neoplastic lesions. This prognostic tool may also be useful in determining whether a more aggressive therapeutic intervention should be used. It is crucial to develop assays that assess biologic activities of altered P53 proteins found in clinical specimens. This, in turn, will allow clinicians to distinguish those probably irrelevant or silent mutations that are acquired by the malignant cell from those that truly contribute to the malignant phenotype.

The RB gene maps to chromosome 13, band 13q14, and encodes the 105-kDa nuclear phosphoprotein described previously. Numerous lines of evidence have confirmed the concept that the **RB gene** is the prototype **tumor suppressor gene.** RB mutations and altered patterns of pRB have been detected in a wide variety of human primary tumors (Cance et al, 1990; Wunder et al, 1991; Cordon-Cardo et al, 1992a; Kornblau et al, 1992; Logothetis et al, 1992; Phillips et al, 1994; Xu et al, 1994). These changes have also been associated with aggressive behavior and poor clinical outcome in specific tumor types, including bladder and lung carcinomas (Cordon-Cardo et al, 1992b; Logothetis et al, 1992; Xu et al, 1994a). Analysis of other neoplastic processes, such as sarcomas, however, suggests that RB alterations are primary events involved in tumorigenesis or early phases of tumor progression (Benedict et al, 1990). An important limitation in the characterization of RB mutations is the lack of hot spots, as those described for TP53. Even though some alterations are found in the "pocket" domain, the pattern of deletions and point mutations for RB is more random than that of TP53. This phenomenon, together with the complexity of the RB gene, offers a challenge for the analysis of molecular aberrations that occur in primary tumors. For all these reasons, it is crucial to conduct in-depth studies of RB alterations. Analyses comparing RB and other tumor suppressor gene abnormalities, using well-characterized groups of patients with long-term follow-up, will allow the evaluation of their critical role as potential tumor markers and possibly aid in the stratification of patients into prognostic categories.

Cyclin-Dependent Kinase Inhibitors Are Negative Regulators

A new family of negative cell cycle regulators has been identified that functions as **Cdk-inhibitory molecules,** and the genes that encode these proteins are designated CKI genes. The mechanism whereby they achieve their function appears to be the **formation of stable complexes that inactivate the catalytically operative units** (Fig. 75–5). The first and probably best-characterized member of this family is **P21** (described previously), which inactivates cyclin E-cdk2; cyclin A-cdk2; and cyclins D1-cdk4, D2-cdk4, and D3-cdk4 complexes (El-Deiry et al, 1993; Harper et al, 1993; Xiong et al, 1993a). As mentioned, these are components of the regulatory kinases that target pRB for phosphorylation. Furthermore, P21 in normal fibroblasts has been found in quaternary complexes containing, in addition to P21, a cyclin, a Cdk, and the proliferating cell nuclear antigen (Zhang et al, 1993). This finding has led to the postulate that P21 could play a dual role in blocking entry into S phase. The P21/WAF1 gene maps to 6p21.1 and encodes a 164–amino acid protein of relative molecular mass (Mr) 18,107. Mutations of this gene appear to be rare events, and only a few have so far been reported. It appears that the rate of P21 gene aberrations is low and that the main mechanism of inactivation may rest at the level of expression because its transcription is directly activated by P53, and TP53 mutations are predominant events in human cancer. Nevertheless, it has been shown that induction of P21 could be accomplished by a P53-independent pathway (Michieli et al, 1994). Serum or individual growth factors, such as platelet-derived growth factor, fibroblast growth factor, and epidermal growth factor, but not insulin-like growth factor, were able to induce P21 in quiescent P53-deficient cells (Fig. 75–6). These results have suggested the existence of two separate pathways for the induction of P21 linked to either DNA damage or cellular mitogens.

Another member of the CKI group is **P16,** which encodes a 148–amino acid protein of Mr 15,845 (Serrano et al, 1993). In contrast to P21, **P16 forms binary complexes specifically with Cdk4 and Cdk6, inhibiting their activity and, by doing so, inhibiting pRB phosphorylation** (see Figs. 75–2 and 75–4). P16, however, does not interact with Cdc2 or Cdk2. The entire P16 sequence is composed of four repeats of an ankyrin consensus motif. Based on the biochemical properties described, **P16 was designated INK4 (*in*hibitor of Cd*k4*)** (Serrano et al, 1993). The **P15/INK4B** gene has been reported, which encodes a protein of 137 amino acids with Mr 14,700, and shown to be a potential effector of transforming growth factor-beta–induced cell cycle arrest

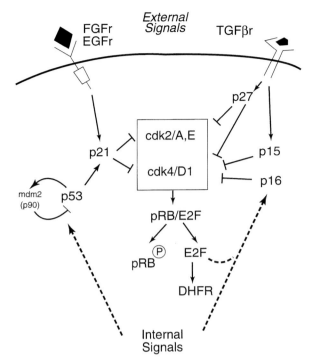

Figure 75–6. Working model of molecular cross-talking between certain internal and external signals and specific cell cycle regulators. These signals exert cell cycle control by directly or indirectly affecting the activity of cyclin-dependent kinases (Cdks). A major path for Cdk regulation is through the Cdk-inhibitors or CKIs, such as P21, P27, P15, and P16. A prominent substrate for the functional cyclin-Cdk complexes is the retinoblastoma protein (pRB). In its underphosphorylated state, pRB forms stable complexes with cellular proteins with transactivation properties, such as E2F. pRB phosphorylation in mid-G1 liberates these bound factors, a number of them being essential for DNA replication (i.e., the enzyme dihydrofolate reductase). Modulation of P27 and P15 activities appears to be mainly mediated by the antimitogenic cytokine transforming growth factor-beta (TGF-β) after binding to its receptor (TGF-βr). P21 is transactivated and mainly controlled by P53 but can also be up-regulated by external signals mediated by certain growth factor receptors, including the fibroblast growth factor receptor (FGFr) and the epidermal growth factor receptor (EGFr). P16 is overexpressed in cells defective in pRB function, and it may participate in a feedback loop wherein repression of P16 expression by pRB may allow Cdk4 to phosphorylate and inhibit pRB. Another important feedback loop is that of P53-mdm2 (or P90), which appears to regulate P53 transcriptional transactivation activity.

(Hannon and Beach, 1994). P15 has substantial homology to P16, and its protein sequence can be also divided into four ankyrin repeats. **P15 has the ability to form binary complexes, to bind and inactivate Cdk4 and Cdk6, inhibiting pRB phosphorylation** (see Figs. 75–2 and 75–4). These two genes map to the short arm of chromosome 9 (9p21), a region that accounts for loss of heterozygosity and homozygous deletions in various human tumor cell lines. Because these genes are also mutated in primary tumors, they are likely to be relevant candidate tumor suppressor genes (see later).

To this rapidly growing group of Cdk inhibitors two new members have been added, P27/Kip1 (Polyak et al, 1994a, 1994b; Toyoshima and Hunter, 1994) and P18 (Guan et al, 1994). P27 is a negative regulator implicated in G_1 phase arrest by transforming growth factor-beta, cell-cell contact, agents that elevate cyclic adenosine monophosphate, and the growth inhibitory drug rapamycin. P27/Kip1 shares sequence

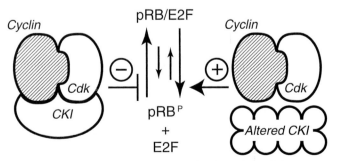

Figure 75–5. Mechanism by which cyclin-dependent inhibitors (CKI) achieve their negative regulation. CKI members, such as P21 and P16, form stable complexes with Cdk proteins and inactivate the catalytically operative units, inhibiting pRB phosphorylation. Altered CKI molecules do not block the activity of cyclin-Cdk complexes, favoring pRB phosphorylation and the release of DNA-binding proteins such as the transcription factor E2F.

homology with P21/WAF, and its encoded product (198 amino acids; Mr 22,257) associates with cyclin E-Cdk2, cyclin A-Cdk2, and cyclin D-Cdk4 complexes, abrogating their activity. Moreover, P27 acts as a stoichiometric inhibitor of G_1 cyclin-Cdks, and even modest changes in the relative levels of P27 can have a major effect on G_1 progression. The authors have mapped P27/Kip1 to 12p12-12p13.1 using a combination of somatic cell hybrid panels and fluorescence in situ hybridization (Ponce-Castaneda et al, 1995). In an extensive search for P27 mutations, the authors and others have not found any structural alteration in the human primary tumors screened (Bullrich et al, 1995; Pietenpol et al, 1995; Ponce-Castaneda et al, 1995).

The cloning of P18 has been reported (Guan et al, 1994). This gene encodes a 168–amino acid protein (Mr 18,116) that is a homologue of P16/INK4A. P18 interacts with Cdk4 and Cdk6 and inhibits the kinase activity of cyclin D-Cdk4 and D-Cdk6 complexes. This novel gene maps to chromosome 1p32, a region that has been reported altered in a variety of tumors, including breast and pancreatic carcinomas (Hainsworth et al, 1991; Bardi et al, 1993) as well as leiomyosarcoma (Sreekantaiah et al, 1993) and neuroblastoma (Schleiermacher et al, 1994). The possible involvement of P18 in these reported abnormalities has yet to be defined.

This family of negative cell cycle regulators can be subdivided into two groups based on their sequence homology. The similarity between P21 and P27 is limited to a 60–amino acid segment in the amino-terminal region with 44% identity. Similar to P21, P27 has a putative bipartite nuclear localization signal near the carboxy terminus. Nevertheless, P27 does not have a zinc-finger motif as P21 does but possesses a consensus cdc2 kinase site. Nonetheless, these two molecules appear to have different regulatory properties because P27 is involved post-transcriptionally in the action of extracellular signals, whereas P21 is mainly regulated by P53 at the level of transcription and may be involved in senescence and cell quiescence.

The other group sharing major structural similarities includes P16, P15, and P18. P16 and P15 contain 82% protein sequence identity, whereas P18 possesses 38% protein sequence identity to P16 and 42% identity to P15. These molecules also have different modes of regulation. P15 is an effector of transforming growth factor-beta–induced cell cycle arrest. In that respect, P15 may be involved in the same pathway of signaling as P27 (see Fig. 75–6). P16 appears to be independent of P53 and membrane signaling pathways (see Fig. 75–6). It has been observed that P16 accumulates in cell lines devoid of pRB (Tam et al, 1994), suggesting that P16 may be under the influence of a transcription factor modulated by pRB.

P16/INK4A/MTS1 and P15/INK4B/MTS2 Are Candidate Tumor Suppressors

Cytogenetic analysis of bladder cancer cells reveals nonrandom chromosomal abnormalities, frequently including monosomy of chromosome 9 (Gibas et al, 1984). Molecular genetic studies of bladder tumors have shown that loss of heterozygosity of chromosome 9 is a frequent mutation occurring in superficial lesions and may be associated with

tumorigenesis in such neoplasms (Olopade et al, 1992; Cairns et al, 1993; Dalbagni et al, 1993). The authors' group has identified two distinct regions containing putative suppressor loci in bladder tumors, mapping to 9p21 and 9q34.1-2 (Orlow et al, 1994). The chromosomal 9p21 region has been found to be mutated in a wide variety of human tumor cell lines. The search for a putative tumor suppressor gene in this region led to the characterization of the so-called **multiple tumor suppressor 1 (MTS1) gene** (Kamb et al, 1994b), which was discovered to be the previously identified P16/INK4A gene. The authors have shown that mutations of the P16/INK4A/MTS1 gene are frequent events in bladder cancer cell lines as well as in clinical samples of bladder tumors (Kamb et al, 1994a, Gruis et al, 1995). **Inactivation of tumor suppressors most often occurs by loss of one allele followed by a point mutation in the remaining allele.** Homozygous deletions of bona fide tumor suppressors are observed only infrequently. One might interpret the unusually high frequency of homozygous P16 deletions as an indication of the existence of a second tumor suppressor locus tightly linked to P16 on 9p21. As discussed previously, the gene encoding P15 lies centromerically adjacent to P16, the two covering a region of approximately 80 kb (Hannon and Beach, 1994; Jen et al, 1994). Jen and colleagues found that P16 and P15 suffer homozygous deletions in a significant percentage of glioblastoma multiforme analyzed, but no intragenic mutations were identified (Jen et al, 1994). These authors concluded that this mutational event may be a more efficient mechanism for simultaneous inactivation of both genes. The occurrence of P16 or P15 alterations has also been reported in lung tumor cell lines and primary lung cancers and shown to affect the non–small cell histologic subtype preferentially (Washimi et al, 1995). Similar to these results, the authors have observed that homozygous **deletions of P16 and P15 are common events in bladder tumors** (Orlow et al, 1994). The authors found P16 or P15 deletions in 18% of tumors analyzed. Taken together, these data support the hypothesis that homozygous deletions may, in fact, be an alternative mechanism of tumor suppressor gene inactivation.

Because the modes of regulation for P16 and P15 are different and include external and internal signals, tumor cells presenting with total deactivation of these two genes may have an advantage for their in vitro expansion. In that respect, an important consideration is the lack of cell contact and transforming growth factor-beta–induced arrest that tumor cells harboring these mutations might possess. Knockout animal models are being developed that will probably reveal the involvement of these molecules in embryogenesis and their potential tumorigenic effects. Further studies are also required using well-characterized cohorts of patients to delineate better the role of P16 and P15 in human cancer.

Reintroduction of Wild-Type TP53 and RB Genes Reverses Tumorigenesis

Studies have documented that the presence of wt P53 products is incompatible with the malignant phenotype in a variety of tumor cell lines. Transfecting wt P53 into rat embryo fibroblasts transformed with a combination of mutant P53 and ras resulted in a decrease in the number of transformed foci (Eliyahu et al, 1989). In another study, wt

TP53 was transduced in T98G human glioblastoma cells and resulted in inhibition of cell cycle progression in exponentially growing cells (Mercer et al, 1990). Casey and associates have shown that expression of wt TP53 was incompatible with cellular growth of MDA-MB-468 and T47-D breast carcinoma cells, which contain mutant TP53 genes (Casey et al, 1991). Suppression of acute leukemia with retroviruses encoding wt P53 was also achieved (Cheng et al, 1992). In addition, in vivo studies showed that tumor volumes were significantly reduced in mice that received peritumoral infiltration with an adenovirus vector carrying wt P53 and that the tumor lesions underwent changes consistent with apoptosis (Liu et al, 1994). More recently, Rosenfeld and colleagues have replaced wt TP53 in the DAOY medulloblastoma cells, which exhibit a point mutation in exon 7, using a defective herpes simplex viral vector carrying wt TP53 (Rosenfeld et al, 1995). The authors observed that after 24 hours, infected DAOY cells accumulated wt P53, produced increased levels of mdm2 protein, and underwent growth arrest and apoptosis.

A series of similar studies have been reported on the replacement of the RB gene in RB-deficient cells from diverse types of human cancers, suppressing their tumorigenic activity. Bookstein and co-workers reported suppression of tumorigenicity of human prostate DU145 carcinoma cells by restoring wt RB using retrovirus-mediated gene transfer (Bookstein et al, 1990). In their study, cells that maintained stable exogenous pRB expression lost the ability to form tumors in nude mice. Zhou and colleagues, however, have pointed out that RB-mediated tumor suppression in RB-defective tumor cells is substantial but often incomplete and that RB replacement has no major effect on cell growth and morphology (Zhou et al, 1994). They have postulated that this partial (incomplete) tumor suppression may reflect the biologic heterogeneity of the tumor cell population and referred to the phenomenon as tumor suppressor resistance (Zhou et al, 1994). They further explored this concept by creating a modified RB gene with enhanced tumor suppression function. These investigators have shown that an N-terminal truncated pRB protein of about 94 kDa exerted surprisingly more potent cell growth suppression as compared to the full-length pRB proteins. Cells failed to enter S phase and displayed multiple changes associated with cellular senescence and apoptosis (Xu et al, 1994b). All of these findings provide new strategies to improve the efficacy of the emerging TP53 and RB tumor suppressor gene replacement therapy.

TUMOR VOLUME AND ABNORMAL GROWTH

Tumor Size and Tumor Doublings

It has been estimated that a 1-g tumor mass contains approximately 1 billion (10^9) cells and occupies a volume of 1 cm^3 (Table 75–3). To the clinician, a 1-cm tumor is frequently thought of as a small "early" tumor; **yet, if one assumes that the tumor develops initially from a single transformed cell, one can calculate that it has already completed 30 cell doublings to reach a 1-g (1-cm^3) size.** A further 10 doublings (total 40) would result in a kilo-

Table 75–3. EFFECT OF HORMONAL THERAPY AND TUMOR STEM CELLS

Tumor Growth Status	Tumor Stem Cell Content	
	Males	*Females*
Parent	1 per 4000	1 per 370,000
Castrate	1 per 70,000	1 per 2,200,000
Recurrent	1 per 200	1 per 800

gram mass (10^{12} cells), which is frequently the maximum tumor burden compatible with life. Thus, at the earliest time of clinical detection, this "small" 1-cm tumor has already completed three quarters of its life span, and considerable opportunity for cell heterogeneity and metastatic potential may have already occurred. To illustrate further, a human breast tumor with a doubling time of 3 months would take apparently 7.5 years to reach a 1-cm^3 size (assuming an origin from a single cell). Furthermore, even assuming some slowing in the growth rate, with increased size resulting in tumor vascularity and necrosis, it can reach a lethal size of approximately 1 kg in just an additional 2.5 years assuming that no effective treatment is administered. This example amply illustrates the difficulty facing the clinician in that despite the small size of a given lesion, the tumor already is "old" with respect to its overall life span and may have already spawned distant unrecognized micrometastasis, which will eventually lead to the death of the patient despite effective therapy to eradicate the primary tumor (Table 75–4).

Tumor Heterogeneity, Spontaneous Resistance to Therapy, and P53

Within a tumor, considerable heterogeneity exists. Cells are found that are de novo resistant to cytotoxics, hormones, or radiation while the surrounding normal tissue remains uniform in its response (Poste and Greig, 1983; Goldie and Coldman, 1984; Pienta et al, 1988). **The likelihood of heterogeneity increases with cell division.**

It becomes more likely that cells resistant to therapy will be found with increasing frequency as the tumor size increases. What needs to be emphasized is that **not every cell division leads to an increase in tumor size.** Most tumors have a large cell loss fraction of cells dying or leaving the reproductive pool of cells, and it is probably a

Table 75–4. RELATIONSHIP BETWEEN TUMOR DOUBLINGS, CELL NUMBER, AND TUMOR SIZE*

Tumor Doublings	Cell Number	Grams of Tumor	Detection
0	0	Nanogram	—
10	10^3	Microgram	—
20	10^6	Milligram	Microscopic
30	10^9	Gram	Palpable
40	10^{12}	Kilogram	Debilitation Death

*Assumes every cell produced proliferates with no cell loss.

mutation that disables the cell death mechanism that is in part responsible for the development of the cell population that is resistant to therapy. The more rounds of division, the more likely mutations are to occur, especially in solid tumors with a high cell loss fraction. An abnormality that could occur is a mutation in P53. P53 is regarded as a protector of the integrity of the DNA. If DNA is damaged, P53 stops the cell cycle and allows for repair, or if the damage is too extensive to repair, it provides for the cell to undergo programmed cell suicide, called apoptosis.

What was not clear is why tumors should be spontaneously resistant to radiation or cytotoxic agents and why that should be related to tumor volume. It has been known for some time that the central area of tumors tended to be **hypoxic.** This is the result of the abnormal vasculature of the tumor, with the outer areas of the tumor being better oxygenated and the central areas being anoxic. **The lack of oxygenation is associated with the induction of apoptosis and P53. If a cell develops a mutated P53, it is not induced to die and thus is more likely to resist cytotoxic chemotherapy and irradiation, less likely to be able to repair cell damage, and more likely to develop more mutations and become more heterogeneous; in such an environment, resistance to hypoxia may function as a selection factor.** To establish that this is what is likely happening in tumor progression, workers used beta-galactosidase as a reporter protein so that the cells could be stained immunohistochemically (Graeber et al, 1996). They transfected cells that lack P53 with the beta-galactosidase and added the P53-negative, beta-galactosidase–positive cells at the level of $\frac{1}{10,000}$ the number of normal cells and repeatedly exposed them to hypoxic conditions. After five exposures, only the cells that lacked P53 were left. This demonstrates how cells can be selected for drug resistance without prior exposure to the therapeutic agent (Fig. 75–7). It can be reasoned that any factor that would protect cells against apoptosis would be similarly selective. Cells that lack P53 are substantially reduced in their sensitivity to most cytotoxic drugs and to the effects of irradiation.

Solid Tumors and Cell-Cell Interactions

Cells of solid tumors grow in an environment of other cells; they not only interact with other tumor cells, but also with diffusible factors from the surrounding stroma and are altered in their activity by contact with basement membranes and the development of support from vascular endothelial cells. These interactions are a composite of growth stimulatory and inhibitory signals. The importance of the stroma in cell interactions is emphasized in the investigations of Cunha et al (1983, 1987). They mixed stroma and epithelium during normal development and demonstrated that if neonatal stroma from the prostate is grown with neonatal bladder epithelial cells the bladder epithelia become prostate-like. If neonatal prostate epithelial cells are grown on bladder mesenchyme, the prostate epithelium becomes bladder epithelium. The importance of the stroma in tumor development is emphasized by the finding that fully transformed **prostatic adenocarcinoma cells are stimulated in their growth by prostatic stroma, and the addition of these stroma to prostatic adenocarcinoma cells implanted into the flank**

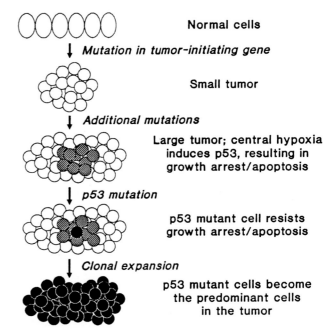

Figure 75–7. Tumor progression that occurs as tumor enlarges with development of tissue anoxia because of a lack of vascularization except at periphery and the lack of the development of lymphatics for drainage. The tumor anoxia results in P53 activation of apoptotic cell death, but mutations in P53 result in lack of cell death, which serves as a selection pressure for mutated P53. (Adapted from Kinzler KW, Vogelstein B: Nature 1996; 379:19–20.)

of animals enhances their ability to form rapidly growing tumors (Camps et al, 1990). Indeed, it has been suggested that the usual mode of tumor transplantation in the animal's flank should not be used but that the transplantable tumors should be placed orthotopically in the tissue of origin because that tissue contains the paracrine-acting factors required for growth that would be more representative of tumors found in patients. The same is likely true for solid tumor metastasis, as both Chackal-Roy and associates and Chung and colleagues have demonstrated that diffusible factors produced by bone marrow cells stimulated prostatic cancer cell growth (Chackal-Roy et al, 1989; Chung et al, 1990). Indeed, it needs to be considered that the tumor which metastasized to the bone is still evolving or progressing. **Metastasis to the bone is not an end in the evolution of the tumor. The bone stroma appears to produce factors that continue to drive the evolution of the metastasis in the bone to a more androgen-independent phenotype** (Thalmann et al, 1994). Aprikian and co-workers observed that P53 expression did not appear to result from the clonal expansion of a founder metastatic cell in bony metastatic deposits but rather that the mutation and progression probably occurred after metastasis to the bone (Aprikian et al, 1994).

Tumor Stem Cell Growth

Tumor Stem Cells

Not every cell in a solid tumor has the capability to grow and form a tumor. This is in contrast to certain leukemias in which every cell has stem cell capability and each cell can regrow a tumor. **Operationally, tumor stem cells are the subset of tumor cells responsible for repopulating the tumor following therapy** (Steel, 1977). Evidence of the pluripotent nature of the tumor stem cell is provided by the observation that a single human colonic adenocarcinoma cell can differentiate into columnar, goblet and entero-endocrine cells in culture (Kirkland, 1988). The altered ability to differentiate can be viewed as a spectrum with greater DNA damage associated with a lesser capacity to differentiate terminally. The concept that the tumor represents a defect in differentiation is supported by the observation that teratocarcinoma cells implanted into a developing embryo can undergo differentiation and behave as normal cells (Illmensee and Mintz, 1976). Thus, it may be possible to restore the normal cell phenotype in a tumor given the right environmental signals.

Assays of Tumor Stem Cells

Cells are examined for their ability to form colonies in soft agar because many normal cells do not grow in soft agar (Hall and Watt, 1989). Some cells form large colonies resulting from many rounds of division, whereas other cells form only small colonies (Hall and Watt, 1989). This suggests that the smaller colonies arose from committed cells with limited reproductive capacity, whereas the larger colonies arose from the true stem cells with unlimited reproductive capacity.

There are a number of assays to approximate the stem cell population of a tumor. Growth in semisolid agar as just described is one method. A unique feature of tumor cells is that if they are transplanted into a suitable host they grow, whereas normal cells do not grow. A proviso here is that some tumors grow when implanted orthotopically but not subcutaneously, further defining the effect of the environment on the clonogenic (stem) cell. In tumor models such as the L1210 leukemia, it takes only the transplantation of a single tumor cell for the animal to develop a tumor and die. Thus, in the L1210 model system, every tumor cell is a tumor stem cell. In most solid tumors, true "stem cells" constitute a small percentage of the total tumor cell populations. Because the number of cells required to form a tumor is often used as an indicator of the number of tumor stem cells present within the tumor, one technique used to determine stem cell number is to implant different numbers of tumor cells and calculate the number of tumor cells required to achieve tumor growth (take) in 50% of the implanted animals. This technique is referred to as the *limiting dilution assay.* Within the region of cell concentrations achieving 1% to 99% "takes," the number of tumor stem cells can be calculated based on Poisson distribution.

Tumor Stem Cell Assay: An Example of the Effect of Androgen Withdrawal on Tumor Stem Cell Content

The limiting dilution assay was used to demonstrate the relative hormonal sensitivity of malignant cells and the effect of castration on the stem cell population by Bruchovsky and colleagues using the androgen-dependent mammary tumor line (Bruchovsky et al, 1990). **In androgen-*dependent* tumors, androgen withdrawal leads to the death of the tumor cell. Conversely, androgen-*sensitive* tumors do not die in the absence of androgen, but androgens stimulate their growth. Androgen-*insensitive* cells are unaffected by androgen levels.**

These investigators transplanted the tumor into nude mice and found a normal growth pattern, with the average tumor attaining the weight of approximately 6 g 20 days after transplantation. Following castration, the tumor lost approximately 90% of its total weight and reached a nadir on approximately day 35. After a short dormant period, the remaining cells again started to grow and by day 80 approximated the tumor weight before castration (Fig. 75–8). In an elegant set of experiments, the Vancouver investigators took cells from the "parent" tumor during tumor growth, from the "castrate" tumor at the time of maximum tumor regression following orchiectomy, and from the cell population of the recurrent tumor at the time when the tumor weight approximated the weight of the parent tumor. They then calculated the stem cell ratios in each population by determining the number of tumors that developed compared with the number of cells inoculated into the animal.

Using this in vivo clonogenic assay, the authors calculated that in the male host, one new tumor developed per 4000 cells inoculated, but it took almost 100 times more cells to develop a single tumor "take" in a female host, indicating the marked effect of hormonal manipulation in the cells derived from the parent tumor (see Table 75–3). When the cells from the "recurrent" tumor, which grew following castration, were injected, there was a marked enrichment of the stem cell ratio. Injecting the "recurrent" cells into the male host resulted in one tumor take per 200 cells inoculated and one per 800 cells inoculated in the female host.

The greatest stem cell ratios occurred using the cell population obtained at the time of maximum tumor regression. In

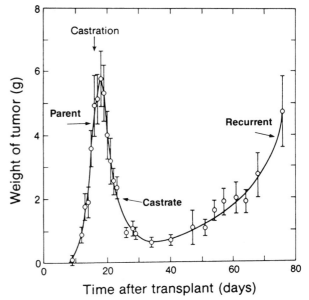

EFFECT OF CASTRATION — SHIONOGI TUMOR

Figure 75–8. Experimental system for obtaining tumor tissue for stem cell quantitation before castration (parent), following castration during tumor regression (castrate), and during tumor regrowth (recurrent). (Adapted from Bruchovsky N, Rennie PS, Coldman AJ, et al: Cancer Res 1990; 50:2275–2287.)

these cells, which were obtained 7 days following castration, it took approximately 70,000 cells to form a single tumor when injected into the male host and 2.2 million cells to form a single tumor when cells from the same population were injected into the female host. These data show a marked depletion of the stem cell population 7 days after castration at the time of maximum tumor regression. Thus, if one were planning additional therapy to augment hormonal manipulation, it seems reasonable that the ideal time to administer the therapy is when the **ratio of stem cells to all cells is at its lowest level.**

With this androgen-sensitive solid tumor, the following was revealed:

1. Not every tumor cell can produce a tumor (i.e., not every cell is a "stem" cell).

2. The "recurrent" tumor, that is, the tumor occurring following castration, appears to be the more aggressive tumor with the highest percentage of stem cells noted. The clinical parallel to this observation would be the apparent increased aggressiveness of prostate cancer recurring after castration or estrogen treatment.

3. The lowest stem cell ratio was observed at the time of maximal regression following castration; hence, theoretically, this would be the optimal time that surgical extirpation of the residual tumor is most likely to be effective in removing all the remaining stem cells.

Although this experiment is an example of the effect of hormonal manipulation, other therapies can be similarly studied following chemotherapy or radiation therapy. The maximum effect of hormone deprivation (castrate population in female) represents a decrease in stem cells of nearly 99.9% and may be considered reasonable monotherapy considering the minimal toxicity. Unless all stem cells are eradicated, however, tumor regrowth is likely. Also, if the stem cell is responsible for tumor regrowth and if only the stem cell represents the true reproductive component of the tumor, one does not have to kill every tumor cell to eradicate the tumor, just eliminate the tumor stem cell. **Lastly, it is likely that the tumor that regrows will be less likely to respond to the original treatment, and a different strategy will be required to treat the resistant tumors.**

In this androgen-sensitive tumor, it has been observed that the recurrent tumor makes a growth factor called fibroblast growth factor. The recurrent tumor that is hormone resistant is making its own growth factor and is not relying on the presence of androgen to provide for the production of the growth factor. Thus, the tumor has become self-sufficient and is self-producing a self-stimulating/death-eliminating growth factor. In human prostate cancer, this is observed fairly early in that many prostate cancers shift from paracrine control and regulation to autocrine regulation (Fig. 75–9). Alternatively, they may also shift to a new paracrine control at their metastatic site.

The stem cell concept has led to an attempt to characterize tumor stem cells to predict which drugs will be useful in the treatment of a patient's malignancy, to develop methods to circumvent resistance, to assess tumor stem cell number as an indicator of patient prognosis, to guide the development of new agents, and to determine the impact of stem cell number on curability. These efforts have had varying degrees of success because of the limitations in understanding of the

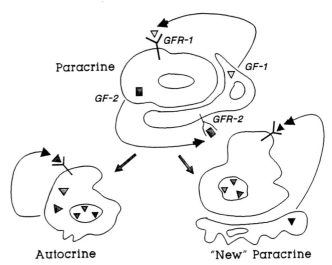

Figure 75–9. Paracrine and autocrine regulation of prostatic growth.

optimal methods for modeling growth conditions experienced by the tumor in the patient.

ANGIOGENESIS

Properties of Angiogenesis

A feature common to many malignancies is the formation of new blood vessels, called angiogenesis. Tumor growth obviously requires a vascular supply. The normal vascular endothelium can be induced to grow in response to injury or to the normal growth processes associated with menstruation or pregnancy. Thus, angiogenesis does not always imply malignancy. The term *angiogenesis* was coined in 1935 to describe the formation of new blood vessels in the placenta (Hertig, 1935). Angiogenesis also may not always appear as the initial step in tumor formation. In cervical neoplasia, angiogenesis typically occurs before the gross appearance of tumor; in breast and bladder carcinoma, a marked increase in angiogenesis appears coincidentally with tumor development; and in melanoma and ovarian carcinoma, angiogenesis develops after tumor formation (Folkman, 1990). Basic fibroblast growth factor stimulates the growth of some tumors and is also angiogenic by stimulating the growth of endothelial cells as well. Basic fibroblast growth factor stimulated the growth of colon tumors when administered to animals receiving implants of tumor cells lacking fibroblast growth factor receptors. The same cells did not produce tumors in the absence of fibroblast growth factor (Folkman, 1990), and this represents further evidence for the importance of angiogenesis in the growth of tumor (Folkman, 1990).

Folkman (1990) has summarized a great amount of evidence for the **angiogenic dependence of tumors:**

1. Tumors grown in isolated perfused organs in which blood vessels do not proliferate are limited to 2 mm³ but expand rapidly to 1 cm³ when transplanted into mice and become vascularized.

2. The growth of experimental tumors implanted in

the avascular cornea is limited until after vascularization, when growth rapidly accelerates.

3. Within a solid tumor, the [³H]thymidine labeling index of tumor cells (which indicates cell growth) decreases with increasing distance of the cell from the nearest open capillary.

4. Carcinoma of the ovary metastasizes to the peritoneal membrane as tiny avascular seeds, which rarely grow beyond a limited size until after vascularization.

5. Angiogenic inhibitors that are not growth suppressive in tissue culture are growth inhibitory in animal models.

6. In transgenic animals that develop carcinoma, large tumors arise from preneoplastic hyperplastic areas that are vascularized.

The identification of angiogenic factors requires the development of reproducible bioassay systems. These systems have focused on visualization and quantitation of the ingrowth of capillaries. These include the implantation of tumor-containing or biopolymer-containing angiogenic molecules into the cornea of the rabbit, rat, or mouse; the chorioallantoic membrane of chick eggs; or the tissue culture growth of vascular endothelial cells (Folkman and Klagsburn, 1987) (Fig. 75–10). Based on these assays, a number of agents with angiogenic as well as antiangiogenic activity have been found. These have been summarized by Tai-Ping and colleagues (1995). **Special mention should be given to vascular endothelial growth factor—as being one of the most specific and potent of the recently discovered angiogenic agents** (Thomas, 1996). **Interestingly, it has been found that vascular endothelial growth factor production is regulated by hypoxia.**

There are a number of inducers and inhibitors of angiogenesis in tissue. In this tightly regulated system, it appears that there are many possible areas in which positive-acting or negative-acting factors could be subverted as part of

Table 75–5. EXAMPLES OF ENDOGENOUS REGULATORS

Activators	Inhibitors
Acidic FGF	Angiostatin
Angiogenin	Cartilage-derived inhibitor
Basic FGF	Thrombospondin
Hepatocyte growth factor	Interferon-α
Interleukin-8	Interferon-β
Placenta growth factor	Platelet factor 4
Transforming growth factor-α	Prolactin fragment
Prostaglandins E₁, E₂	Protamine
Vascular endothelial cell	Tissue inhibitor of metalloproteinase
Growth factor	
Pleotropin	

FGF, Fibroblast growth factor.

tumor progression. The isolation of angiogenic factors was helped by the development of in vitro culturing of endothelial cells to study their growth and motility. Especially potent agents were the fibroblast growth factors. In many tissues, the tissue concentrations of fibroblast growth factors are higher than would be anticipated from the degree of angiogenesis normally found. It appears that basic fibroblast growth factor is bound to both the cytosolic and the extracellular forms of heparan sulfate, which eventually becomes part of the cell matrix. Because it is unlikely that the bound form of fibroblast growth factor is active in angiogenesis, the basic fibroblast growth factor must be released from the extracellular matrix. Heparan sulfate is degraded by heparinase, and the matrix core proteins are degraded by proteinases. Folkman and Klagsburn (1987) observed that the basement membrane basic fibroblast growth factor can be released by heparinase and induce endothelial cell growth. Heparinase may serve two purposes: First, it may serve to release fibroblast growth factor, which diffuses to the endothelial cell and induces chemotaxis toward the site of matrix degradation; second, the residual heparan fragment bound to fibroblast growth factor protects the fibroblast growth factor from degradation by proteolytic enzymes such as plasmin. Although fibroblast growth factor is bound to the heparin fragment, it is still able to activate endothelial cell growth and plasminogen activator production (Folkman, 1990). Many of the angiogenic proteins bind to heparin. Table 75–5 provides a list of endogenous angiogenic molecules and angiogenic inhibitors.

As with the other physical features of cancer, it can be surmised that the angiogenic cells in a tumor arise from normal nononcogenic cells by the accumulation of genetic changes that activate oncogenes and inactivate suppressor genes (Bouck, 1990). Experimentally a transfected oncogene can make a cell angiogenic. Thompson and colleagues have introduced *ras* and *myc* oncogenes into normal epithelial and stromal cells and reconstituted the prostate (Thompson et al, 1989). They observed a tenfold increase in the number of new blood vessels within the prostate. Neoangiogenesis, therefore, may be due to cell cycle–induced synthesis of growth factors. Suppressor gene loss can also influence angiogenesis. Inactivation of a suppressor gene leads to an increase in angiogenic activity that parallels its increase in tumorigenicity (Moroco et al, 1990). **This inhibitor of angiogenic activity is the extracellular protein thrombospondin** (Moroco et al, 1990). Loss of suppressor genes has been

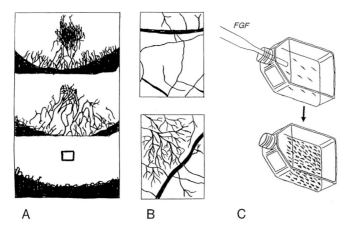

Figure 75–10. Assays used to determine the angiogenic ability test compounds or biologics. *A,* A rabbit iris has been implanted with a tumor tissue, and the neovasculature that has developed to supply the tumor can be seen. *B,* bFGF (basic fibroblast growth factor) has been added to the chicken chorioallantoic membrane (lower) and saline to the upper drawing, and the difference in vascularity 5 days later was determined as highly significant. *C,* Endothelial cells are added to a tissue culture flask. If an endothelial cell growth factor such as bFGF or vascular endothelial cell growth factor is added, there is a large increase in cell number.

correlated with angiogenic activity in many cell systems (Yarden and Ulrich, 1988). **The ability to metastasize often correlates with the amount of tumor vascularization** (Wiedner et al, 1993).

Surgery as a Cause of Metastatic Tumor Growth

Tumors can metastasize and shed, but if the metastases are unable to induce a blood supply they remain dormant. **Some tumors produce factors that are angiogenesis inhibitors, such as angiostatin, which is a 38-kDa fragment of plasminogen** (O'Reilly et al, 1994). O'Reilly and co-workers observed that when the primary tumor was removed, the metastatic deposits were able to induce a vascular supply and grow rapidly. Not all tumors are capable of producing inhibitors of angiogenesis. When a variety of tumors were generated from established cell lines, such as the prostate metastasis–derived PC-3, they were observed to inhibit the growth of angiogenesis in tumors subsequently implanted into the cornea (Chen et al, 1995). **This raises questions concerning tumor treatment in primary cancer patients and suggests that if patients are found to have elevated levels of suppressors before surgery, angiogenesis inhibitors might be considered after surgery to make certain that any metastatic tumors remain dormant.**

Blockade or Enhancement of Irradiation Damage to the Endothelium

Fuks and others have identified that growth factors such as basic fibroblast growth factor protect the endothelial cells from the damaging effects of irradiation in vitro (Fuks et al, 1994). **Fuks and collaborators administered irradiation to regions of the lungs of experimental animals along with basic fibroblast growth factor, and they were able to protect the animals totally from irradiation-induced vascular damage and death.** Damage to the blood vessels of normal tissue is an aspect that limits the dose of irradiation that can be administered to patients, and the administration of bFGF basic fibroblast growth factor may circumvent this limitation to irradiation dose of normal cells. On the same note, Fuks and co-workers have noted that agents that block growth factor activity enhance irradiation-induced apoptotic death of endothelial cells. Thus, it may be possible to increase the sensitivity of irradiation to the tumor while protecting normal tissue. Growth factors signal the cell by signal transduction cascades. An early enzyme in intracellular signal transduction for growth factors involves the activation of protein kinase C. These investigators further observed that indirect activation of protein kinase C-alpha mimicked the effect of basic fibroblast growth factor, whereas inhibition of protein kinase C-alpha blocked the radioprotection afforded by basic fibroblast growth factor (Haimovitz-Friedman et al, 1994). These effects occur at the cell surface. Previously, all irradiation cytotoxicity was thought to be occurring as nuclear DNA-damaging effects. These investigators have identified that irradiation may be activating apoptotic cell death mechanisms via effects on the cell surface.

Table 75–6. INTERSTITIAL PRESSURES IN HUMAN TUMORS

Type of Tumor	Mean Pressure
Normal skin	0.4
Renal cell carcinoma	38.0
Cervical carcinoma	22.8
Colonic liver metastasis	21.0
Breast carcinoma	15.0
Metastatic melanoma	14.3

Data from Jain RK: Sci Am 1994; 270:58–65.

Abnormal Tumor Blood Vessels and Antitumor Drug Therapy

Most therapies targeted against tumors need to reach the tumor through the blood vessels that were generated by the tumor. These vessels tend to be tortuous and abnormal. In addition, **tumors do not generate a lymphatic system.** Thus, the **intratumoral pressure may be much greater than that in the systemic circulation,** resulting in a substantial pressure gradient that works against diffusion into the tumor (Jain, 1994). It is believed that this increased intratumoral pressure is the result of tumors not forming lymphatics. This makes drug delivery and delivery of agents of large molecular size such as antibodies that much more difficult. Jain calculated, as an example, that if a drug is being moved along by convection, the rate of movement is a linear proportion to the distance (i.e., 1, 2, 3, 4), but if moving by diffusion, the rate of movement is proportional to the distance squared (i.e., 1^1, 2^2, 3^3, 4^4) (Table 75–6).

METASTASIS

Metastatic Process

The most clinically devastating biologic alteration of malignant tumors is related to their ability to metastasize and colonize different organs. Many forms of locoregional control are effective, but for the majority of urologic tumors, once they have metastasized the end result is death. This is directly related to the low activity of standard cytotoxic chemotherapy in urologic tumors, testicular tumors being the exception. Some tumors are able to spread by direct extension (e.g., abdominal ovarian carcinomatosis), but invasion and metastatic spread, either hematogenous or vascular, represents the usual mechanisms of tumor spread. Liotta and co-workers have identified the steps involved in the metastatic cascade. (Liotta et al, 1985) (Fig. 75–11).

To metastasize, tumor cells need to disrupt the basement membrane and penetrate into the extracellular matrix. This is followed by invasion of the microvasculature, surviving intravascular circulation and seeding at a distant site (Liotta et al, 1985). More specifically, these processes may be divided as follows. **Tumor cell surface receptors attach to specific components in the matrix,** such as fibronectin or laminin. Laminin is a large glycoprotein found predominantly in the basement membrane, where one end of the molecule binds to type 4 collagen. High concentrations of laminin receptors have been demonstrated in several neoplastic cell lines (Liotta et al, 1985). Interference with the

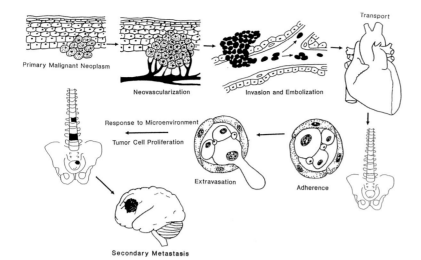

Figure 75–11. The metastatic processes that a cell undertakes to be able to disseminate hematogenously.

laminin receptors' ability to bind matrix has been associated with diminished metastasis in a melanoma model system (Barsky et al, 1984). Normal cells possess laminin receptors, but they appear to be fewer in number compared to homologous cancer cells such as colon (Liotta, 1986). **Second, the matrix needs to be dissolved.** This is done by the elaboration of a variety of proteolytic enzymes. These include the collagenases, in particular, type IV collagenase. Type IV collagen is a major structural component of the basement membrane (Liotta et al, 1980). The implication is that the malignant cell has the ability to degrade the matrix of the endothelial membrane, facilitating its entry into the blood stream. Plasminogen activator activates other proteolytic enzymes and has been proposed to play a major role in the plasminogen activator-plasmin-collagenase cascade. Tumor plasminogen activator activates plasmin, which, in turn, activates collagenase, which then degrades the matrix (Mignatti et al, 1986). This proteolytic activity can be balanced by tissue-specific proteolytic inhibitors that block invasive behavior (Thorgeirsson et al, 1982). The **third** step in the invasion process is **movement of the cells through the attenuated matrix.** Laminin itself may be chemotactic for some tumor cells (McCarthy et al, 1985). Because tumor cells lack lymphatics, the hydrostatic pressure of edema may force tumor cells into the interstitium (Butler et al, 1975). This movement, however, may also be a characteristic associated with the heterogeneity of the transformed cell. Coffey and co-workers examined a series of prostatic tumor cell variants that differed in their metastatic activity by using a video camera to record cell movement in vitro. They demonstrated that the most highly motile cells were the most metastatic (Mohler et al, 1987; Partin et al, 1988). As noted earlier, *ras* oncogenic transformation is often associated with increased motility and metastatic aggressiveness (Partin et al, 1988). A growth factor/receptor/oncogene signaling pathway associated with motility and metastasis is met with a receptor/hepatocyte growth factor/scatter factor. As the name implies, one of the first demonstrations of its action was that it induced motility in cells. Its expression has been found to be up-regulated in metastatic prostatic cancer (Humphrey et al, 1995).

Once the tumor successfully penetrates the endothelial basement membrane, it gains access to the systemic circulation. **Not all tumor cells reaching the circulation, however, survive.** Indeed, even with a highly metastatic melanoma tumor model, only 1% of the injected tumor cells can reach the circulatory system and retain viability (Fidler, 1990). **The tumor cell must also have the ability to leave the circulation and evolve into a metastatic deposit. A cell simply gaining entrance into the circulation does not guarantee metastases.** A clinical example of this fact is in patients with ovarian carcinomatosis, in whom the ascites is often palliated by peritoneovenous shunting. Despite the millions of tumor cells passing through the circulation daily, metastases are rarely seen at autopsy (Tarin et al, 1984).

Because of the specificity and sensitivity of the polymerase chain reaction, a number of investigators are currently revisiting the issue of circulating tumor cells. In most cases, a mRNA marker associated with the specialized function of the cell, such as prostate-specific antigen or prostate-specific membrane antigen, is used to identify the presence of the tumor cell. The mRNA is transcribed by reverse transcriptase into cDNA, and the DNA is then amplified by the polymerase chain reaction. Most groups report being able to detect one prostate cell in 10^6 lymphocytes. The clinical significance of the small numbers of detected tumor cells in the circulation remains to be established. What is needed is a method to determine the biologic potential of these circulating cells (Heston, 1995).

Mechanical Versus Seed and Soil

The metastatic tumor cell may finally be arrested in the capillaries of remote organs. The **mechanical theory** of metastasis suggests that filtration can account for entrapment of large emboli and the eventual generation of metastatic deposits. Indeed, in some situations, it would appear that a metastatic lesion was a passive result with regard to the lymphatic and venous drainage systems (mechanical). When B16 tumor cells are injected, however, and then followed to determine where they lodge, a significant number settle in the liver and spleen, yet invariably it is in the lung that the cells take hold and grow. Such data have provided evidence for the **seed and soil** hypothesis of metastasis first proposed by Paget in 1889. Sugarbaker demonstrated the tissue-specific nature of metastasizing cells when he transplanted ectopic organ grafts and then implanted sarcomas that metastasized strictly to the lungs (Sugarbaker et al, 1971). The only tissues in which there were metastatic deposits observed were in the lungs and ectopic lung tissue; none of the other ectopic tissues demonstrated metastases.

Metastatic site selection can often be determined by cell surface components. Experiments in which the plasma membrane components of cells with different rates of metastasis were reversed show a change to the opposite rate at which they metastasize (Poste and Nicolson, 1980). Factors from the tissue to which a tumor metastasizes (soil) also affect selection. Substances have been isolated from tissues that enhance the rate of metastasis to that site. Terranova and colleagues demonstrated that a variety of malignancies were selectively influenced by extracts from the specific organs to which they metastasize (Terranova et al, 1986). In some cases, inhibitory factors are produced, which prevent growth of metastatic cells, whereas in others growth stimulatory factors are produced, such as bone marrow stroma, which may stimulate the growth of prostatic cancer cells (Chackal-Roy et al, 1989). **The soil not only provides for the growth of the metastatic seed, but also may promote further the evolution of the tumor; Thalmann and co-workers have demonstrated in models of human prostatic carcinoma that bone stroma induces an androgen-resistant state in hormone-sensitive tumors** (Thalmann et al, 1994). Aprikian and colleagues demonstrated that P53 mutations of prostatic cancer in the bone are not clonal and that the P53 mutations occurred after the tumor was established in the bone (Aprikian et al, 1994).

It should not be surprising that tumors vary in their metastatic capability. When a number of highly metastatic tumors were cloned and the clones examined for metastatic potential, there was an incredible range of metastatic expression even in the original tumors, as is shown in Figure 75–12 (Fidler, 1990).

One can also isolate cells that metastasize to different tissues and maintain this feature on repassage and cloning (Fidler, 1990). Primary tumors are also heterogeneous with respect to their organ specificity. Individual cells within a primary tumor also exhibit not only differential abilities to metastasize, but also a differential preference as to the organ that they can colonize (Zetter, 1990). Recognizing the heterogeneous nature of tumors with respect to cellular composition and metastatic propensity enables the physician to appreciate the marked variability in clinical behavior observed in human tumors and underscores the magnitude of the difficulties that need to be surmounted to control the cancer process effectively.

Antimetastatic Genes: Search for Metastasis Suppressors

Autocrine motility factor is a positive-acting factor for tumor motility and metastatic tumor spread. As with positive oncogenes versus tumor suppressor genes, there may be genes that would inhibit the metastatic ability of normal cells, which could be lost during tumor progression. Various groups have sought these suppressor genes using slightly different methodologies, such as differential display and DNA transfer techniques, previously discussed in Chapter 1.

Differential Display

Differential display techniques detect genes that are differentially regulated between two phenotypically different cells (i.e., nonmetastatic tumors versus metastatic tumors) that are derived from the same original cell and otherwise are identical. These techniques are variants on a molecular technique called differential display. When genes are found that differ significantly between the two different phenotypes, those genes are cloned and expressed in the cell type of interest

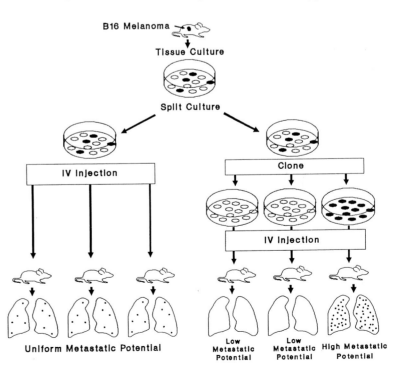

Figure 75–12. In an elegant experiment, Fidler established the clonal heterogeneity that exists in a tumor population. If one takes a tumor, makes a single cell suspension, and injects a constant number of those cells into different animals, a fairly uniform number of metastatic colonies is obtained. If one first takes the tumor, isolates a number of single tumor cells, allows those to grow (clones), and injects cloned cells, some clones produce metastases, whereas others do not. (Adapted from Fidler IJ: Cancer Res 1990; 50:6130–6138.)

(i.e., the purported antimetastatic gene in the metastatic cell), and it is determined whether it suppresses metastasis.

Steeg and colleagues used a series of related rodent melanoma cell lines derived from the K1735 line that differed greatly in their metastatic potential but not in their response to host immune factors, suggesting there were nonimmunologic reasons for their differential metastatic capability (Steeg et al, 1988). They isolated 24 clones differentially expressed between the high and low metastatic cells. In two nonmetastatic clones, the **pNM23** cDNA insert exhibited a consistently greater level of mRNA than that found in five highly metastatic clones (Steeg et al, 1988). These investigators also observed gene expression in several nonmetastatic breast tumors but greatly reduced amounts in metastatic breast tumors. In primary human breast biopsy specimens, 75% of node-negative tumors expressed high levels of NM23. Low-level node-negative tumors were also poorly differentiated and had a low content of nuclear receptors, characteristically predictive of eventual metastatic spread. Indeed, at the time of the report, two of the low-level NM23 tumors had metastasized, whereas none of the high NM23 expressors had metastasized (Bevilacqua et al, 1989). Although NM23 has been found to be a metastasis suppressor for some tumors, such as breast and melanoma, it does not appear to suppress metastasis of all tumors, thus demonstrating that there will likely be a spectrum of metastasis suppressors and probably related to the type of tumor.

DNA Transfer

Another approach to discover antimetastatic genes is to insert chromosomes or chromosome fragments into metastatic cells and determine whether it causes the cells to lose their metastatic behavior selectively, that is, does not affect their rate of growth or ability to form a tumor but makes them no longer able to metastasize. Dong and colleagues have identified a prostate metastasis suppressor on chromosome 11p that they designated as **KAI1** using the technique of microcell DNA transfer, in which a small region of genomic DNA is stably transferred into the cells of interest (Dong et al, 1995). They used metastatic cells that were either prostatic or mammary, and suppression was specific for prostate cells. Expression of this gene did not affect the growth of or immunologic reactivity of the transfected tumor cells. These findings are of special interest because suppressor genes of growth appear to affect all tumor cells. It appears that metastasis suppressors have tissue-restrictive patterns and require a broader-based investigation of tumor types for their discovery.

TUMOR BIOLOGY–BASED THERAPEUTICS

Biology-Based Therapeutics and Rational Drug Development

Cancer therapy has been primarily aimed at developing cytotoxic agents that kill cells. The problem is that the cells may already have a high rate of cell death or have mutations so that they are more resistant to the induction of cell death,

while the body's normal cells still have the same response and are being killed as well or even more so. For the majority of urologic tumors, there is no effective chemotherapy, and even with treatable testicular tumors, patients suffer from the painful side effects of nonspecific cytotoxics. Clearly, effective agents are needed, and those agents need to be selective in their destruction of the tumor. The focus should be shifted from eliminating the tumor to preventing the tumor from occurring in the first place or in keeping it from growing and spreading. Prostate cancer is the number one malignancy of American men, but in other cultures prostate cancer is a minor malignancy, and epidemiologic studies suggest that with alterations in the lifestyle and nutritional habits of American men, the amount of prostate cancer seen could be dramatically reduced.

Nutrition and Lifestyle Changes

There are numerous reports of increased risk for the development of cancer from various environmental and lifestyle factors (Lerman et al, 1989). **Elimination of tobacco products and alterations in nutritional habits such as decreasing the overall caloric intake, especially fats; eating more vegetables such as broccoli, carrots, and tomatoes; and increasing fiber intake have all been recommended** (Lerman et al, 1989; Greenberg et al, 1990; Newmark et al, 1990). These recommendations are not based on the results of large prospective, randomized trials but do have support from numerous retrospective studies and as such require cautious interpretation (Prentice et al, 1989). There are thousands of potential nutritional and chemopreventive agents that need to be investigated. The task here is to identify realistic models that would be useful in predicting agents that can decrease, if not eliminate, the progression of cancer. In a transplantable model of prostate cancer, it was demonstrated that athymic nude mice bearing the transplantable human prostatic cancer LNCaP had a substantial decrease in their rate of growth when their diet was changed from one of high fat to low fat (Wang et al, 1995). As important, however, was the observation that the change in dietary fat did not alter the amount of prostate-specific antigen produced as a function of tumor burden, and thus prostate-specific antigen could be used as a biomarker to monitor the effectiveness of such nutritional interventions.

In the study of breast cancer, the *neu* and *ras* oncogenes have been transfected into embryonic tissue, which is then maintained in the germ line of descendants in model systems referred to as **transgenic** animals. In these, the animals go on to develop breast tumors as they mature and age (Muller et al, 1988). Colon cancer develops in transgenic mice with the deleted in colon cancer mutation (DCC), and the incidence of tumors can be dramatically reduced with dietary manipulation. Development of such models for urologic tumors as has been accomplished for prostatic tumors is needed and should provide a tool for identifying effective prevention strategies.

It has been repeatedly pointed out that the national mortality from cancer continues to increase, and this is likely due to a focus on treatment strategies of cytotoxic elimination of tumor cells. Reliance on this strategy has not been success-

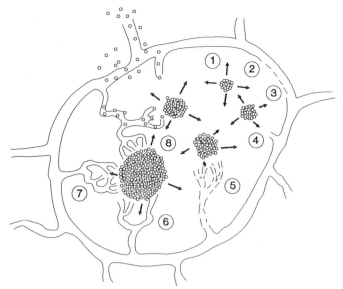

Figure 75–13. Potential therapeutic points of attack of antiangiogenesis agents. Site 1, the production of angiogenic factors, develops antisense oligomers and glucocorticoids. Site 2, the binding of angiogenic factors to their cognate receptors, uses blocking agents such as bFGF antibody, VEGF antibody, PF4, and suramin. Site 3, basement membrane degradation, uses minocycline, PF4, medroxyprogesterone, cartilage-derived inhibitor, and TIMP. Site 4, endothelial cell migration, uses angiostatic steroids, AGM1470, thrombospondin, and 2 methoxyestradiol. Site 5, endothelial cell proliferation, uses angiostatin, penicillamine, AGM1470, IFN-γ, 2-methoxyestradiol, and genistein. Site 6, capillary tube formation, uses IFN-γ, cyclic YISGR peptide, AGM1470, genistein, 2 methoxyestradiol, and integrin $\alpha_5\beta_3$ antagonists. Site 7, basement membrane synthesis, uses angiostatic steroids, GPA1734, and proline analogues. Site 8, metastasis, uses angiostatic steroids, AGM1470, TIMP, and angiostatin. (Adapted from Trends in Pharmacological Sciences; 16; Tai-Ping D, Rhys J, Bicknell R: Controlling the vasculature, antiangiogenesis, and vascular targeting of the gene; 57–66. Copyright 1995, with permission from Elsevier Science Ltd, Elsevier Trends Division, 68 Hills Road, Cambridge, CB2 1LA, UK.)

ful, and it is time to consider alternative strategies of cancer prevention and antipromotion (Beardsley, 1994).

Antimetastatic and Antiangiogenic Agents

Agents that interfere with a cell's ability to form blood vessels or to metastasize are being identified. Areas of intervention are addressed in Figure 75–13.

Antiangiogenic agents have been reviewed (Tai-Ping et al, 1995). Antiangiogenic agents have been divided into two groups: the specific and the nonspecific. The specific angiogenesis inhibitors are those that inhibit the growth of blood vessels without affecting other tissues. One promising agent in this regard is the fumagillin analogue AGM1470. The discovery of this agent is an example of chance favoring the prepared mind. In 1990, Ingber noted that a fungal contaminant in his experiments produced a factor that inhibited endothelial cell growth but was not toxic. This proved to be the secreted antibiotic **fumagillin** from the fungus *Aspergillus fumigatus*. It blocks the growth factor activity of a number of endothelial mitogens apparently without toxicity to other cells. Fumagillin analogues are beginning clinical trials and could provide the specificity and lack of toxicity

required of an agent that will have to be administered for a prolonged period of time. Platelet factor 4 is antiangiogenic but is not specific in that it has anticoagulant properties. It has a heparin-binding site, and when this was engineered out of a recombinant molecule, the modified recombinant protein was no longer an anticoagulant but still inhibited angiogenesis. Platelet factor 4 was effective in a number of preclinical trials and is now being investigated in a number of phase II trials. The use of soluble receptors for vascular endothelial cell growth factor is a means to tie up the growth factor and has demonstrated antiangiogenic activity in preclinical trials. Protease inhibitors that inhibit the proteases responsible for degradation of the basement membrane and allow the invasion of the endothelial cells are also a potential therapeutic tool, and because this step is also involved in invasion and metastases, such a tool would be similarly useful as an antimetastatic agent. There are a number of potential protease inhibitors, and they are described by Tai-Ping and colleagues (1995). Of course, because many of these antiangiogenic agents have differing mechanisms of action, combination approaches may enhance their antitumor activities.

Because of the importance of the cell's ability to extravasate and intravasate and the involvement of the tumor cell's attachment to and degradation of the matrix in the metastatic process, identification of a number of important cell attachment factors is an area of focus. Some have demonstrated that fragments of adhesion molecules, integrins, and others may be able to block metastasis (Albeda and Buck, 1990). Other agents that have shown potential as antimetastatic agents are being tested as well as unique methods to deliver those agents (Roedink and Kroon, 1989; Kohn and Liotta, 1990).

DNA Replacement Therapy

The loss of suppressor genes is associated with the development of malignancies in some systems. The reinsertion of the suppressor gene function with retroviral vectors has been shown to normalize the cell. Thus, having the tumor cells take up normal P53 provides one approach because normal cells should not be affected by such an approach. The question is what if one does not transfect all of the tumor cells. In early studies, it does not appear to matter because the tumor appears to be responsive even if not every cell is transfected (Baker et al, 1990; Bookstein et al, 1990).

Immunotherapy

Tremendous strides have been made in the understanding of the immune mechanisms of tumor recognition and rejection and the potential for breaking tolerance. Transfection of tumor cells with cytokines, the use of antigen-presenting cells such as dendritic cells transfected to express the tumor/tissue antigen, and transfection of altered signaling in cytotoxic T cells by substituting more general antibody recognition units for major histocompatibility complex recognition units all hold out strong promise for generation of specific immune recognition for achieving nontoxic means to eliminate tumors (Pardoll, 1995).

Signal Transduction Inhibitors

It is understood that growth factor signals have to be transduced by the cell so that the DNA can be reproduced. Cell surface molecules such as RAS proteins perform this function. Many of these intracellular membrane-associated factors are anchored by means of farensylation. The farensylation reaction can be interrupted by specific inhibitors, and the signaling mechanism becomes ineffective. These inhibitors have shown promising preclinical antitumor activity while being free of side effects (Gibbs and Oliff, 1994).

Most cytotoxic chemotherapeutic agents and irradiation are active because they activate apoptotic cell death, not solely because they damage DNA. Normally, apoptosis results from a cell balance of growth and death signals. The signal transduction pathways can activate mitogen-activated kinases, MAP kinases (cell proliferation), or stress-activated kinases (cell death), which can cancel each other out or result in cell proliferation or cell death. Theoretically, if one selectively blocked a mitogen-activated kinase pathway, the cell death pathway would predominate and cause cell loss. Such has been reported using prostate cancer models and inhibitors of the nerve growth factor–activated receptor TRK (Dionne et al, 1995).

Toxin Targeting

Potent toxins such as ricin and *Pseudomonas* exotoxin are available. In contrast to the DNA-damaging cytotoxics, these proteins are inhibitors of protein synthesis, and the cell unable to make protein cannot protect itself from its environment and accumulating oxidative damage and dies. These toxins are manipulated so that the regions responsible for binding to the cell have been deleted with a dramatic reduction of nonspecific cytotoxicity. These toxins are then linked to the targeting molecule or genetically engineered to be part of the molecule, to permit selective killing of tumor cells. These toxins are protein synthesis inhibitors. When the toxin is taken up by the cell, it ribosylates the ribosomal initiation factors, leaving them unable to synthesize proteins, resulting in cell death. Because these toxins are enzymes, it requires as little as one molecule per cell to kill the cell (Kohler and Milstein, 1975; Bander, 1987; Frankel, 1988; Olsnes and Sandrig, 1988).

For example, transforming growth factor-alpha is a growth factor expressed in many epithelial cancers and is a ligand for the epidermal growth factor receptor. Molecular engineering has created molecules that combine the transforming growth factor-alpha–binding region and the toxic portion of *Pseudomonas* exotoxin (Heimbrook et al, 1990). This molecule uses the epidermal growth factor receptor for its uptake into cells, and the exotoxin efficiently kills those cells. The problem is finding targets that are limited in expression to the tumor.

CONCLUSION

Strides in molecular and cellular biology have provided tremendous insights into the changes required for a cell to become a cancer. Detection of these changes has already provided for better diagnostic prognostication. Cancerous changes have also been identified that present excellent therapeutic targets and should provide for specificity and lack of toxicity. The future is indeed bright.

REFERENCES

Abramson DH, Ellsworth RM, Kitchin FD, Tung G: Second monocular tumors in retinoblastoma survivors: Are they radiation-induced? Ophthalmology 1984; 91:1351–1355.

Albeda SM, Buck CA: Integrins and other cell adhesion molecules. FASEB J 1990; 4:2868–2880.

Alison MR, Wright NA: Growth kinetics. Rec Results Cancer Res 1981; 41:29–43.

Allred DC, Clark GM, Elledge R, et al: Association of p53 protein expression with tumor cell proliferation rate and clinical outcome in node-negative breast cancer. J Natl Cancer Inst 1993; 85:200–206.

Aprikian AG, Sarkis AS, Fair WR, et al: Immunohistochemical determination of p53 protein nuclear accumulation in prostatic adenocarcinoma. J Urol 1994; 151:1276–1280.

Badalament RA, Hermansen DK, Kimmel M, et al: The sensitivity of bladder wash flow cytometry, bladder wash cytology, and voided cytology in the detection of bladder carcinoma. Cancer 1987; 60:1423–1427.

Baker SJ, Markowitz S, Fearon ER, et al: Suppression of human colorectal carcinoma cell growth by wild type p53. Science 1990; 249:912–915.

Bander NH: Monoclonal antibodies: state of the art. J Urol 1987; 137:603–612.

Bardi G, Johansson B, Pandis N, et al: Karyotypic abnormalities in tumors of the pancreas. Br J Cancer 1993; 67:1106–1112.

Barlogie B: Abnormal cellular DNA content as a marker of neoplasia. Eur J Cancer Clin Oncol 1984; 20:1123–1125.

Barsky SH, Rao CN, Williams JE, et al: Laminin molecular domains which alter metastasis in a murine model. J Clin Invest 1984; 74:843–848.

Beardsley T: A war not won. Sci Am 1994; 270:130–138.

Benedict WF, Xu H-J, Hu S-X, Takahashi R: Role of the retinoblastoma gene in the initiation and progression of human cancer. J Clin Invest 1990; 85:988–993.

Bevilacqua G, Sobel ME, Liotta LA, Steeg PS: Association of low nm23 RNA levels in human primary infiltrating ductal breast carcinomas with lymph node involvement and other histopathological indicators of high metastatic potential. Cancer Res 1989; 49:5185–5190.

Bookstein R, Shew J-Y, Chen PL, et al: Suppression of tumorigenicity of human prostate carcinoma cells by replacing a mutated RB gene. Science 1990; 247:712–715.

Bouck N: Tumor angiogenesis: The role of oncogenes and tumor suppressor genes. Cancer Cells 1990; 2:179–185.

Bruchovsky N, Rennie PS, Coldman AJ, et al: Effects of androgen withdrawal on the stem cell composition of the Shionogi carcinoma. Cancer Res 1990; 50:2275–2287.

Buchkovich K, Duffy LA, Harlow E: The retinoblastoma protein is phosphorylated during specific phases of the cell cycle. Cell 1989; 58:1097–1105.

Bullrich F, MacLachlan TK, Sang N, et al: Chromosomal mapping of members of the cdc2 family of protein kinases, cdk3, cdk6, PISSLRE and PITALRE and a cdk inhibitor, p27[Kip1], to regions involved in human cancer. Cancer Res 1995; 55:1199–1205.

Butler TP, Grantham FH, Gullino PM: Bulk transfer of fluid in the interstitial compartment of mammary tumors. Cancer Res 1975; 35:3084–3088.

Cairns P, Shaw ME, Knowles MA: Initiation of bladder cancer may involve deletion of a tumour-suppressor gene on chromosome 9. Oncogene 1993; 8:1083–1085.

Camps JL, Chang S-M, Hsu TC, et al: Fibroblast-mediated acceleration of human epithelial tumor growth in vivo. Proc Natl Acad Sci USA 1990; 87:75–79.

Cance WG, Brennan MR, Dudas ME, et al: Altered expression of the retinoblastoma gene product in human sarcomas. N Engl J Med 1990; 323:1457–1462.

Casey G, Lo-Hsueh M, Lopez ME, et al: Growth suppression of human breast cancer cells by the introduction of a wild-type p53 gene. Oncogene 1991; 6:1791–1797.

Chackal-Roy M, Niemeyer C, Moore M, Zetter BR: Stimulation of prostatic carcinoma cell growth by factors present in human bone marrow. J Clin Invest 1989; 84:43–50.

Chellappan SP, Hiebert S, Mudryj M, et al: The E2F transcription factor is a cellular target for the RB protein. Cell 1991; 65:1053–1061.

Chen C, Parangi S, Tolentino MJ, Folkman J: A strategy to discover circulating angiogenesis inhibitors generated by human tumors. Cancer Res 1995; 55:4230–4233.

Chen PL, Scully P, Shew J-Y, et al: Phosphorylation of the retinoblastoma gene product is modulated during the cell cycle and cellular differentiation. Cell 1989; 58:1193–1198.

Cheng J, Yee J-K, Yeargin J, et al: Suppression of acute lymphoblastic leukemia by the human wild-type p53 gene. Cancer Res 1992; 52:222–226.

Cho Y, Gorina S, Jeffrey PD, Pavletich NP: Crystal structure of a p53 tumor suppressor-DNA complex: Understanding tumorigenic mutations. Science 1994; 265:346–355.

Chung LWK, Camps JL, Von Eschenbach AC: Cancer Biology II. *In* Chisholm GD, Fair WR, eds: Scientific Foundations of Urology. Oxford, Heinemann Medical Books, 1990, pp 459–473.

Coindre JM, Trojani M, Contesso G, et al: Reproducibility of a histopathological grading system for adult soft tissue sarcoma. Cancer 1986; 58:306–309.

Cordon-Cardo C, Dalbagni G, Richon VM: Significance of the retinoblastoma gene in human cancer. *In* DeVita VT, Hellman S, Rosenberg SA, eds: Principles and Practice of Oncology (Update), Vol 6. Philadelphia, J.B. Lippincott, 1992a, pp 1–9.

Cordon-Cardo C, Wartinger D, Petrylak D, et al: Altered expression of the retinoblastoma gene product: Prognostic indicator in bladder cancer. J Natl Cancer Inst 1992b; 84:1251–1256.

Cunha GR, Chung LWK, Shannon JM, et al: Hormone-inducing morphogenesis and growth: role of mesenchymal epithelial interactions. Recent Prog Horm Res 1983; 39:559–598.

Cunha GR, Donjacour AA, Cooke PS, et al: The endocrinology and developmental biology of the prostate. Endocrinol Rev 1987; 8:338–362.

Czerniak B, Deitch D, Simmons H, et al: Ha-ras gene codon 12 mutations and DNA ploidy in urinary bladder carcinomas. Br J Cancer 1990; 62:762–767.

Dalbagni G, Presti J, Reuter V, et al: Genetic alterations in bladder cancer. Lancet 1993; 324:469–471.

DeCaprio JA, Ludlow JW, Figge J, et al: SV40 large tumor antigen forms a specific complex with the product of the retinoblastoma susceptibility gene. Cell 1988; 54:275–283.

DeFeo-Jones D, Huang PS, Jones RE, et al: Cloning of cDNAs for cellular proteins that bind to the retinoblastoma gene product. Nature 1991; 352:251–254.

Dionne CA, Camoratto A, Jani J, et al: The TRK tyrosine kinase inhibitor CEP-751 inhibits prostate cancer growth. Presented at Breast and Prostate Cancer, Keystone Symposium, Taos, NM, 1995.

Donehower LA, Harvey M, Slagle BL, et al: Mice deficient for p53 are developmentally normal but susceptible to spontaneous tumours. Nature 1992; 356:215–221.

Dong J-T, Lamb PW, Rinker-Schaeffer CW, et al: KAI1, a metastasis suppressor on human chromosome 11p11.2. Science 1995; 268:884–886.

Draetta G, Beach D: Activation of cdc2 protein kinase during mitosis in human cells: Cell cycle-dependent phosphorylation and subunit rearrangement. Cell 1988; 54:17–26.

Drobnjak M, Latres E, Pollack D, et al: Prognostic implications of p53 nuclear overexpression and high proliferation index of Ki-67 in adult soft tissue sarcomas. J Natl Cancer Inst 1994; 86:549–554.

Dunphy WG, Brizuela L, Beach D, Newport J: The Xenopus cdc-2 protein is a component of MPF, a cytoplasmic regulator of mitosis. Cell 1988; 54:423–431.

Dyson H, Howley PM, Munger K, Harlow E: The human papilloma virus-16 E7 oncoprotein is able to bind to the retinoblastoma gene product. Science 1989; 243:934–937.

El-Deiry WS, Tokino T, Velculescu VE, et al: WAF1, a potential mediator of p53 tumor suppression. Cell 1993; 75:817–825.

Eliyahu D, Michalovitz D, Eliyahu S, et al: Wild-type p53 can inhibit oncogene-mediated focus formation. Proc Natl Acad Sci USA 1989; 86:8763–8767.

Esrig D, Elmajian D, Groshen S, et al: Accumulation of nuclear p53 and tumor progression in bladder cancer. N Engl J Med 1994; 331:1259–1264.

Evans T, Rosenthal ET, Youngblom J, et al: Cyclin: A protein specified by maternal mRNA in sea urchin eggs that is destroyed at each cleavage division. Cell 1983; 33:389–396.

Fakharzadeh SS, Trusko SP, George DL: Tumorigenic potential associated with enhanced expression of a gene that is amplified in a mouse tumor cell line. EMBO J 1991; 10:1565–1569.

Fidler IJ: Critical factors in the biology of human cancer metastasis: Twenty-eighth G.H.A. Clowes Award Memorial Lecture. Cancer Res 1990; 50:6130–6138.

Fields S, Jang SK: Presence of a potent transcription activating sequence in the p53 protein. Science 1990; 249:1046–1049.

Folkman J: What is the evidence that tumors are angiogenesis dependent? J Natl Cancer Inst 1990; 82:4–6.

Folkman J, Klagsbrun M: Angiogenic factors. Science 1987; 235:442–447.

Frankel AE, ed: Immunotoxins. Norwell, MA, Kluwer Academic Publishers, 1988.

Frankfurt OS, Greco WR, Slocum HK, et al: Proliferative characteristics of primary and metastatic human solid tumors by DNA flow cytometry. Cytometry 1984; 5:629–635.

Freeman RS, Donoghue DJ: Protein kinases and protooncogenes: Biochemical regulators of the eukaryotic cell cycle. Biochemistry 1991; 30:2293–2302.

Friend SH, Horowitz JM, Gerber MR, et al: Deletions of a DNA sequence in retinoblastomas and mesenchymal tumors: Organization of the sequence and its encoded protein. Proc Natl Acad Sci USA 1987; 84:9059–9063.

Fuks Z, Persaud RS, Alfieri A, et al: Basic fibroblast growth factor protects endothelial cells against radiation-induced programmed cell death in vitro and in vivo. Cancer Res 1994; 54:2582–2590.

Fulker M, Cooper EH, Tanaka T: Proliferation and ultrastructure of papillary transitional cell carcinoma of the human bladder. Cancer 1971; 27:71–82.

Fung Y-K, Murphree AL, T'Ang A, et al: Structural evidence for the authenticity of the human retinoblastoma gene. Science 1987; 236:1657–1661.

Gautier J, Minshull J, Lohka M, et al: Cyclin is a component of maturating-promoting factor from Xenopus. Cell 1990; 60:487–494.

Gibas Z, Prout GR, Connolly JG, et al: Nonrandom chromosomal changes in transitional cell carcinoma of the bladder. Cancer Res 1984; 44:1257–1264.

Gibbs JB, Oliff A: Pharmaceutical research in molecular oncology. Cell 1994; 79:193–198.

Goldie JH, Coldman AJ: The genetic origin of drug resistance in neoplasms: Implications for systemic therapy. Cancer Res 1984; 44:3543–3563.

Gould KL, Nurse P: Tyrosine phosphorylation of the fission yeast cdc2+ protein kinase regulates entry into mitosis. Nature 1989; 342:39–45.

Graeber TG, Osmanian C, Jacks T, et al: Hypoxia-mediated selection of cells with diminished apoptotic potential in solid tumors. Nature 1996; 379:88–91.

Greenberg ER, Baron J, Stukel TA: A clinical trial of beta carotene to prevent basal-cell and squamous-cell cancers of the skin. N Engl J Med 1990; 323:789–795.

Greenblatt MS, Benett WP, Hollstein M, Harris CC: Mutations in the p53 tumor suppressor gene: Clues to cancer etiology and molecular pathogenesis. Cancer Res 1994; 54:4855–4878.

Gruis NA, Weaver-Feldhaus J, Liu Q, et al: The MTS1 and TP53 genes may involve separate pathways of tumorigenesis. Am J Pathol 1995; 146:1199–1206.

Guan K-L, Jenkins CW, Li Y, et al: Growth suppression by p18, a p16$^{INK4/MTS1}$- and p14$^{INK4B/MTS2}$-related CDK6 inhibitor, correlates with wild-type pRB function. Genes Develop 1994; 8:2939–2952.

Haimovitz-Friedman A, Balaban N, McLoughlin M, et al: Protein kinase C mediates basic fibroblast growth factor protection of endothelial cells against radiation-induced apoptosis. Cancer Res 1994; 54:2591–2597.

Hainsworth PJ, Raphael KL, Stillwell RG, et al: Cytogenetic features of twenty-six primary breast cancers. Cancer Genet Cytogenet 1991; 52:205–218.

Hall PA, Levison DA, Wright NA: Assessment of Cell Proliferation in Clinical Practice. London, Springer-Verlag, 1992.

Hall PA, Watt FM: Stem cells: The generation and maintenance of cellular diversity. Development 1989; 106:619–633.

Hannon GJ, Beach D: p15^{INK4B} is a potential effector of TGF-β-induced cell cycle arrest. Nature 1994; 371:257–261.

Hansen MF, Koufos A, Gallie BL, et al: Osteosarcoma and retinoblastoma: A shared chromosomal mechanism revealing recessive predisposition. Proc Natl Acad Sci USA 1985; 82:6216–6220.

Harper JW, Adami GR, Wei N, et al: The p21 cdk-interacting protein Cip1 is a potent inhibitor of G1 cyclin-dependent kinases. Cell 1993; 75:805–816.

Hartwell LH, Kastan MB: Cell cycle control and cancer. Science 1994; 266:1821–1828.

Heim S, Mandahl N, Mitelman F: Genetic convergence and divergence in tumor progression. Cancer Res 1988; 48:5911–5916.

Heimbrook DC, Stirdivant SM, Ahern JD, et al: Transforming growth factor α-*Pseudomonas* exotoxin fusion protein prolongs survival of nude mice bearing tumor xenografts. Proc Natl Acad Sci USA 1990; 87:4687–4706.

Hertig AT: Contrib Embryol 1935; 25:37.

Heston WDW: Detection of hematogenous dissemination of prostatic cancer by RT-PCR with primers specific for prostate specific membrane antigen. Clin Chem 1995; 41:1687–1688.

Humphrey PA, Zhu X, Zamegar R, et al: Hepatocyte growth factor and its receptor (c-MET) in prostatic carcinoma. Am J Pathol 1995; 147:386–396.

Hunter T, Pines J: Cyclins and cancer: II. Cyclin D and CDK inhibitors come of age. Cell 1994; 79:573–582.

Illmensee K, Mintz B: Totipotency and normal differentiation of single teratocarcinoma cells by injection into blastocysts. Proc Natl Acad Sci USA 1976; 73:549–553.

Ingber D, Fujita T, Kishimoto S, et al: Synthetic analogues of fumagillin that inhibit angiogenesis and suppress tumour growth. Nature 1990; 348:555–557.

Jacks T, Fazeli A, Schmitt EM, et al: Effects of an Rb mutation in the mouse. Nature 1992; 359:295–300.

Jain RK: Barriers to drug delivery in solid tumors. Sci Am 1994; 270:58–65.

Jen J, Harper JW, Bigner SH, et al: Deletion of p16 and p15 genes in brain tumors. Cancer Res 1994; 54:6353–6358.

Johnson DJ, Schwarz JK, Cress WD, Nevins JR: Expression of transcription factor E2F1 induces quiescent cells to enter S phase. Nature 1993; 365:349–352.

Kaelin WG Jr, Pallas DC, DeCaprio JA, et al: Identification of cellular proteins that can interact specifically with the T/E1A-binding region of the retinoblastoma gene product. Cell 1991; 64:521–532.

Kamb A, Gruis NA, Weaver-Feldhaus J, Liu Q: A cell cycle regulator potentially involved in genesis of many tumor types. Science 1994a; 264:436–440.

Kamb A, Liu Q, Harshman K, et al: Rates of p16 (MTS1) mutations in primary tumors with 9p loss. Science 1994b; 265:415–417.

Kastan MB, Onkyekwere O, Sidransky D, et al: Participation of p53 protein in the cellular response to DNA damage. Cancer Res 1991; 51:6304–6311.

Kern SE, Pietenpol JA, Thiagalingam S, et al: Oncogenic forms of p53 inhibit p53-regulated gene expression. Science 1992; 256:827–830.

Keyomarsi K, O'Leary N, Molnar G, et al: Cyclin E, a potential prognostic marker for breast cancer. Cancer Res 1994; 54:380–385.

Keyomarsi K, Pardee AB: Redundant cyclin overexpression and gene amplification in breast cancer cells. Proc Natl Acad Sci USA 1993; 90:1112–1116.

King RW, Jackson PK, Kirschner MW: Mitosis in transition. Cell 1994; 79:563–571.

Kirkland SC: Clonal origins of columnar, mucous, and endocrine cell lineages in human colorectal epithelium. Cancer 1988; 61:1359–1363.

Knudson AG Jr: Mutation and cancer: Statistical study of retinoblastoma. Proc Natl Acad Sci USA 1971; 68:820–823.

Kohler G, Milstein C: Continuous cultures of fused cells secreting antibody of predefined specificity. Nature 1975; 256:495–497.

Kohn EC, Liotta LA: L651582: A novel antiproliferative and antimetastasis agent. J Natl Cancer Inst 1990; 82:54–60.

Kornblau SM, Xu H-J, del Giglio A, et al: Clinical implications of decreased retinoblastoma protein expression in acute myelogenous leukemia. Cancer Res 1992; 52:4587–4590.

Koss LG, Wersto RP, Simmons DA, et al: Predictive value of DNA measurements in bladder washings: Comparison of flow cytometry, image cytophotometry, and cytology in patients with a past history of urothelial tumors. Cancer 1989; 64:916–924.

Kovesdi I, Reichel R, Nevins JR: Identification of a cellular transcription factor involved in E1A trans-activation. Cell 1986; 45:219–228.

Lammie GA, Peters G: Chromosome 11q13 abnormalities in human cancer. Cancer Cells (Cold Spring Harbor) 1991; 3:413–420.

Lee E, Chang C-Y, Hu N, et al: Mice deficient for Rb are nonviable and show defects in neurogenesis and hematopoiesis. Nature 1992; 359:270–271.

Lee W-H, Shew J-Y, Hong FD, et al: The retinoblastoma susceptibility gene encodes a nuclear phosphoprotein associated with DNA binding activity. Nature 1987; 329:642–645.

Lerman C, Rimer B, Engstrom PF: Reducing avoidable cancer mortality through prevention and early detection regimes. Cancer Res 1989; 49:4955–4962.

Lewin B: Driving the cell cycle: M phase kinase, its partners, and substrates. Cell 1990; 61:743–752.

Li FP, Fraumeni JF Jr: Rhabdomyosarcoma in children: Epidemiologic study and identification of a familial cancer syndrome. J Natl Cancer Inst 1969; 43:1365–1373.

Linden MD, Torres FX, Kubus J, Zarbo J: Clinical application of morphologic and immunocytochemical assessments of cell proliferation. Am J Clin Pathol 1992; 97:4–13.

Linzer DI, Levine AJ: Characterization of 54K dalton cellular SV40 tumor antigen present in SV40-transformed cells and uninfected embryonal carcinoma cells. Cell 1979; 17:43–52.

Liotta LA: Tumor invasion and metastasis: Role of the extracellular matrix: Rhoads Memorial Award Lecture. Cancer Res 1986; 46:1–7.

Liotta LA, Horan Hand P, Rao CN, et al: Monoclonal antibodies to the human laminin receptor recognize structurally distinct sites. Exp Cell Res 1985; 156:117–126.

Liotta LA, Tryggvason K, Garbisa S, et al: Metastatic potential correlates with enzymatic degradation of basement membrane collagen. Nature 1980; 284:67–68.

Liu T-J, Zhang W-W, Taylor DL, et al: Growth suppression of human head and neck cancer cells by the introduction of a wild-type p53 gene via a recombinant adenovirus. Cancer Res 1994; 54:3662–3667.

Logothetis CJ, Xu H-J, Ro JY, et al: Altered expression of retinoblastoma protein and known prognostic variables in locally advanced bladder cancer. J Natl Cancer Inst 1992; 84:1256–1261.

Lohka ML, Hayes MK, Maller J: Purification of maturation-promoting factor, an intracellular regulator of early mitotic events. Proc Natl Acad Sci USA 1988; 85:3009–3013.

Macartney JC, Camplejohn RS: DNA flow cytometry of non-Hodgkin's lymphomas. Eur J Cancer 1990; 26:635–637.

Malkin D, Jolly RW, Barbier N, et al: Germline mutations of the p53 tumor-suppressor gene in children and young adults with second malignant neoplasms. N Engl J Med 1992; 326:1309–1315.

Malkin D, Li FP, Strong LC, et al: Germ line p53 mutations in a familial syndrome of breast cancer, sarcomas, and other neoplasms. Science 1990; 250:1233–1238.

Masui Y, Markert CL: Cytoplasmic control of nuclear behavior during meiotic maturation of frog oocytes. J Exp Zool 1971; 177:129–145.

McCarthy JB, Basara MJ, Palm SL, et al: The role of cell adhesion proteins—laminin and fibronectin—in the movement of malignant and metastatic cells. Cancer Metastasis Rev 1985; 4:125–152.

Melamed MR, Lindmore T, Mendelsohn ML: Flow Cytometry and Sorting, 2nd ed. New York, Wiley-Liss, 1990.

Mercer WE, Shields MT, Amin M, et al: Negative growth regulation in a glioblastoma tumor cell line that conditionally expresses human wild-type p53. Proc Natl Acad Sci USA 1990; 87:6166–6170.

Merkel DE, McGuire WL: Ploidy, proliferative activity and prognosis: DNA flow cytometry of solid tumors. Cancer 1990; 65:1194–1205.

Michieli P, Chedid M, Lin D, et al: Induction of WAF1/CIP1 by a p53-independent pathway. Cancer Res 1994; 54:3391–3395.

Mignatti P, Robbins E, Rifkin DB: Tumor invasion through the human amniotic membrane: requirement for a proteinase cascade. Cell 1986; 47:487–498.

Mitsudomi T, Oyama T, Kusano T, et al: Mutations of the p53 gene as a predictor of poor prognosis in patients with non-small cell lung cancer. J Natl Cancer Inst 1993; 85:2018–2023.

Mittnacht S, Weinberg RA: G1/S phosphorylation of the retinoblastoma protein is associated with an altered affinity for the nuclear compartment. Cell 1991; 65:381–393.

Mohler JL, Partin AW, Coffey DS: Prediction of metastatic potential by a new grading system of cell motility: Validating in the Dunning r3327 prostatic adenocarcinoma model. J Urol 1987; 138:168–170.

Momand J, Zambetti GP, Olson DC, et al: The mdm-2 oncogene product forms a complex with the p53 protein and inhibits p53-mediated transactivation. Cell 1992; 69:1237–1245.

Morgenbesser SD, Williams BO, Jacks T, DePinho RA: p53-dependent apoptosis produced by Rb-deficiency in the developing mouse lens. Nature 1994; 371:72–74.

Moroco JR, Solt DB, Polverini PS: Sequential loss of suppressor genes for three specific functions during in vivo carcinogenesis. Lab Invest 1990; 63:298–306.

Muller WJ, Simm E, Pattengale PK, et al: Single-step induction of mammary adenocarcinoma in transgenic mice bearing the activated c-*neu* oncogene. Cell 1988; 54:105–115.

Murray AW, Hunt T: The Cell Cycle, An Introduction. New York, Freeman, 1993.

Newmark HL, Lipkin M, Maheshwari N: Colonic hyperplasia and hyper-proliferation induced by a nutritional stress diet with four components of a western-style diet. J Natl Cancer Inst 1990; 82:491–496.

Nurse P: Universal control mechanism in regulating onset of M-phase. Nature 1990; 344:503–508.

Nurse P: Ordering S phase and M phase in the cell cycle. Cell 1994; 79:547–550.

Oliner JD, Kinzler KW, Meltzer PS, et al: Amplification of a gene encoding a p53 associated protein in human sarcomas. Nature 1992; 358:80–83.

Olopade OI, Bohlander SK, Pomykala H, et al: Mapping of the shortest region of overlap of deletions of the short arm of chromosome 9 associated with human neoplasia. Genomics 1992; 14:437–443.

Olsnes S, Sandrig K: How protein toxins enter and kill cells. In Frankel AE, ed: Immunotoxins. Norwell, MA, Kluwer Acad Publ, 1988, pp 39–73.

Ooi A, Herz F, Li S, et al, and the NIH Bladder Network for Bladder Cancer: Ha-ras codon 12 mutation in papillary tumors of the urinary bladder: A retrospective study. Int J Oncol 1994; 4:85–90.

O'Reilly MS, Holmgren L, Shing Y, et al: Angiostatin: A novel inhibitor that mediates the suppression of metastases by Lewis Lung carcinoma. Cell 1994; 79:315–328.

Orlow I, Lianes P, Lacombe L, et al: Chromosome 9 allelic losses and microsatellite alterations in human bladder tumors. Cancer Res 1994; 54:2848–2851.

Paget S: The distribution of secondary growths in cancer of the breast. Lancet 1889; 1:571–592.

Pardoll DM: Paracrine cytokine adjuvants in cancer immunotherapy. Ann Rev Immunol 1995; 13:399–415.

Partin AW, Isaacs JT, Treiger B, Coffey DS: Early cell motility changes associated with an increase in metastatic ability in rat prostatic cancer cells transfected with the v-Harvey-ras oncogene. Cancer Res 1988; 48:6050–6053.

Phillips SMA, Barton CM, Lee SJ, et al: Loss of the retinoblastoma susceptibility gene (RB1) is a frequent and early event in prostatic tumorigenesis. Br J Cancer 1994; 70:1252.

Pienta KJ, Partin AW, Coffey DS: Cancer as a disease of DNA organization and dynamic cell structure. Cancer Res 1988; 49:2525–2532.

Pierce GB, Speers WC: Tumors as caricatures of the process of tissue renewal: Prospects for therapy by directing differentiation. Cancer Res 1988; 48:1996–2004.

Pietenpol JA, Bohlander SK, Sato Y, et al: Assignment of human p27^{Kip1} gene to 12p13 and its analysis in leukemias. Cancer Res 1995; 55:1206–1210.

Polyak K, Kato J-Y, Solomon MJ, et al: p27^{Kip1}, a cyclin-Cdk inhibitor, links transforming growth factor-β and contact inhibition to cell cycle arrest. Genes Develop 1994a; 8:9–22.

Polyak K, Lee M-H, Erdjument-Bromage H, et al: Cloning of p27^{Kip1}, a cyclin-dependent kinase inhibitor and a potential mediator of extracellular antimitogenic signals. Cell 1994b; 78:59–66.

Ponce-Castaneda MV, Lee M-H, Latres E, et al: p27^{Kip1}: Chromosomal mapping to 12p12-12p13.1 and absence of mutations in human tumors. Cancer Res 1995; 55:1211–1214.

Poste G, Greig R: The experimental and clinical implications of cellular heterogeneity in malignant tumors. J Cancer Res Clin Oncol 1983; 106:159–170.

Poste G, Nicolson GL: Arrest and metastasis of blood-borne tumor cells are modified by fusion of plasma membrane vesicles from highly-metastatic cells. Proc Natl Acad Sci USA 1980; 77:399–403.

Prentice RL, Pepe M, Self SG: Dietary fat and breast cancer: A quantitative assessment of the epidemiological literature and a discussion of methodological issues. Cancer Res 1989; 49:3147–3156.

Raber M, Barlogie B: DNA flow cytometry of human solid tumors. In Melamed MR, Lindmore T, Mendelsohn ML, eds: Flow Cytometry and Sorting, 2nd ed. New York, Wiley-Liss, 1990, pp 745–754.

Reed SI: The role of p34 kinases in the G1 to S-phase transition. Ann Rev Cell Biol 1992; 8:529–561.

Richardson HE, Wittenberg C, Cross F, Reed SI: An essential G1 function for cyclin-like proteins in yeast. Cell 1989; 59:1127–1133.

Roedink FH, Kroon AM, eds: Drug Carrier Systems. New York, John Wiley & Sons, 1989.

Rosenfeld MR, Meneses P, Dalmau J, et al: Gene transfer of wild-type p53 results in restoration of tumor suppressor function in a medulloblastoma cell line. Neurology 1995; 45:1533–1539.

Sarkis AS, Dalbagni G, Cordon-Cardo C, et al: Nuclear overexpression of p53 protein in transitional cell bladder carcinoma: A marker for disease progression. J Natl Cancer Inst 1993; 85:53–59.

Sarnow P, Ho YS, Williams J, Levine AJ: Adenovirus E1b-5 58kd tumor antigen and SV40 large tumor antigen are physically associated with the same 54 kd cellular protein in transformed cells. Cell 1982; 28:387–394.

Schauer IE, Siriwardana S, Langan TA, Sclafani RA: Cyclin D1 overexpression vs. retinoblastoma inactivation: Implications for growth control evasion in non-small cell and small cell lung cancer. Proc Natl Acad Sci USA 1994; 91:7827–7831.

Schleiermacher G, Peter M, Michon J, et al: Two distinct deleted regions on the short arm of chromosome 1 in neuroblastoma. Genes Chrom Cancer 1994; 10:275–281.

Serrano M, Hannon GJ, Beach D: A new regulatory motif in cell-cycle control causing specific inhibition of cyclin D/CDK4. Nature 1993; 366:704–707.

Sherr CJ: G1 phase progression: Cycling on cue. Cell 1994; 79:551–555.

Sreekantaiah C, Davis JR, Sandberg AA: Chromosomal abnormalities in leiomyosarcomas. Am J Pathol 1993; 142:293–305.

Steeg PS, Bevilacqua G, Kopper L, et al: Evidence for a novel gene associated with low tumor metastatic potential. J Natl Cancer Inst 1988; 80:200–204.

Steel GG: Growth Kinetics of Tumors. London, Oxford University Press, 1977.

Stenger JE, Mayr GA, Mann K, Tegtmeyer P: Formation of stable p53 homotetramers and multiples of tetramers. Mol Carcinogen 1992; 5:102–106.

Stephenson RA, James BC, Gay H, et al: Flow cytometry of prostatic cancer: Relationship of DNA content to survival. Cancer Res 1987; 47:2504–2509.

Sugarbaker E, Cohen AM, Ketcham AS: Do metastases metastasize? Ann Surg 1971; 174:161–166.

Tai-Ping D, Rhys J, Bicknell R: Controlling the vasculature, anti-angiogenesis and vascular targeting of the gene. TiPS 1995; 16:57–66.

Tam SW, Shay JW, Pagano M: Differential expression and cell cycle regulation of the cyclin-dependent kinase 4 inhibitor p16^{Ink4}. Cancer Res 1994; 54:5816–5820.

Tarin D, Vass ACR, Kettlewell MGW, Price JE: Absence of metastatic sequelae during long-term treatment of malignant ascites by peritoneovenous shunting. Invasion Metast 1984; 4:1–12.

Terranova VP, Hujanen ES, Martin GR: Basement membrane and the invasive activity of metastatic tumor cells. J Natl Cancer Inst 1986; 77:311–316.

Thalmann GN, Anezinis PE, Chang S-M, et al: Androgen-independent cancer progression and bone metastasis in the LNCaP model of human prostatic cancer. Cancer Res 1994; 54:2577–2581.

Thomas KA: Vascular endothelial cell growth factor, a potent and selective angiogenic agent. J Biol Chem 1996; 271:603–606.

Thompson TC, Southgate J, Kitchener G, Land H: Multistage carcinogenesis induced by ras and myc oncogenes in reconstituted organ. Cell 1989; 56:917–930.

Thor AD, Moore DH II, Edgerton SM, et al: Accumulation of p53 tumor suppressor gene protein: An independent marker of prognosis in breast cancers. J Natl Cancer Inst 1992; 84:845–855.

Thorgeirsson UP, Liotta LA, Kalebic T, et al: Effect of neutral protease inhibitors and a chemoattractant on tumor cell invasion in vitro. J Natl Cancer Inst 1982; 69:1049–1054.

Toguchida J, Yamaguchi T, Dayton S, et al: Prevalence and spectrum of germline mutations of the p53 gene among patients with sarcoma. N Engl J Med 1992; 326:1301–1308.

Toyoshima H, Hunter T: p27, a novel inhibitor of G1 cyclin-cdk protein kinase activity, is related to p21. Cell 1994; 78:67–74.

Wang Y, Corr JG, Thaler HT, et al: Decreased growth of established human prostate LNCaP tumors in nude mice fed a low fat diet. J Natl Cancer Inst 1995; 87:1456–1462.

Washimi O, Nagatake M, Osada H, et al: In vivo occurrence of p16 (MTS1) and p15 (MTS2) alterations preferentially in non-small cell lung cancers. Cancer Res 1995; 55:514–517.

Weintraub SJ, Prater CA, Dean C: Retinoblastoma protein switches the E2F site from positive to negative element. Nature 1992; 358:259–261.

Werness BA, Levine AJ, Howley PM: Association of human papillomavirus types 16 and 18 E6 proteins with p53. Science 1990; 248:76–77.

Wheeless LL, Badalament RA, deVere White RW, et al: Consensus review of the clinical utility of DNA cytometry in bladder cancer: Report of the DNA Cytometry Consensus Conference. Cytometry 1993; 14:478–481.

Whyte P, Buchkovich KJ, Horowitz JM, et al: Association between an oncogene and an antioncogene: The adenovirus E1A proteins bind to the retinoblastoma gene product. Nature 1988; 334:124–129.

Wiedner N, Carroll PR, Flax J, et al: Tumor angiogenesis correlates with metastasis in invasive prostate cancer. Am J Pathol 1993; 143:401–409.

Williams BO, Remington L, Albert DM, et al: Cooperative tumorigenic effects of germline mutations in Rb and p53. Nature Genet 1994; 7:480–484.

Willis RA: The Spread of Tumors in the Human Body. London, Butterworth & Co, 1952.

Wunder JS, Czitrom AA, Kandel R, Andrulis IL: Analysis of alterations in the retinoblastoma gene and tumor grade in bone and soft-tissue sarcomas. J Natl Cancer Inst 1991; 83:194–200.

Xiao ZX, Chen J, Levine AJ, et al: Interaction between the retinoblastoma protein and the oncoprotein MDM2. Nature 1995; 375:694–698.

Xiong Y, Hannon GJ, Zhang H, et al: p21 is a universal inhibitor of cyclin kinases. Nature 1993; 366:701–704.

Xu H-J, Quinlan DC, Davidson AG, et al: Altered retinoblastoma protein expression and prognosis in early-stage non-small-cell lung carcinoma. J Natl Cancer Inst 1994a; 86:695–699.

Xu H-J, Xu K, Zhou Y, et al: Enhanced tumor cell growth suppression by an N-terminal truncated retinoblastoma protein. Proc Natl Acad Sci USA 1994b; 91:9837–9841.

Yarden Y, Ulrich A: Growth factor receptor tyrosine kinases. Ann Rev Biochem 1988; 57:443–478.

Zambetti G, Bargonetti J, Walker K, et al: Wild-type p53 mediates positive regulation of gene expression through a specific DNA sequence element. Genes Develop 1992; 6:1143–1152.

Zeng Z-S, Sarkis AS, Zhang Z-F, et al: p53 nuclear overexpression: An independent predictor of survival in lymph node-positive colorectal cancer patients. J Clin Oncol 1994; 12:2043–2050.

Zetter BR: The cellular basis of site-specific metastasis. N Engl J Med 1990; 322:605–612.

Zhang HY, Xiong Y, Beach D: Proliferating cell nuclear antigen and p21 are components of multiple cell cycle kinase complexes. Mol Biol Cell 1993; 4:897–906.

Zhou Y, Li J, Xu K, et al: Further characterization of retinoblastoma gene-mediated cell growth and tumor suppression in human cancer cells. Proc Natl Acad Sci USA 1994; 91:4165–4169.

76
RENAL TUMORS

Arie Belldegrun, M.D.
Jean B. deKernion, M.D.

Historical Considerations

Classification

Benign Renal Tumors
    Cortical Adenoma
    Renal Oncocytoma
    Renal Angiomyolipoma
    Fibroma

    Lipoma
    Other Benign Tumors

Malignant Renal Tumors
    Renal Cell Carcinoma
    Sarcomas of the Kidney
    Lymphoblastoma
    Metastatic Tumors

HISTORICAL CONSIDERATIONS

The evolution of knowledge about renal tumors is in actuality the history of surgical daring in a microcosm. Autopsy information relative to renal disorders was scant. The introduction of nephrectomy and other subsequent surgical interventions for renal diseases provided the clinical information and histopathologic insight that form the bases of current concepts of renal tumors. Thus, the historical data available date back little more than 100 years.

Harris (1882) reported on 100 surgical extirpations of the kidney, a sufficient number to permit some sort of analysis of clinical, surgical, and pathologic features of renal disorders that require surgery. The first documented nephrectomy was apparently accomplished by Wolcott in 1861, who operated with the mistaken assumption that the tumor mass was a hepatoma. In 1867, Spiegelberg removed a kidney incidentally in the course of excising an echinococcus cyst. The first planned nephrectomy was performed by Simon in 1869 for persistent ureteral fistula, and this patient survived with cure of the fistula. One year later (1870), the first planned nephrectomy was successfully accomplished in the United States, by Gilmore in Mobile, AL, as treatment for atrophic pyelonephritis and persistent urinary infection (Glenn, 1980).

With surgical intervention, tissue became available to pathologists for histologic interpretation. Unfortunately, such interpretation was not always accurate, and there were often serious professional differences of opinion. According to Carson (1928), the first accurate gross description of kidney tumors dates to 1826, with Konig's observations. In 1855, Robin examined solid tumors apparently arising in the kid-

ney and concluded that renal carcinoma arose from renal tubular epithelium. This interpretation was confirmed by Waldeyer in 1867. Unfortunately, theoretical and practical considerations of renal tumors were confused by Grawitz (1883), who contended that such apparent renal tumors arose from adrenal rests within the kidney. He introduced the terminology *struma lipomatodes aberrata renis* as descriptive nomenclature for the tumors of clear cells that he believed were derived from the adrenal glands. He based his conclusions not only on the fatty content of the tumors, analogous to that seen in the adrenal glands, but also on the location of the tumors beneath the renal capsule, the approximation to the adrenal glands, the lack of similarity of the cells to uriniferous tubules, and the demonstration of amyloid similar to that seen with adrenal degeneration.

This histogenetic concept was adopted by subsequent investigators, and pathologists of the era readily embraced the idea that renal tumors truly arose from the adrenal glands. In 1894, Lubarch endorsed the idea of a suprarenal origin of renal tumors, and the term *hypernephroid tumors*, indicating origin above the kidneys, was advocated by Birch-Hirschfeld (Birch-Hirschfeld and Doederlein, 1894). This semantic and conceptual mistake led to the introduction of the term *hypernephroma*, which predominates in the literature describing parenchymal tumors of primary renal origin.

Weichselbaum and Greenish (1883) described renal adenomas containing both papillary and alveolar cell types. Some clarification of the histopathology of renal tumors is derived from the work of Albarran and Imbert (1903), and the four-volume contribution of Wolff (1883), written between 1883 and 1928, adds further historical significance to the understanding of renal tumors today (Glenn, 1980).

CLASSIFICATION

An appropriate, simple, and all-inclusive classification of renal tumors has eluded surgical pathologists and urologic surgeons alike over the past century. Even with the elimination of hydronephrosis and various inflammatory tumefactions of the kidney, such as xanthogranulomatous pyelonephritis, from the category, the spectrum of renal tumors remains extremely broad. Various classifications have been adopted in an effort to acknowledge and include the various new growths of diverse causes that can afflict the human kidney.

Certainly the most comprehensive classification of renal tumors is that offered by Deming and Harvard (1970) in a previous edition of this text. They established 11 categories of renal tumors, with multiple subdivisions embracing virtually every known new growth that may involve the kidney—common, uncommon, or rare—including the various renal cystic disorders as well as the perirenal retroperito-

Table 76–1. CLASSIFICATION OF RENAL TUMORS

Tumors of the Renal Capsule	**Neurogenic Tumors**
Fibroma	Neuroblastoma
Leiomyoma	Sympathicoblastoma
Lipoma	Schwannoma
Mixed	
Tumors of the Mature Renal Parenchyma	**Heteroplastic Tissue Tumors**
	Adipose
Adenoma	Smooth muscle
Adenocarcinoma	Adrenal rests
Hypernephroma	Endometriosis
Renal cell cancer	Cartilage
Alveolar carcinoma	Bone
Tumors of the Immature Renal Parenchyma	**Mesenchymal Derivatives**
	Connective tissue
Nephroblastoma (Wilms')	Fibroma
Embryonic carcinoma	Fibrosarcoma
Sarcoma	Osteogenic sarcoma
	Adipose tissue
Epithelial Tumors of the Renal Pelvis	Lipoma
	Liposarcoma
Transitional cell papilloma	Muscle tissue
Transitional cell carcinoma	Leiomyoma
Squamous cell carcinoma	Leiomyosarcoma
Adenocarcinoma	Rhabdomyosarcoma
Cysts	**Pararenal/Perirenal Solid Tumors**
Solitary	Lipoma
Unilateral multiple	Sarcoma
Calyceal	Liposarcoma
Pyogenic	Fibrosarcoma
Calcified	Lymphangiosarcoma
Tubular ectasia	Cancer
Tuberous sclerosis	Teratoma
Cystadenoma	Lymphoblastoma
Papillary cystadenoma	Neuroblastoma
Dermoid	Hodgkin's disease
Pararenal/Perirenal cysts	**Secondary Tumors**
Hydrocele renalis	Cancer
Lymphatic	Sarcoma
Wolffian	Blastoma
Malignant	Granuloma
Vascular Tumors	Thymoma
Hemangioma	Testicular
Hamartoma	Renal
Lymphangioma	

Table 76–2. SIMPLIFIED CLASSIFICATION OF RENAL TUMORS

Benign Tumors

Renal capsule
Renal parenchyma
Vascular tumors
Cystic lesions, dysplasia, hydronephrosis
Heteroplastic, mesenchymal tumors
True oncocytoma

Tumors of Renal Pelvis

Benign papilloma
Transitional and squamous cell carcinomas, adenocarcinomas

Pararenal Tumors

Benign
Malignant

Embryonic Tumors

Nephroblastoma (Wilms' tumor)
Embryonic, mesotheliomatous tumors
Sarcomas

Nephrocarcinoma

Renal cell carcinoma, adenocarcinoma, "hypernephroma"
Papillary cystadenocarcinoma

Other Malignancies

Primary: mesenchymal, hemangiopericytoma, myeloma
Secondary: metastatic lesions

neal tumors that may involve the kidney secondarily. This classification is reproduced here (Table 76–1) because it provides the most succinct presentation of renal tumors, yet retains accuracy and inclusiveness.

An effort must be made, however, to provide a classification that is both complete and uncomplicated, embracing all the lesions that predispose an individual to renal mass or new growth. Such a simplified classification was proposed by Glenn (1980) (Table 76–2). Benign tumors include those of the renal capsule (such as fibroma), renal parenchymatous adenomas, vascular tumors, various cystic lesions and dysplasias, heteroplastic and mesenchymal tumors, and even various hydronephroses. Tumors of the renal pelvis, not a primary consideration here, include benign papillomas as well as transitional, squamous, and adenocarcinomatous malignancies. Perirenal tumors are those that involve the kidney by extension and invasion, and they may be either benign or malignant. Embryonic tumors include predominantly nephroblastoma (Wilms' tumor) and the embryonic or mesotheliomatous carcinomas and sarcomas of childhood. Wilms' tumor, the common renal malignancy of childhood, is addressed elsewhere in this book, as are neuroblastoma, renal cystic disorders, and primary retroperitoneal tumors. Nephrocarcinoma is the generic category that includes adult renal parenchymatous malignancies, primarily the classic hypernephroma and papillary adenocarcinoma. The category of other malignancies embraces the relatively rare mesenchymal malignancies, such as the various sarcomas, hemangiopericytomas, infiltrative malignancies such as myeloma, and secondary or metastatic malignancies manifesting within the renal substance. Oncocytoma has been added to Glenn's original classification.

The true oncocytoma has now been established to be a specific entity with a cell of origin different from that for

Table 76–3. RENAL MASSES CLASSIFIED BY PATHOLOGY

Malignant	Benign	Inflammatory
Renal carcinoma	Simple cyst	Abscess
Lymphoma	Angiomyolipoma	Pyelonephritis
Leiomyosarcoma	Oncocytoma	Xanthogranulomatous pyelonephritis
Hemangiopericytoma	Pseudotumor	Infected renal cyst
Liposarcoma	Reninoma	Tuberculosis
Rhabdomyosarcoma	Pheochromocytoma	Rheumatic granuloma
Schwannoma	Leiomyoma	
Osteosarcoma	Hemangioma	
Fibrous histiocytoma	Cystic nephroma	
Neurofibrosarcoma	Fibroma	
Metastases	Arteriovenous malformation	
Invasion by adjacent neoplasm	Hemangiopericytoma	
Carcinoid	Hibernoma	
Adult Wilms' tumor	Renal artery aneurysm	
Wilms' tumor		
Mesoblastic nephroma		
Leukemia		

renal cell carcinoma, and it is invariably benign (see following discussion). This lesion must be carefully distinguished from renal lesions that have the appearance of oncocytoma, both grossly and microscopically, but that have foci of other than grade I cells.

Another approach has been taken by Barbaric (1994). Renal masses were classified based on pathology (malignant, benign, or inflammatory) (Table 76–3) or based on radiographic appearance (simple cysts, complex cysts, fatty tumors, and others) (Table 76–4). This classification is practical and should assist in the differential diagnosis of renal masses.

BENIGN RENAL TUMORS

Benign renal tumors may arise from any of the multiple cell types within and around the kidney. Renal cysts are perhaps the most common benign renal mass lesions. Approximately 70% of asymptomatic renal mass lesions are simple cysts and are of no clinical significance (Lang, 1973). The major import of most benign lesions lies in either their growth to a large size, creating clinical symptoms, or their differential diagnosis from malignant renal tumors (see following discussion) (Fig. 76–1). Cysts may be single or multiple and unilateral or bilateral.

As discussed later, modern uroradiographic techniques can distinguish renal carcinoma from simple cysts with great accuracy. Occasionally, especially in the case of complex cysts, the true nature of the lesion may be determined only at surgery. It is beyond the scope of this discussion to cite each case report associated with the myriad rare benign tumors; those that are found more commonly and those that are associated with symptoms or bear similarities to malignant tumors are discussed here.

Cortical Adenoma

The existence of benign renal tubular epithelial lesions less than 3 cm in diameter remains controversial. Bell (1950)

Table 76–4. RENAL MASSES CLASSIFIED BY RADIOGRAPHIC APPEARANCE

Simple Cyst	Complex Cyst	Fatty Tumors	All Others
Cyst	Cystic nephroma	Angiomyolipoma	Renal carcinoma
Multiple cysts	Renal carcinoma	Lipoma	Metastases
Peripelvic cyst	Hemorrhagic cyst	Hibernoma	Lymphoma
Calyceal diverticulum	Metastases	Liposarcoma	Sarcomas
	Wilms' tumor		Lobar nephronia
	Infected cyst		Abscess
	Lymphoma		Tuberculosis
	Tuberculosis		Oncocytoma
	Septated cyst		Fibroma
	Renal artery aneurysm		Xanthogranulomatous pyelonephritis
	Arteriovenous malformation		Pheochromocytoma
	Hydrocalyx		Wilms' tumor
			Rheumatic granuloma
			Reninoma
			Leiomyoma
			Hemangioma
			Nephroblastomatosis
			Adenocarcinoma
			Transitional cell carcinoma
			Carcinoid

Adapted from Barbaric ZL: Principles of Genitourinary Radiology, 2nd ed. New York, Thieme Medical Publishers, 1994.

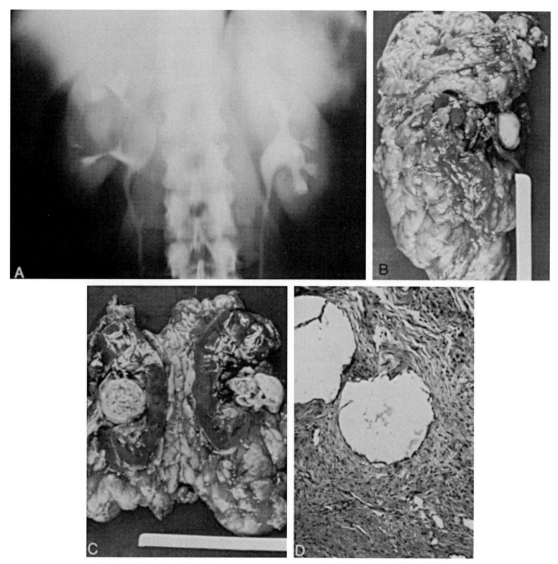

Figure 76–1. *A*, Pyelogram demonstrating a large parapelvic filling defect, which was compound on ultrasonic examination. *B*, A smooth glistening wall of cyst protruding through renal pelvis. *C*, Sagittal section demonstrating laminated, compound cyst. *D*, Microscopic section showing pure cystic nature of the mass.

found a direct correlation between size and malignant potential, noting that tumors less than approximately 3 cm in size had little propensity for metastasis. In his series of 62 tumors less than 3 cm in diameter, however, 3 had metastasized, suggesting that size is not an absolute criterion for metastatic potential. Murphy and Mostofi (1970) concluded that renal adenomas are benign tumors, distinguishable from true adenocarcinomas. An alternative view was presented by Bennington and Beckwith (1975), who argued that all tubular cell adenomas are malignant, simply representing an early stage of renal carcinoma growth, and that there are no clear-cut gross, microscopic ultrastructural or histochemical features to differentiate reliably between these two entities. No definite etiologic factors of renal cortical adenomas have been recognized, but immunohistochemical studies using lectin antibodies suggest an origin from distal tubular epithelium (Fromowitz and Bard, 1990).

Renal adenoma is characterized by uniform basophilic or acidophilic cells with monotous nuclear and cellular characteristics (Presti et al, 1991). The presence of clear cells, mitotic activity, nuclear polymorphism, cell stratification, or necrosis excludes the diagnosis of adenoma. Such lesions, regardless of size, should be considered small renal cell carcinoma (O'Toole et al, 1993). Growth pattern is also quite characteristic. The basophilic cells have a tubulopapillary or purely papillary microarchitecture, and there may be microcyst formations. Both the tubular and the papillary components are lined with a single layer of cells, and although well circumscribed, these lesions tend not to be encapsulated and often merge with adjacent renal parenchyma (Mostofi et al, 1988).

Symptoms are unusual and are observed only when the tumor erodes the collecting system or adjacent vessels. Most renal adenomas are discovered incidentally. The computed tomography (CT) and arteriography characteristics are indistinguishable from those of small renal adenocarcinomas except for the general absence of arteriovenous fistulas, venous pooling, and calcification.

The clinician is often faced with a dilemma when a small, 3-cm renal parenchymal tumor is diagnosed. Although segmental resection or wedge resection may be appropriate, the true tendency for multiplicity is uncertain, and the final characterization of the mass as an adenoma usually awaits careful tissue sectioning. For this reason, most diagnosed renal parenchymal tumors are treated as true renal cell carcinomas.

Renal Oncocytoma

Renal oncocytoma has become a recognized clinical and pathologic entity with almost invariably benign clinical behavior. This tumor is characterized by a histologic pattern of large eosinophilic cells with a granular cytoplasm and typical polygonal form. The nuclei are generally low grade and uniform. Mitoses are rare, and the cells have a benign ultrastructure characterized by a profusion of mitochondria rich in cristae (Fig. 76–2). Electron microscopy demonstrates that the mitochondria of oncocytomas are larger than the mitochondria of other renal cell neoplasms (Weiss et al, 1995). It is important to remember that many renal cell carcinomas have typical oncocytic features and contain eosinophilic granular cells, either alone or in combination with cell-cell neoplastic elements. Differentiation between a typical renal oncocytoma and oncocytic renal cell carcinoma can, therefore, be a somewhat difficult pathologic task based on nuclear morphology. The term *renal oncocytoma* refers only to tumors that contain a population of highly differentiated eosinophilic granular cells or oncocytes.

Grossly the tumors have a typical appearance—usually tan or light brown in color, well circumscribed, round, and encapsulated—and contain a central dense fibrous band with fibrous trabeculae extending out in a stellate pattern. The characteristic central scar is often imaged preoperatively by a CT or magnetic resonance imaging (MRI) examination of the tumor, sometimes even by ultrasound examination, and can serve to suggest the diagnosis of oncocytoma preoperatively. Necrosis and hypervascular areas are absent (Fig. 76–3). The typical cell appearance suggests an origin from the distal renal tubules, in particular, from the interrelated cells of the collecting tubules (Zerban et al, 1987; Nogueira and Bannasch, 1988).

The exact incidence of oncocytoma compared with other renal tumors is unknown; however, current series suggest that 3% to 7% of solid renocortical tumors previously classified as renal cell carcinomas are, in fact, typical renal oncocytomas (Lieber, 1993). Renal oncocytomas occur more commonly in males than in females and have generally the same age incidence as that of renal cell carcinoma.

Oncocytomas vary in size and may be quite large. In collected series, the median size was 6 cm in diameter. They can be found throughout the body and are not necessarily limited to the kidneys. These tumors are typically unifocal, but it is important to remember that in approximately 6% of cases, bilateral oncocytomas can be found. Both synchronous and asynchronous bilateral renal oncocytomas have been reported.

Warfel and Eble (1982) reported a case in which more than 200 small renal oncocytomas were found in bilateral distribution; the specific term *oncocytomastosis* has thus been used to describe this typical entity. Multifocality of renal oncocytomas and coexistence of renal oncocytoma and renal cell carcinoma should be borne in mind when attempting a more conservative surgery (i.e., enucleation or partial nephrectomy). Careful search by radiologic imaging techniques and by direct examination at the time of surgery

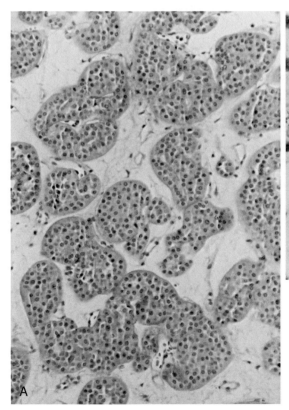
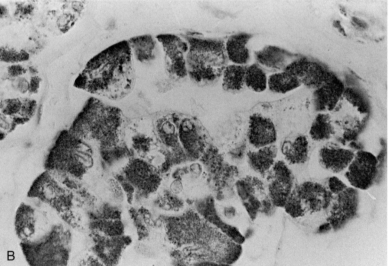

Figure 76–2. *A*, Oncocytoma. Eosinophilic cells with relatively uniform nuclei are arranged in discrete nests separated by edematous fibrovascular septa (hematoxylin and eosin, ×200). *B*, Oncocytoma stained with mES 13 antibody. Intense granular cytoplasmic staining is seen, highlighting the numerous mitochondria (immunoperoxidase, × 400). (From Weiss L, Gelb A, Medeiros J: Adult renal epithelial neoplasms. Am J Clin Pathol 1994; 103(5):625. Copyright 1994, American Society of Clinical Pathologists. Reprinted with permission.)

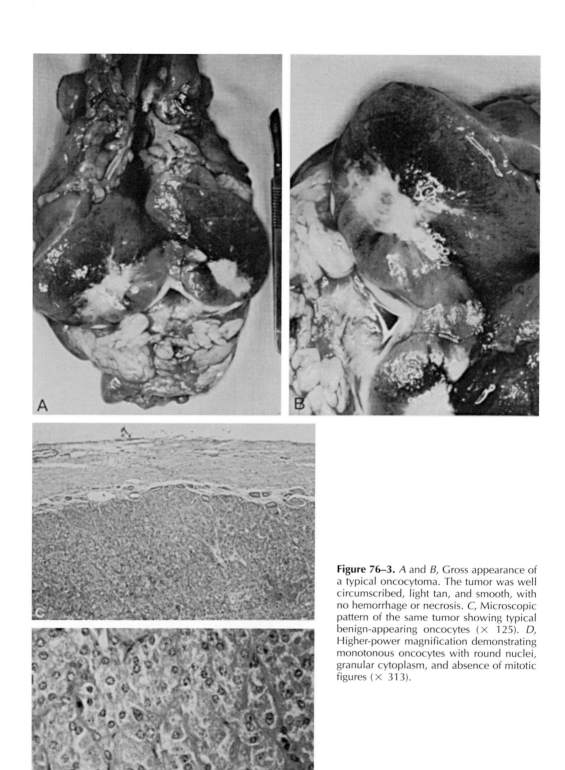

Figure 76–3. *A* and *B*, Gross appearance of a typical oncocytoma. The tumor was well circumscribed, light tan, and smooth, with no hemorrhage or necrosis. *C*, Microscopic pattern of the same tumor showing typical benign-appearing oncocytes ($\times$ 125). *D*, Higher-power magnification demonstrating monotonous oncocytes with round nuclei, granular cytoplasm, and absence of mitotic figures ($\times$ 313).

should thus be performed, so that all tumors can be removed during the same operative procedure.

Oncocytomas are usually asymptomatic, with the majority of tumors being discovered incidentally. Gross hematuria, abdominal pain, flank mass, and microscopic hematuria have all been infrequent findings. Because more ultrasound, CT, and MRI scans are being performed for unrelated conditions, it is anticipated that both renal cell carcinomas and oncocytomas will be discovered earlier, in the asymptomatic stages.

The typical radiographic appearance of the renal oncocytomas has been largely responsible for its identification as a specific clinical entity. The pyelographic appearance is one of a circumscribed solid mass of varying size and location in the kidney. The arterial phase of the angiogram reveals a typical spoke-wheel or stellate pattern seldom associated with venous pooling or arteriovenous fistulas (Bonavita et al, 1981). The typical angiographic picture is not always identified, however, and the angiogram may be indistinguishable from that of a hypovascular renal cell carcinoma. No typical CT scan or specific radionuclide scan has been identified (Davidson et al, 1993). Nuclear DNA ploidy cannot be used to distinguish between benign and malignant neoplasms in the kidney because certain typical oncocytomas have abnormal—tetraploidy or aneuploidy—patterns (Rainwater et al, 1986a, 1986b). Typical cytogenetic and immunologic changes in oncocytomas have been reported, however, including loss of chromosomes 1 and Y (Crotty et al, 1992; Dobin et al, 1992) and loss of HLA class I antigen expression (Licht et al, 1993). Further studies are required to evaluate the strength of these and other molecular markers to differentiate between benign and malignant renal tumors.

The management of renal oncocytomas, therefore, must be influenced by two characteristic features: (1) the unreliability and nonspecificity of current radiographic studies and (2) the presence of malignant elements and oncocytoma cells in the same tumor. Clearly a reliable preoperative diagnosis of renal oncocytoma merits an attempt at more conservative surgery (i.e., partial nephrectomy with frozen section control of the margins of resection). Radical nephrectomy is still the safest method of therapy unless contraindicated by other factors (e.g., solitary kidney, small size, poor renal function). For a relatively young, otherwise healthy patient with a tumor 4 cm diameter or smaller that is well encapsulated by CT and confined to one of the poles of the kidney, renal exploration and partial nephrectomy with a safe parenchymal margin should, however, be considered. Reflexive radical nephrectomy for every solid renocortical lesion should be avoided now because such tumors commonly are being found at an early stage and small size. For elderly patients or patients who are otherwise poor operative risks because of extensive medical problems, *observation treatment* of oncocytomas might be appropriate (Lieber, 1993).

Renal Angiomyolipoma

Renal angiomyolipoma (hamartoma) (Fig. 76–4) is a benign tumor that may occur as an isolated phenomenon or as part of the syndrome associated with tuberous sclerosis. Approximately 50% of patients with the diagnosis of angiomyolipoma have some or all of the other stigmata of tuberous sclerosis. This is a disease that is both hereditary and familial and is characterized by mental retardation, epilepsy, and adenoma sebaceum. In these patients, angiomyolipomas may also be found in the brain, eye, heart, lung, and bone (McCullough et al, 1971). Patients with tuberous sclerosis require careful screening for the presence of renal tumors (Stillwell et al, 1987). They tend to be younger, more likely to have multifocal and bilateral disease, to have more symptoms, and to have larger tumors that are more likely to grow and require surgery (Steiner et al, 1993).

Renal angiomyolipomas are frequently bilateral. They are often yellow and gray and have a propensity for profuse hemorrhage, large size, and multiplicity. Microscopically the

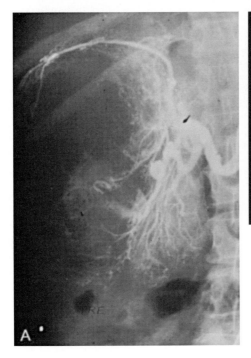

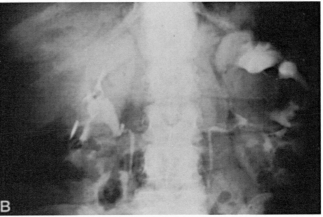

Figure 76–4. *A*, A 60-year-old woman with no evidence of tuberous sclerosis presented with hemorrhage into a large right flank tumor. Exploration and biopsy revealed hamartoma. *B*, Right renal hamartoma is unchanged 1 year after percutaneous angioinfarction. Figure also demonstrates central hamartoma in the left kidney.

Illustration continued on following page

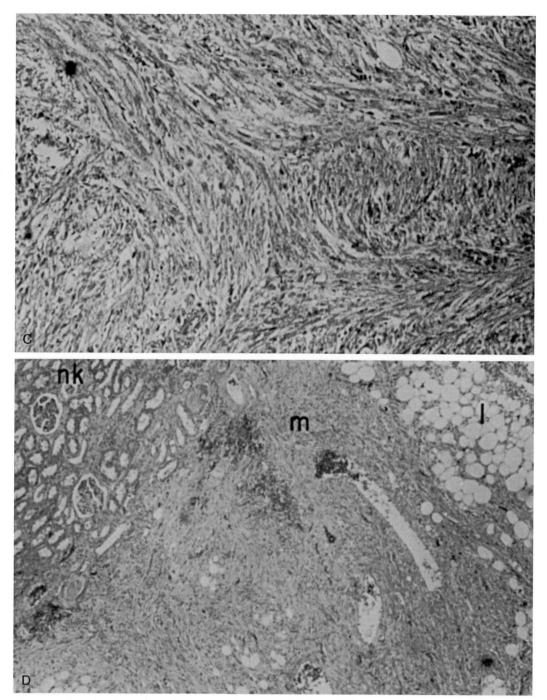

Figure 76–4 *Continued C,* Histologic appearance of fibromyomatous elements of tumor. *D,* Normal kidney (nk) is seen with adjacent myomatous (m) and lipomatous (l) elements of intrinsic tumor, diagnosed as angiofibromyolipoma (hamartoma).

tumor is named for the three primary components: unusual abdominal blood vessels, clusters of adipocytes, and sheets of smooth muscle. Pleomorphism is common, and mitotic figures, although rarely seen, can be prominent (Colvin and Dickersin, 1978). Although there are reports of malignant angiomyolipomas, it is currently believed that extrarenal and lymph node involvement reflects multicentricity rather than metastasis and is not a sufficient criterion for malignancy (Taylor et al, 1989; O'Toole et al, 1993).

The preferred imaging modality for these tumors is CT (Bosniak et al, 1988). The presence of fat is almost charac-

teristic for an angiomyolipoma (Fig. 76–5). On sonography, the tumor is highly echogenic, and on angiography, the tumor is vascular. The angiographic pattern of the tumor is, however, not sufficiently typical to reliably separate it from renal carcinoma. Taylor and co-workers and Blute and co-workers reported on the occasional presence of renal carcinoma in patients with proven angiomyolipoma. It therefore seems prudent to excise surgically tumors that are multiple, that do not have all of the classic characteristics of angiomyolipoma, and that contain calcifications (Blute et al, 1988; Taylor et al, 1989).

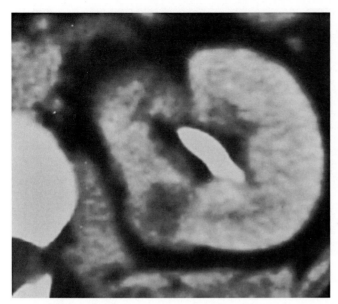

Figure 76–5. Small angiomyolipoma in the left kidney discovered incidentally. Contrast computed tomography scan shows that the mass is composed predominantly of fat.

Angiomyolipomas present clinically in several ways. First, they often are detected incidentally in patients who undergo CT scans for unrelated abdominal problems or in patients with tuberous sclerosis. Second, large tumors may cause local discomfort and gastrointestinal symptoms by compression of the duodenum and stomach. Third, patients may present with sudden pain or hypotension because of massive hemorrhage within the lesions.

The management of angiomyolipoma is controversial, but several generalizations can be made. In their review, Oesterling and associates noted that the size of the lesions was usually associated with propensity for symptoms, especially hemorrhage (Oesterling et al, 1986). Accordingly, based on the world literature of 602 cases and on the review of 13 patients at their institution, they concluded that asymptomatic lesions smaller than 4 cm in diameter may not require therapy but must be observed. Many of these tumors do not increase in size even after many years of follow-up. In a more recent update of the Johns Hopkins series with 35 patients, Steiner and colleagues recommended annual CT or ultrasound studies for patients with isolated small tumors and semiannual follow-up for patients with tumors larger than 4 cm who are asymptomatic or mildly symptomatic (Steiner et al, 1993). If the tumor grows, embolization or renal-sparing surgery should be considered. Patients with large angiomyolipomas and severe symptoms should undergo immediate selective arterial embolization if possible or conservative surgical therapy if embolization is not practical.

Angioinfarction should be the first attempted therapy in any patient having hemorrhage into an angiomyolipoma. The authors' experience has shown, however, that large tumors do not decrease in size after angioinfarction, although bleeding may be prevented (Fig. 76–6). Therefore, patients with large lesions who can undergo excision with preservation of functioning renal tissue should be strongly considered for this approach. Symptomatic lesions that cannot be managed by angioinfarction, multiple lesions that are not all characteristic of angiomyolipoma, and calcification also require exploration and conservative surgical excision when possible.

Fibroma

Fibrous tissue is found in the renal parenchyma, the perinephric tissues, and the renal capsule, and fibromas may arise from any of these structures. Glover and Buck (1982) reviewed the eight reported cases of medullary fibroma and noted that most occurred in women. These are rare tumors that are uniformly benign and occasionally are difficult to distinguish from fibrosarcomas of the retroperitoneum. They are often on the periphery of the kidney and may have to grow to a large size before becoming clinically obvious. Symptoms are rare and are usually associated with either distortion of the collecting system or growth outside the confines of the renal fossa, although hematuria is common in patients with medullary fibromas.

These tumors are large, are adherent to the kidney, and often resemble uterine fibroids. They are microscopically benign, with sheets of fibroblasts or a loose, myxomatous stroma. They are generally hypovascular angiographically but have no specific radiographic characteristics to distinguish them from hypovascular malignant tumors. A radical nephrectomy is usually performed because of the uncertainty of the diagnosis, but awareness of their benign nature warrants partial nephrectomy in selected cases.

Lipoma

Renal lipomas are among the rarest of renal tumors. Their origin is unclear, but they probably originate from fat cells within the renal capsule or parenchyma (Robertson and Hand, 1941). Dineen and colleagues reported a case of lipoma and reviewed the literature, documenting 18 cases of proven intrarenal lipoma (Dineen et al, 1983). This tumor typically occurs in middle-aged women, grows to a large size, and has pain as its presenting symptom, with hematuria occurring in some patients. A malignant potential has been suggested but has not been proven.

The gross characteristics are the same as those of any lipoma. Renal lipomas are confined within the renal capsule, in contrast to perirenal lipomas, which are extracapsular. These tumors have the greasy feeling of all lipomas, pale lobules being interposed with streaks consisting of blood vessels. Microscopically the cells are uniform fat cells with peripherally placed nuclei surrounded by plasma membranes. The treatment is surgical excision, usually requiring total nephrectomy.

Commonly, these lipomas have other cellular elements (Robertson and Hand, 1941) and can be classified as variants of angiomyolipoma. They should not be classified as pure lipomas, but they have the same clinical significance and the same benign course.

Perinephric lipomas are difficult or impossible to separate from intrarenal lipomas and may arise from perinephric fat or adjacent areas of the retroperitoneum (Pfeiffer and Gandin, 1946). These tumors are often huge, and excision without nephrectomy is seldom possible. CT scan should show

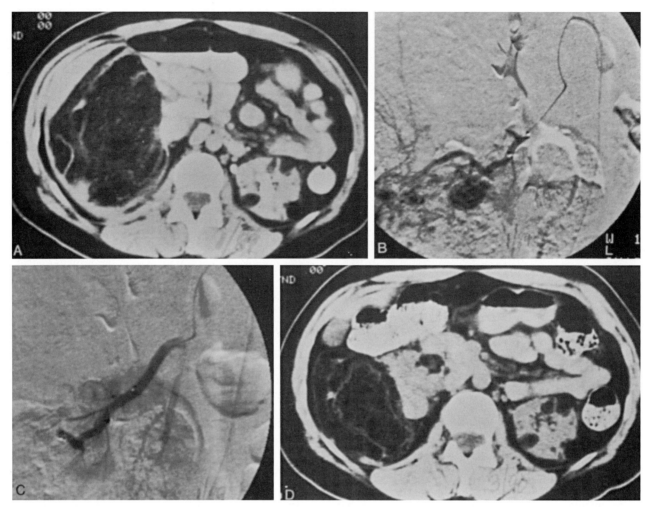

Figure 76–6. *A,* Bilateral multiple angiomyolipomas in a patient with hypotension and a growing right lower quadrant mass, secondary to acute hemorrhage. Computed tomography scan shows a large hematoma in the right perinephric space displacing the kidney anteriorly and medially. *B,* Selective right renal arteriogram shows a large hypervascular mass arising from the lower pole of the right kidney and identifies the bleeding site. Note the multiple tortuous irregular vessels that form the bleeding aneurysms. *C,* Subtraction renal arteriogram following a successful transcatheter, supraselective embolization of the lower pole branch, using steel coils. The upper pole branch was successfully embolized 2 days later. *D,* One-year follow-up postembolization. The right renal antiomyolipoma has only slightly decreased in size, but the hemorrhage at the periphery of the tumor has demonstrated significant reabsorption. Both kidneys are functioning well. The patient resumed normal activity and had no further bleeding episodes.

the typical fat density, allowing preoperative consideration of conservative excision.

Other Benign Tumors

Because the kidney is a complex organ consisting of many cell types within and surrounding the renal capsule, virtually every classification of benign tumor has been reported. Myomas, lymphangiomas, and hemangiomas have been found.

One of the rarest but most fascinating tumors is the functional renin-secreting juxtaglomerular tumor. It was first described by Robertson and co-workers (1967), and approximately ten cases have been described in the literature. These tumors arise from the juxtaglomerular cells in young patients (Orjauvik et al, 1975), who present typically with hypertension, elevated serum renin levels, and hyperaldosteronism. Presence of the tumor is suspected in indivuduals with an extremely high differential renal vein–to–renin ratio with no other obvious cause for hypertension.

Functional renin-secreting juxtaglomerular tumors are typ-

ically small, seldom more than 2 or 3 cm in diameter, and often are not detectable radiographically. Occasionally the segments of the kidney harboring the tumor can be identified by selective renal vein sampling (Bonnin et al, 1977). Grossly the tumors are gray-yellow with hemorrhagic areas; microscopically they are typical hemangiopericytomas. Electron microscopic studies reveal the characteristics of the juxtaglomerular cells, and tumor extracts may be shown to contain high concentrations of renin (Colvin and Dickersin, 1978). This tumor is always benign and should be distinguished from the generally larger, nonfunctional, and sometimes malignant typical renal hemangiopericytoma.

MALIGNANT RENAL TUMORS

Renal Cell Carcinoma

Incidence

Renal cell carcinoma is a relatively rare tumor, accounting for approximately 3% of adult malignancies. Approximately

28,000 new cases of renal carcinoma were predicted to occur in 1995, and an associated 11,000 deaths (Wingo et al, 1995). Little evidence suggests that the tumor is increasing in incidence, although it may be detected in earlier stages than previously.

Renal cell carcinoma is more common among urban dwellers and is more common in males, with a male-to-female ratio of approximately 2:1. Familial renal carcinoma has been reported, affecting as many as five family members. Patients with von Hippel–Lindau disease have a higher incidence of carcinoma (Lauritsen, 1975). Patients with polycystic kidney disease appear to have a predisposition for development of the tumor, although this has not been firmly established. Renal carcinoma is a tumor of adults, occurring primarily in those in their forties to sixties, but it may occasionally occur in younger age groups.

Etiology

Renal cell carcinomas seem to arise from the proximal convoluted tubule, the same cell of origin as that of renal adenomas (Tannenbaum, 1971; Wallace and Nairn, 1972). Although a number of etiologic agents have been identified in animal models (Bennington and Beckwith, 1975), no specific agent has been definitely identified as being causative of human renal carcinoma. Epidemiologic studies have incriminated tobacco, although the specific carcinogen has not been described (Weir and Dunn, 1970; Kantor, 1977). A high incidence of renal carcinoma has been noted in men who smoke pipes or cigars (Kantor, 1977).

In one study, La Vecchia and associates found a 1.7-fold increase in the incidence of renal cell carcinoma among ex-smokers compared with those who never smoked (La Vecchia et al, 1990). A direct and significant dose-risk relationship was observed among current smokers, with a relative risk of 1.1, 1.9, and 2.3 for moderate, intermediate, and heavy smokers, respectively. This trend in risk was statistically significant. The risk was directly related to duration of smoking and inversely related to age at starting. Among ex-smokers, risk was inversely related to time elapsed since stopping. The typical renal cell carcinoma can be produced in the adult Syrian hamster by long-term treatment with diethylstilbestrol (Kirkman and Bacon, 1949), but this hormone has not been shown to cause renal carcinoma in humans.

No definitive relationship between occupational and industrial carcinogens and renal carcinoma has been documented. Male cigarette smokers exposed to industrial contaminants of cadmium have been reported to have a slightly increased risk of developing the tumor (Kolonel, 1976). No other relationship has been reported, although research in this area has been limited. The radiographic agent colloidal thorium dioxide was reported to be associated with a high incidence of renal carcinoma in one study (Wenz, 1967). At the present time, there is a paucity of studies regarding the cause of renal carcinoma, and few hypotheses seem to warrant extensive investigation (Dayal and Wilkinson, 1989).

Molecular Biology and Immunology

CYTOGENETICS

The most consistent chromosomal changes observed in renal cell carcinoma are deletions and translocation involv-

ing the short arm of chromosome 3 (3p). In two families, each member carrying a germ line chromosomal mutation in the form of translocation (3;8) (Cohen et al, 1979) and translocation (3;6) (Kovacs et al, 1989) developed multiple or bilateral renal cancers at an earlier age of onset (40–50 years) than patients with sporadic renal cell carcinoma (60–70 years). The breakpoint on chromosome 3 was localized at the same region (3p13–14.2).

In the early 1980s, scientists at the National Cancer Institute (NCI) initiated studies to identify the gene for kidney cancer. These investigators reported in *Nature* the detection of consistent abnormalities on chromosome 3 in tumor tissue from patients with kidney cancer (Zbar et al, 1987). Subsequent studies by this group and others determined that loss of a segment of chromosome 3 was an early event and was a consistent finding in tumor tissue from patients with sporadic (nonhereditary), clear cell kidney cancer (Anglard et al, 1992; Brooks et al, 1993). These findings suggested that the kidney cancer gene was in this location. Studies were then initiated of the familial form of kidney cancer associated with von Hippel–Lindau disease with the assumption that the same gene might be involved in the origin of both. Von Hippel–Lindau disease is a rare (1 in 36,000 births) familial cancer syndrome in which affected individuals develop tumors in a number of locations. Affected individuals tend to develop bilateral, multifocal renal tumors and cysts, tumors in the cerebellum and spine (hemangioblastomas), retinal hemangiomas, pheochromocytomas, pancreatic islet cell tumors, and epididymal cystadenomas. The kidney cancers that occur in von Hippel–Lindau disease are consistently clear cell renal carcinoma and can advance and metastasize (Linehan et al, 1995). Thirty-five percent to 45% of von Hippel–Lindau disease patients die of kidney cancer if it is not detected and treated early. In 1993, the NCI group reported the discovery of the VHL gene (Latif et al, 1993). More recently, Gnarra and colleagues found mutation of the VHL gene to be a frequent event in clear cell, granular, and sarcomatoid renal carcinoma but not in papillary renal carcinoma (Gnarra et al, 1994). These findings support a molecular classification of clear cell versus papillary kidney cancer with clear cell kidney cancer being characterized by mutation of the VHL gene. The VHL gene has the classic characteristics of a tumor suppressor gene (i.e., a gene whose loss of function is associated with transformation [cancer]).

Molecular activation of proto-oncogenes has also been proposed to explain the observed cytogenetic findings. No single oncogene abnormality, however, has been identified as characteristic of renal cell carcinoma. Overexpression of c-*myc* and epidermal growth factor receptor (EGFR) (c-*erb* B-1) mRNA and underexpression of HER-2 (*erb* B-2) mRNA can be found in the majority of patients with renal cell carcinoma (Yao et al, 1988; Freeman et al, 1989; Weidner et al, 1990). c-Ha-*ras*, c-*fos*, c-*fms*, and f-*raf*-1 expression is elevated in some tumors as well (Slamon et al, 1984; Teyssier et al, 1986; Karthaus et al, 1987; Yao et al, 1988). The significance of these altered patterns of proto-oncogene expression in renal cell carcinoma is currently unfolding with the better understanding of signal transduction pathways. Oka and co-workers demonstrated that the mitogen-activated protein (MAP) kinase pathway, which also involves both Ras and Raf-1 proto-oncogene products, is constitutively activated in a relatively high number of renal tumors (Oka et al, 1995). Moreover, MAP kinase activation was detected more frequently in high-grade renal cell carcinomas than in low-grade tumors. It was therefore suggested that activation of the MAP kinase cascade may play an important role in the carcinogenesis of these tumors and that greater activation of MAP kinase could be associated with increased malignant potential in tumors.

GROWTH FACTORS

Transforming growth factors (TGFs) alpha and beta are two tumor-produced regulatory growth factors that may be related to the development of renal cell carcinoma (Gomella et al, 1989; Linehan et al, 1989). TGF-alpha is known to bind to EGFR, and because both TGF-alpha and EGFR are overexpressed in kidney tumor tissue, it is possible that interaction between TGF-alpha and EGFR plays a role in promoting transformation or proliferation (or both) of kidney neoplasms, perhaps by an autocrine mechanism (Mydlo et al, 1989). TGF-beta is produced in a biologically latent form by human renal cell carcinoma lines in culture, and the addition of exogenous TGF-beta to these cells inhibits their proliferation (Sargent et al, 1989). It appears, therefore, that changes in the production of and response to these stimulatory and inhibitory growth factors may lead to an imbalance of growth control, loss of autocrine growth inhibition, and cancer formation.

MULTIDRUG RESISTANCE

Renal cell carcinoma remains resistant to currently available chemotherapeutic agents. The basis for this multidrug resistance (MDR) in renal cell carcinoma appears to be related to a 170-kD transmembrane glycoprotein (P-glycoprotein, P170) encoded by the MDR1 gene that functions as an energy-dependent drug efflux pump (Fojo et al, 1987; Kakehi et al, 1988). This action results in decreased accumulation within cells of multiple, structurally unrelated, naturally occurring products used as chemotherapeutic agents (Moscow and Cowan, 1988). Cells resistant to chemotherapeutic drugs by virtue of P-glycoprotein expression can be made more sensitive by agents, such as verapamil, amiodarone, quinidine, and cyclosporines, that inhibit the function of the efflux pump and result in increased intracellular concentrations of chemotherapeutic drugs (Kanamaru et al, 1989; Mickisch et al, 1990a; Tsuruo et al, 1984).

A second independent mechanism associated with renal cell carcinoma MDR is the glutathione redox cycle, which is involved in the intracellular binding and detoxification of chemotherapeutic agents and can be inactivated by buthionine sulfoximine (Mickisch et al, 1990b). The transgenic mouse model now provides a useful tool to reverse MDR in vivo and analyze their in vivo toxicity. Clinical trials aiming to inhibit the multidrug transporter and safely overcome MDR are currently underway (Chapman and Goldstein, 1995).

Pathology

Renal cell carcinomas are typically round, varying in size from tumors several centimeters in diameter to tumors that almost fill the abdomen (Fig. 76–7). They generally do not have a true histologic capsule but almost always have a pseudocapsule composed of compressed parenchyma and

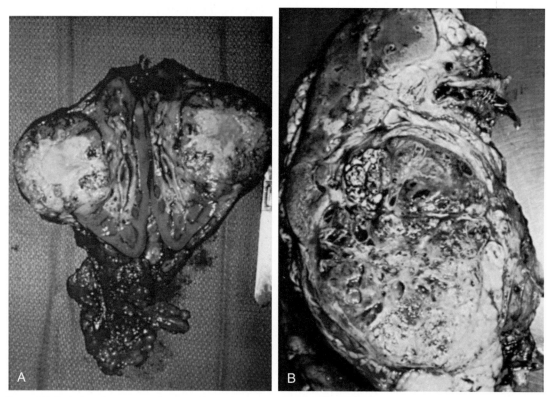

Figure 76–7. *A*, Specimen opened to reveal massive tumor. *B*, Typical renal cell carcinoma with thick pseudocapsule.

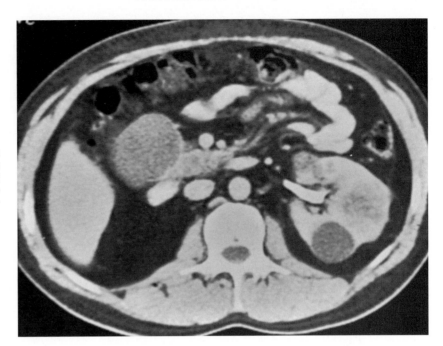

Figure 76–8. Computed tomography scan in a patient with von Hippel–Lindau disease showing multiple pancreatic cysts, posterior renal cyst, and two solid renal tumors in the lateral and anterior aspects (isointense to the cortex representing two renal carcinomas). (Courtesy of Dr. Sachiko Cochran.)

fibrous tissue. The amount of hemorrhage and necrosis varies greatly, but few tumors are uniform in gross appearance. Areas of yellowish or brownish soft tumor are usually interposed between sclerotic bifrontal areas and patches of hemorrhage and necrosis. Multiple cysts are found not infrequently, probably resulting from segmental necrosis and resorption. The collecting system is generally displaced and is often invaded. Gerota's fascia seems to provide a barrier against local spread, but it may be compressed and invaded. Calcification can occur and may be stifled or may occur in a plaque-like arrangement.

Renal carcinoma is typically unilateral, but bilaterality, either synchronous or asynchronous, occurs in approximately 2% of cases (Moertel et al, 1961). Von Hippel–Lindau disease is characteristically associated with the presence of multiple and bilateral renal carcinomas (Fig. 76–8) (Glenn et al, 1990). As noted further on, the tumor frequently extends into the renal vein as a thrombus, which may be propagated for varying distances into the inferior vena cava. The more malignant and larger tumors can invade locally, with extension into the surrounding muscles and direct invasion into adjacent organs.

Electron microscopic studies have identified the proximal tubular cell as the origin of renal cell carcinoma. The proximal tubular cell has multiple surface microvilli, giving the brush border characteristic, and contains a more complex cytoplasm than the more distal tubular cells. The ultrastructural characteristics of the proximal cell are found in varying degrees in most renal carcinomas. Brush borders, however, are usually not fully developed and are present on only some cells.

The origin of the tumor from proximal tubular cells has been supported by a number of investigators (Tannenbaum, 1971; Fisher and Horvat, 1972). Bander and colleagues further refined the derivation of renal cell carcinoma cells by subclassifying the proximal tubular cells using monoclonal antibody (Mo Ab) probes (Bander et al, 1989). They found that in the normal adult kidney, cells of the convoluted portion are URO10 + /URO8 − ; those of the straight portion are URO10 − /URO8 + . Although adult proximal tubular cells demonstrate reciprocal expression of URO10 and URO8, fetal kidney proximal tubule progenitor cells coexpress both antigens (URO10 + /URO8 +). In renal cell carcinoma specimens, 30% of the cells are derived from the proximal convoluted tubule, 18% are derived from the proximal straight tubule, and 50% are derived from proximal tubule progenitor cells (URO10 + /URO8 +). The ultrastructure of the various cell types composing the classic renal carcinoma has been carefully detailed by Colvin and Dickersin (1978).

Although it is unusual to find absolutely pure examples, renal cell carcinomas can be broadly grouped into four histologic types: clear cell, granular cell, tubulopapillary, and sarcomatoid (Murphy, 1989). Based on combined genetic and pathologic characteristics, a new classification of renal tumors was proposed by Kovacs (1993) and extensively reviewed by Weiss and co-workers (1995) (Table 76–5). The clear cell variant of renal cell carcinoma accounts for more than 80% of renal cell neoplasms and is microscopically characterized by sheets, acini, or alveoli of neoplastic cells bounded by a network of delicate vascular sinusoids and reticulin fibers. The clear cells are rounded or polygonal with abundant cytoplasm (Fig. 76–9), which contains cholesterol, cholesterol esters, phospholipids, and glycogen; these sub-

Table 76–5. CLASSIFICATION OF RENAL CELL NEOPLASMS

Oncocytoma
Chromophobe carcinoma
Papillary neoplasm
Adenocarcinoma, not otherwise specified (clear/granular)
Collecting duct carcinoma
Neuroendocrine tumors
   Carcinoid
   Small cell carcinoma

Modified from Kovacs G: Histopathology 1993; 22:1.

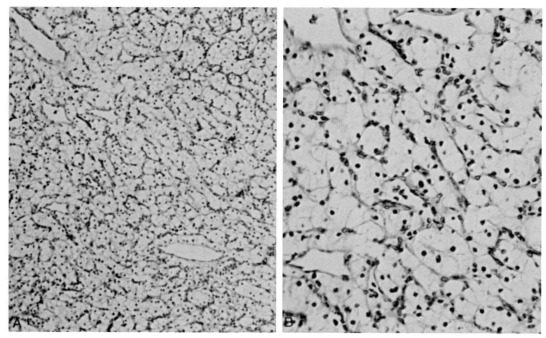

Figure 76–9. *A,* Typical pattern of clear cell carcinoma with small nuclei and clear cytoplasm (× 125). *B,* Higher-power magnification showing pure clear cell pattern (× 313).

stances are largely extracted by the solvents used in routine histologic preparations.

Few tumors contain only clear cells, however; a granular cell (dark cell) component is usually present in varying degrees and may actually compose the major portion of the tumor (Fig. 76–10). Granular cells have eosinophilic cytoplasm and abundant mitochondria. Immunohistochemically, approximately 50% of renal cell carcinomas express vimentin, with high-grade carcinomas more likely than low-

grade carcinomas to be vimentin-positive. Vimentin positivity is more common in sarcomatoid renal cell carcinomas than in neoplasms lacking spindled areas (DeLong et al, 1993). Almost all renal adenocarcinomas express keratin 8 and 18, with a majority of tumors also staining positive for epithelial membrane antigen. The tubulopapillary variant appears to be a histologically distinctive tumor, composing approximately 14% of all renal neoplasms (Fig. 76–11). Macroscopically, this tumor is small, nearly completely en-

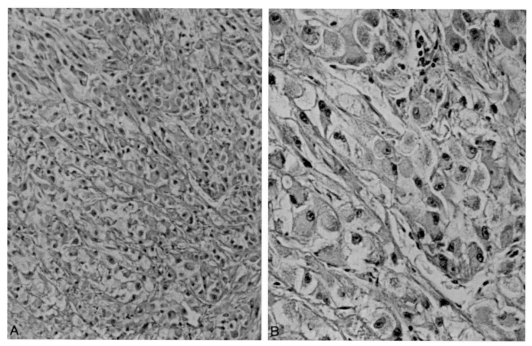

Figure 76–10. *A,* Renal carcinoma showing granular cell pattern with small nuclei and granular cytoplasm (× 125). *B,* Higher-power magnification emphasizing typical granular cell pattern (× 313).

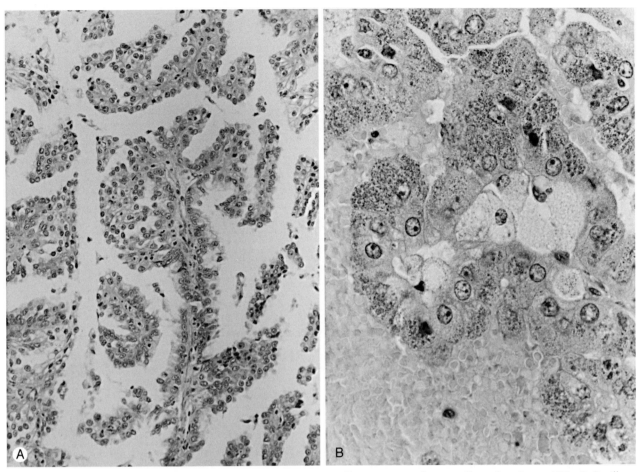

Figure 76–11. *A,* Papillary renal neoplasm. Numerous fine fibrovascular stalks are present (hematoxylin and eosin, × 200). *B,* Papillary renal neoplasm. The stroma is filled with foamy macrophages. Note the hemosiderin pigment in the neoplastic cells lining the stalks (hematoxylin and eosin, × 200). (From Weiss L, Gelb A, Medeiros J: Adult renal epithelial neoplasms. Am J Clin Pathol 1994; 103(5):629. Copyright 1994, American Society of Clinical Pathologists. Reprinted with permission.)

capsulated, and confined to the cortex. In purely papillary neoplasms, significant nuclear anaplasia is uncommon. Ultrastructurally and immunohistochemically, renal papillary neoplasms cannot be distinguished from usual renal adenocarcinomas. Cytogenetically, however, renal papillary neoplasms show a unique pattern, regardless of size, including loss of the Y chromosome along with a trisomy of chromosomes 7 and 17. The sarcomatoid variant of renal cell carcinoma is characterized by a predominantly spindle cell pattern, aggressive behavior, and poor prognosis (Tomera et al, 1983). Spindle cells may resemble pleomorphic mesenchymal cells (Fig. 76–12), and differentiation from fibrosarcoma may be difficult.

Thoenes and colleagues have provided evidence for a new type of renal cell carcinoma—the chromophobe type—which exhibits morphologic and immunohistochemical features of the cortical collecting-duct epithelia (Thoenes et al, 1988). This tumor represents approximately 4% of renal cell neoplasms. Chromophobe cells are characterized by their light (transparent) cytoplasm with a finely reticular, but not empty, appearance. Sometimes a moderately intense eosinophilia is observed. The electron microscopic findings are characteristic and define the entity. The cytoplasm displays abundant reticular structures (microvesicles) poor in glycogen. Preliminary data suggest better survival in patients with the chromophobe rather than the clear cell type of renal cell carcinoma.

A number of investigators have related various types of grading systems to prognosis. It is currently believed that among the microscopic features, assessment of nuclear grade probably has the greatest prognostic significance, and, in contrast to cell type, nuclear grade is a predictor of survival that is independent of pathologic stage (Fuhrman et al, 1982; Kloppel et al, 1986). Within a given stage, however, the microscopic grading seems to have less significance than in some tumors. Nonetheless, tumors with nuclei resembling those of normal cells demonstrate a low malignant potential in contrast to the bizarre heterogeneous nuclei typical of spindle cell tumors, which are associated with a worse prognosis. A great disparity in survival has not been demonstrated between patients whose tumors contain clear cells and patients whose tumors contain granular cells. Tumors composed mainly of spindle cells, however, seem to indicate a worse prognosis for the patient that is independent of nuclear grade (Colvin and Dickersin, 1978).

Nuclear DNA content as measured by image cytometry or flow cytometry has been shown to correlate with tumor behavior (Rainwater et al, 1987). Most reports have confirmed a general relationship between DNA ploidy and nuclear grade with a high percentage of anaplastic tumors

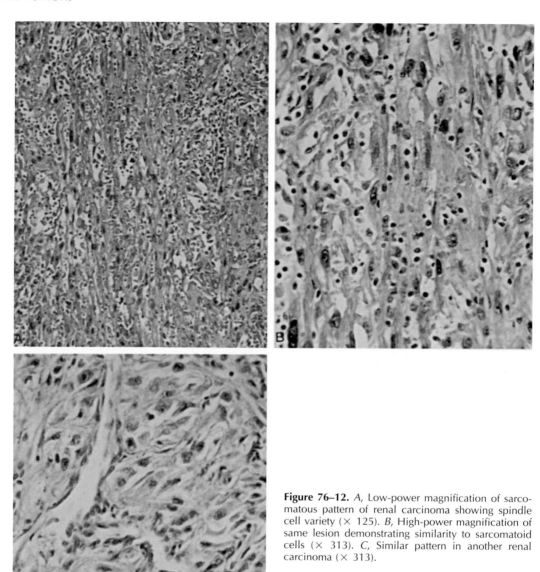

Figure 76–12. *A,* Low-power magnification of sarcomatous pattern of renal carcinoma showing spindle cell variety (× 125). *B,* High-power magnification of same lesion demonstrating similarity to sarcomatoid cells (× 313). *C,* Similar pattern in another renal carcinoma (× 313).

harboring aneuploid cells. Similar correlations have been made between DNA ploidy and the prognoses of patients with various stages of renal cell carcinomas (Grignon et al, 1989). Although measurements of DNA ploidy may be the reflection of tumor heterogeneity and an indication of biologic potential, the clinical value of this technique remains to be determined for renal cell carcinoma (Murphy, 1989).

Clinical Presentation

The human kidney resides in a well-protected environment, and its only expression to the outside environment is through its primary product, the urine. Pain cannot be expected to occur unless the tumor invades surrounding areas or obstructs the outflow of urine owing to hemorrhage and subsequent formation of blood clots. Therefore, it is not surprising that the presenting signs and symptoms are often those related to local invasion or distant metastases.

The classic triad of pain, hematuria, and flank mass is certainly a reliable clinical symptom complex, but it is found in few patients and generally indicates advanced disease. One or two of these symptoms or signs are commonly associated with renal carcinoma (Table 76–6). The most frequent findings are pain or hematuria secondary to the primary tumor, but symptoms owing to metastatic disease probably occur more frequently. Weight loss, fever, night sweats, and the sudden development of a varicocele in the male patient are not uncommon findings. Hypertension is

Table 76–6. INCIDENCE OF SYMPTOMS IN 180 PATIENTS WITH RENAL CELL CARCINOMA

Symptom	Percent
Classic triad	10
Pain	41
Hematuria	38
Mass	24
Weight loss	36
Fever	18
Hypertension	22
Hypercalcemia	6

due to segmental renal artery occlusion or to elaboration of renin or renin-like substances.

Few tumors are associated with such a diversity of paraneoplastic syndromes, some of which may represent the presenting symptoms in patients with renal carcinoma (Sufrin et al, 1989). The normal kidney is involved in the production of prostaglandins, 1,25-dihydroxycholecalciferol, renin, and erythropoietin. Renal malignancies may elaborate these substances in amounts greater than normal and may elaborate parathormone-like factors, glucagon, human chorionic gonadotropin (hCG), and insulin (Pavelic and Popovic, 1981; Mangin et al, 1988).

The most dramatic syndrome is associated with nonmetastatic hepatic dysfunction and is referred to as Staufer syndrome. Patients with this syndrome have abnormal liver function tests, white blood cell loss, fever, and areas of hepatic necrosis without hepatic metastases (Boxer et al, 1978). Renal function returns to normal after nephrectomy in many patients; this is an important prognostic sign because 88% of such patients have survival at least greater than 1 year. Persistence or recurrence of this syndrome is almost invariably associated with recurrence of the tumor.

Hypercalcemia has been reported in up to 10% of patients with renal carcinoma, and the cause is rather obscure. A peptide produced by the tumor that is analogous to the amino-terminal regions of a parathyroid hormone–related protein may be the causative agent (Goldberg et al, 1964; Kemp et al, 1987). Removal of the primary tumor is often associated with a fall in the serum calcium level, although the metastatic sites may elaborate the factor and eventually cause recurrent hypercalcemia. Hypercalcemia may be associated with skeletal metastases.

Hypertension has been associated with renal carcinoma, and elevated renin serum levels were reported in patients with high-stage renal tumors. The levels often fall to normal after nephrectomy (Sufrin et al, 1989). Hypertension in these patients may also be secondary to arteriovenous fistulas within the tumor, hypercalcemia, ureteral obstruction, cerebral metastases, and polycythemia.

Erythropoietin, a glycoprotein elaborated by the renal cortex in response to hypoxia, is a major regulator of erythropoiesis and induces erythrocyte differentiation. Increased levels have been detected in many patients with renal carcinoma, but the mechanism is unclear. This substance may be elaborated by the tumor cells or by the normal renal cells in response to relative hypoxia induced by the tumor (Erslev and Caro, 1986). Tumor production of erythropoietin may identify a subset of individuals with renal cell carcinoma responsive to immunotherapy with interleukin-2 and inter-

feron-alpha (Janik et al, 1993). In 15% to 40% of patients, hypertension is present. The myriad syndromes and their relative incidences are listed in Table 76–7 (Chisholm, 1974).

Radiographic Diagnoses

The rapid evolution of uroradiography has provided the urologist with a number of diagnostic tests designed primarily to determine whether a renal mass lesion exists and to distinguish solid renal mass lesions from the more common benign renal cysts (Fig. 76–13). Controversy exists regarding the reliability of each method and its place in the decision-making process as well as the extent to which each can provide the most cost-effective preoperative information.

With greater use of ultrasound, CT, and MRI, the ability to detect renal tumors earlier and in lower stages has now significantly increased, resulting in better patient survival. Estimates are that approximately two thirds of all locally confined renal tumors are found serendipitously (Konnak and Grossman, 1985; Thompson and Peek, 1988; Levine et al, 1989). Although the traditional intravenous pyelography with infusion nephrotomography remains the primary diagnostic step in many institutions, it is not surprising that many more renal masses are being demonstrated with ultrasound and CT than with urography (Fig. 76–14). Renal tumors that may not be detected with urography because of location, size, or coexisting anatomic abnormality can be detected with increased accuracy with the cross-sectional imaging afforded by CT or the multiple methods of display available with ultrasound (Smith et al, 1989).

Ultrasound evaluation has the advantage of being able to distinguish among solid, cystic, and complex masses. The sonographic criteria for a simple benign cyst include an absence of internal echoes, a smooth and well-defined wall, a good sound transmission, a round or oval shape, and an acoustic shadow arising from the edges of the cyst. Any lesion that on ultrasound is not clearly a simple cyst must be studied further by CT scan.

Solid renal masses have variable echogenicity, ranging from bright echoes to less echogenic than the normal renal parenchyma, no or little through-transmission, poorly demarcated walls, and irregular shape. Small renal parenchymal tumors, however, usually have smooth, well-defined margins and do not cause displacement of the renal sinus or calyces

Table 76–7. INCIDENCE OF SYSTEMIC SYNDROMES IN PATIENTS WITH RENAL CELL CARCINOMA

Effect	Ratio	Percent
Raised erythrocyte sedimentation rate	362/651	55.6
Hypertension	89/237	37.5
Anemia	473/1300	36.3
Cachexia, weight loss	338/979	34.5
Pyrexia	164/954	17.2
Abnormal liver function	65/450	14.4
Raised alkaline phosphatase	64/434	10.1
Hypercalcemia	44/886	4.9
Polycythemia	43/1212	3.5
Neuromyopathy	13/400	3.2
Amyloidosis	12/573	2.0

Adapted from Chisholm GD: Ann NY Acad Sci 1974; 230:403.

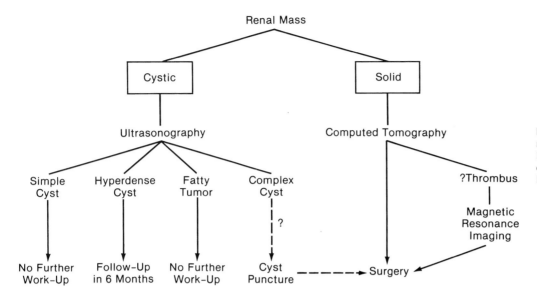

Figure 76–13. Work-up of a renal mass. (Modified from Barbaric ZL: Principles of Genitourinary Radiology. New York, Thieme Medical Publishers Inc., 1991.)

or project significantly beyond the renal contour. Such tumors may simulate normal renal parenchyma, such as a prominent renal column of Bertin or fetal lobation. In these cases, additional studies, such as radionuclide scan or CT scan, help in differentiation (Bosniak and Subramanyam, 1990). Highly echogenic malignant renal masses are rare; most are angiomyolipomas or hemangiomas, which are discussed further in this chapter.

Ultrasound, especially with duplex Doppler technology, can play a role in staging renal carcinoma in some patients. It may serve to diagnose or exclude tumor thrombus or demonstrate the superior extension of a tumor into the inferior vena cava and the right atrium, but it cannot accurately assess regional lymph node involvement. It should, therefore, not be used as the first-line technique but in those cases in which CT causes uncertainty with regard to venous invasion (Newhouse, 1993).

Few purely cystic lesions prove to harbor renal carcinoma. This small group of cystic tumors can be identified in almost every case by CT or by cyst aspiration and injection of contrast material (Bosniak and Subramanyam, 1990) (see Fig. 76–14). Clear fluid that has no malignant cells, low fat and protein content, and low lactic acid dehydrogenase levels, aspirated from a cyst with smooth walls, is almost absolute evidence of the absence of malignancy (Lang, 1977). The only consistent difference between a cyst containing a tumor and a hemorrhagic benign cyst is the presence of malignant cells. Because detection of low-grade tumors may be difficult in aspirated old blood, the presence of blood in a cyst must raise the index of suspicion sufficiently to prompt further diagnostic tests.

CT is the method of choice for detecting and staging renal carcinoma (Fig. 76–15). The development of CT, which offers a number of specific advantages over other methods, has demanded a complete re-evaluation of the traditional approaches to diagnosis (Fig. 76–16). Although infusion of contrast material and ingestion of contrast material are important components, the procedure is less invasive than angiography. Cyst density of the mass lesions can now be accurately measured, usually obviating the need for cystography or cyst puncture. The CT scan is performed as an outpatient procedure, in contrast to angiography, which requires hospitalization. In addition, more thorough staging information is obtained from CT scanning than from any of the other diagnostic methods (Figs. 76–17 through 76–19).

Jaschke and colleagues correlated preoperative staging of 125 renal carcinomas with the angiographic and pathologic findings (Jaschke et al, 1982). The CT scan allows the

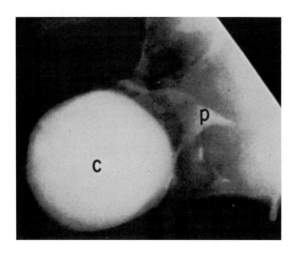

Figure 76–14. Simple renal cyst (c) after needle puncture, aspiration, and instillation of contrast material with simultaneous intravenous pyelogram to opacify renal collecting system (p).

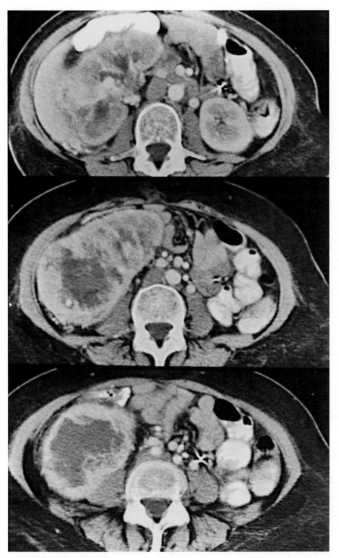

Figure 76–15. Heterogenous-enhancing, right renal carcinoma on contrast-enhancing CT. (From Barbaric Z: Imaging work-up: Is it renal carcinoma and is it operable? Semin Urol Oncol 1996; 14(4):197.)

correct diagnosis of renal vein involvement in 91%, vena caval extension in 97%, perirenal extension in 79%, lymph node metastases in 87%, and extension to adjacent organs in 96% of patients. Richie and co-workers studied not only the staging accuracy but also the diagnostic reliability of CT scan in 45 patients compared with that of the angiography (Richie et al, 1983). The tests were similar in diagnostic accuracy (95% versus 85%) and detection of renal vein extension, but CT scan was more accurate in detection of regional lymph node metastases.

In the excellent article by Lang (1984), the relative accuracy of enhanced CT scan compared with other diagnostic studies was determined in a prospective fashion. In addition to separating cystic from solid lesions accurately, properly performed, enhanced CT can detect tumor extension through the capsule or into surrounding structures. Extension to the renal vein and vena cava can be determined with great accuracy, obviating the need for traditional venacavography. Extension to the regional lymph nodes is a poor prognostic sign, and few patients are cured surgically. CT can detect

extensive regional lymph node involvement in many patients.

From the data presented by Lang (1984), it appears that as a single diagnostic study, CT is the most cost-effective method of evaluating a suspected renal mass lesion and should be the first-line technique for that purpose. Using the rapid-enhancement method suggested by Lang, further staging information seems plausible. Certain pitfalls of CT, however, have also become apparent. Although extension through the capsule is often accurately diagnosed, a number of false-positive findings occur. The test does not detect limited lymph node involvement, and a small but disconcerting number of patients seem to have involved lymph nodes that prove to be normal at surgery. One must be careful today not to deny patients the potential for surgical cure on the basis of these false-positive readings. These patients can then receive adjuvant immunotherapy if needed. Nonetheless, the new-generation CT scanners provide a single test for diagnosis and staging of renal tumors that is minimally invasive and cost-effective.

The role of MRI in the diagnosis and staging of renal cell carcinoma is currently under investigation. Initially, MRI held promise as a means of distinguishing different types of solid renal masses. Subsequent reports have shown that MRI is less sensitive than CT for the discovery of solid lesions less than 3 cm in diameter (Amendola et al, 1988; Hricak et al, 1988; Quint et al, 1988). MRI provides useful information, however, about neoplastic invasion of the renal vein or inferior vena cava without the need for contrast material, and in cases of large, bulky tumors, MRI adds a multidimensional assessment of the tumor extent (Figs. 76–20 and 76–21) (Hricak et al, 1985; Horan et al, 1989; Stewart and Dunnick, 1990). Similar to CT, MRI cannot reliably distinguish between bland and tumor thrombus, stage I and II disease, or hyperplastic and malignant adenopathy.

Selective renal arteriography was the final and definitive diagnostic step in evaluation of renal masses for decades (Fig. 76–22). The emergence of CT, however, has resulted in a marked narrowing of indications for angiography. Because CT gives no information about renal vasculature, angiography remains the primary diagnostic test in the patient with a suspected tumor in the solitary kidney, when parenchymal-sparing procedures are anticipated. Also, although differentiation of primary versus metastatic lesions to the kidney is difficult even with angiography, metastatic lesions are typically hypovascular. This feature can be helpful in selected patients for planning therapy when a metastatic lesion to the kidney is suspected. Lastly, interpretation of some lesions by CT scan may be unclear; angiography, with demonstration of small tumor vessels and other characteristic findings, may assist in ensuring the proper diagnosis.

The classic angiographic picture of renal carcinoma is illustrated in Figure 76–23. Neovascularity, arteriovenous fistulas, pooling of contrast media, and accentuation of capsular vessels are the hallmarks of these tumors. All variations of this angiographic picture may exist, however, and vast hypovascular tumors impose a difficult diagnostic problem. The addition of epinephrine infusion to constrict normal vessels, without constricting tumor vessels, may obviate this difficulty. Properly performed, selected renal arteriography remains an important part of the diagnosis of renal carcinoma in these selected circumstances.

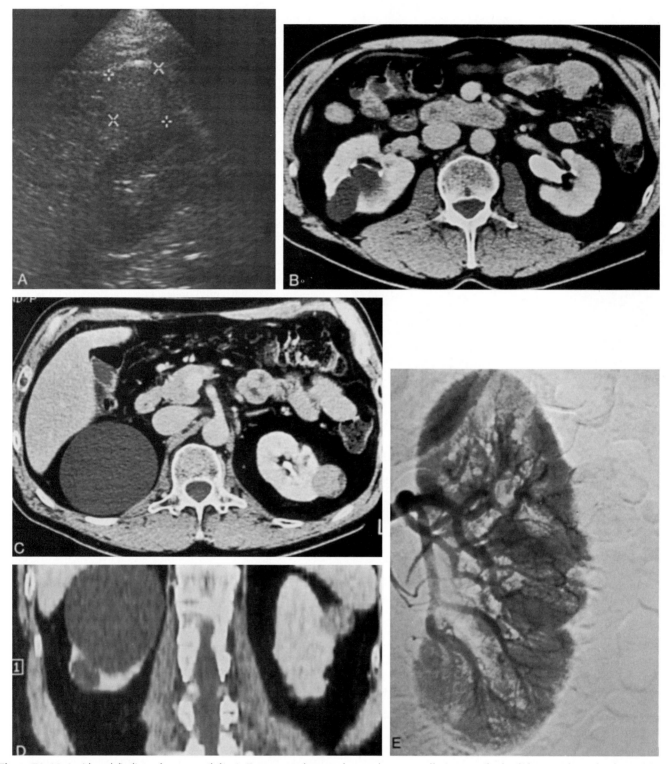

Figure 76–16. Incidental finding of a tumor *(left)*. *A*, Transverse ultrasound scan shows a well-circumscribed solid mass of equal echogenicity to adjacent cortex. *B*, Computed tomography scan reveals small renal calculi and multiple renal cysts in the right kidney. Patient presented with hematuria and right flank pain. *C* and *D*, Different computed tomography cuts of the same patient demonstrating a large right renal cyst and a 3-cm × 3-cm complex renal mass in the lateral aspect of the left kidney. *E*, Selective left renal angiogram reveals an avascular lesion with no evidence of neovascularity. Partial nephrectomy confirmed the mass to be an oncocytoma.

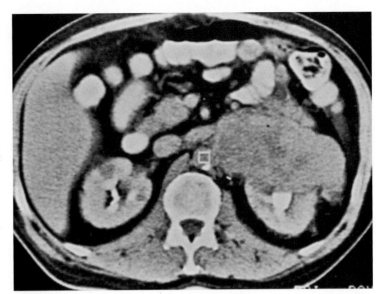

Figure 76–17. Computed tomography scan demonstrating two small cysts in the right kidney and a large solid mass in the left kidney extending over the aorta and filling the left renal vein.

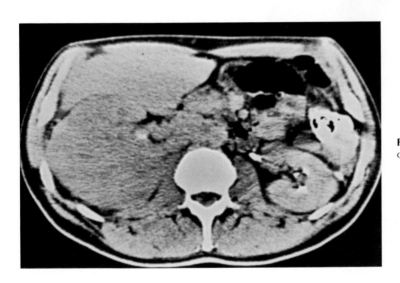

Figure 76–18. Huge right renal cell carcinoma with involvement of pericaval and interaorta-caval lymph nodes proved at surgery.

Figure 76–19. Large right renal mass, mixed solid and cystic on ultrasound. Computed tomography scan demonstrates a renal cell carcinoma with extensive central necrosis and involvement of adjacent lymph nodes.

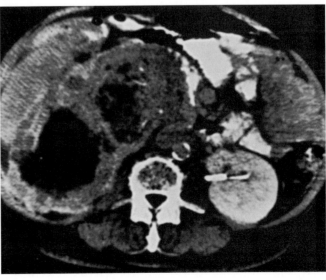

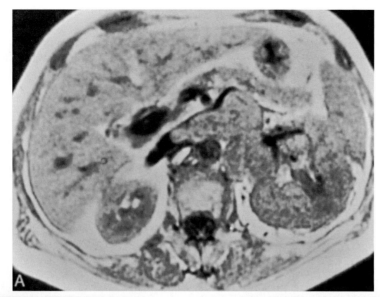

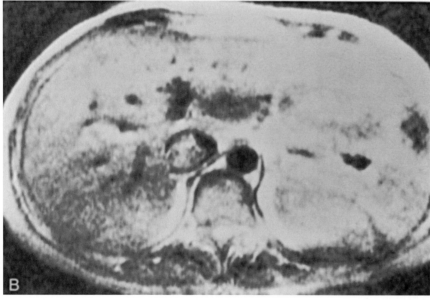

Figure 76–20. *A* and *B*, T1-weighted magnetic resonance spin-echo image displays a large left renal carcinoma extending into the enlarged renal vein and inferior vena cava. (Courtesy of Dr. Sachiko Cochran.)

Staging

The staging system most commonly employed in the United States is Robson's modification of the system of Flocks and Kadesky (Fig. 76–24) (Robson et al, 1968). The limitations of this system become obvious when it is noted that survival of patients with stage II tumor is equal to that of patients with stage III tumor in some series, indicating an inappropriate assignment of prognostic factors. The placement of renal vein, vena cava, and lymph node involvement into the stage III group accounts for this apparent contradiction because of the inclusion of all levels of renal vein extension. Furthermore, the extent of lymphatic metastases is not considered.

The tumor, node, and metastases (TNM) system, proposed by the International Union Against Cancer, is currently preferred by most investigators because it separates venous involvement from nodal invasion and quantitates each and, thus, more explicitly defines the anatomic extent of disease (Table 76–8) (Beahrs, 1992). Tumors extending into the

capsule are grouped with those extending into the vein in the T3 category but are separated by subclasses (T3a, T3b, T3c). The modification of the TNM system proposed by Hermanek and Schrott (1990) appears to provide the best correlation with 5-year survival (Table 76–9). Table 76–10 compares the TNM and the Robson systems.

Clinical staging of renal carcinoma has been mentioned in the discussion of diagnosis. Regional staging with CT is valuable but sometimes misleading, and the true local and regional extent of the tumor is most accurately determined by the pathologist. Evaluation for the presence of distant metastases is important in light of the recognized incurability of patients with metastatic disease. Renal carcinoma blood-borne metastases may be manifested in any organ system, but the most common sites are the lung, liver, subcutaneous tissue, and central nervous system.

The extent of the preoperative evaluation in the asymptomatic patient must emphasize cost-effectiveness. In a study at the authors' institution, no patient with normal liver function tests and a nonpalpable liver was found to have metasta-

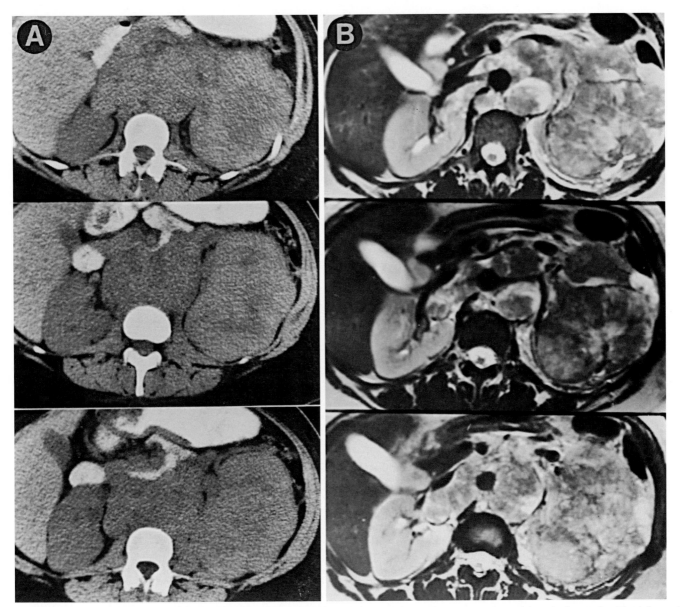

Figure 76–21. *A*, Large, left renal carcinoma as seen on noncontrast CT. There is also massive retroperitoneal lymphadenopathy. The left renal vein and inferior vena cava, and even the aorta, are not identifiable. Intravenous contrast was not administered because of marginal renal failure. Without contrast, it is almost impossible to determine the presence or absence of venous or caval tumor thrombus extension. *B*, On MRI, vessels in the same patient become clearly visible. Massive lymph nodes displace the cava and left renal vein anteriorly. The left renal vein is splayed, but no intraluminal filling defects are present. (From Barbaric Z: Imaging work-up: Is it renal carcinoma and is it operable? Semin Urol Oncol 1996; 14(4):201.)

ses on the radionuclide liver-spleen scan (Lindner et al, 1983). Similarly, no patient without symptoms of skeletal involvement and with normal alkaline phosphatase and serum calcium values had detectable skeletal metastases on radionuclide bone scan. An appropriate preoperative evaluation, therefore, seems to contain a routine chest radiograph, liver function tests, serum calcium measurement, history, and physical examination.

Prognostic Factors

Important prognostic factors in renal cell carcinoma include pathologic stage, tumor size, and nuclear grade. Pathologic stage is the single most important predictor of progno-

sis (Maldazys and deKernion, 1986). Five-year survival rates of 75% for patients in Robson stage 1, 63% for stage 2, 38% for stage 3, and 11% for stage 4 were reported by Guinan and associates and compare favorably with previous studies (Guinan et al, 1995). Tumors greater than 10 cm in size are associated with a poor prognosis, whereas tumors less than 5 cm have a better survival rate than moderate-sized tumors of 5 to 10 cm. Nuclear grade is the most important microscopic feature that independently correlates with survival for all stages of renal cell carcinoma and can also predict survival in patients with stage 1 tumors (Medeiros et al, 1988). The most widely used classification of nuclear grade is the four-tiered system of Fuhrman and colleagues (1982) (Table 76–11). Histologic pattern has not

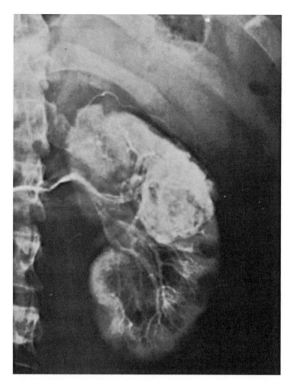

Figure 76–22. Typical arterial phase of selective renal angiogram demonstrating renal carcinoma in solitary kidney as well as multiple small cysts. Typical pattern of puddling of contrast material is noted.

been shown to be an independent prognostic factor, other than renal adenocarcinoma with a sarcomatoid component that carries a poor prognosis.

Nuclear ploidy has also been proposed as a possible prognostic marker. Preliminary DNA flow cytometry data suggest that both prognosis and tumor progression rate may correlate well with nondiploid tumor patterns. Frignon and co-workers observed 37% mortality within 10 years from tumor progression in 19 patients with stage I disease whose tumor was nondiploid versus 8% mortality in 25 patients with diploid

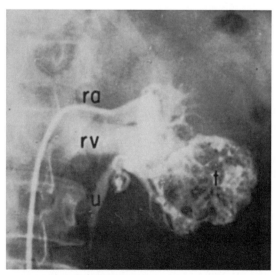

Figure 76–23. Selective renal arteriogram (ra) demonstrating neovascularization of renal tumor (t), early filling of renal vein (rv), and opacification of renal pelvis and ureter (u).

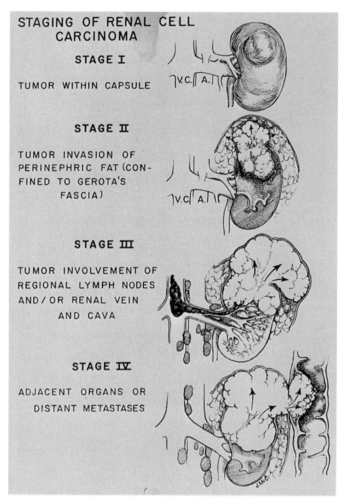

STAGING OF RENAL CELL CARCINOMA

STAGE I
TUMOR WITHIN CAPSULE

STAGE II
TUMOR INVASION OF PERINEPHRIC FAT (CONFINED TO GEROTA'S FASCIA)

STAGE III
TUMOR INVOLVEMENT OF REGIONAL LYMPH NODES AND/OR RENAL VEIN AND CAVA

STAGE IV
ADJACENT ORGANS OR DISTANT METASTASES

Figure 76–24. Staging of nephrocarcinoma as proposed by Holland, in accord with schemes of Robson, Murphy, and Flocks and Kadesky. (From Holland JM: Cancer 1973; 32:1030.)

renal cell carcinomas (Frignon et al, 1989). Studies from the University of California, Los Angeles (UCLA) and from the Mayo Clinic confirm these data, showing a markedly improved survival in patients with metastases whose tumors are diploid compared with those who have aneuploid tumors (deKernion and Huland, 1990).

The factors that have been associated with a poor prognosis in renal cell carcinoma are renal vein involvement, extension to regional lymph nodes, extension through Gerota's fascia, involvement of contiguous organs, and distant metastases (deKernion and Berry, 1980; Maldazys and deKernion, 1986). Although renal vein extension has long been thought to be associated with a poor prognosis (Myers et al, 1968), some studies have failed to show this correlation (Skinner et al, 1972; Selli et al, 1983). This finding may be due to the emphasis on complete excision of the renal veins and on preoperative identification of renal vein extension.

Hoehn and Hermanek (1983) quantitated renal vein extension according to whether the main renal vein was involved or whether only microscopic extension was present. They found a significant increase in local recurrence and metastases in patients with extension into the main renal vein, but no prognostic importance could be attributed to microscopic vein involvement. Golimbu and associates, however, found

Table 76–8. INTERNATIONAL TNM CLASSIFICATION OF RENAL/KIDNEY CARCINOMAS

Definition of TNM

Primary Tumor (T)

TX   Primary tumor cannot be assessed
T0   No evidence of primary tumor
T1   Tumor ≤2.5 cm in greatest dimension limited to the kidney
T2   Tumor >2.5 cm in greatest dimension limited to the kidney
T3   Tumor extends into major veins or invades adrenal gland or perinephric tissues but not beyond Gerota's fascia
    T3a Tumor invades adrenal gland or perinephric tissues but not beyond Gerota's fascia
    T3b Tumor grossly extends into renal vein(s) or vena cava
    T3c Tumor grossly extends into the vena cava above the diaphragm
T4   Tumor invades beyond Gerota's fascia

Regional Lymph Nodes (N)*

NX   Regional lymph nodes cannot be assessed
N0   No regional lymph node metastasis
N1   Metastasis in a single lymph node, ≤2 cm in greatest dimension
N2   Metastasis in a single lymph node, >2 cm but not >5 cm in greatest dimension; or multiple lymph nodes, none >5 cm in greatest dimension
N3   Metastasis in a lymph node >5 cm in greatest dimension

Distant Metastasis (M)

MX   Presence of distant metastasis cannot be assessed
M0   No distant metastasis
M1   Distant metastasis

Stage Grouping

Stage I	T1	N0	M0
Stage II	T2	N0	M0
Stage III	T1	N1	M0
	T2	N1	M0
	T3a	N0, N1	M0
	T3b	N0, N1	M0
Stage IV	T4	Any N	M0
	Any T	N2, N3	M0
	Any T	Any N	M1

*Laterality does not affect the N classification.
From Beahrs OH, ed: American Joint Committee on Cancer: Manual for Staging of Cancer, 4th ed. Philadelphia, J. B. Lippincott, 1992, p 201.

Table 76–10. COMPARISON OF ROBSON AND TNM SYSTEMS FOR STAGING OF RENAL CELL CARCINOMA

	Robson	TNM (1978)
Small tumor, minimal caliceal distortion (confined to renal capsule)	I	T1
Large tumor, caliceal distortion (confined to renal capsule)	I	T2
Tumor extension to perirenal fat or ipsilateral adrenal gland (confined by Gerota's fascia)	II	T3a
Renal vein involvement	IIIa	T3b
Renal vein and vena cava involvement	IIIa	T3c
Vena cava involvement above diaphragm	IIIa	T4b
Single ipsilateral node involved	IIIb	N1
Multiple regional, contralateral, or bilateral nodes involved	IIIb	N2
Fixed regional nodes	IIIb	N3
Juxtaregional nodes involved	IIIb	N4
Combination of IIIa and IIIb	IIIc	T3, 4 N1–4
Spread to contiguous organs except ipsilateral adrenal gland	IVa	T4a
Distant metastases	IVb	M1

vided that the tumor thrombus can be removed completely and no other evidence of locally advanced or metastatic disease is present. Five-year survival rates of 47% to 69% have been reported after complete surgical resection of renal tumors with inferior vena cava involvement in patients with no evidence of metastatic disease. The presence of lymph nodes or perinephric fat involvement in these patients significantly impacts their survival (Skinner et al, 1989; Novick et al, 1990; Thrasher and Paulson, 1993; Swierzewski et al, 1994) (Table 76–12).

Involvement of the regional lymph nodes draining the renal parenchyma is a dire prognostic sign, associated with a 5-year survival rate of 0% to 30% (deKernion, 1980a). The extent of lymphatic dissemination is no doubt important, and those who survive seem to be patients with limited early lymphatic involvement. The implications with respect to the extent of the surgical procedure are discussed later. Invasion through Gerota's fascia and into the perinephric fat decreases the 5-year survival rate to approximately 45% (Skinner et al, 1972; Siminovitch et al, 1983). Tumor extension to contiguous organs is rarely associated with 5-year survival, even after radical surgical excision.

The significance of local tumor persistence or recurrence is reflected in the authors' study of patients with metastatic

no difference in the 5-year survival of patients with either gross or microscopic renal vein invasion (Golimbu et al, 1986).

It appears, therefore, that renal vein invasion alone does not adversely affect survival when associated with an otherwise organ-confined tumor. Similarly, inferior vena cava involvement has only a minimal impact on survival, pro-

Table 76–9. NUMBER (%) OF 5-YEAR SURVIVORS AMONG PATIENTS WITH RENAL CELL CARCINOMA BY ROBSON STAGE OF TUMOR AT NEPHRECTOMY

Author	Total No. of Patients	No. of Patients (%)				Overall Survival No. of Patients (%)
		I	*II*	*III*	*IV*	
Robson et al (1969)	88	32 (66)	14 (64)	24 (42)	9 (11)	79 (52)
Skinner et al (1971)	309	91 (65)	17 (47)	100 (51)	77 (8)	285 (44)
McNichols et al (1981)	506	177 (67)	57 (51)	209 (34)	56 (14)	228 (45)
Selli et al (1983)	115	(93)	(63)	(80)	(13)	(73)
Golimbu et al (1986)	326	52 (88)	39 (67)	73 (40)	88 (2)	252 (41)
Dinney et al (1992)	314	(73)	(68)	(51)	(20)	—
Guinan et al (1995)	2473	1048 (75)	473 (63)	511 (38)	441 (11)	1335 (54)

Modified from Thrasher JB: Urol Clin North Am 1993; 20:247.

Table 76–11. FUHRMAN SYSTEM FOR ASSESSING NUCLEAR GRADE IN RENAL ADENOCARCINOMA

Grade 1	Small (about 10 mm), round, uniform nuclei with inconspicuous or absent nucleoli
Grade 2	Medium-sized (about 15 mm), nuclei with irregularities in outline and small nucleoli (visible under ×400 magnification)
Grade 3	Large (about 20 mm) nuclei with obviously irregular outline and prominent nucleoli
Grade 4	Grade 3 nuclei with the addition of bizarre, often multilobated nuclei possessing heavy chromatin clumps

Modified from Fuhrman SA, et al: Am J Surg Pathol 1982; 6:655–663.

renal carcinoma (deKernion et al, 1978). Those who had incomplete tumor excision because of extension into Gerota's fascia had a much poorer prognosis even than those who developed distant metastases without local tumor recurrence.

Surgical Treatment of Localized Renal Carcinoma

RADICAL NEPHRECTOMY

Surgery remains the only effective method of treatment of primary renal carcinoma, and the objective of the procedure must be to excise all tumor with an adequate surgical margin. Simple nephrectomy was practiced for decades but has been supplanted by radical nephrectomy, which is presumed, although not absolutely proven, to increase the surgical cure rate (Robson, 1963; Patel and Lavengood, 1978).

Although the definition varies, radical nephrectomy generally implies the excision of Gerota's fascia and its contents, including the kidney and the adrenal gland. This approach accomplishes several objectives: (1) The adrenal gland, which is not infrequently involved, is excised; (2) lymphatic metastases, which may diffuse through the perirenal fat, are removed; and (3) a more adequate margin away from the tumor is achieved, especially when the tumor invades the perirenal fat. More adequate renal vein division is also accomplished. Because these appear to be important factors in determining survival, especially invasion of the perinephric fat, cure can be expected to be seriously compromised if microscopic or gross tumor is left in Gerota's fascia. Although the true increase in survival realized by radical nephrectomy versus simple nephrectomy is often debated, radical nephrectomy has become the standard method of surgical therapy.

Regional lymphadenectomy is often added to radical ne-

phrectomy, and increased survival has been attributed to removal of involved lymph nodes (Robson, 1963; Peters, 1980). As noted earlier, regional node extension is an important prognostic factor seldom associated with long-term cure. It is generally impossible to assess the impact of lymph node involvement on survival because other factors usually exist. Survival in patients who have lymph node extension ranges from 5% to 30% at 5 years and 0% to 5% at 10 years, but some investigators have reported improved survival when limited lymph node involvement is successfully resected (Bassil et al, 1985; Golimbu et al, 1986; Thrasher and Paulson, 1993).

Skinner and colleagues found a 17% 10-year survival in those with lymph node involvement (Skinner et al, 1972). The greatest survival—30% of patients alive at 10 years following extensive lymphadenectomy—was reported by Robson (1963). Hulten and co-workers, however, found no survivors when involved regional lymph nodes were excised (Hulten et al, 1969). Pizzocaro and Piva (1990) reported an improved disease-free survival in patients undergoing extensive regional lymphadenectomy. Approximately 20% of patients with positive nodes survived 5 years. Patients were not randomized, however, and the extent and location of the lymph node metastases were not clearly defined. Current data, however, do suggest that some patients can benefit from regional lymphadenectomy, especially the subset of patients with micrometastatic lymph node involvement (Giuliani et al, 1990).

Several characteristics of renal carcinoma argue against a therapeutic role for lymphadenectomy. First, the tumor metastasizes through the blood stream and the lymphatic system with equal frequency, and most patients with positive lymph nodes eventually have blood-borne metastases. Second, the lymphatic drainage of renal carcinoma is variable and may occur anywhere in the retroperitoneum. Third, many patients without metastases to regional lymph nodes develop disseminated metastases (deKernion, 1980a). As pointed out by Marshall and Powell (1982) and confirmed by the authors' own experience, however, most tumors initially metastasize to lymph nodes in the renal hilum or in the paracaval or para-aortic area immediately adjacent to the hilum. Although an occasional patient has distant retroperitoneal lymph nodes as the first site of metastases, one can encompass the most probable first and second drainage areas by performing a limited lymph node dissection—paracaval and interaortacaval for right-sided tumors and para-aortic and interaortacaval for left-sided tumors.

Golimbu and associates were able to show a 10% to 15% increase in the 5-year survival with lymphadenectomy for microscopic disease in patients with stage II cancers and in

Table 76–12. SURVIVAL IN LOCALIZED VERSUS METASTATIC RENAL CELL CARCINOMA WITH IVC INVASION AND COMPLETE RESECTION

Senior Author	N	No Metastases (5 years)	Metastases (5 years)	Median Survival
Skinner et al (1989)	56	47%	0%	4M
Angermeier et al (1990)	43	64%*	11%*	10M*
Thrasher et al (1993)	44	69%	0%	9M
Swierzewski et al (1994)	100	64%	20%	30M

*3 years.

those with renal vein involvement (Golimbu et al, 1986). They evaluated 52 patients who underwent a lymphadenectomy in whom no lymphatic disease was identified and compared their survival with that of 141 patients who had palpably normal retroperitoneal lymph nodes and underwent a radical nephrectomy alone. Lymphadenectomy did not improve survival in patients with stage I disease. Although the practical therapeutic value of lymphadenectomy is still uncertain because of the factors mentioned, it can be accomplished simply and provides valuable staging information.

The surgical technique of radical nephrectomy has been described by a number of investigators (Stewart, 1975; deKernion, 1980b). The surgical approach is guided more by individual preference than by necessity. The transperitoneal approach through a subcostal incision allows early ligation of the renal artery and vein before tumor manipulation. This is an essential technical consideration in the management of renal carcinoma (i.e., early ligation of the artery and vein), and, to be acceptable, any approach must incorporate it. Other transabdominal incisions have also been employed with a similar intent of early ligation of the vessels. For small lower pole tumors, removal of the ipsilateral adrenal gland is probably not routinely necessary, given the actual rarity of adrenal metastases (Robey and Schellhammer, 1986).

The thoracoabdominal incision described by Chute and colleagues is commonly practiced and is especially suitable for large tumors in the upper pole of the kidney (Chute et al, 1949). This technique may include an extraperitoneal or intraperitoneal incision. In many cases, a flank incision through the 11th intercostal space or a supracostal incision allows excellent exposure without entering the pleural cavity and can be performed extraperitoneally. The authors have employed this approach for many small tumors and tumors in the lower pole and have found it to be associated with minimal postoperative morbidity, provided that the costovertebral ligaments of the 11th rib are divided adequately, allowing the rib to be deflected downward (deKernion, 1980b). The urologic surgeon should be skilled in a number of approaches, tailoring the incision to the body habitus of the patient and the size and position of the renal tumor.

Since the advent of sophisticated angiographic methods, preoperative occlusion of the renal artery has been advocated as an adjunct to the surgical procedure. Hemorrhage is reduced, especially in patients with large tumors supplied by many parasitized vessels. The renal vein can be ligated before dissection of the renal artery, and a host immune stimulation has been attributed to renal infarction (Hirsh et al, 1979). A salutary effect on survival has not been demonstrated, however, and the procedure can be associated with complications that may compromise the ability of the patient to tolerate surgery, including pain, ileus, sepsis, and dislocation of the infarcting coil. Early ligation of the renal artery and vein can be safely performed in almost all patients without preoperative infarction, and little evidence suggests that the latter is an appropriate preoperative measure. It may be a reasonable adjunct, however, in patients with large vascular tumors, especially in patients with large caval thrombi.

The long-term outcome following surgical therapy for renal carcinoma depends on many factors, including the tumor stage, grade, and histologic type and the surgical procedure. Data, therefore, are difficult to compare, and the use of various staging systems compounds the problem. Some general statements, however, can be made with respect to the efficacy of radical nephrectomy.

After radical nephrectomy for stage I renal carcinoma, 5-year survival ranges from 60% to 82%, compared with 5-year survival for stage II of 47% to 80% (Robson et al, 1968; Skinner et al, 1972; McNichols et al, 1981; Guinan et al, 1995). In the series reported by Robson (1963), in which all patients underwent radical nephrectomy and extensive lymphadenectomy after careful preoperative selection, the survival of patients with stage II tumors (extension through the capsule) was identical to that for those with stage I disease, presumably because of a more thorough excision of the tumor and a decreased local tumor recurrence. Individuals with stage III tumors have an expected survival of between 35% and 51%, depending on the number of patients included in the category because of renal vein involvement without lymph node extension or extracapsular extension. As mentioned, patients with extension to the contiguous organs have a poor prognostic outlook, and those with distant metastases have virtually no chance of surviving 2 years (Best, 1987).

Radiation therapy has been employed as a preoperative or postoperative surgical adjunct. Several reports showed an increased survival with preoperative radiotherapy (Richie, 1966; Cox et al, 1970). A randomized study conducted by van der Werf-Messing (1973) compared the results of 3000 rad of preoperative therapy with those of no therapy. Five-year survival was not improved, although the onset of local recurrence was postponed. Thus far, no study has demonstrated effectiveness of preoperative radiotherapy for renal carcinoma.

The purpose of postoperative radiotherapy is to sterilize any existing microscopic or gross tumor. A number of studies have used varying doses of radiotherapy to the renal fossa after nephrectomy but have not shown a significantly improved survival (Peeling et al, 1969). Indeed, survival after postoperative radiotherapy was diminished in the study by Finney (1973). For similar reasons, radiotherapy for regional lymph node extension was not proved to be of significant value. Although occasionally a large tumor may be reduced in size by preoperative radiotherapy, no evidence currently exists to support the routine use of radiotherapy in renal carcinoma other than for palliative treatment of skeletal metastases.

RENAL-SPARING SURGERY

Renal cell carcinoma may occur in the patient who has a solitary kidney, the other kidney either being congenitally absent or having been removed for benign disease. Bilateral neoplasms may also occur, either synchronously or asynchronously (Fig. 76–25). A clearer understanding of the renal vasculature and more sophisticated surgical approaches now usually make it possible to excise the tumor, leaving the patient with sufficient parenchyma to maintain life without dialysis. The standard partial nephrectomy in vivo, combined with regional hypothermia, is the most common approach. Autotransplantation following ex vivo excision is now commonplace in many large medical centers. The enthusiasm for this approach has diminished considerably, however, and

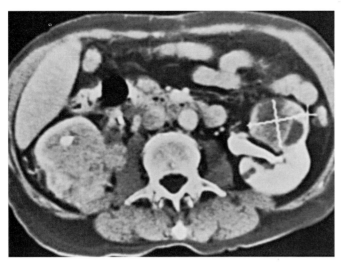

Figure 76–25. Bilateral renal cell carcinoma in a 61-year-old man with microhematuria. The patient underwent partial left nephrectomy and, subsequently, right radical nephrectomy.

most tumors are now excised from the solitary kidney without the need for the "workbench" approach (Morgan and Zincke, 1990).

Excision of tumor in the solitary kidney is associated with excellent long-term cancer-free survival (Licht and Novick, 1993). Initial studies suggested that survival was significantly better in patients with tumor in the solitary kidney than in those with synchronous or asynchronous tumor in the opposite kidney (approximately 70% versus 50%) (Wickham, 1975). A report by Topley and co-workers, however, suggested that 5-year survival was poor only in those with asynchronous bilateral tumors (38%) compared with unilateral tumors in a solitary kidney (71%) and bilateral synchronous tumors (71%) (Topley et al, 1983). This conclusion was supported by the cumulative experience from this institution (Smith et al, 1984). Twenty patients with tumor in the solitary kidney and 18 patients with bilateral renal carcinoma were treated by partial nephrectomy in vivo (21) or by ex vivo incision and autotransplantation (17). Radical nephrectomy with dialysis was the treatment in three patients. A number of conclusions were possible from this study. First, complete removal of the tumor, whether tumor in the solitary kidney or bilateral renal tumors, was associated with a 72% tumor-free survival at 3 years. Second, the survival was independent of whether the patient had tumor in the opposite kidney. Third, overall crude survival for patients with bilateral renal tumors that were completely excised was 57%. Fourth, survival was dependent on the stage of the local tumor. Of patients with stage I tumors, 80% have survived 3 years versus 50% with stage II tumors. Fifth, ex vivo surgery is seldom necessary, and most patients can be adequately managed with regional hypothermia. Sixth, although bilateral nephrectomy with dialysis is seldom necessary, it should be an option offered to selected patients in this modern era of hemodialysis and transplantation.

Conservative surgery with enucleation or partial nephrectomy as a treatment for renal cell carcinoma remains controversial despite good results in terms of local control and disease-free survival (Marshall et al, 1986; Novick et al, 1986; Novick, 1993, 1995). Novick (1995) reported on 216 patients with a follow-up of at least 4 years. The cancer-specific 5-year survival rate was 95% for patients with unilateral tumors, 85% for bilateral synchronous tumors, and 75% for bilateral asynchronous tumors. Cause-specific survival was 95% for patients with stage I tumors versus 79% for patients with stage III tumors. Only 9 (4%) of the 216 patients followed developed local recurrence in the renal remnant without other sites of recurrence. The Mayo Clinic series (Morgan and Zincke, 1990) encompassed 104 patients with overall and cancer-specific 5-year survival rates of 80% and 88%, respectively.

These two large single-center experiences confirmed that most tumors can be successfully excised in situ and that excellent short-term results can be achieved by conservative surgery. The major disadvantage of renal-sparing surgery for renal cell carcinoma is the risk of local tumor recurrence, ranging from 6% to 10%. Some of these local tumor recurrences may, in fact, represent undetected multifocal renal tumors (Campbell et al, 1994). Intraoperative sonography, using a 7.5-MHz transducer with Doppler probe, is a valuable new adjunct in the evaluation and management of these patients and should help to determine the extent of tumor, multicentricity, and associated cysts (Marshall et al, 1992).

Inferior Vena Cava Extension

Propensity for renal carcinoma to invade the renal veins and extend into the main renal vein as a tumor thrombus is well recognized. Continued growth of the thrombus into the vena cava occurs in a small number of cases, usually without direct invasion of the vessel. The importance of delineating the extent of venous involvement is therefore obvious, and inferior venacavogram, CT, or MRI (Fig. 76–26) is essential in preoperative evaluation of renal tumors. Vena cava extension was considered to be a dire prognostic sign in the past, associated with little prospect for surgical cure. Since the recognition of the importance of caval extension and aggressive surgical treatment, however, it is realized that most patients can still be cured surgically (Novick, 1995).

The anatomic and surgical considerations in the patient with vena caval extension have been reviewed by the Lahey Clinic group (Swierzewski et al, 1994). In this excellent report of 100 patients, the 5-year survival following surgical removal of vena cava extension was 64%, and the 10-year survival was 57%. This study and others attest to the wisdom of surgical removal of the vena cava thrombus, even when the tumor extends into the right atrium. The surgical approaches to accomplish vena caval thrombus excision have been thoroughly described (Cummings, 1982; Marshall et al, 1984; Skinner et al, 1989). A limited infracaval extension, once recognized, is managed without difficulty (deKernion and Smith, 1984). Supradiaphragmatic and right atrial extension require an extended operation, however, often with cardiopulmonary bypass. Novick and colleagues reported the Cleveland Clinic experience with cardiopulmonary bypass and deep hypothermic circulatory arrest in 43 patients with large inferior vena cava tumor thrombi (Novick et al, 1990). The 3-year survival rate was 64% with an operative mortality rate of 4.7%. Marshall and associates advocated hypothermia and exsanguination for patients with intracaval extension of thrombi (Marshall et al, 1988). Nine patients were treated, and one postoperative death was reported. Many patients

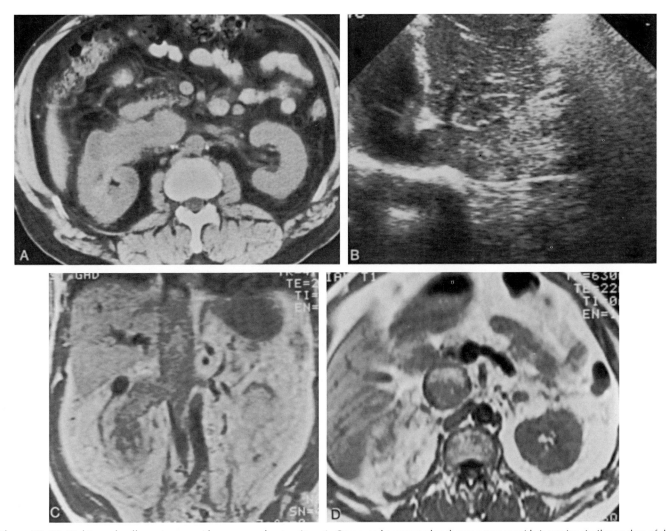

Figure 76–26. Right renal cell carcinoma with vena caval extension. *A,* Computed tomography shows a tumor with intensity similar to that of the normal right kidney. Tumor extends into the enlarged right renal vein and inferior vena cava (IVC). *B,* Longitudinal sonogram displays echogenic tumor in the lumen of the enlarged IVC. *C,* Coronal spin-echo image demonstrated intracaval tumor. The tumor extends proximally as far as the diaphragm but does not enter the thoracic segment of the IVC. *D,* Axial magnetic resonance image. Tumor thrombus is in the IVC.

had local extension, however, and most developed metastatic disease. Foster and colleagues proposed a more simple caval-atrial shunt for extensive thrombi (Foster et al, 1988), but little experience has thus far been reported with this technique.

The current experience indicates that excision of renal carcinoma with caval extension remains the treatment of choice and can be safely performed, even with extension into the right atrium. As reported previously (Cherrie et al, 1982) and confirmed by later studies, however, patients with regional and distant metastases seldom are helped by the radical extension. Long-term survival of a patient who has supradiaphragmatic extension is still uncertain, although some reports suggest that the actual level of propagation of the thrombus has no adverse effect on survival. Application of modern cardiac surgical techniques to minimize intraoperative hemorrhage and to facilitate tumor removal has further improved expected survival after surgery.

Occasionally the tumor may invade the wall of the vena cava. Aggressive resection of the vena cava in these patients appears to provide a survival benefit (Hatcher et al, 1991).

Every attempt should therefore be made to establish negative surgical margins of the involved vena cava with histologic verification by intraoperative frozen sections.

Locally Invasive Renal Carcinoma

The propensity for renal carcinoma to grow to large size locally and to disseminate before diagnosis results in presentation of many patients with large primary tumors that invade adjacent structures. Such patients usually present with pain, generally from invasion of the posterior abdominal wall, nerve roots, or paraspinous muscles. Liver extension is uncommon, and intrahepatic metastases occur more often than local extension. The capsules of large tumors may indent and compress adjacent liver parenchyma but seldom actually grow by direct extension into the liver. Duodenal and pancreatic invasion is an extremely poor prognostic sign, and the authors are not aware of any such patients being surgically cured. The propensity for the tumors to parasitize vessels accounts for the frequent extension into the large bowel, mesentery, and colon.

Because surgical therapy is the only effective management for this type of tumor, extended operations are sometimes indicated. Complete excision of the tumor, including excision of the involved bowel, spleen, or abdominal wall muscles, is essential. En bloc partial hepatectomy is rarely curative but may occasionally be worthwhile.

Partial excision of the large primary tumor, or *debulking*, is seldom, if ever, indicated. Only 12% of patients who underwent incomplete excision of locally extensive tumor were alive at 12 months in a report from this institution (deKernion et al, 1978). Most reports suggest that less than 5% of patients with extension into adjacent viscera survive 5 years after surgery. Ongoing clinical trials with adjuvant immunotherapy regimens might redefine, in the future, the role of debulking surgery in patients with locally advanced disease.

The role of radiation therapy in the treatment of locally extensive carcinoma has been debated. Standard preoperative adjunctive radiotherapy has been shown in several early series to improve survival (Richie, 1966; Cox et al, 1970). A subsequent study by van der Werf-Messing (1973), however, compared results for preoperative therapy of 3000 rad with results for no preoperative therapy. Survival was not influenced at 5 years, although the radiotherapy seemed to delay the time to local renal fossa recurrence. Routine postoperative radiotherapy has not been shown to influence overall survival. When tumor is known to have been left behind in the renal fossa or adjacent structures, postoperative radiotherapy may occasionally retard regrowth of tumor mass. This approach, however, is rarely used today and has largely been replaced by the use of immunotherapy (Belldegrun et al, 1990).

Treatment of Metastatic Renal Carcinoma

CHEMOTHERAPY

The traditional modern management of advanced solid tumors has been with cytotoxic agents. Despite the remarkable advances realized with other tumors, renal cell carcinoma has remained refractory to these agents. A number of drugs have been used as single agents (deKernion and Lindner, 1982). These drugs have been used in various dosage schedules, and responses have been measured by disparate criteria. The lack of therapeutic efficacy, however, is apparent.

Because single agents have generally not been proven to be effective, and because combination therapy depends on the combined efficacy of the agents, responses to combination chemotherapy have been expectedly low. Yagoda and associates reviewed the results of 83 trials involving 4093 patients and found a total response rate of 6%, mostly of short duration (Yagoda et al; 1995). This "background noise" of response clearly documents that renal cell carcinoma is a chemotherapeutically resistant tumor.

The combination of 5-fluorouracil with interleukin-2 (IL-2) and interferon alpha has been described, suggesting an impressive response rate of 46% with 15% complete responses and only moderate toxicity among treated patients (Atzpodien et al, 1993; Sella et al, 1994). If confirmed by larger studies, this combination might offer a promising new role for chemoimmunotherapeutic agents in the treatment of renal cell carcinoma. At this time, new drugs need to be evaluated in carefully constructed prospective clinical trials with the hope of identifying more effective treatment regimens.

HORMONAL THERAPY

The basis for hormone treatment of advanced renal carcinoma was the demonstration of its efficacy against an estrogen-induced clear cell tumor in the adult Syrian hamster (Kirkman and Bacon, 1949). A review of the clinical literature by Bloom (1973) showed an objective response of approximately 15% in patients with metastatic renal carcinoma. This response, however, represented a summary of phase II trials with various methods of patient selection and criteria of response. In a review of 110 patients at the author's institution, no patient had a response to progestational agents (deKernion et al, 1978). Thus, there is little evidence today to support the use of hormonal agents, such as androgens, progestins, and antiestrogens, in this disease. Other hormones, including tamoxifen, are similarly ineffective (Schomburg et al, 1993).

IMMUNOTHERAPY

The theory supporting immunotherapy for metastatic renal carcinoma is that host immune functions play a role in tumor control, and these immune functions can be further stimulated. Immunotherapy can be classifed into active and passive categories. Active immunotherapy refers to the immunization of the tumor-bearing host with materials that attempt to induce in the host a state of immune responsiveness to the tumor. Passive (adoptive) immunotherapy involves the transfer to the tumor-bearing host of active immunologic reagents, such as cells with antitumor reactivity, that can mediate, either directly or indirectly, antitumor effects (Fig. 76–27). The unusual natural history of renal carcinoma, including spontaneous regression, delayed growth of metastatic lesions, and varying tumor doubling times, suggests that host immune factors may be important in the immune surveillance of this tumor.

Most attempts at immunotherapy in the last several decades have involved active immunotherapy using nonspecific immune stimulators, such as bacillus Calmette-Guérin (BCG), *Corynebacterium parvum*, and levamisole, with the hope that a nonspecific increase in human reactivity would concomitantly result in an augmentation of the putative antitumor immunologic response of the tumor-bearing host. Several reports of small numbers of patients treated with BCG (Minton et al, 1976; Montie et al, 1982; Morales et al, 1982), *C. parvum* (McCune et al, 1981), or transfer factor (Bukowski et al, 1979) have noted some benefit. Subsequent randomized trials confirming such benefit have yet to be published.

Xenogeneic immune RNA (probably a stimulator of interferon production) showed initial promise in uncontrolled studies at UCLA (Ramming and deKernion, 1977). Subsequent studies, however, revealed no significant improvement in survival time over controls, and by 4 years, all patients had died of metastatic disease (deKernion and Ramming, 1980). Although Steele and colleagues and Richie and col-

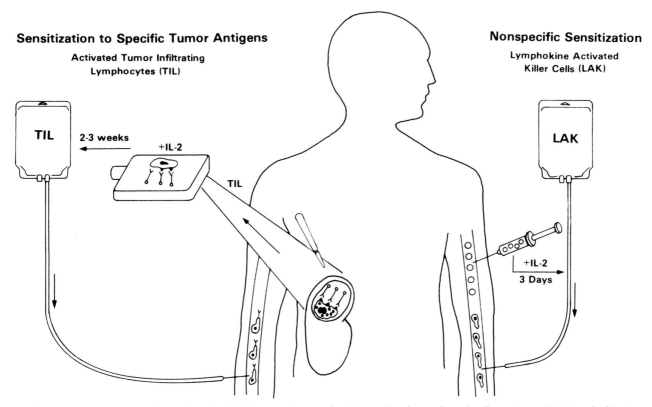

Figure 76–27. Two approaches to the adoptive immunotherapy of patients with advanced renal cell carcinoma. IL-2, interleukin-2.

leagues have reported some responses in patients infused with in vitro, RNA-treated, autologous lymphocytes, the efficacy of RNA administered by any route remains questionable (Richie et al, 1981; Steele et al, 1981).

Coumarin (1,2-benzopyrone) and cimetidine have also been shown to mediate antitumor activity in patients with metastatic renal cell carcinoma (Marshall et al, 1987). A 33% response without any toxicity was achieved in 45 patients treated in a pilot study. Subsequent phase II studies (50 patients) using the same drug and schedule, however, were associated with only a 6% response (Dexeus et al, 1990).

In the past decade, development of recombinant DNA techniques has enabled the production of large quantities of purified lymphokines (cytokines), which are biologic substances involved in the regulation of the immune system. The first of these lymphokines to receive clinical use was *interferon*. The interferons are a family of secreted proteins that were originally characterized by their ability to induce an antiviral state. It has been established that the same proteins that have antiviral activities also have potent antiproliferative and immunomodulatory activities.

The interferons have been divided into antigenically distinct types and classified according to their primary cell of origin or the stimulus for induction. Type I interferons are induced by virus infection in many cell types and include interferon alpha, produced by leukocytes, and interferon beta, produced by fibroblasts. Type II interferon (interferon gamma) is induced by antigen or mitogen in T lymphocytes. In humans, there are more than 30 interferon alpha subspecies, the most important of which is interferon alpha-2.

Recombinant molecular technology has led to the insertion

of human DNA sequence coding for interferon alpha-2 into *Escherichia coli*. The *E. coli* then express large quantities of the molecule, which is purified by chromatography (interferon alpha-2a (Roferon-A), Hoffman LaRoche; interferon alpha-2b (Intron-A), Schering-Plough). A human lymphoblastoid cell line can also be stimulated in vitro to produce a combination of interferon alpha subtypes, which are then purified (Wellferon, Wellcome). Recombinant interferons, in contrast to the natural interferons, are not glycosylated. This does not affect their activity, but it may make them more antigenic.

The interferons have shown some efficacy against a number of human malignancies, including hairy cell leukemia, chronic myelogenous leukemia, T cell lymphoma, and malignant melanoma (Gutterman, 1988). Several studies have been conducted in patients with renal cell carcinoma. In independent studies, deKernion and Lindner (1982) and Quesada and co-workers (1983) reported on the regression of metastatic renal cell carcinoma with a partially purified human interferon alpha preparation. Objective responses, complete and partial, occurred in 16.5% and 26% of patients treated, respectively. Following this initial report, numerous phase II trials with interferon alpha were conducted with a reproducible objective response rate of 15% to 20% and a complete response rate of 1% (Kirkwood et al, 1985; Figlin et al, 1988; Muss et al, 1987; Umeda and Niijima, 1986; Vugrin et al, 1986). Responses appear independent of the interferon alpha preparation used and correlate with those patients who have undergone previous nephrectomy and with those who have had good performance status, a long disease-free interval, and lung-predominant disease.

The survival rate of 84 evaluable patients treated at UCLA

was 49 weeks. Patients with the favorable prognostic variables scored best with slightly higher response rates and a median survival of 155 weeks (Sarna et al, 1987). Combination of interferon with vinblastine resulted in an overall efficacy similar to that achieved by interferon alone, and vinblastine, with its added toxicity, seemed to be unrelated to clinical gain (Figlin et al, 1985). Although interferons have unquestionable activity against renal cell carcinoma, complete responses are rare, and overall survival is not significantly affected. Furthermore, most patients who respond are those with limited metastases, especially those limited to pulmonary metastases. This low level of clinical response indicates the need for further trials with combination interferons and with interferons combined with other agents.

The combination of interferon alpha and interferon gamma demonstrates synergistic activity in vitro and in a murine renal cancer (Renca) model in vivo (Sayers et al, 1990). Because some activity of interferon gamma against human renal cell carcinoma has been documented (Aulitzky et al, 1989), this combination deserves further studies.

The discovery in 1976 by Morgan and colleagues of the T cell growth factor (TCGF) IL-2 revolutionized the field of cancer immunotherapy and altered substantially the prospects for the treatment of renal cell carcinoma. IL-2 is a 15,000-dalton glycoprotein produced in minute quantities by helper T lymphocytes on antigen or antigen-induced activation of resting T cells. In vivo, IL-2 has been shown to generate lymphokine-activated killer (LAK) cells (Belldegrun et al, 1988b), enhance natural killer (NK) cell function, augment alloantigen responsiveness, stimulate growth of T cells with antitumor reactivity, and mediate regression of cancer in experimental animals and in selected patients with advanced cancer (Rosenberg, 1986, 1988a).

In 1985, Rosenberg and co-workers reported the initial NCI results of adoptive cellular therapy with LAK cells plus IL-2 in 25 patients with advanced cancer. In subsequent studies (Rosenberg et al, 1985; Rosenberg, 1988b), 7 of 54 patients with renal cell carcinoma treated experienced complete response and 10 patients had a partial response, for a total of 33% response. Of 38 patients with renal cell carcinoma treated with high-dose bolus IL-2 alone, four complete responses and three partial responses were achieved, for a total of 18.4% response. Responses occurred at a number of different sites, including lung, liver, soft tissue, subcutaneous tissue, and bone. Rosenberg and co-workers updated their overall experience with high-dose bolus IL-2 in 149 patients with metastatic renal cancer (Rosenberg et al, 1994). Ten patients (7%) demonstrated complete regression, and 20 patients (13%) had partial regression. Of the ten patients with complete regression, seven have remained in complete remission from 7 to 76 months after treatment.

Fisher and associates, performing a phase II NCI-sponsored extramural study of the same regimen, reported a 16% objective response in 35 patients with metastatic or unresectable renal cell carcinoma (Fisher et al, 1988). Two patients had complete regression of all tumor, and three additional patients had partial responses with greater than 50% reduction in the total tumor burden. In other studies, the objective responses obtained with IL-2–based immunotherapy were significantly lower than those reported by the

NCI (Parkinson, 1990; Robertson et al, 1990; Parkinson and Sznol, 1995). Nonetheless, there can be no doubt that in some patients with renal cell carcinoma, IL-2 treatment can produce remarkable changes in the natural history of the disease. Because some of these patients have now been clinically disease-free for periods approaching 7 years, it is possible that they have been cured by this therapy. This group, however, represents the minority of patients treated. Only 5% of patients treated with IL-2 respond completely, and an additional 10% to 15% respond partially. Based on careful review of the data presented in these clinical trials, the Food and Drug Administration has approved high-dose IL-2 (aldesleukin (Proleukin), Chiron Therapeutics Inc., Emeryville, CA) for the therapy of good performance status patients with metastatic renal cell carcinoma.

Side effects of IL-2 therapy have been well documented and include fever, chills, malaise, nausea, vomiting, diarrhea, and other constitutional symptoms. The most common serious side effects, however, are primarily renal and cardiopulmonary (Rosenberg et al, 1985). IL-2 therapy induces a prerenal azotemia with hypotension, fluid retention, respiratory distress syndrome, oliguria, and low fractional sodium excretion (Fig. 76–28). Importantly, cessation of IL-2 administration results in a rapid recovery and reversal of almost all side effects. Renal function values return to baseline levels within 7 days in 62% of patients and within 30 days in 95% of patients (Belldegrun et al, 1987, 1989; Taneja et al, 1995). Treatment-related mortality is low at less than 2%.

In an attempt to improve response rates while escaping the toxicity of high-dose treatment, clinical trials are in progress testing the benefit of low-dose IL-2 and an outpatient combination of IL-2 and interferon in this disease (Figlin et al, 1993; Walther et al, 1993; Stadler and Vogelzang, 1995). In experimental murine models, IL-2 and interferon alpha combination resulted in better antitumor effects

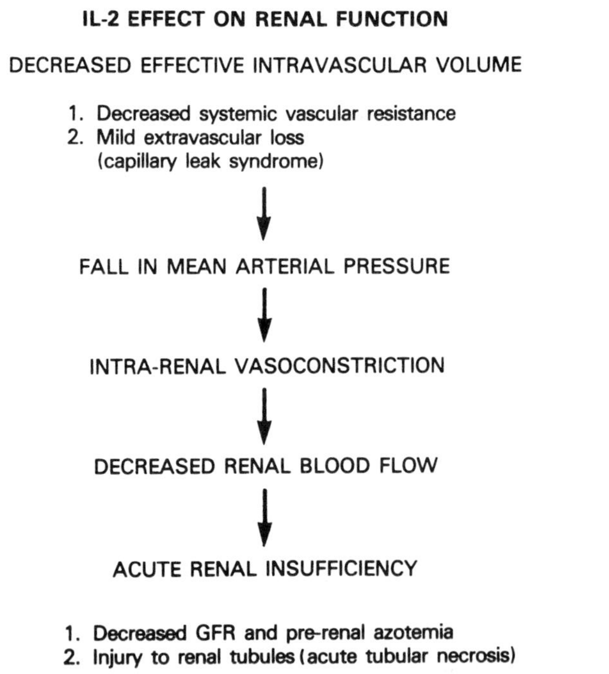

IL-2 EFFECT ON RENAL FUNCTION

DECREASED EFFECTIVE INTRAVASCULAR VOLUME

1. Decreased systemic vascular resistance
2. Mild extravascular loss
   (capillary leak syndrome)

↓

FALL IN MEAN ARTERIAL PRESSURE

↓

INTRA-RENAL VASOCONSTRICTION

↓

DECREASED RENAL BLOOD FLOW

↓

ACUTE RENAL INSUFFICIENCY

1. Decreased GFR and pre-renal azotemia
2. Injury to renal tubules (acute tubular necrosis)

Figure 76–28. Effects of interleukin-2 (IL-2) on renal function. GFR, glomerular filtration rate.

than the administration of either agent alone (Brunda et al, 1987; Cameron et al, 1988).

In the authors' institution, 52 patients with measurable renal cell carcinoma were treated in an outpatient setting with rIL-2 (2 million units m²), by continuous infusion on days 1 through 4, and interferon alpha-2a (Roferon-A) (6 million units m²), by intramuscular or subcutaneous administration on days 1 and 4 of each week (Figlin et al, 1995). Each 4-week treatment period (one course) was followed by a 2-week rest. Four complete (8%) responses and nine (17%) partial responses were observed for a total objective response rate of 25% (Table 27–13). The median duration of response was 17 months among all responders, with duration ranging from 5 to more than 46 months. Little toxicity has been observed, with no deaths and only occasional inpatient hospitalizations. In a similar regimen, Atzpodien and co-workers observed partial tumor regression in 29% of 34 treated patients receiving long-term subcutaneous administration of IL-2 and interferon alpha (Atzpodien et al, 1991).

The most promising new application of IL-2 is with tumor-infiltrating lymphocytes (TILs) (see Fig. 76–27) (Belldegrun and Rosenberg, 1989). TILs are grown selectively from single-cell tumor suspensions cultured in IL-2. After a short period of culture, renal cell carcinoma cells die, and the culture is overgrown by T lymphocytes. This cell population may be expanded in long-term cultures with IL-2 so that about 2 to 3 × 10¹¹ lymphocytes may be reinfused into the patients (Belldegrun et al, 1988a, 1989, 1995).

Whereas LAK cells are mainly activated NK cells, TILs are activated cytotoxic T cells, which show greater specificity in their targets and recirculate and home to tumor masses in a way that LAK cells do not. In experimental systems, TILs are 50 to 100 times as powerful as LAK cells. In addition, TILs, when administered in combination with cyclophosphamide and IL-2, are capable of eradicating advanced bulky tumors against which LAK cells are not effective (Rosenberg et al, 1986).

In a pilot study using TIL, IL-2, and cyclophosphamide to treat 12 patients with metastatic disease, two partial responses to therapy were observed. Pulmonary and mediastinal masses regressed in a patient with melanoma, and a lymph node mass regressed in a patient with renal cell carcinoma (Topalian et al, 1988). In a subsequent study involving 20 patients with metastatic melanoma, Rosenberg (1988c) observed objective responses in 11 patients (55%), including one complete remission. Two of the patients who responded had previously shown no response to LAK cell therapy.

Table 76–13. COMBINATION LOW-DOSE INTERLEUKIN-2 AND INTERFERON THERAPY AT UCLA (n = 52)

Median age (range)	58 (29–79)
Male/female	38/14
Prior nephrectomy	39 (75%)
Pulmonary metastases only	18 (35%)
CR	4 (8%)
CR duration of response (months)	40 + median (24–58 +)
CR survival (months)	50 + median (38 + 62 +)
PR	9 (17%)
PR duration of response (months)	13 median (5–35)
PR survival (months)	31 median (18–56 +)

CR, Complete response; PR, partial response.

Current efforts are in progress to enhance the therapeutic efficacy of TILs. Belldegrun and co-workers reported the UCLA experience with the combination of TILs primed in vivo with interferon, continuous infusion of IL-2, and subcutaneous interferon alpha in patients with advanced renal cell carcinoma (Belldegrun et al, 1993). Three patients (30%) achieved complete responses and continue to be in remission for 60 +, 59 +, and 41 + months. In an attempt to overcome the problem of the heterogeneity of harvested TILs, a collection device has been developed (CELLector, Applied Immune Sciences, Menlo Park, CA) that can separate CD8 + cytolytic T cell population from harvested TILs with a 94% purity. Of the first 48 patients treated by TIL protocol at UCLA, 33 patients received bulk TILs, and 15 were treated with purified CD8 + TILs (Pierce et al, 1995). An overall objective response rate of 33%, including 17% complete responses, has been observed. The duration of response among complete responders ranges up to 43 months with a mean duration of 24 months. A multicenter phase II–III, randomized study is currently in progress to evaluate the safety and efficacy of radical nephrectomy, CD8 + TIL, and IL-2 versus radical nephrectomy and IL-2 in patients with metastatic renal cancer. Given this small and preliminary body of clinical and experimental data, further studies will focus on various forms of combination immunotherapy, which may evolve to be one of the most promising areas of cancer treatment (Fig. 76–29).

Advances in genetic engineering have allowed for the introduction of genes with sustained expression into tumor cells or lymphoid cells (Fig. 76–30). Successful introduction of gene coding for neomycin resistance or for other cytokine genes into human TILs raises the possibility of introducing other programmed genetic materials into TILs that would augment their antitumor properties and be delivered directly to the tumor site. Another strategy in gene therapy of cancer is the construction of tumor vaccines. This approach involves the transfection of tumor cells with genes that render immunogenicity to the tumor (Jaffee and Pardoll, 1995). The rationale for inserting cytokine genes, such as IL-2, interferon, or granulocyte-macrophage colony–stimulating factor, into tumor cells is that sustained local release of high doses of cytokine at the tumor site is critical to the generation of a systemic immune response (Belldegrun et al, 1993). The production of high concentrations of cytokine at tumor sites may directly alter tumor properties associated with invasive and metastatic phenotypes (Hathorn et al, 1994). Phase I clinical trials using genetically modified tumor vaccines are currently ongoing at several institutions around the United States. Although promising, the field of gene therapy for the treatment of human cancer is still in its infancy.

PALLIATIVE OR ADJUNCTIVE NEPHRECTOMY

Approximately 30% of patients have metastases at the time the diagnosis of renal carcinoma is first made, and early reports suggested that removal of the primary lesion induces regression of the metastases. This approach has been widely embraced by urologists and performed for the purpose of both control of symptoms and regression of metastatic sites.

The term *palliative nephrectomy* is best reserved for an operation performed for the control of severe symptoms. This procedure seems to be most effective in patients with

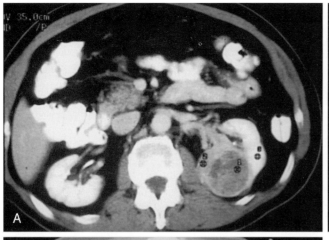

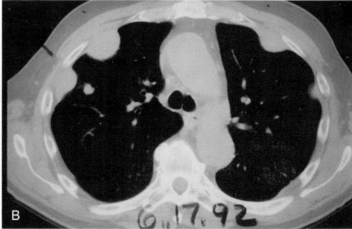

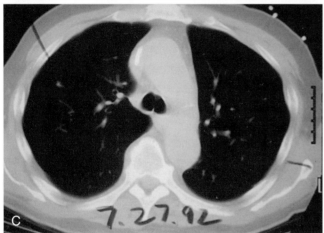

Figure 76–29. Abdominal (A) and pulmonary (B) CT scans demonstrating a left renal tumor and bilateral pulmonary and pleural-based metastasis. This patient underwent left radical nephrectomy and then received a combination of interleukin-2, interferon-alpha, and TIL therapy. Follow-up CT scan of the chest, 6 weeks after initiation of therapy, revealed complete disappearance of all tumors (C). This patient remains in complete clinical remission for over 5 years.

GENE THERAPY OF RENAL CANCER

GENETICALLY ENGINEERED
TUMOR INFILTRATING LYMPHOCYTES (TIL)

TUMOR CELL VACCINE

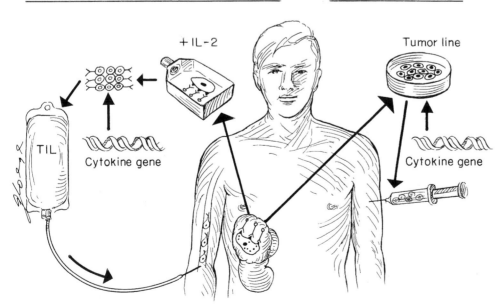

Figure 76–30. Schematic diagram of tumor-infiltrating lymphocytes (TIL) and vaccine production. *Left side,* TIL production. *Right side,* Tumor cell vaccine where tumor cells are transfected with cytokine genes. These cells, now secreting cytokines, are injected or implanted back into the host to stimulate an antitumor immune response. (From Sokoloff M, de-Kernion J, Figlin R, Belldegrun A: Current management of renal cell carcinoma. CA Cancer J Clin 1996; 46:295.)

severe hemorrhage, severe pain, paraneoplastic syndromes, and compression of adjacent viscera. The frequency with which each of these specific symptoms is controlled, however, is unclear, and modern methods, including angioinfarction, seldom make this the only palliative alternative. Patients with metastases at the time of presentation have an average survival of approximately 4 months, and only 10% can be expected to survive 1 year (deKernion et al, 1978). The surgical mortality from the operation must also be superimposed on the potential benefits (Fowler, 1987). Nonetheless, palliative nephrectomy is occasionally warranted for control of severe symptoms, especially profuse hemorrhage.

The term *adjunctive nephrectomy* has been adopted to describe removal of the primary tumor in the patient with metastases, for the purpose of either prolonging survival or causing regression of metastatic lesions. Although a common practice for many years, the procedure has come under more careful scrutiny. The known spontaneous regression of renal tumors has been cited as support for the practice of adjunctive nephrectomy. Regression occurs in renal tumors only rarely, in perhaps 0.4% of patients, or 1 in 250 (Montie et al, 1977). Some reports are even more pessimistic, such as that from the Mayo Clinic, in which no patient underwent regression in the 533 patients reviewed (Myers et al, 1968). Following adjunctive nephrectomy, regression can be expected to occur in less than 1% of patients (Montie et al, 1977). Such regressions are often short-lived, and the mortality rate ranges from 2% to 15%, mainly dependent on patient selection. Furthermore, Oliver (1989) found a 6% spontaneous tumor regression rate despite the absence of any therapeutic intervention in 73 patients with renal cell carcinoma followed systematically for 5 years. Marcus and associates reported on 4 of 91 highly selected patients (4.4%) evaluated at the surgery branch of the NCI who demonstrated spontaneous regression of metastatic renal cancer after removal of the primary tumor. Tumor regression lasted a mean of 24.3 months and was described only in the lungs. On the basis of this information alone, it seems difficult to support routine practice of adjunctive nephrectomy.

Improvement of patient survival by removal of a large primary tumor has also been cited in support of adjunctive nephrectomy. Thus far no study has been reported in which patients were properly stratified and then randomized to undergo adjunctive nephrectomy versus no nephrectomy. In a study from this institution, however, survival of patients undergoing nephrectomy was identical to the survival for the general population of patients with renal carcinoma, suggesting that the nephrectomy alone had minimal impact on the outcome (deKernion et al, 1978).

Adjunctive nephrectomy is, therefore, no longer practiced in many treatment centers on a routine basis, although some investigators still support its application in selected patients (Freed, 1977). Indeed, the procedure may have applications in certain clinical settings. Five-year survival seems to be improved in patients who have excision of solitary renal metastases (Middleton, 1967; O'Dea et al, 1978). It may be appropriate, therefore, to recommend nephrectomy with excision of solitary metastasis in this select group of patients, although micrometastases are likely to be present at other sites. Similarly, as part of an experimental study, adjunctive nephrectomy may be appropriate. One such study requires nephrectomy for the sequestration of TILs from the primary tumor for ultimate biologic therapy. Patients for such protocols are carefully selected based on performance status and degree of metastatic disease to avoid both surgical morbidity and morbidity caused by IL-2–mediated toxicity.

The heterogeneity of renal cell carcinoma and its variable natural history defy therapeutic generalizations. Patients with limited pulmonary metastases, a resectable primary lesion, and a normal performance status seem to have a survival greater than that for others with metastatic disease. In a review of patients at this institution, those in the aforementioned category had a 5-year survival of approximately 30% following adjunctive nephrectomy and various postoperative treatment programs. The impact of the postoperative treatment programs is unclear, but the data indicated that some effect was independent of these systemic therapies.

The impact of adjunctive nephrectomy can also be questioned because a similar group of patients who did not undergo nephrectomy has not been followed. In young healthy patients who meet these specific criteria, however, adjunctive nephrectomy may be appropriate, especially if it is part of a planned treatment program. The role of adjunctive nephrectomy must constantly be reassessed in careful clinical studies (Flanigan, 1989).

Angioinfarction followed by adjunctive nephrectomy was advocated in the past. Review of a large experience using this approach (Swanson et al, 1983; Gottesman et al, 1985; Flanigan, 1987; Kurth et al, 1987), however, does not substantiate its benefit, and it is not indicated as a treatment modality in patients with metastatic disease.

The performance of adjunctive nephrectomy for the purpose of facilitating or instituting experimental immunotherapy is currently an important issue. This indication represents the most valid reason for adjunctive nephrectomy in the presence of metastatic disease. It should be stressed, however, that patients with metastatic renal cell carcinoma who are potential candidates for biologic therapy should be referred to an immunotherapy center for review before the time of nephrectomy. Removing the kidney might constitute an unnecessary procedure in a patient who is not eligible for this type of therapy.

The experience at the National Institutes of Health and elsewhere demonstrated an 11% response rate (9 of 93 patients) at extrarenal sites in patients treated with various IL-2–based regimens with the renal primary in place (Spencer et al, 1992). Strategy was then developed to remove the primary kidney tumor before adoptive immunotherapy if the bulk of the primary kidney tumor was greater than that of the metastatic tumor. The goal was to decrease tumor bulk and to achieve maximum therapeutic response to therapy. This approach has resulted in a beneficial effect of 27% response rate, suggesting that pretreatment nephrectomy might contribute to improved response rates. Nevertheless, the true effect of prior nephrectomy on response to immunotherapy has not been consistently demonstrated, and it remains unclear what influences other factors (performance status, sites of metastases) may have on this effect. Several trials of interferon alpha in metastatic renal cell carcinoma, however, when retrospectively analyzed, have suggested that prior nephrectomy was an independent variable in determining patient response to interferon and was an indicator for better survival (Umeda and Niijima, 1986; Muss et al, 1987; Minasian et al, 1993).

Current analysis of the authors' combined UCLA data suggests a better response rate in the group of patients who underwent nephrectomy within 1 year before the initiation of immunotherapy (Belldegrun et al, 1990). Of 84 evaluable patients, 45 patients were started on interferon therapy within 1 year of the initial diagnosis and nephrectomy. The two groups of patients (nephrectomy versus no nephrectomy) were similar with regard to performance status and lung metastases. Of patients who underwent nephrectomy before immunotherapy, 24.3% responded to interferon compared with 8.3% who did not have prior nephrectomy. The difference was not statistically significant; however, the power of statistical testing was limited by the small number of patients in the nonephrectomy group. An important study currently underway in the Southwestern Oncology Group is evaluating the role of cytoreductive therapy in interferon-treated patients. Clearly a similar study is needed for IL-2–treated patients.

Sarcomas of the Kidney

Sarcomas constitute only about 1% to 3% of malignant tumors of the kidney but increase in incidence with advancing age (Farrow et al, 1968; Saitoh et al, 1982; Spellman et al, 1995). Differentiation from the sarcomatoid variant of renal cell carcinoma is usually difficult or impossible (Vogelzang et al, 1993). The most common presenting signs and symptoms are essentially those of a large renal carcinoma (e.g., pain, a flank mass, and hematuria) (Fig. 76–31).

CT may be helpful in delineating whether a renal mass is parenchymal in origin or whether it originates in the renal sinus or capsule. Otherwise, the density of these tumors mimics that of soft tissue, with the exception of the fat density seen in liposarcoma or osteosarcoma, in which bone may be seen. The findings of tumor originating from renal sinus or capsule or the presence of a mass with fat or bone would be highly suggestive of a renal sarcoma. Absence of retroperitoneal lymphadenopathy in a patient with a large renal tumor is also more compatible with sarcoma than carcinoma (Pollack et al, 1987). Angiographically, these tumors are hypovascular without arteriovenous fistulas (Shirkhoda and Lewis, 1987).

Leiomyosarcomas, originating from smooth muscle cells, are the most common variety, composing about 60% of the total incidence of sarcomas. Sixty-six cases were identified by Niceta and co-workers and were most common in women in their thirties to fifties (Niceta et al, 1974). These tumors tend to compress and displace the kidney rather than invade

it. They usually attain large size and metastasize early and widely throughout the body. Leiomyosarcomas are generally well encapsulated, firm, and multinodular, and they tend to recur locally after resection.

Treatment for leiomyosarcoma, as with any sarcoma, is radical surgical extirpation (Karakousis et al, 1995). This approach is especially important because these tumors can seldom be definitely differentiated from renal adenocarcinoma. Although local and distant recurrence is common, significant prolongation of survival can be achieved only for patients with completely resectable tumors. Prognosis is generally poor despite the use of aggressive chemotherapy or radiotherapy. Two studies have shown significant response rates for ifosfamide-based regimens in patients with advanced, metastatic, or unresectable soft tissue sarcoma (Elias et al, 1989; Antman et al, 1993). Survival, however, was not improved by the use of chemotherapy. At this point, therefore, no recommendations can be made for the routine use of postoperative treatment (Vogelzang et al, 1993).

Osteogenic sarcomas are extremely rare tumors of the kidney. The genesis of such tumors is problematic, and osteogenic differentiation may occur in various sarcomatoid renal cell tumors (Moon et al, 1983; Micolonghi et al, 1984). These tumors contain calcium and are rock-hard or may have sunburst calcification. The presence of extensive calcification in a rather hypovascular tumor should suggest the presence of this rare lesion. The tumor may metastasize to bone and pose a problem as to whether the tumor in the kidney is a metastasis or truly a primary lesion. Biggers and Stewart (1979) reviewed the literature and recorded seven cases, detailing the clinical and pathologic features of the tumor. The poor prognosis was emphasized, and, although radical nephrectomy is the treatment of choice, few patients are cured.

Virtually every other variety of sarcoma has been described in the kidney. *Liposarcomas* represent about 19% of renal sarcomas and are often confused with angiomyolipomas or with large, benign primary lipomas. These tumors occur generally in adults in their forties and fifties and are usually of large size (Economou et al, 1987). They frequently recur locally, and re-excision is usually feasible. Postoperative adjuvant therapy is appropriate when margins are positive, and the authors have seen responses to a combination of radiotherapy, *cis*-platin, and phosphamide. *Carcinosarcoma* of the kidney has been described in several cases and is composed of classic renal cell carcinoma components in addition to fibrosarcomatous elements (Rao et al, 1977). *Fibrosarcoma* has been described and is easily mistaken for

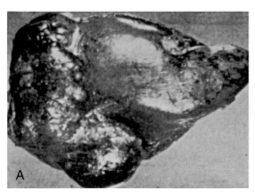
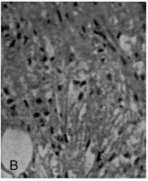

Figure 76–31. Sarcoma of renal capsule. *A,* Massive tumor arising from renal capsule. *B,* Histologic specimen diagnostic of fibrosarcoma.

leiomyoma or leiomyosarcoma (Kansara and Powell, 1980). Fibroxanthosarcoma (Chen, 1979) and *angiosarcoma* (Allred et al, 1981) have also been described.

Rhabdomyosarcoma of the adult, one of the rarest and most malignant renal neoplasms, arises from striated muscle. These tumors are usually large and multinodular with a well-defined capsule. One patient with rhabdomyosarcoma, who was treated in recent years at the authors' institution, died from metastatic disease 14 months after radical nephrectomy.

One of the most thorough studies of the incidence and metastatic pattern of sarcomas was made by Saitoh and colleagues (1982). In 2651 cases of renal tumors, they reported an incidence of sarcomas of 1%; 9 were leiomyosarcoma, 5 were rhabdomyosarcoma, and 5 were fibrosarcoma. The most common sites of metastases were the liver, lymph nodes, and lung.

Surgery is the only potentially curative method of treating these rare tumors. The survival following surgery alone, however, is extremely poor. The success that has been realized by intra-arterial doxorubicin therapy combined with radiation provides at least a testable hypothesis for the adjuvant treatment of these tumors. The patient illustrated in Figure 76–32 had a poorly differentiated sarcoma of the kidney that completely regressed after doxorubicin and external radiotherapy, and the residual fibrous mass was subsequently excised. The patient is free of disease 2 years after surgery. Although adjuvant intravenous doxorubicin after nephrectomy has not been proven to be of value, the current experience suggests that this may be a reasonable approach.

Malignant fibrous histiocytoma is the most common soft tissue sarcoma of late adult life and often occurs in the retroperitoneal space (Goldman et al, 1984). Eight such tumors arising in the kidney have been reported (Scriven et al, 1984). The tumors usually grow to large size and may be clinically and angiographically indistinguishable from renal cell carcinoma. The histology is similar to that of histiocytomas arising in other areas. Therapy is radical nephrectomy, but local recurrence is frequent. Radiotherapy may be effective (Osamura et al, 1978; Raghavaiah et al, 1980).

Hemangiopericytomas, renin-secreting tumors of the kidney, are usually small, benign tumors that produce severe hypertension. These tumors are often histologically hemangiopericytomas (Weiss et al, 1984). Renal and perirenal hemangiopericytoma, however, may exist, may grow to large size, and may develop a malignant potential. Most investigators consider it to be a true sarcomatous lesion.

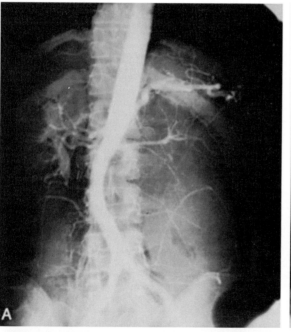

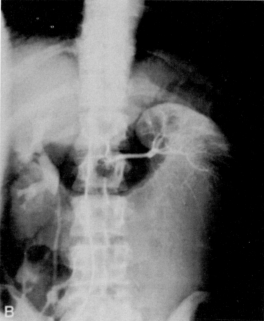

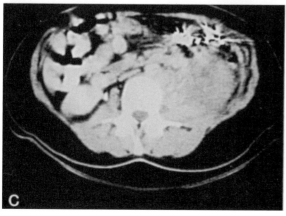

Figure 76–32. *A,* Aortic flush phase demonstrating huge left flank mass in a 36-year-old woman with flank pain. Note aortic displacement. *B,* Selective left renal arteriogram showing typical hypovascular pattern associated with sarcomas. *C,* Computed tomography scan demonstrating the large tumor fixed to the posterior abdominal wall and paraspinous muscles proved to be a poorly differentiated sarcoma by biopsy.

Local or distant metastases have been reported in approximately 15% of patients (Glenn, 1980). Ordonez and co-workers described a hemangiopericytoma extending into the vena cava as a thrombus (Ordonez et al, 1982). DiEsidio and associates reported a retroperitoneal hemangiopericytoma that metastasized to the liver, kidney, and abdominal cavity (DiEsidio et al, 1980). A major concern with these tumors is their profuse vascularity. Smullens and colleagues described catheter embolization of hemangiopericytoma of the retroperitoneum in two cases, which greatly facilitated safe removal (Smullens et al, 1979). When these tumors are confined to the kidney, the most appropriate treatment is radical nephrectomy.

Lymphoblastoma

Malignancies of the lymphoma type, including reticulum cell sarcoma, lymphosarcoma, and leukemia, are uncommon and generally occur in the kidney as only one manifestation of the systemic disease. Knoepp (1956) identified a primary lymphosarcoma of the kidney treated, apparently successfully, with radical nephrectomy. Silber and Chang (1973) also reported a primary lymphoma of the kidney. Leukemia generally involves the kidney in an infiltrative pattern; it can be silent or can produce hematuria, enlarged kidneys, and progressive renal failure. At autopsy, up to 50% of cases with leukemia have renal involvement.

The treatment of these processes is generally the indicated systemic treatment of that particular disease. Nephrectomy is seldom, if ever, indicated except in the case of a solitary lesion or in the patient with severe symptoms, such as uncontrollable hemorrhage.

Because the treatment of these lesions is not the primary purview of the urologist, major concern rests in the diagnosis of renal involvement by these systemic diseases and in their distinction from other renal mass lesions. Hartman and co-workers related pathologic findings with radiologic findings in 21 patients with renal lymphoma (Hartman et al, 1982). The radiographic picture depended on the pattern of involvement and the size, number, and distribution of the lesions. These workers concluded that the lymphoma initially grows between the nephrons and subsequently expands and produces the typical lymphomatous masses.

CT appears to be the method of choice in diagnosing renal lymphoma (Heiken et al, 1983). The initial nodular lesions, which later become confluent, are best detected with contrast medium administration. Four patterns of involvement were documented with CT by Heiken and associates (1983): (1) multiple intraparenchymal nodules, (2) direct contiguous lymph node masses, (3) solitary renal lesions, and (4) diffuse infiltration. Jafri and associates described similar findings in 16 patients with non-Hodgkin's lymphomas of the kidney (Jafri et al, 1982).

CT was accurate in determining the size and location of the tumor and was useful in evaluating the response to systemic therapy. Various patterns of involvement, including solitary nodules, multiple nodules, focal infiltration, diffuse infiltration, contiguous extension, and renal enlargement, were noted. Retroperitoneal adenopathy was identified by CT scan in all of the patients. Others have suggested that the findings of renal infiltration and multiple intraparenchymal

nodules associated with retroperitoneal adenopathy should raise the possibility of renal lymphoma. At the present time, CT appears to be the most reliable way to diagnose renal involvement by lymphoma and to monitor the progress of therapy.

The major diagnostic problem is differentiating a renal lymphoma mass from a renal cell carcinoma. Aspiration biopsy under CT guidance may help in arriving at a histologic diagnosis. Radiologic findings are summarized in Table 76–14 (Barbaric, 1991).

Table 76–14. RADIOLOGIC FINDINGS IN RENAL LYMPHOMA

Computed Tomography	Sonography	Angiography
Multiple renal masses (45%)	Hypoechoic	Hypovascular
Solitary mass (15%)	Anechoic	Capsular artery displacement
Invasion from outside (25%)	No through transmission	
Diffuse infiltration (10%)	Diminished central sinus echoes	Fuzzy renal outline
Perinephric involvement (5%)		

Adapted from Barbaric, ZL: Principles of Genitourinary Radiology, 2nd ed. New York, Thieme Medical Publishers, 1994.

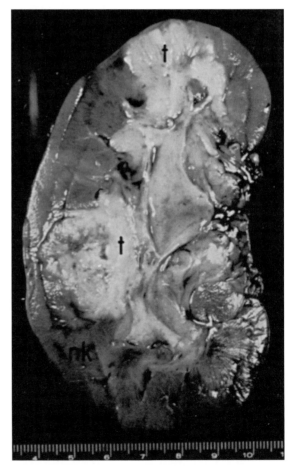

Figure 76–33. Metastatic carcinoma of the kidney from the lung demonstrating the diffuse invasive character of metastatic tumor (t) in normal renal substance (nk).

Metastatic Tumors

The kidney is a frequent site of metastatic deposits from a variety of solid tumors and hematologic malignancies. The high blood flow, profuse vascularity, and "fertile soil" of the renal parenchyma provide a hospitable environment for deposition and growth of malignant cells. Metastases to the kidney are seldom clinically identified and are most often discovered at autopsy. They are, in that sense, often clinically inconsequential because the nature of the metastatic disease militates against the removal of an isolated renal metastasis. In a review of 5000 autopsies, Klinger (1951) found 21 cases of metastases from lung carcinoma (Fig. 76–33). Olsson (1971) reported that 20% of patients dying of lung cancer had renal metastases, 40% of which were bilateral. These tumors are often small and multiple, and it has been estimated that as many as 19,000 persons annually may have lung cancer with secondary renal metastases. Although these tumors seldom are associated with clinical symptoms, massive hemorrhage has been reported (Walther et al, 1979). Virtually every other solid neoplasm may metastasize to the kidney, including ovarian, bowel, and breast malignancies. Lymphoma and lymphoblastoma are among the most common metastatic lesions of the kidney. These tumors usually appear as multiple nodules, but, occasionally, single nodules and diffuse infiltration have been reported (Kyaw and Koehler, 1969).

Metastatic or secondary lesions within the kidney generally produce few symptoms. Flank pain and hematuria may occur. With pyelographic or ultrasonographic identification, it is difficult to distinguish metastatic tumors from primary renal neoplasms. The principal method of detection is CT, and identification often requires a CT-guided aspiration bi-

opsy. The mass on the precontrast scan is almost isodense to the kidney and enhances only slightly on the postcontrast scan (Choyke et al, 1982; Barbaric, 1991). Arteriographically, these tumors are usually round and hypovascular, without the discrete neovascularity and other angiographic characteristics associated with primary renal cell carcinoma (Fig. 76–34).

Whether renal carcinoma frequently metastasizes to the opposite kidney is controversial. The same malignant propensity that caused a tumor in one kidney could be reasonably expected to give rise to another primary lesion in the opposite kidney. The short-term results (cited previously) following excision of tumor in the contralateral kidney (synchronously or asynchronously) seem to be better than survival following excision of a solitary metastasis. No serologic or histologic method, however, has been devised to determine accurately whether such tumors are metastatic or de novo lesions.

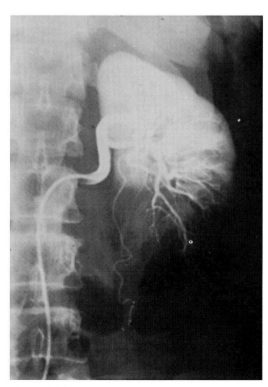

Figure 76–34. Arteriogram demonstrating hypovascular mass in left kidney. A solitary metastasis of lymphoblastoma was confirmed.

REFERENCES

Albarran J, Imbert L: Les Tumeurs du Rein. Paris, Masson et Cie, 1903.

Allred CD, Cathey WJ, McDivitt RW: Primary renal angiosarcoma: A case report. Hum Pathol 1981; 12:665.

Amendola MA, Bree RL, Pollack HM, et al: Small renal cell carcinomas: Resolving a diagnostic dilemma. Radiology 1988; 166:637.

Angermeirer KW, Novick AC, Streem SB, Montie JE: Nephron sparing surgery for renal cell carcinoma with venous involvement. J Urol 1990; 144:1352–1355.

Anglard P, Trahan E, Liu S, et al: Molecular and cellular characterization of human renal cell carcinoma cell lines. Cancer Res 1992; 52:348.

Antman K, Crowley J, Balcerzak SP, et al: An intergroup phase III randomized study of doxorubicin and dacarbazine with or without ifosfamide and mesna in advanced soft tissue and bone sarcomas. J Clin Oncol 1993; 11:1276.

Atzpodien J, Kirchner H, Lopez Hanninen E, et al: Alpha-interferon, interleukin-2, and 5-fluorouracil as a promising biochemotherapy regimen for the management of advanced renal cell carcinoma. Proc Am Soc Clin Oncol 1993; 12:230.

Atzpodien J, Korfer A, Menzel T, et al: Home therapy using recombinant human IL-2 and interferon alpha-2b in patients with metastatic renal cell carcinoma. (Abstract.) Proc Am Soc Clin Oncol 1991; 10:177.

Aulitzky W, Gastl G, Aulitzky WE, et al: Successful treatment of metastatic renal cell carcinoma with a biologically active dose of recombinant interferon-gamma. J Clin Oncol 1989; 7:1875.

Bander NH, Finstad CL, Cordon-Cardo C, et al: Analysis of mouse monoclonal antibody that reacts with a specific region of the human proximal tubule and subsets renal cell carcinomas. Cancer Res 1989; 49:6774.

Barbaric ZL: Genitourinary Radiology. New York, Thieme Medical Publishers, 1991, p 171.

Barbaric ZL: Principles of Genitourinary Radiology, 2nd ed. New York, Thieme Medical Publishers, 1994, p 154.

Bassil B, Dosoretz DE, Prout GR Jr: Validation of the tumor, nodes and metastasis classification of renal cell carcinoma. J Urol 1985; 134:450.

Beahrs OH, ed: American Joint Committee on Cancer: Manual for Staging Cancer, 4th ed. Philadelphia, J. B. Lippincott, 1992, p 201.

Bell ET: Renal Disease, 2nd ed. Philadelphia, Lea & Febiger, 1950, p 435.

Belldegrun A, Dardashti K, Tso CL, et al: The use of cytokines, tumor infiltrating lymphocytes, and gene therapy in the treatment of advanced renal cell carcinoma: The UCLA experience. In Bukowski RM, Finke JH, Klein EA, eds: Biology of Renal Cell Carcinoma. New York, Springer-Verlag, 1995, p 204.

Belldegrun A, Koo AS, Bochner B, et al: Immunotherapy for advanced renal cell cancer: The role of radical nephrectomy. Eur Urol 1990; 18(suppl 2):42.

Belldegrun A, Muul LM, Rosenberg SA: Interleukin-2 expanded tumor infiltrating lymphocytes in human renal cell cancer: Isolation, characterization and antitumor activity. Cancer Res 1988a; 48:206.

Belldegrun A, Pierce W, Kaboo R, et al: Interferon-α primed tumor-infiltrating lymphocytes combined with interleukin-2 and interferon-α as therapy for metastatic renal cell carcinoma. J Urol 1993; 150:1384.

Belldegrun A, Rosenberg SA: Adoptive immunotherapy of urologic tumors. *In* Lepor H, Ratliff TL, eds: Urologic Oncology, Boston, Kluwer Academic Publishers, 1989, p 213.

Belldegrun A, Tso CL, Sakata T, et al: Human renal carcinoma line transfected with interleukin-2 and/or interferon α gene(s): Implications for live cancer vaccines. J Natl Cancer Inst 1993; 85:207.

Belldegrun A, Uppenkamp I, Rosenberg SA: Antitumor reactivity of human lymphokine activated killer (LAK) cells against fresh and cultured preparations of renal cell cancer. J Urol 1988b; 139:150.

Belldegrun A, Webb DE, Austin HA, et al: Effects of interleukin-2 in renal function in patients receiving immunotherapy for advanced cancer. Ann Intern Med 1987; 106:817.

Belldegrun A, Webb DE, Austin HA, et al: Renal toxicity of interleukin-2 administration in patients with metastatic renal cell cancer: Effect of pretherapy nephrectomy. J Urol 1989; 141:499.

Bennington JL, Beckwith JB: Tumors of the Kidney, Renal Pelvis, and Ureter. (Atlas of Tumor Pathology, 2nd series, fascicle 12.) Washington, D.C., Armed Forces Institute of Pathology, 1975.

Best BG: Renal carcinoma: A ten-year review 1971–1980. Br J Urol 1987; 60:100.

Biggers R, Stewart J: Primary renal osteosarcoma. Urology 1979; 13:674.

Birch-Hirschfeld FV, Doederlein A: Zentralbl Krankh Horn Sex Org, Vol. 3, 1894.

Bloom HJ: Hormone induced and spontaneous regression of metastatic renal cancer. Cancer 1973; 32:1006.

Blute ML, Malek RS, Segura JW: Angiomyolipoma: Clinical metamorphosis and concepts for management. J Urol 1988; 139:20.

Bonavita JA, Pollack HM, Banner MP: Renal oncocytoma: Further observations and literature review. Urol Radiol 1981; 2:229.

Bonnin JM, Cain MD, Jose JS, et al: Hypertension due to renin-secreting tumor localized by segmental renal vein sampling. Aust N Z J Med 1977; 7:630.

Bosniak MA, Megibow AJ, Hulnick DH, et al: CT diagnosis of renal angiomyolipoma: The importance of detecting small amounts of fat. AJR 1988; 151:497.

Bosniak MA, Subramanyam BR: Renal parenchymal and capsular tumors in adults. *In* Taveras JM, Ferrucci JT, eds: Radiology—Diagnosis, Imaging, Intervention, Vol 4. Philadelphia, J. B. Lippincott, 1990, p 1.

Boxer RJ, Waisman J, Lieber MM, et al: Non-metastatic hepatic dysfunction associated with renal carcinoma. J Urol 1978; 119:468.

Brooks JD, Bova GS, Marshall FF, Isaacs WB: Tumor suppressor gene allelic loss in human renal cancers. J Urol 1993; 150:1278.

Brunda MJ, Bellantoni D, Sulich V: In vivo antitumor activity of combinations of interferon-α and interleukin-2 in a murine model: Correlation of efficacy with the induction of cytotoxic cells resembling natural killer cells. Int J Cancer 1987; 40:365.

Bukowski RM, Groppe D, Reimer R, et al: Immunotherapy (IT) of metastatic renal cell carcinoma (Abstract C-457). Proc Am Assoc Cancer Res/Am Soc Clin Oncol 1979; 20:402.

Cameron RB, McIntosh JK, Rosenberg SA: Synergistic antitumor effects of combination immunotherapy with recombinant interleukin-2 and a recombinant hybrid alpha-interferon in the treatment of established murine hepatic metastases. Cancer Res 1988; 48:5810.

Campbell SC, Novick AC, Streem S, et al: Complications of nephron-sparing surgery for renal tumors. J Urol 1994; 151:1177.

Carson WJ: Tumors of the kidney: Histologic study. Trans Sect Urol AMA, 1928.

Chapman AE, Goldstein LJ: Multiple drug resistance: Biologic basis and clinical significance in renal cell carcinoma. Semin Oncol 1995; 22:17.

Chen KT: Fibroxanthosarcoma of the kidney. Urology 1979; 13:439.

Cherrie RJ, Goldman DG, Lindner A, deKernion JB: Prognostic implications of vena caval extension of renal cell carcinoma. J Urol 1982; 128:910.

Chisholm GD: Nephrogenic ridge tumors and their syndromes. Ann NY Acad Sci 1974; 230:403.

Choyke PL, White EM, Zeman RK, et al: Renal metastases: Clinicopathologic and radiologic correlation. Radiology 1982; 162:359.

Chute R, Soutter L, Kerr W: The value of thoracoabdominal incision in the removal of kidney tumors. N Engl J Med 1949; 241:951.

Cohen AJ, Li FP, Berg S, et al: Hereditary renal cell carcinoma associated with a chromosomal translocation. N Engl J Med 1979; 301:592.

Colvin RB, Dickersin GR: Pathology of renal tumors. *In* Skinner DG, deKernion JB, eds: Genitourinary Cancer. Philadelphia. W. B. Saunders, 1978, p 84.

Cox CE, Lacy SS, Montgomery WG, Boyce WH: Renal adenocarcinoma: A 28-year review with emphasis on rationale and feasibility of preoperative radiotherapy. J Urol 1970; 105:51.

Crotty TB, Lawrence KM, Moertel CA, et al: Cytogenetic analysis of six renal oncocytomas and a chromophobe cell renal carcinoma: Evidence that − Y, − 1 may be a characteristic anomaly in renal oncocytomas. Cancer Genet Cytogenet 1992; 61:61.

Cummings KB: Surgical management of renal cell carcinoma with extension into the vena cava. *In* Crawford EE, Borden TA, eds: Genitourinary Cancer Surgery. Philadelphia, Lea & Febiger, 1982, p 70.

Davidson AJ, Hayes WS, Hartman DS, et al: Renal oncocytoma and carcinoma: Failure of differentiation with CT. Radiology 1993; 186:693.

Dayal HH, Wilkinson GS: Epidemiology of renal cell cancer. Semin Urol 1989; 3:139.

deKernion JB: Lymphadenectomy for renal cell carcinoma: Therapeutic implications. Urol Clin North Am 1980a; 7:697.

deKernion JB: Radical nephrectomy. *In* Ehrlich RE, ed: Modern Techniques in Surgery. New York, Futura, 1980b, p 1.

deKernion JB, Berry D: The diagnosis and treatment of renal cell carcinoma. Cancer 1980; 45:1947.

deKernion JB, Huland H: The operable renal cell carcinoma: Summary and conclusions. Eur Urol 1990; 18(suppl 2):48.

deKernion JB, Lindner A: Treatment of advanced renal cell carcinoma. *In* Kuss R, Murphy G, Khoury S, Karr J, eds: Proceedings of the First International Symposium on Kidney Tumors. New York, Alan R. Liss, 1982, p 614.

deKernion JB, Ramming KP: The therapy of renal adenocarcinoma with immune RNA. Invest Urol 1980; 17:378.

deKernion JB, Ramming KP, Smith RB: Natural history of metastatic renal cell carcinoma: A computer analysis. J Urol 1978; 120:148.

deKernion JB, Smith RB: The kidney and adrenal glands. *In* Paulson DF, ed: Genitourinary Surgery, Vol 1. New York, Churchill Livingstone, 1984, p 1.

DeLong W, Grignon DJ, Eberwein P, et al: Sarcomatoid renal cell carcinoma: An immunohistochemical study of 18 cases. Arch Pathol Lab Med 1993; 117:636.

Deming CL, Harvard BM: Tumors of the kidney. *In* Campbell MF, Harrison JH, eds: Urology, Vol 2, 3rd ed. Philadelphia, W. B. Saunders, 1970, p 884.

Dexeus F, Logothetics C, Sella A, et al: Phase II study of coumarin and cimetidine in metastatic renal cell carcinoma. J Clin Oncol 1990; 8:325.

DiEsidio M, Gadaleta A, Monina M, Cappelletti V: Retroperitoneal hemangiopericytoma: Presentation of a case with recurrence and multiple metastases. Radiol Med (Torino) 1980; 66:331.

Dineen MK, Venable DD, Misra RP: Pure intrarenal lipoma—report of a case and review of the literature. Presented at the Annual Meeting, Southeastern Section of the American Urologic Association, Miami, Florida, 1983.

Dinney CPN, Awad SA, Gajewski JB, et al: Analysis of imaging modalities, staging systems and prognostic indicators for renal cell carcinoma. Urology 1992; 39:122.

Dobin SM, Harris CP, Reynolds JA, et al: Cytogenetic abnormalities in renal oncocytic neoplasms. Genes Chromosomes Cancer 1992; 4:25.

Economou JS, Lindner A, deKernion JB: Sarcomas of the genitourinary tract. *In* Eilber FR, et al, eds: The Soft Tissue Sarcomas. Orlando, Grune & Stratton, 1987, p 219.

Elias A, Ryan L, Sulkes A, et al: Response to mesna, doxorubicin, ifosfamide, and dacarbazine in 108 patients with metastatic or unresectable sarcoma and no prior chemotherapy. J Clin Oncol 1989; 7:1208.

Erslev AJ, Caro J: Physiologic and molecular biology of erythropoietin. Med Oncol Tumor Pharmacother 1986; 3:159.

Farrow GM, Harrison EG, Utz DC, Remine WH: Sarcomas and sarcomatoid and mixed malignant tumors of the kidney in adults. Cancer 1968; 22:545.

Figlin RA, deKernion JB, Maldazys J, et al: Treatment of renal cell carcinoma with alpha (human leukocyte) interferon and vinblastine in combination: A phase I–II trial. Cancer Treat Rep 1985; 69:263.

Figlin RA, deKernion JB, Mukamel E, et al: Recombinant interferon alpha-2a in metastatic renal cell carcinoma: Assessment of antitumor activity and anti-interferon antibody formation. J Clin Oncol 1988; 6:1604.

Figlin RA, Gitlitz BJ, Belldegrun A: Immunologic approaches to the treatment of cancer. Cancer Inv 1995; 13:339.

Figlin RA, Pierce WC, Belldegrun A: Combination biologic therapy with interleukin-2 and interferon-alpha in the outpatient treatment of metastatic renal cell carcinoma. Semin Oncol 1993; 20:11.

Finney R: The value of radiotherapy in the treatment of hypernephroma—a clinical trial. Br J Urol 1973; 45:258.

Fisher ER, Horvat B: Comparative ultrastructural study of so-called renal adenoma and carcinoma. J Urol 1972; 108:382.

Fisher RI, Coltman CA Jr, Doroshow JH, et al: Metastatic renal cancer treated with interleukin-2 and lymphokine-activated killer cells: A phase II clinical trial. Ann Intern Med 1988; 108:518.

Flanigan RC: The failure of infarction and/or nephrectomy in stage IV renal cell cancer to influence survival or metastatic regression. Urol Clin North Am 1987; 14:757.

Flanigan RC: Role of surgery in metastatic renal cell carcinoma. Semin Urol 1989; 7:191.

Fojo AT, Shen DW, Mickley LA, et al: Intrinsic drug resistance in kidney cancers is associated with expression of a human multidrug resistance gene. J Clin Oncol 1987; 5:1922.

Foster RS, Mahomed Y, Bihrle R, Strup S: Use of a caval-atrial shunt for resection of a caval tumor thrombus in renal cell carcinoma. J Urol 1988; 140:1370.

Fowler JE Jr: Nephrectomy in metastatic renal cell carcinoma. Urol Clin North Am 1987; 14:749.

Freed SZ: Nephrectomy for renal cell carcinoma with metastases. Urology 1977; 9:613.

Freeman MR, Washecka R, Chung LWR: Aberrant expression of epidermal growth factor receptor and HER-2 (erb B-2) messenger RNAs in human renal cancers. Cancer Res 1989; 49:6221.

Frignon DJ, El-Naggar A, Green LK, et al: DNA flow cytometry as a predictor of outcome of stage I renal cell carcinoma. Cancer 1989; 6:1161.

Fromowitz FB, Bard RH: Clinical implications of pathologic subtypes in renal cell carcinoma in humans. Semin Urol 1990; 8:31.

Fuhrman SA, Lasky LC, Limas C: Prognostic significance of morphologic parameters in renal cell carcinoma. Am J Surg Pathol 1982; 6:655.

Giuliani L, Giberti C, Martorama G, et al: Radical extensive surgery for renal cell carcinoma: Long term results and prognostic factors. J Urol 1990; 143:468.

Glenn GM, Choyke PL, Zbar B, Linehan WM: Von Hippel-Lindau disease: Clinical review and molecular genetics. In Anderson EE, ed: Problems in Urologic Surgery: Benign and Malignant Tumors of the Kidney. Philadelphia, J. B. Lippincott, 1990, p 312.

Glenn JF: Renal tumors. In Harrison JH, Gittes RF, Perlmutter AD, et al, eds: Campbell's Urology, 4th ed. Philadelphia, W. B. Saunders, 1980.

Glover SD, Buck AC: Renal medullary fibroma: A case report. J Urol 1982; 127:758.

Gnarra JR, Tory K, Weng Y, et al: Mutation of the VHL tumour suppressor gene in renal carcinoma. Nature Genet 1994; 7:85.

Goldberg MF, Tashjian AH, Order SC, Dammin GJ: Renal adenocarcinoma containing a parathyroid hormone–like substance and associated with marked hypercalcemia. Am J Med 1964; 36:805.

Goldman SM, Hartman DS, Weiss SW: The varied radiographic manifestations of retroperitoneal malignant fibrous histiocytoma revealed through 27 cases. J Urol 1984; 132:337.

Golimbu M, Joshi P, Sperber A, et al: Renal cell carcinoma: Survival and prognostic factors. Urology 1986; 27:291.

Gomella LG, Sargent ER, Wade TP, et al: Expression of transforming growth factor α in normal human adult kidney and enhanced expression of transforming growth factors α and β 1 in renal cell carcinoma. Cancer Res 1989; 49:6972.

Gottesman JE, Crawford ED, Grossman HB, et al: Infarction-nephrectomy for metastatic renal carcinoma. Urology 1985; 25:248.

Grawitz P: Die sogenannten Lipome der Niere. Virchows Arch [A] 1883; 93:39.

Grignon DJ, Ayala AG, El-Naggar A, et al: Renal cell carcinoma: A clinicopathologic and DNA flow cytometric analysis of 103 cases. Cancer 1989; 64:2133.

Guinan PD, Vogelzang NJ, Fremgen AM, et al: Renal cell carcinoma: Tumor size, stage and survival. J Urol 1995; 153:901.

Gutterman J: Overview of advances in the use of biological proteins in human cancer. Semin Oncol 1988; 15(suppl):2.

Harris RP: An analytical examination of 100 cases of extirpations of the kidney. Am J Med Sci 1882; 84:109.

Hartman DS, Davis CJ, Goldman SM, et al: Renal lymphoma: Radiologic-pathologic correlation of 21 cases. Radiology 1982; 144:759.

Hatcher PA, Anderson EE, Paulson DF, et al: Surgical management and prognosis of renal cell carcinoma invading the vena cava. J Urol 1991; 145:20.

Hathorn RW, Tso CL, Kaboo R, et al: In vitro modulation of the invasive and metastatic potentials of human renal cell carcinoma by interleukin-2 and/or interferon-alpha gene transfer. Cancer 1994; 74:1904.

Heiken JP, Gold RP, Schnur MJ, et al: Computed tomography of renal lymphoma with ultrasound correlation. J Comput Assist Tomogr 1983; 7:245.

Hermanek P, Schrott KM: Evaluation of the new tumor, nodes and metastases classification of renal cell carcinoma. J Urol 1990; 144:238.

Hirsh EM, Wallace S, Johnson DE, Bracken RB: Immunological studies in human urological cancer. In Johnson DE, Samuels ML, eds: Cancer of the Genitourinary Tract. New York, Raven Press, 1979, p 47.

Hoehn W, Hermanek P: Invasion of veins in renal cell carcinoma—frequency, correlation and prognosis. Eur Urol 1983; 9:276.

Horan J, Robertson C, Choyke P, et al: The detection of renal carcinoma extension into the renal vein and inferior vena cava: A prospective comparison of venacavography and magnetic resonance imaging. J Urol 1989; 142:943.

Hricak H, Demas BE, Williams RD, et al: Magnetic resonance imaging in the diagnosis and staging of renal and perirenal neoplasms. Radiology 1985; 154:709.

Hricak H, Thoeni RF, Carroll PR, et al: Detection and staging of renal neoplasms: A reassessment of MR imaging. Radiology 1988; 166:643.

Hulten L, Rosencrantz T, Seeman L, et al: Occurrence and localization of lymph node metastases in renal cell carcinoma. Scand J Urol Nephrol 1969; 3:129.

Jaffee EM, Pardoll DM: Gene therapy: Its potential applications in the treatment of renal-cell carcinoma. Semin Oncol 1995; 22:81.

Jafri SZ, Bree RL, Amendola MA, et al: CT of renal and perirenal non-Hodgkin lymphoma. AJR 1982; 138:1101.

Janik JE, Sznol M, Urba WJ, et al: Erythropoietin production: A potential marker for interleukin-2/interferon responsive tumors. Cancer 1993; 72:2656.

Jaschke W, van Kaick G, Peter S, Palmtas H: Accuracy of computed tomography in staging of kidney tumors. Acta Radiol Diagn (Stockh) 1982; 23:593.

Kakehi Y, Kanamaru H, Yoshida O, et al: Measurement of multidrug resistance messenger RNA in urogenital cancers: Elevated expression in renal cell carcinoma is associated with intrinsic drug resistance. J Urol 1988; 139:862.

Kanamaru H, Kakehi Y, Yoshida O, et al: MDR1 RNA levels in human renal cell carcinomas: Correlation with grade and prediction of reversal of doxorubicin resistance by quinidine in tumor explants. J Natl Cancer Inst 1989; 81:844.

Kansara V, Powell I: Fibrosarcoma of the kidney. Urology 1980; 16:419.

Kantor AF: Current concepts in the epidemiology and etiology of primary renal cell carcinoma. J Urol 1977; 117:415.

Karakousis CP, Gerstenbluth R, Kontzoglou K, Driscoll DL: Retroperitoneal sarcomas and their management. Arch Surg 1995; 130:1104.

Karthaus HFM, Bussemakers MJG, Schalken JA, et al: Expression of proto-oncogenes in xenografts of human renal cell carcinomas. Urol Res 1987; 15:349.

Kemp BE, Moseley JM, Rodda CP, et al: Parathyroid hormone–related protein of malignancy: Active synthetic fragments. Science 1987; 238:1568.

Kirkman H, Bacon RL: Renal adenomas and carcinomas in diethylstilbestrol-treated male golden hamsters. Anat Rec 1949; 103:475.

Kirkwood JM, Harris JE, Vera R, et al: A randomized study of low and high doses of leukocyte alpha-interferon in metastatic renal cell carcinoma: The American Cancer Society Collaborative Trial. Cancer Res 1985; 45:863.

Klinger ME: Secondary tumors of the genitourinary tract. J Urol 1951; 65:144.

Kloppel G, Knofel WT, Baisch H, et al: Prognosis of renal cell carcinoma related to nuclear grade, DNA content, and Robson stage. Eur Urol 1986; 12:426.

Knoepp LF: Lymphosarcoma of the kidney. Surgery 1956; 39:510.

Kolonel LN: Association of cadmium with renal cancer. Cancer 1976; 37:1782.

Konnak JW, Grossman HB: Renal cell carcinoma as an incidental finding. J Urol 1985; 134:1094.

Kovacs G: Molecular differential pathology of renal cell tumors. Histopathology 1993; 22:1.

Kovacs G, Brusa P, DeRiese W: Tissue-specific expression of a constitutional 3;6 translocation: Development of multiple bilateral renal cell carcinomas. Int J Cancer 1989; 43:422.

Kurth KH, Debruyne FM, Hall RR, et al: Embolization and postinfarction nephrectomy in patient with primary metastatic renal adenocarcinoma. Eur Urol 1987; 13:251.

Kyaw M, Koehler PR: Renal and perirenal lymphoma: Arteriographic findings. Radiology 1969; 93:1055.

Lang E: Comparison of dynamic and conventional computed tomography, angiography and ultrasonography in the staging of renal cell carcinoma. Cancer 1984; 54:2205.

Lang EK: Roentgenographic assessment of asymptomatic renal lesions. Radiology 1973; 109:257.

Lang EK: Asymptomatic space occupying lesions of the kidney: A programmed sequential approach and its impact on quality and cost of health care. South Med J 1977; 70:277.

Latif F, Tory K, Gnarra J, et al: Identification of the von Hippel-Lindau disease tumor suppressor gene. Science 1993; 260:1317.

Lauritsen JG: Lindau's disease: A study of one family through six generations. Acta Chir Scand 1975; 139:482.

La Vecchia C, Negri E, D'Avanzo B, Franceschi S: Smoking and renal carcinoma. Cancer Res 1990; 50:5231.

Levine E, Huntrakoon M, Wetzel LH: Small renal neoplasms: Clinical, pathologic, and imaging findings. Am J Radiol 1989; 153:69.

Licht MR, Novick AC: Nephron sparing surgery for renal cell carcinoma. J Urol 1993; 149:1.

Licht MR, Novick AC, Tubbs RR, et al: Renal oncocytoma: Clinical and biological correlates. J Urol 1993; 150:1380.

Lieber MM: Renal oncocytoma. Urol Clin North Am 1993; 20:355.

Lindner A, Goldman DG, deKernion JB: Cost effective analysis of prenephrectomy radioisotope scans in renal cell carcinoma. Urology 1983; 22:566.

Linehan WM, Lerman MI, Zbar B: Identification of the VHL gene: Its role in renal carcinoma. JAMA 1995; 273:564–570.

Linehan WM, Robertson CN, Anglard P, et al: Clinical perspective-renal cell carcinoma: Potential biologic and molecular approaches to diagnosis and therapy. In Cancer Cells 7, Molecular Diagnostics of Human Cancer. Cold Spring Harbor Laboratory, 1989, p 59.

Maldazys JD, deKernion JB: Prognostic factors in metastatic renal carcinoma. J Urol 1986; 136:376.

Mangin M, Webb AC, Dreyer BE, et al: Identification of a cDNA encoding a parathyroid hormone–like peptide from a human tumor associated with humoral hypercalcemia of malignancy. Proc Natl Acad Sci USA 1988; 85:597.

Marcus SG, Choyke PL, Reiter R, et al: Regression of metastatic renal cell carcinoma after cytoreductive nephrectomy. J Urol 1993; 150:463.

Marshall F, Powell KC: Lymphadenectomy for renal cell carcinoma: Anatomical and therapeutic considerations. J Urol 1982; 128:677.

Marshall FF, Dietrick DD, Baumgartner WA, Reitz BA: Surgical management of renal cell carcinoma with intracaval neoplastic extension above the hepatic veins. J Urol 1988; 139:116.

Marshall FF, Holdford SS, Hamper UM: Intraoperative sonography of renal tumors. J Urol 1992; 148:1393.

Marshall FF, Reitz BA, Diamond DA: New technique for management of renal cell carcinoma involving right atrium: Hypothermia and cardiac arrest. J Urol 1984; 131:103.

Marshall FF, Taxy JB, Fishman EK, Chang R: The feasibility of surgical enucleation for renal cell carcinoma. J Urol 1986; 135:231.

Marshall ME, Mendelsohn L, Butler K, et al: Treatment of metastatic renal cell carcinoma with coumarin (1,2-benzopyrone) and cimetidine: A pilot study. J Clin Oncol 1987; 6:682.

McCullough DL, Scott R Jr, Seybold HM: Renal angiomyelolipoma (hamartoma): Review of the literature and report of 7 cases. J Urol 1971; 105:32.

McCune CS, Schapira DV, Henshaw EC: Specific immunotherapy of advanced renal carcinoma: Evidence for the polyclonality of metastases. Cancer 1981; 47:1984.

McNichols DW, Segura JW, deWeerd JH: Renal cell carcinoma: Long-term survival and late recurrence. J Urol 1981; 126:17.

Medeiros LJ, Gelb AB, Weiss LM: Renal cell carcinoma: Prognostic significance of morphologic parameters in 121 cases. Cancer 1988; 61:1639.

Mickisch GH, Kossig J, Keilhauer G, et al: Effects of calcium antagonists in multidrug resistant primary human renal cell carcinomas. Cancer Res 1990a; 50:3570.

Mickisch GH, Roehrich K, Koessig J, et al: Mechanisms and modulation of multidrug resistance in primary human renal cell carcinoma. J Urol 1990b; 144:744.

Micolonghi TS, Liang D, Schwartz S: Primary osteogenic sarcoma of the kidney. J Urol 1984; 131:1164.

Middleton RG: Surgery for metastatic renal cell carcinoma. J Urol 1967; 97:973.

Minasian LM, Motzer RJ, Gluck L, et al: Interferon alfa-2A in advanced renal cell carcinoma: Treatment results and survival in 159 patients with long term follow up. J Clin Oncol 1993; 7:1368.

Minton JP, Pennline K, Nawrocki JF, et al: Immunotherapy of human kidney cancer. (Abstract C-258.) Proc Am Assoc Cancer Res Am Soc Clin Oncol 1976; 17:301.

Moertel CG, Dockerty MB, Baggenstoss AH: Multiple primary multiple malignant neoplasms: III. Tumors of multicentric origin. Cancer 1961; 14:238.

Montie JE, Bukowski RM, James RE, et al: A critical review of immunotherapy of disseminated renal adenocarcinoma. J Surg Oncol 1982; 21:5.

Montie JE, Stewart BH, Straffon RA, et al: The role of adjunctive nephrectomy in patients with metastatic renal cell carcinoma. J Urol 1977; 117:272–275.

Moon TD, Dexter DF, Morales A: Synchronous independent primary osteosarcoma and adenocarcinoma of the kidney. Urology 1983; 21:608.

Morales A, Wilson JL, Pater JL, Loeb M: Cytoreductive surgery and systemic bacillus Calmette-Guérin therapy in metastatic renal cancer: A phase II trial. J Urol 1982; 127:230.

Morgan DA, Ruscetti FW, Gallo RG: Selective in vitro growth of T lymphocytes from normal human bone marrows. Science 1976; 193:1007.

Morgan WR, Zincke H: Progression and survival after renal conserving surgery for renal cell carcinoma: Experience in 104 patients and extended follow up. J Urol 1990; 144:852.

Moscow JA, Cowan KH: Multidrug resistance. J Natl Cancer Inst 1988; 80:14.

Mostofi FK, Sesterhenn IA, Davis CJ: Benign tumors of the kidney. In Schroder FH, Kurth KH, Splinter TAW, et al, eds: EORTC Genitourinary Group Monographs: 5. Progress and Controversies in Oncological Urology II. New York, Alan R. Liss, 1988, p 329.

Murphy GP, Mostofi FK: Histologic assessment and clinical prognosis of renal adenoma. J Urol 1970; 103:31.

Murphy WM: Diseases of the kidney. In Urological Pathology. Philadelphia, W. B. Saunders, 1989, p 409.

Muss HB, Costanzi JJ, Leavitt R, et al: Recombinant interferon alpha in renal cell carcinoma: A randomized trial of two routes of administration. J Clin Oncol 1987; 5:286.

Mydlo JH, Michaeli J, Cordon-Cardo C, et al: Expression of transforming growth factor α and epidermal growth factor receptor messenger RNA in neoplastic and nonneoplastic human kidney tissue. Cancer Res 1989; 49:3407.

Myers GH, Fehrenbaker LG, Kellais PP: Prognostic significance of renal vein invasion by hypernephroma. J Urol 1968; 100:420–423.

Newhouse JH: The radiologic evaluation of the patient with renal cancer. Urol Clin North Am 1993; 20:231.

Niceta T, Lavengood RW Jr, Fernandes M: Leiomyosarcoma of kidney. Review of the literature. Urology 1974; 3:270.

Nogueira E, Bannasch P: Cellular origin of rat renal oncocytoma. Lab Invest 1988; 59:337.

Novick AC: Renal-sparing surgery for renal cell carcinoma. Urol Clin North Am 1993; 20:277.

Novick AC: Current surgical approaches, nephron-sparing surgery, and the role of surgery in the integrated immunologic approach to renal cell carcinoma. Semin Oncol 1995; 22:29.

Novick AC, Kaye MC, Cosgrove DM, et al: Experience with cardiopulmonary bypass and deep hypothermic circulatory arrest in the management of retroperitoneal tumors with large vena caval thrombi. Ann Surg 1990; 212:472.

Novick AC, Zincke H, Neaves RJ, Topley HM: Surgical enucleation for renal cell carcinoma. J Urol 1986; 135:235.

O'Dea MJ, Zincke H, Utz DC, Bernatz PE: The treatment of renal cell carcinoma with solitary metastases. J Urol 1978; 120:540.

Oesterling JE, Fishman EK, Goldman SM, Marshall FF: The management of renal angiomyolipoma. J Urol 1986; 135:1121.

Oka H, Chatani Y, Hoshino R, et al: Constitutive activation of mitogen activated protein (MAP) kinases in human renal cell carcinoma. Cancer Res 1995; 55:4182.

Oliver RTD: Surveillance as a possible option for management of metastatic renal cell carcinoma. Semin Urol 1989; 7:149.

Olsson CA: Pulmonary cancer metastatic to the kidney: A common renal neoplasm. J Urol 1971; 105:492.

Ordonez NG, Bracken RB, Strohlein KB: Hemangiopericytoma of the kidney. Urology 1982; 20:191.

Orjauvik OS, Aas M, Fauchald P, et al: Renin-secreting renal tumor with severe hypertension. Acta Med Scand 1975; 197:329.

Osamura RY, Watanabe K, Yoneyama L, Hayashi T: Malignant fibrous histiocytoma of the renal capsule: Light and electron microscopic study of a rare tumor. Virchows Arch [A] 1978; 380:377.

O'Toole KM, Brown M, Hoffmann P: Pathology of benign and malignant kidney tumors. Urol Clin North Am 1993; 20:193.

Parkinson DR: Interleukin-2: Further progress through greater understanding. J Natl Cancer Inst 1990; 82:1374.

Parkinson DR, Sznol M: High-dose interleukin-2 in the therapy of metastatic renal-cell carcinoma. Semin Oncol 1995; 22:61.

Patel NP, Lavengood RW: Renal cell carcinoma: Natural history and results of treatment. J Urol 1978; 119:722.

Pavelic K, Popovic M: Insulin and glucagon secretion by renal adenocarcinoma. Cancer 1981; 48:98.

Peeling WB, Martell B, Shepheard BG: Postoperative irradiation in the treatment of renal cell carcinoma. Br J Urol 1969; 41:23.

Peters P: The role of lymphadenectomy in the management of renal cell carcinoma. Urol Clin North Am 1980; 7:705.

Pfeiffer GE, Gandin MM: Massive perirenal lipoma with report of a case. J Urol 1946; 56:12.

Pierce WC, Belldegrun A, Figlin RA: Cellular therapy: Scientific rationale and clinical results in the treatment of metastatic renal cell carcinoma. Semin Oncol 1995; 22:74.

Pizzocaro G, Piva L: Pros and cons of retroperitoneal lymphadenectomy in operable renal cell carcinoma. Eur Urol 1990; 18(suppl):22.

Pollack HM, Banner MP, Amendola MA: Other malignant neoplasms of the renal parenchyma. Semin Roentgenol 1987; 22:260.

Presti JC, Rao PH, Chen Q, et al: Histopathological, cytogenetic, and molecular characterization of renal cortical tumors. Cancer Res 1991; 51:1544.

Quesada JR, Swanson DA, Trinidade A, et al: Renal cell carcinoma: Antitumor effects of leukocyte interferon. Cancer Res 1983; 43:940.

Quint LE, Glazer GM, Chenevert TL, et al: In vivo and in vitro MR imaging of renal tumors: Histopathologic correlation and pulse sequence optimization. Radiology 1988; 169:359.

Raghavaiah NV, Mayer RF, Hagitt R, Soloway MS: Malignant fibrous histiocytoma of the kidney. J Urol 1980; 123:951.

Rainwater LM, Farrow GM, Hay ID, Lieber MM: Oncocytic tumors of the salivary gland, kidney, and thyroid: Nuclear DNA patterns studied by flow cytometry. Br J Cancer 1986a; 53:799.

Rainwater LM, Farrow GM, Lieber MM: Flow cytometry of renal oncocytoma: Common occurrence of deoxyribonucleic acid polyploidy and aneuploidy. J Urol 1986b; 135:1167.

Rainwater LM, Hosaka Y, Farrow GM, Lieber MW: Well-differentiated clear cell renal carcinoma: Significance of nuclear deoxyribonucleic acid patterns studied by flow cytometry. J Urol 1987; 137:15.

Ramming KP, deKernion JB: Immune RNA therapy for renal cell carcinoma: Survival and immunologic monitoring. Ann Surg 1977; 186:459.

Rao MS, Lotuaco LG, McGregor DH: Carcinosarcoma of the adult kidney. Postgrad Med J 1977; 53:408.

Richie EW: The place of radiotherapy in the management of parenchymal carcinoma. J Urol 1966; 95:313.

Richie JP, Garnick MB, Seltzer S, Bettman MA: Computerized tomography scan for diagnosis and staging of renal cell carcinoma. J Urol 1983; 129:1114.

Richie JP, Wang BS, Steele GD Jr, et al: In vivo and in vitro effects of xenogeneic immune ribonucleic acid in patients with advanced renal cell carcinoma: A phase I study. J Urol 1981; 126:24.

Robertson DN, Linehan WM, Pass HI, et al: Preparative cytoreductive surgery in patients with metastatic renal cell carcinoma treated with adoptive immunotherapy with interleukin-2 or interleukin-2 plus lymphokine activated killer cells. J Urol 1990; 144:614.

Robertson PW, Klidjiian A, Harding LK, et al: Hypertension due to a renin-secreting renal tumor. Am J Med 1967; 43:963.

Robertson TD, Hand JR: Primary intrarenal lipoma of surgical significance. J Urol 1941; 46:458.

Robey EL, Schellhammer PF: The adrenal gland and renal cell carcinoma: Is ipsilateral adrenalectomy a necessary component of radical nephrectomy? J Urol 1986; 135:453.

Robson CJ: Radical nephrectomy for renal cell carcinoma. J Urol 1963; 89:37.

Robson CJ, Churchill BM, Anderson W: The results of radical nephrectomy for renal cell carcinoma. Trans Am Assoc Genitourin Surg 1968; 60:122.

Rosenberg SA: Adoptive immunotherapy of cancer using lymphokine activated killer cells and recombinant interleukin-2. In DeVita VT, Hellman S, Rosenberg SA, eds: Important Advances in Oncology. Philadelphia, J. B. Lippincott, 1986, p 55.

Rosenberg SA: Immunotherapy of patients with advanced cancer using interleukin-2 alone or in combination with lymphokine activated killer cells. In DeVita VT, Hellman S, Rosenberg SA, eds: Important Advances in Oncology. Philadelphia, J. B. Lippincott, 1988a, p 217.

Rosenberg SA: Immunotherapy of cancer using interleukin-2: Current status and future prospects. Immunol Today 1988b; 9:58.

Rosenberg SA: Use of tumor-infiltrating lymphocytes and interleukin-2 in the immunotherapy of patients with metastatic melanoma: A preliminary report. N Engl J Med 1988c; 319:1676.

Rosenberg SA, Lotze MT, Muul LM, et al: Observations on the systemic administration of autologous lymphokine-activated killer cells and recombinant interleukin-2 to patients with metastatic cancer. N Engl J Med 1985; 313:1485.

Rosenberg SA, Spiess P, Lafreniere R: A new approach to the adoptive immunotherapy of cancer using tumor infiltrating lymphocytes. Science 1986; 233:1318.

Rosenberg SA, Yang JC, Topalian SL, et al: Treatment of 283 consecutive patients with metastatic melanoma or renal cell cancer using high-dose bolus interleukin-2. JAMA 1994; 271:907.

Saitoh H, Shimbo T, Wakabayashi T, et al: Metastases of renal sarcoma. Tokai J Exp Clin Med 1982; 7:365.

Sargent ER, Gomella LG, Wade TP, et al: Expression of mRNA for transforming growth factors-alpha and -beta and secretion of transforming growth factor-B in renal cell carcinoma cell lines. Cancer Commun 1989; 1:317.

Sarna G, Figlin R, deKernion J: Interferon in renal cell carcinoma: The UCLA experience. Cancer 1987; 59:610.

Sayers TJ, Wiltrout TA, McCormick K, et al: Antitumor effects of alpha-interferon and gamma-interferon on a murine renal cancer (Renca) in vitro and in vivo. Cancer Res 1990; 50:5414.

Schomburg A, Kirchner H, Fenner M, et al: Lack of therapeutic efficacy of tamoxifen in advanced renal cell carcinoma. Eur J Cancer 1993; 29A:737.

Scriven RR, Thrasher TV, Smith DC, Stewart SC: Primary renal malignant fibrous histiocytoma: A case report and literature review. J Urol 1984; 131:948.

Sella A, Zukiwski A, Robinson E, et al: Interleukin-2 with interferon-α and 5-fluorouracil in patients with metastatic renal cell cancer. (Abstract.) Proc Am Soc Clin Oncol 1994; 13:237.

Selli C, Hinshaw WM, Woodard BH, Paulson DF: Stratification of risk factors in renal cell carcinoma. Cancer 1983; 52:899.

Shirkhoda A, Lewis E: Renal sarcoma and sarcomatoid renal carcinoma: CT and angiographic features. Radiology 1987; 162:353.

Silber SJ, Chang CY: Primary lymphoma of the kidney. J Urol 1973; 110:282.

Siminovitch JM, Montie JE, Straffon RA: Prognostic indicators in renal adenocarcinoma. J Urol 1983; 130:20.

Skinner DG, Pfister RF, Colvin R: Extension of renal cell carcinoma into the vena cava: The rationale for aggressive surgical management. J Urol 1972; 107:711.

Skinner DG, Rand Pritchett T, Lieskovsky G, et al: Vena caval involvement by renal cell carcinoma: Surgical resection provides meaningful long-term survival. Ann Surg 1989; 210:387.

Slamon DJ, deKernion JB, Verma IM, et al: Expression of cellular oncogenes in human malignancies. Science 1984; 224:256.

Smith RB, deKernion JB, Ehrlich RM, et al: Bilateral renal cell carcinoma and renal cell carcinoma in the solitary kidney. J Urol 1984; 132:450.

Smith SJ, Bosniak MA, Megibow AJ, et al: Renal cell carcinoma: Earlier discovery and increased detection. Radiology 1989; 170:699.

Smullens SN, Scotti D, Osterholm J, Weiss A: Preoperative embolization of retroperitoneal angiopericytomas as an aid in their removal. Proc Am Assoc Cancer Res 1979; 20:394.

Spencer WF, Linehan WM, Walther MM, et al: Immunotherapy with interleukin-2 and α-interferon in patients with metastatic renal cell cancer with in situ primary cancers: A pilot study. J Urol 1992; 147:24.

Spellman JE Jr, Driscoll DL, Huben RP: Primary renal sarcoma. Am Surgeon 1995; 61:456.

Stadler WM, Vogelzang NJ: Low-dose interleukin-2 in the treatment of metastatic renal-cell carcinoma. Semin Oncol 1995; 22:67.

Steele G Jr, Wang BS, Richie JP, et al: Results of oncogenic I-RNA therapy in patients with metastatic renal cell carcinoma. Cancer 1981; 47:1286.

Steiner MS, Goldman SM, Fishman EK, et al: The natural history of renal angiomyolipoma. J Urol 1993; 150:1782.

Stewart BH: Radical nephrectomy. *In* Stewart BH, ed: Operative Urology: The Kidney, Adrenal Gland and Retroperitoneum. Baltimore, Williams & Wilkins, 1975, p 114.

Stewart RR, Dunnick NR: Imaging renal neoplasms. Prob Urol 1990; 4:175.

Stillwell TJ, Gomez MR, Kelalis PP: Renal lesions in tuberous sclerosis. J Urol 1987; 138:477.

Sufrin G, Chasan S, Golio A, Murphy GP: Paraneoplastic and serologic syndromes of renal adenocarcinoma. Semin Urol 1989; 7:158.

Swanson DA, Johnson DE, von Eschenbach AC, et al: Angioinfarction plus nephrectomy for metastatic renal cell carcinoma—an update. J Urol 1983; 130:449.

Swierzewski DJ, Swierzewski MJ, Libertino JA: Radical nephrectomy in patients with renal cell carcinoma with venous, vena caval, and atrial extension. Am J Surg 1994; 168:205.

Taneja SS, Pierce W, Figlin R, Belldegrun A: Immunotherapy for renal cell carcinoma: The era of interleukin-2-based treatment. Urology 1995; 45:911.

Tannenbaum M: Ultrastructural pathology of human renal cell tumors. Pathol Annu 1971; 6:259.

Taylor RS, Joseph DB, Kohaut EC, et al: Renal angiomyolipoma associated with lymph node involvement and renal cell carcinoma in patients with tuberous sclerosis. J Urol 1989; 141:930.

Teyssier JR, Dozier HC, Ferre D, et al: Recurrent deletion of the short arm of chromosome 3 in human renal cell carcinoma: Shift of the c-*raf* 1 locus. J Natl Cancer Inst 1986; 7:1187.

Thoenes W, Storkel S, Rumpelt HJ, et al: Chromophobe cell renal carcinoma and its variants: A report on 32 cases. J Pathol 1988; 155:277.

Thompson IM, Peek M: Improvement in survival of patients with renal cell carcinoma: The role of the serendipitously detected tumor. J Urol 1988; 140:487.

Thrasher JB, Paulson DF: Prognostic factors in renal cancer. Urol Clin North Am 1993; 20:247.

Tomera KV, Farrow GM, Lieber MM: Sarcomatoid renal carcinoma. J Urol 1983; 130:657.

Topalian SL, Solomon D, Avis FP, et al: Immunotherapy of patients with advanced cancer using tumor infiltrating lymphocytes and recombinant interleukin-2: A pilot study. J Clin Oncol 1988; 6:839.

Topley M, Novick AC, Montie JE: Long-term results following partial nephrectomy for localized renal adenocarcinoma. Presented at the American Urologic Association Annual Meeting, Las Vegas, 1983.

Tsuruo T, Iida H, Kitatani Y, Tsukagoshi S: Effects of quinidine and related compounds on cytotoxicity and cellular accumulation of vincristine and adriamycin in drug-resistant tumor cells. Cancer Res 1984; 44:4303.

Umeda T, Niijima T: Phase II study of alpha interferon on renal cell carcinoma. Cancer 1986; 58:1231.

van der Werf-Messing B: Carcinoma of the kidney. Cancer 1973; 32:1056.

Vogelzang NJ, Fremgen AM, Guinan PD, et al: Primary renal sarcoma in adults: A natural history and management study by the American Cancer Society, Illinois division. Cancer 1993; 71:804.

Vugrin D, Hood L, Laszlo J: A phase II trial of high-dose human lymphoblastoid alpha interferon in patients with advanced renal carcinoma. J Biol Response Mod 1986; 5:309.

Wallace AC, Nairn RC: Renal tubular antigens in kidney tumors. Cancer 1972; 29:977.

Walther MM, Alexander RB, Weiss GH, et al: Cytoreductive surgery prior to interleukin-2–based therapy in patients with metastatic renal cell carcinoma. Urology 1993; 42:250.

Walther PJ, Marks LS, Stern D, Smith RB: Renal metastasis of adenocarcinoma of the lung: Massive hematuria managed by therapeutic embolization. J Urol 1979, 122:398.

Warfel KA, Eble JN: Renal oncocytomatosis. J Urol 1982; 127:1179.

Weichselbaum A, Greenish RW: Pasadenome der Neire. Med Jahrb Vien Vol 213, 1883.

Weidner U, Peter S, Strohmeyer T, et al: Inverse relationship of epidermal growth factor receptor and HER2/neu gene expression in human renal cell carcinoma. Cancer Res 1990; 50:4504.

Weir JM, Dunn JE Jr: Smoking and mortality: A prospective study. Cancer 1970; 25:105.

Weiss JP, Pollack HM, McCormick JF, et al: Renal hemangiopericytoma: Surgical, radiological and pathological implications. J Urol 1984; 132:337.

Weiss LM, Gelb AB, Medeiros J: Adult renal epithelial neoplasms. Am J Clin Pathol 1995; 103:624.

Wenz W: Tumors of the kidney following retrograde pyelography with colloidal thorium diozide. Ann NY Acad Sci 1967; 145:806.

Wickham JEA: Conservative renal surgery for adenocarcinoma: The place of bench surgery. Br J Urol 1975; 47:25.

Wingo PA, Tong T, Bolden S: Cancer statistics. CA 1995; 45:8.

Wolff J: Die Lehre von der Krebskronsheit: Von den altesten Zeiten bis zur Gagenwart. *In* Adenome der Neire. Med Jahrb Vien Vol 213, 1883.

Yagoda A, Abi-Rached B, Petrylak D: Chemotherapy for advanced renal cell carcinoma: 1983–1993. Semin Oncol 1995; 22:42.

Yao M, Shuin T, Misaki H, et al: Enhanced expression of c-*myc* and epidermal growth factor receptor (c-*erb*B-1) genes in primary human renal cancer. Cancer Res 1988; 48:6753.

Zbar B, Brauch H, Talmadge C, Linehan M: Loss of alleles of loci on the short arm of chromosome 3 in renal cell carcinoma. Nature 1987; 327:721.

Zerban H, Nogueira E, Riedasch G, Bannasch P: Renal oncocytoma: Origin from the collecting duct. Virchows Arch 1987; 52:375.

77
UROTHELIAL TUMORS OF THE URINARY TRACT

Edward M. Messing, M.D.
William Catalona, M.D.

BLADDER CANCER

Bladder cancer is one of the most common diseases treated by urologists. Most bladder cancers are transitional cell carcinomas. These tumors exhibit the entire spectrum of biologic aggressiveness, from benign-behaving, superficial low-grade papillary lesions to highly malignant anaplastic carcinomas. **In practice, however, transitional cell carcinomas tend to occur in two principal forms: low-grade superficial and high-grade invasive cancers.**

BASIC AND CLINICAL BIOLOGY

Although epidemiologic and experimental lines of evidence favor a strong role for chemical carcinogens in the etiology of bladder cancer, many cases arise with no obvious exposure to known carcinogens. It is likely that all malignancies involve aberrations of normal mechanisms regulating cell differentiation and proliferation, often with derangements in the genetic composition of malignant cells. For the overwhelming majority of human malignancies, particularly those arising in middle age or later life, such as bladder cancer, these acquired alterations in DNA often lead to either the induction of oncogenes or the negation of tumor suppressor genes, resulting in a malignantly transformed cell. The effects of the inducing agents, be they viruses, chemical carcinogens, or other chemical or physical stimuli (such as ultraviolet light or radiation), often result from the direct exposure of host cells to these agents. Inherited, acquired, and anatomic factors, however, including those that regulate processes such as metabolism of chemicals and the excretion and delivery of metabolites to potential target cells, help determine which individuals with similar exposures develop malignancies and in which sites. Additionally, because mechanisms usually exist in all cells to repair mutated or miscopied DNA or to effect the death of those cells that contain such altered DNA, escape from such safeguard mechanisms must occur in most, if not all, malignancies. Undoubtedly, all of these influences play important roles in determining who develops bladder cancer.

Bladder cancer often behaves as a field change disease in which the entire urothelium from the renal pelvis to the urethra is susceptible to malignant transformation. The multiple occurrences and reoccurrences of urothelial tumors that are treated by local resection typify this tendency. **Transitional carcinoma cells, however, can also implant and probably migrate to other sites of the urothelium, thus making it difficult to determine whether a recurrent tumor represents an inadequately treated initial one, tumor implantation or migration, or the effects of multifocal carcinogenesis.** Based on data that are presented later, it is likely that all of these factors are important.

EPIDEMIOLOGY

Incidence and Prevalence—Gender and Race

The *incidence* rate of a cancer is defined as the number of new cases diagnosed per 100,000 persons per year. The bladder is the most common site of cancer in the urinary tract. **It is estimated that in 1995, 50,500 new cases of bladder cancer were diagnosed in the United States** (Boring et al, 1995). **Bladder cancer is nearly three times more common among men than women** (Boring et al, 1995). In men, it is the fourth most common cancer after prostate, lung, and colorectal cancer, accounting for 5.5% of all cancer cases (Boring et al, 1995). In women, it is the eighth most common cancer, accounting for 2.3% of all cancers. **Between 1984 and 1993, the number of bladder cancers diagnosed annually in the United States increased by nearly 36% but the increase in new cases was actually 50% higher in men than in women during this interval** (Silverberg, 1985; Miller et al, 1992; Boring et al, 1993).

Because bladder cancer has rarely been found incidentally at autopsy (Marshall, 1956; Resseguie et al, 1978; Kishi et al, 1981), and because the means by which it is diagnosed (cystoscopic inspection and biopsy) have remained constant over the last six decades, one cannot attribute the increased incidence of bladder cancer to technologic innovations (e.g., new laboratory and imaging techniques, mechanical and

2330 UROTHELIAL TUMORS OF THE URINARY TRACT

systematic biopsy methods, needle and cytologic aspiration diagnoses) or changes in health care practice (e.g., organized or ad-lib screening) that may well explain similar or even more dramatic increases in reported incidences of prostatic and breast carcinomas (Silverberg, 1995; Boring et al, 1995). Also, because bladder cancer incidence increases with age in both genders (see later), the greater rise in incidence cases in men seems contrary to what one would expect in view of the longer female life expectancy (roughly 5 years) (National Center for Health Statistics, 1991). **Indeed, for the last 5 years reported (1985–1989), bladder cancer in women had a declining age-adjusted incidence of nearly 2% annually, whereas that in men is rising** (during the same interval, there has been less than a 0.005% increase in average life expectancy in either gender) (National Center for Health Statistics, 1991). **This discrepancy between the genders in the number of new cases of bladder cancer remains particularly surprising because during the past 30 years, women have joined the male workplace and have changed habits that have exposed them to both industrial and environmental carcinogens (such as cigarette smoking) from which they had previously been excluded.** It is possible that genetic (Risch et al, 1995), hormonal (Horn et al, 1995), anatomic (e.g., relative urinary retention in older men because of prostatic enlargement), or other factors may explain this puzzling trend.

Bladder cancer is roughly two times as common among American white men as among black men (Annual Cancer Statistics Review, 1987) **and is only roughly 1.5 times more common among white women than among black women.** There is some evidence that this increased risk in whites is primarily limited to noninvasive cancers (Schairer et al, 1988), implying a later diagnosis of tumors in blacks. Genetic and epidemiologic evidence indicates, however, that blacks may have a more aggressive form of other malignancies such as breast cancer (Shiao et al, 1995), and if this were occurring with bladder cancer, **it might manifest itself as a more advanced stage at presentation, which does occur** (Lynch and Cohen, 1995).

Prevalence is the total number of cancer cases present per 100,000 persons. Because so many patients with bladder cancer experience recurrences but do not die from the disease (see later), **although bladder cancer is only the fourth most common cancer in terms of incidence in American men, it is the second most prevalent malignancy in middle-aged and elderly men (to prostate cancer)** (Feldman et al, 1986).

Mortality—Gender and Race

The *mortality* rate of a cancer is the number of deaths occurring per 100,000 persons per year. **It is estimated that in 1995 there were 11,200 bladder cancer deaths, including 7500 men and 3700 women** (Boring et al, 1995), **making bladder cancer the fifth most common cause of cancer deaths in men.** Bladder cancer accounts for 2.6% of all cancer deaths in men and 1.4% in women. **Men have higher 5-year survival rates than women, with this difference in mortality being particularly impressive in black women (white men, 84%; black men, 71%; white women, 76%; black women, 51% 5-year survival rates)** (Lynch

and Cohen, 1995). **A substantial reason for lower survival rates in blacks of both genders is the lower percentage of black men (65.6%) and black women (56.4%) compared with white men (75.7%) and white women (74.3%) diagnosed with transitional cell carcinoma who have disease confined to the bladder** (Lynch and Cohen, 1995). Factors that may lead to more advanced stage at diagnosis in blacks, particularly black women, include a possible underreporting of superficial cancers, delayed diagnosis, or a more frequent occurrence of more aggressive variants of transitional cell carcinoma in blacks. Insufficient evidence is available to distinguish between these possibilities, although the first is unlikely because of the rarity with which this malignancy goes undiagnosed during life (see later).

Survival by stage at presentation is also more favorable for whites. This may reflect not only more advanced or more aggressive disease within stage categories at diagnosis but also less adequate access to or acceptance of optimal therapies in the black population. The poorer outcome for black Americans again is most extremely manifested **in muscle-invasive disease, with 5-year survival rates of all blacks being less than half that of whites** (Mayer and McWhorter, 1989; Lynch and Cohen, 1995). Finally, although the vast majority of bladder cancers in both genders and races are transitional cell carcinomas, a higher proportion of bladder cancers other than transitional cell carcinomas (primarily squamous cell carcinomas and adenocarcinomas) occurs in blacks (and women), and the relatively poor outcomes from these tumors may explain some of the racial differences in bladder cancer mortality as well.

Since the 1950s, the incidence of bladder cancer has risen for an overall increase of approximately 50% (Annual Cancer Statistics Review, 1987). It is to be anticipated that, with aging of the U.S. population, this trend will continue (see later). **In comparison, there has been a decrease in mortality rate from bladder cancer during this same interval, for an overall decrease of approximately 33%** (Annual Cancer Statistics Review, 1987). Whether this decrease is attributable to a fundamental change in the biology of this disease, alteration in risk factors for different phenotypic variants, better treatments, earlier diagnoses, or a combination of these factors is uncertain. **The reduction in mortality, however, has been achieved primarily in men.** Whether one looks simply at the total number of deaths from this disease annually (11.0% fewer deaths in men and 0.0% in women between 1984 and 1993), the ratio of annual deaths per newly diagnosed cases (0.261 in men in 1984 and 0.166 in 1993 versus 0.324 for women in 1984 and 0.255 in 1993), or the 5-year survival rates previously mentioned, it would appear that women account for a disproportionately high percentage of lives lost from this disease (Silverberg, 1985; Boring et al, 1993). **This is confirmed by the relatively striking reduction in age-adjusted mortality from bladder cancer for the most recent 5 years reported (1985–1989) with more than twice the annual rate reduction in men (−1.3% change annually) than in women (−0.6% change annually)** (Miller et al, 1992). **These age-adjusted trends as well as the greater increase in bladder cancer incidence in men compared with women (see section on incidence) suggest that differences in bladder cancer diagnosis, treatment, or disease characteristics between the sexes, rather than the longer female life**

expectancy, explain the roughly 50% higher mortality from this disease in women.

Age

Bladder cancer can occur at any age—even in children. It is generally a disease of the middle-aged and elderly, **however, with the median ages at diagnosis for transitional cell carcinoma being 69.0 for men and 71.0 for women** (Lynch and Cohen, 1995). **Moreover, the incidence of bladder cancer increases directly with age**—from roughly 130 per 100,000 men and 35 per 100,000 women age 65 to 69 years to 285 per 100,000 and 67 per 100,000 in 85-year-old and older men and women, respectively. Relatively similar trends are found for squamous carcinomas. **Mortality from bladder cancer is also higher in the elderly.** For instance, the ratio of disease-related mortality to incidence rates for Wisconsin men and women age 65 to 70 years is 16% and 24%, whereas that for men and women age 80 and older is 40% and 60% (Cancer in Wisconsin—1992, 1994). Again, whether this increase represents a more aggressive variant of the disease in the elderly, a relatively advanced stage at diagnosis (for both social [patient- and medical provider–driven] and biologic [such as impaired host defenses in the elderly] reasons), or the offering and selection of less aggressive (or successful) therapies in the elderly is uncertain, but probably the increase in mortality is due to a combination of these factors.

In adolescents and adults younger than age 30, bladder cancers tend to express well-differentiated histologies and behave in a more indolent fashion (Benson et al, 1983b). Younger patients appear to have a more favorable prognosis because they present more frequently with superficial low-grade tumors; **however, the risk for disease progression is the same, grade for grade, in younger patients and in older ones** (Wan and Grossman, 1989). As a general rule, patients should be treated on the basis of tumor stage and grade regardless of age (Kurz et al, 1987), although patient comorbidity and other factors obviously influence this decision, particularly in the elderly.

Regional and National Differences

Although the incidence of bladder cancer has been reported to be somewhat higher in the North of the United States than in the South (Cutler and Young, 1975; Morrison, 1984), owing to migrations of elderly populations to the Sun Belt, the incidence is becoming more obscured. Incidence in different countries also differs considerably, with higher rates in Great Britain and the United States than in Japan and Finland (Morrison, 1984). In Hawaii, the incidence is more than twice as high in whites as in those of Japanese descent (Waterhouse et al, 1982). These differences probably reflect combined effects of environmental and hereditary factors.

In the United States, the national Surveillance, Epidemiology, and End Result (SEER) database has provided much of the background information for many epidemiologic studies—particularly in describing trends in incidence and mortality from cancers arising in different sites in different populations. **Unfortunately, in terms of SEER data, blad-**

der cancer has specifically been recognized as having several classification problems that have resulted in confused reporting of in situ, invasive, and papillary and nonpapillary tumors, and there has been no conformation with commonly used grading and staging systems (Lynch et al, 1991). **Because of these problems, distinguishing the influences of biologic, social/economic, and environmental factors in explaining differences in incidence and prognosis of this disease in various age, racial, gender, and demographic groups has been exceedingly difficult to do (as is even defining these differences).** Fortunately a concerted effort is now underway to try to clarify the observed higher mortality in blacks (Howard et al, 1992), which includes actual central pathology review, medical record abstracts, and gathering of risk and exposure information. It is hoped that similar approaches may also be able to decipher intriguing differences in survival among genders, geographic locales, and age groups.

Autopsy Data

In contrast to virtually all other common malignancies, bladder cancer has almost never been reported as an incidental finding at autopsy (Marshall, 1956; Resseguie et al, 1978; Kishi et al, 1981). This is distinctly different from carcinomas of the prostate (Franks, 1954), kidney (Hellstein et al, 1981), and many other sites, in which autopsy cancers actually occur more commonly than the clinically diagnosed entity. Although, in part, this observation may be explained by postmortem urothelial autolysis or erosive effects of indwelling catheters, which might obscure the identification of small malignancies, and is at odds with the occasional experience in which incidental bladder tumors are found during cystoscopic examination for other diseases (Bruskewitz, 1992; Kim and Ignatoff, 1994), **it remains a remarkable observation. It implies that at some point before demise virtually everyone with bladder cancer has the disease diagnosed. Furthermore, it implies that reported differences in incidence rates among people of different genders, races, ages, and locales cannot be explained simply by a failure to diagnose the disease in particular groups. Finally, it implies that the preclinical latency of this tumor (the time between when it is large enough to be seen cystoscopically [or at autopsy] and the time when it actually is symptomatic) must be relatively brief.** The implications of this brief preclinical latency in terms of early detection strategies, including their potential advantages or disadvantages and how often they should be repeated, are considerable (see later).

ETIOLOGY AND RISK FACTORS

Basic Biology

Factors reported to be causally related to bladder cancer's development and progression include occupational exposure to chemicals; cigarette smoking; coffee drinking; ingestion of analgesics or artificial sweeteners; bacterial, parasitic, and viral infections; bladder calculi; and genotoxic chemotherapeutic agents. Data suggest that at least some bladder cancers are carcinogen induced. Carcinogens produce lesions in the DNA of target cells (in this case, the transitional epithelial cells), both initiating and propagating the process of tumorigenesis. It is likely that multiple lesions are required to cause malignant transformation of cells. In experimental systems, classic chemical carcinogenesis may be divided into three processes: *initiation,* in which an irreversible genetic change(s) in stem cells occurs that alone is insufficient to induce and maintain expression of the malignant phenotype; *promotion,* which must follow initiation and induces, either directly or indirectly (Cohen and Elwein, 1991a, 1991b), enough additional genetic changes to effect expression of the malignant phenotype; and *progression,* in which the transformed cells acquire the properties (through genetic and/or epigenetic changes) needed to induce further growth (requiring both mitogenesis and the establishment of a blood supply [angiogenesis]), permit tissue invasion (often through elaboration of basal lamina digesting enzymes and cellular motility), and encourage distant embolism and re-establishment of growth (metastases). In patients, as opposed to experimental systems, the distinctions between these three steps are often blurred. For example, abnormal sensitivity to either exogenous or endogenous mitogens can often not only induce tumor progression (see earlier) but also actually facilitate tumor promotion because further genetic changes are more likely to occur and be perpetuated with more rapid DNA synthesis when those mechanisms that regulate the cell cycle or direct cells with altered DNA to programmed death (apoptosis) are suppressed. Additionally, because the transitional epithelium's microenvironment may affect exposure or sensitivity to carcinogens and mitogens, it may facilitate the development of different genetic alterations to relatively similar chemical insults. Epidemiologic, molecular, and histopathologic evidence confirming that this is often the response to some of the best defined environmental carcinogens—cigarette smoke and industrial chemicals—is presented later.

Oncogenes

Despite these complexities, current oncologic research dictates that genetic changes must occur for malignant transformation to result. Several different potential mechanisms can account for these genetic changes. One involves the induction of oncogenes, altered normal genes that encode for the malignant phenotype, primarily by permitting cells to escape from normal mechanisms of growth control. Oncogenes that have been associated with bladder cancer include those of the ras gene family, including the p21 *ras* oncogene (Visvanathan et al, 1988; Meyers et al, 1989), which at least in some studies has been found to correlate with a higher histologic grade (Viola et al, 1985). Only about 10% of transitional cell carcinomas that have been tested, however, have been found to have ras mutations (Knowles and Williamson, 1993). Another oncogene is *c-myc,* which in different studies has been associated with increased recurrence or progression of superficial bladder cancer (Masters et al, 1988) and with increased tumor stage and grade (DelSenno et al, 1989). The major *c-myc* abnormality, hypomethylation, appears in the gene's flanking and promoting regions (DelSenno et al, 1989), which may ex-

plain its increased expression in most transitional cell cancers (Onodera and Yagihashi, 1995). Another nuclear early-response gene, *c-jun,* under certain circumstances can serve as an oncogene, presumably by coding for the major component of the transcription factor AP-L (Lamph et al, 1988), which plays a role in growth regulation. Tinakos and colleagues assessed *c-jun* expression immunohistochemically in specimens of transitional cell carcinoma and reported that its abnormal expression correlated with invasive stage and increased expression of the receptor for epidermal growth factor (EGF) (which, in turn, has ominous prognostic implications) (Messing, 1990; Tinakos et al, 1994; Mellon et al, 1995).

Tumor Suppressor Genes

Although oncogenes, because they have a positive dominant effect, are easier to detect, **an equally important molecular mechanism in the process of carcinogenesis is the inactivation of genes coding for proteins that regulate cell growth, DNA repair, or apoptosis. Deletions or inactivation of these so-called cancer suppressor genes could encourage unregulated growth or failure to direct DNA-damaged cells to programmed death, ultimately resulting in uncontrolled proliferation of genetically altered clones.** Such proliferation results in genetic instability with DNA copying errors appearing throughout affected cells' genomes. Because multiple short nucleotide sequence repeats are dispersed throughout the normal mammalian genome, searching for DNA replicatory errors in known multiple repeating sequences can be used as a means to screen for malignant cells (Mao et al, 1994), as well as a means of mapping deleted regions of DNA.

For a tumor to result from a suppressor gene alteration, the protein encoded by the gene (the gene product) must be nonfunctional. Hence, both alleles of the gene must be deleted, mutated, or both. Historically, this was most easily recognized by cytogenetic analysis, in which large chromosomal segments or entire chromosomes were missing from karyotypes. Additionally, even in the absence of large enough deletions to be identified cytogenetically, because many genes are polymorphic (i.e., the inherited maternal and paternal alleles differ slightly in genetic code), comparisons of DNA digests from malignant and normal tissues (in which both alleles are retained) can be used to identify deletions of one allele of a specific genetic region (loss of heterozygosity [LOH] of the alleles) in the malignant DNA. Presumably, mutations or small deletions render the product of the retained allele of the gene absent or nonfunctional. **For many of the chromosomal regions known to be deleted from human bladder cancer in a nonrandom fashion (and hence presumably providing the cell with some selective advantage), a suppressor gene has been located in the deleted region, and for several, molecular analysis on the retained gene copy has identified one or several mutations that could render its product nonfunctional or absent.**

Further confirmation of the functional significance of identified deletions and/or mutations of a putative suppressor gene has been done by demonstrating absent or abnormal expression of the gene with molecular studies such as Northern blotting, which uses labeled cDNA probes to detect specific RNA sequences in RNA digests run on gels, or amplification of RNA by converting it back to DNA with reverse transcriptase (RT) and then producing many copies of the newly constructed DNA by an ex vivo technique called polymerase chain reaction (PCR), eventually running the RT-PCR product on a gel and detecting it with a labeled complementary DNA probe. Similarly, proteins can be detected by immunoprecipitation or by immunoblotting a mixture of proteins run on gels with labeled antibodies to the protein of interest (Western blotting). Also, visual approaches (such as in situ hybridization, which anneals labeled c-DNA to specific sequences in tumor cell RNA, or immunohistochemistry) can be used to identify the gene's message (mRNA) or product (protein) in tissue sections.

Three suppressor gene loci have been most closely associated with bladder cancer. These include that of p53 (on chromosome 17p), the retinoblastoma gene (Rb gene) on chromosome 13q, and genes on chromosome 9, at least one of which is likely to be on 9p in region 9p21, where the genes for the p15 and p16 proteins reside.

p53

The p53 gene is the most frequently altered gene in human cancers (Vogelstein, 1990; Harris and Hollstein, 1993). The normal protein, wild type p53 (wt p53), has a variety of functions, including acting as a transcription factor (binds with promoter regions of genes that it induces the transcription of) that suppresses cell proliferation (Vogelstein, 1990) and directing DNA damaged cells toward apoptosis before DNA replication (S-phase of cell cycle) occurs (reviewed in Harris and Hollstein, 1993). Mutations in p53 that have been associated with cancers primarily cause alterations in two regions of the wt p53 molecule—either those that directly alter its DNA binding surface or those that affect its core structure—thus indirectly modifying the DNA binding surface (Cordon-Cardo, 1995). These structural alterations give further credence to the importance of transcriptional regulation as the major way in which wt p53 suppresses tumorigenesis. Crystallographic techniques can now to some degree predict how modifications in the genome will alter the p53 protein's structure and thus predict which mutations or deletions are likely to have functional consequences (Cordon-Cardo, 1995). Because of p53's function of directing cells with genetic abnormalities toward apoptosis, p53 mutations have been associated with genomic instability—and hence progressive development of further mutations (Harris and Hollstein, 1993). Thus, it is not surprising that bladder cancers with p53 abnormalities appear to behave more aggressively (Esrig et al, 1994; Cordon-Cardo, 1995).

Wt p53 normally lasts only briefly in the cell nucleus, whereas mutated forms often accumulate for longer times and hence are more easily detected by immunohistochemistry (Finlay et al, 1988). Several groups have closely correlated p53 accumulation in cell nuclei (immunohistochemical detectability) with genetic mutations in the p53 gene and have employed immunohistology as a fairly simple means of screening cancers to assess whether p53 is mutated. Unfortunately, some important mutations in the p53 gene result in expression of a sufficiently truncated form of the protein (or no protein) so that no nuclear overexpression is seen, a circumstance that is indistinguishable immunohistochemically from one in which wt p53 is expressed (Cordon-Cardo, 1995). Similarly, deletion of both alleles of the gene (homozygous deletion) is also not detectable immunohistochemically.

Retinoblastoma Gene, Its Product, and p16 and p15

The normal protein product of the Rb gene (pRb) is phosphorylated by several of the cyclin-dependent kinases, phosphorylating proteins residing in the cell nucleus, which drive various transitions of the cell cycle. **Phosphorylated pRb dissociates from another protein, the transcription factor E2F, to which it is normally complexed. This permits uncomplexed E2F to bind with promoting regions of several genes whose products induce cells to transit from G1 to S phase (Cordon-Cardo, 1995). Inactivation of pRb through genetic deletion or mutation, therefore, permits cells to go through the G1 → S checkpoint more easily, thus stimulating cell proliferation.**

Similarly, inhibitors of the cyclin-dependent kinases that phosphorylate pRb, dissociating it from E2F, themselves normally serve as regulators of the cell cycle. Such regulators include p15 and p16, proteins coded for on neighboring regions of chromosome 9p, which normally complex with cyclin-dependent kinases 4 and 6, inhibiting the phosphorylation of pRb. Alterations of p16 and p15 proteins thus would permit pRb to become phosphorylated, resulting in uncomplexed E2F driving the G1 → S transition and cellular proliferation. Hence, the presence of mutated or deleted genes coding for p15, p16, or pRb would be expected to result in uninhibited proliferation and perhaps malignant transformation. It is thus not surprising that these genes have all been noted to be bladder cancer suppressor genes.

This was initially demonstrated by nonrandom deletions of chromosomes 13q and 9 in bladder cancers (Vanni et al, 1987; Babu et al, 1989; Hopman et al, 1989; Atkin and Fox, 1990; Tsai et al, 1990) and subsequently confirmed by molecular studies. **Precise molecular analyses have been far more difficult to do for chromosome 9 than for 13q (Rb) or 17p (p53) because most often an entire chromosome is missing (Wheeless et al, 1994). Furthermore, rather than point mutations in the p15 or p16 genes on the retained copy of chromosome 9 (region 9p21), the entire gene regions (often of both p15 and p16) have been deleted (homozygous deletion),** which makes it impossible to detect an abnormality by amplifying malignant cells' DNA (by PCR) and probing with specific p15 or p16 gene sequences for any mutations (Cordon-Cardo, 1995; Williamson et al, 1995) (techniques that have worked successfully for identifying mutations of Rb, p53, and other suppressor genes). Additionally, several authors have data indicating that additional bladder cancer suppressor genes may be located on chromosome 9, including those in the 9q region (Tsai et al, 1990; Spruck et al, 1994; Lin et al, 1995).

Understanding of the normal functions of the products of suspected deleted genes, and particularly their roles in regulating cellular proliferation, has stimulated investigators to try to correlate identified deletions with the known differences in behaviors of the two major types of transitional cell carcinoma: low-grade papillary superficial tumors and high-grade cancers that rapidly become invasive and metastasize. **Through such correlations, several groups have now identified chromosome 9** (Tsai et al, 1990; Spruck et al, 1994) **and p15, p16** (Orlow et al, 1995; Williamson et al, 1995) **deletions as a primary event in the development of low-grade superficial tumors. This would fit nicely with the reported function of p15 and p16 as regulators of cell proliferation because it is known that these malignancies grow quite rapidly (based on both clinical experience and the failure to find them incidentally at autopsy). Alternatively, high-grade cancers are much more commonly associated with p53 abnormalities and chromosome 17p deletions** (Spruck et al, 1994; Gruis et al, 1995). **This again would not be surprising because accumulated genetic errors expected in a cell with a nonfunctioning p53 protein encourage continued genetic instability and selection for aberrant (i.e., aggressive) behavior and anaplastic morphology.** Such abnormalities are beginning to be used to predict future tumor behavior (see later).

Although Rb deletions had initially been reported in primarily aggressive bladder cancers, this did not entirely agree with what is known about pRb's normal function of inhibiting the G1 → S transition of the cell cycle. Indeed, more recent studies correlating LOH analyses for the Rb gene (Ishikawa et al, 1991) with Western blotting (Ishikawa et al, 1991) or immunohistochemistry (Ishikawa et al, 1991; Presti et al, 1991) for pRb protein have reported that from as few as 7% (Ishikawa et al, 1991) to as many as 50% of low-grade and 80% of high-grade bladder tumors (Presti et al, 1991) have abnormal Rb expression. The role or roles of this protein either in the initiation of bladder cancer or in its subsequent progression remain less certain than those of the other two.

Amplification and Overexpression

A third type of carcinogenic genetic mechanism is amplification or overexpression of normal genes that encode for growth factors or their receptors. Messing and Neal and their respective co-workers have independently shown that abnormal expression of the receptor for EGF occurs in bladder cancer cells, and increased expression is associated with more aggressive biologic behavior (Neal et al, 1985; Messing et al, 1987a; Messing, 1990; Neal et al, 1990; Mellon et al, 1995). Because the major ligand for this receptor, EGF, is excreted in urine in high quantities in biologically active forms (Hirata and Orth, 1979; Fuse et al, 1992; Messing and Murphy-Brooks, 1994), abnormally high expression of the EGF receptor may be an example of a cell taking advantage of its unique environment to provide it with a growth advantage. The gene for the EGF receptor is located on chromosome 7, and trisomy 7 is also associated with bladder cancer, particularly with more aggressive disease (Sandberg, 1986; Waldman et al, 1991). Whether these two observations are related is uncertain because even when the protein is overexpressed, amplification of the EGF gene

has not commonly been seen in bladder cancer (Neal et al, 1989).

Alterations in the erbB-2 oncogene, which codes for a growth factor receptor that is functionally and at times anatomically related to that for EGF, have also been associated with a variety of malignancies including bladder cancer (Wright et al, 1991; Swanson et al, 1992; Ding-Wei et al, 1993; Sauter et al, 1993). Sauter and associates found overexpression of the erbB-2 product, p185, in 61 of 141 bladder cancers, but in only 10 of these was amplification of the gene also encountered (Sauter et al, 1993). Ding-Wei and colleagues found 33% of 56 bladder tumors had increased expression of p185 by immunohistochemical detection, which correlated with higher grade, higher stage, and tumor recurrence (Ding-Wei et al, 1993). Not all authors (Wright et al, 1991), however, have found a significant correlation between p185 expression and aggressive bladder cancer behavior. **To date, no specific gene's amplification has been easily correlated with clinical bladder cancers, although abnormal expression of several genes has been.**

Occupational Exposure

Aniline dyes, introduced in the late 1800s to color fabrics, are urothelial carcinogens (Rehn, 1895). Other carcinogens for bladder cancer include the chemicals 2-naphthylamine,4-aminobiphenyl,4-nitrobiphenyl,4-4-diaminobiphenyl (benzidine) and 2-amino-1-naphthol (Morrison and Cole, 1976); combustion gases and soot from coal; possibly chlorinated aliphatic hydrocarbons (Steinbeck et al, 1990); and certain aldehydes such as acrolein, used in chemical dyes and in the rubber and textile industries (Stadler, 1993). **It has been estimated in the past that occupational exposure accounts for roughly 20% of bladder cancer cases in the United States** (Cole et al, 1972), **with long latent periods being typical (i.e., 30–50 years).** This is probably related to cumulative dose, however, and with more intensive exposures, the latent period may well be shortened (Case et al, 1954).

Most bladder carcinogens are aromatic amines. Other potential sources of such compounds are dietary nitrites and nitrates that are acted on by intestinal bacterial flora (Chapman et al, 1981). Also, the metabolites of the amino acid tryptophan have been reported, but not proven, to be potentially carcinogenic. Occupations reported to be associated with an increased risk of bladder cancer include those of autoworkers, painters, truck drivers, drill press operators, leather workers, metal workers, and machinists as well as those that involve organic chemicals such as dry cleaners, paper manufacturers, rope and twine makers, dental technicians, barbers and beauticians, physicians, workers in apparel manufacturing, and plumbers (Morrison, 1984; Malker et al, 1987; Silverman et al, 1989a, 1989b).

Cigarette Smoking

Cigarette smokers have up to a fourfold higher incidence of bladder cancer than nonsmokers (Morrison, 1984; Burch et al, 1989; Clavel et al, 1989). **The risk correlates with the number of cigarettes smoked, the duration of smoking, and the degree of inhalation of the**

smoke. This risk has been observed in both sexes. **Former cigarette smokers have a somewhat reduced incidence of bladder cancer compared with active smokers** (Augustine et al, 1988). The reduction of this risk down to baseline (age adjusted), however, takes at least 20 years following cessation, a period far longer than the reduction of risks for cardiovascular disease and lung cancer takes after smoking has stopped. Other forms of tobacco use are associated with only a slightly higher risk for bladder cancer (Harge et al, 1985; Burch et al, 1989). Although it has been estimated that one third of bladder cancer cases may be related to cigarette smoking (Howe et al, 1980), this figure is clearly complicated by the knowledge that former smokers are also at risk and that the overwhelming majority of American men age 60 and over (who represent 65% to 70% of all patients who develop bladder cancer) have strong smoking histories (Morrison and Cole, 1976).

The specific chemical carcinogen responsible for bladder cancer in cigarette smoke has not been identified. Nitrosamines, 2-naphthylamine, and 4-aminobiphenyl are known to be present, and increased urinary tryptophan metabolites also have been demonstrated in cigarette smokers (Hoffman et al, 1969).

It has long been noted that individuals with seemingly equal exposures to environmental carcinogens (either through occupational exposure or smoking) vary enormously in their risks of developing bladder cancer. Considerable effort for assessing this has focused not only on obtaining precise information about exposures, but also on understanding mechanisms by which purported agents may be carcinogenic, how they reach the bladder, and how humans activate or detoxify them. **Much interest has focused on 4-aminobiphenyl primarily because it is in several industrial chemicals and cigarette smoke. Because acetylation of this agent initiates a detoxifying pathway, measurements of rapid and slow acetylation of substrates metabolized in a similar way to 4-aminobiphenyl, such as sulfamethazine or caffeine, with analysis of acetylated and unacetylated metabolites in urine and blood after a known period of ingestion of the test drug, have been correlated with risk.** Lower and co-workers showed that slow acetylators were more susceptible to developing bladder cancer (Lower et al, 1979). Similar findings have been reported in populations with industrial exposures (Cartwright et al, 1982; Hanke and Krajewska, 1990), although these results have not always been confirmed in studies using other populations, substrates, and techniques (Horai et al, 1989; Miller and Cosgriff, 1983). Complicating matters further is the knowledge that activating as well as detoxifying enzymes exist and that uroepithelial cells contain profiles of these enzymes that differ somewhat from those in the liver. Using a combination of in vitro culture techniques, tissue assays, and acetylator phenotyping, however, workers were able to demonstrate that the acetylator phenotypes in cultured urothelial cells and tissues correlated with those of the entire human being (Pink et al, 1992; Fredrickson et al, 1994).

Because *N*-acetyltransferase 2 (NAT2) appears to be the major acetylating enzyme, investigators have focused on its genetic composition. This is a polymorphic enzyme in which six genetic variants predominate in whites. Of these six alleles, only one produces an enzyme with rapid activity, and hence only individuals homozygous for two rapid alleles

are true rapid acetylators. **Using genetic analyses from white blood cells, Risch and colleagues were able to demonstrate that in bladder cancer patients with and without known industrial or smoking exposures (or both), slow acetylator genotypes predominated as compared to non–bladder cancer controls** (Risch et al, 1995).

In a separate analysis, **Horn and colleagues looked at the role of another enzyme, cytochrome P-450 1A2 (CYP 1A2), which is known to demethylate aromatic amines, thus activating potential carcinogens** (Horn et al, 1995). **As opposed to NAT2, CYP 1A2 is a highly inducible enzyme,** and common environmental chemicals such as caffeine are known inducers. A phenotypic assay of the amount of ^{13}C-labeled carbon dioxide ($^{13}CO_2$) exhaled after ingestion of a known amount of ^{13}C-caffeine (caffeine breath test) can be used to assess the relative activity of CYP 1A2. In a study of normal volunteers, men and parous women had significantly higher amounts of $^{13}CO_2$ in exhaled air on the caffeine breath test than did nulliparous women or parous women taking birth control pills. As expected (because CYP 1A2 is an enzyme inducible by substrate), recent ingestion of caffeine or a strong history of heavy caffeine ingestion both increased $^{13}CO_2$ exhalation as well. **The authors concluded that excessive inducibility and activity of this enzyme in men might predispose them to a greater amount of carcinogen activation and hence a greater bladder cancer risk than women, particularly nulliparous women.** Further studies of populations with bladder cancer patients are necessary to determine if this test has a predictive role. **Preventive strategies to reduce CYP 1A2 inducibility or avoidance strategies to reduce its induction, however, may be useful if this test actually correlates with risk.**

Another enzyme family likely to be important in carcinogen detoxification is the glutathione transferases, particularly glutathione S–transferase M1, encoded for by the polymorphic gene, GSTM1, which occurs in about 50% of the white population. Cigarette smokers who are homozygous for lacking this gene have a 1.8-fold greater risk of developing bladder cancer than smokers who have one or two copies. Nonsmokers who lack this gene, however, have a similar risk of developing bladder cancer as nonsmokers who have it, thus supporting the notion that this gene plays a role in developing smoking-induced bladder cancer (Bell et al, 1993).

Because the molecular adducts resulting from aromatic amine metabolism are believed to mutate DNA in specific ways that potentially affect all areas of the genome, determining the pattern of mutation occurring in known genes in bladder cancer patients may shed light on whether their malignancy arose spontaneously or was induced by a purported chemical carcinogen (Jones et al, 1991). The p53 gene has been focused on particularly, both because its sequence is well established and because of its close association with bladder cancer. The hypothesis guiding these studies is that most common mutations seen spontaneously are transitions at cytosine-phosphate-guanine (CpG) dinucleotides. By assuming that CpG transitions are primarily spontaneous mutations, if these are most of the mutations found in the gene of interest, such mutations would be considered spontaneously induced. Alternatively, because specific carcinogens create specific mutational events, or genetic footprints, finding other types of mutations may indicate a carcinogenic process involving specific agents. When one performs this analysis on tumors associated with p53 mutations, colon carcinomas and leukemias have been shown to have a relatively high rate of predominately spontaneous p53 mutations, whereas small cell carcinomas of the lung appear to have a high proportion of nonspontaneously or exogenously induced mutations (Jones et al, 1991). When this analysis is applied to bladder cancer, an intermediate rate of mutations is seen in which roughly 50% of the mutations are thought to be exogenously produced (Jones et al, 1991). **When comparing p53 mutations in bladder tumors of smokers with those in bladder tumors of patients who have never smoked, however, differences in the types or sites of mutations were not seen, although a higher number of mutations occurred in smokers** (Spruck et al, 1993). **This suggests that smoking might increase the number of mutations in urothelial cells without necessarily directing the site or type of mutation that occurs** (Spruck et al, 1993). **This type of analysis correlates closely with the elegant case-control study of Hayes and co-workers, who found that although exposure to industrial carcinogens and smoking clearly correlated with an increased risk for developing bladder cancer, with the exception of young patients, these exposures did not correlate with any particular bladder cancer phenotype** (Hayes et al, 1993). Thus, assuming that low-grade superficial and high-grade, rapidly invasive transitional cell carcinomas have different fundamental genetic pathways (Spruck et al, 1994; Gruis et al, 1995) (see earlier), the two best-described environmental carcinogenic exposures for bladder cancer predispose for developing each of these genetic alterations in similar proportions to those seen in the nonexposed population.

Coffee and Tea Drinking

Coffee and tea drinking have been implicated in some, but not all, studies in the etiology of bladder cancer (Morrison, 1984; Ciccone and Vineis, 1988; Slattery et al, 1988). This association is complicated because of the widespread consumption of these agents, the use of artificial sweeteners with them, and the history of cigarette smoking as an additional confounder. Indeed, **when cigarette smoking is controlled for, no increased risk with coffee drinking has been found** (Cohen and Johansson, 1992).

Analgesic Abuse

Consumption of large quantities (5–15 kg over a 10-year period) of phenacetin, which has a chemical structure similar to that of the aniline dyes, is associated with an increased risk for transitional cell carcinoma of the renal pelvis and bladder (Piper et al, 1985). The latency period may be longer for bladder tumors than for renal pelvic tumors, for which it may be as long as 25 years (Steffens and Nagel, 1988). A correlation with the use of other analgesics has not been clearly demonstrated (Wahlqvist, 1980; McCredie et al, 1983).

Artificial Sweeteners

Large doses of artificial sweeteners, including saccharin and cyclamates, have been shown in experimental studies to be bladder carcinogens in rodents. These studies are controversial because of the extremely high doses of sweeteners given; because cancer occurred only in animals exposed in utero or in the neonatal period (Sontag, 1980); and because urinary pH in the diet was markedly affected by the doses and electrolyte composition of saccharin given, which, in turn, influenced susceptibility to carcinogenesis (Fukushima et al, 1990; Cohen et al, 1991). **In contrast, case-controlled epidemiologic studies in humans show little evidence for increased risk of bladder cancer in consumers of artificial sweeteners** (Morrison, 1984; Risch et al, 1988). It has been reported that nonsmoking women and heavy-smoking men may have some increased risk associated with the consumption of artificial sweeteners (Hoover and Strasser, 1980).

Chronic Cystitis and Other Infections

Chronic cystitis in the presence of indwelling catheters or calculi is associated with an increased risk for squamous cell carcinoma of the bladder (Kantor et al, 1984; Locke et al, 1985). **Between 2% and 10% of paraplegics with long-term indwelling catheters develop bladder cancer. Approximately 80% of these are squamous carcinomas.**

Similarly, *Schistosoma haematobium* cystitis appears to **be causally related to the development of bladder cancer—often squamous cell carcinoma** (Lucas, 1982). In Egypt, where schistosomiasis is endemic among males, squamous cell carcinoma of the bladder (bilharzial bladder cancer) is the most common malignancy. There is also, however, an increased incidence of transitional cell carcinomas in men with schistosomiasis. **Cystitis-induced bladder cancer from all causes is usually associated with severe, long-term infections.** The mechanisms of carcinogenesis are not understood but may involve formation of nitrite and N-nitroso compounds in the bladder (Tricker et al, 1989)—presumably from parasitic or microbial metabolism of normal urinary constituents (Higgy et al, 1985).

The role of exposure to the human papillomavirus (HPV) in bladder cancer has been evaluated by several groups, with widely divergent findings. Infections with transforming strains of HPV, a DNA virus, are closely associated with squamous cell carcinoma of the uterine cervix and carcinomas of the vagina, female and male urethra, anogenital region, and perhaps penis (Weiner et al, 1992; Weiner and Walther, 1994). Most studies have probed PCR-amplified DNA extracted from tumor tissue with **DNA complementary to known transforming genes present in tumorigenic strains of HPV. These genes code for proteins, which, in turn, bind with or alter the function of cellular proteins known to be important in malignant transformation, including that of the urothelium.** For example, the E5 gene product interacts with the EGF receptor (Zyzak et al, 1994), the E6 gene product binds with and inactivates wt p53 protein (Werness et al, 1990), and the E7 protein binds with and inactivates pRb (Dyson et al, 1989). **Reports**

have indicated that as few as 7% (Maloney et al, 1994; Noel et al, 1994) **to as many as 35% of human bladder cancers are contaminated by HPV DNA** (Lopez-Beltran et al, 1991; Anwar et al, 1992; Furihata et al, 1993; LaRue et al, 1995). Reasons for disparate results are not apparent, although most studies have used specimens of invasive tumors primarily because they provide large amounts of tissue and have more DNA. Studies have not focused on gender or racial differences and have not been correlated with pertinent epidemiologic information, thus further clouding the role of this virus in the development of bladder cancer. **The role of other viral agents in the etiology of transitional cell cancer has been investigated but not established by Fraley and associates** (1976).

Pelvic Irradiation

Women treated with radiotherapy for carcinoma of the uterine cervix have a twofold to fourfold increased risk of developing transitional cell carcinoma of the bladder (Duncan et al, 1977; Sella et al, 1989). These tumors are characteristically high grade and locally advanced at the time of diagnosis (Quilty and Kerr, 1987).

Cyclophosphamide

Patients treated with cyclophosphamide (Cytoxan) have up to a ninefold increased risk of developing bladder cancer, although the relationship has not yet been formally demonstrated in case-controlled epidemiologic studies (Morrison, 1984; O'Keane, 1988; Tuttle et al, 1988). **Most of these tumors are muscle-infiltrating at the time of diagnosis** (Durkee and Benson, 1980). **A urinary metabolite of cyclophosphamide, acrolein, is believed to be responsible for both hemorrhagic cystitis and bladder cancer** (Cohen et al, 1992); **however, the development of hemorrhagic cystitis does not necessarily correlate with the development of bladder cancer** (Pedersen-Bjergaard et al, 1988). **The latent period for cyclophosphamide-induced bladder cancer is relatively short,** ranging from 6 to 13 years. **Studies suggest that the uroprotectant mesna (2-mercaptoethanesulfonic acid) may reduce the risk of bladder cancer** (Habs and Schmahl, 1983). Some authors suggest aggressive therapy on diagnosis (e.g., cystectomy), even when the tumor is still noninvasive, because of the unusually high rate of progression experienced by those in whom cystectomy is withheld.

Tryptophan Metabolites

Bladder cancer patients have been reported to have increased urinary tryptophan metabolite levels (Brown et al, 1969; Wolf, 1973). High levels have been reported to correlate with tumor recurrence rates (Brown et al, 1969; Teulings et al, 1978). Pyridoxine administration normalizes urinary tryptophan metabolite levels in some patients. Moreover, a controlled clinical trial showed that pyridoxine significantly reduced early tumor recurrence rates in patients with super-

ficial bladder cancer (Byar and Blackard, 1977). In this trial, however, tryptophan metabolite levels were not measured.

In contrast, current studies suggest that endogenous tryptophan metabolites do not contribute significantly to the development of bladder cancer (Renwick et al, 1988). Thus, the role, if any, of endogenous metabolites in the etiology of bladder cancer remains controversial.

Heredity

No epidemiologic evidence exists for a hereditary cause in most cases of bladder cancer. Familial clusters of bladder cancer have been reported (Fraumeni and Thomas, 1967; Aherne, 1974; McCullough et al, 1975). More recently, a pedigree with the Lynch syndrome II, an inherited syndrome associated with colorectal cancer without polyposis and with extracolonic cancer sites, has been described in which four male siblings developed transitional cell carcinomas, three of the upper tracts (Lynch et al, 1990). Because all of these individuals were elderly, however, the exact role of this syndrome in developing transitional cell cancer is unclear. In this pedigree, at least one younger individual (31 years old) did develop colon cancer (Greenland et al, 1993). As with other family clusters, an explanation other than inheritance may be similar exposure to the same environmental carcinogens. **An increased risk for bladder cancer among individuals with particular HLA subtypes** (Arce et al, 1978) **and blood group phenotypes** (Orihuela and Shahon, 1987) **has also been reported, although explanations and confirming studies have not been forthcoming.**

Lynch and co-workers also noted an increased risk of developing bladder cancer in relatives of 47 consecutive patients with bladder cancer (Lynch et al, 1987). This risk was significantly higher than the familial risk found for lung cancer, other smoking-related cancers, or nonsmoking-related cancers. This relative risk was quite heterogeneous in that only 3 of 47 families showed markedly increased risk. The authors did not report, however, whether this increased risk in the affected families was related to the fact that relatives of the index case were smokers. This is important because Kantor and associates indicated that the increased familial risk was primarily in relatives who smoked (Kantor et al, 1985). Correlation of familial predisposition, possible exposures, and some of the genotypic/phenotypic analyses discussed earlier (e.g., of GSTM1, NAT2, and CYP 1A2) is required to permit identification of at-risk individuals who may be the best targets for interventions (such as avoidance, prevention, and early detection strategies).

PATHOLOGY

Normal Bladder Urothelium

The urothelium of the normal bladder is transitional cell epithelium, three to seven layers thick. There is a basal cell layer on which rests one or more layers of intermediate cells. The most superficial layer is composed of large flat umbrella cells. The cells of the urothelium are oriented with

2338 UROTHELIAL TUMORS OF THE URINARY TRACT

the long axis of the oval nuclei being perpendicular to the normal basement membrane, giving the urothelium its normal appearance of cellular polarity (Koss et al, 1974). The urothelium rests on the lamina propria basement membrane (Zuk et al, 1989). **In the lamina propria is a tunica muscularis mucosa containing scattered smooth muscle fibers, which are irregularly arranged** (Ro et al, 1987; Keep et al, 1989; Younes et al, 1990; Engel et al, 1992; Hasui et al, 1994; Angulo et al, 1995). Rarely, fat can be seen in the lamina propria, too (Bochner et al, 1995).

Epithelial Hyperplasia and Metaplasia

The term *epithelial hyperplasia* is used to describe an increase in the number of cell layers without nuclear or architectural abnormalities. Urothelial *metaplasia* refers to the bladder lining, often in focal areas, demonstrating a non-transitional epithelial appearance, usually with epidermoid (squamous metaplasia) or glandular (adenomatous metaplasia) development. Squamous metaplasia is a proliferative lesion in which the urothelium is replaced by a mature, non-keratinizing squamous epithelium. It occurs most commonly in the bladder neck and trigone area. Although when it occurs in other regions of the bladder it may be precancerous (Mostofi, 1954), squamous metaplasia of the vaginal type on the trigone of women is a normal variant occurring under hormonal influence (Tyler, 1962). Autopsy studies have shown that squamous metaplasia occurs in the bladder of nearly half of women and fewer than 10% of men (Wiener et al, 1979). **Squamous metaplasia in the absence of cellular atypia or marked keratinization is probably a benign condition in either gender.**

Von Brunn's nests are islands of benign-appearing urothelium situated in the lamina propria. These are believed to result from *inward* proliferation of the basal cells (Patch and Rhea, 1935). **These nests have been reported to be a normal urothelial variant in the supramontanal prostatic urethra** (Kierman and Gafney, 1987) **and occur in 89% of normal bladders at autopsy** (Wiener et al, 1979).

Cystitis cystica is similar to von Brunn's nests except that the center of the nest of urothelium has undergone eosinophilic liquefaction (Kunze et al, 1983). Cystitis cystica also is present in 60% of normal bladders at autopsy (Wiener et al, 1979). It should be distinguished from *cystitis follicularis,* a non-neoplastic response to chronic bacterial infection. Histologically, cystitis follicularis is composed of submucosal lymphoid follicles. Grossly, it appears as punctate yellow submucosal nodules, which have been given the descriptive name bacteriuric bumps.

Cystitis glandularis is similar to cystitis cystica except that the transitional cells have undergone glandular metaplasia. It appears histologically as submucosal nests of columnar epithelial cells surrounding a central liquefied region of cellular degeneration (Mostofi, 1954). **Cystitis glandularis may be a precursor of adenocarcinoma** (Edwards et al, 1972). It has been reported to occur frequently in patients with pelvic lipomatosis (Yalla et al, 1975; Johnson et al, 1980; Gordon et al, 1990). **Cystoscopically, cystitis glandularis may appear as a papillary lesion—although often it is not grossly visible.**

Urothelial Dysplasia

Preneoplastic Proliferative Abnormalities

A variety of changes can occur in the urothelium in response to inflammation and irritation or carcinogens. These changes may be proliferative, metaplastic (see previously), or both.

Atypical hyperplasia is similar to epithelial hyperplasia except that there are also nuclear abnormalities and partial derangement of the umbrella cell layer (Koss et al, 1974). In patients with superficial bladder cancer, the presence of atypia in adjacent urothelium is associated with a 35% to 40% risk of developing invasive disease (Althausen et al, 1976).

Dysplasia

The term *dysplasia* denotes epithelial changes that are intermediate between normal urothelium and carcinoma in situ. There are three categories of dysplasia: mild, moderate, and severe. Dysplastic cells have large, round, notched, basally situated nuclei that do not exhibit the normal epithelial polarity. Dysplastic epithelium does not have an increased number of cell layers or mitotic figures (Murphy and Soloway, 1982). It is difficult to make a sharp distinction between severe dysplasia and carcinoma in situ (Friedell et al, 1986). **As a general rule, mild and moderate dysplasias, even when associated with a history of bladder cancer, warrant careful follow-up but no particular specific therapy, whereas severe dysplasia/carcinoma in situ requires aggressive treatment.**

Inverted Papilloma

An *inverted papilloma* is a benign proliferative lesion caused by chronic inflammation or bladder outlet obstruction. Most commonly, it occurs in the trigone and bladder neck areas in men with prostatitis (DeMeester et al, 1975).

Papillary fronds project into the fibrovascular stroma of the bladder rather than into the bladder lumen. The lesion is usually covered by a thin layer of normal urothelium (Fig. 77–1). Inverted papillomas may contain an area of cystitis cystica or squamous metaplasia.

Two different types of inverted papilloma occur: trabecular and glandular. The trabecular type arises from proliferation of the basal cells. The glandular type is a form of cystitis glandularis arising in the intermediate cells and as such is considered to be potentially a preneoplastic lesion (Kunze et al, 1983).

Rare cases of malignant transformation of inverted papillomas have been reported (Lazarevic and Garret, 1978). **There is a more common association of inverted papilloma, however, occurring in patients with coexistent transitional cell carcinoma elsewhere in the bladder or with histories of such tumors** (Cheon et al, 1995). Because the overlying epithelium is normal, inverted papillomas appear as small raised nodules rather than as papillary or frond-like tumors.

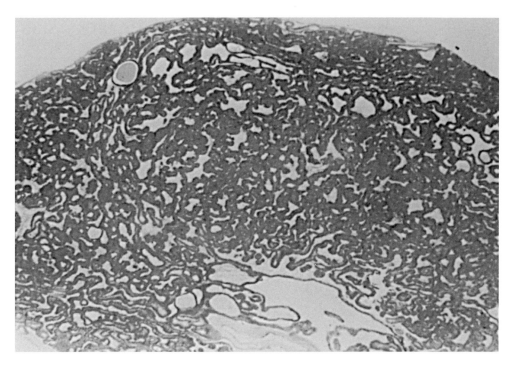

Figure 77–1. Inverted papilloma. (From Mostofi FK, Sobin LH, Tortoni H: Histological Typing of Urinary Bladder Tumors, no. 10. International Histological Classification of Tumors. Geneva, World Health Organization, 1973.)

Nephrogenic Adenoma

Nephrogenic adenoma is a rare lesion that histologically resembles primitive renal collecting tubules. It is a metaplastic response of urothelium to trauma, infection, or radiation therapy. Edema and inflammatory cell infiltration are common, but there is little nuclear atypia or mitotic activity (Navarre et al, 1982). Nephrogenic adenoma is more common in men and is often associated with symptoms of dysuria and urinary frequency. Nephrogenic adenoma also has been reported in children (Kay and Lattanzi, 1985).

Mesonephric adenocarcinoma is the malignant counterpart of nephrogenic adenoma (Schultz et al, 1984). This lesion usually invades through the lamina propria. Radical cystectomy is indicated for muscle-invasive tumors.

Vesical Leukoplakia

Leukoplakia is defined as cornification of a normally noncornified epithelium. The histopathologic criteria include squamous metaplasia with marked keratinization, downward growth of the rete pegs (acanthosis), cellular atypia, and dysplasia (Benson, 1984). Leukoplakia is believed to be a response of the normal urothelium to noxious stimuli and generally is considered a premalignant lesion or a lesion that heralds the presence of malignant disease elsewhere in the bladder (Benson, 1984). Vesical leukoplakia may progress to squamous cell carcinoma in up to 20% of patients (DeKock et al, 1981; Benson, 1984). Leukoplakia is frequently found in patients with chronic cystitis, bladder calculi, long-term indwelling catheters, or schistosomiasis.

Pseudosarcoma (Postoperative Spindle Cell Nodule)

Postoperative spindle cell nodule is a rare lesion resembling a sarcoma of the bladder. It consists of reactive prolif-

eration of spindle cells occurring several months after a lower urinary tract procedure or infection. These lesions have been misinterpreted as being malignant, and radical surgery has been performed inappropriately. Usually, they are confused with leiomyosarcomas (Young and Scully, 1987; Wick et al, 1988; Stark et al, 1989; Huang et al, 1990; Vekemans et al, 1990).

UROTHELIAL CARCINOMA: CARCINOMA IN SITU

Carcinoma in situ may appear as a velvety patch of erythematous mucosa on cystoscopic examination, although quite often it is endoscopically invisible. **Histologically, it consists of poorly differentiated transitional cell carcinoma confined to the urothelium** (Fig. 77–2). Carcinoma in situ may be asymptomatic or may produce severe symptoms of urinary frequency, urgency, and dysuria (Utz et al, 1970; Utz and Farrow, 1984). **Urine cytopathology study results are positive in 80% to 90% of patients with carcinoma in situ because of the poor cohesiveness of the tumor cells.** Carcinoma in situ occurs more commonly in men. **Its symptoms may be mistaken for prostatism, urinary tract infection, neurogenic bladder, or interstitial cystitis.**

Carcinoma in situ occurs only rarely in patients with well-differentiated, superficial bladder tumors, but it is present in 25% or more of patients with high-grade superficial tumors (Koss et al, 1974; Flamm and Dona, 1989). **It portends a poor prognosis.** Patients with carcinoma in situ have higher tumor recurrence rates (Flamm and Dona, 1989); and with just endoscopic resection as treatment, **between 40% and 83% progress to muscle-invasive cancer** (Althausen et al, 1976). **Carcinoma in situ occurs in association with 20% to 75% of high-grade muscle-**

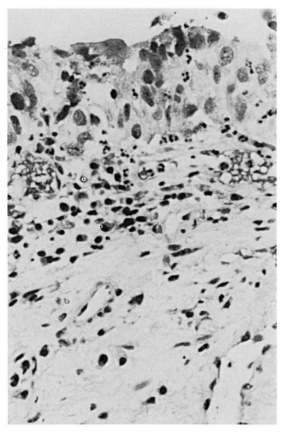

Figure 77–2. Carcinoma in situ. (Courtesy of Louis P. Dehner, M.D.)

invasive cancers (Prout et al, 1983). It is also more common in patients with multiple tumors.

The natural history of carcinoma in situ is not clearly understood. Early in its clinical evolution, it may be asymptomatic; later, it may produce severe symptoms of bladder irritability. **Some patients have protracted courses lasting for more than a decade without developing muscle-invasive bladder cancer** (Riddle et al, 1976; Weinstein et al, 1979). **Others progress rapidly to invasive bladder cancer that has a poor prognosis despite definitive therapy** (Utz et al, 1970).

Some investigators have characterized carcinoma in situ as a peculiar cancer with aggressive morphologic features but having a limited capacity to invade and metastasize (Weinstein et al, 1980). **Patients with marked urinary symptoms generally have a shorter interval preceding the development of muscle-invasive cancer. About 20% of patients treated with cystectomy for diffuse carcinoma in situ are found to have microscopic muscle-invasive cancer** (Farrow et al, 1976).

Besides these clinical associations, a variety of investigative approaches have confirmed the adverse prognostic features of carcinoma in situ and its direct relationship to muscle-invasive cancer. **Cytogenetic (loss of chromosome 17p)** (Olumni et al, 1990; Tsai et al, 1990; Knowles et al, 1994), **molecular genetic** (Sarkis et al, 1993), **and immunohistologic** (Sarkis et al, 1993; Esrig et al, 1994; Sarkis et al, 1994) **studies have shown that a high proportion of both carcinoma in situ and deeply invasive bladder cancer have deletions or mutations (or both) of the p53 gene**

and alterations of its protein product. **This not only supports the contention that carcinoma in situ is a precursor lesion of invasive bladder cancer, but also, to a large degree, eliminates it as a precursor of low-grade papillary tumors, in which p53 abnormalities are almost never found** (Habuchi et al, 1992; Spruck et al, 1994.)

Currently, intravesical therapy has become the preferred primary treatment for carcinoma in situ. Chemotherapeutic agents used include triethylenethiophosphoramide (thiotepa), etoglucid (Epodyl), mitomycin C, doxorubicin (Adriamycin), and epirubicin, with efficacy in eradicating carcinoma in situ reported as approximately 30% (Soloway 1984). **The most effective intravesical therapy for carcinoma in situ is intravesical bacille Calmette-Guérin (BCG) therapy, producing complete regression in approximately 50% to 65% of patients** (Coplen et al, 1990). **Radiation therapy and systemic chemotherapy have been reported to be ineffective in eradicating carcinoma in situ** (Whitmore et al, 1977), although this conclusion was primarily drawn from patients who had concomitant invasive cancer in whom carcinoma in situ lesions elsewhere in the bladder were found at planned cystectomy following preoperative courses of radiation or chemotherapy. It is less clear that pure carcinoma in situ is also refractory to systemic chemotherapy and radiation, although such treatments would probably remain inappropriate in view of the recurrent nature of this entity.

TRANSITIONAL CELL CARCINOMA

Tumor Architecture

More than 90% of bladder cancers are transitional cell carcinomas (see Figs. 77–2 to 77–6). These tumors differ from normal urothelium by having an increased number of epithelial cell layers with papillary foldings of the mucosa, loss of cell polarity, abnormal cell maturation from the basal to superficial layers, giant cells, nuclear crowding, increased nuclear-to-cytoplasmic ratio, prominent nucleoli, clumping of chromatin, and an increased number of mitoses (Koss, 1975). The most significant criteria are the prominent nucleoli, clumping of chromatin, increased cell layers, and loss of cell polarity (Melamed et al, 1960). Some of these same changes can occur in inflammatory, reactive, or regenerative conditions (Mostofi, 1954).

Transitional cell carcinomas manifest a variety of patterns of tumor growth, including papillary, sessile infiltrating, nodular, mixed, and flat intraepithelial growth (carcinoma in situ). Because of the normal undulations of the basal layer of epithelium and because invaginations of the normal urothelium into the submucosa occur as with von Brunn's nests, it is sometimes difficult to demonstrate invasion of the lamina propria (Mostofi, 1954). **Similarly, cancer invasion into the smooth muscle cells of the tunica muscularis mucosa can be mistaken for invasion of the bladder detrusor muscle** (Keep et al, 1989; Younes et al, 1990; Engel et al, 1992), **a particular problem in specimens obtained by endoscopic biopsy or transurethral curettage.**

Transitional epithelium has a great metaplastic potential; therefore, transitional cell carcinomas may contain spindle cell (Young et al., 1988), **squamous cell, or adeno-**

carcinomatous elements. **These elements are present in about one third of bladder cancers, several of which may be exhibited in a single cancer.** Transitional cell carcinomas arise most commonly in the trigone/bladder base area and on the lateral bladder walls; however, they may arise anywhere within the bladder. **Approximately 70% of bladder tumors are papillary, 10% are nodular, and 20% are mixed.**

Tumor Grading

No uniformly accepted grading system for bladder cancer currently exists. **Most commonly used systems are based on the degree of anaplasia of the tumor cells** (Broders 1922; Bergkvist et al, 1965; Mostofi et al, 1973; Koss, 1975) **and group carcinomas into three or four grades corresponding to well differentiated, moderately differentiated, and poorly differentiated tumors.**

A strong correlation exists between tumor grade and tumor stage (Jewett and Strong, 1946), **with most well-differentiated and moderately differentiated tumors being superficial and most poorly differentiated tumors being muscle invasive. Stage for stage, however, there is a significant correlation between tumor grade and prognosis. The correlation between tumor stage and prognosis is even stronger. As Spruck and co-workers have proposed, there are now strong molecular and cytogenetic data to support the well-established clinical impressions that low-grade (all well-differentiated and most moderately differentiated tumors) and high-grade (poorly differentiated) transitional cell carcinomas have fundamentally different origins, with the former losing one or more suppressor genes on chromosome 9 and the latter having p53 abnormalities as early initiating events** (Spruck et al, 1994).

A papilloma (grade 0) is a papillary lesion with a fine fibrovascular core covered by normal bladder mucosa (Friedell et al, 1976) (Fig. 77–3). **Papillomas do not have more than seven epithelial cell layers and no abnormalities in histology.** Well-differentiated (grade I) tumors (Fig. 77–4) have a thin fibrovascular stalk with a thickened urothelium containing more than seven cell layers, with cells exhibiting only slight anaplasia and pleomorphism. There also may be an increased nuclear-to-cytoplasmic ratio and prominence of the nuclear membrane. The disturbance of the base-to-surface cellular maturation is mild, and there are only rare mitotic figures. Moderately differentiated (grade II) tumors (Fig. 77–5) have a wider fibrovascular core, a greater disturbance of the base-to-surface cellular maturation, and a loss of cell polarity. The nuclear-to-cytoplasmic ratio is higher, with more nuclear pleomorphism and prominent nucleoli. Mitotic figures are somewhat more frequent. Poorly differentiated (grade III) tumors (Fig. 77–6) have cells that do not differentiate as they progress from the basement membrane to the surface. Marked nuclear pleomorphism is noted, with a high nuclear-to-cytoplasmic ratio. Mitotic figures may be frequent (Friedell et al, 1980).

Metaplastic Elements

It is not unusual for different tumor types to coexist in the same bladder; however, all epithelial tumors are believed to have a common ancestry in the transitional epithelium. The most frequent combination is a papillary high-grade transitional cell carcinoma with flat carcinoma in situ. **Squamous cell carcinoma elements also are frequently seen with invasive transitional cell carcinoma.** Less common is the combination of adenocarcinoma elements with invasive transitional cell carcinoma (Koss, 1975). **The presence of these metaplastic elements in transitional cell carcinoma does not change the principal classification of the tumor as a transitional cell carcinoma.**

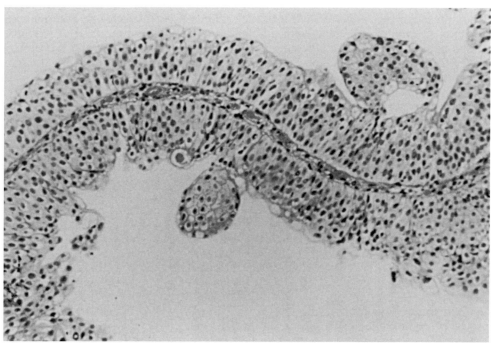

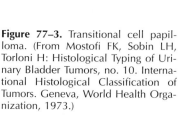

Figure 77–3. Transitional cell papilloma. (From Mostofi FK, Sobin LH, Torloni H: Histological Typing of Urinary Bladder Tumors, no. 10. International Histological Classification of Tumors. Geneva, World Health Organization, 1973.)

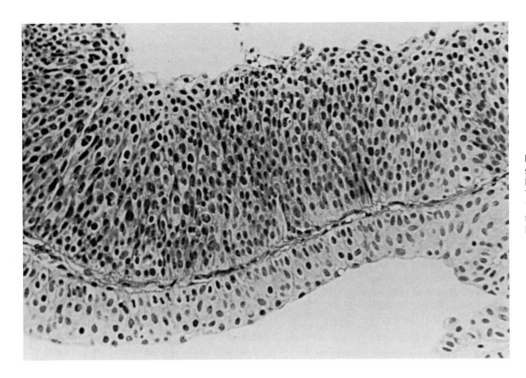

Figure 77–4. Well-differentiated transitional cell carcinoma. (From Mostofi FK, Sobin LH, Torloni H: Histological Typing of Urinary Bladder Tumors, no. 10. International Histological Classification of Tumors. Geneva, World Health Organization, 1973.)

Figure 77–5. Moderately differentiated transitional cell carcinoma. (From Mostofi FK, Sobin LH, Torloni H: Histological Typing of Urinary Bladder Tumors, no. 10. International Histological Classification of Tumors. Geneva, World Health Organization, 1973.)

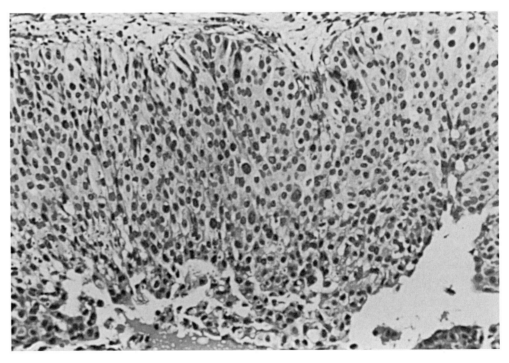

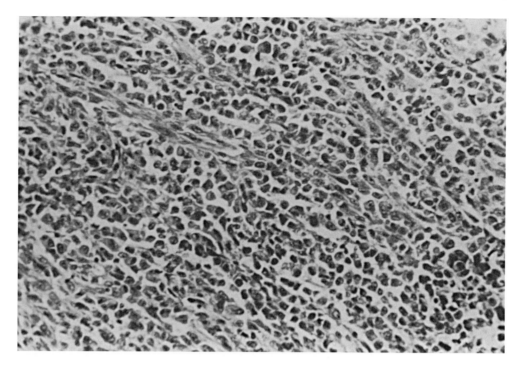

Figure 77–6. Undifferentiated transitional cell carcinoma. (From Mostofi FK, Sobin LH, Torloni H: Histological Typing of Urinary Bladder Tumors, no. 10. International Histological Classification of Tumors. Geneva, World Health Organization, 1973.)

SQUAMOUS CELL CARCINOMA

Etiology

Considerable variability is noted in the prevalence of squamous cell carcinoma of the bladder in different parts of the world. For example, **squamous cell cancer accounts for only 1% of bladder cancers in England** (Costello et al, 1984) **and 3% to 7% in the United States** (Koss, 1975; Kantor et al, 1988; Lynch and Cohen, 1995) **but more than 75% in Egypt** (El-Bolkainy et al, 1981). **About 80% of squamous cell carcinomas in Egypt are associated with chronic infection with _S. haematobium._** These cancers are called bilharzial bladder cancers; they occur in patients who are, on the average, 10 to 20 years younger than patients with transitional carcinoma. **Bilharzial cancers are exophytic, nodular, fungating lesions that usually are well differentiated and have a relatively low incidence of lymph node and distant metastases.** Whether the low incidence of distant metastases is due to capillary and lymphatic fibrosis resulting from chronic schistosomal infection (Ghoneim and Awad, 1980) or the relatively low histologic grade (El-Bolkainy et al, 1981) of these tumors is not clear.

Nonbilharzial squamous cell cancers are usually caused by chronic irritation from urinary calculi, long-term indwelling catheters, chronic urinary infections, or bladder diverticula. As many as 80% of paraplegics have squamous changes in the bladder, and **about 5% develop squamous cell carcinoma** (Broecher et al, 1981; Maruf et al, 1982; Bejany et al, 1987). Cigarette smoking also has been reported to be significantly associated with an increased risk of squamous cell bladder carcinoma (Kantor et al, 1988). **Male predominance is far less striking in squamous cell carcinoma (1.3–1.7:1)** (Lynch and Cohen, 1995). **In general, the prognosis of squamous cell carcinoma is poor because most patients have advanced disease at the time of diagnosis.**

Histology

Squamous cell carcinoma consists, characteristically, of keratinized islands that contain eccentric aggregates of cells called squamous pearls. They may show varying degrees of histologic differentiation (Koss, 1975) (Fig. 77–7). Squamous cell cancers shed keratinized cells into the urine that sometimes can be detected cytologically. **Cytology has been of limited utility, however, in the diagnosis of this tumor, and histologic differentiation far more loosely correlates with prognosis, stage for stage, than it does with transitional cell carcinomas.** Squamous cell cancers are more frequently associated with coexistence of squamous metaplasia than with carcinoma in situ.

Treatment

Squamous cell carcinoma requires aggressive surgical therapy. **Transurethral resection, partial cystectomy, and radiation therapy have not been successful** (Newman et al, 1968; Martin et al, 1989b). Although definitive radiation therapy with salvage cystectomy has been recommended by some (Costello et al, 1984), **the best survival results have been achieved with radical cystectomy with or without planned preoperative radiation therapy** (Ghoneim and Awad, 1980). The true benefit of the planned preoperative radiation therapy has not been clearly established. **Chemotherapy regimens, particularly those developed for transitional cell carcinoma, are not effective for squamous cell carcinoma, either in a pure form or when there are squamous elements in a primarily transitional cell cancer** (Maruf et al, 1982; Logothetis et al, 1988; Sternberg et al, 1989). **Several reports suggest that, stage for stage, the prognosis of squamous cell carcinoma is comparable to that of transitional cell carcinoma** (Johnson et al, 1976; Richie et al, 1976; Faysal and Freiha, 1981). Active or

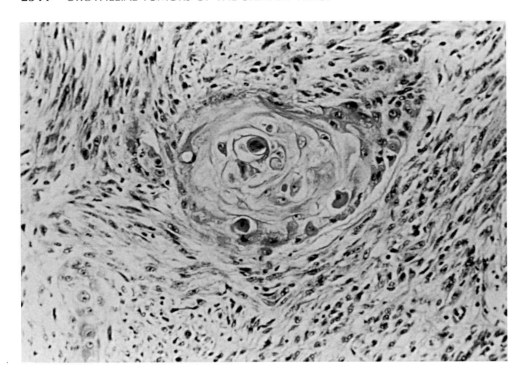

Figure 77-7. Squamous cell carcinoma. (From Mostofi FK, Sobin LH, Torloni H: Histological Typing of Urinary Bladder Tumors, no. 10. International Histological Classification of Tumors. Geneva, World Health Organization, 1973.)

recurrent cancer in the urethra has been reported in about one half of patients with squamous cell carcinoma, suggesting that urethrectomy should be performed routinely in patients undergoing cystectomy (Bejany et al, 1987). It is rare that squamous cell carcinoma in the United States is diagnosed before it is deeply invasive, and hence the issue of the best management for superficial squamous cell carcinoma has not been intensely studied in the United States.

ADENOCARCINOMA

Adenocarcinomas account for less than 2% of primary bladder cancers (Kantor et al, 1988; Lynch and Cohen, 1995). They are classified into three groups: primary vesical, urachal, and metastatic. **Adenocarcinomas also occur in intestinal urinary conduits, augmentations, pouches, and ureterosigmoidostomies** (Husmann and Spence, 1990; Kalble et al, 1990; Spencer and Filmer, 1991). They are discussed in Chapters 100, 101, and 103.

Primary Vesical Adenocarcinoma

Adenocarcinomas of the bladder arise in two common sites: the bladder base area, including the trigone and the immediately adjacent lateral walls; and the dome of the bladder. Adenocarcinomas, however, can occur anywhere in the bladder. **Adenocarcinoma is the most common type of cancer in exstrophic bladders.** These tumors develop in response to chronic inflammation and irritation (Nielson and Nielsen, 1983; Bennett et al, 1984). Adenocarcinoma has also been reported with schistosomiasis (Anderstrom et al, 1983), however, less commonly than squamous cell or transitional cell carcinomas. Other established risk factors have not been well documented except, possibly, coffee drinking (Kantor et al, 1988).

All histologic variants of enteric adenocarcinoma, including signet-ring and colloid carcinoma, may occur in the bladder. Most bladder adenocarcinomas are mucin producing (Koss, 1975). Adenocarcinomas may be papillary or solid. Signet-ring carcinomas characteristically produce linitis plastica of the bladder (Choi et al, 1984; Sheldon et al, 1984; Blute et al, 1989). **Most adenocarcinomas are poorly differentiated and invasive. They are more commonly associated with cystitis glandularis than with carcinoma in situ.**

Radical cystectomy with pelvic lymphadenectomy offers the best chance for cure. Adenocarcinomas are poorly responsive to radiation therapy or cytotoxic chemotherapy—whether they are primary lesions that are pure adenocarcinomas or metaplastic components of transitional cell cancer (Anderstrom et al, 1983; Logothetis et al, 1988; Blute et al, 1989; Sternberg et al, 1989). The generally poor prognosis associated with adenocarcinomas is due primarily to their advanced stage at diagnosis. **There is no evidence to indicate that, stage for stage, their prognosis is markedly different from that of transitional cell carcinoma.**

Urachal Carcinoma

Urachal carcinomas are extremely rare tumors that arise outside the bladder and are usually adenocarcinomas, although they may be primary transitional cell or squamous carcinomas and rarely even sarcomas. **For a tumor to be classified as a urachal carcinoma, there must be a sharp demarcation between the tumor and the adjacent bladder epithelium, with the tumor being located in the bladder wall beneath the normal epithelium** (Mostofi, 1954). Urachal tumors invading through the urothelium and extending into the bladder may be confused with a primary vesical carcinoma (Koss, 1975; Kakizoe et al, 1983).

Urachal carcinomas may extend into the prevesical space. **They may appear with a bloody or mucoid discharge from the umbilicus or produce a mucocele, occurring as a palpable mass.** Many urachal tumors have stippled calcifications on radiographs (Brick et al, 1988; Narumi et al, 1988). Tumors invading the bladder lumen may produce mucus in the urine. **Patients with urachal carcinomas have a worse prognosis than those with primary bladder adenocarcinomas** (Mostofi, 1954). Tumors treated with partial cystectomy have local recurrence rates between 15% and 50% (Magri, 1962). Histologically, these tumors exhibit wider and deeper infiltration of the bladder wall than expected, compromising the results of partial cystectomy (Kakizoe et al, 1983; Sheldon et al, 1984). Normally, therefore, radical cystectomy with en bloc excision of the urachus is the treatment of choice for all except small, well-differentiated urachal carcinomas. Radiation therapy has not been effective in treating these tumors (Sheldon et al, 1984). Urachal carcinomas metastasize to iliac and inguinal lymph nodes, omentum, liver, lung, and bone (Sheldon et al, 1984). Urachal carcinomas are rarely responsive to chemotherapy. Although the general prognosis with urachal carcinoma is poor, Johnson and co-workers reported a 50% survival rate (Johnson et al, 1985).

Metastatic Adenocarcinoma

One of the most common forms of adenocarcinoma of the bladder is metastatic (or invasive) adenocarcinoma (Choi et al, 1984). The primary sites for these tumors include the rectum, stomach, endometrium, breast, prostate, and ovary (Klinger, 1951). Although adenocarcinomatous metastases to the bladder represent only 0.26% of bladder tumors (Klinger, 1951), because of the rareness of primary vesical adenocarcinoma, patients diagnosed with pure adenocarcinomas of the bladder should be evaluated for other primary sites before definitive treatment is undertaken.

ORIGIN AND PATTERNS OF DISSEMINATION OF TRANSITIONAL CELL CARCINOMA

Multicentric Origin

Clinical and urinary tract mapping studies suggest that transitional cell carcinoma is usually a field change disease with tumors arising at different times and sites in the urothelium (polychronotopicity). This suggests a polyclonal etiology of bladder cancer—particularly because recurrences often arise many years after the original tumor(s) (Prout et al, 1992; Thompson et al, 1993). **The phenomenon of late recurrences would be at odds with the competing theory, that recurrences represent clonal seedings of the original tumor, in view of the known rapid growth of even low-grade papillary transitional cell cancers** (Messing et al, 1995b) **and their virtual absence as an incidental finding at autopsy (see previously). Similarly, immunohistochemical and immunocytochemical studies have confirmed that normal-appearing urothelium (histologically and**

cystoscopically) **remote from tumors shares with those tumors altered expression of tumor markers such as G-actin and the receptor for EGF** (Messing, 1990; Rao et al, 1993).

Alternatively, molecular evidence using LOH or gene sequencing analyses, at least at times, indicates a clonal etiology of multiple simultaneous (Sidransky et al, 1992) **or sequential tumors in either the bladder** (Hruban et al, 1994) **or in the upper tracts and bladder** (Harris and Neal, 1992; Lunec et al, 1992). These molecular fingerprinting studies, however, have focused almost exclusively on high-grade invasive transitional cell cancers, which provide the greatest amounts of tissue and in which p53 (for which the DNA sequence is well known) is often mutated. Yet such cancers rarely develop after previously resected superficial tumors (Kaye and Lange, 1982; Hopkins et al, 1983), so that the cases studied, in which index tumors and recurrences have been molecularly analyzed, represent a group (invasive tumors with a history of previous superficial tumors) that comprises a small minority of all transitional cell cancers. Indeed, in part because the specific genetic defects associated with the far more common low-grade superficial papillary tumors either have not been well described or involve complete deletions of both copies of genes such as p16 so that DNA sequencing studies cannot be done, similar fingerprinting analyses have not been performed on much more common types of bladder cancer. **Furthermore, even in the highly selected group in which molecular analyses have been performed, examples of both uniclonal and multiclonal origins have been reported** (Jones, 1994). Certainly, in some cases, multiple tumors are derived from a single cell clone that has disseminated to other sites in the urinary tract by implantation, transepithelial migration, or lymphatic or vascular spread. Whether the frequency of such events is sufficiently common to justify the use of specific genetic analysis of a particular mutation in a gene such as p53 in exfoliated cells as a generalized means to detect tumor recurrence is far less certain. The potentially great sensitivity of this analysis (Hruban et al, 1994) in being able to uncover a single malignant cell out of 10 million nonmalignant cells is counteracted by the potentially high false-negative rate if a multiclonal tumor does arise in an individual patient—something that is known to occur. Further clouding this issue is the fact that a substantial percentage of stage T1 tumors are inadvertently incompletely resected (Klan et al, 1991), leading to the possibility that incomplete treatment, rather than spontaneous or iatrogenic implantation or transepithelial spread, is responsible for purported cases of clonal tumor recurrence.

Patterns of Spread

The process of tumor invasion, in which malignant transitional epithelial cells extend beneath the basal lamina into the connective tissue of the lamina propria and, subsequently, into muscularis propria and perivesical fat, represents the culmination of a variety of biologic processes, which includes stimulation of neovascularization (angiogenesis), proteolysis resulting from elaboration of collagenases, increased cellular motility, proliferation, and escape from local surveillance mechanisms—primarily the immune system. Additionally, because cellular adhesion molecules and other components of the extracellular matrix bind urothelial cells both to each other and to the underlying basal lamina, such connections have to be altered to permit some semblance of cellular disaggregation and local motility. Although these processes are generally shared by all epithelial malignancies that invade, the uniqueness of the urothelium and the microenvironment in which invasion of urothelial carcinoma occurs has been the subject of intense study.

The presence of angiogenic factors excreted in the urine of bladder cancer patients has been recognized for many years (Chodak et al, 1988), and at least some of the substances responsible for such activity, including autocrine motility factor (Guirguis et al, 1988) and acidic and basic fibroblast growth factors (FGFs) (Chopin et al, 1993; Nguyen et al, 1993), have been reported. There is some evidence that the FGFs are produced by urothelial cells (as well as possibly other urinary sources). The source of autocrine motility factor, although presumably the urothelium, is less certain. **Both endothelial cells and malignant transitional epithelial cells appear to contain membrane-bound receptors for these substances** (Chopin et al, 1993; Korman et al, 1995), **thus making it likely that they are involved not only in the formation of new vessels, but also, by serving in an endocrine/paracrine fashion, in the induction of motility in malignant urothelial cells.**

Liu and Liotta and colleagues using several experimental models have shown that malignant transitional epithelial cell lines elaborate proteases, primarily collagenase type IV, that are capable of digesting the connective tissue of the basal lamina and underlying lamina propria (Zuk et al, 1989; Liu and Liotta, 1992). **In specimens of human transitional cell carcinomas, expression of collagenase type IV has been associated with invasive histology** (Liu and Liotta, 1992), thus providing clinical substantiation of implications drawn from experimental models.

Major intracellular adhesion molecules such as E-cadherin and the transmembrane protein family of integrins also appear to be important barriers against invasion that can become disrupted in invasive tumors. This would make sense because these molecules are not only necessary for anchoring epithelial cells to each other and to the basal lamina, but also for cell-cell communication—often regulating the expression and function of membrane-bound growth factor receptors. Reduced expression of E-cadherin has been found in invasive tumors and has been associated with decreased survival of bladder cancer patients (Bringuier et al, 1993). Similarly, the integrin $\alpha_6 \beta_4$, which is normally expressed on the basement membrane surface of cells of the basal urothelial cell layer only, often is expressed diffusely throughout tumors (Grossman et al, 1992). Additionally, in bladder tumors, $\alpha_6 \beta_4$ integrin's normal association with a hemidesmosomal anchoring complex is lost, perhaps explaining defects in the urothelial barrier function that occur with malignancy (Liebert et al, 1994). These events may be particularly important if disruption of the structure or function of integrins, other components of the extracellular matrix, or both also enhance the ability of intraluminal urinary constituents with angiogenic, locomotive, or mitogenic properties to gain unusual access to the interstices of the bladder wall.

As discussed earlier, **abnormal expression or function of receptors for growth factors can, of course, enhance proliferative capacity of malignant cells, a major component of the invasive process.** EGF is a protein mitogen excreted in high concentrations in human urine in a biologically active form (Hirata and Orth, 1979). **Under normal circumstances, receptors for this substance primarily are confined to the basal layer of epithelial cells** (Messing et al, 1987a). **In both transitional and squamous cell carcinomas, however, EGF receptors become expressed not only on basal cells but also on cells of all layers, including those at the luminal surface** (Messing et al, 1987a; Messing, 1990). **This abnormal distribution of the EGF receptor is also seen in dysplastic and normal-appearing urothelium both nearby and remote from transitional cell cancers** (Messing, 1990; Rao et al, 1993). Even tumor cells that invade deeply into the bladder wall still all express the EGF receptor (Messing et al, 1987a; Messing 1990). **Both Messing and Neal and their respective co-workers have independently demonstrated that the degree of expression of the EGF receptor directly correlates with the invasive phenotype** (Messing, 1990; Neal et al, 1990). **Neal and colleagues, with extensive follow-up, have demonstrated that abnormally high expression of the EGF receptor in bladder cancers is an independent predictor of poor survival** (Neal et al, 1990; Mellon et al, 1995).

If the urinary EGF/urothelial EGF receptor interaction is actually important in urothelial tumorigenesis, one would also expect extraction of EGF from urine in patients with active tumors. Indeed, this has been found by several groups (Kristensen et al, 1988; Fuse et al, 1992; Messing and Murphy-Brooks, 1994), **with EGF concentrations in voided urine rising to noncancerous levels in the small number of patients whose urinary EGF has been measured both before and several months after bladder tumor resection** (Fuse et al, 1992). Additionally, other ligands that work through EGF receptors, such as transforming growth factor alpha (TGFα) and heparin-binding EGF-like growth factor (HB-EGF), may also play a role in bladder tumor progression and proliferation and possibly other processes (Cooper et al, 1992; Brown et al, 1993; Freeman et al, 1995b). **Indeed, because ligands for the EGF receptor induce not only mitogenesis but also cellular motility, stimulation of the EGF receptor on malignant urothelial and normal endothelial cells may encourage angiogenesis and malignant cell motility as well as proliferation—all processes important for invasion to occur.**

Histopathology and Clinical Correlates

Local invasion of bladder cancer can occur by three mechanisms (Jewett and Eversole, 1960). The most common is en bloc spread, occurring in about 60% of tumors, characterized by cancer cells invading in a broad front directly beneath the primary mucosal lesion. Tentacle-like (tentacular) invasion occurs in about 25% of tumors, and lateral spread, with tumor cells growing under normal-appearing mucosa, is observed in only about 10%. Malignant urothelial cells entering the lamina propria, and much more commonly the muscularis propria, can gain access to blood vessels and lymphatics through which they may metastasize to regional lymph nodes or distant sites. **The close correlation between muscle invasion and distant metastases was noted 50 years ago by Jewett and Strong (1946), and their work has remained one of the hallmarks of classification, prognosis, and management of this disease. Bladder cancer can also spread locally** to invade adjacent organs, including the prostate, uterus, vagina, ureters, rectum, and intestine.

More than 40% of men undergoing cystectomy for muscle-invasive bladder cancer have involvement of the prostate (Schellhammer et al, 1977; Hardeman et al, 1988; Wishnow and Ro, 1988). In the majority of such cases, the prostatic urethra is the site of involvement, but 6% have stromal involvement without prostatic urethral involvement. Overall, about 40% with prostatic involvement have invasion of the stroma (Wood et al, 1989). **In such patients, there is a high incidence (approximately 80%) of subsequent distant metastases despite seemingly complete local excision of all malignant tissue (e.g., cystoprostatourethrectomy). Because of this finding, it would be justified to consider adjuvant chemotherapy in this group** (neoadjuvant therapy if it is diagnosed preoperatively or when bladder salvage approaches are contemplated) (see later), but the efficacy of chemotherapy in this setting in preventing or delaying the appearance of distant disease has not been conclusively demonstrated. **Coexisting primary adenocarcinoma of the prostate may be present in 25% or more of patients** (Kabalin et al, 1989; Montie et al, 1989).

Tumors arising in bladder diverticula pose a special problem: They can invade directly from the epithelium into the perivesical tissues because bladder diverticula do not have a muscular wall. Often these tumors are treated with simple diverticulectomy or partial cystectomy. Careful mapping studies, however, must be done preoperatively to avoid the relatively poor survival results reported in most series of conservative excision (Faysal and Freiha, 1981). **In incidences of multifocal disease or severe epithelial dysplasia remote from the diverticulum, conservative excision is an unwise choice.**

Metastatic Spread

Roughly 5% of patients with well-differentiated and moderately differentiated superficial papillary cancer and approximately 20% with high-grade superficial disease (including carcinoma in situ) have vascular or lymphatic spread. The former percentage, however, reflects the proportion of patients who ultimately develop distant metastases or succumb to their disease, although many recurrences may have occurred during the interval. **It does not indicate how many had metastases while their tumors remained superficial, and almost all who develop metastases develop muscle-invasive recurrences before, or at the time, metastases are recognized.** Similarly, the latter percentage is based on evaluating cystectomy specimens in the highly selected group of patients with high-grade superficial tumors who fail conservative therapy and ultimately go on to radical cystectomy or eventually die of their malignancy (Freeman et al, 1995a). Presumably, metastases occur with superficial tumors because of invasion into lymphatic and vascular

channels within the lamina propria. **Although, realistically, some patients with superficial malignancies already have developed latent metastases, the vast majority of such individuals have their bladder lesion pathologically understaged and already harbor muscle-invasive lesions** (Freeman et al, 1995a).

Lymphatic Spread

Lymphatic metastases occur earlier and independent of hematogenous metastases in some patients. This may be evidenced in patients with lymph node metastases who are apparently cured with radical cystectomy and pelvic lymphadenectomy (Skinner and Lieskovski, 1984; Grossman and Konnak, 1988; Wishnow and Dmochowski, 1988; Lerner et al, 1993). Autopsy studies have shown that about 25% to 33% of patients dying of bladder cancer do not have pelvic lymph node metastases (Babaian et al, 1980). The most common sites of metastases in bladder cancer are the pelvic lymph nodes, occurring in about 78% of patients with nodal metastases. Among these, the paravesical nodes are involved in 16%, the obturator nodes in 74%, the external iliac nodes in 65%, and presacral nodes in roughly 25%. Juxtaregional common iliac lymph nodes are involved in about 20% of patients—but almost always with involvement of the above-mentioned regional sites as well (Smith and Whitmore, 1981a).

Vascular Spread

The common sites of vascular metastases in bladder cancer are liver, 38%; lung, 36%; bone, 27%; adrenal glands, 21%; and intestine, 13%. Any other organ may be involved (Babaian et al, 1980).

Implantation

Bladder cancer also spreads by implantation in abdominal wounds, denuded urothelium, the resected prostatic fossa, or traumatized urethra (Welden and Soloway, 1975). Implantation occurs more commonly with high-grade tumors (van der Werf-Messing, 1984). Implantation into wound scars can be prevented by giving approximately 10 Gy preoperative radiation, which has been recommended to be administered before performance of partial cystectomy, cystectomy, or cystotomy for interstitial radiation therapy (van der Werf-Messing, 1969). Tumor implantation into the resected prostatic fossa is an infrequent occurrence—but again primarily occurs with high-grade and multiple tumors. Investigators have reported that bladder tumors can be safely resected at the time of transurethral resection of the prostate without conferring a significantly higher risk of tumor cell implantation into the prostate fossa or urethra (Green and Yalowitz, 1972), although this report almost certainly involved a select group of patients, primarily with low-grade papillary malignancies. Avoidance of iatrogenic implantation has been the impetus for the use of immediate postresection intravesical therapy (Oosterlinck et al, 1993), the development of experimental antiadherence agents (See and Chapman, 1987; See et al, 1992; Hyacinthe et al, 1995), and the debate over the risks and benefits of performing random urothelial biopsies at the time of transurethral bladder tumor resection (Kiemeney et al, 1994).

NATURAL HISTORY

In a contemporary U.S. population, **roughly 55% to 60% of all newly diagnosed bladder cancers are well or moderately differentiated, superficial (mucosally confined or lamina propria invading) papillary transitional cell carcinomas** (Messing et al, 1995c). The majority of these patients develop tumor recurrences following endoscopic resection (Althausen et al, 1976; Gilbert et al, 1978; Fitzpatrick et al, 1986; Malmstrom et al, 1987; Prout et al, 1992). **Usually, recurrences of tumors that were well differentiated and superficial at the time of initial diagnosis reflect the characteristics of the initial tumor throughout the life of the patient** (Prout et al, 1992). **However, 16% to 25% recur with higher-grade tumors** (Gilbert et al, 1978; Prout et al, 1992). As discussed earlier, although many recurrences are probably new tumors arising from other areas of dysplastic urothelium, a significant proportion may be true recurrences resulting from inadequate treatment (Klan et al, 1991) or tumor cell implantation (Page et al, 1978; Oosterlinck et al, 1993). **Approximately 10% of patients with superficial papillary tumor subsequently develop invasive or metastatic cancer** (Althausen et al, 1976; Lutzeyer et al, 1982), although this is a distinctly rare event in patients whose initial tumors were grade I and mucosally confined (Prout et al, 1992). Important in understanding these data, however, is that **late and invasive recurrences are not unheard of after a prolonged tumor-free remission (e.g., >5 years) even in those whose index tumors were well differentiated and superficial** (Thompson et al, 1993).

Forty percent to 45% of newly diagnosed bladder cancer patients present with high-grade lesions, more than half of which are muscle invasive or more extensive at the time of diagnosis (Messing et al, 1995c). As discussed earlier, **even those with superficial tumors have high likelihoods of recurrence and far higher chances of developing invasive and metastatic disease than those with low-grade superficial tumors** (Cookson and Sarosdy, 1992; Norming et al, 1992; Freeman et al, 1995a; Messing et al, 1995c). **Thus, clinical evidence would dictate that transitional cell carcinoma has two major variants, low-grade and high-grade disease, which can be determined by routine cystoscopic examination, transurethral resection, and histopathologic analysis.**

Although the use of molecular probes to assess prognosis further remains under continued vigorous study, realistically, only a few provide independent prognostic information over routine cystoscopic and pathologic evaluation. Such markers, however, may also give insight into the biologic processes underlying the dimorphic nature of transitional cell carcinoma. **Because at least the major deleted genes on chromosome 9 primarily deal with cell cycle regulation, and their losses presumably predispose for proliferative lesions but not necessarily genetically unstable, invasive, or metastatic ones, it is not surprising that isolated chromosome 9 abnormalities have mostly been associated**

with papillary and superficial tumors (Tsai et al, 1990; Spruck et al, 1994; Wheeless et al, 1994; Orlow et al, 1995). **Alternatively, abnormalities in p53 functioning, because they not only permit the cell cycle to continue but also prevent cells with abnormal DNA from going into an apoptotic pathway, and hence foster progressive genomic instability** (Harris and Hollstein, 1993), **are more commonly associated with high-grade lesions. These are more likely to continue to undergo further genetic and epigenetic alterations, promoting the processes of invasion and metastasis (see earlier)** (Esrig et al, 1994; Spruck et al, 1994). **Some patients with low-grade tumors, however, eventually develop higher-grade recurrences** (Gilbert et al, 1978; Prout et al, 1992), **and it is not unheard of to have low-grade and high-grade lesions simultaneously in the same patient's bladder. Such an occasional transition in the normally biphasic profile of transitional cell carcinoma is not inconsistent with epidemiologic and molecular data, indicating that there are similarities (and, presumably, common points of origin) between low-grade and high-grade disease** (Messing, 1990; Scheinfeld et al, 1990; Tsai et al, 1990; Hayes et al, 1993; Rao et al, 1993; Golijanin et al, 1995).

Almost 25% of patients with newly diagnosed bladder cancer have muscle-invasive disease, the vast majority being the tumors of high histologic grade (Messing et al, 1995c). **Most patients (85%–92%) with muscle-invasive bladder cancer (both those without and those with histories of previously treated bladder tumors) already have this level of invasion at the time of initial diagnosis** (Kaye and Lange, 1982; Hopkins et al, 1983). Almost 50% of patients with muscle-invasive bladder cancer already have occult distant metastases. This limits the efficacy of local or regional forms of therapy for invasive tumors. **Most patients with occult metastases develop overt clinical evidence of distant metastases within 1 year** (Prout et al, 1979; Babaian et al, 1980).

Nearly all patients with metastatic bladder cancer die within 2 years (Babaian et al, 1980; Loehrer et al, 1992); however, approximately 5% of patients with established metastatic disease have "freak" cancers that run a more indolent clinical course, lasting 5 years or more (Marshall and McCarron, 1977). **Between 10% and 35% of patients with limited regional lymph node metastases survive 5 years or more without evidence of metastases following radical cystectomy and pelvic lymphadenectomy** (LaPlante and Brice, 1973; Smith and Whitmore, 1981a; Skinner and Lieskovsky, 1984; Grossman and Konnak, 1988; Lerner et al, 1993; Freeman et al, 1995a). It is uncertain to what extent these patients represent surgical cures of regional metastatic bladder cancer or simply freak cancers. One must conclude that, at worst, patients with only limited nodal metastases have a more protracted clinical course than those with visceral or osseous metastases, and, at best, **some patients with limited nodal metastases may be cured by local/regional excisional therapy. In patients with extensive nodal metastases, the prospects for cure are poor**—at least without the intervention of systemic chemotherapy (Smith and Whitmore, 1981a).

It should be remembered that many patients with incurable bladder cancer either may not develop severe local symptoms from the primary tumor or may have these symptoms controlled with conservative measures, such as transurethral resection or radiation therapy. It is conceivable that many such patients could retain their bladders even though they may ultimately die from metastatic disease. Thus, in patients with gross nodal metastases (usually visible on preoperative imaging studies) that are biopsy-proven or distant metastases, systemic therapy should probably be initiated before considering extensive local management such as cystectomy or full-dose radiation therapy. The latter two modalities should probably be withheld unless there is a complete or nearly complete response to systemic chemotherapy, when surgical resection of limited metastases (and the primary tumor) can render the patient free of apparent disease.

PROGNOSTIC INDICATORS

Clinical and laboratory tests have been examined as potential means of predicting the clinical course of bladder cancer in individual patients. For these tests to be of prognostic value in the clinical setting, they must add some predictive capacity beyond what standard clinical and pathologic parameters (see later) offer. This usually requires a multivariate analysis to determine each marker's prognostic independence, which, in turn, requires sufficient numbers of samples in the relevant staging and grading categories to permit appropriate statistical analyses to be performed.

Clinical and Pathologic Parameters in Superficial Bladder Cancer

The most clinically useful prognostic parameters for tumor recurrence and subsequent cancer progression in the patient with superficial tumors are tumor grade, depth of tumor penetration (stage), lymphatic invasion, tumor size, urothelial dysplasia or carcinoma in situ in neighboring or distant urothelial areas, papillary or solid tumor architecture, multifocality, and frequency of tumor recurrences (Heney et al, 1983; Fitzpatrick et al, 1986; Wolf and Hojgaard, 1983; Madgar et al, 1988). **The most important among these are tumor grade, stage, and presence of carcinoma in situ.**

Tumor recurrence and progression rates are higher in patients with large (>10 g) or multifocal tumors (Fitzpatrick et al, 1986), high-grade tumors (Heney et al, 1983), tumors with lamina propria invasion (Dalesio et al, 1983), tumors invading lymphatic spaces (Anderstrom et al, 1980; Freeman et al, 1995a), and tumors associated with severe urothelial dysplasia or carcinoma in situ (Althausen et al, 1976). **In patients with lamina propria–invading, grade III transitional cell carcinomas, at least one third exhibit stage progression to muscle invasion** (Gilbert et al, 1978; Jakse et al, 1987), **even with complete endoscopic resection and intravesical therapy with BCG** (Cookson and Sarosdy, 1992; Waples and Messing, 1992).

In patients with diffuse carcinoma in situ, an important prognostic factor is the presence of irritative voiding symptoms (frequency, urgency, dysuria). For example, Riddle and co-workers reported that only 1 of 13 patients who were asymptomatic died of invasive bladder cancer, whereas 15 of 23 with irritative symptoms died of invasive cancer despite definitive radiation therapy or cystectomy (Riddle et al, 1976). **Another important factor is the extent of involvement with carcinoma in situ; those with only focal involvement have a more indolent course than those with diffuse involvement** (Althausen et al, 1976).

Laboratory Parameters

A variety of laboratory parameters also have been evaluated for prognostic significance. Although significant correlations with tumor progression have been demonstrated, these tests have not been adopted into clinical practice yet and currently do not influence treatment decisions in individual patients. It is likely, however, that within the next few years this may well change.

ABH Blood Group Antigens

Patients with type O blood with superficial tumors have a higher incidence of high-grade tumors and cancer progression (Orihuela and Shahon, 1987).

The ABO blood group antigen system consists of carbohydrate antigens that are carried by glycoproteins or glycolipids on blood cells or epithelial cells. The biosynthesis of these carbohydrate antigens is presumed to be controlled by at least five different genes: ABO, Se, H, Le, and X. These genes code for specific transferase enzymes that add the respective carbohydrates to their precursors in a sequential fashion. Studies of expression of blood group antigens on urothelial cells suggest that, **with malignant transformation, bladder cancer cells cease to express the ABH blood group antigens** (Coon et al, 1982; Huben, 1984). **Antigen deletion has correlated with increased recurrence rates and the development of invasive disease** (Malmstrom et al, 1988). The best-documented change has been the deletion of the A and B antigens from patients with type A and B blood, respectively, and the deletion of the H antigen from patients with type O blood (Sheinfeld et al, 1990).

In general, malignant transformation also appears to be associated with enhanced Lewis^x antigen expression (Cordon-Cardo et al, 1988). **This makes Lewis^x antigen expression particularly attractive for the diagnosis of bladder cancer** (because it is a positive test—increased antigen expression—rather than a negative one such as antigen deletion), although **it is likely to be abnormally expressed regardless of tumor grade or stage** (Sheinfeld et al, 1990; Golijanin et al, 1995).

Alterations in blood group antigen expression are due to perturbations of the glycosyltransferase enzymes in the tumor cells or to the use of alternate substrates or competition among the transferases in the altered biosynthetic pathway (Orntoff, 1988). This altered expression not only may be a marker of disease and disease progression but also may have functional significance in that the vast majority of cell surface hormone and growth factor receptors (such as the receptor for EGF, the erbB2 oncogene product, and the receptors for angiogenic substances such as the FGFs and autocrine motility factor) are all transmembrane proteins whose ligand-binding components branch out from the exterior of the cell membrane and are often heavily glycosylated with a variety of carbohydrate moieties. Alterations in glycosylation may well affect ligand binding sites, and other molecular interactions with extracellular matrix structures such as E-cadherin, the integrins, and the glycosaminoglycan layer lining the luminal surface of the superficial urothelial cells.

Thomsen-Friedenreich (T) Antigen Expression

Thomsen-Friedenreich (T) antigen is a cryptic disaccharide present on human erythrocytes, which can be exposed by neuraminidase treatment. T antigen is usually expressed in an unmasked form in bladder cancer cells (Radzikowski et al, 1989; Oda et al, 1990). It is expressed independently of ABH blood group antigens. T antigen expression has been reported to correlate with muscle-invasive disease and is associated with a poor prognosis (Coon et al, 1982; Javadpour, 1984). It has also been reported to be predictive of the response to treatment with BCG and interleukin-2 (Dow et al, 1989), although it is not clear that such is not simply a reflection of tumor aggressiveness.

Other Tumor-Associated Antigens

A variety of transitional cell carcinoma–associated antigens detectable with monoclonal antibodies have shown promise as diagnostic (see later) or prognostic markers. Among the more promising include the antigen M344. This antigenic determinant is on a cytosolic protein of more than 300,000 Da (Cordon-Cardo et al, 1992), is detectable in roughly 70% of superficial bladder tumors, and is rarely found in invasive lesions (Fradet and Cordon-Cardo, 1993). This antigen is also detectable on exfoliated cells and, when found, can often predict further recurrence of bladder cancers at a time when cystoscopic examination is negative (Bonner et al, 1993). A second tumor-associated antigen, T138, also is expressed on exfoliated malignant cells but is associated with decreased survival (Fradet et al, 1990). Another antigen detected by a monoclonal antibody, 19A211, is a sialoglycoprotein in a cytoplasmic protein complex of 100,000 to 200,000 Da (Cordon-Cardo et al, 1992). When it is seen on superficial tumors (it is also found on 25% of normal umbrella cells), it predicts a lower likelihood of tumor recurrence, whereas expression of T138 predicts a significantly higher likelihood (Allard et al, 1995). This was so even when one took into consideration other adverse predictors, such as tumor size, multiplicity, grade, and lamina propria invasion. Other groups have demonstrated that epithelial membrane antigen (EMA) developed more homogeneous staining in bladder tumors associated with poor survival and was more heterogeneously expressed in those associated with improved survival (Lopez-Altran et al, 1993).

Extracellular Matrix and Cell Adhesion Molecules

Fibronectin is a component of the bladder's extracellular matrix that appears primarily in the basement membrane and

submucosa and is absent from the luminal surface of urothelial cells (Pode et al, 1986). **Soluble fibronectin can inhibit BCG's adherence to the vesical wall, which is necessary for it to achieve its antitumor activity** (Ratliff et al, 1991). Because fibronectin can be measured in the urine using an enzyme-linked immunosorbent assay (ELISA), Malmstrom and colleagues correlated urinary fibronectin excretion before and after tumor resection with tumor stage, and response to BCG (Malmstrom et al, 1993). In superficial and superficial muscle-invasive tumors, fibronectin levels changed little but were much higher for deeply invasive malignancies. More importantly, 2 to 4 weeks after seemingly complete transurethral resection, urinary fibronectin excretion decreased sixfold—down to normal levels. Patients receiving BCG therapy who had lower urinary fibronectin levels before the initiation of treatment (but after transurethral resection) had a much higher likelihood of being tumor free at 1 year than those with elevated fibronectin excretion. Although these findings certainly correlate with known mechanisms of BCG activity, the elevated urinary fibronectin levels preceding BCG therapy may have predicted tumor recurrence primarily because they reflected the presence of persistent (although unrecognized) tumor rather than actually predicting lack of BCG responsiveness.

Another extracellular matrix component that is present in the basement membrane of the urothelium is laminin, a 950- to 1000-Da glycoprotein thought to be synthesized by the epithelial or endothelial cells resting on the basement membrane (Foydart et al, 1980). Focal interruption of basal membrane laminin correlated directly with tumor stage (although not with grade), with tumor recurrence rate after endoscopic resection, and with a shorter recurrence-free interval. Additionally, subendothelial (in bladder vessels within the lamina propria) basal membrane laminin disruption was found in all five patients who died of metastatic disease. **Abou Farah and colleagues concluded that disruption of laminin staining in basal laminas of the urothelium and subjacent endothelial structures may identify those cancers with the capacities to invade and metastasize** (Abou Farah et al, 1993). As mentioned earlier, altered expression of two **other extracellular adhesion molecules, E-cadherin and integrin $\alpha_6 \beta_4$ also have been associated with an invasive bladder cancer phenotype** (Bringuier et al, 1993; Liebert et al, 1994).

Growth Factors and Their Receptors

As discussed earlier, several groups have demonstrated that abnormal expression of the receptor for EGF on malignant urothelium correlates with increased tumor aggressiveness (Messing, 1990; Neal et al, 1990; Mellon et al, 1995) **and that in multivariate analysis it is an independent predictor of poor survival from disease** (Mellon et al, 1995). This is a consistent finding despite the considerable variety of reagents and techniques that have been employed to detect this receptor. Unfortunately, in general, it is far easier to detect EGF receptors in frozen tissue sections, thus making the practical utility of this test questionable. Perhaps with the use of antigen retrieval techniques such as microwaving, similar correlations will be possible in formalin-fixed, paraffin-embedded archival tissues, with currently available (or other) anti-EGF receptor antibodies. If such is the case, it is likely that detection of this antigen will enter the realm of routine clinical practice.

Transforming growth factor–betas (TGF-βs) constitute a family of related proteins that include TGF-β1–5, müllerian inhibitory substance, inhibin, and activin (Sporn and Roberts, 1989). **Although TGF-βs were originally found to assist the malignant transformation of rat fibroblasts** (Sporn and Roberts, 1989), **in most cases, they are inhibitors of cellular proliferation, at least in part through stimulating p27 and p15, nuclear proteins that inhibit the phosphorylation of pRb by various cyclin-dependent kinases.** Thus, in many cases, TGF-β activity prevents the uncomplexing of pRb and E2F, impeding cellular proliferation (see earlier) (Cordon-Cardo, 1995). It would therefore be expected that tumors with elevated expression of TGF-βs (particularly TGF-β1) would have slower proliferation and be more indolent than those with reduced expression. This has been found using Northern blotting to detect TGF-β1 and 2 mRNAs by Coombs and colleagues (1993). Alternatively, Miyato and co-workers reported that all types of transitional cell cancers had higher TGF-β1 expression than normal urothelium did (Miyato et al, 1995), but as Coombs and colleagues had found, **TGF-β1 expression was significantly higher in the more indolent tumors than in aggressive ones** (Coombs et al, 1993).

Amplification of the c-erbB2 oncogene is rarely found but when detected has a strong association with progression of bladder cancer. Its overexpression, however, which is far more common than amplification of its gene, has been unrelated to tumor recurrence or progression (Underwood et al, 1995). Underwood and co-workers concluded that expression of this gene may be more useful as a marker of disease than as a prognostic indicator (Underwood et al, 1995). Other authors have found conflicting results as well (see previously).

Chromosomal and Genetic Abnormalities

Chromosomal abnormalities, including increased number of chromosomes, marker chromosomes, and chromosomes of abnormal size or configuration, have also been shown to correlate with an increased risk of tumor recurrence and cancer progression (Gibas and Sandberg, 1984; Sandberg, 1986; Carter et al, 1987; Falor and Ward-Skinner, 1988). Tumor recurrences and cancer progression are most common among patients who have tumors with marker chromosomes and a large proportion of aneuploid tumor cells (Gibas and Sandberg, 1984). Waldman and colleagues have found that particularly an increased number of chromosome 7 correlates with tumor grade and labeling index (as a surrogate for proliferation) (Waldman et al, 1991).

One of the most commonly found chromosomal abnormalities has been deletion of chromosome 9—particularly loss of an entire chromosome. This can be analyzed by image analysis using fluorescence in situ hybridization (FISH) (fluoresceinated DNA probes to various portions of the chromosome are applied and then examined microscopically using computerized technology). **Wheeless and co-workers have demonstrated that having only a single**

copy of chromosome 9 in tumor cells from bladder wash specimens obtained immediately following a 6-week course of BCG correlated well with tumor recurrence and predicted failure of BCG intravesical therapy (Wheeless et al, 1995). This was particularly true when tumors were DNA diploid (see later); DNA aneuploid tumors are usually more likely to recur and progress (see later)—and all had abnormalities of chromosome 9 in this study.

Deletions of chromosome 17p have been associated with tumor progression—presumably because the tumor suppressor gene, p53, is lost with the section of 17p that is deleted. **Others have now looked at increased immunohistochemical detectability of p53 in the nucleus as a surrogate for genetic deletion or mutation (or both)** (Finlay et al, 1988). Esrig and colleagues **demonstrated increased nuclear expression of p53 in formalin-fixed, paraffin-embedded sections of transitional cell carcinomas from patients undergoing cystectomy, correlated with reduced survival and disease progression** (Esrig et al, 1994). This study, however, was composed almost exclusively of high-risk bladder cancer patients, most of whom had invasive or regional disease. Furthermore, **several series have failed to find prognostic value for nuclear immunohistochemical detectability of p53, independent of tumor grade and stage, in patients with superficial bladder tumors** (Lipponen et al, 1993; Gardner et al, 1994; Thomas et al, 1994). **Thus, although its role as a marker of adverse prognosis in superficial tumors is likely, this has not yet been established** (see section on predictors of disease progression in invasive bladder cancer).

Nonrandom losses of chromosome 13q, where the Rb gene is located, have been associated with bladder cancer (Ishikawa et al, 1991; Dalbagni et al, 1993). Mutations or deletions of the Rb gene or its protein product lead to uninhibited proliferation by permitting the cell cycle to go through its G1 → S checkpoint. Initially, loss of pRb function, particularly as determined immunohistochemically as no detectable nuclear staining, had been associated with high-grade, invasive, and poor prognosis disease (Cordon-Cardo et al, 1992; Aprikian et al, 1993; Stadler, 1993). Not all investigators, however, found a significant correlation between lack of pRb expression and poor outcome (Ishikawa et al, 1991; Cordon-Cardo, 1995). Moreover, even those studies reporting a close association with poor prognosis have acknowledged that the majority of even lethal bladder cancers do not lack pRb expression (Cordon-Cardo et al, 1992). Further complicating this matter is that in many of the cases of bladder cancer in which losses of chromosome 13q have been identified, there are no mutations in the remaining copy of the Rb gene and wt pRb is expressed, implying that there may be tumor suppressor genes other than Rb located on chromosome 13q that are important in urothelial tumorigenesis (Ishikawa et al, 1991). **At the current time, therefore, although the biologic importance of pRb deletions or mutations seems likely, the utility of their detection for clinical patient management—and particularly prognosis—remains in question.**

Markers of Proliferation

It has long been recognized that a higher percentage of proliferating cells correlates with tumor aggressivity. Counting mitotic figures per microscopic field has been a standard way of assessing tumor aggressiveness in almost all malignancies. Similarly, various laboratory parameters have been used to assess proliferation. This includes nondiploid fractions in flow cytometric analysis (Wheeless et al, 1994); increased DNA synthesizing S phase fraction on flow cytometry of both exfoliated and formalin fixed cells (Nemoto et al, 1988); immunohistochemical detection of antigens expressed during various phases of the cell cycle, including proliferating cell nuclear antigen (PCNA) (Waldman et al, 1993); and the antigen detected with antibody mib-1, Ki67 (Cohen et al, 1993). Each roughly correlates with cell proliferation or at least DNA synthesis. **Several groups have indicated that increased aneuploid populations and proportion of S phase cells correlate with tumor grade and stage and with a higher likelihood of recurrence, progression, and reduced survival** (Koss et al, 1989; Norming et al, 1992; Wheeless et al, 1993). Increased expression of PCNA or Ki67 (or both) has also been associated with worse prognosis of bladder cancer (Cohen et al, 1993; Waldman et al, 1993), although lack of consensus about appropriate cutoffs and areas of heterogeneity within tumors makes interpretation of results challenging and currently renders the applicability of these tests for individual patient management highly questionable.

DIAGNOSIS

Signs and Symptoms

The most common presenting symptom of bladder cancer is painless hematuria, which occurs in about 85% of patients (Varkarakis et al, 1974). **In reality, nearly all patients with cystoscopically detectable bladder cancer have at least microhematuria if one tests enough urine samples** (Messing and Valencourt, 1990). **Hematuria is often quite intermittent, however, so that a negative result on one or two specimens has little meaning in ruling out the presence of bladder cancer** (Messing et al, 1987b; Messing et al, 1989; Messing and Valencourt, 1990). Thus, if a patient in the bladder cancer age range has unexplained hematuria on a urine specimen (either microscopically or grossly evident), and a "confirmatory" second specimen is free of any hematuria, cystoscopic examination is still usually warranted (Messing et al, 1987b; Messing et al, 1989; Messing et al, 1992). The symptom complex of bladder irritability and urinary frequency, urgency, and dysuria is the second most common presentation and usually is associated with diffuse carcinoma in situ or invasive bladder cancer. **These symptoms, however, almost never occur without (at least) microscopic hematuria.** Other signs and symptoms of bladder cancer include flank pain from ureteral obstruction, lower extremity edema, and a pelvic mass. Rarely, patients present with symptoms of advanced disease, such as weight loss and abdominal or bone pain.

Conventional Microscopic Cytology

Malignant transitional cells can be observed on microscopic examination of the urinary sediment or bladder wash-

ings. Characteristically, tumor cells have large nuclei with irregular, coarsely textured chromatin. **The limitations of microscopic cytology are due to the cytologically normal appearance of cells from well-differentiated tumors, and, because well-differentiated cancer cells are more cohesive, they are not readily shed into the urine. Therefore, microscopic cytology is more sensitive in patients with high-grade tumors or carcinoma in situ. Even in patients with high-grade tumors, however, urinary cytology may be falsely negative in 20%.**

False-positive cytology may occur in 1% to 12% of patients and is usually due to urothelial atypia, inflammation, or changes caused by radiation therapy or chemotherapy (Koshikawa et al, 1989). These changes are frequently observed after several months of therapy and may persist for more than 1 year after the initiation of therapy. **Cytology is not a cost-effective means of screening for bladder cancer unless high-risk populations alone are evaluated** (Gamarra and Zein, 1984). As is discussed below, **because far more surface epithelial cells are present in specimens obtained from bladder washes than through voiding, the former are more useful in the diagnosis of bladder cancer.**

Flow Cytometry

Flow cytometry measures the DNA content of cells. Therefore, it can quantitate the aneuploid cell populations and proliferative activity (percent S-phase cells) in a tumor. With flow cytometry, the isolated cells, whose nuclei are stained with a DNA-binding fluorescent dye, flow through a small tube in which fluorescence is excited by a laser beam. DNA content is measured from fluorescent intensity. **The ability to perform flow cytometry on paraffin-embedded archival tumor tissues allows correlations to be made among flow cytometry parameters, tumor progression, and patient survival.**

For diagnostic purposes, bladder wash specimens usually are required for satisfactory results (Konchuba et al, 1989). Arbitrary limits are required to define normality. For example, if more than 15% of the cells are aneuploid, the cytologic findings are defined as being positive for cancer (Melamed, 1984).

Flow cytometry studies in bladder cancer patients have demonstrated several clinical correlations (Tribukait, 1987; Blomjous et al, 1989; Atallah et al, 1990; Badalament et al, 1990; Wijkstrom and Tribukait, 1990). **Diploid tumors generally tend to be of low grade and low stage, and patients have a favorable prognosis.** Tumors with a triploid to tetraploid chromosome number have unfavorable pathologic characteristics, and patients have a poor prognosis. **Patients with tumors that are tetraploid have a more favorable prognosis than patients with triploid or tetraploid tumors but a worse prognosis than patients with diploid tumors** (Tribukait, 1987; Winkler et al, 1989; Wijkstrom and Tribukait, 1990). **Inflammatory cells can form a hyperdiploid cell fraction, which makes interpretation of standard flow cytometry difficult.**

A correlation exists between proliferative activity, expressed as a percentage of tumor cells in S-phase, and tumor progression. An increased incidence of lymph node metastases occurs in patients with aneuploid tumors and in patients with tumors with greater than 10% S-phase cells. Because S-phase itself represents only a tiny fraction of the entire duration of the cell cycle (Cordon-Cardo, 1995), however, even tumors with aggressive phenotypes are usually not captured with an abundance of their cells in S-phase and may be overlooked by this simple criterion. Tumors with more than one aneuploid cell population also have a higher cancer progression rate. In patients treated with radiation, the presence or persistence of triploid to tetraploid cells is an unfavorable prognostic indicator. In contrast, patients who have cells following radiation therapy that have diploid or tetraploid chromosome complements are likely to have a more favorable response to radiation. It is possible, however, that this simply reflects persistence of aggressive or indolent tumor cells, rather than any effect of radiation.

Flow cytometry can measure multiple parameters simultaneously. For example, cells can be stained for DNA and cytokeratins (a marker for epithelial cells). The flow cytometer can be programmed to measure DNA content only in cells that stain positively for cytokeratins (Hijazi et al, 1989). **This multiparameter approach improves the accuracy of flow cytometry because it makes it possible actually to measure which cells are proliferating in specimens, thus avoiding attributing characteristics to tumor cells that actually belong to nonmalignant cells, such as white blood cells.** Current studies have exploited this type of approach and appear to demonstrate more prognostic significance than either DNA measurements alone or antigen expression measurements alone (Fradet et al, 1990).

In general, flow cytometry has not been found to be more clinically valuable than conventional cytology, although some studies have reported that it is more accurate (Denovic et al, 1982). **Low-grade superficial tumors, which are usually diploid, often produce false-negative results. Aneuploidy is a common feature of high-grade tumors, and thus flow cytometry is especially accurate in patients with carcinoma in situ or high-grade malignancies, in whom 80% to 90% of tumors can be correctly identified** (Melamed, 1984; Badalament et al, 1990). Flow cytometry has not supplanted conventional cytology in managing bladder cancer patients, although advances in preparation and fixation now permit bladder wash specimens to be transported to institutions that commonly use flow cytometry for bladder cancer diagnostic studies.

Despite the correlations mentioned earlier, to predict the likelihood of tumor progression on an individual patient basis, flow cytometry is limited by there being a significant proportion of bladder cancers that progress that are diploid or near-diploid and some aneuploid tumors that do not progress (Tribukait, 1987).

Image Analysis

Quantitative fluorescent image analysis is an automated cytologic technique that analyzes smears of cells on a microscope slide and quantitatively measures DNA content in each cell (Carter et al, 1987). **It combines quantitative biochemical analysis and more subjective visual evaluation of individual cells (whereas cytometry can analyze only a population of cells).**

This technique uses a computer-controlled fluorescence microscope, which automatically scans and images the nucleus of each cell on a slide. The computer quantitates the amount of emitted fluorescence, which is directly proportional to the nucleic acid content, and identifies each cell that contains an abnormal amount of DNA. Thus, a cytotechnologist can focus on each abnormal cell identified by an automatic analyzer for morphologic evaluation. **Because individual cells can be examined by image analysis, this technique can more easily use voided urine specimens than flow cytometry can, as the latter requires a large number of cell populations for its analysis.**

As with flow cytometry, multiparameter image analysis can be performed also. For instance, labeled monoclonal antibodies to various tumor markers used in conjunction with DNA fluorescence can increase the specificity of image analysis for bladder cancer detection. This type of analysis may also serve as a means of monitoring treatment response. **This technique is more sensitive than either standard cytology or flow cytometry** (Parry and Hemstreet, 1988), **and it may be more sensitive especially for detecting low-grade bladder cancer than either conventional cytology or flow cytometry (without reducing specificity)** (Parry and Hemstreet, 1988). Additionally, image analysis can be performed using fluorescently labeled DNA probes to specific chromosomes of interest and can, in conjunction with in situ hybridization, effectively demonstrate that tumors have trisomy of the centromeric region of chromosome 7 (Waldman et al, 1991), loss of various regions (or all) of chromosome 9 (Wheeless et al, 1994), or deletions of chromosome 17p.

Specimen Collection

Saline bladder washes are more accurate than voided urine samples for detecting bladder cancer because the mechanical action of barbotage enhances tumor cell shedding and provides better preserved cells for examination (Trott and Edwards, 1973). In urine that has remained in the bladder for prolonged periods, cellular degeneration occurs. Therefore, first-voided morning specimens should not be sampled for cytology. Urinary tract infection, indwelling catheters, calculi, or bladder instrumentation can also produce artifactual changes in urinary cytology (Gamarra and Zein, 1984). Occasionally, false-positive results can occur in barbotages primarily by shearing off fragments of normal transitional epithelium, which may be mistaken for low-grade bladder tumors. Similarly, osmotic changes in contrast media can also cause difficulties in interpreting cytologic preparations, often resulting in false-positive findings. Also, radiation therapy, intravesical chemotherapy, and intravesical BCG therapy can induce confusing abnormalities.

Perhaps the greatest utility of cytology, cytometry, or image analysis on voided specimens is their capacity to sample areas of the urinary tract other than the bladder that may shed malignant transitional epithelium (such as the renal pelvis, ureter, or prostatic urethra). Additionally, with a diagnosis of a low-grade papillary superficial bladder tumor, positive cytology, cytometry, or image analysis (on either voided or barbotage specimens) for high-grade cells is likely to indicate the presence of cysto-

scopically invisible carcinoma in situ elsewhere in the patient's urinary tract.

EARLY DETECTION

Rationale

All epithelial bladder tumors begin on the urothelial surface, and virtually all patients who succumb to this disease have distant metastases. **Almost all patients who develop metastases, however, have concomitant or prior muscle-invasive bladder cancers** (Jewett and Strong, 1946; Freeman et al, 1995a). **Because 84% to 92% of all patients who have muscle-invasive bladder cancers have cancer at the time of their initial diagnosis** (Kaye and Lange, 1982; Hopkins et al, 1983), management approaches (to be discussed subsequently) for patients with superficial bladder cancers, although critically important to those individuals, are unlikely in themselves to reduce mortality from bladder cancer significantly unless combined with some form of early detection strategy. Conversely, **if bladder cancers can be detected while still confined to the mucosa or lamina propria, they can be treated by relatively nonmorbid (such as endoscopic resection without or with intravesical therapy), highly successful (see later) means. Moreover, even the highly selected subgroup of superficial bladder cancer patients with high-grade malignancies that frequently recur and are refractory to endoscopic and intravesical therapies are cured the overwhelming majority of times with localized therapies** (Freiha, 1990; Malkowicz et al, 1990; Freeman et al, 1995a). **This indicates that even in this selected group with aggressive superficial cancers, distant metastases have rarely occurred. Furthermore, early detection strategies are at least unlikely to hurt individuals in whom tumors are detected because they undoubtedly would have become symptomatic some time during the patient's lifetime, eventually leading to diagnosis and treatment. Were this not the case, far more tumors would be reported as incidental findings on autopsy, as occurs with prostatic** (Franks, 1954) and renal carcinomas (Hellstein et al, 1981).

Bladder Cancer Screening

Biases and Pitfalls

Early detection strategies for chronic diseases such as bladder cancer, besides requiring sensitive and accurate instruments, can be considered of value only if they actually reduce mortality or morbidity from the disease being looked for, compared to what would happen in a comparable population that went unscreened. **In the ideal situation, such demonstrations of efficacy require prospective studies in which survival from the disease is the major end point and in which participants are randomized to standard care or the early detection intervention.** By such a comparison, one can rule out biases in the screening encountered by earlier diagnosis in screenees (and hence a longer time from diagnosis to death even if mortality has not changed at all—*lead time bias*), a tendency to detect more indolent

tumors with longer preclinical durations and clinical courses in the screened group *(length bias sampling)*, a tendency toward overzealous diagnosis of malignancy in the screened population, and a tendency for participants in early detection programs to be more healthy and health conscious *(selection bias)* (summarized in Morrison, 1992). To date, no such prospective, randomized, controlled screening trial for bladder cancer has been carried out.

For early detection to be effective, accurate instruments (screening tools) must be available. In general, particularly for an ostensibly healthy population (albeit at high risk for developing bladder cancer), the screening technique should be inexpensive and nonmorbid. **For instance, cystoscopy and bladder wash cytology are routinely used in screening the individuals at highest risk for developing bladder cancer, those patients with prior histories of superficial bladder tumors. As is discussed subsequently, this policy probably does save lives and bladders. Such techniques, however, although extremely accurate, would be inappropriate (because of patient acceptance, morbidity, and expense) in individuals, even if they were at high risk, who never previously had bladder cancer or had signs or symptoms characteristic of the disease.** In such individuals, non-invasive tests include examining urine for hematuria (Messing et al, 1987b; Britton et al, 1989), examining voided urine for malignant cells with cytology (Gamarra and Zein, 1984) or quantitative fluorescence image analysis (Parry and Hemstreet, 1988), combinations of these methods incorporating marker antigens (Fradet et al, 1990; Sheinfeld et al, 1990; Bonner et al, 1993; Golijanin et al, 1995), or measurements of relevant marker compounds in urine (Chodak et al, 1988; Guirguis et al, 1988; Nguyen et al, 1993; Messing and Murphy-Brooks, 1994). Instruments, however, must be both sensitive (free of false-negative results) and specific (free of false-positive results) and have acceptable positive and negative predictive values (if a test is positive or negative, there is a high likelihood of actually harboring or not having the disease). For example, a test with low specificity, although in itself not that expensive, triggers a diagnostic evaluation and considerable concern on the part of those with false-positive test results that often are unnecessary yet engender considerable expense and possibly morbidity. Alternatively, a test with low sensitivity may lull individuals with false-negative test results (and their physicians) into a false sense of security that may lead both patients and physicians to overlook symptoms caused by the malignancy and actually delay the diagnosis of the cancer beyond when it would have been detected had the patient and physician paid attention to the symptoms, often with tragic consequences (Morrison, 1992). **Unfortunately the vast majority of potentially useful tests for screening have had their sensitivities and specificities assessed on highly biased populations: those with known tumors or histories of tumors or a small number of presumably normal controls often not matched with the bladder cancer population (middle-aged and elderly men with smoking histories) for age, gender, and exposure history. Such characteristics may have little to do with the actual sensitivities and specificities of these tests in a more generalized population in whom only a small fraction actually have bladder tumors.**

Reported Studies

Two major screening studies have been performed on **relatively generalized, geographically defined populations (unselected middle-aged and elderly men) who were not believed to have bladder tumors or urologic malignancies.** Neither study, however, had a prospective, randomized, control population. **Each used multiple hematuria home testings with chemical reagent strips in which participants, solicited from primary care rosters, tested their urine at home repeatedly.** If a test was positive (trace or greater), even once, they were asked to undergo a standard urologic evaluation, which included urinary cytology and cystoscopy. Despite differences in other elements of the evaluation and in the actual testing protocols and solicitation techniques, both Messing (Messing et al, 1989, 1992, 1995b, 1995c) and Britton (Britton et al, 1989, 1992) and their respective collaborators in studies in south-central Wisconsin of the United States and Leeds, England, had similar findings. **In each instance, roughly 20% of participants had hematuria, and in those who underwent a thorough evaluation, 6% to 8% were found to have urothelial cancers; overall, 1.3% of those participating in Wisconsin and 1.2% of those participating in England had bladder cancer diagnosed. Although the follow-up of the British cohort is pending, to date, 9 years after the initiation of the Wisconsin study, not one of the 21 participants in whom bladder cancer was detected by screening has died of their malignancy.**

The percentage of bladder cancers diagnosed through standard clinical presentation in those who were solicited for participation in Wisconsin but elected not to take part in screening was calculated within 18 months of what would have been their final testing date. This represented 1.2% of solicitees who did not take part. **This indicates that those taking part in screening were not more likely to get bladder cancer than those solicited (i.e., self-selection had not occurred)** (Messing et al, 1995c).

A contemporary, geographically similar population who developed bladder cancer but was not screened was also investigated. State tumor registry data were used to compare outcomes, and pathology materials (blocks and slides) were examined in 511 of the 573 cases of men age 50 and over who had bladder cancer newly diagnosed in Wisconsin in 1988 and reported to the state cancer registry. Histologies and outcomes were compared with those of the 21 participants in screening who had bladder cancers diagnosed. **In both screened and unscreened men, roughly the same percentage had low-grade (grade I, II), superficial (epithelial or lamina propria confined) bladder cancers (56.8% of unscreened cases and 52.4% of screened cases). The vast majority of the remaining cancers in both groups were high grade, more than half of which in the unscreened population (nearly 24% of all unscreened cases) were not detected before they invaded the muscularis propria (or deeper), whereas fewer than 5% of screened cases invaded the muscularis propria** (Table 77–1) (Messing et al, 1995c). **Thus, screening had effected a shift of the high-grade tumors to earlier (more superficial) stages at diagnosis. Not surprisingly, mortality was significantly improved in the screened population.** Furthermore, the similarity of the grades of screened and un-

screened cancers made it unlikely that screening-detected tumors were fundamentally different from those normally seen in clinical practice. The fact that those who chose not to participate were diagnosed with a similar percentage of bladder tumors within 18 months of what would have been their final home testing date would also argue against the detection of clinically unimportant tumors by screening, that screening detected cancers that might otherwise have spontaneously regressed, or that bladder tumors have a long preclinical period. Additionally, a similar proportion (1.2%–1.3%) of middle-aged and elderly men who are evaluated for prostatism or prostatic cancer have bladder cancer uncovered at cystoscopy (Bruskewitz, 1992; Kim and Ignatoff, 1994), again indicating that those solicited for the Wisconsin study were not at a higher risk for developing bladder cancer than the general middle-aged and elderly male population in the United States. **The control group in these studies was not a randomized one and hence may well have differed from screening participants in certain risk factors, health awareness, and other comorbidity factors. In the absence of a prospective, randomized trial, however, available information indicates that screening does shift the diagnosis of bladder cancers destined to become invasive to preinvasive stages, which translates into reduced mortality from the disease.**

Furthermore, the Wisconsin group has analyzed the cost-effectiveness of screening and its ability to alter quality of life (Lawrence et al, 1995). When compared with other screening modalities for chronic diseases that have been proven effective in prospective, randomized studies and are well accepted and incorporated into standard medical care, such as fecal occult blood testing for colon cancer, blood pressure checks for hypertension, and mammography for postmenopausal breast cancer, **repetitive chemical reagent strip testing for hematuria offers a favorable cost-effectiveness profile, which extends the longevity of the entire screening population and particularly the bladder cancer patients within it** (Lawrence et al, 1995). **To maximize this benefit, because of the brief preclinical duration of this malignancy, screenings should be repeated on at least an annual basis** (Messing et al, 1995b).

Besides hematuria home testing, other diagnostic technologies have been advocated for bladder cancer screening. Unfortunately, conventional cytology, flow cytometry, and even image analysis have relatively poor sensitivities for well-differentiated and moderately differentiated tumors. This is a serious drawback even though such lesions rarely pose a risk to patients' lives because failure to detect a large proportion of bladder cancers would seriously undermine the confidence both the public and physicians have in the screening modality. **Moreover, missing more than 10% to 20% of high-grade cancers is likely to compromise significantly the major goal of screening, to reduce bladder cancer mortality.** By combining phenotypic antigen expression with cytology (*immunocytology*), multiparameter flow cytometry, or image analysis (see previously), however, specificity would clearly be enhanced, and sensitivity may be as well. Additionally, the excretion of a variety of soluble factors in urine, including growth or motility factors (Guirguis et al, 1988; Nguyen et al, 1993; Messing and Murphy-Brooks, 1994), their receptors (Korman et al, 1995), or other substances (Sarosdy et al, 1995), has been tested in

Table 77–1. COMPARISON OF GRADES AND STAGES OF BLADDER CANCERS DIAGNOSED IN WISCONSIN MEN AGE 50 YEARS AND OLDER IN 1988 VERSUS THOSE OF BLADDER CANCERS DETECTED BY HEMATURIA HOME SCREENING

Bladder Cancer Grade and Stage	Unscreened: New Cases		Screened: New Cases	
	No.	*%*	*No.*	*%*
Low-grade (1,2) superficial (stage Ta, T1)	290*	56.8	11*	52.4
High-grade (3) superficial (stage Ta, T1, TIS)	99†	19.4	9†	42.9
Muscle invasive or greater (stage T2–4 or N+ or M+)	122‡	23.9	1‡	4.8
Totals	511	100.0	21	100.0

*Low-grade superficial unscreened (290 of 511) vs. screened (11 of 21) $P > 0.20$.
†High-grade superficial of all high-grade and/or invasive tumors unscreened (99 of 221) vs. screened (9 of 10) $P = 0.007$.
‡Invasive of all high-grade and/or invasive tumors unscreened (122 of 221) vs. screened (1 of 10) $P = 0.007$.
From Messing EM, Young TB, Hunt VB, et al: Urology 1995; 45:387.

preliminary studies, and some have promise. Finally, because DNA replicating errors may not be adequately repaired in malignantly transformed cells, or such cells may not be appropriately directed toward apoptosis as they normally would be, searching for mutations or copying errors in a number of known repetitive sequences of DNA within the genome of cells exfoliated in voided urine may prove a sensitive means to detect urothelial malignancy (Hruban et al, 1994; Mao et al, 1994). Although none of these methodologies has yet reached clinical practice, examples of the more promising are discussed.

The Lewis^x blood group related antigen is normally absent from urothelial cells in adults except for occasional umbrella cells. Cordon-Cardo and associates noted increased expression of Lewis^x in urothelial carcinoma independent of secretor status, tumor grade, or stage (Cordon-Cardo et al, 1988). **The same investigative group has demonstrated that immunostaining of Lewis^x antigen on epithelial cells from bladder washings could detect tumors with a sensitivity of 86% and specificity of 87%** (Sheinfeld et al, 1990). **Golijanin and colleagues, using a commercially available monoclonal antibody to Lewis^x on cytologic preparations of cells from freshly voided urine specimens, reported a sensitivity in detecting cystoscopically evident bladder tumors on two voidings (considered positive if either one was positive) of 97%, a specificity of 85%, a positive predictive value of 76%, and a negative predictive value of 98%** (Golijanin et al, 1995). **Whether such outstanding results, particularly in terms of sensitivity, could be achieved in populations in which slightly more than 1% (as would occur in most screening studies using general populations) as opposed to 32% (as was present in their cohort of 101 patients, most of whom had histories of recurrent bladder tumors) had bladder cancer is questionable.** Repetition on a larger screening cohort is clearly warranted.

Antigen M344 is expressed on 70% of superficial bladder tumors. Staining for this antigen has been used on exfoliated cells (from bladder washings) to enhance sensitivity, particularly for the group (low-grade superficial tumors) that is generally missed with conventional cytology (Fradet and Cordon-Cardo, 1993). Another antigen, DD23, which is expressed on roughly 80% of bladder tumors regardless of stage and grade and is not seen on normal urothelial cells (Grossman et al, 1992), may again be useful in conjunction with immunocytology or multiparameter image analysis by improving diagnostic sensitivity.

It should be noted that with several of these techniques, what are believed to be false-positive results may simply be the detection of tumors that are not yet cystoscopically visible but will become so within the next 3 to 6 months. This has particularly been found with immunocytologic stainings with M344 (Fradet and Cordon-Cardo, 1993), Lewis^x (Sheinfeld et al, 1992), and conventional cytology (Schwalb et al, 1993).

Excretion of soluble factors in urine, such as autocrine motility factor (Guirguis et al, 1988), autocrine motility factor receptor (Korman et al, 1995), basic FGF (Chodak et al, 1988; Nguyen et al, 1993), EGF (Fuse et al, 1992; Messing and Murphy-Brooks, 1994), and a proprietary bladder tumor antigen (BTA) (Sarosdy et al, 1995), has been found to be abnormal in patients with bladder cancer, with sensitivities reported as high as 80% or higher. None of these, however, has yet reached the level of clinical practice, and they have not been tested in large populations in which bladder cancer is present in only a small proportion of subjects. Furthermore, many have been studied primarily in patients with high-grade tumors, who are often overrepresented in populations available to academic medical centers. Additionally, most of these trials have compared themselves with voided urine cytology (Sheinfeld et al, 1990, 1992; Nguyen et al, 1993; Golijanin et al, 1995; Sarosdy et al, 1995), which has been found to be insufficiently sensitive for routine screening.

Screening Populations with Exposures to Putative Carcinogens

Aside from age and gender, potential screening populations at higher risk than those taking part in the Wisconsin and Leeds studies have been studied. These efforts have primarily focused on workers with prolonged exposure to known or possible carcinogens, including 4,4′-methylenebis (2-chloroanaline) (Ward et al, 1990), beta-naphthylamine (Marsh et al, 1990), alpha-naphthylamine, benzidine, auramine, and magenta (Cartwright, 1990; Mason and Vogler, 1990), using cytology, hematuria chemical reagent strips, quantitative fluorescence image analysis, and cystoscopy. Studies have been limited, despite considerable efforts by investigators, because of a combination of factors, including

incomplete information about previous exposures, changing production standards, and difficulties with compliance and follow-up. At the current time, each study has reported a few patients in whom bladder malignancies have been diagnosed, but the utility of such efforts has not been rigorously assessed. Additionally, the possibility of the chemical exposures themselves effecting abnormal test results without leading to diagnosable malignancy is uncertain.

One of the most impressive industry-based screening programs, **is one testing younger aluminum workers exposed to benzene-soluble coal tar pitch volatiles in Quebec. Researchers have demonstrated that annual urinary cytology examinations have effected a shift of tumors to pre–muscle-invasive stages when compared with historical controls from the 1970s (39% non–muscle-invasive in 1970s versus 63% non–muscle-invasive in 1980s) without any alteration in tumor grade (roughly 40%–45% in both the 1970s and the 1980s groups had high-grade tumors)** (Thériault et al, 1990). Because of lead time issues, and because the unscreened control population has been followed longer, the fact that mortality in the screened group (1980s) was significantly less is not surprising. Considering that 53% of cases in the unscreened population (who were all below age 65) had already died from bladder cancer at the time of the report, however, it is likely that further follow-up will give an indication of whether screening actually saves lives. **This study, of course, does not replace a randomized, prospective, controlled trial (especially because modern workers, more aware of the seriousness of bladder cancer than the 1970s workers, may have sought medical evaluation much sooner than those in the earlier group did, even if they were not being screened) but gives an indication that such workers may be appropriate subjects for screening endeavors.** Perhaps more frequent screening or using different techniques may prove even more beneficial.

Excretory Urography

Excretory urography is indicated in all patients with hematuria or cystoscopic evidence of bladder cancer. Urography is not a sensitive means of detecting bladder tumors, particularly small ones. It is useful, however, in examining the upper urinary tracts for associated urothelial tumors. Large tumors may appear as filling defects in the bladder on the cystogram phase of the urogram. Ureteral obstruction caused by a bladder tumor is usually a sign of a muscle-invasive cancer. Additionally, of course, urography can assess other upper tract abnormalities that may affect management decisions.

Cystoscopy

All patients suspected of having bladder cancer should have careful cystoscopy and bimanual examination. Abnormal areas should be biopsied. Random or selected site mucosal biopsy specimens may also be obtained. **Retrograde pyelography should be performed if the upper tracts are not adequately visualized on the excretory urogram.** If an upper urinary tract lesion is seen, a retro-grade ureteropyelogram obtaining urine samples or saline lavages for cytology or brush biopsies should be performed (see the section on upper tract urothelial tumors).

Resection of Bladder Tumors

The ideal method for resection of a bladder tumor is first to resect the superficial portion of the tumor, sending it to the pathologist as a separate specimen. Then the deep portion along with some underlying bladder muscle is resected and sent as a separate specimen for histologic examination. After the tumor has been completely resected, the resection site is fulgurated. This approach usually enables complete removal of the tumor and provides valuable diagnostic information about the grade and depth of infiltration of the tumor. It has been suggested that resecting low-grade superficial tumors into the muscle layer may unnecessarily increase the potential of bladder perforation and risk muscle-invasive recurrence of tumor implanted in the resected bed (Soloway, 1984).

It is not always necessary to perform a formal resection of superficial low-grade papillary tumors, particularly those that may be difficult to reach with the resectoscope. This is even more the case in patients who have a prior history of recurrent superficial tumors because it is known that the vast majority of recurrences in these instances are also low-grade papillary non-invasive lesions (Prout et al, 1992). It is acceptable to treat these tumors with simple fulguration. The obvious disadvantage of fulguration is that it does not provide tissue for histologic documentation of tumor grade and stage. Laser therapy has also been used for destroying bladder tumors in this clinical setting and has the additional advantage of being able to be performed without spinal or general anesthesia.

It is not always necessary to attempt complete tumor resection in patients with extensive, broad-based sessile tumors, which are almost certain to require cystectomy or partial cystectomy, particularly if a tumor is located in an area that is difficult to reach with the resectoscope. Attempts at complete resection may result in bladder perforation with dissemination of tumor cells. In such cases, it may be more prudent to begin resecting at the margins of the tumor and progress toward its center, **resecting only enough tissue to establish the tumor grade and document muscle invasion. If this approach is taken, it is best accomplished with frozen section confirmation of the adequacy of the biopsy specimens.**

Tumors encroaching on the ureteral orifices should be resected without regard for the orifice; however, it is important not to fulgurate the orifice after the tumor has been resected. When the ureteral orifice is resected, a stent may be left in place for several days to prevent obstruction of the orifice by edema. Some investigators have advocated passing a ureteral catheter first and then resecting around the catheter; however, the ureteral catheter may prevent adequate tumor resection and theoretically could pass malignant cells to the upper urinary tracts that would otherwise not have had an opportunity to reach this locale.

Tumors on the lateral bladder wall may induce stimulation of the obturator nerve during resection, resulting in violent contraction of the adductor muscle of the thigh.

Resections of such tumors should be performed with the patient under general anesthesia with simultaneous intravenous administration of a skeletal muscle relaxant to paralyze the patient adequately to minimize the risk of inadvertent bladder perforation associated with adductor muscle spasm.

Tumors arising in bladder diverticuli often should be biopsied rather than resected. This is so not only because transurethral resection of such tumors is often quite challenging but also because it has a high risk of bladder perforation. In general, patients with tumors in diverticuli are often best treated definitively with either partial or total cystectomy.

Selected Site Mucosal Biopsies

Selected site mucosal biopsies from areas adjacent to the tumor as well as from the opposite bladder wall, bladder dome, trigone, and prostatic urethra have been recommended at the time of resection of the primary tumor. These provide important prognostic information about the likelihood of tumor recurrence, with about 20% to 25% of patients found to have dysplasia or carcinoma in situ on such biopsy specimens (Althausen et al, 1976; Vincente-Rodriguez et al, 1987). Between 30% and 70% of muscle-invasive bladder cancers are associated with carcinoma in situ elsewhere in the bladder. Mufti and Singh (1992) suggested that abnormalities found on mucosal biopsy specimens with a low-grade superficial tumor are particularly predictive of tumor recurrence in patients with solitary tumors. In contrast, some investigators believe that selected site mucosal biopsies are unnecessary (Kiemeney et al, 1994) and even potentially hazardous because they denude the urothelium and may create fertile areas for tumor cell implantation (see section on tumor implantation). Some also believe that urinary or bladder wash cytology are better indicators of the presence of concurrent carcinoma in situ (Harving et al, 1988).

Regardless of the questionable wisdom of obtaining selected site urothelial biopsy specimens for most bladder tumors, these specimens are required if partial cystectomy is contemplated, if urinary cytology indicates the presence of high-grade cancer and cystoscopically no tumors are seen, or if all lesions look like low-grade superficial papillary tumors.

STAGING

Because tumor stage is important in determining therapy, accurate staging of bladder cancer is desirable. Nevertheless, there are considerable staging errors in bladder cancer. Understaging occurs most frequently in patients with high-grade and intermediate-stage tumors, of whom approximately 33% are understaged, and 10% are overstaged (Wijkstrom et al, 1984).

Goals of Staging

Superficial Versus Infiltrating Tumor

The first treatment decision based on tumor stage is whether the patient has a superficial or muscle-invasive

tumor. If it is superficial, more elaborate staging techniques such as bone scan, computed tomography (CT), and so forth are not usually indicated. Such techniques are reserved for patients with documented muscle-invasive bladder cancer because it is very rare for metastases to be associated with superficial disease (Jewett and Strong, 1946; Freeman JA et al, 1995).

The primary transurethral resection of the tumor is the most important test for judging its depth of penetration. Variation occurs in the interpretation of histology sections between different pathologists in assessing the tumor grade and depth of infiltration. Part of the reason for these discrepancies is related to the smooth muscle fibers of the tunica muscularis mucosa in the lamina propria of the bladder wall, which may be confused with detrusor muscle (Abel et al, 1988a, 1988b; Younes et al, 1990). Additionally, on rare occasions, adipose tissue has also been found in the lamina propria, further confusing matters (Bochner et al, 1995). Bimanual physical examination provides little information about whether there is infiltration of the bladder wall or not. In this regard, if the tumor is palpable on bimanual examination before resection, it is usually infiltrating into the muscle or perivesical tissues.

A much finer decision is whether the superficial or deep muscle layers have been penetrated (see later). Despite the time-honored tendency to resect the deepest layers of the ulcer crater after what is believed to be complete tumor resection and to send the curettage material as a separate specimen for histopathologic inspection, the frequent presence of residual cancer found on cystectomy specimens after supposedly complete endoscopic resection would indicate that this technique is often of little value. Thus, although favorable results for conservative management of tumors that invade only the superficial muscularis propria, compared to the deeper layers, have been reported, in the vast majority of cases it is unlikely that this can be reliably distinguished through transurethral resection alone. In an intriguing report, Koraitim and colleagues did think that transurethral ultrasonic assessment using 5.5-MHz probes with 60-, 90-, and 120-degree transducers before and at the end of transurethral resection was helpful in further distinguishing infiltration of superficial versus deep muscle and extravesical spread (Koraitim et al, 1995). One hundred percent sensitivity and more than 98% specificity in distinguishing muscle-invasive from superficial bladder cancers, more than 90% accuracy in distinguishing superficial muscularis invasion from deeper muscle invasion, and 70% positive predictive value in distinguishing vesical-confined from extravesical disease were reported by these authors—certainly far more accurate staging than has been found with other methodologies. Further confirmation of this technique is awaited.

Localized Versus Locally Extensive or Metastatic Tumor

The second treatment decision made based on staging is to identify patients with invasive tumors who may benefit from aggressive, potentially curative therapy. For this purpose, CT scanning, ultrasonography, and magnetic resonance imaging (MRI) have been used to evaluate the local extent of bladder tumors. These staging studies may provide

valuable information, but, with the possible exception of transurethral ultrasonography (Koraitim et al, 1995), **they appear to be inaccurate in determining the presence or absence of microscopic muscle infiltration and minimal extravesical tumor spread** (Koss et al, 1981). **Moreover, postoperative changes produced by the transurethral resection of the primary tumor as well as postirradiation therapy or postchemotherapy fibrosis may also cause difficulties in interpreting CT, MRI, and ultrasound scans.**

Staging Tests

Computed Tomography

In addition to assessing the extent of the primary tumor, **CT scanning also provides information about the presence of pelvic and para-aortic lymphadenopathy and the possible presence of liver or adrenal metastases** (Lantz and Hattery, 1984). To assess the depth of penetration accurately, CT scanning should be done before transurethral resection because artifacts introduced by the resection may be confusing (Husband et al, 1989). Contrast-enhanced CT scanning improves the accuracy of staging (Sager et al, 1987). Studies with spiral CT imaging, however, have not yet been fully assessed to determine if they can improve staging further. **CT scanning is limited in accuracy because it can detect only gross extravesical tumor extension, lymph nodes that are quite enlarged, and liver metastases that are larger than 2 cm in diameter** (Nurmi et al, 1988; Voges et al, 1989). **Enlargement of the lymph nodes does not always indicate metastatic disease.** Furthermore, hepatic lesions, such as cavernous hemangioma, may be confused with liver metastases unless dynamic scanning is performed following injection of contrast material. **CT scans fail to detect nodal metastases in up to 40% of patients having them** (Lantz and Hattery, 1984). Although some workers have questioned the practical utility of using CT scans for local staging of bladder cancer (Nishimura et al, 1988), CT scans are undoubtedly more sensitive than physical examination in evaluating regional and metastatic disease. Also, because of the magnitude of the treatments considered for invasive bladder cancer, it would seem prudent to perform CT scans before embarking on such therapy (see later).

Magnetic Resonance Imaging

MRI scanning is not much more helpful than CT scanning. With few exceptions (Johnson et al, 1990), the resolution of the pelvic and abdominal anatomy with MRI has not been reported to be as good as with CT scanning (Buy et al, 1988; Wood et al, 1988; Husband et al, 1989; Tavares et al, 1990). A double-surface coil may permit more accurate MRI staging of bladder cancer than a conventional coil MRI (Barentsz et al, 1988). With MRI, the possibility of multiplane imaging should theoretically provide better visualization of the anatomy. Soft tissue contrast may be enhanced by use of paramagnetic contrast agents, such as gadolinium-diethylenetriaminepenta-acetic acid complex (Gd-DTPA) (Sohn et al, 1990). In the future, MRI spectros-

copy may also have the capacity to provide information about the states of different tissues, but this possibility has not yet been realized. As might be expected, both CT and MRI scanning are more accurate in advanced tumors (Vock et al, 1982).

One area in which MRI has become particularly useful in clinical management is that it appears to be more sensitive than CT scans and radionuclide bone scans for determining the presence of bone metastases. Thus, if clinical symptoms, pelvic extension on CT scan or bimanual examination, or nuclear bone scan indicates suspicious sites of osseous metastases, MRI may be appropriate in such cases.

Ultrasonography

The potential benefit of transurethral ultrasonography has been reported. The findings of Koraitim and colleagues (1995) (see previously) have been suggested by others (summarized in See and Fuller, 1992). To date, however, this technique has not been adopted into general use. Transabdominal or transrectal sonography has been of minimal value.

Lymphadenectomy

Pelvic lymphadenectomy is the most accurate means of staging bladder cancer patients for regional lymph node involvement. Some patients having only limited nodal metastases below the bifurcation of the common iliac arteries and without invasion of adjacent organs may be cured by pelvic lymphadenectomy (LaPlante and Brice, 1973; Skinner 1982; Grossman and Konnak, 1988; Lerner et al, 1993). The primary regions of lymphatic drainage of the bladder are the perivesical, hypogastric, obturator, external iliac, and presacral lymph nodes (Wishnow et al, 1987). **Perivesical nodes tend to be involved less frequently than the others, thus making it necessary to perform a formal lymphadenectomy if one is to both sample completely and thoroughly remove potentially involved regional nodes.** The common iliac, inguinal, and para-aortic/caval lymph nodes are juxtaregional nodes and serve as secondary landing sites. Lymphadenectomy usually is performed in conjunction with cystectomy rather than as an independent staging procedure. Fine needle aspiration biopsy of enlarged lymph nodes under CT guidance may be performed to document incurable lymph node metastases. Laparoscopic lymphadenectomy seems to have an extremely limited role in the management of most bladder cancer patients, even those with invasive disease who elect bladder salvage approaches with radiation therapy (because of the fairly large field that is irradiated and the current tendency to perform intraperitoneal pelvic laparoscopic surgery, leading to bowel being fixed in the radiation field). It is possible that with refinements of extraperitoneal approaches, in extremely selected high-risk patients, extraperitoneal laparoscopic lymphadenectomy may be of benefit.

The standard staging lymphadenectomy for bladder cancer includes removal of the nodes from the iliac bifurcations through the femoral canals and from the genitofemoral nerves to the bladder pedicles. Some clinicians have routinely performed more extensive node dissections, including

nodes as high as the aortic bifurcation, whereas others have elected not to perform pelvic lymphadenectomy in patients with bladder cancer. The incidence of lymph node involvement correlates with the stage and grade of the tumor, ranging from less than 10% in a highly selected group of high-grade, frequently recurrent, lamina propria–invading tumors to 40% in deeply infiltrating ones. **The potential therapeutic benefit of pelvic lymphadenectomy may be assessed as follows. Of the 10% to 40% of patients who come to cystectomy with lymph node metastases, between 35% and 70% have only limited metastases (one or two nodes below the iliac bifurcations), and 10% to 35% of the latter patients may be cured with cystectomy and pelvic lymphadenectomy. Accordingly, the routine performance of pelvic lymphadenectomy may increase the surgical cure rate by 1% to 10%—although the higher number would probably be more likely. Thus, although the procedure rarely adds more than 30 minutes to surgery and adds almost no additional risk, in elderly patients or those with major comorbid conditions, lymphadenectomy may be omitted without substantially altering the ultimate prospects of cure.**

Chest Radiograph and Computed Tomography Scan

Metastatic evaluation to rule out distant metastases should be performed before proceeding to pelvic lymphadenectomy. The most sensitive means of detecting pulmonary metastasis is chest CT scan; however, CT scans frequently detect small, noncalcified pulmonary lesions, most of which are granulomas. There is a direct correlation between the size of a pulmonary lesion and the likelihood of its being a metastasis. Most noncalcified lesions that are 1 cm or larger are metastases (or primary pulmonary neoplasms). **Because standard films do not have sufficient resolution to demonstrate small granulomas, but rather detect only lesions larger than 1 cm in diameter, routine chest radiographs with or without tomography, rather than CT scans, usually are relied on to rule out pulmonary metastases in bladder cancer patients.**

Bone Scans

Bone scans seldom reveal metastatic disease in patients with normal serum alkaline phosphatase levels (Berger et al, 1981; Brismar and Gustafson, 1988). **A bone scan may be useful, however, as a baseline for future reference.** Thus, the recommended metastatic evaluation for patients with invasive bladder cancer includes a chest radiograph, excretory urogram, abdominal-pelvic CT scan, bone scan, and liver function tests. If any of these suggest the presence of metastases, histologic confirmation should be sought by the least invasive means possible, usually fine needle aspiration biopsy.

Staging Systems

Although two main staging systems of bladder cancer have been in use for some time, the one developed jointly by the International Union Against Cancer (UICC) and the American Joint Committee on Cancer Staging (AJC) (Hermanek and Sobin, 1987) has, to a large degree, replaced the Jewett-Strong (1946) system as modified by Marshall (1956). **In the AJC-UICC system, also termed tumor, node, metastasis (TNM), papillary epithelial confined tumors are classified as stage Ta, and flat in situ carcinomas as Tis. Tumors that have invaded the lamina propria are classified as stage T1. Muscle-invasive tumors, depending on whether there is superficial or deep muscle invasion, are classified as stage T2 or T3a. Tumors that have invaded the perivesical fat are classified as stage T3b. Tumors invading the pelvic viscera, such as the prostatic stroma, rectum, uterus or vagina, or pelvic side walls, are classified as stage T4.** In the AJC-UICC system, the regional lymph nodes from bladder cancer are considered to be the nodes of the true pelvis that lie below the bifurcation of the common iliac arteries. Laterality does not affect the N classification. **N1 denotes a single positive node less than or equal to 2 cm in diameter, N2 denotes a single positive node greater than 2 cm but less than 5 cm in diameter or multiple positive nodes less than 5 cm in diameter, and N3 denotes positive nodes greater than 5 cm in diameter.** The AJC-UICC system does not have a particular stage for juxtaregional lymph nodes, but **distant metastases are designated as M1 and their absence as M0. In patients in whom the nodal or distant status is uncertain, their classification is Nx or Mx.**

SUPERFICIAL BLADDER CANCER (STAGES Ta, T1)

Transurethral Resection or Fulguration

Most patients with superficial bladder cancer can be adequately treated with transurethral resection or fulguration of the tumor. The overall survival rates of these patients are excellent (approximately 70% 5-year overall survival—with most patients who expire doing so from non–bladder cancer causes) (Nichols and Marshall, 1956; Barnes et al, 1967; Prout et al, 1992). **About 10% to 15% of these patients ultimately require more aggressive therapy.**

The incidence of subsequent muscle-invasive tumors is low in patients initially having epithelium confined well-differentiated and moderately differentiated tumors (Prout et al, 1992) but may be as high as 46% in patients initially having lamina propria involvement—particularly if they have high-grade lesions (Cookson and Sarosdy, 1992). Accordingly, **stage T1 tumors should be considered potentially aggressive, particularly if they are high grade** (Abel et al, 1988a; Waples and Messing, 1992). **One of the issues with stage T1 disease is that tumors are often incompletely resected even when the endoscopist thinks that complete resection has been accomplished. In one study from Germany, more than 40% of T1 tumors that were believed to be completely resected were found on re-resection at 6 weeks to have residual disease** (Klan et al, 1991). The efficacy of immediate postresection intravesical therapy (Oosterlinck et al, 1993) may at least in part be explained by this phenomenon.

At the time of initial tumor diagnosis, there is little

doubt that total transurethral resection of all visible disease, with a few notable exceptions mentioned earlier (technically difficult location; very large, almost certain to be deeply invasive malignancy; location within a diverticulum; and so forth), **is appropriate to achieve optimal histologic classification.** For frequently recurrent lesions, particularly if they are low-grade superficial papillary ones or difficult-to-resect lesions, alternative forms of local therapy have been considered. These include photodynamic phototherapy with hematoporphyrin derivatives (HPD), laser therapy, and hydrostatic pressure treatment.

Hematoporphyrin Derivatives

HPD are a mixture of porphyrins that are preferentially concentrated in neoplastic and dysplastic tissues. With irradiation of these tissues with light of the proper wavelength (630 nm), sensitized cells are destroyed through the release of singlet oxygen, causing mitochondrial poisoning. HPD activation by white light also has been used to localize bladder cancer cells. **HPD therapy with subsequent illumination of the bladder with a krypton-ion laser light source has shown effectiveness against superficial tumors or carcinoma in situ (>90% response rate) but not large or invasive tumors** (Benson et al, 1982, 1983; Hisazumi et al, 1983; Benson, 1984; Prout et al, 1987). **The adverse side effects of HPD therapy include generalized cutaneous photosensitivity, which requires the patient to avoid sunlight for 6 to 8 weeks after treatment. Moreover, intense local bladder symptoms lasting 10 to 12 weeks occur in many patients,** and bladder contractures can occur in up to 20% of patients (Nseyo et al, 1987; Harty et al, 1989). It is possible that the occurrence of bladder contractures can be reduced or eliminated by reducing light exposure. HPD therapy is still considered investigational.

Laser Therapy

A variety of lasers have been employed to treat bladder tumors (Smith, 1989). Smith and Dixon (1984) used the argon laser in patients with small superficial bladder tumors and in those with carcinoma in situ. Laser energy is selectively absorbed into vascular tissues, such as tumors. **The argon laser provides 1-mm depth of penetration; therefore, it is safe but can be employed only on small tumors. The neodymium-yttrium-aluminum-garnet (Nd:YAG) laser has a 4- to 15-mm depth of penetration that can destroy larger tumors, but it is also less safe** (Hofstetter et al, 1981). The Nd:YAG laser has been used in the treatment of bladder tumors with good local tumor control within the treated field (5%–10% in-field recurrence rate) (McPhee et al, 1988; Beer et al, 1989), but its proper role in the treatment of bladder cancer is unclear.

Laser treatment of bladder tumors also has been used in selected high-risk patients with muscle-invasive tumors who are either too ill for, or refuse, cystectomy. In these patients, if the tumors are not too large, the Nd:YAG laser may achieve adequate local tumor control (McPhee et al, 1988; Beisland and Sander, 1990).

Laser therapy is theoretically attractive because it can be performed through a small cystoscope using local anesthesia without bleeding or obturator nerve stimulation. The main disadvantage is that limited tumor tissue is obtained for histologic examination. Laser therapy for bladder tumors has not been adopted for general use.

Hydrostatic Pressure Treatment

Hydrostatic pressure treatment was introduced by Helmstein (1972) for treating superficial bladder cancer. With this technique, the bladder is filled with saline under pressure, or a balloon is inserted in the bladder and inflated while the patient is under epidural anesthesia. The balloon pressure is maintained at about the diastolic blood pressure for 5 to 7 hours. This results in necrosis of bladder tumors. **A major complication of this treatment is bladder perforation.** Hydrostatic pressure treatment has also been used for intractable postradiotherapy hemorrhage (Mufti et al, 1990). This treatment has largely been abandoned.

ADJUVANT AND MISCELLANEOUS THERAPIES FOR SUPERFICIAL BLADDER CANCER

A variety of treatments have been employed as adjuvant therapy in patients with superficial bladder cancer to prevent the recurrence and progression of the cancer. These include intravesical chemotherapy; systemic chemotherapy; intravesical immunotherapy with interferon, BCG, and other agents; oral immunotherapy with agents such as bropiramine, an interferon inducer; intravesical biologic therapy with agents such as TP40, a recombinantly synthesized conjugate of TGF-α and *Pseudomonas* exotoxin; chemopreventive strategies with vitamins or polyamine synthesis inhibitors; and other experimental approaches. Other treatments such as radiation, hyperthermia, and hydrostatic pressure have been tested but have not been adopted for general use.

Radiation Therapy

Radiation therapy is rarely appropriate for the treatment of superficial bladder cancer. It does not prevent the occurrence of new tumors (Goffinet et al, 1975) **and may be associated with considerable morbidity, particularly radiation cystitis. Furthermore, conservative management of superficial tumors is so successful, less morbid, and less expensive that it makes little sense to use this modality for most superficial lesions, particularly if there is any possibility that the patient may go on to develop invasive disease (when radiation may be used).** Despite this background, there have been reports on using various forms of radiation for the treatment of superficial tumors. Interstitial radiation therapy has been used to treat superficial tumors in Europe (van der Werf-Messing, 1984). Radon seeds, radioactive gold seeds, and tantalum wires have been used for interstitial radiation therapy. Intercavity radiation therapy using a radium capsule in a catheter (Hewett et al, 1981) and intraoperative electron-beam therapy

combined with conventional fractionated external-beam radiation therapy (Matsumoto et al, 1981; Martinez and Gunderson, 1984) are reported to be effective for superficial bladder cancer. Similarly, Quilty and Kerr (1987) have reported fairly good results for high-grade stage T1 lesions using as little as 50-Gy (usually 67–70 Gy are used for invasive bladder cancers) pelvic external-beam radiotherapy. Several authorities, however, have not found radiotherapy to be effective (summarized in Waples and Messing, 1992). Moreover, at least based on those patients with invasive malignancies who have concomitant carcinoma in situ and undergo radiation therapy, the latter lesion tends to be particularly resistant to radiation. **At this stage, therefore, there is little indication for any patient with a non–muscle-invasive tumor to receive radiation in any form.**

Cystectomy

Total cystectomy is rarely required for patients with superficial bladder cancer except for those with symptomatic, diffuse, unresectable papillary tumors or carcinoma in situ that does not respond to intravesical therapy (Matthews et al, 1984). In appropriately selected patients, survival rates are favorable. **Bracken and associates reported that patients treated with cystectomy with stages Ta and T1 bladder cancer had survival rates comparable to those in the age-matched normal population** (Bracken et al, 1981a). **In patients with high-grade tumors that are highly refractory to conservative therapy, Freeman and colleagues reported roughly an 80% 5-year disease-specific survival, with the vast majority who died from bladder cancer found actually to have had muscle-invasive or more advanced disease at the time of cystectomy** (Freeman et al, 1995a). Indeed, in those patients with high-grade, frequently recurrent superficial tumors or Tis, by the time cystectomy is contemplated, roughly one third actually have microscopic evidence of more extensive disease, and roughly half the patients who are up-staged (to muscle invasion or more) already have extravesical extension or metastases. Not surprisingly, survival is far worse in those patients who are up-staged, thus implying that in some, had cystectomy been performed earlier, it may have been curative. Other authors have had similar findings (Freiha, 1990; Malkowicz et al, 1990; Wishnow et al, 1992).

Intravesical Therapy

Adjuvant intravesical chemotherapy or intravesical immunotherapy is indicated in patients who are at a high risk for tumor recurrence by virtue of having multiple tumors, recurrent tumors, high-grade tumors associated with urothelial atypia, or carcinoma in situ (Rubben et al, 1988). Thiotepa and BCG are the least expensive intravesical agents available. Doxorubicin and interferon alpha have intermediate costs. Mitomycin C is the most expensive. BCG currently appears to be the most effective agent for intravesical use, but the optimum strain and dosage schedule have not been determined. Patients who fail treatment with one intravesical agent may be managed successfully with a different agent. Additionally, there are several experimental agents that have been used for treatment of superficial bladder cancer, which work through biologic mechanisms, including bropirimine (an oral agent), tumor necrosis factor, TP40 (TGF-α–*Pseudomonas* exotoxin), and interleukin-2.

Intravesical or other therapy can also be used to treat existing superficial bladder tumors. Currently, this is reserved primarily for the management of carcinoma in situ (which is often almost impossible to resect endoscopically in its entirety) or the rare patient with so many superficial tumors that endoscopic resection is not feasible yet cystectomy is either not appropriate or not desired by the patient. With these exceptions, however, intravesical therapy is used primarily in an adjuvant form, although this may often be treating existent or persistent disease that is just not yet detectable. **There is a low incidence of developing a secondary hematologic malignancy after intravesical chemotherapy with thiotepa or mitomycin** (Sonneveld et al, 1990).

Triethylenethiophosphoramide (Thiotepa)

Intravesical chemotherapy began in the 1960s with the introduction of intravesical thiotepa (Jones and Swinney, 1961). Before thiotepa, other agents used were silver nitrate, trichloroacetic acid, and podophyllin. **Thiotepa is an alkylating agent that acts by cross-linking nucleic acids and proteins.** Commonly administered doses are 1 mg/ml instilled directly into the bladder and retained for 1 to 2 hours. Often, it is administered in doses of 30 mg in 30 ml of saline or 60 mg in 60 ml. A frequently recommended regimen includes six to eight weekly treatments followed by monthly treatments for 1 year. **Thiotepa has been reported to produce complete tumor remission in approximately 35% of patients and partial remission in approximately 25% of those with existing tumors at initiation of treatment** (Koontz et al, 1981b). **Thiotepa has also been used for prophylaxis against tumor recurrence following complete resection of all visible tumor** (Zincke et al, 1983). **It has been reported to reduce recurrence rates under these circumstances from 73% in patients not receiving a course of thiotepa to 47% at 2 years in those who have. This benefit was observed largely in patients with grade I tumors** (Prout et al, 1983). Moreover, in this study, 16% of patients receiving thiotepa prophylaxis had tumor progression, half of whom developed muscle-invasive disease, and nearly half of those eventually developed distant metastases. **Thiotepa is less valuable for treatment of carcinoma in situ** (Koontz et al, 1981b). In an update of a large, prospective, randomized study with nearly 9 years of follow-up, intravesical thiotepa at a somewhat reduced dose (30 mg in 50 ml of saline), when given immediately after transurethral resection plus once every third month for 1 year, was not found to reduce recurrence rates, time to first recurrence, or failure-free interval, compared with randomized controls receiving no treatment (Medical Research Council Working Party on Urological Cancer, 1994). Because of the relatively low dose of thiotepa used, the failure to employ a more standard treatment schedule (see previously), and the inclusion of a large proportion of patients who now would not be considered candidates for intravesical therapy (newly diagnosed low-grade superficial tumors that are completely

resected), however, this study should not be interpreted as definitively demonstrating absence of efficacy for this agent. **As might be expected, the 7% of patients with grade III stage T1 tumors had a much higher recurrence rate than the remainder of patients regardless of treatment. In another prospective, randomized trial, thiotepa in standard dosage and regimen was shown to be less effective than BCG in the treatment of superficial bladder cancer** (Brosman, 1982). In a separate study, the European Organization for Research and Treatment of Cancer found no differences in terms of recurrence and progression rates in a three-armed therapeutic study in which patients with completely resected recurrent superficial tumors were randomized to receive thiotepa (30 mg in 50 ml of sterile water), doxorubicin (50 mg in 50 ml of water), or *cis*-platin (50 mg in 50 ml of water), weekly for 4 weeks and then monthly thereafter for a year. Thiotepa, however, was better tolerated than the other two drugs, with an occasional anaphylactic reaction occurring with *cis*-platin, and chemical cystitis being most commonly seen with doxorubicin (Bouffioux et al, 1992).

Thiotepa is readily absorbed through the urothelium because of its relatively low molecular weight (198 Da) and causes myelosuppression in 15% to 20% of patients. White blood cell and platelet counts should be obtained before each thiotepa treatment. Based on the above-mentioned Medical Research Council study (1994), despite the low dosage of thiotepa used, a benefit for immediate postresection instillation of thiotepa can hardly be advocated, as some authors have suggested (Soloway, 1983).

Etoglucid (Epodyl)

Etoglucid is available in Europe but not in the United States. **It is an alkylating agent similar to thiotepa with a slightly higher molecular weight (262 Da). Accordingly, it is not as readily absorbed through the urothelium** and causes myelosuppression less frequently than thiotepa. It is administered in a 1% solution weekly for 12 weeks and then monthly thereafter. Etoglucid causes more severe chemical cystitis than thiotepa. Complete responses occur in approximately 45% of patients, and partial responses occur in approximately 35% (Robinson et al, 1977; Lamm, 1983). Etoglucid was reported in a randomized trial to be more effective than transurethral resection alone or transurethral resection with intravesical doxorubicin in preventing tumor recurrences in patients with primary bladder cancers but not in those with recurrent superficial tumors (Kurth et al, 1984). It also has been helpful in treating upper urinary tract superficial tumors (Mathiasen et al, 1988).

Mitomycin C

Mitomycin C is an antibiotic chemotherapeutic agent that acts by inhibiting DNA synthesis. It has a higher molecular weight than thiotepa or etoglucid (334 Da) and, therefore, causes fewer problems with transurothelial absorption. Approximately 1% of instilled mitomycin is absorbed (van Helsdingen et al, 1988). Mitomycin C is effective as primary treatment of previously untreated bladder tumors and has been shown to be effective in patients who have failed prior treatment with thiotepa (Prout et al, 1982; Issell et al, 1984; Stricker et al, 1987). Mitomycin C

is usually administered as dose of 40 mg in 40 ml of saline or water intravesically weekly for 8 weeks followed by monthly maintenance therapy for 1 year. Complete tumor responses occur in about 40% of patients, and partial responses occur in up to another 40% (Prout et al, 1982; Lamm, 1983; Issell et al, 1984). **Mitomycin is reported to be more effective in the treatment of high-grade tumors** (Soloway, 1984). Soloway (1984) reported that 8% of complete responders, 23% of partial responders, and 19% of nonresponders developed muscle-invasive cancer, and 7% died of metastatic bladder cancer. Similar results were reported by Hellstein and co-workers (1990). **The side effects of mitomycin include chemical cystitis (10%–15%) that may lead to bladder contraction, mural calcification** (Drago et al, 1989), **and genital skin rashes (5%–15%).**

Mitomycin C has been reported to prevent the development of invasive bladder cancer in a controversial prospective clinical trial (Huland et al, 1984). In this study, all patients had complete tumor excision and negative cytologic findings before mitomycin C treatment, thus excluding patients with widespread multifocal disease. Moreover, 50% were treated for a solitary primary tumor, and only 29% had high-grade tumors. Others (Denovic et al, 1983; Lockhart et al, 1983) studied mitomycin C prophylaxis in patients with multiple, recurrent, and high-grade tumors and did not confirm Huland and colleagues' low recurrence and progression rates. **In a trial carried out by the Southwest Oncology Group and the Eastern Cooperative Oncology Group in the United States, in patients with recurrent superficial tumors or carcinoma in situ, mitomycin C (20 mg in 20 ml of water) given in weekly instillations for 6 weeks and then monthly for 1 year was found to be significantly less effective in preventing tumor recurrences than BCG (54% recurrences with mitomycin versus 39% for BCG at 10.5 months).** This study was closed before full accrual because of this significant difference between the two treatment arms. Because of the premature closure, the effect of either drug on progression or disease-related survival could not be ascertained (Lamm et al, 1995a).

Doxorubicin (Adriamycin)

Doxorubicin is an antibiotic chemotherapeutic agent. Because of its high molecular weight (580 Da), it is minimally absorbed. A variety of dosage schedules have been followed in the treatment of superficial bladder cancer. A minimal dose of 50 mg should be given for intravesical therapy. Treatment schedules have ranged from three times per week to monthly. Complete responses occur in less than one half of the patients, and partial responses occur in approximately one third. **No significant differences in the response rates of patients with low-grade and high-grade tumors have been reported** (Lundbeck et al, 1983, 1988).

When used for prophylaxis against tumor recurrence, doxorubicin in dosages of 60 to 90 mg given at intervals ranging from every 3 weeks to every 3 months has had mixed results (Nijima et al, 1983; Zincke et al, 1983; Garnick et al, 1984; Kurth et al, 1984). **In a large, multi-institutional Southwest Oncology Group trial, doxorubicin was shown to be significantly less effective than intravesical BCG in the treatment of patients with carcinoma in situ and for prophylaxis against tumor recurrence** (Lamm et al, 1991).

The side effects of doxorubicin include chemical cystitis, which is severe in many patients and may progress to permanent bladder contracture in a small percentage (Kondas et al, 1988).

Epirubicin

Epirubicin is a doxorubicin derivative, an anthracycline analog with somewhat reduced toxicity. In a phase I/II study (not a randomized, prospective, controlled trial), Kurth and co-workers used varying doses of epirubicin in eight weekly instillations (Kurth et al, 1991). Thirteen of 22 evaluable patients (59%) had complete responses. With a mean follow-up of 35 months, however, only 8 of these 13 were alive without recurrences. Roughly one third of evaluable patients had a durable complete response, whereas 18% experienced disease progression. In a separate study carried out by the European Organization for Research and Treatment of Cancer, **patients with completely resected solitary stage Ta or T1 papillary tumors received a single instillation of 80 mg of epirubicin versus water immediately after resection. A significant reduction of recurrence rates to little more than half the rate seen with water alone occurred in those with Ta tumors, particularly those of moderate or a higher grade. It is likely that at least some of this improvement was due to the prevention of recurrent cancer, although the most dramatic benefit was seen at cystoscopy performed 5 to 7 weeks after the resection, which was almost certainly due to eradication of persistent tumor rather than prevention of tumor implantation or prophylaxis against new tumor formation.** This study supports the possibility that epirubicin's major effectiveness might be against cystoscopically invisible cancers already established at the time of first treatment rather than actually preventing implantation. Again, during this study, progression to high-grade cancer, development of distant disease, and death from bladder cancer were not prevented by epirubicin (Oosterlinck et al, 1993).

Epirubicin, which is not yet available in the United States, induced chemical cystitis in fewer than 5% of the patients in Kurth and co-workers' phase I/II study, and one patient developed an allergic reaction (Kurth et al, 1991). **It appeared to be better tolerated than doxorubicin.**

Comparison of Intravesical Chemotherapeutic Agents

All agents for intravesical chemotherapy are about equally effective (Newling, 1990). The possible exception is that mitomycin may be marginally superior to thiotepa in the treatment of patients with stage Ta tumors (Heney et al, 1988) and for high-grade tumors. When used as prophylaxis against tumor recurrence, recurrence rates have been reduced to 30% to 44% compared with about 70% in controls. **Despite the aforementioned study by Huland and coworkers (1984), however, little evidence exists to indicate that any type of intravesical chemotherapy prevents progression to muscle invasion.** From analyzing a variety of randomized, controlled studies that collected progression data, **it appears that patients treated with surgery alone and patients treated with both surgery and intravesical**

chemotherapy experience roughly a 7% chance of developing muscle-invasive disease (7.5% for those receiving intravesical chemotherapy versus 6.9% for those treated by surgery alone) (Lamm et al, 1995b). Other authorities have reached similar conclusions (Herr, 1992; Kilbridge and Kantoff, 1994).

Combination intravesical chemotherapy with both mitomycin C and doxorubicin was no more effective than either drug alone for prophylaxis against tumor recurrence (Ferraris, 1988; Fukui et al, 1989).

Biologic Therapy

Intravesical Bacille Calmette-Guérin Therapy

BCG is an attenuated strain of *Mycobacterium bovis* that has stimulatory effects on immune responses. BCG has been administered intravesically to treat superficial bladder cancer and has emerged as the most effective intravesical agent for this purpose (Catalona and Ratliff, 1990; Martinez-Pineiro et al, 1990). Morales and co-workers first administered BCG to humans, using the Armand-Frappier strain, both intravesically (120 mg in 50 ml saline) and intradermally (5 mg with a Heaf gun) weekly for 6 weeks (Morales et al, 1976). Most subsequent clinical trials have verified the effectiveness of BCG therapy (review by Catalona and Ratliff, 1990). BCG is commonly given in three clinical settings: (1) prophylaxis in tumor-free patients, (2) treatment of residual tumor in patients with papillary transitional cell carcinoma other than carcinoma in situ, and (3) treatment of patients with carcinoma in situ. As with intravesical chemotherapy, the second setting rarely occurs except in clinical trials because under most circumstances visible tumor can be totally resected.

Several strains of BCG have been used, including the Pasteur, Armand-Frappier, Tice, Connaught, Glaxo, Evans, Tokyo, Dutch (RIVM), and Moreau strains. All are derived from the original strain developed at the Pasteur Institute. Some doubt exists about the efficacy of the Glaxo and Dutch strains. The viability of BCG organisms per milligram of vaccine may vary with the strain and from lot to lot with the same strain (Kelley et al, 1985; Cummings et al, 1989). In addition to intravesical instillation, BCG has been administered with intradermal boosters and has been administered orally. All routes of administration have been reported to be effective, but it appears that intradermal immunization is unnecessary. Studies do not confirm the effectiveness of oral BCG (Lamm et al, 1990). Intralesional injections of BCG may be associated with severe anaphylaxis and toxic side effects (Martinez-Pineiro and Muntanola, 1977).

Prospective, randomized trials have shown that BCG is effective for prophylaxis against tumor recurrence (Lamm et al, 1980; Brosman, 1982; Pinsky et al, 1982; Lamm et al, 1991; Herr et al, 1995; Lamm et al, 1995a). Although response rates in studies vary primarily according to entry criteria, a fairly standard example would be that of Lamm and co-workers, who reported that **BCG reduced tumor recurrence rates from 42% in patients treated with transurethral resection alone to 17% in BCG-treated patients (mean follow-up 15 months)** (Lamm et al, 1980). BCG has also been found to be effective in the

treatment of patients who have not responded to intravesical thiotepa (Brosman, 1982; Netto and Lemos, 1983; Brosman, 1984; Schellhammer et al, 1986). Several "head-on-head" studies have also demonstrated significantly greater efficacy of BCG than thiotepa (Brosman, 1982; Netto and Lemos, 1983), doxorubicin (Lamm et al, 1991), and mitomycin C (Lamm et al, 1995a). **Taken together, studies suggest that using BCG for prophylaxis, tumor recurrence rates range from 0 to 41% with most being around 20%, whereas patients not receiving BCG treatments (no treatment, thiotepa, doxorubicin, or mitomycin C) have recurrence rates of 40% to 80%** (Morales and Ersil, 1979; Lamm et al, 1980; Netto and Lemos, 1983; DeKernion et al, 1985; Shinka et al, 1989; Coplen et al, 1990; Lamm et al, 1991; Brosman, 1992; Lamm et al, 1995a).

BCG has also been used to treat residual unresectable cancer, although BCG should *not* be considered a substitute for the resection of resectable tumors (Morales et al, 1981; Brosman, 1984; DeKernion et al, 1985; Schellhammer et al, 1986; Coplen et al, 1990). **Overall, these series show a complete response rate of 58%.** Morales and co-workers advocated initiating BCG therapy within 10 days of tumor resection to take advantage of increasing BCG adherence to the disrupted bladder mucosa (Morales et al, 1981). Early administration of BCG, however, may be associated with a greater risk of severe complications. **It is prudent to wait at least 2 weeks (and probably 3 to 4 weeks) following tumor resection before starting BCG therapy.**

BCG is perhaps most useful in the treatment of patients with carcinoma in situ (Lamm et al, 1982; DeKernion et al, 1985; Herr et al, 1986; Coplen et al, 1990; DeJager et al, 1991; Lamm et al, 1991, 1995a; Herr et al, 1995). In studies with short-term follow-up of 1 or 2 years, BCG induced complete response rates in about 72% of patients. With longer follow-up periods, although more than 50% of patients eventually experienced recurrence (Lamm et al, 1991), median time to BCG treatment failure was more than 3 years as opposed to 5 months in patients receiving doxorubicin (Lamm et al, 1991). The favorable response usually was associated with resolution of urinary irritative symptoms. Intravesical BCG in conjunction with transurethral resection of the prostate may be effective in the treatment of patients with carcinoma in situ involving the prostatic urethral mucosa or prostatic ducts (Hillyard et al, 1988; Bretton et al, 1989).

Long-term studies of BCG therapy have reported favorable responses in 40% to 89% of patients. These studies suggest that patients who fail to respond to initial induction therapy may respond to more intensive regimens (Morales and Nickel, 1986; Sarosdy and Lamm, 1989; Bretton et al, 1990; Coplen et al, 1990; Nadler et al, 1994; Herr et al, 1995). For example, Nadler and associates found that long-term follow-up of patients (mean 74.3 months) yielded 28% tumor-free remissions from a single 6-week course of BCG, but in those who failed and received a second 6-week course of BCG, another 41% had remained tumor-free over a 68-month interval (Nadler et al, 1994). **Overall, therefore, 54% remained tumor-free after one or two courses of BCG. As had been noted previously** (Coplen et al, 1990), **however, those with carcinoma in situ had a somewhat worse chance of responding to the second course of therapy than those with papillary disease without carcinoma**

in situ. Moreover, those with carcinoma in situ at the time of failure to respond had a fourfold greater chance of developing muscle-invasive disease subsequently than those who had papillary tumors at the time of failure (63% versus 16%). Thus, it would seem prudent that those patients who still have carcinoma in situ after the first course of BCG should strongly be considered for more aggressive therapy. Currently, those with papillary tumors at the time of initial failure should probably be considered for a second course of BCG—but those who do not respond to the second course should go on to alternative therapies. The alternative therapy after failure of two courses of BCG depends on the type of tumor present at the time of failure. **If the patient with low-grade, superficial tumors fails to respond, the other conventional conservative treatments are legitimate options. If the patient with high-grade superficial tumors fails to respond, particularly with recurrent high-grade cancers, cystectomy should be considered.**

BCG therapy has been reported to delay tumor progression. A study involving a group of 86 highly refractory patients with stage Ta and T1 tumors, most of whom had carcinoma in situ as well, who were randomized to transurethral resection plus immediate BCG therapy or transurethral resection plus treatment of physician's choice on recurrence, has been updated. **Ten-year progression (to stage T2+)–free rate and disease specific–survival rate were significantly improved in those who had received immediate BCG despite more than half the control patients subsequently crossing over to BCG.** Indeed, in those controls who did cross over to BCG on recurrence, more than 80% did not show tumor progression. **Even in those patients of both arms who did progress ultimately, immediate BCG significantly delayed that event** (Herr et al, 1995). Unfortunately, other randomized, much larger studies comparing BCG with intravesical chemotherapeutic agents contained large proportions of patients who would not be expected to progress regardless of subsequent recurrence (Lamm et al, 1991, 1995a) and, indeed, could not (and did not) confirm unequivocally that BCG prevents progression and improves survival, although it clearly prevented or retarded recurrence.

The value of maintenance BCG has been debated. Two prospective, randomized studies have failed to demonstrate significant benefits from quarterly or monthly maintenance instillations (Badalament et al, 1987; Hudson et al, 1987). The validity of these studies has been questioned because maintenance therapy may have been given to patients treated with suboptimal (6-week course) induction therapy. **In a more recent study, Southwest Oncology Group investigators** (Lamm et al, 1992) **demonstrated that in patients who received a 6-week induction course of Connaught strain BCG and then three weekly BCG instillations at 3 months, 6 months, and every 6 months thereafter for 3 years, the rate of recurrence and time to recurrence were significantly better than in those who received only (and responded to) the initial 6 weeks of BCG.** This benefit was particularly evident for those patients with superficial tumors who did not have carcinoma in situ. The optimum duration to continue maintenance BCG, whether three periodic treatments are the best maintenance regimen, or whether such regimens would be optimal—or even effective—using other BCG strains (or even with the Connaught strain if a longer induction course had been used), however, are all uncertain.

The issue of maintenance instillations, however, also raises questions about BCG's mechanism of action: Is it creating anti–bladder cancer immunity, stimulating already present but latent anti–bladder cancer immunity, or primarily just stimulating immunity to mycobacterial antigens? One would think that if it were the first or second mechanism, except for an occasional booster instillation, particularly if there were a clonal etiology for recurrent bladder cancers, maintenance therapy would not be needed because the hallmarks of both the humoral and the cellular immune systems are memory and enhanced specificity with time. Additionally, the relatively high incidence of upper tract and prostatic urethral cancer in patients who have responded successfully to BCG instillations for bladder tumors, although undoubtedly a reflection of such individuals' high-risk states, seems to be contrary to the concept that BCG is effecting systemic anti–urothelial cancer immunity (Miller et al, 1993; Herr et al, 1995). Alternatively, there can be little doubt that BCG intravesical therapy does induce an inflammatory and an immune response. Work has been done with the elaboration of a variety of cytokines that appear in the urine following BCG instillations, including tumor necrosis factors alpha and beta (Jackson et al, 1995); interleukins 1, 2, 6, and 8 (Fleishman et al, 1989; Bettex-Galland et al, 1991; DeBoeur et al, 1992); interferon gamma (Prescott et al, 1990); and the intracellular adhesion molecule 1 (ICAM-1) (Jackson et al, 1993), all of which can be important regulators and effectors of antitumor immune responses. Whether these reflect nonspecific inflammation, or anti–bladder cancer versus anti-BCG immune responses, however, is less certain.

Regardless of its actual target, intravesical BCG therapy clearly exercises some of its antitumor effects through immune mechanisms (Catalona and Ratliff, 1990; Kavoussi et al, 1990). A weak correlation exists between the skin test reactivity to purified protein derivative and a favorable response to BCG therapy (Brosman, 1982; Lamm et al, 1982). BCG induces a chronic granulomatous response in the bladders of many patients (Morales et al, 1976; Lamm et al, 1980; Schellhammer et al, 1986; Torrance et al, 1988). A marginal correlation has been noted between bladder granuloma formation and a favorable response to BCG therapy. These correlations, however, are weak (Torrance et al, 1988). Some patients who have positive skin test responses and develop bladder granulomas may not respond clinically to BCG therapy. Conversely, some who have negative skin test responses and do not develop granulomas appear to have favorable responses to BCG therapy.

It is known that BCG has to adhere to the bladder tumor and denuded basal lamina for it to be effective (Catalona and Ratliff, 1990) and that adherence to fibronectin may be particularly important (Catalona and Ratliff, 1990). Thus, elevated urinary fibronectin levels (Malmstrom et al, 1993) or conditions (or medicines) that interfere with the clotting cascade adversely affect BCG adherence and reduce the efficacy of BCG immunotherapy.

The reasons for the initial failure to respond to induction regimens may be related to differences in the immune competence of the hosts, differences in vaccine potency, or both (Kelley et al, 1985). **It is believed that at least 10 million organisms are required for therapeutic efficacy.** The recommended doses for various strains of BCG are as follows: Armand-Frappier, 120 mg; Pasteur, 150 mg; Tice, 50 mg; Tokyo, 40 mg; Connaught, 120 mg; and Dutch (RIVM), 120 mg. As with many biologic response modifiers, however, it is not at all clear that a higher dose is necessarily an optimal one. **Indeed, at least one study indicates equal or even greater efficacy for a 50% dose of Pasteur strain BCG (75 mg), with reduction in toxicity** (Pagano et al, 1991). Randomized, prospective studies designed to assess optimal dosing (in terms of efficacy and toxicity) are needed.

Bladder irritability is the main side effect of BCG therapy. It can be relieved to some extent with oral oxybutynin 5 mg thrice daily, and phenazopyridine 200 mg thrice daily. The symptom complex includes dysuria (91%), urinary frequency (90%), hematuria (46%), fever (24%), malaise (18%), nausea (8%), chills (8%), arthralgia (2%), and pruritus (1%). **Granulomatous prostatitis also occurs commonly following BCG therapy** (Oates et al, 1988). **Symptoms severe enough to require antituberculous therapy occur in up to 6% of patients** (Lamm et al, 1986). Systemic BCG infection has been presumed to be responsible for several deaths during treatment (Deresiewicz et al, 1990; Rawls et al, 1990). **Patients having fever persisting more than 48 hours following intravesical BCG therapy and not responding to antipyretics should be treated with oral isoniazid 300 mg daily plus pyridoxine 50 mg daily. Patients with more prolonged or severe systemic symptoms should be treated with isoniazid, pyridoxine, and rifampin 600 mg daily. Ethambutol 1200 mg daily** (Steg et al, 1989) **and cycloserine 250 to 500 mg twice daily should be added to the treatment regimen if the patient appears to be critically ill** (Lamm, 1989; Sakamoto et al, 1989). Corticosteroids (40 mg prednisone daily) have also been recommended for severe reactions, but their value has not been formally tested in humans. These treatment recommendations do not entirely coincide with the current Centers for Disease Control and Prevention recommendations for antituberculosis therapy, but at this time, in the absence of controlled studies of BCG infections, they seem reasonable to follow. **No data exist on the necessary duration of treatment for symptomatic disseminated BCG infections either.** It is possible that a 6-week course of treatment may suffice; however, **it would seem prudent to recommend a 6-month course.** A correlation exists between the intensity of BCG therapy and both its toxicity and results (Morales and Ersil, 1979; Brosman, 1982). Toxicity is also related to the route of administration. Anaphylactic reactions have been reported with intralesional injections, whereas intravesical and oral administration have rarely produced other severe complications. **BCG may be given to patients with vesicoureteral reflux without significantly increased complications** (Bohle et al, 1990). **BCG should not be given to immunocompromised patients and should not be given to patients after traumatic catheterization.** There is no evidence that BCG therapy is contraindicated in patients with valvular heart disease or those with valvular or joint prostheses, although antibiotic prophylaxis for bacterial endocarditis and similar infections should be administered as would normally be done when such patients undergo urethral instrumentation.

Intravesical Interferon

Interferons have antiproliferative, antiangiogenic, and immunostimulatory properties. They have been widely tested as anticancer agents in the treatment of a variety of tumors, including bladder cancer (Williams, 1988). Torti and co-workers reported that intravesical interferon alpha, as primary therapy without prior transurethral excision, resulted in a 25% complete tumor regression rate for patients with papillary tumors, but complete regressions were maintained in only half the patients (Torti et al, 1988). Interferon resulted in complete regression of carcinoma in situ in approximately one third of patients, but again only one half of them (16%) had durable responses. **These durable response rates of 12% for residual papillary disease and 16% for carcinoma in situ are substantially lower than those that have been reported for intravesical chemotherapy or intravesical BCG therapy. Because many of these patients had failed previous instillation regimens, however, the response rates were not as disappointing as it would first seem.**

Recombinant interferon alpha-2b has been effective in some clinical trials in the treatment of carcinoma in situ. A prospective, randomized trial (Glashan, 1990) comparing low-dose (10 million units) with high-dose (100 million units) recombinant interferon alpha-2b weekly for 12 weeks and then monthly for 1 year in patients with carcinoma in situ revealed a 43% complete response rate with the high-dose regimen and a 5% response rate with the low-dose regimen. Complete responses occurred in two of nine patients who had failed to respond to prior intravesical BCG therapy. Complete responses were maintained at least 6 months in 90% of responders. As with other interferon studies, side effects were minimal. As might be surmised from Torti and co-workers' study, **intravesical interferon alpha-2b may be more effective in patients not previously treated with intravesical therapy (67%) than in those failing to respond to intravesical agents (30%)** (Torti et al, 1988). **Alternatively, interferon as prophylaxis of superficial bladder cancers that have been entirely resected was found to be less effective than BCG in terms of tumor recurrence and time to recurrence** (Kalble et al, 1994). Further clinical studies are necessary to compare intravesical interferon with other established treatments for superficial bladder cancer.

Other Immunomodulators

Because of BCG's efficacy and the likelihood that it works through immunomodulatory means, some of the mediators BCG may work through, or substances that induce those mediators, have also been tried in bladder cancer. **Bropiramine is an oral interferon inducer.** In a phase I trial of this agent, Sarosdy and colleagues administered three equal daily doses given at 2-hour intervals for 3 consecutive days, repeated weekly for 12 weeks (Sarosdy et al, 1992). In responders at 12 weeks, the drug was continued for 1 year. **The drug was well tolerated, but particularly impressive was that 5 of 11 patients with carcinoma in situ experienced complete responses and 1 a partial response. At the time of the report, only 1 of the complete responders with carcinoma in situ had experienced a recurrence of carcinoma in situ (at 12 months after initiation of therapy). Because 10 out of the 11 patients with carcinoma in situ had failed either BCG or interferon previously, this would appear to be a potentially promising regimen in BCG failures.** Further studies are now underway.

Tumor necrosis factor has also been found in the urine of BCG-treated patients (see previously) and is known to have antitumorigenic properties. A dose escalation study (200 to 1000 mg) involving nine patients with recurrent superficial bladder cancer who had not previously received intravesical therapy was carried out by the Eastern Cooperative Oncology Group. Patients received weekly instillations for 11 weeks. Toxicity, even at high levels, was minimal, although several patients experienced flu-like symptoms. Eight of the nine patients who had undergone transurethral resections and tumor necrosis factor instillations experienced complete responses at 3 and 6 months. All had relapsed, however, between 7 and 35 months. Because this is a group of patients with frequently recurring previous bladder tumors, such long-term recurrences are not surprising (Glazer et al, 1995). The authors are unaware of any phase II studies with this agent despite its somewhat promising results in this trial.

Interleukin-2 has been useful as an immunomodulator in treating other malignancies, including metastatic renal cell carcinoma. Pizza and colleagues reported complete tumor regression in three of six patients receiving 4000 units of interleukin-2 intralesionally (Pizza et al, 1984). Huland and Huland (1989) observed a complete response in one of four patients with stage T4, Nx, M0 unresected transitional cell carcinoma with continuous intravesical perfusion of interleukin-2 for 5 days, repeated every 4 to 12 weeks. The responder had remained disease-free for 6 months clinically and by biopsy at the time of the report. Again, further testing of this agent in phase II trials or in prospective, controlled studies comparing it with more standard therapies is still forthcoming.

Other Biologic Agents

TP40, a TGF-α–*Pseudomonas* exotoxin hybrid fusion protein, enters cells via the EGF receptor (to which TGF-α binds). After internalization and release into the cytoplasm, the *Pseudomonas* exotoxin-40 domain kills target cells by inhibiting protein synthesis. In in vitro and in animal experiments, TP40 has demonstrated cytotoxicity against a variety of cell lines that express the EGF receptor and against human tumor xenografts bearing EGF receptors in nude mice (Heimbrook et al, 1994). In a dose escalation study of patients with recurrent superficial bladder cancer or carcinoma in situ, **eight of nine evaluable patients with carcinoma in situ exhibited partial or complete responses with weekly instillations of various doses (0.5–9.6 mg) of TP40.** Treatments were not continued beyond 6 to 11 instillations, and only one of the responses (in eight responding patients) was durable. **Perhaps more important is the fact that superficial tumors did not respond even when carcinoma in situ in the same patient did. This implies that TP40 was unable to penetrate beyond a few urothelial cell layers in its current formulation.** Because toxicity was not experienced, maximal tolerated or effective dosages could not be determined. A phase II study to evaluate further efficacy in treating carcinoma in situ has not been carried out. It is important to note, however, that **virtually all patients had been heavily pretreated, with 81% having failed prior BCG** (Goldberg et al, 1995).

Adjuvant Therapy for Superficial Cancers: Conclusions

Because **well-differentiated and moderately differentiated superficial tumors** recur after complete endoscopic resection in roughly 50 percent of patients but rarely progress to more aggressive disease, **it would make sense that intravesical therapy be withheld in such patients until the frequency or multiplicity of recurrences becomes so great that the expense, discomfort, or risk of repeated transurethral resections exceeds that of intravesical therapy.** Alternatively, **because high-grade lesions, particularly Tis or stage T1, have substantial risks of stage progression, intravesical therapy is indicated immediately. Because only BCG has been shown to delay or prevent progression, unless contraindicated, it should be the first agent used.**

CHEMOPREVENTION

Because **patients with superficial bladder cancer are at such high risk for recurrence** yet are usually managed by careful surveillance, they present ideal subjects in whom to test new therapeutic or preventive strategies. Presumably, **approaches that show efficacy in these individuals with high likelihoods of developing more tumors can then be tried in much larger populations who are at some risk for developing, but have never yet had, a bladder tumor.** Approaches that have been tried or are under evaluation include the use of specific vitamins (alone or in combination), polyamine synthesis inhibitors, and other more natural approaches, including dietary alterations that affect urinary constituents.

Vitamins

Vitamin A and its analogues have been considered differentiating agents that have been found experimentally to prevent induced bladder cancer in animals (Sporn et al, 1977). Unfortunately, **two vitamin A analogues, 13-*cis* retinoic acid and tigerson (ethyl-all-*trans*-9 [4-methoxy-2,3,6-trimethylphenol]-3,7-dimethyl-2,4,6,8-nonatetraenoate), were found to be ineffective and actually quite toxic (primarily skin and mucous membrane toxicities) in patients with superficial bladder tumors** (Koontz et al, 1981a; Pedersen et al, 1984).

Vitamins A and E were tested in a well-designed trial in which more than 29,000, 50- to 59-year-old Finnish male smokers without known malignancies of any type were randomized to receive alpha-tocopherol, beta-carotene, a combination of both, or placebo. Neither agent alone nor the two in combination had an influence on bladder cancer development (or for that matter, lung cancer development or mortality). The study has been criticized despite its enormous size (and hence statistical power); dou-

ble-blind, randomized, prospective design; excellent compliance; and extensive follow-up (5–7 years) because some experts have objected to the specific agents used as representatives of the families of compounds they were to test; because their dosages were less than optimal; and because by starting off with patients with an average 720 pack-year history of smoking, the mutagenic events leading to malignancy may have been so far entrenched that even ideal preventive agents were likely to be ineffective (Heinonen et al, 1994). Other analogues of vitamin A are now being considered for new prevention trials.

In a separate study, based on information that vitamin B_6 (pyridoxine) can reduce the level of substituted aminobiphenyls and tryptophan metabolites, which have been found to be carcinogenic in animal bladder cancer (Price and Brown, 1962; Bryan et al, 1964), **patients with resected superficial tumors were randomized to receive 20 mg of pyridoxine daily or placebo. No benefits in terms of time to recurrence or recurrence rates were seen** (Newling et al, 1995). The results of this study are at odds with one previously published in which pyridoxine did reduce the recurrence rate of superficial tumors (Byar and Blackard, 1977).

Megavitamins

Despite the data just presented, based on observations in animal studies and other human tumors implying that vitamins may be beneficial, **Lamm and colleagues have tested high-dose multivitamins (40,000 units vitamin A, 100 mg vitamin B_6, 2000 mg vitamin C, 400 units vitamin E, and 90 mg zinc) versus the recommended daily allowances of these vitamins (RDA), in a high-risk group of patients with superficial bladder cancer who simultaneously received intravesical BCG with or without percutaneous BCG administration** (Lamm et al, 1994). **Patients receiving the "megadose" vitamin regimen did significantly better, with projected 5-year recurrences being reduced from 91% in the RDA group to 41% in the megadose group** (Lamm et al, 1994). **This study has been questioned** because of its small numbers (65 patients—30 in the RDA group and 35 in the megadose vitamin group), its complexity (with patients simultaneously receiving one of two BCG regimens as well as one of the two vitamin regimens), **the relatively poor performance of those in the RDA group who received BCG (20% tumor-free at 3 years and a projected 9% tumor-free at 5 years),** and the relatively mixed histologies and tumor histories of patients (roughly one third had newly diagnosed tumors and roughly one third had carcinoma in situ). A much larger study, testing the value of megadose versus RDA multivitamins in combination with BCG, is planned through the cooperative group mechanism.

Polyamine Synthesis Inhibitors

Induction of activity of the enzyme ornithine dicarboxylase (ODC), which controls the synthesis of the polyamine putrescine and its aminopropyl derivatives, spermidine and spermine, is an integral part of the process of tumor promotion (Boutwell, 1964; Bryan, 1983). In experimental bladder tumors in animals and human bladder cells in culture, induced ODC activity is greater in malignant than in normal urothelium (reviewed in Loprenzi and Messing, 1992). Additionally, in malignant human urothelial tissues, both ODC activities and putrescine concentrations are higher than in normal urothelium (Messing et al, 1995a). Difluoromethylornithine (DFMO), an irreversible inhibitor of ODC, has been shown to inhibit experimentally induced bladder tumors and other experimental malignancies (reviewed in Loprenzi and Messing, 1992). This agent is excreted in high concentrations in a biologically active form in human urine, and in oral doses of up to 1 g per day it is well tolerated for more than 6 to 12 months (Love et al, 1992; Loprenzi et al, 1995). **In these doses, DFMO also decreases bladder tumor ODC activities and putrescine levels to those found in normal urothelium** (Messing et al, 1995a). A randomized phase I/II study has been carried out jointly by the North Central Cancer Treatment Group and Eastern Cooperative Oncology Group in which a mixed group of patients with histories of totally resected superficial bladder cancer received one of four doses of DFMO orally for 1 year (Loprenzi et al, 1995). **The drug was extremely well tolerated in the 76 subjects,** and although no dose-related bladder tumor preventive properties were noted, based on its safety and tolerability as well as its efficacy in preclinical studies, **a prospective, randomized trial of DFMO (1 g/day) versus placebo in patients with totally resected, newly diagnosed low-grade superficial bladder transitional cell carcinomas is planned as an intergroup study.**

Urinary pH

Another therapeutic approach that appears promising is the use of agents or dietary measures that can influence the urinary milieu. By doing so, urothelial exposure to endogenous and environmental tumor promoters, putative carcinogens, and mitogens may be influenced, perhaps altering susceptibility to developing bladder cancer. Fukushima and colleagues noted that saccharine-induced bladder cancer in rats was directly dependent on urinary pH, not occurring in animals with acidic urine (Fukushima et al, 1988a, 1988b, 1990; Sidransky and Messing, 1992). Additionally, it has long been known that receptors for growth factors, including those found in high concentrations in human urine, such as EGF (Fuse et al, 1992; Messing and Murphy-Brooks, 1994) have their ligand-binding properties affected greatly by pH. Considerable reduction in the affinity of the EGF receptor for EGF and TGF-α occurs at a pH of 6.5 and below. This has been demonstrated in vitro in human bladder cancer cells by Messing (1990). In a study in which patients with active bladder tumors or benign prostatic hyperplasia (and without urothelial cancer at cystoscopy) were asked to test the pH of each urination for 1 week with a strip of Nitrazine paper before surgery (transurethral resections of bladder tumors or the prostate), the bladder cancer patients had higher mean, median, minimal, and maximal pH values (Messing and Reznikoff, 1992). Thus, the potential role for urinary acidification as a preventive approach is theoretically attractive. Moreover, this effect may be responsible in part for any antitumor activity of agents such as bropiramine, megadose vitamins, and DFMO.

If any or all of these preventive strategies seem effective in patients with newly diagnosed bladder cancer, it would eventually be reasonable to consider them for populations at risk who have not yet developed bladder cancer. The ideal preventive agent, of course, would be one that is inexpensive, nontoxic, well tolerated in long-term administration, and potentially effective against a variety of malignancies. Vitamins and DFMO certainly have such potentials.

FOLLOW-UP AND UPPER TRACT EVALUATION

The ideal follow-up for patients with superficial bladder cancer after endoscopic resection and treatment is surveillance cystoscopic and cytologic examinations every 3 months for 18 to 24 months after the initial tumor, every 6 months for the 2 years following that, and annually thereafter. There has been considerable debate, however, as to whether such intensive follow-up is needed—particularly for patients with low-grade superficial tumors. Both Gulliford and colleagues (1993) and Abel (1993) have suggested, particularly for patients with solitary stage Ta papillary low-grade tumors that are completely resected and who have negative evaluations at the first 3-month cystoscopy, that far less rigorous surveillance is needed. Both of these groups developed their opinions from data of patients in London, England. It is thus somewhat surprising that Morris and colleagues, also in London, found that **even those patients with superficial tumors who remained tumor-free 2 and 5 years after initial tumor resection had a 43% and 22% chance, respectively, of developing another bladder tumor** (Morris et al, 1995). **The vast majority of these patients had low-grade superficial tumors initially** and would not have remained under surveillance when they ultimately recurred had the recommendations of Gulliford and colleagues (1993) or Abel (1993) been followed. **Even more distressing is the report of Thompson and co-workers, which noted that of 124 patients followed for superficial bladder cancer in the Baltimore Veterans Administration Hospital, 20 went at least 5 years without tumor recurrence and subsequently presented with muscle-invasive cancers** (Thompson et al, 1993). **This report indicates that regardless of the intensity, surveillance probably needs to be continued indefinitely.**

Follow-up cystoscopy can readily be performed as an office procedure. The flexible cystoscope has greatly facilitated patient surveillance. Although Meyhoff and colleagues have reported that a small proportion of tumors in the range of 2 mm or smaller may be overlooked by using flexible cystoscopy (Meyhoff et al, 1988), in a prospective study, Walker and co-workers were unable to find any differences in the sensitivity of rigid versus flexible cystoscopy (Walker et al, 1993). It is likely that with experience, flexible cystoscopy is about as accurate as rigid cystoscopy, although it is clearly more cumbersome to obtain a barbotage specimen through a flexible scope than a rigid one, and at times with the former, a second catheter needs to be passed after the flexible scope is withdrawn to obtain the bladder washing adequately. In this regard, it would seem that **cytologic surveillance, particularly with bladder washings, should accompany every cystoscopic examination.** Certainly, if cystoscopic examination is negative for recurrent disease and the bladder washing is positive, further evaluation, including bladder biopsies, is needed. Similarly, cytology that shows severely dysplastic cells collected during a cystoscopic examination in which only what appears to be low-grade papillary disease is seen would be an indication for relatively compulsive examination of the entire urinary tract, including obtaining many select mucosal biopsy specimens. Even with what appears to be a high-grade tumor at cystoscopy, cytology may provide useful information because completeness of tumor removal can be assessed by obtaining another washing a few weeks after the resection.

How frequently upper tract evaluation needs to be repeated is also unclear. In the absence of vesicoureteral reflux, high-grade superficial cancer or carcinoma in situ, or tumors adjacent to a ureteral orifice, in which the incidences of developing subsequent ureteral or renal pelvic cancers are higher (DeTorres Mateos et al, 1987; Miller et al, 1993). Regular surveillance of the upper tracts, if they were radiologically normal at the time of initial tumor resection, does not need to be intense. Fewer than 5% of patients ever experience renal pelvic or ureteral urothelial cancers (England et al, 1981b; Walzer and Soloway, 1983; Zincke et al, 1984; Smith et al, 1989), with a mean interval to development of upper tract tumors of approximately 70 months (Oldbring et al, 1989; Shinka et al, 1989; Smith et al, 1989).

INVASIVE AND REGIONAL BLADDER CANCER (STAGES T2–T4, N0–N2)

Two essentially different approaches to the treatment of muscle-invasive bladder cancer have been adopted: bladder preservation and bladder reconstruction (Montie, 1990). The goal of bladder preservation is to eradicate the cancer and maintain adequate bladder function. The results of bladder salvage protocols have been reported (Shipley et al, 1988; Wajsman and Klimberg, 1989; Rotman et al, 1990; Roberts et al, 1991; Kaufman et al, 1993; Scher, 1993; Vogelzang et al, 1993; Herr and Scher, 1994; Sumiyoshi et al, 1994). These studies often have focused only on the subgroup of patients who are able to complete the entire treatment protocol, without emphasizing that a patient who still has residual cancer after having undergone the initial radiation therapy and chemotherapy is usually not an ideal candidate for cystectomy. What is known about the responses of bladder cancer to chemotherapy suggests that bladder salvage protocols are best suited for a patient with minimally invasive cancer of pure transitional cell histology. There are no adequate phase III trials comparing bladder salvage protocols with bladder reconstruction protocols.

In the bladder reconstruction approach, the initial treatment is radical cystectomy followed by urinary diversion or reconstruction, adding adjunctive chemotherapy in patients who have pathologic findings suggesting a high risk of recurrence. Advantages of this approach are that it avoids chemotherapy in patients who do not need it, and it provides definitive therapy promptly, avoiding a several-month delay in patients whose cancers are not chemosensitive. The disadvantages are that chemotherapy may not be as well tolerated postoperatively and that some patients may lose their bladders unnecessarily.

Radical cystectomy, the most effective local therapy for patients with bladder cancer, is associated with pelvic recurrence rates of 10% to 20% as compared with recurrence rates of 50% to 70% with definitive radiation therapy alone, definitive chemotherapy alone, or combinations of the two. With the development of continent urinary diversion, orthotopic bladder substitution in both males and females, and nerve (potency)-sparing surgery, the results of bladder reconstruction protocols are more attractive than previously.

Currently, four different types of urinary diversion are used: (1) ileal (or some other intestinal segment) conduit; (2) continent cutaneous diversions such as the Kock or Indiana pouch; (3) continent orthotopic reservoirs to the urethra with ileal, cecal, or sigmoid pouches, which are primarily done in men but occasionally can be performed in women in whom the urethra can be spared; (4) in select patients, cutaneous ureterostomy. **The operative mortality of radical cystectomy has decreased from 20% to between 0.5% and 1%. In comparison, mortality rates associated with chemotherapy range from 2% to 6%.**

TRANSURETHRAL RESECTION

Transurethral resection alone is inadequate therapy for most muscle-invasive bladder cancers (Nichols and Marshall, 1956). Exceptions to this rule are patients with small tumors that have only superficial muscle invasion (stage T2). Barnes and co-workers reported a 40% 5-year survival rate in patients with tumors that infiltrated into but not through the bladder muscle who were treated with transurethral resection alone (Barnes et al, 1967). Current studies have confirmed these early observations. Henry and colleagues reported that 5-year survival rates in patients with stage T2 and T3a bladder tumors treated with transurethral resection alone were better than rates for those treated with preoperative radiation followed by radical cystectomy, radical cystectomy alone, or definitive radiotherapy alone (Henry et al, 1988). In this study, however, patients treated with transurethral resection generally had smaller, less invasive tumors than patients in the other groups. Herr (1987) also reported that appropriately selected patients with muscle-invasive bladder cancer had excellent survival results following transurethral resection, although local recurrences, usually managed by repeat transurethral resection and intravesical BCG, were quite common. Similar results have been found by Solsona and associates (1992).

Transurethral resection as primary therapy should probably be reserved for patients who have small, moderately differentiated tumors with only superficial muscle invasion (stage T2) and for patients who are not medically fit for cystectomy. In all modern studies that have reported good results (Herr, 1987; Henry et al, 1988; Solsona et al, 1992), aggressive re-resection a short time after the initial transurethral resection has been an integral part of the treatment to maximize the possibility of endoscopically clearing all malignancy. It is also possible that some of the more favorable results, in part, are due to confusing muscularis mucosa infiltration in stage T1 tumors with invasion of the muscularis propria.

PARTIAL CYSTECTOMY

As with primary transurethral resection, partial cystectomy must be reserved for a select group of patients—those with solitary muscle-infiltrative tumors with no evidence of carcinoma in situ, history of recent multiple superficial tumors, involvement of the trigone or vesical neck, or cancers in which a tumor-free margin of 1.5 to 2.0 cm cannot be obtained. Preoperatively (at the time of original transurethral biopsy), multiple cold cup biopsy specimens are needed to better assess the feasibility of performing margin-clear surgery as well as to ensure that there is no severe dysplasia in remote urothelial sites. Particularly for tumors lateral to a ureteral orifice, ureteroneocystostomy may be necessary. Some unfavorable reports of local extravesical recurrences or mortality (Faysal and Freiha, 1979, 1981) may have reflected less-than-ideal patient selection, especially in eras when carcinoma in situ was not recognized and select mucosal biopsies not routinely performed. In well-selected patients, however, results superior to those of contemporary cystectomy series (Resnick and O'Connor, 1973; Utz et al, 1973; Brannan et al, 1978; Cummings et al, 1978; Sweeney et al, 1992), presumably because of the highly selected nature of the patients, have been seen. In such patients, local extravesical recurrences are rare with partial cystectomy, and, therefore, attempts to avoid extravesical tumor seeding, such as with preoperative radiotherapy (van der Werf-Messing, 1973) or intravesical instillations of nitrofurantoin or water, are probably unnecessary.

Herr and Scher (1994) have combined preoperative methotrexate, vinblastine, doxorubicin, and cis-platin (MVAC) chemotherapy with partial cystectomy, finding that 17 of 26 patients (65%) were alive beyond 5 years, including 14 (54%) with intact, functioning bladders. Although 12 patients (46%) developed bladder recurrences, 7 of these were superficial. Only 3 of 10 patients with residual muscle-invasive cancer survived 5 years, however, whereas 14 of 16 who had no residual cancer (stage PO), or only carcinoma in situ in their segmental cystectomy specimens, survived 5 years. As with many studies of bladder salvage, however, these 26 patients represented a subgroup of 111 patients who had received a median of four cycles of neoadjuvant chemotherapy and at least one, and at times two, transurethral resections following the transurethral resection of the index tumor, which had preceded the chemotherapy. Thus, this treatment was again confined to a highly select group of patients, and despite this, the results are no better than those of historical partial cystectomy series. It is not clear from this article, however, how many patients who would not have been candidates for partial cystectomy before receiving chemotherapy were capable of undergoing that operation after systemic therapy.

As with transurethral resection alone or other bladder salvage approaches (see later), patients undergoing partial cystectomy with or without neoadjuvant chemotherapy or recurrent transurethral resections must be followed by careful surveillance cystoscopies because intravesical recurrences are quite common (Herr and Scher, 1994).

DEFINITIVE RADIATION THERAPY WITH SALVAGE CYSTECTOMY

Definitive external beam radiation therapy for bladder cancer includes a total tumor dosage of 70 Gy over 7 weeks (35 fractions), with 50 Gy to the pelvis. It has not been proven that pelvic irradiation can control nodal metastses. Representative results of radiation therapy for invasive bladder cancer include 5-year survival rates of about 35% for stage T1, 40% for stage T2, 35% for stage T3a, 20% for stage T3b and T4, and 7% for stage N1,2 (Goffinet et al, 1975; Blandy et al, 1980; Jenkins et al, 1988; Gospodarowicz et al, 1989; Greven et al, 1990). There appears to be no correlation between tumor grade and the responsiveness to radiation therapy (Miller and Johnson, 1973; Goffinet et al, 1975; Wallace and Bloom, 1976), although more poorly differentiated tumors, because they tend to be higher-stage disease, tend to do worse. Many patients in older radiotherapy series were staged by bimanual examination (Miller and Johnson, 1973), thus in part explaining poor results—because patients were understaged. Even in more recent series (Mameghan et al, 1992; Fossa et al, 1993; Pollack et al, 1994), however, results were similar to earlier studies. Moreover, in all, 50% to 70% 5-year bladder recurrence rates were encountered.

Interstitial radiation for invasive bladder tumors as popularized by van der Werf-Messing and colleagues (van der Werf-Messing et al, 1983; van der Werf-Messing and van Putten, 1989), either in combination with partial cystectomy or external-beam radiation, can yield 70% to 80% actuarial disease-specific 5-year survial. In another small study of a select group of seven patients with high-grade, deeply invasive cancer followed a median of 40 months, in which patients underwent open cystotomy and intraoperative iridium implantation after they had received 45 Gy external-beam radiation, five were free of disease and maintained normal bladder function, one was dead of disease, and the other had required a cystectomy but was alive (Grossman et al, 1993). Further follow-up on this group as well as expansion of these techniques to other patients has not yet been reported. This modality remains promising, however, for a select group of individuals with small tumors.

Another technique that had been hoped would offer promise in bladder cancer therapy has been the use of accelerated fractionation. This has become popular for treatment of a variety of tumors with the thought that it could avoid DNA repair and repopulation of clones of cells whose DNA has been damaged by irradiation. It is believed that this process may permit rapidly proliferating tumors to fail to respond to standardly fractionated external-beam radiation. In a pilot study of 24 patients with deeply invasive bladder cancers, Cole and colleagues reported 24-month actuarial local control rates of 56% and actuarial survival rates of 35% (Cole et al, 1992). All but two of the deaths, however, were due to bladder cancer. Significant short-term toxicity was seen but usually resolved rapidly. Delayed urinary or bowel side effects occurred in 27% and 7% of patients, respectively, but were invariably mild. Other studies of this methodology are underway but have not yet been reported.

Clinical trials have also been initiated using fast neutrons to treat bladder cancer in an attempt to improve on the results obtained with photon radiation therapy alone. Neutrons theoretically exhibit biologic properties that may be at least threefold more effective than photons; however, the effectiveness of neutron therapy varies from tissue to tissue. **Trials of neutron therapy for bladder cancer reveal that neutrons are of no greater efficacy than photons and are associated with a higher incidence of serious complications to the bowel and, in some studies, increase treatment-associated death rates** (Russell et al, 1989).

Chemical Radiation Sensitizers

Misonidazole is a radiation sensitizer that has been investigated as a potential means of increasing the effectiveness of radiation therapy for bladder cancer. Early studies suggest a possible benefit; however, results have not been confirmed, and neurotoxicity has been considerable. Radiation sensitizers have not been adopted into general use in the treatment of bladder cancer (Abratt et al, 1987; Bydder et al, 1989). Misonidazole has been recommended for integrated radiation therapy–cystectomy protocols (Ono et al, 1989). *Cis*-platin and 5-fluorouracil are also considered to be potential radiation sensitizers and are discussed subsequently.

Hyperthermia as an Adjunct to Radiation Therapy

Hyperthermia has been combined with radiation therapy with or without chemotherapy to achieve improved tumor response in patients with advanced bladder cancer. This approach has been based on the increased susceptibility of malignant tumors to the toxic effects of hyperthermia (Hall et al, 1974; Kubota et al, 1984). Complete local response has been reported in up to 42% of patients. The toxic side effects are generally greater than those observed in patients treated with conventional radiation therapy or chemotherapy.

Complications of Radiation Therapy

Approximately 70% of patients develop acute self-limiting complications during radiation therapy, including dysuria, urinary frequency, and diarrhea. **Severe, persistent complications occur in less than 10% of patients. One of the most troublesome complications is refractory radiation cystitis, which may require instillations of alum or formalin or even palliative cystectomy. The complications of standard radiation are less than those of neutron therapy or hyperfractionation in the few series reporting these modalities.**

Predictors of Radiation Response

Treatment selection might be facilitated if it were possible to identify patients with radiation-sensitive tumors. Controversial evidence suggests that papillary tumors are more responsive than solid tumors to radiation therapy (Slack and Prout, 1980), but this factor has not been confirmed in all studies (Hall and Heath, 1981; Shipley et al, 1982; Whitmore and Batata, 1985). Other studies have suggested that the presence of squamous elements and the secretion of human chorionic gonadotropin are also associated with a poor response to radiation therapy (Martin et al, 1989a, 1989b).

Vaughan and colleagues have evaluated a method to predict radiotherapeutic response (Vaughan et al, 1993). Hypertonic saline–treated single cell suspensions of tumors release DNA with its supercoiled structure intact. The residual nuclei, or nucleoids, when stained with ethydium bromide at high concentrations, contract as this agent introduces positive supercoiling into individual DNA loops. **Loops that have been damaged by radiation or other insults do not contract, resulting in larger nucleoids.** The variations in size can be assessed by a flow cytometer in which laser light scattered by individual nucleoids can be measured. The authors found that in assessing **tumor cell suspensions treated with 12-Gy irradiation ex vivo and subsequently exposed to hypertonic saline, nucleoids that scattered less light and hence had greater DNA contractility (undamaged DNA or DNA that was damaged and repaired) came from patients who had a much higher likelihood of having residual cancer 6 months after receiving external-beam radiation for bladder cancer than patients whose nucleoids revealed DNA damage and thus greater light scatter. Long-term follow-up was not available,** although it is likely that those patients who were free of the disease at 6 months would eventually survive longer. More problematic, however, is that **it is unlikely, based on the predictive values presented in this article, that this test could be used to predict an individual bladder cancer's radioresistance or radiosensitivity.** Further work with this test and determining the influence of chemotherapy in bladder salvage regimens (see later) on DNA supercoiling is needed before this can be considered a reliable predictor of radiation responsiveness.

Salvage Cystectomy for Radiation Failures

In patients who have incomplete responses to full-course radiation therapy, only 8% to 15% are candidates for salvage cystectomy (Goffinet et al, 1975; Blandy et al, 1980; Goodman et al, 1981). In patients treated with salvage cystectomy, the overall 5-year survival rate is approximately 38%, depending on the pathologic findings in the cystectomy specimen. If no residual tumor is found (indicating that the transurethral resection that diagnosed the recurrence removed the vesical lesion in its entirety), the 5-year survival rate is approximately 70%. When superficial residual tumor is present, 5-year survival is 50%. If deeper infiltrating cancer is present, the 5-year survival rate is only 25% (Blandy et al, 1980; Crawford and Skinner, 1980; Smith and Whitmore, 1981b). The operative morbidity and mortality associated with salvage cystectomy have been reported to be only slightly higher than that associated with primary cystectomy.

Integrated Preoperative Radiation Therapy and Cystectomy

The concept of planned preoperative radiation therapy followed by cystectomy was initiated by Whitmore and co-workers (1977). They proposed the following rationale: (1) Well-oxygenated tumor cells are more susceptible to the effects of radiation therapy, (2) radiation therapy may sterilize peripheral microextensions of tumors as well as regional lymph node metastases, and (3) radiation therapy may preclude the metastatic potential of tumor cells disseminated at the time of cystectomy. In their early experience, 40 Gy was delivered over 4 weeks; however, in 1966, they changed to a short course dosage schedule of 20 Gy delivered in five fractions over 1 week.

Whitmore and colleagues reported on the comparative survival of patients treated with a long course, high dose of radiation, those treated with a short course, low dose of radiation, and a historical group of patients treated with cystectomy alone at their institution between 1949 and 1959 (Whitmore et al, 1977). Marginally better disease-free survival and fewer deaths were noted from tumor recurrences in patients with deeply invasive tumors treated with either course of preoperative radiation. **A variety of subsequent studies, including some that were prospectively randomized, found little** (Miller and Johnson, 1973; Bloom et al, 1982) **or no** (Blackard and Byar, 1972; Prout, 1976; Crawford et al, 1987) **benefit for preoperative radiation therapy over cystectomy alone.**

As first noted by van der Werf-Messing (1973) and subsequently reiterated by Prout (Prout, 1976; Slack and Prout, 1980), patients appeared to do more favorably if, at the time of cystectomy, no tumor or only carcinoma in situ was encountered. As Whitmore and Batata (1985) pointed out, however, because down-staging occurred most frequently among patients with lower-grade, lower-stage tumors and those with pure transitional cell histology, it is possible that the better outlook in such individuals reflected more the indolent nature of the underlying disease process than any therapeutic effect of radiation.

The validity of the concept of integrated therapy came into question in the late 1970s and early 1980s (Vinnicombe and Abercrombie, 1978; Catalona, 1980; Radwin, 1980; Mathur et al, 1981; Montie et al, 1984). The underlying assumptions of the benefits of preoperative radiation therapy, including the validity of the comparision with historical controls, were questioned. The argument for decreased seeding of tumor cells extravesically based on data from patients treated with radium implantation of superficial bladder tumors via open cystotomy, as van der Werf-Messing (1973) had suggested, may not be applicable to patients with invasive bladder cancer undergoing total cystectomy. **If, as reported, two thirds of patients are down-staged by preoperative radiation therapy and the patients who are down-staged have a significant survival advantage, patients as a group treated with preoperative radiation therapy should have a better survival rate than patients not treated with integrated therapy; but, in fact, they do not.**

At the current time, both from controlled studies and from contemporary monomodality cystectomy series, there is little evidence to indicate that integrated preoper- **ative radiation (20 Gy in 1 week or 40 Gy in 4 weeks) followed by cystectomy is more effective than cystectomy alone.** A possible exception to this, based on a randomized, clinical study, is that preoperative radiation may be of benefit in the treatment of patients with stage T3 and T4 bilharzial bladder cancer (Ghoneim and Awad, 1980). Preoperative radiation has also been recommended for the patient with invasive squamous cell carcinoma of the bladder (Swanson et al, 1990).

RADIATION THERAPY AND BLADDER SALVAGE PROTOCOLS

A number of newer strategies attempt to preserve the bladder in patients with invasive cancer. In addition to definitive transurethral resection alone or with partial cystectomy or definitive radiation therapy, bladder salvage protocols include (1) neoadjuvant chemotherapy followed by cystectomy only when "necessary" and (2) neoadjuvant chemotherapy plus radiation therapy followed by cystectomy when necessary. The first approach is discussed under neoadjuvant chemotherapy. With the second approach, patients are treated with a combination of chemotherapeutic regimens, most of which contain cis-platin, vinblastine, and methotrexate (CMV) and 40 Gy of radiation (Shipley et al, 1988). The patient is then re-evaluated, and if there is evidence of complete tumor regression, the radiation therapy is continued for a total dose of 65 Gy in an effort to sterilize the bladder. Patients who failed to have a complete response following 40 Gy of radiation plus two courses of CMV are advised to undergo cystectomy. In a rather complex modification of this treatment protocol in which patients could receive two to four cycles of a modified MVAC regimen, 15 of the initial 29 patients had complete or partial responses to chemotherapy and went on to radiation. All 15 of these patients were alive at subsequent follow-up (median 57 months), although 5 had local recurrences, 4 of whom underwent salvage cystectomy. Two others had metastatic or deeply infiltrative recurrences at the time of follow-up. Thus, of 29 evaluable patients, 15 had radiation therapy following chemotherapy, 9 of whom had functioning bladders and were free of advanced disease. **In this group of 29 patients, therefore, only 9 (29%) had functioning bladders and were likely to survive their disease** (Vogelzang et al, 1993).

In another widely heralded phase II study by Kaufman and colleagues, 53 patients with stage T2–T4, NX, M0 transitional cell carcinoma received two cycles of CMV chemotherapy followed by 40 Gy of pelvic radiotherapy plus cis-platin (cis-platin started the day before radiation therapy and then again 21 days later) (Kaufman et al, 1993). Patients then underwent urologic evaluation, which included bladder biopsy and possible tumor resection. Those with complete responses cytologically and cystoscopically underwent consolidation treatment with an additional 25 Gy radiotherapy to the bladder and another infusion of cis-platin during treatment. **Those with incomplete responses were to undergo cystectomy, although only 8 of 15 such patients actually did. At a median follow-up of 48 months, 24 of 53 patients (45%) were alive without evidence of invasive or metastatic cancer. Of the total of 53 patients, 38% survived with their bladders apparently free of tumor,** although many of these have been followed for far shorter intervals than 48 months, thus making it uncertain how many would actually have tumor-free bladders by the time each of them had been followed for 4 to 5 years. These results are only slightly better than those reported for external-beam radiation (see earlier) or for the combination of *cis*-platin and radiation therapy for invasive bladder cancer (Shipley, 1989; Prout et al, 1991; Chauvet et al, 1993). A perhaps more dismal picture was presented for *cis*-platin plus radiation therapy in a study with long-term follow-up reported by **Raghavan and colleagues (1995) from Australia. In this study of 50 patients, *cis*-platin was given in two courses 3 weeks apart with repeat endoscopic staging after the second course and subsequently consolidation with 60 Gy external-beam radiation (n = 38) or cystectomy (n = 12). Six of the 50 patients (12%) were alive at 10 years, 5 of whom had undergone cystectomy. Intercurrent disease had killed the minority of patients. The 10-year bladder cancer specific mortality rate of patients who underwent radiation was 74%. These long-term results are quite sobering in view of the only modest successes found in the most optimistic series of multidrug chemotherapy plus radiation in bladder salvage regimens at 2 to 4 years of follow-up.**

INTRA-ARTERIAL CHEMOTHERAPY

In a somewhat different approach, various authors have combined intra-arterial chemotherapy with a variety of agents or combination of agents. These were infused via bilateral percutaneously placed femoral artery catheters threaded up to the common iliac arteries, and then the infusion was carried out with femoral artery compression. The rationale for such an undertaking was to deliver high levels of chemotherapy to the tumor itself and to regional lymph nodes. The agents most commonly used, *cis*-platin or doxorubicin (Adriamycin), also have been said to have radiosensitizing or synergistic effects. **In two different studies, Ethan and colleagues found nearly a 90% survival rate at 2 years in 19 patients with *cis*-platin and radiation** (Ethan et al, 1989), **whereas Sumiyoshi and colleagues reported a 72% survival at 5 years with intra-arterial doxorubicin and radiation** (Sumiyoshi et al, 1994). Treatments were usually repeated every 4 weeks for a total of four cycles after the initial 48 hours of treatment. **Comparable or even more favorable results were found by others who administered *cis*-platin–based regimens through intra-arterial routes followed by cystectomy** (Galletti et al, 1989; Jacobs et al, 1989). Follow-up and confirmatory phase III studies are needed to know if intra-arterial therapy has a role in the curative management of bladder cancer. The results of the above-mentioned studies combining intra-arterial chemotherapy infusions with definitive local therapy by either radiation or cystectomy, however, merit further investigation.

SUMMARY

Numerous treatment options are available for patients with invasive bladder cancer. At the current time, **however, pro-**spective, randomized, controlled studies comparing chemotherapy with external-beam radiation versus radiation therapy alone have not found a benefit from the combined approach** (Raghavan et al, 1989; Coppin et al, 1992). **These trials used *cis*-platin alone as the chemotherapy arm, rather than more modern multidrug regimens such as CMV.** Reports from early analyses of phase II studies with *cis*-platin plus radiation therapy (Shipley et al, 1987b, 1988; Saur et al, 1990), **however, were as promising as the more recent reports evaluating multidrug regimens with radiation. Thus, until randomized, prospective trials are completed confirming the benefit of combined modality treatment (multidrug chemotherapy and radiation) versus radiation therapy alone, one should not consider the former as the standard (or best) treatment for invasive bladder cancer in the patient unable or unwilling to undergo cystectomy.**

NEOADJUVANT CHEMOTHERAPY

Most patients with invasive bladder cancer who ultimately die from their disease after local therapy do so from metastases. Therefore, it is believed that the therapeutic limits of regional therapy, such as radical surgery and radiation therapy, have been reached. Effective systemic therapy for distant metastases is needed to improve cure rates. **The rationale for neoadjuvant chemotherapy is that not only it may shrink locally advanced tumors, but also it may eradicate lymph node and distant metastases.**

The principles behind using neoadjuvant chemotherapy as part of a planned multimodality approach, or as a definitive therapy in its own right for advanced localized disease, are as follows: (1) Micrometastases may often be present at the time of first diagnosis. (2) Micrometastases are probably best treated when the volume is minimal. (3) Down-staging of the bladder cancer by neoadjuvant treatment before cystectomy may increase survival benefit. (4) *Cis*-platin may act as a radiation sensitizer. (5) Systemic chemotherapy before radiation therapy may eliminate the reduction in drug access to the tumor that occurs as a result of radiation-induced vascular sclerosis (Raghavan et al, 1989, 1990). Neoadjuvant chemotherapy has been tested largely in patients who present initially with locally advanced tumors with perivesical extension or lymph node metastases. The most promising regimen is the four-drug combination MVAC. Clinical studies with **neoadjuvant MVAC therapy following aggressive transurethral resection of the primary tumor and re-resection of the primary tumor site show about a 50% incidence of clinical complete response and about a 25% to 30% incidence of pathologic complete response** (Scher, 1988; Herr, 1989; McCullough et al, 1989). **The extent to which these responses are caused by the aggressive transurethral resections or the MVAC chemotherapy has not been accurately quantified.** The ultimate effect of neoadjuvant MVAC therapy on long-term disease-free survival is not well documented. It is also uncertain whether patients who clinically have complete responses should be subjected to cystectomy. In this regard, there are significant errors in clinical staging in both directions following MVAC therapy. **Residual masses detected on CT scan may contain fibrosis in only 30% to 40% of inci-**

dences. In comparison, approximately 33% to 40% of patients who have no clinical evidence of residual cancer are found to harbor microscopic tumor if radical excision is performed. Not all studies of neoadjuvant chemotherapy are encouraging (Tannock et al, 1989), and further trials are needed to determine the clinical usefulness of methotrexate-, vinblastine-, and *cis*-platin–containing regimens as definitive therapy or as neoadjuvant treatment in multimodality bladder salvage regimens.

NEOADJUVANT CHEMOTHERAPY AND PARTIAL OR TOTAL CYSTECTOMY

Neoadjuvant chemotherapy has also been used with partial (see section on partial cystectomy) or total cystectomy in patients with invasive bladder cancer. **Single-institution studies of either MVAC or CMV followed by cystectomy or partial cystectomy revealed survival rates that appear little, if any, different from contemporary cystectomy series (Dreicer et al, 1993; Shultz et al, 1994). Similarly, perioperative MVAC with two cycles before cystectomy and two cycles after achieved a durable disease-free status in 50% of patients, results no better than contemporary cystectomy studies (Dreicer et al, 1990).**

Additional benefits attributed to neoadjuvant chemotherapy are, in selected patients, the possibility of avoiding complete cystectomy by downsizing the tumor (Shultz et al, 1994) or permitting the resection of disease that was previously considered unresectable, even in those with metastases (Miller et al, 1993; Shultz et al, 1994). Partial cystectomy was performed in roughly 25% of patients with locally advanced bladder cancer who received neoadjuvant MVAC (although some of these may have been partial cystectomy candidates before receiving chemotherapy) (Shultz et al, 1994), and **in roughly 45% of patients with unresectable tumors (stage T4+), their tumors either shrank (25%) or completely disappeared (20%), permitting cystectomy where it would otherwise not have been feasible (Miller et al, 1993). It should be remembered, however, that these favorable results making otherwise infeasible surgery feasible, were obtained in highly selected patients and cannot be generalized to the much larger pool of all patients with invasive and regionally advanced bladder cancer.**

Currently an intergroup (Southwest Oncology Group and Eastern Cooperative Oncology Group) study is near closure comparing three cycles of MVAC with cystectomy versus cystectomy alone for patients with invasive bladder cancer. Results will determine whether neoadjuvant chemotherapy plus planned cystectomy is a valuable approach, and, if so, which patients are particularly likely to benefit. Until this study is completed and analyzed, however, neoadjuvant chemotherapy should not be considered appropriate standard treatment except perhaps in those individuals with locally or regionally extensive disease in whom complete surgical excision is impossible. The theoretical disadvantages of neoadjuvant chemotherapy are that (1) patients may experience sufficient morbidity to exclude them from subsequent cystectomy; (2) for patients who do not respond, the delay could allow metastases to

occur; and (3) inherent inaccuracy in evaluating the response to neoadjuvant therapy may be misleading, especially in the *clinical complete responders* who then refuse cystectomy. Results from the currently ongoing intergroup study should clarify these concerns.

STANDARD RADICAL CYSTECTOMY

The technique of radical cystectomy and the various forms of urinary diversion are the topics of Chapters 100, 101, and 103 and are discussed here only briefly. In men, the standard operation for muscle-invasive bladder cancer is a radical cystoprostatectomy including pelvic lymphadenectomy (Skinner, 1982) with wide excision of the bladder and prostate along with bladder pedicles and perivesical fat. Total urethrectomy is performed if there is tumor involvement of the prostatic urethra, ducts, or stroma (Lopez-Almansa et al, 1988). **In the absence of tumor involvement of the prostate, urethral recurrences occur in fewer than 5% of patients and urethrectomy is probably not needed.** Standard cystoprostatectomy causes erectile impotence.

In women, the standard operation for invasive bladder cancer is an anterior pelvic exenteration with wide excision of the bladder and urethra in continuity with the uterus, fallopian tubes, ovaries, and anterior wall of the vagina. The operation diminishes the capacity of the vagina but does not preclude postoperative vaginal intercourse in most instances. **The urethra should be removed routinely with cancers involving the bladder neck or trigone, although it may not be necessary in patients with unifocal cancer more than 2 cm from the bladder neck** (Coloby et al, 1994; Stein et al, 1994).

It is important to evaluate the distal ureters, using frozen sections to ensure that there is no evidence of residual cancer. If cancer is found, the ureters should be transected more cephalad to achieve tumor-free margins. Tumor recurrence rates are higher in patients with positive margins (Zincke et al, 1984). In rare circumstances, there may be severe atypia or carcinoma in situ involving the entire length of both upper urinary tracts. In these rare cases, it may not be possible to obtain tumor-free margins, and it may be necessary either to remove the entire affected renal unit or to proceed with ureterointestinal anastomosis despite questionable margins. Linker and Whitmore (1975) and Johnson and co-workers (1989) reported surprisingly low tumor recurrence rates in patients with retained renal units having positive margins for severe dysplasia or Tis.

Nerve-Sparing Radical Cystoprostatectomy

A nerve-sparing modification of the radical cystoprostatectomy that preserves erectile function in the majority of patients was reported by Schlegel and Walsh (1987) (Brendler et al, 1990a). Potency may be more readily preserved in patients in whom the urethra is left intact (Brendler et al, 1990a). Delayed urethrectomy also has been recommended to enhance likelihood of preserving potency. With the nerve-sparing cystectomy, the vesical arteries and bladder pedicles are transected immediately adjacent to the seminal vesicles and ureters to avoid injury to the cephalad portion of the neurovascular bundles.

The advisability of performing nerve-sparing radical cystectomy has been questioned by Pritchett and co-workers, who found lymph nodes in the retained bladder pedicles following nerve-sparing cystoprostatectomy in 60% of patients undergoing cystoprostatectomy (Pritchett et al, 1988). The clinical significance of these lymph nodes remains uncertain. Reported early results with nerve-sparing cystoprostatectomy are favorable (Brendler et al, 1990b).

In patients in whom potency is not preserved, sexual function can usually be restored by intracavernosal injection therapy, vacuum devices, or penile prostheses (Boyd and Schiff, 1989).

Urinary Diversions

A variety of urinary diversions have been used in patients undergoing cystectomy for invasive bladder cancer.

Ureterosigmoidostomy

One of the earliest forms of urinary diversion was ureterosigmoidostomy, which has been largely supplanted by other forms of diversions because of the associated adverse postoperative sequelae. Earlier problems with the ureterosigmoidostomy were related to complications with the ureterocolonic anastomoses. Leadbetter and Clarke (1955) and Goodwin and associates (1953) described antireflux techniques with ureterocolonic anastomoses that reduced the incidence of reflux, but obstruction, urinary stone formation, electrolyte imbalance, and systemic hyperchloremic acidosis still occurred frequently. **Also, colonic neoplasms occurred at the site of the ureterosigmoid anastomosis in nearly 10% of patients living longer than 10 years. These adenocarcinomas are believed to be induced by the carcinogenic action of the combined fecal and urinary streams on the intestinal mucosa** (Husmann and Spence, 1990). Accordingly, other forms of urinary diversion in which the urinary stream is not in continuity with the fecal stream have become more popular.

Intestinal Conduits

The time-honored urinary diversion following radical cystectomy is the ileal conduit popularized by Bricker (1950). Peristomal inflammation, peristomal hernia, stomal stenosis, urinary tract stone disease, ureteroileal anastomotic strictures, pyelonephritis, and upper urinary tract deterioration are the principal complications of the ileal conduit urinary diversion (Sullivan et al, 1980; Bracken et al, 1981b). Virtually all patients find the necessity of wearing an external collecting appliance objectionable, but most adjust to it with time.

In patients with radiation enteritis, a jejunal or transverse colon conduit may be selected. Jejunal conduits are infrequently chosen because of the characteristic metabolic derangement caused by losses of sodium and chloride from the jejunum. Hyperkalemia is quite common. This requires careful metabolic monitoring and management with sodium or bicarbonate replacement. Colon **conduits are more suitable for the performance of nonrefluxing ureterointestinal anastomoses; however, there may be an increased incidence of anastomotic strictures with nonrefluxing ureterointestinal anastomoses.**

Continent Urinary Diversions

An important advance has been the development of continent urinary diversions that do not require an external collection appliance. These techniques use bowel segments to create a reservoir that can be emptied by intermittent catheterization through a continent abdominal stoma or that can be anastomosed to the urethra to form an orthotopic neobladder. Reservoirs that use the ileum alone (Kock pouch) (Skinner et al, 1987) or an ileocecal segment (Mainz pouch [Thuroff et al, 1986], Indiana pouch [Rowland et al, 1987]) and modifications thereof have been the most frequently performed continent urinary diversions. These operations have a high rate of acceptance among patients (Boyd et al, 1987); however, they are technically more demanding than the ileal conduit, and the risk of complications is higher (Kock et al, 1982; Skinner et al, 1984, 1987). The principal complications of these reservoirs include leakage of urine through the anti-incontinence valves, formation of stones within the reservoirs, difficulty in catheterizing the stomas, urinary tract infections, and pouch-ureteral reflux. **Continent diversion can be performed safely in previously radiated patients, but such patients have an increased incidence of urinary leaks and postoperative diarrhea** (Ahlering et al, 1988).

One of the first efforts at neobladder formation was the Camey procedure (Lilien and Camey, 1984), in which a V-shaped loop of ileum is anastomosed on its antimesenteric border directly to the membranous urethra. Because the bowel is not detubularized with this operation, nocturnal incontinence is a significant problem, and daytime incontinence also occurs in some patients. The antireflux mechanism may fail because of the relatively high pressures generated by peristaltic contractions of the tubular ileal loop. Accordingly, the Camey procedure has been largely supplanted by the detubularized ileal or ileocolonic reservoir anastomosed to the urethra (Ghoneim et al, 1987; Marshall, 1988; Kock et al, 1989; Studer et al, 1989; Wenderoth et al, 1990). **With neobladders, patients void using the Valsalva maneuver and relaxation of the urethral sphincter. It is often easier for them to void while sitting.** If the neobladder has adequate capacity (500–800 ml), low internal pressures, and adequate emptying, satisfactory daytime continence can be achieved. **Enuresis is not unusual, however, unless patients awaken themselves in the night to void.** If the neobladder is made too large, incomplete emptying can require the need for intermittent self-catheterization. **Neobladders have been created in women in whom the urethra has been left intact** (Stein et al, 1994). **Long-term follow-up, however, for urethral recurrence in such individuals is still pending.**

An increased reabsorption of methotrexate has been reported in patients with urinary diversions (Wishnow et al, 1989; Fossa et al, 1990). This would appear to be even more of a problem with continent diversions or neobladders in which urine is stored. Concerns also exist about cancer recurring in urinary reservoirs (Filmer and Spencer, 1990). **With any form of urinary diversion in which the urethra** is left in situ, it is important to monitor the patient postoperatively with urinary cytology and urethroscopy.

Complications of Radical Cystectomy and Urinary Diversions

The complication rate of patients undergoing radical cystectomy and urinary diversion is approximately 25% (Skinner et al, 1980; Sullivan et al, 1980). Among the most common complications are wound infections (10%), intestinal obstruction (10%), hemorrhage, thrombophlebitis and venous thrombosis, and cardiopulmonary complications. Rectal injuries have been reported in approximately 4% of patients. In general, if the rectal injury is small, fecal contamination is minimal, and the patient has not undergone irradiation, the rectum can be closed primarily, dilating the external sphincter to allow primary healing with low internal bowel pressures. In other circumstances, a temporary diverting colostomy should be performed (Flechner and Spaulding, 1982). The reoperation rate following cystectomy is about 10% (Wishnow et al, 1989). The mortality rate associated with radical cystectomy in most medical centers has decreased to around 1% (Bracken et al, 1981b).

Efficacy of Cystectomy

Cystectomy remains the most effective means to cure invasive transitional cell carcinoma of the bladder. In representative contemporary series, in patients with vesical contained disease (stage P2, P3a), 5-year actuarial survival and disease-free survival rates have been reported in 65% to 82% (Montie et al, 1984; Freiha, 1990; Pagano et al, 1992; Wishnow et al, 1992). Stage P3b has been reported to have 5-year disease-free survivals of 37% to 61% (Montie et al, 1984; Skinner et al, 1991). Because of a tendency toward clinical understaging, some of the patients discussed in these series would have been characterized as having more superficial tumors, had they been staged only clinically (T stage). This perhaps in part explains the better therapeutic results for cystectomy over multimodality bladder salvage techniques. Even if T stages are used, however, cure rates for stage T2–T3b transitional cell carcinoma by cystectomy are considerably superior to any bladder salvage treatment (Montie et al, 1984).

In a small proportion of patients with microscopic nodal disease (N1 or N2), radical cystectomy with pelvic lymph node dissection may be curative. Five-year survivals in the 30% range have been reported for such patients by several groups (Grossman and Konnak, 1988; Lerner et al, 1993; Vieweg et al, 1994). Other authors, however, have reported a somewhat grimmer prognosis (Smith and Whitmore, 1981a; Zincke et al, 1985; Stockle et al, 1995). The argument about whether pelvic lymphadenectomy should or should not be performed in the presence of nongrossly enlarged nodes has been discussed previously.

Cystectomy remains the best therapy for invasive and regional bladder cancer. Even with cystectomy, however, roughly 18% to 35% of patients with muscle-invasive tumors (stage T2, T3a) eventually died from their malignancy. Local pelvic recurrence rates for even stage T3b and T4 disease are routinely under 12% and are considerably lower for stage T2 and T3a lesions. Thus, it is clear that the vast majority of patients who die from bladder cancer after cystectomy do so from metastases. Indeed, because of the relatively low pelvic recurrence rate and evidence that almost all the patients with pelvic recurrences have concomitant or soon-to-appear disseminated disease as well, it is not surprising that precystectomy radiotherapy does not improve survival over cystectomy alone (Crawford et al, 1987). Alternatively, because of the significant failure rates as a result of metastases, attempts at combining cystectomy with preoperative (neoadjuvant) or postoperative (adjuvant) chemotherapy have been advocated.

ADJUVANT CHEMOTHERAPY

Because of the relatively good outlook for patients with invasive transitional cell carcinoma pathologically confined to the bladder wall (Wishnow et al, 1992), several groups have looked at the role of adjuvant chemotherapy for those with pathologically unfavorable lesions (stage T3b, T4, N1–N3). Studer and colleagues studied patients who underwent cystectomy alone versus those who had cystectomy followed by three courses of cis-platin chemotherapy (90 mg/M²) (Studer et al, 1994). Fifty-four percent in the control group and 57% in the treatment group were alive at 5 years.

Alternatively, in a separate study, a combination regimen, cis-platin 100 mg/M², doxorubicin 60 mg/M², and cyclophosphamide 600 mg/M² (CISCA) repeated every 28 days for four cycles following cystectomy, caused a significant delay in time to progression (4.3 years) compared with time to progression (2.4 years) in prospectively randomized controls who underwent cystectomy and received chemotherapy only on progression. Patients in the CISCA arm also had significant improvement in disease-free survival (70% at 3 years in the treatment group versus 46% in the observation group) (Skinner et al, 1991).

Stockle and colleagues have also carried out a randomized, prospective, controlled study of patients with stages P3b, P4, N1, or N2 transitional cell carcinoma who have undergone cystectomy and pelvic node dissection (Stockle et al, 1995). They found a significant improvement in progression-free survival, from 13% in patients randomized to cystectomy alone to 58% in those who were randomized to adjunctive chemotherapy with MVAC or MVEC (epirubicin replaced Adriamycin) with a minimum follow-up of more than 3 years. This was particularly dramatic for patients with stage N1 disease, in whom 75% of those treated with chemotherapy were free of recurrence at 3 years follow-up, whereas only 25% of those not treated immediately were.

Both of these randomized adjuvant studies have been criticized for several reasons. In the CISCA study, a substantial proportion of patients who were candidates for entry were not entered into the study, perhaps indicating that some degree of selection of participants may have occurred (although the randomization should have corrected for this). Second, statistically significant differences were seen only in disease-free status and not in survival. Third, although there was some improvement in disease-free status for node-negative patients with chemotherapy, **the predominant situation in which chemotherapy appeared to be advantageous was in those who had a single positive lymph node (N1). Ironically, if patients had more than one positive node, there was virtually no advantage for immediate CISCA** (Skinner et al, 1991). In the MVAC/MVEC study, although progression-free survival was clearly superior in patients receiving immediate chemotherapy (58% versus 13%), because 15% of patients in the chemotherapy arm died of causes unrelated to bladder cancer or its treatment (mostly, other smoking-related malignancies), whereas none in the observation arm did (at least in part because so many patients not receiving chemotherapy died rapidly of bladder cancer), significant differences in overall survival (33% of those receiving immediate chemotherapy versus 17% of those on observation—P > .05) were not found. Because the authors stopped the study before reaching their initial accrual goals owing to such dramatic differences in progression rates, this study will not be able to answer whether adjuvant chemotherapy improves survival in patients with regional transitional cell carcinoma after cystectomy. Another criticism of this study is that few of the patients in the observation arm received systemic chemotherapy on progression; if it had been administered, perhaps more survivors would have been seen in the observation arm. Indeed, at least one such individual did appear to be cured with chemotherapy on progression. This further substantiates concerns about drawing definitive conclusions from this study alone (Stockle et al, 1995). Clearly, what is needed are well-designed, large studies of adjuvant chemotherapy in high-risk patients in which those randomized to no treatment after cystectomy receive chemotherapy on progression, and in which survival is the major end point.

PREDICTORS OF DISEASE PROGRESSION IN INVASIVE BLADDER CANCER

Prediction of Lymph Node and Distant Metastases and of Survival

Tumor grade and depth of invasion are the most important factors in predicting the likelihood of lymph node metastases in patients with invasive bladder cancer (Kern, 1984). Nodal metastases are more common in anaplastic tumors and tumors with deep muscle invasion or infiltration into the perivesical fat (Prout et al, 1979; Kern, 1984). A correlation has been found between lymph node metastases and the presence of distant metastases (Prout et al, 1979; Kern, 1984). Distant metastases, however, can occur in the absence of lymph node metastases.

Paraneoplastic Syndromes

Paraneoplastic syndromes, including hypercalcemia, eosinophilia, and leukemoid reaction, occur in patients with metastatic bladder cancer (Block and Whitmore, 1973; Mi-

chel et al, 1984) and are generally associated with a dire prognosis. Each response has been reported in patients without metastases (Bennett et al, 1986).

Predictors of Sensitivity or Resistance to Chemotherapy

A variety of genes, including those coding for the glutathione-S-transferase family of enzymes and the multidrug-resistant gene (MDR) that encodes for p-glycoprotein, have been implicated in resistance to chemotherapy. The MDR gene's product acts as an energy-dependent efflux pump, imparting resistance to several unrelated pharmacologic agents. Unfortunately the response of urothelial cancer to systemic therapy is suboptimal, and because many chemotherapeutic agents act independently of the MDR gene, it is not surprising that at the current time no data exist to substantiate the role of detecting either of these genes in predicting chemotherapeutic responsivity or resistance—particularly to the agents and regimens presently employed for advanced bladder cancer.

p53—Nuclear Expression and Other Molecular Markers of Prognosis

As discussed earlier, the protein encoded for by the tumor suppressor gene p53 is important in controlling cell cycle transition from G1 to S phase through transcriptional regulation and in directing DNA damaged cells to an apoptotic pathway (Finlay et al, 1989; Brecroft et al, 1990; Fields et al, 1990; Hupp et al, 1992; Yui et al, 1992; Cordon-Cardo, 1995). In many cases, mutated forms of the p53 protein are overly stabilized in the nucleus and can therefore be identified immunohistochemically (Finlay et al, 1988). **Indeed, as a general rule in bladder cancer, presence of immunohistochemically detectable p53 in the nucleus of tumor cells correlates well with the presence of p53 mutations by genetic analysis** (Esrig et al, 1993). **Several groups have now reported that nuclear accumulation of p53 in superficial and in invasive bladder cancer correlates with a poor outcome and reduced survival** (Esrig et al, 1994; Sarkis et al, 1995).

In a retrospective analysis of 243 patients who had undergone cystectomy (many of whom had also received preoperative radiation, adjuvant chemotherapy, or both), those with organ-confined bladder cancer and p53 positivity (as defined by at least 10% of tumor cell nuclei having positive p53 immunoreactivity) had significantly worse 5-year survival (24%) and relapse-free (24%) rates than those who had p53-negative tumors (67% 5-year survival and 73% 5-year relapse-free rates). This advantage in 5-year survival and relapse-free rates for patients with p53-negative tumors was not statistically significant for those with extravesical (stage P3b, P4) disease or lymph node metastases (Esrig et al, 1994). Unfortunately, there are problems in extrapolating the results of this study and most others (Sarkis et al, 1995) to the general clinical situation for several reasons. First, **patients have been treated by a variety of means,** which may have had variable impacts on outcome that are impossible to determine retrospectively (and certainly were not clarified in most publications). Furthermore, **methodologies for assessing p53 differ from laboratory to laboratory, including the use of various antibody reagents; staining of frozen versus paraffin-embedded, formalin-fixed tissue; use of a variety of antigen retrieval techniques such as microwaving of tissues; and finally differences in the definition of a p53-positive specimen (cutoffs of 5%, 10%, and 20% positivity have all been proposed). Until some standardization of the methodology to assess and interpret p53 immunopositivity is accomplished, its routine use as a marker of prognosis in bladder cancer should not be considered the standard of care.** For instance, would it be appropriate for a patient with a newly diagnosed grade III stage T1 transitional cell carcinoma to undergo cystectomy rather than intravesical BCG therapy if the tumor was considered to be p53 positive? Similarly, should a patient with stage P2 transitional cell carcinoma of the bladder who has undergone cystectomy receive immediate postoperative adjuvant chemotherapy if the tumor is interpreted as being p53 positive? Currently, critical reading of published data could not support the more aggressive option in either circumstance, although it may well be the appropriate one. Thus, there is an urgent need for methodologic and interpretive standardization and correlation with clinical outcome in well-characterized (grade, stage, all therapeutic interventions, and outcome in terms of progression and survival) cases before the results of this assay should influence the care of any bladder cancer patient not taking part in an experimental study.

With this in mind, there is some intriguing evidence indicating that p53 malfunction (as is often caused by mutation) may modulate a cell's response to chemotherapeutic agents (Lowe et al, 1993). This may account for the report of p53 nuclear immunopositivity predicting a poorer outcome in patients with invasive bladder cancer who underwent neoadjuvant MVAC therapy. Sarkis and colleagues found in their retrospective analysis that 77% of 26 patients with p53-negative tumors who had received neoadjuvant MVAC had long-term survival, whereas only 41% of those with p53-positive tumors who received neoadjuvant MVAC did (Sarkis et al, 1995). In this study, 20% of tumor cells with nuclear immunoreactivity was the cutoff between positivity and negativity. Whether p53 nuclear positivity reflected chemotherapeutic resistance or greater tumor aggressiveness, however, is uncertain.

The only other molecular marker that has yet approached the point where it may influence management recommendations in patients with invasive bladder cancer is immunopositivity for the EGF receptor, which portends significantly worse survival (Mellon et al, 1995). Because clinical bladder cancer studies on the EGF receptor have almost exclusively used frozen tissue sections, however, and it is not certain that immunodetection of this antigen is as consistent after formalin fixation, this test is not yet ready to be applied routinely for the evaluation of most bladder cancer patients.

METASTATIC DISEASE (STAGES N3, M1)
Cytotoxic Chemotherapy

Chemotherapeutic agents that have documented activity against transitional cell carcinoma include *cis*-platin, metho-trexate, vinblastine, and doxorubicin. When provided as single agents, these drugs induce subjective tumor regression in 20% to 30% of patients. Most of these responses are only partial regressions with a duration of about 6 months (Yagoda, 1983; Soloway, 1985).

Combination chemotherapy with three or four of these drugs has been evaluated in clinical trials (Rotman et al, 1990). One of these regimens uses CMV (Harker et al, 1984). **The four-drug combination, MVAC** (Sternberg et al, 1985), **has been the standard regimen in metastatic transitional cell carcinoma for about a decade. In early phase II studies of well-selected patients, these combinations yielded objective response rates of 57% to 70% and complete responses in 30% to 50% of patients.** Response rates decreased, however, in subsequent reports when MVAC was administered to a wider range of patients (Sternberg et al, 1985, 1988, 1989). In a landmark intergroup study in which patients were contributed by Eastern Cooperative Oncology Group, Southwest Oncology Group, the National Cancer Institute of Canada, and the Australian Bladder Cancer Study Group, **269 patients (246 fully evaluable) were randomized to receive MVAC or *cis*-platin for metastatic transitional cell carcinoma** (Loehrer et al, 1992). **Response rates were superior for the MVAC regimen compared with single-agent *cis*-platin (39% versus 12%), and progression-free survival (10.0 versus 4.3 months) and overall survival (12.5 versus 8.2 months) were also significantly greater for the combined regimen. The complete response rate for the MVAC arm, 13%, however, was far worse than what had previously been reported. Toxicity was also quite a bit higher in the MVAC arm, with a 4% drug-related mortality, mostly caused by sepsis, occurring in those receiving the combined regimen,** whereas none was seen in the *cis*-platin arm. Two additional patients who crossed over to MVAC after progressing on *cis*-platin also died of sepsis and renal insufficiency. Thus, although MVAC was clearly superior to single-agent *cis*-platin and did induce a reasonable response rate, results were not nearly as favorable as they had been in smaller phase II studies, and **projected survival in the MVAC arm at 2 years was only 20%.**

Attempts to improve on standard MVAC were given a boost when Gabrilove and associates demonstrated that recombinant leukocyte growth factors such as granulocyte colony-stimulating factor could reduce much of the leukopenia-related toxicity encountered with MVAC (Gabrilove et al, 1988). Several groups added this or similar growth factors to the regimen in the hopes of delivering greater quantities of chemotherapy to the tumor to kill off cells that would otherwise survive standard MVAC. Indeed, **dose intensification with the help of recombinant granulocyte colony-stimulating factor was feasible** (Gabrilove et al, 1988) **and, when tested in a cooperative group setting, seemed to provide a greater response rate (60% complete and partial responses in 35 patients rather than the 39% objective response rate seen for standard MVAC in the large intergroup MVAC versus single-agent *cis*-platin study [Loehrer et al, 1992, 1994]). There was a 23% drug-related mortality rate** (primarily owing to sepsis, although congestive heart failure, respiratory failure, and myocardial infarction also occurred), however, **and median survival was unchanged from that of standard MVAC in**

the intergroup study. Other groups also have had disappointing responses employing recombinant growth factors to intensify MVAC's dose (Seidman et al, 1993; Logothetis et al, 1995).

Although not meant as an improvement over standard or dose-escalated MVAC or CMV, for **patients with advanced transitional cell cancer who were not able to receive *cis*-platin (primarily because of pre-existing renal dysfunction), Bellmunt and colleagues substituted carboplatin (300 mg/M²) for *cis*-platin and administered it with methotrexate and vinblastine** (Bellmunt et al, 1992). They reported a 48% objective response rate in 23 poor-risk patients, with a mean duration of response of 7 months. This regimen and related carboplatin-based ones are now standard systemic therapy in patients who cannot receive MVAC or CMV.

Paclitaxel

Paclitaxel (Taxol) is an antimicrotubular agent with considerable activity in a variety of metastatic cancers of nonurologic origin (McGuire et al, 1989; Holmes et al, 1991; Forastiere, 1993). **Roth and colleagues administered 250 mg/M² of paclitaxel by 24-hour continuous intravenous infusion every 3 weeks to 26 patients with metastatic transitional cell carcinoma** (Roth et al, 1994). **Seven had a complete response and another four a partial response, resulting in a 42% objective response rate in this phase II Eastern Cooperative Oncology Group trial.** At the time of writing, 5 of the 11 responders remained progression-free, with the **major toxicity being granulocytopenic fevers, mucositis, and neuropathy.** Paclitaxel has not yet been tested in patients who have recurred after MVAC therapy or in combination with other agents against bladder cancer.

Ifosfamide

Ifosfamide has been used both alone and in combination with other drugs against a variety of tumors and was tested by the Eastern Cooperative Oncology Group in **patients with metastatic bladder cancer who had previously failed systemic therapy. A 20% response rate was found** in such refractory patients; **five complete responses and six partial responses were seen in 55 pretreated patients** (Witte et al, 1993).

Gallium Nitrate

Gallium nitrate is a heavy metal, as are *cis*-platin and carboplatin. Four of eight patients with metastatic transitional cell carcinoma who had been previously treated with either *cis*-platin or MVAC experienced complete responses to at least two cycles of continuous-infusion gallium nitrate (given for 1 week and repeated every 21 days). **Significant toxicity, however, occurred, with severe hypocalcemia and hypomagnesemia being identified in almost all patients** (Seligman and Crawford, 1991). To reduce toxicity, shorter courses of continuous-infusion gallium nitrate were tried in patients with metastatic transitional cell

carcinoma who had failed MVAC in a combined dose-escalation and phase II trial. **At least 350 mg/M²/day were required to see any responses.** Objective responses (all partial) were seen in 17.4% of patients who received this or higher doses (Seidman et al, 1991). Toxicity was less severe, and when seen it was encountered only at the higher continuous infusion doses used by Seligman and Crawford (1991).

Encouraged by these findings, the Eastern Cooperative Oncology Group carried out a phase II trial of a combination of **vinblastine, ifosfamide, and gallium nitrate (VIG) in 27 patients with metastatic urothelial cancer who had not received systemic therapy for their metastatic lesions but could have received prior neoadjuvant or adjuvant chemotherapy.** Despite using granulocyte colony-stimulating factor, leukopenia and granulocytopenic fevers occurred in more than a quarter of the patients, and dosages had to be reduced in elderly patients with prior histories of pelvic irradiation, *cis*-platin therapy, or prior nephrectomy. **Sixty-seven percent of the 27 patients, however, achieved an objective response, including 41% complete responses and 26% partial responses.** Clearly, therefore, this combined regimen appears to have considerable activity in this disease even with the inclusion of some individuals who had received previous chemotherapy (Einhorn et al, 1994). **This response rate, however, although impressive, is no different from those initially reported a decade ago for the CMV and MVAC regimens in their initial phase II studies of well-selected patients** (Harker et al, 1984; Sternberg et al, 1985). **Because of this, it would be hard to justify the use of any of these agents or regimens in place of standard or dose-escalated MVAC in patients with metastatic transitional cell carcinoma in standard clinical practice.** Clearly, however, a randomized, prospective trial needs to be carried out comparing VIG or a paclitaxel-containing regimen with standard or dose-escalated MVAC to determine the best available regimen.

Additional issues need to be resolved concerning chemotherapy for patients with advanced bladder cancer. Because individuals who have been rendered complete responders to agents and regimens such as MVAC, VIG, and paclitaxel almost always eventually experience recurrence of their disease (Connor et al, 1989; Loehrer et al, 1992; Einhorn et al, 1994; Roth et al, 1994), the possibility of maintenance chemotherapy, a concept that is out of favor in the treatment of many other tumors, may be appropriate in this instance. Similarly, because nearly half the individuals treated with neoadjuvant MVAC who experience clinical complete responses and subsequently undergo cystectomy are found on careful histologic inspection to have residual invasive cancer in their bladders, it is almost certain that the same is occurring in those with metastatic disease who are complete responders. Should such individuals undergo further surgery of the bladder if it is still in place or of sites where metastases had been? Also, should those individuals who are partial responders or have stable disease after systemic therapy and are rendered complete responders by surgical excision undergo further immediate chemotherapy?

Immunotherapy for Metastatic Bladder Cancer

Approaches to metastatic urothelial cancer other than through systemic chemotherapy have been primarily reserved for palliative endeavors (see next). Because bladder cancer is known to be an immunoresponsive disease (see section on BCG) and because immunomodulators have been effective in shrinking locally advanced disease (Pizza et al, 1984; West et al, 1987; Huland and Huland, 1989), the possibility that systemic immunotherapy may be effective in metastatic bladder cancer has been proposed. Unfortunately, recombinant interleukin-2 infusions and reinfusion of lymphocytes stimulated in vitro with recombinant interleukin-2 (lymphocyte activated killer cells) have not been demonstrated to be effective in patients with regionally advanced or metastatic urothelial cancer (Hermann et al, 1992). At the current time, it appears that systemic chemotherapy is a more promising approach in this disease.

PALLIATIVE THERAPY FOR PATIENTS WITH ADVANCED BLADDER CANCER

Palliative Radiation Therapy

Radiation therapy in doses of 30 to 35 Gy given in 10 fractions often is effective in relieving pain from osseous metastases. Pain relief is usually prompt. It is advisable to use prophylactic radiation in minimally symptomatic metastases involving weight-bearing bones, such as the spine or the femoral neck. Internal fixation may be required for the prevention or treatment of pathologic fractures.

Palliative radiation therapy in doses of 40 to 45 Gy may be effective in controlling local symptoms from the primary tumor, but doses of radiation in this range also can aggravate the local symptoms produced by the primary tumor, such as urgency, frequency, hematuria, and dysuria.

Intravesical Alum or Formalin Instillations

A 1% alum solution may be effective in treating hemorrhage from radiation cystitis (Ostroff and Chenault, 1982). **The solution may be instilled with continuous bladder irrigation without the need for anesthesia and is generally well tolerated.** Occasionally, discontinuation may be required because of symptoms of vesical pain and irritability. Danger of possible seizures from aluminum toxicity has been reported in patients with diminished renal function (Kavoussi et al, 1986).

Formalin is a 37% solution of formaldehyde gas dissolved in water. Formalin solution in concentrations of 1% to 10% (0.37%–3.7% formaldehyde gas) has been given in bladder instillations to control hemorrhage from advanced bladder tumors or radiation cystitis (Brown, 1970). Formalin solution is exceedingly irritating to the bladder and, thus, **requires general or regional anesthesia for intravesical instillation.** Because a 10% formalin solution (3.7% formaldehyde gas) may cause fibrosis and obstruction of the ureteral orifices, formalin instillations should begin with a 1% solution and be repeated with a 4% and then a 10% solution, if necessary. **A cystogram should be performed before instillation to rule out vesicoureteral reflux. If reflux is present, Fogarty catheters should be passed up both ureters, and the patient should be tilted into the head-up position to protect the upper urinary tracts from the toxic effects of formalin** (Fall and Pettersson, 1979). The formalin solution is instilled into the bladder and maintained in contact with the urothelium for 5 to 30 minutes.

Hyperbaric Oxygen

Hyperbaric oxygen has been advocated for hemorrhagic cystitis caused by a variety of lesions, including bladder cancer (Norkool et al, 1993). There are only a limited number of facilities in the United States with appropriate equipment for this treatment, and often 30 to 60 days of therapy are needed. Furthermore, success is by no means guaranteed. If bladder cancer itself is the cause of severe hematuria, in view of the extremely rapid growth of this disease (see section on screening), especially in an individual with metastases who probably has only a brief time left to live, it is hard to see how hyperbaric oxygen therapy would play a role in such a patient's management. If an individual has received prior radiation therapy, however, and has severe hemorrhagic cystitis in the absence of cytologically, cystoscopically, and histologically detectable malignancy and other conservative means fail, hyperbaric oxygen can be attempted. If this is to be done, care must be taken to make certain that recurrent cancer is not present.

Palliative Hypogastric Artery Embolization and Palliative Cystectomy

Life-threatening hemorrhage rarely occurs from hemorrhagic cystitis or uncontrolled bladder tumors. If it does and if fulguration, laser treatment, or intravesical alum or formalin instillation fails to control the hemorrhage, it may be necessary to perform transfemoral percutaneous hypogastric artery embolization (Carmignani et al, 1980). If hypogastric embolization fails to control the hemorrhage, palliative cystectomy may be required as a last resort. As an alternative, urinary diversion, either through surgical or percutaneous routes, has been effective in anecdotal situations in stopping hemorrhagic cystitis from nonmalignant causes. If persistent cancer in the bladder is the cause of hematuria, however, it is unlikely that urinary diversion in itself will provide satisfactory management.

NONUROTHELIAL TUMORS OF THE BLADDER

Small-Cell Carcinoma

It is believed that small-cell carcinomas of the bladder are derived from neuroendocrine stem cells. Small-cell carcinoma may be mixed with elements of transitional cell carcinoma in the same tumor. Another possible source of small-cell carcinoma is the dendritic cells in the normal urothelium. Small-cell carcinomas exhibit neuroendocrine markers, such as staining positively for neuron-specific enolase. Small-cell carcinomas are usually biologically aggressive tumors with early vascular and muscle invasion. **Patients with small-cell carcinoma should be evaluated for a primary small-cell carcinoma of the lung, or prostate, which may have metastasized or spread to the bladder** (Swanson et al, 1988). There are isolated reports of favorable responses to chemotherapy for small-cell carcinoma of the bladder (Davis et al, 1989), and, **similar to small-cell carcinomas of other sites, most respond to *cis*-platin–based therapy. In virtually all cases, however, treatment with chemotherapy or radiation is ultimately ineffective** (Mills et al, 1987).

Carcinosarcoma

Carcinosarcomas are highly malignant tumors containing both malignant mesenchymal and epithelial elements. The mesenchymal elements are usually chondrosarcoma or osteosarcoma (Koss, 1975; Young, 1987). The epithelial elements may be transitional cell carcinoma, squamous cell carcinoma, or adenocarcinoma. These tumors are rare, usually occurring in middle-aged men. The common presenting symptom is gross, painless hematuria. **The prognosis is uniformly poor despite aggressive treatment with cystoprostatectomy. For example, in one series, the 5-year survival rate was only 20%** (Sen et al, 1985). **Carcinosarcomas are resistant to radiation therapy and chemotherapy** (Schoborg et al, 1980; Uyama and Moriwaki, 1981).

Some bladder cancers exhibit a prominent spindle cell component and are sometimes referred to as sarcomatoid carcinomas. These are also aggressive tumors with a poor prognosis but should not be confused with true carcinosarcoma (Young et al, 1988). Similarly, sarcomatoid inflammatory reactions may sometimes be confused with carcinosarcomas. Because of the benign nature of these lesions, it is of utmost importance to distinguish them from true carcinosarcomas. As mentioned earlier, pseudosarcomatoid reactions almost invariably occur in patients who have had bladder surgical procedures or severe infections within the past 6 months.

Metastatic Carcinoma

The bladder may be secondarily involved by cancers from virtually any other primary site. The most common primary sites are prostate, ovary, uterus, lung, breast, kidney, and stomach as well as primary melanoma, lymphoma, and leukemia (Koss, 1975).

NONEPITHELIAL BLADDER TUMORS

The three categories of nonepithelial bladder tumors are (1) primitive connective tissue tumors, including leiomyosarcoma, rhabdomyosarcoma, chondrosarcoma, osteosarcoma, liposarcoma, and granular cell myoblastoma; (2) tumors of non–connective tissue origin, including angiosarcoma, neurosarcoma, neurofibroma, pheochromocytoma, melanoma, and so forth; and (3) secondary nonepithelial tumors, includ-

ing lymphoma, leukemia, plasmacytoma, and myeloma (Rosi et al, 1983). Approximately 1% to 5% of all bladder tumors are nonepithelial in origin. The most common nonepithelial bladder tumors are reviewed here.

Neurofibroma

A neurofibroma is a benign tumor of the nerve sheath resulting from overgrowth of Schwann's cells. Multiple neurofibromas may occur as an inherited autosomal dominant trait of variable penetrance (neurofibromatosis) (Torres and Bennett, 1966). In the bladder, neurofibromas arise from the ganglia of the bladder wall and may occur as either solitary lesions or plexiform lesions. Vesical neurofibromatosis often becomes clinically manifested in children with symptoms of urinary tract obstruction, urinary incontinence, vesical irritability, or pelvic mass (Clark et al, 1977). Conservative management should be attempted unless there is severe urinary tract obstruction or unless symptoms become incapacitating. Rarely, bladder neurofibromas may undergo malignant degeneration to form neurofibrosarcoma (Clark et al, 1977).

Pheochromocytoma

Bladder pheochromocytomas account for less than 1% of all bladder tumors and less than 1% of all pheochromocytomas (Albores-Saavedra et al, 1969). They arise from paraganglionic cells within the bladder wall, usually in the region of the trigone (Koss, 1975). There is no sex predilection, and the peak age incidences are in the teens through the thirties. **About 10% of pheochromocytomas are malignant and have the capacity to metastasize to the regional lymph nodes or distant sites. Malignancy is determined more by the clinical behavior than the histologic features of the tumor. Most pheochromocytomas in the bladder are hormonally active, causing paroxysms of hypertension on filling and emptying of the bladder in two thirds of patients.** The classic symptom of micturitional syncope has been attributed to this entity. **Hematuria develops in only about one half of patients.**

On cystoscopic examination, the tumor appears as a submucosal nodule covered by intact urothelium. Histologically, the tumors are composed of nests of polyhedral cells with eosinophilic cytoplasm. **Partial cystectomy with complete excision of the tumor is the treatment of choice. Transurethral resection is generally contraindicated because it may precipitate a hypertensive crisis.** The histologic features of benign pheochromocytoma cannot be distinguished from its malignant counterpart (Koss, 1975). The regional lymph nodes should also be evaluated preoperatively with CT scans and gross inspection at the time of operation. If lymph node metastases are suspected preoperatively, arteriography may reveal hypervascular lesions. **Pelvic lymphadenectomy should be performed if lymph node metastases are present. As with metabolically active pheochromocytomas in other sites, appropriate preoperative adrenergic blockade is mandatory to avoid intraoperative hypertensive crisis,** although following tumor removal, hypotension may be challenging to manage. **Lifelong**

follow-up is required after removing a bladder pheochro-mocytoma because late metastases may occur, often her-alded by return of endocrine manifestations (DeKlerk et al, 1975).

Primary Lymphoma

Primary bladder lymphoma arises in the submucosal lymphoid follicles (Koss, 1975) and is the second most common type of nonepithelial bladder tumor (Binkovitz et al, 1988). **The peak age is 40 to 60 years old, and women are affected more often than men.** All histologic types of malignant lymphomas occur in the bladder. **Radia-tion therapy is the preferred treatment for localized pri-mary bladder lymphomas.** Approximately 50% of patients survive 5 years with radiation therapy (Koss, 1975). **With contemporary chemotherapy, the survival rate may be as high as 65%.**

Plasmacytoma, Granular Cell Myoblastoma, Malignant Melanoma, Choriocarcinoma, and Yolk Sac Tumor

These rare primary bladder tumors exhibit the same char-acteristics as their counterparts in other sites of the body and are managed in a similar fashion.

Sarcoma

Malignant connective tissue tumors containing cell types that are normally present in the bladder include angiosar-coma and leiomyosarcoma. Those that contain tissues not normally present in the bladder include rhabdomyosarcoma, liposarcoma, chondrosarcoma, and osteosarcoma. **Sarcomas of the bladder account for less than 1% of all malignant bladder tumors.** It is believed that sarcomas other than angiosarcomas and leiomyosarcomas arise from pluripoten-tial mesenchymal tissues of the bladder wall.

Angiosarcoma

Angiosarcomas are extremely rare tumors that arise within the bladder wall. Histologically, they contain dilated vascular channels with prominent papillary endothelial proliferation (Koss, 1975). If the tumor has not metastasized, radical cystectomy is the treatment of choice.

Leiomyosarcoma

Leiomyosarcoma is the most common malignant mes-enchymal tumor of the bladder occurring in adults. It is twice as common in men as in women. **Grossly, it appears as a submucosal nodule or ulcerating mass.** Histologically, spindle cells are arranged in parallel bundles. **The presence of nuclear abnormalities distinguishes a leiomyosarcoma from a benign leiomyoma. Leiomyosarcomas may some-times be amenable to treatment with partial cystectomy, but survival results may be compromised when conserva-tive options are performed for larger extensive tumors** (Swartz et al, 1985). **Total cystectomy has yielded a 5-year survival rate of 65%** (Tsukamoto and Lieber, 1991). Benign leiomyomas may be treated with simple enucleation or local excision (Vargas and Mendez, 1983; Teran and Gambrell, 1989; Kabalin et al, 1990).

Rhabdomyosarcoma

Rhabdomyosarcomas may occur at any age but are most common in young children. Embryonal rhabdomyo-sarcomas in children characteristically produce polypoid lesions in the base of the bladder, giving rise to the descriptive term *sarcoma botryoides.* These are described in Chapter 74.

Adult rhabdomyosarcomas include three cell types: spin-dle cell, alveolar cell, and giant cell. These aggressive tumors respond poorly to radiation therapy or chemotherapy, and, in general, the prognosis is poor (Koss, 1975; Tsukamoto and Lieber, 1991). The rare benign counterpart of rhabdo-myosarcoma, called rhabdomyoma, is treated with conserva-tive excision alone.

Other Sarcomas

The extremely rare liposarcomas, chondrosarcomas, and osteosarcomas that occur in the bladder may occur alone or with malignant epithelial elements such as a carcinosarcoma. The most effective treatment for these tumors is total cystec-tomy, although wide segmental excision may be effective for small localized lesions (MacKenzie et al, 1971; Wilson et al, 1979; Rosi et al, 1983; Ahlering et al, 1988b). The prognosis of patients with bladder sarcomas is generally poor regardless of treatment.

UROTHELIAL TUMORS OF THE RENAL PELVIS AND URETER

EPIDEMIOLOGY

Upper urinary tract epithelial tumors involving the renal pelvis are relatively uncommon. National incidence and mor-tality statistics for the United States on renal pelvis tumors are limited because they are grouped along with renal cell carcinoma (Annual Cancer Statistics Review, 1987). **Renal pelvis tumors account for approximately 10% of all renal tumors and about 5% of all urothelial tumors** (Fraley, 1978). **Ureteral tumors are even more uncommon, oc-**

curring with one quarter the incidence of renal pelvis tumors (Huben et al, 1988). **Epidemiologic statistics are more readily available on ureteral tumors, however, because they are classified separately.**

Ureteral tumors are roughly three times more common in men than in women and twice as common in whites as in blacks. The peak incidence in white men is 10 cases per 100,000 per year and occurs in the 75- to 79-year-old age range (Annual Cancer Statistics Review, 1987). The incidence of upper urinary tract tumors is increasing, and because, as with bladder cancer, upper tract tumors are rarely if ever diagnosed on autopsy (Resseguie et al, 1978), this likely reflects a true increase. One explanation for this might be the aging population. Upper tract urothelial tumors rarely occur before the age of 40, the peak incidence being in the fifties, sixties, and seventies. The mean age of occurrence is 65 years (Anderstrom et al, 1989).

ASSOCIATION WITH BALKAN NEPHROPATHY

The preceding statistics are dramatically different in areas plagued by the Balkan endemic nephropathy. This illness, which is characterized by a degenerative interstitial nephropathy, seems to be confined to rural areas of Balkan countries. **In families afflicted with Balkan endemic nephropathy, a much higher incidence of upper tract transitional cell carcinoma is seen.** Petkovic (1975) reported that the incidence rates for some villages affected by Balkan endemic nephropathy were 100 to 200 times greater than for similar nearby towns. **Despite these impressive increases in the incidence of upper tract transitional cell tumors, bladder cancer incidence in these regions remains unchanged. These tumors are generally low grade and more often multiple and bilateral than upper tract transitional cell cancers of other etiologies** (Petkovic, 1975; Radovanovic et al, 1985).

This nephropathy, although familial, is not obviously inherited. It may affect many people living in the same house, but the pattern of its genetic transmission or susceptibility, if one exists, is not clear (Petkovic, 1975; Radovanovic et al, 1985). As a result, family members who leave home at an early age may not be affected, whereas those who join the family may contract the illness. In addition, those afflicted may also be at an increased risk for developing non–urinary tract cancers (Radovanovic et al, 1985). **Environmental agents have not been identified.**

Because of these tumors' relatively indolent behavior and frequent multiplicity and bilaterality as well as the underlying endemic nephropathy causing some degree of renal impairment, this syndrome has necessitated the adoption of conservative renal-sparing surgery in many patients. This has provided an impetus to use conservative treatment of upper tract urothelial cancers in other clinical settings.

ETIOLOGY AND RISK FACTORS

Many factors have been shown to contribute to the development of upper tract urothelial tumors. Besides age, gender, and race, the most important of these is cigarette smoking. In addition, analgesics, coffee consumption, cyclophosphamide treatment, exposure to occupational carcinogens, history of urinary tract infections and stones, and inherited tendencies have been implicated in their etiology.

Smoking

Cigarette smoking is the agent most strongly associated with an increased risk of developing upper tract transitional cell cancers, with studies reporting a greater than threefold increase in risk. The risk also appears to be higher for ureteral than renal pelvic cancers and higher for renal pelvic than bladder cancer (Jensen et al, 1988; McLaughlin et al, 1992). A strong dose-response relationship exists between the total amount of tobacco smoked and the risk of developing tumors. McLaughlin and co-workers reported a 7.2-fold increased risk in long-term (≥45 years) smokers (McLaughlin et al, 1992). They also estimated that 70% of all upper tract tumors in men and 40% in women are caused by smoking. There are, however, conflicting data on risks conferred by depth of inhalation and smoking filtered versus unfiltered cigarettes (Jensen et al, 1988; McLaughlin et al, 1992). **Unfortunately, as with bladder cancer and in contrast to other smoking-related diseases, the risk declines only partially on permanent cessation of smoking. Thus, although cessation of smoking for more than 10 years resulted in a 50% to 60% reduction in risk, former smokers still had approximately twice the risk of developing upper tract urothelial cancer as similarly aged persons who never smoked of** (Ross et al, 1989; McLaughlin et al, 1992).

Coffee Drinking

Heavy coffee consumption has also been found to carry with it an increased risk for upper tract cancers. Ross and associates reported that individuals who drank more than seven cups of coffee per day had a relative risk of 1.8 for developing these tumors (Ross et al, 1989). **There was, however, a strong association with cigarette smoking, and after control for this, the risk decreased to 1.3** (Ross et al, 1989).

Analgesics

A well-documented, significant increased risk for upper tract urothelial tumors is analgesic abuse (Morrison, 1984; McCredie et al, 1986). Steffens and Nagel (1988) reported that 22% of patients with renal pelvic tumors and 11% with ureteral tumors gave a history of phenacetin abuse. The latency period ranged from 24 to 26 years. **McCredie and co-workers have also shown that renal papillary necrosis and phenacetin abuse are independent, but synergistic, risk factors** (McCredie et al, 1986). **The results showed that, alone, papillary necrosis and phenacetin abuse resulted in a relative risk of 6.9 and 3.6, respectively. Together, the risk increased 20-fold.** These numbers, however, are estimated because the control population was based on an autopsy study. **Long-term exposure to analgesics induces a nephropathy that is associated with up to a 70% incidence of upper urinary tract transitional cell carcinoma** (Johansson and Wahlqvist, 1979). In the urinary tract, **analgesic abuse induces the thickening of basement membranes around subepithelial capillaries, called capillarosclerosis. This finding is pathognomonic for analgesic abuse and has been reported in 15% of patients with renal pelvis and ureteral tumors** (Palvio et al, 1987). This finding, then, in a kidney removed for transitional cell carcinoma or biopsied for some other reason, should raise the clinician's suspicion for excessive analgesic use and the increased risk of upper tract transitional cell cancer that it carries. It should also prompt the clinician to question the patient more intensely about analgesic ingestion and should encourage the immediate institution of avoidance of phenacetin-based analgesics and possibly other high-risk activities, such as smoking.

It is believed that the risks associated with several exposures are at least additive, and after adjustment for smoking and high-risk occupational exposure, the relative risk for upper tract urothelial tumors for analgesic abusers was 2.4 for men and 4.2 for women. A dose-effect relationship was observed for phenacetin and aspirin, although, based on metabolism, phenacetin is probably the more important agent (Jensen et al, 1989).

Occupational Factors

Occupational exposures are known to be common etiologic factors in carcinoma of the bladder and contribute to the development of upper tract cancers. Significant increased risk for renal pelvic and ureteral tumors has been reported for those employed in the chemical, petrochemical, and plastics industries (relative risk = 4) and for those exposed to coal, coke (relative risk = 4), asphalt, and tar (relative risk = 5.5) (Jensen et al, 1988).

Chronic Infections, Irritation, and Calculi

Chronic bacterial infection associated with urinary calculi and obstruction predisposes individuals to squamous cell carcinoma or, less commonly, to urothelial adenocarcinoma (Godec and Murrah, 1985; Li and Cheung, 1987; Spires et al, 1993). Additionally, hydronephrosis is suspected to be an independent etiologic factor in the pathogenesis of adenocarcinoma of the renal pelvis (Godec and Murrah, 1985; Spires et al, 1993). Schistosomiasis involving the ureter is associated with squamous cell carcinoma of the ureter, as it is in the bladder, although to a lesser extent.

Cyclophosphamide

Cyclophosphamide, an alkylating chemotherapeutic agent that is known to confer an increased risk for developing bladder cancer, has also been related to upper tract urothelial tumors (Brenner and Schellhammer, 1987).

One of the metabolites of cyclophosphamide, acrolein, is believed to be the causative agent (Cohen et al, 1992). **As with bladder malignancies, tumors induced by this agent are generally high grade and aggressive** (Brenner and Schellhammer, 1987).

Heredity

Upper tract transitional cell carcinoma has been reported in several familial cancer syndromes (Frischer et al, 1985; Orphali et al, 1986; Lynch et al, 1990). **The Lynch syndrome II, which is characterized by the early onset of proximal colonic tumors without polyposis, numerous synchronous and metachronous colon tumors, and extracolonic cancers (most frequently of the endometrium)** (Greenland et al, 1993), **may also include an increased risk for developing upper tract transitional cell cancer.** Lynch and colleagues described four Lynch syndrome II families in which ureteral cancer developed in six family members (Lynch et al, 1990). In contrast to nonhereditary transitional cell carcinoma, they found a younger age of onset (55 years) and a female predominance. An increase in upper tract tumors was also noted by Greenland and associates in their study of four male siblings in a Lynch syndrome II family (Greenland et al, 1993).

LOCATION AND DISTRIBUTION OF TUMORS

Bilateral involvement (synchronous or metachronous) occurs in 2% to 5% of sporadic upper tract transitional cell carcinomas (Babaian and Johnson, 1980; Murphy et al, 1981). **Upper tract cancers occur in 2% to 4% of patients with bladder cancer** (Oldbring et al, 1989a) **except in occupational bladder cancer, in which case the incidence was reported to be as high as 13%** (Shinka et al, 1988). **The mean interval between the bladder tumor and the upper tract tumor has been reported to be as long as 70 months with a range of 40 to 170 months** (Shinka et al, 1988; Oldbring et al, 1989a). **Although the performance of routine excretory urography for follow-up of upper tract urinary cancers in bladder cancer patients is controversial, patients with multiple tumors, recurrent tumors, and tumors near or involving ureteral orifices are appropriate candidates for repeat upper tract monitoring.**

Approximately 30% to 75% of patients with upper tract urothelial tumors have bladder tumors at some time (Kakizoe et al, 1980; Abercrombie et al, 1988; Huben et al, 1988; Anderstrom et al, 1989). **This high incidence of subsequent bladder cancer suggests the need for routine follow-up cystoscopy in patients with upper tract cancers.** The explanation for the disparity between the relatively low incidence of subsequent upper tract tumors in patients with bladder cancer and the relatively high incidence of subsequent bladder tumors in patients with upper tract tumors may be related to seeding of tumor cells downstream or to the fact that bladder mucosa has a longer exposure time to urinary carcinogens than the renal pelvis and ureter because the former functions as a reservoir and the latter as conduits.

Shedding some light on this issue has been the ability to do *molecular fingerprinting,* in which specific mutations in the p53 gene found in upper tract tumors have been identified in bladder tumors that have subsequently developed in the same patients (Harris and Neal, 1992). These studies, however, have almost exclusively investigated patients with high-grade invasive tumors (the ones that tend to have p53 mutations) in whom the recurrences were fairly rapid. Whether such is the case for the more commonly found low-grade papillary tumors is not known, and, in view of the absence of molecular markers of low-grade papillary transitional cell carcinoma in which DNA sequencing of a specifically mutated suppressor gene or oncogene could be performed (see section on origins and patterns of dissemination of transitional cell carcinoma), such studies are impossible to do currently. Another explanation for the much higher incidence of lower tract tumors is that there are many more urothelial cells to serve as potential targets for carcinogens in the bladder than in either or both upper tracts. Thus, if carcinogenic events are relatively random, the bladder would far more commonly be involved.

Ureteral tumors are located most commonly in the lower ureter and least commonly in the upper ureter (Anderstrom et al, 1989). Babaian and Johnson (1980) reported that 73% of ureteral tumors were in the distal ureter, 24% in the mid-ureter, and 3% in the proximal ureter. This information again may be a reflection of implantation, but from at least a clinical point of view **it makes it mandatory to remove the most distal portion of the ureter when one is considering excising the kidney and ureter for a urothelial tumor higher up in the collecting system.**

Several investigators have reported on histologic mapping studies of upper tract urothelial tumors (Heney et al, 1981; McCarron et al, 1982; Mahadevia et al, 1983). These studies revealed associated urothelial changes ranging from hyperplasia to dysplasia to frank carcinoma in situ in a substantial proportion of patients. In the renal pelvis, carcinoma in situ may be patchy in distribution and extend into the collecting ducts of the kidney (Mahadevia et al, 1983), which limits the potential efficacy of conservative surgery for renal pelvic tumors. These changes are more frequently associated with higher-grade tumors. **More severe urothelial histologic changes are associated with a greater risk for tumor recurrence in the distal ureter and bladder and with a poorer overall prognosis. Because of the diffuseness of these changes, which are often invisible on gross inspection** (McCarron et al, 1982) **(and often on endoscopic inspection as well), local excision of any ureteral tumor that is not low grade and solitary must be approached with a great deal of caution.**

PATHOLOGY

Transitional Cell Carcinoma

Transitional cell carcinoma accounts for more than 90% of upper tract urothelial tumors. Histopathologic features are similar to those of transitional cell carcinomas of the bladder.

Squamous Cell Carcinoma

Squamous cell carcinomas account for 0.7% to 7% of upper tract tumors (Babaian and Johnson, 1980; Blacker et

al, 1985). Typically, these are moderately to poorly differentiated tumors, which occur approximately six times more frequently in the renal pelvis than in the ureter (Petersen, 1992). **They are frequently associated with infected staghorn calculi that have been present for a long duration.** Patients characteristically present with advanced disease. The response to treatment with surgery, radiation therapy, or chemotherapy is poor (Grabstald et al, 1971; Li and Cheung, 1987).

Adenocarcinoma

Adenocarcinoma of the renal pelvis is an extremely rare tumor, representing less than 1% of all renal pelvis tumors. **As with squamous cell carcinoma, adenocarcinoma usually is associated with calculi, long-term obstruction, and inflammation** (Stein et al, 1988; Spires et al, 1993). Spires and co-workers found a total of 59 cases in reviewing the English language literature (Spires et al, 1993). They subdivided these tumors into tubulovillous, mucinous, and papillary nonintestinal categories. The first two types resemble intestinal adenocarcinoma and constitute 93% of cases. Tubulovillous adenocarcinoma resembles colon carcinoma, with mucin-secreting columnar or goblet cells lining glandular acini, although extracellular mucus is not a dominant feature. Mucinous adenocarcinoma, as the name suggests, is characterized by intestinal-like cells with much mucus production. Finally, papillary nonintestinal tumors have no stainable mucin. They have fibrovascular stalks lined by cuboidal cells. This variety tends to occur in younger individuals and is not necessarily associated with infection. Of the two intestinal-type tumors, mucinous adenocarcinoma tends to have a better prognosis and occur more commonly in an elderly population. Papillary adenocarcinoma occurring in the ureter may represent the malignant counterpart of nephrogenic adenoma of the ureter (Kim et al, 1988).

Inverted Papilloma

Inverted papillomas occur in the upper urinary tract as well as in the bladder. Their gross, endoscopic, and histologic appearance is identical to those found in the bladder. The urothelium overlying inverted papillomas can be normal, attenuated, or hyperplastic, and foci of squamous metaplasia as well as cystic areas may be seen (Kyriakos and Royce, 1989; Grainger et al, 1990; Petersen, 1992). Although generally considered benign tumors, some have been associated with malignant change (Stower et al, 1990). **In fact, Grainger and colleagues reported an 18% incidence of malignancy within inverted papillomas of the ureter** (Grainger et al, 1990). **Additionally, both upper tract and bladder inverted papillomas often occur in association with other urothelial carcinomas, both synchronously and asynchronously** (Renfer et al, 1988; Schultz and Boyle, 1988; Kyriakos and Royce, 1989). **These findings, then, suggest that patients with inverted papillomas of the upper urinary tract should be followed closely for upper urinary tract and bladder transitional cell carcinomas.**

Nonurothelial Tumors of the Upper Urinary Tract

Rarely, sarcomas, including leiomyosarcoma (Madgar et al, 1988) and carcinosarcoma (Byard et al, 1987; Fleming, 1987); leiomyomas (Zaitoon, 1986); neurofibromas (Varela-Duran et al, 1987); small-cell carcinomas (Essenfeld et al, 1990); plasmacytomas (Igel et al, 1991); angiosarcomas (Coup, 1988); and fibroepithelial polyps (Musselman and Kay, 1986; Blank et al, 1987), occur in the upper urinary tract. **These tumors behave similarly to their counterparts in the bladder. For most, surgical excision is the preferred treatment.**

NATURAL HISTORY

Patterns of Spread

Transitional cell carcinoma of the upper urinary tract may spread by direct invasion into the renal parenchyma or surrounding structures, by epithelial extension (either direct extension or seeding), by lymphatic invasion, or by vascular invasion (Jitsukawa et al, 1985). **High-grade tumors demonstrate a greater propensity to spread.** Davis and co-workers reported that invasion of the renal hilar tissues by renal pelvis tumors had a greater predictive value for metastases (95%) than vascular (83%) or lymphatic (77%) invasion did (Davis et al, 1987).

Epithelial Spread

Evidence exists that tumor cells seed along the epithelial surface from cephalad to caudad in the urinary tract (Johnson and Babaian, 1979). **This finding is supported by clinical studies documenting a high incidence of recurrences in the ureteral stump of patients treated with nephrectomy and incomplete ureterectomy for renal pelvis tumors and by the occurrences of bladder tumors in the region of the ipsilateral ureteral orifice of patients with upper tract tumors. Johnson and Babaian (1979) reported that transitional cell carcinoma rarely develops subsequently in the upper urinary tract above the level of resection of a ureteral tumor.** Amar and Das (1985), however, reported that upper tract tumors developed in 6.4% of bladder cancer patients with vesicoureteral reflux as compared with only 0.4% of patients without reflux. Others have supported this finding (DeTorres Mateos et al, 1987). This observation, however, was not confirmed by Mukamel and co-workers in patients routinely treated with thiotepa instillations (Mukamel et al, 1985). An alternative explanation for the findings of Amar and Das and DeTorres Mateos and colleagues may be that the patients with "upper tract recurrences" might have had pre-existing undetected upper tract tumors that seeded down through the ureteral orifice, producing bladder tumors that required resection of the ureteral orifice to excise them completely. As mentioned earlier, **with high-grade tumors that have p53 abnormalities, in at least certain instances, sequential downward seeding has been confirmed by relatively irrefutable molecular techniques** (Harris and Neal, 1992).

Lymphatic Extension

The most common sites of lymphatic extension from upper tract tumors are the para-aortic, para-caval, and ipsilateral common iliac and pelvic lymph nodes (Batata et al, 1975), depending on the location of the primary tumor. **In view of the rather diffuse distribution of urothelial atypia and carcinoma in situ concomitant with obvious ipsilateral upper tract tumors** (Heney et al, 1981; McCarron et al, 1982; Nocks et al, 1982; Mahadevia et al, 1983), however, **if lymphadenectomy is to be performed for those transitional cell cancers that have even a modest chance of involving the nodes (i.e., moderately and poorly differentiated ones), extensive dissections involving nodes surrounding the great vessel, common iliac, and pelvic vessels on the ipsilateral side should probably be performed with the standard nephroureterectomy and bladder cuff excision.**

Hematogenous Dissemination

Venous extension into the renal veins and vena cava may occur with renal pelvic tumors as it does with renal cell carcinoma (Jitsukawa et al, 1985; Geiger et al, 1986). Surgical excision is the preferred treatment if there is no evidence of metastatic disease. The most common sites of hematogenous metastases from upper tract tumors are the liver, lung, and bone (Batata et al, 1975). **In general, transitional cell cancers of the upper tract are relatively hypovascular on angiography (see later).**

DIAGNOSTIC INDICATORS

Tumor Stage and Grade

Tumor stage and grade clinically are the most useful prognostic variables (Guinan et al, 1992; Terrell et al, 1995). Tumor grade and stage match in 83% of patients (Huben et al, 1988). Of the two, tumor stage is the more accurate predictor of prognosis. **Huben and colleagues reported that the median survival for low-grade tumors was 67 months but for high-grade tumors was only 14 months** (Huben et al, 1988). **Similarly, the median survival for low-stage tumors was 97 months and for high-stage tumors was 13 months.** The grading systems used are similar to those for bladder transitional cell carcinoma.

As with bladder cancer, the TNM staging system is currently used (Spiessl et al, 1989). In the current staging system, Tis represents carcinoma in situ; Ta tumors are epithelial confined and usually papillary; T1 tumors invade the lamina propria; T2 tumors invade the muscularis propria; T3 tumors invade the peripelvic/periureteral tissue or invade the renal parenchyma; and T4 tumors involve contiguous organs. Regional nodal metastases are N1 if there is only one involved node that is less than or equal to 2 cm in diameter, N2 if there is one positive node greater than 2 cm but less than 5 cm in diameter or multiple positive nodes less than 5 cm in diameter, and N3 if there are positive nodes greater than 5 cm in diameter. M1 refers to hematogenous or distant nodal metastases. **Guinan and coworkers, however,** suggested that in reviewing the Illinois tumor registry data, stage T3 renal pelvic carcinomas had a far better prognosis than stage T3 ureteral carcinomas, in part because the renal parenchyma may serve as a barrier against further dissemination (Guinan et al, 1992). Further complicating the issue was the rather detailed analysis by **Fujimoto and colleagues, who found that patients with renal pelvic cancers that had microscopic involvement of the collecting duct** with or without minimal renal parenchymal invasion **or with minimal microscopic invasion of the renal parenchyma (<5 mm extension)** with no collecting duct involvement **had a far better prognosis than those with extensive parenchymal extension** (Fujimoto et al, 1995). Only 8% of the former group (intraductular extension or minimal parenchymal involvement) succumbed to their disease, whereas 88% of those with extensive parenchymal involvement died of transitional cell carcinoma. **Thus, staging systems that distinguish between the presence of, and degree of, renal parenchymal involvement may be valuable.**

The distribution of tumor stages and grades differs in various published series (Bloom et al, 1970; Babaian and Johnson, 1980; Zoretic and Gonzales, 1983; Huben et al, 1988; Anderstrom et al, 1989; Zungri et al, 1990). **The majority, however, are low-grade, low-stage transitional cell carcinomas.**

Molecular Markers of Prognosis

In addition to standard clinical and histologic parameters (grade, stage, architecture, size, and multiplicity), molecular markers have begun to be applied to assess the prognosis of upper tract transitional cell cancers, although in most instances none have yet significantly affected clinical management decisions.

ABH Blood Group and Thomsen-Friedenreich (T) Antigen Expression

ABH blood group antigen expression has been reported to be of prognostic significance in upper tract urothelial tumors, as it is in bladder cancer. T antigen expression, however, was reported not to correlate with prognosis (Kagawa et al, 1985).

DNA Flow Cytometry

Flow DNA analysis correlates with the malignant potential of upper tract urothelial tumors. Oldbring and associates reported that all grade III tumors and 50% of grade II tumors were aneuploid (Oldbring et al, 1989). Others have confirmed these findings (Blute et al, 1988; Badalament et al, 1990; Corrado et al, 1991; Miyakawa et al, 1994). In a long-term study, Blute and co-workers found a correlation between tumor cell DNA ploidy, grade, stage, and clinical outcome (Blute et al, 1988). This was particularly of value in low-grade, low-stage tumors, in which an aneuploid pattern portended decreased survival (Blute et al, 1988). Although Corrado and associates also found a correlation between ploidy and survival, in contrast to Blute and co-workers, they saw no difference in survival based on ploidy in patients with low-grade or low-stage transitional cell carcinomas (Corrado et al, 1991).

DNA Synthesizing (S-Phase) Fraction

Studies by Nemoto and colleagues measuring the S-phase fraction of renal pelvis and ureteral tumors with bromodeoxyuridine labeling revealed that all low-grade tumors had an S-phase fraction of less than 10% (Nemoto et al, 1989). The average S-phase fraction for noninvasive tumors was 9.7% and for invasive tumors was 20.9%. They concluded that an S-phase fraction of greater than 10% indicated an aggressive tumor with potential for invasion and may be associated with a high probability of short-term relapse. In a more recent study, Miyakawa and associates used multivariate analysis to identify the most informative combination of prognostic factors (Miyakawa et al, 1994). **They found stage to be the most important factor predicting survival followed by grade and bromodeoxyuridine labeling index. The 3-year survival for patients with a low (<10%) bromodeoxyuridine-labeled cell index was 82.4%, compared with 16.4% in those with a high (>10%) index.**

Abnormalities in p53

Mutations in the p53 gene have been shown to correlate with an increased risk of recurrence and a decreased overall survival in patients with transitional cell carcinoma of the bladder (see previously). Although many studies have indicated an independent predictive value for p53 abnormalities (Esrig et al, 1994; Sarkis et al, 1994), not all groups concur that this is an independent prognostic variable (Lipponen, 1993; Thomas et al, 1993; Gardner et al, 1994; Vet et al, 1994). **Terrell and colleagues, in studying upper tract tumors, found no additional prognostic value for p53 abnormalities as detected immunohistochemically over that conferred by grade and stage** (Terrell et al, 1995). As with bladder cancer, it is likely that p53 mutations and malfunctions have an important role to play in tumor development and progression that can be useful for predicting outcome, but until there is standardization of the ways to detect these mutations and to interpret results, the findings of p53 studies should not influence management decisions for upper tract urothelial tumors.

Other Markers

Other markers that have been studied in transitional cell carcinoma of the bladder have also been found in some patients with upper tract tumors. These include chromosomal abnormalities (particularly trisomy of chromosome 7) (Sandberg et al, 1986; Gibas et al, 1987) and abnormal expression of the EGF receptor (Messing et al, 1987; Messing, 1990). In general, these markers occur or are expressed in similar conditions as they are with bladder transitional cell carcinomas, but data are not available to demonstrate their clinical utility as diagnostic or prognostic tools that can assist in the management of upper tract transitional cell carcinoma.

SIGNS AND SYMPTOMS

The most common presenting symptom or sign of upper tract urothelial tumors is gross or microscopic hema-

turia, occurring in more than 75% of patients (Bloom et al, 1970; Murphy et al, 1981). As with bladder cancer, it is likely that if enough voidings were examined, microhematuria would be present in all cases of upper tract urothelial tumors (Messing and Valencourt, 1990). Visible hematuria throughout urination suggests bleeding is from the upper urinary tracts or bladder. Long thin clots that are "casts" of the ureter imply an upper tract source.

Flank pain occurs in up to 30% of patients and usually is dull because of gradual obstruction and distention of the collecting system. Acute colic, however, occurs from passage of blood clots, which acutely obstruct the collecting system. In some studies, 10% to 15% of patients are asymptomatic, with the tumor diagnosed as an incidental finding on an imaging study obtained for other reasons. A small proportion of patients present with symptoms of advanced disease, including abdominal or flank mass, weight loss, anorexia, and bone pain. **As with bladder cancer, however, almost all upper tract tumors become clinically diagnosed at some point during life because they are virtually never found at autopsy in the absence of a known history of suspicious symptoms or a prior history of transitional cell carcinomas** (Resseguie et al, 1978).

DIAGNOSIS

Imaging Studies

Excretory Urography

Upper tract urothelial tumors usually are diagnosed as radiolucent filling defects on excretory or retrograde urography (Fein and McClennan, 1986). The differential diagnosis includes overlying bowel gas, external compression of the collecting system by a crossing vessel, blood clot, radiolucent stone, sloughed renal papilla, or fungus ball. Other less common possibilities include fibroepithelial polyp (Blank et al, 1987), air bubble, granuloma, leukoplakia, malacoplakia, hemangioma, renal tuberculosis, cholesteatoma, and leiomyoma.

Approximately 50% to 75% of patients have a filling defect (Murphy et al, 1981), **which is characteristically irregular and in continuity with the wall of the collecting system.** In the kidney, the tumor may produce incomplete filling or nonfilling of a renal infundibulum or calyx. **In 10% to 30% of patients, the tumor causes obstruction or nonvisualization of the collecting system** (Babaian and Johnson, 1980). **This finding is usually associated with a greater degree of invasiveness** (Bloom et al, 1970).

It is important to study carefully the contralateral upper urinary tract for subtle filling defects because its status may play an important role in treatment planning. It is also important to evaluate the entirety of both ureters on the composite of films to make certain that additional lesions are not present on either side.

Retrograde Urography

Retrograde urography may provide better visualization of the collecting system than excretory urography. **Contrast materials should be diluted by one third to one half to** avoid obscuring subtle filling defects by too dense contrast. Contrast materials should be injected through a bulb-tip ureteral catheter to fill the entire renal pelvis and ureter. At times, considerable pressure is needed for contrast to pass cephalad to obstructing lesions; however, extravasation and certainly perforation of the collecting system should be avoided. Although specific details of the collecting system may not always be as easily visualized under fluoroscopic guidance as they are with standard radiographs, the former may be helpful in avoiding extravasation. Additionally, because endoscopic evaluation of the upper tract is often useful in the work-up and management of ureteral and renal pelvic tumors, for convenience sake, radiographic imaging under fluoroscopic control can be performed as the initial part of the ureteroscopic procedure.

Because hyperosmotic contrast material may alter the cellular detail and make cytologic studies more difficult to interpret, nonionic contrast material may be preferable for retrograde studies. **Retrograde ureteropyelography is particularly helpful in patients with high-grade obstructions or with poor visualization or nonvisualization on excretory urography. Overall, retrograde urography is accurate in establishing the diagnosis of urothelial cancer with greater than 75% accuracy** (Murphy et al, 1981).

After retrograde urography, a ureteral catheter can be passed into the upper urinary tract to collect urine for cytologic studies and to obtain saline barbotage specimens or to perform brush biopsies of the lesion (see later). Sometimes these specimens could be as simply obtained, however, through a ureteroscope.

Antegrade Pyelography

Antegrade pyelography is not advisable in patients suspected of having upper tract transitional cell carcinoma because of the risk of seeding tumor cells along the needle tract. In exceptional clinical circumstances, however, such as when a patient has a nonvisualizing kidney and it is not possible to perform a retrograde study, antegrade pyelography may be required to determine the cause of the obstruction. This should be done as a procedure of last resort, however, because complete obstruction is more likely to be associated with a high-grade tumor, for which the risk of tumor cell seeding is even greater. **In these situations, CT scanning may reveal a soft tissue mass within the collecting system and obviate the need for such a study.**

Computed Tomography

CT is useful both in the diagnosis and in the staging of upper tract urothelial tumors (Baghdassarian Gatewood et al, 1982; Lantz and Hattery, 1984; Milestone et al, 1990). Because CT is more sensitive than conventional radiography in visualizing minimally radiopaque substances, it can demonstrate low concentrations of contrast agents in the urine excreted by poorly functioning kidneys. Thus, CT may delineate a collecting system tumor better than excretory urography in some instances (Kenney and Stanley, 1987). In comparison, small tumors may be overlooked on CT scans, owing to volume averaging.

Uric acid stones, which are radiolucent on standard urography, are opaque on CT scans because their radio-

density is usually greater than 100 HU (range 80–250 HU) (Lantz and Hattery, 1984). **Transitional cell carcinomas are recognized as soft tissue masses with an average density of 46 HU and a range of 10 to 70 HU** (Lantz and Hattery, 1984). **To evaluate such masses, however, and indeed, whenever CT is used to evaluate hematuria or renal lesions, it should be performed without intravenous contrast material first followed by intravenous contrast injection. Transitional cell cancers are usually relatively hypovascular (particularly compared with renal cell carcinoma) and do not usually have increased density following intravenous contrast injection.**

Large, infiltrating renal pelvis tumors may be difficult to distinguish from renal cell carcinomas. On CT, transitional cell carcinomas have a low attenuation relative to normal renal parenchyma. CT scans also can reveal necrosis or spontaneous hemorrhage within tumors (Bree et al, 1990), although this obviously could occur with either transitional cell or renal cell carcinomas.

CT evaluation of squamous cell carcinoma of the upper urinary tract generally reveals a tumor with extraluminal extension, as opposed to transitional cell carcinoma, which is predominantly intraluminal. **Additionally, in four of five patients with upper tract squamous cell carcinomas reported by Narumi and colleagues, these tumors were associated with a stone** (Narumi et al, 1989). Therefore, squamous cell carcinoma should be considered in the differential diagnosis in patients with CT evidence of an infiltrating tumor associated with a calculus.

Ultrasonography

Ultrasonography may also be helpful in distinguishing between a urothelial tumor and radiolucent calculus, but ultrasonography is generally of little value in the definitive diagnosis or staging of upper tract urothelial tumors.

Magnetic Resonance Imaging

MRI has not been reported to offer any material advantage over CT scanning in the diagnosis and staging of patients with upper tract urothelial tumors (Milestone et al, 1990).

Cystoscopy

Because of the high incidence of associated bladder tumors in patients with upper tract transitional cell carcinoma, cystoscopy is mandatory to rule out coexistent bladder lesions. If performed at the time of bleeding, cystoscopy may also be helpful in localizing the upper tract from which bleeding is arising.

Cytopathology

A voided urine specimen for cytopathology is the most convenient, least invasive means of obtaining cells from the urinary tract for cytologic evaluation. Precautions for collecting samples for cytology are presented in the section on bladder cancer. **Even under ideal circumstances, however, voided urine samples for cytopathology provide an insensitive test for establishing the diagnosis of upper tract urothelial tumors.** With low-grade tumors, the cytology is read as normal in up to 80% of patients (Grace et al, 1967). **As with bladder cancers, there is a correlation between tumor grade and positive cytology results.** Accordingly, some workers have reported that urinary cytology is of little help in diagnosing primary tumors of the renal pelvis or ureter (Nielsen and Ostri, 1988). Murphy and associates reported that cytology was accurate in 45% of patients with grade II tumors, in 78% with grade III tumors, and in 83% with grade IV tumors. Many of these patients, however, also had concomitant bladder tumors (Murphy et al, 1981). Even if the voided cytology finding is positive in a patient with an upper tract filling defect, one cannot be absolutely certain of the site of origin of the malignant cells.

Ureteral catheterization for collection of urine directly from the upper urinary tract provides more accurate cytologic results (Hawtrey, 1971; Sarnacki et al, 1971; Zincke et al, 1976) **but is still associated with substantial false-negative (22%–35%) and false-positive (at least in part because of the use of hyperosmotic contrast material) findings.** Saline washes provide better cell yields because hydraulic forces release loosely adherent cells from the urothelium and improve the accuracy of cytology results.

Gill and co-workers introduced the concept of brush biopsy to establish the diagnosis of upper tract urothelial tumors (Gill et al, 1973). With this technique, a fine brush mounted on the end of a guide wire is passed through a ureteral catheter into the collecting system and, under fluoroscopic guidance, is manipulated adjacent to the filling defect (Gittes, 1984). The lesion is then sampled by moving the brush back and forth within the ureteral catheter. The brush is removed through the catheter, and the sample (brushings) is sent for cytologic examination. Brush biopsies have a high positive predictive value (approaching 100%) when they are read as being conclusive or suspicious for malignancy or when they show severely dysplastic cells. Brushings that show atypical cells have a positive predictive value of 75%. **Sheline and colleagues reported that brush biopsy had a sensitivity of 91%, a specificity of 88%, and an accuracy of 89%** (Sheline et al, 1989). **Blute and associates reported a 78% overall accuracy** (Blute et al, 1981). In general, brush biopsies are well tolerated with minimal complications; however, severe complications, including massive hemorrhage in the upper urinary tracts and ureteral perforation, have been reported (Blute et al, 1981). The risk of spreading tumor cells to areas of the ureteral mucosa denuded by the manipulations associated with the brush biopsy also must be borne in mind. Gittes (1984) reported that brush biopsies are not indicated in patients with radiographically obvious lesions, in those with positive upper tract cytology findings, or in those with no visible lesion. **If endoscopic (ureteroscopic or nephroscopic) evaluation is planned, cup or brush biopsies can be performed under direct vision, and hence there would be little reason to perform them through a retrogradely placed ureteral catheter.**

Ureteroscopy and Nephroscopy

Currently, with the development of rigid and flexible ureteroscopes, ureteroscopy has been used increasingly in establishing the diagnosis of upper tract urothelial tumors. **Streem and co-workers reported that ureteropyeloscopy increased the diagnostic accuracy of the standard diagnostic regimen from 58% to 83%** (Streem et al, 1986). **Similarly, Blute and colleagues reported that the diagnosis of renal pelvic tumors was accurately made in 86% of cases and of ureteral tumors in 90% by ureteropyeloscopy** (Blute et al, 1989). **The complication rate in this series was 7%.** The major concerns about performing ureteroscopy in patients with upper tract urothelial tumors include a risk of ureteral perforation with extravasation of tumor cells, denudation of the ureteral mucosa facilitating implantation of tumor cells, and development of complete ureteral disruption or stricture formation. Additionally, Lim and colleagues reported the possible complication of pyelo-venous-lymphatic migration of transitional carcinoma cells after ureteropyeloscopy (Lim et al, 1993).

Small endoscopic biopsy forceps are available for performing biopsies through a ureteroscope. **These forceps obtain small tissue fragments that may be difficult for the pathologist to interpret. Nonetheless, the characteristic endoscopic appearance of a transitional cell carcinoma usually is sufficient to establish the correct diagnosis. Indeed, the combination of typical radiographic and endoscopic findings of transitional cell carcinoma, even in the face of negative cytology or biopsy specimens should persuade one to plan treatment approaches for upper tract transitional cell carcinoma.** Besides problems with sampling errors, it should be remembered that not all radiographically visible lesions are accessible to endoscopic inspection and that even trivial amounts of hematuria can sufficiently cloud visibility (even with the use of hypoosmotic irrigants such as sterile water) to the point where accurate inspection becomes impossible. Therefore, **there is a risk of undergrading and understaging as well as the inability to exclude small tumors at other sites. Furthermore, because of potential complications and the fact that it is an invasive procedure requiring full anesthesia, diagnostic ureteroscopy should be reserved for patients in whom the diagnosis remains in doubt after using conventional diagnostic techniques and for those in whom the treatment would be influenced by the results of ureteroscopy.**

Nephroscopy through an open pyelotomy incision or a percutaneous nephrostomy tube has been reported as a valid diagnostic technique and as a means of treating upper tract urothelial tumors (Gittes, 1984; Streem et al, 1986; Woodhouse et al, 1986; Smith et al, 1987a; Nolan et al, 1988; Orihuela and Smith, 1988; Blute et al, 1989; Tasca and Zattoni, 1990). **Tumor cell implantations in the retroperitoneum and nephrostomy tube tract, however, have been reported following these procedures** (Tomara et al, 1982; Huang et al, 1995).

STAGING

The TNM staging system proposed by the AJC-UICC (Spiessl et al, 1989) and potential limitations concerning collecting ductular and renal parenchymal spread have been described earlier.

METASTATIC EVALUATION

CT scanning is helpful in determining the local extent of the primary tumor as well as in evaluating metastases. CT scanning can demonstrate extension into the renal parenchyma or periureteral soft tissue, venous involvement, lymph node involvement, or liver metastases (Lantz and Hattery, 1984; Milestone et al, 1990; McCoy et al, 1991; Badalament et al, 1992). **Results have been disappointing, however, when CT staging is compared with pathologic staging.** For example, CT is incapable of distinguishing Ta from T2 lesions (Lantz and Hattery, 1984; Milestone et al, 1990; McCoy et al, 1991; Badalament et al, 1992). Moreover, **the accuracy of detecting fat invasion** (McCoy et al, 1991) **and periureteral extension** (Badalament et al, 1992) **is restricted to tumors with massive extension. Similarly, CT often fails to detect multifocal lesions. These limitations of CT staging must be remembered when planning conservative therapy for upper tract tumors.**

Other useful tests for metastatic evaluation include chest radiography (rather than chest CT; see discussion of bladder cancer), bone scan (see discussion of bladder cancer), and liver function tests. In patients with compromised renal function, it is advisable to obtain a creatinine clearance and at times a renal scan to determine split renal function. These results may have a bearing on whether nephron-sparing surgery or nephrectomy is performed.

TREATMENT

As with bladder cancer, upper tract tumors are virtually never found incidentally at autopsy (Resseguie et al, 1978), indicating that some symptoms or signs eventually lead to diagnosis within a brief period of time. **Hence, once diagnosed, some sort of treatment is mandatory.** Current data suggest that the following generalizations are valid concerning the treatment of upper tract urothelial tumors. **Patients with low-grade, low-stage tumors do well with either conservative or radical surgery. Patients with intermediate-grade tumors do better with radical surgery. Patients with high-grade, high-stage tumors do poorly with either conservative or radical surgery. With conservative surgery, tumor recurrence rates in the retained ipsilateral collecting system vary from 7% to 60%, depending on the tumor grade and multifocality. There is little evidence, however, that these ipsilateral recurrences directly compromise patient survival.**

These generalizations are supported by an experience in which only 1 of 15 (7%) patients with grade I tumors treated with conservative resections had a recurrence in the ipsilateral ureter. The 5-year survival was 88% for radical surgery and 75% for conservative surgery for grade I tumors. **Of patients with grade II tumors, 8 of 29 (28%) treated with conservative resection had ipsilateral recurrences. The 2-year survival was 90% for radical surgery versus 46% for conservative surgery.** No patient with a grade III or IV tumor had an ipsilateral recurrence, probably because of short survival in all patients. **Contralateral recurrences occurred in less than 2% of patients** (Murphy et al, 1980, 1981). These data provide the basis for the following general treatment guidelines. Most renal pelvis tumors should be treated with total nephroureterectomy. **Upper ureteral and midureteral tumors should be treated with segmental resections if they are solitary and low-grade lesions and with total nephroureterectomy if they are multifocal or moderately or poorly differentiated. Distal ureteral tumors should be treated by distal ureterectomy and ureteroneocystostomy assuming no evidence of multifocality. Because of the aforementioned mapping studies** (McCarron et al, 1982; Nocks et al, 1982), **however, it is not entirely certain that a patient with a distal high-grade ureteral tumor should undergo simple local excision because, if the patient was fortunate enough to survive several years, the likelihood of high-grade ipsilateral recurrences might be enormous. Similarly, tumor spill in such cases, because of the high likelihood of severe urothelial dysplasia elsewhere in the retained ureter, would be considerable. Conservative resections are especially appropriate for solitary or functionally dominant kidneys; bilateral tumors; or small polypoid, low-grade ureteral tumors.** In the rare patient with bilateral diffuse tumors (or diffuse tumors in a solitary kidney), bilateral nephrectomy with hemodialysis and possible subsequent renal transplantation may be a preferable treatment option to attempts at conservative surgery, endoscopic management, or topical therapy.

Patients with only positive cytologic findings of the upper tract and normal radiographic and endoscopic examinations should be followed closely with excretory or retrograde urography and should *not* be treated blindly.

Total Nephroureterectomy

The traditional treatment for upper tract urothelial tumors is total nephroureterectomy with excision of a cuff of bladder (Anderstrom et al, 1989). This is **based on many studies that have demonstrated a high incidence (30%–75%) of subsequent tumor recurrence in the ureteral stump or around the ipsilateral ureteral orifice in patients treated with more conservative operations** (Bloom et al, 1970; Kakizoe et al, 1980; Mullen and Kovacs, 1980). Further studies have demonstrated that conservative surgery is acceptable in selected patients (Mufti et al, 1989; Zungri et al, 1990). **Whether nephroureterectomy is performed through one or two incisions, it is important to avoid transection of the ureter simply to facilitate the operation. The potential of tumor spill for all but low-grade tumors is sufficiently great on ureteral transection during the open operation that it should be avoided. Additionally, unless patients have a recent history of bladder tumors, an anterior cystotomy should be performed to ensure removal of the entire distal and intramural ureter and vesical epithelium immediately adjacent to the orifice. Furthermore, the anterior cystotomy permits easy identification of the contralateral ureteral orifice, thus making it less likely to sustain injury.** The surgical technique of total nephroureterectomy is discussed in Chapters 97 and 98.

Johansson and Wahlqvist (1979) recommended performing an extra-Gerotal radical nephroureterectomy with adrenalectomy and retroperitoneal lymphadenectomy for upper tract transitional cell carcinomas. In their

series, the 5-year survival was 84% with radical operation and only 51% with conventional nephroureterectomy—with **the principal difference in prognosis being observed in patients with high-stage tumors in whom the radical operation produced a 74% survival compared with a 37% survival with conservative surgery.** These were not concurrently treated series, however, thus bringing into question the comparability of each group, and many patients in the study had analgesic abuse, which theoretically could have influenced the results. Similar results were reported by Zungri and associates (1990).

With the presence of lymph node involvement, only a relatively small percentage of patients are cured with nephroureterectomy and extensive lymphadenectomy (Johansson and Wahlqvist, 1979; Heney et al, 1981). Certainly the scope of the operation is considerable, necessitating removing tissue around the ipsilateral great vessel from cephalad to the renal hilum to the deep pelvis. **If data from transitional cell carcinoma of the bladder can be extrapolated to upper tract transitional cell carcinoma, however, patients with microscopic nodal involvement may be cured by surgery alone, and adjuvant chemotherapy may be particularly beneficial for this group (see section on bladder cancer). Thus, at least for healthy individuals (who are likely to tolerate well the additional scope of the surgery) with moderately or poorly differentiated tumors or high-stage tumors, extensive lymphadenectomy would seem reasonable.** Currently, however, as with bladder cancer, for those in whom the extra time or scope of lymphadenectomy might be more risky, the marginal additional benefit would not justify its performance. **Representative 5-year survival results for total nephroureterectomy reported by Batata and co-workers were for stage Tis, Ta, T1, 91%; stage T2, 43%; stage T3 or T4 or N1 or N2, 23%; and stage N3 or M1, 0%** (Batata et al, 1975).

Conservative Excision

The concept of conservative excision for upper tract urothelial tumors was first introduced by Vest (1945); however, this concept was generally ignored until the early 1970s, when favorable results of conservative surgery were reported in patients with Balkan nephropathy. Most evidence suggests that for low-grade, low-stage tumors, equivalent results are achieved with conservative excision or nephroureterectomy (Murphy et al, 1980; Zoretic and Gonzales, 1983; Anderstrom et al, 1989). Zoretic and Gonzales (1983) reported on 16 patients who underwent segmental resections for ureteral tumors. The 5-year survival rate was 71% with a ureteral recurrence rate of 6%. Mufti and co-workers reported that the survival of patients treated with conservative resection was greater than 90% (Mufti et al, 1989). When urothelium was left behind after conservative resection, however, there was a 22% recurrence rate on the same side, noted almost exclusively in patients with multifocal tumors. Bazeed and associates reported tumor recurrences in four of nine (44%) patients treated with local excision, four of whom had normal contralateral kidneys (Bazeed et al; 1986). All recurrences were reported to be successfully treated with repeat local excisions.

Other series have reported **tumor recurrence rates ranging from 25% to 40% with segmental resection or local excision** (Ghazi et al, 1979; Wallace et al, 1981; Hatch et al, 1988). **The recurrence rates following conservative resection of renal pelvis tumors are higher than those following conservative resection of ureteral tumors** (Mazeman, 1976; Zincke and Neves, 1984). For obvious anatomic reasons, renal pelvic tumors are more difficult to excise completely with conservative surgery than are ureteral tumors.

Partial nephrectomy also has been reported in patients with transitional cell carcinoma of the renal pelvis. **Ziegelbaum and colleagues (1987) reported tumor recurrence in 38% of patients treated with a variety of different conservative surgical procedures for upper tract urothelial tumors, and only 46% of patients were tumor-free at the time of their report. These investigators recommended conservative surgery only in situations in which it was necessary to avoid renal failure.**

For distal ureteral tumors, particularly for well-differentiated or moderately differentiated lesions, even if they are of higher stage, distal ureterectomy, removing a cuff of bladder with ureteral reimplantation using a psoas hitch or Boari flap if necessary, is likely to be as successful as total nephroureterectomy. Although for high-grade tumors, a strong argument for total nephroureterectomy and bladder cuff excision could be made because of the usual multifocality of the lesions, data concerning tumor recurrence and local seeding with distal ureterectomy are sparse. This is probably because many high-grade lesions are so extensive that because of ipsilateral renal dysfunction, obvious multifocality, or difficulty in obtaining negative proximal ureteral margins, suitable candidates for local excision with high-grade tumors are quite rare (Johnson and Babaian, 1979).

Endoscopic Treatment

The rationale for endoscopic treatment of upper tract urothelial tumors is the same as that for endoscopic management of superficial bladder tumors. The principal differences are related to the logistic difficulties encountered in gaining access to the upper urinary tract and in performing the manipulations necessary to ablate the tumors. Another major consideration is the relative thinness of the wall of the upper urinary collecting system, which makes it more susceptible to perforation and extravasation of tumor cells. Also, the small diameter of the upper urinary tract makes it more susceptible to obstruction by relatively minor degrees of post-treatment edema or fibrosis. Finally, in view of both the high ipsilateral recurrence rates reported for conservative open surgical excision and the technical issues that make it difficult if not impossible to be assured of the completeness of local excision, it is obvious that frequent surveillance of upper tract tumors managed endoscopically is required. Endoscopic examinations would, of course, have to be done with patients fully anesthetized, something that is unnecessary for surveillance of patients with cystoscopically resected bladder tumors.

Technical aspects of endoscopic treatment of upper tract urothelial tumors are discussed in Chapters 93 and 94. Essentially, ureteroscopic or percutaneous approaches are the primary options available.

Ureteroscopic Treatment

Because of the risk of tumor spillage and extra–urinary tract implantation, the ureteroscopic approach is generally the preferred one in endoscopic management of upper tract tumors. Huffman and colleagues initially reported their results on eight patients with localized low-grade tumors managed ureteroscopically (Huffman et al, 1985). Three of these patients had multiple recurrences, which were easily managed with endoscopic fulguration. **Their series demonstrates the necessity of rigorous follow-up, with the eight patients having undergone a total of 45 procedures over an average follow-up of 21 months.** Blute and associates noted a recurrence in 1 of 5 ureteroscopically managed renal pelvis and 2 of 13 ureteral tumors (Blute et al, 1989). Grossman and co-workers reported on eight patients managed ureteroscopically, of which two required a subsequent open procedure (Grossman et al, 1992). Of the remaining six, three experienced recurrences in the series. Most recurrences were low-grade, papillary tumors. Grossman and co-workers used the Nd:YAG laser for most of their treatments, and no strictures or serious complications were noted. **The overall major complication rate of ureteroscopic management of upper tract tumors is reported by Blute and associates (1989) at 7%,** although **Schmeller and Hofstetter (1989) claimed that ureteral strictures occurred in more than one third of patients with long-term follow-up. They suggested this high stricture incidence might be reduced with greater reliance on lasers.**

Because of the high recurrence rates and potential tumor multifocality, rigorous follow-up is needed after ureteroscopic treatment of upper tract tumors. **Several authorities have suggested that this may have to be done ureteroscopically, an approach that normally would not be feasible without repeated full anesthetics** (Huffman et al, 1985; Segura, 1992).

Percutaneous Treatment

The advantage of percutaneous treatment of renal pelvic tumors, despite the potential risks of bleeding, tumor implantation, and tumor spillage (Tomera et al, 1982; Huang et al, 1995), **is that it permits the use of larger scopes that facilitate endoscopic manipulations. Second, under special circumstances, instillations of topical therapies can be easily administered if a nephrostomy tube is left in place. Orihuela and Smith (1988) reported recurrences in 5 of 11 patients treated with percutaneous management but none for patients with solitary, low-grade superficial transitional cell carcinomas. By leaving the percutaneous nephrostomy tube in place, the authors also recommended a second-look procedure to ensure complete tumor removal and treatment of any suspicious areas with the Nd:YAG laser.** Similar results from smaller series have been reported by others (Blute et al, 1989; Tasca and Zattoni, 1990). It must be remembered, however, that each of these series contained highly selected patients, not only because patient preference, other comorbid medical conditions, and the status of the contralateral renal unit all may have mandated conservative or even endoscopic treatment, but also because the size, number, and location of tumors made them amenable to percutaneous assessment and treatment, while still permitting placement of radiologic guide wires and other instruments antegradely down the ureter and into the bladder for full endoscopic control. **As a general rule, in the presence of a normal contralateral kidney and collecting system, this approach should probably be restricted to patients with small, solitary, low-grade tumors not amenable to ureteroscopic excision, as recommended by Tasca and Zattoni (1990).**

Instillation Therapy

Limited information is available about instillation therapy for upper tract urothelial tumors. Smith and colleagues (1987b) reported on intravesical mitomycin C to treat distal ureteral tumors in patients with vesicoureteral reflux. De-Kock and Breytenbach (1986) reported on local excision and instillation of thiotepa into the upper urinary tracts with beneficial effects and no adverse side effects. Powder and colleagues also instilled thiotepa and reported their anecdotal favorable experience with this agent (Powder et al, 1984). Also, responses have been noted for topical treatment with BCG, including the treatment of carcinoma in situ (Herr 1985; Smith et al, 1987a; Studer et al, 1989; Ramsey and Soloway, 1990). BCG demonstrated efficacy in this clinical setting, but there are reports of some patients developing sepsis (Studer et al, 1989; Ramsey and Soloway, 1990). **It is obvious that currently the indications and success rate for topical therapy of upper tract tumors are not known.** Furthermore, besides sepsis, other potential complications include collecting system scarring and obstruction (particularly with BCG and mitomycin) and systemic absorption (with all agents). Although these adverse effects have not been widely reported, current series are far too small to make their absence from the literature a validation of the safety of this technique. **Perhaps the most appropriate place for this form of therapy should be in patients with multiple superficial tumors or carcinoma in situ of the upper urinary tract who also have limited renal function or bilateral disease. In general, instillations should be performed via a nephrostomy tube rather than retrogradely through a ureteral catheter, to reduce the likelihood of sepsis and to improve contact time of the topical agent with the urothelium.**

Although not an instillation agent, the oral interferon inducer bropiramine has been administered on a compassionate-use basis to patients with upper tract urothelial cancer who had contraindications to surgical, endoscopic, or instillation therapies. Results are currently anecdotal, but a number of successes have been claimed.

Radiation Therapy

In patients with upper tract urothelial tumors, radiation therapy has been largely employed as a postoperative adjuvant in those patients considered, based on pathologic inspection, to be at high risk for local recurrence. In this clinical setting, radiation therapy has been reported to be of some benefit (Brookland and Richter, 1985; Cozad et al, 1992). **In two contemporary studies** (Brookland and Richter, 1985; Cozad et al, 1992), **a total of 20 patients who underwent extirpative surgery for stage T3 disease received postoperative radiation in doses of 37 to 60 Gy. Reduced local recurrence rates and** modest **improvement in median survival were seen in the treatment groups compared with nonrandomized patients treated with surgery alone.** No statistically significant difference was noted in 5-year survival, however. Among other problems with this treatment are the potential difficulties with irradiating a large tumor bed, particularly if radiation doses approaching those considered therapeutic for transitional cell cancer (60–70 Gy) are to be achieved. Potential toxicity to neighboring structures—particularly small intestine, spinal cord, and kidney (if conservative surgery had been performed)—must be kept in mind, and in general, limited fields and reduced doses have been used. **The role of radiation therapy, then, in the treatment of upper tract urothelial tumors is still ill-defined, but there appears to be some benefit in the adjuvant setting for high-grade or invasive lesions, at least in terms of local control.** Additionally, radiation therapy also is effective for palliation of painful osseous metastases (see section on bladder cancer).

Systemic Chemotherapy

The chemotherapeutic regimens for the treatment of upper tract urothelial tumors are the same as those used for treatment of bladder cancer. Because of the rarity of these tumors, no large series have been reported. The long-term results of MVAC chemotherapy for urothelial cancer have been disappointing, with durable complete responses being reported in as few as 5% to 10% of patients; as many as 41% experienced neutropenic sepsis, and 2% to 4% suffered treatment-related mortality (Tannock et al, 1989). This has led to a search for more effective regimens (see section on bladder cancer). **Extrapolation of possible benefits of adjuvant chemotherapy from the bladder cancer experience with stage T3, T4, or N-positive upper tract urothelial tumors after surgical resection** (Skinner et al, 1991; Stockel et al, 1995) **may be appropriate, but this almost certainly will never be confirmed by prospective, randomized, controlled trials, owing to the rarity of upper tract tumors.**

Angiofarction

Angiographic infarction is rarely used in the treatment of renal pelvic tumors but may have a role in selected patients with symptomatic primary tumors who either have incurable distant metastases or, because of comorbidity, are not candidates for immediate nephrectomy (Jacobs et al, 1981). **This technique has been reported to be effective as a short-term remedy** (Jacobs et al, 1981) **despite the normally hypovascular angiographic appearance of these tumors.**

REFERENCES

Bladder Cancer

Abel PD: Follow-up of patients with superficial transitional cell carcinoma of the bladder: Case for a change in policy. Br J Urol 1993; 72:125.

Abel PD, Hall RR, Williams G: Should pT1 transitional cell cancers of the bladder still be classified as superficial? Br J Urol 1988a; 62:235.

Abel PD, Henderson D, Bennett MK, et al: Differing interpretations by pathologists of the pT category and grade of transitional cell cancer of the bladder. Br J Urol 1988b; 62:339.

Abou Farah KMM, Janknegt RA, Kester ADM, Arenz JW: Value of immunohistochemical lamenin staining in transitional cell carcinoma of the human bladder. Urol Int 1993; 50:133.

Abratt RP, Barnes DR, Potin AR, et al: Radical radiation and oral and intravesical misonidazole for bladder cancer. Int J Radiat Oncol Biol Phys 1987; 13:1053.

Aherne G: Retinoblastoma associated with other primary malignant tumors. Trans Ophthalmol Soc UK 1974; 94:938.

Ahlering TE, Kanellos A, Boyd SD, et al: A comparative study of perioperative complications with Kock pouch urinary diversion in highly irradiated versus nonirradiated patients. J Urol 1988a; 139:1202.

Ahlering TE, Weintraub P, Skinner DG: Management of adult sarcomas of the bladder and prostate. J Urol 1988b; 140:1397.

Albores-Saavedra J, Maldonado ME, Ibarra J, et al: Pheochromocytoma of the urinary bladder. Cancer 1969; 23:1110.

Allard P, Fradet Y, Tzui B, et al: Tumor associated antigens as prognostic factors for recurrence in 382 patients with primary transitional cell carcinoma of the bladder. Clin Cancer Res 1995; 1:1195.

Althausen AF, Prout GR Jr, Daly JJ: Noninvasive papillary carcinoma of the bladder associated with carcinoma in situ. J Urol 1976; 116:575.

Anderstrom C, Johansson S, Nilsson S: The significance of lamina propria invasion on the prognosis of patients with bladder tumors. J Urol 1980; 124:23.

Anderstrom C, Johansson SL, von Schultz L: Primary adenocarcinoma of the urinary bladder: A clinicopathologic and prognostic study. Cancer 1983; 52:1273.

Angulo JC, Lopez JI, Grignon DJ, Sanchez-Chapado M: Muscularis mucosa differentiates two populations with different prognosis in stage T1 bladder cancer. Urology 1995; 45:47.

Annual Cancer Statistics Review: Including Cancer Trends: 1950–1985. Bethesda, MD, National Cancer Institute, U.S. Department of Health and Human Services, NIH publication no. 88-2789, 1987.

Anwar K, Phil M, Naiki H, et al: High frequency of human papillomavirus infection in carcinoma of the urinary bladder. Cancer 1992; 70:1967.

Aprikian AG, Sarkis AS, Reuter VE, et al: Biologic markers of prognosis in transitional cell carcinoma of the bladder: Current concepts. Semin Urol 1993; 11:137.

Arce S, Lopez R, Almaguer M, et al: HLA-antigens and transitional cell carcinoma. Mater Med Pol 1978; 10:98.

Atein JP, Stenzl A, Esrig D, et al: Lower urinary tract reconstruction following cystectomy in women using the Kock ileal reservoir with bilateral ureteroileal urethrostomy: Initial clinical experience. J Urol 1994; 152:1404.

Atkin NB, Fox MF: 5q deletion: The sole chromosome change in a carcinoma of the bladder. Cancer Genet Cytogenet 1990; 46:129.

Augustine A, Hebert JR, Kabat GC, et al: Bladder cancer in relation to cigarette smoking. Cancer Res 1988; 48:4405.

Babaian RJ, Johnson DE, Llamas L, et al: Metastases from transitional cell carcinoma of the urinary bladder. Urology 1980; 16:142.

Babu VR, Miles BJ, Cerney JC, et al: Chromosome 21q22 deletion: A specific chromosome change in a new bladder cancer subgroup. Cancer Genet Cytogenet 1989; 38:127.

Badalament RA, Herr HW, Wong GY, et al: A prospective randomized trial of maintenance versus nonmaintenance intravesical bacillus Calmette-Guerin therapy of superficial bladder cancer. J Clin Oncol 1987; 5:441.

Badalament RA, O'Toole RV, Keyhani-Rofagha S, et al: Flow cytometric analysis of primary and metastatic bladder cancer. J Urol 1990; 143:912.

Barentsz JO, Lemmens JA, Ruijs SH, et al: Carcinoma of the urinary bladder: MR imaging with a double surface coil. AJR 1988; 151:107.

Barnes RW, Bergman RT, Hadley HT, et al: Control of bladder tumors by endoscopic surgery. J Urol 1967; 97:864.

Beer M, Jocham D, Beer A, et al: Adjuvant laser treatment of bladder cancer: 8 years experience with the Nd-YAG laser 1064 nm. Br J Urol 1989; 63:476.

Beisland HO, Sander S: Neodymium-YAG laser irradiation of stage T2 muscle-invasive bladder cancer: Long-term results. Br J Urol 1990; 65:24.

Bejany EC, Lockhart JL, Rhamy RK: Malignant vesical tumors following spinal cord injury. J Urol 1987; 138:1390.

Bell D, Taylor JA, Paulson DF, et al: Genetic risk and carcinogen exposure: A common inherited defect on the carcinogen-metabolism gene glutathione S-transferase M1(GST M1) that increases susceptibility to bladder cancer. J Natl Cancer Inst 1993; 85:1159.

Bellmunt J, Albanell J, Gallego OS, et al: Carboplatin, methotrexate, and vinblastine in patients with bladder cancer who are ineligible for cisplatin-based chemotherapy. Cancer 1992; 70:1974.

Bennett JK, Wheatley JK, Walton KN: 10-year experience with adenocarcinoma of the bladder. J Urol 1984; 131:262.

Bennett JK, Wheatley JK, Walton KN: Nonmetastatic bladder cancer associated with hypercalcemia, thrombocytosis and leukemoid reaction. J Urol 1986; 135:47.

Benson RC Jr: Endoscopic management of bladder cancer with hematoporphyrin derivative phototherapy. Urol Clin North Am 1984; 11:637.

Benson RC Jr, Farrow GM, Kinsey JH, et al: Detection and localization of in situ carcinoma of the bladder with hematoporphyrin derivative. Mayo Clin Proc 1982; 57:548.

Benson RC Jr, Kinsey JH, Cortese DA, et al: Treatment of transitional cell carcinoma of the bladder with hematoporphyrin derivative phototherapy. J Urol 1983a; 130:1090.

Benson RC Jr, Swanson SK, Farrow GM: Relationship of leukoplakia to urothelial malignancy. J Urol 1984; 131:507.

Benson RC Jr, Tomera KM, Kelalis PP: Transitional cell carcinomas of the bladder in children and adolescents. J Urol 1983b; 130:54.

Berger GL, Sadlowsky RW, Sharp JR, et al: Lack of value of routine postoperative bone and liver scans in cystectomy candidates. J Urol 1981; 125:637.

Bergkvist A, Ljungqvist A, Moberger G: Classification of bladder tumours based on the cellular pattern: Preliminary report of a clinical-pathological study of 300 cases with a minimum follow-up of eight years. Acta Chir Scand 1965; 130:371.

Bettex-Galland M, Studer UE, Walls A, et al: Neutrophil activating peptide 1/interleukin 8 detection in human urine during acute bladder inflammation caused by transurethral resection of superficial cancer and bacillus Calmette Guerin. Eur Urol 1991; 19:171.

Binkovitz LA, Hattery RR, LeRoy AJ: Primary lymphoma of the bladder. Urol Radiol 1988; 9:231.

Blackard CE, Byar DP: Results of a clinical trial of surgery and radiation in stages II and III carcinoma of the bladder. J Urol 1972; 108:875.

Blandy JP, England HR, Evans SJW, et al: T3 bladder cancer: The case for salvage cystectomy. Br J Urol 1980; 52:506.

Block NL, Whitmore WF Jr: Leukemoid reaction, thrombocytosis, and hypercalcemia associated with bladder cancer. J Urol 1973; 110:660.

Blomjous CEM, Schipper NW, Vos W, et al: Comparison of quantitative and classic prognosticators in urinary bladder carcinoma: A multivariate analysis of DNA flow cytometric, nuclear morphometric and clinicopathologic features. Virch Arch [A] 1989; 415:421.

Bloom HJG, Hendry WF, Wallace DM, et al: Treatment of T3 bladder cancer: Controlled trial of preoperative radiotherapy and radical cystectomy versus radical radiotherapy. Br J Urol 1982; 54:136.

Blute ML, Engen DE, Travis WD, et al: Primary signet ring cell adenocarcinoma of the bladder. J Urol 1989; 141:17.

Bochner BH, Nichols PW, Skinner DG: Overstaging of transitional cell carcinoma: Clinical significance of lamina propria fat within the urinary bladder. Urology 1995; 45:528.

Bohle A, Schuller J, Knipper A, et al: Bacillus Calmette-Guerin treatment and vesicorenal reflux. Eur Urol 1990; 17:125.

Bonner RB, Hemstreet GP 3d, Fradet Y, et al: Bladder cancer risk assessment with quantitative fluorescence image analysis of tumor markers in exfoliated bladder cells. Cancer 1993; 72:2461.

Boring CC, Squires TS, Tong T: Cancer statistics, 1993. Cancer J Clin 1993; 43:7.

Boring CC, Squires TS, Tong T, et al: Cancer statistics—1995. Cancer J Clin 1995; 45:2.

Bouffioux CH, Denis L, Oosterlinck W, et al: Adjuvant chemotherapy of recurrent superficial transitional cell carcinoma: Results of a European Organization for Research on Treatment of Cancer randomized trial comparing intravesical instillation of thiotepa, doxorubicin and cisplatin. J Urol 1992; 148:297.

Boutwell RK: Some biological aspects of skin carcinogenesis. Prog Exp Tumor Res 1964; 4:207.

Boyd SD, Feinberg SM, Skinner DG, et al: Quality of life survey of urinary diversion patients: Comparison of ileal conduits versus continent Kock ileal reservoirs. J Urol 1987; 138:1386.

Boyd SD, Schiff WM: Inflatable penile prostheses in patients undergoing cystoprostatectomy with urethrectomy. J Urol 1989; 141:60.

Bracken RB, McDonald MW, Johnson DE: Cystectomy for superficial bladder cancer. Urology 1981a; 28:459.

Bracken RB, McDonald M, Johnson DE: Complications of single-stage radical cystectomy and ileal conduit. Urology 1981b; 17:141.

Brannan W, Oschrer MG, Fuselier HA, et al: Partial cystectomy in the treatment of transitional cell carcinoma of the bladder. J Urol 1978; 119:213.

Brecroft L, Wu H, Lozano G, et al: Transcriptional activation by wild-type but not transforming mutants of the p53 anti-oncogene. Science 1990; 249:1049.

Brendler CB, Schlegel PN, Walsh PC: Urethrectomy with preservation of potency. J Urol 1990a; 144:270.

Brendler CB, Steinberg GD, Marshall FF, et al: Local recurrence and survival following nerve-sparing radical cystoprostatectomy. J Urol 1990b; 144:1137.

Bretton PR, Herr HW, Kimmel M, et al: The response of patients with superficial bladder cancer to a second course of intravesical bacillus Calmette-Guerin. J Urol 1990; 143:710.

Bretton PR, Herr HW, Whitmore WF Jr, et al: Intravesical bacillus Calmette-Guerin therapy for in situ transitional cell carcinoma involving the prostatic urethra. J Urol 1989; 141:853.

Brick SH, Friedman AC, Pollack HM, et al: Urachal carcinoma: CT findings. Radiology 1988; 169:377.

Bricker EM: Bladder substitution after pelvic evisceration. Surg Clin North Am 1950; 30:1511.

Bringuier PP, Umbas R, Schaafsma HE, et al: Decreased E-cadherin immunoreactivity correlates with poor survival in patients with bladder tumors. Cancer Res 1993; 53:3241.

Brismar J, Gustafson T: Bone scintigraphy in staging of bladder carcinoma. Acta Radiol 1988; 29:251.

Britton JP, Dowell AC, Whelan P: Dipstick hematuria and bladder cancer in men over 60: Results of a community study. BMJ 1989; 299:1010.

Britton JP, Dowell AC, Whelan P, Harris CM: A community study of bladder cancer screening by the detection of occult urinary bleeding. J Urol 1992; 148:788.

Broders AC: Epithelioma of the genitourinary organs. Ann Surg 1922; 75:574.

Broecher BH, Klein FA, Hackler RH: Cancer of the bladder in spinal cord injury patients. J Urol 1981; 125:196.

Brosman SA: Experience with bacillus Calmette-Guerin in patients with superficial bladder carcinoma. J Urol 1982; 128:27.

Brosman SA: BCG in the management of superficial bladder cancer. Urology 1984; 23(suppl):82.

Brown LF, Berse B, Jackman RW, et al: Increased expression of vascular permeability factor (vascular endothelial growth factor) and its receptors in kidney and bladder carcinomas. Am J Pathol 1993; 143:1255.

Brown RB: Experiences with intravesical formalin administration in advanced carcinoma of the bladder. Br J Urol 1970; 42:738.

Brown RR, Price JM, Friedell GH, et al: Tryptophan metabolism in patients with bladder cancer: Geographic differences. J Natl Cancer Inst 1969; 43:295.

Bruskewitz RC: Veteran's Administration randomized benign prostatic hypertrophy study. J Urol 1992; 147(part 2):107A.

Bryan GT: Chemical carcinogenesis in human subjects. In Kahn SD, Love RR, Sherman C Jr, Chakravorty R, eds: Concepts in Cancer Medicine. New York, Grune & Stratton, 1983, pp 45–66.

Bryan GT, Brown RR, Price JM: Mouse bladder carcinogenicity of certain tryptophan metabolites and other nitrogen compounds suspended in cholesterol. Cancer Res 1964; 24:596.

Burch JD, Rohan TE, Howe GR, et al: Risk of bladder cancer by source and type of tobacco exposure: A case-control study. Int J Cancer 1989; 44:622.

Buy JN, Moss AA, Guinet C, et al: MR staging of bladder carcinoma: Correlation with pathologic findings. Radiology 1988; 169:695.

Byar D, Blackard C: Comparisons of placebo, pyridoxine, and topical thiotepa in preventing recurrence of stage I bladder cancer. Urology 1977; 10:556.

Bydder PV, Burry AF, Gowland S, et al: A controlled trial of misonidazole in the curative treatment of infiltrating bladder cancer. Australas Radiol 1989; 33:8.

Cairns P, Tokino K, Eby Y, Sidransky D: Homozygous deletions of 9p21 in primary human bladder tumors detected by comparative multiplex polymerase chain reaction. Cancer Res 1994; 54:1422.

Cancer in Wisconsin—1988. Madison, Wisconsin Dept. Health and Social Services, Division of Health, Center for Health Statistics, 1989.

Cancer in Wisconsin—1992. Madison, Wisconsin Dept. Health and Social Services, Division of Health, Center for Health Statistics, 1994.

Carmignani G, Belgrano E, Puppo P, et al: Transcatheter embolization of the hypogastric arteries in cases of bladder hemorrhage from advanced pelvic cancers: Follow-up in 9 cases. J Urol 1980; 124:196.

Carter HB, Amberson JB, Bander NH, et al: Newer diagnostic techniques for bladder cancer. Urol Clin North Am 1987; 14:763.

Cartwright RA: Bladder cancer screening in the United Kingdom. J Occup Med 1990; 32:878.

Cartwright RA, Glashau RW, Rogers HJ, et al: Role of N-acetyltransferase phenotypes in bladder carcinogenesis: A pharmacogenetic epidemiologic approach to bladder cancer. Lancet 1982; 2:842.

Case RAM, Hosker ME, McDonald DB, et al: Tumors of the urinary bladder in workmen engaged in the manufacture and use of certain dyestuff intermediates in the British chemical industry. Br J Ind Med 1954; 11:75.

Catalona WJ: Bladder carcinoma. J Urol 1980; 123:35.

Catalona WJ, Hudson MA, Gillen DP, et al: Risks and benefits of repeated courses of intravesical bacillus Calmette-Guerin therapy for superficial bladder cancer. J Urol 1987; 137:220.

Catalona WJ, Ratliff TL: Bacillus Calmette-Guerin and superficial bladder cancer: Clinical experience and mechanism of action. Surg Ann 1990; 22:363.

Chapman JW, Connolly JG, Rosenbaum L: Occupational bladder cancer: A case-control study. In Connolly JG, ed: Carcinoma of the Bladder. New York, Raven Press, 1981, p 45.

Chauvet B, Brewer Y, Felix-Faure C, et al: Combined radiation therapy and cisplatin for locally advanced carcinoma of the urinary bladder. Cancer 1993; 72:2213.

Cheon J, Kim HK, Yoon DK, Koh SK: Malignant inverted papilloma of the bladder: The histopathological aspect of malignant potential of the inverted papilloma. J Korean Med Sci 1995; 10:103.

Chetsanga C, Malmstrom PU, Gyllenstein U, et al: Low incidence of human papillomavirus type 16 DNA in bladder tumor detected by the polymerase chain reaction. Cancer 1992; 69:1208.

Chodak GW, Hospelhorn V, Judge SM, et al: Increased levels of fibroblast growth factor–like activity in urine from patients with bladder or kidney cancer. Cancer Res 1988; 48:2083.

Choi H, Lamb S, Pintar K, et al: Primary signet-ring cell carcinoma of the urinary bladder. Cancer 1984; 53:1985.

Chopin DK, Caruelle J-P, Columbel M, et al: Increased immunodetection of acidic fibroblast growth factor in bladder cancer, detectable murine. J Urol 1993; 150:1126.

Ciccone G, Vineis P: Coffee drinking and bladder cancer. Cancer Lett 1988; 41:45.

Clark SS, Marlett MM, Prudencio RF, et al: Neurofibromatosis of the bladder in children: Case report and literature review. J Urol 1977; 118:654.

Clavel J, Cordier S, Bocon-Gibod L, et al: Tobacco and bladder cancer in males: Increased risk for inhalers and smokers of black tobacco. Int J Cancer 1989; 44:605.

Cohen MB, Waldman FM, Carroll PR, et al: Comparison of five histopathologic methods to assess cellular proliferation in transitional cell carcinoma of the urinary bladder. Hum Pathol 1993; 24:772.

Cohen SM, Ellwein LB: Cell proliferation and bladder tumor promotion. In: Progress in Clinical and Biological Research, Vol. 369: Chemically Induced Cell Proliferation. New York, Wiley-Liss, 1991a, pp 347–355.

Cohen SM, Ellwein LB: Genetic errors, cell proliferation, and carcinogenesis. Cancer Res 1991b; 51:6493.

Cohen SM, Ellwein LB, Okamura T, et al: Comparative bladder tumor promoting activity of sodium saccharin, sodium ascorbate, related acids, and calcium salts in rats. Cancer Res 1991c; 51:1766.

Cohen SM, Garland EM, St. John M, et al: Acrolein initiates rat urinary bladder carcinogenesis. Cancer Res 1992; 52:3577.

Cohen SM, Johansson SL: Epidemiology and etiology of bladder cancer. Urol Clin North Am 1992; 3:421.

Cole DJ, Durrant DR, Roberts JT, et al: A pilot study of accelerated fractionation in the radiotherapy of invasive carcinoma of the bladder. Br J Radiol 1992; 65:792.

Cole P, Hoover R, Friedell GH: Occupation and cancer of the lower urinary tract. Cancer 1972; 29:1250.

Coloby PJ, Kakizoe T, Tobisu K-I, Sakamoto M-I: Urethral involvement in female bladder cancer patients: Mapping of 47 consecutive cystourethrectomy specimens. J Urol 1994; 152:1437.

Connor JP, Olsson CA, Benson MC, et al: Long-term follow-up in patients treated with methotrexate, vinblastine, doxorubicin, and cisplatin (M-VAC) for transitional cell carcinoma of urinary bladder: Cause for concern. Urology 1989; 34:353.

Cookson MS, Sarosdy MF: Management of stage T_1 superficial bladder cancer with intravesical bacillus Calmette-Guerin therapy. J Urol 1992; 148:797.

Coombs LM, Pigott DA, Eydman DA, et al: Reduced expression of TGFβ is associated with advanced disease in transitional cell carcinoma. Br J Cancer 1993; 67(3):578–584.

Coon JS, Weinstein RS, Summers JL: Blood group precursor T-antigen expression in human urinary bladder carcinoma. Am J Clin Pathol 1982; 77:692.

Cooper CS, See WA, Crist SA: Urine from iatrogenically traumatized bladders promotes transitional carcinoma cell growth in a manner consistent with a growth factor dependent mechanism. J Urol 1992; 147:262A.

Coplen DE, Marcus MD, Myers JA, et al: Long-term follow-up of patients treated with 1 or 2, 6-week courses of intravesical bacillus Calmette-Guerin: Analysis of possible predictors of response free tumor. J Urol 1990; 144:652.

Coppin C, Gospodarowicz M, Dixon P, et al: Improved local control of invasive bladder cancer by concurrent cisplatin and preoperative or radical radiation. Proc Am Soc Clin Oncol 1992; 11:198A.

Cordon-Cardo C: Mutation of cell cycle regulators—biological and clinical implications for human neoplasia. Am J Pathol 1995; 147:545–560.

Cordon-Cardo C, Reuter VE, Lloyd KO, et al: Blood group-related antigens in human urothelium: Enhanced expression of Le^x and Le^y determinants in urothelial carcinoma. Cancer Res 1988; 48:4113.

Cordon-Cardo C, Wartinger D, Petrylak D, et al: Altered expression of the retinoblastoma gene product: Prognostic indicator in bladder cancer. J Natl Cancer Inst 1992; 84:1251.

Cordon-Cardo C, Wartinger DD, Melamed MR, et al: Immunopathologic analysis of human bladder cancer—characterization of two new antigens associated with low grade superficial bladder tumors. Am J Pathol 1992; 140:375.

Costello AJ, Tiptaft RC, England HR, et al: Squamous cell carcinoma of the bladder. Urology 1984; 23:234.

Crawford ED, Das S, Smith JA: Preoperative radiation therapy in the treatment of bladder cancer. Urol Clin North Am 1987; 14:781.

Crawford ED, Skinner DG: Salvage cystectomy after irradiation failure. J Urol 1980; 123:32.

Cummings JA, Hargreave TB, Webb JM, et al: Intravesical Evans bacille Calmette-Guerin in the treatment of carcinoma in situ. Br J Urol 1989; 63:259.

Cummings KB, Mason JT, Correa RJ, et al: Segmental resection in the management of bladder carcinoma. J Urol 1978; 119:56.

Cutler SH, Young JL Jr, eds: Third National Cancer Survey: Incidence Data. J NCI Mongr 41, 1975.

Dalbagni G, Presti J, Reuter V, et al: Genetic alterations in bladder cancer. Lancet 1993; 342:469.

Dalesio O, Schulman CC, Sylvester R, et al: Prognostic factors in superficial bladder tumors: A study of the European Organization for Research on the Treatment of Cancer. Genitourinary Tract Cancer Cooperative Group. J Urol 1983; 129:730.

Davis MP, Murthy MSN, Simon J, et al: Successful management of small cell carcinoma of the bladder with cisplatin and etoposide. J Urol 1989; 142:817.

DeBoeur EC, DeJong WH, Sternberg PA, et al: Induction of interleukin 1 (Il-1), Il2, Il6 and tumor necrosis factor during intravesical immunotherapy with Bacillus Calmette Guerin in superficial bladder cancer. Cancer Immunol Immunother 1992; 34:306.

DeJager R, Guinan P, Lamm DL, et al: Long-term complete remission in bladder carcinoma in situ with intravesical Tice Bacillus Calmette Guerin—overview analysis of six phase II clinical trials. Urology 1991; 38:507.

DeKernion JB, Huang M, Lindner A, et al: The management of superficial bladder tumors and carcinoma in situ with intravesical bacille Calmette-Guerin (BCG). J Urol 1985; 133:598.

DeKlerk DP, Catalona WJ, Nime FA, et al: Malignant pheochromocytoma of the bladder: The late development of renal cell carcinoma. J Urol 1975; 113:864.

DeKock MLS, Anderson CK, Clark PB: Vesical leukoplakia progressing to squamous cell carcinoma in women. Br J Urol 1981; 53:316.

DelSenno L, Maestri I, Piva R, et al: Differential hypomethylation of c-myc protooncogene in bladder cancers at different stages and grades. J Urol 1989; 142:146.

DeMeester LJ, Farrow GM, Utz DC: Inverted papillomas of the urinary bladder. Cancer 1975; 36:505.

Denovic M, Bovier R, Sarkissian J, et al: Intravesical instillation of mitomycin C in the prophylactic treatment of recurring superficial transitional cell carcinoma of the bladder. Br J Urol 1983; 55:382.

Denovic M, Darzynkiewicz A, Kostryrka-Claps ML, et al: Flow cytometry of low stage bladder tumors. Cancer 1982; 48:109.

Deresiewicz RL, Stone RM, Aster JC: Fatal disseminated mycobacterial infection following intravesical bacillus Calmette-Guerin. J Urol 1990; 144:1331.

DeTorres Mateos JA, Banus Gassol JM, Palou-Redorta J, et al: Vesicorenal reflux and upper urinary tract transitional cell carcinoma after transurethral resection of recurrent superficial bladder carcinoma. J Urol 1987; 138:49.

Ding-Wei Y, Jia-Fu Z, Yong-Jiang M: Correlation between the expression of oncogenes ras and c-erb B-2 and the biological behavior of bladder tumors. Urol Res 1993; 21:39.

Dow JA, di Sant' Agnese PA, Cockett ATK: Expression of blood group precursor T antigen as a prognostic marker for human bladder cancer treated by bacillus Calmette-Guerin and interleukin-2. J Urol 1989; 142:978.

Drago PC, Badalament RA, Lucas J, Drago JR: Bladder wall calcification after intravesical mitomycin C treatment of superficial bladder cancer. J Urol 1989; 142:171.

Dreicer R, Kollomergen TA, Smith RF, et al: Neoadjuvant cisplatin, methotrexate, and vinblastine for muscle invasive bladder cancer: Long-term follow-up. J Urol 1993; 150:849.

Dreicer R, Messing EM, Loehrer PJ, Trump DL: Perioperative methotrexate, vinblastine, doxorubicin and cisplatin (M-VAC) for poor risk transitional cell carcinoma of the bladder: An Eastern Cooperative Oncology Group pilot study. J Urol 1990; 144:1123.

Duncan RE, Bennett DW, Evans AT, et al: Radiation-induced bladder tumors. J Urol 1977; 118:43.

Durkee C, Benson R Jr: Bladder cancer following administration of cyclophosphamide. Urology 1980; 16:145.

Dyson N, Howley PM, Munger K, Harlow E: The human papillomavirus 16 E7 oncoprotein is able to bind the retinoblastoma gene product. Science (Washington) 1989; 243:934.

Edwards PD, Hurm RA, Jaeschke WH: Conversion of cystitis glandularis to adenocarcinoma. J Urol 1972; 108:56.

Einhorn LH, Roth BJ, Ansari R, et al: Phase II trial of vinblastine, ifosfamide and gallium combination chemotherapy in metastatic urothelial carcinoma. J Clin Oncol 1994; 12:2271.

El-Bolkainy MN, Mokhtar NM, Ghoneim MA, et al: The impact of schistosomiasis on the pathology of bladder carcinoma. Cancer 1981; 48:2643.

Engel P, Amagnostaki L, Braendstrup O: The muscularis mucosae of the human urinary bladder—implications for tumor staging on biopsies. Scand J Urol Nephrol 1992; 26:249.

England HR, Molland EA, Oliver RTD, et al: Systemic cyclophosphamide in flat carcinoma in situ of the bladder. In Oliver RTD, Hendry WF, Bloom HJG, eds: Bladder Cancer: Principles of Combination Therapy. London, Butterworths, 1981a, p 97.

England HR, Paris AMJ, Blandy JP: The correlation of T1 bladder tumor history with prognosis and follow-up requirements. Br J Urol 1981b; 53:593.

Esrig D, Elmajian D, Groshen S, et al: Accumulation of nuclear p53 and tumor progression in bladder cancer. N Engl J Med 1994; 331:1259.

Esrig E, Spruck CH, Nichols PW, et al: p53 nucleoprotein expression correlates with mutations in the p53 gene, tumor grade, and stage in bladder cancer. J Pathol 1993; 143:1390.

Ethan L, Stuart D, Dangoux C, et al: Intraarterial cisplatin and concurrent radiation for locally advanced bladder cancer. J Clin Oncol 1989; 7:230.

Fall M, Pettersson S: Ureteral complications after intravesical formalin instillation. J Urol 1979; 122:160.

Falor WH, Ward-Skinner RM: The importance of marker chromosomes in superficial transitional cell carcinoma of the bladder: 50 patients followed up to 17 years. J Urol 1988; 139:929.

Farrow GM, Utz DC, Rife CC: Morphological and clinical observations of patients with early bladder cancer treated with total cystectomy. Cancer Res 1976; 36:2495.

Faysal MH, Freiha FS: Evaluation of partial cystectomy for carcinoma of the bladder. Urology 1979; 14:352.

Faysal MH, Freiha FS: Primary neoplasm in vesical diverticula. Br J Urol 1981; 53:141.

Feldman AR, Kessler L, Myers MH, Naughton MD: The prevalence of cancer: Estimates based on the Connecticut Tumor Registry. N Engl J Med 1986; 315:1394.

Ferraris V: Doxorubicin plus mitomycin C regimen in the prophylactic treatment of superficial bladder tumors. Cancer 1988; 62:1055.

Fields S, Jang SK: Presence of a potent transcription activating sequence in the p53 protein. Science 1990; 249:1046.

Filmer RB, Spencer JR: Malignancies in bladder augmentations and intestinal conduits. J Urol 1990; 143:671.

Finlay CA, Heinz PW, Levine AJ, et al: The p53 protooncogene can act as a suppressor of transformation. Cell 1989; 57:1083.

Finlay CA, Heinz PW, Tan TH, et al: Activating mutations for transformation by p53 producer gene products that forms an HSC-70-p53 complex with an altered half-life. Mol Cell Biol 1988; 8:531.

Fitzpatrick JM, West AB, Butler MR, et al: Superficial bladder tumors (stage pTa, grades 1 and 2): The importance of recurrence pattern following initial resection. J Urol 1986; 135:920.

Flamm J, Dona S: The significance of bladder quadrant biopsies in patients with primary superficial bladder cancer. Eur Urol 1989; 16:81.

Flechner SM, Spaulding JT: Management of rectal injury during cystectomy. Urology 1982; 19:143.

Fleishman JD, Toosi Z, Ellner JJ, et al: Urinary interleukins in patients receiving intravesical Bacillus Calmette Guerin therapy for superficial bladder cancer. Cancer 1989; 64:1447.

Forastiere, AA: Use of paclitaxel (Taxol) in squamous cell carcinoma of the head and neck. Semin Oncol 1993; 20:55.

Fossa SD, Heilo A, Bormer O: Unexpectedly high serum methotrexate levels in cystectomized bladder cancer patients with an ileal conduit treated with intermediate doses of the drug. J Urol 1990; 143:498.

Fossa SD, Woehere H, Aass N, et al: Definitive radiation therapy of muscle invasive bladder cancer: A retrospective analysis. Cancer 1993; 72:3036.

Foydart JM, Bere EW, Year M, et al: Distribution in immunoelectron microscopic localization of laminin: A non-collagenous basement membrane glycoprotein. Lab Invest 1980; 42:336.

Fradet Y, Cordon-Cardo C: Critical appraisal of tumor markers in bladder cancer. Semin Urol 1993; 11:145.

Fradet Y, Tardif M, Bourget L, et al: Clinical cancer progression in urinary bladder tumors evaluated by multiparameter flow cytometry with monoclonal antibodies. Cancer Res 1990; 50:432.

Fraley EE, Lange PH, Hakala TR: Recent studies on the immunobiology and biology of human urothelial tumors. Urol Clin North Am 1976; 3:31.

Franks LM: Latent carcinoma of the prostate. J Pathol Bacteriol 1954; 68:603.

Fraumeni JF Jr, Thomas LB: Malignant bladder tumors in a man and his three sons. JAMA 1967; 201:507.

Fredrickson SM, Messing EM, Reznikoff CA, Swaminathan S: Relationships between *in vivo* acetylator phenotypes and cytosolic *N*-acetyltransferase and O-acetyltransferase activities in human uroepithelial cells. Cancer Epidemiol Biomark Prev 1994; 3:25.

Freeman JA, Esrig DE, Stein JP, et al: Radical cystectomy for high risk patients with superficial bladder cancer in the era of orthotopic urinary reconstruction. Cancer 1995a; 76:833.

Freeman MR, Schenck FX, Soker S, et al: Human urothelial cells secrete and are regulated by heparin-binding epidermal growth factor-like growth factor (HB-EGF). J Urol 1995b; 153:307A.

Freiha FS: Treatment options for patients with invasive bladder cancer with special reference to bladder substitution with the Stanford pouch. Monogr Urol 1990; 11:34.

Friedell GH, Bell JR, Burney SW, et al: Histopathology and classification of urinary bladder carcinoma. Urol Clin North Am 1976; 3:53.

Friedell GH, Parija GC, Nagy GK, et al: The pathology of human bladder cancer. Cancer 1980; 45:1823.

Friedell GH, Soloway MS, Hilgar AG, et al: Summary of workshop on carcinoma in situ of the bladder. J Urol 1986; 136:1047.

Fujimoto K, Yamada Y, Okajima E, et al: Frequent association of p53 gene mutation in invasive bladder cancer. Cancer Res 1992; 52:1393.

Fukui I, Sekine H, Kihara K, et al: Intravesical combination chemotherapy with mitomycin C and doxorubicin for carcinoma in situ of the bladder. J Urol 1989; 141:531.

Fukushima S, Imaida K, Shibata M, et al: L-ascorbic acid amplification of second-stage bladder carcinogenesis promotion by NaHCO₃. Cancer Res 1988a; 48:6317.

Fukushima S, Shibata M, Shirai T, et al: Roles of urinary sodium ion

concentration and pH in promotion by ascorbic acid of urinary bladder carcinogenesis in rats. Cancer Res 1986; 46:1623.

Fukushima S, Tamano S, Shibata M-A, et al: The role of urinary pH and sodium concentration in the promotion stage of two-stage carcinogenesis of the rat urinary bladder. Carcinogenesis 1988b; 9:1203.

Fukushima S, Uwagawa S, Shirai T, et al: Synergism by sodium L-ascorbic acid for sodium saccharin promotion of rat two-stage bladder carcinogenesis. Cancer Res 1990; 50:4195.

Furihata M, Inoue K, Ohtsuki Y, et al: High risk human papillomavirus infections in overexpression of p53 protein as prognostic indicators in transitional cell carcinoma of the urinary bladder. Cancer Res 1993; 53:4823.

Fuse H, Mizuno I, Sakamoto M, Karayama T: Epidermal growth factor in the urine from the patients with urothelial tumors. Urol Int 1992; 48:261.

Gabrilove JL, Jakubowski A, Scher H, et al: Effect of granulocyte colony-stimulating factor on neutropenia and associated morbidity due to chemotherapy for transitional cell carcinoma of the urothelium. N Engl J Med 1988; 318:1414.

Galletti TP, Pontes JE, Montie J, et al: Neoadjuvant intraarterial chemotherapy in the treatment of advanced transitional cell carcinoma of the bladder: Results and findings. J Urol 1989; 142:1212.

Gamarra MC, Zein T: Cytologic spectrum of bladder cancer. Urology 1984; 23:23.

Gardner RA, Walsh MD, Allen V, et al: Immunohistological expression of p53 in primary pT1 transitional cell bladder cancer in relation to tumor progression. Br J Urol 1994; 73:526.

Garnick MB, Schade D, Israel M, et al: Intravesical doxorubicin for prophylaxis in the management of recurrent superficial bladder carcinoma. J Urol 1984; 131:43.

Ghoneim MA, Awad HK: Results of treatment in carcinoma of the bilharzial bladder. J Urol 1980; 123:850.

Ghoneim MA, Kock NG, Lycke G, et al: An appliance-free, sphincter-controlled bladder substitute: The urethral Kock pouch. J Urol 1987; 138:1150.

Gibas Z, Sandberg AA: Chromosomal rearrangements in bladder cancer. Urology 1984; 23:3.

Gilbert HA, Logan JL, Lagan AR, et al: The natural history of papillary transitional cell carcinoma of the bladder and its treatment in an unselected population on the basis of histologic grading. J Urol 1978; 119:486.

Glashan RW: A randomized controlled study of intravesical α-2b-interferon in carcinoma in situ of the bladder. J Urol 1990; 144:658.

Glazer DB, Bahnson RR, McLeod DG, et al: Intravesical recombinant tumor necrosis factor in the treatment of superficial bladder cancer: An Eastern Cooperative Oncology Group Study. J Urol 1995; 154:66.

Goffinet DR, Schneider MJ, Glatstein EJ, et al: Bladder cancer: Results of radiation therapy in 384 patients. Radiology 1975; 117:149.

Goldberg MR, Heimbrook DC, Russo P, et al: Phase I clinical study of the recombinant oncotoxin TP40 in superficial bladder cancer. Clin Cancer Res 1995; 1:57.

Golijanin D, Sherman Y, Shapiro A, Pode D: Detection of bladder tumors by immunostaining of the Lewisˣ antigen in cells from voided urine. Urology 1995; 46:173.

Goodman GB, Hislop TG, Elwood JM, et al: Conservation of bladder function in patients with invasive bladder cancer treated by definitive irradiation and selective cystectomy. Int J Radiat Oncol Biol Phys 1981; 7:569.

Goodwin WE, Harris AP, Kaufman JJ, et al: Open, transcolonic ureterointestinal anastomosis: A new approach. Surg Gynecol Obstet 1953; 97:295.

Gordon NS, Sinclair RA, Snow RM: Pelvic lipomatosis with cystitis cystica, cystitis glandularis and adenocarcinoma of the bladder. First reported case. Aust N Z J Surg 1990; 60:229.

Gospodarowicz MK, Hawkins NV, Rawlings GA, et al: Radical radiotherapy for muscle invasive transitional cell carcinoma of the bladder: Failure analysis. J Urol 1989; 142:1448.

Green LF, Yalowitz PA: The advisability of concomitant transurethral excision of vesical neoplasm and prostatic hyperplasia. J Urol 1972; 107:445.

Greenland JE, Weston PMT, Wallace DMA: Familial transitional cell carcinoma and the Lynch syndrome II. Br J Urol 1993; 72:177.

Greven KM, Solin LJ, Hanks GE: Prognostic factors in patients with bladder carcinoma treated with definitive irradiation. Cancer 1990; 65:908.

Grossman HB, Konnak JW: Is radical cystectomy indicated in patients with regional lymphatic metastases? Urology 1988; 31:214.

Grossman HB, Sandler HM, Perez-Tamayo C: Treatment of T3a bladder cancer with irradium implant. Urology 1993; 41:217.

Grossman, HB, Washington RW, Carey TE, Liebert M: Alterations in antigen expression in superficial bladder cancer. J Cell Biochem 1992; 161(suppl):63.

Gruis NA, Weaver-Feldhaus J, Liu Q, et al: Genetic evidence in melanoma and bladder cancers that p16 and p53 function in separate pathways of tumor suppression. Am J Pathol 1995; 146:1199.

Guinan P, Vogelzang NJ, Randozzo R, et al: Renal pelvic cancer: A review of 611 patients treated in Illinois 1975–1985. Urology 1993; 40:393.

Guirguis R, Schiffmann E, Lui B, et al: Detection of autocrine motility factor in urine as a marker of bladder cancer. J Natl Cancer Inst 1988; 80:1203.

Gulliford MC, Burney PGJ, Petruckitch A: Can efficiency of follow-up of superficial bladder cancer be increased? Ann Roy Coll Surg Engl 1993; 75:57.

Habs MR, Schmahl D: Prevention of urinary bladder tumors in cyclophosphamide-treated rats by additional medication with uroprotectors sodium 2-mercaptoethane sulfonate (Mesna) and disodium 2.2'-dithio-bis-ethane sulfonate (Dimesna). Cancer 1983; 51:606.

Habuchi T, Ogawa O, Kakehi Y, et al: Allelic loss of chromosome 17p in urothelial cancer: Strong association with invasive phenotype. J Urol 1992; 148:1595.

Hajazi A, Devoneck M, Bouvier R, et al: Flow cytometry study of cytokeratin 18 expression according to tumor grade and deoxyribonucleic acid content in human bladder tumors. J Urol 1989; 141:522.

Hall RR, Heath AB: Radiotherapy and cystectomy for T3 bladder carcinoma. Br J Urol 1981; 53:598.

Hall RR, Schade ROK, Swinney J: Effect of hyperthermia on bladder cancer. BMJ 1974; 2:593.

Hanke J, Krajewska B: Acetylation phenotypes and bladder cancer. J Occup Med 1990; 32:917.

Hardeman SW, Perry A, Soloway MS: Transitional cell carcinoma of the prostate following intravesical therapy for transitional cell carcinoma of the bladder. J Urol 1988; 140:289.

Harge P, Hoover R, Kantor A: Bladder cancer risks and pipes, cigars and smokeless tobacco. Cancer 1985; 55:901.

Harker WG, Freiha FS, Shortliffe L, et al: Cisplatin, methotrexate, and vinblastine (CMV) for metastatic transitional cell carcinoma of the urinary tract (TCC): Chemotherapy evaluation of complete response by site. Proc Am Soc Clin Oncol 1984; 3:Abstract C-6773:160.

Harris AL, Neal DE: Bladder cancer-field versus clonal origin. N Engl J Med 1992; 326:759.

Harris CC, Hollstein M: Clinical implications of the p53 tumor-suppressor gene. N Engl J Med 1993; 329:1318.

Harty JI, Amin M, Wieman TJ, et al: Complications of whole bladder dihematoporphyrin ether photodynamic therapy. J Urol 1989; 141:1341.

Harving N, Wolf H, Melsen F: Positive urinary cytology after tumor resection: An indicator for concomitant carcinoma in situ. J Urol 1988; 140:495.

Hasui Y, Osada Y, Kitada S, Nishi S: Significance of invasion to the muscularis mucosal on the progression of superficial bladder cancer. Urology 1994; 43:782.

Hayes RB, Friedell GH, Zahm SH, Cole P: Are the known bladder cancer risk-factors associated with more advanced bladder cancer? Cancer Causes Control 1993; 4:157.

Heimbrook DC, Stirdivant SM, Ahern JD, et al: Transforming growth factor α-pseudomonas exotoxin fusion protein prolongs survival of nude mice bearing tumor xenografts. Proc Natl Acad Sci USA 1994; 87:4697.

Heinonen OP, Albanes D, the Alpha-Tocopherol, Beta Carotene Cancer Prevention Study Group: The effect of vitamin E and beta carotene on the incidence of lung cancer and other cancers in male smokers. N Engl J Med 1994; 330:1029.

Hellstein S, Berg T, Wehlin L: Unrecognized renal cell carcinoma: Clinical and diagnostic aspects. Scand J Urol Nephrol 1981; 15:269.

Hellstein S, Mansson W, Henrikson H, et al: Intravesical mitomycin C for carcinoma in situ of the urinary bladder. Scand J Urol Nephrol 1990; 24:35.

Helmstein K: Treatment of bladder carcinoma by a hydrostatic pressure technique. Br J Urol 1972; 44:434.

Heney NM, Ahmed S, Flanagan M, et al: Superficial bladder cancer: Progression and recurrence. J Urol 1983; 130:1083.

Heney NM, Koontz WW, Barton B, et al: Intravesical thiotepa versus mitomycin C in patients with T_A, T_1 and T_{IS} transitional cell carcinoma of the bladder: A phase III prospective randomized study. J Urol 1988; 140:1390.

Henry K, Miller J, Mori M, et al: Comparison of transurethral resection to radical therapies for stage B bladder tumors. J Urol 1988; 140:964.

Hermanek P, Sobin LH, eds: UICC-International Union Against Cancer TNM Classification of Malignant Tumors, 4th ed. Heidelberg, Springer-Verlag, 1987, p 135.

Hermann GG, Gertsen PF, von der Masse H, et al: Recombinant interleukin 2 and lymphokine activated killer cell treatment of advanced bladder cancer: Clinical results and immunological effects. Cancer Res 1992; 52:726.

Herr HW: Conservative management of muscle-infiltrating bladder cancer: Prospective experience. J Urol 1987; 138:1162.

Herr HW: Neoadjuvant chemotherapy for invasive bladder cancer. Semin Surg Oncol 1989; 5:266.

Herr HW: Intravesical therapy. Hematol Oncol Clin North Am 1992; 6:117.

Herr HW, Pinsky CM, Whitmore WF Jr, et al: Long-term effect of intravesical bacillus Calmette-Guerin on flat carcinoma in situ of the bladder. J Urol 1986; 135:265.

Herr HW, Scher HI: Neoadjuvant chemotherapy and partial cystectomy for invasive bladder cancer. J Clin Oncol 1994; 12:975.

Herr HW, Schwalb DM, Zhang Z-F, et al: Intravesical Bacillus Calmette Guerin prevents tumor progression and death from superficial bladder cancer: 10-year follow-up of a prospective randomized trial. J Clin Oncol 1995; 13:1404.

Hewett CB, Babiszewski JF, Antunez AR: Update on intracavitary radiation in the treatment of bladder tumors. J Urol 1981; 126:323.

Higgy NA, Verma AK, Erturk E, Bryan GT: Augmentation of N-butyl-N-(4-hydroxybutyl) nitrosamine (BHBN) bladder carcinogenicity in Fischer 344 female rats by urinary infection. Proc Annu Meet Am Assoc Cancer Res 1985; 26:118.

Hijazi A, Devoneck M, Bouvier R, et al: Flow cytometry study of cytokeratin 18 expression according to tumor grade and deoxyribonucleic acid content in human bladder tumors. J Urol 1989; 141:522.

Hillyard RW Jr, Ladaga L, Schellhammer PF: Superficial transitional cell carcinoma of the bladder associated with mucosal involvement of the prostatic urethra: Results of treatment with intravesical bacillus Calmette-Guerin. J Urol 1988; 139:290.

Hirata Y, Orth DN: Epidermal growth factor (urogastrone) in human fluids: Size heterogeneity. J Clin Endocrinol Metab 1979; 48:673.

Hisazumi H, Misahi T, Myosi N: Photoradiation therapy of bladder tumors. J Urol 1983; 130:685.

Hoffman D, Masuda Y, Wynder EL: Alpha-naphthylamine and beta-naphthylamine in cigarette smoke. Nature 1969; 221:254.

Hofstetter A, Frank F, Keditsch E, et al: Endoscopic neodymium-YAG laser application for destroying bladder tumors. Eur Urol 1981; 7:278.

Holmes FA, Walters RS, Theriault RL, et al: Phase II trial of Taxol, an active drug in the treatment of metastatic breast cancer. J Natl Cancer Inst 1991; 83:1797.

Hoover R, Strasser PH: Artifical sweeteners and human bladder cancer. Lancet 1980; 1:837.

Hopkins SC, Ford KS, Soloway MS: Invasive bladder cancer: Support for screening. J Urol 1983; 130:61.

Hopman AHN, Poddighe PJ, Smeets AWB, et al: Detection of numerical chromosome aberrations in bladder cancer by in situ hybridization. Am J Clin Pathol 1989; 135:1105.

Horai Y, Fujita K, Ishizaki T: Genetically determined N-acetylation and oxidation capacities in Japanese patients with non-occupational urinary bladder cancer. Eur J Clin Pharmacol 1989; 37:581.

Horn EP, Tucker MA, Lambert G, et al: A study of gender-based cytochrome P450 1A2 variability: A possible mechanism for the male excess of bladder cancer. Cancer Epidemiol Biomark Prev 1995; 4:529.

Howard J, Hankey BF, Greenberg RS, et al: A collaborative study of differences in the survival rates of black patients and white patients with cancer. Cancer 1992; 69:2349.

Howe GR, Burch JD, Miller AB, et al: Tobacco use, occupation, coffee, various nutrients, and bladder cancer. J Natl Cancer Inst 1980; 64:701.

Hruban RH, van der Riet P, Erozan YS, Sidransky D: Brief report: Molecular biology and the early detection of carcinoma of the bladder—the case of Hubert H. Humphrey. N Engl J Med 1994; 330:1276.

Huang W-L, Ro JY, Griguon DJ, et al: Postoperative spindle cell nodule of the prostate and bladder. J Urol 1990; 143:824.

Huben RP: Tumor markers in bladder cancer. Urology 1984; 23:10.

Hudson MA, Ratliff TL, Gillen DP, et al: Single course versus maintenance bacillus Calmette-Guerin therapy for superficial bladder tumors: A prospective randomized trial. J Urol 1987; 138:295.

Huland E, Huland H: Local continuous high dose interleukin-2: A new therapeutic model for the treatment of advanced bladder carcinoma. Cancer Res 1989; 49:5469.

Huland H, Otto U, Droese M, et al: Long-term mitomycin C instillation after transurethral resection of superficial bladder carcinoma: Influence on recurrence, progression, and survival. J Urol 1984; 132:27.

Hupp TR, Meek DW, Midgley CA, et al: Regulation of the specific DNA binding function of p53. Cell 1992; 71:875.

Husband JE, Olliff JF, Williams MP, et al: Bladder cancer: Staging with CT and MR imaging. Radiology 1989; 173:435.

Husmann DA, Spence HM: Current status of tumor of the bowel following ureterosigmoidoscopy: A review. J Urol 1990; 144:607.

Hyacinthe LM, Jarrett TW, Gordon CS, et al: Inhibition of bladder tumor cell implantation in cauterized urothelium, without inhibition of healing, by a fibronectin-related peptide (GRGDS). Ann Surg Oncol 1995; 2:450.

Ishikawa J, Xu H, Hu S, et al: Inactivation of the retinoblastoma gene in human bladder and renal cell carcinomas. Cancer Res 1991; 51:5736.

Issell BF, Prout GR Jr, Soloway MS, et al: Mitomycin C intravesical therapy in noninvasive bladder cancer after failure on thiotepa. Cancer 1984; 53:1025.

Jackson AM, Alexandrof AB, Gribbon SC, et al: Expression and shedding of ICAM-1 in bladder cancer and its immunotherapy. Int J Cancer 1993; 55:921.

Jackson AM, Alexandrof AB, Prescott S, James K: Production of urinary tumor necrosis factors and soluble tumor necrosis factor receptors in bladder cancer patients after bacillus Calmette-Guerin immunotherapy. Cancer Immunol Immunother 1995; 40:119.

Jacobs JA, Ring EJ, Wein AJ: New indications for renal infarction. J Urol 1981; 125:243.

Jacobs SC, Menashe DS, Mewissen MW, et al: Intraarterial cisplatin infusion in the management of transitional cell carcinoma of the bladder. Cancer 1989; 64:388.

Jakse G, Loidl W, Seeber G, et al: Stage T1, grade 3 transitional cell carcinoma of the bladder: An unfavorable tumor? J Urol 1987; 137:39.

Javadpour N: Multiple cell markers in bladder cancer: Principles and clinical practice. Urol Clin North Am 1984; 11:609.

Jenkins BJ, Caulfield MJ, Fowler CG, et al: Reappraisal of the role of radical radiotherapy and salvage cystectomy in the treatment of invasive (T2, T3) bladder cancer. Br J Urol 1988; 62:343.

Jensen OM, Knudsen JB, McLaughlin JK, et al: The Copenhagen case-control study of renal pelvis and ureter cancer: Role of smoking and occupational exposures. Int J Cancer 1988; 41:557.

Jewett HJ, Eversole SL: Carcinoma of the bladder: Characteristic modes of local invasion. J Urol 1960; 83:383.

Jewett HJ, Strong GH: Infiltrating carcinoma of the bladder: Relation of depth of penetration of the bladder wall to incidence of local extension and metastases. J Urol 1946; 55:366.

Johnson DE, Hodge GB, Abdul-Karim FW, et al: Urachal carcinoma. Urology 1985; 26:218.

Johnson DE, Schoenwald MB, Ayala AG, et al: Squamous cell carcinoma of the bladder. J Urol 1976; 115:542.

Johnson DE, Wishnow KI, Tenney D: Are frozen-section examinations of ureteral margins required for all patients undergoing radical cystectomy for bladder cancer? Urology 1989; 33:451.

Johnson OL, Bracken RB, Ayala AG: Vesical adenocarcinoma occurring in patients with pelvic lipomatosis. Urology 1980; 15:280.

Johnson RJ, Carrington BM, Jenkins JP, et al: Accuracy in staging carcinoma of the bladder by magnetic resonance imaging. Clin Radiol 1990; 41:258.

Jones HC, Swinney J: Thiotepa in the treatment of tumors of the bladder. Lancet 1961; 2:615.

Jones PA: Molecular basis for disease—transitional cell carcinoma. Presented at Society of Urologic Oncology Annual Meeting, San Francisco, CA, May 14, 1994. J Urol 1994; 151:63A.

Jones PA, Buckley JD, Henderson BE, et al: From gene to carcinogen: A rapidly evolving field in molecular epidemiology. Cancer Res 1991; 51:3617.

Kabalin JN, Freiha FS, Niebel JD: Leiomyoma of the bladder: Report of 2 cases and demonstration of ultrasonic appearance. Urology 1990; 35:210.

Kabalin JN, McNeal JE, Price HM, et al: Unsuspected adenocarcinoma of the prostate in patients undergoing cystoprostatectomy for other causes: Incidence, histology and morphometric observations. J Urol 1989; 141:1091.

Kakizoe T, Matsumoto K, Audoh M, et al: Adenocarcinoma of the urachus: Report of 7 cases and review of the literature. Urology 1983; 21:360.

Kalble T, Beer M, Staehler G: Intravesical prophylaxis with BCG versus interferon A for superficial bladder cancer. J Urol 1994; 151:233A.

Kalble T, Tricker AR, Friedel P, et al: Ureterosigmoidostomy: Long-term results, risk of carcinoma and etiological factors for carcinogenesis. J Urol 1990; 144:1110.

Kantor AF, Hartge P, Hoover RN, et al: Urinary tract infection and risk of bladder cancer. Am J Epidemiol 1984; 119:510.

Kantor AF, Hartge P, Hoover RN, et al: Epidemiological characteristics of squamous cell carcinoma and adenocarcinoma of the bladder. Cancer Res 1988; 48:3853.

Kantor AF, Hartge P, Hoover RN, Fraumeni JF: Familial and environmental interactions in bladder cancer risk. Int J Cancer 1985; 35:703.

Kaufman DS, Shipley WU, Greffen PP, et al: Selective bladder preservation by combination treatment of invasive bladder cancer. N Engl J Med 1993; 329:1377.

Kavoussi LR, Brown EJ, Ritchey JK, et al: Fibronectin-mediated Calmette-Guerin bacillus attachment to murine bladder mucosa. J Clin Invest 1990; 85:62.

Kavoussi LR, Gelstein LD, Andriole GL: Encephalopathy and an elevated serum aluminum level in a patient receiving intravesical alum irrigation for severe urinary hemorrhage. J Urol 1986; 136:665.

Kay R, Lattanzi C: Nephrogenic adenoma in children. J Urol 1985; 133:99.

Kaye KW, Lange PH: Mode of presentation of invasive bladder cancer: Reassessment of the problem. J Urol 1982; 128:31.

Keep JC, Piehl M, Miller A, et al: Invasive carcinomas of the urinary bladder: Evaluation of tunica muscularis mucosae involvement. Am J Clin Pathol 1989; 91:575.

Kelley DR, Ratliff TR, Catalona WJ, et al: Intravesical BCG therapy for superficial bladder cancer: Effect of BCG viability on treatment results. J Urol 1985; 134:48.

Kern WH: The grade and pathologic stage of bladder cancer. Cancer 1984; 53:1185.

Kiemeney LALM, Witjes JA, Heijbrock RP, et al: Should random urothelial biopsies be taken from patients with primary superficial bladder cancer? A decision analysis. Br J Urol 1994; 73:164.

Kierman M, Gafney EF: Brunn's nests and glandular metaplasia: Normal urothelial variants in the supramontanal prostatic urethra. J Urol 1987; 137:877.

Kilbridge KL, Kantoff P: Intravesical therapy for superficial bladder cancer: Is it a wash? J Clin Oncol 1994; 12:1.

Kim ED, Ignatoff JM: Unsuspected bladder carcinoma in patients undergoing radical prostatectomy. J Urol 1994; 152:397.

Kishi K, Hirota T, Matsumoto K, et al: Carcinoma of the bladder: A clinical and pathological analysis of 87 autopsy cases. J Urol 1981; 125:36.

Klan R, Loy V, Huland H: Residual tumor discovered in routine second transurethral resection in patients with stage T1 transitional cell carcinoma of the bladder. J Urol 1991; 146:316.

Klinger ME: Secondary tumors of the genitourinary tract. J Urol 1951; 65:144.

Knowles MA, Elder PA, Williamson M, et al: Allelotype of human bladder cancer. Cancer Res 1994; 54:531.

Knowles MA, Williamson M: Mutation of H-ras is infrequent in bladder cancer: Confirmation by single-strand conformation polymorphism analysis, designed restriction fragment length polymorphisms, and direct sequencing. Cancer Res 1993; 53:133.

Kock NG, Ghoneim MA, Lycke KG, et al: Replacement of the bladder by the urethral Kock pouch: Functional results, urodynamics and radiological features. J Urol 1989; 141:1111.

Kock NG, Nilson AE, Nilsson LO, et al: Urinary diversion via continent ileal reservoir: Clinical results in 12 patients. J Urol 1982; 128:469.

Konchuba AM, Schellhammer PF, Alexander JP, et al: Flow cytometric study comparing paired bladder washing and voided urine for bladder cancer detection. Urology 1989; 33:89.

Kondas J, Szentgyorgyi E, Szoke D: Local adriamycin treatment for prevention of recurrence of superficial bladder tumors. Int Urol Nephrol 1988; 20:611.

Koontz W, Flannigan M, Ahmed S, et al: Chemoprevention of bladder cancer with 13-cis retinoic acid. Proceedings of First International Conference on Bladder Cancer, Mt. Fuji, Japan, 1981a.

Koontz WW, Prout GR Jr, Smith W, et al: The use of intravesical thiotepa in the management of non-invasive carcinoma of the bladder. J Urol 1981b; 125:307.

Koraitim M, Kamal B, Metwally N, Zaky Y: Transurethral ultrasonic assessment of bladder carcinoma: Its value and limitations. J Urol 1995; 154:375.

Korman HJ, Peabody JO, Cerry JC, et al: Autocrine motility factor receptor as a possible urine marker for transitional cell carcinoma of the bladder. J Urol 1996; 155:347–349.

Koshikawa T, Leyh H, Schenck U: Difficulties in evaluating urinary specimens after local mitomycin therapy of bladder cancer. Diagn Cytopathol 1989; 5:117.

Koss JC, Arger PH, Coleman BG, et al: CT staging of bladder carcinoma. AJR 1981; 137:359.

Koss LG: Tumors of the urinary bladder. In Atlas of Tumor Pathology, Second Series, Fascicle 11. Washington, D.C., Armed Forces Institute of Pathology, 1975, p 1.

Koss LG, Esperanza MT, Robbins MA: Mapping cancerous and precancerous bladder changes: A study of the urothelium in ten surgically removed bladders. JAMA 1974; 227:281.

Koss LG, Wersto RP, Simmons DA, et al: Predictive value of DNA measurements in bladder washings: Comparison of flow cytometry, image cytophotometry, and cytology in patients with a past history of urothelial tumors. Cancer 1989; 64:916.

Kristensen JK, Lose G, Lund F, Nexo E: Epidermal growth factor in urine from patients with urinary bladder tumors. Eur Urol 1988; 14:313.

Kubota Y, Shuin T, Miura T, et al: Treatment of bladder cancer with a combination of hyperthermia, radiation and bleomycin. Cancer 1984; 53:199.

Kunze E, Schauer A, Schmitt M: Histology and histogenesis of two different types of inverted urothelial papillomas. Cancer 1983; 51:348.

Kurth KH, Schroder FH, Tunn U, et al: Adjuvant chemotherapy of superficial transitional cell bladder carcinoma: Preliminary results of a European Organization for Research on Treatment of Cancer randomized trial comparing doxorubicin hydrochloride, ethoglucid and transurethral resection alone. J Urol 1984; 132:258.

Kurth K, Vijgh WJ, ten Kate F, et al: Phase I/II study of intravesical epirubicin in patients with carcinoma in situ of the bladder. J Urol 1991; 146:1508.

Kurz KR, Pitts WR, Vaughan ED Jr: The natural history of patients less than 40 years old with bladder tumors. J Urol 1987; 137:395.

Lamm DL: Intravesical therapy of superficial bladder cancer. AUA Update 1983; 2:2.

Lamm DL, Blumenstein BA, Crawford ED, et al: A randomized trial of intravesical doxorubicin and immunotherapy with bacille Calmette-Guerin for transitional cell carcinoma of the bladder. N Engl J Med 1991; 325:1205.

Lamm DL, Blumenstein BA, Crawford ED, et al: Randomized intergroup comparison of bacillus Calmette-Guerin immunotherapy and mitomycin C chemotherapy prophylaxis in superficial transitional cell carcinoma of the bladder. Urol Oncol 1995a; 1:119.

Lamm DL, Crawford ED, Blumenstein BA, et al: Maintenance BCG immunotherapy of superficial bladder cancer: A randomized prospective Southwest Oncology Group study. J Urol 1992; 147:247A.

Lamm DL, DeHaven JI, Shriver J, et al: A randomized prospective comparison of oral versus intravesical and percutaneous bacillus Calmette-Guerin for superficial bladder cancer. J Urol 1990; 144:65.

Lamm DL, Riggs DR, Shriver JS, et al: Megadose vitamins in bladder cancer: A double-blind clinical trial. J Urol 1994; 151:21.

Lamm DL, Riggs DR, Traynelis CL, Nyseo NS: Apparent failure of current intravesical chemotherapy prophylaxis to influence the longterm course of superficial transitional cell carcinoma of the bladder. J Urol 1995b; 153:1444.

Lamm DL, Stogdill VD, Stogdill BJ, et al: Complications of bacillus Calmette-Guerin immunotherapy in 1,278 patients with bladder cancer. J Urol 1986; 135:272.

Lamm DL, Thor DE, Harris SC, et al: Bacillus Calmette-Guerin immunotherapy of superficial bladder cancer. J Urol 1980; 124:38.

Lamm DL, Thor DE, Stogdill VD, et al: Bladder cancer immunotherapy. J Urol 1982; 128:931.

Lamph W, Walmsley P, Gassone-Corsi P, Verma I: Induction of proto-oncogene JUN/AP-1 by serum and TPA. Nature 1988; 334:629.

Lantz EJ, Hattery RR: Diagnostic imaging of urothelial cancer. Urol Clin North Am 1984; 11:576.

LaPlante M, Brice M II: The upper limits of hopeful application of radical cystectomy for vesical carcinoma: Does nodal metastasis always indicate incurability? J Urol 1973; 109:261.

LaRue H, Simoneau M, Fradet Y: Human papillomavirus in transitional cell carcinoma of the urinary bladder. Clin Cancer Res 1995; 1:435.

Lawrence WF, Messing EM, Bram LL: Cost-effectiveness of screening for bladder cancer using chemical reagent strips to detect microscopic hematuria. J Urol 1995; 153:477A.

Lazarevic B, Garret R: Inverted papilloma and papillary transitional cell carcinoma of urinary bladder. Cancer 1978; 42:1904.

Leadbetter WF, Clarke BG: Five years experience with ureteroenterostomy by combined technique. J Urol 1955; 73:67.

Lerner SP, Skinner DG, Lieskovski G, et al: The rationale for en bloc pelvic lymph node dissection for bladder cancer patients with nodal metastases: Long-term results. J Urol 1993; 149:758.

Liebert M, Washington RW, Wedemeyer G, et al: Loss of α6β4 integrin and collagen VII in bladder cancer. Am J Pathol 1994; 144:787.

Lilien OM, Camey M: 25-year experience with replacement of human bladder (Camey procedure). J Urol 1984; 132:886.

Lin C-W, Zhang D-S, Kwiatkowski DJ, et al: Potential location of a bladder tumor suppressor gene on chromosome 9q at 9q13 to 9q22.1. Urol Oncol 1995; 1:88.

Linker DG, Whitmore WF Jr: Ureteral carcinoma in situ. J Urol 1975; 113:777.

Lipponen PK: Over-expression of p53 nuclear oncoprotein in transitional-cell bladder cancer and its prognostic value. Int J Cancer 1993; 53:365.

Liu SC-S, Liotta LA: Biochemistry of bladder cancer invasion and metastases: Clinical implications. Urol Clin North Am 1992; 19:621.

Locke JL, Hill DE, Walzer Y: Incidence of squamous cell carcinoma in patients with long-term catheter drainage. J Urol 1985; 133:1034.

Lockhart JL, Chaikin L, Bondhus MJ, et al: Prostatic recurrences in the management of superficial bladder tumors. J Urol 1983; 130:256.

Loehrer PJ, Einhorn LH, Elson PJ, et al: A randomized comparison of cisplatin alone or in combination with methotrexate, vinblastine, and doxorubicin in patients with metastatic urothelial carcinoma: A cooperative group study. J Clin Oncol 1992; 10:1066.

Loehrer PJ, Elson P, Dreicer R, et al: Escalated dosages of methotrexate, vinblastine, doxorubicin, and cisplatin plus recombinant human granulocyte colony-stimulating factor in advanced urothelial carcinoma: An Eastern Cooperative Oncology Group trial. J Clin Oncol 1994; 12:483.

Logothetis CJ, Dexeus FH, Chong C, et al: Cisplatin, cyclophosphamide and doxorubicin chemotherapy for unresectable urothelial tumors: The M. D. Anderson experience. J Urol 1989; 141:33.

Logothetis CJ, Finn LD, Smith T, et al: Escalated MVAC with or without recombinant human granulocyte-macrophage colony-stimulating factor for the initial treatment of advanced malignant urothelial tumors: Results of a randomized trial. J Clin Oncol 1995; 13:2272.

Logothetis CJ, Johnson DE, Chong C, et al: Adjuvant cyclophosphamide, doxorubicin, and cisplatin chemotherapy for bladder cancer: An update. J Clin Oncol 1988; 6:1590.

Lopez-Almansa M, Molina R, Huben RP: Transitional cell carcinoma of the urethra in men after radical cystectomy for bladder cancer: Is prophylactic urethrectomy indicated? Br J Urol 1988; 61:507.

Lopez-Altran A, Groghan GA, Groghan I, Jotea JF: Cell and tumor marker immunohistochemistry in transitional cell carcinoma of the bladder. Urol Int 1993; 50:61.

Lopez-Beltran A, Carrusco-Aznar JC, Reymundo C, et al: Bladder cancer survival and human papilloma virus infection: Immunohistochemistry and in situ hybridization. In Olsson CA, ed: Oncogenes and Molecular Genetics of Urological Tumors. New York, Churchill Livingstone, 1991, pp 83–89.

Loprenzi CL, Messing EM: A prospective clinical trial of defluoromethylornithine (DFMO) in patients with resected superficial bladder cancer. J Cell Biochem 1992; 161(suppl):153.

Loprenzi CL, Messing EM, O'Fallon JR, et al: Toxicity evaluation of difluoromethylornithine (DFMO): Doses for chemoprevention trials. Cancer Epi Biomarkers 1996; 5:371.

Love R, Carbone P, Verma A, et al: Phase I study of difluoromethylornithine (DFMO): A chemopreventive agent. Proc Am Assoc Cancer Res 1992; 33:207.

Lowe SW, Rouley HE, Jacks T, et al: p53 dependent apoptosis modulates the cytotoxicity of anticancer agents. Cell 1993; 74:957.

Lower GM Jr, Nilsson T, Nelson CE, et al: N-acetyltransferase phenotype and risk in urinary bladder cancer: Approaches in molecular epidemiology: Preliminary results in Sweden and Denmark. Environ Health Perspect 1979; 29:71.

Lucas SB: Squamous cell carcinoma of the bladder and schistosomiasis. East Afr Med J 1982; 59:345.

Lundbeck F, Mogensen P, Jeppersen N: Intravesical therapy of noninvasive bladder tumors with doxorubicin and urokinase. J Urol 1983; 130:1087.

Lundbeck R, Brunn E, Finnerup B, et al: Intravesical therapy of noninvasive bladder tumors (stage Ta) with doxorubicin: Initial treatment results and the long-term course. J Urol 1988; 139:1212.

Lunec J, Challen C, Wright C, et al: Amplification of c-erbB2 and mutation of p53 in concomitant transitional carcinomas of renal pelvis and urinary bladder. Lancet 1992; 339:439.

Lutzeyer W, Rubben H, Dahm H: Prognostic parameters in superficial bladder cancer: An analysis of 315 cases. J Urol 1982; 127:250.

Lynch CF, Cohen MB: Urinary system. Cancer 1995; 75(suppl):316.

Lynch CF, Platz CE, Jones MP, Gazzaniga JM: Cancer registry problems in classifying bladder cancer. J Natl Cancer Inst 1991; 83:429.

Lynch HT, Ens JA, Lynch JF: The Lynch syndrome II and urological malignancies. J Urol 1990; 143:24.

Lynch HT, Kimberling WJ, Lynch JF, Brennan K: Familial bladder cancer in an oncology clinic. Cancer Genet Cytogenet 1987; 27:161.

Mackenzie AR, Sharma TC, Whitmore WF Jr, et al: Non-extirpative treatment of myosarcomas of the bladder and prostate. Cancer 1971; 28:329.

Madgar I, Goldwasser B, Nativ O, et al: Long-term follow-up of patients less than 30 years old with transitional cell carcinoma of the bladder. J Urol 1988; 139:933.

Magri J: Partial cystectomy: Review of 104 cases. Br J Urol 1962; 34:74.

Malker HS, McLaughlin JK, Silverman DT, et al: Occupational risks for bladder cancer among men in Sweden. Cancer Res 1987; 47:6763.

Malkowicz SB, Nichols P, Lieskovsky G, et al: The role of radical cystectomy in the management of high grade superficial bladder cancer (PA, PI, PIS, and P2). J Urol 1990; 144:641.

Malmstrom PU, Busch C, Norlen BJ: Recurrence, progression and survival in bladder cancer: A retrospective analysis of 232 patients with greater than or equal to 5-year follow-up. Scand J Urol Nephrol 1987; 21:185.

Malmstrom PU, Busch C, Norlen BJ, et al: Expression of ABH blood group isoantigen as a prognostic factor in transitional cell bladder carcinoma. Scand J Urol Nephrol 1988; 22:265.

Malmstrom PU, Larssen A, Johansson S: Urinary fibronectin in diagnosis and follow-up of patients with urinary bladder cancer. Br J Urol 1993; 72:307.

Maloney KE, Weiner JS, Walther PJ: Oncogenic human papillomaviruses are rarely associated with squamous cell carcinoma of the bladder: Evaluation by differential polymerase chain reaction. J Urol 1994; 154:360.

Mameghan H, Fischer RI, Watt WH, et al: The management of invasive transitional cell carcinoma of the bladder. Cancer 1992; 69:2771.

Mao L, Lee DJ, Tockman MS, et al: Microsatellite alterations as clonal markers for the detection of human cancer. Proc Natl Acad Sci USA 1994; 91:9871.

Marsh GM, Callahan C, Ravlock J, et al: A protocol for bladder cancer screening and medical surveillance among high risk groups: The Drake health registry experience. J Occup Med 1990; 32:881.

Marshall FF: Creation of an ileocolic bladder after cystectomy. J Urol 1988; 139:1264.

Marshall VF: Symposium on bladder tumors: Current clinical problems regarding bladder tumors. Cancer 1956; 9:543.

Marshall VF, McCarron JP Jr: The curability of vesical cancer: Greater now or then? Cancer Res 1977; 37:753.

Martin JE, Jenkins BJ, Zuk RJ, et al: Clinical importance of squamous metaplasia in invasive transitional cell carcinoma of the bladder. J Clin Pathol 1989a; 42:250.

Martin JE, Jenkins BJ, Zuk RJ, et al: Human chorionic gonadotrophin expression and histological findings as predictors of response to radiotherapy in carcinoma of the bladder. Virchows Arch [A] 1989b; 414:273.

Martinez A, Gunderson LL: Intraoperative radiation therapy for bladder cancer. Urol Clin North Am 1984; 11:693.

Martinez-Pineiro JA, Jimenez Leon J, Martinez-Pineiro L Jr, et al: Bacillus Calmette-Guerin versus doxorubicin versus thiotepa: A randomized prospective study in 202 patients with superficial bladder cancer. J Urol 1990; 143:502.

Martinez-Pineiro JA, Muntanola P: Nonspecific immunotherapy with BCG vaccine in bladder tumors: A preliminary report. Eur Urol 1977; 3:11.

Maruf NJ, Godec CJ, Strom RL, et al: Unusual therapeutic response of massive squamous cell carcinoma of the bladder to aggressive radiation and surgery. J Urol 1982; 128:1313.

Mason TJ, Vogler WY: Bladder cancer screening at the Dupont Chamber Works: A new initiative. J Occup Med 1990; 32:874.

Masters JR, Vesey SG, Mumm CF, et al: C-myc oncoprotein levels in bladder cancer. Urol Res 1988; 16:341.

Mathiasen H, Frimodt-Moller PC, Nielsen HV: Ureteropyeloscopic tumour treatment. Scand J Urol Nephrol 1988; 110:201.

Mathur VK, Krahn HP, Ramse ER: Total cystectomy for bladder cancer. J Urol 1981; 125:784.

Matsumoto K, Kakizoe T, Mikuriza S, et al: Clinical evaluation of intraoperative radiotherapy for carcinoma of the urinary bladder. Cancer 1981; 47:509.

Matthews PN, Madden M, Bidgood KA, et al: The clinical pathological features of metastatic superficial papillary bladder cancer. J Urol 1984; 132:904.

Mayer WJ, McWhorter WP: Black white differences in non-treatment of bladder cancer patients and implications for survival. Am J Public Health 1989; 79:772.

McCredie M, Stewart JH, Ford JM, et al: Phenacetin-containing analgesics and cancer of the bladder or renal pelvis in women. Br J Urol 1983; 55:220.

McCullough DL, Cooper RM, Yeaman LD, et al: Neoadjuvant treatment of stages T2 to bladder cancer with cis-platinum, cyclophosphamide and doxorubicin. J Urol 1989; 141:849.

McCullough DL, Lamm DL, McLaughlin AP III, et al: Familial transitional cell carcinoma of the bladder. J Urol 1975; 113:269.

McGuire WP, Rowinsky EK, Rosenshein NB, et al: Taxol: A unique antineoplastic agent with significant activity in advanced ovarian epithelial neoplasms. Ann Intern Med 1989; 111:273.

McLaughlin JK, Silverman DT, Hsing AW, et al: Cigarette smoking and cancers of the renal pelvis and ureter. Cancer Res 1992; 52:254.

McPhee MS, Arnfield MR, Tulip J, et al: Neodymium:YAG laser therapy for infiltrating bladder cancer. J Urol 1988; 140:44.

Medical Research Council Working Party on Urologic Cancer, Subgroup on Superficial Bladder Cancer: The effect of intravesical thiotepa on tumor recurrence after endoscopic treatment of newly diagnosed superficial bladder cancer: A further report with long-term follow-up of the Medical Research Council's randomized trial. Br J Urol 1994; 73:632.

Melamed MR: Flow cytometry of the urinary bladder. Urol Clin North Am 1984; 11:599.

Melamed MR, Koss LG, Ricci A, et al: Cytohistological observations on developing carcinoma of the urinary bladder in man. Cancer 1960; 13:67.

Mellon K, Wright C, Kelly P, et al: Long-term outcome related to epidermal growth factor receptor status in bladder cancer. J Urol 1995; 153:919.

Messing EM: Clinical implications of the expression of epidermal growth factor receptors in human transitional cell carcinoma. Cancer Res 1990; 50:2530.

Messing EM, Hanson P, Ulrich P, Erturk E: Epidermal growth factor-interactions with normal and malignant urothelium: In vitro and in situ studies. J Urol 1987a; 138:1329.

Messing EM, Murphy-Brooks N: Recovery of epidermal growth factor in voided urine of patients with bladder cancer. Urology 1994; 44:502.

Messing EM, Reznikoff CA: Epidermal growth factor and its receptor: Markers of—and targets for—chemoprevention of bladder cancer. J Cell Biochem 1992; 161(suppl):56.

Messing EM, Tutsch K, Storer B, et al: Ornithine decarboxylase (ODC) blockade—a potential approach to bladder cancer (BC) prevention. Presented at the Northeast Section American Urological Association 47th Annual Meeting, Cairo, Egypt, 1995a.

Messing EM, Valencourt A: Hematuria screening for bladder cancer. J Occup Med 1990; 32:838.

Messing EM, Young TB, Hunt VB, et al: The significance of asymptomatic microhematuria in men 50 or more years old: Findings of a home screening study using urinary dipsticks. J Urol 1987b; 137:919.

Messing EM, Young TB, Hunt VB, et al: Urinary tract cancers found by home screening with hematuria dipsticks in healthy men over 50 years of age. Cancer 1989; 64:2361.

Messing EM, Young TB, Hunt VB, et al: Home screening for hematuria: Results of a multiclinic study. J Urol 1992; 148:289.

Messing EM, Young TB, Hunt VB, et al: Comparison of bladder cancer outcome in men undergoing hematuria home screening versus those with standard clinical presentations. Urology 1995c; 45:387.

Messing EM, Young TB, Hunt VB, et al: Hematuria home screening: Repeat testing results. J Urol 1995b; 154:57.

Meyers FJ, Gumerlock PH, Kokoris SP, et al: Human bladder and colon carcinomas contain activated ras p21: Specific detection of twelfth codon mutants. Cancer 1989; 63:2177.

Meyhoff HH, Andersen JT, Klarskov P, et al: Flexible fiberoptic versus conventional cystourethroscopy in bladder tumor patients: A prospective study. Scand J Urol Nephrol 1988; 110:237.

Michel F, Gattegno B, Meyrier A, et al: Paraneoplastic hypercalcemia associated with bladder carcinoma: Report of 2 cases. J Urol 1984; 131:753.

Miller BA, Gloeckler-Reis LA, Hanbey BF, et al: Cancer statistics review Bethesda, MD, 1973–1989. National Cancer Institute, U.S. Department of Health and Human Services, NIH publication no. 92-2789, 1992.

Miller EB, Eure GR, Schellhammer PF: Upper tract transitional cell carcinoma following treatment of superficial bladder cancer with BCG. Urology 1993; 42:26.

Miller LS, Johnson DE: Megavoltage irradiation for bladder cancer: Alone, postoperative or preoperative. *In* Proceedings of the Seventh National Cancer Conference. Philadelphia, J. B. Lippincott, 1973, p 771.

Miller ME, Cosgriff JM: Acetylator phenotype in human bladder cancer. J Urol 1983; 130:65.

Miller RS, Freiha FS, Reese JH, et al: Cisplatin, methotrexate, and vinblastine plus surgery restaging for patients with advanced transitional cell carcinoma of the urothelium. J Urol 1993; 150:65.

Mills SE, Wolfe JT, Weiss MA, et al: Small cell undifferentiated carcinoma of the urinary bladder: A light-microscopic, immunocytochemical, and ultrastructural study of 12 cases. Am J Surg Pathol 1987; 11:606.

Miyato H, Kubota Y, Shuin T, et al: Expression of transforming growth factor β1 in human bladder cancer. Cancer 1995; 75:2565.

Montie JE: High-stage bladder cancer: Bladder preservation or reconstruction. Cleve Clin J Med 1990; 57:280.

Montie JE, Straffon RA, Stewart BH: Radical cystectomy without radiation therapy for carcinoma of the bladder. J Urol 1984; 131:477.

Montie JE, Wood DP Jr, Pontes JE, et al: Adenocarcinoma of the prostate in cystoprostatectomy specimens removed for bladder cancer. Cancer 1989; 63:381.

Morales A, Eidinger D, Bruce AW: Intracavitary Bacillus Calmette-Guerin in the treatment of superficial bladder tumors. J Urol 1976; 116:180.

Morales A, Ersil A: Prophylaxis of recurrent bladder cancer with bacillus Calmette-Guerin. *In* Johnson DE, Samuels ML, eds: Cancer of the Genitourinary Tract. New York, Raven Press, 1979, p 121.

Morales A, Nickel JC: Immunotherapy of superficial bladder cancer with BCG. World J Urol 1986; 3:209.

Morales A, Ottenhof P, Emerson L: Treatment of residual noninfiltrating bladder cancer with bacillus Calmette-Guerin. J Urol 1981; 125:649.

Morris SB, Gordon EM, Shera RJ, Woodhouse CRI: Superficial bladder cancer: How long should a tumor-free patient have check cystoscopies? Br J Urol 1995; 75:193.

Morrison AS: Advances in the etiology of urothelial cancer. Urol Clin North Am 1984; 11:557.

Morrison AS: Early detection: Sensitivity and lead time. *In:* Screening in Chronic Disease, 2nd ed. New York, Oxford University Press, 1992, pp 43–73.

Morrison AS, Cole P: Epidemiology of bladder cancer. Urol Clin North Am 1976; 3:13.

Mostofi, FK: Potentialities of bladder epithelium. J Urol 1954; 71:715.

Mostofi FK, Sobin LH, Torloni H: Histological Typing of Urinary Bladder Tumors (International Histologic Classification of Tumors, No. 10). Geneva, World Health Organization, 1973.

Mufti GR, Singh M: Value of random mucosal biopsies in the management of superficial bladder cancer. Eur Urol 1992; 22:288.

Mufti GR, Virdi JS, Singh M: Reappraisal of hydrostatic pressure treatment for intractable postradiotherapy vesical hemorrhage. Urology 1990; 35:9.

Murphy WM, Soloway MS: Urothelial dysplasia. J Urol 1982; 127:849.

Nadler B, Catalona WJ, Hudson MA, Ratliff TL: Durability of the tumor-free response for intravesical bacillus Calmette Guerin therapy. J Urol 1994; 152:367.

Narumi Y, Sato T, Kuriyama K, et al: Vesical dome tumors: Significance of extravesical extension on CT. Radiology 1988; 169:83.

National Center for Health Statistics: Health United States 1990. Hyattsville, MD, U.S. Department of Health and Human Services, DHHS publication no. PHS 91-1232, 1991.

Navarre RJ Jr, Loening SA, Platz C. et al: Nephrogenic adenoma: A report of 9 cases and review of the literature. J Urol 1982; 127:775.

Neal DE, Marsh C, Bennett MK, et al: Epidermal-growth-factor receptors in human bladder cancer: Comparison of invasive and superficial tumours. Lancet 1985; 16:366.

Neal DE, Sharples L, Smith K, et al: The epidermal growth factor receptor and the prognosis of bladder cancer. Cancer 1990; 65:1619.

Neal DE, Smith K, Fennelly JA, et al: Epidermal growth factor receptor in human bladder cancer: A comparison of immunohistochemistry and ligand binding. J Urol 1989; 41:517.

Nemoto R, Uchida K, Hattori K, et al: S-phase fraction of human bladder tumor measured in situ with bromodeoxyuridine labeling. J Urol 1988; 139:286.

Netto NR Jr, Lemos GC: A comparison of treatment methods for the prophylaxis of recurrent superficial bladder tumors. J Urol 1983; 129:33.

Newling D: Intravesical therapy in the management of superficial transitional cell carcinoma of the bladder: Experience of the EORTC group. Br J Cancer 1990; 61:497.

Newling DWW, Robinson MRG, Smith PH, et al: Tryptophan metabolites, pyridoxine (vitamine B₆) and their influence on the recurrence rate of superficial bladder cancer. Eur Urol 1995; 27:110.

Newman DM, Brown JR, Jay AC, et al: Squamous cell carcinoma of the bladder. J Urol 1968; 100:470.

Nguyen M, Hiroyaki W, Budson AE, et al: Elevated levels of angiogenic peptide basic fibroblast growth factor in urine of bladder cancer patients. J Natl Cancer Inst 1993; 85:241.

Nichols JA, Marshall VF: The treatment of bladder carcinoma by local excision and fulguration. Cancer 1956; 9:559.

Nielsen K, Nielsen KK: Adenocarcinoma in exstrophy of the bladder—the last case in Scandinavia? A case report and review of the literature. J Urol 1983; 130:1180.

Nijima T, Koiso K, Akaza H, The Japanese Urological Cancer Research Group for Adriamycin: Randomized clinical trial on chemoprophylaxis of recurrence in cases of superficial bladder cancer. Cancer Chemother Pharmacol 1983; 11(suppl):79.

Nishimura K, Hida S, Nishio Y: The validity of magnetic resonance imaging (MRI) in the staging of bladder cancer: Comparison with computed tomography (CT) and transurethral ultrasonography (US). Jpn J Clin Oncol 1988; 18:217.

Nocks BN, Heney NM, Daily JJ, et al: Transitional cell carcinoma of renal pelvis. Urology 1982; 19:472.

Noel JC Thiry L, Verhest A, et al: Transitional cell carcinoma of the bladder: Evaluation of the role of human papillomaviruses. Urology 1994; 44:671.

Norkool DN, Hampson NB, Gibbons RP, Weissman RM: Hyperbaric oxygen therapy for radiation induced hemorrhagic cystitis. J Urol 1993; 150:332.

Norming U, Tribukait B, Gustavsson H, et al: Deoxyribonucleic acid profile on tumor progression in primary carcinoma in situ of the bladder: A study of 63 patients with grade III lesions. J Urol 1992a; 147:11.

Norming U, Tribukait B, Nyman CR, et al: Prognostic significance of mucosal aneuploidy in stage Ta/T1 grade 3 carcinoma of the bladder. J Urol 1992b; 148:1420.

Nseyo UO, Dougherty TJ, Sullivan L: Photodynamic therapy in the management of resistant lower urinary tract carcinoma. Cancer 1987; 60:3113.

Nurmi M, Kateyuo K, Puntala P: Reliability of CT in preoperative evaluation of bladder carcinoma. Scand J Urol Nephrol 1988; 22:125.

Oates RD, Stilmant MM, Freedlund MC, et al: Granulomatous prostatitis following bacillus Calmette-Guerin immunotherapy of bladder cancer. J Urol 1988; 140:751.

Oda H, Oda T, Okada H, et al: Flow cytometric evaluation of Thomsen-Friedenreich antigen on transitional cell cancer using monoclonal antibody. Urol Res 1990; 18:107.

O'Keane JC: Carcinoma of the urinary bladder after treatment with cyclophosphamide. N Engl J Med 1988; 319:871.

Oldbring J, Glifberg I, Mikulowski P, et al: Carcinoma of the renal pelvis and ureter following bladder carcinoma: Frequency, risk factors and clinicopathological findings. J Urol 1989; 141:1311.

Olumni AF, Tsai YC, Nichols PW, et al: Allelic loss of chromosome 17 p distinguishes high grade from low grade transitional cell carcinomas of the bladder. Cancer Res 1990; 50:7081.

Ono K, Akuta K, Takaasi M, et al: Effect of misonidazole in preoperative irradiation for bladder cancer followed by total cystectomy. Radiat Med 1989; 7:105.

Onodera T, Yagihashi S: c-myc, c-erbB-1 and c-erbB-2 expressions in urinary tract cancers. J Urol 1995, in press.

Oosterlinck W, Kurth KH, Schroder F, et al: A prospective European Organization for Research and Treatment of Cancer Genitourinary Group randomized trial comparing transurethral resection followed by a single intravesical instillation of epirubicin or water in single Ta, T1 papillary carcinoma of the bladder. J Urol 1993; 149:749.

Orihuela E, Shahon RS: Influence of blood group type on the natural history of superficial bladder cancer. J Urol 1987; 138:758.

Orlow I, Lacombe L, Hannon GJ, et al: Deletion of the p16 (INK4A/MTS1/CDKN2) and p15 (1NK4B/MTS2) genes in human bladder cancer. J Natl Cancer Inst 1995; 20:1499.

Orntoff FF: Activity of the human blood group ABO, Se, H, Le and X gene-encoded glycosyltransferases in normal and malignant bladder urothelium. Cancer Res 1988; 48:4427.

Ostroff EB, Chenault OW Jr: Alum irrigation for the control of massive bladder hemorrhage. J Urol 1982; 128:929.

Pagano F, Bassi P, Galetti TP, et al: Results of contemporary radical cystectomy for invasive bladder cancer: A clinicopathological study with an emphasis on the inadequacy of the tumor, nodes and metastases classification. J Urol 1992; 145:45.

Pagano F, Bassi P, Milani C, et al: A low dose bacillus Calmette Guerin regimen in superficial bladder cancer therapy: Is it effective? J Urol 1991; 146:32.

Page BH, Levison VB, Curwen MP: The site of recurrence of noninfiltrating bladder tumors. Br J Urol 1978; 50:237.

Parry WL, Hemstreet GP III: Cancer detection by quantitative fluorescence image analysis. J Urol 1988; 139:270.

Patch FS, Rhea LJ: The genesis and development of Brunn's nests and their relationship to cystitis cystica, glandularis and primary adenocarcinoma of the bladder. Can Med Assoc J 1935; 33:597.

Pedersen-Bjergaard J, Ersboll J, Hansen VL, et al: Carcinoma of the bladder after treatment with cyclophosphamide for non-Hodgkin's lymphoma. N Engl J Med 1988; 318:1028.

Pedersen H, Wolf H, Jensen SK, et al: Administration of a retinoid as prophylaxis of recurrent non-invasive bladder tumors. Scand J Urol Nephrol 1984; 18:121.

Pink JC, Messing EM, Reznikoff CA, et al: Correlation between N-acetyltransferase activities in uroepithelial and in vivo acetylator phenotype. Drug Met Dispos 1992; 20:559.

Pinsky CM, Camacho FJ, Kerr D, et al: Treatment of superficial bladder cancer with intravesical BCG. In Terry WD, Rosenberg SA, eds: Immunotherapy of Human Cancer. New York, Elsevier North Holland, 1982, p 309.

Piper JM, Tonascia J, Metanoski GM: Heavy phenacetin use and bladder cancer in women aged 20 to 49 years. N Engl J Med 1985; 313:292.

Pizza G, Severini G, Menniti D, et al: Tumour regression after intralesional injection of interleukin-2 (IL-2) in bladder cancer: Preliminary report. Int J Cancer 1984; 34:359.

Pode DO, Alone Y, Horowitz AT, et al: The mechanism of human bladder tumor implantation in an in vitro model. J Urol 1986; 136:482.

Pollack A, Zagar GK, Swanson DA: Muscle invasive bladder cancer treated with external beam radiotherapy: Prognostic factors. Int J Rad Oncol Biophys 1994; 30:267.

Powder JR, Mosberg WH, Pierpoint RZ: Bilateral primary carcinoma of the ureter: Topical and ureteral thiotepa. J Urol 1984; 132:349.

Prescott S, James A, Hargreave TB, Chisholm GD: Radioimmunoassay detection of interferon-gamma in urine after intravesical BCG therapy. J Urol 1990; 144:1248.

Presti JC, Reuter V, Galan T, et al: Molecular genetic alterations in superficial and locally advanced human bladder cancer. Cancer Res 1991; 51:5405.

Price JM, Brown RR: Studies of etiology of carcinoma of the urinary bladder. Acta Unio Int Carcirum 1962; 8:684.

Pritchett TR, Schieff WM, Klatt E, et al: The potency-sparing radical cystectomy: Does it compromise the completeness of the cancer resection? J Urol 1988; 140:1400.

Prout GR Jr: The surgical management of bladder carcinoma. Urol Clin North Am 1976; 3:149.

Prout GR, Barton BA, Griffin PP, Friedell G: Treated history of noninvasive grade 1 transitional cell cancer. J Urol 1992; 148:1413.

Prout GR Jr, Griffin PP, Nocks BN, et al: Intravesical therapy of low stage bladder carcinoma with mitomycin C: Comparison of results in untreated and previously treated patients. J Urol 1982; 127:1096.

Prout GR Jr, Griffin PP, Shipley WU: Bladder carcinoma as a systemic disease. Cancer 1979; 42:2532.

Prout GR Jr, Koontz WW Jr, Coombs J, et al: Long-term fate of 90 patients with superficial bladder cancer randomly assigned to receive or not to receive thiotepa. J Urol 1983; 130:677.

Prout GR Jr, Lin CW, Benson R Jr, et al: Photodynamic therapy with hematoporphyrin derivative in the treatment of superficial transitional-cell carcinoma of the bladder. N Engl J Med 1987; 317:1251.

Prout HR, Shipley WU, Kaufman DS, et al: Interval report of a phase I–II study utilizing multiple modalities in the treatment of invasive bladder cancer. Urol Clin North Am 1991; 18:547.

Quilty PM, Kerr GR: Bladder cancer following low- or high-dose pelvic irradiation. Clin Radiol 1987; 38:583.

Radwin HM: Invasive transitional cell carcinoma of the bladder: Is there a place for preoperative radiotherapy? Urol Clin North Am 1980; 7:551.

Radzikowski CZ, Steuden I, Wiedlocha A, et al: The Thomsen-Friedenreich antigen on human urothelial cell lines detectable by peanut lectin and monoclonal antibody raised against human glycophorin A. Anticancer Res 1989; 9:103.

Raghavan D, Boyer M, Rodgers J, et al: Initial intravenous cisplatin therapy

for invasive bladder cancer: Minimum follow-up of ten years. Urol Oncol 1995.

Raghavan D, Shipley WU, Garnick MB, et al: Biology in management of bladder cancer. N Engl J Med 1990; 322:1129.

Raghavan D, Wallace MA, Sandeman T, et al: First randomized trials of pre-emptive (neoadjuvant) intravenous (IV cisplatin CDDP) for invasive transitional cell carcinoma of the bladder (TCCB) (Abstract). Proc Am Soc Clin Oncol 1989; 8:133.

Rao JY, Hemstreet GP III, Hurst RE, et al: Alterations in phenotypic biochemical markers in bladder epithelium during tumorigenesis. Proc Natl Acad Sci USA 1993; 90:8287.

Ratliff TL, Hudson MA, Catalona WJ: Strategy for improving therapy of superficial bladder cancer. World J Urol 1991; 9:95.

Rawls WH, Lamm DL, Lowe BA, et al: Fatal sepsis following intravesical bacillus Calmette-Guerin administration for bladder cancer. J Urol 1990; 144:1328.

Rehn L: Ueber blasentrumoren bei fuchsinarbeitern. Arch Kind Chir 1895; 50:588.

Renfer LG, Kelley J, Belville WD: Inverted papilloma of the urinary tract: Histogenesis, recurrence, and associated malignancy. J Urol 1988; 140:832.

Renwick AG, Thakrar A, Lawrie CA, et al: Microbial amino acid metabolites and bladder cancer: No evidence of promoting activity in man. Hum Toxicol 1988; 7:267.

Resnick MI, O'Connor VJ Jr: Segmental resection for carcinoma of the bladder: Review of 102 patients. J Urol 1973; 109:1007.

Resseguie LT, Nobrega FT, Farrow GM, et al: Epidemiology of renal and ureteral cancer in Rochester, Minnesota, 1950–1974, with special reference to clinical and pathologic features. Mayo Clin Proc 1978; 53:503.

Richie JP, Waisman J, Skinner DG, et al: Squamous cell carcinoma of the bladder: Treatment by radical cystectomy. J Urol 1976; 115:670.

Riddle PR, Chisholm GD, Trott PA, et al: Flat carcinoma in situ of bladder. Br J Urol 1976; 47:829.

Risch A, Wallace DMA, Sim E: Slow N-acetylation genotype is a susceptibility factor in occupational and smoking related bladder cancer. Human Mol Genet 1995; 4:231.

Risch HA, Burch JD, Miller AB, et al: Dietary factors and the incidence of cancer in the urinary bladder. Am J Epidemiol 1988; 127:1179.

Ro JY, Ayala AG, El-Naggar A: Muscularis mucosa of urinary bladder: Importance for staging and treatment. Am J Surg Pathol 1987; 11:668.

Roberts JT, Fossa SD, Richards B, et al: Results of a Medical Research Council phase II study of low-dose cisplatin and methotrexate in the primary treatment of locally advanced (T3 and T4) transitional cell carcinoma of the bladder. Br J Urol 1991; 68:162.

Robinson MRG, Sheltz MB, Richards B, et al: Intravesical epodyl in the management of bladder tumors: Combined experience of the Yorkshire Urological Cancer Research Group. J Urol 1977; 118:972.

Rosi P, Selli C, Carini M, et al: Myxoid liposarcoma of the bladder. J Urol 1983; 130:560.

Ross RK, Paganini-Hill A, Landolph J, et al: Analgesics, cigarette smoking, and other risk factors for cancer of the renal pelvis and ureter. Cancer Res 1989; 49:1045.

Roth BJ, Dreicer R, Einhorn LH, et al: Significant activity of paclitaxel in advanced transitional cell carcinoma of the urothelium: A phase II trial of the Eastern Cooperative Oncology Group (E1892). J Clin Oncol 1994; 12:2264.

Rotman M, Aziz H, Porrazzo M, et al: Treatment of advanced transitional cell carcinoma of the bladder with irradiation and concomitant 5-fluorouracil infusion. Int J Radiat Oncol Biol Phys 1990; 18:1131.

Rowland RG, Mitchell ME, Bihrle R, et al: Indiana continent urinary reservoir. J Urol 1987; 137:1136.

Rubben H, Lutzeyer W, Fischer N, et al: Natural history and treatment of low and high risk superficial bladder tumors. J Urol 1988; 139:283.

Russell KJ, Laramore, GE, Griffin TW, et al: The fast neutron radiotherapy for treatment of carcinoma of the urinary bladder. Am J Clin Oncol 1989; 12:301.

Sager EM, Talle K, Fossa SD, et al: Contrast-enhanced computed tomography to show perivesical extension in bladder carcinoma. Acta Radiol 1987; 28:307.

Sakamoto GD, Burden J, Fisher D: Systemic bacillus Calmette-Guerin infection after transurethral administration for superficial bladder cancer. J Urol 1989; 142:1073.

Sandberg AA: Chromosome changes in bladder cancer: Clinical and other correlations. Cancer Genet Cytogenet 1986; 19:163.

Sarkis AS, Bajarin DF, Reuter VE, et al: Prognostic value of p53 nuclear overexpression in patients with invasive bladder cancer treated with neoadjuvant MVAC. J Clin Oncol 1995; 13:1384.

Sarkis AS, Dalbagni G, Cordon-Cardo C, et al: Nuclear overexpression of p53 protein in transitional cell carcinoma: A marker for disease progression. J Natl Cancer Inst 1993; 85:53.

Sarkis AS, Dalbagni G, Cordon-Cardo C, et al: Association of p53 nuclear overexpression and tumor progression in carcinoma in situ of the bladder. J Urol 1994; 152:388.

Sarosdy MF, De Vere White RW, Soloway MS, et al: Results of a multicenter trial using the bladder tumor antigen test to monitor for and diagnose recurrent bladder cancer. J Urol 1995; 154:379.

Sarosdy MF, Lamm DL: Long-term results of intravesical bacillus Calmette-Guerin therapy for superficial bladder cancer. J Urol 1989; 142:719.

Sarosdy MF, Lamm DL, Williams RD, et al: Phase I trial of oral bropirimine in superficial bladder cancer. J Urol 1992; 147:31.

Saur R, Donst J, Altendorf-Hoffman A, et al: Radiotherapy with or without cisplatin in bladder cancer. Int J Radiat Oncol Biophys 1990; 19:687.

Sauter G, Moch D, Carroll P, et al: Heterogeneity of erbB-2 gene amplification in bladder cancer. Cancer Res 1993; 53:2199.

Schairer C, Harge P, Hoover RN, et al: Racial differences in bladder cancer risk: A case-control study. Am J Epidemiol 1988; 128:1027.

Schellhammer PF, Bean MA, Whitmore WF Jr: Prostatic involvement by transitional cell carcinoma: Pathogenesis, patterns and prognosis. J Urol 1977; 118:399.

Schellhammer PF, Ladago LE, Fillion MB: Bacillus Calmette-Guerin (BCG) for superficial transitional cell carcinoma (TCC) of the bladder. J Urol 1986; 135:261.

Scher HI: New approaches to the treatment of bladder cancer. N Engl J Med 1993; 329:1420.

Scher HI, Yagoda A, Herr HW, et al: Neoadjuvant M-VAC (methotrexate, vinblastine, doxorubicin and cisplatin) effect on the primary bladder lesion. J Urol 1988; 139:470.

Schlegel PN, Walsh PC: Neuroanatomical approach to radical cystoprostatectomy with preservation of sexual function. J Urol 1987; 138:1402.

Schoborg TW, Saffos RO, Rodriguez AP, et al: Carcinosarcoma of the bladder. J Urol 1980; 124:724.

Schultz RE, Bloch MJ, Tomaszewski JE, et al: Mesonephric adenocarcinoma of the bladder. J Urol 1984; 132:263.

Schwalb DM, Herr HW, Fair WR: The management of clinically unconfirmed positive urinary cytology. J Urol 1993; 150:1751.

See WA, Chapman J: Heparin prevention of tumor cell adherence and implantation on injured urothelial surfaces. J Urol 1987; 138:182.

See WA, Fuller JR: Staging of advanced bladder cancer: Current concepts and pitfalls. Urol Clin North Am 1992; 19:663.

See WA, Rahlf D, Crist S: In vitro particulated urines to fibronectin: Correlation to in vivo particulated adherence to sites of bladder injury. J Urol 1992; 147:1416.

Segura JW: Ureteroscopic treatment of urothelial carcinoma of the ureter and renal pelvis (Editorial). J Urol 1992; 148:277.

Seidman AD, Scher HI, Galrielove JL: Dose intensification of MVAC with recombinant granulocyte colony stimulating factors—initial therapy in advanced urothelial cancer. J Clin Oncol 1993; 11:408.

Seidman AD, Scher HI, Heinemann MH, et al: Continuous infusion gallium nitrate for patients with advanced refractory urothelial tract tumors. Cancer 1991; 68:2561.

Seligman PA, Crawford ED: Treatment of advanced transitional cell carcinoma of the bladder with continuous-infusion gallium nitrate. J Natl Cancer Inst 1991; 83:1582.

Sella A, Dexeus FH, Chong C, et al: Radiation therapy–associated invasive bladder tumors. Urology 1989; 33:185.

Sen SE, Malek RS, Farrow GM, et al: Sarcoma and carcinosarcoma of the bladder in adults. J Urol 1985; 133:29.

Sheinfeld J, Reuter VE, Melamed MR, et al: Enhanced bladder cancer detection with the Lewis X antigen as a marker of neoplastic transformation. J Urol 1990; 143:285.

Sheinfeld J, Reuter VE, Sarkis AS, Cordon-Cardo C: Blood group antigens in normal and neoplastic urothelium. J Cell Biochem 1992; 161(suppl):50.

Sheldon CA, Clayman RV, Gonzalez R, et al: Malignant urachal lesions. J Urol 1984; 131:1.

Shiao Y-H, Chen VW, Scheer WD, et al: Racial disparity in the association of p53 gene alterations with breast cancer survival. Cancer Res 1995; 55:1485.

Shinka T, Hirano A, Uekado Y, et al: Intravesical bacillus Calmette-Guerin treatment for superficial bladder tumors. Br J Urol 1989; 63:610.

Shipley WU: Cisplatin and external beam radiation in patients with invasive bladder cancer. Int J Radiat Oncol Biophys 1989; 16:1649.

Shipley WU, Cummings KB, Coombs LJ: 4,000 Rad pre-op radiation followed by prompt radial cystectomy for invasive bladder cancer: A prospective study of patient tolerance and pathologic downstaging. J Urol 1982; 127:48.

Shipley WU, Kaufman SD, Prout GR Jr: Intraoperative radiation therapy in patients with bladder cancer: A review of techniques allowing improved tumor doses and providing high cure rates without loss of bladder function. Cancer 1987a; 60:1485.

Shipley WU, Kaufman SD, Prout GR Jr: The role of radiation therapy and chemotherapy in the treatment of invasive carcinoma of the urinary bladder. Semin Oncol 1988; 15:390.

Shipley WU, Prout GR, Einstein AB: Treatment of invasive bladder cancer by cisplatin and radiation in patients unsuited for surgery. JAMA 1987b; 258:931.

Shultz PK, Herr HW, Zhang Z-F, et al: Neoadjuvant chemotherapy for invasive bladder cancer: Prognostic factors for survival of patients treated with MVAC with five year follow-up. J Clin Oncol 1994; 12:1394.

Sidransky D, Frost P, Von Eschenbach A, et al: Clonal origin of bladder cancer. N Engl J Med 1992; 326:737.

Sidransky D, Messing E: Molecular genetics and biochemical mechanisms in bladder cancer. Urol Clin North Am 1992; 19:629.

Sidransky D, Von Eschenbach A, Tsai Y, et al: Identification of p53 gene mutations in bladder cancer and urine samples. Science (Washington) 1991; 252:706.

Silverberg E: Cancer statistics 1985. Cancer J Clin 1985; 35:19.

Silverman DT, Levin LI, Hoover RN, et al: Occupational risks of bladder cancer in the United States: I. White men. J Natl Cancer Inst 1989a; 81:1472.

Silverman DT, Levin LI, Hoover RN: Occupational risks of bladder cancer in the United States: II. Nonwhite men. J Natl Cancer Inst 1989b; 81:1480.

Skinner DG: Management of invasive bladder cancer: A meticulous pelvic node dissection can make a difference. J Urol 1982; 128:34.

Skinner DG, Boyd SD, Lieskovsky G: An update on the Kock pouch for continent urinary diversion. Urol Clin North Am 1987; 14:789.

Skinner DG, Crawford ED, Kaufman JJ: Complications of radical cystectomy for carcinoma of the bladder. J Urol 1980; 123:640.

Skinner DG, Daniels JR, Russell CA, et al: The role of adjuvant chemotherapy following cystectomy for invasive bladder cancer: A prospective comparative trial. J Urol 1991; 145:459.

Skinner DG, Lieskovsky G: Contemporary cystectomy with pelvic node dissection compared to preoperative radiation therapy plus cystectomy in management of invasive bladder cancer. J Urol 1984; 131:1069.

Skinner DG, Lieskovsky G, Boyd SD: Technique of creation of a continent internal ileal reservoir (Kock pouch) for urinary diversion. Urol Clin North Am 1984; 11:741.

Slack NH, Prout GR Jr: The heterogeneity of invasive bladder carcinoma and different responses to treatment. J Urol 1980; 123:644.

Slattery ML, West DW, Robinson LM: Fluid intake and bladder cancer in Utah. Int J Cancer 1988; 42:17.

Smith H, Weaver D, Barjenbruch O, et al: Routine excretory urography in follow-up of superficial transitional cell carcinoma of bladder. Urology 1989; 34:193.

Smith JA Jr: Current concepts in laser treatment of bladder cancer. Prog Clin Biol Res 1989; 303:463.

Smith JA Jr, Dixon JA: Argon laser phototherapy of superficial transitional cell carcinoma of the bladder. J Urol 1984; 131:655.

Smith JA Jr, Whitmore WF Jr: Regional lymph node metastases from bladder cancer. J Urol 1981a; 126:591.

Smith JA Jr, Whitmore WF Jr: Salvage cystectomy for bladder cancer after failure of definitive irradiation. J Urol 1981b; 125:643.

Sohn M, Neuerburg J, Teufl F, et al: Gadolinium-enhanced magnetic resonance imaging in the staging of urinary bladder neoplasms. Urol Int 1990; 45:142.

Soloway MS: Intravesical and systemic chemotherapy in the management of superficial bladder cancer. Urol Clin North Am 1984; 11:623.

Soloway MS: Learning to integrate systemic chemotherapy into a treatment plan for patients with advanced bladder cancer. J Urol 1985; 133:440.

Soloway MS, Einstein A, Corder MP, et al: A comparison of cisplatin and the combination of cisplatin and cyclophosphamide in advanced urothelial cancer: A National Bladder Cancer Collaborative Group A Study. Cancer 1983; 52:767.

Solsona E, Iborra I, Ricos JV, et al: Feasibility of transurethral resection for muscle infiltrating carcinoma of the bladder: Prospective study. J Urol 1992; 147:1513.

Sonneveld P, Kurth KH, Hagemyer A, et al: Secondary hematologic neoplasm after intravesical chemotherapy for superficial bladder carcinoma. Cancer 1990; 65:23.

Sontag JM: Experimental identification of genitourinary carcinogens. Urol Clin North Am 1980; 7:803.

Spencer JR, Filmer RB: Malignancy associated with urinary tract reconstruction using enteric segments. In Lepor H, Lawson RK, eds: Urologic Oncology V. Norwell MA, Kluwer Academic Publishers, 1991, pp 75–87.

Sporn MB, Roberts AB: Transforming growth factor-β: Multiple actions and potential clinical applications. JAMA 1989; 262:938.

Sporn MB, Squire RA, Brown CC, Smith JM: 13-cis retinoic acid: Inhibition of bladder carcinogenesis in the rat. Science 1977; 195:487.

Spruck CH III, Ohneseit PF, Gonzales-Zulueta M, et al: Two molecular pathways to transitional cell carcinoma of the bladder. Cancer Res 1994; 54:784.

Spruck CH, Rideout WM, Olumi AF, et al: Distinct pattern of p53 mutations in bladder cancer: Relationship to tobacco usage. Cancer Res 1993; 53:1162.

Stadler WM: Molecular events in the initiation and progression of bladder cancer. Int J Oncol 1993; 3:549.

Stadler WM, Sherman J, Bohlander SK, et al: Homozygous deletions within chromosomal bands 9p21–22 in bladder cancer. Cancer Res 1994; 54:2060.

Stark GL, Feddersen R, Lowe BA, et al: Inflammatory pseudotumor (pseudosarcoma) of the bladder. J Urol 1989; 141:610.

Steffens J, Nagel R: Tumours of the renal pelvis and ureter: Observations in 170 patients. Br J Urol 1988; 61:277.

Steg A, Leleu C, Debre B, et al: Systemic bacillus Calmette-Guerin infection: "BCGitis" in patients treated by intravesical bacillus Calmette-Guerin therapy for bladder cancer. Eur Urol 1989; 16:161.

Stein JP, Stenzl A, Esrig D, et al: Lower urinary tract reconstruction following cystectomy in women using the Kock ileal reservoir with bilateral ureteroileal urethrostomy: Initial clinical experience. J Urol 1994; 152:1404.

Steinbeck G, Plato N, Norell SE, et al: Urothelial cancer and some industry-related chemicals: An evaluation of the epidemiologic literature. Am J Ind Med 1990; 17:371.

Sternberg CN, Yagoda A, Scher HI, et al: Preliminary results of M-VAC (methotrexate, vinblastine, doxorubicin and cisplatin) for transitional cell carcinoma of the urothelium. J Urol 1985; 133:403.

Sternberg CN, Yagoda A, Scher HI, et al: M-VAC (methotrexate, vinblastine, doxorubicin and cisplatin) for advanced transitional cell carcinoma of the urothelium. J Urol 1988; 139:461.

Sternberg CN, Yagoda A, Scher HI, et al: Methotrexate, doxorubicin and cisplatin for advanced transitional cell carcinoma of the urothelium: Efficacy and patterns of response and relapse. Cancer 1989; 64:2448.

Stockle M, Meyenburg W, Wellek S, et al: Adjuvant polychemotherapy of nonorgan-confined bladder cancer after radical cystectomy revisited: Long-term results of a controlled prospective study and further clinical experience. J Urol 1995; 153:47.

Stricker PD, Grant AB, Hosken BM, et al: Topical mitomycin C therapy for carcinoma of the bladder. J Urol 1987; 138:1164.

Studer UE, Ackermann D, Casanova GA, et al: Three years experience with an ileal low pressure bladder substitute. Br J Urol 1989; 63:43.

Studer UE, Bacchi M, Biedermann C, et al: Adjuvant cisplatin chemotherapy following cystectomy for bladder cancer: Results of a prospective randomized trial. J Urol 1994; 152:81.

Sullivan JW, Grabstald H, Whitmore WF Jr: Complications of ureteroileal conduit with radical cystectomy: Review of 336 cases. J Urol 1980; 124:797.

Sumiyoshi Y, Yokota K, Akeyama M, et al: Intraarterial doxorubicin chemotherapy in combination with low dose radiotherapy for the treatment of locally advanced transitional cell carcinoma of the bladder. J Urol 1994; 152:362.

Swanson DA, Liles A, Zagars GK: Preoperative irradiation and radical cystectomy for stages T2 and T3 squamous cell carcinoma of the bladder. J Urol 1990; 143:37.

Swanson PE, Frierson HF, Wick MR: c-erbB-2 (HER-2/neu) oncopeptide immunoreactivity in localized, high grade transitional cell carcinoma of the bladder. Mod Pathol 1992; 5:531.

Swanson TE, Brooks R, Pearse H, et al: Small cell carcinoma of the urinary bladder. Urology 1988; 32:558.

Swartz DA, Johnson DE, Ayala AG, et al: Bladder leiomyosarcoma: A review of 10 cases with 5-year follow-up. J Urol 1985; 133:200.

Sweeney P, Kursh ED, Resnick MI: Partial cystectomy. Urol Clin North Am 1992; 19:701.

Tannock I, Gospodarowicz M, Connolly J, et al: M-VAC (methotrexate, vinblastine, doxorubicin and cisplatin) chemotherapy for transitional cell carcinoma: The Princess Margaret Hospital experience. J Urol 1989; 142:289.

Tavares NJ, Demas BE, Hricak H: MR imaging of bladder neoplasms: Correlation with pathologic staging. Urol Radiol 1990; 12:27.

Teran AZ, Gambrell RD Jr: Leiomyoma of the bladder: Case report and review of the literature. Int J Fertil 1989; 34:289.

Terrell RB, Cheville JC, See WA, Cohen MB: Histopathologic features and p53 nuclear protein staining as predictors of survival and tumor recurrence in patients with transitional cell carcinoma of renal pelvis. J Urol 1995; 154:1342.

Teulings FAG, Peters HA, Hop WCJ, et al: A new aspect of the urinary excretion of tryptophan metabolites in patients with cancer of the bladder. Int J Cancer 1978; 21:140.

Thériault GP, Tremblay CG, Armstrong BG: Bladder cancer screening among primary aluminum production workers in Quebec. J Occup Med 1990; 32:869.

Theuer CP, Fitzgerald DJ, Pastan I: A recombinant form of pseudomonas exotoxin A containing transforming growth factor alpha near its carboxyl terminus for the treatment of bladder cancer. J Urol 1993; 149:1626.

Thomas DJ, Robinson MC, Charlton R, et al: p53 expression ploidy and progression in pT1 transitional cell carcinoma of the bladder. Br J Urol 1994; 73:533.

Thompson RA, Campbell EW Jr, Kramer HC, et al: Late invasive recurrence despite long-term surveillance for superficial bladder cancer. J Urol 1993; 149:1010.

Thuroff JW, Alken P, Riedmiller H, et al: The Mainz pouch (mixed augmentation, ileum and cecum) for bladder augmentation and continent diversion. J Urol 1986; 137:17.

Tinakos DG, Mellon K, Anderson JJ, et al: c-jun oncogene expression in transectional cell carcinoma. Br J Urol 1994; 74:757.

Torrence RJ, Kavoussi LR, Catalona WJ, et al: Prognostic factors in patients treated with intravesical bacillus Calmette-Guerin for superficial bladder cancer. J Urol 1988; 139:941.

Torres H, Bennett MJ: Neurofibromatosis of the bladder: Case report and review of the literature. J Urol 1966; 96:910.

Torti F, Shortliffe LD, Williams RD, et al: Alpha interferon and superficial bladder cancer: A Northern California Oncology Group Study. J Clin Oncol 1988; 6:476.

Tribukait B: Flow cytometry in assessing the clinical aggressiveness of genitourinary neoplasms. World J Urol 1987; 5:108.

Tricker AR, Mostafa MH, Spiegelhalder B, et al: Urinary excretion of nitrate, nitrite and N-nitroso compounds in schistosomiasis and bilharzial bladder cancer patients. Carcinogenesis 1989; 10:547.

Trott PA, Edwards L: Comparison of bladder washings and urine cytology in the diagnosis of bladder cancer. J Urol 1973; 110:664.

Tsai YC, Nichols PW, Hiti AL, et al: Allelic losses of chromosomes 9, 11, and 17 in human bladder cancer. Cancer Res 1990; 50:44.

Tsukamoto T, Lieber MM: Sarcomas of the kidney, urinary bladder, prostate, spermatic cord paratestis and testis in adults. In Raaf JH, ed: Management of Soft Tissue Sarcomas. Chicago, Year Book Medical Publishers, 1991.

Tuttle TM, Williams GM, Marshall FF: Evidence for cyclophosphamide-induced transitional cell carcinoma in a renal transplant patient. J Urol 1988; 140:1009.

Tyler DE: Stratified squamous epithelium in the vesical trigone and urethra: Findings correlated with menstrual cycle and age. Am J Anat 1962; 111:319.

Underwood M, Bartlett J, Reeves J, et al: c-erbB2 gene amplification: A molecular marker of recurrent bladder tumors? Cancer Res 1995; 55:2422.

Utz DC, Farrow GM: Carcinoma in situ of the urinary tract. Urol Clin North Am 1984; 11:735.

Utz DC, Hanash KA, Farrow GM: The plight of the patient with carcinoma in situ of the bladder. J Urol 1970; 103:160.

Utz DC, Schmitz SE, Fugelso PD, et al: A clinicopathologic evaluation of partial cystectomy for carcinoma of the urinary bladder. Cancer 1973; 32:1075.

Uyama T, Moriwaki S: Carcinosarcoma of urinary bladder. Urology 1981; 18:191.

van der Werf-Messing B: Carcinoma of the bladder treated by suprapubic radium implants: The value of additional external irradiation. Eur J Urol 1969; 5:277.

van der Werf-Messing B: Carcinoma of the bladder treated by preoperative radiation followed by cystectomy. Cancer 1973; 32:1084.

van der Werf-Messing BHP: Carcinoma of the urinary bladder treated by interstitial radiotherapy. Urol Clin North Am 1984; 11:659.

van der Werf-Messing B, Mennen RS, Hopp WCJ: Cancer of the urinary bladder category T2, T3, NX, M0 treated by interstitial radium implant: Second report. Int J Radiat Oncol Biophys 1983; 9:481.

van der Werf-Messing BH, van Putten WL: Carcinoma of the urinary bladder category T2, T3, NX, M0 treated by 40 Gy external irradiation followed by cesium 137 implant at reduced dose (50%). Int J Radiat Oncol Biol Phys 1989; 16:369.

van Helsdingen PJ, Rikken CH, Sleeboom HP, et al: Mitomycin C resorption following repeated intravesical instillations using different instillation times. Urol Int 1988; 43:42.

Vanni R, Peretti D, Scarpa RM, et al: Cytogenetics of bladder cancer: Rearrangements of the short arm of chromosome 11. Cancer Detect Prev 1987; 10:401.

Vargas AD, Mendez R: Leiomyoma of the bladder. Urology 1983; 21:308.

Vaughan AT, Anderson P, Wallace MA, et al: Local control of T2/3 transitional cell carcinoma of bladder is correlated to differences in DNA supercoiling: Evidence for two discrete tumor populations. Cancer Res 1993; 53:2300.

Vekemans K, Vanneste A, Van Oyen P, et al: Postoperative spindle cell nodule of bladder. Urology 1990; 35:342.

Vieweg J, Whitmore WF, Herr HW, et al: Thorough pelvic lymphadenectomy and radical cystectomy of lymph node positive bladder cancer: The Memorial Sloan-Kettering Cancer Center experience. Cancer 1994; 73:3020.

Vincente-Rodriguez J, Chechile G, Algaba F, et al: Value of random endoscopic biopsy of the diagnosis of bladder carcinoma in situ. Eur Urol 1987; 13:150.

Vinnicombe J, Abercrombie GF: Total cystectomy—a review. Br J Urol 1978; 50:488.

Viola MV, Fromowitz F, Oravez S, et al: Ras oncogene p21 expression is increased in premalignant lesions of high grade bladder carcinomas. J Exp Med 1985; 161:1213.

Visvanathan KV, Pocock RD, Summerhayes IC: Preferential and novel activation of H-ras in human bladder. Oncogene Res 1988; 3:77.

Vock P, Haertel M, Fuchs WA, et al: Computed tomography in staging of carcinoma of the urinary bladder. Br J Urol 1982; 54:158.

Vogelstein B: A deadly inheritance. Nature (London) 1990; 348:681.

Vogelzang NJ, Meir JA, Awan AM, et al: Methotrexate, vinblastine, doxorubicin, and cisplatin followed by radiotherapy or surgery for muscle invasive bladder cancer: The University of Chicago experience. J Urol 1993; 149:753.

Voges GE, Tauschke E, Stockle M, et al: Computerized tomography: An unreliable method for accurate staging of bladder tumors in patients who are candidates for radical cystectomy. J Urol 1989; 142:972.

Wahlqvist L: Chemical carcinogenesis—a review and personal observations with special reference to the role of tobacco and phenacetin in the production of urothelial tumors. In Pavone-Maculoso M, et al, eds: Bladder Tumors and Other Topics in Urological Oncology. New York, Plenum Press, 1980, p 47.

Wajsman Z, Klimberg IW: Treatment alternatives for invasive bladder cancer. Semin Surg Oncol 1989; 5:272.

Waldman FM, Carroll PR, Cohen MB, et al: 5-Bromodeoxyuridine incorporation and PCNA expression as measures of cell proliferation in transitional cell carcinoma of the urinary bladder. Mod Pathol 1993; 6:20.

Waldman FM, Carroll PR, Kerschmann R, et al: Centromeric copy number of chromosome 7 is strongly correlated with tumor grade and labeling index in human bladder cancer. Cancer Res 1991; 51:3807.

Walker L, Liston T-B, Lloyd Davies RW: Does flexible cystoscopy miss more tumours than rod-lens examination? Br J Urol 1993; 72:449.

Wallace DM, Bloom HJG: The management of deeply infiltrating (T₃) bladder carcinoma: Controlled trial of radical radiotherapy and radical cystectomy (first report). Br J Urol 1976; 48:587.

Walzer Y, Soloway MS: Should the follow-up of patients with bladder cancer include routine excretory urography? J Urol 1983; 130:672.

Wan J, Grossman HB: Bladder carcinoma in patients age 40 years or younger. Cancer 1989; 64:178.

Waples MJ, Messing EM: The management of stage T₁, grade 3 transitional cell carcinoma of the bladder. In Lytton B, ed: Advances in Urology, Vol 5. St. Louis, Mosby-Year Book, 1992, p 33.

Ward E, Halperin W, Thun M: Screening workers exposed to 4,4¹-methylenebis (2 chloroanaline) for bladder cancer by cystoscopy. J Occup Med 1990; 32:865.

Waterhouse J, Muir C, Shanmugartanam K, et al: Cancer Incidence in Five Continents, Vol 4. Lyon, International Agency for Research on Cancer, 1982.

Weiner JS, Liu ET, Walther PJ: Oncogenic human papillomavirus type 16 is associated with squamous cell carcinoma of the male urethra. Cancer Res 1992; 52:5018.

Weiner JS, Walther PJ: A high association of oncogenic human papillomaviruses with carcinomas of the female urethra: Polymerase chain reaction–based analysis of multiple histological types. J Urol 1994; 151:49.

Weinstein RS, Alroy J, Farrow GM, et al: Blood group isoantigen deletion in carcinoma in situ of the urinary bladder. Cancer 1979; 43:661.

Weinstein RS, Miller AW III, Pauli BV: Carcinoma in situ: Comment on the pathobiology of a paradox. Urol Clin North Am 1980; 7:523.

Weldon TE, Soloway MS: Susceptibility of urothelium to neoplastic cellular implantation. Urology 1975; 5:824.

Wenderoth UK, Bachor R, Egghart G, et al: The ileal neobladder: Experience and results of more than 100 consecutive cases. J Urol 1990; 143:492.

Werness BA, Levine AJ, Howley PM: Association of human papilloma virus types 16 and 18 E6 proteins with p53. Science 1990; 248:76.

West WH, Taner W, Yannelli JR, et al: Constant infusion recombinant interleukin 2 in adoptive immunotherapy of bladder cancer. N Engl J Med 1987; 316:898.

Wheeless LL, Badalament RA, deVere White RW, et al: Consensus review of the clinical utility of DNA cytometry in bladder cancer: Report of the DNA Cytometry Consensus Conference. Cytometry 1993; 14:478.

Wheeless LL, Morreale JF, O'Connell MJ, et al: Predictive value of aberrations of chromosome 9 following bacillus Calmette-Guerin (BCG) therapy in bladder cancer. J Urol 1996, submitted.

Wheeless LL, Reeder JR, Han R, et al: Bladder irrigation specimens—assayed by fluorescence in situ hybridization to interphase nuclei. Cytometry 1994; 17:319.

Whitmore WF Jr, Batata M: Status of integrated irradiation and cystectomy for bladder cancer. Urol Clin North Am 1985; 11:681.

Whitmore WF Jr, Batata MA, Hilaris BS, et al: A comparative study of two preoperative radiation regimens with cystectomy for bladder cancer. Cancer 1977; 40:1077.

Wick MR, Brown BA, Young RH, et al: Spindle-cell proliferations of the urinary tract: An immunohistochemical study. Am J Surg Pathol 1988; 12:379.

Wiener DP, Koss LG, Sablay B, et al: The prevalence and significance of Brunn's nests, cystitis cystica and squamous metaplasia in normal bladders. J Urol 1979; 122:317.

Wijkstrom H, Edsmyr F, Lundh B: The value of preoperative classification according to the TNM system. Eur Urol 1984; 10:101.

Wijkstrom H, Tribukait B: Deoxyribonucleic acid flow cytometry in predicting response to radical radiotherapy of bladder cancer. J Urol 1990; 144:646.

Williams RD: Intravesical interferon alpha in the treatment of superficial bladder cancer. Semin Oncol 1988; 15:10.

Williamson M, Elder PA, Shaw ME, Knowles MA: p16 (CDKN2) is a major deletion target at 9p21 in bladder cancer. Hum Mol Genet 1995; 4:1569.

Wilson TM, Fauver HE, Weigel JW: Leiomyosarcoma of urinary bladder. Urology 1979; 13:565.

Winkler HZ, Nativ O, Hosaka Y, et al: Nuclear deoxyribonucleic acid ploidy in squamous cell bladder cancer. J Urol 1989; 141:297.

Wishnow KI, Dmochowski R: Pelvic recurrence after radical cystectomy without preoperative radiation. J Urol 1988; 140:42.

Wishnow KI, Johnson DE, Dmochowski R, et al: Ileal conduit in era of systemic chemotherapy. Urology 1989; 33:358.

Wishnow KI, Johnson DE, Ro JY, et al: Incidence, extent, and location of unsuspected pelvic lymph node metastases in patients undergoing radical cystectomy for bladder cancer. J Urol 1987; 137:408.

Wishnow KI, Levinson AK, Johnson DE, et al: Stage B (P₂/₃ₐ/N₀) transitional cell carcinoma of the bladder highly curable by radical cystectomy. Urology 1992; 39:12.

Wishnow KI, Ro JY: Importance of early treatment of transitional cell carcinoma of prostate duct. Urology 1988; 32:11.

Witte R, Loehrer P, Dreicer R, et al: Ifosfamide in advanced urothelial carcinoma: An ECOG trial. Proc Am Soc Clin Oncol 1993; 12:230.

Wolf H: Studies on the role of tryptophan metabolites in the genesis of bladder cancer. Acta Clin Scand 1973; 433(suppl):154.

Wolf H, Hojgaard K: Urothelial dysplasia concomitant with bladder tumors as a determinant factor for future new recurrences. Lancet 1983; 2:134.

Wood DP, Montie JE, Pontes JE, et al: The role of magnetic resonance imaging in the staging of bladder carcinoma. J Urol 1988; 140:741.

Wood DP, Montie JE, Pontes JE, et al: Transitional cell carcinoma of the prostate in cystoprostatectomy specimens removed for bladder cancer. J Urol 1989; 141:346.

Woodhouse CRJ, Kallette MJ, Bloom HJG: Percutaneous renal surgery and local radiotherapy in the management of renal pelvic transitional cell carcinoma. Br J Urol 1986; 58:245.

Wright C, Mellin K, Johnston P, et al: Expression of p53, c-erbB-2 and the epidermal growth factor receptor in transitional cell carcinoma of the human urinary bladder. Br J Cancer 1991; 63:967.

Yagoda A: Chemotherapy for advanced urothelial cancer. Semin Urol 1983; 1:60.

Yalla AV, Ivker M, Burros HM, et al: Cystitis glandularis with perivesical lipomatosis: Frequent association of two unusual proliferative conditions. Urology 1975; 5:383.

Younes M, Sussman J, True L: The usefulness of the level of the muscularis mucosae in the staging of invasive transitional cell carcinoma of the urinary bladder. Cancer 1990; 66:543.

Young RH: Carcinosarcoma of the urinary bladder. Cancer 1987; 59:1333.

Young RH, Scully RE: Pseudosarcomatous lesions of the urinary bladder, prostate gland, and urethra: A report of three cases and review of the literature. Arch Pathol Lab Med 1987; 111:354.

Young RH, Wick MR, Mills SE: Sarcomatoid carcinoma of the urinary bladder: A clinicopathologic analysis of 12 cases and review of the literature. Am J Clin Pathol 1988; 90:653.

Yui Y, Tanisky MA, Bischoff FZ, et al: Wild-type p53 restores cell cycle control and inhibits gene amplification in cells with mutant p53 alleles. Cell 1992; 70:937.

Zincke H, Garbeff PJ, Beahrs JR: Upper urinary tract transitional cell cancer after radical cystectomy for bladder cancer. J Urol 1984; 131:50.

Zincke H, Patterson DE, Utz DC, Benson RC Jr: Pelvic lymphadenectomy and radical cystectomy for transitional cell carcinoma of the bladder with pelvic node disease. Br J Urol 1985; 57:156.

Zincke H, Utz DC, Taylor WF, et al: Influence of thiotepa and doxorubicin instillation at time of transurethral surgical treatment of bladder cancer on tumor recurrence: A prospective, randomized, double-blind, controlled trial. J Urol 1983; 129:505.

Zuk RJ, Baithun SI, Martin JE, et al: The immunocytochemical demonstration of basement membrane deposition in transitional cell carcinoma of the bladder. Virchows Arch [A] 1989; 414:447.

Zyzak LL, MacDonald LM, Batova A, et al: Increased levels and constitutive tyrosine phosphorylation of the epidermal growth factor receptor contribute to autonomous growth of human papillomavirus type 16 immortalized human keratinocytes. Cell Growth Differ 1994; 5:537.

Urothelial Tumors of the Renal Pelvis and Ureter

Abercrombie GF, Eardley I, Payne SR, et al: Modified nephroureterectomy: Long-term follow-up with particular reference to subsequent bladder tumours. Br J Urol 1988; 61:198.

Amar AD, Das S: Upper urinary tract transitional cell carcinoma in patients with bladder carcinoma and associated vesicoureteral reflux. J Urol 1985; 133:468.

Anderstrom C, Johansson SL, Pettersson S, et al: Carcinoma of the ureter: A clinicopathologic study of 49 cases. J Urol 1989; 142:280.

Annual Cancer Statistics Review: Including Cancer Trends: 1950–1985. Bethesda, MD, National Cancer Institute, U.S. Department of Health and Human Services, NIH Publication no. 88-2789, 1987.

Babaian RJ, Johnson DE: Primary carcinoma of the ureter. J Urol 1980; 123:357.

Badalament RA, Bennett WF, Bova JG, et al: Computed tomography of primary transitional cell carcinoma of upper urinary tracts. Urology 1992; 40:71.

Badalament RA, O'Toole RV, Kenworthy P, et al: Prognostic factors in patients with primary transitional cell carcinoma of the upper urinary tract. J Urol 1990; 144:859.

Baghdassarian Gatewood OM, Goldman SM, Marshal FF, et al: Computerized tomography in the diagnosis of carcinoma of the kidney. J Urol 1982; 127:876.

Batata MA, Whitmore WF Jr, Milaris BS, et al: Primary carcinoma of the ureter: A prognostic study. Cancer 1975; 35:1626.

Bazeed MA, Scharfe T, Becht E, et al: Local excision of urothelial cancer of the upper urinary tract. Eur Urol 1986; 12:89.

Blacker EJ, Johnson DE, Abdul-Karim FW, et al: Squamous cell carcinoma of renal pelvis. Urology 1985; 25:124.

Blank C, Lissmer L, Kaneti J, et al: Fibroepithelial polyp of the renal pelvis. J Urol, 1987; 137:962.

Bloom NA, Vidone RA, Lytton B: Primary carcinoma of the ureter: A report of 102 new cases. J Urol 1970; 103:590.

Blute ML, Segura JW, Patterson DE, et al: Impact of endourology on diagnosis and management of upper urinary tract urothelial cancer. J Urol 1989; 141:1298.

Blute ML, Tsushima K, Farrow GM, et al: Transitional cell carcinoma of the renal pelvis: Nuclear deoxyribonucleic acid ploidy studied by flow cytometry. J Urol 1988; 140:944.

Blute RD Jr, Gittes RR, Gittes RF: Renal brush biopsy: Survey of indications, techniques and results. J Urol 1981; 126:146.

Bree RL, Schultz SR, Hayes R: Large infiltrating renal transitional cell carcinomas: CT and ultrasound features. J Comput Assist Tomogr 1990; 14:381.

Brenner DW, Schellhammer PF: Upper tract urothelial malignancy after cyclophosphamide therapy: A case report and literature review. J Urol 1987; 137:1226.

Brookland RK, Richter MP: The postoperative irradiation of transitional cell carcinoma of the renal pelvis ureter. J Urol 1985; 133:952.

Byard RW, Bell MEA, Alkan M: Primary carcinosarcoma: A rare cause of unilateral ureteral obstruction. J Urol 1987; 137:732.

Cohen SM, Garland EM, St. John M, et al: Acrolein initiates rat urinary bladder carcinogenesis. Cancer Res 1992; 52:3577.

Corrado F, Ferri C, Mannini D, et al: Transitional cell carcinoma of the upper urinary tract: Evaluation of prognostic factors by histopathology and flow cytometric analysis. J Urol 1991; 145:1159.

Coup AJ: Angiosarcoma of the ureter. Br J Urol 1988; 62:275.

Cozad SC, Smalley SR, Austenfeld M: Adjuvant radiotherapy in high stage transitional cell carcinoma of the renal pelvis and ureter. In J Radiat Oncol Biol Phys 1992; 24:743.

Davis BW, Hough AJ, Gardner WA: Renal pelvic carcinoma: Morphological correlates of metastatic behavior. J Urol 1987; 137:857.

DeKock ML, Breytenbach IH: Local excision and topical thiotepa in the treatment of transitional cell carcinoma of the renal pelvis: A case report. J Urol 1986; 135:566.

DeTorres Mateos JA, Banus Gassol JM, Palou Redorta J, et al: Vesicorenal reflux and upper urinary tract transitional cell carcinoma after transurethral resection of recurrent superficial bladder carcinoma. J Urol 1987; 138:49.

Esrig D, Elmajian D, Groshen S, et al: Accumulation of nuclear p53 and tumor progression in bladder cancer. N Engl J Med 1994; 331:1259.

Essenfeld H, Manivel JC, Benedetto P, et al: Small cell carcinoma of the renal pelvis: A clinicopathological, morphological and immunohistochemical study of 2 cases. J Urol 1990; 144:344.

Fein AB, McClennan BL: Solitary filling defects of the ureter. Semin Roentgenol 1986; 21:201.

Fleming S: Carcinosarcoma (mixed mesodermal tumor) of the ureter. J Urol 1987; 138:1234.

Fraley EE: Cancer of the renal pelvis. In Skinner, DG, deKernion JB, eds: Genitourinary Cancer. Philadelphia, W. B. Saunders, 1978, p 134.

Frischer Z, Waltzer WC, Gonder MJ: Bilateral transitional cell carcinoma of the renal pelvis in the cancer family syndrome. J Urol 1985; 134:1197.

Fujimoto H, Tobisu K, Sakamoto M, et al: Intraductal tumor involvement and renal parenchymal invasion of transitional cell carcinoma in the renal pelvis. J Urol 1995; 153:57.

Gardner RA, Walsh MD, Allen V, et al: Immunohistological expression of p53 in primary pT1 transitional cell bladder cancer in relation to tumor progression. Br J Urol 1994; 73:526.

Geiger J, Fong Q, Fay R: Transitional cell carcinoma of renal pelvis with invasion of renal vein and thrombosis of subhepatic inferior vena cava. Urology 1986; 28:52.

Ghazi MR, Morales PA, Al-Askari S: Primary carcinoma of ureter: Report of 27 new cases. Urology 1979; 14:18.

Gibas Z, Griffin CA, Emanuel BS: Trisomy 7 and i(5p) in a transitional cell carcinoma of the ureter. Cancer Genet Cytogenet 1987; 25:369.

Gill WB, Lu CT, Thomsen S: Retrograde brushing: A new technique for obtaining histologic and cytologic material from ureteral, renal pelvic and renal calyceal lesions. J Urol 1973; 109:573.

Gittes RF: Retrograde brushing and nephroscopy in the diagnosis of upper-tract urothelial cancer. Urol Clin North Am 1984; 11:617.

Godec CJ, Murrah VA: Simultaneous occurrence of transitional cell carcinoma and urothelial adenocarcinoma associated with xanthogranulomatous pyelonephritis. Urology 1985; 26:412.

Grabstald H, Whitmore WF, Melamed MR: Renal pelvic tumors. JAMA 1971; 218:845.

Grace DA, Taylor WN, Taylor JN, et al: Carcinoma of the renal pelvis: A 15-year review. J Urol 1967; 98:566.

Grainger R, Gikas PW, Grossman HB: Urothelial carcinoma occurring within an inverted papilloma of the ureter. J Urol 1990; 143:802.

Greenland JE, Weston PMT, Wallace DMA: Familial transitional cell carcinoma and the Lynch syndrome II. Br J Urol 1993; 72:177.

Grossman HB, Schwartz SL, Konnak JW: Ureteroscopic treatment of urothelial carcinoma of the ureter and renal pelvis. J Urol 1992; 148:275.

Guinan P, Vogelzang NJ, Randozzo R, et al: Renal pelvic cancer: A review of 611 patients treated in Illinois 1975–1985. Urology 1992; 40:393.

Harris AL, Neal DE: Bladder cancer-field versus clonal origin. N Engl J Med 1992; 326:759.

Hatch TR, Hefty TR, Barry JM: Time-related recurrence rates in patients with upper tract transitional cell carcinoma. J Urol 1988; 140:40.

Hawtrey CE: Fifty-two cases of primary ureteral carcinoma: A clinical-pathologic study. J Urol 1971; 105:188.

Heney NM, Nocks BN, Daly JJ, et al: Prognostic factors in carcinoma of the ureter. J Urol 1981; 125:632.

Herr HW: Durable response of a carcinoma in situ of the renal pelvis to topical bacillus Calmette-Guerin. J Urol 1985; 134:531.

Huang A, Low RK, deVere White R: Nephrostomy tract tumor seeding following percutaneous manipulation of a ureteral carcinoma. J Urol 1995; 153:1041.

Huben RP, Mounzer AM, Murphy GP: Tumor grade and stage as prognostic variables in upper tract urothelial tumors. Cancer 1988; 62:2016.

Huffman JL, Bagley DH, Lyon ES, et al: Endoscopic diagnosis and treatment of upper-tract urothelial tumors: A preliminary report. Cancer 1985; 55:1422.

Igel TC, Engen DE, Banks PM, et al: Renal plasmacytoma: Mayo Clinic experience and review of the literature. Urology 1991; 37:385.

Jacobs JA, Ring EJ, Wein AJ: New indications for renal infarction. J Urol 1981; 125:243.

Jensen OM, Knudsen JB, McLaughlin JK, et al: The Copenhagen case-control study of renal pelvis and ureter cancer: Role of smoking and occupational exposures. Int J Cancer 1988; 41:557.

Jensen OM, Knudsen JB, Tomasson H, et al: The Copenhagen case-control study of renal pelvis and ureter cancer: Role of analgesics. Int J Cancer 1989; 44:965.

Jitsukawa S, Nakamura K, Nakayama M, et al: Transitional cell carcinoma of kidney extending into renal vein and inferior vena cava. Urology 1985; 25:310.

Johansson S, Wahlqvist L: A prognostic study of urothelial renal pelvic tumors: Comparison between the prognosis of patients treated with infrafascial nephrectomy and perifascial nephroureterectomy. Cancer 1979; 43:2525.

Johnson DE, Babaian RJ: Conservative management for noninvasive distal ureteral carcinoma. Urology 1979; 13:365.

Kagawa S, Takigawa H, Ghazizadeh M, et al: Immunohistological detection of T antigen and ABH blood group antigens in upper urinary tract tumours. Br J Urol 1985; 57:386.

Kakizoe T, Fujita J, Murase T, et al: Transitional cell carcinoma of the bladder in patients with renal pelvic and ureteral cancer. J Urol 1980; 124:17.

Kenney PJ, Stanley RJ: Computed tomography of ureteral tumors. J Comput Assist Tomogr 1987; 11:102.

Kim YI, Yoon DH, Lee SW, et al: Multicentric papillary adenocarcinoma of the renal pelvis and ureter: Report of a case with ultrastructural study. Cancer 1988; 62:2402.

Kyriakos M, Royce RK: Multiple simultaneous inverted papillomas of the upper urinary tract. Cancer 1989; 63:368.

Lantz EJ, Hattery RR: Diagnostic imaging of urothelial cancer. Urol Clin North Am 1984; 11:567.

Li MK, Cheung WL: Squamous cell carcinoma of the renal pelvis. J Urol 1987; 138:269.

Lipponen PK: Over-expression of p53 nuclear oncoprotein in transitional-cell bladder cancer and its prognostic value. Int J Cancer 1993; 53:365.

Lim DJ, Shattuck MC, Cook WA: Pyelovenous lymphatic migration of transitional cell carcinoma following flexible ureterorenoscopy. J Urol 1993; 149:109.

Lynch HT, Ens JA, Lynch JF: The Lynch syndrome II and urological malignancies. J Urol 1990; 143:24.

Madgar I, Goldwasser B, Czerniak A, et al: Leiomyosarcoma of the ureter. Eur Urol 1988; 14:487.

Mahadevia PA, Karwa GL, Koss LG: Mapping of urothelium in carcinomas of the renal pelvis and ureter: A report of nine cases. Cancer 1983; 51:890.

Mazeman E: Tumours of the upper urinary tract, calyces, renal pelvis and ureter. Eur Urol 1976; 2:120.

McCarron JP Jr, Chasko SB, Gray GF Jr: Systematic mapping of nephroureterectomy specimens removed for urothelial cancer: Pathological findings and clinical correlations. J Urol 1982; 128:243.

McCoy JG, Honda H, Reznicek M, et al: Computerized tomography for detection and staging of localized and pathologically defined upper tract urothelial tumors. J Urol 1991; 146:1500.

McCredie M, Stewart JH, Carter JJ, et al: Phenacetin and papillary necrosis: Independent risk factors for renal pelvic cancer. Kidney Int 1986; 30:81.

McLaughlin JK, Silverman DT, Hsing AW, et al: Cigarette smoking and cancers of the renal pelvis and ureter. Cancer Res 1992; 52:254.

Messing EM: Clinical implications of the expression of epidermal growth factor receptors in human transitional cell carcinoma. Cancer Res 1990; 50:2530.

Messing EM, Hanson P, Ulrich P, et al: Epidermal growth factor—interactions with normal and malignant urothelium: In vivo and in situ studies. J Urol 1987; 138:1329.

Messing EM, Valencourt A. Hematuria screening for bladder cancer. J Occup Med 1990; 32:838.

Milestone B, Freidman AC, Seidmon EJ, et al: Staging of ureteral transitional cell carcinoma by CT and MRI. Urology 1990; 36:346.

Miyakawa A, Tachibana M, Nakashima J, et al: Flow cytometric bromodeoxyuridine/deoxyribonucleic acid bivariate analysis for predicting tumor invasiveness of upper tract urothelial cancer. J Urol 1994; 152:76.

Morrison AS: Advances in the etiology of urothelial cancer. Urol Clin North Am 1984; 11:557.

Mufti GR, Gove JR, Badenoch DF, et al: Transitional cell carcinoma of the renal pelvis and ureter. Br J Urol 1989; 63:135.

Mukamel E, Nissenkorn I, Glanz I, et al: Upper tract tumours in patients with vesico-ureteral reflux and recurrent bladder tumours. Eur Urol 1985; 11:6.

Mullen JB, Kovacs K: Primary carcinoma of the ureteral stump: A case report and a review of the literature. J Urol 1980; 123:113.

Murphy DM, Zincke H, Furlow WL: Primary grade I transitional cell carcinoma of the renal pelvis and ureter. J Urol 1980; 123:629.

Murphy DM, Zincke H, Furlow WL: Management of high grade transitional cell cancer of the upper urinary tract. J Urol 1981; 135:25.

Musselman P, Kay R: The spectrum of urinary tract polyps in children. J Urol 1986; 136:476.

Narumi Y, Sato T, Hor S, et al: Squamous cell carcinoma of the uroepithelium: CT evaluation. Radiology 1989; 173:853.

Nemoto R, Hattori K, Sasaki A, et al: Estimations of the S-phase fraction in situ in transitional cell carcinoma of the renal pelvis and ureter with bromodeoxyuridine labelling. Br J Urol 1989; 64:339.

Nielsen K, Ostri P: Primary tumors of the renal pelvis: Evaluation of clinical and pathological features in a consecutive series of 10 years. J Urol 1988; 140:19.

Nocks BN, Heney NM, Daily JJ, et al: Transitional cell carcinoma of renal pelvis. Urology 1982; 19:472.

Nolan RL, Nickel JC, Froud PJ: Percutaneous endourologic approach for transitional cell carcinoma of the renal pelvis. Urol Radiol 1988; 9:217.

Oldbring J, Glifberg I, Mikulowski P, et al: Carcinoma of the renal pelvis and ureter following bladder carcinoma: Frequency risk factors and clinicopathological findings. J Urol 1989a; 41:1311.

Oldbring J, Hellsten S, Lindholm K, et al: Flow DNA analysis in the characterization of carcinoma of the renal pelvis and ureter. Cancer 1989b; 64:2141.

Orihuela E, Smith AD: Percutaneous treatment of transitional cell carcinoma of the upper urinary tract. Urol Clin North Am 1988; 15:425.

Orphali SL, Shols GW, Hagewood T, et al: Familial transitional cell carcinoma of renal pelvis and upper ureter. Urology 1986; 27:394.

Palvio DH, Andersen JC, Falk E: Transitional cell tumor of the renal pelvis and ureter associated with capillarosclerosis indicating analgesic abuse. Cancer 1987; 59:972.

Petersen RO: Urologic Pathology, 2nd ed. Philadelphia, J. B. Lippincott, 1992.

Petkovic SD: Epidemiology and treatment of renal pelvic and ureteral tumors. J Urol 1975; 114:858.

Powder JR, Mosberg WH, Pierpoint RZ: Bilateral primary carcinoma of the ureter: Topical and ureteral thiotepa. J Urol 1984; 132:349.

Radovanovic Z, Krajinovic S, Jankovic S, et al: Family history of cancer among cases of upper urothelial tumours in the Balkan nephropathy area. J Cancer Res Clin Oncol 1985; 110:181.

Ramsey JC, Soloway MS: Instillation of bacillus Calmette-Guerin into the renal pelvis of a solitary kidney for the treatment of transitional cell carcinoma. J Urol 1990; 143:1220.

Renfer LG, Kelley J, Belville WD: Inverted papilloma of the urinary tract: Histogenesis, recurrence, and associated malignancy. J Urol 1988; 140:832.

Resseguie LT, Nobrega FT, Farrow GM, et al: Epidemiology of renal and ureteral cancer in Rochester, Minnesota, 1950–1974, with special reference to clinical and pathologic features. Mayo Clin Proc 1978; 53:503.

Ross RK, Paganini-Hill A, Landolph J, et al: Analgesics, cigarette smoking, and other risk factors for cancer of the renal pelvis and ureter. Cancer Res 1989; 49:1045.

Sandberg AA, Berger CS, Haddad FS, et al: Chromosome change in transitional cell carcinoma of ureter. Cancer Genet Cytogenet 1986; 19:335.

Sarkis AS, Dalbagni G, Cordon-Cardo C, et al: Association of p53 nuclear overexpression and tumor progression in carcinoma in situ of the bladder. J Urol 1994; 152:388.

Sarnacki CT, McCormack LJ, Kiser WS, et al: Urinary cytology and the clinical diagnosis of urinary tract malignancy: A clinicopathologic study of 1,400 patients. J Urol 1971; 106:761.

Schemeller NT, Hofstetter AG: Laser treatment of ureteral tumors. J Urol 1989; 141:840.

Schultz RE, Boyle DE: Inverted papilloma of renal pelvis associated with contralateral ureteral malignancy and bladder recurrence. J Urol 1988; 139:111.

Segura JW: Ureteroscopic treatment of urothelial carcinoma of the ureter and renal pelvis (Editorial). J Urol 1992; 148:277.

Sheline M, Amendola MA, Pollack HM, et al: Fluoroscopically guided retrograde brush biopsy in the diagnosis of transitional cell carcinoma of the upper urinary tract: Results in 45 patients. AJR 1989; 153:313.

Shinka T, Uekado Y, Aoshi H, et al: Occurrence of uroepithelial tumors of the upper urinary tract after the initial diagnosis of bladder cancer. J Urol 1988; 140:745.

Skinner DG, Daniels JR, Russell CA, et al: The role of adjuvant chemotherapy following cystectomy for invasive bladder cancer: A prospective comparative trial. J Urol 1991; 145:459.

Smith AY, Orihuela E, Crowley AR: Percutaneous management of renal pelvic tumors: A treatment option in selected cases. J Urol 1987a; 137:852.

Smith AY, Vitale PJ, Lowe BA, et al: Treatment of superficial papillary transitional cell carcinoma of the ureter by vesicoureteral reflux of mitomycin C. J Urol 1987b; 138:1231.

Spiessl B, Beahrs OH, Hermanek P, et al: Renal pelvis and ureter. *In* Spiessl B, Beahrs OH, Hermanek P, et al, eds: UICC TNM Atlas Illustrated Guide to the TNM/p TNM Classification of Malignant Tumours. Berlin, Springer-Verlag, 1989, p 260.

Spires SE, Banks ER, Cibull ML, et al: Adenocarcinoma of renal pelvis. Arch Pathol Lab Med 1993; 117:1156.

Steffens J, Nagel R: Tumours of the renal pelvis and ureter: Observations in 170 patients. Br J Urol 1988; 61:277.

Stein A, Sova Y, Lurie M, et al: Adenocarcinoma of the renal pelvis: Report of two cases, one with simultaneous transitional cell carcinoma of the bladder. Urol Int 1988; 43:299.

Stockle M, Meyenburg W, Wellek S, et al: Adjuvant polychemotherapy of nonorgan-confined bladder cancer after radical cystectomy revisited: Long-term results of a controlled prospective study and further clinical experience. J Urol 1995; 153:47.

Stower MJ, MacIver AG, Gingell JC, et al: Inverted papilloma of the ureter with malignant change. Br J Urol 1990; 65:13.

Streem SB, Pontes JE, Novick AC, et al: Ureteropyeloscopy in the evaluation of upper tract filling defects. J Urol 1986; 136:388.

Studer UE, Casanova G, Kraft R, et al: Percutaneous bacillus Calmette-Guerin perfusion of the upper urinary tract for carcinoma in situ. J Urol 1989; 142:975.

Tannock I, Gospodarowicz M, Connolly J, et al: M-VAC (methotrexate, vinblastine, doxorubicin and cisplatin) chemotherapy for transitional cell carcinoma: The Princess Margaret Hospital experience. J Urol 1989; 142:28.

Tasca A, Zattoni F: The case for a percutaneous approach to transitional cell carcinoma of the renal pelvis. J Urol 1990; 143:902.

Terrell RB, Cheville JC, See WA, Cohen MB: Histopathologic features and p53 nuclear protein staining as predictors of survival and tumor recurrence in patients with transitional cell carcinoma of renal pelvis. J Urol 1995; 154:1342.

Thomas DJ, Robinson MC, Charlton R, et al: p53 expression, ploidy and progression in pT1 transitional cell carcinoma of the bladder. Br J Urol 1994; 73:533.

Tomera KM, Leary FJ, Zincke H: Pyeloscopy in ureter tumors. J Urol 1982; 127:1088.

Varela-Duran J, Urdiales-Viedma M, Taboada-Blanco F, et al: Neurofibroma of the ureter. J Urol 1987; 138:1425.

Vest SA: Conservative surgery in certain benign tumors of the ureter. J Urol 1945; 53:97.

Vet JAM, Bringuier PP, Poddighe PJ, et al: p53 mutations have no additional prognostic value over stage in bladder cancer. Br J Cancer 1994; 70:496.

Wallace DMA, Wallace DM, Whitfield HN, et al: The late results of conservative surgery for upper tract urothelial carcinomas. Br J Urol 1981; 53:537.

Woodhouse CRJ, Kallette MJ, Bloom HJG: Percutaneous renal surgery and local radiotherapy in the management of renal pelvic transitional cell carcinoma. Br J Urol 1986; 58:245.

Zaitoon MM: Leiomyoma of ureter. Urology 1986; 28:50.

Ziegelbaum M, Novick AC, Streem SB, et al: Conservative surgery for transitional cell carcinoma of the renal pelvis. J Urol 1987; 138:1146.

Zincke H, Aguilo JJ, Farrow GM, et al: Significance of urinary cytology in the early detection of transitional cell cancer of the upper urinary tract. J Urol 1976; 166:781.

Zincke H, Neves RJ: Feasibility of conservative surgery for transitional cell cancer of the upper urinary tract. Urol Clin North Am 1984; 11:717.

Zoretic S, Gonzales J: Primary carcinoma of the ureters. Urology 1983; 21:354.

Zungri E, Chechile G, Algaba F, et al: Treatment of transitional cell carcinoma of the ureter: Is the controversy justified? Eur Urol 1990; 17:276.

78
NEOPLASMS OF THE TESTIS

Jerome P. Richie, M.D.

Testicular cancer, although relatively rare, represents the most common malignancy in males in the 15- to 35-year-old age group and evokes widespread interest for several reasons. Testicular cancer has become one of the most curable solid neoplasms and serves as a paradigm for the multimodal treatment of malignancies. The dramatic improvement in survival resulting from the combination of effective diagnostic techniques, improved tumor markers, effective multidrug chemotherapeutic regimens, and modifications of surgical technique has led to a decrease in patient mortality from greater than 50% before 1970 to less than 10% in 1996. With the availability of effective treatment even for patients with advanced disease, attention has been turned to reduction of morbidity by altering therapeutic pro-tocols in selected subsets of patients. These changes in treatment philosophy are based on the knowledge of effective backup should alternative methods of treatment fail.

Testicular cancer is one of the few neoplasms associated with accurate serum markers, human beta-subunit chorionic gonadotropin (beta HCG) and alpha-fetoprotein (AFP). These accurate tumor markers allow careful follow-up with intervention earlier in the course of disease. Additional characteristics of testicular tumors that favor successful therapeutic manipulation include origin from germ cells, which are generally sensitive to both radiation therapy and a wide variety of chemotherapeutic agents; the capacity for differentiation into histologically more benign counterparts; rapid rate of growth; predictable, systematic pattern of spread; and occurrence in young individuals without comorbid disease who may tolerate multimodal treatment. **Nonetheless, it is of interest that in patients whose tumors arise outside the testicle (extragonadal germ cell tumors), the prognosis with similar treatment is approximately half that which can be expected in those patients with tumors of primary germ cell origin.**

The burgeoning field of molecular biology holds promise for the identification of intracellular changes that alter the kinetics of growth of normal testicular cells. Whereas in the 1980s cell surface antigens and morphologic characteristics could be evaluated, the potential for better understanding and possible elucidation of the etiology of testicular cancer may well be achieved in the not-too-distant future.

CLASSIFICATION

Histology

The testis is covered by a series of tunics that are acquired during descent from the genital ridge in the retroperitoneum through the inguinal canal into the scrotum. These tunics include the tunica vaginalis, the internal spermatic fascia, the cremasteric fascia, the external spermatic fascia, and the scrotum with skin and dartos tunic. The testicular tubules, arranged in a series of lobules, have a dense fascial covering called the tunica albuginea. On its posterior surface, the tunica albuginea is invaginated into the body of the testis to form the mediastinum testis. The mediastinum sends septae into the testis, dividing into lobules. The upper pole of the testis has a vestigial remnant, the appendix testis. On the posterior surface of the testis, the adnexal structures are the epididymis, vas deferens, and spermatic cord.

The normal testis is composed of seminiferous tubules arranged in 200 to 350 lobules, which converge at the mediastinum testis where they connect with 12 to 20 efferent ducts that drain into the globus major of the epididymis. The tubuli recti coalesce in the mediastinum to form the rete testis, which merges into the efferent ductules that traverse the testis to enter the globus major of the epididymis.

The seminiferous tubules contain two cell populations, the supporting, or Sertoli, cells and the spermatogenic cells, called spermatogonia. The supporting Sertoli cells line the basement membrane of the tubules and envelop the germ cells as they pass through various stages of spermatogenesis. The stroma between the seminiferous tubules is connective tissue in which the interstitial cells of Leydig are arranged in clusters. **These cells are the androgen-producing cells that are essential for spermatogenesis to occur.** The majority of primary neoplasms of the testis arise from germinal elements, accounting for 90% to 95% of all testicular neoplasms. The nongerminal elements, accounting for roughly 5% of all primary testicular neoplasms, include neoplasms arising from gonadal stroma, mesenchymal structures, and ducts in addition to other miscellaneous lesions. Metastatic tumors to the testis are distinctly uncommon, although involvement by neoplasms of the reticuloendothelial system may occur.

The blood supply to the testis is derived from the site of origin near the genital ridge. The internal spermatic arteries arise from the aorta below the renal arteries and course through the spermatic cord directly to the testis. The artery to the vas deferens anastomoses with the internal spermatic artery. Venous drainage from the testis starts at the pampiniform plexus of the spermatic cord. This plexus, at the internal ring, joins to form the spermatic vein and drains into the vena cava on the right and the left renal vein on the left. Lymphatics tend to follow the cord to the area of the lumbar lymphatics around the area of the great vessels.

The appendages of the testis and epididymis are embryologic remnants. **The appendix testis, a remnant of the müllerian duct, represents the only müllerian remnant in the area of the testis.** The remaining appendages include the appendix epididymis and paradidymis, which arise from the mesonephric or wolffian duct. The appendix epididymis is attached to the globus major of the epididymis. The paradidymis is attached at the junction of the epididymis and vas deferens. The appendix testis is found in 90% of patients at autopsy; the appendix epididymis is present in roughly 33% of patients.

Histologic classifications, grading systems, and staging evaluations have traditionally provided a major clinical basis for therapeutic decisions (Table 78–1). Morphologic descriptions provide standardized means of identifying a given tumor and, in conjunction with past clinical experience, of estimating its potential for local growth or distant metastases, or both. Clinical and surgical staging indicates the extent to which a given tumor's potential has been realized at the time of evaluation. Although histologic and staging systems play important roles in treatment selection, grading schema have not been uniformly employed. There have been at least six

Table 78–1. HISTOLOGIC CLASSIFICATION

I. Primary neoplasms
  A. Germinal neoplasms (demonstrating one or more of the following components)
    1. Seminoma
      a. Classic (typical) seminoma
      b. Anaplastic seminoma
      c. Spermatocytic seminoma
    2. Embryonal carcinoma
    3. Teratoma (with or without malignant transformation)
      a. Mature
      b. Immature
    4. Choriocarcinoma
    5. Yolk sac tumor (endodermal sinus tumor; embryonal adenocarcinoma of the prepubertal testis)
  B. Nongerminal neoplasms
    1. Specialized gonadal stromal neoplasms
      a. Leydig cell tumor
      b. Other gonadal stromal tumor
    2. Gonadoblastoma
    3. Miscellaneous neoplasms
      a. Adenocarcinoma of the rete testis
      b. Mesenchymal neoplasms
      c. Carcinoid
      d. Adrenal rest "tumor"
II. Secondary neoplasms
  A. Reticuloendothelial neoplasms
  B. Metastases
III. Paratesticular neoplasms
  A. Adenomatoid
  B. Cystadenoma of epididymis
  C. Mesenchymal neoplasms
  D. Mesothelioma
  E. Metastases

major attempts since 1940 to classify germinal tumors with a clinical basis that is meaningful for therapeutic decisions. A major distinction between the British and American systems is the fact that the British refer to all nonseminomatous germ cell tumors as malignant teratomas of one cell type or another, whereas American pathologists generally prefer the term *embryonal carcinoma* for the more undifferentiated form of teratoma. Nonetheless, these classifications can be correlated (Table 78–2). Freidman and Moore (1946) provided one of the first generally accepted histologic classifications; this system, later modified by Dixon and Moore (1952) and Mostofi (1973), has become the North American standard classification. Teilum (1959) suggested the incorporation of the endodermal sinus tumor (infantile embryonal type) in the germ cell category (Pierce, 1975). Mostofi and Price (1973) subdivided teratomas into mature and immature varieties and coined the term *polyembryoma*. The British Testicular Tumour Panel (Pugh and Cameron, 1976) formalized the English version of testicular tumor nomenclature. The World Health Organization (Mostofi and Sobin, 1977) modified the earlier system of Mostofi and Price (1973) by including the term *yolk sac* and by subdividing the embryonal carcinoma with teratoma category. The commonly used histologic classifications are summarized and compared in Tables 78–1 and 78–2.

Carcinoma in Situ

The early detection of preneoplastic change could improve survival for many tumors including testicular cancer. Controversy exists, however, concerning the premalignant alteration of intratubular germ cell neoplasia with the development of frank malignancy. One of the champions of intratubular germ cell neoplasia has been Skakkebaek. Skakkebaek (1972) described the occurrence of intratubular germ cells that are atypical in nature when seen on testicular biopsy from infertile men. In one of his series, four of six patients with intratubular germ cell neoplasia developed "invasive tumor" between 1 and 5 years after initial biopsy (Skakkebaek, 1978). One problem, however, is that *invasive* as defined by his methodology involves invasion of the basement membrane. This is distinctly different from the standard germ cell tumor that is seen in a patient with a palpable mass within the testis.

To investigate the preinvasive phase of adult germ cell tumors detected in childhood, Parkinson and associates evaluated 70 testicular biopsy specimens taken at orchidopexy with follow-up data available (Parkinson et al, 1994). Carcinoma in situ was seen in only 1 of the 70 biopsy specimens, and this preceded appearance of a teratoma by 4 years. Carcinoma in situ was not seen in biopsy specimens 11 and 22 years before tumor diagnosis, raising questions about the extent to which appearance of testicular biopsy specimens during orchidopexy can exclude the development of a tumor in adult life (Parkinson et al, 1994).

The rate of intratubular germ cell neoplasia is well defined and described. How to deal with this problem remains in question, as does in what percentage of patients clinically apparent testicular tumors will develop.

Experimental Models

Teratocarcinomas contain primitive malignant cells and embryonal carcinoma cells as well as various tissues that are partially or fully differentiated, including cartilage, bone, muscle, respiratory, and transitional epithelium. This admixture of tissues suggests the capability of differentiation or dedifferentiation. In fact, murine embryonal carcinoma cells, when placed in a mouse blastocyst, may differentiate in an orderly fashion and participate in the creation of a normal mouse. These studies emphasize the effect of the environment on the development of the malignant or normal cell. In the embryonal carcinoma cell, both neoplasia and embryogenesis come together, allowing the embryonal carcinoma cell and the blastocyst to serve as a model for tumor-host interactions.

Teratoma or teratocarcinoma rarely develops spontaneously in mice. With careful inbreeding of strains with low frequency, however, strains such as the 129-TERSv have been obtained in which up to 30% of male offspring have spontaneous congenital testicular teratocarcinoma. Stevens (1967) developed and successfully manipulated a testicular

Table 78–2. GERM CELL NOMENCLATURE

Friedman and Moore (1946)	Mostofi and Price (1973)	British (Pugh and Cameron, 1976)	Mostofi and Sobin (1977)
Seminoma	Seminoma (typical) Spermatocytic Anaplastic	Seminoma Spermatocytic —	Seminoma Spermatocytic —
Teratoma	Teratoma Mature Immature With malignant transformation	Teratoma differentiated (TD)	Teratoma Mature Immature With malignant transformation
Teratocarcinoma	Embryonal carcinoma with teratoma	Malignant teratoma—intermediate (MTI)	Embryonal carcinoma and teratoma
Embryonal carcinoma	Embryonal carcinoma—adult Polyembryoma	Malignant teratoma—undifferentiated (MTU)	Embryonal carcinoma (adult type)
Chorioepithelioma	Choriocarcinoma with or without embryonal carcinoma and/or teratoma	Malignant teratoma—trophoblastic (MTT)	Choriocarcinoma with or without embryonal carcinoma and/or teratoma
—	Embryonal carcinoma (juvenile type)	Yolk sac tumor	Yolk sac tumor (endodermal sinus tumor)

teratoma line in a strain of the 129 mice. The tumors are first visible as embryonic cell clusters within the seminiferous tubules as early as day 14 of fetal development. Unfortunately, this murine model has been of limited value because the tumors can rarely be sustained by serial transplantation in the new hosts. In this model, more primitive-appearing embryonal cells occasionally persisted, and if these were implanted within the peritoneal cavity, yolk sac tumors and "embryoid bodies" were produced.

In the 129 strain mice, Stevens also found microscopic teratomas in the genital ridges. By transplantation of the genital ridge of appropriate strains of fetal mice into the testes of syngeneic adult mice, teratomas and teratocarcinomas can develop. The Stevens model is effective in producing teratocarcinomas between the twelfth and sixteenth day of development with an approximately 80% rate of tumor production (Stevens, 1968). The grafts, however, fail if ridge transplantation is attempted to other sites outside the scrotum. Also, some strains of mice that are susceptible to embryo-derived tumors do not form tumors when genital ridges are transplanted. For example, the strain A-HE—with a low rate of incidence of spontaneous tumors—allows genital ridge transplantation to be successful at about an 80% rate. In other strains with no germ cells in the genital ridge, however, transplantation fails to produce tumors. Thus, the importance of genetic predisposition as well as environmental factors and timing sequences in oncogenesis is apparent.

Primordial germ cells, early embryos, and embryonal carcinoma cells share similar characteristics, including (1) pluripotency, (2) ultrastructural appearance, (3) alkaline phosphatase content, (4) formation of embryoid bodies, and (5) surface antigens. During the process of differentiation, these features become altered. Artz and Jacob (1974) noted that some cell surface antigens remain unchanged, whereas others, notably histocompatibility antigens, do not make their appearance until primitive elements have matured into adult forms.

Molecular Biology

Tumorigenesis of testicular tumors includes differentiation of primordial germ cells to a variety of mature-type tumors. The question of the role of proto-oncogenes in this tumorigenic mechanism has been evaluated by many authors. Shuin and co-workers examined 15 proto-oncogenes in primary germ cell tumors with Northern blot analyses (Shuin et al, 1994). Ninety-four percent of seminomas and 83% of embryonal carcinomas had N-*myc* expression but not c-*erb*B-1 and c-*erb*B-2. Interestingly, immature teratomas did have a high level of c-*erb*B-1 expression. c-Ki-*ras* or N-*ras* was observed in all histologic subgroups as well as normal testes, suggesting that proto-oncogene expression may be switched during differentiation (Shuin et al, 1994).

Genomic imprinting was investigated by a comparison of specimens of normal testicular tissue and testicular tumor from 20 patients, 10 of whom had seminoma. Testicular germ cell tumors show consistent expression of both parental alleles of the H19 and IGF2 genes, suggesting that imprinting has either been erased or subjected to relaxation effect (van Gurp et al, 1994). C-kit proto-oncogene expression has been reported in seminoma but not in nonsemino-

matous testicular germ cell tumors by Northern blot analysis (Strohmeyer et al, 1995).

The role of P53 in adult germ cell testicular tumors has been controversial. P53 immunostaining was evaluated to see if it would serve as a clinically useful tumor marker. Seminoma and nonseminomatous germ cell tumors reveal P53 expression in 90% and 94% of cases, respectively, with a trend toward decreased P53 expression with advanced stage of seminoma. P53 immunostaining did seem to correlate with stage of disease but was not as useful as vascular invasion or percent of embryonal carcinoma in detecting aggressiveness of the tumor (Lewis et al, 1994). Peng and associates, however, looked for mutations in coding sequences of P53 using denaturant gel electrophoresis and single-strand conformational polymorphism analysis (Peng et al, 1993). No mutations were found in 22 germ cell cancers of the testis or in germ line DNA of 17 members of the testis cancer family, in striking contrast to most other human cancers. The authors concluded that P53 is not likely to play an important role in the development of germ cell cancers of the testis (Peng et al, 1993). This work was further substantiated by Schenkman and colleagues, who examined 30 primary testicular tissues looking specifically for P53 mutations in exons 5–8. Only one patient with seminoma had a silent mutation at codon 140 (Schenkman et al, 1995).

GERM CELL NEOPLASM

Epidemiology

Incidence

Approximately 5500 new cases related to testicular cancer are reported in the United States annually (Wingo et al, 1995). Estimates indicate that for American white males, the lifetime probability of developing testicular cancer is approximately 0.2%, or 1 in 500 (Zdeb, 1977). **The average annual age-adjusted incidence rate for American males from 1969 to 1971 was 3.7 per 100,000—nearly twice the rate of 2.0 per 100,000 from 1937 to 1939.** The average rate among American black males is 0.9 per 100,000, unchanged in the last 40 years.

Similar trends have been noted in Denmark, where the age-adjusted incidence rose from 3.4 to 6.4 per 100,000 between 1945 and 1970 (Clemmesen, 1974). Data compiled by Muir and Nectoux (1979) indicate considerable variability in the worldwide incidence of adult germ cell tumors. The average annual rate (age-adjusted) is highest in Scandinavia (Denmark, Norway), Switzerland, Germany, and New Zealand; is intermediate in the United States and Great Britain; and is low in Africa and Asia. In data collected by Clemmesen (1974), the age-adjusted rate rose from 3.2 to 6.7 per 100,000 in Copenhagen between 1943 and 1967. Prevalence rates in Copenhagen were double those of rural Denmark during the same period.

Age

Peak incidences of testicular tumors occur in late adolescence to early adulthood (20–40 years), in late adulthood (over 60 years), and in infancy (0–10 years). **Overall the highest incidence is noted in young adults, making these neoplasms the most common solid tumors of men between 20 and 34 years of age and the second most common from age 35 to 40 in the United States and Great Britain. Seminoma is rare below the age of 10 and above the age of 60, but it is the most common histologic type overall with a peak incidence between the ages of 35 and 39 years.** Spermatocytic seminoma (approximately 10% of seminomas) occurs most often in patients over the age of 50 years. Embryonal carcinoma and teratocarcinoma occur predominantly between the ages of 25 and 35 years. Choriocarcinoma (1%–2% of germ cell tumors) occurs more often in the 20- to 30-year age group. Yolk sac tumors are the predominant lesions of infancy and childhood but are frequently found in combination with other germ cell elements in young adults. Histologically benign pure teratoma occurs most often in the pediatric age group but frequently appears in combination with other elements in adulthood. Malignant testicular lymphomas are predominantly tumors of men over 50 years of age.

Racial Factors

Variable incidence rates are noted between different ethnic groups within a given geographic region. The incidence of testicular tumors in American blacks is approximately one-third that in American whites but 10 times that in African blacks. In Israel, Jews have at least an eightfold higher incidence of testis tumors in comparison with non-Jews. In Hawaii, the incidence among Filipino/Japanese sectors is approximately one tenth that of the Chinese/white/native Hawaiian populations.

Graham and Gibson (1972) presented data indicating a higher incidence among professional men. Mack and Henderson (1980) noted higher incidence rates in upper and middle socioeconomic classes of whites in Los Angeles County. Although similar trends have been noted in American blacks (Ross et al, 1979), the rate is still less than one third that of whites of comparable social status.

Genetic Factors

Although a relatively higher incidence of testicular tumors has been reported in twins, brothers, and family members, the evidence for a predominant genetic influence is not overwhelming (Johnson, 1976). In nearly 7000 sets of twins from the Danish Twin Registry, Harvald and Hauge (1963) found no higher incidence of cancer in twins than was expected in the general population. Nicholson and Harland (1995) reported that one third of all testis cancer patients are genetically predisposed to disease, likely a homozygous (recessive) inheritance of a single predisposing gene. The 2% to 3% incidence of bilateral tumors may suggest the potential importance of genetic (or congenital) factors.

Laterality and Bilaterality

Testicular neoplasms appear to be slightly more common in the right testis than in the left, similar to the slightly greater incidence of right-sided cryptorchidism. **Approximately 2% to 3% of testicular tumors are bilateral,** occurring either simultaneously or successively. If secondary testicular tumors are excluded, the incidence of bilateral tumors is between 1% and 2.8% of all cases of germinal neoplasms (Sokal et al, 1980). Similar rather than different histology in the two testes predominates with bilateral tumors. Bach and co-workers tabulated the histology in 337 cases of bilateral testicular tumors (Bach et al, 1983). Bilateral seminoma was the most common histologic type (48%); bilateral similar nonseminomas were found in 15%; germinal tumors with different histology were present in 15%; and nongerminal tumors with similar histology occurred in 22%. A history of cryptorchidism (unilateral or bilateral) in nearly half of these men is consistent with observations that bilateral dysgenesis occurs frequently in unilateral maldescent (Sohval, 1956). Long-term surveillance of patients with a history of cryptorchidism or previous orchiectomy for a germ cell tumor is mandatory.

Frequency of Histologic Types

Germinal tumors constitute between 90% and 95% of all primary testicular malignancies. Variability in the reported frequency of histologic types may reflect true differences in the incidence of such tumors. It is possible, however, that such variations merely reflect demographic differences, variance of histologic interpretations, or other unquantified selection factors. The overall incidence rates have been tabulated as follows: **seminoma, 40%; embryonal carcinoma, 20% to 25%; teratocarcinoma, 25% to 30%; teratoma, 5% to 10%; and pure choriocarcinoma, 1%.** When combined histologic patterns (more than one histologic pattern) are considered as a separate entity, the frequency approximates as follows: seminoma, 30%; embryonal carcinoma, 30%; teratoma, 10%; teratocarcinoma, 25%; choriocarcinoma, 1%; and combined patterns (e.g., seminoma plus embryonal carcinoma, embryonal carcinoma plus choriocarcinoma), 15% (Mostofi, 1973).

Etiology

Experimental and clinical evidence supports the importance of congenital factors in the etiology of germ cell tumors. During development, the primordial germ cell may be altered by environmental factors, resulting in disturbed differentiation. The germ cell is conceivably detained from normal development by cryptorchidism, gonadal dysgenesis, or hereditary predisposition or by chemical carcinogens, trauma, or orchitis. The teratocarcinoma tumor model (Stevens, 1968) suggests the crucial influence of temporal relationships on normal versus abnormal differentiation.

Congenital Causes: Cryptorchidism

LeComete (1851) is credited with the initial observation that testicular maldescent and tumor formation are interrelated (Grove, 1954). Pooled data from several large series indicate that approximately 7% to 10% of patients with testicular tumors have a prior history of cryptorchidism (Whitaker, 1970). Mostofi (1973) lists five possible, but unquantified, factors that may play a causative role in the cryptorchid/malignant testis: abnormal germ cell morphology, elevated temperature, interference with blood supply, endocrine dysfunction, and gonadal dysgenesis.

The exact incidence of cryptorchidism is unknown because much of the relevant information on testicular maldescent includes data on patients with retractile testes. From accumulated series, Scorer and Farrington (1971) estimate that approximately 4.3% of neonates, 0.8% of infants and children, and 0.7% of adults over the age of 18 years (army selectees) harbor a truly cryptorchid testis. In reviewing more than 7000 cases of testicular tumor, Gilbert and Hamilton (1940) found a history of cryptorchidism in 840 men (12%). Based on the observed incidence of cryptorchidism in military inductees (0.23%, roughly 1 in 500), they calculated the estimated risk of tumorigenesis in a man with a history of maldescent to be 48 times that of men with normally descended testes. **More recent epidemiologic studies have reported the relative risk of testicular cancer in patients with cryptorchidism to be much lower: 3 to 14 times the normal expected incidence** (Henderson et al, 1979; Schottenfeld et al, 1980; Farrer et al, 1985).

Between 5% and 10% of patients with a history of cryptorchidism develop malignancy in the contralateral, normally descended gonad. This observation is consistent with the findings of Berthelsen and colleagues (1982). They have provided biopsy data in 250 patients with testis cancer relative to the contralateral testis. Carcinoma in situ was found in 13 (5.2%), representing one third of patients with atrophy of the remaining testis and one fifth of patients with a history of cryptorchidism. Two of the patients (10%) with contralateral carcinoma in situ subsequently developed a second testis cancer. Campbell (1942) noted that roughly 25% of patients with bilateral cryptorchidism and a history of testis cancer were subject to the risk of a second germ cell tumor.

Campbell (1942) indicated that nearly half of patients with malignancy associated with cryptorchidism have impalpable abdominal testes. Although the anatomic position (inguinal versus abdominal) may play a role in determining the degree of gonadal damage (and the risk of subsequent tumor formation), the relative influence on the cryptorchid testis may depend largely on the observer (Gilbert, 1940).

Ultrastructural abnormalities of the spermatogonia and Sertoli cells are readily apparent in the cryptorchid testis by the age of 3 years. Cellular degeneration is followed by progressive fibrosis, destruction of the basement membrane, and deposition of myelin and lipids (Mengel et al, 1982). Consideration of these histologic changes and other social factors has favored the practice of early orchiopexy. Such a philosophy, however, has not completely prevented tumor formation in the testis (Martin, 1979; Batata et al, 1982).

Acquired Causes

TRAUMA. Although trauma is considered a contributing factor in zinc-induced or copper-induced fowl teratomas, there is little to suggest a cause-and-effect relationship in humans (Carleton et al, 1953). Most investigators conclude that trauma to the enlarged testis is an event that prompts medical evaluation rather than being a causative factor.

HORMONES. Sex hormone fluctuations may contribute to the development of testicular tumors in experimental animals and humans. The administration of estrogen to preg-

nant mice may cause maldescent and dysgenesis of the testis in the offspring (Nomura and Kanzak, 1977). Similar findings have been noted in the male offspring of women exposed to diethylstilbestrol (Cosgrove et al, 1977) or oral contraceptives (Rothman and Louik, 1978). Exogenous estrogen administration has also been linked to the induction of Leydig cell tumors. Epidemiologic studies found relative risk rates ranging from 2.8% to 5.3% for testicular tumor in the male progeny of diethylstilbestrol-treated mothers (Schottenfeld et al, 1980; Henderson et al, 1983).

ATROPHY. Nonspecific or mumps-associated atrophy of the testis has been suggested as a potential causative factor in testicular cancer. Gilbert (1944) collected 80 cases of testicular tumors occurring in patients with a history of nonspecific atrophy and 24 additional cases related to a previous history of mumps orchitis among 5500 cases of testicular tumors. Although a causative role for atrophy remains speculative, it is tempting to invoke local hormonal imbalance as a possible cause for malignant transformation.

Pathogenesis and Natural History

Local growth characteristics and patterns of spread have been well defined by the clinical observation of patients with germinal testicular tumors. Following malignant transformation, intratubular carcinoma in situ extends beyond the basement membrane and may eventually replace most of the testicular parenchyma. Local involvement of the epididymis or spermatic cord is hindered by the tunica albuginea, and, seemingly as a consequence, lymphatic or hematogenous spread may occur first. Approximately half of patients with nonseminomatous tumors present with disseminated disease (Bosl et al, 1981). **Involvement of the epididymis or cord may lead to pelvic and inguinal lymph node metastasis, whereas tumors confined to the testis proper usually spread to retroperitoneal nodes.** Hematogenous spread to lung, bone, or liver occurs either by direct vascular invasion or indirectly from previously established lymphatic metastasis, by way of the thoracic duct and subclavian veins or other lymphaticovenous communications. The natural history of germinal testis tumors has been the subject of numerous treatises and appears sufficiently well defined to permit the following generalizations (Whitmore, 1968):

1. Complete spontaneous regressions are rare.

2. All germinal testis tumors in adults should be regarded as malignant. Although the infantile teratoma may be regarded as benign, teratoma of the adult testis may be associated with vascular invasion microscopically and a definite mortality risk in patients treated with orchiectomy alone (as high as 29%, according to Mostofi and Price [1973]). Clinical experience has shown that retroperitoneal teratoma in the adult, whether resulting from maturation of embryonal carcinoma or from regression of the embryonal carcinoma component of a teratocarcinoma (spontaneous or induced), may be accompanied by unrelenting local growth and ultimate fatality (Hong et al, 1977).

3. The tunica albuginea is a natural barrier to expansile local growth. Extension through this dense membrane occurs at the testicular mediastinum, where the blood vessels, lymphatics, nerves, and efferent tubules exit the testis proper.

Local involvement of the epididymis or spermatic cord occurs in 10% to 15% of cases and increases the risks of lymphatic or blood-borne metastasis.

4. Lymphatic metastasis is common to all forms of germinal testis tumors, although pure choriocarcinoma almost uniformly disseminates by means of vascular invasion as well. The spermatic cord contains four to eight lymphatic channels that traverse the inguinal canal and retroperitoneal space. As the spermatic vessels cross ventral to the ureter, these lymphatics fan out medially and drain into the retroperitoneal lymph node chain. The primary drainage of the right testis is usually located within the group of lymph nodes in the interaortocaval region at the level of the second vertebral body; the first echelon of nodes draining the left testis is located in the para-aortic region in the compartment bounded by the left ureter, the left renal vein, the aorta, and the origin of the inferior mesenteric artery. Subsequent cephalad drainage is to the cisterna chyli, thoracic duct, and supraclavicular nodes (usually left), but retrograde spread may occur to common, external, and inguinal lymph nodes. Although the thoracic duct–subclavian vein juncture is the major site of communication, other lymphaticovenous communications may be occasioned by massive retroperitoneal lymph node deposits. Furthermore, it has been demonstrated by spermatic lymphangiography that testicular lymphatics can rarely communicate directly with the thoracic duct, bypassing the retroperitoneal nodes. Lymphatics of the epididymis drain into the external iliac chain, affording locally extensive testicular tumors access to pelvic lymph nodes. Inguinal node metastasis may result from scrotal involvement by the primary tumor, prior inguinal or scrotal surgery, or retrograde lymphatic spread secondary to massive retroperitoneal lymph node deposits.

5. Extranodal distant metastasis results from either direct vascular invasion or tumor emboli from lymphatic metastasis via major thoracoabdominal channels or minor lymphaticovenous communications. Most, but not all, blood-borne metastases occur following lymph node involvement. This is of obvious practical importance in treatment and prognosis. Despite surgical excision of negative retroperitoneal lymph nodes, the distant failure rate is approximately 5% (Whitmore, 1973). In programs reserving further treatment following inguinal orchiectomy for clinical stage A nonseminoma patients, approximately 30% fail, most with retroperitoneal lymph node metastasis (80% of failures) and the remainder with extralymphatic distant metastasis (20% of failures) independent of retroperitoneal deposits (Duchesne et al, 1990). Primary and secondary deposits of nongerminal tumors frequently vary histologically. Pure seminomas, however, rarely metastasize as another form of germinal tumor; nonseminomas rarely metastasize as pure seminomas unless the primary lesion has combined histology containing seminomatous elements (Ray et al, 1974). Although the clinical incidence of nonseminomatous metastasis from an apparently pure seminoma is less than 10%, 30% to 45% of patients dying from apparently pure seminoma harbor nonseminomatous metastases (Bredael et al, 1982).

With the exception of seminoma, the growth rate among germ cell tumors tends to be high. **Doubling times calculated on the basis of serial chest radiographs usually range from 10 to 30 days.** Alterations in the production of tumor marker substances (beta HCG, AFP, lactic acid dehydrogenase [LDH]) are in keeping with rapid metabolic activity and growth. The anticipated rapid demise of patients failing treatment has been confirmed by clinical observation; 85% of patients dying from germ cell tumors do so within 2 years and the majority of the remainder within 3 years. Because of a sometimes indolent course, seminoma may recur from 2 to 10 years following apparently successful initial management.

Because of the short natural history of germinal tumors, it has become customary to regard 2-year survival as an end point for judging the effectiveness of therapy. With the evolution of multimodal therapy, surviving patients may not be actually cured of their neoplasm, and a disease-free interval of 5 years may be a more appropriate yardstick for assessing curability. Longer followup after chemotherapy is mandatory, however, because relapse has been noted up to 10 years after treatment.

Clinical Manifestations

In general, survival in patients with germ cell tumors is related to the stage at presentation and therefore the amount of tumor burden as well as the effectiveness of subsequent treatment. Those patients who present with advanced disease (stage III) generally have a much poorer prognosis than do those with disease confined to the testis or with regional nodal involvement only. Delay in diagnosis of 1 to 2 months or more is not uncommon in these patients. Delay in diagnosis seems to be related directly to patient factors such as ignorance, denial, and fear as well as physician factors such as misdiagnosis. Almost half of patients present with metastatic disease (Bosl et al, 1981). **The need clearly exists for patient education through programs such as advocation of testicular self-examination. Only through these widespread public health techniques will the knowledge of testicular tumors be promulgated so that diagnosis can occur earlier.** Physician-related causes still remain major factors in delay of treatment, emphasizing the need for continuing education. It is of interest that denial is such a strong force in patients with testicular tumor. Some of these patients present with masses as large as a grapefruit within the scrotal contents.

Signs and Symptoms

The usual presentation of a testicular tumor is a nodule or painless swelling of one gonad. This may be noted incidentally by the patient or by his sexual partner. The classic description is that of a lump, swelling, or hardness of the testis. Approximately 30% to 40% of patients may complain of a dull ache or a heavy sensation in the lower abdomen, anal area, or scrotum. **In approximately 10% of patients, acute pain is the presenting symptom.** Occasionally, patients with a previously small atrophic testis note enlargement. On rare occasions, infertility may be the presenting complaint (Skakkebaek, 1972). Acute onset of pain is rare unless there is associated epididymitis or bleeding within the tumor.

In approximately 10% of patients, the presenting man-

ifestations may be due to metastases, including a neck mass (supraclavicular lymph node metastasis); respiratory symptoms, such as cough or dyspnea (pulmonary metastasis); gastrointestinal disturbances, such as anorexia, nausea, vomiting, or hemorrhage (retroduodenal metastasis); lumbar back pain (bulky retroperitoneal disease involving the psoas muscle or nerve roots); bone pain (skeletal metastasis); central and peripheral nervous system manifestations (cerebral, spinal cord, or peripheral root involvement); or unilateral or bilateral lower extremity swelling (iliac or caval venous obstruction or thrombosis).

Gynecomastia, seen in about 5% of patients with testicular germ cell tumors, may be regarded as a systemic endocrine manifestation of these neoplasms. Gynecomastia may or may not be associated with elevated levels of HCG, human chorionic somatomammotropin, prolactin, estrogens, or androgens. Relationships between gynecomastia, the morphologic characteristics of the primary tumor, and endocrine abnormalities remain incompletely defined.

Physical Examination

Physical examination of the testis is performed by bimanual examination of the scrotal contents, beginning with the normal contralateral testis. This provides a baseline and allows the examiner to appreciate the relative size, contour, and consistency of the normal testis as well as the suspected gonad. Physical examination of the testis is performed by careful palpation of the testis between the thumb and first two fingers of the examining hand. The normal testis is homogeneous in consistency, freely movable, and separable from the epididymis. Any firm, hard, or fixed area within the substance of the tunica albuginea should be considered suspicious until proved otherwise. Further appreciation of the suspected tumor should be directed toward possible involvement of the cord, scrotal investments, or skin. In general, seminoma tends to expand within the testis as a painless, rubbery enlargement. Embryonal carcinoma or teratocarcinoma may produce an irregular, rather than discrete mass, although this distinction is not always easily appreciated.

Testicular tumors tend to remain ovoid, being limited by the tough investing tunica albuginea. In 10% to 15% of patients, spread to the epididymis or cord may occur. A hydrocele may be present and increase the difficulty in appreciation of a testicular neoplasm. **Ultrasonography of the scrotum is a rapid, reliable technique to exclude hydrocele or epididymitis and should be used in patients if there is any suspicion of testicular tumor.**

Physical examination should include palpation of the abdomen for evidence of nodal disease or visceral involvement. Routine assessment of the supraclavicular lymph nodes may reveal adenopathy in patients with advanced disease. Examination of the chest may disclose gynecomastia or the presence of respiratory tract involvement.

Rarely, patients present with advanced disease without a recognizable primary in the testis. Some of these may be extragonadal germ cell tumors, with an inherently worse prognosis. Others, however, may represent a small primary testicular tumor with large extragonadal metastases. **Palpa-**

tion of the testes is important to exclude primary germ cell tumor in origin. In patients with a diagnosis of "extragonadal" germ cell tumor, ultrasound of the testis is mandatory to be certain one is not dealing with a primary germ cell tumor.

Differential Diagnosis

The differential diagnosis of a testicular mass includes testicular torsion, epididymitis, or epididymo-orchitis. Less common problems include hydrocele, hernia, hematoma, spermatocele, or syphilitic gumma. **In any patient with a solid, firm, intratesticular mass, testicular cancer must be the considered diagnosis until proved otherwise.** In patients in whom the diagnosis is unclear or in whom a hydrocele precludes adequate examination, ultrasonography of the scrotal contents should be used as an important second step. **Ultrasonography of the scrotum is basically an extension of the physical examination. Any hypoechoic area within the tunica albuginea is markedly suspicious for testicular cancer.** With the advent of scrotal ultrasonography and its general availability throughout the United States, the delay in diagnosis from confusion with epididymitis should be markedly reduced.

Imaging Studies

Immersion and high-resolution ultrasonography may aid in the clinical evaluation of scrotal masses (Friedrich et al, 1981; Richie et al, 1982). Intrascrotal fluid collections are no barrier to the examination of the underlying testicular parenchyma by ultrasonography. In patients with palpably normal genitalia and evidence of extragonadal germ cell malignancy, sonography has been reported to be successful in identifying occult testicular neoplasms (Glazer et al, 1982).

CLINICAL STAGING

Once the diagnosis of the germ cell neoplasm has been established by radical orchiectomy, clinical staging is necessary to define further treatment modalities. Staging evaluations should take into account the pathologic examination of the primary specimen, history, and physical findings as well as a variety of other diagnostic modalities. Clinical staging attempts to define the extent of disease at the time of diagnosis as well as during the course of treatment and at subsequent follow-up evaluation. **The accuracy of clinical assessment is imperative if the physician is to be able to make a logical decision about therapy. The importance of clinical staging cannot be overemphasized; this knowledge allows the orderly decision of appropriate treatment as well as reasonable expectations for prognosis. With the advent of alternative treatment protocols for patients with clinical low-stage testicular cancer, the impact of staging and its accuracy is even more critical.**

Sites of Metastases

For staging to be effective and complete, familiarity is necessary with the likely routes of spread and usual sites for metastasis from primary germ cell tumors. **The majority of testicular cancers spread through the lymphatics in an orderly fashion, although vascular dissemination can take place early in some tumors. The primary lymphatic drainage from the right testicle is to the interaortal caval lymph nodes primarily and subsequently to precaval, preaortic, and paracaval lymph nodes. Once the interaortal caval nodes are involved, there tends to be spread to the left para-aortic area, more commonly from right to left side.** Subsequent drainage can go to the left common iliac and left external iliac nodes once extensive involvement occurs in the left para-aortic region. **The primary drainage of the left testis is to the left para-aortic nodes just below the level of the left renal vein and subsequently to preaortic nodes. Cross-metastases occur more commonly in patients with right-sided tumors because of the lymphatic drainage from right to left.** Iliac lymph nodes may be involved primarily when the tumor has invaded the epididymis or spermatic cord and secondarily when para-aortic disease is present. **Inguinal metastases may occur if the tunica albuginea has been invaded or when previous surgery, such as inguinal herniorrhaphy or orchiopexy, has altered the normal lymphatic flow.** Although the suprahilar area was thought to be involved commonly in patients with more extensive retroperitoneal nodal involvement, in actuality, the lymphatics tend to follow the aorta below the crus of the diaphragm into the retrocrural space. Landing sites for minimal, moderate, or extensive disease have been well worked out and reported by Donohue and associates (1982).

Distant spread of testicular cancer occurs most commonly to the pulmonary region with intraparenchymal pulmonary involvement. Subsequent spread may be noted to liver, viscera, brain, or bone (Johnson et al, 1976). In general, bone metastases are encountered rather late in the course of disease. Central nervous system metastases may be understaged.

Staging Systems

The predictable mode of metastasis in patients with germ cell tumors, along with technologic advances in imaging and biochemical marker assays, has improved the accuracy of initial clinical evaluations, although they are far from perfect. A variety of clinical staging systems have been advocated over the past 40 years. For testicular tumors, the system proposed by Boden and Gibb in 1951 has been the mainstay of clinical staging. This ABC system has been refined by Skinner (1976) with subclassification of regional nodal involvement into B1, B2, and B3. Refinement in staging methods and treatment has led to the development of many substages with different prognostic and therapeutic importance. More commonly used clinical staging systems are listed in Table 78–3. **It should be noted that these clinical staging systems are based on noninvasive diagnostic techniques.** Pathologic staging systems, based on retroperitoneal lymph node dissection, are detailed in Table 78–4. Confusion exists because of differences among these clinical and pathologic staging systems, making the interinstitutional comparisons sometimes difficult.

Findings noted at orchiectomy, predominantly histologic findings in the primary tumor, plus physical examination, radiologic procedures, and laboratory studies are essential in assessing clinical stage of disease. Radiologic procedures can include chest x-ray study, intravenous urography, lymphangiography, computed tomography (CT) scan, and magnetic resonance imaging scan. Laboratory studies include tumor markers, beta HCG, AFP, and a multiple screening analysis. Metastases may be assessed not only clinically but also by surgical methods. Some investigators have advocated routine supraclavicular lymph node biopsy

Table 78–3. CLINICAL STAGING SYSTEMS

Boden/Gibb Stage	MSKCC	Royal Marsden Hospital	M. D. Anderson Hospital	American Joint Committee
A (I) Tumor confined to testis	A	I	I	TX unknown status T0 no evidence primary T1 confined to testis T2 beyond tunica T3 invades rete testis or epididymis T4a invades cord T4b invades scrotum
B (II) Spread to regional nodes	B1 <5 cm	IIA <2 cm	IIA negative lymphangiogram/positive nodes	
	B2 >5 cm B3 >10 cm ("bulky")	IIB >2, <5 cm IIC >5 cm	IIB positive lymphangiogram N/A	
C (III) Spread beyond retroperitoneal nodes	CIII	III Supraclavicular (SCN) or mediastinal involvement IV Extralymphatic metastasis		

Table 78–4. PATHOLOGIC STAGING SYSTEMS

Skinner	Walter Reed	TNM
A	I	N-0
Confined to testis		
B		
Spread to retroperitoneum		
B$_1$	IA	N-1, N-2A
<6 positive nodes, no node >2 cm, no extranodal extension		
B$_2$	IIB	N-2B
>6 positive nodes, any node >2 cm		
B$_3$	IIC	N-3
Massive retroperitoneal disease		
C	III	M+
Metastatic		

for staging patients with testicular tumors (Fowler et al, 1979). The relative lack of yield of subclinical metastases along with the potential morbidity of this procedure contraindicates routine supraclavicular node biopsy in patients without a palpable supraclavicular mass (Lynch and Richie, 1980).

Staging classifications should have several purposes: the decision for proper therapy, the evaluation of treatment results, and the capability of comparing results of therapy from a variety of institutions regionally and internationally. Staging systems should be used in tumors with similar biologic characteristics; thus, a clinical staging system for seminoma has been developed as well as one for nonseminomatous germ cell tumors. **Although numerous staging classifications are currently used, the majority are a modification or extension of the one originally proposed by Boden and Gibb in 1951. These investigators separated extent of disease into three stages: stage I, tumor limited to the testis with no evidence of spread through the capsule or to the spermatic cord; stage II, with clinical or radiologic evidence of tumor extension beyond the testicle but contained within the regional lymph nodes; and stage III, disseminated disease above the diaphragm or visceral disease.** A variety of systems has been developed related to differences in treatment among various centers, differences in methods used to assess the extent of disease, and differences in the needs among various treating specialties responsible for these patients. A convenient dividing point for staging systems is those patients with seminomas and those with nonseminomatous tumors. Patients with pure seminoma are usually staged by clinical means, whereas staging may employ surgical techniques in patients with nonseminomatous tumors.

Findings at Orchiectomy

Radical or inguinal orchiectomy, with early clamping of the spermatic cord at the deep inguinal ring, effectively removes a primary tumor and allows staging in patients with testicular cancer. The orchiectomy specimen should be processed carefully to ensure that all elements within the tumor are recognized and that the histologic diagnosis is reasonably accurate. Of equal import is determination of the local extent of tumor. **The pathologist should record**

whether the tumor is confined within the body of the testis (stage T1), extends beyond the tunica albuginea (stage T2), involves the rete testis or epididymis (stage T3), or invades either the spermatic cord (stage T4-A) or the scrotal wall (stage T4-B). The histologic report should also determine whether lymphatic or vascular invasion is seen within the tumor mass as well as the percentage of subtypes of tumors present.

The extent of staging is determined in part by decisions for therapy; for example, if surveillance protocols are to be considered, every effort should be made to exclude patients with any evidence of retroperitoneal disease. If retroperitoneal lymphadenectomy is likely to be elected as the primary treatment for low-stage, nonseminomatous tumors, efforts should be directed toward delineation of regional nodal versus distant metastases.

Imaging Studies

Chest X-Ray Study

Posteroanterior and lateral chest x-ray studies should be the initial radiographic procedure performed. These x-ray films provide the minimal assessment of the lung parenchyma and mediastinal structures. Whole-lung tomography is not obtained routinely at the Brigham & Women's Hospital and the Dana-Farber Cancer Institute. In a study of 120 whole-lung tomography scans performed, whole-lung tomography altered the therapeutic decision in only 4 of 120 patients (Jochelson et al, 1984).

Chest CT scans provide more sensitive evaluations of the thorax and may increase the detection of pulmonary metastases. Chest CT, however, delineates lesions as small as 2 mm in size. Approximately 70% of these small lesions turn out to be benign processes. Thus, if CT scanning is used, a critical high index of suspicion should be present, with recognition that small lesions may, in fact, be benign and not related to the primary testicular cancer. See and Hoxie (1993) evaluated the added benefit of chest CT. They found in patients with negative abdominal CT scan that chest CT failed to increase diagnostic sensitivity above chest x-ray study alone. In patients with abnormal abdominal CT scans, however, chest CT identified abnormalities missed on routine standard chest x-ray study alone.

Computed Tomography

Abdominal CT scans have been touted as being the most effective means to identify retroperitoneal lymph node involvement. CT scanning has replaced intravenous urography and pedal lymphangiography as the procedure of choice for evaluation of the retroperitoneum. Pedal lymphangiography has an error rate of roughly 25% false-negative and 10% false-positive results. Given the overall inaccuracy coupled with its invasive nature, lymphangiography is no longer needed for staging purposes (Bussar-Maatz and Weissbach, 1993). CT has largely supplanted intravenous pyelography in visualization of the kidneys and course of the ureters and is much more sensitive in the detection of extensive retroperitoneal disease. Abdominal CT scans, especially with third-generation and fourth-generation scanners, can

identify small lymph node deposits less than 2 cm in diameter in the upper para-aortic regions. CT scanning provides a generally accurate three-dimensional estimate of tumor size and involvement of soft tissue structures and regional viscera. **In addition, CT provides a view of the retrocrural space in the para-aortic region above the crus of the diaphragm, an important site of metastasis. CT scanning, however, is not sufficiently accurate to distinguish fibrosis, teratoma, or malignancy by size criteria alone** (Stomper et al, 1985).

Tumor Markers

Germinal testis tumors are among a select group of neoplasms identified as producing so-called marker proteins that are relatively specific and readily measurable in minute quantities using highly sensitive radioimmunoassay technology. Applied to the study of body fluids and tissue sections, these biochemical markers theoretically may be capable of detecting small tumor burdens (10^5 cells) that are not detectable by currently available imaging techniques (Bagshawe and Searle, 1977). **The study of biochemical marker substances, particularly AFP and HCG, is clinically useful in the diagnosis, staging, and monitoring of treatment response in patients with germ cell neoplasms and may be useful as a prognostic index.** Germ cell tumor markers belong to two main classes: (1) oncofetal substances associated with embryonic development (AFP and HCG) and (2) certain cellular enzymes, such as LDH and placental alkaline phosphatase (PLAP).

The production by germ cell tumors of oncofetal substances provides evidence that oncogenesis and ontogenesis are closely related. AFP is a dominant serum protein of the early embryo, and HCG is a secretory product of the placenta. During normal maturation of the fetus, both products fall to barely detectable levels soon after birth. **The production of AFP and HCG by trophoblastic and syncytiotrophoblastic cells, respectively, within germ cell neoplasms implies the re-expression of repressed genes (presumably lost during differentiation) or malignant transformation of a pluripotential cell that has retained the ability to differentiate into cells capable of producing oncofetal proteins** (Abelev, 1974; Uriel, 1979).

Alpha-Fetoprotein

AFP is a single-chain glycoprotein (molecular weight approximately 70,000) first demonstrated by Bergstrand and Czar (1954) in normal human fetal serum. In the fetus, AFP is a major serum binding protein produced by the fetal yolk sac, liver, and gastrointestinal tract. **The highest concentrations noted during the twelfth to fourteenth weeks of gestation gradually decline so that 1 year following birth, AFP is detectable only at low levels (<40 ng/ml).** In 1963, Abelev and colleagues detected AFP in mouse embryos and in the sera of mice with chemically induced liver tumors. Further investigation led to the discovery of elevated levels in humans with hepatomas and testis tumors. **The metabolic half-life of AFP in humans is between 5 and 7 days, a fact useful in evaluating treatment response.**

After the first 6 weeks of postnatal life, an elevated AFP may be detected in association with a number of malignancies (testis, liver, pancreas, stomach, lung), normal pregnancy, benign liver disease, ataxia telangiectasia, and tyrosinemia. In endodermal sinus (or yolk sac) tumors, immunofluorescent methods indicate that the epithelial lining of the cysts and tubules is the site of the synthesis of AFP (Teilum et al, 1975). **AFP may be produced by pure embryonal carcinoma, teratocarcinoma, yolk sac tumor, or combined tumors but not by pure choriocarcinoma or pure seminoma** (Javadpour, 1980a, 1980b). Taken together, these observations indicate that yolk sac elements are not always recognizable by conventional light microscopy in individuals with elevated serum AFP owing to germ cell tumors. Binding studies with lectins have shown that AFP produced in the fetal liver has a different molecular structure from that produced in yolk sac tumors, a characteristic that may discriminate benign from malignant liver disease (Ruoslahti et al, 1978).

Human Chorionic Gonadotropin

This glycoprotein (molecular weight 38,000) is composed of alpha and beta polypeptide chains and is normally produced by trophoblastic tissue. Pituitary hormones (luteinizing hormone, follicle-stimulating hormone, thyroid-stimulating hormone) possess alpha subunits closely resembling that of HCG. The beta subunit of HCG is structurally and antigenically distinct from that of the pituitary hormones and allows the production of specific antibodies against the purified beta HCG subunit used in radioimmunoassay techniques (Vaitukaitis, 1979).

During pregnancy, HCG is secreted by the placenta for the maintenance of the corpus luteum. Zondek (1930) was the first to demonstrate that HCG is detectable in the sera of some patients with germ cell tumors. An elevated HCG may also be demonstrated in various other malignancies (liver, pancreas, stomach, lung, breast, kidney, bladder) and perhaps in marijuana smokers. **In germ cell tumors, syncytiotrophoblastic cells have been found responsible for the production of HCG. Some of the radioimmunoassay techniques for HCG variously cross react with luteinizing hormone, and, accordingly, caution should be exercised with patients whose luteinizing hormone may be physiologically elevated (e.g., postcastration).**

The serum half-life of HCG is between 24 and 36 hours, but the individual subunits are cleared much more rapidly (20 minutes for the alpha subunit and 45 minutes for the beta subunit). All patients with choriocarcinoma and 40% to 60% of patients with embryonal carcinoma are expected to have elevated serum levels of HCG. **Approximately 5% to 10% of patients with "pure" seminoma have detectable levels of HCG (usually below the level of 500 ng/ml), apparently produced by the syncytiotrophoblast-like giant cells occurring in some seminomas.**

Clinical Applications of Alpha-Fetoprotein and Human Chorionic Gonadotropin

Among patients with nonseminomatous testis tumors, approximately 50% to 70% have elevated levels of AFP and approximately 40% to 60% have elevated levels of HCG

when sensitive radioimmunoassay techniques are used. If both markers are measured simultaneously, approximately 90% of patients have elevations of one or both marker substances (Barzell and Whitmore, 1979; Fraley et al, 1979; Javadpour, 1980a). These values are derived from patient populations comprising clinical stages I, II, and III tumors. In patients with clinical stage I tumors only, the incidence of positive markers is lower.

Clinical Staging Accuracy

The overall sensitivity of any test or marker varies with the amount of tumor burden. Determinations of AFP and HCG, in concert with other staging modalities, have helped reduce the understaging error in germ cell tumors to a level of 10% to 15%. **Expressed another way, approximately 10% to 15% of patients with nonseminomatous germ cell tumors can be expected to have normal marker levels even at advanced stages of disease.** Although large numbers of patients with clinical stage I nonseminoma have not had markers drawn before orchiectomy, data from the University of Minnesota suggest that roughly two thirds have elevated levels of AFP or HCG or both (Lange and Raghavan, 1983). Up to 90% of such patients are expected to produce marker substances in the presence of advanced disease.

Following orchiectomy, persistent elevation of one or both markers suggests residual tumor, and although a rapid normalization of previously elevated marker(s) conceivably represents elimination of tumor, this is not categorically the case. In patients with disease clinically confined to the testis (clinical stage I), approximately 30% develop metastatic disease while under surveillance despite negative tumor markers immediately following inguinal orchiectomy. Similarly a persistent marker elevation following a technically satisfactory retroperitoneal lymph node dissection indicates the presence of residual disease (stage III), whereas normal values do not categorically exclude the possibility of future recurrence.

Monitoring Therapeutic Response

The rate of tumor marker decline relative to expected marker half-life following treatment has been proposed as a prognostic index. Patients whose values decline according to negative half-lives following treatment appear more likely to be disease-free than those whose marker decline is slower or whose markers never return to normal levels (Lange and Raghavan, 1983). Serial determinations of AFP and HCG closely reflect the effectiveness of therapy in patients with testicular tumors. The rate of marker decline following treatment (surgery, irradiation, chemotherapy) is proportional to the decrease in tumor burden and viability. Following apparently successful treatment, serologic relapse may precede clinical detection by an appreciable but unquantified interval. Alternative therapy may be initiated when minimal tumor burden is thereby perceived.

Following treatment of metastatic disease with irradiation, systemic drugs, or surgery, persistent marker elevation indicates an incomplete response. Because of a therapeutic lag following irradiation or chemotherapy, definition of the "expected" rate of decline and subsequent normalization of markers remains somewhat uncertain; no clear end point of tumor destruction can be identified. Such an end point has been precisely defined for surgery, in that serum markers should fall immediately according to half-life, if such a procedure eradicates the tumor. Nevertheless, marker determinations do act as guidelines following primary chemotherapy or irradiation. Clinical experience has shown that if a patient with advanced disease fails to achieve normalization of tumor markers following aggressive combination chemotherapy, attempts at surgical excision almost uniformly fail. Normalization of marker levels after treatment cannot be equated with the absence of residual disease. **Between 10% and 20% of patients receiving combined systemic chemotherapy for bulky metastatic disease, and subsequently subjected to retroperitoneal lymph node dissection, have viable tumor confirmed histologically despite normal preoperative tumor marker levels.** Similarly, failure to achieve normal levels of AFP and beta HCG following definitive irradiation indicates persistent tumor.

Histologic Diagnosis

Classification of germ cell neoplasms according to morphologic appearance is invaluable in treatment selection. The broad distinction between seminomas and nonseminomas has been particularly important in determining management strategies for retroperitoneal lymph node metastasis. In that germ cell tumors arise from pluripotential cells, a variety of elements may inhabit a given primary tumor or its secondary metastatic sites. Ray and co-workers noted that in the majority of patients (71 of 75, or 95%), a primary tumor containing embryonal carcinoma and seminoma either metastasized as pure embryonal carcinoma or combined with other elements but rarely metastasized as pure seminoma (2 of 75, or 3%) (Ray et al, 1974). Heterogeneity among germ cell neoplasms is an expected consequence of their pluripotential origin. Biochemical marker "probes" can provide a means of delineating tumor heterogeneity, which may be useful in treatment selection.

Relative to seminoma, the detection of an elevated AFP strongly suggests the presence of a nonseminomatous element. Step sections of the primary tumor may further define the source of the marker abnormality. Metastatic disease accompanied by an elevated serum AFP from a pure seminoma indicates a nonseminomatous element, and treatment plans should be restructured accordingly. **Parenthetically, 30% to 45% of patients dying with seminoma are found to have elements of nonseminomatous histology at autopsy. It is generally accepted that between 5% and 10% of patients with "pure" seminoma have mild elevation of HCG because of the presence of syncytiotrophoblastic giant cell forms.** If step sections of the primary tumor fail to disclose nonseminomatous elements, conventional therapy is justified. **If the HCG normalizes after orchiectomy, patients should be treated as having pure seminoma. Current clinical evidence has indicated that HCG levels as high as 500 ng/ml may be found in association with a pure seminoma, although such an occurrence is rare.**

Prognostic Value

Heterogeneity within nonseminomatous tumors is indicated by differences in growth rate, metastatic potential, and

response to therapy and survival. The identification of factors associated with a poor prognosis or high risk provides a basis for altering therapeutic guidelines. Analyses concerning the prognostic implications of elevated marker values are conflicting. The degree of AFP or HCG elevation does appear directly proportional to the amount of tumor burden (stage and number of metastatic sites). The importance attached to the elevation of one tumor marker or another is not readily appreciated unless all potential variables are subjected to multivariate analysis. In studying interrelationships between tumor histology, tumor markers, tumor burden, and number of metastatic sites, **Bosl and colleagues identified elevation of HCG, LDH, or both and number of metastatic sites as the most important prognostic factors in determining survival in patients with germ cell tumors** (Bosl et al, 1983). Elevation of either tumor marker associated with multiple sites of metastasis implies a high risk of treatment failure despite the use of aggressive multidrug chemotherapy regimens.

Lactic Acid Dehydrogenase

LDH is a ubiquitous cellular enzyme (molecular weight 134,000) with particularly high levels detectable in smooth, cardiac, and skeletal muscles; liver; kidney; and brain. Elevation of serum LDH or one of its isoenzymes (LDH I–IV) has been reported useful in monitoring the treatment of germ cell tumors. **Because of its low specificity (high false-positive rate), serum LDH levels must be correlated with other clinical findings in making therapeutic decisions.**

In evaluating experience with serum LDH as a tumor marker for nonseminomatous germ cell tumors, **Boyle and Samuels (1977) reported a direct relationship between tumor burden and LDH levels.** Increased LDH values were noted in 7 of 92 (8%) patients with stage I disease, 15 of 42 (32%) with stage II, and 57 of 70 (81%) with stage III. Recurrence rates in patients with stage I and II disease were higher—15 of 22 (77%) if pretreatment LDH values were elevated—than in those with normal levels—42 of 112 (40%). The first fraction (LDH-I) as determined by agar-gel electrophoresis was responsible for LDH elevation in 25 of 29 patients studied. Skinner and Scardino (1980) found that an elevated LDH may be the sole biochemical abnormality in as many as 10% of patients with persistent or recurrent nonseminomatous tumors. Serum LDH may be even more useful as a marker substance in the surveillance of patients with advanced seminoma. In reviewing their experience in patients with advanced "pure" seminoma, Stanton and associates found elevation of LDH in 21 of 26 patients (81) (Stanton et al, 1983). LDH seems to be most useful as a marker for "bulk" tissue.

Placental Alkaline Phosphatase and Gamma-Glutamyl Transpeptidase

PLAP is a fetal isoenzyme structurally different from adult alkaline phosphatase. **Small studies using enzyme-linked immunoabsorbent assays indicate that as many as 40% of patients with advanced disease have elevated levels of PLAP** (Javadpour, 1983). Gamma-glutamyl transpeptidase (GGT) is a hepatocellular enzyme frequently elevated in benign or neoplastic diseases of the liver. Its presence has been documented in humans in the early placenta, normal testis, and seminal fluid and in sacrococcygeal teratocarcinoma and testicular seminoma (Krishnaswamy et al, 1977). Javadpour (1983) found that one third of patients with active seminomas had elevated levels of GGT. Although the individual sensitivity of PLAP and GGT is low, simultaneous determinations revealed elevation of one or both in 25 of 30 patients (80%) considered to have active disease. CD30 antigen has been evaluated as a possible marker for embryonal carcinoma, with detection of soluble CD30 molecule noted in a high percentage of patients with embryonal carcinoma but not other testicular germ cell tumors (Latza et al, 1995).

Other Prognostic Factors

Because of the importance of distinguishing stage I non-seminomatous germ cell tumors from those that have spread to the retroperitoneum or beyond, a variety of additional techniques have been advocated. Moul and co-workers analyzed 92 patients for factors to distinguish stage I from occult stage II disease (Moul et al, 1994). With multivariate logistic regression analysis, vascular invasion and percentage of embryonal carcinoma remained significant; a model using these variables was accurate 86% of the time. Albers and colleagues used immunohistochemical staining for a proliferation marker (MIB-1) to assess growth fraction in combination with histopathology to predict pathologic stage (Albers et al, 1995). The authors recommended a combined approach using absolute volume of embryonal carcinoma and MIB-1 immunostaining to define an extremely low-risk group for occult metastatic disease.

Based on the work of Folkman and description of angiogenesis as a predictor of prognosis, Olivarez and co-workers conducted a blinded review in 65 clinical stage A testis cancer patients to evaluate usefulness of angiogenesis (Olivarez et al, 1994). The authors found that angiogenesis measured by quantitation of microvessel counts using factor VIII staining is significantly predictive of occult nodal metastatic disease by a univariate analysis. This study needs prospective evaluation for confirmation.

Treatment

Principal treatment strategies for patients with germ cell tumor of the testis have evolved from conceptions of tumor natural history, clinical staging (assessment of the extent of disease), and effectiveness of treatment (alteration of natural history). Analysis of tumor histology and of the frequency and pattern of spread indicates some predictable features of germ cell neoplasms. Pathologic stage is a function of disease progression, and clinical staging is an application of the methods available for assessment of pathologic stage. Selection of treatment alternatives depends on the relative advantages and disadvantages of different regimens. **Multimodal therapy has been largely credited with treatment successes, but the current accuracy of clinical staging, the ability to recognize failure early, and the high probability of successful treatment of such failures have**

prompted investigations aimed at reducing the therapeutic burden.

Each of the major treatment alternatives—surgery, irradiation, and chemotherapy—has a particular but imperfectly defined role in the management of testicular tumors. **As a means of establishing local control, inguinal or "radical" orchiectomy is clearly preferred. Such a procedure provides histologic diagnosis and local staging information (P-category); controls the neoplasm locally with virtually 100% effectiveness, the rare exception usually being attributable to iatrogenic influence; results in the cure of patients with tumor confined to the testis; and is accomplished with minimal morbidity and virtually no mortality.** Surgical excision of a retained spermatic cord remnant or of the "contaminated" scrotum is recommended following scrotal violation or tumor spillage, although additional irradiation of groin and ipsilateral hemiscrotum suffices when pure seminoma is diagnosed. **Because more than half of patients with testicular tumors present with metastatic disease, further treatment following orchiectomy is usual.**

Clinical staging in addition to treatment of the retroperitoneal lymph nodes is a logical next step if no evidence of disease is detected in supradiaphragmatic or extralymphatic sites. It is now generally acknowledged that the majority of patients with large retroperitoneal metastatic deposits are best managed by chemotherapy initially.

Histologic diagnosis is a major factor in the natural history of testicular neoplasms. Between 65% and 85% of all seminomas are clinically confined to the testis, whereas 60% to 70% of nonseminomas present with recognizable metastatic disease. Both the relatively low rate of spread and the radiosensitivity have made radiation therapy the most widely accepted form of treatment for seminomas following inguinal orchiectomy. Radiation therapy, principally in Europe, and surgical excision, in North America, have been employed in the management of regional lymph node metastasis from nonseminomas.

SEMINOMA

Seminoma is the most common histologic testis tumor in adults and accounts for approximately 60% to 65% of all germ cell tumors of the testis. **The established treatment for low-stage seminoma has been inguinal orchiectomy followed by therapeutic or adjuvant radiation therapy** (Figure 78–1). This treatment represents a highly effective method of treating low-stage disease with minimal morbidity; with the advent of multidrug chemotherapy for cure of patients with more disseminated disease, the overall cure rate for all stages exceeds 90%.

Seminoma is sensitive to radiation therapy and usually presents at an early stage. **Approximately 75% of patients with seminoma present with stage I disease, and in this group, greater than 95% survival should routinely be anticipated.** Postorchiectomy external beam radiation therapy to the retroperitoneal lymph nodes achieves high cure rates for these patients.

The optimum treatment of patients who present with distant metastases or bulk retroperitoneal disease is chemotherapy initially. The role of salvage chemotherapy, surgical removal, or radiation therapy in the clinical

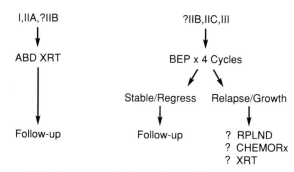

Therapy of Patients with Seminoma

Figure 78–1. Treatment plan for patients with pure seminoma. BEP, bleomycin, etoposide, and *cis*-platin; ABD XRT, abdominal radiation therapy; RPLND, retroperitoneal lymph node dissection; CHEMORx, chemotherapy; XRT, radiation therapy.

situations in which there are persistent radiographic masses remains controversial. Controversy exists about the treatment of bulk stage II disease as well.

Autopsy studies in patients dying with seminoma reveal that liver and lung involvement is common, seen in approximately 75% of patients. Bone and brain metastases are seen in 50% and 25% of patients. **Of major importance is the fact that roughly one third of patients with histologically pure seminoma of the testes who ultimately die of the disease are found to harbor nonseminomatous elements in metastatic sites** (Bredael et al, 1982).

Because seminoma occurs in a young population, and because surgical extirpation, radiation therapy, and multidrug chemotherapy all have salient benefits, treatment should be aimed not only at consideration of cure, but also at attempted maintenance of fertility and avoidance of potentially harmful long-term sequelae. Although the role of irradiation therapy is unquestioned in patients with low-stage disease, it has become apparent that survival in patients with nonseminomatous germ cell tumors now parallels or exceeds that of patients with seminoma when compared stage-for-stage, especially for patients with advanced-stage disease. Analyses of treatment failures have exposed a number of controversial issues in the management of patients with seminomatous tumor. An obligation exists to explore integrated therapeutic regimens in patients with more advanced disease and attempt to reduce treatment burden in others.

Clinical Staging

Staging evaluation by physical examination, radiographic studies, and biochemical marker determinations indicates that approximately 75% of seminomas are confined to the testis at the time of clinical presentation. Between 10% and 15% harbor metastatic disease in regional retroperitoneal lymph nodes, and no more than 5% to 10% have advanced to juxtaregional lymph node or visceral metastases. **Data on the incidence of retroperitoneal lymph node involvement in clinical stage I seminoma are sparse but suggest that roughly 15% of patients with negative history, physical examination, and intravenous pyelography have nodal**

metastasis documented by retroperitoneal lymphadenectomy (Whitmore, 1968). **Owing to the recognized effectiveness of radiation therapy, improved staging methods, and favorable natural history, few advocate lymph node dissection in patients with stage I seminoma.**

Following inguinal orchiectomy, determination of serum tumor markers may provide additional clinicopathologic information relative to treatment selection for patients with "pure" seminomas. Although no ideal tumor marker exists for seminoma, determination of AFP and HCG supplements the histologic characterization of all germ cell tumors. **An elevated AFP virtually excludes a diagnosis of pure seminoma in that step sectioning of the primary tumor or histologic examination of secondary deposits almost uniformly discloses nonseminomatous elements. An elevated HCG level occurs in 5% to 10% of pure seminomas,** although levels over 1000 ng/ml have not been reported (Javadpour et al, 1978). **Syncytiotrophoblastic giant cell elements responsible for the production of beta HCG have been detected by immunoperoxidase techniques. A specific predictive value of an elevated beta HCG level has not been noted; however, patients in whom the beta HCG level does not normalize should generally be treated as if they have nonseminomatous elements.**

After radical orchiectomy, clinical evaluation for possible extragonadal metastatic disease should include postorchiectomy serum tumor markers, chest x-ray study, and retroperitoneal CT scan. In the past, bipedal lymphangiography was recommended for patients with pure seminoma. This recommendation had been based on recommended treatment to one portal higher than lymphatic involvement occurred. Thus, if the lymphangiogram was positive, patients were treated with supplemental mediastinal and supraclavicular nodal radiation. **With the advent of effective chemotherapy for salvage, radiation therapy above the diaphragm should be avoided. Therefore, the need for lymphangiography has diminished substantially.** Some centers, however, still advocate routine use of lymphangiography for patients with seminoma to increase the amount of radiation therapy to the retroperitoneum.

The system of Boden and Gibb (1951) has been modified through the years as clinical staging procedures have become more precise and have been more precisely correlated with treatment results. **For the most part, extent of disease has been defined by three clinical stages: stage I, tumor confined to the testis with or without epididymis, spermatic cord, or both; stage II, metastasis present in retroperitoneal lymph nodes only; and stage III, spread beyond retroperitoneal lymph nodes. Currently, most workers** subdivide stage II into II-A (nonbulky retroperitoneal deposits) and II-B (palpable or radiographically bulky [>10 cm diameter] retroperitoneal disease). Others distinguish between supradiaphragmatic lymph node metastasis (stage III) and visceral involvement (stage IV). A comparison between various staging systems in common use is shown in Table 78–5.

Histology

Three subtypes of pure seminomas have been described: classic, anaplastic, and spermatocytic. The histologic and biochemical properties, natural history, and response to therapy of these subtypes have been characterized.

Several histopathologic characteristics of the primary tumor have been evaluated with regard to prognostic features as well as predictive value for likelihood of metastatic involvement (Hoeltl et al, 1987). **Unfortunately, however, no significant predictors have been identified that reliably detail the likelihood of metastatic involvement. Because most patients are treated with retroperitoneal irradiation, and surgical confirmation is not obtained, a small difference with these risk factors would not be identified.**

Typical Seminoma

Typical or classic seminoma accounts for 82% to 85% of all seminomas, occurring most commonly in men in their thirties but not uncommonly in men in their forties or fifties. Seminoma rarely, if ever, occurs in the adolescent or infant population but may occur in patients over the age of 60 years. Histologically, it is composed of islands or sheets of relatively large cells with clear cytoplasm and densely staining nuclei. **Syncytiotrophoblastic elements occur in 10% to 15% and lymphocytic infiltration in approximately 20%. The incidence of syncytiotrophoblastic elements corresponds to the frequency of beta HCG production. The slower growth rate of seminomas may be inferred from the observation that treatment failures may become evident 2 to 10 years following apparently adequate irradiation of metastatic sites.**

Anaplastic Seminoma

This accounts for between 5% and 10% of all seminomas and has an age distribution similar to that of the typical subtype. Despite its rarity, discrimination of anaplastic semi-

Table 78–5. COMPARISON OF CLINICAL STAGING SYSTEMS IN SEMINOMA

Clinical Extent of Disease	Walter Reed (Maier and Sulak, 1973)	M. D. Anderson (Doornbos et al, 1975)	Royal Marsden (Peckham, 1982)	UCLA (Crawford et al, 1983)
Testis/cord	I-A (II-B = I-A but positive RPLND)	I	I	I
Retroperitoneal nodes	II	II-A <10 cm	II-a <2 cm II-b 2–5 cm	II-A <2 cm II-B 2–10 cm
Nodes above diaphragm	III	III	III	III
Viscera	III	III	IV	III

RPLND, Retroperitoneal lymph node dissection.

noma is noteworthy because up to 30% of patients dying with seminoma have an anaplastic morphology. **A number of features suggest that anaplastic seminoma is a more aggressive and potentially more lethal variant of the typical seminoma. These characteristics include (1) greater mitotic activity, (2) a higher rate of local invasion, (3) an increased rate of metastatic spread, and (4) a higher rate of tumor marker production (beta HCG).**

Histologically, anaplastic seminoma is typified by increased mitotic activity (three or more mitoses per high-power field), nuclear pleomorphism, and cellular anaplasia (Mostofi and Price, 1973). Morphologically, histiocytic lymphoma and embryonal carcinoma may closely resemble anaplastic seminoma. Relative to the rate of metastasis, Percarpio and associates noted in a series of 77 patients with anaplastic seminoma that 19 (25%) had clinical evidence of stage II disease (Percarpio et al, 1979). Shulman and co-workers reported a similar incidence of metastatic disease (29%), a relatively high rate of extragonadal extension (46%), and an unexpectedly high rate (36%) of elevated beta HCG in 14 patients with anaplastic seminoma (Shulman et al, 1983).

The less favorable results of treatment for patients with anaplastic seminoma may merely reflect a greater metastatic potential; there is no difference from classic seminoma when patients are treated appropriately and compared stage-for-stage. Analyses of treatment results indicate that inguinal orchiectomy plus radiation therapy is equally effective in controlling anaplastic and classic seminoma.

Spermatocytic Seminoma

This lesion is composed of cells varying in size with deeply pigmented cytoplasm and rounded nuclei containing characteristic filamentous chromatin. The cells closely resemble different phases of maturing spermatogonia. Spermatocytic seminoma accounts for 2% to 12% of all seminomas, and nearly half occur in men over age 50. Bilateral tumors have been reported, but no cases have occurred in conjunction with cryptorchidism. The association of spermatocytic seminoma with other nonseminomatous tumors is rare.

The metastatic potential of spermatocytic seminoma is extremely low, and prognosis is accordingly favorable. Reviews by Thackray and Crane (1976) and Weitzner (1979) document no cases of metastatic disease. When histologic and staging evaluations have confirmed the diagnosis and the fact that disease is limited to the testis, treatment beyond inguinal orchiectomy appears unwarranted.

Treatment

The natural history and radiosensitivity of seminoma favor megavoltage irradiation in relatively modest amounts as the treatment of choice in the vast majority of patients following inguinal orchiectomy. Because the staging error may be 15% to 25% for stage I seminoma, any treatment (or lack of it) should produce a cure in 75% of patients or better. **The overall effectiveness of radiation therapy is confirmed, however, in that 2500 to 3500 cGy delivered over a 3-**week period to the periaortic and ipsilateral inguinopelvic lymph nodes results in 5-year survival rates of 90% to 95%. In stage II disease, 5-year survival rates of roughly 80% are anticipated following therapeutic retroperitoneal irradiation with or without additional treatment of the mediastinum. Deposits in supradiaphragmatic nodes or distant sites and bulky abdominal disease respond less favorably to primary radiation therapy, which by itself yields survival rates as low as 20% to 30%. **Evidence indicates that seminoma is exquisitely sensitive to various chemotherapy regimens, particularly platinum-based ones, with response rates of 60% to 100% being reported.**

Stages I and II-A

In stage I and low-volume stage II seminoma, irradiation of para-aortic and inguinal pelvic lymphatics is delivered through anterior and posterior parallel opposing fields. The retroperitoneal lymph node groups included in radiation treatment fields are the ipsilateral external iliac, the bilateral common iliac, the paracaval, and the para-aortic nodes superiorly, including coverage of the cisterna chyli. CT scanning is useful in planning and simulation of treatment fields. The exact field depends on characteristics of the individual patient as well as the equipment used. The para-aortic field is bounded superiorly by the origin of the thoracic duct and includes the anterior surface of the eleventh or tenth thoracic vertebra anteriorly to the internal inguinal ring and inguinal excision, laterally to include the ipsilateral renal hilum, more generously on the left side than on the right. The contralateral para-aortic nodes are treated on an individual basis. The pelvic segment stretches from the fourth lumbar vertebra to the inguinal ligament and includes the orchiectomy scar. In patients with retained spermatic cord remnant or contaminated scrotum, the field may be widened considerably.

In patients with a history of herniorrhaphy or prior orchiopexy, with potential alteration in lymphatic drainage, the inferior portion of the field should include the contralateral inguinal region as well. The contralateral testis should be shielded.

Fields are treated with conventional fractionation of 150 cGY per day, 5 days per week including both anterior and posterior fields treated on a daily basis. Elective supradiaphragmatic irradiation for patients with stage I neoplasm is not recommended. Prophylactic treatment of the mediastinum or supraclavicular area is not indicated.

Treatment Results: Stage I

Patients with stage I seminoma treated with postorchiectomy radiation therapy enjoy outstanding 5-year survival rates approximating 95%. Five-year disease-free survival rates roughly equate with cure in that late relapses with death are exceedingly rare beyond that time frame. Results for disease-free survival in patients with postorchiectomy radiation therapy in clinical stages I and II seminoma are presented in Table 78–6. Routine survival rates above 95% are to be expected in patients with clinical stage I seminoma. This survival rate does not seem altered by the addition of prophylactic mediastinal irradiation. In fact, prophylactic mediastinal irradiation has been discontinued in the majority of institutions (Thomas et al, 1982). **With the advent of**

Table 78–6. RADIATION THERAPY IN CLINICAL STAGES I AND II SEMINOMA (DISEASE-FREE SURVIVAL)

Author	Stage I		Stage II		Years Follow-up (A/C)
	No. Patients	Survival (%)	No. Patients	Survival (%)	
Maier and Sulak (1973)	284	97	34	91	5 (A)
Earle et al (1973)	71	100	27	85	5 (A)
Peckham and McElwain (1974)	78	98	27	93	4 (A)
Doornbos et al (1975)	79	94	48	77	3 (C)
Blandy (1976)	98	93	35	71	5 (A)
van der Werf-Messing (1976)	91	100	67	85	5 (A)
Batata et al (1979)	227	88	53	62	5 (C)
Dosoretz et al (1981)	135	97	18	92	5 (A)
Thomas et al (1982)	338	94	86	74	5 (A)

A, Actuarial survival; C, crude survival.

effective chemotherapy against disseminated disease, mediastinal or supradiaphragmatic irradiation could potentially compromise the patient's ability to receive effective therapy (Loehrer et al, 1987).

Treatment Results: Stage II

Patients with clinical stage II seminoma treated with postorchiectomy radiation therapy enjoy 5-year survival rates of approximately 80% with a range of 70% to 92% (see Table 78–6). This subset of patients creates increasing controversy in the decision for radiation therapy versus combination chemotherapy as primary treatment. Treatment results are reported depending on the staging system used. Some centers designate stage IIA as less than 10 cm in diameter and stage IIB as greater than 10 cm in diameter. Other centers use different definitions for bulk retroperitoneal disease. Certainly, patients with masses less than 5 cm enjoy a reasonably good 5-year survival with radiation therapy alone. Patients with stage IIA disease have enjoyed survival rates above 90%, which statistically does not differ from patients with stage I disease. For patients with stage IIB disease treated by extended radiation therapy alone, approximately one third of patients develop metastatic disease outside the treated fields. In a study from the Royal Marsden Hospital, 10% of patients with stage IIA, defined as retroperitoneal metastases less than 2 cm, relapsed; 18% of patients with nodes less than 5 cm relapsed; and 38% of patients with nodes greater than 5 cm relapsed (Peckham et al, 1981).

Treatment Results: Advanced Seminoma

The overall disease-free survival in patients with stage IIB or greater disease treated with abdominal irradiation is only approximately 50%. Radiation therapy was the treatment of choice for patients with advanced seminoma before the advent of platinum-based combination chemotherapy (Table 78–7). Patients relapsed with equal frequency in the abdomen or in distant sites regardless of whether prophylactic mediastinal or supraclavicular irradiation was used. Patients who relapse might be salvaged with radiation therapy, although the response rate is poor.

Before the 1970s, alkylating agents were used against

metastatic seminoma. **The combination of *cis*-platin, vinblastine, and bleomycin has been found to be effective against disseminated testicular seminoma as well as nonseminomatous tumors. More than 90% of patients who present with stage III disease achieve a complete response to chemotherapy alone, and approximately 90% of the responders remain disease-free during follow-up evaluation to 4 years** (Table 78–8).

Response rates seem to be somewhat better when *cis*-platin-based chemotherapy is given as the primary treatment with no prior radiation, but reasonable results can be obtained for relapse after initial irradiation. Extensive prior irradiation can have an impact on the amount of chemotherapy received as well as the response rate. Thus, response rates seem to be higher in patients treated with chemotherapy than in those treated with primary radiation therapy alone. One difficulty in patients with advanced seminoma treated with *cis*-platin combination chemotherapy is the lack of complete resolution of radiographic masses on CT scan. Controversy exists about the need for further treatment as opposed to observation. **Attempts to remove bulk residual disease after chemotherapy for seminoma are fraught with difficulty. Because seminoma involves the retroperitoneum as a fibrotic process similar to retroperitoneal fibrosis, clean retroperitoneal dissection is rarely achieved. In most patients explored after chemotherapy, only residual necrosis or fibrosis is found.** In a Sloan-

Table 78–7. RADIATION THERAPY IN CLINICAL STAGES II-B AND III SEMINOMA (DISEASE-FREE SURVIVAL)

Author	Stage II-B		Stage III	
	No. Patients	Survival (%)	No. Patients	Survival (%)
Maier and Sulak (1973)	—	—	18	17
Doornbos et al (1975)	22	61	14	21
Blandy (1976)	—	—	17	12
van der Werf-Messing (1976)	21	75	30	43
Smith (1978)	7	29	14	14
Batata et al (1979)	—	—	24	42
Dosoretz et al (1981)	7	43	9	44
Thomas et al (1982)	46	48	20	32
Green et al (1983)	18	94*	—	—

*5/18 lost to follow-up <2 years.

Table 78–8. PRIMARY CHEMOTHERAPY FOR ADVANCED SEMINOMA

Author	Regimen	Patients	Prior Irradiation No. (%)	Follow-up CR + PR	NED (%)	Months
Einhorn and Williams (1980)	PVB (A)	19	13 (68)	12 + 7	11 (58)	19
Vugrin et al (1981)*	DDP + Cy	9	6 (67)	5 + 4	7 (78)	19
Morse et al (1983)*	VAB VI	22	8 (38)	9 + 10	17 (77)	17
Wajsman et al (1983)	DDP + VBPr/VP-16	12	4 (33)	12	12 (100)	—
Crawford et al (1983)†	VAC	16	1 (7)	15	15 (94)	48
Mencel et al (1994)	VAB-VI/EP	140		105 + 25	120 (86)	43
Fossa et al (1995)	VIP	42		26 + 11	36 (90)	36

*Series contains patients with extragonadal primary tumors and patients who received additional surgery with or without radiation therapy.
†15/16 patients received radiation therapy following chemotherapy.
CR + PR, Complete response plus partial response; NED, no evidence of disease.

Kettering study, however, in a review of patients with bulky stage II or III seminoma in which the residual mass was 3 cm or greater, residual viable tumor was found in approximately 50% of patients (Motzer et al, 1987).

Both irradiation and chemotherapy are highly effective against pure seminoma. Natural history of seminoma generally favors a minimal therapeutic burden, which justifies radiation therapy after orchiectomy in the majority of patients (see Fig. 78–1). **In patients with bulk or advanced disease, however, initial treatment should be *cis*-platin-based chemotherapy, with surgery or radiation therapy reserved for treatment failures.**

Because of the effectiveness of chemotherapy, surveillance has been advocated by certain centers (Duchesne et al, 1990; Oliver et al, 1990).

It would seem that patients with advanced seminoma have a chemosensitive tumor with potential cure with chemotherapy that is comparable to that seen with patients with nonseminomatous germ cell tumors. More than 85% of patients have achieved continuous disease-free status with *cis*-platin combination chemotherapy. **Therefore, multidrug, *cis*-platin-based chemotherapy should be used initially in patients with advanced seminoma and no further treatment in patients with radiographic complete responses. With residual mass, close careful observation is favored as opposed to consolidation with radiation therapy or surgical excision** (Fossa et al, 1987). **Although surveillance can be considered in patients following orchiectomy for stage I seminoma, the excellent results with minimal morbidity and toxicity from low-dose, retroperitoneal irradiation make this the treatment of choice.** Long-term late clinical effects of irradiation are minimal. In a study of 104 patients followed long-term, there were no serious acute toxic effects or late complications. Six patients developed second malignancies at a mean of 10 years after treatment, none of which was considered to be radiation induced (van Rooy and Sagerman, 1994).

NONSEMINOMA

Tumors designated as nonseminoma include those that are histologically composed of embryonal carcinoma, teratoma, choriocarcinoma, and yolk sac elements alone or in various combinations. **Tumors containing both seminomatous and nonseminomatous elements are generally regarded as nonseminomas, a consideration that may have practical bearing on treatment selection.** Aside from morphologic differences, distinctions between seminoma and nonseminoma are made relative to natural behavior, clinical staging, and treatment strategies.

Natural History

Clinical evidence is strong that nonseminomas follow a potentially less favorable natural history than do pure seminomas. Depending to some degree on referral patterns and staging criteria, 50% to 70% of patients with nonseminoma, but only 20% to 30% of those with seminoma, present with metastatic disease at the time of diagnosis. The first echelon of spread for all germ cell tumors is most commonly the retroperitoneal lymph nodes. Evidence for this generalization stems from postmortem and clinical experiences. Autopsy studies indicate that roughly three quarters of patients dying with germ cell tumors have a concomitant or prior history of retroperitoneal nodal and parenchymal metastases despite therapeutic retroperitoneal irradiation or lymphadenectomy. **After retroperitoneal lymph nodes, the lungs are the next most common site of spread.** This observation is evident from autopsy studies and from the follow-up of patients after lymph node dissection, in that lung metastasis represents the most frequently recognized site of treatment failure regardless of lymph node status. **Next in frequency of spread are liver, brain, bone, and kidney, although almost any site may be involved.**

Clinical Staging

The natural history and frequency of disease dissemination favor the accurate clinical staging of nonseminomatous tumors. The rapid development of precise imaging techniques and tumor-indexing substances frequently produced by nonseminomas also foster staging accuracy. **The principal differences between staging systems for seminomas and nonseminomas relate to the roles of surgical lymph node sampling and serum tumor markers.**

Histology

Embryonal carcinoma is generally discovered as a small, rounded but irregular mass invading the tunica vaginalis and not infrequently involving contiguous cord structures. The cut surface reveals a variegated, grayish white, fleshy tumor, often with areas of necrosis or hemorrhage and a poorly defined capsule. The typical histologic appearance is that of distinctly malignant epithelioid cells arranged in glands or tubules. The cell borders are usually indistinct, the cytoplasm pale or vacuolated, and the nuclei rounded with coarse chromatin and one or more large nucleoli. Pleomorphism, mitotic figures, and giant cells are features common to these highly malignant tumors.

Pure choriocarcinoma may occur as a palpable nodule, the size depending on the extent of local hemorrhage. **Patients with pure choriocarcinoma may present with evidence of advanced distant metastasis and what seems a paradoxically small intratesticular lesion that may not distort the normal testicular size or shape.** Central hemorrhage with viable grayish white tumor at the periphery may be seen on the cut surface if the lesion can be demonstrated grossly. **Microscopically, two distinct and appropriately oriented cell types must be demonstrated to satisfy the histologic diagnosis of choriocarcinoma—syncytiotrophoblasts and cytotrophoblasts. The syncytiotrophoblasts may be large multinucleated cells containing abundant, often vacuolated, eosinophilic cytoplasm and large, hyperchromatic, irregular nuclei. Less commonly, the syncytial elements may be spindle-shaped and contain one large dark-staining nucleus. The cytotrophoblasts are closely packed, intermediate-sized, uniform cells with a distinct cell border, clear cytoplasm, and a single vesicular nucleus.**

Teratoma contains more than one germ cell layer in various stages of maturation and differentiation. **"Mature" elements resemble benign structures derived from normal ectoderm, entoderm, and mesoderm. "Immature" teratoma consists of undifferentiated primitive tissues from each of the three germ cell layers.** Grossly the tumors are usually large, lobulated, and nonhomogeneous in consistency. The cut surface may reveal variably sized cysts containing gelatinous, mucinous, or hyalinized material interspersed with islands of solid tissue often containing cartilage or bone. Histologically the cysts may be lined by squamous, cuboidal, columnar, or transitional epithelium; the solid component may contain any combination of cartilage; bone; intestinal, pancreatic, or liver tissue; smooth or skeletal muscle; and neural or connective tissue elements. On rare occasions, malignant changes may be recognized in such differentiated tissues, justifying the designation *malignant teratoma.*

Yolk sac tumor is the most common testis tumor of infants and children. In adults, it occurs most frequently in combination with other histologic types and is presumably responsible for the production of AFP. The terms *endodermal sinus tumor, adenocarcinoma of the infantile testis, juvenile embryonal carcinoma,* and *orchioblastoma* are used synonymously. In its pure form, the lesion has a homogeneous yellowish, mucinous appearance. Microscopically the tumor is composed of epithelioid cells that form glandular and ductal structures arranged in columns, papillary projections, or solid islands within a primitive mesenchymal stroma. The individual epithelial tumor cells may be columnar, cuboidal, or flat, with poorly defined cell borders and vacuolated cytoplasm containing glycogen and fat. The large, irregularly shaped nuclei contain one or more promi-

nent nucleoli and variable amounts of chromatin. **Embryoid bodies, a common finding in yolk sac tumors, resemble 1- to 2-week-old embryos. These ovoid structures, commonly measuring less than 1 mm in diameter, consist of a cavity surrounded by loose mesenchyme containing syncytiotrophoblasts and cytotrophoblasts.**

In classifying more than 6000 testis tumors, Mostofi (1973) found that in roughly 40% more than one histologic pattern was identified. Because of its frequent occurrence (24% of testis tumors), the combination of teratoma and embryonal carcinoma, termed *teratocarcinoma,* is usually classified as a specific entity. Teratocarcinomas are frequently large and frequently disseminated. Metastatic deposits associated with teratomas usually contain embryonal carcinoma (80%) and, less frequently, teratoma or choriocarcinoma. The bisected tumor exhibits cysts, typical of teratoma, within the solid, sometimes hemorrhagic stroma containing embryonal elements.

The pluripotential nature of germ cell tumors, and in particular nonseminomatous tumors, is evident from the varied histologic patterns of metastasis, more than half of which display different morphologies in primary versus metastatic sites, although pure choriocarcinoma invariably spreads unaltered. Although postmortem studies indicate that 30% to 45% of patients dying with seminoma harbor nonseminomatous metastases, the converse is rarely documented.

Treatment: Stage I

Removal of the testis via an inguinal approach, the so-called radical orchiectomy, remains the definitive procedure for pathologic diagnosis as well as local treatment of testicular neoplasms. Morbidity is minimal, and mortality should be virtually zero while allowing 100% local control. **Transscrotal biopsy is to be condemned.** The inguinal approach permits early control of the vascular and lymphatic supply as well as en bloc removal of the testis with all its tunics.

In patients with nonseminomatous germ cell tumor, following inguinal orchiectomy, the accuracy of clinical staging is critical as a determinant for further treatment selection. Because of the inexactitude of clinical staging, retroperitoneal lymphadenectomy remains the mainstay of surgical therapy in patients with nonseminomatous germ cell tumors (Table 78–9). These tumors generally spread to the retroperitoneal lymph nodes before further dissemination, and the primary landing sites are well identified. After spread to the retroperitoneum, the next most common site of metastasis is to the lungs, which can be identified early with plain radiographs. Furthermore, these tumors often produce beta HCG or AFP, both of which are measurable in the serum at nanogram levels.

Historical Perspectives

Anatomic studies at the turn of the century by Most (1898) and Cuneo (1901) as well as later work by Jamieson and Dobson (1910) and Rouviere (1938) demonstrated the lymphatic drainage of the testis with the primary echelon of drainage for right-sided tumors to be interaortal caval and for left-sided tumors to be left para-aortic and preaortic

Table 78–9. TWO- TO FIVE-YEAR SURVIVAL AFTER ORCHIECTOMY AND RETROPERITONEAL LYMPH NODE DISSECTION IN PATHOLOGIC STAGE I NONSEMINOMATOUS GERM CELL TUMORS

Author	No Evidence of Disease		Years Follow-up
	Number	*(%)*	
Whitmore (1970)	50/58	86	5
Walsh et al (1971)	24/25	96	3
Bradfield et al (1973)	28/40	70	3
Staubitz et al (1974)	42/45	93	3
Johnson et al (1976)	65/72	90	5
Skinner (1976)*	39/43	91	2
Donohue et al (1978)	27/30	90	3
Fraley et al (1979)	28/28	100	2
Bredael et al (1983)†	126/138	91	3
Total	429/479	Average 90	

*Adjuvant actinomycin D.
†30 patients received adjuvant chemotherapy.

nodes. There exists some cross-over, especially from right to left. **These anatomic studies provided the basis for regional control after establishing local control by orchiectomy.** The first site of metastasis in patients with nonseminomatous tumors is generally the retroperitoneal lymph nodes (90%). In approximately 10% of patients, the first site of metastasis is outside the borders of a standard retroperitoneal lymph node dissection. **Thorough excision of the retroperitoneal lymph nodes remains the epitome or gold standard of staging. Although noninvasive staging techniques are somewhat accurate, 20% to 25% of patients with clinical stage I disease are understaged by all available modalities of nonsurgical staging. The cure rate for patients with pathologically confirmed stage I disease is roughly 95% with surgery alone. The 5% to 10% of patients who may relapse following negative retroperitoneal lymph node dissection for stage I disease have a high cure rate with salvage chemotherapy.**

The 5% to 10% of patients who relapse generally do so within the first 2 years after diagnosis. Thus, careful follow-up is necessary for the first 2 years, generally with monthly chest x-ray studies and tumor markers for the first year and every other month for the second year. Because relapse beyond 2 years is rare, these patients can be followed annually for the next several years. Patients who relapse generally do so in the lungs, suggesting hematogenous spread that preceded lymphatic dissemination. Recurrences in the retroperitoneum have been recognized rarely in patients who previously had a negative lymph node dissection.

Retroperitoneal lymph node dissection was established as a primary therapy for nonseminomatous germ cell tumors by Lewis in 1948. Kimbrough and Cook (1953) fostered inguinal orchiectomy plus retroperitoneal lymphadenectomy as the preferred local regional treatment for patients with testis tumors. In Europe, conversely, radiation therapy was used as a primary means for sterilizing nodal deposits. Lewis reported a 46% 5-year survival among 28 patients treated with lymphadenectomy or radiation therapy, or both, after orchiectomy.

A variety of surgical approaches have been advocated for retroperitoneal lymphadenectomy. **Cooper and associates popularized the transthoracic approach in 1950** (Cooper et al, 1950). **Staubitz and colleagues (1974) and Whitmore (1979) used the transabdominal approach.** The question of bilateral suprahilar dissection was raised by Donohue and associates (1982). This led to important mapping studies for the distribution of retroperitoneal lymph node metastases in patients with minimal, moderate, or advanced retroperitoneal disease. This mapping has allowed tailoring of the surgical procedure to the amount of retroperitoneal adenopathy that is present.

Retroperitoneal lymph node dissection, via a transabdominal or thoracoabdominal approach, is a generally well-tolerated, 3- to 4-hour procedure with negligible mortality and minimal morbidity. The mortality rate is less than 1%. Morbidity ranges from 5% to 25%, usually related to atelectasis, pneumonitis, ileus, lymphocele, or pancreatitis.

Fertility After Retroperitoneal Lymph Node Dissection

Semen quality as an indicator of potential fertility has been studied by many investigators before, during, and after various treatments for testicular cancer. **Approximately 50% to 60% of men are reportedly subfertile at the time of diagnosis of a nonseminomatous germ cell tumor. Controversy exists as to whether spermatogenesis is impaired before the clinical manifestation of testicular cancer or whether semen quality is impaired as a result of diagnosis or initial therapy (or both).** Nonetheless, in a large proportion of patients, spermatogenesis impairment may be reversible.

EMISSION AND EJACULATION. Before 1980, a high incidence of infertility was noted following retroperitoneal lymph node dissection in patients with testicular cancer. This infertility was largely due to either failure of seminal emission or retrograde ejaculation secondary to damage to the sympathetic nerve fibers involved in ejaculation.

Early descriptions of retroperitoneal lymphadenectomy included a complete bilateral dissection from above the renal hilar area bilaterally, encompassing both ureters down to where each ureter crossed the common iliac artery. Retroperitoneal tissue was removed both anterior to and posterior to the great vessels to remove all nodal bearing tissue completely. **Thorough removal of all lymphatic tissue was considered essential because of the lack of effective alternative therapies.** Indeed, retroperitoneal lymph node dissection using the previous template has been curative in patients with minimal nodal involvement, even without the use of adjunctive chemotherapy. **With the development of effective combination *cis*-platin–based chemotherapy, testicular cancer has become one of the most curable of all genitourinary tumors. As survival rates have improved, the long-term effects of infertility resulting from retroperitoneal lymph node dissection have assumed greater importance. A major impetus for close observation or surveillance therapy has been the long-term effect of ejaculatory compromise and infertility in patients with low-stage testicular cancer.**

MODIFIED RETROPERITONEAL LYMPH NODE DISSECTION. In the early 1980s, Narayan and associates published an important paper concerning ejaculation after extended retroperitoneal lymph node dissection (Narayan et al, 1982). **This paper showed that modification of surgical boundaries could allow return of ejaculation in approximately half of patients with low-stage testicular cancer following retroperitoneal lymph node dissection.** Even with more extensive dissections for stage BII or BIII retroperitoneal involvement, ejaculatory capability returned in approximately one third of patients.

Richie (1990) reported a prospective study of modified lymph node dissection in 85 patients with clinical stage I nonseminomatous germ cell tumor of the testis. The dissection is bilateral above the level of the inferior mesenteric artery but unilateral below the inferior mesenteric artery. The technique involves a thoracoabdominal approach through the ipsilateral side with mobilization of the peritoneal envelope completely. Once the peritoneum is peeled from the posterior rectus fascia, an incision is made in the peritoneum and palpation carried out to be certain there is no bulk disease or more extensive disease that would preclude retroperitoneal rather than transperitoneal lymphadenectomy. By peeling the peritoneal envelope and remaining in a retroperitoneal fashion, along with preservation of the inferior mesenteric artery, injury to the contralateral side of the aorta and great vessels below the inferior mesenteric artery is avoided (Figs. 78–2 and 78–3).

Thus, for a right-sided tumor, the dissection encompasses the renal hilar area bilaterally to the level of the

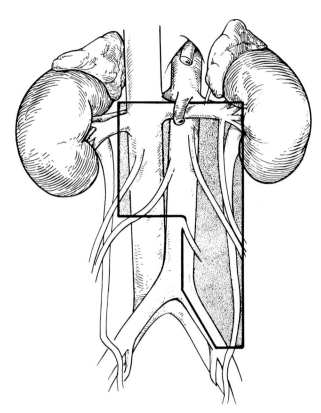

Figure 78–3. Template for modified left-sided retroperitoneal lymph node dissection. The right-sided border is near the right margin of the inferior vena cava.

left ureter or gonadal vein. On the left side, dissection is carried down to the level of the inferior mesenteric artery, then across to the right side and down the right side of the aorta encompassing the right common iliac artery. All nodal bearing tissue in the interaortal caval area is removed, and posteriorly the margin is the anterior spinous ligament. Both sympathetic chains are preserved. On the right side, the dissection is carried along the right renal hilar area to the level of the right ureter and down to where the ureter crosses the common iliac artery. The ipsilateral spermatic vessels are removed to the level of the deep inguinal ring and the previously ligated stump of the cord (see Fig. 78–2).

For left-sided dissection, a similar dissection is performed with the exception of the right lateral margin (see Fig. 78–3). Because nodal spread tends to be from right to left, dissection is carried only to the lateral margin of the inferior vena cava rather than all the way over to the right ureter. **This dissection is bilateral above the inferior mesenteric artery and unilateral below the inferior mesenteric artery.**

The final pathology report of the 85 patients who underwent modified retroperitoneal lymph node dissection indicated stage A cancer in 64 patients and stage BI cancer in 21 patients. As of this writing, patients had been followed from 12 to 84 months with a median of 38 months. Seven patients relapsed, all with pulmonary metastases. All patients have been salvaged with chemotherapy and remain free of disease. **There have been no retroperitoneal recurrences other than one retrocrural recurrence.**

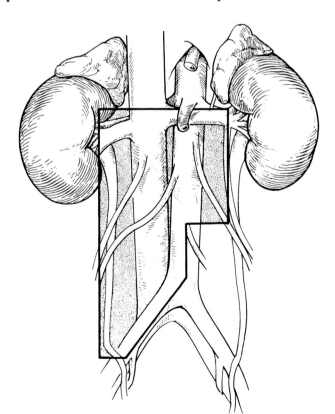

Figure 78–2. Template for modified right-sided retroperitoneal lymph node dissection. The dissection is complete above the level of the inferior mesenteric artery but limited to the unilateral/ipsilateral side below the level of the inferior mesenteric artery.

With respect to preservation of ejaculatory function, 75 of 85 patients have reported spontaneous return of antegrade ejaculation, usually within 1 month postoperatively. An additional five patients have been converted to antegrade ejaculation with imipramine (Tofranil). **Thus, 80 of 85 patients (94%) have recovered antegrade ejaculation, either spontaneously or with medication.** Five patients remain with retrograde ejaculation, as documented by sperm in the urine after ejaculation. Sperm counts have been obtained in 65 patients. The counts range from a low of 2×10^6/ml to a high of 120×10^6/ml. Volume has ranged from 0.5 to 4.5 ml. Most patients report that post–node dissection ejaculate volume is approximately one half that of pre–node dissection ejaculate volume. There have been 11 pregnancies for this group of patients.

The template or boundary method or retroperitoneal lymph node dissection has significant advantages. By use of this technique, a complete bilateral dissection can be performed in the area most likely to be involved with retroperitoneal nodal disease, yet modification in a less likely area can spare some of the ejaculatory consequences. This type of procedure is universally transferable to surgeons with some experience in performance of retroperitoneal lymph node dissection and requires no additional new skills or techniques of identification. The aforementioned technique represents a therapeutically and diagnostically sound method for treatment of patients with pathologic stage A and BI disease, with preservation of ejaculation in more than 90% of patients.

Various centers have described modifications of retroperitoneal lymph node dissection with a variety of techniques to preserve ejaculation. Donohue and associates reported modifications with preservation of ejaculation in two thirds of patients with right-sided tumors and one third of those with left-sided tumors (Donohue et al, 1990). Pizzocaro and co-workers reported on unilateral retroperitoneal lymph node dissection with excellent preservation of ejaculation (Pizzocaro et al, 1986). Ninety percent of patients with stage A and BI testicular cancer had preservation of ejaculation, whereas only 23% of patients with stage BII had preservation of ejaculation (Donohue et al, 1990).

Attempts have been made to identify individual retroperitoneal sympathetic nerves responsible for antegrade ejaculation. **Jewett and Torbey (1988) describe early experience with nerve-sparing techniques with excellent return of ejaculation. Likewise, Donohue and associates have performed a similar procedure with excellent return of ejaculation** (Donohue et al, 1990). **These techniques involve removal of nodal bearing tissue from around the postganglionic fibers.** The techniques are somewhat more time-consuming and may require a steeper learning curve as well. Nonetheless, ejaculation can be preserved in 100% of patients and fertility noted in 75% of patients using these techniques (Foster et al, 1994).

Laparoscopy to perform retroperitoneal lymph node dissection has been described but has a steep learning curve and may not completely remove all of the retroperitoneal nodal tissue (Gerber et al, 1994).

Radiation Therapy

Megavoltage irradiation has been available since the 1950s and in common use since the 1960s, by which time retroperitoneal lymph node dissection had already become established, especially in the United States. Radiation therapy of the retroperitoneum in patients with clinical stage I nonseminomatous germ cell tumors remains accepted practice in many treatment centers outside North America. **The main objections to the use of retroperitoneal lymph node irradiation have been the inaccuracy of clinical staging of the retroperitoneal lymph nodes; the resultant lack of survival data that could be reasonably compared with surgical data; and the concern that, in the event of postirradiation relapse, the prior irradiation might preclude adequate chemotherapy or surgical excision.** Modern staging techniques have reduced the false-negative staging error in clinical stage I to approximately 20%. In patients with clinical stage I disease subjected to retroperitoneal lymph node dissection, 10% to 15% harbor undetected nodal metastasis, and another 5% to 10% relapse following surgery, almost always in extranodal sites. The tumoricidal dose for nonseminomatous germ cell tumors ranges between 4000 and 5000 cGy, far in excess of that required to sterilize seminoma. A dose of 4000 to 4500 cGy delivered in 4 to 5 weeks to the para-aortic and ipsilateral pelvic lymph nodes is the recommended radiation standard in clinical stage I nonseminoma. **The long-term complications of para-aortic irradiation include radiation enteritis, bowel obstruction, and bone marrow suppression, with a reported frequency of between 5% and 10%. Secondary malignancy has been reported following abdominal radiation therapy for Hodgkin's disease, but such reports following treatment for testis tumors are anecdotal.**

The overall success rate of radiation therapy in the treatment of clinical stage I nonseminoma in terms of 5-year survival is between 80% and 95% when chemotherapy is used to treat relapses (Table 78–10). Relapse rates following radiation therapy for clinical stage I are as high as 24% (14 of 59), 3% within the irradiated volume and 21% outside (Raghavan et al, 1982).

Surveillance

If staging modalities were sufficiently accurate to identify patients whose disease is truly confined to the testis,

Table 78–10. SURVIVAL AFTER ORCHIECTOMY AND RADIOTHERAPY FOR CLINICAL STAGES I AND II NONSEMINOMATOUS GERM CELL TUMORS (2–5 YEARS)

Author	Stage I (%)		Stage II (%)		Total (%)	
Battermann et al (1973)	24/30	(80)	6/19	(32)	30/49	(61)
Tyrell and Peckham (1976)	73/88	(84)	14/29	(48)	87/117	(74)
van der Werf-Messing (1976)*	26/29	(90)	16/35	(46)	42/64	(66)
Maier and Mittemeyer (1977)	25/29	(86)	9/11	(82)	34/40	(85)
Peckham et al (1981)†	37/39	(95)	17/21	(81)	54/60	(90)
Blandy et al (1983)	125/162 (77)		—		125/162 (77)	
Total	310/377 (82)		62/115 (54)		372/492 (76)	

*Extrapolated from actuarial tables.
†Includes patients treated successfully for relapse and patients in stage II treated primarily with preirradiation chemotherapy.

orchiectomy alone should yield survival results equal to therapeutic strategies that incorporate treatment of the regional lymph nodes. With the inaccuracies of staging, however, retroperitoneal lymph node dissection remains the only modality that can accurately delineate pathologic stage I from pathologic stage II testicular cancer. Clinical understaging approximates 25% even in the best of series. Nonetheless, approximately 70% of patients who undergo retroperitoneal lymph node dissection are found to have pathologic stage I disease and, therefore, receive no therapeutic benefit from the operation. Additionally, 5% to 10% of patients relapse outside of the field of the retroperitoneal node dissection.

With the advent of effective chemotherapy, coupled with concerns about the need for retroperitoneal lymph node dissection in all patients with clinical stage I testicular cancer as well as the complications of loss of ejaculation and infertility, postorchiectomy observation or surveillance has a certain appeal. **Several large surveillance programs have been undertaken throughout the world. In several of the largest series, detailed in Table 78–11, the relapse rate is approximately 30%. Unfortunately the death rate in those patients who relapse has been 7%, or 1.8% of the entire series.** Even with monitoring, 80% of relapses are noted at more advanced stage compared to those patients who undergo retroperitoneal lymph node dissection and who tend to relapse with pulmonary metastases at a lower stage of advanced disease (Rowland et al, 1982). Considering that the majority of these patients have favorable factors in order to enter a surveillance protocol, death rates should be exceedingly rare in this subset of patients.

An additional concern about surveillance is the extraordinary period of time necessary to follow patients. At least two reports have appeared of late relapses, 6 and 9 years, for patients with nonseminomatous germ cell tumor on surveillance protocols (Hurley and Libertino, 1995; McCrystal et al, 1995). In addition to potential problems with inadequate follow-up, imaging study difficulties, and higher mortality with relapse, one must factor in the increased cost and labor for longer surveillance periods.

As more experience has been generated, patient selection should identify those individuals at low risk for metastases in whom close observation could be elected. These patients require meticulous evaluation before entering a well-designed and well-managed surveillance protocol. Staging

should be carried out compulsively in selected patients with no evidence of suspicious nodes or pulmonary masses.

Several series have evaluated prognostic factors associated with relapse (Dunphy et al, 1988; Fung et al, 1988). Patients with a significant percentage of embryonal carcinoma in the primary are believed to be at high risk of relapse. The local T stage or extent of involvement of the tumor is also an important prognostic factor. Patients with invasion of the epididymis or tunica albuginea (T2 or greater) have a higher rate of relapse. Finally and most importantly, the presence of vascular or lymphatic invasion is significantly associated with relapse.

In patients in whom surveillance therapy is elected, this should be considered an active form of treatment with careful follow-up being mandatory. **Physical examination, chest x-ray studies, and tumor marker studies are performed monthly for the first year, every 2 months for the second year, and every 3 to 6 months thereafter. Because of the difficulty with assessment of the retroperitoneum, CT scan should be performed approximately every 2 to 3 months for the first 2 years and at least every 6 months thereafter. Surveillance is necessary for a minimum of 5 years and possibly 10 years following orchiectomy.**

Treatment: Stage II (Spread to Retroperitoneal Lymph Nodes)

Surgical Treatment

The potential advantages of retroperitoneal lymph node dissection in the treatment of testis cancer stem from the fact that retroperitoneal deposits are usually the first and frequently the sole evidence of extragonadal spread. Such therapy is capable of eradicating resectable disease in more than half of patients with stage II tumors. Analysis of different surgical experiences reveals that several uncontrolled variables exist. These include the clinical staging accuracy, the extent and quality of node dissection, the criteria of surgical resectability, the pathologic examination of surgical specimen, and the use of adjuvant or salvage (for recurrent disease) chemotherapy.

A variety of surgical approaches to retroperitoneal lymphadenectomy have been explored. Thoracoabdominal and midline transperitoneal exposures are in common use today. The usual distribution of nodal metastasis as determined by anatomic studies, surgical exploration, and lymphangiography extends from the superior border of the renal vessels around the aorta and vena cava to each ureter laterally and along the common iliac vessels to just beyond their bifurcations. The extent of lymph node dissection is individualized from the following considerations: (1) serum tumor marker levels after orchiectomy, (2) lymphangiographic or abdominal CT interpretations, and (3) findings at laparotomy. Positive markers following orchiectomy or positive radiographic studies indicate the need for a complete bilateral lymphadenectomy. **Clinical experience has shown that surgical exploration alone is more than 90% accurate in assessing the presence or absence of lymph node metastasis. When suspicious lymph nodes are encountered at laparotomy, a complete bilateral lymphadenectomy is recommended, although nerve-sparing techniques can be**

Table 78–11. SURVEILLANCE STUDIES IN PATIENTS WITH CLINICAL STAGE I NONSEMINOMATOUS GERM CELL TUMOR

Series	No. of Patients	No. Relapsed (%)	No. Dead
Read et al (1983)	45	11 (24)	0
Johnson et al (1984)	36	12 (33)	2
Pizzocaro et al (1986)	85	23 (27)	1
Freedman et al (1987)	259	70 (27)	3
Gelderman et al (1987)	54	11 (20)	0
Rorth et al (1987)	79	24 (30)	2
Raghavan et al (1988)	46	13 (28)	2
Sogani et al (1988)	45	10 (22)	2
Thompson et al (1988)	36	12 (33)	2
Total	685	186 (27)	14 (8%)

used. **Suprarenal nodal metastasis occurs infrequently in the absence of advanced infrarenal disease.** Routine suprahilar lymph node dissection in the absence of palpable metastasis in this region has not demonstrably improved local control rates. **When serum markers, CT scan, and laparotomy are collectively negative, a modified bilateral dissection may be performed.**

Since first popularized by Lewis (1948), retroperitoneal lymph node dissection has been used with varying success to treat regional metastasis from testis cancer. Retroperitoneal lymph node dissection is certainly capable of controlling regional node metastasis in selected patients. The majority of surgical series furnish little information relating the frequency of relapse and curability to the size, number, site, or histology of the nodal metastasis. Surgicopathologic correlation according to criteria in Table 78–12 may provide some relevant data.

Chemotherapy

The high relapse and unresectability rates in patients with bulky retroperitoneal disease, coupled with the demonstrated effectiveness of multidrug regimens in treating disseminated cancer, prompted the use of chemotherapy as initial therapy for those with advanced nodal or pulmonary metastases during the mid-1970s (Fig. 78–4). Almost simultaneously, advances in clinical staging identified patients who might benefit from such a strategy. **Because chemotherapy was so effective in treating disseminated disease, it appeared prudent to redefine the role of surgery following primary chemotherapy.** This question was approached by systematically administering combination-drug therapy and then subjecting patients to surgical excision of residual disease, if such were judged feasible. **The results from different institutions using varying drug combinations and techniques of lymphadenectomy indicated that chemotherapy is capable of sterilizing bulky disease, with resultant tumor necrosis and fibrosis, in roughly one third of cases.** Another 20%, however, harbored residual malignant elements, and the remainder harbored teratoma. Survival was excellent in patients with necrotic or fibrosed tumor and in those with teratoma or completely resected viable cancer. Complete resection was rarely feasible in patients with persistently elevated serum markers following chemotherapy. Negative post-treatment serum markers did not exclude the possible existence of a histologically viable cancer.

The recognition of teratoma within surgically excised residual masses following combination chemotherapy for advanced disease is a relatively recent phenomenon (Merrin et al, 1975; Hong et al, 1977). **The surgical removal of benign "mature" or "immature" teratoma should be accomplished for five reasons: (1) Preoperative studies cannot rule out the possibility of residual malignancy; (2) pathologic examination may not detect small malignant foci within an apparently benign mass; (3) expansion of benign solid and cystic teratomatous elements may compromise vital organ function; (4) teratoma may exist as or degenerate into a malignant sarcomatous form; and (5) chemotherapy and radiation therapy are ineffective against benign or malignant teratoma.**

In earlier series, roughly one third of patients with advanced nonseminomatous germ cell tumors who have normal serum tumor markers following preoperative cytoreductive chemotherapy have a malignant component within the excised residual tissues (Einhorn et al, 1981; Vugrin et al, 1981). In 1995, approximately 10% of patients had residual malignancy. Although pathologic techniques vary, it is unlikely that step-sectioning is routine in the assessment of all resected material, implying that a malignant element may be missed by sampling error. **Logothetis and colleagues described the "growing teratoma syndrome" after observing the enlargement of teratomatous deposits during or after chemotherapy** (Logothetis et al, 1982). **Although the early recognition and resection of teratoma have been accompanied by an excellent prognosis, untreated disease may possess a lethal potential by virtue of continued local growth or from putative subsequent malignant transformation of histologically benign components. These considerations, together with the inability to distinguish between teratoma and carcinoma and the uncertain natural history of untreated teratoma, warrant surgical resection of residual masses following chemocytoreduction.** Although irradiation may have favorable effects in such a setting, relevant pathologic data are wanting.

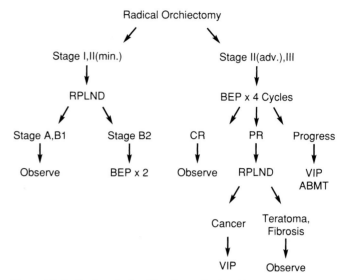

Figure 78–4. Treatment algorithm for patients with nonseminomatous germ cell testicular tumors (NSGCT). RPLND, retroperitoneal lymph node dissection; BEP, bleomycin, etoposide, and *cis*-platin; VIP, vinblastine, ifosfamide and *cis*-platin; ABMT, autologous bone marrow transplantation; CR, complete response; PR, partial response.

Table 78–12. PATHOLOGIC STAGING OF NONSEMINOMATOUS GERM CELL TUMORS

Stage	Description of Retroperitoneal Nodes
I (A)	Negative
II (B)	Positive
N-1	Microscopic involvement
N-2	Nodes grossly involved
A (B₁)	<5 nodes involved with none >2 cm diameter
B (B₂)	>5 nodes involved and/or nodes >2 cm diameter
N-3	Extranodal extension (gross or microscopic), resectable
N-4 (B₃)	Incompletely resected/unresectable disease

Surgical excision of residual nodal tissue or extranodal masses following treatment with multidrug chemotherapy is recommended. If chemotherapy is given initially for pulmonary metastasis alone (when pretreatment studies fail to demonstrate significant retroperitoneal disease) and there is no serologic or radiographic evidence of neoplasm after therapy, surveillance without retroperitoneal lymph node dissection may be undertaken but with an apparently substantial risk.

Controversy exists about the role of retroperitoneal lymphadenectomy versus primary chemotherapy in patients with clinical stage B or stage II testis cancer. The author's preference is to use chemotherapy or primary treatment for patients with nodes larger than 3 cm in diameter. It is apparent that both retroperitoneal lymph node dissection and chemotherapy are similarly effective for clinical low-volume stage II nonseminomatous germ cell tumors. In a review by Donohue and associates, 174 patients considered to have clinical stage B disease underwent retroperitoneal lymph node dissection (Donohue et al, 1995). Twenty-three percent actually had pathologic stage A disease. Sixty-five percent of the pathologic stage B cancer patients were cured by retroperitoneal lymph node dissection alone, indicating that surgery has diagnostic and therapeutic import. Relapsers were uniformly salvaged with chemotherapy. From a cost analysis, using the Indiana University experience, overall direct costs for 100 patients undergoing primary retroperitoneal lymph node dissection were compared with direct costs for 100 patients receiving primary chemotherapy for low-volume stage II disease (Baniel et al, 1995). The overall 5-year costs of retroperitoneal lymph node dissection were significantly less than the costs of primary chemotherapy, although the two options did not differ in terms of survival or quality of life.

Radiation Therapy

An alternative approach to patients with clinical stage II nonseminomatous germ cell tumors is lymph node irradiation. This approach had been fairly routine outside of the United States before the development of effective chemotherapy and routine abdominal CT scan. This approach was abandoned in most institutions because of a lack of evidence that prophylactic irradiation was effective. No randomized prospective study had been successfully completed comparing radiotherapy with any other modality when this approach was largely abandoned. It fell into disuse along with the development of effective chemotherapy.

The efficacy of lymph node irradiation still remains in question, although one randomized study that has reached maturity now exists. Between 1980 and 1984, 153 patients with clinical stage I nonseminoma were randomized after orchiectomy to either prophylactic irradiation or observation. With a minimal follow-up of 5 years, 23 of 85 (27%) of the patients who were observed relapsed, with 14 of the 23 (61%) relapsing primarily in the retroperitoneum. Only 11 of 68 (16%) patients treated with irradiation relapsed, with 0 of 11 (0%) relapsing in the retroperitoneum. All patients in both groups who relapsed were salvaged with chemotherapy with the exception of one patient in the irradiation-treated group. These data suggest that irradiation can be an effective modality for low-stage nonseminoma, and the failure to demonstrate its efficacy previously may be due to a high proportion of understaged patients in historical controls not evaluated by CT scanning. If, however, "prophylactic" irradiation is effective, it appears that less than 50% of those patients with retroperitoneal disease truly benefit from this therapy. Similar to retroperitoneal lymph node dissection, prophylactic irradiation likely eradicates disease in the retroperitoneum; however, disease coexists outside of the retroperitoneum in a large proportion of these patients. In contrast to retroperitoneal lymph node dissection, irradiation gives no information regarding the need for adjuvant chemotherapy. Furthermore, many patients are treated unnecessarily (although the morbidity is low), and for those patients who relapse, there is potentially a greater likelihood of morbid consequences from chemotherapy.

The evolution of effective multidrug regimens has changed the attitudes of both radiation and surgical oncologists. Many radiotherapists now recommend the use of chemotherapy as initial treatment for (1) nodal metastasis clinically judged larger than 2 cm in diameter, (2) supradiaphragmatic node involvement, and (3) extralymphatic spread. Supplementary irradiation is then delivered to initially large nodal deposits, with surgical excision being reserved for selected patients with residual masses (Peckham et al, 1981). The main drawback of such an approach is that if relapse occurs following radiation therapy for small-volume disease or following an integrated scheme, the effectiveness of chemotherapy may be undermined by cumulative myelosuppression. Furthermore, surgical treatment of focally persistent disease may be complicated by prior irradiation.

Treatment: Stage III

Before the 1970s, advanced stages of testicular cancer were treated with chemotherapy, albeit with modest response rates. Li and co-workers described the so-called triple therapy consisting of chlorambucil, methotrexate, and actinomycin-D for patients with disseminated testicular cancer (Li et al, 1960). They reported a 50% objective response rate and a 5% to 10% complete response rate with chemotherapy based predominantly on actinomycin-D. Subsequently, MacKenzie (1966) reviewed the Sloan-Kettering Memorial experience in 154 patients with disseminated nonseminomatous germ cell tumor and concluded that actinomycin-D was the most effective and active agent, either alone or in combination with the above-mentioned agents. During the 1960s, additional agents such as mithramycin, vinblastine, and bleomycin were also shown to be active in this disease (Kennedy, 1970). Samuels and Howe (1970) were among the first to recognize the utility of vinblastine in the treatment of patients with disseminated testicular cancer. They reported four complete responses in 21 patients with advanced disease using this regimen. In 1972, investigators at Sloan-Kettering used the combination of vinblastine, actinomycin-D, and bleomycin (VAB-1) with partial remission in 19% and complete response in 19% (Wittes et al, 1976). With the above-mentioned regimens, response rate was generally in the order of 10% to 15% with at least a 50% relapse rate.

The concept of combination of vinblastine with bleomycin was initially described by Samuels and associates at M. D. Anderson (Samuels et al, 1975). Although intermittent therapy was used initially, Samuels and associates switched to continuous infusion bleomycin in combination with vinblastine in 1973 (Samuels et al, 1976). This so-called VB III regimen of continuous infusion resulted in overall response rates in the 60% range.

Cis-platin, arguably the single most active agent in the treatment of testicular cancer, was identified initially on studies of agents that inhibit bacterial replication (Rosenberg et al, 1965). Nephrotoxicity and ototoxicity were potential problems, although doses of 20 mg/m² could be given with adequate hydration.

Vinblastine–Actinomycin-D–Bleomycin Protocols

Beginning in 1972, the Sloan-Kettering Memorial group began using combination chemotherapy with vinblastine plus actinomycin-D plus bleomycin (VAB) resulting in 19% complete response and 19% partial response rates (Wittes et al, 1976). From 1974 to 1975, *cis*-platin was added to continuous infusion bleomycin (VAB-II) (Cheng et al, 1978). These authors reported a 50% complete response and 34% partial response rate; 12 (24%) patients remained alive and disease-free. A number of patients were subjected to second-look surgical procedures following VAB-II chemotherapy.

The 50% relapse rate in patients who had achieved complete response with VAB-II led to the inauguration of the VAB-III regimen from 1975 through 1976. Modifications in the protocol with the addition of cyclophosphamide to the induction phase and adriamycin to the maintenance schedule resulted in 61% overall complete response, but the durable complete response rate was only 44% (Cvitkovic et al, 1978). VAB-III involved two major inductions spaced approximately 6 months apart. In September 1976, additional modifications resulted in the VAB-IV combination, with the complete response rate of 80%; 50% of 48 patients remained disease-free (Cvitkovic et al, 1978). In 1977, patients with poor prognostic features such as bulky retroperitoneal metastases; liver, brain, or multiple sites of involvement; and high elevations of serum tumor markers underwent a more intensive VAB-IV regimen. The complete response rate, however, was only 47%, and toxicity was quite severe. This regimen was abandoned in 1978.

The VAB-VI regimen was initiated in 1979 and accrued 166 patients by 1982. This regimen was a major departure from prior VAB programs. *Cis*-platin was given monthly for three courses at a dose of 120 mg/m² along with vinblastine 4 mg/m², cyclophosphamide 600 mg/m², actinomycin 1 mg/m², and bleomycin 30 units. This regimen was repeated every 4 weeks for three cycles with bleomycin held on the third cycle. Interval between inductions was shortened, and chlorambucil was omitted. Maintenance therapy was compared with no maintenance therapy in a randomized study. Complete response rate was 57%. Overall relapse was 12% (Bosl et al, 1986).

Cis-platin–Vinblastine–Bleomycin Studies

One of the major contributors to the development of combination chemotherapy for patients with disseminated testicular cancer has been the group at Indiana University, headed by Einhorn. **Beginning in 1974, *cis*-platin was added to the standard two-drug regimen of vinblastine and bleomycin (PVB)** (Einhorn and Donohue, 1977). Originally, this consisted of *cis*-platin 20 mg/m² every 3 weeks, vinblastine 0.2 mg/kg on days 1 and 2 every 3 weeks, and bleomycin 30 units intravenous push. This cycle was repeated four times. Saline hydration was used to prevent nephrotoxicity. **In the early trial, complete response was achieved in 70%, and virtually 100% objective response rate was noted.**

Because of toxicity with high-dose vinblastine, specifically myalgias, neuropathy, and ileus, a second randomized, prospective trial was introduced to study the standard PVB regimen with a lower dose of vinblastine (0.3 mg/kg total dose). Maintenance vinblastine was used for 2 years after achievement of response. In this trial, there was no significant difference in efficacy with the lower vinblastine dosage with or without the addition of adriamycin (Einhorn and Williams, 1980b). **Thus, the lower dose of vinblastine, 0.3 mg/kg, was shown to be equally effective with long-term, durable response rates.**

Beginning in 1978, a third-generation study was performed in a randomized, prospective fashion comparing four cycles of PVB chemotherapy versus four cycles with maintenance vinblastine. This study confirmed the fact that cure rates could be achieved with four cycles of chemotherapy without the need for maintenance (Einhorn et al, 1980a). Overall, 80% of patients on this study were alive and disease-free with follow-up greater than 5 years.

Etoposide (VP-16) has single-agent activity in patients with testicular cancer. Because of the toxicity, especially neuromuscular, with vinblastine, VP-16 was studied in a randomized, prospective trial under the auspices of the Southeastern Cancer Study Group (Williams et al, 1987a). **In this multi-institutional trial, 121 patients were treated with PVB with a 61% complete remission rate. A total of 123 patients were treated with bleomycin, *cis*-platin, and VP-16 with a 60% complete remission rate.** Including patients rendered disease-free after resection of teratoma, 74% were disease-free in the PVB group versus 83% in the *cis*-platin, bleomycin, and VP-16 group. Toxicity was similar in both arms. **Thus, bleomycin, etoposide (VP-16), and platinum (BEP) would seem to be a superior combination chemotherapy and has become the standard treatment for patients with disseminated germ cell tumor** (Table 78–13).

Randomized studies have compared three cycles versus four cycles of BEP. The response rate is equivalent in both groups. **Thus, for patients without adverse risk factors** (see later), **three cycles of BEP chemotherapy should suffice.** A prospective, randomized trial compared three cycles of etoposide plus *cis*-platin (EP) versus three cycles of BEP. Although response rates were initially similar, a greater number of treatment failures, including persistent carcinoma and relapses from complete remission, occurred in the EP arm. Therefore, in a three-cycle regimen, the addition of bleomycin is an essential component of therapy (Loehrer et al, 1995).

Adjuvant Chemotherapy

Surgical excision has been the standard treatment for patients with clinical stage I or low stage II nonseminoma-

Table 78–13. STANDARD CHEMOTHERAPY FOR
NONSEMINOMATOUS GERM CELL TUMORS

Chemotherapy	Dose	Days	Toxicity
BEP (per cycle)			
Bleomycin	30 units	2, 9, 16	Pulmonary fibrosis
Etoposide (VP-16)	100 mg/m²	1–5	Myelosuppression
			Alopecia
			Renal insufficiency (mild)
			Secondary leukemia
Cis-platin	20 mg/m²	1–5	Renal insufficiency
			Nausea, vomiting
			Neuropathy
VIP (per cycle)			
VP-16 (etoposide)	75 mg/m²	1–5	Myelosuppression
			Alopecia
			Renal insufficiency (mild)
			Secondary leukemia
Ifosfamide	1.2 g/m²	1–5	Hemorrhagic cystitis
Cis-platin	20 mg/m²	1–5	Renal insufficiency
			Nausea, vomiting
			Neuropathy
Mesna	240 mg/m² q4h × 3		

tous germ cell tumors. **At issue is whether adjuvant chemotherapy is necessary in patients with disease in the retroperitoneum that has been resected completely.** In patients with pathologic stage II nonseminomatous germ cell tumors, controversy exists concerning the role of adjunctive chemotherapy. Two-year disease-free survival rate for such patients is 60% to 80%, indicating that 20% to 40% of these patients experience recurrence, usually in the lungs. These patients can be salvaged with three or four cycles of combination chemotherapy.

A national intergroup study published by Williams and associates reported a 48% relapse rate for patients with any positive nodes who were observed following retroperitoneal lymphadenectomy (Williams et al, 1987b). **This relapse rate was compared with a 2% relapse rate in patients who received two cycles of adjuvant chemotherapy, either VAB-VI or PVB, postoperatively.** This study included all patients with positive retroperitoneal lymph nodes dissected, from stage N1 to N3. There was no difference in relapse rate among patients with nodal stages: 40% for N1, 53% for N2a, and 60% for N2b.

In a review of 39 patients who underwent retroperitoneal lymph node dissection at the Brigham & Women's Hospital for pathologic stage BI disease, with fewer than six positive nodes and no node greater than 2 cm, only 3 of 39 patients relapsed with a median follow-up of 3.5 years (Richie and Kantoff, 1991). Thus, for patients with minimal retroperitoneal disease, resected completely, careful follow-up is recommended. For patients with more extensive disease, adjuvant chemotherapy with two cycles can be initiated relatively shortly after retroperitoneal lymph node dissection. The other alternative is careful follow-up with three or four cycles of chemotherapy to be used at the time of relapse. Two cycles of cis-platin–based adjuvant chemotherapy almost always prevents relapse.

Salvage Chemotherapy

Cis-platin combination chemotherapy effects cure in approximately 70% of patients with disseminated germ cell tumors. In patients in whom serum markers have normalized after three cycles of chemotherapy, residual masses should be resected surgically. The operative procedures for surgical resection are more extensive and are covered in a separate chapter. **Surgeons should be aware of potential bleomycin-related complications, especially pulmonary fibrosis.** Barneveld and colleagues reported 8 of 93 patients with evidence of bleomycin pneumonitis, one of whom died from bleomycin toxicity (Barneveld et al, 1987). **Bleomycin toxicity can be minimized by careful monitoring intraoperatively and postoperatively, reduction in the forced inspiratory oxygen (<0.25), and restriction of free water intraoperatively and immediately postoperatively.**

In patients with residual cancer that has been resected after chemotherapy, or more commonly in patients who do not respond to the traditional courses of induction therapy, salvage therapy with different agents is available and should be considered (see Fig. 78–4). In patients who show evidence of progression during cis-platin combination chemotherapy, salvage chemotherapy with cis-platin should not be used. In patients whose disease progresses after having received cis-platin, cis-platin may still be useful and should be considered in salvage regimens.

Ifosfamide is an active agent in patients with testicular cancer with a 22% single-agent response rate (Wheeler et al, 1986). **Ifosfamide in combination with vinblastine and cis-platin (VIP regimen) has achieved an approximate 30% disease-free status in patients who have failed initial chemotherapy regimens** (see Table 78–13) (Lauer et al, 1987). **In patients who receive ifosfamide, mesna should be used before starting ifosfamide to prevent the complication of hemorrhagic cystitis.** In patients who have initially received vinblastine, VP-16 should be used in the VIP regimen. In patients who receive VP-16, vinblastine should be used.

Third-line chemotherapy for patients who have not responded to first-line and second-line therapy includes autologous bone marrow transplantation with high-dose chemotherapy regimens. Carboplatin, an agent with activity similar to cis-platin, has myelosuppression as its dose-limiting toxicity. Therefore, carboplatin can be used in lieu of cis-platin in patients who are undergoing autologous bone marrow transplantation. Early salvage therapy using autologous bone marrow support including carboplatin has resulted in complete response in 9 of 18 and partial response in 6 of 18 patients in a relatively small series of first relapse (Broun et al, 1994).

Management of High-Risk Testicular Cancer Patients

Patients with stage C nonseminomatous testicular cancer can be subdivided into patients whose cancer responds to standard chemotherapy and patients whose cancer responds to more aggressive chemotherapy. The Indiana University staging system detailed in Table 78–14 has proven to be a workable model with therapeutic advantages. Patients with minimal or moderate disease do well with standard chemotherapy, with response rates in the 91% to 95% category (Birch et al, 1986). Patients with advanced disease, however, had only a 53% therapeutic response. Therefore, more ag-

Table 78–14. INDIANA UNIVERSITY STAGING SYSTEM FOR DISSEMINATED TESTICULAR CANCER

Minimal Extent

Elevated markers only
Cervical nodes (±nonpalpable retroperitoneal nodes)
Unresectable nonpalpable retroperitoneal disease
<five pulmonary metastases per lung field *and* largest <2 cm
   (±nonpalpable retroperitoneal nodes)

Moderate Extent

Palpable abdominal mass only (no supradiaphragmatic disease)
Moderate pulmonary metastases: 5–10 metastases per lung field and largest <3 cm or solitary pulmonary metastasis of any size >2 cm (±nonpalpable retroperitoneal disease)

Advanced Extent

Advanced pulmonary metastases: primary mediastinal nonseminomatous germ cell tumor or >10 pulmonary metastases per lung field, or multiple pulmonary metastases
Palpable abdominal mass plus supradiaphragmatic disease
Liver, bone, or central nervous system metastases

gressive chemotherapy should be used in patients with advanced-extent disease according to this category.

High-dose chemotherapy and autologous bone marrow transplantation can be used in patients with poor-prognosis tumors, resulting in a complete response rate of 35% to 45% and long-term survival in about 25% (Barnett et al, 1993; Lotz et al, 1995).

EXTRAGONADAL TUMORS

Primary tumors of extragonadal origin are rare, with fewer than 1000 cases described in the literature. Distinction between a primary extragonadal germ cell tumor (EGT) and metastatic disease from an undetected testis primary tumor may be difficult but has obviously important clinical implications. **Surgical and autopsy series have confirmed the absence of a "burned-out" testicular primary lesion in a number of cases, laying to rest some of the skepticism surrounding the diagnosis of EGT in the past** (Luna and Valenzuela-Tamariz, 1976). More recently, testicular ultrasonography has emerged as a sensitive technique for the detection of tiny neoplasms a few millimeters in size within the clinically normal testis. **Although the exact incidence of EGTs is unknown, clinical data suggest that roughly 3% to 5% of all germ cell tumors are of extragonadal origin.**

The most common sites of origin are, in decreasing order of frequency, the mediastinum, retroperitoneum, sacrococcygeal region, and pineal gland, although many unusual sources have also been reported. Two schools of thought exist as to the origin of these neoplasms: (1) displacement of primitive germ cells during early embryonic migration from the yolk sac entoderm and (2) persistence of pluripotential cells in sequestered primitive rests during early somatic development. The theory of misplaced germ cells holds that during ontogeny, migration through the retroperitoneum is misdirected cephalad to the mediastinum and pineal gland or caudad to the sacrococcygeal region, rather than to the genital ridges. The alternative hypothesis maintains that primitive pluripotential cells may be dislocated during early embryogenesis (blastema or morula phase). A

germ cell rest in the third brachial cleft, for example, could result in a mediastinal tumor, which, interestingly, often resembles a thymoma histologically.

Males are affected predominantly, although a female predominance has been noted with sacrococcygeal lesions. With the exception of sacrococcygeal tumors in the newborn, these tumors generally lack encapsulation, in contrast to their testicular counterparts, and tend to invade or envelope contiguous structures. **The majority of adults with EGTs present with advanced local disease and distant metastases.** These tumors most commonly spread to regional lymph nodes, lung, liver, and bone. **Histologically, all germ cell types are represented, with pure seminoma accounting for roughly half of the tumors in the mediastinum and retroperitoneum.** In general, sacrococcygeal tumors of the newborn and young adult are functionally and histologically benign, whereas tumors discovered during infancy prove malignant in about half of the cases.

EGTs may reach a large size with no or relatively few symptoms. Diagnosis of mediastinal EGT is most commonly established in patients during their twenties, with or without signs and symptoms of chest pain, cough, or dyspnea. Patients with primary retroperitoneal tumors may present with abdominal or back pain, a palpable mass, vascular obstruction, or other vague constitutional symptoms. **Sacrococcygeal tumors are most often diagnosed in the neonate (1 in 40,000 births) and less frequently during infancy or adulthood, with findings of a palpable mass, skin discoloration or hairy nevus, or bowel or urinary obstruction.** Tumors of the pineal gland occur in children and young adults, producing symptoms of increased intracranial pressure (headache, visual impairment), oculomotor dysfunction (diplopia, ptosis), hearing loss, hypopituitarism (abnormal menses), and hypothalamic disturbances (diabetes insipidus).

Complete local excision of mediastinal or retroperitoneal tumors is rarely feasible because of frequent local extension and high rates of metastatic disease. In reviewing 30 cases of primary mediastinal tumors, Martini and associates found only 4 of 30 patients who presented with no metastasis (Martini et al, 1974). Three of these four had pure seminoma. In the 10 patients with pure seminoma, only 4 were long-term survivors following surgery or radiotherapy. Of 20 patients with elements of embryonal carcinoma, only 1 was alive at 20 months following surgery, radiotherapy, and chemotherapy. Sterchi and Cordell (1975) reviewed 108 patients with mediastinal seminoma, finding a 5-year survival rate of 58% following primary radiation therapy or surgery. The Memorial Sloan-Kettering experience with 21 cases of extragonadal seminoma was reviewed with primary *cis*-platin–based chemotherapy; only 1 patient died of metastatic disease, with the remainder disease-free at 19+ to 46+ months' follow-up. **Patients with primary retroperitoneal seminoma appear equally responsive to intensive chemotherapy regimens (Stanton et al, 1983). In contrast, patients with nonseminomatous EGT have done poorly despite surgery, radiotherapy, and chemotherapy** (Recondo and Libshitz, 1978; Reynolds et al, 1979). **Disappointingly, only 2 of 18 patients treated at Memorial Sloan-Kettering with successive VAB protocols have achieved complete remission.** Although Garnick and colleagues (1983) reported similar results, those of Hainsworth and co-workers (1982), using the PVB regimen, were superior. The reason for this apparent discrepancy remains unclear.

Wide local excision is the treatment of choice for sacrococcygeal tumors, in that the majority are benign. Limited experience renders uncertain the advisability of adjunctive irradiation or chemotherapy for malignant tumors. Radical excisions for pineal tumors have been disappointing from the standpoints of local control and operative morbidity. Such procedures have been largely abandoned in favor of primary radiation therapy, although a cerebrospinal fluid shunt may be required (Cole, 1971).

OTHER TESTIS NEOPLASMS

Under the designation "other testis neoplasms" are included a heterogeneous group of tumors of relatively infrequent occurrence. Together, they constitute between 5% and 10% of all testis tumors.

Sex Cord–Mesenchyme Tumors (Gonadal Stromal Tumors; Sex Cord–Stromal Tumors)

Both semantic and histogenetic uncertainties have contributed to the continuing difficulties in the classification of such lesions. Distinguishing between hyperplasia and benign and malignant tumors has added to the problems of classification. Teilum (1946, 1971) was principally responsible for calling attention to this group of tumors and for emphasizing the comparative pathology of the analogous ovarian and testicular neoplasms. **The cell type, architecture, and degree of differentiation of these tumors may closely duplicate the supporting tissues in the gonads of either sex. In the testis, the microscopic appearance may be that of undifferentiated gonadal stroma, a Sertoli cell tumor in germ cell–free seminiferous tubules, or a Leydig cell tumor. More rarely, tumors that are apparently composed of granulosa cells or theca cells occur.**

Interstitial Cell Lesions (Leydig Cell Tumors)

Varying degrees of apparent focal or diffuse interstitial cell hyperplasia may be noted with a variety of conditions associated with seminiferous tubule atrophy. To what extent these represent absolute or relative increases in interstitial cells may be difficult to assess. **Interstitial cell tumors, the most common of the sex cord–mesenchyme lesions, make up between 1% and 3% of all testis tumors.** Although the majority have been recognized in men between the ages of 20 and 60 years, approximately one fourth have been reported before puberty.

The etiology of Leydig cell tumors is unknown. In contrast to germ cell tumors, there appears to be no association with cryptorchidism. The experimental production of Leydig cell tumors in mice following chronic estrogen administration or following intrasplenic testicular autografting is consistent with a hormonal basis.

The lesions are generally small, yellow-to-brown, and well circumscribed and rarely exhibit hemorrhage or necrosis. Microscopically the tumors consist of relatively uniform, polyhedral, closely packed cells with round, slightly eccentric nuclei and eosinophilic granular cytoplasm with lipoid vacuoles, brownish pigmentation, and occasional characteristic inclusions known as Reinke crystals. Pleomorphism with large and bizarre cell forms may occur, and mitotic figures may or may not be identified. **None of these features appears to be consistently related to malignant potential.** Furthermore, limited observations suggest that ultrastructural features do not categorically distinguish between normal and neoplastic Leydig cells, whether benign or malignant.

Approximately 10% of interstitial cell tumors are malignant, but there are no consistently reliable histologic criteria for making this judgment. Large size, extensive necrosis, gross or microscopic evidence of infiltration, invasion of blood vessels, and excessive mitotic activity are all features that suggest the possibility of malignancy, but metastasis is generally regarded as the only reliable criterion of malignancy. Similar to other testis tumors, malignant lesions may involve retroperitoneal lymph nodes, lung, and bone. Of importance is the observation that malignancy is nonexistent in the prepubertal age group.

CLINICAL PRESENTATION. In the prepubertal cases (average age 5 years), presenting manifestations are usually those of isosexual precocity with prominent external genitalia, mature masculine voice, and pubic hair growth. Hormonal assays in such patients have been few and generally incomplete or have been carried out by antiquated techniques. **Increased testosterone production is usually demonstrable, and urinary 17-ketosteroid output may or may not be elevated. Virilizing types of congenital adrenocortical hyperplasia may also produce the endocrine signs and symptoms of interstitial cell tumors, so differential tests must be carried out to clarify the diagnosis.** Such tests include estimation of urinary 17-hydroxysteroid and 17-ketosteroid levels as well as plasma cortisol before and after adrenocorticotropic hormone stimulation and dexamethasone suppression. Because interstitial cell carcinomas have been shown to possess 21-hydroxylase activity and to be capable of forming cortisol and hydroxylating steroids at the 11-beta position, it is clear that interstitial cell tumors may possess some of the same functional activities as adrenocortical tissue. The similar embryologic origin of interstitial cells and adrenocortical cells and the occurrence of adrenal rests in the testis complicate interpretation. The paradox of the tumor's arising in the interstitial cells of a prepubertal testis and behaving metabolically similar to its adult counterpart, in conjunction with cells in the normal prepubertal testis containing enzymes capable of producing testosterone, explains the occurrence of spermatogenesis in the seminiferous tubules more remote from the tumor.

In adults, the majority of reported cases have shown manifestations of endocrine imbalance, although some do not. The endocrinologic manifestations may precede the palpable testis mass, which is the most common presenting feature. In the remaining adult cases, symptoms of a feminizing nature, such as impotence, decreased libido, and gynecomastia, may occur. The slow progression of these neoplasms is suggested by the long duration

of gynecomastia, which may precede recognition of the testicular mass. In contrast to the situation with adult germ cell tumors, the duration of gynecomastia with adult interstitial cell tumors has ranged from 6 months to 10 years and averages more than 3 years. Elevation of urinary and plasma estrogens in association with this tumor is relatively common. Lockhart and colleagues reported a nonfunctioning interstitial cell tumor of the testis of a malignant type in which there was neither clinical nor chemical manifestation of endocrinopathy (Lockhart et al, 1976). Hormonal disturbance, therefore, is not an essential feature. In cases in which a testicular swelling is not clinically apparent, Gabrilove and associates performed selective venous catheterization and measurement of the testicular venous effluent to assess gynecomastia of obscure etiology (Gabrilove et al, 1975). Measurement of AFP and beta HCG may be helpful in differential diagnosis. **Occasionally, magnetic resonance imaging detects a small nonpalpable Leydig cell tumor not seen by ultrasonography** (Kaufman et al, 1990). Other considerations in the differential diagnosis include feminizing adrenocortical disorders, Klinefelter's syndrome, and other feminizing testicular disorders.

TREATMENT. **Radical inguinal orchiectomy is the initial procedure of choice. With documentation of Leydig cell tumor, endocrinologic studies and further clinical staging evaluations are indicated. In the event of histopathologic suspicion of malignancy, lymphangiogram, CT scan, or ultrasound (alone or in combination) of the retroperitoneum is indicated to seek retroperitoneal adenopathy.** As with germ cell tumors of the adult testis, spread to the lung, liver, or supradiaphragmatic lymph nodes is possible. The potential production of hormones by metastatic tumor invites exploration of these substances as markers for metastatic disease, but data are lacking. Urinary estrogens, androgens, corticoids, and pregnanediol have each demonstrated abnormalities based on the metabolic activity of different interstitial cell tumors. **Retroperitoneal lymph node dissection has been recommended as routine in patients whose interstitial cell tumors appear histologically or biochemically malignant. Total experience with any form of therapy, however, is limited by the small number of patients who have been treated, although the existing data suggest the relative radioresistance of this tumor.** Ortho-para-DDD has been used with evidence of benefit in some patients (Azer and Braumstein, 1981). A variety of chemotherapeutic agents, including *cis*-platin, vinblastine, bleomycin, cyclophosphamide, doxorubicin, and vincristine, have been used in various combination regimens without convincing benefit, but experience is limited. Experimental evidence of estrogen receptors in various mouse Leydig cell tumor lines provides an experimental basis for trials of endocrine therapy (Sato et al, 1978). In addition, inhibition of mitochondrial protein synthesis with concomitant arrest of in vivo growth of solid Leydig cell tumors in rats by oxytetracycline has been reported (van der Bogert et al, 1983).

The prognosis for Leydig cell tumors is good because of their generally benign nature. The persistence of virilizing and feminizing features following orchiectomy is not necessarily an indication of malignancy because these changes are to some extent irreversible. As might be anticipated from the characterization of malignancy (i.e.,

metastasis), the average survival time from surgery for patients with a malignant Leydig cell tumor is approximately 3 years.

Sertoli Cell Tumors (Androblastoma; Gonadal Stromal Tumor; Sertoli Cell–Mesenchyme Tumor)

Nodules of immature seminiferous tubules with lumens lined by undifferentiated cells are found not infrequently in cryptorchid testes and in roughly one fourth of patients with testicular feminization. Such lesions were formerly considered tubular adenomas, but it seems probable that they are not neoplastic, and malignant change appears not to have been reported.

True Sertoli cell–mesenchyme tumors constitute less than 1% of all testicular tumors and may occur in any age group, including infancy. Although rare in humans, they are the most common testicular tumor in dogs. The majority of Sertoli cell tumors are benign, but approximately 10% have proved malignant based on the currently accepted criterion of malignancy—the demonstration of metastasis. As with Leydig cell tumors, definitive histologic criteria of malignancy remain to be established.

The etiology of these tumors has not been determined. The majority have arisen in apparently normal intrascrotal testes, although occurrence in maldescended or cryptorchid testes has been reported.

Grossly, these tumors vary in size from 1 cm to more than 20 cm. The cut surface is usually gray-white to creamy yellow, with a uniform consistency interrupted by cystic change that becomes increasingly evident with increasing tumor size. The benign lesions are usually well-circumscribed, whereas the malignant lesions tend to be larger and less well demarcated. Invasion of paratesticular structures may occur and is suggestive of malignancy.

The precise origin of these tumors remains somewhat uncertain, although derivation from the primitive gonadal mesenchyme is suspected. A diversity of microscopic appearances is evident not only between tumors, but also between different areas within the same tumor. **The essential diagnostic features include epithelial elements resembling Sertoli cells and varying amounts of stroma. The amount and organization of these two components have led to various attempts to subclassify the tumors.** The epithelial element, on the one hand, may be arranged in tubules with or without lumens and lined by radially arranged cells in one or multiple layers; on the other hand, the epithelial cells may form columns or sheets of trabeculae growing between stromal elements. The stromal elements may be scant, or the tumor may be largely composed of stroma resembling a fibroma but containing strands of epithelial cells. Secretory material forming Call-Exner–like bodies are occasionally seen within tubules, the morphologic appearance resembling that of granulosa cell tumors. Furthermore, the stromal elements may be sufficiently well differentiated to be recognizable as Leydig cells. **The enormous potential for variation both in stromal and epithelial components and in degrees of differentiation accounts for the wide range of morphologic appearances described for these lesions and contributes to the difficulty in their classification.**

Although large size, poor tumor demarcation, invasion

of adjacent structures, blood vessel and lymphatic invasion, and increased mitotic activity are all suggestive of a malignant potential, as with Leydig cell tumors, the designation of malignancy can be made with certainty only in the presence of metastasis.

CLINICAL PRESENTATION. The presenting signs and symptoms are those of testicular mass with or without pain and with or without gynecomastia. Although the lesions have been reported in all age groups, approximately one third of the recorded patients have been 12 years old or younger. About one third of the patients have had gynecomastia. Gynecomastia in the presence of a testis tumor in the prepubertal age group is an important finding in differential diagnosis because feminization in boys with Leydig cell tumors is always superimposed on virilism.

Studies of the endocrinologic activity of these tumors have been uncommon. Gynecomastia is presumably a consequence of estrogen production, but whether the Sertoli cells or the stromal elements are responsible for estrogen production remains to some extent uncertain. Gabrilove and colleagues reported an elevated plasma testosterone value in association with some virilizing features in a young patient with Sertoli cell tumor (Gabrilove et al, 1975).

TREATMENT. Radical orchiectomy is the initial procedure of choice and is, of course, curative in the 90% of cases that are benign. In the small proportion of patients in whom malignancy has been demonstrated by the presence of metastasis, retroperitoneal lymph node involvement has been common, and retroperitoneal lymph node dissection has been performed with apparent therapeutic success (Rosvoll and Woodard, 1968). The course of the disease, even in patients with metastasis, may be protracted compared with that of patients with metastatic germ cell tumors. Lung and bone metastasis may occur and warrants the inclusion of chest films and bone scans in the staging evaluation. The value of radiation therapy and chemotherapy in the management of patients with this disease is uncertain. Although hormone production is a potential marker for follow-up in patients with apparently malignant tumors, clinical evidence on this point is lacking.

Gonadoblastoma (Tumors of Dysgenetic Gonads; Mixed Germ Cell Tumor; Gonadocytoma)

These rare tumors, occurring almost exclusively in patients with some form of gonadal dysgenesis, constitute approximately 0.5% of all testis neoplasms and occur in all age groups from infancy to beyond 70 years, although the majority have occurred in individuals under 30 years of age.

Grossly the lesions may be unilateral or bilateral and may vary in size from microscopic to greater than 20 cm in diameter. Aggressive growth may replace and obscure the nature of the gonad from which the tumor arose, and lesions weighing more than 1000 g have been reported. The tumors generally are round, with a smooth, slightly lobulated surface, and vary from soft and fleshy to firm or hard in consistency. Calcified areas are frequent and probably reflect the extensive spontaneous retrogressive changes common with these lesions. The cut surface is grayish white to yellow but may vary considerably, depending on the histologic makeup of the tumor.

Although gonadoblastomas are currently regarded as neoplasms, the possibility that they represent hamartomas or nodular hyperplasia in response to pituitary gonadotropins has been suggested. First clearly described by Scully (1953), the tumors consist of three elements: Sertoli cells, interstitial tissue, and germ cells, the proportions of which show considerable variation. In about half of such tumors, germ cell overgrowth, with the evolution of what is readily recognized as seminoma, or germ cell element(s) with histologic features of embryonal carcinoma, teratoma, choriocarcinoma, or yolk sac tumor may occur. Throughout the tubules, characteristic Call-Exner bodies may be identified, consisting of periodic acid–Schiff–positive material similar to that seen in the basement membrane of the tubules.

Clinical Presentation

The clinical manifestations of patients with this tumor are the consequence of three factors: (1) the usual concurrence of gonadal dysgenesis with resultant abnormalities in the external genitalia and gonads; (2) the presence of germ cells with malignant potential; and (3) the endocrine function of the gonadal stromal components of the tumor, usually with the production of androgen. Although interstitial cells may not be evident by light microscopy, a steroidogenic potential of the tumor may exist. Furthermore, demonstration of Leydig cells in the tumor does not necessarily dictate virilism, either because the resultant steroids may be biologically inactive or because the end organs may be defective. The usual appearance is that of solid tubules of varying size containing germ cells in close association with Sertoli cells and of mature interstitial cells evident between the tubules.

The germ cells of gonadoblastoma are similar to those of seminoma, and if germ cell proliferation occurs, it may progress from an in situ stage to invasive germinoma (seminoma), referred to as gonadoblastoma with germinoma (seminoma).

Approximately four fifths of patients with gonadoblastoma are phenotypic females, usually presenting with primary amenorrhea and sometimes with a lower abdominal mass. The remainder are phenotypic males, almost always presenting with cryptorchidism, hypospadias, and some female internal genitalia. Gonadoblastoma, however, has been described in an anatomically normal male (Talerman, 1972). In the phenotypic females, the breasts are small, the internal genitalia hypoplastic, and the gonads usually of the streak type. Sex chromatin is negative, and the chromosome analysis usually shows XY or XO or XO/XY patterns. Virilization in the phenotypic female usually manifests as hypertrophy of the clitoris. In the phenotypic male, gynecomastia may occasionally be present, and there is usually hypospadias, some female internal genitalia, and dysgenetic testes usually located in the abdomen or inguinal region; sex chromatin is negative, and the chromosome pattern is XY or XO/XY.

In general, 90% of patients with gonadal dysgenesis and gonadoblastoma are chromatin negative, and more than half have an XY karyotype, with the remainder demonstrating mosaicism. The external sex organs of patients with gonadoblastoma show a wide range of appearances ranging from normal to completely ambiguous. The secondary sex organs usually consist of a hypoplastic uterus and two normal or slightly hypoplastic fallopian tubes. Male internal sex organs, such as epididymis, vas deferens, and prostate, are found sometimes in phenotypic virilized females and always in phenotypic male pseudohermaphrodites.

Treatment

Radical orchiectomy is the first step in therapy, and the high incidence of bilaterality (50%) argues for contralateral gonadectomy when gonadal dysgenesis is present. The prognosis is excellent for patients with gonadoblastoma or gonadoblastoma with germinoma. In the presence of seminoma or other germ cell types, clinical staging employing the techniques used for the staging of germ cell tumors of the adult testis may be indicated, although experience is too limited to justify categorical recommendations. As with germ cell tumors of the adult testis, therapy may logically be based on tumor histology and the results of clinical staging.

Neoplasms of Mesenchymal Origin

A variety of neoplasms derived from mesenchymal elements may arise on the tunica albuginea or, more rarely, within the testis. Included are benign fibroma, angioma, neurofibroma, and leiomyoma. Occurring as painless masses, they are of concern chiefly because of the possibility of a malignant tumor. Differential diagnosis includes abnormalities of the testicular appendages, fibrous pseudotumors, adenomatoid tumors, and non-neoplastic cystic lesions. Varying from minute "shot-like" lesions on the surface of the testis to masses of several centimeters, the reported lesions have been variously treated by local excision or orchiectomy.

Malignant mesothelioma may arise from any site on the mesothelial membrane—pleura, peritoneum, pericardium, or tunica vaginalis. Fewer than 20 cases involving the tunica vaginalis have been reported. The lesion occurs in patients from 21 to 78 years of age, and the usual presentation is with a hydrocele. Radical orchiectomy is indicated for local control, but local recurrence and abdominal and pulmonary metastases may ensue. Limited experience suggests that surgery and irradiation may be of some value in controlling intra-abdominal metastasis. The value of chemotherapy remains to be defined, although doxorubicin appears active.

Miscellaneous Primary Non–Germ Cell Tumors

The testis may be the primary site of a number of tumors of unrelated histogenesis and varied pathologic type.

Epidermoid Cyst

Representing an estimated 1% of testis tumors (Shah et al, 1981), approximately half of epidermoid cysts occur in the twenties and most of the remainder between the teens and thirties. Grossly, these lesions present as round, sharply circumscribed, firm, and encapsulated intratesticular nodules; the cut surface reveals a grayish white to yellowish, cheesy, amorphous mass. Microscopically the wall is composed of dense fibrous tissue lined by stratified squamous keratinized epithelium, desquamations from which, with degeneration and microcalcification, make up the amorphous interior.

Although the histogenesis remains uncertain, a common thesis is that the tumor represents a monolayer teratoma. Such a histogenesis is circumstantially supported by the age and racial incidences of such tumors and by the occasional association with cryptorchidism. This histogenesis, in turn, supports the use of radical orchiectomy as the usual treatment because the possibility of other germ cell elements in association with such lesions can be excluded only by careful microscopic examination. **Nevertheless, the clinical behavior of these tumors has been consistently benign; apparently, no instance of associated, clinically unrecognized but microscopically confirmed germ cell tumor has been reported.** Rare instances of bilaterality have been reported (as with germ cell tumors) (Forrest and Whitmore, 1984). **Testicular ultrasonography may demonstrate a well-circumscribed lesion with a solid central core and may aid in the distinction from a germ cell tumor. Although most have been managed by radical orchiectomy, local excision in a small number of patients appears to have been equally successful.** The weakness in the latter approach stems from uncertainty in clinical diagnosis and the potential risks of spillage of a germ cell tumor.

Adenocarcinoma of the Rete Testis

These rare but highly malignant tumors occur uniformly in adults, over a wide age range (20–80 years). Jacobellis and co-workers reported only the nineteenth case (Jacobellis et al, 1981). **The usual presentation is a painless scrotal mass, commonly with an associated hydrocele.** Pathologic evaluation reveals a multicystic papillary adenocarcinoma composed of small cuboidal cells with elongated nuclei and scanty cytoplasm, presumably arising from the rete tubules of the testicular mediastinum. **Despite radical orchiectomy, half of the patients die within 1 year from the time of diagnosis.** Metastasis has occurred in inguinal and retroperitoneal lymph nodes, lungs, bone, and liver. The observation that retroperitoneal deposits may represent the sole site of metastasis supports the rationale of retroperitoneal lymphadenectomy in the absence of distant metastasis. Irradiation and chemotherapy with methotrexate, 5-fluorouracil, actinomycin D, or cyclophosphamide in the treatment of metastasis have been of limited, if any, benefit.

Adrenal Rest Tumors

The association of bilateral testis tumors with congenital adrenal hyperplasia and the remission of both endocrine manifestations and tumors following appropriate corticoid treatment call attention to these unusual lesions. Whether they represent neoplasms or hyperplasia and whether they derive from "normal" adrenal rests or from abnormal interstitial cells remain uncertain in some cases.

Kirkland and associates suggested that luteinizing hormones may contribute to the growth of these tumors because high serum luteinizing hormone may be seen in association with incomplete suppression of adrenal steroid secretion, and there is evidence of gonadotropin secretion with testicular tumors in some patients with congenital adrenal hyperplasia (Kirkland et al, 1977). **Nevertheless, these tumors are primarily dependent on adrenocorticotropic hormone for growth and steroid secretion; the most likely circumstance is that they may arise from the adrenocortical rests that may occur normally in the testis but that are abnormally stimulated in the syndrome of congenital adrenal hyperplasia.** Recognition of congenital adrenal hyperplasia and appropriate medical treatment may obviate surgical treatment of the testis "tumors."

Adenomatoid Tumors (Angiomatoid Tumors of the Endothelium; Adenofibroma; Mesothelioma; Lymphangioma; Adenofibromyoma; Adenoma)

These lesions are characteristically small benign tumors peculiar to the genital tract of males and females. They consist of a fibrous stroma in which disoriented spaces of epithelial cells occur, resembling endothelium, epithelium, or mesothelium. Histogenesis remains debatable; although the lesion occurs primarily in the epididymis in the male, occasional instances of tumor confined to the testis have been reported.

Carcinoid

Carcinoid is uncommon outside the gastrointestinal tract. Nearly 150 cases of carcinoid in the ovary have been recorded as well as 23 in the testis, 17 of which were primary and 6 metastatic (Talerman et al, 1978). On gross pathologic examination, the tumors have been circumscribed and limited to the testis, with diameters ranging up to 8 cm. Microscopically the tumors are composed of islands, nests, or discrete masses of round, oval, or polygonal cells separated by fibrous strands and exhibiting a solid acinar structure. Although most of the reported cases have been pure carcinoids, a few have arisen in association with teratoma. In primary ovarian carcinoids, the majority have arisen in association with teratoma. The histogenesis of these tumors remains uncertain, but one-sided development of a teratoma or origin from argentaffin or enterochromaffin cells within the gonad are the alternatives. **A slow, progressive, painless testicular enlargement is the most frequent presentation.** Although minimal symptoms suggestive of carcinoid syndrome were noted in one patient, estimations of serum serotonin and 5-hydroxyindoleacetic acid have not been performed preoperatively. **Treatment has been inguinal orchiectomy, which apparently has been curative in patients with primary testicular carcinoid.** In contrast, patients with metastatic carcinoid to the testis have a poor prognosis.

Secondary Tumors of the Testis

Lymphoma

Testicular involvement by lymphoma may be (1) a manifestation of primary extranodal disease, (2) the initial manifestation of clinically occult nodal disease, or (3) a later manifestation of disseminated nodal lymphoma. **Accounting for about 5% of all testis tumors, these lesions constitute the most common secondary neoplasms of the testis and the most frequent of all testis tumors in patients over 50 years of age. The median age of occurrence is approximately 60 years.** Primary lymphoma of the testis may occur in children; eight cases in patients ranging from 2 to 12 years of age were reviewed by Weitzner and Gropp (1976).

Grossly the testis is diffusely enlarged, usually to a diameter of 4 to 5 cm or more, bulging with a granular gray to light tan to pink solid tumor. Foci of hemorrhage and necrosis may be evident, and there may be gross extension to the epididymis or cord. **Microscopically, all varieties of reticuloendothelial neoplasms, including Hodgkin's disease, have been described in the testis. The vast majority, however, are diffuse; of these, most are histiocytic** (74%), according to the Rappaport classification, or large noncleaved (70%), according to the Lukes and Collins classification. **Diffuse replacement of the normal architecture is the rule, with focal sparing of the seminiferous tubules.**

Malignant lymphoma confined to the testis at the time of clinical onset of disease is rare compared with the frequency with which the gonadal mass represents the initial clinical manifestation of occult or apparent nodal disease. When lymph node disease is limited to the regional nodes, however, it is possible that the neoplasm arose in the gonad and metastasized to the regional nodes. The pattern of dissemination of testicular lymphomas is similar to that of testicular germ cell tumors. In autopsy cases, a pattern of pulmonary nodules not contiguous to the mediastinum or hilum strongly suggests a propensity of testicular lymphomas to spread by the hematogenous route, consistent with the observation of vascular invasion not infrequently seen in patients with testicular lymphoma.

A poor prognosis may be anticipated when there is evidence of generalized disease within a year after diagnosis. **As with lymphomas elsewhere, patients with poorly differentiated lymphocytic types tend to survive longer than those with the histiocytic type.** Disease-free survivals of 60 months or longer in patients with testicular lymphoma treated by orchiectomy alone provide strong circumstantial evidence that a true primary testicular lymphoma occurs occasionally. Even patients whose disease seems to be limited to the gonads after clinical and surgical staging, however, may still have a short survival time. Patients who have no clinical evidence of systemic spread 1 year after therapy have a high probability of cure. Whether the long-term survival following orchiectomy alone is a reflection of a cured primary testicular tumor or of a spontaneous regression or prolonged remission of a generalized disease remains debatable.

A common clinical presentation is a painless enlargement of the testis, although about one fourth of patients present with generalized constitutional symptoms, includ-

ing weight loss, weakness, and anorexia. **Bilateral tumors occur in almost half of patients, simultaneously in roughly 10%, and metachronously in the remainder.**

Investigation may include a complete blood count, peripheral smears, bone marrow studies, chest x-ray, bone scan, CT scan or intravenous pyelogram, lymphogram, and liver and spleen scans. **There appears to be a high probability of generalized disease if para-aortic nodes are involved, indicating the importance of retroperitoneal staging.** Although radical orchiectomy provides the diagnosis and initial treatment, once the diagnosis of lymphoma has been established, referral to a medical oncologist is advisable for staging evaluation and decisions about further treatment.

Survival is poor with bilateral disease and poor in patients presenting with lymphoma at other sites and later experiencing a testicular relapse, but among patients with disease apparently confined to the testis, Turner and colleagues reported 8 of 14 to be alive and well for 7 to 87 months (mean 2.5 years) (Turner et al, 1981).

Leukemic Infiltration of the Testis

The testicle appears to be a prime initial site of relapse in boys with acute lymphocytic leukemia. Stoffel and colleagues reported an 8% incidence of extramedullary involvement of the testis in children with acute leukemia, the majority of patients being in complete remission at the time of testicular enlargement (Stoffel et al, 1975). The interval from testicular involvement to death ranges from 5 to 27 months, with a median of 9 months. Kuo and associates reported seven children who developed testicular swelling during bone marrow remission in whom needle biopsy was used to confirm leukemic infiltration (Kuo et al, 1976).

The leukemic infiltration occurs mainly in the interstitial spaces, with destruction of the tubules by infiltration in advanced cases. Enlargement is bilateral in 50% of cases and is commonly associated with scrotal discoloration. **Testicular irradiation with doses of 1200 cGy over 6 to 8 days is clinically successful in local control. Because of the frequency of bilateral involvement microscopically, bilateral irradiation seems advisable even with apparent unilateral involvement.** Almost all patients can be expected to develop subsequent marrow relapse, despite control of testicular involvement by irradiation, unless effective systemic chemotherapy is given.

Biopsy is essential to the diagnosis, orchiectomy is probably unwarranted, and the treatment of choice is testicular irradiation with 2000 cGy in 10 fractions plus reinstitution of adjunctive chemotherapy or reinduction therapy for children who relapse in the testis while on chemotherapy. The prognosis of boys who undergo such a bout of testicular infiltration is guarded.

Metastatic Tumors

Approximately 200 cases of metastatic carcinoma to the testis have been reported. In the vast majority, it is discovered incidentally at autopsy in patients dying of widespread metastatic disease. In rare circumstances, a metastatic focus in the testis may be the presenting feature of an occult neoplasm or the first evidence of a recurrent, previously diagnosed and treated neoplasm.

The usual pathologic feature of secondary testicular cancers is the microscopic demonstration of neoplastic cells in the interstitium, with relative sparing of the tubules. The route of dissemination to the testis may be hematogenous, lymphatic, or by direct invasion from contiguous masses. Renal adenocarcinoma may involve the testis via the spermatic vessels; rarely, dropped metastasis from a diffuse intra-abdominal malignancy can involve the cord and testis via a patent processus vaginalis. Retrograde extension through the vas deferens presumably may be a source as well. **The common primary sources in decreasing order of frequency are prostate, lung, gastrointestinal tract, melanoma, and kidney.** A relatively high incidence of prostatic lesions reflects in part the frequency with which carcinoma of the prostate occurs and the use of orchiectomy in its treatment. Metastatic tumors to the testis occur later in life, usually in the fifties or sixties, in contrast to primary testicular tumors. Metastasis has been bilateral in a small proportion of cases. Approximately 2.5% of lymphomas are found in the testis in metastatic fashion.

TUMORS OF TESTICULAR ADNEXA

Epithelial Tumors

Epithelial tumors of the testicular adnexal structures are rare, even though the epididymis and paratesticular tissues may be involved by extensions from primary germinal cell testicular tumors. With the exception of cystadenomas of the epididymis, the majority of tumors involving the testicular adnexal structures are of mesenchymal origin.

Adenomatoid Tumors

Adenomatoid tumors are the most common tumors of the paratesticular tissues, accounting for approximately 30% of all paratesticular tumors. In the male, they are located in a restricted anatomic distribution of the epididymis, testicular tunics, and rarely the spermatic cord; in the female, they have been described in the uterus and fallopian tubes and rarely the ovary. In the male, the majority of these tumors arise in or adjacent to the lower or upper pole of the epididymis, with a slightly higher incidence in the lower pole.

The majority of these tumors occur in individuals in their twenties or thirties, but cases have been seen ranging from 20 to 80 years of age. Clinically, adenomatoid tumors present as a small, solid, asymptomatic mass generally found on routine examination. These rounded, discrete masses lie anywhere in the epididymis and may be embedded in the testicular tunics. An occasional patient presents with mild pain or discomfort in association with the nodule. Most of these tumors have been present for several years without obvious change in size. These tumors uniformly behave in a benign fashion.

On gross examination, the tumors are small, ranging from 0.5 to 5 cm in diameter. The tumors are usually attached to the testicular tunics. On sectioning, the tumors appear uniformly white, yellow, or tan with a fibrous appearance.

On microscopic examination, there are two different elements: epithelium-like cells and fibrous stroma. The epithelium-like cells are usually arranged in a framework of poorly delineated spaces sometimes with flattened or cuboidal cells.

A fairly common feature of adenomatoid tumors is the presence of vacuoles within the epithelial cells (Mostofi and Price, 1973). **The vacuoles may range in size from minute to large and may, in fact, replace most of the cytoplasm of the cell.** The nuclei show marked uniformity in size and chromatin distribution. Nuclei are generally round or oval and centrally placed with a single nucleolus present. The cytoplasm is acidophilic and finely granular. The stroma ranges from loose tissue to dense collagenized tissue with occasional hyalinization. Variations in the amount of stroma are common.

The origin of this tumor is unknown. Some pathologists have considered this to be a reaction to injury or inflammation. Jackson (1958) as well as other authors has suggested that adenomatoid tumor may be of mesothelial origin, predominantly on the basis of histology. Occasional misclassification of adenomatoid tumors has been reported as mesothelioma. Others have suggested that adenomatoid tumors are of endothelial origin and may represent a specialized hemangioma or lymphangioma. Ultrastructural findings by Marcus and Lynn (1970) failed to confirm any similarities to hemangioma. These authors found morphologic similarity to pleural mesotheliomas.

These tumors behave in a benign fashion, and there has never been a documented case of metastasis. Cellular atypia and local invasion have been observed occasionally. **Nonetheless, the long history of these tumors and the absence of distant metastases suggest a benign nature. Treatment, therefore, is surgical excision** (Sóderström and Leidberg, 1966).

Mesothelioma

Paratesticular mesothelioma is more common in older individuals but may be encountered in any age group including children. Usually the tumor presents as a firm, painless scrotal mass in association with a hydrocele. Gradual enlargement of the hydrocele or sometimes the mass itself is seen in approximately 50% of patients. Most of these patients are treated by orchiectomy.

On gross examination, there is a poorly demarcated lesion, whitish or yellowish with intermittent firm, shaggy, and friable areas. Microscopically, there is a background of papillary and solid structures against densely fibrous fibroconnective tissue. The complex structure has papillary processes combined with solid sheets of cells. Tumor cells tend to have a generous amount of cytoplasm and poorly defined cytoplasmic borders. Nuclei are often vesicular with a single small nucleolus. Mitotic activity is usually absent. Calcifications may be seen scattered throughout these neoplastic structures. Solid mesotheliomas may have small or rather extensive areas of spindle-shaped cells resembling sarcomas. This feature, although devoid of clinical significance, may lead to an erroneous diagnosis of soft tissue sarcoma. Psam-

moma bodies are sometimes found within papillary areas within the tumor.

Approximately 15% of testicular mesotheliomas have been documented to result in metastatic involvement of inguinal lymph nodes or abdominal structures (Kasdon, 1969). The pure papillary tumors nearly always prove benign. Those of a more complex structure, however, may recur and may develop multiple recurrences or even metastases.

Clinical management should consist of adequate surgical excision with follow-up examination and local biopsy if a metastatic focus is suspected (Hollands et al, 1982). Antman and associates reported a patient in whom conservative management failed (Antman et al, 1984). Limited experience with chemotherapy and radiation therapy in these rare tumors has not produced any conclusions. Staging includes CT scans of the chest and abdomen and rarely laparotomy if there is clinical suspicion of recurrent disease.

Cystadenoma

Cystadenoma of the epididymis corresponds to benign epithelial hyperplasia. Sherrick described the first case in 1956, and about 20 cases have been the subjects of subsequent reports. **Approximately one third of the cases are bilateral and may be seen as part of von Hippel–Lindau disease.** The tumor occurs most often in young adults and produces either minimal local discomfort or no symptoms. When seen in the elderly individual, it is frequently an incidental finding at the time of orchiectomy.

On gross examination, the lesion is partially cystic ranging from 1.5 to 5 cm in diameter. The cut section may be multicystic, well encapsulated, or circumscribed. The wall is studded by one or several nodules of epithelial cells arranged in small glands and papillary structures. Many of the glands are lined by columnar and ciliated cells, many of which display a vacuolated or clear cytoplasm. Staining shows abundant glycogen as well as stainable lipids in the clear cells. This pattern is similar to that of renal cell carcinoma, and distinction from metastases of renal cell carcinoma may be difficult.

Paratesticular Tumors

There are occasional reports of purely testicular mesenchymal tumors (one-sided teratomas) (Davis, 1962), but for the most part, the overwhelming majority of mesenchymal tumors in this area arise from paratesticular structures, although sometimes it may be difficult to determine whether the primary origin was the spermatic cord, the epididymis, or the tunica vaginalis.

Most series agree that rhabdomyosarcoma in its juvenile form probably accounts for approximately 40% of all paratesticular tumors, benign and malignant. Leiomyosarcoma appears to be the second most common lesion in this area, followed by occasional occurrences of fibrosarcoma, liposarcoma, and undifferentiated mesenchymal tumors, which complete the spectrum of this group. Cooperative study groups have described some of their results with these tumors as well. One is dependent on this sort of accrual because the rarity of the tumor makes certain conclusions about therapy still tentative. In one report (Kingston et al, 1983), four boys with primary paratesticular tumors were seen. There are now late relapses, defined as recurrence or tumor persistence 2 years after the diagnosis and treatment. This should be kept in mind for follow-up evaluation of such tumors.

Rhabdomyosarcoma

Paratesticular rhabdomyosarcoma occurs predominantly in children and adolescents and, with some exceptions, is most commonly seen during the first two decades of life. Clinically, this tumor usually presents as a large interscrotal mass that compresses the testis and the epididymis, sometimes reaching the external inguinal ring; the location varies somewhat, depending on the exact point of origin. On gross inspection, it can appear circumscribed, but on microscopic examination, it often extends well beyond the margin seen by the naked eye. The cut surface is solid, grayish white, and firm and is rarely hemorrhagic. Some patches of necrosis can be noted, especially around the central portion of the lesion.

The microscopic features of paratesticular rhabdomyosarcoma are largely characterized by pronounced variation from case to case and even within the same tumor. Most of them show more than one pattern of the spectrum, ranging from totally undifferentiated mesenchymal elements to the distinctive features of skeletal muscle fibers. It is characteristic to find a combination of various patterns containing an admixture of cellular elements accurately described by Patton and Horn (1962).

Some paratesticular rhabdomyosarcomas are partially or predominantly arranged in an "alveolar" fashion identical with the distinctive pattern frequently seen in other locations that was first designated as *alveolar rhabdomyosarcoma* by Riopelle and Thériault (1956) and is currently accepted as a variant of embryonal rhabdomyosarcoma.

Riehle and Venkatachalam (1982) make the point that has often been made about other sarcomas—that electron microscopic diagnosis assisted frequently in sorting out aberrations, variance, and, particularly, identification of the sarcoma in question. Electron microscopy has been successfully used to identify the cytoplasmic myofilaments and Z bands in a paratesticular rhabdomyosarcoma. This, of course, applies to paratesticular tumors as well.

Testicular and Paratesticular Tumor Management

The primary testicular or paratesticular tumor should be removed by inguinal orchiectomy with high ligation of the cord. The primary lymphatic drainage of the testis and the cord courses through lymphatics parallel to the testicular vessels; these intercommunicate with para-aortic nodes at the level of the renal vessels. The lower para-aortic and iliac nodes serve as a route of lymphatic spread when the primary spermatic lymphatics have become occluded by fibrosis or tumor. Several papers discussing these tumors have recommended routine retroperitoneal lymph node dissection (Ghavimi et al, 1973; Johnson, 1975). The fact that rhabdomyosarcoma is the most common malignant sperma-

tic cord tumor has been reaffirmed. A 5-year survival rate of 75%, using multimodal treatment, remains the current goal. Current adjuvant therapy is as follows.

RADIOTHERAPY. Cobalt 60 teletherapy can be delivered in a total tumor dose of 4000 to 6000 cGy over a period of 5 to 8 weeks through ports extending well beyond the known confines of the tumor. Dose and port size are determined by the primary site and extent of the tumor and by the age of the patient. Radiotherapy can be used for local tumors even when the tumor is generalized.

CHEMOTHERAPY. Chemotherapy with vincristine (1.5 mg/m^2), cyclophosphamide (300 mg/m^2), and dactinomycin (0.4 mg/m^2) is used. A report by Ghavimi and co-workers describes 29 children younger than 15 years of age with embryonal rhabdomyosarcoma who were treated according to a multidisciplinary protocol, which consisted of surgical removal of the tumor, if possible, followed by chemotherapy and by radiation therapy in patients with gross or microscopic residual disease (Ghavimi et al, 1973). Radiation therapy was given in a dose in the 4500- to 7000-cGy range. Additional new trials of chemotherapy consisted of cycles of sequential administration of dactinomycin, doxorubicin (Adriamycin), vincristine, and cyclophosphamide, with obligatory periods of rest. The drug therapy was continued for 2 years. In addition, at the present time, early phase II trials are also employing a method of intravenous administration of methyl-CCNU (semustine) that appears promising.

Tumor stage and site are now considered important prognostic indicators. Grosfeld and colleagues state that chemotherapy improves survival in stage I (91%) and stage II (86%) tumors and may shrink bulky stage III tumors, allowing less radical procedures in certain selective sites, particularly the urinary tract (Grosfeld et al, 1983). It is still true, however, that survival is poor in stage III, with 35% survival, and dismal in stage IV, with 5.2% survival, despite combined therapy. Relapses are generally fatal despite attempts at second-look resection, altered chemotherapy, and radiation (Grosfeld et al, 1983).

Leiomyosarcoma

Smooth muscle tumors of the spermatic cord and epididymis are rare, and their exact incidence is difficult to determine: first, because the clinical and histologic differences between benign smooth muscle tumors and malignant ones are slight and, second, because some adenomatoid tumors are erroneously classified as leiomyomas, especially those that exhibit a significant component of smooth muscle (Wilson, 1949). **Most cases of benign and malignant smooth muscle tumors described in the literature are in patients ranging in age from their forties to seventies.** Ninety percent of extratesticular tumors occurring within the scrotum are found in the spermatic cord. Of the latter, 30% are malignant, and 70% are benign. Of the malignant variety, the majority are mesenchymal sarcomas (i.e., fibrosarcoma, myxosarcoma, liposarcoma, rhabdomyosarcomaa, and leiomyosarcoma). There are more than 25 cases reported of leiomyosarcoma of the spermatic cord. Local invasion of the adjacent tissues was found in 5 of the 13 cases in which this detail was described. The first recurrence was usually local, in the scrotum or at the distal spermatic stump. This feature was described in six cases.

Distant spread has been hematogenous in a large number of cases (i.e., in tumors of humerus, liver, ileum, and lung). Autopsies were not done in many cases, however, and the clincal finding of abdominally palpable masses probably represented metastatic disease in the para-aortic lymph nodes. The ratio of the number of cases in which hematogenous spread was known to have occurred to the number with known lymphatic spread is 6:2. These facts, at least, support the opinion of Strong (1942) and of others who believe that the spread is as frequently hematogenous as lymphatic. The importance of electron microscopy in the documentation of these particular tumors, as contrasted to light microscopy, has been emphasized (Gaffney et al, 1984).

The philosophy and planning of treatment have been greatly affected by the mode of spread. It is agreed that all cases of tumor of the spermatic cord should be explored, and the growth should be removed. If it is benign, simple excision is all that is necessary. The standard therapy for leiomyosarcoma has been radical orchiectomy in which a high ligation of the cord is carried out. Owing to the high incidence of hematogenous spread, the surgeon should carry out early clamping of the cord to prevent escape of tumor cells.

Electron microscopy is extremely helpful in the differentiation of the type of testicular sacrcoma. Although at present management may not be radically changed, depending on the histologic description, there are differences as to the extent of dissection of the nodes. In children and adolescents, the complications of node dissection have been minimal, although these obviously have to be considered as well as in adults (Waters et al, 1982). Particularly important for children and adolescents is a discussion with the parents concerning obvious difficulties with fertility in the future. This aspect has been addressed but chiefly in adult patients (Lipshultz, 1982). The additional use of tumor markers must be further explored in these entities, and experience at the present time is limited in contrast to what might be called adult testis tumors (Vugrin et al, 1982).

Miscellaneous Mesenchymal Tumors of the Spermatic Cord

Isolated cases of other mesenchymal tumors of the spermatic cord, including liposarcoma, lipoma, fibrosarcoma, and myxochondrosarcoma, have been recorded. **Liposarcoma is probably the most significant one in this group because of its greater frequency.** Samellas (1964), in his review of 112 tumors of the spermatic cord, added one case of his own to three cases already reported, and Gowing and Morgan (1964) found two cases in their review of paratesticular tumors of connective tissue.

On histologic examination, liposarcomas of the spermatic cord and of the scrotal area show essentially the same features as those described in other soft tissue sites, although most of the recorded cases just mentioned were predominantly characterized as well differentiated. The Armed Forces Institute of Pathology collected 14 paratesticular liposarcomas that also appear to show this tendency to be well differentiated. In most cases, they appear as a discrete nodular mass, sometimes attaining a large size, frequently located near the spermatic cord and entirely separate from the testicle.

On histologic examination, mesenchymal tumors of the spermatic cord are characterized by the presence of a rather uniform pattern of interwoven bundles of long spindle-shaped cells with blunt-ended nuclei and with cytoplasmic myofibrils extending along their longitudinal axis. Leiomyoma is distinguished from leiomyosarcoma based on occasional or absent mitotic figures and uniform cellular arrangement. Approximately 70% of those tumors considered malignant on initial histologic examination either recur or metastasize (or both), regardless of their location.

Malignant neoplasms arising within the spermatic cord are uncommon, with 161 cases reported in the literature (Arlen et al, 1969). Sporadic cases have continued to appear, but the cumulative number remains relatively small. Although Banowsky and Shultz (1970) have described 19 histologic types of sarcoma originating from the spermatic cord and the tunics, none was classified as neurofibrosarcoma. Johnson and associates have described such a case (Johnson et al, 1975).

REFERENCES

Classification

Artz K, Jacob R: Absence of serologically detectable H2 on primitive teratocarcinoma cells in culture. Transplantation 1974; 17:632.

Dixon FJ, Moore RA: Tumors of the Male Sex Organs. Fascicle 32. Washington, DC, Armed Forces Institute of Pathology, 1952.

Freidman NB, Moore RA: Tumors of the testis: A report on 922 cases. Milit Surg 1946; 99:57.

Lewis DJ, Sesterhenn IA, McCarthy WF, Moul JW: Immunohistochemical expression of P53 tumor suppressor gene protein in adult germ cell testis tumors: Clinical correlation in stage I disease. J Urol 1994; 152:418.

Mostofi FK: Testicular tumors: Epidemiologic, etiologic and pathologic features. Cancer 1973; 32:1186.

Mostofi FK, Price EB: Tumors of the male genital system. In Atlas of Tumor Pathology, Second Series. Fascicle 8. Washington, DC, Armed Forces Institute of Pathology, 1973.

Mostofi FK, Sobin LH: International Histological Classification of Tumors of Testes (No. 16). Geneva, World Health Organization, 1977.

Parkinson MC, Swerdlow AJ, Pike MC: Carcinoma in situ in boys with cryptorchidism: When can it be detected? Br J Urol 1994; 73:431.

Peng HQ, Hogg D, Malkin D, et al: Mutations of the p53 gene do not occur in testis cancer. Cancer Res 1993; 53:3574.

Pierce GB: Teratocarcinoma: Introduction and perspectives. In Sherman MI, Solter D, eds: Teratomas and Differentiation. New York, Academic Press, 1975, pp 3–12.

Pugh RCB, Cameron K: Teratoma. In Pugh RCB, ed: Pathology of the Testis. Oxford, Blackwell Scientific Publications, 1976, pp 199–244.

Schenkman NS, Sesterhenn IA, Washington L: Increased p53 protein does not correlate to p53 gene mutations in microdissected human testicular germ cell tumors. J Urol 1995; 154:617.

Shuin T, Misaki H, Kubota Y: Differential expression of proto-oncogenes in human germ cell tumors of the testis. Cancer 1994; 73:1721.

Skakkebaek NE: Possible carcinoma in situ of the testis. Lancet 1972; 2:516.

Skakkebaek NE: Carcinoma in situ of the testis: Frequency in relationship to invasive germ cell tumors in infertile men. Histopathology 1978; 2:157.

Stevens LC: Origin of testicular teratomas from primordial germ cells in mice. J Natl Cancer Inst 1967; 38:549.

Stevens LC: The development of teratomas from intratesticular grafts of tubal mouse eggs. J Embryol Exp Morphol 1968; 20:329.

Strohmeyer T, Reese D, Press M: Expression of the c-kit proto-oncogene and its ligand stem cell factor (SCF) in normal and malignant human testicular tissue. J Urol 1995; 153:511.

Teilum G: Endodermal sinus tumors of ovary and testis: Comparative morphogenesis of so-called mesonephroma ovarie (Schiller) and extraembryonic structure of rat placenta. Cancer 1959; 12:1092.

van Gurp RJ, Oosterhuis JW, Kalscheuer V: Biallelic expression of the H19 and IGF2 genes in human testicular germ cell tumors. J Natl Cancer Inst 1994; 86:1070.

Germ Cell Neoplasm

Bach DW, Weissbech L, Hartlapp JH: Bilateral testicular tumors. J Oncol 1983; 129:989.

Batata MA, Chu FCH, Hilaris BS, et al: Testicular cancer in cryptorchids. Cancer 1982; 49:1023.

Berthelsen JG, Skakkebaek NE, Sorensen BC, Mogensen P: Screening for carcinoma in situ of the contralateral testis in patients with germinal testicular cancer. Br Med J 1982; 285:1683.

Bosl GJ, Vogelzang NJ, Goldman A, et al: Impact of delay in diagnosis on clinical stage of testicular cancer. Lancet 1981; 2:970.

Bredael JJ, Vugrin D, Whitmore WF Jr: Autopsy findings in 154 patients with germ cell tumors of the testis. Cancer 1982; 50:548.

Campbell HE: Incidence of malignant growth of the undescended testicle. Arch Surg 1942; 44:353.

Carleton RL, Freidman NB, Bomge EJ: Experimental teratomas of the testis. Cancer 1953; 6:464.

Clemmesen J: Statistical studies in malignant neoplasms. Microbiol Scand 1974; 247(suppl):1.

Cosgrove MD, Benton B, Henderson BE: Male genitourinary abnormalities and maternal diethylstilbestrol. J Urol 1977; 117:220.

Duchesne GM, Horwich A, Dearnaley DP, et al: Orchidectomy alone for Stage I seminoma of the testis. Cancer 1990; 65:1115.

Farrer JH, Walker AH, Rajfer J: Management of the postpubertal cryptorchid testis: A statistical review. J Urol 1985; 134:1071.

Friedrich M, Claussen CD, Felix R: Immersion ultrasound of testicular pathology. Radiography 1981; 141:235.

Gilbert JB: Tumors of the testis following mumps orchitis: Case report and review of 24 cases. J Urol 1944; 51:296.

Gilbert JB, Hamilton JB: Studies in malignant testis tumors: Incidence and nature of tumors in ectopic testis. Surg Gynecol Obstet 1940; 71:731.

Glazer HS, Lee JKT, Melson GL, McClennan BC: Sonographic detection of occult testicular neoplasms. Am J Radiol 1982; 138:67.

Graham S, Gibson R: Social epidemiology of cancer of the testis. Cancer 1972; 29:1324.

Grove JS: The cryptorchid problem. J Urol 1954; 71:735.

Harvald B, Hauge M: Heredity of cancer elucidated by a study of unselected twins. JAMA 1963; 186:749.

Henderson BE, Benton B, Jing J, et al: Risk factors for cancer of the testis in young men. J Cancer 1979; 3:598.

Henderson BE, Ross RK, Pike MC, Depue RH: Epidemiology of testis cancer. In Skinner DG, ed: Urological Cancer. New York, Grune & Stratton, 1983, pp 237–250.

Hong WK, Wittes RE, Hajdu ST, et al: The evolution of mature teratoma from malignant testicular tumors. Cancer 1977; 40:2987.

Johnson DE: Epidemiology of testicular tumors. In Johnson DE, ed: Testicular Tumors, 2nd ed. Flushing, NY, Medical Examination Publishing Co, 1976, pp 37–46.

Mack TM, Henderson BE: Cancer Registries for Special and General Uses. US–USSR monograph, NIH pub. no. 80–2044 7–61, Bethesda, Maryland, U.S. Dept. of Health and Human Services, National Cancer Institute, 1980.

Martin DC: Germinal cell tumors of the testis after orchiopexy. J Urol 1979; 121:42.

Mengel W, Wronecki K, Schroeder J, Zimmermann FA: Histopathology of the cryptorchid testis. Urol Clin North Am 1982; 9:331.

Mostofi FK: Testicular tumors: Epidemiologic, etiologic and pathologic features. Cancer 1973; 32:1186.

Mostofi FK, Price EB: Tumors of the male genital system. In Atlas of Tumor Pathology, Second Series. Fascicle 8. Washington, DC, Armed Forces Institute of Pathology, 1973.

Muir CS, Nectoux J: Epidemiology of cancer of the testis and penis. Natl Cancer Inst Monogr 1979; 53:157.

Nicholson PW, Harland SJ: Inheritance and testicular cancer. Br J Cancer 1995; 71:421.

Nomura T, Kanzak T: Induction of urogenital anomalies and some tumor in the progeny of mice receiving diethylstilbestrol during pregnancy. Cancer Res 1977; 37:1099.

Ray B, Hajou SI, Whitmore WF Jr: Distribution of retroperitoneal lymph node metastases in testicular germinal tumors. Cancer 1974; 33:340–348.

Richie JP, Birnholz J, Garnick MB: Ultrasonography as a diagnostic adjunct for the evaluation of masses in the scrotum. Surg Gynecol Obstet 1982; 154:695.

Ross RK, McCurtis JW, Henderson BF, et al: Descriptive epidemiology of testicular and prostatic cancer in Los Angeles. Br J Cancer 1979; 39:284.

Rothman KJ, Louik C: Oral contraceptives and birth defects. N Engl J Med 1978; 299:522.

Schottenfeld D, Warshauer ME, Sherlock S, et al: The epidemiology of testicular cancer in young adults. Am J Epidemiol 1980; 112:232.

Scorer CC, Farrington GH: Congenital Deformities of the Testis and Epididymis. New York, Appleton-Century-Crofts, 1971.

Skakkebaek NE: Possible carcinoma in situ of the testis. Lancet 1972; 2:516.

Sohval AR: Testicular dysgenesis in relation to neoplasm of the testicle. J Urol 1956; 75:285.

Sokal M, Peckham MJ, Hendry WF: Bilateral germ cell tumours of the testis. Br J Urol 1980; 5:158.

Stevens LC: The development of teratomas from intratesticular grafts of tubal mouse eggs. J Embryol Exp Morphol 1968; 20:329.

Whitaker RH: Management of the undescended testis. Br J Hosp Med 1970; 4:25.

Whitmore WF Jr: The treatment of germinal tumors of the testis. In Proceedings of the Sixth National Cancer Conference. Philadelphia, J. B. Lippincott, 1968, pp 347–355.

Whitmore WF Jr: Germinal tumors of the testis. In Proceedings of the Seventh National Cancer Conference. Philadelphia, J. B. Lippincott, 1973, pp 485–499.

Wingo PA, Tong T, Bolden S: Cancer statistics, 1995. Cancer J Clin 1995; 45:8–30.

Zdeb MS: The probability of developing cancer. Am J Epidemiol 1977; 106:6.

Clinical Staging

Abelev GI: Alpha-fetoprotein as a marker of embryo-specific differentiation in normal and tumor tissue. Transplant Rev 1974; 20:3.

Abelev GI, Perova SD, Kramkova NI, et al: Production of embryonal alpha I globulin by transplantable mouse hepatomas. Transplantation 1963; 1:174.

Albers P, Miller GA, Orazi A: Immunohistochemical assessment of tumor proliferation and volume of embryonal carcinoma identify patients with clinical stage A nonseminomatous testicular germ cell tumor at low risk for occult metastasis. Cancer 1995; 75:844.

Bagshawe KD, Searle F: Tumour markers. In Marks CN, Hales CN, eds: Essays in Medical Biochemistry, Vol 3. London, Biochemical Society, 1977, pp 25–74.

Barzell WE, Whitmore WF Jr: Clinical significance of biological markers: Memorial Hospital experience. Semin Oncol 1979; 6:48.

Bergstrand CG, Czar B: Demonstration of new protein from carcinoma of the colon. J Urol 1954; 72:712.

Boden G, Gibb R: Radiotherapy and testicular neoplasms. Lancet 1951; 2:1195.

Bosl GJ, Geller NL, Cirrincione C, et al: Multivariate analysis of prognostic variables in patients with metastatic testicular cancer. Cancer Res 1983; 43:3404.

Boyle LE, Samuels ML: Serum LDH activity and isoenzyme patterns in nonseminomatous germinal (NSG) testis tumors. Proc Am Soc Clin Oncol 1977; 18:278.

Bussar-Maatz R, Weissbach L: Retroperitoneal lymph node staging of testicular tumours: TNM Study Group. Br J Urol 1993; 72:234.

Donohue JP, Zachary JM, Maynard BR: Distribution of nodal metastases in non-seminomatous testis cancer. J Urol 1982; 128:315.

Fowler JE Jr, McLeod DG, Stutzman RE: Critical appraisal of routine supraclavicular lymph node biopsy in staging of testicular tumors. Urology 1979; 14:230.

Fraley EE, Lange PH, Kennedy BJ: Germ-cell testicular cancer in adults. N Engl J Med 301:1370, 1979.

Javadpour N: The role of biologic tumour markers in testicular cancer. Cancer 1980a; 45:1755.

Javadpour N: Significance of elevated serum alpha-fetoproteins (AFP) in seminoma. Cancer 1980b; 45:2166.

Javadpour N: Multiple biochemical tumour markers in testicular cancer. Cancer 1983; 52:887.

Jochelson M, Garnick MB, Balikian J, Richie JP: The efficacy of routine whole lung tomography in germ cell tumors. Cancer 1984; 54:1007.

Johnson DE, Appelt G, Samuels MC, Luna M: Metastases from testicular carcinoma. Urology 1976; 8:234.

Krishnaswamy PR, Tate S, Meister A: Gamma-glutamyl transpeptidase of human seminal fluid. Life Sci 1977; 20:681.

Lange PH, Raghavan D: Clinical application of tumor markers in testicular cancer. *In* Donohue JP, ed: Testis Tumor. Baltimore, Williams & Wilkins, 1983, pp 111–130.

Latza U, Foss HD, Durkop H: CD30 antigen in embryonal carcinoma and embryogenesis and release of the soluble molecule. Am J Pathol 1995; 146:463.

Lynch DF, Richie JP: Supraclavicular node biopsy in staging testis tumors. J Urol 1980; 123:39.

Moul JW, McCarthy WF, Fernandez EB: Percentage of embryonal carcinoma and of vascular invasion predicts pathological stage in clinical stage I nonseminomatous testicular cancer. Cancer Res 1994; 54:362.

Olivarez D, Ulbright T, DeRiese W: Neovascularization in clinical stage A testicular germ cell tumor: Prediction of metastatic disease. Cancer Res 1994; 54:2800.

Ray B, Hajou SI, Whitmore WF Jr: Distribution of retroperitoneal lymph node metastases in testicular germinal tumors. Cancer 1974; 33:340–348.

Ruoslahti E, Engvall E, Pakkala A, Seppala M: Developmental changes in carbohydrate moiety of human alpha-fetoprotein. Int J Cancer 1978; 22:515.

See WA, Hoxie L: Chest staging in testis cancer patients: Imaging modality selection based upon risk assessment as determined by abdominal computerized tomography scan results. J Urol 1993; 150:874.

Skinner DG: Nonseminomatous testis tumors: A plan of management based on 96 patients to improve survival in all stages by combined therapeutic modalities. J Urol 1976; 115:65.

Skinner DG, Scardino PT: Relevance of biochemical tumor markers and lymphadenectomy in management of nonseminomatous testis tumors: Current perspective. J Urol 1980; 123:378.

Stanton GF, Bosl GJ, Vugrin D, et al: Treatment of patients with advanced seminoma with cyclophosphamide, bleomycin, actinomycin D, vinblastine and cis-platin (VAB-6) (Abstract C-551). Proc Am Soc Clin Oncol 1983; 2:1.

Stomper PC, Jochelson MS, Garnick MB, Richie JP: Residual abdominal masses following chemotherapy for nonseminomatous testicular cancer: Correlation of CT and histology. AJR 1985; 145:743.

Teilum G, Albrechtsen R, Norgaard-Pederson B: The histogenetic embryologic basis for reappearance of alpha-fetoprotein in endodermal sinus tumors (yolk sac tumors) and teratoma. Acta Pathol Microbiol Scand 1975; 83:80.

Uriel J: Retrodifferentiation and the fetal patterns of gene expression in cancer. Adv Cancer Res 1979; 29:127.

Vaitukaitis JL: Human chorionic gonadotropin: A hormone secreted for many reasons. N Engl J Med 1979; 301:324.

Zondek B: Versuch einer biologischen (Hormonalen) diagnostik beim malignen hodentumor. Chirug 1930; 2:1072.

Seminoma

Batata MA, Chu FCH, Hilaris BS, et al: Radiation therapy role in testicular germinomas. Adv Med Oncol 1979; 6:279.

Blandy JP: Urology, Vol 2. Oxford, Blackwell Scientific Publications, 1976.

Boden G, Gibb R: Radiotherapy and testicular neoplasms. Lancet 1951; 2:1195.

Bredael JJ, Vugrin D, Whitmore WF Jr: Autopsy findings in 154 patients with germ cell tumors of the testis. Cancer 1982; 50:548.

Crawford ED, Smith RB, deKernion JB: Treatment of advanced seminoma with preradiation therapy. J Urol 1983; 19:75.

Doornbos JF, Hussey DH, Johnson DE: Radiotherapy for pure seminoma of the testis. Radiology 1975; 116:401.

Dosoretz DE, Shipley WU, Blitzer PH, et al: Megavoltage irradiation for pure testicular seminoma: Results and patterns of failure. Cancer 1981; 48:2184.

Duchesne GM, Horwich A, Dearnaley DP, et al: Orchidectomy alone for Stage I seminoma of the testis. Cancer 1990; 65:1115.

Earle JD, Bagshaw MA, Kaplan HS: Supervoltage radiation therapy of the testicular tumors. AJR 1973; 117:653.

Einhorn LH, Williams SD: Chemotherapy of disseminated seminoma. Cancer Clin Trials 1980; 3:307.

Fossa S, Borge L, Aass N, et al: The treatment of advanced metastatic seminoma: Experience in 55 cases. J Clin Oncol 1987; 5:1071.

Fossa SD, Droz JP, Stoter G: Cisplatin, vincristine and ifosfamide combination chemotherapy of metastatic seminoma: Results of EORTC trial 30874. EORTC GU Group. Br J Cancer 1995; 71:619.

Green N, Broth E, George FW, et al: Radiation therapy in bulky seminoma. Urology 1983; 21:467.

Hoeltl W, Kosak D, Paunt J, et al: Testicular cancer: Prognostic implications of vascular invasion. J Urol 1987; 137:683.

Javadpour N, McIntire KR, Waldmann TA: Human chorionic gonadotropin (hCG) and alpha-fetoprotein (AFP) in sera and tumor cells of patients with testicular seminoma. Cancer 1978; 42:2768.

Loehrer PJ, Birch R, Williams SD, et al: Chemotherapy of metastatic seminoma: The Southeastern Cancer Study Group Experience. J Clin Oncol 1987; 5:1212.

Maier JG, Sulak MH: Radiation therapy in malignant testis tumors: Part I. Seminoma. Cancer 1973; 32:1212.

Mencel PJ, Motzer RJ, Mazumdar M: Advanced seminoma: Treatment results, survival, and prognostic factors in 142 patients. J Clin Oncol 1994; 12:120.

Morse MJ, Herr HW, Sogani PC, et al: Surgical exploration of metastatic seminoma following VAB-6 chemotherapy (Abstract C-559). Proc Am Soc Clin Oncol 1983; 2:143.

Mostofi FK, Price EB: Tumors of the male genital system. *In* Atlas of Tumor Pathology, Second Series. Fascicle 8. Washington, DC, Armed Forces Institute of Pathology, 1973.

Motzer R, Bosl G, Heelen R, et al: Residual mass: An indication for surgery in patients with advanced seminoma following systemic chemotherapy. J Clin Oncol 1987; 5:1064.

Oliver RT, Lore S, Ong J: Alternatives to radiotherapy in the management of seminoma. Br J Urol 1990; 65:61.

Peckham MJ: Testicular tumours, investigation and staging: General aspects and staging classifications. *In* Peckham MJ, ed: The Management of Testicular Tumours. Chicago, Year Book Medical Publishers, 1982, pp 89–101.

Peckham MJ, Barrett A, McElwain TJ, et al: Nonseminoma germ cell tumours (malignant teratoma) of the testis: Results of treatment and an analysis of prognostic factors. Br J Urol 1981; 53:162.

Peckham MJ, McElwain TJ: Radiotherapy of testicular tumors. Proc R Soc Med 1974; 67:100.

Percarpio B, Clements JC, McLeod DG, et al: Anaplastic seminoma: An analysis of 77 patients. Cancer 1979; 43:2510.

Shulman Y, Ware S, Al-Askari S, Morales P: Anaplastic seminoma. Urology 1983; 21:379.

Smith RB: Management of testicular seminoma. *In* Skinner DG, deKernion JB, eds: Genitourinary Cancer. Philadelphia, W. B. Saunders, 1978, pp 460–469.

Thackray AC, Crane WAJ: Seminoma. *In* Pugh RCB, ed: Pathology of the Testis. Oxford, Blackwell Scientific Publications, 1976.

Thomas GM, Rider WD, Dembo AJ, et al: Seminoma of the testis: Results of treatment and patterns of failure after radiation therapy. Int J Radiat Oncol Biol Phys 1982; 8:165.

van der Werf-Messing B: Radiotherapeutic treatment of testicular tumors. Int J Radiat Oncol Biol Phys 1976; 1:235.

van Rooy EM, Sagerman RH: Long-term evaluation of postorchiectomy irradiation for stage I seminoma. Radiology 1994; 191:857.

Vugrin D, Whitmore WF Jr, Batata M: Chemotherapy of disseminated seminoma with combination of cis-diamminedichloroplatinum (II) and cyclophosphamide. Cancer Clin Trials 1981; 4:42.

Wajsman Z, Beckley SA, Pontes JE: Changing concepts in the treatment of advanced seminomatous tumors. J Urol 1983; 129:303.

Weitzner S: Spermatocytic seminoma. Urology 1979; 6:74.

Whitmore WF Jr: The treatment of germinal tumors of the testis. *In* Proceedings of the Sixth National Cancer Conference. Philadelphia, J. B. Lippincott, 1968, pp 347–355.

Nonseminoma

Baniel J, Roth BJ, Foster RS: Cost and risk benefit in the management of clinical stage II nonseminomatous testicular tumors. Cancer 1995; 75:2897.

Barnett MJ, Coppin CM, Murray N: High-dose chemotherapy and autologous bone marrow transplantation for patients with poor prognosis nonseminomatous germ cell tumours. Br J Cancer 1993; 68:594.

Barneveld PW, Sleijfer DT, VanderMark TW, et al: Natural course of bleomycin-induced pneumonitis. Am Rev Respir Dis 1987; 135:48.

Battermann JJ, Delemarre JFM, Hart AAM, et al: Testicular tumors: A retrospective study. Arch Chir Neerl 1973; 25:457.

Birch R, Williams SD, Cohn A, et al: Prognostic factors for a favorable outcome in disseminated germ cell tumors. J Clin Oncol 1986; 4:400.

Blandy JP, Oliver RTD, Hope-Stone HF: A British approach to the management of patients with testicular tumors. Testes Tumors 1983; 7:207.

Bosl GJ, Gluckman R, Geller NL, et al: VAB-VI: An effective chemotherapy regimen for patients with germ cell tumors. J Clin Oncol 1986; 4:1493.

Bradfield JS, Hagen RO, Ytredal DO: Carcinoma of the testis: An analysis of 104 cases with germinal tumors of the testis other than seminoma. Cancer 1973; 31:633.

Bredael JJ, Vugrin D, Whitmore WF Jr: Recurrences in surgical stage I non-seminomatous germ cell tumors of the testis. J Urol 1983; 130:476.

Broun ER, Nichols CR, Turns M: Early salvage therapy for germ cell cancer using high dose chemotherapy with autologous bone marrow support. Cancer 1994; 73:1716.

Cheng E, Cvitkovic E, Wittes RE, Golbey RB: Germ cell tumors: VAB II in metastatic testicular cancer. Cancer 1978; 42:1262.

Cooper JF, Leadbetter WF, Chute R: The thoracoabdominal approach for retroperitoneal gland dissection: Its application to testis tumors. Surg Gynecol Obstet 1950; 90:46.

Cuneo B: Note sur les lymphatiques du testicle. Bull Soc Anat (Paris) 1901; 76:105.

Cvitkovic E, Wittes R, Golbey R, et al: Primary combination chemotherapy for metastatic or unresectable germ cell tumors. Proc Am Assoc Cancer Res 1978; 19:174.

Donohue JP, Einhorn LH, Perez JM: Improved management of nonseminomatous testis tumor. Cancer 1978; 42:2903.

Donohue JP, Foster RS, Rowland RG, et al: Nerve-sparing retroperitoneal lymphadenectomy with preservation of ejaculation. J Urol 1990; 144:287.

Donohue JP, Thornhill JA, Foster RS: The role of retroperitoneal lymphadenectomy in clinical stage B testis cancer: The Indiana University experience (1965–1989). J Urol 1995; 153:85.

Donohue JP, Zachary JM, Maynard BR: Distribution of nodal metastases in non-seminomatous testis cancer. J Urol 1982; 128:315.

Dunphy CH, Ayala AG, Swanson DA, et al: Clinical stage I nonseminomatous and mixed germ cell tumors of the testis: A clinicopathologic study of 93 patients on a surveillance protocol after orchiectomy alone. Cancer 1988; 62:1202–1206.

Einhorn LH, Donohue JP: Cis-diamminedichloroplatinum, vinblastine, and bleomycin combination chemotherapy in disseminated testicular cancer. Ann Intern Med 1977; 87:293.

Einhorn LH, Williams SD: Chemotherapy of disseminated testicular cancer. Cancer 1980a; 46:1339.

Einhorn LH, Williams SD: Chemotherapy of disseminated seminoma. Cancer Clin Trials 1980b; 3:307.

Einhorn LH, Williams SD, Troner M, et al: The role of maintenance therapy in disseminated testicular cancer. N Engl J Med 1981; 305:727.

Foster RS, McNulty A, Rubin LR: The fertility of patients with clinical stage I testis cancer managed by nerve sparing retroperitoneal lymph node dissection. J Urol 1994; 152:1139.

Fraley EE, Lange PH, Kennedy BJ: Germ-cell testicular cancer in adults. N Engl J Med 1979; 301:1370.

Freedman LS, Jones WG, Peckham MJ, et al: Histopathology in the prediction of relapse of patients with stage I testicular teratoma treated by orchidectomy alone. Lancet 1987; 2:294.

Fung CY, Kalish LA, Brodsky GL, et al: Stage I nonseminomatous germ cell testicular tumor: Prediction of metastatic potential by primary histopathology. J Clin Oncol 1988; 6:1467–1473.

Gelderman WAH, Koops HS, Sleijfer DF, et al: Orchidectomy alone in stage I non-seminomatous testicular germ cell tumor. Cancer 1987; 59:578.

Gerber GS, Bissada NK, Hulbert JC: Laparoscopic retroperitoneal lymphadenectomy: Multi-institutional analysis. J Urol 1994; 152:1188.

Hong WK, Wittes RE, Hajdu ST, et al: The evolution of mature teratoma from malignant testicular tumors. Cancer 1977; 40:2987.

Hurley LJ, Libertino JA: Recurrence of a nonseminomatous germ cell tumor 9 years postoperatively: Is surveillance alone acceptable? J Urol 1995; 153:1060.

Jamieson JK, Dobson JF: The lymphatics of the testicle. Lancet 1910; 1:493.

Jewett MAS, Torbey C: Nerve-sparing techniques in retroperitoneal lymphadenectomy in patients with low-stage testicular cancer. Semin Urol 1988; 6:233.

Johnson DE, Appelt G, Samuels MC, Luna M: Metastases from testicular carcinoma. Urology 1976; 8:234.

Johnson DE, Lo RK, von Eschenbach AC, et al: Surveillance alone for patients with clinical stage I non-seminomatous germ cell tumors of the testis: Preliminary results. J Urol 1984; 131:491.

Kennedy BJ: Mithramycin therapy in advanced testicular neoplasms. Cancer 1970; 26:755.

Kimbrough JC, Cook FE Jr: Carcinoma of the testis. JAMA 1953; 153:1436.

Lauer RL, Roth B, Loehrer PJ, et al: Cis-platinum plus ifosfamide plus either VP-16 or vinblastine as third-line therapy for metastatic testicular cancer. Proc Am Soc Clin Oncol 1987; 6:99.

Lewis LG: Testis tumor: Report on 250 cases. J Urol 1948; 59:763.

Li MC, Whitmore WF Jr, Golbey R, Grabstald H: Effects of combined drug therapy on metastatic cancer of the testis. JAMA 1960; 174:1291.

Loehrer PJ Sr, Johnson D, Elson P: Importance of bleomycin in favorable-prognosis disseminated germ cell tumors: An Eastern Cooperative Oncology Group trial. J Clin Oncol 1995; 13:470.

Logothetis CJ, Samuels MC, Trindade A, Johnson DE: The growing teratoma syndrome. Cancer 1982; 50:1629.

Lotz JP, Andre T, Donsimoni R: High dose chemotherapy with ifosfamide, carboplatin, and etoposide combined with autologous bone marrow transplantation for the treatment of poor-prognosis germ cell tumors and metastatic trophoblastic disease in adults. Cancer 1995; 75:874.

MacKenzie AR: The chemotherapy of metastatic seminoma. J Urol 1966; 96:790.

Maier JG, Mittemeyer BT: Carcinoma of the testis. Cancer 1977; 39:981.

McCrystal MR, Zwi LJ, Harvey VJ: Late seminomatous relapse of a mixed germ cell tumor of the testis on intensive surveillance. J Urol 1995; 153:1057.

Merrin C, Baumastner G, Wajsman Z: Benign transformation of testicular carcinoma by chemotherapy. Lancet 1975; 2:43.

Most H: Uber malique loden ges chwulste und ihremetastatasin. Arch Pathol Anat 1898; 54:235.

Mostofi FK: Testicular tumors: Epidemiologic, etiologic and pathologic features. Cancer 1973; 32:1186.

Narayan P, Lange PH, Fraley EE: Ejaculation and fertility after extended retroperitoneal lymph node dissection for testicular cancer. J Urol 1982; 127:685.

Peckham MJ, Barrett A, McElwain TJ, et al: Nonseminoma germ cell tumours (malignant teratoma) of the testis: Results of treatment and an analysis of prognostic factors. Br J Urol 1981; 53:162.

Pizzocaro G, Zanoni F, Milani A, et al: Orchiectomy alone in clinical stage I non-seminomatous testis cancer: A critical appraisal. J Clin Oncol 1986; 4:35.

Raghavan D, Colls B, Levi J, et al: Surveillance for stage I non-seminomatous germ cell tumours of the testis: The optimal protocol has not yet been defined. Br J Urol 1988; 61:522.

Raghavan D, Peckham MJ, Heyderman E, et al: Prognostic factors in clinical Stage I non-seminomatous germ-cell tumours of the testis. Br J Cancer 1982; 45:167.

Read G, Johnson RJ, Wilkinson PM, et al: Prospective study on follow-up alone in stage I teratoma of the testis. Br Med J 1983; 287:1503.

Richie JP: Modified retroperitoneal lymphadenectomy for clinical stage I testicular cancer. J Urol 1990; 144:1160.

Richie JP, Kantoff P: Is adjuvant chemotherapy necessary for patients with stage B_1 testicular cancer? J Clin Oncol 1991; 9:1393–1396.

Rorth M, von der Maase H, Nielsen ES, et al: Orchidectomy alone versus orchidectomy plus radiotherapy in stage I non-seminomatous testicular cancer: A randomized study by the Danish Carcinoma Study Group. Int J Androl 1987; 10:255.

Rosenberg B, VanCamp L, Krigas T: Inhibition of cell division in E-coli by electrolysis products from a platinum electrode. Nature 1965; 205:678.

Rouviere H: Anatomy of the Human Lymphatic System (trans MJ Tobias). Ann Arbor, MI, Edwards Bros, 1938.

Rowland RG, Weisman D, Williams S, et al: Accuracy of preoperative staging in Stage A and B non-seminomatous germ cell testis tumors. J Urol 1982; 127:718.

Samuels ML, Howe CD: Vinblastine and the management of testicular cancer. Cancer 1970; 25:1009.

Samuels ML, Johnson DE, Holoye PY: Continuous intravenous bleomycin therapy with vinblastine in stage III testicular neoplasia. Cancer Chemother Rep 1975; 59:563.

Samuels ML, Lanzotti VJ, Holoye PY, et al: Combination chemotherapy and germinal cell tumors. Cancer Treat Rev 1976; 3:185–204.

Skinner DG: Nonseminomatous testis tumors: A plan of management based on 96 patients to improve survival in all stages by combined therapeutic modalities. J Urol 1976; 115:65.

Sogani PC, Whitmore WF Jr, Herr HW, et al: Long-term experience with orchiectomy alone in treatment of clinical stage I non-seminomatous germ cell tumour of the testis. J Urol 1988; 133:246A.

Staubitz WJ, Early KS, Magoss IV, Murphy GP: Surgical management of testis tumors. J Urol 1974; 111:205.

Thompson PI, Nixon J, Harvey VJ: Disease relapse in patients with stage I non-seminomatous germ cell tumor of the testis on active surveillance. J Clin Oncol 1988; 6:1597.

Tyrell CJ, Peckham MJ: The response of lymph node metastasis of testicular teratoma to radiation therapy. Br J Urol 1976; 48:363.

van der Werf-Messing B: Radiotherapeutic treatment of testicular tumors. Int J Radiat Oncol Biol Phys 1976; 1:235.

Vugrin D, Whitmore WF Jr, Batata M: Chemotherapy of disseminated seminoma with combination of cis-diamminedichloroplatinum (II) and cyclophosphamide. Cancer Clin Trials 1981; 4:42.

Walsh PC, Kaufman JJ, Coulson WF, Goodwin WE: Retroperitoneal lymphadenectomy for testicular tumors. JAMA 1971; 217:309.

Wheeler BM, Loehrer PJ, Williams SD, Einhorn LH: Ifosphamide and refractory germ cell tumors. J Clin Oncol 1986; 4:28.

Whitmore WF Jr: Germinal tumors of the testis. In Proceedings of the Sixth National Cancer Conference. Philadelphia, J. B. Lippincott, 1970, pp 219–221.

Whitmore WF Jr: Surgical treatment of adult germinal testis tumors. Semin Oncol 1979; 6:55.

Williams SD, Birch R, Einhorn LH, et al: Treatment of disseminated germ cell tumors with cis-platinum, bleomycin and either vinblastine and etoposide. N Engl J Med 1987a; 316:1435.

Williams SD, Stablain DM, Einhorn LH, et al: Immediate adjuvant chemotherapy versus observation with treatment at relapse in pathologic Stage II testicular cancer. N Engl J Med 1987b; 317:1433.

Wittes RE, Yagoda A, Silvay O, et al: Chemotherapy of germ cell tumors of the testis. Cancer 1976; 37:637.

Extragonadal Tumors

Cole H: Tumours in the region of the pineal. Clin Radiol 1971; 22:110.

Garnick MB, Canellos GP, Richie JP: Treatment and surgical staging of testicular and primary extragonadal germ cell cancer. JAMA 1983; 250:1733–1741.

Hainsworth JD, Einhorn LH, Williams SD, et al: Advanced extragonadal germ cell tumors: Successful treatment with combination chemotherapy. Ann Intern Med 1982; 97:7.

Luna MA, Valenzuela-Tamariz J: Germ cell tumors of the mediastinum: Post-mortem findings. Am J Clin Pathol 1976; 65:450.

Martini N, Golbey RB, Hajdu SI, et al: Primary mediastinal germ cell tumors. Cancer 1974; 33:763.

Recondo J, Libshitz HI: Mediastinal extragonadal germ cell tumors. Urology 1978; 11:369.

Reynolds TF, Tagoda A, Vugrin D, Golbey RB: Chemotherapy of mediastinal germ cell tumors. Semin Oncol 1979; 6:113.

Stanton GF, Bosl GJ, Vugrin D, et al: Treatment of patients with advanced seminoma with cyclophosphamide, bleomycin, actinomycin D, vinblastine and cis-platin (VAB-6). (Abstract C-551). Proc Am Soc Clin Oncol 1983; 2:1.

Sterchi M, Cordell AR: Seminoma of the anterior mediastinum. Ann Thorac Surg 1975; 19:371.

Other Testis Neoplasms

Azer PC, Braumstein GD: Malignant Leydig cell tumor. Cancer 1981; 47:1251.

Forrest JB, Whitmore WF Jr: Bilateral synchronous epidermoid cysts. World J Urol 1984; 2:76.

Gabrilove JL, Nicolis GL, Mitty HA, Sohval AR: Feminizing interstitial cell tumor of the testis: Personal observations and a review of the literature. Cancer 1975; 35:1184.

Jacobellis U, Ricco R, Ruotolo G: Adenocarcinoma of the rete testis 21 years after orchiopexy: Case report and review of the literature. J Urol 1981; 125:429.

Kaufman E, Akiya F, Foucar E, et al: Virilization due to Leydig cell tumor diagnosis by magnetic resonance imaging: Case management report. Clin Pediatr 1990; 29:414.

Kirkland RT, Kirkland JL, Keenan BS, et al: Bilateral testicular tumors in congenital adrenal hyperplasia. J Clin Endocrinol Metab 1977; 44:367.

Kuo TT, Tschang TP, Chu JY: Testicular relapse in childhood acute lymphocytic leukemia during bone marrow remission. Cancer 1976; 38:6204.

Lockhart JL, Dalton DL, Vollmer RT, Glenn JF: Nonfunctioning interstitial cell carcinoma of the testis. Urology 1976; 8:392.

Muller K: Cancer Testis Thesis. Copenhagen, Munksgaard, 1962.

Rosvoll RV, Woodard JR: Malignant Sertoli cell tumor of the testis. Cancer 1968; 22:8.

Sato B, Huseby RA, Samuels LT: Characterization of estrogen receptors in various mouse Leydig cell tumor lines. Cancer Res 1978; 38:2842.

Scully RE: Gonadoblastoma: A gonadal tumor related to the dysgerminoma (seminoma) and capable of sex-hormone production. Cancer 1953; 6:455.

Shah KH, Maxted WC, Chun B: Epidermoid cysts of the testis. Cancer 1981; 47:577.

Stoffel TJ, Nesbit ME, Levitt SH: Extramedullary involvement of the testis in childhood leukemia. Cancer 1975; 35:1203.

Talerman A: A distinctive gonadal neoplasm related to gonadoblastoma. Cancer 1972; 30:1219.

Talerman A, Gramata S, Miranda S, Okagaka T: Primary carcinoid tumor of the testis. Cancer 1978; 42:2696.

Teilum G: Arrhenoblastoma-androblastoma: Homologous ovarian and testicular tumors. Acta Pathol Microbiol Scand 1946; 23:252.

Teilum G: Special Tumors of Ovary and Testis and Related Extragonadal lesions. Philadelphia, J. B. Lippincott, 1971.

Turner RR, Colby TV, MacKintosh FR: Testicular lymphomas. Cancer 1981; 48:2095.

van der Bogert C, Dontje BHJ, Kroon AM: Arrest in in vivo growth of a solid Leydig cell tumor by prolonged inhibition of mitochondrial protein synthesis. Cancer Res 1983; 43:2247.

Weitzner S, Gropp A: A primary reticulum cell sarcoma of the testis in a 12-year old. Cancer 1976; 37:935.

Tumors of Testicular Adnexa

Antman K, Cohen S, Dimitrov NV, et al: Malignant mesothelioma of the tunica vaginalis testis. J Clin Oncol 1984; 2:447.

Arlen M, Grabstald H, Whitmore WF Jr: Malignant tumors of the spermatic cord. Cancer 1969; 23:525.

Banowsky LH, Shultz GN: Sarcoma of the spermatic cord and tunics: Review of the literature, case report and discussion of the role of retroperitoneal lymph node dissection. J Urol 1970; 103:628.

Davis AE Jr: Rhabdomyosarcoma of the testicle. J Urol 1962; 87:148.

Gaffney EF, Harte PJ, Browne HJ: Paratesticular leiomyosarcoma: An ultrastructural study. J Urol 1984; 133:133.

Ghavimi F, Exelby PR, D'Angio GJ, et al: Proceedings: Combination therapy of urogenital embryonal rhabdomyosarcoma in children. Cancer 1973; 32:1178.

Grosfeld JL, Weber TR, Weetman RM, Baener RL: Rhabdomyosarcoma in childhood: Analysis of survival in 98 cases. J Pediatr Surg 1983; 18:141.

Gowing NF, Morgan AD: Paratesticular tumors of connective tissue and muscle. Br J Urol 1964; 36:78.

Hollands MJ, Dottori V, Nash AG: Malignant mesothelioma of the tunica vaginalis testis. Eur Urol 1982; 8:121.

Jackson JR: The histogenesis of the "adenomatoid" tumor of the genital tract. Cancer 1958; 11:337.

Johnson DE: Trends in surgery for childhood rhabdomyosarcoma. Cancer 1975; 35:916.

Johnson DE, Kaesler KE, Mackay BM, Ayala AG: Neurofibrosarcoma of the spermatic cord. Urology 1975; 5:680.

Kasdon EJ: Malignant mesothelioma of the tunica vaginalis propria testis: Report of two cases. Cancer 1969; 23:1144.

Kingston JE, McElwain TJ, Malpas JS: Childhood rhabdomyosarcoma: Experience of the Children's Solid Tumor Group. Br J Cancer 1983; 48:195.

Lipshultz LI: Management of infertility following treatment for testicular carcinoma. Cancer Bull 1982; 34:31.

Marcus JB, Lynn JA: Ultrastructural comparison of an adenomatoid tumor, lymphangioma, hemangioma and mesothelioma. Cancer 1970; 25:171.

Mostofi FK, Price EB: Tumors of the male genital system. In Atlas of Tumor Pathology, Second Series. Fascicle 8. Washington, DC, Armed Forces Institute of Pathology, 1973.

Patton RB, Horn RC Jr: Rhabdomyosarcoma: Clinical and pathological features and comparison with human fetal and embryonal skeletal muscle. Surgery 1962; 52:572.

Riehle RA, Venkatachalam H: Electron microscopy in diagnosis of adult paratesticular rhabdomyosarcoma. Urology 1982; 19: 658–661.

Riopelle JL, Thériault JP: Sur une forme meconnue de sarcoma des parties molles: Le rhabdomyosarcome alvJolaire. Ann Anat Pathol (Paris) 1956; 1:88.

Samellas W: Malignant neoplasms of spermatic cord: Liposarcoma. NY State J Med 1964; 64:1213.

Sherrick JC: Papillary cystadenoma of the epididymis. Cancer 1956; 9:403.

Söderström J, Leidberg CF: Malignant "adenomatoid" tumour of the epididymis. Acta Pathol Microbiol Scand 1966; 67:165.

Strong GH: Lipomyxoma of the spermatic cord: Case report and review of literature. J Urol 1942; 48:527.

Vugrin D, Whitmore WF Jr, Nisselbaum J, Watson RC: Correlation of serum tumor markers and lymphangiography with degrees of nodal involvement in surgical Stage II testis cancer. J Urol 1982; 127:683.

Waters WB, Garnick MB, Richie JP: Complications of retroperitoneal lymphadenectomy in the management of nonseminomatous tumors of the testis. Surg Gynecol Obstet 1982; 154:501.

Wilson WW: Adenomatoid leiomyoma of the epididymis. Br J Surg 1949; 37:240.

79
TUMORS OF THE PENIS

Donald F. Lynch, Jr., M.D.
Paul F. Schellhammer, M.D.

Penile malignancies are uncommon tumors that are often devastating for the patient and diagnostically and therapeutically challenging for the urologist. Any discussion of penile cancer must first begin by addressing both benign and malignant tumors of the penis. **Some penile lesions are strictly benign, whereas others have the potential to evolve into malignancies.** A description of these lesions establishes their anatomic, etiologic, and histologic relationship to squamous cell carcinoma, which is the most common malignant tumor of the penis, as well as other malignancies that involve the penis. Management of benign disease as well as current therapy of local, regional, and metastatic disease is discussed.

BENIGN LESIONS

Benign Noncutaneous Lesions

Congenital inclusion cysts have occurred in the penoscrotal raphe (Cole and Helwig, 1976). Acquired inclusion cysts from circumcision or trauma are more common. Retention cysts arise from the sebaceous glands located on the mucosal surface of the prepuce and on the skin of the penile shaft. Retention cysts may arise in the parameatal area as a result of obstruction of the urethral glands (Shiraki, 1975). Syringomas—benign tumors of the sweat glands—may become large and symptomatic (Lipshutz et al, 1991; Sola Casas et al, 1993). Neurilemomas have been reported in the frenulum (Chan et al, 1993).

Benign tumors of the supporting structures include angiomas, fibromas, neuromas, lipomas, and myomas. Angiomas are usually superficial and appear most frequently as punctate reddish papules or macules on the corona. They resemble the small angiokeratomas found on the scrotum. Neuromas present as firm, whitish papules at the corona or frenulum (Montgomery et al, 1990).

Penile masses and deformities, or pseudotumors, may develop following self-administered injections or implantation of foreign bodies (Nitidandhaprabhas, 1975). Testosterone in oil (Zalar et al, 1969) and other common oils (Engelman et al, 1974) have been applied to or injected into the penis, producing a destructive lipogranulomatous process that may grossly mimic carcinoma. Pyogenic granuloma may arise at the site of self-injection in impotence therapy (Summers, 1990).

Occasionally, phlebitis, lymphangitis, and angiitis may produce subcutaneous cords or nodules in the penis (Grossman et al, 1965; Ball and Pickett, 1975).

When a diagnosis is in question, all benign lesions are best treated with local excision and thorough histologic evaluation to rule out malignancy.

Benign Cutaneous Lesions

Pearly penile papules, hirsute papillomas, and coronal papillae are normal and commonly encountered lesions of the glans penis. They occur in about 15% of postpubertal men and are more common in uncircumcised males (Neinstein and Goldenring, 1984). These lesions present as linear, curved, or irregular rows of conical or globular excrescences, varying from white to yellow to red, arranged along the coronal sulcus. They are considered acral angiofibromas. When larger than usual, they may be mistaken for condyloma acuminatum (Evans and Patten, 1990). Treatment is usually unnecessary, but when indicated, lesions have responded to fulguration with the carbon dioxide (CO_2) laser (Magid and Garden, 1989). These lesions have not been associated with malignancy (Tannenbaum and Becker, 1965; Ferenczy et al, 1991).

Zoon's balanitis is characterized by a shiny, erythematous plaque or erosion, which on biopsy demonstrates normal cell layers but a dense plasma cell infiltrate. It most commonly involves the glans but may involve the prepuce. Treatment is by circumcision, although reports exist of successful management with the CO_2 laser (Baldwin and Geronemus, 1989).

The full range of rashes and ulceration due to irritation, allergy, or infection must be considered in the differential diagnosis of the cutaneous lesion.

PREMALIGNANT CUTANEOUS LESIONS

Some histologically benign penile lesions have been recognized as having malignant potential or close association with the development of squamous carcinoma. In one large series, 42% of patients with squamous cell cancer

had a history of pre-existing penile lesions (Bouchot et al, 1989). Although the incidence of progression of these lesions to squamous cell carcinoma is not known, all have been associated with the disease.

Cutaneous Horn

The penile cutaneous horn is a rare lesion. It usually develops over a pre-existing skin lesion—wart, nevus, traumatic abrasion, or malignancy—and is characterized by overgrowth and cornification of the epithelium, which forms a solid protuberance. Microscopically, extreme hyperkeratosis, dyskeratosis, and acanthosis are noted. Treatment consists of surgical excision with a margin of normal tissue about the base of the horn. These lesions may recur and may demonstrate malignant change on subsequent biopsy, even when initial histology is benign (Fields et al, 1987). **Because this tumor may evolve into a carcinoma or may develop as a result of an underlying carcinoma, careful histologic evaluation of the base and close follow-up of the excision site are essential (Pressman et al, 1962; Hassan et al, 1967).**

Pseudoepitheliomatous Micaceous and Keratotic Balanitis

These unusual lesions present as hyperkeratotic, micaceous growths on the glans and may have some of the microscopic features of verrucous carcinoma. They tend to recur and may represent an early form of verrucous carcinoma (Jenkins and Jakubovic, 1988; Gray and Ansell, 1990). Treatment includes excision, laser ablation, and cryotherapy. These lesions require aggressive treatment and close follow-up. Fibrosarcoma of the glans following treatment of a pseudoepitheliomatous micaceous and keratotic balanitis lesion with cryotherapy has been reported (Irvine et al, 1987).

Balanitis Xerotica Obliterans

This is a genital variation of lichen sclerosis et atrophicus that presents as a whitish patch on the prepuce or glans, often involving the meatus and sometimes extending into the fossa navicularis. The lesions may be multiple and may assume a mosaic appearance. The meatus may appear white, indurated, and edematous. Glandular erosions, fissures, and meatal stenosis may occur. The disorder is most common in uncircumcised men and occurs most commonly in middle-aged men but does occur in boys (McKay et al, 1975). Symptoms include pain, local penile discomfort, pruritus, painful erections, and urinary obstruction (Bainbridge et al, 1971).

Histologically, these lesions show atrophic epidermis with loss of the rete pegs and homogenization of collagen on the upper third of the dermis, combined with a zone of lymphocytic and histiocytic infiltration. They resemble the lesions of lichen sclerosis et atrophicus found elsewhere (Laymon and Freeman, 1944). **There are reports documenting the association of balanitis xerotica obliterans with squamous** cell carcinoma as well as the development of carcinoma long after a lesion of balanitis xerotica obliterans has been treated (Laymon and Freeman, 1944; Bart and Kopf, 1978; Jamieson et al, 1986; Dore et al, 1990).

Treatment consists of topical steroid cream, injectable steroids, and surgical excision. Meatal stenosis is a common problem often requiring repeated dilations, steroid injection, or even formal meatoplasty (Poynter and Levy, 1967). Close follow-up is essential, with biopsy if a change in clinical appearance occurs.

Leukoplakia

These lesions present as solitary or multiple whitish plaques, often involving the meatus. Histologically, there is hyperkeratosis, parakeratosis, and hypertrophy of the rete pegs with dermal edema and lymphocytic infiltration. Careful microscopic examination is necessary to determine the presence of malignancy.

Treatment involves elimination of chronic irritation, and circumcision may be indicated. Surgical excision and radiation have been used in the treatment of leukoplakia. **This disorder has been associated with both in situ squamous cell cancer and verrucous carcinoma of the penis** (Hanash et al, 1970; Reece and Koontz, 1975; Bain and Geronemus, 1989). Because of this close relationship with carcinoma, close follow-up of the excision site, with periodic biopsy of incompletely excised lesions, is necessary to detect early malignant change.

VIRUS-RELATED DERMATOLOGIC LESIONS

There is increasing evidence to suggest that a number of penile lesions share a common viral etiology. **Condyloma acuminatum, bowenoid papulosis, and Kaposi's sarcoma appear to be related to infection with human papillomavirus (HPV).**

Condyloma Acuminatum

Condylomata acuminata are soft, papillomatous growths generally considered to be benign. Also known as "genital warts" or "venereal warts," they have a predilection for the moist, glabrous areas of the body and the mucocutaneous surfaces of the perineal and genital areas. The lesions are soft and friable and may occur singly on a pedicle or in a moruloid cluster on a broad base. These lesions are rare before puberty (Redman and Meachum, 1973; Copulsky et al, 1975) and when encountered may suggest sexual abuse (Handly et al, 1993).

In the male, condylomata occur most commonly on the glans, the penile shaft, and the prepuce. The meatus should also be carefully inspected. Lesions recur frequently, both in new and in previously treated sites. Approximately 5% of patients demonstrate urethral involvement, which may extend to the prostatic urethra (Culp et al, 1944). Rarely, extreme involvement of the urethra may require ure-

throplasty (Feneley et al, 1992). Bladder involvement, although rare, is extremely difficult to treat effectively (Bissada et al, 1974).

Microscopically, condylomata acuminata demonstrate an outer layer of keratinized tissue covering papillary fronds, which are supported by connective tissue stroma. The epithelial layer consists of well-ordered rows of squamous cells. Usually a dermal lymphocytic infiltrate is present. **Treatment of these lesions with podophyllin may induce histologic changes suggestive of carcinoma** (King and Sullivan, 1947). **Preliminary biopsy of large lesions that appear to be condylomata acuminata should therefore precede any treatment with topical podophyllin.**

Interest in genital condylomata has increased dramatically, stimulated by increased understanding of the relationship between HPV infection and certain human cancers. The terms *genital condyloma, venereal warts, genital warts,* and *genital HPV infection* all refer to a sexually transmitted disease caused by HPV. Although HPV is not a reportable sexually transmitted disease, a current estimate puts the number of new infections at 500,000 to 1 million annually. Prevalence figures are unknown (Stone, 1989). **HPV infection is recognized as the principal etiologic agent in cervical dysplasia and cervical cancer** (Lancaster et al, 1986).

Finally, significant numbers of male partners of women with cervical condylomata have lesions not identified by simple inspection (Sedlacek et al, 1986).

On histologic examination, the koilocyte—a cell characterized by an empty cavity surrounding an atypical nucleus—is pathognomonic for HPV infection (Schneider, 1989). DNA hybridization techniques have been used to identify and classify infection, and some 40 subtypes of HPV virus have been identified (Lowhagen et al, 1993). **Viral types 6, 11, and 42 to 44 are associated with gross condylomata and low-grade dysplasia. Types 16, 18, 31, 33, 35, and 39 have a higher association with malignancy** (Smotkin, 1989). Although such viral typing has been largely a research tool, it is being developed as a means of identifying potentially aggressive lesions and assisting in treatment planning (Carpiniello et al, 1990; Noel et al, 1992).

Subclinical disease may be detected by the application of 5% acetic acid solution to the penis, followed by inspection with a magnifying glass. Lesions turn white, and flat lesions, often invisible on regular inspection, may be detected. These "aceto-white" lesions are not always due to HPV, and biopsy must be performed to confirm the diagnosis (Krebs, 1989a). Careful inspection of the base of the shaft, the scrotum, and the inguinal folds is essential. The meatus should be examined, and if lesions are present, urethroscopy should be performed (Culp et al, 1944; Barrasso et al, 1987).

Topical treatment of condylomata with either podophyllin or trichloroacetic acid is well established and often successful with small lesions. A 0.5% to 1% solution of podophyllin is applied weekly for 2 to 6 weeks (Culp et al, 1944; Kinghorn et al, 1993). Because normal skin can be disrupted by podophyllin, careful supervision of such treatment is suggested, although self-application protocols have been successfully employed (Edwards et al, 1988). Circumcision removes preputial lesions, gains exposure for treatment, and allows post-treatment monitoring. Fulguration and excision may be advisable to avoid large areas of maceration, ulceration, and secondary infection.

Surgical laser therapy has been used extensively in the management of condylomata and is covered in a subsequent section in this chapter. Surgical therapy using a pediatric resectoscope may be helpful in debulking large intraurethral lesions. The lowest power required to resect the lesions should be used, and electrocautery should be minimized to avoid the development of urethral stricture.

Intraurethral lesions may be extremely difficult to treat. 5-Fluorouracil cream applied weekly for 3 weeks has been successful in eliminating urethral lesions (Bissada et al, 1974; Dretler and Klein, 1975; Boxer and Skinner, 1977). Care must be taken to work the cream down the urethra and to avoid exposure of the scrotal skin. Use of a scrotal support or zinc oxide cream may be helpful. The addition of 5-fluorouracil cream to laser therapy did not improve the success rate (Carpiniello et al, 1987).

Various interferons have been used in condyloma treatment (Geffen et al, 1984). A randomized study has shown that short-term intralesional interferon alpha-2b has activity against condyloma (Eron et al, 1986). The outcome of studies using other interferons has been less clear (Zouboulis et al, 1991). Interferon therapy continues to be reserved for extensive and recalcitrant lesions (Krebs, 1989a, 1989b; Ferenczy, 1990).

HPV infection is common and potentially carcinogenic. Condylomata have been associated with squamous cell carcinoma of the penis (Beggs and Spratt, 1961; Dawson et al, 1965; Rhatigan et al, 1972). Malignant transformation of condyloma to squamous cell carcinoma has been reported (Boxer and Skinner, 1977; Coetzee, 1977; Malek et al, 1993). Condylomata acuminata located in the perianal, scrotal, and oral areas have undergone malignant degeneration (Siegel, 1962; Burmer et al, 1993). An increased incidence of penile intraepithelial neoplasia has been found in the male partners of women with cervical intraepithelial neoplasia (Barrasso et al, 1987). HPV infection has been implicated in the development of bowenoid papulosis. The role of HPV in the transformation of condylomatous lesions to malignancy is undergoing careful study.

Bowenoid Papulosis

Carcinoma in situ of the penis has been well recognized since its first description by Queyrat in 1911. Bowenoid papulosis, a condition having a similar histologic appearance to carcinoma in situ but having a benign course, was described by Kopf and Bart in 1977.

Bowenoid papulosis presents as multiple papules on the penile skin or female vulva, usually during the teens or twenties. The lesions are usually pigmented and range from 0.2 to 3.0 cm in diameter, and smaller lesions may coalesce into larger ones (Patterson et al, 1986). Pigmented lesions present on the penile skin, whereas glanular lesions tend to be flat papules (Gross et al, 1985). Diagnosis is confirmed by biopsy (Peters and Perry, 1981). Histologically, these lesions meet all the criteria of carcinoma in situ but display differing growth patterns relative to flat, endophytic, or exophytic clinical appearance (Wade et al, 1978; Peters and Perry, 1981; Gross et al, 1985; Patterson et al, 1986). DNA

sequences suggestive of HPV 16 have been found in specimens of bowenoid papulosis, and a causative role for HPV is suspected (Gross et al, 1985). **Although histologically this condition is a carcinoma in situ, the clinical course of bowenoid papulosis is invariably benign.**

Treatment has included electrodesiccation, cryotherapy, laser fulguration, topical 5-fluorouracil cream, and excision with skin grafting.

Kaposi's Sarcoma

Kaposi's sarcoma, first described in 1972, is a tumor of the reticuloendothelial system (Kaposi, 1982). It presents as a cutaneous neovascular lesion, a raised, painful, bleeding papule or ulcer with bluish discoloration. Histologically the tumor is vasoformative with endothelial proliferation and spindle cell formation.

Initially, Kaposi's sarcoma occurred rarely in Europe and North America. It was characterized by a slowly progressive tumor affecting the lower extremities of older men, usually of Eastern European Jewish or Italian descent. Kaposi's sarcoma was also found in other populations: young black African men and patients receiving immunosuppressive therapy. The disease is now closely linked with patients having acquired immunodeficiency syndrome (AIDS) and takes a much more aggressive clinical course in this group.

Kaposi's sarcoma is now subcategorized as follows: (1) classic Kaposi's sarcoma, which occurs in patients without known immunodeficiency and has an indolent and rarely fatal course; (2) immunosuppressive treatment–related Kaposi's sarcoma, which occurs in a patient receiving immunosuppressive therapy for organ transplantation or other indications and which is often reversed with dosage modification of the immunosuppressive agents; (3) African Kaposi's sarcoma, which occurs in young men and which may be indolent or aggressive in course; and (4) epidemic Kaposi's sarcoma, which occurs in patients with AIDS.

The classic and immunosuppressive forms of the disease are considered nonepidemic. Nonepidemic Kaposi's sarcoma limited to penile involvement should be aggressively treated because it is rarely associated with diffuse organ involvement. Localized surgical excision or small-field external beam or electron beam radiation has been effective (Lands et al, 1992). With wider areas of involvement, partial penectomy is indicated. In the immunosuppressed patient, Kaposi's sarcoma often regresses with the discontinuation of immunosuppressive therapy. If regression does not occur, local excision or radiation should be considered. Systemic management for multisystem involvement has employed interferon and cytotoxic therapy (National Cancer Institute Position Statement, 1990).

In the patient with AIDS, the underlying immunodeficiency predisposes the host to Kaposi's sarcoma by a factor of 7000 (Miles, 1994). The first case of AIDS epidemic Kaposi's sarcoma was reported in 1981 (Friedman Kien, 1981) and the first with penile involvement in 1986 (Seftel et al, 1986). Subsequently, Kaposi's sarcoma of the penis has become a relatively common lesion in the patient with AIDS. Penile involvement is more common in homosexual men than in others with AIDS. In the first 1000 cases

of AIDS reported by the Centers for Disease Control and Prevention, incidence of penile Kaposi's sarcoma was 44% in homosexual and bisexual patients compared with only 16% in intravenous drug abusers with AIDS and 0% of hemophiliac patients with AIDS (Bayne and Wise, 1988; Jaffe et al, 1983). Some studies have found epidemic Kaposi's sarcoma in patients who are HIV-negative, which suggests that certain sexual practices and a separate sexually transmitted agent may be responsible for this form of the disease (Miles, 1994).

Kaposi's sarcoma may be the presenting sign of the disease in many AIDS patients; however, early involvement of the penis is rare in this group (Grunwald et al, 1994). Treatment is directed toward palliation (Lowe et al, 1989). Glans penis or corpus spongiosum involvement may produce urethral obstruction, necessitating proximal urethrostomy. This treatment usually allows voiding in the upright position. With large lesions involving the penis, partial or total penectomy may be necessary. Radiation therapy and use of the neodymium:yttrium aluminum garnet (Nd:YAG) laser to alleviate distal urethral obstruction have also been reported (Wishnow and Johnson, 1988).

BUSCHKE-LÖWENSTEIN TUMOR (VERRUCOUS CARCINOMA, GIANT CONDYLOMA ACUMINATUM)

The Buschke-Löwenstein tumor was initially described by Buschke and Löwenstein in 1925, and later by Löwenstein in 1939 in the United States. Ackerman described a histologically similar tumor presenting in the oral cavity (Ackerman, 1948). Verrucous carcinomas of the larynx, vulva, and penis were described by Goethals and colleagues (Goethals et al, 1968). **Although verrucous carcinomas of nonpenile sites do metastasize, metastasis from the Buschke-Löwenstein tumor is distinctly rare.** Rather the Buschke-Löwenstein tumor invades locally, destroying adjacent tissues and producing urethral erosion and fistulization. This aggressive growth, combined with bleeding, discharge, and odor, prompts the patient to seek medical evaluation and treatment.

The true incidence of the Buschke-Löwenstein tumor is unknown, but it is probably higher than reported because many cases have been labeled as low-grade squamous carcinoma of the penis. Retrospective analyses of several reports have revealed a number of cases of verrucous cancer or giant condylomata under the category of low-grade squamous cell carcinomas (Davies, 1965; Hanash et al, 1970).

The Buschke-Löwenstein tumor differs from condyloma acuminatum in that condylomata, regardless of size, always remain superficial and never invade adjacent tissue. The Buschke-Löwenstein tumor displaces, invades, and destroys adjacent structures by compression. Aside from this unrestrained local growth, it demonstrates no signs of malignant change on histologic examination. Microscopically the tumor forms a luxuriant mass composed of broad, rounded rete pegs, often extending far into underlying tissue. The pegs are composed of well-differentiated squamous cells that show no cellular anaplasia. These epithelial pegs are characteristically surrounded by a dense band of acute and chronic inflammatory cells. As with condyloma acuminatum, the cause may be viral (Dawson et

al, 1965; Ubben et al, 1979). HPV 6 and 11 have been identified in these tumors (Boshart and zur Hausen, 1986).

Lymph node metastases are rare with verrucous carcinoma (Ackerman, 1948; Davies, 1965; Seixas et al, 1994), **and their presence probably reflects malignant degeneration in the primary lesion.** Such changes are known to occur in verrucous carcinoma of nonpenile sites (Davies, 1965; Dawson et al, 1965). Anecdotal cases of malignant degeneration in association with penile carcinoma have been reported (Youngberg et al, 1983).

Either excisional biopsy or multiple deep biopsy specimens are required to distinguish the lesion from true penile carcinoma. Treatment consists of excision, sparing as much of the penis as possible. Large lesions may necessitate total penectomy. Recurrence is common, and close follow-up is essential. Topical therapy with either podophyllin or 5-fluorouracil has been unsuccessful, probably because the characteristic thickened stratum corneum is impervious to the medication (Bruns et al, 1975).

Radiation therapy is ineffective and has been associated with subsequent rapid malignant changes when used with verrucous carcinomas in other locations (Lepow and Leffler, 1960; Kraus and Perez-Mesa, 1966; Proffitt et al, 1970). Bleomycin has been used in both a primary and an adjunctive mode for verrucous carcinoma (Misma and Matunalea, 1972). Successful treatment of a Buschke-Löwenstein tumor with systemic interferon therapy combined with Nd:YAG laser therapy has been reported (Gilbert and Beckert, 1990).

SQUAMOUS CELL CARCINOMA

Carcinoma in Situ (Erythroplasia of Queyrat, Bowen's Disease)

Carcinoma in situ of the penis is referred to by urologists and dermatologists as erythroplasia of Queyrat if it involves the glans penis, prepuce, or penile shaft and as Bowen's disease if it involves the remainder of the genitalia or perineal region. This nomenclature has served to separate carcinoma in situ from the mainstream of thinking and reporting of penile carcinoma. The epidemiology and natural history of this lesion, however, parallel that of early carcinoma of the penis, and carcinoma in situ can progress to invasive carcinoma.

The erythroplasia originally described by Queyrat in 1911 consists of a red, velvety, well-marginated lesion of the glans penis or, less frequently, the prepuce of the uncircumcised male (Aragona et al, 1985). It may ulcerate and may be associated with discharge and pain.

On histologic examination, the normal mucosa is replaced by atypical hyperplastic cells characterized by disorientation, vacuolation, multiple hyperchromatic nuclei, and mitotic figures at all levels. The epithelial rete extend into the submucosa and appear elongated, broadened, and bulbous. The submucosa shows capillary proliferation and ectasia with a surrounding inflammatory infiltrate, usually rich in plasma cells. These microscopic features distinguish erythroplasia of Queyrat from chronic localized balanitis. HPV has been identified in penile carcinoma in situ (Pfister and Haneke, 1984).

Intraepithelial neoplasm of the skin associated with a high occurrence of subsequent internal malignancy was described as a distinct entity by Bowen in 1912. When Bowen's disease involves the penis, it is called erythroplasia of Queyrat: Histologically the two conditions are similar (Graham and Helwig, 1973). Both tumors are characterized by the noninvasive changes of carcinoma in situ. **Visceral malignancy is not associated with erythroplasia of Queyrat, and case-controlled studies have shown no association of Bowen's disease with internal malignancy** (Epstein, 1960). **Penile cancer does not warrant a specific search for internal malignancy.**

Treatment is based on proper histopathologic confirmation of the malignancy with multiple biopsy specimens of adequate depth to determine the presence of invasion. When lesions are small and noninvasive, local excision that spares penile anatomy and function is satisfactory. Circumcision adequately treats preputial lesions. Fulguration may be successful but often results in recurrences. Radiation therapy has successfully eradicated these tumors, and well-planned, appropriately delivered radiation results in minimal morbidity (Kelley et al, 1974; Grabstald and Kelley, 1980).

Topical 5-fluorouracil as the 5% base causes denudation of malignant and premalignant areas while preserving normal skin. Cosmetic results are excellent (Dillaha et al, 1965; Hueser and Pugh, 1969; Lewis and Bendl, 1971; Graham and Helwig, 1973; Goette, 1974). Systemic absorption of 5-fluorouracil is minimal. There are reports of successful treatment with Nd:YAG laser (Landthaler et al, 1986), CO_2 laser (Rosemberg and Fuller, 1980), and liquid nitrogen (Madej and Meyza, 1982; Mortimer et al, 1983) with excellent control and cosmetic outcome.

Invasive Carcinoma

Incidence

Penile carcinoma accounts for 0.4% to 0.6% of all malignancies among males in the United States and Europe; it may constitute up to 10% of malignancies in males in some African and South American countries (Gloeckler-Ries et al, 1990). **It is a disease of older men, with an abrupt increase in incidence around age 60, peaking around age 80** (Persky, 1977). In two studies, the mean age was 58 years (Gursel et al, 1973) and 55 years (Derrick et al, 1973). The tumor is not unusual in younger men: In one large series, 22% of patients were younger than 40, and 7% were younger than 30 (Dean, 1935). The disease has also been reported in children (Kini, 1944; Narasimharao et al, 1985). Although some series have shown no racial predisposition (Beggs and Spratt, 1961), others have noted a 2:1 preponderance for blacks (Muir and Nectoux, 1979). This may represent a difference in the frequency of neonatal circumcision in these two populations rather than a genetic predilection for the tumor.

Etiology

The incidence of carcinoma of the penis varies markedly with the hygienic standards and the cultural and religious practices of different countries. **Circumcision has been well established as a prophylactic measure that virtually eliminates the occurrence of penile carcinoma. The development of the tumor in uncircumcised men has been attributed to the chronic irritative effects of smegma, a by-product of bacterial action on desquamated cells that are within the preputial sac. Such exposure is accentuated by phimosis, which is found in 25% to 75% of patients reported in most large series.**

Although definitive evidence that smegma is a carcinogen has not been established (Reddy and Baruah, 1963), its relationship to the development of penile carcinoma has been widely observed (Plaut and Kohn-Speyer, 1947; Pratt-Thomas et al, 1956). Although the development of carcinoma of the scrotum has a clear relationship with chemical carcinogens (coal dust, tar, paraffin), a similar relationship between penile carcinoma and these same chemicals does not exist, although exposure of the penis must be similar.

Carcinoma of the penis is so rare among the Jewish population that its occurrence warrants comment (Licklider, 1961). Neonatal circumcision is a universal practice in this population. Similarly, in the United States, where neonatal circumcision is widely practiced, penile cancer composes less than 1% of male malignancies. Among the uncircumcised tribes of Africa and within the uncircumcised Asian cultures, penile cancer may amount to 10% to 20% of all male malignancies (Dodge, 1965; Narayana et al, 1982). In Paraguay, penile carcinoma is the most common malignancy (Lynch and Krush, 1969), and in areas of Brazil, it may constitute 17% of all male malignancies (Ornellas et al, 1994). In India, carcinoma of the penis is extremely rare among the neonatally circumcised Jewish population but somewhat more common among Muslims who practice prepubertal circumcision. It is quite common among the uncircumcised Christian and Hindu population (Paymaster and Gangadharan, 1967).

Data from most large series show that the tumor is rare among neonatally circumcised individuals but more frequent when circumcision is delayed until puberty (Frew et al, 1967; Gursel et al, 1973; Johnson et al, 1973). **Adult circumcision appears to offer little or no protection from subsequent development of the disease** (Thomas and Small, 1963). This suggests that some period of exposure to smegma may account for the decreased effectiveness of pubertal circumcision and negligible protective effect of adult circumcision.

Routine neonatal circumcision has been criticized (Morgan, 1965; Preston, 1970), and in the 1971 edition of Standards and Recommendations of Hospital Care of Newborn Infants by the Committee on the Fetus and Newborn of the American Academy of Pediatrics, it was stated that "there are no valid medical indications for circumcision in the neonatal period." This view was reiterated by an ad hoc task force of this committee in 1975, and in 1983 by both the American Academy of Pediatrics and the American College of Obstetrics and Gynecology in Guidelines to Perinatal Care (Schoen et al, 1989).

Since the 1975 report, however, new evidence has suggested possible medical benefit from neonatal circumcision. Data now suggest that the incidence of urinary tract infection in male infants may be reduced when neonatal circumcision is performed. Additional information has been published concerning the relationship of circumcision to sexually trans-

mitted diseases and, in turn, the relationship of viral sexually transmitted diseases to cancer of the penis and cervix (Burmer et al, 1993). In 1988, the Task Force (Schoen et al, 1989) revised its stance as follows: "Newborn circumcision has potential medical benefits and advantages as well as disadvantages and risks. When circumcision is being considered, the benefits and risks should be explained to the parents and informed consent obtained."

Circumcision may not be as important in countries where good hygiene is practical and soap and clean water are readily available. Any argument against circumcision must consider that penile carcinoma represents the only neoplasm for which there exists a predictable and simple means of prophylaxis that spares the organ at risk (Dagher et al, 1973) and must now consider the findings of the task force regarding infection.

Although a history of trauma may predate the development of carcinoma of the penis, it is thought this finding is coincidental rather than causal (Hanash et al, 1970). The development of carcinoma in the scarred penile shaft after mutilating circumcision, however, has been reported as a distinct entity (Bissada et al, 1986). No consistent etiologic relationship of penile cancer to venereal disease—syphilis, granuloma inguinale, and chancroid—has been found, and association of these diseases with penile cancer is probably coincidental (Schrek and Lenowitz, 1947).

The role of viral infection in the etiology of penile cancer is an area of intense interest. Both penile and cervical carcinoma have been related to herpesvirus infection. A threefold to eightfold increase in the incidence of cervical carcinoma among the sexual partners of patients with penile carcinoma has been documented in several studies (Goldberg et al, 1979). Other series have failed to demonstrate such a relationship (Redd et al, 1977). Penile cancer has also been associated with sexually transmitted HPV: A study from Brazil demonstrated HPV 18 DNA sequences in 7 of 18 cases (Villa and Lopes, 1986). Although a marked increase in squamous cancers has been observed in the renal transplant population, only one case of penile cancer in a renal transplant recipient has been reported (Previte et al, 1979).

Natural History

Carcinoma of the penis usually begins with a small lesion, which gradually extends to involve the entire glans, shaft, and corpora. The lesion may be papillary and exophytic or flat and ulcerative; if untreated, penile autoamputation may occur. The rates of growth of the papillary and ulcerative lesions are quite similar, but the flat, ulcerative tumor has a tendency toward earlier nodal metastasis and is associated with poorer 5-year survival rates (Dean, 1935; Marcial et al, 1962; Ornellas et al, 1994). Lesions larger than 5 cm (Beggs and Spratt, 1961) and those extending over 75% of the shaft (Staubitz et al, 1955) are also associated with an increased incidence of metastases and a decreased survival rate. Others, however, have not found a consistent relationship between lesion size, presence of metastases, and decreased survival (Ekstrom and Edsmyr, 1958; Puras et al, 1978).

Buck's fascia acts as a temporary natural barrier to local extension of the tumor, protecting the corporeal bodies from invasion. Penetration of Buck's fascia and the tunica albuginea permits invasion of the vascular corpora and estab-lishes the potential for vascular dissemination. Urethral and bladder involvement are rare (Riveros and Gorostiaga, 1962; Thomas and Small, 1963).

Metastases to the regional femoral and iliac nodes are the earliest route of dissemination from penile carcinoma. A detailed description of lymphatic drainage of the penis is found elsewhere in this text and is well documented in the literature (Dewire and Lepor, 1992). Briefly the lymphatics of the prepuce form a connecting network that joins with the lymphatics from the skin of the shaft. These tributaries drain into the superficial inguinal nodes (the nodes external to the fascia lata). The lymphatics of the glans join the lymphatics draining the corporeal bodies, and they form a collar of connecting channels at the base of the penis that drain by way of the superficial nodes. The superficial nodes drain to the deep inguinal nodes (those deep to the fascia lata); from there, drainage is to the pelvic nodes (external iliac, internal iliac, and obturator). Penile lymphangiogram studies demonstrate a consistent pattern of drainage that proceeds from superficial inguinal to deep inguinal to pelvic nodes sites without evidence of skip drainage (Cabanas, 1977; Cabanas, 1992). Multiple cross-connections exist at all levels of drainage, so that penile lymphatic drainage is bilateral to both inguinal areas.

Metastatic enlargement of the regional nodes eventually leads to skin necrosis; chronic infection; and death from inanition, sepsis, or hemorrhage secondary to erosion into the femoral vessels. **Clinically detectable distant metastatic lesions to the lung, liver, bone, or brain are uncommon and are reported as occurring in 1% to 10% of most large series** (Staubitz et al, 1955; Beggs and Spratt, 1961; Riveros and Gorostiaga, 1962; Derrick et al, 1973; Johnson et al, 1973; Kossow et al, 1973; Puras et al, 1978). Such metastases usually occur late in the course of the disease after the local lesion has been treated. Distant metastases in the absence of regional node metastases are unusual.

Carcinoma of the penis is characterized by a relentless progressive course, causing death for the majority of untreated patients within 2 years (Beggs and Spratt, 1961; Skinner et al, 1972; Derrick et al, 1973). Rarely, long-term survival occurs, even with advanced local disease and regional node metastases (Furlong and Uhle, 1953; Beggs and Spratt, 1961). **No report of spontaneous remission of carcinoma of the penis is known.** About 5% to 15% of patients have been reported to develop a second primary neoplasm (Beggs and Spratt, 1961; Buddington et al, 1963; Gursel et al, 1973), and one series reported secondary carcinoma in 17% of patients (Hubbell et al, 1988).

Modes of Presentation

Signs

The penile lesion itself usually alerts the patient to the presence of a penile cancer. The presentation ranges from relatively subtle induration or small excrescence to a small papule, pustule, warty growth, or more luxuriant exophytic lesion. It may appear as a shallow erosion or deep excavated ulcer with elevated or rolled-in edges. Phimosis may obscure a lesion and allow for a tumor to progress silently. Eventually, erosion through the prepuce, foul preputial odor, and discharge with or without bleeding call attention to the disease.

Penile tumors may present anywhere on the penis but occur most commonly on the glans (48%) and prepuce (21%). Other tumors involve both glans and prepuce (9%), coronal sulcus (6%), and shaft (less than 2%) (Sufrin and Huben, 1991). This distribution of lesions may be due to the glans, coronal sulcus, and interior prepuce being constantly exposed to smegma and other irritants within the prepuce, whereas the shaft and meatus are not.

Rarely a mass, ulceration, suppuration, or hemorrhage may present in the inguinal area because of the presence of nodal metastases from a lesion concealed within a phimotic foreskin. Urinary retention or urethral fistula owing to local corporeal involvement are rare presenting signs.

Symptoms

Pain does not develop in proportion to the extent of the local destructive process and usually is not a presenting complaint. Weakness, weight loss, fatigue, and systemic malaise occur secondary to chronic suppuration. Occasionally, significant blood loss from the penile lesion, the nodal lesion, or both may occur. Because local and regional disease are usually far advanced by the time distant metastases occur, presenting symptoms referable to such metastases are rare.

Diagnosis

Delay

Patients with cancer of the penis, more than patients with other types of cancer, seem to delay seeking medical attention (Lynch and Krush, 1969). In large series, from 15% to 50% of patients have been noted to delay medical care for more than a year (Dean, 1935; Buddington et al, 1963; Hardner et al, 1972; Gursel et al, 1973). Explanations include embarrassment, guilt, fear, ignorance, and personal neglect. This level of denial is substantial, given that the penis is observed and handled on a daily basis.

Delay in initiating treatment on the part of the physician may also be considerable. Although some studies show that the difference in survival rates between patients who present early and those who present later is negligible (Ekstrom and Edsmyr, 1958; Johnson et al, 1973), other series show decreased survival with longer delay (Hardner et al, 1972). It appears logical that earlier diagnosis and treatment should improve outcome.

Examination

At presentation, the majority of lesions are confined to the penis (Skinner et al, 1972; Derrick et al, 1973; Johnson et al, 1973). The penile lesion is assessed with regards to size, location, fixation, and involvement of the corporeal bodies. Inspection of the base of the penis and scrotum is necessary to rule out extension into these areas. Rectal and bimanual examination provide information about perineal body involvement and the presence of a pelvic mass. Careful bilateral palpation of the inguinal area for adenopathy is of extreme importance.

Biopsy

Confirmation of the diagnosis of carcinoma of the penis and assessment of the depth of invasion of the lesion by microscopic examination of a biopsy specimen are mandatory before the initiation of any therapy. Biopsy may be a separate procedure from definitive surgical treatment. Frequently a dorsal slit is necessary to gain adequate exposure of the lesion for satisfactory biopsy. No harmful effects related to tumor dissemination from biopsy of the penis have been reported (Ekstrom and Edsmyr, 1958). An alternative approach to treatment is biopsy with frozen section confirmation followed by partial or total penectomy. Full informed consent must be obtained before the procedure.

Histology

The majority of tumors of the penis are squamous cell carcinomas demonstrating keratinization, epithelial pearl formation, and various degrees of mitotic activity. The normal rete pegs are disrupted. Invasive lesions penetrate the basement membrane and surrounding structures.

Grading

Most malignancies of the penis are of low grade (Staubitz et al, 1955; Murrell and Williams, 1965). Lack of correlation between grade and survival has been noted by a number of investigators (Staubitz et al, 1955; Beggs and Spratt, 1961; Edwards and Sawyers, 1968; Kuruvilla et al, 1971; Hardner et al, 1972; Johnson et al, 1973). Other series report reduced survival among patients with anaplastic tumors (Ekstrom and Edsmyr, 1958; Marcial et al, 1962; Frew et al, 1967; Hanash et al, 1970; Puras et al, 1978). Two reviews emphasized the association of high-grade disease with regional nodal metastases (Fraley et al, 1989; Ravi, 1993). No relationship between the degree of infiltration with plasma cells, lymphocytes, or eosinophils has been established (Kuruvilla et al, 1971).

Loss of cell surface blood group antigens has been associated with invasion and metastases (Prasad and Veliath, 1986). DNA ploidy determination using archival pathology material has been related to prognosis in a number of urogenital and nonurologic tumors. Aneuploidy may predict disease of greater biologic potential for growth and metastases. Ploidy analysis of squamous cell carcinoma of the penis is limited to a small number of patients, and its ability to predict tumor behavior appears limited (Hoofnagle et al, 1990; Yu et al, 1992).

The strongest prognostic indicator for survival continues to be the presence or absence of nodal metastases (Ravi, 1993).

Laboratory Studies

Laboratory studies in patients with penile cancer are usually normal. Anemia, leukocytosis, and hypoalbuminemia may be present in patients with chronic illness, malnutrition, and extensive suppuration at the area of the primary and inguinal metastatic sites. Azotemia may develop secondary to urethral or ureteral obstruction.

Hypercalcemia without detectable osseous metastases has been associated with penile cancer (Anderson and

Glenn, 1965; Rudd et al, 1972). In a review from Memorial Sloan-Kettering Cancer Center (Sklaroff and Yagoda, 1982), 17 of 81 patients (20.9%) were hypercalcemic. Hypercalcemia seems to be largely a function of the bulk of the disease. It is often associated with inguinal metastases and may resolve following excision of involved inguinal nodes (Block et al, 1973). Parahormonal substances may be produced by both tumor and metastases (Malakoff and Schmidt, 1975). Medical treatment of hypercalcemia includes saline hydration and administration of diuretics, steroids, calcitonin, and mithramycin (Linderman and Papper, 1975).

Radiologic Studies

Distant metastases are rarely identified on radiographic examination or scanning. Intravenous pyelography is generally negative unless massive retroperitoneal nodes are present. Lymphangiography has previously been used most productively in the localization of inguinal and pelvic nodes to direct needle biopsy but because of irregular and inconsistent filling has limited usefulness. Although lymphangiography can opacify the three major nodal groups—external iliac, common iliac, and obturator nodes—the hypogastric and presacral nodes are generally not seen. The technical difficulty of the procedure, combined with increased availability of computed tomography (CT) scanning and magnetic resonance imaging (MRI), has made lymphangiography now largely obsolete in this disease.

The development of new imaging modalities has improved primary and secondary staging and follow-up of penile cancers and enhanced the role of imaging in the diagnosis and assessment of this disease. Both ultrasonography and MRI of the penis have proven to be quite effective in the assessment of the extent of the local lesion. Ultrasonography may evaluate the inguinal nodes as well as delineate the extent of the primary in the penile shaft preoperatively, so as to assist with treatment planning (Yamashita and Ogawa, 1989; Dorak et al, 1992; Horenblas et al, 1994). MRI can produce sharp images of the penile structures and demonstrate corporeal involvement and local extension with an accuracy of more than 80% (Kawada et al, 1994; Vapnek et al, 1992). CT of the groins may be helpful in identifying enlarged inguinal nodes in obese patients or in patients with prior surgery in the groins. CT-guided fine needle aspiration of enlarged inguinal or pelvic nodes may modify or avoid groin dissection in selected patients. CT of the penis is not effective in the evaluation of primary penile lesions.

Staging

Currently, no universal staging system for carcinoma of the penis exists, although systems suggested by Jackson and the Union Internationale Contre le Cancer (UICC) tumor, nodes, metastases (TNM) systems are most commonly employed (Jackson, 1966; Baker and Watson, 1975; Burgers et al, 1992). Accurate assessment of the extent of the primary tumor as well as identification of regional and distant metastatic disease are necessary in directing appropriate initial therapy and assessing end results. Clinical evaluation for the presence of inguinal metastases is subject to considerable inaccuracy.

The Jackson and UICC staging systems are outlined in Figure 79–1 and Tables 79–1, 79–2, and 79–3. Differences

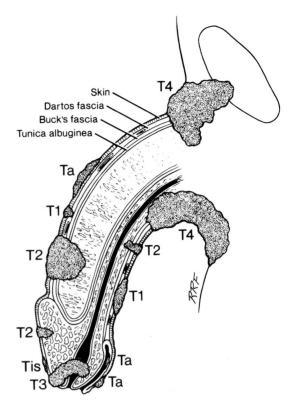

Figure 79–1. Because treatment decisions for inguinal node dissections are currently based on the characteristics of the primary lesion (see Treatment of Inguinal Nodes), a careful assessment of the depth of invasion of the primary is required. This diagram illustrates the importance of depth of invasion in assigning tumor (T) stage.

in the systems often make direct comparisons of results impossible. In the Jackson system, characteristics of the initial primary lesion—confined to the epidermis, superficial or invasive, small or large, limited to the glans or involving other structures—are not stated (Table 79–1). The nature and extent of nodal metastases are also not specified. Additionally, histologic criteria are not addressed, although the tumor grade and extent of invasion may be critical in formulating treatment or prognosis. In the Jackson system, a description of the lesion and its histologic features should supplement the tumor stage designation. The TNM system is more precise in describing the tumor and degree of invasion. The diagnostic criteria for TNM staging are listed in Tables 79–1 and 79–3 and Figure 79–1.

Differential Diagnosis

A number of penile lesions must be considered in the differential diagnosis of penile carcinoma. They include

Table 79–1. CLASSIFICATION FOR CARCINOMA OF THE PENIS

Stage I (A)	Tumors confined to glans, prepuce, or both
Stage II (B)	Tumors extending onto shaft of penis
Stage III (C)	Tumors with inguinal metastasis that are operable
Stage IV (D)	Tumors involving adjacent structure; tumors associated with inoperable inguinal metastasis or distant metastasis

Adapted from Jackson SM: Br J Surg 1966; 53:33. Published by Blackwell Science Ltd.

Table 79–2. TNM CLASSIFICATION OF PENILE CARCINOMA

Primary Tumor (T)

TX	Primary tumor cannot be assessed
T0	No evidence of primary tumor
Tis	Carcinoma-in-situ
Ta	Noninvasive verrucous carcinoma
T1	Tumor invades subepithelial connective tissue
T2	Tumor invades corpus spongiosum or cavernosum
T3	Tumor invades urethra or prostate
T4	Tumor invades other adjacent structures

Regional Lymph Nodes (N)

NX	Regional lymph nodes cannot be assessed
N0	No regional lymph node metastasis
N1	Metastasis in a single, superficial, inguinal lymph node
N2	Metastasis in multiple or bilateral superficial inguinal lymph nodes
N3	Metastasis in deep inguinal or pelvic lymph node(s), unilateral or bilateral

Distant Metastases (M)

MX	Presence of distant metastasis cannot be assessed
M0	No distant metastases
M1	Distant metastases

Adapted from Union Internationale Contre le Cancer (UICC): TNM Atlas: Illustrated Guide to the TNM/pTNM-Classification of Malignant Tumours, 3rd ed. New York, Springer-Verlag, 1989, pp. 237–244; and American Joint Committee on Cancer: Manual Staging for Cancer, 3rd ed. Philadelphia, J. B. Lippincott, 1988, pp. 189–191.

some of the lesions previously discussed—condyloma acuminatum, Buschke-Löwenstein tumor—as well as a number of inflammatory lesions—chancre, chancroid, herpes, lymphogranuloma venereum, granuloma inguinale, and tuberculosis. These diseases can be identified by appropriate skin tests, tissue studies, serologic examinations, cultures, or specialized attaining techniques.

TREATMENT OF THE PRIMARY NEOPLASM

The gold standard of therapy for penile cancer is partial or total penectomy. The low incidence of distant metastases, the significant morbidity that can result from untreated local disease, and the success of long-term palliation and survival even with advanced local disease

Table 79–3. MINIMAL DIAGNOSTIC CRITERIA FOR CARCINOMA OF THE PENIS

Primary Tumor (T)
Clinical examination
Incisional-excisional biopsy of lesion and histologic examination for grade and depth of invasion

Regional and Juxtaregional Lymph Nodes (N)
Clinical examination
CT scan
Superficial inguinal node dissection for high-grade or invasive histology
Lymphangiography and aspiration cytology (optional)

Distant Metastases (M)
Clinical examination
Chest radiograph, CT scan
MRI, bone scan (optional)
Biochemical determinations (liver functions, calcium)

CT, Computed tomography; MRI, magnetic resonance imaging.

support aggressive local therapy whenever possible. The disfigurement that occurs with penile amputation has encouraged efforts toward organ-sparing techniques employing partial excision or Mohs' micrographic surgery (MMS) as well as nonsurgical techniques employing x-ray, laser, or cryodestruction. The necessary goal of any treatment is complete destruction of the primary tumor.

Conventional Surgical Treatment

In selected cases with small lesions involving only the prepuce, complete tumor excision may be accomplished by circumcision (Ekstrom and Edsmyr, 1958). Circumcision alone is frequently followed by tumor recurrence (Marcial et al, 1962; Hardner et al, 1972; Gursel et al, 1973; Skinner et al, 1973). Two series have documented postcircumcision recurrence of 50% (Narayana et al, 1982) and 32% (McDougal et al, 1986).

For lesions involving the glans and distal shaft, even when apparently superficial, partial amputation with a 2-cm margin proximal to the tumor is necessary to minimize local recurrence. Frozen section of the proximal margin is recommended for confirmation of a tumor-free margin of resection. Following this guideline, recurrent tumor at the line of resection is rare, even with deep corporeal invasion, because tumor is spread by embolic metastases and not by lymphatic permeation (DeKernion et al, 1973; Ekstrom and Edsmyr, 1958; Hardner et al, 1972; DeKernion et al, 1973).

McDougal and associates reported no local recurrences following total penectomy and a 6% local recurrence rate after partial penectomy (McDougal et al, 1986). Local wedge resection has been associated with recurrences of up to 50% (Jensen, 1977). Adequate partial penectomy in the absence of inguinal nodes can provide 5-year survival rates of 70% to 80%. The residual penile stump is usually serviceable for upright micturition and sexual function.

If the tumor involves the penile shaft so that resection does not provide a 2-cm margin or if an adequate phallic stump to allow voiding in the standing position cannot be achieved, total penectomy with perineal urethrostomy is preferable. This procedure allows the patient to void in the sitting position (Fig. 79–2). In the rare circumstance in which a tumor of penile shaft skin involves epidermis only, excision of the skin and subcutaneous tissue may provide satisfactory control of the tumor (Fig. 79–3) (Grabstald, 1970). When the tumor involves scrotum or pubis (stage T4), or with fixed inguinal nodes (N3), hemipelvectomy followed by combination chemotherapy may warrant consideration in the carefully selected patient (Fig. 79–4) (Block et al, 1973).

Mohs' Micrographic Surgery

MMS is a method of removing skin cancer by excising tissue in thin layers. MMS includes color coding of excised specimens with tissue dyes, accurate orientation of excised tissue through construction of tissue maps, and microscopic examination of the horizontal frozen sections. The technique, first introduced in 1941 by Mohs, was described as micro-

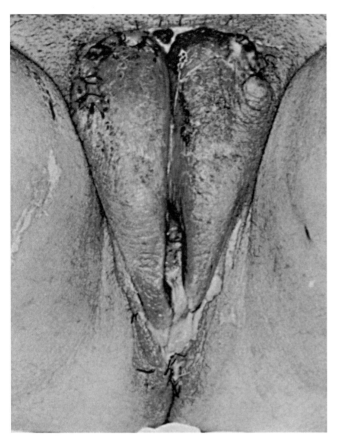

Figure 79–2. Appearance of the perineum following total penectomy and partial scrotectomy with formation of a perineal urethrostomy.

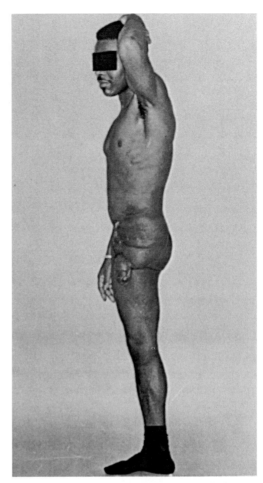

Figure 79–4. Hemipelvectomy. This young patient had invasive carcinoma with inguinal node metastases, but no evidence of positive juxtaregional nodes or distant metastases.

scopically controlled chemosurgery. The term *chemosurgery* has been replaced by MMS, a more descriptive term.

MMS is a much more time-consuming modality than many of the traditional tissue-sparing techniques. The American College of Mohs Micrographic Surgery frowns on the use of additional personnel for the examination of these carefully prepared sections. They state that "the precise accuracy of MMS can be obtained only if the Mohs micro-

graphic surgeon is responsible for all of the steps in the process. Variations from the technique or extra steps involving additional personnel may introduce errors which reduce the cure rate" (Cottel et al, 1988; Mohs et al, 1992).

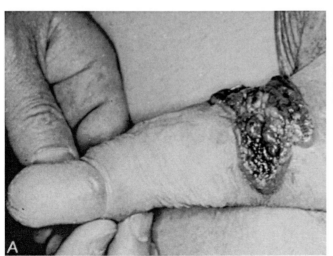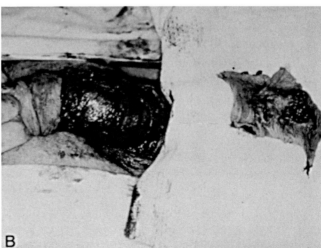

Figure 79–3. *A,* Erosive but superficial lesion of the proximal shaft skin. This lesion was treated by sleeve resection of the skin with preservation of the penis. *B,* Postresection appearance. Excised skin is to the right of the picture.

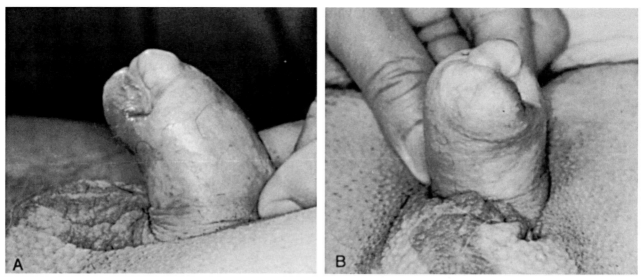

Figure 79–5. *A* and *B,* Two views of the glans and distal shaft following Mohs' micrographic surgery (MMS). The glans is small and deformed, and the coronal margin is almost totally absent. Note the stenotic urethral meatus.

The capability of MMS to trace out silent tumorous "extensions" with a cure rate equivalent to the more radical surgical techniques, while allowing the maximum preservation of normal, uninvolved tissue, makes it an attractive modality for the treatment of some carcinomas of the penis. In the Mohs series and other series, MMS seems to be ideally suited for small, distally located carcinomas (Mohs et al, 1985; Brown et al, 1987; Mohs et al, 1992). Mohs reported a 100% cure rate in the lesions he treated that were less than 1 cm in diameter but only a 50% cure rate in lesions that were greater than 3 cm.

After MMS, the areas of excision are allowed to heal by secondary intention, and meatal stenosis can be a complication. Meatal stenosis is treated by standard techniques with island flaps to reconstruct the meatus or a Y-V advancement technique to relieve the stenosis. In the majority of patients treated with MMS, patients have adequate functional shaft length; in many, however, the glans penis is misshapen or totally absent (Fig. 79–5). These patients may seek reconstructive surgery, which is often difficult to perform.

Often the appearance of the distal shaft of the penis can be improved by recreating a coronal margin. This can be accomplished by placing a split-thickness skin graft into a small circumcising groove, thus providing a pigmented line mimicking the coronal margin. A further cosmetic effort is achieved by tubing and burying the split-thickness graft, which can provide tissue contour variance along with a pigmentation difference. It is difficult to recreate the bulky shape of the normal glans penis. The ventral fascial flap with a skin island, described by Jordan (1987) for reconstruction of the fossa navicularis, has been employed in a limited number of patients to provide bulk on the distal end of the penis (Figs. 79–6 through 79–9).

Similar to most methods to control local tumor, MMS does not represent a panacea. **For small lesions and in selected patients, however, MMS appears to provide cure rates at least equal to those associated with partial penectomy, while leaving the patient with less long-term functional and cosmetic disability.** The reconstructive surgeon is often faced with a delicate dilemma in patients who have

had MMS for larger lesions. These patients have essentially undergone partial penectomy, and it is difficult to achieve a satisfactory result with minor reconstructive techniques. The more aggressive techniques of total phallic reconstruction, however, often do not provide an acceptable option to the patient.

Radiation Therapy

Primary radiation therapy allows for preservation of penile structure and function in carefully selected pa-

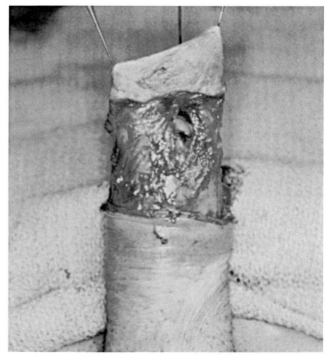

Figure 79–6. A transverse ventral skin island is elevated on a dartos fascia pedicle. The fascia pedicle is buttonholed, allowing transposition of the flap to the dorsum of the penis.

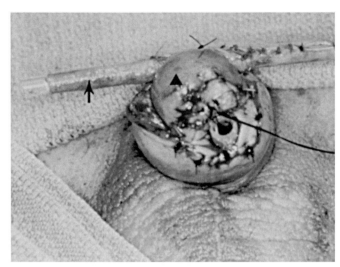

Figure 79–7. The placement of a tubed skin graft *(arrow)* for coronoplasty is illustrated. Note the transverse skin island *(dart)* transposed to the dorsum of the penis.

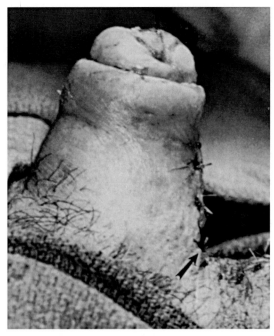

Figure 79–9. Later postoperative result illustrating the appearance of the coronal margin with the improved bulk of the glans penis. Not infrequently, the patient so treated requires a release of the penoscrotal tethering, as has been done here *(arrow)*.

tients. In reality, the number of patients for whom this treatment is appropriate is small. Advances in surgical therapy—laser therapy, MMS, and reconstructive surgery—can provide excellent surgical treatment while minimizing functional loss and avoiding the considerable complications associated with radiation therapy. Among elderly patients, preservation of an esthetic anatomic structure and sexual function are often of secondary importance.

There are significant disadvantages to radiation therapy. Squamous cell carcinoma is characteristically radioresistant, and the dosage required to sterilize the tumor (i.e., 6000 rad) may cause urethral fistula, stricture, or stenosis, with or without penile necrosis, pain, and edema (Kelley et al, 1974). **In some instances, secondary penectomy may be required** (Duncan and Jackson, 1972).

Infection is frequently associated with newly diagnosed

penile cancer, and this markedly decreases the therapeutic effect of radiation while increasing the risk of damage to the radiosensitive penile tissue (Murrell and Williams, 1965).

Additionally, radiation therapy is usually administered over a period of 3 to 6 weeks and is followed by several months of morbidity. This may pose a formidable burden in elderly patients. By contrast, partial penectomy offers a prompt and effective treatment, with relatively few side effects limiting activity in the postoperative period.

Finally, it must be accepted that should radiation therapy

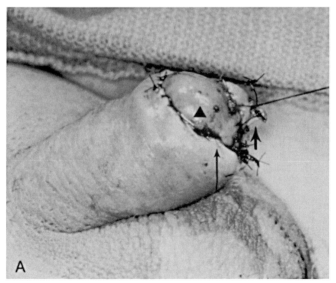
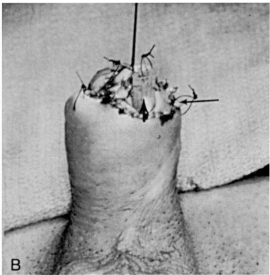

Figure 79–8. *A* and *B,* Appearance of the immediate postoperative result with the stenting urethral catheter *(short arrow)* and buried stenting tube *(long arrow)* for the first-stage coronoplasty. The transverse ventral skin island that has been transposed to the dorsum of the penis provides bulk and dorsal "glans" *(arrowhead).*

fail, prompt penectomy must be done to avoid jeopardizing survival. Careful long-term follow-up is essential to detect recurrence promptly, and it must be recognized that recurrence may occur relatively late. In one series, 7 of 11 recurrences were detected after 2 years (63%) and 2 (18%) after 5 years (Mazeron et al, 1984). Close follow-up may be difficult in a group of patients whose reliability is often poor and who have often neglected a markedly symptomatic primary lesion for an extended period of time before seeking treatment. Furthermore, distinguishing postirradiation ulcer, scar, and fibrosis from possible recurrent carcinoma is often impossible, and repeated biopsies of the lesions may be required.

Radiation therapy may be considered in a select group of patients: (1) young individuals presenting with small (2–3 cm), superficial, exophytic, noninvasive lesions on the glans or coronal sulcus; (2) patients refusing surgery as an initial form of treatment; and (3) patients with inoperable tumor or distant metastases who require local therapy to the primary tumor but who express a desire to retain the penis. Radiation may be considered after a course of topical 5-fluorouracil cream has failed in the treatment of carcinoma in situ. Before radiation therapy, circumcision or dorsal slit is necessary to expose the lesion, allow resolution of any surface infection, and prevent maceration and preputial edema.

The success of radiation therapy in the treatment of penile cancers is difficult to assess because of the relative rarity of these tumors, the variability of treatment within single series, and the variations between different series. Treatment schedules, total radiation dosages, and modality—external beam (Jackson, 1966), electron beam (Kelley et al, 1974), radium mold (Jackson, 1966), and interstitial therapy (Pierquin et al, 1971; Delannes et al, 1992; Gerbaulet and Lambin, 1992)—vary considerably.

Radiation therapy to select, small, superficial lesions is quite successful. A 90% rate of control of the primary tumor among 20 patients treated with megavoltage radiation has been reported (Duncan and Jackson, 1972). The dosages employed—5000 to 5700 rad over 3 weeks—produced significant complications, however: penile necrosis in 10% of patients and urethral stricture in 30%.

The most successful series employing radiation therapy is that reported by Memorial Sloan-Kettering Cancer Center (Kelley et al, 1974). Using electron beam therapy, a 100% success rate in controlling lesions in ten carefully selected patients was achieved clinically and confirmed histologically by means of negative post-treatment biopsy specimens. In one patient, carcinoma developed at another penile site, suggesting a new primary tumor. Nine patients retained sexual function. The most common complication was urethral stricture in four patients (Grabstald and Kelley, 1980). A series from the M. D. Anderson Hospital and Tumor Institute also reports good control of smaller lesions without significant morbidity (Haile and Delclos, 1980), and similar success with well-selected cases has been reported by other centers (Raynal et al, 1977; Salaverria et al, 1979; Daly et al, 1982; Mazeron et al, 1984; McLean et al, 1993). Gerbaulet and Lambin, using interstitial iridium implants, report successful local control in 82% of 109 patients, with long-term survivals of 75% to 80% in patients with tumor-free regional lymph nodes (Gerbaulet and Lambin, 1992).

When radiation therapy is employed as the initial treatment for penile carcinoma, control of the primary lesions occurs with much less frequency than when surgery is primarily employed (Table 79–4). A patient's prognosis is not altered if surgery is promptly performed when radiation fails to control the carcinoma (Murrell and Williams, 1965). Jackson (1966), however, did show that nodal metastases develop more frequently during or after a course of radiation therapy than after surgery; this suggests the potential for metastases to occur during or following a course of unsuccessful radiation therapy.

Small, superficial tumors respond well to radiotherapy, and, with careful planning, complications can be minimized. The treatment of larger, invasive malignancies is less successful, may be associated with severe local complications, and theoretically may provide an interval

Table 79–4. SURGERY REQUIRED AFTER RADIATION THERAPY FOR CARCINOMA OF THE PENIS

Series	Number of Patients	Amputation for Recurrent or Persistent Disease, or Both (%)*	Other Surgery (%)	Total (%)
Lederman, 1953	48	35	—	35
Murrell & Williams, 1965	92	48	—	48
Jackson, 1966	58	51	—	51
Knudsen & Brennhovd, 1967	145	62	6†	68
Almgard & Edsmyr, 1973	33	52	18‡	70
Engelstad, 1948	64	45§	8†	53
Raynal et al, 1977	45	22	8†	30
Salaverria et al, 1979	13	23	—	23
Haile & Delclos, 1980	20	10	10†	20
Daly et al, 1982	22	5	10†	15
Sagerman et al, 1984	15	40	—	40
Mazeron et al, 1984	50	20	10	30
Fossa et al, 1987	11	33	—	33
McLean et al, 1993	26	19	12†	31
Suchaud et al, 1989	53	42	—	42

*Difference from 100% indicates cure from radiation alone.
†Penectomy for radiation complications.
‡Local excision or electrocoagulation of recurrent neoplasm.
§Includes seven radiation therapy failures not having further surgery.

during which metastatic dissemination may occur. Other untoward effects of radiation include testicular damage and secondary neoplasia (Lederman, 1953; Prescott and Mainwaring, 1990; Fukunaga et al, 1994). In the case of a sexually active young patient with an invasive lesion, surgical amputation followed by penile reconstruction (see later) rather than primary radiation therapy should be considered.

LASER SURGERY IN PENILE LESIONS

Laser Technology

Over the past 10 years, the use of laser therapy to treat genital lesions has evolved substantially. **Laser therapy has been employed to treat many benign and premalignant penile lesions as well as stage Tis, Ta, T1, and some T2 penile cancers. Potential advantages of laser therapy in penile cancer are destruction of the lesion with preservation of normal structure and function.** Several disadvantages exist, however, which are especially apparent when laser therapy is used to treat larger lesions. Depth of laser destruction may be difficult to determine, and histologic documentation of the depth of malignant penetration may not be available. Therefore, it is imperative to stage the tumor adequately with deep biopsy specimens before using laser therapy. In the properly selected patient, however, laser therapy offers an excellent treatment option.

Currently, four different types of lasers are used in the treatment of penile lesions: CO_2, Nd:YAG, argon, and potassium titanyl phosphate (KTP). The CO_2 laser has a wavelength of 10,600 nm. The beam energy is absorbed by intracellular water, which is then heated to a high temperature. This results in vaporization of the tissue being treated. The beam penetrates only the outermost 0.01 mm of tissue. The CO_2 laser thus produces a "scalpel" effect limited to the surface of the tissue under treatment. This laser can coagulate only small blood vessels (<0.5 mm), so it is not effective in producing hemostasis. The beam is directed along a system of mirrors and cannot be used in a liquid medium, precluding its use with a cystoscope. For small superficial lesions, however, it can be quite effective.

The Nd:YAG laser has a wavelength of 1060 nm and produces tissue penetration, depending on the power used, of 3 to 6 mm, making it ideal for treating superficial skin lesions. It can coagulate vessels up to 5 mm in diameter effectively. There is a 20% to 30% "forward scatter" of energy, which may inadvertently produce tissue changes beyond the immediate field of treatment. This laser beam is delivered via a fiberoptic bundle and may be used in water or urine effectively. Additionally, sapphire-tipped fibers for direct contact applications have been developed that allow for a "scalpel" effect, allowing this laser to be used on larger lesions.

Both the argon and KTP lasers have similar wavelengths (488–515 nm for argon and 532 nm for KTP), which are maximally absorbed in tissue pigments such as hemoglobin and melanin. Both beams have less tissue-penetrating ability than the CO_2 laser but can be transmitted via a fiberoptic delivery system and used through a cystoscope. They are employed most successfully in the treatment of pigmented lesions, particularly those that are highly vascular, such as hemangiomas (Carpiniello and Schoenberg, 1991; Jiminez-Cruz and Osca, 1993).

Laser Management of Benign Penile Lesions

Condyloma Acuminatum

Condylomata acuminata or venereal warts are readily treated with both CO_2 and Nd:YAG lasers; however, the risk of recurrence may be higher than some original reports have suggested, and close follow-up with magnified penile surface scanning using loupe lenses and 5% acetic acid solution to accentuate the presence of subclinical areas of involvement is recommended (Graversen et al, 1990; Krogh et al, 1990; Carpiniello and Schoenberg, 1991). Combination therapy using laser surgery and interferon therapy may provide more durable disease-free intervals (Reichman et al, 1988; Hockley et al, 1989). Excellent cosmetic control of condylomata can be achieved with the Nd:YAG laser (15 watts power) applied to the lesion and a 0.5 to 1 cm circumferential area (Carpiniello and Schoenberg, 1991). The CO_2 laser set at 5 watts of power also achieves an excellent cosmetic result but may not provide tissue penetration deep enough to sterilize the tissue of residual viral infection.

Other Benign Lesions

Both CO_2 and Nd:YAG lasers have been used in the successful management of balanitis xerotica obliterans (Rosemberg et al, 1982), pearly penile papules (Magid and Garden, 1989), and Zoon's balanitis (Baldwin and Geronemus, 1989). Both Nd:YAG and argon lasers have successfully treated glanular hemangiomas (Jiminez-Cruz and Osca, 1993) as well as small scrotal hemangiomas. Generally the Nd:YAG laser is set to 15 watts, and the skin surrounding the lesion is cooled during treatment to prevent damage to normal structures. The CO_2 laser is employed at a setting of 5 watts.

Management of Premalignant Lesions, Carcinoma in Situ, and Squamous Cell Carcinoma

Premalignant Lesions and Carcinoma in Situ

Treatment of Tis tumors (Bowen's disease, erythroplasia of Queyrat, bowenoid papulosis) can be achieved using any of the common surgical lasers. Several reports have documented the ability of the CO_2 laser to treat these lesions (Rosemberg and Fuller, 1980; Bandieramonte et al, 1987). Because these lesions are superficial, are often multifocal, and require precise treatment, the CO_2 laser and the operating microscope are the ideal approach. In addition, 5% acetic acid staining may be helpful in delineating the full extent of the lesion (Greenbaum et al, 1989). The

Nd:YAG laser has also been used successfully in the treatment of Tis tumors (Malloy et al, 1988).

Penile Cancers

Treatment of T1 and T2 tumors has not been as uniformly successful. Several different techniques have been used, employing both CO_2 and Nd:YAG lasers. The most aggressive use of the CO_2 laser has been reported by Bandieramonte and co-workers (1987, 1988). Total resection of the surface of the glans penis was carried out for T1 tumor. By using a short pulse with a high peak power at the base of the lesion and around the meatus, precise excision providing a specimen for pathologic examination can be achieved.

Despite magnification, positive surgical margins have been noted, and a 15% recurrence rate has been reported (Bandieramonte et al, 1988). The Nd:YAG laser has received more widespread attention either as primary therapy or as an adjunct to excision. By using the focusing handpiece and iced saline irrigation, six of nine patients with T1 tumors were tumor-free with a mean follow-up of 26 months. Tumors were not completely destroyed in two patients with T2 disease (Malloy et al, 1988). Laser excision with the aid of a sapphire tip, followed by laser coagulation of the base in stage T1 and T2 tumors, was associated with an 81% tumor-free rate with a mean follow-up of 17 months (Boon, 1988). Von Eschenbach and associates reported similar success in a group of 10 patients with superficial or microscopically invasive tumors treated with the Nd:YAG laser and followed for a mean of 32 months. One patient died of unrelated causes and was free of tumor, and two patients required retreatment for recurrent tumors (one at 7 months and one at 15 months) but were subsequently free of disease (Von Eschenbach et al, 1991).

The Nd:YAG laser may be effective in the management of penile Kaposi's sarcoma when a symptomatic lesion develops or when meatal obstruction develops (Wishnow and Johnson, 1988).

TREATMENT OF INGUINAL NODES

The prognosis for patients with carcinoma of the penis is markedly worsened by the presence of inguinal metastases. This finding affects the prognosis of the disease more than tumor grade, gross appearance, or morphologic or microscopic patterns of the tumor. Nodal metastases are more frequently associated with high-grade lesions or invasive histology.

In contrast to other genitourinary tumors for which there is no effective systemic treatment, systematic lymphadenectomy is curative in about 50% of cases and should be undertaken. Also avoided are late complications of bulky inguinal disease—ulceration, infection, and vascular compromise.

Patients with penile carcinoma and palpable lymphadenopathy require control of the primary tumor, followed by re-evaluation of the inguinal nodes 2 to 6 weeks after the nodal inflammatory response from infection has been controlled. This interval for antibiotic treatment not only serves to permit more accurate assessment of the cause of lymphadenopathy (inflammatory versus neoplastic), but also markedly reduces the potential operative morbidity secondary to sepsis and may reduce long-term morbidity as well.

Surgical Treatment

There are several controversial issues regarding the treatment of regional lymph nodes. (1) Should lymphadenectomy be performed for a patient with palpable inguinal lymphadenopathy that is persistent after treatment of the primary penile lesion and following a course of antibiotics sufficient to allow nodal inflammation secondary to infection to subside? (2) Should lymphadenectomy be performed on a prophylactic or adjunctive basis in a patient with clinically negative inguinal nodes? (3) Should lymphadenectomy be performed bilaterally if only unilateral nodes are palpable, or should node dissections be limited to the side of palpable abnormality? (4) Should lymphadenectomy be extended to the pelvic lymph nodes, unilaterally or bilaterally, or should it be restricted to the inguinal lymph node area?

Because penile cancer is a rare disease, it is impossible to conduct adequate prospective, randomized trials to resolve the issues surrounding the management of regional nodes. Using historical and retrospective data from the literature, the above-listed questions are subsequently addressed. Although treatment guidelines can be developed from retrospective analysis, treatment must often be individualized to meet the requirements of the particular case.

The technical aspects of surgical therapy are discussed at length in Chapter 108. Inguinal dissections may involve biopsy of the sentinel nodes, an extended biopsy of the sentinel nodes and immediate surrounding nodal tissue, or more formal inguinal dissections. Superficial inguinal node dissections excise the nodes superficial to the fascia lata, and the more extensive classic dissection, which is accompanied by significant postoperative complications, has been modified at some centers to spare the saphenous vein and reduce the boundaries of dissection in an attempt to reduce sequelae (Catalona, 1988). Deep inguinal node dissection removes those nodes deep to the fascia lata, whereas iliac or pelvic lymphadenectomy removes the external iliac and obturator nodes. Total inguinal lymphadenectomy includes superficial and deep inguinal lymphadenectomies plus pelvic lymphadenectomy.

Should lymphadenectomy be performed in the presence of clinically palpable inguinal nodes after appropriate treatment of the primary lesion and subsidence of inflammation? This question can be answered affirmatively. Evidence to support this statement is based on the following findings: Patients with penile carcinomas and inguinal metastases who do not undergo treatment rarely survive 2 years and almost never survive 5 years. No spontaneous regression of penile carcinoma has been reported. **Twenty percent to 50% of patients with clinically palpable adenopathy and histologically proven inguinal node metastases who are treated by inguinal lymphadenectomy, however, achieve a 5-year disease-free survival** (Table 79–5). When extent of nodal disease has been identified, patients with limited node involvement fare even better.

Srinivas and associates from Memorial Sloan-Kettering Cancer Center reported an 82% 5-year survival for patients

Table 79–5. CARCINOMA OF THE PENIS—PROGNOSTIC INDICATORS FOR SURVIVAL

Series	Number of Patients	Percent with Palpable Nodes	Clinically and Pathologic Characteristics of Inguinal Adenopathy		5-Year Survival Rates (%)	
			Percent Clinically False-Positive (Nodes Palpable, Histologic Findings Negative)	Percent Clinically False-Negative (Nodes Palpable, Histologic Findings Positive)	Inguinal Nodes Negative on Histologic or Repeated Physical Examination	Inguinal Nodes Resected and Positive on Histologic Examination of Adenectomy Specimen
Ekstrom & Edsmyr, 1958	229	33	48	—	80[a]	42
Beggs & Spratt, 1961	88	35	36	20	72.5	45
Thomas & Small, 1963	190	—	64	20	—	26
Edwards & Sawyers, 1968	77	—	—	0	68	25
Hanash et al, 1970	169	—	58[b]	2[b]	77[c]	—
Kuruvilla et al, 1971	153	39	63	10	69	33
Hardner et al, 1972	100	42	41[b]	16[b]	—	—
Gursel et al, 1973	64	53	60[b]	—	58	—
Skinner et al, 1972	34	29	40	—	75 / 87[d]	20 / 50[d]
DeKernion et al, 1973	48	54	38[b]	—	84[e]	55[e]
Derrick et al, 1973	87	29	52	—	53 / 76[d]	22 / 55[d]
Johnson et al, 1973	153	—	—	—	64.4	21.8
Kossow et al, 1973	100	51	49	25	—	—[f]
Puras et al, 1978	576	82	47	38[b]	89	67[g] / 29[h]
Cabanas, 1977	80	96	65	100	90	70[i] / 50[j] / 20[k]
Fossa et al, 1987	79	—	—	13	90	80[l] / 20[m]
Srinivas et al, 1987	199	63	14[n]	18	74	82[o] / 54[p] / 40[q] / 12[r]
McDougal et al, 1986	65	—	—	66	100	83[s] / 66[t] / 38[u]
Young et al, 1991	34	24	27	42	77	0
Horenblas et al, 1993	110	36	26	40	100	38
Ravi, 1993	201	53	8	16	95	81[v] / 50[w] / 86[x] / 60[y]
Ornellas et al, 1994	414	50	51[y]	39	87	29
Theodorescu et al, 1995	40	70	35	—	46	45
Puras-Baez et al, 1995	272	—	—	—	89	38

[a]Majority of patients received prophylactic or preoperative radiotherapy to inguinal area.
[b]Histologic classification based on node biopsy, not node dissection.
[c]Corrected 5-year survival; i.e., patients dying before 5 years without evidence of disease are excluded.
[d]Patients dying free of cancer before 5 years are considered surgical cures.
[e]Three-year survival.
[f]Omitted.
[g]Positive findings in inguinofemoral nodes.
[h]Positive findings in inguinofemoral and pelvic nodes.
[i]Single inguinal node with positive findings.
[j]More than one inguinal node with positive findings.
[k]Three-year survival with positive findings in inguinal and pelvic nodes.
[l]N1–2.
[m]N3.
[n]After antibiotic therapy.
[o]One node positive.
[p]One to six nodes positive.
[q]Greater than six nodes positive.
[r]Bilateral nodes positive.
[s]Adjunctive adenectomy.
[t]Immediate therapeutic adenectomy.
[u]Delayed therapeutic adenectomy.
[v]One to three positive nodes.
[w]More than three positive nodes.
[x]Unilateral.
[y]Some lymph node dissection done without antibiotic pretreatment.

Table 79–6. FIVE-YEAR SURVIVAL RELATED TO EXTENT OF NODAL METASTASIS

Series	Number of Patients	Number of Positive Nodes	
		≤2	>2
Fraley et al, 1989	31	15/17 (88%)	1/14 (7%)
Johnson & Lo, 1984a	22	6/7 (85%)*	2/15 (13%)
Srinivas et al, 1987	119	5/6 (82%)	7/34 (20%)
			9/16 (54%)†
Fossa et al, 1987	18	11/12 (88%)‡	2/6 (33%)§
Ravi, 1993	21	47/58 (81%)‖	5/10 (50%)¶
Horenblas et al, 1994	110	5/15 (67%)	9/23 (39%)

*Approximate.
†A subset with one to six positive nodes.
‡N1–2.
§N3.
‖One to three positive nodes.
¶More than three positive nodes.

having a single node at lymphadenectomy (Srinivas et al, 1987). Another large series from the Norwegian Radium Hospital reported an 88% 5-year survival following lymphadenectomy for patients with minimal nodal metastases (Fossa et al, 1987). Several other series have confirmed favorable survival rates in the face of minimal nodal disease (Table 79–6) (Beggs and Spratt, 1961; Johnson and Lo, 1984a; Fraley et al, 1989; Ornellas et al, 1994; Ravi, 1993).

Only 50% of patients presenting with palpable lymphadenopathy actually have metastatic disease, the remainder having lymph node enlargement secondary to inflammation. Persistent adenopathy following treatment of the primary lesion and 4 to 6 weeks of antibiotic therapy is most often due to metastatic disease. Similarly the development of new adenopathy during follow-up is much more likely to be due to tumor than inflammatory response. In the Memorial Sloan-Kettering Cancer Center series cited previously, 66 of 76 patients (86%) with palpable adenopathy after 6 weeks of antibiotic therapy had pathologically positive nodes. A study by Ornellas and associates from Brazil confirmed a 70% incidence of metastases in patients with clinically positive nodes following antibiotic treatment (Ornellas et al, 1994).

Should complete inguinal lymphadenectomy be routinely performed in patients with clinically negative groin examination findings at the time of presentation of the primary lesion? This question invites the greatest amount of controversy. As noted, the cure rate with inguinal lymphadenectomy when nodes are positive for malignancy may be as high as 80%. A cure rate of this magnitude with surgery in the face of regional nodal metastases parallels the urologist's experience with testicular cancer, in which retroperitoneal lymphadenectomy provides cure in many patients with positive regional nodes. In contrast, for other common genitourinary malignancies—bladder, prostate, and kidney—surgical cure in the face of regional nodal metastases is rare. Given that node dissection can cure metastatic penile cancer, why is there debate over whether the procedure should be performed, especially given that regional node dissections are often advocated in other malignancies when evidence of their efficacy is marginal at best?

The reluctance to advocate automatic ilioinguinal lymphadenectomy in all patients with penile cancer stems from the substantial morbidity that the procedure produces, as opposed to the relatively limited postoperative morbidity of pelvic or retroperitoneal lymphadenectomies. Early complications of phlebitis, pulmonary embolism, wound infection, and flap necrosis as well as permanent and disabling lymphedema of the scrotum and lower limbs are frequent after both inguinal and ilioinguinal node dissections (Fig. 79–10) (Skinner et al, 1972; Johnson and Lo, 1984b; McDougal et al, 1986; Fraley et al, 1989). In recent years, postoperative complications have been reduced by improved preoperative and postoperative care; advances in surgical technique; and preservation of the dermis, Scarpa's fascia, and the saphenous vein as well as modification of the extent of the dissection (Catalona, 1988). Furthermore, experience has suggested that lymphadenectomy in the setting of microscopic disease may be less likely to produce complications than node dissection in the presence of bulky nodal metastases (Fraley et al, 1989; Ornellas et al, 1994).

Mortality after inguinal lymphadenectomy has been reported only in association with surgery done concomitantly with penectomy and was related to sepsis. Mortality has not been reported when lymphadenectomy was delayed several weeks after amputation (Ekstrom and Edsmyr, 1958). An operative mortality of 3.3% was reported in early series (Beggs and Spratt, 1961). Johnson and Lo (1984b) and others (Ornellas et al, 1994; Ravi, 1993) have reported no mortality in more recent series. Postoperative mortality should be less than 1%.

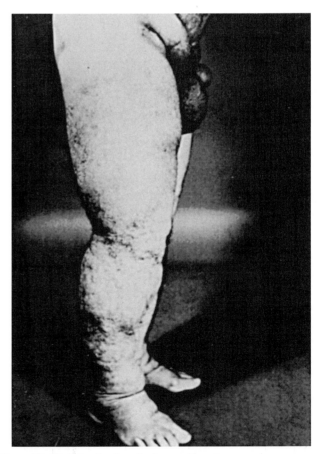

Figure 79–10. Extensive lymphedema with cutaneous changes secondary to recurrent lymphangitis and phlebitis.

The significant postoperative morbidity associated with ilioinguinal lymphadenectomy warrants serious consideration and represents a significant issue in determining the role of prophylactic or adjunctive lymphadenectomy in the absence of palpable nodes. **The incidence of metastases to the inguinal nodes in patients presenting with penile tumors and clinically negative groin examinations has been reported at 2% to 25%. Several large series have reported high false-negative rates of 38%** (Puras et al, 1978) **and 39%** (Ornellas et al, 1994), **particularly when obesity or changes in the inguinal area—scar or postsurgical induration—make accurate assessment impossible.**

The incidence of metastases to clinically normal nodes is based on information derived from both complete node dissections and limited lymph node biopsies. Because some patients subsequently develop positive nodes after initial limited dissections or selected biopsy findings are negative and because the detection of metastases on pathologically submitted material depends on the number of sections per node examined—that is, how diligently the pathologist looks for tumor—the incidence rates for false-negative clinical examinations represent the minimum. These patients with clinically negative but histologically positive nodes are at risk for death from penile cancer. One review calculated that 17% of patients who presented initially with negative nodes died of disease (Catalona, 1980).

The curative benefit of lymphadenectomy in the presence of grossly palpable nodes involved with tumor has been established. It is logical to presume that a lymphadenectomy performed in the setting of microscopic nodal disease would confer an even greater survival advantage. Reports from the Ellis Fischel State Cancer Hospital in Columbia, Missouri, however, demonstrated no apparent reduction in 5-year survival rates among those patients with negative nodes initially who were carefully followed and later, when adenopathy appeared, underwent therapeutic node dissection (Lesser and Schwartz, 1955). The 5-year survival in this group paralleled that of patients presenting with metastatic lymphadenopathy initially who were treated with immediate node dissection (Baker et al, 1976). This expectant treatment policy was also supported by Frew and colleagues (1967). Given these findings, it is difficult to justify a broad recommendation for lymph node dissection to patients with negative clinical inguinal examinations, for whom the procedure is not therapeutic in approximately 75% of cases.

Unfortunately, most series have not analyzed separately survival of patients after lymphadenectomy with clinically impalpable nodes that are positive for neoplasm on histologic examination. Four studies have compared 5-year disease-free survival among patients presenting with clinically negative inguinal lymph nodes who had either immediate adjunctive or delayed therapeutic lymphadenectomy.

McDougal and co-workers reported a series of 23 patients with invasive primary lesions and non-palpable nodes (McDougal et al, 1986). Nine patients were treated with immediate adjunctive lymph node dissection (6 were positive), and 14 were treated with surveillance and delayed lymph node dissection. The 5-year survival in the node-positive immediate adjunctive lymphadenectomy group was 88% (five of six), whereas in the surveillance plus delayed lymphadenectomy group, the 5-year survival was 38%. Only one patient in the surveillance group, however, had node

dissection. Presumptively the other patients had progressed to inoperable local tumor or distant disease before clinical manifestation of lymphadenopathy, emphasizing the role of careful, frequent follow-up and the difficulty of enforcing it. A third subset in this series had palpable nodes at presentation and had immediate therapeutic lymph node dissection with 10 of 15 patients (66%) surviving 5 years (McDougal et al, 1986). The best results were from immediate adjunctive lymph node dissection (88%), with the next best from immediate therapeutic lymphadenectomy (66%). The worst results were from the surveillance and delayed lymphadenectomy group (38%), in which dissection was delayed until palpable nodes developed. The interval of opportunity for cure in this third group appears to have been lost.

Fraley and colleagues reported that immediate adjunctive lymphadenectomy resulted in a 5-year disease-free survival in 6 of 9 (66%) node-positive patients compared with 1 of 12 patients (8%) in whom the groins had been followed and then treated by delayed lymphadenectomy when nodal enlargement occurred (Fraley et al, 1989). Although only two of six immediate lymphadenectomy patients had more than two positive nodes, all of the patients treated by delayed lymph node dissection had three or more positive nodes.

A series from the M. D. Anderson Hospital compared 5-year disease-free survival for 14 patients with early adjunctive lymphadenectomy for clinically impalpable but histologically node-positive disease with that for 8 patients who were followed and later had lymphadenectomy when clinical nodal enlargement appeared (Johnson and Lo, 1984a). The primary tumors were of similar stage. The 5-year disease-free survival was 57% for early lymphadenectomy compared with 13% for delayed node dissection. Of note, the number of involved nodes in the immediate lymphadenectomy group (median = 2) was half that of the delayed lymphadenectomy group (median = 4), and no patient with more than two positive nodes survived more than 5 years.

In a large series from Brazil, Ornellas and associates reported a 62% 5-year disease-free survival in 102 patients undergoing immediate lymphadenectomy but only 8% in 42 patients followed until suspicious nodes occurred and then subjected to delayed inguinal lymphadenectomy (Ornellas et al, 1994). The 5-year disease-free survival of patients in this series who initially had clinically negative nodes and had immediate lymphadenectomy was contingent on the results of lymphadenectomy: 87% with pathologically negative nodes versus 29% with positive nodes.

Other studies supporting early lymphadenectomy include one by Puras and associates from Puerto Rico that showed the highest 5-year survival in patients undergoing surgical removal of the primary tumor followed within 1 month by routine lymphadenectomy (Puras et al, 1978). Another study from Uruguay (Cabanas, 1977) reported improved survival by using early node biopsy followed by prompt complete node dissection if the biopsy specimen was positive. Information from several series supports improved survival with resection of low-volume nodal disease. Adjunctive or early lymphadenectomy gives greater assurance that surgical intervention occurs when tumor volume is small (Table 79–6) (Fossa et al, 1987; Srinivas et al, 1987; Fraley et al, 1989; Johnson and Lo, 1984a; Ravi, 1993).

It is important to identify indicators that predict for increased risk of nodal involvement so as to be able to select patients who are most likely to harbor subclinical metastases.

Primary tumor stage assessment is of paramount importance (DeKernion et al, 1973; McDougal et al, 1986). **Lesions that invade through the basement membrane of the penile integument are more likely to be associated with nodal metastases, and proposals have been made for ilioinguinal node dissection in medically suited patients with clinically negative nodes, whose primary lesion is invasive** (DeKernion et al, 1973; Catalona, 1980; McDougal et al, 1986; Horenblas et al, 1993; Lubke and Thompson, 1993).

Grade can provide information about the likelihood of nodal metastases (Fraley et al, 1989; Horenblas et al, 1993). Fraley's study of tumor grade and relationship to nodal metastases showed a higher correlation than do most series: One of 19 patients with well-differentiated tumor, 5 of 19 patients with moderately differentiated tumor, and all 16 patients with poorly differentiated tumor developed nodal metastases. Horenblas and associates also showed close correlation of tumor differentiation and nodal metastases: Nine of 11 (82%) of grade 3 tumor patients and 13 of 28 (46%) with grade 2 tumors showed nodal metastases, whereas 17 of 59 (29%) of those with grade 1 lesions had nodal involvement.

Sentinel node biopsy, limited node dissection superficial to the fascia lata, and aspiration cytology are staging procedures that are less extensive than complete inguinal lymphadenectomy but that can provide useful information. The concept of sentinel node biopsy as described by Cabanas is predicated on detailed penile lymphangiographic studies that have demonstrated consistent drainage of the penile lymphatics into a sentinel node or group of nodes located superomedial to the junction of the saphenous and femoral veins in the area of the superficial epigastric vein (Cabanas, 1977). In this series, when this sentinel node was negative for tumor, metastases to other ilioinguinal lymph nodes did not occur. Metastases to this node indicated the need for a complete superficial and deep inguinal dissection.

The accuracy of the sentinel node histology to identify inguinal node metastases has been questioned by a number of reports (DeKernion et al, 1973; Perenetti et al, 1980; Wespes et al, 1986). Because nodal metastases became palpable within 1 year of negative sentinel node biopsy in some patients in these series, a false-negative biopsy result must be presumed. In one large series, 5 of 82 (6%) sentinel node-negative groins in 5 of 41 patients (12%) with negative sentinel node biopsy subsequently developed inguinal node metastases (Fossa et al, 1987). In Cabanas' series, 3 of 31 patients with negative sentinel nodes died of disease, suggesting a false-negative rate for identifying metastases of 10% (Cabanas, 1977). McDougal and associates reported a 50% false-negative rate with inguinal node biopsy (McDougal et al, 1986). A report by Pettaway and colleagues from M. D. Anderson Cancer Center confirms that extended sentinel node biopsy is associated with a false-negative rate of 17% (Pettaway et al, 1995).

Superficial inguinal node dissection has been proposed for the patient without palpable inguinal lymphadenopathy. Superficial node dissection involves removal of those nodes superficial to the fascia lata (see Chapter 108). Total lymphadenectomy—that is, removal also of those nodes deep to the fascia lata contained within the femoral triangle—is then performed if the superficial nodes are positive (DeKernion et al, 1973).

The advantages of the superficial dissection are that it provides more information than does biopsy of a single node, it avoids the possibility of misidentifying the sentinel node, and it is associated with minimal morbidity. The incidence of positive nodes deep to the fascia lata in the absence of positive superficial inguinal nodes is not known, but two series have shown no incidence of positive nodes deep to the fascia lata unless superficial nodes were also positive (Pompeo et al, 1995; Puras-Baez et al, 1995). **Although corporeal lymphatics have been presumed occasionally to drain directly into the deep inguinal nodes, clinical evidence supports the superficial nodes as the first echelon of metastasis and an accurate marker for deep and more proximal node involvement.** Also, penile lymphatic studies show no evidence by lymphangiography of direct pelvic node drainage (Riveros et al, 1967).

Experience with aspiration cytology is limited, and most information is derived from a single large series (Scappini et al, 1986). The procedure requires pedal or penile lymphangiography for nodal localization, followed by aspiration under fluoroscopic or CT scan guidance. Multiple nodes must be sampled (e.g., 170 node chains in 29 patients in this series). Of 20 patients who had lymphadenectomy for histologic confirmation, there was complete agreement between aspiration cytology and histologic results. Two of nine patients, however, whose cytology was negative subsequently died of metastatic disease—a presumptive 20% false-negative result. This finding and the technical difficulty with lymphangiography make aspiration less practical than sentinel biopsy or limited superficial node dissection. Direct aspiration of palpable inguinal nodes, however, if positive, can provide immediate information with which to advise patients regarding further treatment.

Should inguinal lymphadenectomy be bilateral rather than unilateral for patients presenting with unilateral adenopathy at initial presentation of the primary tumor? The answer to this question is yes. **The anatomic crossover of penile lymphatics is well established, and bilateral drainage is the rule. Bilateral lymphadenectomy is recommended in patients presenting with unilateral palpable adenopathy in conjunction with the primary lesion.** The contralateral node dissection may be limited to the area superficial to the fascia lata if no histologic evidence of positive superficial nodes is found. Clinical support for a bilateral procedure is based on the finding of contralateral metastases in more than 50% of patients so treated, even if the contralateral nodal region appears negative to palpation (Ekstrom and Edsmyr, 1958).

Should bilateral inguinal lymphadenectomy be performed in patients who present with unilateral lymphadenopathy sometime after the initial presentation and treatment of the primary tumor? The answer to this question would logically appear to be yes based on the data provided in the preceding paragraph. It is generally believed, however, that a bilateral node dissection in this setting is not necessary. The recommendation of unilateral rather than bilateral node dissection with delayed unilateral lymphadenopathy is supported by the elapsed disease-free observation on the normal side.

If one assumes that nodal metastases enlarge at the same rate, nodal metastases, if present in both groins, should be clinically palpable at approximately the same time. The absence of clinical adenopathy on one side dictates a higher probability of freedom from disease on that side (Ekstrom and Edsmyr, 1958). This situation, however, should occur much less frequently than in the past because of identification of high-risk patients for immediate bilateral lymphadenectomy. **The low-risk patients with superficial, well-differentiated lesions who are selected for expectant treatment will probably have a less than 10% incidence of nodal metastases after treatment of the primary tumor** (Hardner et al, 1972; DeKernion et al, 1973; McDougal et al, 1986).

Should pelvic lymphadenectomy be performed in patients with positive inguinal metastases? The therapeutic gain of adding a pelvic node dissection to inguinal dissections has not been determined. Information is limited about the frequency of pelvic node metastases in the setting of positive or negative inguinal nodes. **Horenblas and colleagues found increased probability of pelvic nodal involvement when two or more positive inguinal nodes were encountered** (Horenblas et al, 1993). Histologic evaluation of pelvic nodes has demonstrated metastatic spread in two of four patients undergoing staging laparotomy (Uehling, 1973). Iliac nodes have been found to be positive for tumor metastases in 5 of 13 patients (35%) at autopsy (Gursel et al, 1973), in 15 of 45 patients (30%) (Riveros and Gorostiaga, 1962), in 9 of 30 patients (29%) with positive inguinal nodes (Puras et al, 1978), and in 11 of 75 (15%) of patients with positive inguinal nodes (Srinivas et al, 1987).

Puras and colleagues found no evidence of positive iliac nodes among 40 patients having ilioinguinal node dissection and negative inguinal nodes (Puras et al, 1978). Srinivas and associates related extent of inguinal metastases to iliac metastases (Srinivas et al, 1987). Only 1 of 16 patients (6%) with fewer than six positive inguinal nodes had iliac metastases, whereas 10 of 27 patients (37%) with more than six positive inguinal nodes had iliac node metastases. Srinivas and associates (1987) and Horenblas and colleagues (1993) reported no instance of positive pelvic nodes in the absence of positive inguinal nodes. Similarly, Ravi (1993) also found no instances of positive pelvic nodes when inguinal nodes were negative but found positive pelvic nodes in 17 of 75 patients (22%) with one to three positive inguinal nodes and in 13 of 23 patients (57%) with more than three positive inguinal nodes.

Survival of patients with positive iliac nodes is limited. Of 11 patients in the Srinivas series, none survived to 3 years, and most died within 7 months (Srinivas et al, 1987). Similarly, none of the 30 patients reported by Ravi (1993) to have positive iliac nodes survived 5 years. Given the grim outlook for most patients with pelvic nodal metastases, specific recommendations against pelvic node dissection have appeared (Hanash et al, 1970). **Until more information is available, a definitive statement about the advisability of pelvic node dissection is not possible. However, because involvement of pelvic nodes on microscopic examination may occur with some frequency, because survival with positive pelvic nodes has been documented** (Cabanas, 1977; DeKernion et al, 1973; Puras et al, 1980) (see Table 79–1), **and because duration of survival has been lengthened after iliac node dissection** (Hardner et al, 1972), **the procedure is reasonable for the young man who is**

otherwise a good surgical risk. The finding of pelvic nodal metastases also identifies a group of patients for whom adjuvant chemotherapy is a consideration.

Information specifying the location of positive nodes found at dissection (femoral, iliac, bilateral, unilateral) and the number of nodes involved with tumor on histologic examination is generally unavailable. A larger body of data relating the pattern and extent of nodal metastases to patient survival will aid in accurately defining the natural history of node-positive penile carcinoma and identifying indications for extent of lymphadenectomy.

Several options for treatment of inguinal nodes are proposed. Because staging systems are imprecise, a description of the location, extent of invasion, and histologic grade of a lesion is required (Fig. 79–11).

Tis, Ta, T1: N0M0 (Jackson Stage I, II)

This stage describes flat and exophytic lesions that involve only the glans mucosa, shaft skin, or submucosa. These penile neoplasms, in the absence of palpable adenopathy, are likely to involve nodal metastases in less than 10% of cases (DeKernion et al, 1973; McDougal et al, 1986; Horenblas et al, 1993) and after treatment of the primary tumor may be followed with periodic examination of the inguinal area. The subsequent appearance of unilateral lymphadenopathy provides the indication for unilateral superficial and deep inguinal node dissection as determined by the histology of the inguinal nodes and the patient's medical condition. A contralateral superficial lymphadenectomy is also a consideration. If contralateral dissection is not performed and lymphadenopathy later presents on the opposite side, a superficial and deep dissection should be undertaken. **Because most inguinal metastases occur within the 2- or 3-year interval following initial therapy** (Beggs and Spratt, 1961; Derrick et al, 1973; Johnson et al, 1973; Horenblas et al, 1993), **this period of risk must be closely supervised with examinations at 2- to 3-month intervals.**

The patient should be taught careful self-examination of the inguinal areas for early detection of metastases. Inguinal metastases may occur even after several years, so the patient should continue to be followed indefinitely. Such a program requires close cooperation of the patient—a formidable responsibility in a group of patients who have historically demonstrated unreliability and lack of compliance. In the past, approximately 20% of stage I patients were expected to develop inguinal metastases (Whitmore, 1970). This group, however, included patients with stage I invasive glans lesions who would now be selected for immediate lymphadenectomy. Immediate assessment of the inguinal nodes by bilateral superficial node dissection with further dissection as dictated by histology is another option for treating superficial penile lesions, especially in a young patient.

Recent studies suggest that patients with grade 2 or 3 lesions should undergo immediate prophylactic inguinal lymphadenectomy, regardless of the stage of the primary tumor, and that surveillance of such patients may compromise survival by delaying surgery (Theodorescu et al, 1996; McDougal, 1995). These studies also suggest a higher relapse rate in patients with grade 1 tumors than previously noted, suggesting that early prophylactic node dissection may also be indicated in many of these patients.

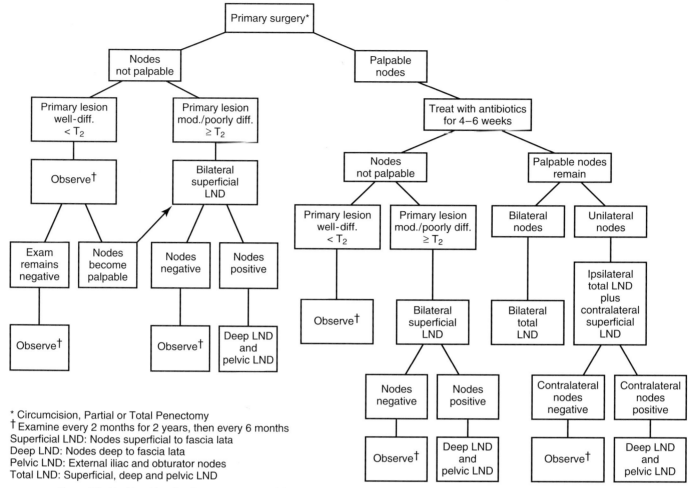

Figure 79–11. Algorithm for the management of the inguinal nodes following diagnosis of squamous carcinoma of the penis.

Stage T2, T3 N0M0 (Jackson Stage I, II)

These lesions, although limited to the glans or shaft, demonstrate invasion of Buck's fascia, tunica albuginea, or corporeal bodies. The incidence of nodal metastases increases significantly in the presence of a tumor that invades the corporeal tissue. Nodes were positive in 17 of 25 (68%) invasive penile carcinomas (DeKernion et al, 1973) and in 6 of 9 (66%) of invasive tumors in the absence of palpable lymphadenopathy (McDougal et al, 1986). Therefore, immediate bilateral adjunctive lymph node dissection is indicated. The decision whether to limit dissection to the nodes superficial to the fascia lata, if all such nodes are negative on frozen section, or to perform both a superficial and a deep inguinal node dissection is a matter of personal preference. With strong evidence that "skip" metastases do not occur, however, and that negative superficial nodes predict for negative deep nodes, the deep lymphadenectomy may be omitted if the superficial dissection is negative. Employing the limited boundary technique described by Catalona (1988) to maximize staging accuracy and therapeutic value and minimize morbidity should be considered.

Stage Tis, Ta, T1–3, N1–3, M0 (Jackson Stage III)

If bilateral lymphadenopathy persists following adequate antibiotic therapy, bilateral radical inguinal node dissections are recommended. If lymphadenopathy is unilateral, metastases necessitating complete inguinal node dissection are anticipated in approximately 50% of the clinically normal contralateral groins. A superficial node dissection only, if histology is negative, may be considered for the normal contralateral groin, or a deep node dissection with limited boundaries may be used. If lymphadenopathy resolves with antibiotic therapy, the decision for adjunctive lymphadenectomy is based on primary tumor stage, as discussed later.

Stage Any T, Any N, M1; T4; Inoperable N (Jackson Stage IV)

This category includes patients with distant metastases, inguinal lymphadenopathy that is inoperable because of invasion and fixation, and extensive adjacent organ invasion. Treatment is often limited to palliative chemotherapy or radiotherapy, but aggressive combined modality therapy with chemotherapy and surgery—especially for the young patient—is warranted. **In selected patients with fixed nodes but no distant metastases, neoadjuvant chemotherapy (see later) followed by inguinal and pelvic lymphadenectomy with consideration of hemipelvectomy or hemicorporectomy is an option. Prior staging laparotomy is necessary to exclude abdominal visceral disease or high common iliac or para-aortic nodal metastases.**

Radiation Therapy

Assessment of the treatment of the inguinal area by primary radiation therapy is hampered by the uncertainty arising from the inaccuracy of clinical staging and the frequent lack of histologic confirmation of nodal metastases. Objections to the treatment of inguinal node metastases are that the inguinal areas tolerate radiation poorly and are subject to skin maceration and ulceration. Infectious lymphadenopathy reduces the effectiveness of radiation therapy and exacerbates complications. The perilymphatic fat that frequently surrounds nodes may act as a protective barrier to the effective radiation treatment of intranodal metastatic deposits (Harlin, 1952). Information about the use of radiation therapy as a primary mode for the treatment of penile carcinoma comes primarily from Europe.

The adjunctive or therapeutic use of radiation in treatment is controversial. Even if metastases are documented by node biopsy, the efficacy of subsequent radiation is impossible to judge because all tumor may have been removed by the biopsy. In one series, 70% of nodal metastases involved a single node, and survival in this group was 70% (Cabanas, 1977). Radiotherapy for inguinal metastases documented by histologic examination has been compared with surgery for the node-positive groin. A 50% 5-year survival rate was observed among the surgically treated group, and a 25% 5-year survival rate was observed among the irradiated group (Staubitz et al, 1955). Other series report that radiation to the inguinal areas has not proved therapeutically effective (Murrell and Williams, 1965; Jensen, 1977).

Several Scandinavian centers have delivered radiation therapy to inguinal nodes as well as to the primary tumor in all cases of penile carcinoma; surgical lymphadenectomy followed if palpable nodes persisted or appeared subsequently (Engelstad, 1948; Ekstrom and Edsmyr, 1958).

Ravi (1993) reported on 201 patients of whom 106 had clinically metastatic inguinal lymphadenopathy. Patients with inguinal nodes greater than 4 cm received 4000 rad radiation before undergoing node dissection. Perinodal infiltration, believed to have an adverse impact on survival, was found in 14 of 43 (33%) of nonirradiated groins but in only 3 of 34 (9%) of radiated groins.

In a series of 130 patients initially having clinically impalpable nodes but treated with adjuvant radiation therapy, 18 subsequently developed palpable nodal disease requiring lymphadenectomy, and another 11 patients had metastases but no surgery. Therefore, 29 of 130 (22%) of men who received prophylactic groin irradiation subsequently developed inguinal metastases (Ekstrom and Edsmyr, 1958).

Murrell and Williams (1965) found that 3 of 11 patients (25%) who received radiation therapy to the inguinal area without initially palpable nodes subsequently developed inguinal metastases. These percentages closely approximate the incidence of subclinical metastases that are encountered if node dissection is performed when the clinical examination is normal (see Table 79–5), and they suggest that radiation therapy did not alter the course of the disease. Furthermore, the clinical evaluation of the groin following radiation therapy is difficult, and the complications encountered with groin dissection after radiation can be significant.

Lastly the 5-year survival rate for patients with prophylactically irradiated groins followed as necessary by lymphadenectomy differs little from that for patients having surgery alone. Although a large, randomized, controlled study might definitely answer the question of efficacy of radiation therapy for inguinal metastases, both microscopic and macroscopic, it is unlikely that such a study could be realized. Present information identifies surgical therapy for inguinal metastasis as superior to radiation therapy.

Radiation therapy may be considered in patients presenting with inoperable fixed and ulcerative inguinal lymph nodes. Occasionally, radiation to these areas is well tolerated, may result in significant palliation, and may postpone local complications for prolonged periods (Furlong and Uhle, 1953; Staubitz et al, 1955; Vaeth et al, 1970).

Radiation therapy to the inguinal area is not as effective therapeutically as lymph node dissection, but it may be used for palliation in the situation of inoperable nodes. Our policy has been not to combine preoperative radiation therapy with inguinal lymphadenectomy, but others have used the combination (Engelstad, 1948; Ekstrom and Edsmyr, 1958; Horenblas et al, 1993; Ravi, 1993).

Chemotherapy

Because of the relative rarity of penile carcinomas, experience with their chemotherapeutic management is limited. The use of topical 5-fluorouracil in superficial and precancerous lesions has already been discussed. It has been used as a continuous intravenous infusion in combination with *cis*-platin in a limited number of patients. Only three other drugs have been employed to any extent: *cis*-platin, bleomycin, and methotrexate. Experience with combination chemotherapy is quite limited.

Because single-agent *cis*-platin had demonstrated response in squamous carcinomas of the head and neck and elsewhere, it was used in two separate trials in advanced penile cancer. In a study from Memorial Sloan-Kettering Cancer Center, 13 patients with extensive disease and either prior radiotherapy or chemotherapy were treated with 70 to 120 mg/m^2 every 21 days. Three patients (23%) demonstrated partial responses (Ahmed et al, 1984). Gagliano and associates from the Southwest Oncology Group treated 26 patients—12 of whom had had prior radiation—with low-dose (50 mg/m^2) *cis*-platin and observed a 15% response rate of limited duration (Gagliano et al, 1989).

Initial favorable reports from Japan suggested that bleomycin appeared to be effective in the treatment of penile and scrotal cancer. Ichikawa and associates reported a 50% response in 24 previously untreated patients with squamous carcinoma of the penis (Ichikawa et al, 1969; Ichikawa, 1977). A similar report from Uganda documents partial or complete tumor regression in 45% of treated patients (Kyalwazi et al, 1974). A review of 90 patients from the world literature demonstrated similar responses (Eisenberger, 1992).

Methotrexate produced partial responses in 8 of 13 patients (61%) treated at Memorial Sloan-Kettering Cancer Center (Ahmed et al, 1984). Five patients were treated with high-dose therapy with folinic acid rescue, and eight were treated with low-dose intravenous therapy (30–40 mg/m^2/week). Methotrexate has been shown to be effective in other reports (Mills, 1972; Garnick et al, 1979).

Combination vincristine, bleomycin, and methotrexate (VBM) was administered in 12 weekly treatments to 17 patients as either a neoadjuvant (5 patients) or postoperative (12 patients) treatment program at the Milan National Tumor Institute. The patients treated with adjuvant therapy were at high risk: Nine showed extranodal tumor growth, five had pelvic nodal involvement, and five had bilateral metastases. At follow-up ranging between 18 and 102 months, only one relapse had occurred (Pizzocaro and Piva, 1988). A more recent report from this center further confirms the value of adjuvant chemotherapy. Of 56 node-positive patients treated with adjuvant VBM, 82% of the 25 patients receiving adjuvant VBM therapy survived 5 years compared with 37% of 31 patients treated with surgery alone (Pizzocaro et al, 1995). Hussein and associates used a combination of 5-fluorouracil and *cis*-platin in six patients—five with penile and one with urethral squamous cell carcinoma. The five patients with penile cancer had partial responses, whereas the patient with urethral cancer had complete disappearance of tumor (Hussein et al, 1990).

VBM has also been used neoadjuvantly, with partial responses noted in three of five patients with extremely large (6–11 cm) nodal metastases. These three patients subsequently were completely resected and were free of tumor at intervals ranging from 20 to 72 months. In another neoadjuvant study, four patients with stage III tumors were treated with a regimen of *cis*-platin and 5-fluorouracil and resected. Two patients showed no residual tumor in the lymphadenectomy specimen, and disease had not recurred in any patient 6 to 40 months following surgery (Fisher et al, 1990).

The rarity of penile carcinoma in the United States makes it difficult to conduct successful phase II and III chemotherapy trials. This information will need to come from trials conducted in South America, Africa, or Asia. Studies must be designed to determine which agents will be most useful as (1) neoadjuvant therapy in stage III disease; (2) adjuvant therapy when pathologic evaluation of the nodes reveals extensive inguinal metastases or pelvic metastases, which predict for diminished survival (Johnson and Lo, 1984a; Srinivas et al, 1987; Fraley et al, 1989; Eisenberger, 1992); and (3) palliative chemotherapy in patients with locally inoperable tumor or distant metastases.

Combined Therapy

Combined modality programs using chemotherapy plus surgery or radiotherapy have been employed with encouraging results in treatment of squamous cell carcinomas of both the larynx and the anus (Eisenberger, 1992; Pedrick et al, 1993). Similar strategies may be helpful in minimizing the disfigurement and functional loss associated with penile amputative surgery in selected cases. **Combined modality approaches have been employed with some success in patients presenting with unresectable disease to convert the tumor to a potentially resectable lesion** (Abratt et al, 1989; Germiyanoglu et al, 1993). Again the low incidence of these tumors necessitates evaluation of treatment protocols by means of multi-institutional cooperative studies with international scope (Table 79–7).

Table 79–7. COMBINATION CHEMOTHERAPY FOR PENILE CANCER

VBM (8–12 Weekly Courses)

Vincristine	1 mg	IV	Day 1
Bleomycin	15 mg	IM	6 and 24 hours after vincristine
Methotrexate	30 mg	PO	Day 3

Principal toxicities
  Vincristine: alopecia, neurotoxicity
  Bleomycin: mucositis, pneumonitis
  Methotrexate: myelosuppression (nadir 7–14 days), mucositis,
    nausea/vomiting

PF (4 Courses at Intervals of 3 Weeks)

Cis-Platinum	100 mg/m²	IV	Day 1
5-Fluorouracil	1.0 g/m²	Continuous IV infusion	Day 1

Principal toxicities
  Cis-Platinum: myelosuppression (nadir 18–23 days), nephrotoxicity,
    neurotoxicity, ototoxicity, severe nausea/vomiting
  5-Fluorouracil: myelosuppression (nadir 7–14 days), mucositis,
    dermatitis

Data from Pizzocaro G, Piva L, Nicolai N: J Urol 1995; 153:246A.

RECONSTRUCTION OF THE PENIS FOLLOWING PENECTOMY AND EMASCULATION

Partial Penectomy

The patient who has undergone partial penectomy, after proven to be cancer free, has the option of penile reconstruction. **Free flap reconstruction of the penis with a radial forearm flap would, in most centers, be considered the modality of choice** (Chang and Hwang, 1984; Devine et al, 1987; Gilbert et al, 1987; Gilbert et al, 1988). Modifications of the forearm flap (Biemer, 1988; Farrow et al, 1989) have enhanced the versatility of microvascular free transfer reconstruction of the penis. Additionally the upper lateral arm flap has proved to be useful for reconstruction of the penis. This flap has thin, relatively nonhirsute skin with dependable blood supply and cutaneous innervation. Because these flaps have dependable innervation, which can be elevated with the flap, they can provide phallic reconstructive covering with erogenous sensibility. Because sensation must be present before prosthesis placement, this sensibility serves a purpose beyond sexual gratification. The patient who has undergone partial penectomy has proved to be an optimal candidate for reconstruction and subsequent prosthetic placement.

The remaining proximal corporeal bodies serve well to seat the prostheses, and the distal corpora are constructed with a vascular graft material, usually Gore-Tex, which allows for tissue ingrowth and stability.

It is emphasized that partial penectomy for carcinoma of the penis should not be avoided for strictly cosmetic concerns because modern penile reconstructive surgery can provide excellent cosmetic results as well as good functional results following successful prosthetic placement.

Total Penectomy

Phallic reconstruction following total loss of the penis presents genitourinary surgery with one of its greatest challenges. **The anatomy and physiology of the erectile tissues (i.e., corpora cavernosa) are unique and are not reproducible by the transfer of other human tissues.** The earlier attempts at phallic construction or reconstruction consisted of the "tube within a tube" concept, using a tubed abdominal flap for the urethra, enclosed within another covering flap of abdominal skin. The "phallus" was transferred to the area of the penis by sequential steps of delay. Such reconstructions were often unsuccessful because of the multiple procedures involved; often a "little bit of phallus" was lost with every step of delay. Additionally the phallus lacked sensibility and had suboptimal esthetic appearance.

Direct cutaneous arterialized flaps (superficial groin flap), superficial perineal artery flap, and musculocutaneous flaps (gracilis, rectus femoris, and rectus abdominis) have been used with moderate success in phallic reconstruction. Although these local flaps ostensibly diminished the number of reconstructive stages, they too were insensate, tended to atrophy, and were attended with multiple steps to "restore" the cosmetic appearance.

Newer concepts in microsurgical reconstruction have improved both the function and the appearance of the neophallus. **Ideally, phallic construction or reconstruction should address the following requirements: (1) a one-stage microsurgical procedure, (2) creation of a competent urethra to achieve normal voiding, (3) restoration of a phallus that has both tactile and erogenous sensibility, (4) a phallus with enough bulk to allow implantation of a prosthetic stiffener for vaginal penetration, and (5) esthetic acceptance by the patient.** A number of donor sites have been used in an effort to address all of these optimal requirements. As microvascular free tissue transfer has evolved, these requirements have been more realistically attainable.

For the patient following total penectomy, successful reconstruction of a phallus using microvascular transfer is now technically straightforward. Prosthetic placement, however, is somewhat more difficult in that total reconstruction of the corporeal body is a necessity. Gore-Tex has served well at this center for "corporeal" reconstruction. The Gore-Tex corpora allows for tissue ingrowth, thus limiting migration of the prosthetic elements. Additionally the Gore-Tex sleeves can be anchored in the perineum to the ischial tuberosities and to the pubis, stabilizing the devices. This stabilization allows for better rigidity and limits migration of the prosthetic elements. In that the Gore-Tex is placed to allow for tissue ingrowth and anchoring only, the thin stretch Gore-Tex grafts serve well and limit the amount of foreign body placed.

Cooperation between the urologist and the plastic surgeon continues to allow for refinements in the techniques of "free" flap phallic construction. Experience with microneurovascular tissue transfers has demonstrated that successful one-stage phallic construction or reconstruction is possible.

Inguinal Reconstruction Following Node Dissection

Changes in the technique of lymph node dissection and the incisions employed have limited the complications seen previously following that procedure. Previously, flaps were elevated on the dermal and subdermal blood supply, and tissue loss was a frequent occurrence. The realization that skin lymphatics are not involved in the metastatic path led to an alteration in the plane of dissection. Now the dissection is carried deep to Scarpa's fascia, thus lessening the insult to the skin. The transposition of the sartorius muscle over the vessels has minimized the incidence of vascular erosion and thrombosis. Nonetheless, wound problems still occur, and certain patients require the excision of a wide area of skin because of the mass of metastatic tumor contained in the superficial groin nodes.

The majority of wound problems are secondary to the loss of skin at the edge of the wound. These skin problems arise because the blood supply to the skin of the lower leg is for the most part musculocutaneous or fasciocutaneous in distribution (McCraw and Dibbell, 1977; McCraw et al, 1977). With the elevation of the skin without the underlying muscle or fascia, the deep perforator vessels are divided, and the skin flaps are left to survive as random flaps. In some instances, the flap elevation exceeds the cutaneous vascular territory. The superior aspect of the wound represents a "tidal zone" between the cuticular vascular territory of the circumflex iliac artery and musculocutaneous vascular territories of the venous thigh flaps (Brown et al, 1975; Hester et al, 1984; Cormack and Lamberty, 1985) (Fig. 79–12). The inferior extent of dissection is clearly in a musculocutaneous vascular area and, if aggressive, creates a random flap that exceeds the vascularity of the dermal plexuses. In most instances, only a small amount of superficial skin is lost, and these areas can be easily covered with split-thickness skin grafting. With deeper skin loss or in cases requiring the excision of a large area of skin with the specimen, however, more substantial tissue transfer is required. A number of local flaps are available for transposition into these tissue defects. The gracilis musculocutaneous unit is totally expendable and easily transposed into a groin defect (Orticochea, 1972a; Orticochea, 1972b).

For dissections requiring larger flaps, the tensor fascia lata flap represents an excellent tissue transfer unit (Nahai et al, 1979; Nahai, 1980). The tensor fascia lata flap is easily transposed to the groin, and its large size and bulk make it an ideal choice for coverage of large defects. To insure reliability of the flap tip, it is beneficial to include to the rectus lateralis with the flap.

The inferiorly based rectus abdominis musculocutaneous flap also represents an excellent transfer unit for groin and perineal defects (Taylor et al, 1984). The contralateral inferior rectus abdominis muscle flap can be transposed across the infrapubic space to the opposite groin without difficulty, if the ipsilateral flap is not usable. The location of the flap pedicle combined with the placement of the skin paddle over the umbilicus makes this unit mechanically most efficient. The transversely oriented inferior rectus abdominis flap offers another excellent option for groin or perineal coverage.

If the inferior based rectus abdominis flap is unavailable, however, omental flaps represent a valuable option (Arnold et al, 1983). Their rich arterial supply has been shown to impart neovascularity in the host site. The lymphatic abundance in the flap also helps in the control of infection and reabsorption of extracellular fluid (McCraw and Arnold, 1986; Bunkis and Walton, 1990; Hoffman and Trengove-Jones, 1990; Samson, 1990; Taylor et al, 1990; Trier, 1990).

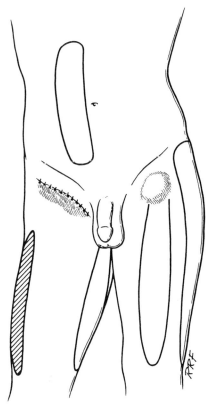

Figure 79–12. Flaps useful in groin coverage. On the left, the tensor fasciae latae musculocutaneous transfer unit is outlined on the lateral part of the leg. The biceps femoris musculocutaneous unit is illustrated on the anterior thigh. On the right, the vastus lateralis muscle flap is illustrated on the lateral leg. The vastus can be included with the tensor fasciae latae unit, thus making the cutaneous tip more reliable. The gracilis musculocutaneous unit is illustrated medially. On the abdomen is illustrated the vertical rectus abdominis muscle flap. This flap can be transposed to the ipsilateral or the contralateral groin. On the right groin is illustrated the tidal zone of skin loss following lymph node dissection; on the left groin is illustrated a bulky tumor, which may require en bloc skin removal with the node dissection.

The omental flap provides an excellent graft host bed and thus can be used in association with split-thickness skin grafts. When available, the flaps described here are invariably sufficient to cover both the femoral vessels and the groin defect.

NONSQUAMOUS MALIGNANCY

Melanoma and basal cell carcinoma rarely occur on the penis, presumably because the organ's skin is protected from exposure to the sun. Malignancies arising from the supporting structures of the penis are also quite rare and include any combination of tumors of smooth or striated muscle or of fibrous, fatty, or vascular tissue. Information about appropriate treatment of these malignancies is derived from the review of single case reports and small series (Belville and Cohen, 1992).

Basal Cell Carcinoma

Although basal cell carcinoma is frequently encountered on other cutaneous surfaces, it is rare on the penis.

Fewer than 15 cases have been well documented (Goldminz et al, 1989). **Treatment is by local excision, which is virtually always curative** (Hall et al, 1968; Goldminz et al, 1989). No instances of metastases or local recurrence following local excision have been reported.

A benign variant of basal cell carcinoma, the premalignant fibroepithelioma of Pinkus, has been reported to occur on the penile shaft (Heymann et al, 1983). Diagnosis is made at excisional biopsy. Excision has been uniformly curative.

Melanoma

Fewer than 60 cases of melanoma of the penis have been reported. Of 1200 melanomas treated at Memorial Sloan-Kettering Cancer Center, only two were of penile origin (Das Gupta and Grabstald, 1965). At the M. D. Anderson Cancer Center, less than 1% of all primary penile cancers were malignant melanomas (Johnson and Ayala, 1973). **Melanoma presents as a blue-black or reddish brown pigmented papule, plaque, or ulceration on the glans penis. It occurs on the prepuce less frequently.** Diagnosis is made by histologic examination of biopsy specimens, which demonstrate atypical junctional cell activity with displacement of pigmented cells into the dermis.

Prognostic characteristics that have been found significant for melanoma in other sites, such as depth of invasion and thickness of the tumor, have not been applied to penile lesions because experience with these lesions is so limited. When this information is available, local excision might be possible in select cases (Martin et al, 1988). Distant metastatic spread has been found in 60% of patients studied (Abeshouse, 1958; Johnson et al, 1973). Hematogenous metastases occur by means of the vascular structures of the corporeal bodies; lymphatic spread to the regional lymphatic ilioinguinal nodes occurs by lymphatic permeation.

Surgery is the primary mode of treatment, with radiotherapy and chemotherapy being of only adjunctive or palliative benefit. For stage I melanoma (localized lesion without metastases) and stage II melanoma (metastases confined to one regional area), adequate excision of the primary tumor by partial or total penile amputation together with en bloc bilateral ilioinguinal node dissection offers the greatest prospect for cure (Johnson et al, 1973; Bracken and Diokno, 1974; Manivel and Fraley, 1988). The prognosis for patients with this neoplasm is poor, however, with few reported 5-year survivors (Wheelock and Clark, 1943; Reid, 1957) because of the frequency of metastases occurring beyond the confines of surgical resection.

Sarcomas

Primary mesenchymal tumors of the penis are rare. A thorough review of 46 such tumors from the Armed Forces Institute of Pathology revealed an equal number of benign and malignant lesions (Dehner and Smith, 1970). The patients ranged in age from newborn to the seventies. The presenting signs and symptoms of subcutaneous mass, penile pain and enlargement, priapism, and urinary obstruction were the same for both benign and malignant lesions. A

sarcoma has been reported to "masquerade" as a Peyronie's plaque (Moore et al, 1975).

Malignant lesions were found more frequently on the proximal shaft; benign lesions were more often located distally. The most common malignant lesions were those of vascular origin (hemangioepithelioma), followed in frequency by those of neural, myogenic, and fibrous origin (Ashley and Edwards, 1957). Single case reports of sarcomatous lesions have been published, for example, malignant fibrous histiocytoma (Parsons and Fox, 1988), angiosarcoma (Rasbridge and Parry, 1989), and epithelioid sarcoma (Leviav et al, 1988).

Sarcomas have been classified as superficial when they arise from the integumentary supporting structures and as deep when they develop from the corporeal body supporting structures (Pratt and Ross, 1969). Wide local surface excision and partial penile amputation for the superficial tumors have been suggested and used successfully in isolated case reports (Pak et al, 1986; Dalkin and Zaontz, 1989). Total penile amputation has been reserved for tumors of deep corporeal origin. **Local recurrences, however, are characteristic of sarcomas** (Dehner and Smith, 1970). To avoid local recurrences, a total amputation, even for superficial malignancies of any cell type, should be considered.

Regional metastases are rare. Unless adenopathy is palpable, node dissections are not recommended (Hutcheson et al, 1969). Distant metastases have also been unusual (Dehner and Smith, 1970). This supports aggressive local treatment in anticipation of cure. Radiation therapy and chemotherapy have not been used extensively enough to comment on their efficacy.

Paget's Disease

Paget's disease of the penis is extremely rare. Fewer than 15 cases have been reported (Mitsudo et al, 1981). It appears grossly as an erythematous, eczematoid, well-demarcated area that cannot be clinically distinguished from erythroplasia of Queyrat, Bowen's disease, or carcinoma in situ of the penis. Clinical presentation includes local discomfort, pruritus, and occasionally a serosanguineous discharge. On microscopic examination, identification is clearly made by the presence of large, round or oval, clear-staining hydropic cells with hypochromatic nuclei (i.e., Paget cells).

Paget's disease may often herald a deeply-seated carcinoma with Paget cells moving through ducts or lymphatics to the epidermal surface. In the penis, a sweat gland carcinoma (Mitsudo et al, 1981) or periurethral gland adenocarcinoma (Jenkins, 1989) may be the primary neoplasm. Complete local surgical excision of the skin and subcutaneous tissue is the recommended form of therapy. If inguinal adenopathy is present, radical node dissection is advised (Hagan et al, 1975). Careful observation for recurrence at the margins is necessary.

Lymphoreticular Malignancy

Primary lymphoreticular malignancy rarely occurs on the penis (Dehner and Smith, 1970). **Leukemia may infiltrate the corpora, resulting in priapism** (Pochedly et al,

1974). **When lymphomatous infiltration of the penis is diagnosed, a thorough search for systemic disease is necessary.** If the penile lesion is indeed a primary tumor, treatment with systemic chemotherapy may be used. It is the most effective therapy for local disease, for potential occult deposits that may exist elsewhere, and for preservation of form and function (Marks et al, 1988). Local low-dose irradiation has also been reported to be successful (Stewart et al, 1985).

Kaposi's sarcoma, usually a cutaneous manifestation of a generalized lymphoreticular disorder, may produce genital lesions and is now most frequently associated with AIDS (see earlier).

Metastases

Metastatic lesions to the penis are unusual. Approximately 200 cases have been reported in the literature. Their infrequency is somewhat puzzling when one considers the rich blood and lymphatic supply to the organ and its proximity to the bladder, prostate, and rectum—areas frequently involved with neoplasm. From these three organs, the majority of metastatic penile lesions originate (Abeshouse, 1958). Renal and respiratory neoplasms have also metastasized to the penis. The most likely routes of spread are by direct extension, retrograde venous and lymphatic transport, and arterial embolism.

The most frequent sign of penile metastasis is priapism: Penile swelling, nodularity, and ulceration have also been reported (McCrea and Tobias, 1958; Abeshouse and Abeshouse, 1961; Weitzner, 1971). Urinary obstruction and hematuria may occur. The most common histologic feature of penile invasion by metastatic lesions is the replacement of one or both corpora cavernosa, which explains the frequent occurrence of priapism. Solitary cutaneous, preputial, and glanular deposits are less common.

The differential diagnosis includes idiopathic priapism; venereal or other infectious ulcerations; tuberculosis; Peyronie's plaque; and primary, benign, or malignant tumors.

Penile metastases represent an advanced form of virulent disease and usually appear rather rapidly after recognition and treatment of the primary lesion (Abeshouse and Abeshouse, 1961; Hayes and Young, 1967; Mukamel et al, 1987). On rare occasions, a long period may elapse between the treatment of the primary lesion and the appearance of penile metastases (Abeshouse and Abeshouse, 1961), or the penile lesion may occur as the initial and only site of metastasis.

Because of the association of a penile metastatic lesion with advanced disease, survival after its presentation is limited, and the majority of patients die within 1 year (Mukamel et al, 1987; Robey and Schelhammer, 1984). Successful treatment may occasionally be possible in the case of solitary nodules or localized distal penile involvement if complete excision by partial amputation succeeds in removing the entire area of malignant infiltration (Spaulding and Whitmore, 1978). The prospect for surgical cure is minimal if proximal corporeal invasion is present. Penectomy is occasionally indicated after failure of other modalities to palliate intractable pain (Mukamel et al, 1987). Pain can also be managed by dorsal nerve section (Hill and

Khalid, 1988). Treatment with radiation therapy has been generally unsuccessful, and chemotherapy has not been employed in a sufficient number of cases to warrant definitive recommendations.

ACKNOWLEDGMENTS

We wish to acknowledge Dr. Harry Grabstald, who directed our efforts in the previous three editions, and Drs. Gerald H. Jordan and Steven M. Schlossberg, who contributed the section on reconstruction of the penis. We are grateful to Mrs. Linda Engler and Mrs. Lynn Vass for manuscript preparation.

REFERENCES

Abeshouse BS: Primary and secondary melanoma of the genitourinary tract. South Med J 1958; 51:994.

Abeshouse BS, Abeshouse GA: Metastatic tumors of the penis: A review of the literature and a report of two cases. J Urol 1961; 86:99.

Abratt RP: The treatment of bilateral ulcerated lymph node metastases from carcinoma of the penis. Cancer 1984; 54:1720–1722.

Abratt RP, Barnes RD, Pontin AR: The treatment of clinically fixed inguinal lymph node metastases from carcinoma of the penis by chemotherapy and surgery. Eur J Surg Oncol 1989; 15:285–286.

Ackerman LV: Verrucous carcinoma of the oral cavity. Surgery 1948; 23:670.

Ahmed T, Sklaroff R, Yagoda A: Sequential trials of methotrexate, cisplatin and bleomycin for penile cancer. J Urol 1984; 132:465–468.

Almgard LE, Edsmyr F: Radiotherapy in treatment of patients with carcinoma of the penis. Scand J Urol Nephrol 1973; 7:1.

Anderson EE, Glenn JF: Penile malignancy and hypercalcemia. JAMA 1965; 192:128.

Aragona F, Serretta V, Marconi A, et al: Queyrat's erythroplasia of the prepuce: A case-report. Acta Chir Belg 1985; 85:303.

Arnold PG, Witzke DJ, Irons GB, Woods JE: Use of omental transposition flaps for soft-tissue reconstruction. Ann Plast Surg 1983; 11:508.

Ashley DJB, Edwards EC: Sarcoma of the penis: Leiomyosarcoma of the penis: Report of a case with a review of the literature of sarcoma of the penis. Br J Surg 1957; 43:170.

Bahmer FA, Tang DE, Payeur-Kirsch M: Treatment of large condylomata of the penis with the neodymium-YAG-laser. Acta Dermatol Venereol (Stockh) 1984; 64:361–363.

Bain L, Geronemus R: The association of lichen planus of the penis with squamous cell carcinoma in situ and with verrucous squamous carcinoma. J Dermatol Surg Oncol 1989; 15:413–415.

Bainbridge DR, Whitaker RH, Shepheard BGF: Balanitis xerotica obliterans and urinary obstruction. Br J Urol 1971; 43:487.

Baker BH, Spratt JS, Perez-Mesa C, et al: Carcinoma of the penis. J Urol 1976; 116:458.

Baker BH, Watson FR: Staging carcinoma of the penis. J Surg Oncol 1975; 7:243.

Baldwin HE, Geronemus RG: The treatment of Zoon's balanitis with the CO_2 laser. J Dermatol Surg Oncol 1989; 15:491–499.

Ball TP, Pickett JD: Traumatic lymphangitis of penis. Urology 1975; 6:594.

Bandieramonte G, Lepera P, Marchesini R, et al: Laser microsurgery of superficial lesions of the penis. J Urol 1987; 138:315.

Bandieramonte G, Santoro O, Boracchi P, et al: Total resection of glans penis surface by CO_2 laser microsurgery. Acta Oncol 1988; 27:575.

Barrasso R, De Brux J, Croissant O, Orth G: High prevalence of papillomavirus-associated penile intraepithelial neoplasia in sexual partners of women with cervical intraepithelial neoplasia. N Engl J Med 1987; 317:916.

Bart RS, Kopf AW: Squamous cell carcinoma arising in balanitis xerotica obliterans. J Dermatol Surg Oncol 1978; 4:556–561.

Bayne D, Wise GJ: Kaposi sarcoma of the penis and genitalia: A disease of our times. Urology 1988; 31:22.

Beggs JH, Spratt JS: Epidermoid carcinoma of the penis. J Urol 1961; 91:166.

Belville WD, Cohen JA: Secondary penile malignancies: The spectrum of presentation. J Surg Oncol 1992; 51:134–137.

Biemer E: Penile construction by the radial arm flap. Clin Plast Surg 1988; 15:425.

Bissada NK, Cole AT, Fried FA: Extensive condylomas acuminata of the entire male urethra and the bladder. J Urol 1974; 112:201.

Bissada NK, Morcos RR, El-Senoussi M: Post-circumcision carcinoma of the penis: I. Clinical aspects. J Urol 1986; 135:283.

Block NL, Rosen P, Whitmore WF: Hemipelvectomy for advanced penile cancer. J Urol 1973; 110:703.

Blum RH, Carter SK, Agre K: A clinical review of bleomycin—a new antineoplastic agent. Cancer 1973; 31:903.

Boon TA: Sapphire probe laser surgery for localized carcinoma of the penis. Eur J Surg Oncol 1988; 14:193.

Boshart M, zur Hausen H: Human papillomaviruses (HPV) in Buschke-Lowenstein tumors: Physical state of the DNA and identification of a tandem duplication in the non-coding region of a HPV 6-subtype. J Virol 1986; 58:963.

Bouchot O, Auvigne J, Peuvrel P, et al: Management of regional lymph nodes in carcinoma of the penis. Eur Urol 1989; 16:410.

Bowen J: Precancerous dermatoses: A review of two cases of chronic atypical epithelial proliferation. J Cutan Dis 1912; 30:241.

Boxer RJ, Skinner DG: Condylomata acuminata and squamous cell carcinoma. Urology 1977; 9:72.

Bracken RB, Diokno AC: Melanoma of the penis and the urethra: 2 case reports and review of the literature. J Urol 1974; 111:198.

Brown MD, Zachary CB, Grekin RC, Swanson NA: Penile tumors: Their management by Mohs micrographic surgery. J Dermatol Surg Oncol 1987; 13:1163.

Brown RG, Vasconez LO, Jurkiewicz MJ: Transverse abdominal flaps and the deep epigastric arcade. Plast Reconstr Surg 1975; 55:416.

Bruns TNC, Lauvetz RJ, Kerr ES, Ross G: Buschke-Lowenstein giant condylomas: Pitfalls in management. Urology 1975; 5:773.

Buddington WT, Kickham CJE, Smith WE: An assessment of malignant disease of the penis. J Urol 1963; 89:442.

Bunkis J, Walton RL: The rectus abdominis flap for groin defects. In Strauch B, Vasconez LO, Hall-Findlay EJ, eds: Grabb's Encyclopedia of Flaps, Vol III. Boston, Little, Brown, 1990, pp 1410–1415.

Burgers JK, Badalament RA, Drago JR: Penile cancer: Clinical presentation, diagnosis, and staging. Urol Clin North Am 1992; 19:247–256.

Burmer GC, True LD, Krieger JN: Squamous cell carcinoma of the scrotum associated with human papillomaviruses. J Urol 1993; 149:374–377.

Buschke A, Lowenstein L: Uber carcinomahnliche condylomata acuminata des penis. Klin Wochenschr 1925; 4:1726.

Cabanas R: An approach to the treatment of penile carcinoma. Cancer 1977; 39:456.

Cabanas RM: Anatomy and biopsy of the sentinel lymph nodes. Urol Clin North Am 1992; 19:267–276.

Carpiniello VL, Malloy TR, Sedlacek TV, Zderic SA: Results of carbon dioxide laser therapy and topical 5-fluorouracil treatment for subclinical condyloma found by magnified penile surface scanning. J Urol 1988; 140:53.

Carpiniello VL, Schoenberg M: Laser treatment of condyloma and other external genital lesions. Semin Urol 1991; 9:175–179.

Carpiniello VL, Schoenberg M, Malloy TR: Long-term follow-up of subclinical human papillomavirus infection treated with the carbon dioxide laser and intraurethral 5-fluorouracil: A treatment protocol. J Urol 1990; 143:726.

Carpiniello VL, Zderic SA, Malloy TR, Sedlacek TV: Carbon dioxide laser therapy of subclinical condyloma found by magnified penile surface scanning. Urology 1987; 24:608.

Catalona WJ: Role of lymphadenectomy in carcinoma of the penis. Urol Clin North Am 1980; 7:785.

Catalona WJ: Modified inguinal lymphadenectomy for carcinoma of the penis with preservation of saphenous veins: Technique and preliminary results. J Urol 1988; 140:306.

Chan WP, Chaing SS, Huang AH, Lin CN: Penile frenulum neurilemoma: A rare and unusual genitourinary tumor. J Urol 1993; 144:136–137.

Chang TS, Hwang WY: Forearm flap in one-stage reconstruction of the penis. Plast Reconstr Surg 1984; 74:251.

Coetzee T: Condyloma acuminatum. South Afr J Surg 1977; 15:75.

Cole LA, Helwig EB: Mucoid cysts of the penile skin. J Urol 1976; 115:397.

Copulsky J, Whitehead ED, Orkin LA: Condyloma acuminata in a three-year-old boy. Urology 1975; 5:372.

Cormack GC, Lamberty BGH: The blood supply of thigh skin. Plast Reconstr Surg 1985; 75:342.

Cottel WJ, Bailin PL, Albom MJ, et al: Essentials of Mohs micrographic surgery. J Dermatol Surg Oncol 1988; 14:11.

Culp OS, Magid MA, Kaplan IW: Podophyllin treatment of condylomata acuminata. J Urol 1944; 51:655.

Dagher R, Selzer ML, Lapides J: Carcinoma of the penis and the anti-circumcision crusade. J Urol 1973; 110:79.

Dalkin B, Zaontz MR: Rhabdomyosarcoma of the penis in children. J Urol 1989; 141:908.

Daly NJ, Douchez J, Combes PF: Treatment of carcinoma of the penis by iridium 192 wire implant. Int J Radiat Oncol Biol Phys 1982; 8:1239.

Das Gupta T, Grabstald H: Melanoma of the genitourinary tract. J Urol 1965; 93:607.

Davies SW: Giant condyloma acuminata: Incidence among cases diagnosed as carcinoma of the penis. J Clin Pathol 1965; 18:142.

Dawson DF, Duckworth JK, Bernhardt H, Young JM: Giant condyloma and verrucous carcinoma of the genital area. Arch Pathol 1965; 79:225.

Dean AL: Epithelioma of the penis. J Urol 1935; 33:252.

Dehner LP, Smith BH: Soft tissue tumors of the penis. Cancer 1970; 25:1431.

DeKernion JB, Tynbery P, Persky L, Fegen JP: Carcinoma of the penis. Cancer 1973; 32:1256.

Delannes M, Malavaud B, Douchez J, et al: Iridium-192 interstitial therapy for squamous cell carcinoma of the penis. Int J Radiat Oncol Biol Phys 1992; 24:479–483.

Derrick FC, Lynch KM, Kretkowski RC, Yarbrough WJ: Epidermoid carcinoma of the penis: Computer analysis of 87 cases. J Urol 1973; 110:303.

Devine PC, Winslow BH, Jordan GH, et al: Reconstructive phallic surgery. In Libertino JA, ed: Pediatric and Adult Reconstructive Urologic Surgery, 2nd ed. Baltimore, Williams & Wilkins, 1987, p 552.

Dewire D, Lepor H: Anatomic considerations of the penis and its lymphatic drainage. Urol Clin North Am 1992; 19:211–219.

Dillaha CJ, Jansen T, Honeycutt WM, Holt GA: Further studies with topical 5-fluorouracil. Arch Dermatol 1965; 92:410.

Dodge OG: Carcinoma of the penis in East Africans. Br J Urol 1965; 37:223.

Dorak AC, Ozkan GA, Tamac NI, Saray A: Ultrasonography in the recognition of penile cancer. J Clin Ultrasound 1992; 20:624–626.

Dore B, Irani J, Aubert J: Carcinoma of the penis in lichen sclerosis et atrophicus: A case report. Eur Urol 1990; 18:153–155.

Dretler SP, Klein LA: The eradication of intraurethral condyloma acuminata with 5-fluorouracil cream. J Urol 1975; 113:195.

Duncan W, Jackson SM: The treatment of early cancer of the penis with megavoltage x-rays. Clin Radiol 1972; 23:246.

Edsmyr F, Andersson L, Esposti P: Combined bleomycin and radiation therapy in carcinoma of the penis. Cancer 1985; 56:257.

Edwards A, Atma-Ram A, Thin RN: Podophyllotoxin 0.5% v podophyllin 20% to treat penile warts. Genitourin Med 1988; 64:263–265.

Edwards RH, Sawyers JL: The management of carcinoma of the penis. South Med J 1968; 61:843.

Eisenberger MA: Chemotherapy for carcinomas of the penis and urethra. Urol Clin North Am 1992; 19:333–338.

Ekstrom T, Edsmyr F: Cancer of the penis: A clinical study of 229 cases. Acta Chir Scand 1958; 115:25.

El-Demiry MIM, Oliver RTD, Hope-Stone NF, Blandy JP: Reappraisal of the role of radiotherapy and surgery in the management of carcinoma of the penis. Br J Urol 1984; 56:724–728.

Engelman ER, Herr HW, Ravera J: Lipogranulomatosis of external genitalis. Urology 1974; 3:358.

Engelstad RB: Treatment of cancer of the penis at the Norwegian Radium Hospital. AJR 1948; 60:801.

Epstein E: Association of Bowen's disease with visceral cancer. Arch Dermatol 1960; 82:349.

Eron LJ, Judson F, Tucker S, et al: Interferon therapy for condylomata acuminata. N Engl J Med 1986; 315:1059.

Evans D, Patten JJ: Misdiagnosis of coronal papillae. Med J Aust 1990; 152:109.

Ewalt DH, McConnell JD: Penile neoplasms—30 year experience 1958–1988. (Abstract 651.) J Urol 1990; 143:351A.

Farrow GA, Boyd JB, Semple JL: Total reconstruction of the penis employing the "cricket bat flap" single stage forearm free graft. (Abstract 77.) J Urol 1989; 141:52A.

Feneley MR, Liu S, Miller PD, Kirby RS: Urethroplasty for condylomata acuminata throughout the urethra. Br J Urol 1992; 69:218–219.

Ferenczy A: Strategies to eradicate genital HPV infection in men. Contemp Urol 1990; 2:19.

Ferenczy A, Richart RM, Wright TC: Pearly penile papules: Absence of human papillomavirus DNA by the polymerase chain reaction. Obstet Gynecol 1991; 78:118–122.

Fields T, Drylie D, Wilson J: Malignant evolution of penile horn. J Urol 1987; 30:65–66.

Fisher HAG: Management of penile carcinoma: The case for selective application of inguinal lymph node dissection in stages T1–T4. Semin Urol 1993; 11:74–79.

Fisher HAG, Barada JH, Horton J, VonRoemeling RL: Neoadjuvant therapy with Cisplatin and 5-Fluorouracil for Stage III squamous cell carcinoma of the penis. (Abstract 653.) J Urol 1990; 143:352A.

Fossa SD, Hall KS, Johannessen MB, et al: Carcinoma of the penis: Experience at the Norwegian Radium Hospital 1974–1985. Eur Urol 1987; 13:372.

Fraley EE, Zhang G, Manivel C, Niehans GA: The role of ilioinguinal lymphadenectomy and significance of histological differentiation in treatment of carcinoma of the penis. J Urol 1989; 142:1478–1482.

Frew IDO, Jefferies JD, Swiney J: Carcinoma of the penis. Br J Urol 1967; 39:398.

Friedman Kien AE: Disseminated Kaposi's sarcoma syndrome in young homosexual men. J Am Acad Dermatol 1981; 5:468.

Fukunaga M, Yokoi K, Miyazawa Y, et al: Penile verrucous carcinoma with anaplastic transformation following radiotherapy: A case report with human papillomavirus typing and flow cytometric DNA studies. Am J Surg Pathol 1994; 18:501–505.

Furlong JH, Uhle CAW: Cancer of penis: A report of eighty-eight cases. J Urol 1953; 60:550.

Gagliano RG, Blumenstein BA, Crawford ED, et al: Cis-diamminedichloro-platinum in the treatment of advanced epidermoid carcinoma of the penis: A Southwest Oncology Group. J Urol 1989; 141:66.

Garnick MB, Skarin AT, Steele GD: Metastatic carcinoma of the penis: Complete remission after high dose methotrexate chemotherapy. J Urol 1979; 122:265–266.

Geffen JR, Klein RJ, Friedman Kien AE: Intralesional administration of large doses of human leukocyte interferon for the treatment of condylomata acuminata. J Infect Dis 1984; 150:612–615.

Gerbaulet A, Lambin P: Radiation therapy of cancer of the penis. Urol Clin North Am 1992; 19:325–332.

Germiyanoglu C, Horasanli K, Erol D, Altug U: Treatment of clinically fixed lymph node metastases from carcinoma of the penis by chemotherapy and surgery. Int Urol Nephrol 1993; 25:475–478.

Gilbert DA, Horton CE, Terzis JK, et al: New concepts in phallic reconstruction. Ann Plast Surg 1987; 18:128.

Gilbert DA, Williams MW, Horton CE, et al: Phallic reinnervation via the pudendal nerve. J Urol 1988; 140:295.

Gilbert P, Beckert R: Combination chemotherapy for penile giant Buschke-Lowenstein condyloma. Urol Int 1990; 45:122–124.

Gloeckler-Ries LA, Hankey BF, Edwards BK, eds: Cancer Statistics Review 1973–1987. In National Cancer Institute, National Institutes of Health Publication No. 90-2789. Bethesda, National Institutes of Health, 1990.

Goethals PL, Harrison EG, Denne KD: Verrucous carcinoma of the oral cavity. Am J Surg 1968; 106:845–849.

Goette DK: Erythroplasia of Queyrat. Arch Dermatol 1974; 110:271.

Goldberg HM, Pell-Ilderton R, Daw E, Saleh N: Concurrent squamous cell carcinoma of the cervix and penis in a married couple. Br J Obstet Gynaecol 1979; 86:585.

Goldminz D, Scott G, Klaus S: Penile basal cell carcinoma: Report of a case and review of the literature. J Am Acad Dermatol 1989; 20:1094.

Grabstald H: Carcinoma of the penis involving skin of base. J Urol 1970; 104:438.

Grabstald H, Kelley CD: Radiation therapy of penile cancer. Urology 1980; 15:575.

Graham JH, Helwig EB: Erythroplasia of Queyrat. Cancer 1973; 32:1396.

Graversen PH, Bagi P, Rosenkilde P: Laser treatment of recurrent urethral condylomata acuminata in men. Scand J Urol Nephrol 1990; 24:163–166.

Gray MR, Ansell ID: Pseudo-epitheliomatous hyperkeratotic and micaceous balanitis: Evidence for regarding it as pre-malignant. Br J Urol 1990; 66:103–105.

Greenbaum SS, Glogan R, Stegman SJ, Tromovitch TA: Carbon dioxide laser treatment of erythroplasia of Queyrat. J Dermatol Surg Oncol 1989; 15:747–750.

Gross G, Hagedorn M, Ikenberg H, et al: Bowenoid papulosis: Presence of human papillomavirus (HPV) structural antigens and of HPV 16-related DNA sequences. Arch Dermatol 1985; 121:858.

Grossman LA, Kaplan HJ, Grossman M, Ownby FD: Thrombosis of the penis: Interesting facet of thromboangiitis obliterans. JAMA 1965; 192:329.

Grunwald MH, Amichai B, Halevy S: Purplish penile papule as a presenting sign of Kaposi's sarcoma. Br J Urol 1994; 74:517.

Gursel EO, Georgountzos C, Uson AC, et al: Penile cancer. Urology 1973; 1:569.

Hagan KW, Braren V, Viner NA, et al: Extramammary Paget's disease in the scrotal and inguinal areas. J Urol 1975; 114:154.

Haile K, Delclos L: The place of radiation therapy in the treatment of carcinoma of the distal end of the penis. Cancer 1980; 45:1980.

Hall TC, Britt DB, Woodhead DM: Basal cell carcinoma of the penis. J Urol 1968; 99:314.

Hanash KA, Furlow WL, Utz DC, Harrison EG: Carcinoma of the penis: A clinicopathologic study. J Urol 1970; 104:291.

Handly J, Dinsmore W, Maw R, et al: Condyloma lesions in children. Int J STD AIDS 1993; 4:271–279.

Hardner GJ, Bhanalaph T, Murphy GP, et al: Carcinoma of the penis: Analysis of therapy in 100 consecutive cases. J Urol 1972; 108:428.

Harlin JC: Carcinoma of the penis. J Urol 1952; 67:326.

Hassan AA, Orteza AM, Milam DF: Penile horn: Review of literature with 3 case reports. J Urol 1967; 97:315.

Hayes WT, Young JM: Metastatic carcinoma of the penis. J Chronic Dis 1967; 20:891.

Hester TR Jr, Nahai F, Beegle PE, Bostwick J III: Blood supply of the abdomen revisited, with emphasis on the superficial inferior epigastric artery. Plast Reconstr Surg 1984; 74:657.

Heymann WR, Soifer I, Burk PG: Penile premalignant fibroepithelioma of Pinkus. Cutis 1983; 31:519–521.

Hill JT, Khalid MA: Point of technique—penile denervation. Br J Urol 1988; 61:167.

Hockley NM, Bihrle R, Bennett RM, Curry JM: Congenital genitourinary hemangiomas in a patient with the Klippel-Trenaunay syndrome: Management with the Nd:YAG laser. J Urol 1989; 141:940–941.

Hoffman WY, Trengove-Jones G: The rectus femoris flap. In Strauch B, Vasconez LO, Hall-Findlay EJ, eds: Grabb's Encyclopedia of Flaps, Vol III. Boston, Little, Brown, 1990, pp 1408–1409.

Hofstetter A, Frank F: Laser use in urology. In Dixon JA, ed: Surgical Application of Lasers. Chicago, Year Book Medical Publishers, 1983, pp 146–162.

Hoofnagle RF, Mahin EJ, Lamm DL, Kandzari SJ: Deoxyribonucleic acid flow cytometry of squamous cell carcinoma of the penis. (Abstract 654.) J Urol 1990; 143:352A.

Horenblas S, Kroger R, Gallee MP, et al: Ultrasound in squamous cell carcinoma of the penis: A useful addition to clinical staging? A comparison of ultrasound with histopathology. Urology 1994; 43:702–707.

Horenblas S, Van Tinteren H, Delemarre JFM, et al: Squamous cell carcinoma of the penis: III. Treatment of regional lymph nodes. J Urol 1993; 149:492–497.

Hubbell CR, Rabin VR, Mora RG: Cancer of the skin with blacks: V. A review of 175 black patients with squamous cell carcinoma of the penis. J Am Acad Dermatol 1988; 18:292–298.

Hueser JN, Pugh RP: Erythroplasia of Queyrat treated with topical 5-fluorouracil. J Urol 1969; 102:595.

Hussein A, Benefetto P, Sridhar KS: Chemotherapy with cisplatin and 5-fluorouracil for penile and urethral squamous cell cancers. Cancer 1990; 65:433–438.

Hutcheson JB, Wittaker WW, Fronstin MH: Leiomyosarcoma of the penis: Case report and review of literature. J Urol 1969; 101:874.

Ichikawa T: Chemotherapy of penis carcinoma. Rec Results Cancer Res 1977; 60:140–156.

Ichikawa T, Nakano I, Hirokawa I: Bleomycin treatment of the tumors of penis and scrotum. J Urol 1969; 102:699.

Irvine C, Anderson JR, Pye RJ: Micaceous and keratotic pseudoepitheliomatous balanitis and rapidly fatal fibrosarcoma of the penis occurring in the same patient. Br J Dermatol 1987; 116:719–721.

Jackson SM: The treatment of carcinoma of the penis. Br J Surg 1966; 53:33.

Jaffe HW, Bregman DJ, Selik RM: Acquired immunodeficiency syndrome in the United States: The first one thousand cases. J Infect Dis 1983; 148:339.

Jamieson NV, Bullock KN, Barker THW: Adenosquamous carcinoma of the penis associated with balanitis xerotica obliterans. Br J Urol 1986; 58:730–731.

Jenkins D Jr, Jakubovic HR: Pseudoepitheliomatous, keratotic, micaceous balanitis: A clinical lesion with two histologic subsets: Hyperplastic dystrophy and verrucous carcinoma. J Am Acad Dermatol 1988; 18:419–423.

Jenkins IL: Extra-mammary Paget's disease of the penis. Br J Urol 1989; 63:103.

Jensen MS: Cancer of the penis in Denmark 1942 to 1962 (511 cases). Dan Med Bull 1977; 24:66.

Jiminez-Cruz JF, Osca JM: Laser treatment of glans penis hemangioma. Eur Urol 1993; 24:81–83.

Johnson DE, Ayala AG: Primary melanoma of penis. Urology 1973; 2:174.

Johnson DE, Fuerst DE, Ayala AG: Carcinoma of the penis: Experience in 153 cases. Urology 1973; 1:404.

Johnson DE, Lo RK: Complications of groin dissection in penile carcinoma: Experience with 101 lymphadenectomies. Urology 1984a; 24:312.

Johnson DE, Lo RK: Management of regional lymph nodes in penile carcinoma: Five-year results following therapeutic groin dissections. Urol 1984b; 24:308–311.

Jordan GH: Reconstruction of the fossa navicularis. J Urol 1987; 138:102.

Kaposi M: Idiopathic multiple pigmented sarcoma of the skin. (Reprinted from Arch Derm Syphil 4:265, 1892.) Cancer 1982; 32:342.

Kaushal V, Sharma SC: Carcinoma of the penis: A 12-year review. Acta Oncol 1987; 26:413–417.

Kawada T, Hashimoto K, Tokunaga T, et al: Two cases of penile cancer: Magnetic resonance imaging in the evaluation of tumor extension. J Urol 1994; 152:963–965.

Kelley CD, Arthur K, Rogoff E, Grabstald H: Radiation therapy of penile cancer. Urology 1974; 4:571.

King LS, Sullivan M: Effects of podophyllin and of colchicine on normal skin, on condyloma acuminatum and on verruca vulgaris. Arch Pathol 1947; 43:374.

Kinghorn GR, McMillan A, Mulcahy F, et al: An open comparative study of the efficacy of 0.5% podophyllotoxin lotion and 0.25% podophyllotoxin solution in the treatment of condylomata acuminata in males and females. Int J STD AIDS 1993; 4:194–199.

Kini MG: Cancer of the penis in a child, aged two years. Ind Med Gaz 1944; 79:66.

Kleiman H, Lancaster Y: Condyloma acuminata of the bladder. J Urol 1962; 88:52.

Knudsen OS, Brennhovd IO: Radiotherapy in the treatment of the primary tumor in penile cancer. Acta Chir Scand 1967; 133:69.

Kopf AW, Bart RS: Tumor conference number 11: Multiple bowenoid papulosis of the penis: A new entity? J Dermatol Surg Oncol 1977; 3:265.

Kossow JH, Hotchkiss RS, Morales PA: Carcinoma of penis treated surgically: Analysis of 100 cases. Urology 1973; 2:169.

Kraus FT, Perez-Mesa C: Verrucous carcinoma: Clinical and pathologic study of 105 cases involving oral cavity, larynx and genitalia. Cancer 1966; 19:26.

Krebs HB: Genital HPV infections. Clin Obstet Gynecol 1989a; 32:180.

Krebs HB: Management strategies. Clin Obstet Gynecol 1989b; 32:200.

Krebs HB, Schneider V: Human papillomavirus-associated lesions of the penis: Colposcopy, cytology, and histology. Obstet Gynecol 1987; 70:299.

Kriegmair M, Rothenberger KH, Spitzenpfeil E, et al: Neodym-YAG-laser treatment for carcinoma of the penis. (Abstract 650.) J Urol 1990; 143:351A.

Krogh J, Beuke HP, Miskowiak J, et al: Long-term results of carbon dioxide laser treatment of meatal condylomata acuminata. Br J Urol 1990; 65:621–623.

Kuruvilla JT, Garlick FH, Mammen KE: Results of surgical treatment of carcinoma of the penis. Aust NZ J Surg 1971; 41:157.

Kyalwazi SK, Bhana D: Bleomycin in penile carcinoma. East Afr Med J 1973; 50:331.

Kyalwazi SK, Bhana D, Harrison NW: Carcinoma of the penis and bleomycin therapy in Uganda. Br J Urol 1974; 46:689–696.

Lancaster WD, Castellano C, Santos C, et al: Human papillomavirus deoxyribonucleic acid in cervical carcinoma from primary and metastatic sites. Am J Obstet Gynecol 1986; 154:115.

Lands RH, Ange D, Hartman DL: Radiation therapy for classic Kaposi's sarcoma presenting only on the glans penis. J Urol 1992; 147:468–470.

Landthaler M, Haina D, Brunner R, et al: Laser therapy of bowenoid papulosis and Bowen's disease. J Dermatol Surg Oncol 1986; 12:1253.

Laymon CW, Freeman C: Relationship of balanitis xerotica obliterans to lichen sclerosus et atrophicus. Arch Dermatol Syph 1944; 49:57.

Lederman M: Radiotherapy of cancer of the penis. Br J Urol 1953; 25:224.

Lenk S, Oesterwitz H, Audring H: Laser surgery in superficial penile tumors. Int Urol Nephrol 1991; 23:357–363.

Lepow H, Leffler N: Giant condylomata acuminata (Buschke-Lowenstein tumor): Report of two cases. J Urol 1960; 83:853.

Lesser JH, Schwarz H II: External genital carcinoma: Results of treatment at Ellis Fischel State Cancer Hospital. Cancer 1955; 8:1021.

Leviav A, Devine PC, Schellhammer PF, Horton CE: Epithelioid sarcoma of the penis. Clin Plast Surg 1988; 15:489.

Levine RU, Crum CP, Herman E, et al: Cervical papillomavirus infection and intraepithelial neoplasia: A study of male sexual partners. Obstet Gynecol 1984; 64:16.

Lewis RJ, Bendl BJ: Erythroplasia of Queyrat: Report of a patient successfully treated with topical 5-fluorouracil. Can Med Assoc J 1971; 104:148.

Licklider S: Jewish penile carcinoma. J Urol 1961; 86:98.

Linderman RD, Papper S: Therapy of fluid and electrolyte disorders. Ann Intern Med 1975; 82:64.

Lipshutz RL, Kantor GR, Vonderheid EC: Multiple penile syringomas mimicking verrucae. Int J Dermatol 1991; 30:69.

Lowe FC, Lattimer G, Metroka CE: Kaposi's sarcoma of the penis in patients with acquired immunodeficiency syndrome. J Urol 1989; 142:1475.

Lowenstein LW: Carcinoma-like condylomata acuminata of the penis. Med Clin North Am 1939; 5:789.

Lowhagen GB, Bolmstedt A, Ryd W, Voog E: The prevalence of "high-risk" HPV types in penile condyloma-like lesions: Correlation between HPV type and morphology. Genitourin Med 1993; 69:87–90.

Lubke WL, Thompson IM: The case for inguinal lymph node dissection in the treatment of T2–T4, N0 penile cancer. Semin Urol 1993; 11:80–84.

Lynch HT, Krush AJ: Delay factors in detection of cancer of the penis. Nebr State Med J 1969; 54:360.

Madej G, Meyza J: Cryosurgery of penile carcinoma. Oncology 1982; 39:350.

Magid M, Garden JM: Pearly penile papules: Treatment with the carbon dioxide laser. J Dermatol Surg Oncol 1989; 15:552–554.

Malakoff AF, Schmidt JD: Metastatic carcinoma of penis complicated by hypercalcemia. Urology 1975; 5:519.

Malek RS: Laser treatment of premalignant and malignant squamous cell lesions of the penis. Lasers Surg Med 1992; 12:246–253.

Malek RS, Goellner JR, Smith TF, et al: Human papillomavirus infection and intraepithelial, in situ, and invasive carcinoma of penis. Urology 1993; 42:159–170.

Malloy TR, Wein AJ, Carpiniello VL: Carcinoma of the penis treated with neodymium YAG laser. Urology 1988; 31:26.

Manivel JC, Fraley EE: Malignant melanoma of the penis and male urethra: 4 case reports and literature review. J Urol 1988; 139:813.

Marcial VA, Figueroa-Colon J, Marcial-Rojas RA, Colon JE: Carcinoma of the penis. Radiology 1962; 79:209.

Marks D, Crosthwaite A, Varigos G, et al: Therapy of primary diffuse large cell lymphoma of the penis with preservation of function. J Urol 1988; 139:1057.

Martin RW III, Russell RC, Trautmann VF, Klingler WG: Conservative excision of penile melanoma. Ann Plast Surg 1988; 20:266–269.

Mazeron JJ, Langlois D, Lobo PA, et al: Interstitial radiation therapy for carcinoma of the penis using iridium 192 wires: The Henri Mondor experience (1970–1979). Int J Radiat Oncol Biol Phys 1984; 10:1891.

McCraw JB, Arnold PG: McCraw and Arnold's Atlas of Muscle and Musculocutaneous Flaps. Norfolk, VA, Hampton Press Publishing, 1986.

McCraw JB, Dibbell DG: Experimental definition of independent myocutaneous vascular territories. Plast Reconstr Surg 1977; 60:212.

McCraw JB, Dibbell DG, Carraway JH: Clinical definition of independent myocutaneous vascular territories. Plast Reconstr Surg 1977; 60:341.

McCrea LW, Tobias GL: Metastatic disease of the penis. J Urol 1958; 80:489.

McDougal WS: Carcinoma of the penis: Improved survival by early regional lymphadenectomy based on the histologic grade and depth of the primary lesion. J Urol 1995; 134:1364–1369.

McDougal WS, Kirchner FK Jr, Edwards RH, Killion LT: Treatment of carcinoma of the penis: The case of primary lymphadenectomy. J Urol 1986; 136:38.

McKay DL, Fuqua F, Weinberg AG: Balanitis xerotica obliterans in children. J Urol 1975; 114:773.

McLean M, Akl AM, Warde P, et al: The results of primary radiation therapy in the management of squamous cell carcinoma of the penis. Int J Radiat Oncol Biol Phys 1993; 25:623–628.

Mikhail GR: Cancers, precancers, and pseudocancers on the male genitalia: A review of clinical appearances, histopathology, and management. J Dermatol Surg Oncol 1980; 6:1027–1038.

Miles SA: Pathogenesis of HIV-related Kaposi's sarcoma. Curr Opin Oncol 1994; 6:497–502.

Mills EED: Intermittent intravenous methotrexate in the treatment of advanced epidermoid carcinoma. S Afr Med J 1972; 46:398.

Misma Y, Matunalea M: Effect of bleomycin on benign and malignant cutaneous tumors. Acta Dermatol Venereol (Stockh) 1972; 52:211.

Mitsudo S, Nakanishi I, Koss LG: Paget's disease of the penis and adjacent skin. Arch Pathol Lab Med 1981; 105:518.

Mohs FE: Chemosurgery: A microscopically controlled method of cancer excision. Arch Surg 1941; 42:279.

Mohs FE, Snow SN, Larson PO: Mohs' micrographic surgery for penile tumors. Urol Clin North Am 1992; 19:291–304.

Mohs FE, Snow SN, Messing EM, Kuglitsch ME: Microscopically controlled surgery in the treatment of carcinoma of the penis. J Urol 1985; 133:961.

Montgomery BS, Fletcher CD, Palfrey EL, Lloyd-Davies RW: Traumatic neuroma of the penis. Br J Urol 1990; 65:420–421.

Moore SW, Wheeler JE, Hefter LG: Epithelioid sarcoma masquerading as Peyronie's disease. Cancer 1975; 35:1706.

Morgan WKC: The rape of the phallus. JAMA 1965; 193:223.

Mortimer PS, Sonnex TS, Dawber RPR: Cryotherapy for multicentric pigmented Bowen's disease. Clin Exp Dermatol 1983; 8:319.

Muir CS, Nectoux J: Epidemiology of cancer of the testis and penis. Natl Cancer Inst Monogr 1979; 53:157–161.

Mukamel E, Farrer J, Smith RB, deKernion JB: Metastatic carcinoma of penis: When is total penectomy indicated? Urology 1987; 24:15.

Murrell DS, Williams JL: Radiotherapy in the treatment of carcinoma of the penis. Br J Urol 1965; 37:211.

Nahai F: The tensor fascia lata flap. Clin Plast Surg 1980; 7:51.

Nahai F, Hill HL, Hester TR: Experiences with the tensor fascia lata flap. Plast Reconstr Surg 1979; 63:788.

Narasimharao KL, Chatterjee H, Veliath AJ: Penile carcinoma in the first decade of life. Br J Urol 1985; 57:358.

Narayana AS, Olney LE, Loening SA, et al: Carcinoma of the penis: Analysis of 219 cases. Cancer 1982; 49:2185.

National Cancer Institute (NCI) Position Statement: Kaposi's sarcoma. In PDQ, Physician Data Query (Database). Bethesda, MD, National Cancer Institute, 1990, pp 1–11.

Neinstein LS, Goldenring J: Pink pearly papules: An epidemiologic study. J Pediatr 1984; 105:594.

Nickel WR, Plumb RT: Nonvenereal sclerosing lymphangitis of penis. Arch Dermatol 1962; 86:761.

Nitidandhaprabhas P: Artificial penile nodules: Case reports from Thailand. Br J Urol 1975; 47:463.

Noel JC, Vandenbossche M, Peny MO, et al: Verrucous carcinoma of the penis: Importance of human papillomavirus typing for diagnosis and therapeutic decision. Eur Urol 1992; 22:83–85.

Ornellas AA, Correia AL, Marota A, Seixas ALC: Surgical treatment of invasive squamous cell carcinoma of the penis: Retrospective analysis of 350 cases. J Urol 1994; 151:1244–1247.

Ornellas AA, Seixas ALC, DeMoraes JA: Analysis of 200 lymphadenectomies in patients with penile carcinoma. J Urol 1991; 146:330–332.

Ornellas AA, Seixas AL, Marota A, et al: Surgical treatment of invasive squamous cell carcinoma of the penis. J Urol 1994; 151:1244–1249.

Orticochea M: Musculo-cutaneous flap method: Immediate and heroic substitute for the method of delay. Br J Plast Surg 1972a; 25:106.

Orticochea M: New method of total reconstruction of the penis. Br J Plast Surg 1972b; 25:347.

Pak K, Sakaguchi N, Takayama H, Tomoyoshi T: Rhabdomyosarcoma of the penis. J Urol 1986; 136:438.

Parsons MA, Fox M: Malignant fibrous histiocytoma of the penis. Eur Urol 1988; 14:75.

Patterson JW, Kao GF, Graham JH, Helwig EB: Bowenoid papulosis: A clinicopathologic study with ultrastructural observations. Cancer 1986; 57:823.

Paymaster JC, Gangadharan P: Cancer of the penis in India. J Urol 1967; 97:110.

Pedrick TJ, Wheeler W, Riemenschneider H: Combined modality therapy for locally advanced penile squamous cell carcinoma. Am J Clin Oncol 1993; 16:501–505.

Pereira-Bringel PJ, de Andrade Arruda R: 5-Fluorouracil cream 5% in the treatment of intraurethral condylomata acuminata. Br J Urol 1982; 54:295.

Perinetti EP, Crane DC, Catalona WJ: Unreliability of sentinel lymph node biopsy for staging penile carcinoma. J Urol 1980; 124:734.

Persky L: Epidemiology of cancer of the penis. Rec Results Cancer Res 1977; 60:97–109.

Peters BS, Perry HO: Bowenoid papules of the penis. J Urol 1981; 126:482.

Pettaway CA, Pisters LL, von Eschenbach AC, et al: Sentinel lymph node biopsy for penile squamous carcinoma: The M. D. Anderson Cancer Center 9-year experience. J Urol 1995; 153:246A.

Pfister H, Haneke E: Demonstration of human papillomavirus type 2 DNA in Bowen's disease. Arch Dermatol Res 1984; 276:123.

Pierquin B, Chassagne D, Cox JD: Toward consistent local control of certain malignant tumors. Radiology 1971; 99:661.

Pizzocaro G, Piva L: Adjuvant and neoadjuvant vincristine, bleomycin, and methotrexate for inguinal metastases from squamous cell carcinoma of the penis. Acta Oncol 1988; 27:823–824.

Pizzocaro G, Piva L, Nicolai N: Improved management of nodal metastases of squamous cell carcinoma (SCC) of the penis. J Urol 1995; 153:246A.

Plaut A, Kohn-Speyer AC: The carcinogenic action of smegma. Science 1947; 195:391.

Pochedly C, Mehta A, Feingold E: Priapism with hyperacute stem-cell leukemia. NY State J Med 1974; 75:540.

Pompeo AC, Mesquita JL, Junior WA, et al: Staged inguinal lymphadenectomy (SIL) for carcinoma of the penis (CP): 13 years prospective study of 50 patients. J Urol 1995; 153:246A.

Poynter JH, Levy J: Balanitis xerotica obliterans: Effective treatment with topical and sublesional steroids. Br J Urol 1967; 39:420.

Prasad KR, Veliath AJ: Cell surface blood group antigens in carcinoma of the penis. Appl Pathol 1986; 4:192.

Pratt RM, Ross RTA: Leiomyosarcoma of the penis. Br J Surg 1969; 56:870.

Pratt-Thomas HR, Heins HC, Latham E, et al: The carcinogenic effect of human smegma: An experimental study. Cancer 1956; 9:671.

Prescott RJ, Mainwaring AR: Irradiation-induced penile angiosarcoma. Postgrad Med J 1990; 66:576–579.

Pressman D, Rolnick D, Turbow B: Penile horn. Am J Surg 1962; 104:640.

Preston EN: Whither the foreskin? A consideration of routine neonatal circumcision. JAMA 1970; 213:1853.

Previte SR, Karian S, Cho SI, Austen G Jr: Penile carcinoma in renal transplant recipient. Urology 1979; 13:298.

Proffitt SD, Spooner TR, Kosek JC: Origin of undifferentiated neoplasm from verrucous epidermal carcinoma of oral cavity following irradiation. Cancer 1970; 26:389.

Puras A, Fortuno R, Gonzalez-Flores B, Sotolongo A: Staging lymphadenectomy in the treatment of carcinoma of the penis. Proc Kimbrough Urol Semin 1980; 14:15.

Puras A, Gonzalez-Flores B, Furtuno B, et al: Treatment of carcinoma of the penis. Proc Kimbrough Urol Semin 1978; 12:143.

Puras-Baez A, Rivera-Herrera J, Miranda G, et al: Role of superficial inguinal lymphadenectomy in carcinoma of the penis. J Urol 1995; 153:246A.

Queyrat L: Erythroplasie du gland. Soc Franc Dermatol Syphilol 1911; 22:378.

Rasbridge SA, Parry JRW: Angiosarcoma of the penis. Br J Urol 1989; 63:440.

Ravi R: Correlation between the extent of nodal involvement and survival following groin dissection for carcinoma of the penis. Br J Urol 1993; 72:817–819.

Raynal M, Chassagne D, Baillet F, Pierquin B: Endocuritherapy of penis cancer. Rec Results Cancer Res 1977; 60:135.

Reddy CR, Rao TG, Venkatarathnam G, et al: A study of 80 patients with penile carcinoma combined with cervical biopsy study of their wives. Int Surg 1977; 62:549.

Reddy DG, Baruah IKSM: Carcinogenic action of human smegma. Arch Pathol 1963; 75:414.

Redman JF, Meacham KR: Condyloma acuminata of the urethral meatus in children. J Pediatr Surg 1973; 8:939.

Reece RW, Koontz WW Jr: Leukoplakia of the urinary tract: A review. J Urol 1975; 114:165.

Reichman R, Oakes D, Banner W: Treatment of condyloma acuminata with three different interferons administered interlesionally: A double-blind, placebo-controlled trial. Ann Intern Med 1988; 108:675–679.

Reid JD: Melanosarcoma of the penis. Cancer 1957; 10:359.

Revuz J, Clerici T: Penile melanosis. J Am Acad Dermatol 1989; 20:567–570.

Rhatigan RM, Jimenez S, Chopskie EJ: Condyloma acuminatum and carcinoma of the penis. South Med J 1972; 65:423.

Rheinschild GW, Olsen BS: Balanitis xerotica obliterans. J Urol 1970; 104:860.

Riveros M, Garcia R, Cabanas R: Lymphadenography of the dorsal lymphatics of the penis. Cancer 1967; 20:2026.

Riveros M, Gorostiaga R: Cancer of the penis. Arch Surg 1962; 85:377.

Robey EL, Schelhammer PF: Four cases of metastases to the penis and a review of the literature. J Urol 1984; 132:992.

Rosemberg SK, Fuller TA: Carbon dioxide rapid superpulsed laser treatment of erythroplasia of queyrat. Urology 1980; 16:181.

Rosemberg SK, Jacobs H, Fuller T: Some guidelines in the treatment of urethral condylomata with carbon dioxide laser. J Urol 1982; 127:906.

Rothenberger KH: Value of the neodymium-YAG laser in the therapy of penile carcinoma. Eur Urol 1986; 12:34.

Rubenstein M, Wolff SM: Penile nodules as a major manifestation of subacute angiitis. Arch Intern Med 1964; 114:449.

Rudd FV, Rott RK, Skoglund RW, Ansell JS: Tumor-induced hypercalcemia. J Urol 1972; 107:986.

Sagerman RH, Yu WS, Chung CT, Puranik A: External beam irradiation of cancer of the penis. Radiology 1984; 152:183.

Sakoda R, Oka M, Nakashima K: Leukoplakia of the penis: Bleomycin treatment. Br J Urol 1978; 50:355–356.

Salaverria JC, Hope-Stone HF, Paris AMI, et al: Conservative treatment of carcinoma of the penis. Br J Urol 1979; 51:32.

Samson RH: Omental flap for coverage of exposed groin vessels. In Strauch B, Vasconez LO, Hall-Findlay EJ, eds: Grabb's Encyclopedia of Flaps, Vol III. Boston, Little, Brown, 1990, pp 1404–1407.

Sand PK, Bowen LW, Blischke SO, Ostergard DR: Evaluation of male consorts of women with genital human papillomavirus infection. Obstet Gynecol 1986; 68:679.

Scappini P, Piscioli F, Pusiol T, et al: Penile cancer: Aspiration biopsy cytology for staging. Cancer 1986; 58:1526–1533.

Schneider V: Microscopic diagnosis of HPV infection. Clin Obstet Gynecol 1989; 32:148.

Schoen EJ, Anderson G, Bohon C, et al: Task force on circumcision, report of the task force on circumcision. Pediatrics 1989; 84:388.

Schrek R, Lenowitz H: Etiologic factors in carcinoma of penis. Cancer Res 1947; 7:180.

Schultz RE, Miller JW, MacDonald GR, et al: Clinical and molecular evaluation of acetowhite genital lesions in men. J Urol 1990; 143:920.

Sedlacek TV, Cunnane M, Carpiniello V: Colposcopy in the diagnosis of penile condyloma. Am J Obstet Gynecol 1986; 154:494.

Seftel AD, Sadick NS, Waldbaum RS: Kaposi's sarcoma of the penis in a patient with the acquired immune deficiency syndrome. J Urol 1986; 136:673.

Seixas ALC, Ornellas AA, Marota A, et al: Verrucous carcinoma of the penis: Retrospective analysis of 32 cases. J Urol 1994; 152:1476–1479.

Shiraki IW: Parameatal cysts of the glans penis: A report of nine cases. J Urol 1975; 114:544.

Siegel A: Malignant transformation of condyloma acuminatum. Am J Surg 1962; 103:613.

Skinner DG, Leadbetter WF, Kelley SB: The surgical management of squamous cell carcinoma of the penis. J Urol 1972; 107:273.

Sklaroff RB, Yagoda A: Cis-diamminodichloride platinum II (DDP) in the treatment of penile carcinoma. Cancer 1979; 44:1563.

Sklaroff RB, Yagoda A: Methotrexate in the treatment of penile carcinoma. Cancer 1980; 45:214.

Sklaroff RB, Yagoda A: Penile cancer: Natural history and therapy. In Spiers AS, ed: Chemotherapy and Urological Malignancy. New York, Springer-Verlag, 1982, pp 98–105.

Smetana HF, Bernhard W: Sclerosing lipogranuloma. Arch Pathol 1950; 50:296.

Smotkin D: Virology of human papillomavirus. Clin Obstet Gynecol 1989; 32:117.

Sola Casas MA, Soto de Del as J, Redondo Bellon P, Quintanilla Gutirrez E: Syringomas localized to the penis. Clin Exp Dermatol 1993; 18:384–385.

Sonnex TS, Ralfs IG, Plaza de Lanza M, Dawber RPR: Treatment of erythroplasia of Queyrat with liquid nitrogen cryosurgery. Br J Dermatol 1982; 106:581.

Spaulding JT, Whitmore WF Jr: Extended total excision of prostatic adenocarcinoma. J Urol 1978; 120:188.

Srinivas V, Morse MJ, Herr HW, et al: Penile cancer: Relation of extent of nodal metastasis to survival. J Urol 1987; 137:880–882.

Staubitz WJ, Melbourne HL, Oberkircher OJ: Carcinoma of the penis. Cancer 1955; 8:371.

Stein BS: Laser treatment of condylomata acuminata. J Urol 1986; 136:593.

Stewart AL, Grieve RJ, Banerjee SS: Primary lymphoma of the penis. Eur J Surg Oncol 1985; 11:179.

Stone KM: Epidemiologic aspects of genital HPV infection. Clin Obstet Gynecol 1989; 32:112.

Suchaud JP, Kantor G, Richaud P: Curietherapie des cancers de la verge: Analyse d'une serie de 53 cas. J Urol (Paris) 1989; 95:27–31.

Sufrin G, Huben R: Benign and malignant lesions of the penis. In Gillenwater JY, ed: Adult and Pediatric Urology, 2nd ed. Chicago, Year Book Medical Publishers, 1991, p 1643.

Summers JL: Pyogenic granuloma: An unusual complication of papaverine injection therapy for impotence. J Urol 1990; 143:1227–1228.

Tannenbaum MH, Becker SW: Papillae of the corona of the glans penis. J Urol 1965; 93:391.

Taylor GI, Corlett RJ, Boyd JB: The versatile deep inferior epigastric (inferior rectus abdominis) flap. Br J Plast Surg 1984; 37:330.

Taylor GI, Corlett RJ, Boyd JB: The deep inferior epigastric artery island rectus musculocutaneous flap. In Strauch B, Vasconez LO, Hall-Findlay EJ, eds: Grabb's Encyclopedia of Flaps, Vol III. Boston, Little, Brown, 1990, pp 1416–1420.

Theodorescu D, Fair WR, Herr HW, et al: Expectant management of patients with T1-4N0M0 penile cancer. J Urol 1995; 153:247A.

Theodorescu D, Russo P, Zhang ZF, et al: Outcomes of initial surveillance of invasive squamous cell carcinoma of the penis and negative nodes. J Urol 1996; 155:1626–1631

Thomas JA, Small CS: Carcinoma of the penis in southern India. J Urol 1963; 160:520.

Trier WC: Local skin flaps. In Strauch B, Vasconez LO, Hall-Findlay EJ, eds: Grabb's Encyclopedia of Flaps, Vol III. Boston, Little, Brown, 1990, pp 1393–1395.

Ubben K, Kryzek R, Ostrow R: Human papillomavirus DNA detected in two verrucous carcinomas. J Invest Dermatol 1979; 22:195–210.

Uehling DT: Staging laparotomy for carcinoma of penis. J Urol 1973; 110:213.

Vaeth JM, Green JP, Lowry RO: Radiation therapy of carcinoma of the penis. AJR Rad Ther Nucl Med 1970; 108:130.

Vapnek JM, Hricak H, Carroll PR: Recent advances in imaging studies for staging of penile and urethral carcinoma. Urol Clin North Am 1992; 19:257–266.

Villa LL, Lopes A: Human papillomavirus DNA sequences in penile carcinomas in Brazil. Int J Cancer 1986; 37:853.

Von Eschenbach AC, Johnson DE, Wishnow KI, et al: Results of laser therapy for carcinoma of the penis: Organ preservation. Prog Clin Biol Res 1991; 370:407–412.

Wade TR, Kopf AW, Ackerman AB: Bowenoid papulosis of the penis. Cancer 1978; 42:1890.

Weitzner S: Secondary carcinoma in the penis: Report of three cases and literature review. Am Surg 1971; 37:563.

Wespes E, Simon J, Schulman CC: Cabanas' approach: Is sentinal node biopsy reliable for staging of penile carcinoma? Urology 1986; 28:278.

Wheelock MC, Clark PJ: Sarcoma of penis. J Urol 1943; 49:478.

Whitmore WF: Tumors of the penis, urethra, scrotum, and testes. In Campbell MF, Harrison HH, eds: Urology, 3rd ed. Philadelphia, W. B. Saunders, 1970, pp 1190–1129.

Wishnow KI, Johnson DE: Effective outpatient treatment of Kaposi's sarcoma of the urethral meatus using the neodymium: YAG laser. Lasers Surg Med 1988; 8:428.

Yamashita T, Ogawa A: Ultrasound in penile cancer. Urol Radiol 1989; 11:174–183.

Young MJ, Reda DJ, Waters WB: Penile carcinoma: A twenty-five year experience. Urology 1991; 38:529–532.

Youngberg GA, Thornthwaite JT, Inoshita T: Cytologically malignant squamous-cell carcinoma arising in a verrucous carcinoma of the penis. J Dermatol Surg Oncol 1983; 9:474.

Yu DS, Chang SY, Ma CP: DNA ploidy, S-phase fraction, and cytomorphometry in relation to survival of human penile cancer. Urol Int 1992; 48:265–269.

Zalar JA, Knode RE, Mir JA: Lipogranuloma of the penis. J Urol 1969; 102:75.

Zelickson AS, Prawer SE: Bowenoid papulosis of the penis: Demonstration of intranuclear viral-like particles. Am J Dermatopathol 1980; 2:305.

Zouboulis CC, Stadler R, Ikenberg H, Orfanos CE: Short-term systemic recombinant interferon-gamma treatment is ineffective in recalcitrant condylomata acuminata. J Am Acad Dermatol 1991; 24:302–303.

XI
CARCINOMA OF THE PROSTATE

80
ETIOLOGY, EPIDEMIOLOGY, AND PREVENTION OF CARCINOMA OF THE PROSTATE

Kenneth J. Pienta, M.D.

Etiology
Cell Kinetics
Germ Line Mutations
DNA Methylation
Tumor Suppressor Genes and Oncogenes
Androgen Receptor Mutations
Growth Factors and Epithelial-Stromal Interactions

Epidemiology
Descriptive Epidemiology

Definitive Risk Factors
Probable Risk Factors
Potential Risk Factors

Prevention Strategies
Screening Strategies
Avoidance of Risk Factors
Chemoprevention

Summary

In 1995, there were approximately 244,000 new cases and 44,000 deaths from prostate cancer—numbers that will continue to rise as the population ages (Carter and Coffey, 1990; Wingo et al, 1995). Ninety-five percent of prostate cancer is diagnosed in men between 45 and 89 years of age with a median age of diagnosis of 72 years. The epidemiology of prostate cancer in men is similar to that of breast cancer in women (Table 80–1). Both cancers are the most commonly diagnosed as well as the second leading cause of cancer death after lung cancer in their respective sexes. At least in their early stages, they both

Table 80–1. COMPARISON OF PROSTATE AND BREAST CANCER

Disease	Prostate Cancer	Breast Cancer
1995 incidence	244,000	182,000
Percentage of new cancer cases	36%	32%
1995 deaths	40,400	46,000
Percentage of cancer deaths	14%	18%
Probability of developing	1 in 6 (lifetime)	1 in 8 (lifetime)
Selected risk factors	Age, family history	Age, family history
Hormone dependent	Early disease	Early disease

appear to be hormone dependent, and the incidence of both rises dramatically with age. Men and women with a positive family history have a higher likelihood of developing disease, often at a younger age than their counterparts with no history of cancer in the family. Because approximately 50% of patients diagnosed with these cancers develop metastatic and therefore incurable disease, prevention of cancer development is a life-saving and cost-effective health strategy. The development of successful cancer prevention strategies is facilitated by an understanding of the etiology of the disease, knowledge of factors that contribute to the carcinogenic process, and subsequent development of effective intervention measures.

ETIOLOGY

Considerable progress has been made to begin to define the molecular events that contribute to the transformation of a normal prostate epithelial cell to a metastatic, androgen-independent cancer cell (Fig. 80–1). Although the multistep nature of carcinogenesis has been demonstrated for many human cancers, the elucidation of individual steps involved in prostate cell transformation has proven more elusive, and only recently have investigators started to identify the

2489

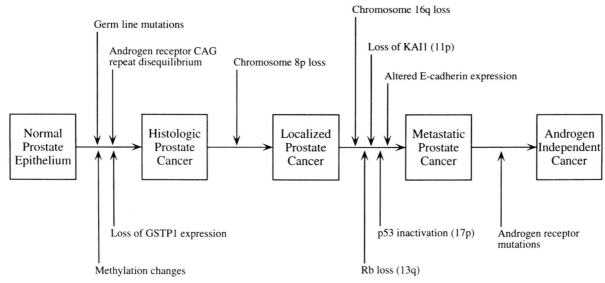

Figure 80–1. A summary of genetic alterations associated with the progression of prostate cancer. (Adapted from Isaacs WB, Bova GS, Morton RA, et al: Cancer 1995; 75:2004–2012. By permission of Wiley-Liss, a division of John Wiley and Sons, Inc. © 1995.)

oncogenes and tumor suppressor genes involved in prostate carcinogenesis. **Prostate cancer is unique among the solid tumors because it essentially exists in two forms: a histologic or latent form, which can be identified in approximately 30% of men over the age of 50 and 60% to 70% of men over the age of 80, and the clinically evident form, which affects approximately one out of six American men in their lifetimes** (Carter and Coffey, 1990; Wingo et al, 1995).

Cell Kinetics

The growth of prostate cancer depends on the rate of cells proliferating balanced by the rate of cells dying. Normal prostate glandular epithelial cells have a low, balanced rate of cell proliferation and death, which results in a steady-state condition in which there is no net growth, although the epithelial cells are constantly being replaced with a turnover time of approximately 500 days (Berges et al, 1995). Transformation of these cells into high-grade prostatic intraepithelial neoplastic (PIN) cells, a probable precursor lesion for at least a subset of prostate carcinomas, involves an increase in cell proliferation and cell death, resulting in increased cell turnover and increasing their risk for further genetic changes. Further transformation to prostate carcinoma appears to involve a decrease in the percentage of cells dying, resulting in net growth of the cancer lesions with doubling times of 33 to 126 days (Berges et al, 1995).

Germ Line Mutations

Several steps of the prostate carcinogenesis pathway have been identified (see Fig. 80–1). **Approximately 9% of all prostate cancers and 45% of cases in men younger than 55 years of age can be attributed to a cancer susceptibility gene that is inherited in a mendelian fashion as a rare autosomal dominant allele** (Carter et al, 1992). These studies suggest that a germ line mutation may be important

in at least a subset of prostate cancers and may be critically important to understanding carcinogenesis events because this gene may contribute to the evolution of clinically evident cancer at a younger age.

It has been postulated that **the strength of the response of the androgen receptor to androgens is inversely dependent on the length of the CAG microsatellites located in the 5′ promoter region of the gene** (Irvine et al, 1995). The shorter the length of the microsatellite in the germ line, the more responsive the cell would be to androgen, thus promoting growth. Black men have a higher prevalence of shorter CAG alleles than their white counterparts, and white patients with prostate cancer have a higher prevalence of short alleles as compared to controls. These data as well as that of others suggest a potential association between microsatellite length within the androgen receptor gene and prostate cancer development.

DNA Methylation

An early event in solid tumor carcinogenesis appears to be alterations in DNA methylation, and prostate cancer is no exception to this. Hypermethylation of genomic areas rich in CpG nucleotide "islands" has been associated with gene inactivation. Hypermethylation of an area of chromosome 17p may possibly lead to inactivation of a tumor suppressor gene at that site (Isaacs et al, 1995). The promoter region of the glutathione s-transferase pi gene, an enzyme that plays a critical role in detoxification of free radicals thereby protecting DNA from damage, is methylated and inactivated in prostate cancer tissue but not in normal tissue (Lee et al, 1994). Loss of glutathione s-transferase pi could, therefore, lead to increased mutation susceptibility of prostate cells.

Tumor Suppressor Genes and Oncogenes

The loss of several potential tumor suppressor genes has been demonstrated to occur as later events in prostate cell transformation. **Loss of heterozygosity (LOH) studies that identify areas of consistent chromosomal deletion have identified potential tumor suppressor genes on chromosomes 8p, 10q, 13q, 16q, 17p, and 18q. Almost 70% of patients with clinically localized prostate cancer can be shown to have deletions of chromosome 8p22** (Macoska et al, 1994). **Thirty-six percent of patients with localized disease and 60% of patients with metastatic tumors demonstrated deletions on chromosome 16q, the site of the putative tumor suppressor gene E-cadherin** (Isaacs et al, 1995). E-cadherin is a cell surface molecule that mediates epithelial cell-cell interactions and adhesion. Loss of E-cadherin expression correlates with increased invasive potential, and preliminary studies have demonstrated that aberrant E-cadherin expression is a predictor of disease progression and poor overall survival (Umbas et al, 1994).

The role of other tumor suppressor genes and oncogenes continues to be defined. Although the activation of specific oncogenes has not been implicated in prostate carcinogenesis of American men, studies have suggested that approximately 25% of tumors from Japanese men harbor mutations in the ras oncogene (Anwar et al, 1992). Loss of the retinoblastoma gene located on chromosome 13q appears to play a role in approximately 25% of prostate cancers (Bookstein et al, 1990). The inactivation of KAI1, a metastasis suppressor gene for prostate cancer located on 11p, may play a role in the transition from localized to metastatic disease (Dong et al, 1995). The importance of chromosome 17p, the site of the p53 gene as well as other potential tumor suppressor genes, is also becoming more clear. The p53 gene encodes a protein that arrests the cell cycle at G1 to permit DNA repair. Inactivation of the gene, therefore, creates an environment in which DNA damage is not repaired and creates a cell environment permissive to mutation and proliferation. **Although p53 mutations do not appear to be common in low-grade, clinically localized cancers, as many as 50% of high-grade, metastatic tumors appear to harbor mutant p53,** and mutations in this gene may be associated with the transition to hormone refractory disease (Navone et al, 1993).

Androgen Receptor Mutations

Few mutations in the androgen receptor have been consistently identified in primary tumors; however, it appears that approximately 50% of metastatic androgen-independent cells obtained from bone marrow of patients carry mutations in the androgen receptor (Taplin et al, 1995). It has been postulated that mutations in the androgen receptor may provide a selective growth advantage to prostate cancer cells after androgen ablation. These mutations may allow the androgen receptor to respond to other growth factors, such as insulin-like growth factor–1 or keratinocyte growth factor (Tenniswood et al, 1992; Yan et al, 1992; Cohen et al, 1994a). These growth factors may bind to a mutated, promiscuous androgen receptor and cause activation even after the cells have become androgen resistant.

Growth Factors and Epithelial-Stromal Interactions

In addition to their potential role in activating mutated androgen receptors, growth factors have been demonstrated

to contribute to the control of normal and cancerous prostate growth. **Transforming growth factor-beta, epidermal growth factor, platelet-derived growth factor, and neuroendocrine peptides have all been demonstrated to be modulators of prostate epithelial cell proliferation, differentiation, and invasiveness** (Hoosein et al, 1993; Cohen et al, 1994b; Fudge et al, 1994; Steiner et al, 1994). The effects of these growth factors are mediated in part by the interaction of epithelial cells with the stromal cells that surround them. The stromal or mesenchymal cells of the prostate produce many of these growth factors that act on the epithelial cells in a paracrine fashion (Gleave et al, 1991). **It has been demonstrated that bone cells produce selected growth factors which stimulate the proliferation of prostate cells and that prostate cells produce factors which stimulate bone formation,** thereby potentially explaining why prostate cancer preferentially metastasizes to bone.

EPIDEMIOLOGY

Descriptive Epidemiology

The age-adjusted incidence and death rates from prostate cancer vary dramatically from country to country as well as between racial-ethnic groups (Fig. 80–2). **In 1989, the incidence rates were highest in blacks (149/100,000 person-years), intermediate in U.S. whites (107/100,000 person-years), and lowest in Orientals (Japanese [39/100,000 person-years] and Chinese [28/100,000 person-years])** (Taylor et al, 1994; Irvine et al, 1995). While the incidence rates are increasing yearly, these variations continue to persist. Clinically apparent disease is rare under the age of 50 and increases dramatically with age. **The age-adjusted incidence rate is 21 per 100,000 person-years for U.S. whites under age 65 and 819 per 100,000 person-years for those over 65.**

Between 1973 and 1989, the age-adjusted U.S. incidence rates of prostate cancer have increased at approximately 2.7 per 100,000 yearly (Fig. 80–3). This rise was attributed to an aging population and in part to the increased use of transurethral resection of the prostate yielding more stage A disease. Improvements in ultrasound and biopsy techniques also may have contributed to finding more prostate cancer in the community. **Between 1989 and 1991, incidence rates rose by 23.5 per 100,000** (Demers et al, 1994). It has been demonstrated that the use of prostate-specific antigen (PSA) as a screening tool contributed to the rise in prostate cancer incidence rates since it came into widespread clinical use in the 1990s (Potosky et al, 1995). This can be explained in part by the detection by PSA of cancers across all age groups that had previously not been detected by more conventional means and is reflected in the dramatic increase in the detection of localized as compared to regional and metastatic prostate cancers (Demers et al, 1994). It was expected that the incidence rates for prostate cancer would start to level off as these prevalent cancers were detected, and in 1993, the age-adjusted incidence rates of invasive prostate cancer fell in white men. The fact that the incidence rates have not decreased in black men is most likely secondary to the lower rates of screening in the black

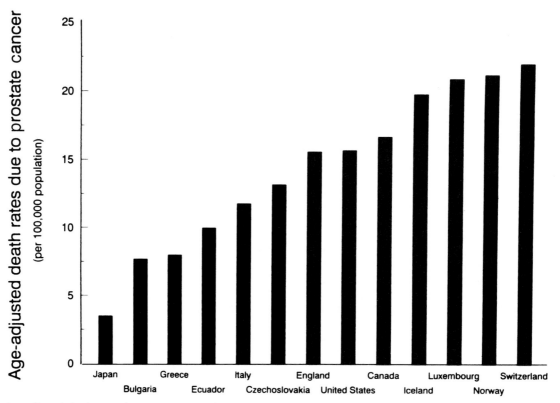

Figure 80–2. Age-adjusted death rates due to prostate cancer per 100,000 population in various countries. (From Boring CC, Squires TS, Tong T: CA Cancer J Clin 1992; 42:19–39.)

population. **The mortality from prostate cancer has also been rising, albeit at a slower rate. This increase is most likely secondary to the fact that men are living longer and experiencing less cardiovascular mortality.** Over the last decade, men over the age of 65 have shown the greatest annual rise in mortality from prostate cancer.

Age-Adjusted Incidence Rates of Invasive Prostate Cancers, All Stages Combined

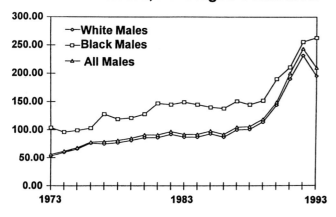

Figure 80–3. Prostate cancer incidence rates for the years 1973 to 1993. Rates are shown for the tricounty metropolitan Detroit area as measured by the Surveillance, Epidemiology, and End Results (SEER) program (NO1-CN-05225). Rates are per 100,000, are age-adjusted to the 1970 U.S. standard population, and are representative of new cancer cases diagnosed in a given year.

Definitive Risk Factors

Age

The prevalence of prostate cancer continues to increase with age, and after age 50, both incidence and mortality rates from prostate cancer increase at a near exponential rate (Fig. 80–4). Prostate cancer increases faster with age than any other major cancer, and with an aging population, the impact of prostate cancer will continue to increase in the future. The probability of developing prostate cancer is less than 1 in 10,000 in men aged less than 39 years, 1 in 103 for men aged 40 to 59 years, and 1 in 8 for men 60 to 79 years (Wingo et al, 1995).

Family History

Several studies have suggested that the incidence of prostate cancer in male relatives of prostate cancer patients is increased (Spitz et al, 1991; Carter et al, 1992, 1993). A form of early-onset prostate cancer may be inherited in an autosomal dominant fashion of a rare high-risk allele, accounting for approximately 9% of all prostate cancers and 45% of cases in men younger than 55 years of age (Carter et al, 1992). **The risk of a man's developing prostate cancer depends on the age of onset of prostate cancer and the number of affected relatives** (Table 80–2) (Carter et al, 1993). The father or brother of a proband diagnosed with prostate cancer at age 50 years with an additional first-degree relative affected carries a relative risk of 7.0 for developing prostate cancer as compared to a brother or father

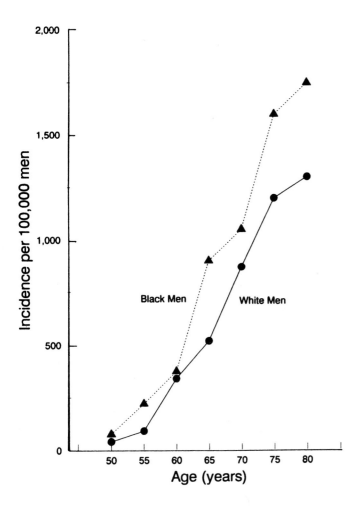

Figure 80–4. Incidence rates by age and race for invasive prostate cancer. Rates are shown for the tricounty metropolitan Detroit area as measured by the Surveillance, Epidemiology, and End Results (SEER) program (NO1-CN-05225). Rates are per 100,000 and are age-adjusted to the 1970 U.S. standard population. (From Pienta KJ, Esper PS: Ann Intern Med 1993; 118:793–803.)

of a proband diagnosed at age 70 years with no additional affected relatives (Carter et al, 1993). Investigators at Johns Hopkins have subdivided patients into three groups: hereditary, familial, and sporadic. The hereditary group is defined as (1) a cluster of three or more affected relatives within any nuclear family, (2) the occurrence of prostate cancer in each of three generations in the proband's paternal or maternal lineage, or (3) a cluster of two relatives affected at 55

Table 80–2. FAMILY HISTORY AND RISK OF PROSTATE CANCER

Age of Onset, Years	Additional Relatives	Relative Risk
70	None	1.0
60	None	1.5
50	None	2.0
70	1 or more	4.0
60	1 or more	5.0
50	1 or more	7.0

Adapted from Carter BS, Bova GS, Beaty TH, et al: J Urol 1993; 150:797–802.

years old or less. A recent study has provided the first convincing evidence for a major susceptibility locus on chromosome 1. This study of 91 families from North America and Sweden demonstrated significant linkage to the long arm of chromosome 1 (1q24–25). Allowing for heterogeneity, the multipoint lod score reached 5.43. Approximately 30% to 40% of hereditary cases may be caused by this mutation (Smith et al, 1996).

Race

There is a wide variation in the reported incidence of clinical prostate cancer between different ethnic groups. It is clear from both incidence and mortality data that the incidence of clinical prostate cancer is low in Oriental men and higher in Scandinavian men (Pienta and Esper, 1993). **Black men living in the United States have a higher incidence rate of clinical prostate cancer than white men** of similar education and socioeconomic classes (Baquet et al, 1991). The age-adjusted invasive prostate cancer incidence rates in the tri-county metropolitan Detroit area, as measured by the Surveillance, Epidemiology, and End Results program database in 1990, demonstrated a 30% greater incidence among black compared with white men, continuing a trend observed over the last several years (Demers et al, 1994). Black men have a higher incidence of prostate cancer at all ages (see Fig. 80–4). Furthermore, **black men are routinely diagnosed with later stage disease, and survival rates, even when corrected for stage, are uniformly lower for black men.** The 5-year survival rates for all stages of prostate cancer are 62% for black men and 72% for white men.

Probable Risk Factors

Dietary Fat

The idea that the risk of prostate cancer is enhanced by high intake of fat has been the subject of many studies and much heated debate; however, **dietary fat appears to stand out as an important risk factor** (Kolonel et al, 1983; West et al, 1991; Giovannucci et al, 1993; Whittemore et al, 1995). It has been hypothesized that dietary patterns could alter the production of sexual hormones and affect the risk of cancer within the prostate gland. This hypothesis has implications not only for the intake of dietary fat, but also for the fat-soluble vitamins, such as vitamins A, D, and E, as well as associated trace nutrients, such as zinc. Studies have revealed differences between the fat content of diets in high-risk and low-risk areas, and it has been found that prostate cancer deaths from 32 countries were highly correlated with total fat consumption, a finding similar to that for breast cancer (Armstrong and Doll, 1975; Rose et al, 1986). **The diet of Japanese men, for example, has much less fat content than that of U.S. men; as the fat content of the Japanese diet has increased toward westernized levels, the incidence of prostate cancer in Japan has started to rise.** Japanese men who move to the United States, furthermore, carry a risk of developing prostate cancer that is intermediate between the low risk in Japan and the high risk in the United States (Shimizu et al, 1991).

Hormones

The prostate is an androgen-dependent organ. **Testosterone is necessary for normal prostate epithelium to grow, and early prostate cancer has been shown to be endocrine dependent** (Montie and Pienta, 1994). The interaction of steroid hormones with the development of prostate cancer is poorly understood; however, a low-fat, high-fiber diet has been shown to affect male sex hormone metabolism by decreasing circulating testosterone (Adlercreutz, 1990). It has been suggested that altered hormone metabolism may play a role in the progression of prostate cancer from histologic to clinically significant form (Hamalainen et al, 1984). Higher circulating levels of testosterone in prostate cancer patients have not been consistently observed, however, and other hormones, especially prolactin and estrogen, may play an undefined role in prostate metabolism (Wynder et al, 1984). It has been demonstrated that young black men have serum testosterone levels that are approximately 15% higher than their white counterparts, and this difference may be enough to explain the increased risk of prostate cancer in black men (Ross et al, 1986). In a related study comparing American and Japanese men, American men had different levels of testosterone metabolizing enzymes than their Japanese counterparts (Ross et al, 1992). Clearly, hormones play an important role in normal and cancerous prostate physiology; however, their relationship to prostate cancer risk is still undefined.

Potential Risk Factors

Vasectomy

Several large retrospective and prospective studies have suggested that vasectomy may increase the risk of prostate cancer 1.2-fold to 2-fold, especially if vasectomy was performed at a young age (<35 years old) (Giovannucci et al, 1993a, 1993b; Hayes et al., 1993). These findings, however, have been vigorously debated. First, there are few plausible biologic explanations for this relationship (Howards, 1993). Second, the methodology of the published studies has been seriously questioned (DerSimonian et al, 1993). Third, several other studies have not demonstrated a link between prostate cancer and prior vasectomy (Sidney, 1987; Rosenberg et al, 1994). Notably a case-control study of 1642 cancer patients and 1636 control subjects revealed no increased prostate cancer risk associated with vasectomy (John et al, 1995). **If vasectomy is associated with an increased risk of prostate cancer, the risk appears to be low.**

Cadmium

Cadmium is a trace mineral found in cigarette smoke and alkaline batteries. People working in the welding and electroplating occupations are exposed to high levels of cadmium. **Several studies have demonstrated a weak association between cadmium exposure and prostate cancer risk** (Kipling and Waterhouse, 1967; Lemen et al, 1976; Elghany et al, 1990). It has been suggested that cadmium increases the risk of prostate cancer by interacting with zinc, a necessary trace element in multiple intracellular metabolic pathways of which the prostate contains high amounts (Kerr et al, 1960).

Vitamin A

Vitamin A or retinol is a fat-soluble vitamin that is essential for normal differentiation of epithelial cells, physiologic growth, visual function, and reproduction. Vitamin A deficiency has been related to the development of several different tumors in experimental model systems, and supplementary retinoids have decreased the number of experimentally induced prostate cancers in animal studies (Pienta et al, 1993). Several studies have reported an increased risk of prostate cancer with increased vitamin A intake, whereas other studies have contradicted these results (Hirayama, 1979; Kolonel et al, 1987; Ohno et al, 1988; Mettlin et al, 1989; Mills et al, 1989). In Japan and other low-risk areas, the major source of vitamin A is from vegetables, whereas the major source of vitamin A in high-risk areas such as the United States appears to be from animal fat. Therefore, **the risk of prostate cancer associated with vitamin A intake may actually be a reflection of the higher risk associated with high animal fat intake.**

Vitamin D

It has been demonstrated that prostate cancer is more common in Northern countries as compared with those closer to the equator (Hanchette and Schwartz, 1992). **Prostate cancer mortality rates in the United States are inversely proportional to ultraviolet radiation, which is necessary for the synthesis of vitamin D** (Skowronski et al, 1995). In the laboratory, vitamin D has been demonstrated to induce differentiation as well as to slow the growth of prostate cancer cells. Further studies are being undertaken to determine the association between vitamin D and the risk of developing prostate cancer.

PREVENTION STRATEGIES

An understanding of the steps involved in malignant transformation as well as the factors identified through epidemiologic and laboratory studies that may influence these steps allows the application of prevention strategies, many of which are already in use.

Screening Strategies

Few screening strategies to detect cancer have been clearly shown to be beneficial, and detection of prostate cancer is no exception. **Prostate cancer screening has continued to grow in popularity, fueled by the belief that detection of the cancer early through digital rectal examination or PSA leads to the identification of organ-confined, curable tumors** (Scardino, 1989). To date, no trial has been completed to determine whether screening for prostate cancer saves lives. Eventually, data from screening programs such as Prostate Cancer Awareness Week should identify the utility and value of prostate cancer screening programs. Currently the American Cancer Society and the American

Urological Association recommend digital rectal examination and a PSA blood test annually starting at age 50.

Avoidance of Risk Factors

Although avoidance of known risk factors, such as smoking for lung cancer, is clearly desirable and a method to decrease incidence and mortality from a given disease, this strategy cannot be currently employed for prostate cancer. The known risk factors of age, race, and family history cannot be avoided. Avoidance of potential risk factors may be possible. For example, men could decrease fat intake in the diet if this factor is proven to be true a risk factor for the development of carcinoma of the prostate.

Chemoprevention

Chemoprevention agents can be classified into several major types based on their presumed mode of intervention and include inhibitors of initiation, antipromotional agents, and inhibitors of progression (Boone et al, 1990). **Because of the long period over which prostate cancer appears to develop, the chemoprevention or chemosuppression of prostate cancer growth appears to be a real possibility.** Finasteride (Proscar), an agent that inhibits the conversion of testosterone to its prostatic active metabolite dihydrotestosterone, is now in active clinical trials (Brawley and Thompson, 1994). Finasteride, in theory, could interfere with the promotional effects of testosterone on prostate cells. Other agents, such as the retinoids, are under development as differentiation and antiprogression agents (Pollard et al, 1991).

SUMMARY

After the age of 50, both the incidence and the mortality rates from prostate cancer rise almost exponentially. In 1986, the average life expectancy of the an American white man aged 65 years was 14.8 years; at age 70, 11.7 years; at age 75, 9.1 years; and at age 80, 6.9 years. The median survival for white men aged 65 to 69 diagnosed with local prostate cancer is 9.6 years and for men aged 75 to 79, 5.3 years (Pienta et al, 1995). **Prostate cancer, the second leading cause of cancer death in men after lung cancer, shortens life expectancy dramatically.** Prostate cancer develops as a result of an interplay of genetic and epigenetic factors. Understanding of how these factors interact within the prostate will allow the investigation of prevention strategies for prostate cancer as well as help define who will benefit from treatment (Scardino et al, 1992).

REFERENCES

Carter HB, Coffey DS: The prostate: An increasing medical problem. Prostate 1990; 16:39–48.
Wingo PA, Tong T, Bolden S: Cancer statistics, 1995. Cancer J Clin 1995; 45:8–31.

Etiology

Carter HB, Coffey DS: The prostate: An increasing medical problem. Prostate 1990; 16:39–48.
Wingo PA, Tong T, Bolden S: Cancer statistics, 1995. Cancer J Clin 1995; 45:8–31.

Cell Kinetics

Berges RR, Vukanovic J, Epstein JI, et al: Implication of cell kinetic changes during the progression of human prostate cancer. Clin Cancer Res 1995; 1:473–480.

Germ Line Mutations

Carter BS, Beaty TH, Steinberg GD, et al: Mendelian inheritance of familial prostate cancer. Proc Natl Acad Sci 1992; 89:3367–3371.
Irvine RA, Yu MC, Ross RK, Coetzee GA: The CAG and GGC microsatellites of the androgen receptor gene are in linkage disequilibrium in men with prostate cancer. Cancer Res 1995; 55:1937–1940.
Smith JR, Freije D, Carpten JD, et al: Major susceptibility locus for prostate cancer on chromosome 1, suggested by a genome-wide search. Science 1996; 274:1371–1374.

DNA Methylation

Isaacs WB, Bova GS, Morton RA, et al: Molecular genetics and chromosomal alterations in prostate cancer. Cancer 1995; 75:2004–2012.
Lee WH, Morton RA, Epstein JI, et al: Cytidine methylation of regulatory sequences near the pi class glutathione S-transferase gene accompanies human prostatic carcinogenesis. Proc Natl Acad Sci USA 1994; 91:11733–11737.

Tumor Suppressor Genes and Oncogenes

Anwar K, Nakakuki K, Shiraishi T, et al: Presence of ras oncogene mutations and human papilloma virus DNA in human prostate carcinoma. Cancer Res 1992; 52:5991–5996.
Bookstein R, Rio P, Madreperla S, et al: Promoter deletion and loss of retinoblastoma gene expression in human prostate carcinoma. Proc Natl Acad Sci USA 1990; 87:7762–7767.
Dong JT, Lamb PW, Rinker-Schaeffer CW, et al: KAI1, a metastasis suppressor gene for prostate cancer on human chromosome 11p11.2. Science 1995; 268:884–886.
Isaacs WB, Bova GS, Morton RA, et al: Molecular genetics and chromosomal alterations in prostate cancer. Cancer 1995; 75:2004–2012.
Macoska JA, Trybus TM, Sakr WA, et al: Fluorescence in situ hybridization analysis of 8p allelic loss and chromosomal instability in human prostate cancer. Cancer Res 1994; 54:3824–3830.
Navone NM, Troncoso P, Pisters LL, et al: p53 protein accumulation and gene mutation in the progression of human prostate carcinoma. J Natl Cancer Inst 1993; 85:1657–1669.
Umbas R, Isaacs WB, Bringuier PP, et al: Decreased E-cadherin expression is associated with poor prognosis in patients with prostate cancer. Cancer Res 1994; 54:3929–3933.

Androgen Receptor Mutations

Cohen P, Peehl DM, Graves HC, Rosenfeld RG: Biological effects of prostate specific antigen as an insulin-like growth factor binding protein-3 protease. J Endocrinol 1994a; 142:407–415.
Taplin ME, Bubley GJ, Shuster TD, et al: Mutation of the androgen-receptor gene in metastatic androgen-independent prostate cancer. N Engl J Med 1995; 332:1393–1398.
Tenniswood MP, Guenette RS, Lakins J, et al: Active cell death in hormone-dependent tissues. Cancer Metast Rev 1992; 11:197–220.
Yan G, Fukabori Y, Nikolaropoulos S, et al: Heparin-binding keratinocyte growth factor is a candidate stromal-to-epithelial-cell andromedin. Mol Endocrinol 1992; 6:2123–2128.

Growth Factors and Epithelial-Stromal Interactions

Cohen DW, Simak R, Fair WR, et al: Expression of transforming growth factor-alpha and the epidermal growth factor receptor in human prostate tissues. J Urol 1994b; 152:2120–2124.
Fudge K, Wang CY, Stearns ME: Immunohistochemistry analysis of plate-

let-derived growth factor A and B chains and platelet-derived growth factor alpha and beta receptor expression in benign prostatic hyperplasia and Gleason-graded human prostate adenocarcinomas. Mod Pathol 1994; 7:549–554.

Gleave M, Hsieh JT, Gao CA, et al: Acceleration of human prostate cancer growth in vivo by factors produced by prostate and bone fibroblasts. Cancer Res 1991; 51:3753–3761.

Hoosein NM, Logothetis CJ, Chung LW: Differential effects of peptide hormones bombesin, vasoactive intestinal polypeptide and somatostatin analog RC-160 on the invasive capacity of human prostatic carcinoma cells. J Urol 1993; 149:1209–1213.

Steiner MS, Zhou ZZ, Tonb DC, Barrack ER: Expression of transforming growth factor-beta 1 in prostate cancer. Endocrinology 1994; 135:2240–2247.

Epidemiology

Descriptive Epidemiology

Boring CC, Squires TS, Tong T: Cancer statistics, 1992. Cancer 1992; 42:19–39.

Demers RY, Swanson GM, Weiss LK, Kau TY: Increasing incidence of cancer of the prostate. Arch Intern Med 1994; 154:1211–1216.

Irvine RA, Yu MC, Ross RK, Coetzee GA: The CAG and GGC microsatellites of the androgen receptor gene are in linkage disequilibrium in men with prostate cancer. Cancer Res 1995; 55:1937–1940.

Potosky AL, Miller BA, Albertsen PC, Kramer BS: The role of increasing detection in the rising incidence of prostate cancer. JAMA 1995; 273:548–552.

Taylor JD, Holmes TM, Swanson GM: Descriptive epidemiology of prostate cancer in metropolitan Detroit. Cancer 1994; 73:1704–1707.

Definitive Risk Factors

Baquet CR, Horm JW, Gibbs T, Greenwald P: Socioeconomic factors and cancer incidence among blacks and whites. J Natl Cancer Inst 1991; 83:551–557.

Carter BS, Beaty TH, Steinberg GD, et al: Mendelian inheritance of familial prostate cancer. Proc Natl Acad Sci 1992; 89:3367–3371.

Carter BS, Bova GS, Beaty TH, et al: Hereditary prostate cancer: Epidemiologic and clinical features. J Urol 1993; 150:797–802.

Demers RY, Swanson GM, Weiss LK, Kau TY: Increasing incidence of cancer of the prostate. Arch Intern Med 1994; 154:1211–1216.

Pienta KJ, Esper PS: Risk factors for prostate cancer. Ann Intern Med 1993; 118:793–803.

Spitz MR, Currier RD, Fueger JJ, et al: Familial patterns of prostate cancer: A case control analysis. J Urol 1991; 146:1305–1307.

Wingo PA, Tong T, Bolden S: Cancer statistics, 1995. Cancer J Clin 1995; 45:8–31.

Probable Risk Factors

Adlercreutz H: Western diet and western diseases: Some hormonal and biochemical mechanisms and associations. Scand J Clin Lab Invest 1990; 50(suppl):3–23.

Armstrong B, Doll R: Environmental factors and cancer incidence and mortality in different countries with special reference to dietary practices. Int J Cancer 1975; 15:617–631.

Giovannucci E, Rimm EB, Colditz GA, et al: A prospective study of dietary fat and prostate cancer. J Natl Cancer Inst 1993; 85:1571–1579.

Hamalainen E, Adlercreutz H, Puska P, Pietinen P: Diet and serum hormones in healthy men. J Steroid Biochem 1984; 20:459–464.

Kolonel LN, Nomura AMY, Hinds MW, et al: Role of diet in cancer incidence in Hawaii. Cancer Res 1983; 43(suppl):2397–2402.

Montie JE, Pienta KJ: A review of the role of androgenic hormones in the pathogenesis of benign prostatic hypertrophy and prostate cancer. Urology 1994; 43:892–899.

Rose DP, Boyar AP, Wynder EL: International comparisons of mortality rates for cancer of the breast, ovary, prostate, and colon, and per capita food consumption. Cancer 1986; 58:2363–2371.

Ross RK, Bernstein L, Judd H, et al: Serum testosterone levels in healthy young black and white men. J Natl Cancer Inst 1986; 76:45–48.

Ross RK, Bernstein L, Lobo RA, et al: 5-alpha-reductase activity and risk of prostate cancer among Japanese and US white and black males. Lancet 1992; 339:887–889.

Shimizu H, Ross RK, Bernstein L, et al: Cancers of the prostate and breast among Japanese and white immigrants in Los Angeles County. Br J Cancer 1991; 63:963–966.

West DW, Slattery ML, Robison LM, et al: Adult dietary intake and prostate cancer risk in Utah: A case-control study with special emphasis on aggressive tumors. Cancer Causes Cont 1991; 2:84–94.

Whittemore AS, Kolonel LN, Wu AH, et al: Prostate cancer in relation to diet, physical activity, and body size in blacks, whites, and Asians in the United States and Canada. J Natl Cancer Inst 1995; 87:652–661.

Wynder EL, Laakso K, Sotarauta M, Rose DP: Metabolic epidemiology of prostatic cancer. Prostate 1984; 5:47–53.

Potential Risk Factors

DerSimonian R, Clemens J, Spirtas R, Perlman J: Vasectomy and prostate cancer risk: Methodological review of the evidence. J Clin Epidemiol 1993; 46:163–172.

Elghany NA, Schumacher MC, Slattery ML, et al: Occupation, cadmium exposure, and prostate cancer. Epidemiology 1990; 1:107–115.

Giovannucci E, Ascherio A, Rimm EB, et al: A prospective cohort study of vasectomy and prostate cancer in US men. JAMA 1993a; 269:873–877.

Giovannucci E, Tosteson TD, Speizer FE, et al: A retrospective cohort study of vasectomy and prostate cancer in US men. JAMA 1993b; 269:878–882.

Hanchette CL, Schwartz GG: Geographic patterns of prostate cancer: Evidence for a protective effect of ultraviolet radiation. Cancer 1992; 70:2861–2869.

Hayes RB, Pottern LM, Greenberg R, et al: Vasectomy and prostate cancer in US blacks and whites. Am J Epidemiol 1993; 137:263–269.

Hirayama T: Epidemiology of prostate cancer with special reference to the role of diet. Natl Canc Inst Monogr 1979; 53:149–155.

Howards SS: Possible biologic mechanisms for a relationship between vasectomy and prostatic cancer. Eur J Cancer 1993; 29A:1060–1062.

John EM, Whittemore AS, Wu AH, et al: Vasectomy and prostate cancer: Results from a multiethnic case-control study. J Natl Cancer Inst 1995; 87:662–669.

Kerr WK, Keresteci AG, Mayoh H: The distribution of zinc within the human prostate. Cancer 1960; 13:550–554.

Kipling MD, Waterhouse JAH: Cadmium and prostatic carcinoma. Lancet 1967; 1:730–731.

Kolonel LN, Hankin JH, Yoshizawa CN: Vitamin A and prostate cancer in elderly men: Enhancement of risk. Cancer Res 1987; 47:2982–2985.

Lemen RA, Lee JS, Wagoner JK, Blejer HP: Cancer mortality among cadmium production workers. Ann NY Acad Sci 1976; 271:273–279.

Mettlin C, Selenskas S, Natarajan N, Huben R: Beta-carotene and animal fats and their relationship to prostate cancer risk: A case-control study. Cancer 1989; 64:605–612.

Mills PK, Beeson WL, Phillips RL, Fraser GE: Cohort study of diet, lifestyle, and prostate cancer in Adventist men. Cancer 1989; 64:598–604.

Ohno Y, Yoshida O, Oishi K, et al: Dietary beta-carotene and cancer of the prostate: A case-control study in Kyoto, Japan. Cancer Res 1988; 48:1331–1336.

Pienta KJ, Nguyen NM, Lehr JE: Treatment of low volume prostate cancer in the rat with the synthetic retinoid fenretinide (4HPR). Cancer Res 1993; 53:224–226.

Rosenberg L, Palmer JR, Zauber AG, et al: The relation of vasectomy to the risk of cancer. Am J Epidemiol 1994; 140:431–438.

Sidney S: Vasectomy and the risk of prostatic cancer and benign prostatic hypertrophy. J Urol 1987; 138:795–797.

Skowronski RJ, Peehl DM, Feldman D: Actions of vitamin D3 analogs on human prostate cancer cell lines: Comparison with 1,25-dihydroxyvitamin D3. Endocrinology 1995; 136:20–26.

Prevention Strategies

Boone CW, Kelloff GJ, Malone WF: Identification of candidate cancer chemopreventive agents and their evaluation in animal models and human clinical trials. Cancer Res 1990; 50:2–9.

Brawley OW, Thompson IM: Chemoprevention of prostate cancer. Urology 1994; 43:594–599.

Pollard M, Luckert PH, Sporn MB: Prevention of primary prostate cancer by n-4-hydroxyphenyl retinamide. Cancer Res 1991; 51:3610–3611.

Scardino PT: Early detection of prostate cancer. Urol Clin North Am 1989; 16:635–655.

Summary

Pienta KJ, Demers R, Hoff M, et al: Effect of age and race on the survival of men with prostate cancer in the metropolitan Detroit tricounty area, 1973 to 1987. Urology 1995; 45:93–101.

Scardino PT, Weaver R, Hudson MA: Early detection of prostate cancer. Human Pathol 1992; 23:211–222.

81
PATHOLOGY OF ADENOCARCINOMA OF THE PROSTATE

Jonathan I. Epstein, M.D.

The role of the pathologist in assessing adenocarcinomas of the prostate has assumed greater importance over the last few years. The availability of postoperative serum prostate-specific antigen (PSA) levels as a sensitive indicator of progression following surgery has provided the impetus to correlate pathologic findings with progression following radical prostatectomy. The second major role pathologists play is in the diagnosis of adenocarcinoma of the prostate. With the advent of the thin needle biopsy gun and screening with serum PSA, there has been a dramatic increase in the number of needle biopsies performed to rule out adenocarcinoma of the prostate. With these samples, pathologists are challenged to make diagnoses on limited tissue as well as to accurately grade and quantify tumor.

This chapter covers the pathology of adenocarcinoma of the prostate from its precursor lesions to invasive carcinomas, from needle biopsies to radical prostatectomies. In particular, practical points of pathology that are critical for urologists to know for the management of patients are emphasized.

PROSTATIC INTRAEPITHELIAL NEOPLASIA

Prostatic intraepithelial neoplasia (PIN) consists of architecturally benign prostatic acini or ducts lined by cytologically atypical cells. Initially, this lesion was termed *intraductal dysplasia,* with PIN1 equal to mild dysplasia, PIN2 equal to moderate dysplasia, and PIN3 equal to severe dysplasia (McNeal and Bostwick, 1986). Most authorities use the term

high-grade PIN to encompass both PIN2 and PIN3 and *low-grade PIN* for PIN1 (Fig. 81–1).

Low-grade PIN should not be commented on in diagnostic reports. First, pathologists cannot reproducibly distinguish between low-grade PIN and benign prostate tissue (Epstein et al, 1995). Second, when low-grade PIN is diagnosed on needle biopsy, these patients are at no greater risk of having carcinoma on repeat biopsy (Brawer et al, 1991; Stahl et al, 1994). There are two reasons why PIN2 and PIN3 should be combined as high-grade PIN. First, there is

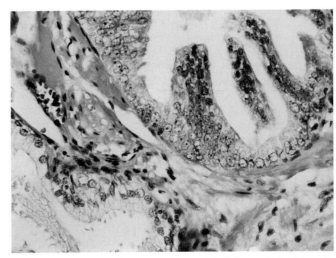

Figure 81–1. High-grade prostatic intraepithelial neoplasia. Note the cytologically atypical cells with prominent nucleoli in the architecturally benign gland, contrasted to benign gland *(lower left).*

much interobserver variability in the distinction between PIN2 and PIN3 (Epstein, 1995). The other reason is that the finding of either PIN2 or PIN3 on needle biopsy is associated with the same risk of carcinoma on subsequent biopsy (Weinstein and Epstein, 1993).

In prostates with carcinoma, there is an increase in the size and number of high-grade PIN foci as compared with prostates without carcinoma. Also, with increasing amounts of high-grade PIN, there are a greater number of multifocal carcinomas (McNeal and Bostwick, 1986; Epstein, 1994). Several studies have also noted an increase of high-grade PIN in the peripheral zone of the prostate, corresponding to the site of origin for most adenocarcinomas of the prostate. There is a growing body of data demonstrating that the expression of various biomarkers in high-grade PIN are either (1) the same in high-grade PIN and carcinoma, as opposed to benign prostate tissue, or (2) intermediate between benign tissue and carcinoma. All of the above-mentioned findings are expected if high-grade PIN is a precursor lesion to carcinoma of the prostate (Epstein, 1994).

High-grade PIN is most critical when found on needle biopsy. In a consecutive series of sextant biopsies performed at Johns Hopkins Hospital, the incidence of high-grade PIN without carcinoma on needle biopsy material was 2%. **When high-grade PIN is found on needle biopsy, there is a 30% to 50% risk of finding carcinoma on subsequent biopsies** (Brawer et al, 1991; Shinohara et al, 1993; Weinstein and Epstein, 1993; Davidson et al, 1994). The presence of an abnormal rectal examination or an abnormal ultrasound scan does not discriminate which patients are more likely to have carcinoma on follow-up biopsies (Weinstein and Epstein, 1993); high-grade PIN may appear indistinguishable from cancer as a hypoechoic lesion (Hamper et al, 1991). In men with high-grade PIN on needle biopsy, the one finding that increases the likelihood that there is an unsampled carcinoma is an elevated serum PSA density (Weinstein and Epstein, 1993); **PIN by itself does not give rise to elevated serum PSA values** (Ronnette et al, 1993). **Repeat biopsy should be performed when high-grade PIN is found on needle biopsy.** The significance of finding high-grade PIN on transurethral resection of the prostate is more controversial because there are no follow-up studies in the literature. Some pathologists recommend that needle biopsies be performed on patients who have high-grade PIN on transurethral resection of the prostate, although others recommend needle biopsies only in younger men (Epstein et al, 1995).

Histologically, PIN can be confused with several benign entities as well as ductal and acinar (ordinary) adenocarcinoma of the prostate. There are also some histologic patterns that to some pathologists are diagnostic of high-grade PIN, yet to others represent high-grade PIN and associated adenocarcinoma (Epstein et al, 1995). Ploidy does not discriminate between high-grade PIN and infiltrating cancer (Baretton et al, 1994).

The one piece of evidence available for premalignant lesions in other organs that is lacking in the prostate is the natural history of high-grade PIN. With the prostate, there is currently no such capability of monitoring a PIN focus to determine whether there is not already infiltrating carcinoma at that site or, when infiltrating carcinoma evolves, whether it has done so in the immediate vicinity of the PIN focus. Because when high-grade PIN is found on biopsy material

we do not know what percentage of patients develop infiltrating carcinoma over a given follow-up interval, most authorities do not use the term *carcinoma in situ of the prostate*. Also, some data raise questions about the relationship of PIN to carcinoma. The majority of prostates with early carcinomas lack any high-grade PIN. Also, when PIN is present in glands with early carcinomas, the PIN is often not adjacent to the carcinoma (Sakr et al, 1993). **It appears that high-grade PIN is a precursor lesion to many peripheral intermediate-grade to high-grade adenocarcinomas of the prostate. PIN need not be present, however, for carcinoma to arise.** Low-grade carcinomas, especially those present within the transition zone, are not closely related to high-grade PIN (Epstein, 1994).

ADENOCARCINOMA

Location

In clinical stage T2 carcinomas and in 85% of non-palpable tumors diagnosed on needle biopsy (stage T1c), the major tumor mass is peripheral in location up against the edge of the prostate (McNeal, 1969; Byar et al, 1972; Epstein et al, 1994b). In the remaining cases, tumors are predominantly located in the transition zone (i.e., periurethrally or anteriorly). Tumors that appear to be unilateral on rectal examination are bilateral in approximately 70% of cases when examined pathologically. **Adenocarcinoma of the prostate is multifocal in more than 85% of cases** (Byar et al, 1972). In many of these cases of bilateral or multifocal tumor, the other tumors are small, low grade, and clinically insignificant.

Spread of Tumor

Although the prostate lacks a discrete histologic capsule, the term *capsular penetration* is a convenient method of describing tumor that has extended out of the prostate into periprostatic soft tissue. Some authors use the term *capsular invasion* when they believe that the capsule is infiltrated by tumor but the tumor does not extend out of the prostate. **Because there is no such entity as the prostatic capsule, the term *capsular invasion* makes no sense.** Peripherally located adenocarcinomas of the prostate tend to extend out of the prostate via perineural space invasion (Villers et al, 1989). **Perineural invasion by itself does not worsen prognosis because perineural invasion merely represents extension of tumor along a plane of decreased resistance and not invasion into lymphatics** (Hassan and Maksem, 1980). Capsular penetration preferentially occurs posteriorly and posterolaterally, paralleling the location of most adenocarcinomas.

Further local spread of tumor may lead to seminal vesicle invasion, which is diagnosed when tumor extends into the muscular wall of the seminal vesicle. The most common route of seminal vesicle invasion is by tumor penetration of the prostatic capsule at the base of the gland with growth and extension into peri–seminal vesicle soft tissue and eventually into the seminal vesicles. Less commonly, there may be direct extension through the ejaculatory ducts into the seminal vesicles or direct extension from the base of the prostate into the wall of the seminal vesicles. Least commonly, there may be discrete metastases to the seminal vesicle, which one study found to have a better prognosis (Ohori et al, 1993). Local spread of prostate cancer may also involve the rectum, where it may be difficult to distinguish from a rectal primary (Fry et al, 1979).

The most frequent sites of metastatic prostate carcinoma are lymph node metastases, followed by bone metastases. Prostate cancer may present with metastases to the left supradiaphragmatic lymph nodes. Lung metastases from prostate carcinoma are extremely common at autopsy, and almost all cases have bone involvement as well (Varkarakis et al, 1974). Metastatic lesions usually take the form of multiple small nodules or diffuse lymphatic spread rather than large metastatic deposits. Clinically, prostate carcinoma metastatic to the lung is usually asymptomatic. Following in frequency after lymph nodes, bones, and lung, the next most common regions of spread of prostate cancer at autopsy are bladder, liver, and adrenal (Saitoh et al, 1984). A not uncommon site of metastatic prostate carcinoma diagnosed premortem is the testis (Haupt et al, 1984).

Tumor Volume

In general, the size of a prostate cancer correlates with its extent (McNeal, 1992). Capsular penetration is uncommon in tumors less than 0.5 ml. Tumors that are less than 4 ml uncommonly reveal lymph node metastases or seminal vesicle invasion. Tumor volume is also proportional to the grade (see later). The location and grade of the tumor also modulate the effect of tumor volume (Christensen et al, 1991; McNeal, 1992). For example, **transition zone tumors in general penetrate the capsule at larger volumes than peripheral zone tumors, as a result of their lower grade and greater distance from the edge of the gland.**

Grade

Although numerous grading systems exist for the evaluation of prostatic adenocarcinoma, the Gleason grading system is the most widely accepted (Gleason et al, 1974). **The Gleason system is based on the glandular pattern of the tumor as identified at relatively low magnification (Fig. 81–2). Cytologic features play no role in the grade of the tumor. Both the primary (predominant) and the secondary (second most prevalent) architectural patterns are identified and assigned a grade from 1 to 5, with 1 the most differentiated and 5 the least differentiated. When Gleason compared his grading system with survival rates, it was noted that in tumors with two distinct tumor patterns the observed number of deaths generally fell in between the number expected based on the primary pattern and that based on the secondary pattern.** Because both the primary and the secondary patterns were influential in predicting prognosis, a Gleason sum resulted, obtained by the addition of the primary and secondary grade. If a tumor had only one histologic pattern, for uniformity the primary and secondary patterns were given the same grade. Gleason sums range from 2 (1 + 1 = 2), which represents tumors uniformly composed of Gleason pattern 1 tumor, to 10 (5 + 5 = 10), which represents totally undifferentiated tumors. Synonyms for Gleason sum are *combined Gleason grade* and *Gleason score*. Pathologists may assign only a Gleason pattern rather than a Gleason sum in cases with limited adenocarcinoma of the prostate on needle biopsy. It should be made perfectly clear by the pathologist, however, that he or she is assigning only a pattern and not a sum. Cases in which the pathologist signs out a case as Gleason grade 4 (i.e., Gleason pattern 4) may be misconstrued as Gleason sum 4. Consequently, the author prefers to assign both a primary and a secondary pattern even when presented with limited cancer so as not to give rise to any confusion.

The other most commonly used system is a three-grade system corresponding to tumors that are well, moderately well, and poorly differentiated. The disadvantage of the 1-to-3 system is that although Gleason sum 2 to 4 might be equated with grade 1 tumor, and Gleason sum 8–10 might be equated with grade 3 tumor, one cannot consider Gleason sum 5 to 7 tumor as grade 2. **Gleason sum 7 tumors have a significantly worse prognosis than Gleason sum 5 to 6 cancers, although they are not as aggressive as Gleason sum 8 to 10 cancers.** Although some tumors with Gleason

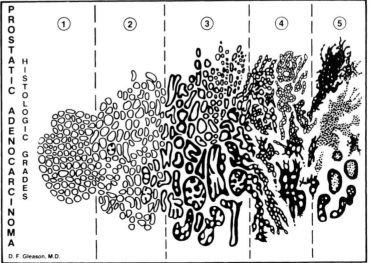

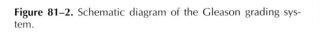

Figure 81–2. Schematic diagram of the Gleason grading system.

score 5 to 6 may be followed conservatively, most urologists treat Gleason sum 7 cancers definitively. Using the 1-to-3 grading scheme, this distinction is lost.

Gleason pattern 1 and pattern 2 tumors are composed of relatively circumscribed nodules of uniform, single, separate, closely packed, medium-sized glands. Some investigators have coined the term *clear cell carcinoma*. The author believes that this term is not necessary because it merely describes low-grade carcinomas, which often have pale cytoplasm. Gleason pattern 3 tumor infiltrates in and among the non-neoplastic prostate, and the glands have marked variation in size and shape with smaller glands than seen in Gleason pattern 1 or 2. Gleason pattern 4 glands are no longer single and separate as seen in patterns 1 to 3. In Gleason pattern 4, one may also see large irregular cribriform glands as opposed to the smoothly circumscribed smaller nodules of cribriform Gleason pattern 3. **It is important to recognize Gleason pattern 4 tumor because tumors with this pattern have a significantly worse prognosis than those with pure Gleason pattern 3** (McNeal et al, 1990a; Epstein et al, 1996). Gleason pattern 5 tumor shows no glandular differentiation, composed of solid sheets, cords, single cells, or solid nests of tumor with central comedonecrosis. A common diagnostic problem is in differentiating on transurethral resection of the prostate between a poorly differentiated transitional cell carcinoma of the bladder and a Gleason pattern 5 prostatic adenocarcinoma. **Because in some cases antisera to PSA is more sensitive in identifying prostatic tumors, and prostate-specific acid phosphatase (PSAP) gives superior results in other cases, both antisera should be used in establishing if the tumor is of prostatic origin.** Even when both PSA and PSAP are employed, the lack of immunoreactivity in a poorly differentiated tumor within the prostate, especially if present in limited amount, does not exclude the diagnosis of a poorly differentiated prostatic adenocarcinoma. With only a few exceptions, immunoperoxidase staining for PSA and PSAP is specific for prostatic tissue (Epstein, 1993).

There is good interobserver and intraobserver reproducibility using the Gleason system, with agreements to within 1 Gleason sum of more than 80% and 90%, respectively (Harada et al, 1977; Bain et al, 1982). One of the most frequent causes of discordant grading is the grading of tumors that straddle two grades. The Gleason grade on biopsy material has also been shown to correlate fairly well with that of the subsequent prostatectomy (Garnett et al, 1984; Mills and Fowler, 1986; Bostwick, 1994; Spires et al, 1994). Undergrading of the needle biopsy is more a problem than overgrading and to some extent is unavoidable because of sampling error. An error, which is frequently avoidable, is to grade the tumor on biopsy as Gleason sum 2 to 4 with the subsequent prostatectomy showing predominantly Gleason pattern 3 tumor resulting in a Gleason sum of 6 (Bostwick, 1994). Gleason sum 2 to 4 should be diagnosed only in approximately 3% of needle biopsy specimens; this incidence correlates well with the incidence of low-grade carcinoma at radical prostatectomy.

The ultimate value of any grading system is its prognostic ability. Both Gleason's data with 2911 patients and subsequent studies with long-term follow-up have demonstrated a good correlation between Gleason sum and prognosis (Gleason et al, 1977; Sogani et al, 1985). When stage of disease is factored in with the grade, prognostication is enhanced (Gleason et al, 1977). The Gleason grade of tumor at radical prostatectomy and the preoperative Gleason grade also correlate with final pathologic stage (Table 81–1) (Oesterling et al, 1987).

No advantage has been demonstrated for grading systems that account for nuclear anaplasia over that of the Gleason system (Gaeta et al, 1986). The measurement of nuclear morphology using a computerized image analysis system, however, enhances prognostication to that provided by the Gleason system (Partin et al, 1992).

After several years, some men with low-grade cancers develop high-grade tumor (Brawn, 1983). It is unclear whether the residual low-grade cancer progressed or whether there was subsequent development of multifocal, more aggressive tumor. Although in general larger tumors are high grade and small tumors low grade, exceptions occur (Epstein et al, 1994a). There is a tendency to hypothesize that tumors begin as low-grade tumors and on reaching a certain size dedifferentiate into higher-grade lesions, accounting for the relationship between size and grade. Alternatively, high-grade tumors may be high grade at their inception yet because of their rapid growth are detected at an advanced size. Similarly, low-grade tumors may evolve so slowly that they tend to be detected at lower volumes.

Needle Biopsy Specimens

Processing

When biopsy specimens are taken from different areas of the prostate, they should be submitted to pathology in separate containers. This way, if the pathologist diagnoses an atypical focus on one core, the urologist can direct sampling at the time of repeat biopsy into the atypical region.

Differential Diagnosis

The underdiagnosis of limited adenocarcinoma of the prostate on needle biopsy is one of the most frequent problems in prostate pathology (Epstein et al, 1995). It is not uncommon to have several needle biopsy cores of prostatic tissue in which there are only a few malignant glands, which may be difficult to diagnose. There are also numerous benign mimickers of adenocarcinoma of the prostate (Epstein et al, 1995). In some of these cases, the use of antibodies to high-molecular-weight cytokeratin may resolve the diagnosis (Wojno and Epstein, 1995; Kahane et al, 1995). Benign glands contain basal cells and are labeled with these antibod-

Table 81–1. CORRELATION OF GLEASON SUM WITH PATHOLOGY AT RADICAL PROSTATECTOMY

Pathology	Gleason Sum			
	5	6	7	8–10
Established capsular penetration	16%	24%	62%	85%
Positive margins	20%	29%	48%	59%
Mean tumor volume	2.2	2.7	5.1	4.0
Seminal vesicle invasion	1%	4%	17%	48%
Lymph node metastases	1%	2%	12%	24%

ies, whereas prostate cancer shows no staining. In certain cases, there are findings suspicious of but not diagnostic of carcinoma. The percent of such atypical cases varies depending on the material and the threshold for diagnosing limited cancer. In a review of sextant biopsies performed at Johns Hopkins, 3.7% of cases were atypical yet not diagnostic of cancers. In a review of several regional community hospitals, the author found that the atypical rate averaged approximately 6%. **Pathologists should sign out atypical cases descriptively as a "focus of atypical glands" rather than use ambiguous terminology such as "atypical hyperplasia."** A comment should be added in the report describing why the focus is suspicious for cancer yet not diagnostic with a recommendation for repeat biopsy. In this way, there is no confusion in the urologist's mind that he or she is dealing with a lesion that is likely to be infiltrating cancer, yet the pathologist is not comfortable establishing the diagnosis. If repeat biopsy is negative, this does not exclude the presence of carcinoma because prostatic needle biopsies are associated with fairly high false-negative rates (Keetch et al, 1994). Numerous cases have been seen in which the first biopsy specimen was called atypical and a repeat biopsy specimen was entirely benign, whereas on review of the initial biopsy specimen, it was diagnostic of cancer. It is incumbent on the pathologist in these cases to have the initial biopsy specimen sent off for consultation or try to resolve the initial biopsy results with ancillary techniques such as immunoperoxidase with antibodies to high-molecular-weight keratin. **Approximately 90% of cases that are initially signed out as atypical can be resolved more definitively following consultation.**

Prognosis

It is important to recognize limited adenocarcinoma of the prostate because there is often no correlation between the amount of cancer seen on the needle biopsy and the amount of tumor present within the prostate. When less than 3 mm of cancer is present on one core and the cancer is not high grade (Gleason score <7), 21% of the radical prostatectomy specimens still have moderate or advanced tumor (Epstein et al, 1994b). Similarly, when there is low-grade tumor (Gleason score 2–4) on needle biopsy, 55% of the prostates contain moderate or advanced tumor (Epstein et al, 1994b). These findings reflect a sampling problem in which more extensive or higher-grade tumor may be missed on the needle biopsy specimen. By combining the needle biopsy grade and serum PSA values (Partin et al, 1993) or the needle biopsy grade, needle tumor volume, and serum PSA density measurements (Epstein et al, 1994b), the extent of tumor within the prostate can be more accurately predicted.

The finding of perineural invasion on needle biopsy is associated with more than a 95% likelihood of finding capsular penetration in the corresponding radical prostatectomy specimen (Bastacky et al, 1993). The finding of extra-prostatic spread on needle biopsy is uncommon.

The performance of ploidy studies on needle biopsy specimens is controversial for several reasons. Arguments against performance of ploidy on needle biopsy specimens include a lack of independent prognostication beyond that of grade, DNA heterogeneity, and whether the results of ploidy would change clinical management (Shankey et al, 1993; Adolfsson, 1994). Support for ploidy being performed on needle biopsy specimens comes from Ross and colleagues, who found ploidy of prostate cancer on needle biopsy specimen was prognostic, independent of grade (Ross et al, 1994).

Transurethral Resection Specimens

Processing

The system that is gaining widespread acceptance is based on the percentage of the specimen involved by tumor, with 5% being the cutoff between stage T1a and T1b (Cantrell et al, 1981). All stage T1b tumors are detected by processing between six and eight cassettes of a transurethral resection specimen. By processing 8 to 10 cassettes, more than 90% of stage T1a lesions are identified (Newman et al, 1982; Murphy et al, 1986; Vollmer, 1986; Rohr, 1987). Depending on the institution, all transurethral resection tissues may be examined in relatively young men (≤65 years), in whom aggressive therapy for stage T1a disease might be pursued.

Differential Diagnosis

One of the most common lesions that may be confused with low-grade adenocarcinoma is adenosis (atypical adenomatous hyperplasia) (Gaudin and Epstein, 1994). In the author's institution, 1.6% of benign transurethral resection specimens and 0.8% of all needle biopsy specimens contain adenosis. It is characteristically found in the transition zone of the prostate, frequently multifocal, and most often as an incidental finding in transurethral resections performed for urinary obstruction. **Although adenosis mimics carcinoma, there is no conclusive evidence suggesting that patients with adenosis have an increased risk of harboring or developing adenocarcinoma of the prostate.**

Prognosis

The prognostic significance of cancer found on transurethral resection is discussed in Chapter 85.

Radical Prostatectomy Specimens

Assessment

Within institutions that are not totally embedding radical prostatectomy specimens, sampling techniques exist that provide accurate pathologic staging (Hall et al, 1992). **Whole mount sectioning of the prostate provides more esthetically pleasing sections for teaching and publications, yet the information obtained using routine sections is identical.** In a minority of cases, routinely processed, thinly sliced sections identify positive margins not identified using thicker slices of tissue that are necessary for whole mount processing.

If the urologist plans on aborting radical prostatectomy when lymph nodes are positive, the pathologist should freeze representative nodes because approximately two thirds of microscopic metastases can be identified with random frozen sections (Epstein et al, 1986). For urologists who perform radical prostatectomy in the face of microscopic metastases for local control, it has been demonstrated that men with Gleason sum less than 8 on needle biopsy specimens have a relatively prolonged interval before distant metastases appear; the pathologist need not examine the nodes at frozen section in these cases because these urologists proceed with surgery even if nodal metastases are found. In patients with combined Gleason grades of 8 to 10 on needle biopsy specimens, it has been shown that if the lymph nodes are involved, these men do not benefit from radical surgery, whereas if the nodes are free of tumor, cure following radical prostatectomy is possible (Sgrignoli et al, 1994). Consequently, in men with Gleason sum 8 to 10 on biopsy specimen, all the nodes are examined at the time of surgery and the urologist aborts the prostatectomy if the nodes are positive. Other features that have correlated with prognosis are the extent of nodal metastases as well as the grade and ploidy of the nodal metastases (Winkler et al, 1988). The author routinely submits all of the tissue removed during lymphadenectomy because the modified lymphadenectomy contains relatively scant tissue, and in 5% of cases with lymph node metastases, the only metastases have been present in a small lymph node, which was unidentifiable grossly (Epstein et al, 1986).

Prognosis

The author updated an evaluation of 721 men (mean follow-up 6.5 years) after radical prostatectomy. Progression was defined as an elevated postoperative serum PSA level, local failure, or distant metastases. **Only 25% of men with seminal vesicle invasion and none with lymph node metastases are free of progression at 10 years following radical prostatectomy** (Epstein, 1996). The presence of capsular penetration and its extent also influence progression (Table 81–2). Pathologists frequently underdiagnose capsular penetration. When tumor penetrates the prostatic gland, it induces a dense desmoplastic response in the periprostatic adipose tissue, where it can be difficult to judge whether the tumor has extended out of the gland or is within the fibrous tissue of the prostate. Posterior, posterolateral, and lateral regions account for 18%, 17%, and 4% of positive margins in the author's material. These sites parallel the location of most stage T2 carcinomas. In particular, these sites are disproportionately involved toward the apex (Stamey et al, 1990; Epstein et al, 1996). **Only approximately 50% of men with positive margins progress after radical prostatectomy (see Table 81–2)** (Epstein et al, 1996). A major source of this discrepancy is that even in cases in which margins histologically appear to be positive, additional tissue removed from the site does not always show tumor (Epstein, 1990). Artifactually positive margins relate to the scant tissue surrounding the prostate, which may easily be disrupted during surgery or the pathologic evaluation of the gland.

In a multivariate analysis, Gleason grade, capsular penetration, and margins of resection were all strong independent predictors of progression (elevated postoperative serum PSA level). A more refined prognostication is not needed for men with Gleason sum 2 to 4 because almost all these men are

Table 81–2. KAPLAN-MEIER ESTIMATES OF RISK OF PROGRESSION WITH NEGATIVE SEMINAL VESICLES AND NEGATIVE LYMPH NODES

Prostatectomy Pathology	5 Years Post-Prostatectomy (%)	10 Years Post-Prostatectomy (%)
Gleason sum 2–4	0	4
Gleason sum 5–6	3	19
Gleason sum 7	25	50
Gleason sum 8–10	43	66
OC	0	17
FCP	10	33
ECP	24	43
MAR −	6	22
MAR +	27	46
Gleason sum 5–6 (OC & MAR −)*	1	8
Gleason sum 5–6 (FCP & MAR ±) or (ECP & MAR −)*	2	23
Gleason sum 5–6 (ECP & MAR +)*	15	28
Gleason sum 7 (OC & MAR −)	3	32
Gleason sum 7 (FCP & MAR ±) or (ECP & MAR −)	17	52
Gleason sum 7 (ECP & MAR +)	50	58

*Excluding tumors with Gleason pattern 4.
OC, Organ confined; FCP, focal capsular penetration; ECP, established capsular penetration; MAR −, margins negative; MAR +, margins positive; MAR ±, margins positive or negative.

cured by surgery (see Table 81–2). Men with Gleason sum 8 to 10 have a poor prognosis following prostatectomy (see Table 81–2), with nodal metastases as the major prognostic determinant. Of cases with negative seminal vesicles and lymph nodes, men with Gleason sum 5 to 7 account for 88% of tumors removed by radical prostatectomy and have an indeterminate prognosis (see Table 81–2). These cases can be stratified into prognostic groups depending on the status of capsular penetration and margins. There are relatively few men with Gleason sum 7 tumor who have been followed to 10 years; it is unclear whether the long-term progression rates seen in Table 81–2 are accurate for this group or whether the greater differences in prognosis seen at 5 years will persist at 10 years.

Tumor volume correlates well with pathologic stage and Gleason grade in clinical stage T2 cancers (McNeal et al, 1990b). **The author found, however, that tumor volume does not independently predict post–radical prostatectomy progression once grade and pathologic stage are accounted for** (Epstein et al, 1993a). **Consequently, it is not essential that tumor volume be calculated for clinical purposes in radical prostatectomy specimens.** Rather, there should be some overall subjective indication of tumor volume to identify cases with minute amount of tumor with an excellent prognosis and those with extensive tumor and a worse prognosis.

The evaluation of ploidy on radical prostatectomy specimens is controversial for the same reasons as is ploidy on needle biopsy specimens, as described previously. The strongest data to support the prognostic importance of ploidy are in patients undergoing radical prostatectomy with pelvic node metastases (Winkler et al, 1988).

Subtypes of Prostate Carcinoma

Mucinous adenocarcinoma of the prostate gland is one of the least common morphologic variants of prostatic carcinoma (Epstein and Lieberman, 1985) (Fig. 81–3A). It has an aggressive biologic behavior and, similar to nonmucinous prostate carcinoma, has a propensity to develop bone metastases and increased serum PSAP and PSA levels with advanced disease.

Even in ordinary adenocarcinomas of the prostate without light microscopic evidence of neuroendocrine differentiation, almost one half show neuroendocrine differentiation when evaluated with immunohistochemistry for multiple neuroendocrine markers (di Santagnese, 1992). Most of these neuroendocrine cells contain serotonin and less frequently contain calcitonin, somatostatin, or human chorionic gonadotropin. The majority of these cases have no evidence of ectopic hormonal secretion clinically. It is controversial whether the extent of neuroendocrine differentiation in ordinary prostate cancer affects prognosis. Small cell carcinomas of the pros-

tate are identical to small cell carcinomas of the lung (Tetu et al, 1987). In approximately 50% of the cases, the tumors are mixed small cell carcinoma and adenocarcinoma of the prostate (Fig. 81–3B). Although most small cell tumors of the prostate lack clinically evident hormone production, they account for the majority of prostatic tumors with clinically evident adrenocorticotropic hormone or antidiuretic hormone production. The average survival of patients with small cell carcinoma of the prostate is less than a year. There is no difference in prognosis between patients with pure small cell carcinomas and those with mixed glandular and small cell carcinomas.

Between 0.4% and 0.8% of prostatic adenocarcinomas arise from prostatic ducts (Epstein and Woodruff, 1986; Christensen et al, 1991). When prostatic duct adenocarcinomas arise in the large primary periurethral prostatic ducts, they may grow as an exophytic lesion into the urethra, most commonly in and around the verumontanum and give rise to either obstructive symptoms or hematuria (Fig. 81–3C). Tumors arising in the more peripheral prostatic ducts may present similar to ordinary (acinar) adenocarcinoma of the prostate. Tumors are often underestimated clinically because rectal examination and serum PSA levels may be normal. Most prostatic duct adenocarcinomas are advanced stage at presentation and have an aggressive course.

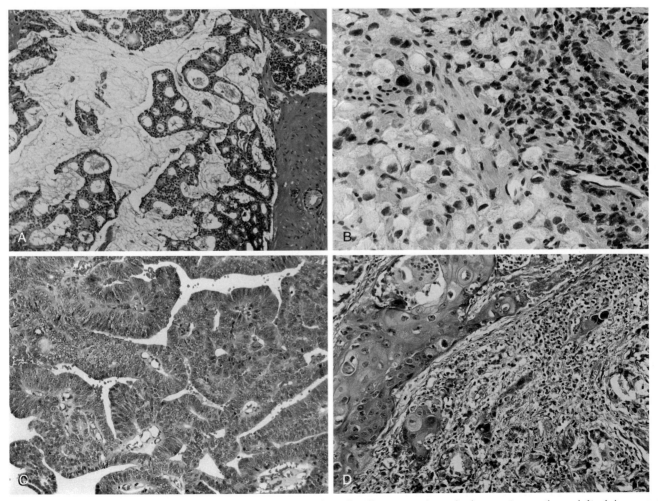

Figure 81–3. *A,* Mucinous adenocarcinoma of the prostate. *B,* Mixed small cell *(upper right)* and adenocarcinoma *(lower left)* of the prostate. *C,* Ductal adenocarcinoma of the prostate. *D,* Adenosquamous carcinoma of the prostate.

Pure primary squamous carcinoma of the prostate is rare and is associated with a poor survival (Little et al, 1993). These tumors develop osteolytic metastases, do not respond to estrogen therapy, and do not develop elevated serum acid phosphatase levels with metastatic disease. More commonly, squamous differentiation occurs in the primary and metastatic deposits of adenocarcinomas that have been treated with estrogen therapy (Fig. 81–3*D*).

Sarcomas of the prostate account for 0.1% to 0.2% of all malignant prostatic tumors. Rhabdomyosarcoma is the most frequent mesenchymal tumor within the prostate and is seen almost exclusively in childhood (see Chapter 74). Leiomyosarcomas are the most common sarcomas involving the prostate in adults (Smith and Dehner, 1972; Christoffersen, 1973; Narayana et al, 1978). There are two benign reactive spindle cell lesions, which may simulate a leiomyosarcoma. One may rarely occur following recent transurethral resection, and the other occurs without a history of transurethral resection (Proppe et al, 1984; Sahin et al, 1991). Carcinosarcomas have also been reported within the prostate and have a dismal prognosis (Lauwers et al, 1993).

Primary prostatic lymphoma without lymph node involvement appears to be much less common than secondary infiltration of the prostate (Bostwick and Mann, 1985). The most common form of leukemic involvement of the prostate is that of chronic lymphocytic leukemia, although monocytic, granulocytic, and lymphoblastic leukemias have also been described in the prostate (Dajai and Burke, 1976).

REFERENCES

Adolfsson J: Prognostic value of deoxyribonucleic acid content in prostate cancer: A review of current results. Int J Cancer 1994; 58:211–216.

Ayala AG, Ro JY, Babaian R, et al: The prostatic capsule: Does it exist? Its importance in the staging and treatment of prostatic carcinoma. Am J Surg Pathol 1989; 13:21–27.

Bain GO, Koch M, Hanson J: Feasibility of grading prostatic carcinomas. Arch Pathol Lab Med 1982; 106:265–267.

Baretton GB, Vogt T, Blasenbreu S, Löhrs U: Comparison of DNA ploidy in prostatic intraepithelial neoplasia and invasive carcinoma of the prostate: An image cytometric study. Hum Pathol 1994; 25:506–513.

Bastacky SI, Walsh PC, Epstein JI: Relationship between perineural tumor invasion on needle biopsy and radical prostatectomy capsular penetration in clinical stage B adenocarcinoma of the prostate. Am J Surg Pathol 1993; 17:336–341.

Bostwick DG: Gleason grading of prostatic needle biopsies: Correlation with grade in 316 matched prostatectomies. Am J Surg Pathol 1994; 18:796–803.

Bostwick DG, Mann RB: Malignant lymphoma involving the prostate: A study of 13 cases. Cancer 1985; 56:2932–2938.

Brawer MK, Bigler SA, Sohlberg OE, et al: Significance of prostatic intraepithelial neoplasia on prostate needle biopsy. Urology 1991; 38:103–107.

Brawn PN: The dedifferentiation of prostate carcinoma. Cancer 1983; 52:246–251.

Byar DP, Mostofi FK, Veterans Administrative Cooperative Urologic Research Groups: Carcinoma of the prostate: Prognostic evaluation of certain pathologic features in 208 radical prostatectomies. Cancer 1972; 30:5–13.

Cantrell BB, DeKlerk DP, Eggleston JC, et al: Pathological factors that influence prognosis in stage A prostatic cancer: The influence of extent versus grade. J Urol 1981; 125:516–520.

Catalona WJ, Stein AJ: Accuracy of frozen section detection of lymph node metastases in prostatic carcinoma. J Urol 1982; 127:460–461.

Christensen WN, Partin AW, Walsh PC, Epstein JI: Pathologic findings in stage A2 prostate cancer: Relation of tumor volume, grade and location to pathologic stage. Cancer 1990; 65:1021–1027.

Christensen WN, Steinberg WN, Walsh PC, Epstein JI: Prostatic duct adenocarcinoma: Findings at radical prostatectomy. Cancer 1991; 67:2118–2124.

Christoffersen J: Leiomyosarcoma of the prostate: 6 new cases and a survey of the literature. Acta Chir Scand 1973; 433(suppl):75–84.

Dajai YF, Burke M: Leukemic infiltration of the prostate: A case study and clinicopathologic review. Cancer 1976; 38:2442–2446.

Davidson D, Bostwick DG, Qian J, et al: Prostatic intraepithelial neoplasia is a risk factor for adenocarcinoma: Predictive accuracy in needle biopsies. J Urol 1995; 154:1295–1299.

di Santagnese PA: Neuroendocrine differentiation in human prostatic carcinoma. Hum Pathol 1992; 23:287–296.

Donahue RE, Mani JH, Whitesel JA, et al: Pelvic lymph node dissection: Guide to patient management in clinically locally confined adenocarcinoma of prostate. Urology 1982; 20:559–565.

Epstein JI: Evaluation of radical prostatectomy capsular margins of resection: The significance of margins designated as negative, closely approaching, and positive. Am J Surg Pathol 1990; 14:626–632.

Epstein JI: PSAP and PSA as immunohistochemical markers. Urol Clin North Am 1993; 20:757–770.

Epstein JI: Prostatic intraepithelial neoplasia. Adv Anat Pathol 1994; 1:123–134.

Epstein JI. Diagnostic criteria of limited adenocarcinoma of the prostate on needle biopsy. Hum Pathol 1995; 26:223–229.

Epstein JI, Carmichael MJ, Partin AW: Small high grade adenocarcinomas of the prostate in radical prostatectomy specimens performed for non-palpable disease: Pathogenic and clinical implications. J Urol 1994a; 151:1587–1592.

Epstein JI, Carmichael M, Partin AW, Walsh PC: Is tumor volume an independent predictor of progression following radical prostatectomy? A multivariate analysis of 185 clinical stage B adenocarcinomas of the prostate with five years follow-up. J Urol 1993a; 149:1478–1481.

Epstein JI, Grignon DJ, Humphrey PA, et al: Interobserver reproducibility in the diagnosis of prostatic intraepithelial neoplasia. Am J Surg Pathol 1995; 19:873–886.

Epstein JI, Lieberman P: Mucinous adenocarcinomas of the prostate gland. Am J Surg Pathol 1985; 9:299–307.

Epstein JI, Oesterling JE, Eggleston JC, Walsh PC: Frozen section detection of lymph node metastases in prostatic carcinoma: Accuracy in grossly uninvolved pelvic lymphadenectomy specimens. J Urol 1986; 136:1234–1237.

Epstein JI, Partin AW, Sauvageot J, Walsh PC: Prediction of progression following radical prostatectomy: A multivariate analysis of 721 men with long-term follow-up. Am J Surg Pathol 1996; 20:286–292.

Epstein JI, Walsh PC, Carmichael M, Brendler CB: Pathological and clinical findings to predict tumor extent of non-palpable (stage T1c) prostate cancer. JAMA 1994b; 271:368–374.

Epstein JI, Woodruff J: Prostatic carcinomas with endometrioid features: A light microscopic and immunohistochemical study of ten cases. Cancer 1986; 57:111–119.

Fry DE, Amin M, Harbrecht PJ: Rectal obstruction secondary to carcinoma of the prostate. Ann Surg 1979; 189:488–492.

Gaeta JF, Englander LC, Murphy GP: Comparative evaluation of the National Prostatic Cancer Treatment Group and Gleason systems for pathologic grading of primary prostatic cancer. Urology 1986; 27:306–308.

Garnett JE, Oyasu R, Grayhack JT: The accuracy of diagnostic biopsy specimens in predicting tumor grades by Gleason's classification of radical prostatectomy specimens. J Urol 1984; 131:690–693.

Gaudin PB, Epstein JI: Adenosis of the prostate: Histologic features in transurethral resection specimens. Am J Surg Pathol 1994; 18:863–870.

Gleason DF, Mellinger GT, Veterans Administration Cooperative Urological Research Group: Prediction of prognosis for prostatic adenocarcinoma by combined histologic grading and clinical staging. J Urol 1974; 111:58–64.

Gleason DF, Veterans Administration Cooperative Urological Research Group: Histologic grading and clinical staging of prostatic carcinoma. *In* Tannenbaum M, ed: Urologic Pathology: The Prostate. Philadelphia, Lea & Febiger, 1977, pp 171–197.

Greene DR, Wheeler TM, Egawa S, et al: A comparison of the morphological features of cancer arising in the transition zone and in the peripheral zone of the prostate. J Urol 1991; 146:1069–1076.

Hall GS, Kramer CE, Epstein JI: Evaluation of radical prostatectomy specimens: A comparative analysis of various sampling methods. Am J Surg Pathol 1992; 16:315–324.

Hamper UM, Sheth S, Walsh PC, et al: Stage B adenocarcinoma of the prostate: Transrectal US and pathologic peripheral zone lesions. Radiology 1991; 180:101–104.

Harada M, Mostofi FK, Corle DK, et al: Preliminary studies of histologic prognosis in cancer of the prostate. Cancer Treat Rep 1977; 61:223–224.

Hassan MO, Maksem J: The prostatic perineural space and its relation to tumor spread. Am J Surg Pathol 1980; 4:143–148.

Haupt HM, Mann RB, Trump DL, Abeloff MD: Metastatic carcinoma involving the testis: Clinical and pathologic distinction from primary testicular neoplasms. Cancer 1984; 54:709–714.

Kahane H, Sharp JW, Shuman GB, et al: Utilization of high molecular weight cytokeratin on prostate needle biopsies in an independent laboratory. Urology 1995; 45:981–986.

Keetch DW, Catalona WJ, Smith DS: Serial prostatic biopsies in men with persistently elevated serum prostate specific antigen values. J Urol 1994; 151:1571–1574.

Keetch DW, Humphrey P, Stahl D, Smith DS, Catalona WJ: Morphometric analysis and clinical followup of isolated prostatic intraepithelial neoplasia in needle biopsy of the prostate. J Urol 1995; 154:347–351.

Larsen MP, Carter HB, Epstein JI: Can stage A1 tumor extent be predicted by transurethral resection tumor volume, per cent, or grade? A study of 64 stage A1 radical prostatectomies with comparison to prostates removed for stage A2 and B disease. J Urol 1991; 146:1059–1063.

Lauwers GY, Schevchuk M, Armenakas N, Reuter VE: Carcinosarcoma of the prostate. Am J Surg Pathol 1993; 17:342–349.

Lee F, Torp-Pedersen ST, Carroll JT, et al: Use of transrectal ultrasound and prostate-specific antigen in diagnosis of prostatic intra-epithelial neoplasia. Urology 1989; 34(suppl):4–8.

Little NA, Wiener JS, Walther PJ, et al: Squamous cell carcinoma of the prostate: 2 cases of a rare malignancy and review of the literature. J Urol 1993; 149:137–139.

McNeal JE: Origin and development of carcinoma in the prostate. Cancer 1969; 23:24–34.

McNeal JE, Bostwick DG: Intraductal dysplasia: A pre-malignant lesion of the prostate. Hum Pathol 1986; 17:64–71.

McNeal JE, Villers AA, Redwine EA, et al: Histologic differentiation, cancer volume, and pelvic lymph node metastasis in adenocarcinoma of the prostate. Cancer 1990a; 66:1225–1233.

McNeal JE, Villers AA, Redwine EA, et al: Histologic differentiation, cancer volume, and pelvic lymph node metastasis in adenocarcinoma of the prostate. Cancer 1990b; 66:1225–1233.

McNeal JE, Villers A, Redwine EA, et al: Microcarcinoma in the prostate: Its association with duct-acinar dysplasia. Hum Pathol 1991; 22:644–652.

McNeal JE: Cancer volume and site of origin of adenocarcinoma of the prostate: Relationship to local and distant spread. Hum Pathol 1992; 23:258–266.

Mills SE, Fowler JE: Gleason histologic grading of prostatic carcinoma: Correlations between biopsy and prostatectomy specimens. Cancer 1986; 53:346–349.

Murphy WM, Dean PJ, Brasfield JA, Tatum L: Incidental carcinoma of the prostate: How much sampling is adequate? Am J Surg Pathol 1986; 10:170–174.

Narayana AS, Loening S, Weimar GW, Culp DA: Sarcoma of the bladder and prostate. J Urol 1978; 119:72–76.

Newman AJ, Graham MA, Carlton CE, Lieman S: Incidental carcinoma of the prostate at the time of transurethral resection: Importance of evaluating every chip. J Urol 1982; 128:948–950.

Oesterling JE, Brendler CB, Epstein JI, et al: Correlation of clinical stage, serum prostatic acid phosphatase, and pre-operative Gleason grade with final pathologic stage in 275 patients with clinically localized adenocarcinoma of the prostate. J Urol 1987; 138:92–98.

Ohori M, Scardino PT, Lapin SL, et al: The mechanisms and prognostic significance of seminal vesicle involvement by prostate cancer. Am J Surg Pathol 1993; 17:1252–1261.

Partin AW, Steinberg GD, Pitcock RV, et al: Use of nuclear morphometry, Gleason histologic scoring, clinical stage and age to predict disease-free survival among patients with prostate cancer. Cancer 1992; 70:161–168.

Partin AW, Yoo J, Carter HB, et al: The use of prostate specific antigen, clinical stage and Gleason score to predict pathological stage in men with localized prostate cancer. J Urol 1993; 150:110–114.

Proppe KH, Scully RE, Rosai J: Postoperative spindle cell nodules of genitourinary tract resembling sarcoma. Am J Surg Pathol 1984; 8:101–108.

Rohr LR: Incidental adenocarcinoma in transurethral resections of the prostate: Partial versus complete microscopic examination. Am J Surg Pathol 1987; 11:53–58.

Ronnette BM, CarMichael MJ, Carter HB, Epstein JI: Does prostatic intraepithelial neoplasia result in elevated serum prostate specific antigen levels? J Urol 1993; 150:386–389.

Ross JS, Figge H, Bui HX, et al: Prediction of pathologic stage and post-prostatectomy disease recurrence by DNA ploidy analysis of initial prostatic cancer needle biopsy specimens. Cancer 1994; 74:2811–2818.

Sahin AA, Ro JY, El-Naggar AK, et al: Pseudosarcomatous fibromyxoid tumor of the prostate: A case report with immunohistochemical, electron microscopic, and DNA flow cytometric analysis. Am J Clin Pathol 1991; 96:253–258.

Saitoh H, Hida M, Shimbo T, et al: Metastatic patterns of prostatic cancer: Correlation between sites and number of organs involved. Cancer 1984; 54:3078–3084.

Sakr WA, Haas GP, Cassin BF, et al: The frequency of carcinoma and intraepithelial neoplasia of the prostate in young male patients. J Urol 1993; 150:379–385.

Sands ME, Zagars GK, Pollack A, Von Eschenbach AC: Serum prostate-specific antigen, clinical stage, and pathologic grade, and the incidence of nodal metastases in prostate cancer. Urology 1994; 44:215–220.

Sgrignoli AR, Walsh PC, Steinberg GD, et al: Prognostic factors in men with stage D1 prostate cancer: Identification of patients less likely to benefit from radical surgery. J Urol 1994; 152:1077–1081.

Shankey TV, Kallioniemi OP, Koslowski JM, et al: Consensus review of the clinical utility of DNA content cytometry in prostate laser. Cytometry 1993; 14:497–500.

Shinohara K, Aboseif S, Narayan P, et al: Prostatic intraepithelial neoplasia: Its significance and correlation with adenocarcinoma of the prostate. J Urol 1993; 149:263A.

Smith BH, Dehner LP: Sarcoma of the prostate gland. Am J Clin Pathol 1972; 58:43–50.

Smith JA, Seaman JP, Gleidman JB, Middleton RG: Pelvic lymph node metastases from prostate cancer: Influence of tumor grade and stage in 452 consecutive patients. J Urol 1983; 130:290–292.

Sogani PC, Israel A, Lieberman PH, et al: Gleason grading of prostate cancer: A predictor of survival. Urology 1985; 25:223–227.

Spires SE, Cibull ML, Wood DP Jr, et al: Gleason histologic grading in prostatic carcinoma: Correlation of 18-gauge core biopsy with prostatectomy. Arch Pathol Lab Med 1994; 118:705–708.

Stamey TA, Villers AA, McNeal JE, et al: Positive surgical margins at radical prostatectomy: Importance of the apical dissection. J Urol 1990; 143:1166–1173.

Tetu B, Ro JY, Ayala AG, et al: Small cell carcinoma of prostate: Part 1. A clinicopathologic study of 20 cases. Cancer 1987; 59:1803–1809.

Varkarakis MJ, Winterberger AR, Gaeta J, et al: Lung metastases in prostatic carcinoma. Urology 1974; 3:447–452.

Villers AA, McNeal JE, Redwine EA, et al: The role of perineural space invasion in the local spread of prostatic adenocarcinoma. J Urol 1989; 142:763–768.

Vollmer RT: Prostate cancer and chip specimens: Complete versus partial sampling. Hum Pathol 1986; 17:285–290.

Weinstein MH, Epstein JI: Significance of high grade prostatic intraepithelial neoplasia (PIN) on needle biopsy. Hum Pathol 1993; 24:624–629.

Winkler HZ, Rainwater LM, Myers RP, et al: Stage D1 prostatic adenocarcinoma: Significance of nuclear DNA patterns studied by flow cytometry. Mayo Clin Proc 1988; 63:103–112.

Wojno KJ, Epstein JI: The utility of basal cell specific anti-cytokeratin antibody (34 beta E12) in the diagnosis of prostate cancer: A review of 228 cases. Am J Surg Pathol 1995; 19:251–260.

82

ULTRASONOGRAPHY OF THE PROSTATE AND BIOPSY

Michael K. Brawer, M.D.
Michael P. Chetner, M.D.

Transrectal ultrasonography (TRUS) of the prostate has revolutionized the ability to examine this organ. Perhaps more so than in other urologic applications of this imaging modality, ultrasonography of the prostate has served to extend the possibilities of the physical examination. Although there are a myriad of indications for ultrasonography of the prostate, the most common application is the evaluation of a man for the presence of prostatic carcinoma. In this regard, TRUS is most commonly performed in conjunction with prostatic needle biopsy. This rapid, generally well-tolerated procedure with low morbidity, in conjunction with the development of serum assays for prostate-specific antigen (PSA), has resulted in the impressive contemporary change in the manner and stage presentation of men with prostatic carcinoma.

INDICATIONS FOR TRANSRECTAL ULTRASONOGRAPHY

Generally the indication for prostate ultrasonography and biopsy is either an abnormality on digital rectal examination (DRE) or elevation in the serum PSA level. Occasionally, men undergo TRUS owing to symptoms of bladder outlet obstruction or constitutional symptoms suggestive of metastatic prostate carcinoma. TRUS has many other indications, including the evaluation of complicated urinary tract infections, work-up of certain types of infertility, and evaluation of men with unusual pelvic symptoms. These and other applications are described elsewhere in this text.

TRUS provides excellent visualization of the prostate. This, and the ability to direct the biopsy needle precisely into regions of interest or to provide uniform spatial separation of the areas sampled, has resulted in performance of most prostate biopsies under ultrasound guidance today. Indeed, in many settings, this has become the standard of care. TRUS has been demonstrated to identify many nonpalpable malignancies (Lee et al, 1988; Cooner et al, 1990; Mettlin et al, 1994). Few data are available, however, on the comparable yield of digitally directed biopsy versus those under TRUS guidance. Weaver and associates (1991) performed biopsies under both ultrasound and digital guidance in 51 men with palpable prostatic abnormality. They noted carcinoma in nine of the patients on digitally directed biopsy. In contrast, 23 men had carcinoma detected when biopsies were performed under ultrasound guidance. Each of the men who had positive digitally guided biopsy results had carcinoma also detected on the ultrasound-guided procedure. Lippman and colleagues (1992) observed carcinoma on TRUS biopsy in 9% of men with negative digitally guided biopsy results.

APPROACHES TO PROSTATE ULTRASONOGRAPHY

There are many approaches to imaging the prostate using diagnostic ultrasound. These include transabdominal, transperineal, endourethral, and endorectal or transrectal. Both the transabdominal and the transperineal approaches have the advantage of not requiring specialized equipment or patient preparation. Transabdominal ultrasonography also allows for imaging of the other abdominal organs. These approaches are severely limited, however, in their ability to provide useful diagnostic information as compared with the transrectal approach. Therefore, they are rarely used for imaging the prostate, the most common application being the patient without a rectum (i.e., post–abdominal perineal resection). In this instance, a transperineal approach may be the best method of imaging and directing biopsies of the prostate (Lee, 1993).

TRUS is the most widely used method. It allows excellent visualization of the prostate and seminal vesicles and can provide useful information about pathologic processes. Conventional transducers allow for biopsy guidance either transperineally or transrectally. Since the initial reports of TRUS of the prostate by Wild and Reid (1955), there have been substantial technologic advances that improve the diagnostic capabilities of this modality.

INSTRUMENTS FOR PROSTATE ULTRASONOGRAPHY

An organized or systematic approach to imaging the prostate is necessary and requires viewing the gland in both the transverse and the sagittal planes. Advances in transducer technology have allowed biplanar transducers to be developed, and a single probe can now image the gland in both the transverse and the sagittal planes. The single probe can have two perpendicularly positioned transducers or a single transducer that can rotate. Some transrectal probes use an "end-fire" transducer, which provides both a transverse and a sagittal view by rotating the probe through 90 degrees.

Early probes used relatively low-frequency transducers, less than 4 MHz (Resnick et al, 1978; Rifkin et al, 1986; Rifkin, 1987a). These transducers did not provide the sharp imagery of the 5- to 8-MHz transducers used currently in most transrectal probes. These higher-frequency transducers have sharply focused near-field images and improved transverse and sagittal resolution. Optimization of the transducer frequency has intrinsic limitations. Higher-frequency transducers have greater tissue resolution but decreased ability to penetrate distally (anteriorly). In contrast, lower-frequency transducers are able to image the anterior portion of the prostate better but do so with a poorer-quality image. Some manufacturers have developed probes that afford frequency

adjustment; however, these have not been clearly demonstrated to provide improved clinical outcome. Early instrumentation incorporated a water balloon to provide a standoff between the anterior rectal wall; however, in general because of complications associated with these instruments, particularly when biopsy is performed, most sonographers currently employ probes that do not necessitate this. The probe should be covered with a latex condom sheath. To lessen the chance of contamination, the authors incorporated two sheaths: one beneath the biopsy guide and one over the biopsy guide with sonographic gel placed between the two to lessen the likelihood of air-induced artifact. Transducer design also varies among manufacturers. Basically, three modalities are used: radial arrays, in which the transducer rotates 360 degrees; sector arrays, in which there is an oscillation (right-left or cephalad-caudad); and linear arrays, in which a series of piezoelectric crystals are placed in a line, and each crystal fires and then receives in a sequential order. Each of these technologies has advantages and disadvantages.

COLOR DOPPLER

All urologists are aware of the vascularity of the prostate gland and surrounding structures. The neurovascular bundles and dorsal vein complex can be easily identified on TRUS. Flow can be identified in these vessels using color Doppler. Scattered flow can be identified throughout the prostate, but usually the flow patterns cannot distinguish between the various anatomic zones described by McNeal (1981). Cancer has been identified as having increased flow within the lesion or adjacent to the tumor (McNeal, 1981).

This increased blood flow is consistent with the observation that prostate cancer has a twofold increase in microvessel density as compared to benign prostatic tissue (Bigler et al, 1993). The quantitation of microvessel density has been shown to provide a unique indicator of pathologic stage as well as progression in prostatic cancer (Weidner et al, 1993; Brawer et al, 1994; Deering et al, 1994; Hall et al, 1994; Siegal et al, 1995).

Both initial and more recent experience with color flow Doppler of the prostate failed to demonstrate a significant advantage over traditional TRUS in detecting carcinoma (Kelly and Lees, 1993; Rifkin and Sudakoff, 1993). Although increased flow was associated with cancerous lesions on TRUS, both benign prostatic hyperplasia and prostatitis also demonstrated diffusely abnormal flow. Objective parameters such as resistive index and spectral wave form analysis failed to identify specific prostate pathology, although subjectively the authors believed that color flow Doppler may yet prove to be a useful adjunct (Rifkin and Sudakoff, 1993). Kelly and Lee (1993) demonstrated that color flow Doppler increased the positive predictive value of TRUS but at the expense of diminished sensitivity. The exact role of color flow Doppler as an adjunct to standard TRUS is as yet ill defined. It has been demonstrated to enhance detection of residual carcinoma after radical prostatectomy (Smith et al, 1995).

COMPUTER ENHANCEMENT AND THREE-DIMENSIONAL TRANSRECTAL ULTRASOUND AND AUTOMATIC VOLUME ASSESSMENT

Two groups of investigators have used a computer-driven motor during standard TRUS to provide three-dimensional reconstruction of the gland (Sehgal et al, 1992, 1994; Downey et al, 1995). Sehgal and colleagues (1994) used digitized TRUS information and computer post-processing to provide a three-dimensional view of the gland as well as volume determination. This method was accurate and significantly faster than planimetric measurements (Sehgal et al, 1994). The same group has used this method of prostate imaging for interstitial seed irradiation treatment of prostate cancer. They believed the three-dimensional imaging enhanced seed placement during treatment and allowed for uniform dosimetry (Sehgal et al, 1994). Downey and co-workers suggested that three-dimensional TRUS not only allowed for more accurate volume measurements, but also enhanced detection of prostate cancer, with improved sensitivity and specificity (Downey et al, 1995). Chin and co-workers (1995) have also used three-dimensional TRUS to enhance their protocol for cryoablation of the prostate. The authors believed that the three-dimensional TRUS enhanced placement of the cryoprobes and allowed more accurate monitoring of the ice ball as it progressed through the prostate gland (Chin et al, 1995). Aarnink and colleagues reported on an edge detection method to calculate prostate volume automatically (Aarnink et al, 1995). They observed an excellent correlation to volume estimate based on planimetry.

TRUS has revolutionized the urologist's ability to image the prostate. Biopsy guidance in patients suspected of having carcinoma and its use in conjunction with cryotherapy and brachytherapy are well established. Undoubtedly, improvements in instrumentation, and particularly computer image enhancement, will provide further advances.

PATIENT PREPARATION

Informed consent is obtained by the physician. A DRE should be performed before insertion of the probe. The DRE allows for identification of palpable abnormalities in the prostate and allows the clinician to rule out significant rectal pathology, such as a rectal cancer, thrombosed hemorrhoids, proctitis, anal fissures, or other rectal or anal pathology that might preclude the insertion of the endorectal probe.

In general, TRUS of the prostate is extremely well tolerated (Kenny and Brawer, 1989; Torp-Pedersen et al, 1989; Sohlberg et al, 1991; Aus et al, 1993; Collins et al, 1993; Hammerer and Huland, 1994; Resnick and Selzman, 1994; Santucci and Brawer, 1994). **No anesthetic is required even when biopsy is undertaken. The significant complication rate should be less than 1%** (Torp-Pedersen et al, 1991; Sohlberg et al, 1991; Aus et al, 1993; Santucci and Brawer, 1994). Three reports have tabulated the risk (Kenny and Brawer, 1989; Collins et al, 1993; Hammerer and Huland, 1994). Hematuria occurs commonly (14%–58%) as does hematospermia (6%–28%).

For purely diagnostic TRUS, little preparation is necessary. A cleansing enema removes feces and gas from the rectum, which might mechanically interfere with the study. **Prophylactic antibiotics are essential if biopsy is to be performed.** Most urologists recommend an oral fluoroquinolone, administered approximately 2 hours before the procedure (Torp-Pedersen, 1989; Aus et al, 1993; Santucci and Brawer, 1994). The oral antibiotic prophylaxis is continued for 24 to 48 hours after prostate biopsy. In addition, the authors ensure adequate antimicrobial tissue levels by administering an aminoglycoside intramuscularly.

The authors prefer the left lateral decubitus position for TRUS (Santucci and Brawer, 1994). This posture allows for easy insertion of the rectal probe while allowing the patient to relax during the study. The knee-chest position is also applicable, but patients find this uncomfortable for prolonged periods of time. The lithotomy position is occasionally employed because it allows for concomitant abdominal examination and cystoscopy but requires a special table with leg supports and again may be more uncomfortable for the patient.

TRANSRECTAL ULTRASOUND PROCEDURE

After insertion of the transducer, the authors optimize the console settings to provide a uniform midgray image of the normal peripheral zone. This is exceedingly important because the echogenicity of this area serves as the standard by which other areas in the prostate are classified as hypoechoic, isoechoic, or hyperechoic. The procedure is performed initially using transverse imaging and begun at the base of the urinary bladder. Transverse images are then obtained through the seminal vesicles, and care is taken to visualize their insertion into the ejaculatory duct area. Imaging is then carried out rotating the transducer clockwise and counterclockwise to provide optimum imaging of the entire prostate. In general, the largest transverse image of the prostate is visible at approximately the level of the verumontanum, and it is in this area that transverse and anterior-posterior measurements are performed. Transverse images are then carried distally through the apex of the prostate into the urogenital diaphragm.

Following completion of transverse imaging, the biplanar transducer is repositioned or the console setting selected to provide sagittal imaging. Alternatively a sagittal transducer is introduced. Sagittal imaging is begun on the right side of the gland and the transducer is rotated medially through the midsagittal section. Care is taken in the midsagittal plane to measure the prostate if this is part of the procedure. In the sagittal plane, cephalocaudal as well as anterior-posterior dimensioning of the prostate is provided—the latter has been shown to be more reproducible than the anterior-posterior transverse measurement. The left side of the prostate is similarly studied.

Anechoic lesions are classically represented by fluid-filled cysts. Hypoechoic areas are those that result in less reflection of the sound images than the normal peripheral zone. Isoechoic areas have a sonographic appearance indistinguishable from that of the previously selected normal peripheral zone. Finally, hyperechoic lesions (dramatically characterized by calcifications) are those

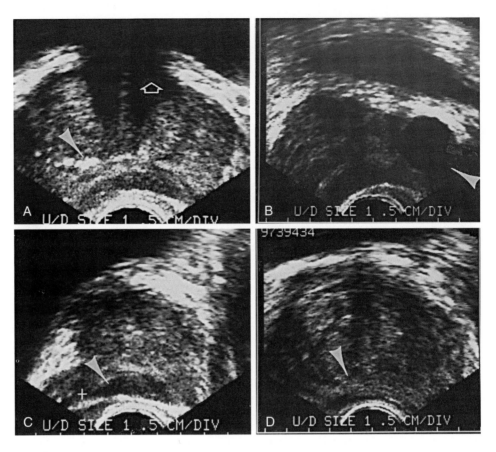

Figure 82–1. Typical sonographic appearance of prostatic lesions. *A,* Transverse transrectal ultrasonography demonstrating calcification at surgical capsule *(arrowhead)* and anterior shadowing *(open arrow)*. *B,* Large intraprostatic cyst *(arrowhead)* demonstrating lack of internal echoes and increased through-transmission (anteriorly). *C,* A hypoechoic peripheral zone lesion *(arrowhead),* which on biopsy revealed a Gleason 3+3 adenocarcinoma. *D,* Transrectal ultrasonography image of a man with extensive benign prostatic hypertrophy demonstrating the heterogeneity of the image in the transition zone and compression of the peripheral zone posteriorly. The subtle demarcation between the peripheral and transition zone (surgical capsule) is illustrated by the arrowhead.

with an acoustic impedance far greater than the normal peripheral zone, resulting in virtually all of the sound energy being reflected. Figure 82–1 demonstrates the appearance of typical prostatic entities.

Throughout imaging, lesions of interest should be thoroughly evaluated by rotating the transducer so that these are shown in the midfield portion of the sound arc. This provides optimal resolution and characterization. During this procedure, adjustment of the console controls may allow refinement of the image.

Because the primary indication for ultrasonography is the evaluation of a man for the potential of prostate cancer, care is taken to search for clues to this diagnosis. **The most important finding is a hypoechoic peripheral zone lesion.** As such, any area within the peripheral zone that is more echopenic than the previously identified normal peripheral zone is considered suspect. **More subtle indications of carcinoma, including bulging or irregularity of the prostatic capsule, extension of hypoechoic areas from the central zone into the seminal vesicle, or any area corresponding to an abnormality on DRE, are carefully evaluated.**

TRANSRECTAL ULTRASOUND BIOPSY

The authors use a modification of the systematic sector approach first described by Hodge and colleagues (1989b). **Biopsies are performed from the base, midgland, and apex of both sides of the prostate** (Fig. 82–2). **If a hypoechoic peripheral zone lesion is noted within one of these**

six sectors, the transducer is positioned so that the biopsy sample will be of the largest possible diameter of the lesion. If no hypoechoic peripheral zone lesion is identified, the biopsy samples are obtained in such a way to maximize the sampling of the peripheral zone in each sector. Owing to compression of the peripheral zone by expansion of the transition zone, laterally placed parasagittal biopsies are performed (Fig. 82–3).

Transition zone biopsies are performed when indicated in a random fashion. Generally two to four biopsy specimens are obtained without regard to echogenicity because no clear pattern of ultrasound has been recognized for transition zone carcinoma. The authors simply insert the biopsy needle through the peripheral zone before "firing" the device. Patients should be cautioned that these biopsies are often associated with greater discomfort.

DETERMINING PROSTATE VOLUME

TRUS estimation of prostate volume is widely employed to calculate PSA density (the quotient of serum PSA divided by the prostate volume) and in planning brachytherapy and cryotherapy. There are two methods for determining prostatic volume (Terris and Stamey, 1987). The first employs a mathematical formula for calculating the volume and assumes the prostate to be ellipsoid, spherical, or a prolate spheroid (Littrup et al, 1991). The formula for determining prostate volume assuming the prostate to be a prolate ellipsoid is: (anterior-posterior diameter) × (transverse diameter) × (sagittal diameter) × π/6 (Terris and Stamey, 1987).

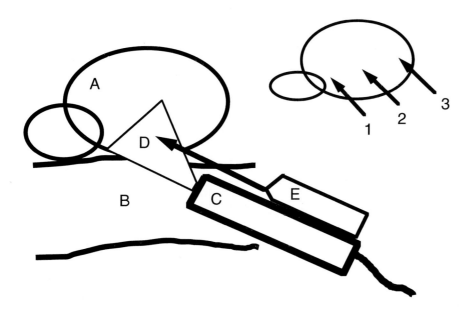

Figure 82–2. Sagittal schematic of ultrasound-guided biopsy: prostate (A), rectal lumen (B), ultrasound probe (C), sound wave (D), and biopsy device (E). *Inset:* Biopsies are directed toward base (1), midgland (2), and apex (3) in systematic sector fashion.

The formula volume calculation assuming the gland to be spherical is: (diameter)^3 × π/6 (Terris and Stamey, 1987). Terris and Stamey (1987) suggested that this formula was most accurate with prostate glands greater than 80 g. The more accurate formula for prostate volume calculation in glands less than 80 g is: (major axis diameter)^2 × minor axis diameter × π/6, that of a prolate spheroid (Terris and Stamey, 1987). Planimetric methods require calculating the cross-sectional area in 2- to 5-mm step sections (using a stepper attachment) along the prostate and then calculating the overall volume (Littrup et al, 1991). This is a slow, arduous process. It is, however, perhaps more accurate than "calculated" estimates (Terris and Stamey, 1987; Littrup et al, 1991).

TRANSRECTAL ULTRASOUND FINDINGS

The ultrasound anatomy is strikingly different in the man less than 40 years of age from that observed in older men. In the young, the central and peripheral zones make up the bulk of the gland. As men age and expansion of the

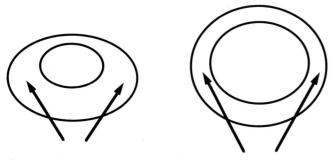

Figure 82–3. Parasagittal direction of biopsy needle to maximize sampling of peripheral zone tissue. *Left,* Normal prostate; *right,* prostate with large transition zone consistent with benign prostatic hypertrophy. Note that expansion of transition zone results in compression of the peripheral zone, particularly in the midline, necessitating more lateral placement of the biopsy needle.

transition zone with benign prostatic hyperplasia occurs, there is compression of the central and particularly the peripheral zone (Watanabe, 1991). In men without benign prostatic hyperplasia, there is a central hypoechoic region that is composed of the periurethral glands, the normal transition zone, and the smooth muscle internal sphincter. This hypoechoic area extends, in the midline, from the bladder neck down to the level of the verumontanum (Watanabe, 1991).

The prostate almost universally enlarges with aging owing to benign prostatic hyperplasia, and this is readily apparent on TRUS (Watanabe, 1991). **With expansion of the transition zone, the central and peripheral zones are compressed.** Zonal demarcation develops, and the surgical capsule (the compressed tissue demarcating the boundary between the benign prostatic hyperplasia adenoma and the normal prostate) becomes evident. Often, punctate calcifications can be identified along the surgical capsule on TRUS and help separate the transition zone from the central and peripheral zones. These echoes correspond to calcification of corpora amylacea. The echogenic pattern of benign prostatic hyperplasia can vary significantly and can range from hyperechoic through isoechoic to hypoechoic in appearance (Rifkin, 1987b). Often, cysts can be identified on TRUS that are usually located centrally, within the transition zone. Their appearance is identical to the ultrasound appearance of cysts elsewhere in the body. They appear hypoechoic with no internal echoes and increased through transmission of the sound resulting in posterior wall enhancement (Hamper et al, 1990).

The echogenic pattern of typical prostatic carcinoma was a widely debated topic (King et al, 1973; Resnick et al, 1977; Rifkin et al, 1986) until **Lee and co-workers clearly demonstrated that the most common appearance for cancer is a hypoechoic peripheral zone lesion** (Lee et al, 1986). Lee's findings countered those of previous investigators who reported that most cancers were hyperechoic. This discrepancy may have been a result of the use of lower-frequency transducers in the earlier studies with their inherent difficulty in lesion resolution.

Although it is widely accepted that most carcinomas are

hypoechoic (see Fig. 82–1), the histologic factors that give rise to this in a malignancy remain unclear. Some investigators (Salo et al, 1987; Miller, 1989; Shinohara et al, 1989) have claimed that hypoechogenicity is related to sound reflection at the interface with the carcinoma and supporting stroma. In this regard, it has been observed by some that the grade of carcinoma correlates with the degree of hypoechogenicity. The decreased echogenicity in higher-grade carcinoma may result from close packing of malignant acini with scant intervening stroma.

The recognition first by Lee and co-workers that hypoechoic peripheral zone lesions were the most common presentation for prostatic carcinoma provided great impetus for the application of TRUS to detecting nonpalpable carcinoma (Lee et al, 1986). In a screening cohort of 784 men, Lee and colleagues noted that TRUS was twice as sensitive as DRE (Lee et al, 1988). It should be noted that half of these men had had a normal DRE within the past year.

A number of investigators have reported on the yield of carcinoma in men undergoing ultrasound-guided biopsies either alone or in conjunction with DRE and serum PSA level. Table 82–1 displays the results of studies of TRUS as the initial test in screening. As is apparent, variability exists with regard to the observed detection rate (1.7%–20.6%) and the positive predictive value (6.8%–58.3%). This high degree of variability suggests that the patient population differed in prostate cancer. Of greater importance, the authors believe these data illustrate the subjectivity of this procedure.

Carter and associates were the first to suggest the relative lack of sensitivity with TRUS when they observed that only 54% of carcinomas identified on the nonclinically suspicious side of the prostate could be visualized with ultrasound in men who underwent radical prostatectomy (Carter et al, 1989). Others have reported similar results, observing that 20% to 40% of prostate cancers are isoechoic or nonvisible on ultrasound (Table 82–2) (Dahnert, 1986; Salo et al, 1987b; Carter et al, 1989; Ellis and Brawer, 1994; Ellis et al, 1994).

The lack of specificity of the classic sonographic findings of carcinoma has been observed by numerous investigators (Lange and Brawer, 1988; Lee et al, 1989a, 1989b; Hammerer et al, 1992; Stilmant and Kuligowska, 1993). Lee and colleagues have shown that hypoechoic peripheral zone

Table 82–2. PREVALENCE OF ISOECHOIC CARCINOMA

Reference	Isoechoic Cancer (%)
Ellis and Brawer, 1994	35
Carter et al, 1989	42
Shinohara et al, 1989	32

lesion on biopsy may reveal **normal prostate, acute or chronic prostatitis, atrophy, prostatic infarct, or prostatic intraepithelial neoplasia** (Lee FL, 1989). Hodge and associates performed ultrasound-guided biopsy using both the directed and the systematic approach in 136 men (Hodge et al, 1989b). Among the 83 cancers detected, only 3 would have been missed if no directed biopsies were performed. The importance of the systematic sector approach as opposed to directed biopsies that sample only areas of abnormality on ultrasound has been confirmed by the authors (Ellis and Brawer, 1994) as well as others (Dahnert et al, 1986; Salo et al, 1987; Carter et al, 1989; Billebaud et al, 1990).

SEATTLE EXPERIENCE WITH TRANSRECTAL ULTRASOUND–GUIDED BIOPSY

Between April 4, 1989, and April 11, 1995, 2197 individuals underwent ultrasound-guided biopsy at the University of Washington or the Seattle VA Medical Center. The procedures were performed by one of three urology attending physicians or senior residents with attending supervision. TRUS was performed with a Bruel & Kjaer 1846 scanner and 7.0-MHz end-fire transducer (Bruel & Kjaer, Marlborough, MA). All biopsies were performed in a systematic sector approach with specimens taken from the base, midgland, and apex of the right and left sides. The 18-gauge Biopty instrument (Bard Urologic, Covington, GA) was used.

Portions of this series have been previously published (Brawer et al, 1992, 1993a, 1993b; Ellis et al, 1994; Ellis and Brawer, 1994, 1995). Indications for ultrasound-guided biopsy included an abnormality on DRE, a PSA greater than 4.0 ng/ml, a 20% annualized increase in serum PSA, men seeking alternative treatment to transurethral resection for symptomatic benign prostatic hyperplasia, and a few men presenting with constitutional symptoms or imaging evidence of advanced prostatic carcinoma without a prior diagnosis.

Each of the six systematic sector needle biopsy samples was submitted separately for pathologic examination. Carcinomas were graded according to the method of Gleason (Gleason and Mellinger, 1974). Biopsy samples demonstrating prostatic intraepithelial neoplasia (Brawer, 1992) or atypia were catalogued as benign.

Using this protocol, 2197 men have undergone biopsy. A total of 304 men have undergone more than one biopsy: 252 men have undergone two biopsies, and 52 have undergone three or more. For this review, each biopsy is tabulated as a separate experience. The ultrasound findings are available from 2036 men. Complete data including results of DRE, a prebiopsy PSA determination from the authors' laboratory,

Table 82–1. RESULTS OF PROSTATE CANCER SCREENING BY TRANSRECTAL ULTRASOUND

Reference	No. of Cancers/No. of Subjects Screened (Detection Rate) (%)	No. of Cancers/No. of Biopsies (Positive Predictive Value) (%)
Catalona et al, 1994	153/1167 (13.1)	153/540 (28)
Cooner et al, 1990	263/1807 (14.6)	263/835 (31.5)
Devonec et al, 1988	42/213 (19.7)	42/132 (31.8)
Fritzsche et al, 1983	41/228 (18.0)	41/121 (33.9)
Hunter et al, 1989	29/508 (5.7)	29/119 (24.4)
Lee et al, 1988	20/748 (2.7)	20/64 (31.3)
McWhorter et al, 1992	7/34 (20.6)	7/12 (58.3)
Mettlin et al, 1994	44/2425 (1.8)	44/290 (15.2)
Perrin et al, 1980	11/666 (1.7)	11/162 (6.8)
Ragde et al, 1989	50/765 (6.5)	50/138 (36.2)
Rifkin et al, 1986	3/112 (2.7)	3/8 (37.5)

Table 82–3. TRANSRECTAL ULTRASOUND BIOPSY YIELD AND PATIENT AGE

Age (Years)	Biopsy	Series (%)	CAP	CAP in Decade (%)	Total Cancer in this Decade (%)
41–50	42	2.0	8	19.0	1.5
51–60	261	12.5	55	21.1	10.6
61–70	978	47.0	230	23.5	44.5
71–80	756	36.3	198	26.2	38.3
81–90	46	2.2	26	56.5	5.0
Total	2083*	100	517	24.8	100

*Patient age not recorded in 114 patients.
CAP, Prostatic carcinoma.

and sonography results are available in 1359. The mean patient age was 66.8 ± 2.3 years.

Carcinoma was detected in 542 of the men undergoing initial biopsy (24.7%). Of the 252 men undergoing a second biopsy, 43 demonstrated carcinoma (17.1%), and among the 52 undergoing more than two procedures, 8 demonstrated cancer (15.4%). Interestingly, the positive biopsy rate has remained essentially constant throughout the authors' experience. After the first 1001 patients underwent this protocol, the authors reported carcinoma in 253 (25.3%) (Ellis et al, 1994). As noted, over the entire biopsy experience, carcinoma has been found in 24.7% of the men. As expected, the positive biopsy rate increased with increasing patient age. Table 82–3 demonstrates the yield per decade.

Table 82–4 demonstrates the biopsies performed and yield for abnormalities in PSA, DRE, and TRUS. **As is apparent, the positive predictive value ranged from 43.8% in men who had abnormality on all three tests to 9.5% in men who had no abnormality.** These latter men generally underwent biopsy owing to a significant change in their PSA level from a prior measurement. Of note, the cancer detection in these latter individuals was greater than among those with an abnormality on DRE. Table 82–4 also demonstrates the increasing yield in the setting of peripheral zone hypoechoism compared with those men without sonographic abnormality. **The reader should note, however, the significant**

Table 82–4. POSITIVE PREDICTIVE VALUE FOR VARIOUS COMBINATIONS OF PROSTATE-SPECIFIC ANTIGEN, DIGITAL RECTAL EXAMINATION, AND TRANSRECTAL ULTRASOUND

PSA*	DRE†	TRUS‡	CAP/Biopsy (%)
Pos	Pos	Pos	218/498 (43.8)
Pos	Pos	Neg	20/110 (18.2)
Pos	Neg	Pos	26/95 (27.4)
Pos	Neg	Neg	20/84 (23.8)
Neg	Pos	Pos	51/369 (13.8)
Neg	Pos	Neg	7/122 (5.7)
Neg	Neg	Pos	7/54 (13.0)
Neg	Neg	Neg	4/42 (9.5)

*PSA >4.0 ng/ml.
†DRE >0.
‡Any hypoechoic peripheral zone lesion (see text for details).
PSA, Prostate-specific antigen; DRE, digital rectal examination; TRUS, transrectal ultrasound; CAP, prostatic carcinoma; Pos, positive; Neg, negative.

number of men without sonographic abnormality that harbored cancer: **51 of 373 (13.7%).** In each combination, an additional abnormal test resulted in enhanced yield of cancer (P<.001 chi square), with the exception of the addition of a sonographic abnormality in men with a normal DRE and a PSA greater than 4.0 ng/ml.

Figure 82–4 demonstrates the receiver operating characteristic curve for each of the three primary diagnostic tests for prostatic carcinoma: DRE, serum PSA, and TRUS. In this depiction of data, a movement of the curve to the upper left or an increase of the area under the curve indicates a superior test. **The best single predictor of carcinoma is the PSA level.**

Figures 82–5 and 82–6 demonstrate the influence of the ultrasound findings within individuals. Figure 82–5 shows that **although 85.6% of the patients with carcinoma had a sonographic abnormality in at least one of the areas revealing cancer, 14.4% had their only cancer found in sonographically normal areas.** Figure 82–6 illustrates the lack of specificity of a normal ultrasound scan on a per-patient basis. Of the men, 75.2% had at least one area of sonographic abnormality. Among these, 70.9% failed to demonstrate carcinoma on biopsy. In contrast, among **the 24.8% of men who had no hypoechoic peripheral zone lesion on ultrasound, almost 15% had cancer.**

The sonographic finding of a hypoechoic peripheral zone lesion demonstrates a sensitivity of carcinoma of 85.5, specificity of 28.4, positive predictive value of 29.0, negative predictive value of 85.2, and overall accuracy of 43.0. These performance characteristics indicate that although most men with carcinoma have at least one area of hypoechoism in the peripheral zone, a significant cohort does not. This underscores the need for obtaining biopsy samples of the normal-appearing peripheral zone (systematic sector approach).

Table 82–5 demonstrates the findings in each of the six sectors. Hypoechoic peripheral zone lesions were more commonly found in the base of the gland, which may reflect difficulty in differentiating the juxtaposition of the ejaculatory duct, the seminal vesicle, and the prostate itself. When a

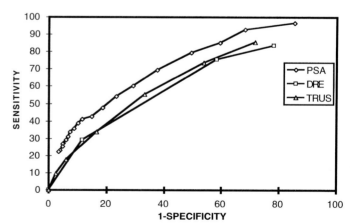

Figure 82–4. Receiver operating characteristic curve comparing transrectal ultrasonography (TRUS), prostate-specific antigen (PSA), and digital rectal examination (DRE). For this analysis, the number of hypoechoic peripheral zone lesions is tabulated from 0 to 6. DRE is graded on the following sale: 0 (normal examination) to 3 (indicating a gland strongly suspicious for malignancy).

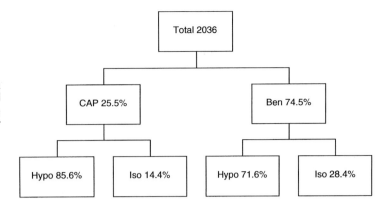

Figure 82–5. Results of Seattle ultrasound-guided biopsy as a reflection of histology. Yield of transrectal ultrasonography–guided pelvic node biopsy by patient. CAP, prostatic carcinoma; BEN, benign; Hypo, hypoechoic peripheral zone lesion; Iso, no hypo-echoic peripheral zone lesion.

sector was hypoechoic as shown, the cancer was slightly more commonly found in the midgland position bilaterally. Sectors that were isoechoic had relatively uniform yields of cancer.

IMPORTANCE OF ISOECHOIC CARCINOMA

Although the authors' findings demonstrate the frequent discovery of carcinoma in sonographically normal prostates, few data exist on the nature of such tumors. The potential pathologic basis of echogenicity has been discussed earlier. Previously the authors have reported findings of surgical staging in 107 men from ultrasound-guided biopsy series (Table 82–6) (Ellis and Brawer, 1994). As is apparent, there is no difference between those 32 men who had only isoe-choic cancers from the 75 who had at least one hypoechoic sector demonstrating cancer in pathologic stage. These observations indicate that a significant proportion of men have their only cancer detected in areas that are normal on ultrasound, and these appear to be of similar malignant potential as classic hypoechoic cancers.

REPEAT TRANSRECTAL ULTRASOUND BIOPSY

One area of ongoing investigation surrounds the determination of who should undergo repeat ultrasound-guided biopsy after an initial negative result. Historical studies with digitally directed biopsy have demonstrated a significant false-negative result of prostate biopsy. Among 639 patients

with initially negative directed biopsy results compiled from six series, carcinoma was eventually diagnosed in 82 (12.8%) (Fortunoff, 1962; Sika and Lindquist, 1963; Bertelsen, 1966; Hoskins and Mellinger, 1966; Zincke et al, 1973; Ostroff et al, 1975).

Three reports on the yield of carcinoma on ultrasound-guided biopsy following negative digitally performed biopsy have been published. The authors observed carcinoma in 11 of 22 (50.0%) patients undergoing ultrasound-guided biopsy following initial negative digitally guided biopsy results (Brawer and Nagle, 1989). Hodge and co-workers noted similar results, with 23 of 42 patients (53.5%) demonstrating carcinoma on negative digitally guided biopsy (Hodge et al, 1989a), and Rifkin observed a 39.3% positive biopsy experience in such patients (Rifkin et al, 1991).

The recognition that the majority of prostate cancers arise in the peripheral zone and the difficulty in evaluating the transition zone have resulted in most biopsies being directed primarily into the former. Stamey and associates described **significant yield of cancer in men undergoing transition zone biopsies** (Stamey et al, 1993). Subsequent to this finding, the Stanford group (Lui et al, 1995) went on to evaluate transition zone biopsies in several clinical scenarios. In one group of 26 men who had a palpable abnormality on DRE and an elevated PSA, 61.5% had positive biopsy specimens of the transition zone; however, in no case were only the transition zone biopsy specimens positive. A second group of 49 men had sonographic abnormalities in the transition zone, and 15 (30.6%) demonstrated positive biopsy specimens, including 2 (13.3%) who had their only cancer found in the transition zone. **The third group included 65 men who had a normal DRE and an elevated PSA. Twenty-**

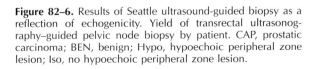
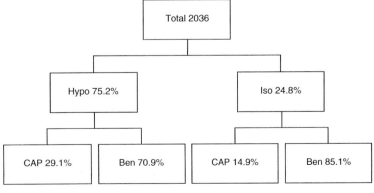

Figure 82–6. Results of Seattle ultrasound-guided biopsy as a reflection of echogenicity. Yield of transrectal ultrasonography–guided pelvic node biopsy by patient. CAP, prostatic carcinoma; BEN, benign; Hypo, hypoechoic peripheral zone lesion; Iso, no hypoechoic peripheral zone lesion.

Table 82–5. SECTOR ECHOGENICITY AND CANCER YIELD

Sector	Hypo (%)	Hypo CAP (%)	Iso CAP (%)	CAP (%)
Rt apex	31.5	17.1	8.0	10.8
Rt mid	28.9	22.6	8.2	12.4
Rt base	44.2	17.4	7.4	11.8
Lt apex	33.2	16.2	8.1	10.8
Lt mid	30.7	23.2	8.7	13.1
Lt base	41.4	20.3	8.8	13.6

Hypo, Hypoechoic peripheral zone lesion; CAP, prostatic carcinoma; Iso, isoechoic sector; Rt, right; Lt, left.

four (36.9%) demonstrated carcinoma in the transition zone, and a third of them (8 men) demonstrated their only cancer in the transition zone. Finally, 47 men who were clinically suspicious of harboring prostate cancer but had no cancer on prior biopsy were examined. Seventeen (36.1%) had cancer, including nine (19.1%) of these demonstrating cancer uniquely in the transition zone. These authors concluded that in select cases transition zone biopsies may be indicated.

General indications for repeat biopsy have included atypia or a lesion suspicious for malignancy but without fulfilling all of the criteria that would allow the pathologist to make a diagnosis of malignancy. Prostatic intraepithelial neoplasia fulfills the majority of the criteria for premalignant condition (Brawer, 1992). The authors have previously described their experience of repeat biopsy in 21 men who had prostatic intraepithelial neoplasia noted on initial prostate needle biopsy specimens (Brawer et al, 1991). **All 10 patients with high-grade prostatic intraepithelial neoplasia had carcinoma on repeat biopsy.** In contrast, only 2 of 11 men (18.2%) with low-grade prostatic intraepithelial neoplasia had cancer on the repeat biopsy. It should be noted that in this series the initial biopsies were directed, sampling only hypoechoic lesions on ultrasound. Garnett and Oyasu (1989) observed carcinoma in **62.5% of men with high-grade prostatic intraepithelial neoplasia when they performed repeat biopsy.** Shephard and colleagues, in an update of their experience from Washington University, noted carcinoma in **24 of 59 men (40.6%) with prostatic intraepithelial neoplasia on initial biopsy** (Shephard et al, 1995).

These latter authors had performed systematic sector biopsies during the initial biopsy procedure. Owing to the juxtaposition of prostatic intraepithelial neoplasia to invasive carcinoma and the frequent association of these two entities, fewer cancers were missed with the systematic sector approach on the initial biopsy. This may explain the decreased rate of carcinoma in this series. In 62.5%, the prostatic intraepithelial neoplasia was ipsilateral to the cancer. In

16.7%, however, it was found contralaterally. In five cases, cancer was bilateral.

The authors have reported on their experience with 100 men undergoing repeat ultrasound-guided biopsy after negative systematic sector biopsy (Table 82–7) (Ellis and Brawer, 1995). Carcinoma was detected in 20 of the patients. Carcinoma was noted in 10 of the 69 patients who had had no evidence of prostatic intraepithelial neoplasia or atypia on the initial biopsy (14.5%), in 5 of 17 (29.4%) who had an initial diagnosis of atypia, and in all 5 with high-grade prostatic intraepithelial neoplasia on initial biopsy. Of note, none of the men with low-grade prostatic intraepithelial neoplasia had carcinoma on repeat biopsy.

TRANSRECTAL ULTRASOUND AND STAGING

Accurate clinical staging of prostate cancer is critical before a treatment decision is made. Clinical stage has an impact on the treatment options, and TRUS can provide additional information beyond that provided by DRE and serum PSA alone. PSA, PSA density, and other modalities as they relate to staging are discussed elsewhere in this text.

It is appropriate that the TRUS study be reviewed with initial attention to the overall shape and symmetry of the gland. A bulky lesion would obviously lead to asymmetry and change the margins of the gland on TRUS (Hamper and Sheth, 1993). **Discontinuity of the capsule as seen on the TRUS image can identify locally extensive disease** (Pontes et al, 1985). Pontes and associates demonstrated TRUS to be highly sensitive in detecting capsular involvement (89%) but were unable to differentiate clearly between capsular penetration and higher stages with extensive localized disease (Pontes et al, 1985). Table 82–8 demonstrates the results of several TRUS-based staging studies. As is readily apparent, there is great variability in the performance reported by these authors, undoubtedly a reflection of different patient selection criteria, variable pathologic analysis, and, perhaps most importantly, the tremendous subjectivity of this approach.

Lee and colleagues described a **trapezoidal area bounded by the apex of the prostate (superior and anterior), the rectal wall (posteriorly), the urethra (inferior and anterior), and the rectourethralis muscle (inferior). With local apical extension, the trapezoidal area identified on TRUS is obliterated** (Lee et al, 1989b).

Tumor volume plays an important role in pathologic stage (McNeal et al, 1980; Dhom, 1983; Scardino et al, 1989). When tumor volume exceeds 3 cm³, invasion beyond the capsule or into the seminal vesicles is common. **Unfortunately, accurate estimation of tumor volume has not been afforded by TRUS, owing to factors such as lack of definition of tumor edge, the infiltrating nature of cancers, and the isoechoic appearance of many tumors. TRUS can accurately identify the neurovascular bundles, but its ability to detect invasion along these bundles is variable** (Hamper et al, 1990). **Hamper and associates were able to detect neurovascular bundle involvement with a sensitivity of 66% and a specificity of 78%** (Hamper et al, 1990). **They concluded that TRUS lacked the**

Table 82–6. PATHOLOGIC STAGE AND ECHOGENICITY

TRUS	OC	C1	C2	C3	D1	Total
Hypoechoic CAP	22 (29)	17 (23)	22 (29)	5 (7)	9 (12)	75 (70)
Isoechoic CAP	14 (44)	5 (16)	8 (25)	1 (3)	4 (13)	32 (30)
Total	36 (34)	22 (21)	30 (28)	13 (12)	13 (12)	107

TRUS, Transrectal ultrasound; OC, organ confined; C1, capsular penetration; C2, positive margin; C3, seminal vesicle extension; D1, pelvic lymph node metastases; CAP, prostatic carcinoma.
Data from Ellis WJ, Brawer MK: J Urol 1994; 152:2304–2307.

Table 82–7. RESULTS OF INITIAL AND SUBSEQUENT BIOPSIES

Initial Biopsy (no.)	Normal	Atypia	PIN I	PIN II	PIN III	CAP	CAP (%)
Normal (69)	52	5	1	1	0	10	14.5
Atypia (17)	10	1	0	1	0	5	29.4
PIN							
Grade I (9)	4	0	5	0	0	0	0
Grade II (3)	0	0	0	0	0	3	100
Grade III (2)	0	0	0	0	0	2	100
Total	66	6	6	2	0	20	20.0

PIN, Prostatic intraepithelial neoplasia; CAP, prostatic carcinoma.
Data from Ellis WJ, Brawer MK: J Urol 1995; 153:1496–1498.

resolution to predict invasion along the neurovascular bundles accurately.

Extension of tumor into the seminal vesicles can also be identified by TRUS. Again, Lee and associates defined the normal anatomy at the junction of the seminal vesicles, the ejaculatory ducts, and the prostate (Lee et al, 1989b). Loss of this normal "beak" formation suggests invasion of cancer.

In general, staging studies have demonstrated understaging more commonly than overstaging when ultrasonography is compared to the radical prostatectomy specimen. Owing to limits of resolution and the realization that the majority of pathologic upstaging is microscopic, the limitation of TRUS is probably to be expected.

Table 82–8. SENSITIVITY AND SPECIFICITY OF TRANSRECTAL ULTRASOUND IN DETECTING EXTRAPROSTATIC SPREAD OF CANCER

Source	Sensitivity (%)	Specificity (%)	Staging
All Sites of Extraprostatic Disease			
Wolf et al, 1992	51	92	Pathologic
Palken et al, 1990	5	100	Pathologic
Rifkin et al, 1990	66	46	Clinical
Andriole et al, 1989	38	90	Pathologic
Salo et al, 1987b	67	97	Pathologic
Scardino et al, 1989	89	76	Pathologic
Hardeman et al, 1989	54	54	Pathologic
Perrapato et al, 1989	71	91	Pathologic
Lee et al, 1985	39	61	Clinical
Seminal Vesicle Involvement			
Wolf et al, 1992	57	100	Pathologic
Palken et al, 1990	5	100	Pathologic
Andriole et al, 1989	20	100	Pathologic
Salo et al, 1987b	29	100	Pathologic
Scardino et al, 1989	92	100	Pathologic
Hardeman et al, 1989	60	89	Pathologic
Pontes et al, 1985	33	100	Pathologic
Lee et al, 1985	31	69	Clinical
Capsular Penetration			
Wolf et al, 1992	51	92	Pathologic
Palken et al, 1990	0	100	Pathologic
Andriole et al, 1989	50	90	Pathologic
Ebert et al, 1991	53	71	Pathologic
Salo et al, 1987b	86	94	Pathologic
Hardeman et al, 1989	54	58	Pathologic
Pontes et al, 1985	59	78	Pathologic
Lee et al, 1985	27	73	Clinical

Data from Santucci RA, Brawer MK: Semin Urol 1994; 12:252–264.

Scardino and associates (1989) as well as Resnick and colleagues (1994) provided evidence critical of the validity of TRUS-based staging. Scardino and associates demonstrated that extraprostatic tumor spread was accurate in only 20% of cases (Scardino et al, 1989). Resnick and colleagues provided evidence of significant inter-observer variability when comparing TRUS studies (Resnick et al, 1994).

TRUS-guided staging biopsies have been suggested by several authors (Hodge et al, 1989a; Lee et al, 1989b). Lee and co-workers recommended staging TRUS-guided biopsies at the apex and at the junction of the prostate with the seminal vesicles (the trapezoid and "beak" areas previously decribed) (Lee et al, 1989b). Hodge and associates performed biopsies in 20 patients with abnormal seminal vesicles on TRUS and identified tumor extension in 14 (70%) (Hodge et al, 1989a). Eighteen percent of the 40 patients with normal seminal vesicles on TRUS, however, were found to have tumor invasion on post–radical prostatectomy pathology (Hodge et al, 1989a). Takayama and associates observed similar positive seminal vesicle biopsy rates but noted no seminal vesicle cancer in 13 radical prostatectomy specimens from men with negative seminal vesicle biopsy specimens (Takayama et al, 1994).

MONITORING THERAPY

TRUS has the ability to provide consistent images of the prostate and is also capable of assessing prostatic volume. These characteristics make TRUS applicable in the follow-up of patients after treatment of prostatic carcinoma.

TRUS has been used in following men after endocrine therapy, radiation therapy, and cryotherapy. In these settings, although some authors have demonstrated a correlation of clinical response and change in TRUS imaging, others have not.

Perhaps the largest experience in post–radical prostatectomy ultrasound and biopsy is that updated by Shinohara and co-workers (1994). These authors performed ultrasound-guided biopsy of the prostatic fossa in 112 men 3 months to 137 months following radical prostatectomy with detectable PSA. They noted carcinoma in 46 patients (41.1%). The most common site of recurrence was at the perianastomotic region.

TRUS has revolutionized the ability to provide imaging and, most importantly, simplified biopsy of the prostate. Its utility in providing useful staging information is doubtful with current instrumentation. Undoubtedly, with technologic advances, applications for this technology will expand.

REFERENCES

Aarnink RG, Huynen AL, Giesen RJB, et al: Automated prostate volume determination with ultrasonographic imaging. J Urol 1995; 153:1549–1554.

Andriole GL, Coplen DE, Mikkelson DJ, et al: Sonographic and pathological staging of patients with clinically localized prostate cancer. J Urol 1989; 142:1259–1261.

Aus G, Hermansson GG, Hugosson J, et al: Transrectal ultrasound examination of the prostate: Complications and acceptance by patients. Br J Urol 1993; 71:457–459.

Bertelsen S: Transrectal needle biopsy of the prostate. Acta Chir Scand 1966; 357:226–231.

Bigler SA, Deering RE, Brawer MK: Comparison of microscopic vascularity in benign and malignant prostate tissue. Hum Pathol 1993; 24:220–226.

Billebaud T, Sibert A, Dauge MC, et al: The value of ultrasound-guided multiple systematic biopsies in the early diagnosis of cancer of the prostate. Ann Urol (Paris) 1990; 24:524–529.

Brawer MK: PIN: A premalignant lesion. Human Pathol 1992; 23: 242–248.

Brawer MK, Beattie J, Wener MH: PSA as the initial test in prostate carcinoma screening: Results of the third year. J Urol 1993a; 149 (Suppl):299A.

Brawer MK, Beattie J, Wener MH, et al: Screening for prostatic carcinoma with PSA: Results of the second year. J Urol 1993b; 150:106–109.

Brawer MK, Chetner MP, Beatie J, et al: Screening for prostatic carcinoma with PSA. J Urol 1992; 147:841–845.

Brawer MK, Deering RE, Brown M, et al: Predictors of pathologic stage in prostatic carcinoma: The role of neovascularity. Cancer 1994; 73:678–687.

Brawer MK, Nagle RB: Transrectal ultrasound guided prostate needle biopsy following negative digitally guided biopsy. J Urol 1989; 141:278A.

Brawer MK, Nagle RB, Bigler SA, et al: Significance of PIN on prostate needle biopsy. Urology 1991; 38:103–107.

Carter HB, Hamper UM, Sheth S, et al: Evaluation of transrectal ultrasound in the early detection of prostate cancer. J Urol 1989; 142:1008–1010.

Catalona WJ, Richie JP, Ahmann FR, et al: Comparison of DRE and serum PSA in the early detection of prostate cancer: Results of a multicenter clinical trial of 6,630 men. J Urol 1994; 151:1283–1290.

Chin JL, Downey DB, Onik G, et al: Three dimensional ultrasound guided cryoablation of the prostate. Can J Urol 1995; 2:A66.

Collins GN, Lloyd SN, Hehir M, McKelvie GB: Multiple transrectal ultrasound-guided prostatic biopsies—true morbidity and patient acceptance. Br J Urol 1993; 71:460–463.

Cooner WH, Mosley RB, Rutherford CL Jr, et al: Prostate cancer detection in a clinical urological practice by ultrasonography, digital rectal examination and prostate specific antigen. J Urol 1990; 143:1146–1152.

Dahnert WF, Hamper UM, Eggleston JC, et al: Prostatic evaluation by transrectal sonography with histopathologic correlation: The echopenic appearance of early carcinoma. Radiology 1986; 158:97–102.

Deering RE, Bigler SA, Brown M, Brawer MK: Microvascularity in BPH. J Urol 1994; 151(Suppl):314A.

Devonec M, Chapeleon JY, Cathignol D: Comparison of the diagnostic value of sonography and rectal examination in cancer of the prostate. Eur Urol 1988; 14:189–195.

Dhom G: Epidemiologic aspects of latent and clinically manifest carcinoma of the prostate. J Cancer Res Clin Oncol 1983; 106:210–218.

Downey DB, Chin JL, Elliott TL, et al: Three dimensional US imaging of prostate cancer: Histo-pathologic correlation. Can J Urol 1995; 2:A31.

Ebert T, Schmitz-Drager B, Burrig K, et al: Accuracy of imaging modalities in staging the local extent of prostate cancer. Urol Clin North Am 1991; 18:453–457.

Ellis WJ, Brawer MK: The significance of isoechoic prostatic carcinoma. J Urol 1994; 152:2304–2307.

Ellis WJ, Brawer MK: Repeat prostate needle biopsy: Who needs it? J Urol 1995; 153:1496–1498.

Ellis WJ, Chetner M, Preston S, Brawer MK: Diagnosis of prostatic carcinoma: The yield of serum PSA, DRE and TRUS. J Urol 1994; 152:1520–1525.

Fortunoff S: Needle biopsy of the prostate: A review of 346 biopsies. J Urol 1962; 87:159.

Fritzsche PJ, Axford PO, Ching VC, et al: Correlation of transrectal sonographic findings in patients with suspected and unsuspected prostatic disease. J Urol 1983; 30:272–274.

Garnett JE, Oyasu R: The urologic evaluation of atypical prostatic hyperplasia. Urology 1989; 34:66–69.

Gleason DF, Mellinger GT: The Veterans Administration Cooperative Urological Research Group: Prediction of prognosis for prostatic carcinoma by combined histological grading and clinical staging. J Urol 1974; 111:58–64.

Hall MC, Troncoso P, Pollack A, et al: Significance of tumor angiogenesis in clinically localized prostate carcinoma treated with external beam radiotherapy. Urology 1994; 44:869–875.

Hammerer P, Huland H: Systematic sextant biopsies in 651 patients referred for prostate evaluation. J Urol 1994; 151:99–102.

Hammerer P, Loy V, Dieringer J, Huland H: Prostate cancer in nonurological patients with normal prostates on DRE. J Urol 1992; 147:833–836.

Hamper UM, Epstein JI, Sheth S, et al: Cystic lesions of the prostate gland: A sonographic-pathologic correlation. J Ultrasound Med 1990a; 9:395–402.

Hamper UM, Sheth S: Prostate ultrasonography. Semin Roentgenol 1993; 38:57–73.

Hamper UM, Sheth S, Walsh PC, et al: Carcinoma of the prostate: Value of transrectal sonography to detect extension into the neurovascular bundle. AJR 1990b; 155:1015–1019.

Hardeman SW, Causey JQ, Hickey DP, et al: Transrectal ultrasound for staging prior to radical prostatectomy. Urology 1989; 34:175–180.

Hodge KK, McNeal JE, Stamey TA: Ultrasound guided transrectal core biopsies of the palpably abnormal prostate. J Urol 1989a; 142:66–70.

Hodge KK, McNeal SE, Terris MK, Stamey TA: Random systematic versus directed ultrasound-guided transrectal core biopsies of the prostate. J Urol 1989b; 142:71–74.

Hoskins JH, Mellinger GT: Needle biopsy of the prostate. GP 1966; 34:88–92.

Hunter PT, Butler SA, Hodge GB, et al: Detection of prostatic cancer using transrectal ultrasound and sonographically guided biopsy in 1410 symptomatic men. J Endourol 1989; 3:167.

Kelly IM, Lees WR, Rickards D: Prostate cancer and the role of color Doppler US. Radiology 1993; 189:153–156.

Kenny JN, Brawer MK: Complications of transrectal ultrasound guided prostate needle biopsy. J Urol 1989; 141(Suppl): 503A.

King WW, Wilkiemeyer RM, Boyce WH, McKinney WM: Current status of prostatic ultrasonography. JAMA 1973; 226:444–447.

Lange PH, Brawer MK: Prostatic acid phosphatase and PSA in the era of transrectal ultrasonography. In Resnick MI, Watanabe H, Karr JP, eds: Diagnostic Ultrasound of the Prostate. Bethesda, Elsevier Science Publishing Co, 1989.

Lee F, Gray J, McCleary R: Transrectal ultrasound in the diagnosis of prostate cancer: Location, echogenicity, histopathology and staging. Prostate 1985; 7:117–129.

Lee F, Littrup PJ, Torp-Pedersen ST, et al: Prostate cancer: Comparison of transrectal US and DRE for screening. Radiology 1988; 168:389–394.

Lee F, Torp-Pedersen ST, McLeary RD: Diagnosis of prostate cancer by transrectal ultrasound. Urol Clin North Am 1989a; 16:663–673.

Lee F, Torp-Pedersen ST, Siders DB, et al: Transrectal ultrasonography in the diagnosis and staging of prostatic carcinoma. Radiology 1989b; 170:609.

Lee FL, Torp-Pedersen ST, Carroll JT, et al: Use of transrectal ultrasound and prostate-specific antigen in diagnosis of prostatic intraepithelial neoplasia. Urology 1989; 34(Suppl):4–8.

Lee FR, Gray JM, McLeary RD, et al: Prostatic evaluation by transrectal sonography: Criteria for diagnosis of early carcinoma. Radiology 1986; 158:91–95.

Lee JY: Technical tip: Transperineal ultrasound guided needle biopsy of the prostate in the postproctocolectomy patient. J Endourol 1993; 7:75–77.

Lippman HR, Ghiatas AA, Sarosdy MF: Systematic transrectal ultrasound guided prostate needle biopsy after negative digitally directed prostate biopsy. J Urol 1992; 147:827–829.

Littrup PJ, Kane RA, Williams CR, et al: Determination of prostate volume with TRUS for cancer screening: Part I. Comparison with PSA assays. Radiology 1991; 178:537–542.

Lui PD, Terris MK, McNeal JE, Stamey TA: Indications for ultrasound guided transition zone biopsies in the detection of prostate cancer. J Urol 1995; 153:1000–1003.

McNeal JE: The zonal anatomy of the prostate. Prostate 1981; 2:35–49.

McNeal JE, Bostwick DG, Kindrachuk RA, et al: Patterns of progression in prostatic cancer. Lancet 1980; 1:60–63.

McWhorter WP, Hernandez AD, Meikle AW, et al: A screening study prostate cancer in high risk families. J Urol 1992; 148:826–828.

Mettlin C, Littrup PJ, Kane RA, et al: Relative sensitivity and specificity of serum PSA level compared with age-referenced PSA, PSA density and PSA change. Cancer 1994a; 74:1615–1620.

Mettlin C, Murphy GP, Lee F, et al: Characteristics of prostate cancers detected in a multimodality early detection program. Cancer 1994b; 72:1701–1708.

Miller GJ: Histopathology of prostate cancer: Prediction of malignant behavior and correlation with ultrasonography. Urology 1989; 33:18–26.

Ostroff EG, Almario J, Kramer H: Transrectal needle method for biopsy of the prostate: Review of 90 cases. Am Surg 1975; 41:659–661.

Palken M, Cobb OE, Warren BH: Prostate cancer: Correlation of DRE, TRUS, and PSA levels with tumor volumes in radical prostatectomy specimens. J Urol 1990; 143:1155–1162.

Perrapato SD, Carothers GG, Maatman TJ, et al: Comparing clinical staging plus transrectal ultrasound with surgical-pathologic staging of prostate cancer. Urology 1989; 33:103–105.

Perrin P, Mouriquand P, Monsallier M, et al: Irradiation of carcinoma of the prostate localized to the pelvis: Analysis of tumor response and prognosis. Int J Radiat Oncol Biol Phys 1980; 6:555.

Pontes JE, Eisenkraft S, Watanabe H, et al: Preoperative evaluation of localized prostatic carcinoma by transrectal ultrasonography. J Urol 1985; 134:289–291.

Ragde H, Bagley CM, Aldpae HC: Screening for prostatic cancer with high-resolution ultrasound. J Endourol 1989; 3:115.

Resnick MI, Smith JA, Scardino PT, et al: Transrectal prostate ultrasonography—variability of interpretation. J Urol 1994; 151(Suppl):503A.

Resnick MI, Selzman AA: Transrectal ultrasound and prostate biopsy. Semin Urol 1994; 12:265–273.

Resnick MI, Willard JW, Boyce WH. Recent progress in ultrasonography of the bladder and prostate. J Urol 1977; 4:444–446.

Resnick MI, Willard JW, Boyce WH: Ultrasonic evaluation of the prostatic nodule. J Urol 1978; 120:86–89.

Rifkin M, Zerhouni E, Gatsonis C, et al: Comparison of magnetic resonance imaging and ultrasonography in staging early prostate cancer: Results of a multi-institutional cooperative trial. N Engl J Med 1990; 323:621–626.

Rifkin MD: Endorectal sonography of the prostate: clinical implications. AJR 1987a; 148:1137–1142.

Rifkin MD: Prostate imaging. Radiology 1987b; 165:220.

Rifkin MD, Alexander AA, Pisarchick J, Matteucci T: Palpable masses in the prostate: Superior accuracy of ultrasound guided biopsy compared with accuracy of digitally guided biopsy. Radiology 1991; 179:41–42.

Rifkin MD, Friedland GW, Shortliffe L: Prostatic evaluation by transrectal ultrasonography: Detection of carcinoma. Radiology 1986; 158:85–90.

Rifkin MD, Sudakoff GS, Alexander AA: Prostate: Techniques, results and potential applications of color Doppler US scanning. Radiology 1993; 186:509–513.

Salo JO, Kivisaari L, Rannikko S, et al: Relationship between PSA, prostate volume, and age in the benign prostate. Br J Urol 1987a; 71:445–450.

Salo JO, Rannikko S, Makinen J, Lehtonen T: Echogenic structure of prostatic cancer imaged on radical prostatectomy specimens. Prostate 1987b; 10:1–9.

Santucci RA, Brawer MK: Correlation of PSA and ultrasonography in the evaluation of patients with carcinoma of the prostate. Semin Urol 1994; 12:252–264.

Scardino PT, Shinohara K, Wheeler TM, et al: Staging of prostate cancer: Value of ultrasonography. Urol Clin North Am 1989; 16:713–734.

Sehgal CM, Broderick GA, Whittington R, et al: Three dimensional US and volumetric assessment of the prostate. Radiology 1994; 192:274–278.

Sehgal CM, Fodor L, Arger PH: Three dimensional reconstruction of ultrasonic images of human prostate. J Ultrasound Med 1992; 25(Suppl):11.

Shephard D, Keetch DW, Stahl D, Humphrey PA: Rebiopsy strategy in men with isolated prostatic intraepithelial neoplasia on prostate needle biopsy. J Urol 1995; 153(Suppl):420A.

Shinohara K, Presti JC Jr, Ingerman A: Local recurrence after radical prostatectomy: Characteristics in size, location, and PSA. J Urol 1994; 151(Suppl):256A.

Shinohara K, Scardino PT, Carter SSC, Wheeler TM: Pathologic basis of the sonographic appearance of the normal and malignant prostate. Urol Clin North Am 1989; 16:675–691.

Siegal JA, Yu E, Brawer MK: Topography of neovascularity in human prostate carcinoma. Cancer 1995; 75:2545–2551.

Sika JV, Lindquist HD: Relationship of needle biopsy diagnosis of prostate to clinical signs of prostatic cancer: An evaluation of 300 cases. J Urol 1963; 89:737.

Smith RC, Sudakoff GS, Rukstalis DB, Brendler CB: Early experience with color Doppler imaging during transrectal ultrasound of prostatic fossa following prostatectomy. J Urol 1995; 153(Suppl):501.

Sohlberg OE, Chetner MP, Ploch N, Brawer MK: Prostatic abscess after transrectal ultrasound guided biopsy. J Urol 1991; 146:420–422.

Stamey TA, Dietrick DD, Issa MM: Large, organ confined, impalpable transition zone prostate cancer: Association with metastatic levels of prostate specific antigen. J Urol 1993; 149:510–515.

Stilmant MM, Kuligowska E: Transrectal ultrasound screening for prostatic adenocarcinoma with histopathologic correlation. Cancer 1993; 71:2041–2047.

Takayama TK, Tisdale E, Bigler S, et al: Indication for seminal vesicle biopsy in the evaluation of prostate carcinoma. J Urol 1994; 151(Suppl):503A.

Terris MK, Stamey TA: Determination of prostate volume by transrectal ultrasound. J Urol 1987; 145:984.

Torp-Pedersen S, Lee F, Littrup PJ, et al: Transrectal biopsy of the prostate guided with US: Longitudinal and multiplaner scanning. Radiology 1989; 170:23–27.

Watanabe H: Transrectal sonography: A personal review and recent advances. Scand J Urol Nephrol 1991; 137:75–83.

Weaver RP, Noble MJ, Weigel JW: Correlation of ultrasound guided and digitally directed transrectal biopsies of palpable prostatic abnormalities. J Urol 1991; 145:516–518.

Weidner N, Carroll PR, Flax J, et al: Tumor angiogenesis correlates with metastasis in invasive prostate carcinoma. Am J Pathol 1993; 143:401–409.

Wild JJ, Reid JM: Echographic tissue diagnosis. Proceedings at the Fourth Annual Conference on Ultrasound Therapy, Philadelphia, 1955.

Wolf JS Jr, Shinohara K, Narayan P: Staging of prostate cancer: Accuracy of transrectal ultrasound enhanced by PSA. Br J Urol 1992; 70:534–541.

Zincke H, Campbell JT, Utz DC, et al: Confidence in the negative transrectal needle biopsy. Surg Gynecol Obstet 1973; 136:78–80.

83
DIAGNOSIS AND STAGING OF PROSTATE CANCER

H. Ballentine Carter, M.D.
Alan W. Partin, M.D., Ph.D.

Detection of Prostate Cancer

Diagnostic Modalities
Digital Rectal Examination
Prostate-Specific Antigen
Transrectal Ultrasound–Directed Prostate Biopsy

Staging of Prostate Cancer
Classification Systems
Clinical and Pathologic Staging
Staging Modalities

The histologic diagnosis of prostate cancer is made, in the majority of cases, by prostatic needle biopsy. Prostate cancer rarely causes symptoms until advanced. Thus, suspicion of prostate cancer resulting in a recommendation for prostatic biopsy is most often raised by abnormalities found on digital rectal examination (DRE) or serum prostate-specific antigen (PSA) elevations. Although there is controversy about the benefits of early diagnosis (Litwin and deKernion, 1994), it has been demonstrated that an early diagnosis of prostate cancer is best achieved using a combination of DRE and PSA to assess the risk that prostate cancer is present (Catalona et al, 1994b; Littrup et al, 1994; Stone et al, 1994; Bangma et al, 1995). Transrectal ultrasound (TRUS)–guided, systematic needle biopsy is the most reliable method at present to ensure accurate sampling of prostatic tissue (Hodge et al, 1989) in those men at high risk for harboring prostatic cancer based on DRE and PSA findings.

The goal of cancer staging is to determine the extent of disease as precisely as possible to assess prognosis and guide management recommendations. The local extent of disease determined by DRE (T stage), the serum PSA level before prostatic biopsy, and the grade of the tumor correlate directly with the pathologic extent of disease and are useful in the staging evaluation of men with adenocarcinoma of the prostate (Partin et al, 1993c; Bluestein et al, 1994). Currently no imaging studies capable of reliably identifying early extra-prostatic spread of disease are available (Rifkin et al, 1990). Less invasive methods of lymph node sampling (laparoscopic lymphadenectomy) have been used to detect metastatic disease in men judged to be at high risk of harboring lymph node metastases based on preliminary evaluation with DRE, serum PSA, and tumor grade.

DETECTION OF PROSTATE CANCER

Prostate cancer rarely causes symptoms early in the course of the disease because the majority of adenocarcinomas arise in the periphery of the gland distant from the urethra. The presence of symptoms as a result of prostate cancer suggests locally advanced or metastatic disease. Growth of prostate cancer into the urethra or bladder neck can result in obstructive voiding symptoms (e.g., hesitancy, decreased force of stream, intermittency) and irritative voiding symptoms (e.g., frequency, nocturia, urgency, urge incontinence). Local progression of disease and obstruction of the ejaculatory ducts can result in hematospermia and the finding of decreased ejaculate volume. Impotence can be a manifestation of prostate cancer that has spread outside the prostatic capsule to involve the branches of the pelvic plexus (neurovascular bundle) responsible for innervation of the corpora cavernosa.

Metastatic disease involving the axial or appendicular skeleton can cause bone pain or anemia from replacement of the bone marrow. Lower extremity edema can result from cancerous involvement of the pelvic lymph nodes and compression of the iliac veins. Less common findings from metastatic disease may include malignant retroperitoneal fibrosis from dissemination of cancer cells along the periureteral lymphatics, paraneoplastic syndromes from ectopic hormone production, and disseminated intravascular coagulation.

Although the patient with prostate cancer may present with voiding symptoms suggestive of prostate disease as well as signs and symptoms related to metastatic disease, the vast majority of men diagnosed with prostate cancer are initially suspected of having the disease based on DRE abnormalities or serum PSA elevations. Changes in prostate cancer screening have reduced the proportion of patients with prostate cancer detected because of symptoms suggestive of advanced disease (Gilliland et al, 1994). The proportion of cases diagnosed in men presenting with obstruction, retention, and pain decreased, whereas the proportion of cases diagnosed in men with milder voiding symptoms increased threefold between 1973 and 1991 (Gilliland et al, 1994). This trend is likely to continue with increasing use of serum PSA for diagnosis of prostatic cancer in asymptomatic men.

The routine use of DRE and PSA testing in asymptomatic men, as a means of reducing prostate cancer mortality by earlier detection and treatment, is controversial (Litwin and deKernion, 1994; Barry et al, 1995a). The American Cancer Society (Mettlin et al, 1993) and the American Urological Association recommend the routine use of DRE and PSA in asymptomatic men over age 50. The Canadian Task Force on the Periodic Health Examination (1991; Feightner, 1994) and the U.S. Preventive Services Task Force (1989) do not support routine use of PSA for prostate cancer screening. Arguments for prostate cancer screening are based on the belief that early detection decreases disease mortality, as follows: (1) There is no effective treatment for prostate cancer that is advanced. (2) Simple tests (DRE and PSA) used together result in the increased detection of organ-confined prostate cancer. (3) Effective treatment is available for prostate cancer that is confined to the prostate. Arguments against prostate cancer screening are based on the belief that early detection could result in more overall harm than improvement of health in large populations, as follows: (1) There is a lack of evidence based on randomized trials that aggressive treatment for early prostate cancer is beneficial through documentation that treated and untreated men with early disease have significantly different outcomes. (2) PSA testing may result in excessive, unnecessary further evaluations that are cost prohibitive without proving that screening reduces prostate cancer mortality. (3) The morbidity of treatment is considered excessive (Barry et al, 1995b). A definitive answer to this controversy that is based on a well-designed randomized trial is not available at present (Kramer et al, 1993).

DIAGNOSTIC MODALITIES

The triad of DRE, serum PSA, and TRUS-directed prostatic biopsy is used in the early detection of prostate cancer. **DRE and serum PSA are the most useful first-line tests for assessing the risk that prostate cancer is present in an individual** (Catalona et al, 1994b; Littrup et al, 1994; Stone et al, 1994; Bangma et al, 1995). TRUS is not recommended as a first-line screening test because of low predictive value for early prostate cancer (Carter et al, 1989; Ellis et al, 1994; Flanigan et al, 1994) and high cost of examination.

Digital Rectal Examination

Jewett (1956) reported that approximately 50% of suspicious lesions on DRE actually represented cancer on prostate biopsy. The positive predictive value for DRE (the probability that cancer is present if the test is positive) in current studies ranges from 21% to 53%, depending on the degree of suspicion for cancer and whether the population studied is referral or screened (Cooner et al, 1990; Catalona et al, 1994b; Ellis et al, 1994; Stone et al, 1994). **Because of the significant risk of prostate cancer, prostate biopsy is recommended for all men who have DRE abnormalities, regardless of the PSA level, because 25% of men with cancer have PSA levels less than 4.0 ng/ml.**

In both screened and nonscreened populations, DRE misses from 23% to 45% of the cancers that are subsequently found with prostatic biopsies done for serum PSA elevations or TRUS abnormalities (Cooner et al, 1990; Catalona et al, 1994b; Ellis et al, 1994). In addition, prostate cancers detected by DRE in screened and nonscreened populations of men are pathologically advanced in more than 50% of men (Thompson et al, 1987; Epstein et al, 1994a). Before the availability of PSA testing, physicians relied solely on DRE for early detection of prostate cancer. **DRE is a test with only fair reproducibility in the hands of experienced examiners** (Smith and Catalona, 1995) **that misses a substantial proportion of cancers and detects most cancers at a more advanced pathologic stage, when treatment is less likely to be effective.** Seventy-five percent of 366 men in the Physicians Health Study, who were diagnosed with prostate cancer in an era when DRE was the primary diagnostic method available ultimately died of prostatic cancer (Gann et al, 1995).

Prostate-Specific Antigen

PSA, a member of the kallikrein gene family (McCormack et al, 1995), is a serine protease produced by the prostatic epithelium and periurethral glands in the male. The gene encoding PSA is on chromosome 19, and DNA sequencing has been performed (Lundwall and Lilja, 1987). PSA is secreted into seminal fluid in high concentration (mg/ml), in which it is involved in liquefaction of the seminal coagulum (Lilja, 1985; McGee and Herr, 1988), and is found normally in low concentration in sera (ng/ml). PSA within sera circulates in both bound and unbound forms. Most PSA in sera is complexed to antiproteases within sera; alpha$_1$-antichymotrypsin (ACT) and alpha$_2$-macroglobulin (MG) primarily (Christensson et al, 1990; Lilja et al, 1991; Stenman et al, 1991). The serum protease inhibitors binding PSA are present in large excess compared to serum PSA, and therefore all enzymatically active PSA should be complexed. Binding of free PSA to ACT inactivates the protease, but the complex of PSA-ACT remains immunodetectable by current assays. Binding of PSA by MG still allows some proteolytic activity but renders the PSA-MG complex undetectable by current assays (Christensson et al, 1990). Free PSA without proteolytic activity is probably rendered inactive within the prostatic epithelial cell before release into the sera. This free inactive PSA does not form complexes with antiproteases, circulates unbound in sera, and is immunodetectable by current assays (Lilja et al, 1991). Thus, free unbound PSA and PSA-ACT are detectable by PSA assays and are thought to represent the total PSA reported using current assays (see also Chapter 45). Measurement of the different molecular forms of PSA within sera—bound and unbound—is currently being evaluated as a means of improving prostate cancer detection (see later on).

The clearance of complexed PSA from sera is thought to be through the liver because the size of the complexed PSA is too large for glomerular filtration, and other protease complexes are cleared by hepatic mechanisms (Pizzo et al, 1988). The serum half-life of PSA calculated after removal of all prostate tissue is 2 to 3 days (Stamey et al, 1987; Oesterling et al, 1988). Thus, several weeks may be necessary for PSA to become undetectable after radical prostatectomy. Studies evaluating clearance rates of free PSA from sera suggest a shorter half-life of 2 to 3 hours (Bjork et al, 1995), and clearance may be through the kidneys by glomerular filtration.

PSA expression is strongly influenced by androgens (Young et al, 1991; Henttu et al, 1992). Immunohistochemical detection of PSA within the prostate is characterized by bimodal peaks between 0 and 6 months and after 10 years, correlating directly with testosterone levels (Goldfarb et al, 1986). Serum PSA becomes detectable at puberty with increases in luteinizing hormone and testosterone (Vieira et al, 1994).

Serum PSA elevations occur as a result of disruption of the normal prostatic architecture that allows PSA to diffuse into the prostatic tissue and gain access to the circulation. This can occur in the setting of prostate disease and with prostate manipulation (prostate massage, prostate biopsy) (Stamey et al, 1987). Prostatic trauma such as occurs after prostatic biopsy can result in a "leak" of PSA into the circulation that may require more than 4 weeks for return to baseline values (Yuan et al, 1992). DRE as performed in an outpatient setting can lead to increases in serum PSA. The change in PSA after DRE, however, would not appear to be clinically significant because the change is within the error of the assay and rarely causes false-positive test results (Chybowski et al, 1992; Crawford et al, 1992). An evaluation of 100 men between the ages of 20 and 35 suggests that ejaculation can lead to a significant decrease in serum PSA measured 1 day after ejaculation (Westphal et al, 1995), confirming the findings of an earlier pilot study (Simak et al, 1993). A history of sexual activity may be important in the interpretation of serum PSA levels.

The presence of prostate disease (prostate cancer, benign prostatic hyperplasia [BPH], and prostatitis) is the most important factor affecting serum levels of PSA (Wang et al, 1981; Ercole et al, 1987; Robles et al, 1988). PSA elevations may indicate the presence of prostate disease, but not all men with prostate disease have elevated PSA levels. Furthermore, PSA elevations are not specific for cancer.

Prostate-directed treatment (for both BPH and cancer) can lower serum PSA by decreasing the volume of prostatic epithelium available for PSA production and by decreasing the amount of PSA produced per cell. Manipulation of the hormonal environment for treatment of cancer and BPH with orchiectomy, luteinizing hormone–releasing hormone analogues, and finasteride (Proscar); radiotherapy for cancer; and surgical ablation of prostate tissue for BPH or cancer can lead to reductions in serum PSA. Finasteride, a 5-alpha-reductase inhibitor, has been shown to lower PSA levels by 50% after 12 months of treatment (Guess et al, 1993). Men who are to be treated with finasteride should have a baseline

PSA measurement before initiation of treatment and should be followed with serial PSA measurements. If PSA does not decrease by 50%, or there is a rise in PSA when the patient is taking finasteride, these men should be suspected of having an occult prostate cancer. Interpretation of PSA values should always take into account the presence of prostate disease, previous diagnostic procedures, or treatments directed at the prostate gland.

Historical information and clinical aspects of PSA as a prostate tumor marker have been reviewed (Oesterling, 1991; Armbruster, 1993; Carter, 1994; Partin and Oesterling, 1994). PSA can be accurately measured in sera by immunoassay. Available assays differ, however, with respect to assay standardization (Vessella and Lange, 1993), and different assays detect free and bound forms of PSA in sera to variable degrees (Zhou et al, 1993; Sokoloff et al, 1994). These issues have been addressed (Stamey, 1995), but the clinical significance of assay differences with respect to prostate cancer detection has not been completely evaluated. The Tandem assay (Hybritech, San Diego, CA) with a reference range of 0.0 to 3.99 ng/ml has been used for measurement of serum PSA in the majority of studies evaluating PSA and prostate cancer detection.

It was initially believed that PSA would not be useful in prostate cancer detection because of overlap in serum levels between men with BPH and those with cancer (Stamey et al, 1987). Earlier studies suggested that 21% to 86% of men with BPH had PSA elevations (Stamey et al, 1987; Oesterling et al, 1988; Hudson et al, 1989). Numerous studies, however, have documented the validity of PSA as a method for assessing the risk that prostate cancer is present (Cooner et al, 1990; Catalona et al, 1991; Brawer et al, 1992; Labrie et al, 1992; Catalona et al, 1994b; Ellis et al, 1994; Littrup et al, 1994; Stone et al, 1994; Gann et al, 1995). **Routine use of PSA increases the detection of prostate cancer over that of DRE, improves the predictive value of the DRE for cancer, and increases the detection of prostate cancers that are organ confined yet significant in terms of size and grade.**

Evaluation of prostate cancer detection methods in both screened and nonscreened populations of men has shown that **PSA is the single test with the highest positive predictive value for cancer.** If serum PSA is elevated, a greater proportion of men actually have cancer found at biopsy when compared to an abnormality on DRE or TRUS (Catalona et al, 1994b; Ellis et al, 1994; Stone et al, 1994). In addition, although DRE and TRUS are dependent on the examiner, PSA is an objective measure of prostate cancer risk. The risk of prostate cancer is directly related to the PSA level (Cooner et al, 1990). Although there are differences between studies with regard to population selection and biopsy protocols, among screened populations the approximate chance of cancer on biopsy is 1 in 50 for men with PSA levels below 4.0 ng/ml (Labrie et al, 1992), 1 in 3 for PSA of 4.0 ng/ml or greater, 1 in 4 for PSA of 4.0 to 10.0 ng/ml, and 1 in 2 to 2 in 3 for PSA greater than 10 ng/ml (Catalona et al, 1991; Labrie et al, 1992; Brawer et al, 1992; Catalona et al, 1993; Catalona et al, 1994b; Stone et al, 1994; Littrup et al, 1994). A comparison of PSA and mammography in terms of cancer detection reveals that a man over age 50 with a PSA abnormality is twice as likely to harbor cancer than is

Table 83–1. CHANCE OF CANCER AS A FUNCTION OF SERUM PROSTATE-SPECIFIC ANTIGEN LEVEL AND DIGITAL RECTAL EXAMINATION FINDINGS

| Study | Chance of Cancer on Biopsy (%): PSA <4.0 ng/ml | | Chance of Cancer on Biopsy (%): PSA >4.0 ng/ml | |
	Negative DRE	Positive DRE	Negative DRE	Positive DRE
Cooner et al, 1990	9	17	25	62
Hammerer and Huland, 1994	4	21	12	72
Ellis et al, 1994	6	13	24	42
Catalona et al, 1994b	—	10	32	49

PSA, Prostate-specific antigen; DRE, digital rectal examination.

a woman over age 50 who has an abnormal mammogram (Kerlikowske et al, 1993).

PSA increases the predictive value of the DRE for cancer (Cooner et al, 1990; Catalona et al, 1994b; Ellis et al, 1994; Hammerer and Huland, 1994). Table 83–1 shows the chance of cancer as a function of PSA level in men with a normal and with an abnormal DRE in studies of screened and nonscreened populations. Because of the substantial risk of cancer in men with PSA elevations, prostate biopsy is recommended regardless of the findings on DRE. **Although PSA has the highest positive predictive value for prostate cancer, use of PSA without DRE is not recommended because 25% of men with prostate cancers have PSA levels less than 4.0 ng/ml.**

The most effective method for early detection of prostate cancer is the combined use of DRE and PSA to assess prostate cancer risk. When DRE and PSA are used as screening tests for prostate cancer detection, detection rates are higher with PSA compared to DRE and highest with a combination of the two tests (Table 83–2) (Catalona et al, 1994b; Littrup et al, 1994; Stone et al, 1994). Of 264 cancers detected in a screening study of 6630 men (Catalona et al, 1994b), 18% of the cancers would have been missed if PSA had been used alone, and 45% of the cancers would have been missed if DRE had been used alone (see Table 83–2). Because DRE and PSA do not always detect the same cancers, the tests are complementary in terms of cancer detection.

PSA testing increases the lead time for prostate cancer diagnosis. Thus, the use of PSA results in detection of prostate cancers that are more often confined to the prostate when compared to cancers discovered by DRE testing alone.

Table 83–2. CANCER DETECTION WITH SERUM PROSTATE-SPECIFIC ANTIGEN AND DIGITAL RECTAL EXAMINATION

Method of Detection	Cancer Detection Rate (%) Among 6630 Men	No. of Cancers Detected (%), n = 264
DRE	3.2	48 (18)
PSA	4.6	118 (45)
DRE/PSA	5.8	98 (37)

DRE, Digital rectal examination; PSA, prostate-specific antigen.
Adapted from Catalona WJ, Richie JP, Ahmann FR, et al: J Urol 1994; 151;1283–1290.

This has been confirmed by both longitudinal and cross-sectional studies. Longitudinal studies using frozen sera samples to analyze PSA levels years before the diagnosis of prostate cancer suggest that the cancers detected with DRE in the pre-PSA era (which are most often advanced at diagnosis) could have been detected earlier with PSA testing (Carter et al, 1992; Helzlsouer et al, 1992; Stenman et al, 1994; Gann et al, 1995; Tibblin et al, 1995). Data from the Baltimore Longitudinal Study of Aging (BLSA) (Shock et al, 1984) using multiple frozen sera samples have allowed comparison of serial PSA measurements in men who were ultimately diagnosed with prostate cancer and men without the disease (Fig. 83–1). These data reveal that men with prostate cancer have higher PSA levels than men without prostate cancer years before conventional diagnosis with DRE. Within the BLSA population, use of a PSA cutoff of 4.0 ng/ml as a detection criterion could have increased the lead time of diagnosis on average 4 years among the 48 men who were ultimately diagnosed with prostate cancer. Data from the Physicians Health Study using only one PSA measurement made on frozen sera collected before prostate cancer diagnosis demonstrated that an average lead time of 5.5 years could have been provided by PSA testing with a 4.0-ng/ml cutoff (Gann et al, 1995). In a similar study using a single frozen serum sample before the diagnosis of prostate cancer, a PSA exceeding 4.0 ng/ml was associated with a 20-fold excess risk of prostate cancer over the 6 years after the sera sample was obtained (Tibblin et al, 1995). Thus, PSA testing would appear to result in discovery of prostate cancer earlier in the natural history of the disease.

Cross-sectional studies evaluating the extent of disease

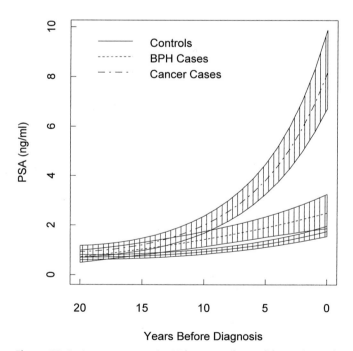

Figure 83–1. Average curves (±95th percentile confidence intervals) of prostate-specific antigen (PSA) levels (ng/ml) as a function of years before diagnosis for 48 men with prostate cancer, 39 men with histologically diagnosed benign prostatic hyperplasia (BPH), and 243 men without a history of prostate disease. All subjects had at least three repeat measurements within 10 years of diagnosis or exclusion of disease. Average number of repeat PSA measurements: cancer subjects, 7; BPH subjects, 6; subjects without prostate disease, 5.

after radical prostatectomy in men diagnosed by PSA testing support the increased lead time provided by PSA testing. In a PSA-based prostate cancer screening study, 57% of men who were referred primarily for evaluation of DRE abnormalities (nonscreened) had clinically or pathologically advanced disease, compared with 37% and 29% of those men with prostate cancer discovered by initial and serial PSA-based screening, respectively (Catalona et al, 1993). When a PSA cutoff of 4.0 ng/ml and an abnormal DRE were used together as screening criteria for prostate cancer, pathologically organ-confined disease was found in 71% of men who underwent surgery for prostate cancer (Catalona et al, 1994b). In contrast, when DRE has been used alone to screen for prostate cancer, organ-confined disease has been found in less than 50% of men undergoing surgery (Thompson et al, 1987; Mueller ct al, 1988; Chodak et al, 1989). Thus, the addition of PSA testing to DRE leads to detection of a greater proportion of pathologically confined cancers compared with cancer detection by DRE alone.

More than 80% to 90% of cancers detected with PSA testing are considered significant based on the size and grade of the cancer. Epstein and associates evaluated the pathologic features of PSA-detected prostate cancers using tumor size, grade, and pathologic stage as surrogates for biologic aggressiveness (Epstein et al, 1994a, 1994b). They discovered that PSA-detected cancers (stage T1c) more closely resemble DRE-detected cancers (stage B or T2) than the smallest cancers detected by transurethral resection (stage A1 or T1a), which are often managed expectantly. Other investigators have demonstrated the similarity between PSA-detected and DRE-detected prostate cancers in terms of size and grade (Stormont et al, 1993; Ohori et al, 1994b; Skaletsky et al, 1994). The cross-sectional data indicating the significance of PSA-detected prostate cancers are supported by longitudinal studies.

Gann and associates evaluated the ability of a single PSA measurement, made on a frozen serum sample at baseline, to detect 366 cancer cases that later arose in men enrolled in the Physicians Health Study (Gann et al, 1995). In this case-control study, cancers were detected after baseline blood sampling by DRE before the availability of PSA testing. Measurement of PSA using the baseline frozen serum sample revealed that a PSA cutoff of 4.0 ng/ml could have detected 73% of the cancers that arose within 4 years of PSA measurement, with a specificity among controls of greater than 90%. Seventy-five percent of these 366 men with prostate cancer in this study eventually died of prostate cancer. These longitudinal data suggest that a PSA cutoff of 4.0 ng/ml has high validity for detection of prostate cancers that are life-threatening. Thus, available cross-sectional and longitudinal data provide evidence that most PSA-detected cancers are significant cancers in terms of biologic potential.

Recognizing that PSA elevations are common in aging men because of the high prevalence of BPH, investigation has focused on methods of improving the ability of the PSA test to distinguish between men with BPH and men with cancer. Adjusting PSA levels for patient age or age-specific PSA (Collins et al, 1993; Dalkin et al, 1993; Oesterling et al, 1993), adjusting the PSA level for prostate volume or PSA density (Babaian et al, 1990; Littrup et al, 1991; Benson et al, 1992a, 1992b; Bazinet et al, 1994; Rommel et al, 1994), and evaluating rate of change in PSA or PSA velocity

(Carter et al, 1992, 1995a; Smith and Catalona, 1994) all have been evaluated as methods of improving the predictive value of PSA for cancer. With the advent of specific assays for quantitating PSA molecular forms, the measurement of free, unbound PSA has been evaluated as a method of distinguishing between BPH and cancer (Catalona et al, 1995; Luderer et al, 1995; Partin et al, 1995a).

Age-Specific Prostate-Specific Antigen Reference Ranges

Oesterling and associates evaluated a large cohort of men of all ages without prostate cancer and used the 95th percentile of PSA to establish normal age-specific reference ranges: age 40 to 50 years, 0 to 2.5 ng/ml; age 50 to 60, 0 to 3.5 ng/ml; age 60 to 70, 0 to 4.5 ng/ml; age 70 to 80, 0 to 6.5 ng/ml (Oesterling et al, 1993). PSA increases with age primarily because of increases in prostate size, and age-adjustment of PSA is a means of accounting for this size increase with age. It has been suggested that age adjustment of PSA—compared to the use of a single PSA cutoff for all ages—may lead to increased cancer detection in younger men more likely to benefit from treatment and minimize unnecessary evaluations in older men less likely to benefit from treatment (Oesterling et al, 1993, 1995; El-Galley et al, 1995). Other studies suggest that age adjustment of PSA provides no advantage in terms of cancer detection over the use of a single PSA cutoff of 4.0 ng/ml (Catalona et al, 1994a; Littrup et al, 1994; Mettlin et al, 1994). At present, the data suggest that a cutoff point of 4.0 ng/ml—using the Tandem assay (Hybritech, San Diego, CA)—is an effective threshold for maximizing prostate cancer detection and minimizing unnecessary biopsies in men between the ages of 50 and 70. The optimal PSA threshold—the cutoff that results in detection of clinically significant cancers in those men who would most likely benefit from treatment—is not known. For younger individuals, a greater index of suspicion is warranted at PSA levels below 4.0 ng/ml because the relative risk of cancer is increased even at PSA levels between 2.0 and 4.0 ng/ml (Gann et al, 1995), and these men have the most to gain from a diagnosis of prostate cancer (Gronberg et al, 1994). A greater suspicion of prostate cancer at lower PSA levels is especially important in the setting of known risk factors of positive family history and black race. The use of higher PSA thresholds among older men, who are less likely to benefit from prostate cancer treatment, should take into consideration the overall health and life expectancy of the individual. Issues that need to be addressed include the optimal PSA threshold for nonequivalent assays and the optimal tradeoff between detection of cancer (sensitivity) and unnecessary evaluations (specificity), which may differ among individuals depending on patient age and overall health.

Prostate-Specific Antigen Density

The majority of men with PSA elevations (>80%) have serum levels in the range of 4.0 to 10.0 ng/ml (Catalona et al, 1994b). In these men, the most likely reason for the PSA elevation is prostate enlargement—not prostate cancer—because of the high prevalence of BPH in the population. Benson and colleagues suggested that adjusting PSA for ultrasound-determined prostate size—by calculating the quotient of PSA and prostate volume—could help distinguish between men with PSA elevations caused by BPH and those caused by prostate cancer (Benson et al, 1992a, 1992b). A direct relationship between PSA density (PSAD) and the chance of cancer has been documented (Seaman et al, 1993; Bazinet et al, 1994; Rommel et al, 1994), and a PSAD of 0.15 or greater has been proposed as a threshold for recommending prostate biopsy in men with PSA levels between 4.0 and 10.0 ng/ml and no suspicion of cancer on DRE or TRUS (Seaman et al, 1993; Bazinet et al, 1994). The usefulness of PSAD in prostate cancer detection has not been confirmed in all studies. Catalona and associates found that half of the cancers detected in men with PSA levels between 4.0 and 10.0 ng/ml—and a normal DRE and TRUS—would have been missed using a PSAD of 0.15 as a threshold for biopsy (Catalona et al, 1994c). Brawer and colleagues found that PSAD did not enhance the ability of PSA level alone to predict the presence of cancer in men with PSA values of 4.0 to 10.0 ng/ml and a normal DRE (Brawer et al, 1993). The finding of higher PSAD among groups of men with positive biopsy results—when compared with men with negative biopsy results—may be because prostate cancers are more likely to be found using sextant biopsies in men with smaller prostate volumes (Uzzo et al, 1995).

The conflicting results among investigators using PSAD to predict cancer have been addressed by Cooner (1994). There is variation in the amount of epithelium (source of PSA) between prostates of similar size, and at present there is no noninvasive method for determining how much epithelium is contributing to overall PSA. In addition, there is variability in the shape of prostates, which limits the use of a common volume equation for calculating prostate size. The major determinant of serum PSA in men without prostate cancer is the transition zone epithelium, not the epithelium of the peripheral zone of the prostate (Lepor et al, 1994). Because BPH represents an enlargement of the transition zone—and serum PSA levels are primarily a reflection of transition zone histology in men with BPH—adjusting PSA for transition zone volume may help distinguish between BPH and prostate cancer (Kalish et al, 1994). Although PSAD is an imperfect predictor of cancer, it is an additional method of risk assessment with potential usefulness for counseling men with intermediate PSA levels (4.0–10.0 ng/ml) about the need for prostate biopsy (Benson, 1994).

Prostate-Specific Antigen Velocity

Substantial changes or variability in serum PSA can occur between measurements in the presence or absence of prostate cancer (Carter et al, 1992; Riehmann et al, 1993; Carter et al, 1995b; Stamey et al, 1995). The short-term changes in PSA between repeated measurements are primarily due to physiologic variation (Komatsu et al, 1996). The changes in serum PSA can be adjusted (corrected) for the elapsed time between the measurements, a concept known as PSA velocity or rate of change in PSA. Using frozen sera to measure PSA years before the diagnosis of prostate disease in men with and without prostate cancer, Carter and associates showed that a rate of change in PSA more than 0.75 ng/ml

per year was a specific marker for the presence of prostate cancer and that men with cancer had significantly more rapid rates of rise in PSA than men without prostate cancer at a time (5 years before diagnosis) when PSA levels were not elevated (Carter et al, 1992). In that study, 72% of men with cancer and 5% of men without cancer had a PSA velocity of more than 0.75 ng/ml per year. In a large prospective screening study, the cancer detection rate was 47% among men with a PSA velocity more than 0.75 ng/ml per year compared with 11% among men with a PSA velocity less than 0.75 ng/ml per year (Smith and Catalona, 1994). In addition, less than 5% of men without a history of prostate cancer have a PSA velocity more than 0.75 ng/ml per year (95th percentile for PSA velocity), supporting the specificity of rate of change in PSA as a marker for the presence of cancer (Carter et al, 1995b). The minimal length of follow-up time over which changes in PSA should be adjusted—for PSA velocity to be useful in cancer detection—has been calculated in separate studies to be 18 months (Smith and Catalona, 1994; Carter et al, 1995a). Furthermore, evaluation of three repeated PSA measurements, to determine an average rate of change in PSA, appears to optimize the accuracy of PSA velocity for cancer detection (Carter et al, 1992; Carter et al, 1995b).

Molecular Forms of Prostate-Specific Antigen

The discovery that PSA exists in bound and unbound molecular forms within sera and the development of assays to measure molecular forms of PSA may improve the ability of the PSA test to predict the presence of cancer (McCormack et al, 1995). It has been shown that men with prostate cancer have a greater fraction of serum PSA complexed to ACT—lower percentage of total PSA that is free—than men without prostate cancer (Christensson et al, 1993; Leinonen et al, 1993; Lilja, 1993; Stenman et al, 1994), possibly because more ACT is produced by cancerous compared to noncancerous epithelial cells (Bjartell et al, 1993; Bjork et al, 1994). Christensson and associates measured free and total PSA fractions in men with and without prostate cancer and found that a free/total PSA cutoff of 0.18 or less (18% free/total PSA) significantly improved the ability to distinguish between cancer and noncancer subjects, compared to the use of total PSA alone (Christensson et al, 1993). In the intermediate PSA range between 4.0 and 10.0 ng/ml, Catalona and co-workers found that the percentage of free PSA provided independent predictive information about the presence or absence of cancer above that provided by other clinical indices, including age, total PSA, DRE results, and prostate size (Catalona et al, 1995). The percent free PSA cutoff that optimizes sensitivity and specificity for cancer detection depends on prostate size because overlap in the percentage of free PSA is greatest among men without cancer who have enlarged prostates and those men with cancer in the setting of prostate enlargement (Catalona et al, 1995). Maintaining a sensitivity for cancer detection of 90% among men with PSA levels between 4.0 and 10.0 ng/ml and a nonsuspicious DRE, Catalona and co-workers found that a free PSA cutoff of 23% or less would have eliminated 31% of unnecessary biopsies in men with prostate glands larger than 40 cm³, whereas a free PSA cutoff of 14% or less would have eliminated 79% of unnecessary biopsies in men with prostate glands less than 40 cm³ (Catalona et al, 1995). Thus, assays for measurement of PSA molecular forms have the potential for further categorization of those men with intermediate PSA elevations into low-risk and high-risk groups that could result in a marked reduction of unnecessary prostate biopsies (Catalona et al, 1995; Luderer et al, 1995; Partin et al, 1995a).

PSA has the highest positive predictive value of any test for prostate cancer. Prostate cancers detected by PSA testing are comparable to DRE-detected cancers in terms of size and grade. In screening studies, the majority of cancers detected by DRE are pathologically advanced. In contrast, the majority of prostate cancers detected with a combination of DRE and PSA screening are pathologically confined to the prostate. The role of PSA in the detection of prostate cancer is evolving with continued evaluation of methods to distinguish better between men with and without prostate cancer.

Transrectal Ultrasound–Directed Prostate Biopsy

Enthusiasm for using ultrasound to identify early prostate cancers by detection of hypoechoic lesions has not been proven with longer follow-up (see Chapter 82). Studies have confirmed the inability of TRUS to localize early prostate cancer (Ellis et al, 1994; Flanigan et al, 1994). Flanigan and associates found that only 18% of 855 sonographically suspicious quadrants actually contained cancer on biopsy, whereas 65% of quadrants containing cancer were not sonographically suspicious (Flanigan et al, 1994). In another study, analysis of 6006 sectors biopsied revealed that 17% of hypoechoic sectors contained cancer, whereas 37% of sectors containing cancer were not suspicious by ultrasound (Ellis et al, 1994). **The limitations of TRUS in prostate cancer detection are that most hypoechoic lesions found on TRUS are not cancer, and 50% of nonpalpable cancers more than 1 cm in greatest dimension are not visualized by ultrasound** (Carter et al, 1989). **Although hypoechoic areas on TRUS are more than twice as likely to contain cancer as isoechoic areas** (Ellis et al, 1994; Hammerer and Huland, 1994), **25% to 50% of cancers would be missed if only hypoechoic areas were biopsied. Therefore, any patient with a DRE suspicious for cancer or a PSA elevation should undergo prostate biopsy regardless of TRUS findings if an early diagnosis of cancer would result in a recommendation for treatment.**

Because TRUS is not an accurate method for localizing early prostate cancer, it is not recommended as a first-line screening tool. The primary role of TRUS in the detection of prostate cancer was originally outlined by Cooner and associates (1990). **The major role of TRUS is to ensure accurate wide-area sampling of prostate tissue in men at higher risk of harboring cancer.** This is best accomplished by targeted biopsy of TRUS-suspicious lesions and systematic biopsy of areas without hypoechoic lesions (Hodge et al, 1989).

STAGING OF PROSTATE CANCER

After the diagnosis of adenocarcinoma of the prostate has been histologically confirmed, an accurate assessment of the stage—or extent—of the disease should be made. **The goals in staging of prostate cancer are twofold: (1) to evaluate prognosis and (2) to direct therapy rationally based on the extent of disease.** The extent of disease correlates directly with prognosis in men with newly diagnosed prostate cancer. Treatment directed at eradication of the primary tumor is not likely to affect prognosis when the disease is no longer confined because adjuvant therapy capable of eradicating extraprostatic disease is unavailable. Thus, an accurate assessment of disease extent is pivotol when counseling the patient with newly diagnosed prostate cancer. The available modalities for assessing disease extent in men with prostate cancer are DRE, serum tumor markers, histologic grade, radiographic imaging, and pelvic lymphadenectomy. Pretreatment staging, although not uniformly reproducible, provides a means of distinguishing among clinically localized, locally advanced, and metastatic disease and helps accomplish the stated goals.

Classification Systems

The first and most widely used clinical staging classification system for prostate cancer was introduced by Whitmore (1956) and later modified by Jewett (1975). The tumor, node, and metastases (TNM) system for staging prostate cancer was adopted in 1975 by the American Joint Committee for Cancer Staging and End Results Reporting (Wallace et al, 1975; Beahrs and Myers, 1983; Beahrs et al, 1988; Schroder et al, 1992). In 1992, the American Joint Committee on Cancer and the International Union Against Cancer adopted a new TNM classification system for prostate cancer (Beahrs et al, 1992; International Union Against Cancer, 1992; Schroeder et al, 1992). Table 83–3 compares the Whitmore-Jewett and TNM classifications—the most commonly used staging systems for prostate cancer.

The TNM clinical staging system states that any nonpalpable lesion identified by imaging should be classified as a T2 lesion. If a nonpalpable prostate cancer is detected by needle biopsy because of a PSA elevation—and a hypoechoic lesion is found on TRUS at the time of biopsy—the TNM classification of this lesion is T2. Ohori and co-workers found that 33 nonpalpable/nonvisible tumors detected because of a PSA elevation (T1c) had tumor volumes similar to those of patients with T1b and T2a disease but were significantly smaller than those of patients with T2b, T2c, and T3 disease (Ohori et al, 1994b). Tumors that were visible on TRUS but not palpable (n = 42) were not significantly different in terms of tumor volume when compared with T2 tumors that were not visible on ultrasound (n = 20). Although the aforementioned findings support the classification of nonpalpable cancers detected by ultrasound into the T2 category, this area is controversial. Epstein and colleagues found that TRUS findings were not predictive of tumor extent in a study of PSA-detected (nonpalpable) cancers (Epstein et al, 1994b), and similar findings were reported by Ferguson and associates (1995). Realizing that most hypoechoic lesions do not represent cancer and that many significant cancers are not seen

Table 83–3. PROSTATE CANCER STAGING SYSTEMS

TNM	Description	Whitmore-Jewett	Description
TX	Primary tumor cannot be assessed	None*	None
T0	No evidence of primary tumor	None	None
T1	Clinically unapparent tumor—not palpable or visible by imaging	A	Same as TNM
T1a	Tumor found incidentally in tissue removed at TUR; 5% or less of tissue is cancerous	A1	Same as TNM
T1b	Tumor found incidentally at TUR; more than 5% of tissue is cancerous	A2	Same as TNM
T1c	Tumor identified by prostate needle biopsy because of PSA elevation	None	None
T2	Palpable tumor confined within the prostate	B	Same as TNM
T2a	Tumor involves half of a lobe or less	B1N	Tumor involves half of a lobe or less; surrounded by normal tissue
T2b	Tumor involves more than half of a lobe, but not both lobes	B1	Tumor involves less than one lobe
T2c	Tumor involves both lobes	B2	Tumor involves one entire lobe or more
T3	Palpable tumor extending through prostate capsule and/or involving seminal vesicle(s)	C1	Tumor <6 cm in diameter
T3a	Unilateral extracapsular extension	C1	Same as TNM
T3b	Bilateral extracapsular extension	C1	Same as TNM
T3c	Tumor invades seminal vesicle(s)	C1	Same as TNM
T4	Tumor is fixed or invades adjacent structures other than seminal vesicles	C2	Tumor ≥6 cm in diameter
T4a	Tumor invades bladder neck and/or external sphincter and/or rectum	C2	Same as TNM
T4b	Tumor invades levator muscles and/or is fixed to pelvic wall	C2	Same as TNM
N+	Involvement of regional lymph nodes	D1	Same as TNM
None	None	D0	Elevation of prostatic acid phosphatase only (enzymatic assay)
NX	Regional lymph nodes cannot be assessed	None	None
N0	No regional lymph node metastases	None	None
N1	Metastasis in a single regional lymph node, ≤2 cm in greatest dimension	D1	Same as TNM
N2	Metastasis in a single regional lymph node, >2 cm but not >5 cm in greatest dimension, or multiple regional lymph nodes, none >5 cm in greatest dimension	D1	Same as TNM
N3	Metastasis in a regional lymph node >5 cm in greatest dimension	D1	Same as TNM
M+	Distant metastatic spread	D2	Same as TNM
MX	Presence of distant metastases cannot be assessed	None	None
M0	No distant metastases	None	None
M1	Distant metastases	D2	Same as TNM
M1a	Involvement of nonregional lymph nodes	D2	Same as TNM
M1b	Involvement of bone(s)	D2	Same as TNM
M1c	Involvement of other distant sites	D2	Same as TNM
None	None	D3	Hormone refractory disease

*None = No comparable category.
TUR, Transurethral resection; PSA, prostate-specific antigen.

by TRUS, it seems unlikely that identification of a lesion using today's imaging techniques will provide useful separation of nonpalpable tumors.

Clinical and Pathologic Staging

Clinical stage refers to an assessment of the extent of disease determined by DRE, serum tumor markers, tumor grade, and imaging modalities. Determination of the local extent of disease—primarily by DRE—is referred to as T stage (see Table 83–3). Pathologic stage is a more accurate representation of the extent of disease within and beyond the prostate that is described following histologic examination of

the pelvic lymph nodes and prostate after removal of these tissues. Pathologic staging is more useful than clinical staging in the prediction of prognosis because tumor volume, surgical margin status, extent of extracapsular spread, and involvement of seminal vesicles and pelvic lymph nodes can be determined. For this reason alone, accurate survival comparisons between nonsurgical and surgical therapies will continue to be limited (Benson and Olson, 1989).

There is no currently accepted pathologic staging system for prostate cancer. Based on evaluation of radical prostatectomy specimens, pathologic stage is classified as organ confined or non–organ confined. Subclassifications, based on the presence of cancer within the periprostatic tissue, seminal vesicles, and pelvic lymph nodes, have been proposed as follows: (1) organ confined when disease is confined within the prostatic capsule, (2) capsular penetration when disease extends beyond the prostatic capsule into periprostatic tissue but does not involve the seminal vesicles, (3) seminal vesicle involvement when disease extends beyond the prostatic capsule into the muscular wall of the seminal vesicles, and (4) involvement of the pelvic lymph nodes. The probability of a man's remaining free of disease diminishes with each increase in pathologic stage of disease. Table 83–4 describes the distribution of pathologic stages in several large radical prostatectomy series.

The important pathologic criteria that are predictive of prognosis after radical prostatectomy are tumor grade; surgical margin status; and presence of extracapsular disease, seminal vesicle invasion, or involvement of pelvic lymph nodes. The presence of a positive surgical margin or the presence of high-grade tumor (Gleason score ≥7) in the setting of extraprostatic disease is associated with a higher probability of residual disease after surgical removal of the prostate (Epstein, 1990; Epstein et al, 1993a, 1993b; Frazier et al, 1993; Partin et al, 1993a, 1993b; reviewed by Montie, 1990; Ohori et al, 1995). The Gleason histologic grade has independent prognostic significance for those men with extracapsular disease (Epstein et al, 1993a, 1993b). Epstein and co-workers demonstrated a significant difference in the actuarial PSA recurrence of a group of men with extracapsular penetration—without seminal vesicle or lymph node involvement—who had Gleason scores less than 7 when compared with those men with Gleason scores 7 or greater and the same pathologic stage (Epstein et al, 1993a). They also demonstrated marked differences in actuarial PSA recurrence following radical prostatectomy in men with "focal" capsular penetration (fewer than three glands beyond the capsule) when compared with those with "established" capsular penetration (three or more glands beyond the capsule) (Epstein et al, 1993a).

The finding of seminal vesicle invasion or lymph node metastases on pathologic evaluation after radical prostatectomy is associated with a low probability of total eradication of tumor and a high probability of distant failure (Jewett, 1975; Walsh and Jewett, 1980; Partin et al, 1993b; Catalona and Smith, 1994). Biopsy of the seminal vesicles has been recommended by some investigators as a means to improve staging before treatment (Terris et al, 1993; Vallancien et al, 1994; Stone et al, 1995). Seminal vesicle invasion can occur either through direct extension or through hematogenous spread (Villers et al, 1989, 1990). Wheeler (1989) suggested subclassification of seminal vesicle involvement into three types based on mechanisms of tumor spread: type 1, extension from prostate to seminal vesicles along the ejaculatory complex; type 2, invasion across the prostatic capsule into the muscular coat of the seminal vesicle from without; and type 3, hematogenous spread without involvement of the ejaculatory complex or adjacent extracapsular cancer. The prognostic significance of this subclassification has not been evaluated.

Staging Modalities

The methods in common use for assessing the extent of prostate cancer include DRE for determination of T stage, serum tumor markers, histologic grading, radiologic imaging, and surgical lymphadenectomy. A discussion of prostate cancer grading systems, radiologic imaging of the prostate, and surgical lymphadenectomy can be found in other chapters.

Digital Rectal Examination

The DRE is routinely used to evaluate the local extent of prostate cancer. Whitmore (1956) was the first to use "palpability" of prostate cancers for staging, and Jewett (1975) was the first to subclassify the local extent of the tumor based on the DRE. Because DRE is subjective, however, both understaging and overstaging are found when the pathologic extent of disease is correlated with DRE findings.

Earlier studies involving small groups of men in whom extraprostatic disease spread had been expected on DRE—and who subsequently underwent radical prostatectomy—confirmed the clinical impression in only 25% of the cases (Turner and Belt, 1957; Byar et al, 1972). **Histologic evaluation of surgical specimens after radical prostatectomy for presumed organ-confined disease demonstrates a significant degree of understaging by DRE** (Walsh and Jewett, 1980). Table 83–5 is a composite of

Table 83–4. DISTRIBUTION OF PATHOLOGIC STAGES IN RADICAL PROSTATECTOMY SERIES

Study	Organ Confined, No. (%)	Capsular Penetration, No. (%)	Seminal Vesicles, No. (%)	Lymph Nodal Status, No. (%)
Partin et al, 1993b; Johns Hopkins, 1982–1991 (N = 955)	356 (37)	462 (48)	66 (7)	71 (7)
Catalona and Smith, 1994; Washington University, 1983–1993 (N = 925)	590 (64)	227 (25)	86 (9)	22 (2)
Ohori et al, 1994a; Baylor College of Medicine, 1983–1993 (N = 500)	226 (45)	161 (32)	83 (17)	30 (6)
Zincke et al, 1994; Mayo Clinic 1966–1991 (N = 3170)	1497 (47)	1339 (42)*	Not listed	334 (11)

*Includes some with positive seminal vesicles.

Table 83–5. COMPARISON OF CLINICAL AND PATHOLOGIC STAGES IN RADICAL PROSTATECTOMY SERIES

Reference	No. of Patients	Organ Confined, No. (%)	Non–organ Confined, No. (%)
T1a			
Partin et al, 1993c; Johns Hopkins University	31	31 (100)	—
Catalona and Bigg, 1990; Washington University	13	13 (100)	—
Zincke et al, 1994; Mayo Clinic	49	44 (90)	5 (10)
Total	93	88 (94)	5 (6)
T1b			
Partin et al, 1993c; Johns Hopkins University	71	50 (70)	21 (30)
Catalona and Bigg, 1990; Washington University	40	26 (65)	14 (35)
Zincke et al, 1994; Mayo Clinic	177	120 (68)	57 (32)
Total	288	196 (68)	92 (32)
T1c (nonpalpable)			
Epstein et al, 1994a; Johns Hopkins University	157	80 (51)	77 (49)
Paulson, 1994; Duke University	142	81 (57)	61 (43)
Total	299	161 (54)	138 (46)
T2			
Partin et al, 1993c; Johns Hopkins University	565	294 (52)	271 (48)
Paulson, 1994; Duke University	131	49 (37)	64 (63)
Zincke et al, 1994; Mayo Clinic	2944	1333 (45)	1289 (55)
Catalona and Bigg, 1990; Washington University	197	103 (52)	94 (48)
Total	3837	1779 (46)	1718 (54)
T3a			
Partin et al, 1993c; Johns Hopkins University	36	7 (19)	26 (81)

several radical prostatectomy series in which understaging, or false-negative prediction of organ-confined status by DRE, could be determined. In these series, an increasing percentage of understaged tumors is seen with increasing clinical stage.

The sensitivity and specificity of DRE in determining organ-confined status were evaluated in a large series (Partin et al, 1993c) in which all DREs and radical prostatectomies were performed by one urologist, with pathologic evaluations completed by a single pathologist. Within this series of 565 men in whom the DRE suggested organ-confined disease (T2), 52% actually had organ-confined disease, 31% had capsular penetration, and the remaining 17% had either seminal vesicle or lymph node involvement. Within the same series, of the 36 men in whom extraprostatic disease was suspected on DRE (T3a), 19% had organ-confined disease, 36% had capsular penetration, and 45% had involvement of either the seminal vesicles or the lymph nodes. This represents a sensitivity of 52% and a specificity of 81% for prediction of organ-confined disease by DRE alone.

Serum Tumor Markers

Two prostatic tumor markers—serum prostatic acid phosphatase (PAP) and serum PSA—have been used as indicators of disease extent in prostate cancer. The lower sensitivity of PAP compared to PSA in the prediction of advanced disease and the close correlation between PSA and extent of disease have led some experts to question the need for measurement of PAP in men with newly diagnosed prostate cancer.

PROSTATIC ACID PHOSPHATASE. See reviews by Heller (1987), Romas and Kwan (1993), and Lowe and Trauzzi (1993). Before the availability of PSA, PAP was the serum marker used most often for staging prostate cancer. Enzymatic phosphatase activity is widely distributed in various human tissues and organs. The isoenzymes detected by assays that measure PAP are not found exclusively in the prostate. Thus, although PAP activity is 1000-fold greater in the prostate than in any other tissue, PAP is not prostate specific because detectable levels are noted even after removal of all prostate tissue. In addition to prostatic manipulation and disease, a variety of medical conditions can cause PAP elevations, including malignancies and renal, skeletal, and liver diseases.

In terms of prostate cancer staging, PAP elevations are directly related to the extent (stage) of disease (Heller, 1987). Radioimmunoassays for measurement of PAP are more sensitive but less specific than enzymatic assays as a marker of advanced disease. The enzymatic assay using thymolpthalein monophosphate as a substrate for hydrolysis of PAP (Roy enzymatic assay) is a specific assay for the presence of advanced disease in the absence of other diseases that cause acid phosphatase elevations. Numerous studies have documented the close relationship between advanced disease and enzymatic elevations of PAP (Whitesel et al, 1984; Bahnson and Catalona, 1987; Oesterling et al, 1987). Abnormal PAP values (Roy enzymatic assay) and values in the upper half of the normal range suggest a high likelihood (>80%) of extraprostatic disease (Bahnson and Catalona, 1987; Oesterling et al, 1987). A normal enzymatic PAP level, however, is not highly predictive for the absence of extraprostatic disease.

In the PSA era, use of PAP in staging has a limited role because of the closer relationship between PSA and disease extent (Stamey et al, 1987). PAP rarely adds additional information in those men who are considered to have clinically localized prostate cancer based on the results of DRE, PSA, and Gleason grade (Burnett et al, 1992).

PROSTATE-SPECIFIC ANTIGEN. Numerous studies have shown that for groups of men with prostate cancer, serum PSA correlates directly with advancing clinical and pathologic stage (Ercole et al, 1987; Stamey et al, 1987; Oesterling et al, 1988; Hudson et al, 1989; Haapianen et al, 1990; Partin et al, 1990; Rainwater et al, 1990; Catalona et al, 1991; Partin et al, 1993c). **In most cases, however, PSA level alone does not provide accurate staging information for the individual patient because of overlap in PSA levels between stages.** PSA is directly related to the volume of cancer present (Stamey et al, 1987), but other variables influence the overall PSA level. The preoperative interpretation of serum PSA as it relates to tumor extent is confounded by both the volume of BPH tissue present and the tumor grade, both of which influence serum PSA levels in men with prostatic cancer (Partin et al, 1990).

The contribution of BPH to overall serum PSA has been estimated to be 0.3 ng/ml per gram of BPH tissue (Stamey et al, 1987) using the Yang Pros-Check polyclonal immunoassay (Bellevue, WA). The Yang polyclonal and Tandem monoclonal assays (Hybritech, San Diego, CA) are not equivalent, but in general the Yang assay gives values 1.4 to 1.9 times higher than the Tandem assay (Graves et al, 1990). This conversion would yield an estimated 0.15 ng/ml of PSA per gram of BPH tissue using the monoclonal assay—the PSA density cutoff that is most often used to distinguish between BPH and cancer. An accurate assessment of the BPH contribution to overall serum PSA is not possible for a given individual because (1) the epithelial component of BPH is the source of PSA, (2) there is a variable amount of epithelium and stroma within BPH tissue, and (3) no noninvasive methods are available for distinguishing between epithelium and stroma within BPH tissue. Partin and colleagues have shown that men with disease at a more advanced stage have higher-grade, higher-volume tumors that produce less PSA per gram of tumor (Partin et al, 1990). The heterogeneity of prostate cancer with respect to tumor grade prevents an accurate assessment of the effect of grade on overall serum PSA before treatment.

The confounding variables of BPH and tumor grade result in the overlap of serum PSA levels between stages, which hinders the prediction of final pathologic stage using PSA

alone for most patients. **As general guidelines, the majority of men (70%–80%) with PSA values less than 4.0 ng/ml have pathologically organ-confined disease; more than 50% of men with PSA levels greater than 10.0 ng/ml already have established capsular penetration; and most men (75%) with serum PSA levels greater than 50 ng/ml have positive pelvic lymph nodes** (Partin et al, 1990, 1993c). Approximately 60% of men with clinically localized prostate cancer, however, have serum PSA levels between 4.0 and 50.0 ng/ml (Partin et al, 1990), a large group of men for whom PSA is of limited use for preoperative staging when used alone. Table 83–6 shows the relationship between serum PSA and pathologic stage in a radical prostatectomy series.

Histologic Grade

Many histologic grading systems for prostate cancer have been introduced to help predict pathologic stage and prognosis (Utz and Farrow, 1969; Mostofi, 1976; Gleason et al, 1977; Harada et al, 1977; Geata et al, 1980; Brawn et al, 1982). The most commonly used histologic grading system for prostate cancer is the Gleason system (Gleason and the VACURG, 1977; Gleason, 1966), which has been shown to correlate directly with the pathologic extent of disease. Table 83–7 shows the distribution of Gleason scores determined on prostate biopsy before treatment, as a function of final pathologic stage for 703 men who underwent surgery for clinically localized prostate cancer (Partin et al, 1993c).

The pathologic criteria and method for determining the Gleason grade of a prostatic tumor is discussed in detail in Chapter 81. The Gleason grading system is based on a low-power microscopic description of the architectural criteria of the cancer (Gleason and the VACURG, 1977; Gleason, 1966). A Gleason grade (or pattern) of 1 to 5 is assigned as a primary grade (the pattern occupying the greatest area of the specimen) and a secondary grade (the pattern occupying the second largest area of the specimen). A Gleason sum (2–10) is determined by adding the primary grade to the secondary grade. **The presence of Gleason pattern 4 or greater (primary or secondary) or a Gleason sum of 7 or greater is predictive of a poorer prognosis** (Stein et al, 1991, 1992; Epstein et al, 1993a, 1993b; Partin et al, 1993b; Ohori et al, 1994a; Zincke et al, 1994). The importance of histologic grading is supported by multivariate analyses (Partin et al, 1993c, 1995b; Epstein et al, 1993a, 1993b, 1994a, 1994b, 1995; Blackwell et al, 1994; Irwin and Trapasso, 1994; Miller and Cygan, 1994; Sands et al, 1994; Sgrignoli

Table 83–6. PATHOLOGIC STAGE AS A FUNCTION OF PREOPERATIVE PROSTATE-SPECIFIC ANTIGEN LEVEL

PSA Level	No.	Organ Confined, No. (%)	Non–organ Confined, No. (%)
0.0–4.0 ng/ml	284	211 (75)	73 (25)
4.0–10.0 ng/ml	246	131 (53)	115 (47)
>10.0 ng/ml	173	50 (28)	123 (72)

PSA, Prostate-specific antigen.
Data from Partin AW, Yoo JK, Carter HB, et al: J Urol 1993; 150:110–114.

Table 83–7. DISTRIBUTION OF GLEASON SCORE BY PATHOLOGIC STAGE IN 703 MEN WITH CLINICALLY LOCALIZED PROSTATE CANCER

Gleason Score	No. Patients, (%)	Pathologic Stage			
		Organ-Confined Disease, No. (%)	Established Capsular Penetration, No. (%)	Positive Seminal Vesicles, No. (%)	Positive Lymph Nodes,* No. (%)
2–4	64 (9)	49 (77)	12 (19)	2 (3)	1 (1)
5	168 (24)	116 (69)	43 (26)	3 (2)	6 (4)
6	303 (43)	173 (57)	89 (30)	16 (5)	25 (8)
7	130 (19)	39 (30)	50 (38)	15 (12)	26 (20)
8–10	38 (5)	5 (13)	9 (24)	8 (21)	16 (42)
Total	703 (100)	382 (54)	203 (29)	44 (6)	74 (11)

*Includes patients who did not undergo radical prostatectomy because of positive lymph nodes at pelvic lymph node dissection.
Adapted from Partin AW, Yoo JK, Carter HB, et al: J Urol 1993; 150:110–114.

et al, 1994; Zeitman et al, 1994; CarMichael et al, 1995; D'Amico et al, 1995; Terris et al, 1995) of prognostic criteria for men with clinically localized disease that demonstrates Gleason sum (or grade) as a strong predictor of disease extent. Epstein and associates have suggested that all new prognostic indicators should be compared with the Gleason sum (grade) and proven to provide statistically independent predictive information before being considered clinically useful (Epstein et al, 1993a, 1993b, 1994a, 1994b, 1995).

Combined Use of Clinical Data to Predict Pathologic Stage

When used alone, the prognostic value of any clinical criterion used to predict tumor extent is limited for the individual patient with prostate cancer. **The staging accuracy for prostate cancer can be significantly enhanced by combining the parameters of local disease extent (T stage), serum PSA level, and Gleason grade from the prostate biopsy specimen** (Humphrey et al, 1991; Kleer et al, 1993; Kleer and Oesterling, 1993; Partin et al, 1993c; Bluestein et al, 1994). Probability tables, based on the parameters of preoperative clinical stage, serum PSA level, and Gleason sum, have been constructed from large numbers of men who have undergone radical prostatectomy with precise determination of the pathologic stage. In Tables 83–8 and 83–9, numbers within the nomogram represent the percent probability of having a given final pathologic stage based on logistic regression analyses for all three variables combined; dashes represent data categories in which insufficient data existed to calculate a probability. This information is useful in counseling men with newly diagnosed prostate cancer about treatment alternatives and probability of complete eradication of tumor. As examples, a man with a serum PSA of 3.0 ng/ml who has a clinical stage T2a cancer with a Gleason score of 5 has an 81% chance of having organ-confined disease, whereas a man with a serum PSA of 15 ng/ml who has a clinical stage T1c cancer and a Gleason score of 7 has only a 24% chance of having organ-confined disease.

Imaging

Bone scintigraphy (radionuclide bone scan), intravenous urography, magnetic resonance imaging (MRI), computed tomography (CT), and TRUS have been evaluated as methods for staging prostate cancer (Schaffer and Pendergrass, 1976; Paulson, 1979; Lee and Siders, 1990; Yang and Yang, 1990). These techniques are also discussed elsewhere in this text. For an imaging modality to be clinically useful for staging prostate cancer, the modality must reliably distinguish organ-confined disease from disease that has spread beyond the confines of the prostate gland (locally or distantly) and is thus not amenable to a curative approach.

Intravenous urography is not recommended for men with newly diagnosed prostate cancer as part of the staging evaluation. In those men with associated hematuria, intravenous urography may be useful in further evaluation of the upper urinary tract.

Bone survey films (skeletal radiography) are insensitive as a method to screen for the presence of bone metastases. Lachman (1955) and Lentle and co-workers (1974) demonstrated that greater than 50% of the bone density must be replaced by tumor before standard radiographic imaging methods identify distant spread. Skeletal radiography is recommended only for confirmation of a positive bone scan in men in whom bony metastases are not suspected at initial evaluation.

Bone scintigraphy (radionuclide bone scan) provides the most sensitive method for detecting bone metastases (Schaffer and Pendergrass, 1976; Gerber and Chodak, 1991; Terris et al, 1991). Of those men who are believed to be free of metastatic disease by bone survey, at least 25% demonstrate skeletal disease by bone scan (Paulson, 1979). False-negative results occur in 8% of patients undergoing metastatic evaluation for prostate cancer (Ball and Maynard, 1979). A positive bone scan is not specific for prostate cancer and should be confirmed by a bone survey if positive in men in whom bone metastases are unexpected. A bone scan is also a method of screening for urinary tract obstruction, obviating the need for further evaluation of the upper urinary tract in men with prostate cancer (Narayan et al, 1988).

Routine use of the radionuclide bone scan for prostate cancer staging has come into question with the advent of PSA testing because the probability of a positive scan is low in men with a PSA less than 10 ng/ml and no bone pain. Data using PSA as part of the staging evaluation for men with prostate cancer have suggested that the radionuclide bone scan may not be cost-effective (Chybowski et al, 1991). A negative radionuclide bone scan, however, provides valuable information before treatment as follows: upper urinary tract imaging to ensure bilateral renal function and a baseline

Table 83–8. MULTIVARIATE LOGISTIC REGRESSION ANALYSIS FOR PREDICTION OF PATHOLOGIC STAGE USING PROSTATE-SPECIFIC ANTIGEN, GLEASON SCORE, AND CLINICAL STAGE (TNM): PREDICTION OF ORGAN-CONFINED DISEASE (PERCENT)

	Prostate-Specific Antigen Level (ng/ml)													
	0.0–4.0 Clinical Stage							4.1–10.0 Clinical Stage						
Score	T1a	T1b	T1c	T2a	T2b	T2c	T3a	T1a	T1b	T1c	T2a	T2b	T2c	T3a
2–4	100	85	92	88	76	82	—	100	78	82	83	67	71	—
5	100	78	81	81	67	73	—	100	70	71	73	56	64	43
6	100	68	69	72	54	60	42	100	53	59	62	44	48	33
7	—	54	55	61	41	46	—	100	39	43	51	32	37	26
8–10	—	—	—	48	31	—	—	—	32	31	39	22	25	12

	Prostate-Specific Antigen Level (ng/ml)													
	10.0–20.0 Clinical Stage							>20 Clinical Stage						
Score	T1a	T1b	T1c	T2a	T2b	T2c	T3a	T1a	T1b	T1c	T2a	T2b	T2c	T3a
2–4	100	—	—	61	52	—	—	—	—	33	20	7	—	—
5	100	49	55	58	43	37	26	—	—	24	32	—	3	—
6	—	36	41	44	28	37	19	—	—	22	14	1	4	5
7	—	24	24	36	19	24	14	—	—	7	18	4	5	3
8–10	—	11	—	29	14	15	9	—	—	3	3	—	2	2

evaluation for comparison after treatment in men who later complain of bone pain (i.e., differential diagnosis of arthritis versus metastatic disease). Whether the additional cost of bone scan is justified for men with lower PSA levels is controversial.

TRUS is an insensitive method for detecting local extension of tumor (Rifkin et al, 1990). Some experts believe that TRUS adds additional staging information over that gained with DRE. The TRUS characteristics suggesting disease extension are covered in Chapter 82.

Pelvic imaging with CT or MRI for detection of local extension of disease or the presence of lymph node metastases is not routinely useful because of low sensitivity (Rifkin et al, 1990; Tempany et al, 1994; Wolf et al, 1995). **Pelvic imaging for lymph node assessment may be warranted in men at higher risk of metastases when sus-**

Table 83–9. MULTIVARIATE LOGISTIC REGRESSION ANALYSIS FOR PREDICTION OF PATHOLOGIC STAGE USING PROSTATE-SPECIFIC ANTIGEN, GLEASON SCORE, AND CLINICAL STAGE (TNM): PREDICTION OF LYMPH NODAL STATUS (PERCENT)

	Prostate-Specific Antigen Level (ng/ml)													
	0.0–4.0 Clinical Stage							4.1–10.0 Clinical Stage						
Score	T1a	T1b	T1c	T2a	T2b	T2c	T3a	T1a	T1b	T1c	T2a	T2b	T2c	T3a
2–4	0	2	<1	1	2	4	—	0	2	1	1	2	5	—
5	0	4	1	2	4	8	—	0	4	1	2	5	10	8
6	0	8	2	3	9	17	15	0	9	2	4	11	19	16
7	—	15	2	7	18	31	—	0	18	3	8	20	34	28
8–10	—	—	—	13	32	—	—	—	30	5	15	35	53	50

	Prostate-Specific Antigen Level (ngm/ml)													
	10.1–20.0 Clinical Stage							>20 Clinical Stage						
Score	T1a	T1b	T1c	T2a	T2b	T2c	T3a	T1a	T1b	T1c	T2a	T2b	T2c	T3a
2–4	0	—	—	1	3	—	—	—	—	6	2	7	—	—
5	0	5	3	2	6	13	11	—	—	9	3	—	29	—
6	—	11	4	5	13	22	20	—	—	8	9	18	53	31
7	—	21	7	9	24	39	35	—	—	24	11	44	62	55
8–10	—	41	—	17	40	59	54	—	—	41	35	76	73	65

pected by locally advanced disease on DRE, marked PSA elevations (>20 ng/ml), or the presence of poorly differentiated cancer on needle biopsy. Wolf and colleagues suggest, based on decision analysis, that the probability of lymph node metastases would need to be greater than 30% for pelvic imaging to be cost-effective (Wolf et al, 1995). Individuals at high risk for pelvic lymph node disease can be identified using probability tables as previously described (see Table 83–9). The majority of men found to have prostate cancer with PSA testing and DRE, excluding those with poorly differentiated tumors, do not benefit from pelvic imaging. Table 83–10 summarizes statistical data from a variety of studies evaluating TRUS, CT, and MRI for prostate cancer staging.

Pelvic Lymph Node Dissection

The status of the pelvic lymph nodes provides important information with respect to management because a curative

Table 83–10. PREDICTION OF PATHOLOGIC STAGE BY IMAGING TECHNIQUES

Reference	No. of Men	Sensitivity	Specificity
Extracapsular Penetration			
TRUS			
Rifkin et al, 1990	219	66	46
Andriole et al, 1989	64	50	90
Pontes et al, 1985	31	89	50
Salo et al, 1987a	38	86	94
CT			
Hricak et al, 1987	46	55	73
Platt et al, 1987	32	75	60
MRI			
Rifkin et al, 1990	194	77	57
Hricak et al, 1987	46	35–75	81–88
Bezzi et al, 1988	37	44	81
Seminal Vesicle Involvement			
TRUS			
Andriole et al, 1989	64	20	100
Pontes et al, 1985	31	100	85
Salo et al, 1987a	38	29	100
CT			
Salo et al, 1987a	38	36	96
Platt et al, 1987	32	33	60
MRI			
Bezzi et al, 1988	37	83	88
Biondetti et al, 1987	29	50	97
Lymph Nodal Involvement			
CT			
Hricak et al, 1987	46	22	—
Platt et al, 1987	32	0	96
Weinerman et al, 1983	32	66	90
Giri et al, 1982	12	80	86
Levine et al, 1981	15	100	87
Golimbu et al, 1981	46	70	93
MRI			
Hricak et al, 1987	46	44	—
Bezzi et al, 1988	51	69	95
Biondetti et al, 1987	18	67	100

Adapted from Gishman JR, de Vere White RW: *In* Krane RJ, Siroky MB, Fitzpatrick JM, eds: Clinical Urology. Philadelphia, J. B. Lippincott, 1994, pp 947–948.

approach has a low probability of success in the setting of lymph node metastases. The prevalence of pelvic lymph node metastases correlates directly with T stage, serum PSA levels, and histologic grade (Partin et al, 1993c). Studies have demonstrated that 5% to 12% of men who present with clinically localized prostate cancer are found to have either gross or microscopic lymph node metastases (Catalona and Bigg, 1990; Petros and Catalona, 1992; Danella et al, 1993; Partin et al, 1993c; Zincke et al, 1994). These data contrast markedly with data from prostatectomy series from the 1980s in which more than 20% of men thought to have clinically localized disease were found to have lymph node metastases at prostatectomy (Donohue et al, 1981, 1982). The decreasing prevalence of men presenting with pelvic lymph node metastases can be attributed primarily to earlier detection of cancer with PSA testing and TRUS biopsy, a phenomenon known as stage migration (Petros and Catalona, 1992; Danella et al, 1993; Partin and Oesterling, 1994).

Surgical removal and histologic examination of the pelvic lymph nodes provides the most accurate staging information relative to pelvic lymph node status. Pelvic lymph node dissection (PLND) has been routinely performed in conjunction with radical prostatectomy and can now be performed laparoscopically (the surgical technique of laparoscopic PLND is covered elsewhere in this text). The indication for laparoscopic PLND is a high suspicion of lymph node metastases based on the finding of (1) enlarged pelvic lymph nodes by pelvic imaging, (2) prebiopsy serum PSA level above 20 ng/ml, (3) poorly differentiated tumor on needle biopsy of the prostate (Gleason score 8–10) (Sgrignoli et al, 1994), or (4) palpable locally advanced tumor. Some authors believe that PLND—at the time of radical prostatectomy—is unecessary for men at low risk of having pelvic lymph node metastases based on preoperative parameters of T stage, serum PSA, and tumor grade (Kerbl et al, 1993; Bluestein et al, 1994; Narayan et al, 1994).

Molecular Staging of Prostate Cancer

All current, noninvasive staging techniques are limited by an inability to detect microscopic spread of prostatic cancer. The emphasis on earlier detection of disease with PSA testing has resulted in decreasing numbers of men who are diagnosed with grossly metastatic disease detectable by current imaging methods. More sensitive staging techniques—referred to as molecular staging—have focused on the detection of circulating prostate cancer cells in the peripheral blood. If circulating prostate cancer cells are present in peripheral blood, they can be identified indirectly by reverse transcription of circulating PSA mRNA to complementary DNA and amplification of DNA coding for PSA by polymerase chain reaction (RT-PCR). Thus, a positive PCR assay for PSA using peripheral blood suggests the presence of circulating prostate cells because the genetic message (mRNA) for PSA is prostate specific.

Moreno and co-workers used PCR analysis to evaluate blood from 12 patients with stage D prostate cancer and 17 controls (Moreno et al, 1992). PCR analysis was negative in all controls, whereas 4 of 12 cancer cases had positive PCR assays, suggesting the presence of circulating prostate cancer cells in the blood stream. Using a sensitive PCR technique for circulating PSA message, Katz and associates found that the results of the PCR assay better predicted pathologic stage among men undergoing radical prostatectomy than all other currently used predictors, including PSA and Gleason score (Katz et al, 1994). In addition, the PCR assay for PSA was a stronger predictor of pathologic stage among men with clinically localized disease who underwent radical prostatectomy than a PCR assay for prostate-specific membrane antigen (PSMA)—a prostate epithelial transmembrane glycoprotein (Cama et al, 1995). Direct comparisons of PCR assays for PSA and PSMA among men with metastatic prostate cancer have revealed a greater percentage of positive PCR-PSA assays in one study (Cama et al, 1995) and a greater percentage of positive PCR-PSMA assays in another study (Israeli et al, 1995). These results suggest that the sensitivity of these assays for detecting circulating cancer cells differs among investigators. PCR analysis for PSA has been found to be negative in men with no evidence of prostate cancer and in women. Thus, a positive PCR-PSA assay appears to be specific for prostate cancer cells and correlates directly with the pathologic extent of the cancer. False-positive PCR assays could result if very sensitive assays detect low levels of PSA—or "PSA like"—RNA in nonprostate cells within the circulation (Smith et al, 1995). One in 4 of 65 men with localized prostate cancer who underwent radical prostatectomy and had specimen-confined disease had a positive PCR-PSA assay in the study by Katz et al (1994). These men would be denied surgery if one concludes that circulating prostate cancer cells are synonymous with incurable disease. The ability of circulating prostate cancer cells—detected by PCR assays—to establish distant metastases is not yet known. Until the significance of a positive PCR assay is known by long-term follow-up, men with localized prostate cancer who have the potential for cure should not be denied curative treatment based on a PCR assay.

REFERENCES

Altwein JE, Leitenberger A, Ar R: Value of computed tomography and lymphography for the demonstration of pelvic lymph node metastases in prostatic cancer. Urol Int 1984; 39:178–183.

Andriole GL, Coplen DE, Mikkelsen DJ, Catalona WJ: Sonographic and pathological staging of patients with clinically localized prostate cancer. J Urol 1989; 142:1259–1261.

Armbruster DA: Prostate-specific antigen: Biochemistry, analytical methods, and clinical application. Clin Chem 1993; 39:181–195.

Babaian RJ, Fritsche HA, Evans RB: Prostate-specific antigen and prostate gland volume: Correlation and clinical application. J Clin Lab Anal 1990; 4:135–137.

Bahnson RR, Catalona WJ: Adverse implications of acid phosphatase levels in the upper range of normal. J Urol 1987; 137:427–430.

Ball JD, Maynard CD: Nuclear imaging in urology. Urol Clin North Am 1979; 6:321–342.

Bangma CH, Kranse R, Blijenberg BG, Schroeder FH: The value of screening tests in the detection of prostate cancer: Part I. Results of a retrospective evaluation of 1726 men. Urology 1995; 46:773–778.

Barry MJ, Fleming C, Coley CM, et al: Should Medicare provide reimbursement for prostate-specific antigen testing for early detection of prostate cancer? Part I. Framing the debate. Urology 1995a; 46:2–13.

Barry MJ, Fleming C, Coley CM, et al: Should Medicare provide reimbursement for prostate-specific antigen testing for early detection of prostate cancer? Part IV. Estimating the risks and benefits of an early detection program. Urology 1995b; 46:445–461.

Bazinet M, Meshref AW, Trudel C, et al: Prospective evaluation of prostate-specific antigen density and systematic biopsies for early detection of prostatic carcinoma. Urology 1994; 43:44–52.

Beahrs OH, Henson DE, Hutter RVP: Manual for Staging of Cancer, 3rd ed. Philadelphia, J. B. Lippincott, 1988.

Beahrs OH, Henson DE, Hutter RVP, Kennedy BJ: Manual for Staging of Cancer, 4th ed. Philadelphia, J. B. Lippincott, 1992, pp 181–186.

Beahrs OH, Myers MH: American Joint Committee on Cancer: Manual for Staging of Cancer, 2nd ed. Philadelphia, J. B. Lippincott, 1983, pp 159–164.

Benson MC: Prostate specific antigen (Editorial). J Urol 1994; 152:2046–2048.

Benson MC, Olson CA: The staging and grading of prostatic cancer. In Fitzpatrick JM, Krane RJ, eds: The Prostate. New York, Churchill Livingstone, 1989, pp 261–272.

Benson MC, Whang IS, Olsson CA, et al: Use of prostate specific antigen density to enhance predictive value of intermediate levels of serum prostate specific antigen. J Urol 1992a; 147:817–821.

Benson MC, Whang IS, Pantuck A, et al: Prostate specific antigen density: Means of distinguishing benign prostatic hypertrophy and prostate cancer. J Urol 1992b; 147:815–816.

Bezzi M, Kressel HY, Allen KS, et al: Prostatic carcinoma: Staging with MR at 1.5 T. Radiology 1988; 169:339–346.

Biondetti PR, Lee JKT, Ling D, Catalona WJ: Clinical stage B prostate carcinoma: Staging with MR imaging. Radiology 1987; 162:325–329.

Bjartell A, Bjork T, Matikainen MT, et al: Production of alpha₁-antichymotrypsin by PSA-containing cells of human prostate epithelium. Urology 1993; 42:502–510.

Bjork T, Abrahamsson P-A, Lilja H, et al: Rates of clearance of free and complexed forms of PSA in serum after radical prostatectomy and transurethral microwave therapy. J Urol 1995; 153:295A.

Bjork T, Bjartell A, Abrahamsson PA, et al: Alpha₁-antichymotrypsin production in PSA-producing cells is common in prostate cancer but rare in benign prostatic hyperplasia. Urology 1994; 43:427–434.

Blackwell KL, Bostwick DG, Myers RP, et al: Combining prostate specific antigen with cancer and gland volume to predict more reliably pathological stage: The influence of prostate specific antigen cancer density. J Urol 1994; 151:1566–1570.

Bluestein DL, Bostwick DG, Bergstralh EJ, Oesterling JE: Eliminating the need for bilateral pelvic lymphadenectomy in select patients with prostate cancer. J Urol 1994; 151:1315–1320.

Brawer MK, Aramburu EAG, Chen GL, et al: The inability of prostate specific antigen index to enhance the predictive value of prostate specific antigen in the diagnosis of prostatic carcinoma. J Urol 1993; 150:369–373.

Brawer MK, Chetner MP, Beatie J, et al: Screening for prostatic carcinoma with prostate specific antigen. J Urol 1992; 147:841–845.

Brawn PN, Ayala AG, Von Eschenbach AC, et al: Histologic grading study of prostate adenocarcinoma: The development of a new system and comparison with other methods—a preliminary study. Cancer 1982; 49:525–532.

Burnett AL, Chan DW, Brendler CB, Walsh PC: The value of serum enzymatic acid phosphatase in the staging of localized prostate cancer. J Urol 1992; 148:1832–1834.

Byar DP, Mostofi FK, the Veterans Administration Cooperative Urological Research Group: Carcinoma of the prostate: Prognostic evaluation of certain pathological features in 208 radical prostatectomies examined by step-section technique. Cancer 1972; 30:5–13.

Cama C, Olsson CA, Raffo AJ, et al: Molecular staging of prostate cancer: II. Comparison of application of enhanced reverse transcriptase polymerase chain reaction assay for prostate specific antigen versus prostate specific membrane antigen. J Urol 1995; 153:1373.

Canadian Task Force on the Periodic Health Examination: Periodic health examination, 1991 update: 3. Secondary prevention of prostate cancer. Can Med Assoc J 1991; 145:413–428.

CarMichael M, Veltri RW, Partin AW, et al: Deoxyribonucleic acid ploidy analysis as a predictor of recurrence following radical prostatectomy for stage T2 disease. J Urol 1995; 153:1015–1019.

Carter HB: Current status of PSA in the management of prostate cancer. In Cameron JL, ed: Advances in Surgery, Vol 27. Chicago, Mosby-Year Book, 1994, pp 81–95.

Carter HB, Hamper UM, Sheth S, et al: Evaluation of transrectal ultrasound in the diagnosis of prostate cancer. J Urol 1989; 142:1008–1010.

Carter HB, Pearson JD, Metter JE, et al: Longitudinal evaluation of prostate specific antigen levels in men with and without prostate disease. JAMA 1992; 267:2215–2220.

Carter HB, Pearson JD, Morrell CH, et al: What is the shortest time interval over which PSA velocity should be measured? J Urol 1995a; 153:419A.

Carter HB, Pearson JD, Waclawiw Z, et al: Prostate-specific antigen variability in men without prostate cancer: The effect of sampling interval and number of repeat measurements on prostate-specific antigen velocity. Urology 1995b; 45:591–596.

Catalona WJ, Bigg SW: Nerve-sparing radical prostatectomy: Evaluation of results after 250 patients. J Urol 1990; 143:538–544.

Catalona WJ, Hudson MA, Scardino PT, et al: Selection of optimal prostate specific antigen cutoffs for early detection of prostate cancer: Receiver operating characteristic curves. J Urol 1994a; 152:2037–2042.

Catalona WJ, Richie JP, Ahmann FR, et al: Comparison of digital rectal examination and serum prostate specific antigen in the early detection of prostate cancer: Results of a multicenter clinical trial of 6630 men. J Urol 1994b; 151:1283–1290.

Catalona WJ, Richie JP, DeKernion JB, et al: Comparison of prostate specific antigen concentration versus prostate specific antigen density in the early detection of prostate cancer: Receiver operating characteristic curves. J Urol 1994c; 152:2031–2036.

Catalona WJ, Smith DJ: Five-year tumor recurrence rates after anatomic radical retropubic prostatectomy for prostate cancer. J Urol 1994; 152:1837–1842.

Catalona WJ, Smith DS, Ratliff TL, Basler JW: Detection of organ-confined prostate cancer is increased through prostate-specific antigen based screening. JAMA 1993; 270:948–954.

Catalona WJ, Smith DS, Ratliff TL, et al: Measurement of prostate-specific antigen in serum as a screening test for prostate cancer. N Engl J Med 1991; 324:1156–1161.

Catalona WJ, Smith DS, Wolfert RL, et al: Evaluation of percentage of free serum prostate-specific antigen to improve specificity of prostate cancer screening. JAMA 1995; 274:1214–1220.

Catalona WJ, Whitmore WF Jr: New staging systems for prostate cancer (Editorial). J Urol 1989; 142:1302–1304.

Chodak GW, Keller P, Schoenberg HW: Assessment of screening for prostate cancer using the digital rectal examination. J Urol 1989; 141:1136–1138.

Christensson A, Bjork T, Nilsson O, et al: Serum prostate-specific antigen complexed to alpha₁-antichymotrypsin as an indicator of prostate cancer. J Urol 1993; 150:100–105.

Christensson A, Laurell CB, Lilja H: Enzymatic activity of prostate-specific antigen and its reactions with extracellular serine proteinase inhibitors. Eur J Biochem 1990; 194:755–763.

Chybowski FM, Bergstralh EJ, Oesterling JE: The effect of digital rectal examination on the serum prostate specific antigen concentration: Results of a randomized study. J Urol 1992; 148:83–86.

Chybowski FM, Larson-Keller JJ, Bergstralh EJ, Oesterling JE: Predicting radionuclide bone scan findings in patients with newly diagnosed untreated prostate cancer: Prostate specific antigen is superior to all other clinical parameters. J Urol 1991; 145:313–318.

Collins GN, Lee RJ, McKelvie GB, et al: Relationship between prostate specific antigen, prostate volume and age in the benign prostate. Br J Urol 1993; 71:445–550.

Cooner WH: Prostate cancer (Editorial). J Urol 1994; 151:103–104.

Cooner WH, Mosley BR, Rutherford CL Jr, et al: Prostate cancer detection in a clinical urologic practice by ultrasonography, digital rectal examination and prostate specific antigen. J Urol 1990; 143:1146–1154.

Crawford ED, Schutz MJ, Clejan S, et al: The effect of digital rectal examination on prostate-specific antigen levels. JAMA 1992; 267:2227–2228.

Dalkin BL, Ahmann FR, Kopp JB: Prostate specific antigen levels in men older than 50 years without clinical evidence of prostatic carcinoma. J Urol 1993; 150:1837–1839.

D'Amico AV, Whittington R, Malkowicz SB, et al: A multivariate analysis of clinical and pathological factors that predict for prostate specific antigen failure after radical prostatectomy for prostate cancer. J Urol 1995; 154:131–138.

Danella JF, deKernion JB, Smith RB, Steckel J: The contemporary incidence of lymph node metastases in prostate cancer: Implications for laparoscopic lymph node dissection. J Urol 1993; 149:1488–1491.

Donohue RE, Fauver HE, Whitesel JA, et al: Prostatic carcinoma: Influence of tumor grade on results of pelvic lymphadenectomy. Urology 1981; 17:435–440.

Donohue RE, Mani JH, Whitesel JA, et al: Pelvic lymph node dissection: Guide to patient management in clinically localized adenocarcinoma of prostate. Urology 1982; 20:559–565.

El-Galley RES, Petros JA, Sanders WH, et al: Normal range prostate-specific antigen versus age-specific prostate-specific antigen in screening prostate adenocarcinoma. Urology 1995; 46:200–204.

Ellis WJ, Chetner MP, Preston SD, Brawer MK: Diagnosis of prostatic carcinoma: The yield of serum prostate specific antigen, digital rectal examination and transrectal ultrasonography. J Urol 1994; 52:1520–1525.

Emory TH, Reinke DB, Hill AL, Lange PH: Use of CT to reduce understaging in prostate cancer: Comparison with conventional staging techniques. AJR 1983; 141:351–354.

Epstein JI: Evaluation of radical prostatectomy capsular margins of resection: The significance of margins designated as negative, closely approaching and positive. Am J Surg Pathol 1990; 14:626–632.

Epstein JI: PSA and PAP as immunohistochemical markers in prostate cancer. Urol Clin North Am 1993; 20:757–770.

Epstein JI, CarMichael M, Partin AW: OA-519 (Fatty acid synthase) as an independent predictor of pathologic stage in adenocarcinoma of the prostate. Urology 1995; 45:81–86.

Epstein JI, CarMichael MJ, Pizov G, Walsh PC: Influence of capsular penetration on progression following radical prostatectomy: A study of 196 cases with long-term follow-up. J Urol 1993a; 150:135–141.

Epstein JI, Pizov G, Walsh PC: Correlation of pathologic findings with progression after radical retropubic prostatectomy. Cancer 1993b; 71:3582–3593.

Epstein JI, Walsh PC, Brendler CB: Radical prostatectomy for impalpable prostate cancer: The Johns Hopkins experience with tumors found on transurethral resection (stages T1a and T1b) and on needle biopsy (stage T1c). J Urol 1994a; 152:1721–1729.

Epstein JI, Walsh PC, Carmichael M, Brendler CB: Pathologic and clinical findings to predict tumor extent of non-palpable (stage T1c) prostate cancer. JAMA 1994b; 271:368–374.

Ercole CJ, Lange PH, Mathiesen M, et al: Prostate-specific antigen and prostatic acid phosphatase in the monitoring and staging of patients with prostatic cancer. J Urol 1987; 138:1181–1184.

Feightner JW: The early detection and treatment of prostate cancer: The perspective of the Canadian Task Force on the Periodic Health Examination. J Urol 1994; 152:1682–1684.

Ferguson JK, Bostwick DG, Suman V, et al: Prostate-specific antigen detected prostate cancer: Pathological characteristics of ultrasound visible versus ultrasound invisible tumors. Eur Urol 1995; 27:8–12.

Flanigan RC, Catalona WJ, Richie JP, et al: Accuracy of digital rectal examination and transrectal ultrasonography in localizing prostate cancer. J Urol 1994; 152:1506–1509.

Frazier A, Robertson JE, Humphrey PA, Paulson DF: Is prostate-specific antigen of clinical importance in evaluating outcome after radical prostatectomy. J Urol 1993; 149:516–518.

Gann PH, Hennekens CH, Stampfer MJ: A prospective evaluation of plasma prostate-specific antigen for detection of prostatic cancer. JAMA 1995; 273:289–294.

Geata JF, Asirwatham JE, Miller G, Murphy GP: Histologic grading of primary prostatic cancer: A new approach to an old problem. J Urol 1980; 123:689–693.

Gerber G, Chodak GW: Assessment of value of routine bone scans in patients with newly diagnosed prostate cancer. Urology 1991; 37:418–422.

Gilliland F, Becker TM, Smith A, et al: Trends in prostate cancer incidence and mortality in New Mexico are consistent with an increase in effective screening. Cancer Epidemiol Biol Prev 1994; 3:105–111.

Giri PG, Walsh JW, Hazra TA, et al: Role of computed tomography in the evaluation and management of carcinoma of the prostate. Int J Radiat Oncol Biol Phys 1982; 8:283–287.

Gleason DF: Classification of prostatic carcinoma. Cancer Chemother Rep 1966; 50:125–128.

Gleason DF, the VACURG: Histological grading and clinical staging of prostatic carcinoma. In Tannenbaum M, ed: Urologic Pathology: The Prostate. Philadelphia, Lea & Febiger, 1977, pp 171–197.

Goldfarb DA, Stein BS, Shamszadeh M, Petersen RO: Age-related changes in tissue levels of prostatic acid phosphatase and prostate specific antigen. J Urol 1986; 136:1266–1269.

Golimbu M, Morales P, Al-Askari S, Shulman Y: CAT scanning and staging of prostate cancer. Urology 1981; 23:505–508.

Graves HCB, Wehner N, Stamey TA: Comparison of a polyclonal and monoclonal immunoassay for PSA: Need for an international antigen standard. J Urol 1990; 144:1516–1522.

Gronberg H, Damber J-E, Jonsson H, Lenner P: Patient age as a prognostic factor in prostate cancer. J Urol 1994; 152:892–895.

Guess HA, Heyse JF, Gormley GJ, et al: Effect of finasteride on serum PSA concentration in men with benign prostatic hyperplasia: Results from the North American Phase III Clinical Trial. Urol Clin North Am 1993; 20:627–636.

Haapianen RK, Permi EJ, Rannikko SAS, et al: Prostate tumor markers as an aid in staging of prostate cancer. Br J Urol 1990; 65:264–267.

Hammerer P, Huland H: Systematic sextant biopsies in 651 patients referred for prostate evaluation. J Urol 1994; 151:99–102.

Harada M, Mostofi FK, Corle DK, et al: Preliminary studies of histologic prognosis in cancer of the prostate. Cancer Treat Rep 1977; 61:223–225.

Heller JE: Prostatic acid phosphatase: Its current clinical status. J Urol 1987; 137:1091–1103.

Helzlsouer KJ, Newby J, Comstock GW: Prostate-specific antigen levels and subsequent prostate cancer: Potential for screening. Cancer Epidemiol Biomark Prev 1992; 1:537–540.

Henttu P, Liao S, Vihko P: Androgens up-regulate the human prostate-specific antigen messenger ribonucleic acid (mRNA) but down-regulate the prostatic acid phosphatase mRNA in the LNCaP cell line. Endocrinology 1992; 130:766–772.

Hodge KK, McNeal JE, Terris MK, Stamey TA: Random systematic versus directed ultrasound guided transrectal core biopsies of the prostate. J Urol 1989; 142:71–75.

Hricak H, Dooms GC, Jeffrey RB, et al: Prostatic carcinoma: Staging by clinical assessment, CT, and MRI. Radiology 1987; 162:331–336.

Hudson MA, Bahnson RR, Catalona WJ: Clinical use of prostate-specific antigen in patients with prostate cancer. J Urol 1989; 142:1011–1017.

Humphrey PA, Walther PJ, Currin SM, Vollmer RT: Histologic grade, DNA ploidy, and intraglandular tumor extent as indicators of tumor progression of clinical stage B prostate carcinoma. Am J Surg Pathol 1991; 15:1165–1170.

International Union Against Cancer: Urological tumours: Prostate. *In* Hermanek P, Sobin LH, eds: TNM Classification of Malignant Tumors, 4th ed, 2nd rev. Berlin, Springer-Verlag, 1992, pp 141–144.

Irwin MB, Trapasso JG: Identification of insignificant prostate cancers: Analysis of preoperative parameters. Urology 1994; 44:862–868.

Israeli RS, Miller WH Jr, Su SL, et al: Sensitive detection of prostatic hematogenous tumor cell dissemination using prostate specific antigen and prostate specific membrane-derived primers in the polymerase chain reaction. J Urol 1995; 153:573–577.

Jewett HJ: Significance of the palpable prostatic nodule. JAMA 1956; 160:838.

Jewett HJ: The present status of radical prostatectomy for stages A and B prostatic cancer. Urol Clin North Am 1975; 2:105–124.

Kalish J, Cooner WH, Graham SD: Serum PSA adjusted for volume of transition zone (PSAT) is more accurate than PSA adjusted for total gland volume (PSAD) in detecting adenocarcinoma of the prostate. Urology 1994; 43:601–606.

Katz AE, Olsson CA, Raffo AJ, et al: Molecular staging of prostate cancer with the use of an enhanced reverse transcriptase-PCR assay. Urology 1994; 43:765–775.

Kerbl K, Clayman RV, Petros JA, et al: Staging pelvic lymphadenectomy for prostate cancer: A comparison of laparoscopic and open techniques. Urology 1993; 150:396–398.

Kerlikowske K, Grady D, Barclay J, et al: Positive predictive value of screening mammography by age and family history of breast cancer. JAMA 1993; 270:2444–2450.

Kleer E, Larson-Keller JJ, Zinke H, Oesterling JE: Ability of pre-operative serum prostate-specific antigen value to predict pathologic stage and DNA ploidy. Urology 1993; 41:207–216.

Kleer E, Oesterling JE: Prostate-specific antigen and staging of localized prostate cancer. Urol Clin North Am 1993; 20:675–704.

Komatsu K, Wehner N, Prestigiacomo AF, Chen Z, Stamey TA: Physiologic (intraindividual) variation of serum prostate-specific antigen in 814 men from a screening population. Urology 1996; 47:343–346.

Kramer BS, Brown ML, Prorok PC, et al: Prostate cancer screening: What we know and what we need to know. Ann Intern Med 1993; 119:914–923.

Labrie F, Dupont A, Suburu R, et al: Serum prostate specific antigen as pre-screening test for protate cancer. J Urol 1992; 147:846–852.

Lachman E: Osteoporosis: The potentialities and limitations of its roentgenologic diagnosis. AJR Radium Ther Nucl Med 1955; 74:712–725.

Lange PH, Erole CJ, Lightner DJ, et al: The value of serum prostate-specific antigen determinations before and after radical prostatectomy. J Urol 1989; 141:873–879.

Lee F, Siders DB: Prostate cancer: Staging by transrectal ultrasonography. *In* Resnick MI, ed: Prostatic Ultrasonography. Philadelphia, B. C. Decker, 1990, pp 85–95.

Leinonen J, Lovgren T, Vornanen T, Stenman UH: Double-label time-resolved immunofluorometric assay of prostate-specific antigen and of its complex with alpha-1-antichymotrypsin. Clin Chem 1993; 39:2098–2103.

Lentle BC, McGowan DG, Dierich H: Technetium-99m polyphosphate bone scanning in carcinoma of the prostate. Br J Urol 1974; 46:543–548.

Lepor H, Wang B, Shapiro E: Relationship between prostatic epithelial volume and serum prostate-specific antigen levels. Urology 1994; 44:199–205.

Levine MS, Arger PH, Coleman BG, et al: Detecting lymphatic metastases from prostatic carcinoma: Superiority of CT. AJR 1981; 137:207–211.

Lilja H: A kallikrein-like serine protease in prostatic fluid cleaves the predominant seminal vesicle protein. J Clin Invest 1985; 76:1899–1903.

Lilja H: Significance of different molecular forms of serum PSA: The free, non-complexed form of PSA versus that complexed to alpha-1-antichymotrypsin. Urol Clin North Am 1993; 20:681–686.

Lilja H, Christensson A, Dahlen U, et al: Prostate-specific antigen in human serum occurs predominantly in complex with alpha$_1$-antichymotrypsin. Clin Chem 1991; 37:1618–1625.

Littrup PJ, Kane RA, Mettlin CJ, et al: Cost-effective prostate cancer detection. Cancer 1994; 74:3146–3158.

Littrup PJ, Kane RA, Williams CR, et al: Determination of prostate volume with transrectal US for cancer screening. Radiology 1991; 178:537–542.

Litwin MS, deKernion JB: Perspectives on the problem of prostate cancer (Editorial). J Urol 1994; 152:1680–1681.

Lowe FC, Trauzzi SJ: Prostatic acid phosphatase in 1993. Urol Clin North Am 1993; 20:589–595.

Luderer AA, Chen Y-T, Soriano TF, et al: Measurement of the proportion of free to total prostate-specific antigen improves diagnostic performance of prostate-specific antigen in the diagnostic gray zone of total prostate-specific antigen. Urology 1995; 146:187–194.

Lundwall A, Lilja H: Molecular cloning of human prostate specific antigen cDNA. FEBS Letters 1987; 214:317–322.

McCormack RT, Rittenhouse HG, Finlay JA, et al: Molecular forms of prostate-specific antigen and the human kallikrein gene family: A new era. Urology 1995; 45:729–744.

McGee RS, Herr JC: Human seminal vesicle-specific antigen is a substrate for prostate-specific antigen (or P-30). Biol Reprod 1988; 39:499–510.

Mettlin C, Jones G, Averette H, et al: Defining and updating the American Cancer Society guidelines for the cancer-related checkup: Prostate and endometrial cancers. Cancer 1993; 43:42.

Mettlin C, Littrup PJ, Kane RA, et al: Relative sensitivity and specificity of serum prostate specific antigen (PSA) level compared with age-referenced PSA, PSA density, and PSA change. Cancer 1994; 74:1615–1620.

Miller GJ, Cygan JM: Morphology of prostate cancer: The effects of multifocality on histological grade, tumor volume and capsular penetration. J Urol 1994; 152:1709–1713.

Montie JE: Significance and treatment of positive margins or seminal vesicle invasion after radical prostatectomy. Urol Clin North Am 1990; 17:803–812.

Moreno JG, Croce CM, Fischer R, et al: Detection of hematogenous micrometastasis in patients with prostate cancer. Cancer Res 1992; 52:6110–6112.

Morton RA, Steiner MS, Walsh PC: Cancer control following anatomical radical prostatectomy: An interim report. J Urol 1991; 145:1197–1200.

Mostofi FK: Problems of grading carcinoma of the prostate. Semin Oncol 1976; 3:161–169.

Mueller EJ, Crain TW, Thompson IA, Rodriguez FR: An evaluation of serial digital rectal examinations in screening for prostate cancer. J Urol 1988; 140:1445–1447.

Narayan P, Fournier G, Gajendran V, et al: Utility of preoperative serum prostate-specific antigen concentration and biopsy Gleason score in predicting risk of pelvic lymph node metastases in prostate cancer. Urology 1994; 44:519–524.

Narayan P, Lillian D, Hellstrom W, et al: The benefits of combining early radionuclide renal scintigraphy with routine bone scans in patients with prostate cancer. J Urol 1988; 140:1448–1451.

Oesterling JE: Prostate specific antigen: A critical assessment of the most useful tumor marker for adenocarcinoma of the prostate. J Urol 1991; 145:907–923.

Oesterling JE, Brendler CB, Epstein JI, et al: Correlation of clinical stage, serum prostatic acid phosphatase and preoperative Gleason grade with final pathological stage in 275 patients with clinically localized adenocarcinoma of the prostate. J Urol 1987; 138:92–98.

Oesterling JE, Chan DW, Epstein JI, et al: Prostate specific antigen in the preoperative and postoperative evaluation of localized prostatic cancer treated with radical prostatectomy. J Urol 1988; 139:766–772.

Oesterling JE, Jacobsen SJ, Chute CG, et al: Serum prostate-specific antigen in a community-based population of healthy men: Establishment of age-specific reference ranges. JAMA 1993; 270:860–864.

Oesterling JE, Jacobsen SJ, Cooner WH: The use of age-specific reference ranges for serum prostate specific antigen in men 60 years old or older. J Urol 1995; 153:1160–1163.

Ohori M, Goad JR, Wheeler TM, et al: Can radical prostatectomy alter the progression of poorly differentiated prostate cancer. J Urol 1994a; 152:1843–1849.

Ohori M, Wheeler TM, Kattan MW, et al: Prognostic significance of positive surgical margins in radical prostatectomy specimens. J Urol 1995; 154:1818–1824.

Ohori M, Wheeler TM, Scardino PT: The new American Joint Committee on Cancer and International Union Against Cancer TNM classification of prostate cancer: Clinicopathologic correlations. Cancer 1994b; 73:104–114.

Partin AW, Borland RN, Epstein JI, Brendler CB: Influence of established capsular penetration on prognosis in men with clinically localized prostate cancer. J Urol 1993a; 150:135–141.

Partin AW, Carter HB, Chan DW, et al: Prostate specific antigen in the staging of localized prostate cancer: Influence of tumor differentiation, tumor volume and benign hyperplasia. J Urol 1990; 143:747–752.

Partin AW, Kelly CA, Subong ENP, et al: Measurement of the ratio of free PSA to total PSA improves prostate cancer detection for men with total PSA levels between 4.0–10.0 ng/ml (Abstract no. 266). J Urol 1995a; 153:295A.

Partin AW, Oesterling JE: The clinical usefulness of prostate specific antigen: Update 1994. J Urol 1994; 152:1358–1368.

Partin AW, Piantadosi S, Sanda MG, et al: Selection of men at high risk for disease recurrence for experimental adjuvant therapy following radical prostatectomy. Urology 1995b; 45:831–838.

Partin AW, Pound CR, Clemens JQ, et al: Prostate-specific antigen after anatomic radical prostatectomy: The Johns Hopkins experience after ten years. Urol Clin North Am 1993b; 20:713–725.

Partin AW, Yoo JK, Carter HB, et al: The use of prostate-specific antigen, clinical stage and Gleason score to predict pathological stage in men with localized prostate cancer. J Urol 1993c; 150:110–114.

Paulson DF: The impact of current staging procedures in assessing disease extent of prostatic adenocarcinoma. J Urol 1979; 121:300–302.

Paulson DF: Impact of radical prostatectomy in the management of clinically localized disease. J Urol 1994; 152:1826–1830.

Petros JA, Catalona WJ: Lower incidence of unsuspected lymph node metastases in 512 consecutive patients with clinically localized prostate cancer. J Urol 1992; 147:1574–1575.

Pizzo SV, Mast AE, Feldman SR, Salvesen G: In vivo catabolism of α_1-antichymotrypsin is mediated by the serpin receptor which binds α_1-proteinase inhibitor, antithrombin II and heparin cofactor II. Biochem Biophys Acta 1988; 967:158–162.

Platt JF, Bree RI, Schwab RE: The accuracy of CT in the staging of carcinoma of the prostate. AJR 1987; 149:315.

Pontes JE, Eisenkraft S, Watanabe H, et al: Preoperative evaluation of localized prostate cancer by transrectal ultrasonography. J Urol 1985; 134:289.

Price JM, Davidson AJ: Computed tomography in the evaluation of the suspected carcinomatous prostate. Urol Radiol 1979; 1:38–51.

Rainwater LM, Morgan WR, Klee GG, Zinke H: Prostate-specific antigen testing in untreated and treated prostatic adenocarcinoma. Mayo Clin Proc 1990; 65:1118–1126.

Riehmann M, Rhodes PR, Cook TD, et al: Analysis of variation in prostate-specific antigen values. Urology 1993; 42:390–397.

Rifkin MD, Zerhouni EA, Gatsonis CA, et al: Comparison of magnetic resonance imaging and ultrasonography in staging early prostate cancer: Results of a multi-institutional cooperative trial. N Engl J Med 1990; 323:621–626.

Robles JM, Morell AR, Redorta JP, et al: Clinical behavior of prostatic specific antigen and prostatic acid phosphatase: A comparative study. Eur Urol 1988; 14:360–366.

Romas NA, Kwan DJ: Prostatic acid phosphatase. Urol Clin North Am 1993; 20:581–588.

Rommel FM, Agusta VE, Breslin JA, et al: Use of prostate specific antigen and prostate specific antigen density in diagnosis of prostate cancer in community based urology practice. J Urol 1994; 151:88–93.

Roy AV, Brower ME, Hayden JE: Sodium thymolphthalein monophosphate: A new acid phosphatase substrate with greater specificity for the prostatic enzyme in serum. Clin Chem 1971; 17:1093–1102.

Salo JO, Kivisarri L, Rannikko S, Lehtonen T: CT and transrectal ultrasound in the assessment of local extension of prostatic cancer before radical retropubic prostatectomy. J Urol 1987a; 137:435.

Salo JO, Rannikko S, Makinen J, Lehtonen T: Echogenic structure of prostatic cancer imaged on radical prostatectomy specimens. Prostate 1987b; 10:1–9.

Sands EM, Zagars GK, Pollack A, vonEschenbach AC: Serum prostate-specific antigen, clinical stage, pathological grade, and the incidence of nodal metastases in prostate cancer. Urology 1994; 44:215–220.

Sawczuk IS, deVere White R, Gold RP, Olson CA: Sensitivity of computed tomography in evaluation of pelvic lymph node metastases from carcinoma of bladder and prostate. Urology 1983; 21:81–84.

Schaffer DL, Pendergrass HP: Comparison of enzyme, clinical, pathological, radiographic and radionuclide methods of detecting bone metastases from carcinoma of the prostate. Radiology 1976; 121:431–434.

Schroder FH, Hermanek P, Denis L, et al: The TNM classification of prostate cancer. Prostate 1992; 4(Suppl):129–138.

Seaman E, Whang M, Olsson CA, et al: Prostate-specific antigen density (PSAD): Role in patient evaluation and management. Urol Clin North Am 1993; 20:653–663.

Sgrignoli AR, Walsh PC, Steinberg GD, et al: Prognostic factors in men with stage D1 prostate cancer: Identification of patients less likely to have prolonged survival after radical prostatectomy. J Urol 1994; 152:1077–1081.

Shock NW, Greulich RC, Andres R, et al: Normal Human Aging: The Baltimore Longitudinal Study of Aging. Washington, D.C., U.S. Government Printing Office (NIH publication no. 84–2450), 1984.

Simak R, Madersbacher S, Zhang Z-F, Maier U: The impact of ejaculation on serum prostate specific antigen. J Urol 1993; 150:895–897.

Skaletsky R, Koch MO, Eckstein CW, et al: Tumor volume and stage in carcinoma of the prostate detected by elevations in prostate specific antigen. J Urol 1994; 152:129–131.

Smith DS, Catalona WJ: Rate of change in serum prostate specific antigen levels as a method for prostate cancer detection. J Urol 1994; 152:1163–1167.

Smith DS, Catalona WJ: Interexaminer variability of digital rectal examination in detecting prostate cancer. Urology 1995; 45:70–74.

Smith MR, Biggar S, Hussain M: Prostate-specific antigen messenger RNA is expressed in non-prostate cells: Implications for detection of micrometastases. Cancer Res 1995; 55:2640–2644.

Sokoloff RL, Armour KW, Wolfert RL, et al: Immunoassay analytical recovery of prostate-specific antigen purified from seminal fluid. Clin Chem 1994; 40:1029.

Spiessl B, Hermanek P, Scheibe O, Wagner G: Prostate. In TNM Atlas: Illustrated Guide to the Classification of Malignant Tumours, 2nd ed. New York, Springer-Verlag, 1982, p 180.

Stamey TA: Second Stanford Conference on international standardization of prostate-specific antigen immunoassays: September 1 and 2, 1994. Urology 1995; 45:173–184.

Stamey TA, Yang N, Hay AR, et al: Prostate-specific antigen as a serum marker for adenocarcinoma of the prostate. N Engl J Med 1987; 317:909–916.

Stein A, deKernion JB, Dorey F: Prostatic specific antigen related to clinical status 1 to 14 years after radical retropubic prostatectomy. Br J Urol 1991; 67:626–631.

Stein A, deKernion JB, Smith RB, et al: Prostatic specific antigen after radical prostatectomy in patients with organ confined and locally extensive prostate cancer. J Urol 1992; 147:942–946.

Stenman UH, Hakama M, Knekt P, et al: Serum concentrations of prostate specific antigen and its complex with α-1-antichymotrypsin before diagnosis of prostate cancer. Lancet 1994; 344:1594–1598.

Stenman UH, Leinonen J, Alfthan H, et al: A complex between prostate-specific antigen and alpha$_1$-antichymotrypsin is the major form of prostate-specific antigen in serum of patients with prostatic cancer: Assay of the complex improves clinical sensitivity for cancer. Cancer Res 1991; 51:222–226.

Stone NN, DeAntoni EP, Crawford ED: Screening for prostate cancer by digital rectal examination and prostate-specific antigen: Results of prostate cancer awareness week, 1989–1992. Urology 1994; 44:18–25.

Stone NN, Stock RG, Unger P: Indications for seminal vesicle biopsy and laparoscopic pelvic lymph node dissection in men with localized carcinoma of the prostate. J Urol 1995; 154:1392–1396.

Stormont TJ, Farrow GM, Myers RP, et al: Clinical stage B0 or T1c prostate cancer: Nonpalpable disease identified by elevated serum prostate-specific antigen concentration. Urology 1993; 41:3–8.

Tempany CM, Zhou X, Zerhouni EA, et al: Staging of prostate cancer: Results of Radiology Diagnostic Oncology Group Project comparison of three MR imaging techniques. Radiology 1994; 192:47–54.

Terris MK, Haney DJ, Johnstone IM, et al: Prediction of prostate cancer volume using prostate-specific antigen levels, transrectal ultrasound and systematic sextant biopsies. Urology 1995; 45:75–80.

Terris MK, Klonecke AS, McDougall IR, Stamey TA: Utilization of bone scans in conjunction with prostate-specific antigen levels in the surveillance for recurrence of adenocarcinoma after radical prostatectomy. J Nucl Med 1991; 32:1713–1717.

Terris MK, McNeal JE, Freiha FS, Stamey TA: Efficacy of transrectal ultrasound-guided seminal vesicle biopsies in the detection of seminal vesicle invasion by prostate cancer. J Urol 1993; 149:1035–1039.

Thompson IM, Rounder JB, Teague JL, et al: Impact of routine screening for adenocarcinoma of the prostate on stage distribution. J Urol 1987; 137:424–426.

Tibblin G, Welin L, Bergstrom R, et al: The value of prostate specific antigen in early diagnosis of prostate cancer: The study of men born in 1913. J Urol 1995; 154:1386–1389.

Turner RD, Belt EA: A study of 229 consecutive cases of total perineal prostatectomy for cancer of the prostate. J Urol 1957; 77:62–77.

U.S. Preventive Services Task Force: Guide to Clinical Preventive Services: An Assessment of the Effectiveness of 169 Interventions. Baltimore, Williams & Wilkins, 1989, p 63.

Utz DC, Farrow GM: Pathologic differentiation and prognosis of prostatic carcinoma. JAMA 1969; 209:1701–1703.

Uzzo RG, Wei JT, Waldbaum RS, et al: The influence of prostate size on cancer detection. Urology 1995; 46:831–836.

Vallancien G, Bochereau G, Wetzel O, et al: Influence of preoperative positive vesicle biopsy on the staging of prostatic cancer. J Urol 1994; 152:1152–1156.

Vessella RL, Lange PH: Issues in the assessment of PSA immunoassay. Urol Clin North Am 1993; 20:607–619.

Vieira JGH, Nishida SK, Pereira AB, et al: Serum levels of prostate-specific antigen in normal boys throughout puberty. J Clin Endocrinol Metab 1994; 78:1185–1187.

Villers AA, McNeal JE, Redwine EA, et al: The role of perineural space invasion in the local spread of prostatic adenocarcinoma. J Urol 1989; 142:763–768.

Villers AA, McNeal JE, Redwine EA, et al: Pathogenesis and biological significance of seminal vesicle invasion in prostatic adenocarcinoma. J Urol 1990; 143:1183–1187.

Wallace DM, Chisolm GD, Hendry WF: TNM classification for urological tumors (UICC)—1974. Br J Urol 1975; 47:1–12.

Walsh PC, Jewett HJ: Radical surgery for prostatic cancer. Cancer 1980; 45(Suppl):1906–1911.

Walsh PC, Partin AW, Epstein JI: Cancer control and quality of life following anatomical radical retropubic prostatectomy: Results at ten years. J Urol 1994; 152:1831–1836.

Wang MC, Papsidero LD, Kuriyama M, et al: Prostate antigen: A new potential marker for prostate cancer. Prostate 1981; 2:89–96.

Weinerman PM, Arger PH, Coleman BG, et al: Pelvic adenopathy from bladder and prostate carcinoma: Detection by rapid sequence computed tomography. AJR 1983; 140:95–99.

Weinerman PM, Arger PH, Pollack HM: CT evaluation of bladder and prostate neoplasms. Urol Radiol 1982; 4:105–118.

Westphal J, Heidenreich A, Zumbe J, Engelmann UH: The impact of ejaculation on serum PSA. J Urol 1995; 153:464A.

Wheeler TM: Anatomic considerations in carcinoma of the prostate. Urol Clin North Am 1989; 16:623–634.

Whitesel JA, Donohue RE, Mani JH, et al: Acid phosphatase: Its influence on the management of carcinoma of the prostate. J Urol 1984; 131:70–72.

Whitmore WF Jr: Hormone therapy in prostate cancer. Am J Med 1956; 21:697–713.

Whitmore WF Jr, Catalona WJ, Grayhack JT, et al: Organ systems program staging classification for prostate cancer. *In* Coffey DS, Resnick MI, Dorr FA, Karr JP, eds: A Multidisciplinary Analysis of Controversies in the Management of Prostate Cancer. New York, Plenum Press, 1988, pp 295–297.

Wolf JS Jr, Cher M, Dall'era M, et al: The use and accuracy of cross-sectional imaging and fine needle aspiration cytology for detection of pelvic lymph node metastases before radical prostatectomy. J Urol 1995; 153:993–999.

Yang A, Yang S: MRI and CT of the prostate gland. *In* Goldman SM, Gatewood OMB, eds: CT and MRI of the Genitourinary Tract. New York, Churchill Livingstone, 1990, pp 157–184.

Young CYF, Montgomery BT, Andrews PE, et al: Hormonal regulation of prostate-specific antigen messenger RNA in human prostatic adenocarcinoma cell line LNCaP. Cancer Res 1991; 51:3748–3752.

Yuan JJJ, Coplen DE, Petros JA, et al: Effects of rectal examination, prostatic massage, ultrasonography and needle biopsy on serum prostate specific antigen levels. J Urol 1992; 147:810–814.

Zagars GK, Sherman NE, Babaian RJ: Prostate-specific antigen after external beam radiation therapy in prostate cancer. Cancer 1992; 67:412–420.

Zeitman AL, Edelstein RA, Coen JJ, et al: Radical prostatectomy for adenocarcinoma of the prostate: The influence of preoperative and pathologic findings on biochemical disease-free outcome. Urology 1994; 43:828–833.

Zhou AM, Tewari PC, Bluestein BI, et al: Multiple forms of prostate-specific antigen in serum: Differences in immunorecognition by monoclonal and polyclonal assays. Clin Chem 1993; 39:2483–2491.

Zincke H, Oesterling JE, Blute ML, et al: Long-term (15 years) results after radical prostatectomy for clinically localized (stage T2c or lower) prostate cancer. J Urol 1994; 152:1850–1857.

84
THE NATURAL HISTORY OF LOCALIZED PROSTATE CANCER: A GUIDE TO THERAPY

Patrick C. Walsh, M.D.

Longitudinal Studies of Serum Prostate-Specific Antigen

Results with Deferred Treatment
Individual Series
Combined Series
Decision Analysis

Results with Ineffective Treatments

Results Following Radical Prostatectomy

Summary

At present, prostate cancer is the most common cancer diagnosed in men in the United States and the second most common cause of cancer death. Over the past decade, there have been a number of major advances in the diagnosis and treatment of the disorder. Through the use of digital rectal examination, prostate-specific antigen (PSA) testing, and improved biopsy techniques, it is now possible to diagnose prostate cancer in more men at an earlier curable stage. Furthermore, through the use of anatomic studies, the morbidity of radical prostatectomy has been reduced, making this form of management more acceptable to patients and to their physicians. Recognizing, however, that prostate cancer is most frequently diagnosed in older men and often has a long protracted course, many question whether any treatment is actually necessary.

To answer this question, some have proposed long-term prospective, randomized trials comparing early diagnosis with active therapy versus no treatment (watchful waiting). Data from these clinical trials, however, will not be available for many years, long after most urologists who are practicing today have retired. Therefore, it is necessary to provide some additional guidance to urologists who are practicing today and to the patients they are treating. To provide this answer, the natural history of untreated localized prostate cancer and its impact on the quality and duration of survival in affected patients should be examined.

In 1994, it was estimated that there were 200,000 new cases of prostate cancer diagnosed and 38,000 prostate can-

cer deaths (Boring et al, 1994) (Fig. 84–1). **The ratio of death rate to incidence inferred from these statistics suggests that approximately 20% of men with clinical diagnoses of prostate cancer die from the disease. The true percentage is most likely higher.** In Sweden, where the incidence rates have been stable for many years and have not been influenced by PSA testing and where prostate cancer is not treated with curative intent, 55% of men with prostate cancer die from the disease (Gronberg et al, in press). Some are surprised by these facts and have the impression that less than 1% of men with the disease die from it. For example, Stamey (1983) is often quoted as saying that only one of 380 men with prostate cancer dies from it. His interpretation of the data is flawed in two ways. The annual death rate was used but was divided by the prevalence of the disease (the number of men who are alive today with prostate cancer) rather than the incidence (the number of new cases per year). Even if his calculation were correct, this statistic would have little meaning if one wished to estimate what percentage of men with *clinical* prostate cancer would eventually die from the disease. In Stamey's calculation, the prevalence of the disease was based on the assumption that 30% to 50% of all men over the age of 50 have prostate cancer. Because there is no form of early detection sensitive enough to diagnose all incidental microscopic tumors, this calculation is meaningless.

There is widespread acceptance that breast cancer is an important cause of death in women. For comparison, in

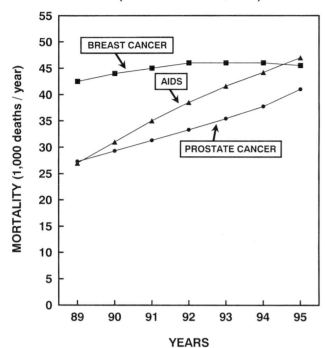

MORTALITY
(Thousand Deaths / Year)

Figure 84–1. Mortality from breast cancer, AIDS, and prostate cancer in the United States during the years 1989 through 1995. (Data from Breast Cancer and Prostate Cancer Mortality: Cancer Facts and Figures. Atlanta, American Cancer Society, 1989–1995 editions, AIDS Mortality, HIV/AIDS Surveillance Report. Atlanta, Centers for Disease Control, 1994 [based on graph on cover for AIDS-opportunistic illness incidence].)

1994, there were an estimated 182,000 new cases of breast cancer, and 48,000 women died from the disease (Boring et al, 1994). The ratio of death rate to incidence inferred from these statistics suggests that **approximately 25% of women with clinical diagnoses of breast cancer die of the disease, a number that closely approximates the percentage of men with prostate cancer who die from that disease. Furthermore, deaths from prostate cancer are increasing by 2% to 3% per year because fewer men are dying of cardiovascular disease.** All these statistics suggest that death from prostate cancer is common and that it produces a significant burden of suffering for men who die of the disease.

Although death from prostate cancer is common, there is a major unanswered question: **Is it possible to reduce deaths from prostate cancer through efforts at early diagnosis and aggressive treatment?** In other words, does localized prostate cancer progress at a rate fast enough to kill most men if it is left untreated? Unfortunately, there are no well-performed studies that compare active therapy with no treatment. Insight into the natural history of the disease, however, can be inferred from a number of sources: (1) longitudinal studies of serum PSA, (2) the results of deferred treatment, (3) the results from ineffective treatments (i.e., interstitial radiotherapy); and (4) the profile of men who die following radical prostatectomy.

LONGITUDINAL STUDIES OF SERUM PROSTATE-SPECIFIC ANTIGEN

Longitudinal studies of serum PSA provide a retrospective evaluation of progression of tumor in men with prostate cancer. The most comprehensive study is derived from the Baltimore Longitudinal Study of Aging, which is an ongoing prospective study of the National Institute of Aging, Bethesda, Maryland. Participants in this study are community-dwelling volunteers who return approximately every 2 years for physical examinations and a battery of physiologic, psychologic, and medical tests. During these visits, fasting and nonfasting serum samples are stored. Carter and associates measured PSA in men with normal prostates, benign prostatic hyperplasia (BPH), local or regional prostate cancer, and metastatic prostate cancer using sera stored for an average of 17 years before diagnosis (Carter et al, 1992a). Fifteen years before diagnosis, men with metastatic prostate cancer had serum PSA levels significantly greater than the controls, men with BPH, or men with localized prostate cancer. In addition, the yearly rate of change of PSA in these patients was also significantly greater (Fig. 84–2). At an average of 9 years before the diagnosis of metastatic disease, PSA was increasing exponentially (Carter et al, 1992b). **These data indicate that men with metastatic disease already had unrecognized advanced disease at least 10 years before diagnosis. This suggests that death rates within the first decade after the diagnosis of prostate cancer do not measure the efficacy of any form of treatment. Rather, death rates 10 years after therapy merely reflect the number of patients with pre-existing advanced disease who were subjected needlessly to treatment.**

This study and the one by Gann and co-workers also indicate that **the lead time in diagnosis associated with PSA testing averages 4 to 5 years** (Gann et al, 1995). **Thus, when using historical series to project cancer-specific survival rates today, this 4- to 5-year lead time should be factored in.**

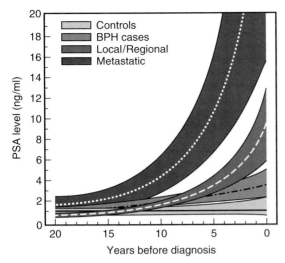

Figure 84–2. Summary of longitudinal evaluation of prostate-specific antigen (PSA) levels in men with and without prostate disease. Average curves (±95% confidence intervals) of PSA levels as a function of years before diagnosis for three diagnostic groups estimated from a mixed-effects model assuming an age of diagnosis of 75 years. (From Carter HB, Pearson JD, Metter EJ, et al: Longitudinal evaluation of prostate-specific antigen levels in men with and without prostate disease. JAMA 267:2215–2220, 1992. Copyright 1992, American Medical Association.)

RESULTS WITH DEFERRED TREATMENT

Individual Series

There are four major series reporting long-term results following deferred therapy. **The first two suffer from selection bias.** Whitmore and colleagues selected 75 men out of a pool of 4000 patients seen during his career (Whitmore et al, 1991). **Johansson and co-workers reported on 223 of 306 eligible men** (Johansson et al, 1992). **Also, for the first 2 years of that study, which contributes the patients with the longest follow-up, only patients with grade 1 (well-differentiated) disease were treated conservatively.** In subsequent years, patients with grade 2 (moderate) and grade 3 (poorly differentiated) disease were randomized to radiation or delayed therapy, and only the patients with deferred treatment were analyzed. The follow-up of Johansson's patients was also questionable. One patient who was reported to have died progression free was found at autopsy to have died from prostate cancer. Furthermore, because the diagnosis was frequently made by cytology, it is entirely possible that some of these patients did not even have cancer. Servoll and co-workers found, in their early experience with radical retropubic prostatectomies, that two of their patients mistakenly underwent surgery because of false-positive cytology results (Servoll et al, 1992). They subsequently adopted transrectal core biopsies before performing surgery.

The progression-free, metastasis-free, and cancer-specific survival rates are reported in Table 84–1. At 5 and 10 years, they are remarkably similar. As indicated previously, however, death rates at 5 and 10 years have little meaning. Johansson concluded that with further follow-up it was unlikely that the results would change. It is difficult to reconcile

this low rate of progression with the fact that Sweden has one of the highest rates of death from prostate cancer in the world.

Aus (1994) performed a retrospective analysis of 536 patients with known diagnoses of prostate cancer who died in Goteborg, Sweden, during the years between 1988 and 1990. In this way, he avoided selection bias by including all patients. The follow-up between diagnosis and death was as long as 25 years in some cases. **His study made two important points: First, the duration of follow-up is crucial in assessing the impact of localized prostate cancer on cancer-specific survival. For example, in patients who had no metastases at diagnosis and survived more than 10 years, 63% eventually died from prostate cancer.** In a further analysis of the data, it was shown that the mortality from prostate cancer does not decline after 10 years of follow-up but continues up to 25 years after the diagnosis; this was true for all stages and grades (Hugosson et al, 1995). **Second, he found that the median cancer-specific survival for well-differentiated or low-stage tumors (T2a) was approximately 15 years.** These data are consistent with the findings in Whitmore's series, in which cancer-specific survival at 15 years was only 68% (Whitmore et al, 1991). **Aus (1994) concluded that 15 years was the earliest time when cancer-specific mortality analysis had any significance.** He also emphasized the importance of age at diagnosis. **In men less than 65 years old with nonmetastatic cancer at the time of diagnosis, 75% died from prostate cancer when managed with noncurative intent.** In another study from Sweden, the age at diagnosis was also demonstrated to be an important prognostic factor (Gronberg et al, 1994). For example, in patients with grade 1 tumors, the years of life lost to prostate cancer ranged from 11 years in men 45 to 55 years to 1.2 years in patients 75 to 80. These studies may explain Johansson and colleagues' (1992) low estimates of rates of death. Their patients had an average age of 72 years at diagnosis, and follow-up evaluation did not extend beyond 10 years.

Using data from the Connecticut Tumor Registry, Albertsen and colleagues analyzed the long-term outcome (av-

Table 84–1. RESULTS OF DEFERRED THERAPY: INDIVIDUAL INSTITUTIONS

	Johansson et al, 1992	Whitmore et al, 1991
Patients studied	223	75
Total patients	306	4000
Mean age (y)	72	66
Mean follow-up (y)	10	11
Grade 1	66%	28%
Grade 3	4%	1%
Hormonal treatment	39%	24%
Progression-free survival		
5 y	68%	—
10 y	53%	—
Metastatic disease		
5 y	10%	0–18%
10 y	17%	20–55%
Cancer-specific survival		
5 y	94%	100%
10 y	87%	84%
15 y		68%

erage follow-up 15.5 years) of 451 men with T1 and T2 tumors who were managed with immediate or delayed hormonal therapy (Albertsen et al, 1995). **Death from prostate cancer at 15 years occurred in 9% of men with Gleason 2 to 4 score tumors, 28% with Gleason 5 to 7 score tumors, and 51% with Gleason 8 to 10 score tumors. They estimated that the maximum lost life expectancy for men with Gleason score 5 to 7 tumors was 4 to 5 years and for men with Gleason score 8 to 10 tumors 6 to 8 years.** Although the survival of men with low Gleason score tumors was not significantly different from that of the general population, these tumors were present in only 10% of men in this study and today are rarely diagnosed by needle biopsies. **The 28% death rate from prostate cancer in men with Gleason score 5 to 7 tumors study represents the probability that a 65- to 75-year-old man will die from prostatic cancer, and not from something else, within 15 years. If one had asked what percent of men who lived 15 years will die of prostate cancer, the answer is 46%.**

Recognizing that most men with localized cancer present with moderately well differentiated tumors, these studies suggest that when managed with noncurative intent, approximately 50% of men who live 15 years will die of the disease.

Combined Series

Two studies evaluated the literature and summarized the results. In 1993, Adolfsson and colleagues analyzed studies since 1980 that reported the results of radical prostatectomy, external radiation therapy, and deferred treatment for localized prostate cancer. **They found that the disease-specific survival at 10 years was 83% for deferred therapy, 93% for radical prostatectomy, and 62% for external radiotherapy.**

In 1994, Chodak and associates performed a pooled analysis of 823 case records from six nonrandomized studies published since 1985 of men treated conservatively for clinically localized prostate cancer. Rather than relying on the published reports, however, they participated with the primary investigators who were obtaining the raw data for analysis, thus extending the follow-up and guaranteeing more-or-less uniform inclusion of patients. All were highly selected series. In addition to the Johansson and Whitmore series, Moskovitz and co-workers (1987) excluded 38% of patients, and Jones (1992) reported on only 233 of 312 observed patients. As further evidence for this selection bias, 60% of all patients in the combined series had grade 1 tumors. Accepting the fact that this study evaluated only patients who were hand picked to do well, **the metastatic rates at 10 years and 15 years were substantial** (Table 84–2). **Recognizing that the median survival of men with metastatic disease is 2 to 3 years, the projected survival of men with grade 2 disease corresponds closely with the 15-year findings of Whitmore, Albertsen, and Aus. Many of the patients in the Chodak series, however, received hormonal therapy at the time of progression. For this reason, the time to the appearance of metastatic disease in many patients was delayed. This caveat must be recognized when performing decision analysis.** These data can-

Table 84–2. PERCENT OF MEN WITH LOCALIZED PROSTATE CANCER TREATED CONSERVATIVELY WHO DEVELOPED METASTASES AT 10 AND 15 YEARS: A POOLED ANALYSIS

Histologic Grade	Metastases	
	10 y	15 y
1	19	40
2	42	70
3	74	85

Adapted from Chodak GW, Thisted RA, Gerber GS, et al: N Engl J Med 1994; 330:242–248. Copyright 1994. Massachusetts Medical Society. All rights reserved.

not be used to project median rates of survival of 2 to 3 years after the diagnosis of metastatic disease. These estimates refer only to patients who are hormonally naive. Most patients with hormone-refractory metastatic disease have a life span that averages only 12 months.

Decision Analysis

Decision analysis is a relatively new field of outcomes research that integrates information from multiple sources to characterize the efficacy of medical interventions. These studies can be useful in predicting the therapeutic benefit derived from early intervention and treatment. Fleming and associates analyzed the influence of radical prostatectomy on survival in a Medicare population of men using the Markov model (Fleming et al, 1993). In this statistic technique, estimations of the likelihood of progression to metastatic disease are derived from reviews of the literature. Once a metastatic rate has been established, the rate of death from cancer can be predicted. By assigning various levels of efficacy for treatment, the impact of any form of treatment on survival can be estimated. Furthermore, survival advantage can be modified on the basis of quality of life issues.

In the Fleming study, metastatic rates were estimated based on four watchful waiting series composed mainly of stage A (T1) patients (Byar et al, 1972; Haapiainen et al, 1986; Johansson et al, 1989; Zhang et al, 1991). **Although the authors readily admitted that stage A cancers had a lower rate of metastasis than palpable cancers** (Wasson et al, 1993), **they ignored this fact in their analysis.** Based on these stage A series, they estimated the mean metastatic rate at 10 years to be 2.7% (0%–10% range) for grade 1 disease, 13% (3%–57%) for grade 2 disease, and 42% (0%–80%) for grade 3 disease. **When these rates are compared to the pooled analysis of Chodak and associates, they are unrealistically low. They were then used, however, to estimate progression to death from prostate cancer. Clearly, with use of low rates of metastasis, the model predicts that few men will die. Thus, intervention would have little impact on survival.**

The efficacy of radical prostatectomy was arbitrarily based on the assumption that all patients with organ-confined disease were cured, and all patients with capsular penetration were not cured. Radical prostatectomy was then further stratified into higher estimates of treatment efficacy based on pathologic findings in men with stage A disease and lower efficacy based on an evaluation of one study of men with clinical stage A2 or B cancer; however, in this study, only 16% of men with capsular penetration developed metastatic disease (Fowler and Mills, 1985). To account for diminished quality of life from complications of treatment, survival advantages were reduced by an arbitrary amount determined by "a consensus of clinicians involved in outcome research and treatment of prostate cancer." Death from metastatic disease was considered the least important outcome. Impotence and incontinence were assigned values more important than death from metastases; all elderly men were considered to be potent preoperatively, and there was no recognition that potency could be restored postoperatively.

In a study by the same group, men who underwent radical prostatectomy were questioned about the impact of incontinence and impotence on their quality of life (Fowler et al, 1995). This study showed that, despite problems with incontinence and impotence, men who underwent radical prostatectomy scored high on quality of life measures and reported feeling positive about the results (81%) and would choose surgical treatment again (89%). If the investigators had carried out this study first, the reduction in survival based on reductions in quality of life would have been much less. They did not reduce quality of life in men with watchful waiting owing to worry and anxiety about progression of disease. **Using this model, the authors concluded that in patients with well-differentiated tumors treatment at best offers limited benefit in terms of quality-adjusted life expectancy and may result in harm to the patient. In patients with moderate or poorly differentiated tumors, using the most optimistic assumptions in patients aged 60 to 65 years, treatment offered less than a 1-year improvement in quality-adjusted life expectancy. In patients over age 70, invasive treatment generally appeared to be harmful. These findings led the authors to conclude that the choice of watchful waiting is a reasonable alternative to invasive treatment for men with localized prostate cancer.**

Subsequently, **this study was critiqued by Beck and coworkers (1994). Using the same model, they used the rates of progression obtained from the publication of Chodak and associates (1994) and rates of progression in men treated with interstitial radioactive iodine (¹²⁵I) reported by Fuks and colleagues (1991). Using these rates of progression, the survival advantage for well-differentiated lesions (with quality of life adjustments) went from −0.3 years to 1 to 1.8 years, for moderately differentiated lesions from +0.3 years to 2.4 to 2.9 years, and for poorly differentiated lesions from 1 to 2.3 to 2.7 years** (Table 84–3). It is unclear why Fleming and co-workers used the low rates of progression that they selected and did not include the available 15-year review data cited by Chodak in a publication that came out less than 1 year later. **Clearly, with use of more realistic rates of progression, the benefit of radical prostatectomy is increased from 3 months to 2 to 3 years. When the observations are extended out to 15 years, they are also consistent with Albertsen's estimation of 4 to 8 years in loss of life expectancy** (Albertsen et al, 1995).

Another decision analysis was published by Krahn and associates (1994). This article used Johansson's data and the Fleming Markov model. The authors asked whether screening for prostate cancer with digital rectal examination, PSA,

Table 84–3. ESTIMATED SURVIVAL BENEFIT (WITH QUALITY OF LIFE ADJUSTMENTS) FROM THE MARKOV MODEL USING THREE DIFFERENT METASTATIC RATES

	Estimated Benefit of Therapy (y)		
Histologic Grade	Fleming et al, 1993	Chodak et al, 1994	Fuks et al, 1991
Well	−0.34	+1.01	+1.81
Moderate	+0.33	+2.41	+2.94
Poor	+1.00	+2.68	+2.34

From Beck JR, Kattan MW, Miles BJ: J Urol 1994; 152:1894–1899.

and transrectal ultrasound would have a net health benefit on all men if screening were carried out *once* in asymptomatic men 50 to 70 years of age. Survival was reduced based on quality of life considerations. Furthermore, survival benefit was averaged out over all 50- to 70-year-old men who were screened. The authors found that life expectancy was increased by 0.6 to 1.7 days per patient screened for 50- and 70-year-old men. When quality of life was considered, however, there was a net loss of 3 to 13 days. This article was severely flawed for many reasons. First, it used Johansson's unrealistic rates of progression. Also, it looked at screening only once through the population; screening once during a lifetime for any tumor is not a recommended practice. Furthermore, the first time a population is screened, it is more likely to detect asymptomatic advanced disease in patients who are unlikely to benefit from definitive therapy. Thus, by using low rates of progression and a screening process that picks up advanced disease, the authors artificially created a system in which treatment was unlikely to benefit the patient. Their quality of life assessment, similar to Fleming's, was based on the judgment of 10 physicians and had no patient input. Incontinence following surgery and deaths from prostate cancer were given virtually equal weight. Finally, they took the reduced survival benefit and divided it by the number of all men aged 50 to 70 to estimate the net health benefit. In fact, there is no test (blood pressure, nonfasting cholesterol, mammography) that could be performed once in any population of patients and result in an overall lengthening of life for all patients screened. **Without a positive control, the results of this study are meaningless.** Furthermore, the authors never clearly stated that the life expectancy changes that they estimated in days represented net health benefit to each man screened rather than benefit to individual patients who were diagnosed with cancer.

RESULTS WITH INEFFECTIVE TREATMENTS

A major flaw in watchful waiting series is the selection of patients who are not comparable with men who are candidates for radical prostatectomy. Typically, they are older and have small, well-differentiated tumors. To obtain a better estimation of the natural history of localized prostate cancer, the results following ineffective forms of treatment can be used. Interstitial radiation therapy, as practiced more than a decade ago using interstitial ¹²⁵I or radioactive gold seeds, has proven to be ineffective in controlling localized prostate cancer in a larger number of patients. **Thus, the long-term results from those ineffective forms of treatment provide another means to evaluate the natural history of prostate cancer.** Indeed, in many respects, the findings are more applicable than those derived from deferred therapy series because most patients underwent surgical staging of the pelvic lymph nodes, and the clinical stage and grade of these patients more closely approximate the profile of men who undergo radical prostatectomy. Indeed, these may be the most representative groups of untreated patients to be used for comparison with radical prostatectomy.

The results of two large series with long-term results have been reported. **Fuks and colleagues reviewed the long-term results in patients treated with ^{125}I implantation** (Fuks et al, 1991). Between the years 1970 and 1985, 679 patients underwent treatment. The mean age was 61 years, and the mean follow-up was 97 months. The clinical stage at presentation was T2 in 590 (87%) and T3 in 87 (13%). The histologic grade was low in 249 (37%), moderate in 362 (53%), high in 41 (6%), and unknown in 4%. All patients underwent a staging pelvic lymph node dissection, and **only the 679 patients with negative lymph nodes were used in this analysis. The 5- and 10-year actuarial progression-free likelihoods were 68% and 44%, respectively. Even in the most favorable subset of patients, the results were not good; at 10 years, metastases had developed in 25% of the node-negative T2a patients, 45% of the T2b patients, and 55% of the T2c patients.** Metastases had also developed in 30% of the patients with grade 1 disease, 50% of the patients with grade 2 disease, and 70% of the patients with grade 3 disease. The authors noted that "these data suggest that the existence and regrowth of local residual disease in localized prostate cancer promotes an enhanced spread of metastatic disease and that early and complete eradication of the primary tumor is required if long-term cure is to be achieved." Although the authors did not provide information on death from prostate cancer, they did state that "as of the 10th year after implantation, the actuarial curves for distant metastases-free survival and for overall survival were essentially identical, consistent with the fact that distant metastases are incurable, invariably leading to death in otherwise surviving patients."

Lerner and co-workers analyzed the results on 360 patients who underwent staging pelvic lymphadenectomy and a course of combined interstitial radioactive gold seeds and external beam radiotherapy between the years 1966 and 1979 (Lerner et al, 1991). In patients with negative pelvic lymph nodes, the risk of dying from prostate cancer at 10 years was $13 \pm 7\%$ for patients with stage T1b and T2 tumors. These results correspond closely to those of Johansson and associates (1992) and Whitmore and colleagues (1991).

RESULTS FOLLOWING RADICAL PROSTATECTOMY

The natural history of untreated localized prostate cancer has been reviewed in an effort to provide a baseline for analyzing what happens when prostate cancer is left un-

treated and how that compares with the results of radical prostatectomy. In an effort to make this comparison, the results of 561 patients from the Johns Hopkins Hospital who were considered to be candidates for radical prostatectomy during 1975 to 1987 are summarized in Table 84–4 (Walsh and Partin, 1994). The results are subdivided into all 561 patients who presented for radical prostatectomy and the 501 patients who underwent surgery and had negative lymph nodes at staging pelvic lymphadenectomy; 60 men were excluded from radical prostatectomy because of the finding of positive lymph nodes on frozen section. Comparable information from the series of Johansson and colleagues (1992) and Fuks and co-workers (1991) are presented in the same table. Although radical prostatectomy series are frequently criticized because of favorable selection, the series by Johansson and associates is also favorably selected. Indeed, the Johns Hopkins radical prostatectomy series has more high-grade lesions included than the series by Johansson and associates or Fuks and co-workers. **In comparing the 10-year actuarial progression-free survival likelihood, 69% of all patients at Johns Hopkins who were candidates for radical prostatectomy were progression free, compared with only 53% of Johansson's patients and 44% of the patients who were treated with interstitial ^{125}I. When the patients with negative lymph nodes at Johns Hopkins are compared with the patients with negative lymph nodes studied by Fuks and associates, the 10-year actuarial progression-free survivals are 79% and 44%, respectively. These data strongly suggest that patients who undergo radical prostatectomy are more likely to be progression free at 10 years than the most highly selected group of untreated patients** (Johansson et al, 1992) **or comparable patients managed with ineffective therapy** (Fuks et al, 1991).

It is interesting to analyze the pathologic stage of the patients who died within the first 10 years following radical prostatectomy. In virtually all cases, the patients had pathologically advanced disease: In 93% there was capsular penetration; in 67% there was seminal vesicle involvement; and in 40%, the lymph nodes contained tumor on permanent section (but not on frozen section). Similarly, most patients had high-grade disease: 57% had Gleason scores of 8 to 10, 33% had Gleason score 7, and only 10% had Gleason score 6. These data once again support the notion that patients with apparently localized disease who died within the first 10 years of diagnosis were understaged and had more advanced disease than was anticipated.

SUMMARY

The natural history of localized prostate cancer has been evaluated on the basis of data from longitudinal studies of serum PSA and the long-term follow-up of deferred treatment, ineffective treatment, and radical prostatectomy. The following conclusions can be made.

Age at diagnosis is the major factor that influences cancer-specific death rates in untreated men. Studies from Sweden have shown that if men younger than age 65 are left untreated, 75% eventually die from the disease.

Cancer-specific rates of death at 10 years are meaning-

Table 84–4. COMPARISON OF 561 MEN (JOHNS HOPKINS) WHO WERE SUBJECTED TO STAGING PELVIC LYMPHADENECTOMY WITH (501) OR WITHOUT (60) RADICAL PROSTATECTOMY AND THE SERIES OF JOHANSSON ET AL AND FUKS ET AL*

Category	Johns Hopkins (All)	Johns Hopkins (LN negative)	Johansson et al, 1992	Fuks et al, 1991
Dates	6/75–12/87	Same	3/77–2/84	1970–1985
No. patients	561	501	223	679
Mean follow-up	75 (12–192) mo	74 (12–192) mo	123 (81–165) mo	97 mo
Mean age	59	59	72	61
Stage				
T1	80 (14%)	75 (15%)	106 (47%)	—
T2	481 (86%)	476 (85%)	117 (53%)	T2 590 (87%)
				T3 87 (13%)
Grade				
Well	60 (11%)	57 (12%)	148 (66%)	249 (37%)
Moderate	367 (70%)	343 (72%)	66 (30%)	362 (53%)
Poor	103 (19%)	74 (16%)	9 (4%)	41 (6%)
Total local progression	T1 1	T1 1	T1 14	T1 —
	T2 23	T2 20	T2 36	T2 44%
	All 24 (4%)	All 21 (4%)	All 50 (22%)	
Total distant progression	T1 5	T1 3	T1 12	T1 —
	T2 60	T2 30	T2 14	T2 34%
	All 65 (12%)	All 33 (6.6%)	All 26 (12%)	
Total death from prostate cancer	T1 1	T1 1	T1 9	T1 —
	T2 25	T2 12	T2 (10)	T2 —
	All 26 (5%)	All 13 (3%)	All 19 (9%)	
5-y actuarial progression-free† likelihood	93 (89–94)‡	94 (91–96)	68 (61–75)	68
10-y actuarial progression-free likelihood	69 (59–76)	79 (70–86)	53 (44–62)	44

*Statistical comparison: Progression-free likelihood: Johns Hopkins (all) and Johansson: 5-y P < .001; 10-year P < .05. Johns Hopkins (all) and Johns Hopkins (lymph node [LN] negative): 5-y NS: 10-y P < .05.
†Progression-free—local or distant recurrence.
‡Percent likelihood (95% confidence intervals).
Adapted from Walsh PC, Partin AW: In DeVita VT Jr, et al, eds.: Important Advances in Oncology, Philadelphia, J. B. Lippincott, 1994, pp 211–223.

less and cannot be used as a measure of efficacy of any form of treatment for localized prostate cancer. Rates of death at 10 years merely reflect the number of patients with advanced disease who were subjected to treatment needlessly. This conclusion is based on the pattern of progression of PSA in patients with known metastatic disease, the long-term results from deferred therapy for the treatment of localized prostate cancer, and the pathologic stage of men who die within the first 10 years following radical prostatectomy.

Fifteen years is the earliest time when cancer-specific mortality analysis has any significance. Recognizing that most men with localized prostate cancer present with moderately well differentiated tumors, it can be estimated that when managed conservatively 45% to 50% of the men who live 15 years will die of prostate cancer.

Metastasis-free progression at 10 years is a reasonable early end point for judging efficacy of treatment for localized prostate cancer. This end point, however, is reliable only if hormonal therapy is withheld until patients develop established metastases. Early hormonal therapy at the time of local progression can delay this end point artificially. Series using early hormonal therapy cannot be evaluated.

The lead time in diagnosis associated with PSA testing averages 4 to 5 years. Thus, when using historical series to project cancer-specific or metastases-free survival rates today, this 5-year lead time must be factored in.

Death from untreated localized prostate cancer occurs only after a protracted course. This has several important clinical implications. There is no need to treat localized prostate cancer aggressively in men with limited life spans. Because men are now living longer, however, physicians who care for men with prostate cancer need better instruments to evaluate potential life span. Also, because progression and death from localized prostate cancer occur after such a protracted course, it is likely that there is a reasonable window of opportunity for early diagnosis and cure while the disease is still localized. This conclusion is based on the retrospective evaluation of PSA in men with localized prostate cancer, which appears consistent with progression evolving from localized disease. Although it is likely that definitive treatment of localized prostate cancer will improve cancer-specific survival, it was not possible to evaluate this possibility in the past because men with localized prostate cancer were rarely identified at a curable stage. Today, however, with improved screening techniques, it is possible to diagnose prostate cancer at an earlier curable stage. The prospective evaluation of treatment for localized prostate cancer should now be possible through rigorously designed trials involving young men who will live long enough to provide an answer to the question.

REFERENCES

Adolfsson J, Steineck G, Whitmore WF Jr: Recent results of management of palpable clinically localized prostate cancer. Cancer 1993; 72:43–55.

Albertsen PC, Fryback DG, Storer BE, et al: Long-term survival among men with conservatively treated localized prostate cancer. JAMA 1995; 274:626.

Aus G: Prostate cancer: Mortality and morbidity after non-curative treatment with aspects on diagnosis and treatment. Scand J Urol Nephrol 1994; 167(suppl):1–41.

Beck JR, Kattan MW, Miles BJ: A critique of the decision analysis for clinically localized prostate cancer. J Urol 1994; 152:1894–1899.

Boring CC, Squires TS, Tong T: Cancer statistics 1994. Cancer 1994; 44:7.

Byar DP, VA Administration Cooperative Urological Research Group: Survival of patients with incidentally found microscopic cancer of the prostate: Results of a clinical trial of conservative treatment. J Urol 1972; 108:908–913.

Cann PH, Hennekens, Stampfer MJ: A prospected evaluation of plasma prostate-specific antigen for detection of prostate cancer. JAMA 1995; 273:289–294.

Carter HB, Morrell CH, Pearson JD, et al: Estimation of prostatic growth using serial prostate-specific antigen measurements in men with and without prostate disease. Cancer Res 1992a; 52:3323–3328.

Carter HB, Pearson JD, Metter EJ, et al: Longitudinal evaluation of prostate-specific antigen levels in men with and without prostate disease. JAMA 1992b; 267:2215–2220.

Chodak GW, Thisted RA, Gerber GS, et al: Results of conservative management of clinically localized prostate cancer. N Engl J Med 1994; 330:242–248.

Fleming C, Wasson JH, Albertsen PC, et al: A decision analysis of alternative treatment strategies for clinically localized prostate cancer. JAMA 1993; 269:2650–2658.

Fowler FJ Jr, Barry MS, Lu-Yao G, et al: The effect of radical prostatectomy for prostate cancer on patient quality of life: Results from a Medicare Survey. Urology 1995; 45:1007–1015.

Fowler JE, Mills SE: Operable prostatic carcinoma: Correlations among clinical stage, pathologic stage, Gleason histologic score, and early disease-free survival. J Urol 1985; 13:49–52.

Fuks Z, Leibel SA, Wallner KE, et al: The effect of local control on metastatic dissemination in carcinoma of the prostate: Long-term results in patients treated with ^{125}implantation. Int J Radiat Oncol Biol Phys 1991; 21:537–547.

Gann PH, Hennekens CH, Stampfer MJ: A prospective evaluation of plasma prostate-specific antigen for detection of prostate cancer. JAMA 1995; 273:289–294.

Gronberg H, Damber JE, Jonsson H, Lenner P: Patient age as a prognostic factor in prostate cancer. J Urol 1994; 152:892–895.

Gronberg H, Damber L, Jonsson H, Damber JE: Prostate cancer mortality in northern Sweden with special reference to tumor grade and patient age. J Urol Submitted.

Haapiainen R, Rannikko S, Makinen J, Alfthan O: T_0 carcinoma of the prostate: Influence of tumor extent and histologic grade on prognosis of untreated patients. Eur Urol 1986; 12:16–20.

Hugosson J, Aus G, Bergdahl C, Bergdahl S: Prostate cancer mortality in patients surviving more than 10 years after diagnosis. J Urol 1995; 154: 2115.

Johansson JE, Adami H-O, Andersson SO, et al: Natural history of localized prostatic cancer. A population-based study of 223 untreated patients. Lancet 1989; 1:799–803.

Johansson JE, Adami H-O, Andersson SO, et al: High 10-year survival rate in patients with early, untreated prostatic cancer. JAMA 1992; 267:2191–2196.

Jones GW: Prospective, conservative management of localized prostate cancer. Cancer 1992; 70(suppl):307–310.

Krahn MD, Mahoney JE, Eckman MH, et al: Screening for prostate cancer: A decision analytic view. JAMA 1994; 272:773–780.

Lerner SP, Seale-Hawkins C, Carlton CE Jr, Scardino PT: The risk of dying of prostate cancer in patients with clinically localized disease. J Urol 1991; 146:1040–1045.

Moskovitz B, Nitecki S, Levin DR: Cancer of the prostate: Is there a need for aggressive treatment? Urol Int 1987; 42:49–52.

Servoll E, Halvorsen OJ, Haukaas S, Hoisaeter PA: Radical retropubic prostatectomy: Our experience with the first 54 patients. Scand J Urol Nephrol 1992; 26:231–234.

Stamey TA: Cancer of the prostate. An analysis of some important contributions and dilemmas. Monographs in Urology 1983; 4:68–92.

Walsh PC, Partin AW: Treatment of early stage prostate cancer: Radical prostatectomy. In DeVita VT Jr, Hellman S, Rosenberg SA (eds): Important Advances in Oncology. Philadelphia, J. B. Lippincott, 1994, pp 211–223.

Wasson JH, Cushman CC, Bruskewitz RC, et al: A structured literature review of treatment for localized prostate cancer. Arch Fam Med 1993; 2487–2493.

Whitmore WF Jr, Warner JA, Thompson IM Jr: Expectant management of localized prostatic cancer. Cancer 1991; 67:1091–1096.

Zhang G, Wasserman NF, Sidi AA, et al: Long-term followup results after expectant management of stage A_1 prostatic cancer. J Urol 1991; 146:99–103.

85
RADICAL PROSTATECTOMY

James A. Eastham, M.D.
Peter T. Scardino, M.D.

The prostate has become the leading site of internal malignancy in men and the second most common cause of cancer death. It is estimated that more than 317,100 men will be diagnosed with prostate cancer in the United States in 1996, and 41,400 will die of this disease (Parker et al, 1996). Because the incidence of prostate cancer increases more rapidly with age than any other cancer and the average age of American men is increasing, the number of men with prostate cancer and the number of deaths from the disease are expected to rise steadily into the next century. Prostate cancer will cause the death of 3% of all men alive today who are greater than 50 years old. It will also cause many men to suffer serious complications from local growth or distant metastases as well as from complications of treatment.

Despite its epidemic proportions, prostate cancer evokes enormous controversy because of its unusual biologic features and, until recently, because of the lack of firm data about the natural history of the disease. Prostate cancer is relatively slow growing, with doubling times for local tumors estimated at 2 to 4 years. Because the disease often strikes elderly men with high comorbidity rates, the risks to life and health posed by the cancer itself have been difficult to quantify. Prospective, randomized, controlled trials to establish whether early detection (PLCO) or treatment (PIVOT) of localized prostate cancer will decrease the mortality rate from the disease have not yet been completed (Gohagan et al, 1994; Wilt and Brawer, 1994). Until such studies are completed in 10 to 15 years, the decision whether

to treat aggressively or conservatively must be made with the best available evidence.

RATIONALE FOR SURGICAL TREATMENT

Clinical Importance of Cancers Detected with Currently Available Tests

When the prostate gland is evaluated at autopsy in men 50 years of age or older who have no clinical evidence of cancer, adenocarcinoma is identified in approximately 30% of cases (Franks, 1954; McNeal, 1969). Yet, the lifetime risk of developing a clinically detected prostate cancer is 10% (Seidman et al, 1985). This discrepancy between the high prevalence of prostate cancer found at autopsy and the lower incidence of clinical cancer raises the question concerning which prostate cancers might best be managed without immediate treatment. Specifically, are cancers that are identified solely on the basis of an elevated serum prostate-specific antigen (PSA) clinically indolent, or are these tumors significant but diagnosed at an earlier stage?

To evaluate this question, a study was conducted at the authors' institution to compare the pathologic features of impalpable prostate cancers detected by an elevated serum PSA (stage T1c), prostate cancers that were palpable on digital rectal examination (DRE), and prostate cancers found

Table 85–1. PERCENT OF CANCERS DETECTED CLINICALLY (RADICAL PROSTATECTOMY SERIES) AND INCIDENTALLY (CYSTOPROSTATECTOMY SERIES) THAT WERE INDOLENT, CLINICALLY IMPORTANT BUT CURABLE, AND ADVANCED

Cancer	No.	Group (%)		
		*Indolent**	*Curable†*	*Advanced‡*
Cystoprostatectomy series	90	78	22	0
Radical prostatectomy series	301	9	62	29
Palpable tumors	246	8	58	34
Impalpable, elevated PSA	55	13	76	11
Elevated PSA only (impalpable, nonvisible)	29	17	79	11

*Indolent: Tumors ≤0.5 cm³ confined to the prostate gland with no primary or secondary Gleason grade 4 or 5.

†Curable: Tumors >0.5 cm³ or poorly differentiated (primary or secondary Gleason grade 4 or 5) cancers confined to the prostate or with microscopic extracapsular extension. 5-year nonprogression rate 87 ± 7%.

‡Advanced: Any tumor, regardless of volume or grade, with extensive extracapsular extension (to the surgical margin), seminal vesicle invasion, or lymph node metastases. 5-year nonprogression rate 46 ± 14%.

PSA, Prostate-specific antigen.

incidentally at cystoprostatectomy for bladder cancer (Ohori et al, 1994b) (Table 85–1). Cancer was diagnosed in 55 patients solely on the basis of an elevated serum PSA (stage T1c). Their tumors were often high grade (55% had a primary or secondary Gleason grade of 4 or 5) and frequently extended outside the prostate (40%). These tumors, however, had a more favorable profile than the group of 246 patients with tumors palpable on DRE. Only 11% of stage T1c tumors had advanced pathologic features compared with 34% of palpable cancers (P <.001), whereas the proportion of indolent cancers changed insignificantly from 13% to 8%. This profile is in sharp contrast to that of the cystoprostatectomy series (see Table 85–1), in which 78% of the prostate cancers were considered indolent, and none had advanced pathologic features. Similar findings have been reported by other institutions (Table 85–2). **Most prostate cancers detected solely on the basis of an elevated PSA are clinically important and are more likely to be curable with radical prostatectomy than palpable tumors.**

Although the majority of prostate cancers detected with currently available tests are clinically important, efforts must be made to identify indolent cancers. In an attempt to identify patients who have unimportant (indolent) tumors that may not require intervention, Epstein and associates examined preoperative clinical and pathologic features in 157 men with stage T1c prostate cancer who underwent radical prostatectomy and correlated those findings with the pathologic features of the tumor specimen (Epstein et al, 1994). **Their model for predicting an "insignificant" tumor was (1) PSA density 0.1 or less, no Gleason grade of 4 or 5 in the biopsy specimen, fewer than three biopsy cores involved (minimum of three cores obtained), and no core with greater than 50% involvement with cancer; or (2) PSA density of 0.15 or less, no Gleason grade of 4 or 5 in the biopsy specimen, and less than 3 mm cancer on only one prostate biopsy sample (minimum of three cores).** This model had a positive predictive value of 95% and a negative predictive value of 66%. These investigators were able to predict 73% of cases of insignificant tumors (tumor volume <0.2 cc, Gleason sum <7, organ confined). Similarly, Goto and co-workers evaluated 170 patients who had six or more systematic needle biopsies. An algorithm that predicted a 75% probability of an unimportant cancer (<0.5 cc, confined, no Gleason grade 4 or 5) was a PSA density less than 0.1, no Gleason grade 4 or 5, and less than 2 mm cancer in a single specimen (Goto et al, 1996).

Slow But Inevitable Progression of Clinically Detected Cancer

The natural history of localized prostate cancer and a guide to therapy are presented in detail in Chapter 84. Until recently, the natural history of localized prostate cancer was not well documented. Two large series, however, have been published that document the long-term risk of development of metastases and of death from prostate cancer in men with clinically localized cancers treated conservatively (Chodak et al, 1994; Albertsen et al, 1995).

In a pooled analysis of 828 patients from six medical centers around the world, Chodak and colleagues documented that the risk of metastases at 10 years was 19% for well-differentiated, 42% for moderately differentiated, and 74% for poorly differentiated cancers (Fig. 85–1). Although the confidence intervals were broad beyond 10 years, it is evident from the curves in Figure 85–1 that metastases continue to develop for long periods of time. In Chodak's series, the cancer-specific mortality rate at 10 years (13%) was identical for well-differentiated and moderately differentiated tumors, which reflects the inadequacy of that time interval to document the full impact on mortality of a local-

Table 85–2. PERCENTAGE OF INDOLENT (CLINICALLY UNIMPORTANT) PROSTATE CANCERS DETECTED IN PATIENTS UNDERGOING RADICAL PROSTATECTOMY FOR CLINICALLY LOCALIZED PROSTATE CANCER

Series	Stage	No.	% Indolent Cancers	Definition
Smith and Catalona, 1994	T1–2	816	3	Impalpable, focal, no Gleason grade 3, 4, or 5
Ohori et al, 1994b	T1–2	301	9	Tumor volume <0.5 cm³, confined, no Gleason grade 4 or 5
	T1c	55	13	
	T1c*	29	17	
Epstein et al, 1994	T1c	157	16	Tumor volume <0.2 cm³, confined, no Gleason grade 4 or 5
			27	Volume <0.5 cm³, confined, no Gleason grade 4 or 5

*Impalpable, not visible on ultrasound.

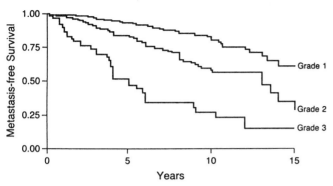

Figure 85–1. Metastasis-free survival among untreated patients with localized prostate cancer, according to tumor grade. (From Chodak GW, Thisted RA, Gerber GS, et al: N Engl J Med 330:242–248, 1994. Copyright 1994, Massachusetts Medical Society. Reprinted by permission of *The New England Journal of Medicine*.)

ized prostate cancer. For poorly differentiated tumors, 66% had died of prostate cancer by 10 years.

Albertsen and colleagues reported the results of a population-based study in Connecticut of 451 men between the ages of 65 and 75 with clinically localized prostate cancer treated conservatively (Albertsen et al, 1995). The cancer specific mortality rate at 10 years was 9% for well-differentiated, 24% for moderately differentiated, and 46% for poorly differentiated cancers. When compared to age-matched controls, men with localized prostate cancer (whose mean age was 70.9 years) lost an estimated 3.8 to 5.2 years of life (Table 85–3). Although the authors emphasized that men with well-differentiated tumors (Gleason sum 2–4) survived as long as age-matched controls, this favorable group included only 9% of the patient population. The remaining 91%, who had moderately or poorly differentiated tumors, experienced a markedly shortened survival with conservative treatment (see Table 85–3).

Some prostate cancers progress slowly and present little risk to the overall health of the patient. These cancers almost always fall into the T1a classification or occasionally T1b-T2, which is small, focal, and well differentiated. **Most clinically detected prostate cancers are not indolent, however, and pose a threat to health and life expectancy**

except in elderly men or those with serious comorbid conditions.

Surgical Treatment Effective if Cancer Detected Early

Overall Recurrence After Radical Prostatectomy

After radical prostatectomy, serum PSA, measured by standard clinical assays, should decline to undetectable levels. Although recurrence of prostate cancer after radical prostatectomy has been documented rarely in patients with an undetectable PSA level (Goldrath and Messing, 1989; Takayama et al, 1992; Leibman et al, 1995; Oefelein et al, 1995), a detectable and rising PSA level almost always precedes clinical recurrence, usually by 3 to 5 years (Abi-Aas et al, 1992; Paulson, 1994). Therefore, treatment outcomes and cancer control should be based primarily on postoperative monitoring of the serum PSA.

After a cancer has been treated, the risk of tumor recurrence during each year of follow-up (the *hazard rate*) can be calculated. A high hazard rate early after definitive therapy for a localized cancer is largely due to understaging, whereas a high or rising hazard rate several years after treatment suggests that the local tumor had not been eradicated and continues to shed metastases. The authors calculated the hazard rate for progression by PSA after radical prostatectomy for a cohort of 611 men with clinically localized prostate cancer followed for 1 to 125 months (Table 85–4) (Dillioglugil et al, 1995a; 1996a; 1996b). No patient received adjuvant therapy before relapse—defined as a PSA 0.4 ng/ml and rising. Recurrence of prostate cancer was documented in 69 (17%) patients, but no recurrences were documented beyond 6 years after surgery. The hazard rate was highest during the first year of follow-up and then

Table 85–3. LIFE EXPECTANCY OBSERVED IN A POPULATION-BASED STUDY IN CONNECTICUT COMPARING MEN TREATED CONSERVATIVELY FOR CLINICALLY LOCALIZED PROSTATE CANCER (cT1–T2NXM0), OVERALL AND BY GLEASON SCORE, WITH LIFE EXPECTANCY FROM THE GENERAL POPULATION*

	Life Expectancy (years)		
	Age 65	*Age 70*	*Age 75*
General population	15.8	12.7	10.0
Patients with T1–2 PCa	10.6	8.2	6.2
Gleason score			
2–4	16.1	13.0	10.2
5–7	11.3	8.8	6.7
8–10	7.9	5.9	4.4

*Except for Gleason score 2–4, which composed only 9% of the study population, men with prostate cancer experienced a markedly shortened life expectancy, even at age 70 and 75.
Adapted from Albertsen et al, 1995.

Table 85–4. ACTUARIAL NONPROGRESSION RATES AND RISK OF PROGRESSION EACH YEAR FOR 611 T1–2NXM0 PATIENTS TREATED WITH RADICAL PROSTATECTOMY ALONE (NO HORMONAL OR RADIOTHERAPY) AND FOLLOWED EVERY 6 TO 12 MONTHS WITH PROSTATE-SPECIFIC ANTIGEN FOR 1–125.5 (MEDIAN 23.9, MEAN 30.3) MONTHS*

Year	Total No.	Recurrence	Censored†	HR%	95% CI
1	611	45	171	9.0	6.3–11.5
2	395	19	93	5.6	3.1–8.1
3	283	8	72	3.3	1.0–5.6
4	203	6	74	3.7	0.7–6.6
5	123	4	38	3.9	0.8–7.8
6	81	1	34	1.6	0–4.7
7	46	0	18	0	—
8	28	0	12	0	—
9	16	0	9	0	—
10	7	0	6	0	—
11	1	0	1	0	—

*Note that 6.4% had positive lymph nodes and another 11.3% had seminal vesicle invasion (pT3c) (Dillioglugil et al, 1996a).
†Patients lost to follow-up.
HR, Hazard rate.

Table 85–5. PROGRESSION-FREE RATE, DETERMINED BY PROSTATE-SPECIFIC ANTIGEN, AFTER
RADICAL RETROPUBIC PROSTATECTOMY

Group	No. Patients	Stage	Years	PSA Nonprogression (%) 5 Years	10 Years
Partin et al, 1993a	894*	T1–2NX	1982–91	83	70
Trapasso et al, 1994	601†	T1–2N0	1972–92	69	47
	425†	T1–2N0	1987–92	80	—
Zincke et al, 1994	3170*	T1–2NX	1966–91	70	52
	3170†	T1–2NX	1966–91	77	54
Catalona and Smith, 1994	925‡	T1–2NX	1983–93	78	—
Baylor (unpublished data)	672†	T1–2NX	1983–95	80	78

*Progression defined as a serum PSA >0.2 ng/ml.
†Progression defined as a serum PSA >0.4 ng/ml.
‡Progression defined as a serum PSA >0.6 ng/ml.
PSA, Prostate-specific antigen.

steadily declined after 5 years, suggesting that failure after radical prostatectomy is largely due to understaging. Consequently the nonprogression rate 5 years after surgery is a reasonable estimate of the fraction of patients who will remain disease-free.

The actuarial nonprogression rates after radical retropubic prostatectomy from several series, summarized in Table 85–5, show that about 80% of patients at 5 years and 70% at 10 years have no evidence of cancer documented by an undetectable PSA level. The data from Baylor (unpublished data) are based on 672 patients with clinically localized prostate cancer (T1–2NXM0) who underwent radical retropubic prostatectomy between 1983 and 1995 (Fig. 85–2A). No patient received postoperative irradiation or hormonal therapy before PSA recurrence. The actuarial 5- and 10-year nonprogression rates for these patients were 80% and 78%.

Clinical Prognostic Factors

Freedom from progression after radical prostatectomy is related to several well-established clinical prognostic factors, including clinical stage, Gleason grade in the biopsy speci-

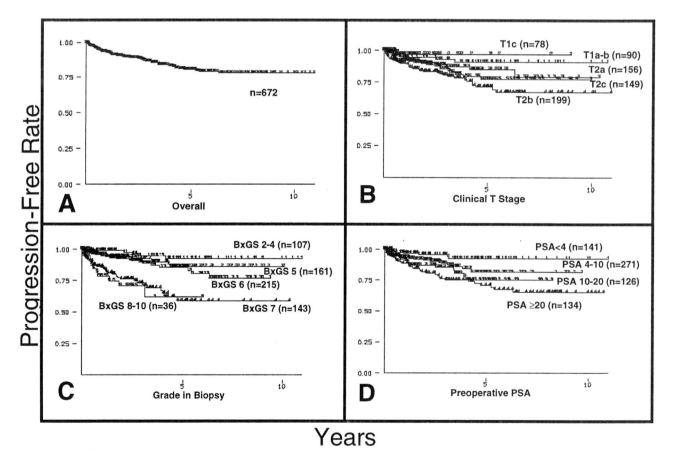

Figure 85–2. Probability of serum prostate-specific antigen (PSA) recurrence after radical prostatectomy for the overall group *(A)* and based on clinical stage *(B)*, biopsy Gleason sum (BxGS) *(C)*, and preoperative PSA *(D)*.

men, and serum PSA levels (Table 85–6). Figure 85–2 shows the actuarial nonprogression rates in the authors' series of 672 patients. **As clinical stage increased, so did the risk of disease recurrence.** Note that patients with tumors found solely on the basis of an elevated serum PSA (Stage T1c, 78 patients) had a 97% PSA nonprogression rate at 5 years in this series, similar to the 99% to 100% nonprogression rates reported by others (see Table 85–6).

PSA nonprogression rates at 5 years following radical prostatectomy according to the Gleason score of the preoperative needle biopsy of the prostate are summarized in Table 85–6. **As the tumor becomes more poorly differentiated, the likelihood of disease recurrence increases.** In the authors' series, 662 men had biopsy Gleason scores available. Of these, 107 had well-differentiated cancers (Gleason score 2, 3, or 4), whereas 36 had poorly differentiated tumors (Gleason score 8, 9, or 10). The remainder of the patients had Gleason score 5 (161 men), 6 (215 men), or 7 (143 men). There was a marked decrease in the probability of nonprogression with more poorly differentiated cancers (Fig. 85–2C). Note that patients with Gleason score 6 or less fared similarly well, whereas those with Gleason score 7 had a prognosis similar to those with Gleason score 8 to 10.

Table 85–6. ACTUARIAL (PSA-BASED) 5-YEAR NONPROGRESSION RATES (%) AFTER RADICAL PROSTATECTOMY FOR CLINICAL STAGE T1–2NXM0 PROSTATE CANCER ACCORDING TO CLINICAL STAGE, BIOPSY GLEASON SCORE, PREOPERATIVE SERUM PROSTATE-SPECIFIC ANTIGEN, AND PATHOLOGIC STAGE

	Partin et al, 1993a	Catalona and Smith, 1994	Zincke et al, 1994	Baylor
No. Patients	894	925	3170	672
Clinical Stage				
T1a	100	89[a]	85[e]	91[a]
T1b	91			
T1c	100	99		97
T2a	87	85[b]	81	85
T2b	71		74[f]	71
T2c	69			78
Gleason Score				
2–4	98	91	93[g]	92
5	92	89[c]	80[h]	86
6	85			85
7	62			59
8–10	46	74	60[i]	57
Preoperative PSA				
0–4	92	95		93
4.1–10.0	83	93		81
10.1–20.0	56	71[d]		74
>20.0	45			71
Pathologic Stage				
Organ confined	97	91	—	95
Extracapsular extension	—	—	—	81
Seminal vesicle invasion	47	—	—	40
Positive lymph node(s)	15	—	—	35

[a]Includes T1a and T1b.
[b]Includes T2a and T2b.
[c]Includes Gleason scores 5–7.
[d]Includes PSA >10.
[e]Includes T1a, T1b, and T1c.
[f]Includes T2b and T2c.
[g]Includes Gleason scores ≤3.
[h]Includes Gleason scores 4–6.
[i]Includes Gleason scores ≥7.
PSA, Prostate-specific antigen.

Table 85–7. MULTIVARIATE ANALYSIS OF CLINICAL PROGNOSTIC FACTORS FOR RECURRENCE AFTER RADICAL PROSTATECTOMY*

	P
Preoperative PSA	.0041
Primary biopsy Gleason grade	.0054
Secondary biopsy Gleason grade	.0262
PSA density	NS
Ultrasound tumor volume	NS
Ultrasound visibility	NS
Elevated prostatic acid phosphatase	NS
Abnormal digital rectal examination	NS
Age	NS
Race	NS
UICC stage†	NS

*n = 728; no adjuvant therapy; end point was clinical or PSA recurrence.
†Spiessl et al, 1992.
PSA, Prostate-specific antigen.

Freedom from PSA progression as a function of preoperative serum PSA is shown in Table 85–6. Among the authors' group of 672 men, 141 had a serum PSA within the normal range (≤4.0 ng/ml), 271 had a PSA of 4.1 to 10 ng/ml, 126 had a PSA of 10 to 20 ng/ml, and 134 had a value greater than 20 (see Fig. 85–2D). **Preoperative serum PSA levels are highly predictive of the risk of progression after radical prostatectomy.**

In a multivariate analysis of clinical prognostic factors, including age, race, clinical stage, Gleason score, serum PSA levels, PSA density, palpability on DRE, and visibility on ultrasound, the primary Gleason grade in the biopsy specimen was the most powerful prognostic factor followed by the secondary grade and the preoperative PSA level (Table 85–7). None of the other variables, including the TNM stage, added significantly to the model predicting prognosis (Eastham et al, 1996c).

Pathologic Prognostic Factors

In addition to clinical factors, more precise prognostic information can be gained from a detailed analysis of the radical prostatectomy specimen. The single most powerful prognostic factor, considering all clinical and pathologic factors in a multivariate analysis, is the pathologic stage of the cancer (Fig. 85–3) (Epstein et al, 1993; Stapleton et al, 1996a). **For patients with prostate cancer pathologically confined to the prostate, 5-year disease-free recurrence measured by serum PSA is excellent (>90%).** The prognosis is particularly poor when the cancer involves the seminal vesicles or pelvic lymph nodes (see Table 85–6). Note, however, that microscopic extracapsular extension is much more favorable. In the authors' series, 81% of such patients are disease-free at 5 years (see Fig. 85–3).

Similar to the results for Gleason score in the preoperative prostate biopsy, the Gleason score in the radical prostatectomy specimen also correlated with disease progression. Again, those with Gleason score 2 to 4, 5, and 6 had a similarly favorable prognosis, and those with Gleason score 8 to 10 fared poorly. Those with a Gleason score of 7, however, had an intermediate prognosis (see Fig. 85–3C), in contrast to those with a biopsy score of 7 (see Fig. 85–2C),

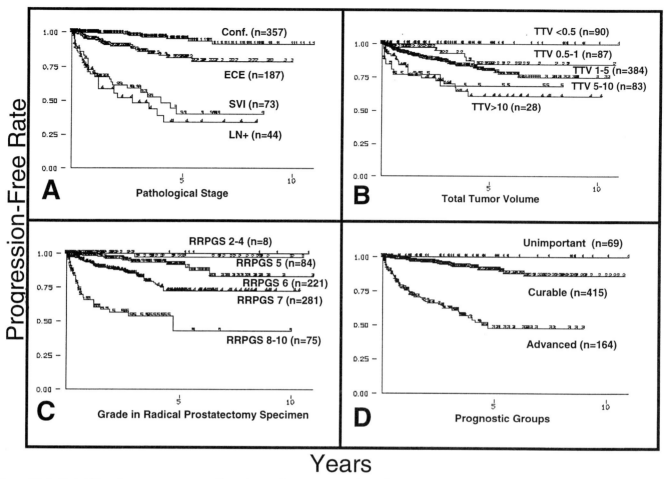

Figure 85–3. Probability of serum prostate-specific antigen (PSA) recurrence after radical prostatectomy based on pathologic stage (*A*), total tumor volume (TTV) (*B*), Gleason sum in the surgical specimen (*C*), and prognostic groups (*D*). ECE, extracapsular extension; conf, confined; SVI, seminal vesicle invasion; LN, positive lymph nodes; RRPGS, radical retropubic prostatectomy Gleason score.

suggesting that the volume or percent of Gleason grade 4 or 5 cancer is an important prognostic feature (McNeal et al, 1990).

Depending on the pathologic features of the tumor in the radical prostatectomy specimen, patients can be classified as having an indolent, curable, or advanced prostate cancer (see Table 85–1 for definitions). By assigning patients to one of these three prognostic groups, overall risk of progression can be assessed (see Fig. 85–3*D*). This classification has implications for therapeutic decision making, such that indolent cancers, if recognized preoperatively, might be treated conservatively except in young men, whereas advanced cancers would be excellent candidates for adjuvant therapy, if an effective adjuvant were available. In the authors' series of 648 patients, 69 (11%) were considered to have indolent cancers and none progressed. There were 415 patients whose tumor had pathologic features consistent with a clinically important but curable cancer. This group also fared well with a nonprogression rate of 90% at 5 years. Patients whose tumors had advanced pathologic features (n = 164, 25%) did poorly, with only 48% disease-free at 5 years (Ohori et al, 1994b).

Perhaps the most convincing evidence that surgical removal of the prostate can interrupt the natural history of the disease is the long-term results of surgery for high-grade cancers (Ohori et al, 1994a). In a reanalysis of an earlier published series, the authors followed 174 patients with Gleason score 7 to 10 cancer in the needle biopsy specimen. In 32%, the cancer was confined to the prostate pathologically, and only one patient has progressed with follow-up ranging from 1 to 8 years. If the cancer extended outside the prostate, however, progression occurred rapidly (Fig. 85–4).

In a multivariate analysis of clinical and pathologic prognostic factors (Table 85–8), pathologic stage was the dominant factor, followed by the Gleason grade in the radical prostatectomy specimen. The only other significant factor was total tumor volume (see Fig. 85–3*B*), which added marginally to the predictive model in the multivariate analysis (see Table 85–8) and, therefore, does not need to be measured in routine clinical practice. Preoperative PSA, PSA density, or any other clinical factor did not add significant prognostic information to that available from a thorough pathologic examination of the prostatectomy specimen (Stapleton et al, 1996a).

Locally Advanced (Clinical Stage T3) Cancers

The results of definitive treatment, whether radiotherapy or radical prostatectomy, for clinical stage T3 prostate cancer

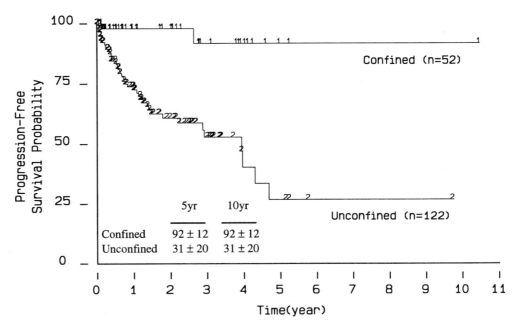

Figure 85–4. Progression-free survival probability by pathologic stage (confined versus unconfined) after radical prostatectomy for 174 patients with a clinically localized (cT1-2NXM0), poorly differentiated (Gleason sum 7–10) cancer on biopsy (P = .0001). Note that 30% (n = 52) of patients had a cancer confined to the prostate pathologically and only two cases have progressed.

are poor. When a cancer extends palpably outside the prostate into the lateral sulci or seminal vesicles, up to 50% of patients have lymph node metastases (Gervasi et al, 1989). Even in patients considered to have small T3 cancers, seminal vesicle invasion is identified pathologically in 67%, and 20% have lymph node metastases (Ohori et al, 1994b). Only 30% of the authors' patients with clinical stage T3 cancers are free of PSA recurrence at 5 years. Although there may be some palliative benefit with removal of the primary tumor, no studies are available that document such benefit. Regardless of the local therapy employed, patient survival is ultimately determined by the response to hormonal therapy and is 25% to 50% less than age-matched men in the general population (Epstein and Hanks, 1992; Morgan et al, 1993).

Neoadjuvant androgen deprivation does not alter the long-term recurrence rate in men with clinical stage T3 prostate cancer. Cher and associates treated 26 selected patients with clinical stage T3 prostate cancers with 3 to 4 months of neoadjuvant hormonal therapy followed by radical prostatectomy and pelvic lymphadenectomy (Cher et al, 1995). Despite significant decreases in the volume of the prostate (35%) and the tumor (50%), decreases in serum PSA levels (96%), and a low rate of positive surgical margins (31%), 69% of the patients had evidence of disease recurrence within 20 to 48 (mean 33) months, a result similar to surgical series without neoadjuvant therapy.

Treatment Safety

Early Complications

Historically, hemorrhage has been the most common intraoperative complication during radical prostatectomy. The procedure frequently resulted in substantial blood loss and the need for transfusions. With the accurate description of the dorsal vein complex and periprostatic anatomy by Reiner and Walsh (1979), surgeons have been able to reduce intraoperative blood loss. With a bloodless operative field, the surgeon can focus on complete removal of the cancer, particularly during dissection of the apex of the prostate; selective preservation of the neurovascular bundles; and precise construction of the vesicourethral anastomosis (Goad and Scardino, 1994; Walsh, 1996).

The estimated blood loss during radical prostatectomy from several large centers is summarized in Table 85–9. Through careful attention to control of the dorsal vein complex and meticulous dissection and control of the many small vessels surrounding the seminal vesicles, the authors have substantially reduced intraoperative blood loss. At present, 75% of the authors' patients lose less than 1000 ml. This reduction in blood loss, together with a more stringent transfusion policy, has decreased the use of allogeneic blood to 10% of patients who do not donate autologous blood (Goad et al, 1995). The same transfusion criteria are applied

Table 85–8. MULTIVARIATE ANALYSIS OF PROGNOSTIC FACTORS AFTER RADICAL PROSTATECTOMY*

	P
Seminal vesicle invasion	< .0001
Gleason primary grade (4 or 5)	< .0001
Lymph node involvement	.0027
Gleason secondary grade (4 or 5)	.0097
Positive surgical margin	.0225
Pathologic tumor volume	.0400
Extracapsular extension	.0475
Preoperative PSA	NS
PSA density	NS
Ultrasound tumor volume	NS
Primary biopsy Gleason grade	NS
Secondary biopsy Gleason grade	NS
Elevated prostatic acid phosphatase	NS
Abnormal digital rectal examination	NS
Age	NS
UICC stage†	NS

*n = 728; no adjuvant therapy; end point was clinical or PSA recurrence.
†Spiessl et al, 1992.
PSA, Prostate-specific antigen.

Table 85–9. ESTIMATED BLOOD LOSS IN PATIENTS UNDERGOING RADICAL RETROPUBIC PROSTATECTOMY

Series	No.	Mean Estimated Blood Loss (ml)	Range (ml)
Rainwater and Segura, 1990	316	1020	100–4320
Kavoussi et al, 1991	65*	1420	200–2500
	65†	1605	250–3500
Frazier et al, 1992	122‡	565	150–1850
	51	2000	600–10,000
Leandri et al, 1992	220	300	100–1500
Zincke et al, 1994	1728	600	—
Baylor (unpublished data)	954	800	150–5000

*With temporary internal iliac artery occlusion.
†Without temporary internal iliac artery occlusion.
‡Radical perineal prostatectomy.

to nondonors and donors. Only 21% of autologous blood units donated were transfused. With a blood loss less than 1000 ml, most patients do not require transfusion. The authors do not routinely request preoperative autologous donation, which results in a substantial cost savings (Eastham et al, 1996b).

Intraoperative complications are less frequent now than in previous decades. In a review of all Medicare patients undergoing radical prostatectomy in 1990, Mark (1994) reported an operative mortality, defined as death within 30 days of surgery, of 0.5% (33 of 7052 patients). Operative mortality from several large medical centers occurred in only 11 (0.3%) of 3834 men (Table 85–10). Rectal injury during radical prostatectomy occurs in less than 1% of patients. Prior pelvic irradiation, prior rectal surgery, and prior transurethral resection of the prostate have been cited as predis-

posing factors for rectal injury (McLaren et al, 1993). The injury occurs most commonly with division of the rectourethralis muscle during the apical dissection. In the event of a rectal injury, repair should not be undertaken until after the prostatectomy has been completed. The injury is usually repaired in two layers and the anal sphincter dilated at the end of the procedure. A segment of omentum may be placed between the vesicourethral anastomosis and rectum to reduce the risk of fistula formation (Borland and Walsh, 1992). Routine colostomy is not necessary. Temporary diversion of the fecal stream, however, should be considered for a patient with prior pelvic irradiation.

Deep venous thrombosis and pulmonary embolism occur in about 1.1% and 1.3% of patients undergoing radical prostatectomy (see Table 85–10). Controversy exists regarding the role of anticoagulants and sequential pneumatic compression devices in the prevention of these complications. Numerous studies have suggested that sequential pneumatic compression devices are effective in preventing thromboembolic complications. Caprini and associates showed that the evidence of deep venous thrombosis detected by fibrinogen uptake was decreased from 21% in control patients to 3% in patients wearing a sequential pneumatic compression device (Caprini et al, 1983). Other studies evaluating urologic patients undergoing pelvic surgery have also suggested a benefit of sequential pneumatic compression devices in reducing the incidence of deep venous thrombosis (Coe et al, 1978; Hansberry et al, 1991). In one series, however, Cisek and Walsh (1993) found no difference in the incidence of clinically detected pulmonary embolism or deep venous thrombosis in the 30-day period following radical prostatectomy for patients whose treatment included the use of sequential pneumatic compression devices compared with those whose treatment did not. This study differed from

Table 85–10. PERIOPERATIVE COMPLICATIONS AND MORTALITY OF RADICAL RETROPUBIC PROSTATECTOMY IN CONTEMPORARY SERIES*

Complications	Washington University (Andriole et al, 1994) (n = 1324) No.	%	Mayo Clinic (Lerner et al, 1995) (n = 1000) No.	%	Ulm (Hautman et al, 1994) (n = 418) No.	%	Toulouse (Leandri et al, 1992) (n = 620) No.	%	Baylor (Dillioglugil et al, 1996c) (n = 472) No.	%	Overall (n = 3834) No.	%
Mortality	3	0.2	0	0.0	5	1.2	1	0.2	2	0.4	11/3834	0.3
Rectal injury	3	0.2	6	0.6	11	2.9	3	0.5	3	0.6	26/3834	0.7
Colostomy	—	—	0	0.0	—	—	—	—	0	0.0	0	0.0
Ureteral injury	—	—	—	—	1	0.2	0	0.0	1	0.2	2/1510	0.1
Myocardial infarction	9	0.7	7	0.7	3	0.7	1	0.2	2	0.4	22/3834	0.6
Pulmonary embolism	22	1.7	6	0.6	6	1.4	5	0.8	5	1.0	44/3834	1.1
Thrombophlebitis/deep venous thrombosis	8	0.6	14	1.4	7	1.7	14	2.3	6	1.3	49/3834	1.3
Sepsis	—	—	2	0.5	—	—	1	0.2	3	0.6	6/2092	0.3
Wound infection or dehiscence	17	1.3	9	0.9	11	2.6	6	1.0	14	2.9	57/3834	1.5
Lymphocele	—	—	—	—	28	6.7†	14	2.3‡	10	2.1†	52/1510	3.4
Prolonged fluid leak§	8	0.6	—	—	—	—	—	—	3	0.6	11/1796	0.6
Premature catheter loss	4	0.3	—	—	—	—	—	—	7	1.5	11/1796	0.6
Anastomotic stricture	—	—	87	8.7	37	8.6	3	0.5	42	9.0	169/2510	6.7

*Note that complications are not mutually exclusive, that is, one patient may have had more than one complication.
†All lymphoceles.
‡Surgically drained lymphoceles.
§Urine or lymph.
— signifies unavailable data.
From Dillioglugil et al: J Urol 1996c; submitted.

previous investigations in that clinical events rather than fibrinogen/platelet scanning were used. More importantly, this last study included a longer period of follow-up and large numbers of patients. **The majority of patients suffered a deep venous thrombosis or pulmonary embolism after discharge from the hospital. As hospital stay following radical prostatectomy continues to decrease, patients should be well informed about the signs and symptoms of deep venous thrombosis and pulmonary embolism to avoid delays in diagnosis and treatment.**

Subcutaneous low-dose heparin has been shown to be effective in reducing the incidence of both deep venous thrombosis and pulmonary embolism in urologic patients. Its routine use following major surgical procedures has been limited primarily because of concerns about an increased risk of hemorrhagic complications. Low-molecular-weight heparin, however, has been shown to be equally effective in preventing deep venous thrombosis and pulmonary embolism as standard heparin, but has not been associated with an increased risk of hemorrhagic complications (Fricker et al, 1988). Whether or not it will prove useful after radical prostatectomy is unknown.

Late Complications

Overall, the risk of mortality or serious morbidity after radical prostatectomy in recent series is remarkably low (see Table 85–10). Anastomotic stricture has been reported in 0.5% to 9% of patients following radical prostatectomy (see Table 85–10), with one series reporting strictures in 17.5% of 456 patients (Geary et al, 1995). Prior transurethral resection of the prostate, excessive intraoperative blood loss, and urinary extravasation at the anastomotic site may contribute to stricture development (Surya et al, 1990). Any factor that interferes with mucosa-to-mucosa apposition increases the risk of stricture. Simple dilation is usually effective over the long-term only in minimal filmy strictures. Most anastomotic strictures require cold knife incision or periodic dilation to maintain an adequate urine flow.

Urinary incontinence remains one of the most troubling side effects following radical prostatectomy. Although an anatomic approach to the procedure has resulted in a decrease in the incidence of incontinence, reported rates of this complication vary widely (Table 85–11). The American College of Surgeons Committee on Cancer surveyed 484

Table 85–11. INCIDENCE OF INCONTINENCE AFTER RADICAL PROSTATECTOMY

Series from Centers of Excellence	Incontinence No.	(%)	Definition of Incontinence
Steiner et al, 1991	593	8	Leaks with moderate activity
Leandri et al, 1992	398	5	Leaks with moderate activity
Zincke et al, 1994	1728	5	Requires 3 or more pads per day
Catalona, 1995	925	6	No pads
Geary et al, 1995	458	20	Requires pads
Eastham et al, 1996	581	9	Leaks with moderate activity
Series from Patient Surveys			
Fowler et al, 1993	738	31	Pads or clamps
Murphy et al, 1994	1796	19	Requires pads
Litwin et al, 1995	98	25	"Bother" score

hospitals to evaluate the status of patients who had undergone radical prostatectomy in the United States (Murphy et al, 1994). Of 1796 men who were continent preoperatively, 330 (19%) wore pads on a daily basis, and 3.6% were totally incontinent after surgery. Fowler and colleagues reported that 31% of a sample population of Medicare patients who underwent radical prostatectomy from 1988 to 1990 reported some degree of wetness (Fowler et al, 1993). In contrast, **most centers with broad expertise in radical prostatectomy report that less than 10% of patients are incontinent after surgery** (see Table 85–11). Despite the relatively high rates of urinary incontinence reported in population surveys, the majority of these patients were minimally bothered by this complication and were highly satisfied with their treatment (Litwin et al, 1995).

The authors reviewed their data to identify risk factors associated with incontinence after radical retropubic prostatectomy. For their most recent 390 patients, the median time to recovery of continence was 1.5 months (Fig. 85–5). At 1 year, 92% were dry, and at 2 years, 95% were dry. Using multivariate analysis, the authors evaluated whether or not clinical or pathologic stage, the size of the prostate, operative blood loss, the presence of palpable tumor near the apex, postoperative hemorrhage, patient age, patient weight, history of transurethral resection of the prostate, or development of an anastomotic stricture affected urinary continence after surgery. **The age of the patient and whether or not an anastomotic stricture developed each influenced the recovery of continence. Patients with clinical stage T1a or T1b, those over age 65, and those who developed a stricture were at greater risk for incontinence.**

Recovery of continence is also sensitive to surgical technique (Goad and Scardino, 1994; Eastham et al, 1996a), which may, in addition to the risk factors listed previously, explain the wide variation in recovery of continence in different series (see Table 85–11). In 1990, the authors revised their technique to avoid retraction on the urethra during the prostatectomy, to place the anastomotic sutures through a small bite of urethra and a large bite of the lateral pelvic fascia surrounding the oversewn dorsal vein complex, and to form a fully everted (stomatized) bladder neck. This change resulted in a marked improvement in continence (see Fig. 85–5).

Patients should be encouraged to perform pelvic floor (Kegel) exercises after catheter removal. Combining this technique with biofeedback may be beneficial in some patients with mild stress incontinence. **Improvement in continence is common up to 1 year and may occur up to 2 years following surgery** (Leandri et al, 1992; Eastham et al, 1996a). The physiologic mechanism for this delayed return of continence is unclear, but from a clinical standpoint, **it is best to defer invasive treatments for incontinence for at least 1 year after prostatectomy.**

In men with persistent incontinence following radical prostatectomy, a cause should be sought. The possibility that a bladder neck contracture may be impeding the recovery of urinary control should be considered. **Patients with a bladder neck contracture usually have a dribbling urinary stream or symptoms of overflow incontinence. Flexible cystoscopy can be used to evaluate the anastomotic site after ultrasound measurement of postvoid residual urine. If no anastomotic stricture is identified, urody-**

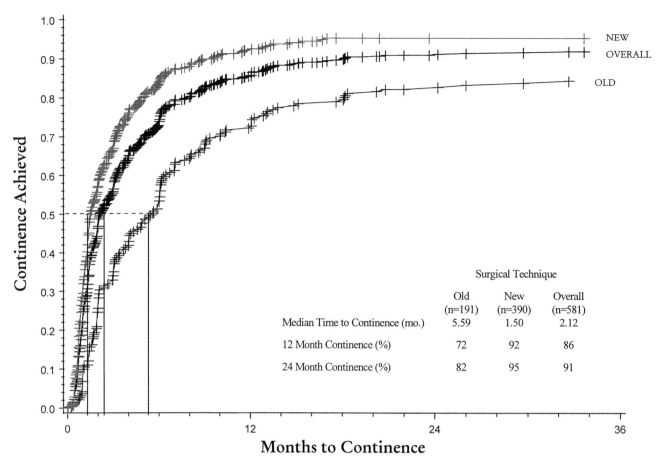

Figure 85–5. Time to return of continence for the entire group of 581 patients and for the old and new anastomotic techniques (see text for description). For 390 patients who had the new technique, median time to continence was 1.5 months, and 95% were continent by 24 months.

namic evaluation is warranted (Foote et al, 1991; Goluboff et al, 1995). **Some men have bladder dysfunction rather than pure sphincteric injury.** Treatment decisions should be based on urodynamic findings: Patients with bladder dysfunction should be treated medically, whereas those with sphincteric damage are best treated surgically.

Return of erections after radical prostatectomy has been correlated with patient age, pathologic tumor stage, and extent of preservation of the neurovascular bundles (Table 85–12). Quinlan and colleagues evaluated 503 potent men between the ages of 34 and 72 years who underwent radical retropubic prostatectomy (Quinlan et al, 1991). For men under the age of 50, 90% were potent if one or both neurovascular bundles were preserved. For men 50 years of age

or older, potency was better if both neurovascular bundles were preserved. Catalona (1995) reported similar results: 63% of patients retained potency with bilateral neurovascular bundle preservation compared with only 41% of men with unilateral nerve-sparing surgery. Pathologic stage also influences the return of erections after radical prostatectomy. Quinlan and associates reported that 70% of men with pathologically confined prostate cancer were able to have erections if both neurovascular bundles were preserved compared with only 50% of patients with seminal vesicle involvement (Quinlan et al, 1991). The less satisfactory preservation of potency in men with pathologically advanced tumors results from a wider dissection to encompass the tumor.

Data on the recovery of potency after radical prostatectomy appear to be quite different if one compares results from centers of excellence to population surveys. The American College of Surgeons Committee on Cancer (Murphy et al, 1994) reported that only 27% of patients recovered potency, although the median age (65–69 years) and pathologic stage (39% C or D) were higher than those reported by Quinlan and associates (1991) and Catalona (1995). Also, the potency status of these men before the operation was not known. Litwin and colleagues used a validated quality of life survey to assess sexual function in 214 men treated with watchful waiting, radiotherapy, or radical prostatectomy (Litwin et al, 1995). Again, prior potency status was not documented. In the surgical group, nerve-sparing was not used routinely, yet 29% recovered normal erections com-

Table 85–12. POTENCY FOLLOWING BILATERAL NERVE-SPARING RADICAL RETROPUBIC PROSTATECTOMY

Age	Quinlan et al, 1991*	Leandri et al, 1992†	Catalona, 1995*
<50	90%		
50–59	82%	76%‡	75%‡
60–69	69%	72%	60%
≥70	22%	20%	50%

*Potency at 18 months.
†Potency at 12 months.
‡Includes patients ≤59.

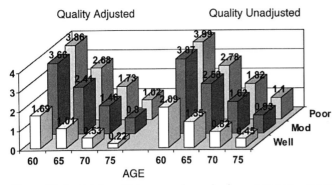

Figure 85–6. Net benefit in years for radical prostatectomy versus watchful waiting for the treatment of clinically localized prostate cancer. (From Kattan MW, Miles BJ, Beck JR, Scardino PT: J Urol 1995;153:390A.)

pared with 36% treated with radiotherapy (Litwin et al, 1995). These data and the authors' experience confirm that erectile function can be preserved after radical prostatectomy, but the probability of recovery depends on the potency status before the operation, the age of the patient, the stage of the tumor, and the preservation of the neurovascular bundles (Stapleton et al, 1996b). The results are sensitive to subtle variations in surgical technique (Walsh, 1994; Stapleton and Scardino, 1996).

INDICATIONS AND CONTRAINDICATIONS

Radical prostatectomy should be reserved for men who are likely to be cured and will live long enough to benefit from the cure. As has been learned from attempts to simulate the outcome of treatment using decision-analysis models (Fleming et al, 1993; Beck et al, 1994), the factors that influence the risk-to-benefit ratio include the age and health of the patient, the nature of the cancer (the risk of metastasis over time if left untreated), the probability that surgery will cure the cancer, and the complications of surgery. Because of the protracted course of prostate cancer, the age and comorbid conditions of the patient are critical determinants of the benefits of treatment (Kattan et al, submitted) (see

Table 85–3; Fig. 85–6). Albertsen and co-workers clearly documented the impact of comorbidity on survival for 65- to 75-year-old men (Albertsen et al, 1995), while also demonstrating the profound shortening of life expectancy for those with a moderately or poorly differentiated cancer treated conservatively (see Table 85–3). Although the efficacy and complication rate of treatment are important factors in the decision-analysis model, the dominant features are the metastatic rate of the cancer and the age and life expectancy of the patient (Beck et al, 1994). If the metastatic rate of the cancer is judged to be low, neither screening with PSA nor treatment (with radiotherapy or surgery) appears beneficial except for young men with poorly differentiated cancers (Fleming et al, 1993; Krahn et al, 1994). If the metastatic rate is higher, however, as reported in comprehensive, multi-institutional pooled analyses (Chodak, 1994; Chodak et al, 1994), the impact on mortality of the untreated disease is greater, and the benefits of treatment, in terms of life years gained, are clearer even when adjusted for the complications of treatment (see Fig. 85–6) (Beck et al, 1994; Kattan et al, 1995). When the overall survival rate of a 65-year-old man with a T1–2NXM0 prostate cancer (any grade) treated with surgery is compared in a decision-analysis model with one managed conservatively, the 15-year survival rate is 41% versus 29% (Fig. 85–7).

Age and Health

In choosing therapy for an individual patient with clinically localized prostate cancer, the age and general health of the patient remain critically important because of the well-established protracted course of the disease. Mortality from a localized cancer left untreated is not likely to occur for 8 to 10 years, yet the risk of death from cancer continues to increase for at least 15 to 20 years or more (Chodak et al, 1994; Albertsen et al, 1995; Aus et al, 1995; Dillioglugil et al, 1996a). In 1989, the average life expectancy of a 70-year-old man was 12.1 years, and for a 75-year-old man it was less than 10 years. Thus, the potential benefits of therapy decrease rapidly as men age.

Chronologic age, however, is only one factor that influences life expectancy. Prostate cancer frequently occurs in older men who have associated comorbid conditions. Con-

Figure 85–7. Survival rates (all causes) by treatment estimated in a decision-analysis model 5, 10, and 15 years after diagnosis of a clinically localized (T1-2NXM0) prostate cancer, all grades combined. (From Beck JR, Kattan MW, Miles BJ: J Urol 1994;152:1894–1899.)

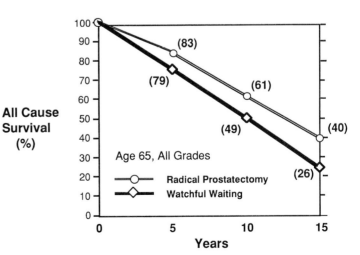

versely, some older patients are in excellent physical condition and have a life expectancy greater than average for their age group. Therefore, an arbitrary age should not be set at which a patient would no longer be considered a surgical candidate. Clinical judgment informed by a thorough assessment of the life expectancy of the individual patient with prostate cancer allows the physician to explain to the patient fully about the risks and benefits of conservative management as well as active intervention, so that the patient can make a well-informed decision about the management of his disease.

Selection of Patients by Clinical Prognostic Factors

Prostate-Specific Antigen

Serum PSA levels increase proportionally with advancing clinical stage (reviewed in Oesterling, 1991). Using a polyclonal PSA assay, Stamey and Kabalin (1989) were able to distinguish the various clinical stages in a cohort of 209 patients but could not distinguish stage B2 from B3 or stage C from D1. In most studies, considerable overlap is present among all clinical stages (Ohori et al, 1994c).

As with clinical stage, there is a correlation between advanced pathologic stage and increasing serum PSA levels but with considerable overlap between preoperative PSA and pathologic stage (reviewed in Oesterling, 1991). Higher preoperative serum PSA levels are not always associated with advanced pathologic features (established extracapsular extension, seminal vesicle invasion, positive lymph nodes), and lower values do not necessarily suggest organ-confined disease. Stamey and co-workers reported three patients with high PSA levels (150–456 ng/ml) who had a large transition zone cancer confined to the prostate (Stamey et al, 1993). Therefore, **PSA cannot definitively distinguish the stage of the cancer in an individual patient and cannot be used alone as a contraindication to definitive treatment.**

Gleason Grade

Although radical prostatectomy has been shown to result in excellent long-term cancer-specific survival (Gibbons et al, 1989; Partin, 1994a; Zincke et al, 1994), several investigators have questioned the need for early definitive treatment (Fleming et al, 1993; Chodak et al, 1994), suggesting that conservative management of patients with clinically localized well-differentiated or moderately differentiated cancers poses little risk of death from cancer within 10 to 15 years. Indeed, Albertsen and colleagues found little impact of a well-differentiated cancer on the mortality of men age 65 to 75 years (see Table 85–3), but these were largely early-stage (T1a with a few T2) cancers and made up only 9% of the patient population (Albertsen et al, 1995). Watchful waiting—conservative management—has been widely recommended for elderly men or those with a life expectancy less than 10 years as well as for some men with a longer life expectancy who have a small, focal, well-differentiated cancer (Johansson et al, 1992; Mettlin et al, 1993).

In contrast, poorly differentiated tumors progress rapidly and have a high cancer-specific mortality rate within 10

years when managed conservatively. Even with definitive treatment, poorly differentiated cancers have a poor prognosis because they have usually spread beyond the prostate at the time of diagnosis. With early detection, however, many high-grade cancers are being found while still confined to the prostate, and the prognosis for such cancers is excellent (see Fig. 85–4) (Ohori et al, 1994b). Although Gleason grade is an important prognostic factor, it cannot be used categorically to determine prognosis or to justify management.

Clinical Stage

Clinical stage also influences the outcome after radical prostatectomy, but within the substages considered localized (T1-2NX) it has not proven to be a powerful independent prognostic factor. The prognosis for patients with locally advanced (T3) tumors is poor because most patients already have occult metastases. When a cancer extends palpably beyond the prostate into the lateral sulci or seminal vesicles, lymph node metastases are present in 30% to 50% of patients (Gervasi et al, 1989). Even in carefully selected patients with small T3 cancers, seminal vesicle invasion is present in 67% and lymph node metastases in 20% (Ohori et al, 1994c). With the exception of an increased risk of impotence, the prostate can be removed with no greater morbidity for T3 cancers than for T1-2 lesions. Although there may be some palliative benefit of removing a T3 tumor, no studies are available that document such benefit.

Radical Prostatectomy in Patients with Lymph Node Metastases

Before the widespread use of serum PSA, the incidence of pelvic lymph node metastases at the time of radical prostatectomy for clinically localized prostate cancer was in excess of 20% (Fowler and Whitmore, 1981; Smith et al, 1983; Gervasi et al, 1989). **In more recent series, however, the incidence of pelvic lymph node metastases was 5% to 7%** (Danella et al, 1993; Petros and Catalona, 1992). With such a low probability of metastases, it has been difficult to identify subsets of patients whose risk of metastases is significantly higher or lower than the population as a whole. Analyzing pooled data from several institutions, Rees and co-workers proposed an algorithm for identifying men with a low probability of lymph node metastases (Rees et al, 1995). If the PSA was 5 or less, or Gleason score 5 or less, or PSA 25 or less and Gleason score 7 or less and the DRE negative, only 1 of 246 patients had metastases in the pelvic lymphadenectomy specimen (Rees et al, 1995). Others have attempted similar analyses (Bluestein et al, 1994; Partin et al, 1993b), but the applicability to modern series is confounded by the much lower rate of lymph node metastases currently encountered (Stapleton et al, 1996a).

In fact, it would be reasonably accurate to assume that all patients with clinically localized (T1-2NXM0) cancers have negative pelvic lymph nodes (false-negative rate 5%–7%). Consequently, some have questioned the need to perform routine pelvic lymphadenectomy in patients undergoing radical prostatectomy. Despite these concerns, the presence of lymph node metastases has powerful prognostic implications (see Tables 85–6 and 85–8) and should be determined if feasible without increasing the morbidity of treatment. No patient with documented positive nodes treated with surgery or radiotherapy alone (no hormonal therapy) has remained free of progression (documented by PSA) for 10 years (Gervasi et al, 1989; Partin et al, 1994b). Currently, **the authors do not recommend routine pelvic lymphadenectomy before definitive radiotherapy or radical perineal prostatectomy** except in unusual patients with high-grade, high-stage cancers and a markedly elevated serum PSA level, whose probability of having nodal metastases is judged to be 30% or greater. This is the only group of patients for whom staging computed tomography (CT) or magnetic resonance imaging (MRI) scans of the pelvis are indicated to detect the rare gross nodal metastases that can be confirmed by fine needle biopsy and a node dissection avoided. If the CT or MRI scans are normal, a laparoscopic pelvic lymphadenectomy or minilaparotomy (Hortopan et al, 1995) is indicated. If the nodes are negative, the patient is treated with definitive radiotherapy or radical perineal prostatectomy. If the nodes are positive, immediate or deferred hormonal therapy (androgen ablation) is instituted and local therapy avoided except for the rare patient who develops clinical local progression.

Grossly positive nodes are encountered in less than a third of patients with positive nodes (Gervasi et al, 1989), no more than 1% to 2% of candidates for radical prostatectomy, so **CT scans and MRI studies of the pelvis are not indicated as routine staging procedures in men with clinically localized prostate cancer.** When these patients are treated with radical retropubic prostatectomy, pelvic lymphadenectomy is performed routinely because it does not increase the morbidity of the procedure. Historically, the lymph nodes have been submitted for frozen section examination, and if metastases were found, the prostatectomy was abandoned. Today, it is clear that radical prostatectomy provides excellent local control, and the complication rate is low. Many surgeons, therefore, recommend removal of the prostate unless the nodes are grossly involved by cancer. **The authors no longer perform frozen sections routinely but proceed with the radical prostatectomy** as scheduled if the lymph nodes appear grossly normal.

Of course, some 5% to 7% of patients so treated are found to have lymph nodal metastases on permanent histologic evaluation. The optimal management of these patients remains controversial: whether to begin hormonal therapy immediately or to monitor the course of the disease and delay hormonal therapy until the PSA level begins to rise or until clinical recurrence is documented. There is no role for radiotherapy in these patients. The controversy about the timing of hormonal therapy revolves around the question of whether immediate hormonal therapy prolongs survival. There is no question that immediate therapy delays the appearance of biochemical or clinical progression (Zincke, 1989). Claims have been made, based on uncontrolled studies, that immediate therapy prolongs overall survival (Zincke, 1989, 1990; Zincke et al, 1992; Cheng et al, 1994). No randomized trial has addressed this issue, and there is no physiologic basis to support this claim. With the early indication of disease progression provided by PSA, there seems little rationale for instituting hormonal therapy immediately rather than waiting for an unequivocal rise in the serum PSA

level. Certainly, patients should be carefully informed and given the opportunity to delay therapy if they choose.

Neoadjuvant Androgen Ablation

Because of the high probability of extension outside the prostate in clinically localized prostate cancers that are presumed to be confined to the gland, attempts have been made to reduce the pathologic stage and the rate of positive surgical margins with neoadjuvant androgen ablation. In five randomized, prospective, controlled clinical trials, **neoadjuvant hormonal therapy reduced the rate of positive surgical margins from an average of 47% (range 38%–64%) to an average of 22% (range 13%–34%),** reduced the preoperative serum PSA levels by 96% (range 90%–99%), and reduced prostate volume by 34% (range 12%–52%) (Labrie et al, 1993; Debruyne et al, 1994; Dillioglugil et al, 1995b; Goldenberg et al, 1995; Soloway et al, 1995; Van Poppel et al, 1995; Abbas and Scardino, 1996). Whether such dramatic effects represent only the expected reduction in tumor volume with androgen ablation, an artifactual reduction in the rate of positive surgical margins, and **whether these effects will translate into a benefit in long-term disease control or survival remains uncertain because of the relatively short follow-up in the reported trials.** In fact, preliminary results indicate no difference in the progression rate between treated and untreated patients.

Certainly the rate of positive margins in these trials is unacceptably high. In a review of 7596 patients treated with radical prostatectomy reported in eight series, the positive surgical margin rate was 25% (range 14%–41%) (Abbas and Scardino, 1996). The rate of positive margins clearly depends on surgical technique (Stamey et al, 1990; Ohori et al, 1995). With no change in pathologic stage or tumor volume over the past 10 years, the authors reduced the rate of positive margins in their radical prostatectomy series from 24% to 8% (Ohori et al, 1995) by adjusting the extent of the resection of periprostatic tissue (including the neurovascular bundles) to the size and location of the cancer (Goad and Scardino, 1994). Neoadjuvant hormonal therapy often causes periprostatic fibrosis, obscuring normal tissue planes, and shrinks the tumor mass, making it difficult to palpate during the operation. The surgeon is left with little to guide the extent of dissection and the degree of resection of the neurovascular bundles. Whether potency can be preserved successfully after hormonal therapy remains to be seen. Hormonal therapy does not make the operation easier or reduce blood loss or the risk of transfusions. There are disadvantages to neoadjuvant hormonal therapy. Until the benefits, in disease-free interval or survival, are clear, hormonal therapy should not be used as a substitute for optimal surgical technique.

Treatment of Rising Prostate-Specific Antigen After Radical Prostatectomy

Serum PSA levels should become undetectable after radical prostatectomy. With rare exceptions (Leibman et al, 1995; Oefelein et al, 1995), the PSA level begins to rise 3 to 6 years before recurrence is detected by standard clinical tests (bone scan, acid phosphatase, symptoms). It is not clear, however, how and when patients with a rising PSA level should be treated.

Because standard PSA assays were not designed to be accurate at low levels, the physician must first verify that the PSA level is consistently rising. A conservative definition of PSA progression is a level 0.4 ng/ml and rising on at least two subsequent occasions. Rarely, minimal elevations in PSA can result from unresected benign prostatic tissue (Foster et al, 1993; Fowler et al, 1995), in which case the PSA usually rises, then levels off. In contrast, cancer typically causes a steady continuing rise. Treatment depends on whether the recurrence is local or distant. Bone scans usually show no abnormality in these patients. Unless there is a mass palpable in the prostatic fossa, the site of recurrence is difficult to document.

Local recurrence is more likely in men with a low-grade, low pathologic stage cancer and a PSA level that becomes undetectable after the operation and begins to rise slowly months or years later (reviewed in Ferguson and Oesterling, 1994; Danella et al, 1993; Partin et al, 1994b). With local recurrence, PSA first becomes detectable, on average, some 3 years later than with distant recurrence. The authors perform ultrasound-guided needle biopsies of the anastomotic area to document local recurrence. Although a positive biopsy result is not mandatory before radiotherapy, with a positive biopsy local irradiation therapy can be given with confidence. If the biopsy result is negative, the authors carefully follow PSA levels and repeat the biopsy in 6 to 12 months because postoperative adjuvant radiotherapy may cause troublesome proctitis as well as decrease the chance of recovering continence and potency. The efficacy of radiation therapy for patients with presumed local recurrence detected by a rising PSA level after radical prostatectomy has been investigated. There is a transient decrease in the serum PSA in 53% to 64% of men. Although several authors report no subsequent disease progression in small series (Lange et al, 1990; Schild et al, 1992), Partin and associates found undetectable serum PSA for longer than 2 years in only 10% (Partin et al, 1994b). Some of these patients subsequently developed clinical local recurrence despite radiation therapy, suggesting that irradiation is not always effective in eliminating the local tumor.

The benefit of immediate adjuvant radiation therapy for men at increased risk of local recurrence (extracapsular extension, positive margins, seminal vesicle invasion) has been debated for years. In some studies, the risk of subsequent local recurrence was reduced substantially, but there was no effect on distant metastases or cancer-specific survival (Gibbons et al, 1986). This issue is being addressed in a National Cancer Institute–supported intergroup prospective clinical trial led by the Southwest Oncology Group. Pending the outcome of this trial, there is little rationale for treating microscopic extracapsular extension with adjuvant radiotherapy routinely because 81% remain free of progression with surgery alone (see Table 85–6). Those with seminal vesicle invasion typically recur with distant metastases rather than locally (D'Amico et al, 1995). Adjuvant radiotherapy (in those with an undetectable PSA level) seems most appropriate for patients with positive surgical margins in the absence of seminal vesicle invasion and lymph node metastases because cancer cells may have been left within the field of irradiation. **Only 40% to 50% of patients with a positive**

surgical margin who do not receive immediate radiation therapy, however, develop an elevated PSA level within 5 years (Epstein et al, 1993; Ohori et al, 1995). **Although a significant risk factor for recurrence** (see Table 85–8), **positive surgical margins do not mean that the cancer is destined to recur or that local tumor has been left behind.** In radical prostatectomy specimens in which the surgical margin was considered positive, Epstein (1990) removed the adjacent neurovascular bundle and only 60% contained tumor.

For patients whose pathologic stage and grade and rate of rise in PSA point to distant recurrence, hormonal therapy is more appropriate than irradiation therapy. Androgen ablation may be initiated immediately or delayed until symptomatic recurrence is imminent. There is no evidence for a survival benefit with early therapy, but most patients insist on treatment in the face of a rapidly rising PSA.

Salvage Radical Prostatectomy

Radical prostatectomy has been used successfully to eradicate locally recurrent cancer after definitive radiotherapy, but complications are common. The authors reviewed 39 salvage radical prostatectomies for locally recurrent prostate cancer, defined as a positive biopsy result in conjunction with an increasing serum PSA level and no evidence of metastases (Rogers et al, 1995). Mean estimated blood loss, transfusion requirements, and average hospital stay were significantly greater than for standard radical prostatectomy patients. **Rectal injuries occurred in 15% of patients, whereas 27% developed anastomotic strictures. Urinary incontinence persisted in 58%.** A total of 21 patients (54%) had pathologically advanced disease, which was defined as seminal vesicle invasion, lymph node metastases, or both. **Preoperative serum PSA levels, but not clinical stage or biopsy grade, correlated positively with pathologic stage. If the preoperative PSA was less than 10 ng/ml, only 15% of the patients had advanced pathologic features, compared with 86% if the PSA was greater than 10 ng/ml.**

When PSA levels were used to detect recurrence after salvage prostatectomy, the actuarial nonprogression rates at 5 and 8 years were 55% and 33%, respectively (Fig. 85–8). The 5-year actuarial nonprogression rate was 100% for patients with organ-confined cancer, 71% for those with extracapsular extension, and 28% for those with seminal vesicle invasion. Stage for stage, these results were similar to the results of standard radical prostatectomy (Table 85–13). Among patients with a PSA level less than 10 ng/ml, the actuarial nonprogression rate at 4 years was 50% compared with 29% for patients with a PSA level greater than 10 ng/ml (P <.05) (Rogers et al, 1995). Salvage prostatectomy, although technically challenging, provides excellent local control of radiorecurrent cancer and can eradicate the disease in a high proportion of patients treated when the cancer is confined to the prostate or immediate periprostatic tissue. As for standard prostatectomy, patient selection is of utmost importance. Patients should be in good health with a life expectancy greater than 10 years, have a local tumor proven by biopsy, and have no evidence of metastatic disease. Most

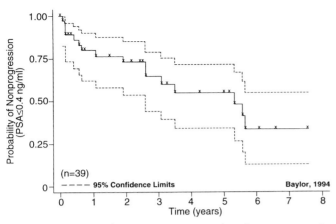

Figure 85–8. Actuarial nonprogression rates based on postoperative prostate-specific antigen (PSA) levels after salvage prostatectomy. Progression was defined as PSA level of 0.4 ng/ml and increasing. (From Rogers E, Ohori M, Kassabian VS, et al: J Urol 1995;153:104–110.)

importantly, candidates for salvage prostatectomy should be treated before the PSA level rises above 10 ng/ml.

CONCLUSIONS

Men diagnosed with clinically localized prostate cancer should be considered for definitive treatment if they are in good general health and have a life expectancy of 10 years or longer. Assessing the benefits of active treatment with radical prostatectomy versus conservative management depends on accurate estimations of the life expectancy (age and health) of the patient; the risk that the cancer will metastasize each year if left untreated (indicated most accurately by the grade and PSA level); the probability that surgical excision will eradicate the cancer and prevent metastases; and the frequency, intensity,

and bother of complications from the surgical procedure and from the cancer itself. Decision analysis models provide a tool to quantitate the degree of benefit (or harm) and will become more useful as the quality of the information about each of these factors improves. The experience with radical prostatectomy reported in the past 5 years clearly documents that this operation effectively eradicates the cancer in a large proportion of patients. This operation is generally accompanied by low morbidity and mortality, but recovery of continence and potency are remarkably sensitive to fine details in surgical technique. It remains a challenge to the finest skills of modern surgeons to perform radical prostatectomy without blood transfusions, with complete removal of the cancer and negative surgical margins in all patients, and with preservation of continence and erectile function in those patients continent and potent before the operation.

REFERENCES

Abbas F, Scardino PT: Why neoadjuvant androgen deprivation prior to radical prostatectomy is unnecessary. Urol Clin North Am 1996; 23:587–604.

Abi-Aas AS, MacFarlane MT, Stein A, deKernion JB: Detection of local recurrence after radical prostatectomy by prostate specific antigen and transrectal ultrasound. J Urol 1992; 147:952–955.

Adolfsson J, Steineck G, Whitmore WF: Recent results of management of palpable clinically localized prostate cancer. Cancer 1993; 72:310–322.

Albertsen PC, Fryback DG, Storer BE, Kolon TF: Long-term survival among men with conservatively treated localized prostate cancer. JAMA 1995; 274:626–631.

Andriole GL, Smith DS, Rao G, et al: Early complications of contemporary anatomical radical retropubic prostatectomy. J Urol 1994; 152:1858–1860.

Andros AE, Danesghari F, Crawford ED: Neoadjuvant hormonal therapy in stage C adenocarcinoma of the prostate. Clin Invest Med 1993; 16:510–515.

Aus G: Mortality and morbidity after non-curative treatment with aspects on diagnosis and treatment. Scand J Urol Nephrol 1994; 167(suppl):1–41.

Aus G, Hugosson J, Norlen L: Long-term survival and mortality in prostate cancer treated with noncurative intent. J Urol 1995; 154:460–465.

Beck JR, Kattan MW, Miles BJ: A critique of the decision analysis for clinically localized prostate cancer. J Urol 1994; 152:1894–1899.

Bluestein DL, Bostwick DG, Bergstralh EJ, Oesterling JE: Eliminating the need for bilateral pelvic lymphadenectomy in select patients with prostate cancer. J Urol 1994; 151:1315–1320.

Borland RN, Walsh PC: The management of rectal injury during radical retropubic prostatectomy. J Urol 1992; 147:905–907.

Caprini JA, Chuker JL, Zuckerman L, et al: Thrombosis prophylaxis using external compression. Surg Gynecol Obstet 1983; 156:599–604.

Catalona WJ: Surgical management of prostate cancer. Cancer 1995; 75:1903–1908.

Catalona WJ, Smith DS: 5-year tumor recurrence rates after anatomical radical retropubic prostatectomy for prostate cancer. J Urol 1994; 152:1837–1842.

Cheng WS, Bergstralh EJ, Frydenberg M, Zincke H: Prostate-specific antigen levels after radical prostatectomy and immediate adjuvant hormonal treatment for stage D1 prostate cancer are predictive of early disease outcome. Eur Urol 1994; 25:189–193.

Cher ML, Shinohara K, Breslin S, et al: High failure rate associated with long-term follow-up of neoadjuvant androgen deprivation followed by radical prostatectomy for stage C prostate cancer. Br J Urol 1995; 75:771–777.

Chodak GW: The role of watchful waiting in the management of localized prostate cancer. J Urol 1994; 152:1766–1768.

Chodak GW, Thisted RA, Gerber GS, et al: Results of conservative management of clinically localized prostate cancer. N Engl J Med 1994; 330:246–248.

Cisek LJ, Walsh PC: Thromboembolic complications following radical

Table 85–13. COMPARISON OF 5-YEAR ACTUARIAL NONPROGRESSION RATES (UNDETECTABLE SERUM PROSTATE SPECIFIC ANTIGEN LEVEL) IN 39 PATIENTS TREATED WITH RADICAL PROSTATECTOMY AFTER RADIOTHERAPY (SALVAGE) AND 500 PATIENTS TREATED WITH RADICAL PROSTATECTOMY WITH NO PRIOR THERAPY (STANDARD)

| | Mean Nonprogression Rates (95% CI) | | | |
| | Salvage | | Standard | |
	N	%	N	%
Total	39	55 ± 20	500	76 ± 5
Preoperative PSA				
<10	13	50 ± 50	300	82 ± 8
≥10	14	29 ± 26	140	64 ± 12
Pathologic Stage				
pT1–2 (confined)	8	100	226	94 ± 4
pT3a,b (ECE)	10	71 ± 34	157	75 ± 10
pT3c (SVI) or LN+	21	28 ± 24	94	44 ± 12
Positive surgical margins	15	46 ± 32	83	61 ± 16

From Rogers E, Ohori M, Kassabian VS, et al: J Urol 1995; 153:104–110.
ECE, Extracapsular extension; LN+, positive lymph nodes.

retropubic prostatectomy: Influence of external sequential pneumatic compression devices. Urology 1993; 42:406–408.

Coe NP, Collins RE, Klein LA, et al: Prevention of deep venous thrombosis in urological patients: A controlled, randomized trial of low-dose heparin and external pneumatic compression boots. Surgery 1978; 83:230–234.

D'Amico AV, Whittington R, Malkowicz SB, et al: A multivariate analysis of clinical and pathological factors that predict for prostate specific antigen failure after radical prostatectomy for prostate cancer. J Urol 1995; 154:131–138.

Danella JF, deKernion JB, Smith RB, Steckel J: The contemporary incidence of lymph node metastases in prostate cancer: Implications for laparoscopic lymph node dissection. J Urol 1993a; 149:1488–1491.

Danella J, Steckel J, Dorey F, et al: Detectable prostate specific antigen levels following radical retropubic prostatectomy: Relationship of doubling time to clinical recurrence. J Urol 1993b; 149:A447.

Debruyne FMJ, Witjes WPJ, Schulman CC, et al, the European Study Group on Neoadjuvant Treatment: A multicentric trial of combined neoadjuvant androgen blockade with zoladex and flutamide prior to radical prostatectomy in prostate cancer. Eur Urol 1994; 26:4.

Dillioglugil O, Leibman BD, Kattan MW, et al: Hazard rates (HR) for progression, determined by PSA, after radical prostatectomy (RP) for T1-2 prostate cancer (Abstract 649). J Urol 1995a; 153:391A.

Dillioglugil O, Leibman BD, Kattan MW, et al: Hazard rates for progression after radical prostatectomy for clinically localized prostate cancer. J Urol 1996a, submitted.

Dillioglugil O, Leibman BD, Kattan MW, Scardino PT: Comparative long-term outcomes after various management strategies for T1-2 prostate cancer: A hazard rate (HR) analysis (Abstract 988). J Urol 1996b; 155:558A.

Dillioglugil O, Leibman BD, Leibman N, et al: Perioperative complications and morbidity of radical retropubic prostatectomy. J Urol 1996c; submitted.

Dillioglugil O, Miles BJ, Scardino PT: Current controversies in the management of localized prostate cancer. Eur Urol 1995b; 28:85–101.

Eastham JA, Kattan MW, Rogers E, et al: Risk factors for urinary incontinence after radical retropubic prostatectomy. J Urol 1996a; 156:1707–1713.

Eastham JA, Scardino PT, Yawn DH, et al: Preoperative autologous blood donation in radical retropubic prostatectomy: A cost-effectiveness analysis. J Urol 1996b, submitted.

Eastham JA, Stapleton AMF, Kattan MW, et al: Development of a nomogram predicting disease recurrence following radical prostatectomy for prostate cancer. Urol 1996c; in preparation.

Egawa S, Shoji K, Mikitoshi G, et al: Long-term impact of conservative management of localized prostate cancer. Urology 1993; 42:520–527.

Epstein BE, Hanks GE: Prostate cancer: Evaluation and radiotherapeutic management. Cancer J Clin 1992; 42:223–240.

Epstein JI: Evaluation of radical prostatectomy capsular margins of resection: The significance of margins designated as negative, closely approaching, and positive. Am J Surg Pathol 1990; 14:626–632.

Epstein JI, Pizov G, Walsh PC: Correlation of pathologic findings with progression after radical retropubic prostatectomy. Cancer 1993; 71:3582–3593.

Epstein JI, Walsh PC, Brendler CB: Radical prostatectomy for impalpable prostate cancer: The Johns Hopkins experience with tumors found on transurethral resection (stages T1a and T1b) and on needle biopsy (stage T1c). J Urol 1994; 152:1721–1729.

Fair WR, Aprikian AG, Cohen D, et al: Use of neoadjuvant androgen deprivation therapy in clinically localized prostate cancer. Clin Invest Med 1993; 16:516–522.

Ferguson JK, Oesterling JE: Patient evaluation if prostate-specific antigen becomes elevated following radical prostatectomy or radiation therapy. Urol Clin North Am 1994; 21:677–685.

Fleming C, Wasson JH, Albertsen PC, et al, for the Prostate Patient Outcomes Research Team: A decision analysis of alternative treatment strategies for clinically localized prostate cancer. JAMA 1993; 269:2650–2658.

Foote J, Yun S, Leach GE: Postprostatectomy incontinence: Pathophysiology, evaluation, and management. Urol Clin North Am 1991; 18:229–241.

Foster LS, Jajodia P, Fournier G Jr, et al: The value of prostate specific antigen and transrectal ultrasound guided biopsy in detecting prostatic fossa recurrences following radical prostatectomy. J Urol 1993; 149:1024–1028.

Fowler FJ Jr, Barry MJ, Lu-Yao G, et al: Patient-reported complications and follow-up treatment after radical prostatectomy. Urology 1993; 42:622–629.

Fowler JE Jr, Brooks J, Pandey P, Seaver LE: Variable histology of anastomotic biopsies with detectable prostate specific antigen after radical prostatectomy. J Urol 1995; 153:1011–1014.

Fowler JE Jr, Whitmore WF Jr: The incidence and extent of pelvic lymph node metastases in apparently localized prostatic cancer. Cancer 1981; 47:2941–2945.

Franks LM: Latent carcinoma of the prostate. J Pathol Bacteriol 1954; 68:603–616.

Frazier HA, Robertson JE, Humphrey PA, Paulson DF: Is prostate specific antigen of clinical importance in evaluating outcome after radical prostatectomy. J Urol 1993; 149:516–518.

Frazier HA, Robertson JE, Paulson DF: Radical prostatectomy: The pros and cons of the perineal versus the retropubic approach. J Urol 1992; 147:888–890.

Fricker JP, Vergnes Y, Schach R, et al: Low dose heparin versus low molecular weight heparin (Kabi 2165, Fragmin) in the prophylaxis of thromboembolic complications of abdominal oncological surgery. Eur J Clin Invest 1988; 18:561–567.

Geary ES, Dendinger TE, Freiha FS, Stamey TA: Incontinence and vesical neck strictures following radical retropubic prostatectomy. Urology 1995; 45:1000–1006.

Gervasi LA, Mata J, Easley JD, et al: Prognostic significance of lymph nodal metastases in prostate cancer. J Urol 1989; 142:332–336.

Gibbons RP, Cole BS, Richardson RG, et al: Adjuvant radiotherapy following radical prostatectomy: Results and complications. J Urol 1986; 135:65–68.

Gibbons RP, Correa RJ Jr, Branner GE, Weissman RM: Total prostatectomy for clinically localized prostate cancer: Long-term results. J Urol 1989; 141:564–566.

Goad JR, Eastham JA, Fitzgerald KB, et al: Radical retropubic prostatectomy: Limited benefit of autologous blood donation. J Urol 1995; 154:2103–2109.

Goad JR, Scardino PT: Modifications in the technique of radical retropubic prostatectomy to minimize blood loss. Atlas Urol Clin North Am 1994; 2:65–80.

Gohagan JK, Prorok PC, Kramer BS, Cornett JE: Prostate cancer screening in prostate, lung, colorectal and ovarian cancer screening trial of National Cancer Institute. J Urol 1994; 152:1905–1909.

Goldenberg SL, Klotz LH, Jewett MAS, et al, the Canadian Urologic Oncology Group: Randomized controlled study of neoadjuvant reversible androgen withdrawal therapy with cyproterone acetate in the surgical management of localized prostate cancer (Abstract 103). J Urol 1995; 254A.

Goldrath DE, Messing EM: Prostate specific antigen: Not detectable despite tumor progression after radical prostatectomy. J Urol 1989; 142:1082–1083.

Goluboff ET, Chang DT, Olsson CA, Kaplan SA: Urodynamics and the etiology of post-prostatectomy urinary incontinence: The initial Columbia experience. J Urol 1995; 153:1034–1037.

Goto Y, Ohori M, Arakawa A, et al: Distinguishing clinically important from unimportant prostate cancers before treatment: Value of systematic biopsies. J Urol 1996; 156:1059–1063.

Hansberry KL, Thompson IM Jr, Bauman J, et al: A prospective comparison of thromboembolic stockings, external sequential pneumatic compression stockings, and heparin sodium/dihydroergotamine mesylate for the prevention of thromboembolic complications in urologic surgery. J Urol 1991; 145:1205–1208.

Hautman RE, Sauter TW, Wenderoth UK: Radical retropubic prostatectomy: Morbidity and urinary continence in 418 consecutive cases. Urology 1994; 43:47–51.

Hortopan S, Partin AW, Carter HB, Marshall FF: "Minilap" incision for radical retropubic prostatectomy (RRP): Report of first 107 cases with respect to extent of lymphadenectomy and surgical margin status (Abstract 622). J Urol 1995; 153:384A.

Johansson JE, Adami HO, Andersson SO, et al: High 10-year survival rate in patients with early, untreated prostatic cancer. JAMA 1992; 267:2191–2196.

Kattan MW, Cowen ME, Miles BJ: A decision analysis for treatment of clinically localized prostate cancer. J Gen Intern Med; submitted.

Kattan MW, Miles BJ, Beck JR, Scardino PT: A reexamination of the decision analysis for clinically localized prostate cancer: Age and grade comparisons (Abstract 646). J Urol 1995; 153:390A.

Kavoussi LR, Myers JA, Catalona WJ: Effect of temporary occlusion of hypogastric arteries on blood loss during radical retropubic prostatectomy. J Urol 1991; 146:362–365.

Krahn MD, Mahoney JE, Eckman MH, et al: Screening for prostate cancer: A decision analytic view. JAMA 1994; 272:773–780.

Labrie F, Dupont A, Cusan L, et al: Downstaging of localized prostate cancer by neoadjuvant therapy with flutamide and lupron: The first controlled and randomized trial. Clin Invest Med 1993; 16:499–509.

Lange PH, Lightner DJ, Medini E, et al: The effect of radiation therapy after radical prostatectomy in patients with elevated prostate specific antigen levels. J Urol 1990; 144:927–933.

Leandri P, Rossignol G, Gautier J-R, Ramon J: Radical retropubic prostatectomy: Morbidity and quality of life: Experience with 620 consecutive cases. J Urol 1992; 147:883–887.

Leibman BD, Dilioglugil O, Wheeler TM, Scardino PT: Distant metastasis after radical prostatectomy in patients without an elevated serum prostate specific antigen level. Cancer 1995; 76:2530–2534.

Lerner SE, Blute ML, Lieber MM, Zincke H: Morbidity of contemporary radical retropubic prostatectomy for localized prostate cancer. Oncology 1995; 9:379–382.

Litwin MS, Hays RD, Fink A, et al: Quality-of-life outcomes in men treated for localized prostate cancer. JAMA 1995; 273:129–135.

Mark DH: Mortality of patients after radical prostatectomy: Analysis of recent Medicare claims. J Urol 1994; 152:896–898.

McLaren RH, Barrett DM, Zincke H: Rectal injury occurring at radical retropubic prostatectomy for prostate cancer etiology and treatment. Urology 1993; 42:401–405.

McNeal JE: Origin and development of carcinoma of the prostate. Cancer 1969; 23:24–34.

McNeal JE, Villers AA, Redwine EA, et al: Histologic differentiation, cancer volume, and pelvic lymph node metastasis in adenocarcinoma of the prostate. Cancer 1990; 66:1225–1233.

Mettlin C, Jones GW, Murphy GP: Trends in prostate cancer care in the United States, 1974–1990: Observations from the patient care evaluation studies of the American College of Surgeons Commission on Cancer. Cancer J Clin 1993; 43:83–91.

Morgan WR, Bergstrahl EJ, Zincke H: Long term evaluation of radical prostatectomy as treatment for clinical stage C (T3) prostate cancer. Urology 1993; 41:113–120.

Murphy GP, Mettlin C, Menck H, et al: National patterns of prostate cancer treatment by radical prostatectomy: Results of a survey by the American College of Surgeons Committee on Cancer. J Urol 1994; 152:1817–1819.

Oefelein MG, Smith N, Carter M, et al: The incidence of prostate cancer progression with undetectable serum prostate specific antigen in a series of 394 radical prostatectomies. J Urol 1995; 154:2128–2131.

Oesterling JE: Prostate specific antigen: A critical assessment of the most useful tumor marker for adenocarcinoma of the prostate. J Urol 1991; 145:907–923.

Ohori M, Goad JR, Wheeler TM, et al: Can radical prostatectomy alter the progression of poorly differentiated prostate cancer? J Urol 1994a; 152:1843–1846.

Ohori M, Wheeler TM, Dunn JK, Stamey TA, et al: The pathological features and prognosis of prostate cancer detectable with current diagnostic tests. J Urol 1994b; 152:1714–1720.

Ohori M, Wheeler TM, Scardino PT: The new American Joint Committee on Cancer and International Union Against Cancer TNM classification of prostate cancer. Cancer 1994c; 73:104–114.

Ohori M, Wheeler TM, Kattan MW, et al: Prognostic significance of positive surgical margins in radical prostatectomy specimens. J Urol 1995; 154:1818–1824.

Parker SL, Tone T, Bolden S, Wingo PA: Cancer statistics, 1996. Cancer J Clin 1996; 46:5–27.

Partin AW, Lee BR, Carmichael M, et al: Radical prostatectomy for high grade disease: A reevaluation 1994. J Urol 1994a; 151:1583–1586.

Partin AW, Pearson JD, Landis PK, et al: Evaluation of serum prostate-specific antigen velocity after radical prostatectomy to distinguish local recurrence from distant metastases. Urology 1994b; 43:649–659.

Partin AW, Pound CR, Clemens JQ, et al: Serum PSA after anatomic radical prostatectomy. Urol Clin North Am 1993a; 20:713–725.

Partin AW, Yoo J, Carter HB, et al: The use of prostate specific antigen, clinical stage and Gleason score to predict pathological stage in men with localized prostate cancer. J Urol 1993b; 150:110–114.

Paulson DF: Impact of radical prostatectomy in the management of clinically localized disease. J Urol 1994; 152:1826–1830.

Petros JA, Catalona WJ: Lower incidence of unsuspected lymph node metastases in 521 consecutive patients with clinically localized prostate cancer. J Urol 1992; 147:1574–1575.

Quinlan DM, Epstein JI, Carter BS, Walsh PC: Sexual function following radical prostatectomy: Influence of preservation of neurovascular bundles. J Urol 1991; 145:998–1002.

Rainwater LM, Segura JW: Technical considerations in radical retropubic prostatectomy: Blood loss after ligation of dorsal venous complex. J Urol 1990; 143:1163–1165.

Rees MA, McHugh TA, Dorr RP, et al: Assessment of the utility of bone scan, CT scan and lymph node dissection in staging of patients with newly diagnosed prostate cancer (Abstract 495). J Urol 1995; 352A.

Reiner WG, Walsh PC: An anatomic approach to the surgical management of the dorsal vein and Santorini's plexus during radical retropubic prostatectomy. J Urol 1979; 121:198–200.

Rogers E, Ohori M, Kassabian VS, et al: Salvage radical prostatectomy: Outcomes measured by serum prostate specific antigen levels. J Urol 1995; 153:104–110.

Schild SE, Buskirk SJ, Robinow JS, et al: The results of radiotherapy for isolated elevation of serum PSA levels following radical prostatectomy. Int J Radiat Oncol Biol Phys 1992; 23:141–145.

Seidman H, Mushinski MH, Geib SK: Probabilities of eventually developing or dying of cancer: United States 1985. Cancer 1985; 35:35–56.

Smith DS, Catalona WJ: Nature of prostate cancer detected through prostate specific antigen based screening. J Urol 1994; 152:1732–1736.

Smith JA, Seamen JP, Gleidman JB, Middleton RG: Pelvic lymph node metastasis from prostate cancer: Influence of tumor grade and stage in 452 consecutive patients. J Urol 1983; 130:290–292.

Solomon MH, McHugh TA, Dorr RP, et al: Hormone ablation therapy as neoadjuvant treatment to radical prostatectomy. Clin Invest Med 1993; 16:532–538.

Soloway MS, Sharifi R, Wajsman Z, et al, for the Lupron Depot Neoadjuvant Prostate Cancer Study Group: Randomized prospective study comparing radical prostatectomy alone versus radical prostatectomy preceded by androgen blockade in clinical stage B2 (T2bNxM0) prostate cancer. J Urol 1995; 154:424–428.

Spiessl B, Beahrs OH, Hermanek P, et al, eds: TNM Atlas: Illustrated Guide to the TNM/pTNM Classification of Malignant Tumours. Berlin, Springer-Verlag, 1992.

Stamey TA, Dietrick DD, Issa MM: Large, organ confined, impalpable transition zone prostate cancer: Association with metastatic levels of prostate specific antigen. J Urol 1993; 149:510–515.

Stamey TA, Kabalin JN: Prostate specific antigen in the diagnosis and treatment of adenocarcinoma of the prostate: I. Untreated patients. J Urol 1989; 141:1070–1075.

Stamey TA, Villers AA, McNeal JE, et al: Positive surgical margins at radical prostatectomy: Importance of the apical dissection. J Urol 1990; 143:1166–1173.

Stapleton AMF, Kattan MW, Eastham JA, et al: Prognosis after radical prostatectomy for clinically localized prostate cancer: A multivariate analysis of clinical and pathologic factors. J Urol 1996a, in preparation.

Stapleton AMF, Kattan MW, Palapattu GS, Scardino PT: The impact of surgical technique and other factors on potency following radical retropubic prostatectomy. J Urol 1996b, in preparation.

Stapleton AMF, Scardino PT: Nerve-sparing radical retropubic prostatectomy. In Krane RJ, Fitzpatrick J, Siroky MB, eds: Operative Urology. London, Churchill Livingstone, 1996, in press.

Stein A, deKernion JB, Smith RB, et al: Prostate specific antigen levels after radical prostatectomy in patients with organ confined and locally extensive prostate cancer. J Urol 1992; 147:942–946.

Steiner MS, Morton RA, Walsh PC: Impact of anatomical radical prostatectomy on urinary continence. J Urol 1991; 145:512–515.

Surya BV, Provet J, Johanson K-E, Brown J: Anastomotic strictures following radical prostatectomy: Risk factors and management. J Urol 1990; 143:755–758.

Takayama T, Krieger JN, True LD, Lange PH: Recurrent prostate cancer despite undetectable prostate specific antigen. J Urol 1992; 148:1541–1542.

Trapasso JG, deKernion JB, Smith RB, Dorey F: The incidence and significance of detectable levels of serum prostate specific antigen after radical prostatectomy. J Urol 1994; 152:1821–1825.

Van Poppel H, De Ridder D, Elgamal AA, et al, members of the Belgian Uro-oncological Study Group: Neoadjuvant hormonal therapy before radical prostatectomy decreases the number of positive surgical margins in stage T2 prostate cancer: Interim results of a prospective randomized trial. J Urol 1995; 154:429–434.

Walsh PC: Technique of vesicourethral anastomosis may influence recovery of sexual function following radical prostatectomy. Atlas Urol Clin North Am 1994; 2:59–64.

Walsh PC: Anatomical radical retropubic prostatectomy. *In* Walsh PC, Retik AB, Stamey TA, Vaughan ED Jr, eds: Campbell's Urology, 7th ed. Philadelphia, W. B. Saunders, 1996, pp 2565–2588.

Wilt TJ, Brawer MK: Prostate Cancer Intervention Versus Observation Trial: Randomized trial comparing radical prostatectomy versus expectant management for treatment of localized prostate cancer. J Urol 1994; 152:1910–1914.

Zincke H: Extended experience with surgical treatment of stage D1 adenocarcinoma of prostate: Significant influence of immediate adjuvant hormonal treatment (orchiectomy) on outcome. Urology 1989; 33:27–36.

Zincke H: Combined surgery and immediate adjuvant hormonal treatment for stage D1 adenocarcinoma of the prostate: Mayo Clinic experience. Semin Urol 1990; 8:175–183.

Zincke H, Bergstralh EJ, Larson-Keller JJ, et al: Stage D1 prostate cancer treated by radical prostatectomy and adjuvant hormonal treatment: Evidence for favorable survival in patients with DNA diploid tumors. Cancer 1992; 70:311–323.

Zincke H, Oesterling JE, Blute ML, et al: Long-term (15 years) results after radical prostatectomy for clinically localized (stage T2c or lower) prostate cancer. J Urol 1994; 152:1850–1857.

86
ANATOMIC RADICAL RETROPUBIC PROSTATECTOMY

Patrick C. Walsh, M.D.

The retropubic approach to radical prostatectomy was pioneered by Millin in 1947. Over the next decade, this technique was adopted by others and modified (Lich et al, 1949; Memmelaar, 1949; Chute, 1954; Ansell, 1959; Campbell, 1959) but never gained widespread popularity because of the significant complications of bleeding, incontinence, and impotence.

Over the past 20 years, a series of anatomic discoveries have improved the surgeon's ability to remove all tumor and substantially reduced perioperative morbidity. Delineation of the anatomy of the dorsal vein complex improved hemostasis and allowed precise anatomic dissection in a relatively bloodless field. With an understanding of the anatomy of the pelvic plexus and its branches to the corpora cavernosa, modifications in surgical technique made it possible to preserve sexual function. Improvements in understanding of periprostatic anatomy have achieved wider margins of excision. Technical refinements in the apical dissection and vesicourethral anastomosis arise directly from improved understanding of the pelvic floor musculature.

In my opinion, radical retropubic prostatectomy is one of the most difficult operations in the field of urology. **The three goals of the surgeons, in order of importance, are cancer control, preservation of urinary control, and preservation of sexual function.** Great skill and experience in the selection of surgical candidates and operative technique are necessary to achieve all three. This chapter summarizes my 20 years' experience with the hope that it will shorten the reader's learning curve. A videotape illustrating this technique is also available (Walsh, 1997).

ARTERIAL AND VENOUS ANATOMY

The prostate receives arterial blood supply from the inferior vesical artery. According to Flocks (1937), after the inferior vesical artery provides small branches to the seminal vesicle and the base of the bladder and prostate, the artery terminates in two large groups of prostatic vessels: the urethral and capsular groups (Fig. 86–1). The urethral vessels enter the prostate at the posterolateral vesicoprostatic junction and supply the vesical neck and

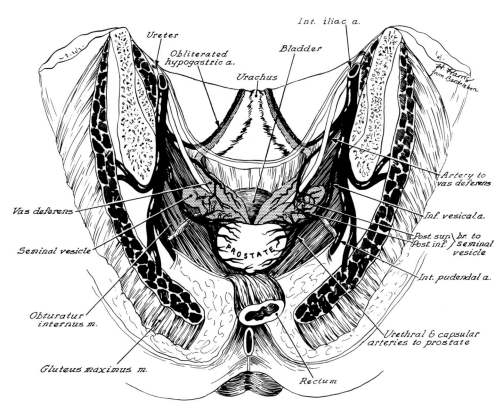

Figure 86–1. Posterior view of the arterial supply to the prostate. The rectum has been removed to expose the posterior surface of the prostate and pelvis. (From Weyrauch HM: Surgery of the Prostate. Philadelphia, W. B. Saunders, 1959.)

ARTERIAL SUPPLY OF PROSTATE.

periurethral portion of the gland. **The capsular branches run along the pelvic sidewall in the lateral pelvic fascia posterolateral to the prostate, providing branches that course ventrally and dorsally to supply the outer portion of the prostate.** The capsular vessels terminate as a small cluster of vessels that supply the pelvic floor. Histologically the capsular arteries and veins are surrounded by an extensive network of nerves (Walsh and Donker, 1982; Walsh et al, 1983; Lue et al, 1984; Lepor et al, 1985). **These capsular vessels provide the macroscopic landmark that aids in the identification of the microscopic branches of the pelvic plexus that innervate the corpora cavernosa.**

The veins of the prostate drain into the plexus of Santorini. It is necessary to have a complete understanding of these veins to avoid excessive bleeding and to ensure a bloodless field when exposing the membranous urethra and apex of the prostate. **The deep dorsal vein leaves the penis under Buck's fascia between the corpora cavernosa and penetrates the urogenital diaphragm, dividing into three major branches: the superficial branch and the right and left lateral venous plexuses** (Fig. 86–2) (Reiner and Walsh, 1979). The superficial branch, which travels between the puboprostatic ligaments, is the centrally located vein overlying the bladder neck and prostate. This vein is easily visualized early in retropubic operations and has communicating branches over the bladder itself and into the endopelvic fascia. The superficial branch lies outside the anterior prostatic fascia.

The common trunk and lateral venous plexuses are covered and concealed by the prostatic and endopelvic fasciae. The lateral venous plexuses traverse posterolaterally (see Fig. 86–2) and communicate freely with the pudendal, obtur-

ator, and vesical plexuses. Near the puboprostatic ligaments, small branches from the lateral plexus often penetrate the pelvic sidewall musculature and communicate with the internal pudendal vein. The lateral plexus interconnects with other venous systems to form the inferior vesical vein, which empties into the internal iliac vein. With the complex of veins and plexuses anastomosing freely, any laceration of these rather friable structures can lead to considerable blood loss.

The major arterial supply to the corpora cavernosa is derived from the internal pudendal artery. **Pudendal arteries, however, can arise from the obturator, inferior vesical, and superior vesical arteries. Because these aberrant branches travel along the lower part of the bladder and anterolateral surface of the prostate, they are divided during radical prostatectomy.** This may compromise arterial supply to the penis, especially in older patients with borderline penile blood flow (Breza et al, 1989; Polascik and Walsh, 1995).

PELVIC PLEXUS

The autonomic innervation of the pelvic organs and external genitalia arises from the pelvic plexus, which is formed by parasympathetic visceral efferent preganglionic fibers that arise from the sacral center (S2–S4) and sympathetic fibers from the thoracolumbar center (Tll–L2) (Fig. 86–3) (Walsh and Donker, 1982; Lue et al, 1984; Lepor et al, 1985; Schlegel and Walsh, 1987). The pelvic plexus in humans is located retroperitoneally beside the rectum 5 to 11 cm from the anal verge and forms a fenestrated rectangular plate that is situated in the sagittal plane with its midpoint located at the level of the tip of the seminal vesicle.

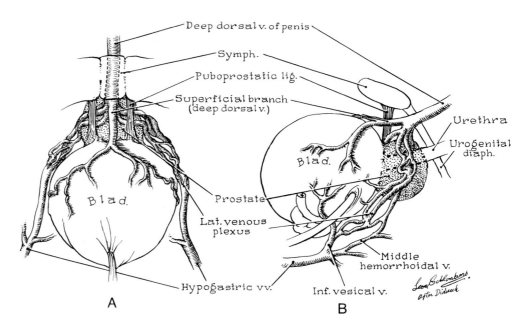

Figure 86–2. Santorini's venous plexus. *A,* View of trifurcation of the dorsal vein of the penis with the patient in the supine position. Relationship of venous branches to puboprostatic ligaments is depicted. *B,* Lateral view shows anatomic relationship at trifurcation. In this schematic illustration, the lateral pelvic fascia has been removed. In reality, these structures are never visualized in this skeletonized manner because they are encased by the pelvic fascia. (From Reiner WG, Walsh PC: J Urol 121:198, 1979. Copyright 1979, Williams & Wilkins.)

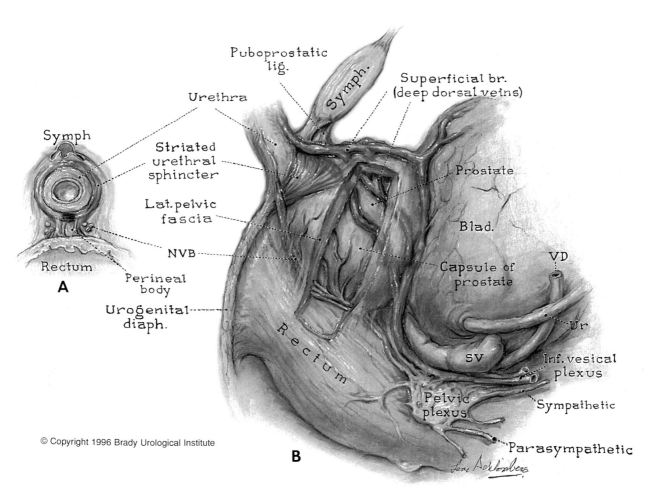

© Copyright 1996 Brady Urological Institute

Figure 86–3. *A,* Cross section of the urethra just distal to the apex of the prostate demonstrating the inner circular layer of smooth muscle, the outer striated urethral sphincter, and the perineal body (central tendon of the perineum). *B,* Anatomic relationship of the prostate to the pelvic fascia (window of fascia removed to illustrate prostatic capsule), pelvic plexus, and neurovascular bundle (NVB). Note the attachment of the striated urethral sphincter to the apex of the prostate. (Copyright 1996, Brady Urological Institute.)

The branches of the inferior vesical artery and vein that supply the bladder and prostate perforate the pelvic plexus. For this reason, ligation of the so-called lateral pedicle in its midportion not only interrupts the vessels, but also transects the nerve supply to the prostate, urethra, and corpora cavernosa. The pelvic plexus provides visceral branches that innervate the bladder, ureter, seminal vesicles, prostate, rectum, membranous urethra, and corpora cavernosa. In addition, branches that contain somatic motor axons travel through the pelvic plexus to supply the levator ani, coccygeus, and striated urethral musculature. **The nerves innervating the prostate travel outside the capsule of the prostate and Denonvilliers' fascia until they perforate the capsule, where they enter the prostate.**

The branches to the membranous urethra and corpora cavernosa also travel outside the prostatic capsule in the lateral pelvic fascia dorsolaterally between the prostate and rectum (see Fig. 86–3). The neurovascular bundles are located in the lateral pelvic fascia *between* the prostatic and levator fasciae (Fig. 86–4). At the level of the membranous urethra, they travel at 3 and 9 o'clock. After piercing the urogenital diaphragm, they pass behind the dorsal penile artery and dorsal penile nerve before entering the corpora cavernosa (Walsh and Donker, 1982). **Although these nerves are microscopic, their anatomic location can be estimated intraoperatively by using the capsular vessels as a landmark. For this reason, throughout the remainder of the chapter this structure is referred to as the neurovascular bundle** (see Fig. 86–3).

PELVIC FASCIA

The prostate is covered with three distinct, separate fascial layers: Denonvilliers' fascia, the prostatic fascia, and the levator fascia (see Figs. 86–3 and 86–4). Denonvilliers' fascia is a filmy delicate layer of connective tissue that is located between the anterior wall of the rectum and prostate.

This fascial layer extends cranially to cover the posterior surface of the seminal vesicles and lies snugly against the posterior prostatic capsule. This fascia is most prominent and dense near the base of the prostate and seminal vesicles and thins dramatically as it extends caudally to its termination at the striated urethral sphincter. Microscopically, it is impossible to discern a posterior and anterior layer to this fascia (Jewett et al, 1972). For this reason, one must excise this fascia completely to obtain an adequate surgical margin.

In addition to Denonvilliers' fascia, the prostate is also invested with the prostatic and levator fasciae. Anteriorly and anterolaterally the prostatic fascia is in direct continuity with the true capsule of the prostate. The major tributaries of the dorsal vein of the penis and Santorini's plexus travel within the anterior prostatic fascia (see Figs. 86–3 and 86–4). Laterally the prostatic fascia fuses with the levator fascia, which covers the pelvic musculature, to form the lateral pelvic fascia (see Fig. 86–4) (Myers, 1991, 1994). Posterolaterally the levator fascia separates from the prostate to travel immediately adjacent to the pelvic musculature surrounding the rectum. **The prostate receives its blood supply and autonomic innervation between the layers of the levator fascia and prostatic fascia** (see Fig. 86–4).

In an effort to avoid injury to the dorsal vein of the penis and Santorini's plexus during radical perineal prostatectomy, the lateral and anterior pelvic fasciae are reflected off the prostate. This accounts for the reduced blood loss associated with radical perineal prostatectomy. In performing radical retropubic prostatectomy, the prostate is approached from outside these fascial investments. For this reason, the dorsal vein complex must be ligated, and the lateral pelvic fascia must be divided.

STRIATED URETHRAL SPHINCTER

The external sphincter, at the level of the membranous urethra, is often depicted as a sandwich of muscles in the

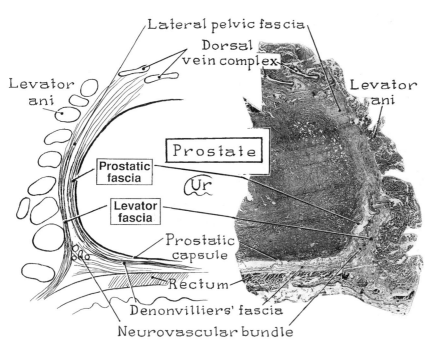

Figure 86–4. Cross section through an adult prostate demonstrating the anatomic relationships of the lateral pelvic fascia, Denonvilliers' fascia, and neurovascular bundle. Note how the neurovascular bundle is located between the two layers of lateral pelvic fascia—the levator fascia and the prostatic fascia. (Copyright 1996, Brady Urological Institute.)

© Copyright 1996 Brady Urological Institute

horizontal plane. Oelrich (1980) has demonstrated clearly, however, that the striated urethral sphincter with its surrounding fascia is a vertically oriented tubular sheath that surrounds the membranous urethra. In utero, this sphincter extends without interruption from the bladder to the perineal membrane. As the prostate develops from the urethra, it invades and thins the sphincter muscle causing a reduction or atrophy of some of the muscle.

In the adult, the fibers at the apex of the prostate are horseshoe-shaped and form a tubular striated sphincter surrounding the membranous urethra. In the midline posteriorly, the edges fuse with the perineal body (also called the central tendon of the perineum) (see Fig. 86–3; Fig. 86–5). Thus, as Myers (1987) has shown, the prostate does not rest on a flat transverse urogenital diaphragm like an apple on a shelf, with no striated muscle proximal to the apex. Rather, the external striated sphincter is more tubular and has broad attachments over the fascia of the prostate near the apex. This has important implications in the apical dissection and reconstruction of the urethra for preservation of urinary control postoperatively (Walsh et al, 1990).

The striated sphincter contains fatigue-resistant, slow-twitch fibers that are responsible for passive urinary control. Active continence is achieved by voluntary contraction of the levator ani musculature, which surrounds the apex of the prostate and membranous urethra. Some fibers of the levator ani (levator urethrae; pubourethralis) surround the proximal urethra and apex of the prostate and insert into the perineal body in the midline posteriorly (Myers, 1991). **The pudendal nerve provides the major nerve supply to the striated sphincter and levator ani.** When patients are instructed to perform sphincter exercises postoperatively, they are actually contracting the levator ani musculature. Because the striated urethral sphincter has similar innervation, however, they are exercising this important muscle as well. In addition, somatic motor nerves traveling through the pelvic plexus provide additional innervation to the pelvic floor musculature (Zvara et al, 1994).

SURGICAL TECHNIQUE

Preoperative Preparation

Surgery is deferred for 6 to 8 weeks after the needle biopsy of the prostate and 12 weeks after transurethral resection of the prostate. This delay enables inflammatory adhesions or hematoma to resolve so that the anatomic relationships between the prostate and surrounding structures return to a near normal state before surgery. This is especially important if one hopes to preserve the neurovascular bundles intraoperatively and avoid rectal injury.

During this delay, patients may be offered the opportunity to donate 2 or 3 units of autologous blood. Patients should avoid taking aspirin or nonsteroidal anti-inflammatory agents, which interfere with platelet function, while donating blood and immediately before surgery. The patients have a Fleet enema on the morning of surgery and are admitted to the hospital on that day.

Special Instruments

In contrast to radical perineal prostatectomy, radical retropubic prostatectomy requires few special instruments. A fiberoptic headlight is most useful because much of the procedure is performed beneath the pubis in an area where visualization can be difficult. A standard Balfour retractor with a malleable center blade is useful during the lymph node dissection and is necessary during the radical prostatectomy to provide cranial and posterior retraction on the peritoneum and bladder. Coagulating forceps, vessel loops, McDougal clamp (Pilling, Research Triangle Park, NC), Yu-Holtgrewe malleable blade (Grieshaber, Inc., Norridge, IL), and bulldog clamps are the only other specialized instruments that should be available.

Anesthesia, Incision, and Lymphadenectomy

A spinal or epidural anesthetic is preferable for this procedure. **Regional anesthesia is associated with less blood loss and a lower frequency of pulmonary emboli** (Peters and Walsh, 1985; Shir et al, 1995). The patient is placed in the supine position with the table broken at the umbilicus to extend the distance between the pubis and umbilicus. The table is then tilted in the Trendelenburg position until the legs are almost parallel to the floor (Fig. 86–6).

The skin is prepared and draped in the usual way. A No. 16 Silastic Foley catheter is passed into the bladder, inflated with 30 ml of saline, and connected to sterile closed continu-

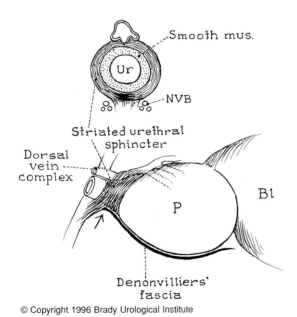

© Copyright 1996 Brady Urological Institute

Figure 86–5. Schematic illustration of the striated urethral sphincter and its relationship to the dorsal vein complex, smooth musculature of the urethra, and neurovascular bundles. *Arrow* points to the site where the striated urethral sphincter is sharply divided posteriorly at the perineal body. Note that this area is anterior to the neurovascular bundles and that it is the distal site of attachment of Denonvilliers' fascia. Sharp division at this point enables the surgeon to identify the correct plane on the anterior surface of the rectum, maintaining all layers of Denonvilliers' fascia on the prostate. (Copyright 1996, Brady Urological Institute.)

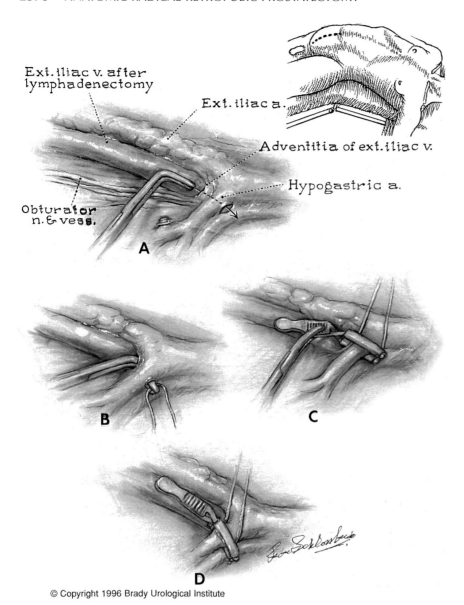

Ext. iliac v. after lymphadenectomy

Ext. iliac a.

Adventitia of ext. iliac v.

Hypogastric a.

Obturator n. & vess.

A

B

C

D

© Copyright 1996 Brady Urological Institute

Figure 86–6. *Inset,* View of the patient on the operative table with the table broken in the midline. *A,* View of the right pelvis following completion of the staging lymph node dissection. Note that the fibrofatty tissue overlying the external iliac artery has not been disturbed. In preparation for placement of the bulldog clamp on the hypogastric artery, the adventitia over the external iliac vein has been elevated. *B,* The right-angle clamp is easily passed immediately anterior to the external iliac vein beneath the hypogastric artery. This maneuver provides a bloodless plane through which a vessel loop is passed. *C* and *D,* Placement of the bulldog clamp on the hypogastric artery. (Copyright 1996, Brady Urological Institute.)

ous drainage. The use of a No. 16 Fr catheter facilitates passing the McDougal clamp when dividing the dorsal vein complex, placing sutures in the mucosa of the urethra, and releasing the neurovascular bundles. A right-handed surgeon always stands on the left side of the patient.

A midline extraperitoneal lower abdominal incision is made extending from the pubis to the umbilicus. The rectus muscles are separated in the midline, and the transversalis fascia is opened sharply to expose the space of Retzius. The anterior fascia is incised down to the pubis, and the posterior fascia is divided above the semicircular line to the umbilicus. Laterally the peritoneum is mobilized off the external iliac vessels to the bifurcation of the common iliac artery. **Care is taken to preserve the soft tissue covering the external iliac artery that contains the lymphatics, which drain the lower extremity. Interruption of these lymphatics may lead to lower extremity edema and lymphocele formation.** This maneuver is accomplished without dividing the vas deferens. Next a self-retaining Balfour retractor is placed. Exposure is facilitated by using a narrow malleable blade

attached to the Balfour retractor to displace the peritoneum superiorly and a deep Deaver retractor to retract the bladder medially.

Previously, when the vas deferens was routinely divided, some men complained of persistent testicular pain, which I attributed to excessive traction on the spermatic cord during this maneuver. If the vas deferens is not divided, however, the traction on the spermatic cord is absorbed by the vas deferens, and persistent testalgia is rare.

A pelvic lymph node dissection is performed before the radical prostatectomy. Lymphadenectomy is considered a staging and not a therapeutic procedure. Its value is to identify those patients with occult metastases to pelvic lymph nodes in whom a radical prostatectomy would be of little benefit. The dissection is initiated on the ipsilateral side of the major tumor in the prostate by dividing the adventitia over the external iliac vein (see Fig. 86–6). The lymphatics overlying the external iliac artery are preserved. The dissection proceeds out to the pelvic sidewall and then inferiorly to the femoral canal, where the lymphatic channels are

ligated at a convenient point. There is no need to remove the node of Cloquet. The dissection then proceeds superiorly along the pelvic sidewall to the bifurcation of the common iliac artery, where the lymph nodes in the angle between the external iliac and hypogastric arteries are removed. Next the obturator lymph nodes are removed with care to avoid injury to the obturator nerve. The obturator artery and vein are usually left undisturbed and are not ligated unless excessive bleeding occurs. At the completion of the dissection, the vasculature in the hypogastric and obturator fossa should be neatly skeletonized (see Fig. 86–6). A similar procedure is performed on the opposite side. **If the patient has a well-differentiated to moderately well-differentiated tumor (Gleason score ≤7) and the lymph nodes are normal to palpation, frozen section analysis is not performed** (Sgrignoli et al, 1994). To reduce blood loss during the remainder of the procedure, the hypogastric arteries are encircled with vessel loops, and bulldog clamps are placed proximal to the origin of the obliterated umbilical artery.

Incision in Endopelvic Fascia

At this point, a malleable blade with a notch (Yu-Holtgrewe blade) is positioned to retract the bladder superiorly (Fig. 86–7). Excellent exposure of the anterior surface of the prostate is achieved by positioning the balloon on the Foley catheter in the dome of the bladder beneath the Yu-Holtgrewe malleable blade. The fibroadipose tissue covering the prostate is carefully dissected away to expose the pelvic fascia, puboprostatic ligaments, and superficial branch of the dorsal vein.

The endopelvic fascia is entered where it reflects over the pelvic sidewall, well away from its attachments to the bladder and prostate (see Fig. 86–7). The point of incision is where the fascia is transparent, revealing the underlying levator ani musculature. After the fascia has been opened, one can usually visualize the bulging lateral venous plexus of Santorini, which is located medially. Therefore, **an incision in the endopelvic fascia too close to the bladder or the prostate risks laceration of these veins with potential severe blood loss.** Beneath this venous complex lie the prostatic arteries and the branches of the pelvic plexus that course toward the prostate, urethra, and corpora cavernosa.

The incision in the endopelvic fascia is then carefully extended in an anteromedial direction toward the puboprostatic ligaments. This allows the surgeon to palpate the lateral surface of the prostate. At this point, one often encounters small arterial and venous branches from the pudendal vessels, which perforate the pelvic musculature to supply the prostate. These vessels should be ligated with clips to avoid coagulation injury to the pudendal artery and nerve, which are located just deep to this muscle as they travel along the pubic ramus (see Fig. 86–7). Using finger dissection, the fibers of the levator ani musculature are released from the lateral surface of the prostate down to the apex of the prostate.

Division of Puboprostatic Ligaments

The fibrofatty tissue covering the superficial branch of the dorsal vein and puboprostatic ligaments is gently teased away to prepare for division of the ligaments without injuring the superficial branch of the dorsal vein. Care must be taken to dissect the superficial branch away from the medial edge of the ligaments before dividing them (Fig. 86–8). After all fibrofatty tissue has been removed, a sponge stick is used to displace the prostate posteriorly, and the scissors are used to divide each ligament in their midpoint. As each ligament is released, the space between the prostate and pubis opens exposing more of the ligament (see Fig. 86–8). The puboprostatic ligaments are not just discrete bands of fascia that fix the prostate to the pubis but rather pyramid-shaped structures that are part of a larger urethral suspensory mechanism that attaches the membranous urethra to the pubic bone (Steiner, 1994). **Every effort should be made to preserve the pubourethral component.**

The dissection should continue down far enough to expose the anterior surface of the dorsal vein complex at

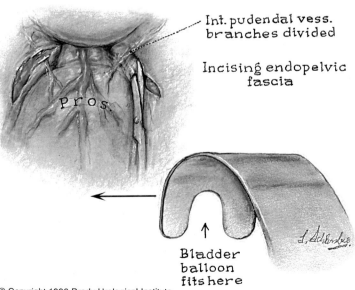

Figure 86–7. The bladder is displaced superiorly using the Yu-Holtgrewe blade with the balloon of the Foley catheter inside the groove of the retractor. The incision in the endopelvic fascia is made at the junction with the pelvic sidewall well away from the prostate and bladder. Anteriorly, near the puboprostatic ligaments, small arterial and venous branches from the internal pudendal vessels are often encountered. These are clipped and divided. (Copyright 1996, Brady Urological Institute.)

© Copyright 1996 Brady Urological Institute

Dissection of
puboprostatic
lig.

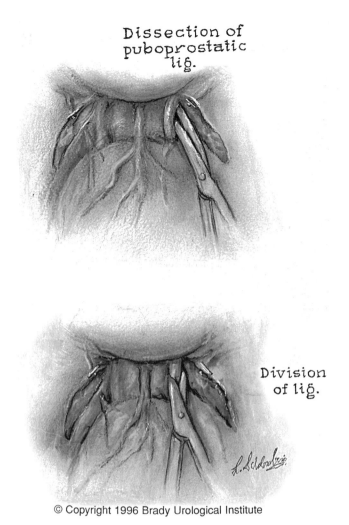

Division
of lig.

© Copyright 1996 Brady Urological Institute

Figure 86–8. Division of the puboprostatic ligaments. The endopelvic fascia is divided up to the edge of the puboprostatic ligament. Using a sponge stick to displace the prostate posteriorly, the puboprostatic ligament is divided sharply at its midpoint from lateral to medial with care not to damage the superficial branch of the dorsal vein or enter the anterior prostatic fasica. (Copyright 1996, Brady Urological Institute.)

the point where it is to be divided. **Attempts to divide the ligaments beyond this point risk excessive bleeding and may result in inadequate anterior fixation of the distal urethral segment.** With the puboprostatic ligaments transected, the superficial branch of the dorsal vein is readily apparent in the midline over the bladder neck. This vein should be displaced carefully from the undersurface of the pubis and coagulated.

Division of Dorsal Vein Complex

Just beyond the apex of the prostate, the lateral wall of the urethra can be identified by palpating the indwelling catheter. Anterior to the catheter is a thick complex composed of the main trunk of the dorsal vein, the striated urethral sphincter, and surrounding pelvic fascia (Fig. 86–9). If these structures are not easily identifiable, it is likely that the levator ani musculature has not been released adequately from the lateral surface of the prostate (see Fig. 86–12). The attachments must be released before the McDougal clamp is

passed (see later). Recognizing that the striated urethral sphincter is a tubular structure that surrounds the urethra and is part of the dorsal vein complex, I attempt to preserve as much of this complex as possible on the anterior surface of the urethra. With the use of a No. 16 Fr Foley catheter, there is more space between the urethra and venous complex, making this maneuver easier. The complex is identified by palpating its distinct, sharp, shelf-like edge just anterior to the urethra. **Using gentle pressure, the lateral pelvic fascia is perforated with a McDougal clamp, and the clamp is passed through the avascular plane between the anterior surface of the urethra and the posterior surface of the dorsal vein complex.** At this level, the complex with its associated fascia and striated urethral sphincter is 1 to 2 cm thick. **Care must be taken to avoid fracturing the apex of the prostate or entering the anterior surface of the prostate; the correct plane is between the dorsal vein complex and the urethra.** To identify the correct plane, the clamp should be pressed gently against the anterior surface of the urethra. After several attempts, the correct plane can be identified, and eventually the tell-tale "pop" can be felt. Because the neurovascular bundles are posterior to the urethra, they cannot be damaged during this maneuver.

Using a sponge stick to displace the prostate posteriorly, the dorsal vein complex is placed on traction providing ample room for division. This maneuver is necessary to provide adequate space on the right side. The jaws of the McDougal clamp are opened before division (Fig. 86–10). **Using a No. 15 blade on a long handle, the complex is divided without ligation. If the McDougal clamp is under**

McDougal clamp passes
beneath dorsal v. complex
& thru ant. striated sphincter

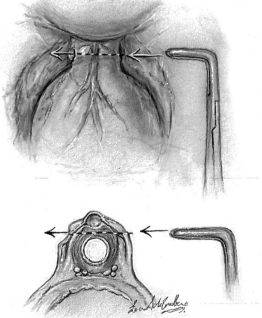

© Copyright 1996 Brady Urological Institute

Figure 86–9. Division of the dorsal vein complex. The McDougal clamp is passed anterior to the urethra through the lateral pelvic fascia and striated sphincter beneath the dorsal vein complex. (Copyright 1996, Brady Urological Institute.)

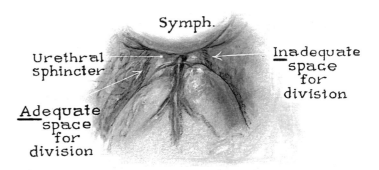

Symph.

Urethral
sphincter

Inadequate
space
for
division

Adequate
space
for
division

Figure 86–10. Downward displacement of the prostate using the sponge stick is necessary to widen the space on the anterior dorsal vein complex, especially on the right side, facilitating sharp division of the complex. (Copyright 1996, Brady Urological Institute.)

© Copyright 1996 Brady Urological Institute

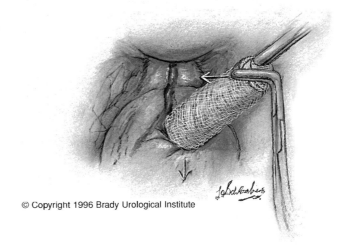

Correct angle
for division
of striated
urethral
sphincter

Incorrect angle
for division
of striated
urethral
sphincter

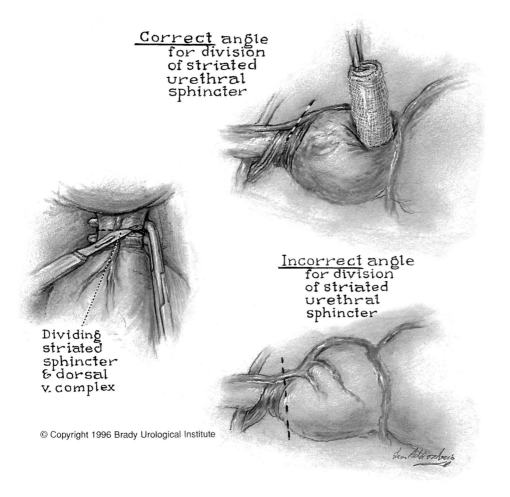

Dividing
striated
sphincter
& dorsal
v. complex

© Copyright 1996 Brady Urological Institute

Figure 86–11. Anterior and lateral view demonstrating the correct oblique angle for division of the striated urethral sphincter and dorsal vein complex leaving ample soft tissue on the anterior surface of the prostate. A more perpendicular incision enters the anterior surface of the prostate. (Copyright 1996, Brady Urological Institute.)

the entire complex, it is possible to divide the complex completely without much blood loss. I begin dividing the complex superficially using the sponge stick to displace the prostate. In this way, the knife can be used to "palpate" the anterior surface of the prostate to make certain that ample soft tissue remains on the anterior surface of the prostate as the incision deepens. During this process, the surgeon should be conscious of the correct angle for division of the striated urethral sphincter. The knife should be directed in an oblique fashion on the anterior surface of the prostate toward the urethra (Fig. 86–11). By dividing the complex in this way, the anterior component of the striated sphinter should be well preserved. **If the angle of the incision is perpendicular, the anterior apical portion of the prostate can be entered. This occurs most often when the levator ani musculature has not been released adequately at the apex of the prostate** (Fig. 86–12). When this occurs, the correct plane between the dorsal vein complex and the urethra is not identified, and the initial incision is made into the apex of the prostate. By not ligating the dorsal vein and by using the aforementioned technique, however, the texture of the tissue can be recognized as prostate. At that point, the levator fibers should be released from the prostate and the incision redirected (see Fig. 86–12).

Once the surgeon has mastered this technique, it is possi-

ble to divide the dorsal vein complex without using the McDougal clamp. The puboprostatic ligaments should be divided down to the junction of the anterior prostatic fascia with the dorsal vein complex, but no farther. Using the sponge stick to push the prostate posteriorly, a 3–0 Monocryl suture is passed superficially around the dorsal vein complex just distal to the apex of the prostate (Fig. 86–13). Next, using the Metzenbaum scissors, the complex is divided down to the urethra. This technique produces less disruption of the distal urethral mechanism, resulting in the earlier return of continence.

Absolute control of venous bleeding from the dorsal vein complex is mandatory so that the remainder of the procedure can be performed in a bloodless field. To achieve hemostasis, a running 3–0 Monocryl suture on a 5/8 circle needle is used to oversew the superficial edges of the striated urethral sphincter/dorsal vein complex (Fig. 86–14). **In placing these sutures in the left side of the complex, the surgeon should face the head of the table and hold the needle driver against the pubis perpendicular to the patient.** If the needle driver is held loosely, the superficial edges of the complex can be easily approximated forming a hood over the anterior urethra. Circumflex veins are often present at the posterior edge of the complex at 5 and 7 o'clock. For this reason, this running suture should extend into both corners posteriorly. At the completion of this maneuver,

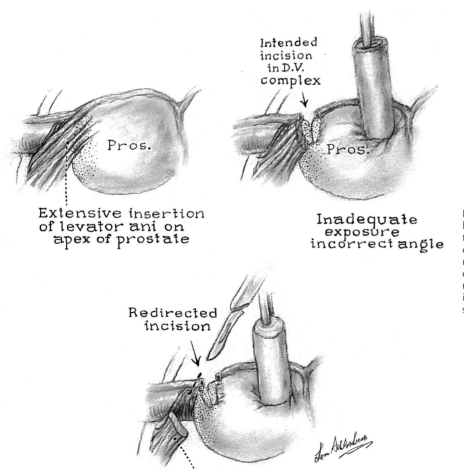

Extensive insertion
of levator ani on
apex of prostate

Intended
incision
in D.V.
complex

Pros.

Pros.

Inadequate
exposure
incorrect angle

Redirected
incision

Release of
levator ani

Figure 86–12. Upper illustrations demonstrate how failure to release the insertion of the levator ani musculature on the apex of the prostate can lead to inadvertent incision into the anterior apex of the prostate. The lower illustration demonstrates how this can be corrected by releasing the musculature and redirecting the incision. (Copyright 1996, Brady Urological Institute.)

© Copyright 1996 Brady Urological Institute

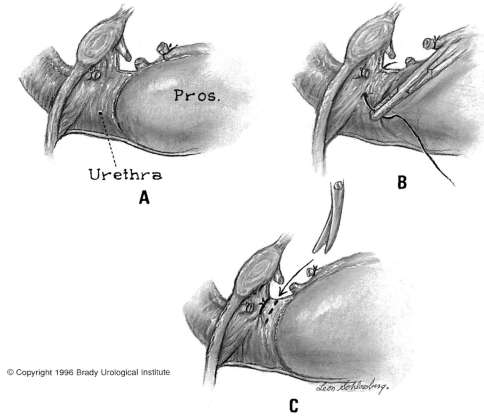

Figure 86–13. *A*, The puboprostatic ligament is divided down to the junction of the anterior prostatic fascia with the dorsal vein complex, but no farther. *B*, The dorsal vein complex is ligated superficially just distal to the apex with a 3–0 Monocryl suture. *C*, The dorsal vein complex is divided with the Metzenbaum scissors.

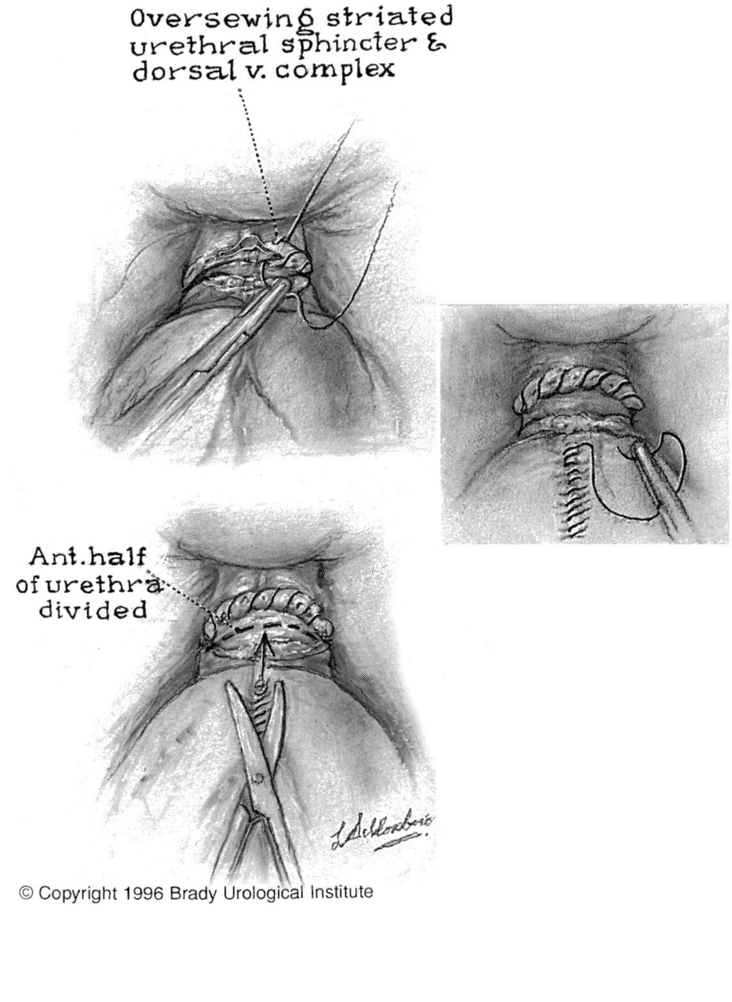

© Copyright 1996 Brady Urological Institute

Oversewing striated urethral sphincter & dorsal v. complex

Ant. half of urethra divided

Figure 86–14. A hemostatic horizontal running suture ligature is used to oversew the distal striated urethral sphincter and dorsal vein complex. Note that the suture extends into both posterolateral angles to control bleeding from circumflex veins. The proximal dorsal vein complex over the prostate is also oversewn. Once hemostasis has been perfected, the anterior two thirds of the urethra is divided at a point distal to the apex to provide an adequate surgical margin. (Copyright 1996, Brady Urological Institute.)

© Copyright 1996 Brady Urological Institute

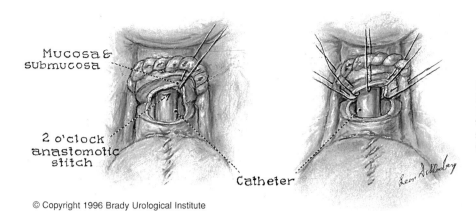

© Copyright 1996 Brady Urological Institute

Figure 86–15. Using 3–0 Monocryl sutures on a 5/8 circle tapered needle, sutures are placed at 12-, 2-, 5-, 7-, and 10-o'clock positions. Care is taken to incorporate just the edge of the striated sphincter and urethral mucosa and submucosa. (Copyright 1996, Brady Urological Institute.)

hemostasis should be excellent. Finally, to avoid backbleeding from the anterior surface of the prostate, the proximal divided venous complex on the anterior surface of the prostate is oversewn with a running 2–0 chromic suture. While the dorsal vein/striated urethral complex is being oversewn, this backbleeding is usually controlled by the sponge stick. Alternatively, before the complex is divided, a figure-of-eight 2–0 chromic catgut suture can be placed in the anterior surface of the prostate to discourage bleeding. At this point, the anesthesiologist is requested to give the patient an ampule of indigo carmine dye to aid later in identification of the ureteral orifices.

Division of Urethra

By gently displacing the prostate posteriorly with a sponge stick, the prostatourethral junction should be well visualized. Using scissors, the anterior two thirds of the urethra is divided with care to avoid damage to the Foley catheter (see Fig. 86–14). This provides excellent exposure for placement

of five sutures in the distal urethral segment at 12, 2, 5, 7, and 10 o'clock (Fig. 86–15). Using 3–0 Monocryl on a 5/8 circle tapered needle, **the needle should incorporate just the edge of the striated sphincter and the urethral mucosa and submucosa.** Deeper sutures might compromise the functional integrity of the striated sphincter or smooth muscle of the urethra, both of which appear to be important for the ultimate return of urinary control. As stated earlier, to place these sutures the surgeon should face the head of the table and hold the needle driver against the pubis perpendicular to the patient. Initially the suture is placed in the mucosa and submucosa of the urethra at 2 o'clock and then into the edge of the striated sphincter. By using a No. 16 Fr catheter, the mucosa is easily identified. The smooth muscle should not be incorporated in this stitch because stitches in the smooth muscle delay the recovery of urinary control. Once the mucosa has been elevated by the 2-o'clock stitch, the remaining sutures are more easily placed. For a right-handed surgeon, it is easiest to place the 7-o'clock and 10-o'clock sutures from the outside of the lumen to the inside. The other three sutures are more easily placed beginning first on

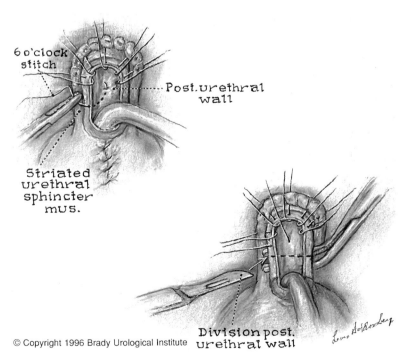

© Copyright 1996 Brady Urological Institute

Figure 86–16. The Foley catheter has been clamped and divided. The 6-o'clock suture is placed from outside to inside through the smooth muscle, submucosa, and mucosa of the urethra. Next the posterior wall of the urethra is divided. (Copyright 1996, Brady Urological Institute.)

the luminal surface and then proceeding outside. In performing the final anastomosis, a French eye needle can be used to place these latter three sutures through the lumen of the bladder. The sutures are covered with towels to avoid inadvertent traction or displacement.

After placing the sutures, the balloon is released from beneath the malleable blade, and the catheter is clamped and divided. The 6-o'clock suture is placed through the mucosa and submucosa of the urethra, from the outside to the inside (Fig. 86–16). The posterior band of urethra is now divided to expose the posterior portion of the striated urethral sphincter complex. The posterior sphincter complex is composed of skeletal muscle and fibrous tissue and when viewed laterally represents the junction of the apex of the prostate, Denonvilliers' fascia, and central tendon of the perineum (see Fig. 86–5). **Identification and precise division of this complex are most important in (1) obtaining adequate margins of resection for apical lesions, (2) identifying the correct plane on the anterior wall of the rectum to ensure that all layers of Denonvilliers' fascia are excised, (3) avoiding blunt trauma to the neurovascular bundles that are located immediately posteriorly, and (4) preserving urinary continence.** Recall that the perineal body stabilizes the striated urethral sphincter and levator urethrae. **Damage to the perineal body may give rise to a flail sphincter, thus resulting in incontinence.**

To divide the posterior portion of the sphincter safely, a right-angle clamp is passed immediately beneath the left edge of this complex. **This plane is usually not difficult to find if one slides the clamp along the outside edge of the glistening fascia covering the lateral surface of the prostate at the apex** (Fig. 86–17). Because the neurovascular bundle is beneath this glistening fascia, the right-angle clamp travels immediately anterior to the neurovascular bundle (see Fig. 86–5). The left border of the complex is then divided with scissors. Next, the right-angle clamp is placed beneath the right edge of the complex and the complex is divided

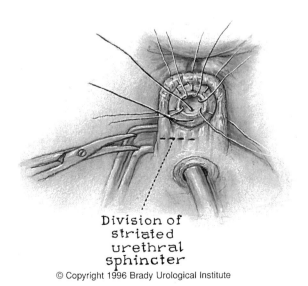

Division of striated urethral sphincter

© Copyright 1996 Brady Urological Institute

Figure 86–17. A right-angle clamp is passed beneath the left edge of the complex. The correct plane is identified by sliding the right angle along the outside glistening fascia covering the lateral surface of the prostate at the apex. The left border of the complex is divided with scissors. (Copyright 1996, Brady Urological Institute.)

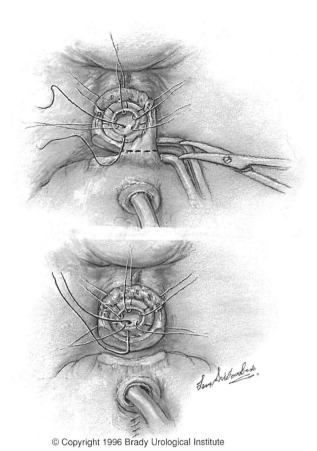

© Copyright 1996 Brady Urological Institute

Figure 86–18. *Top,* A right-angle clamp is passed easily beneath the right edge of the striated urethral sphincter complex, anterior to the neurovascular bundle. *Bottom,* The complex has been completely divided. (Copyright 1996, Brady Urological Institute.)

(Fig. 86–18). It is necessary to divide the complex from each side because if one tries to divide the entire complex from one side, the contralateral neurovascular bundle may be damaged. Finally, the central component of the complex is divided. This often is surprisingly thick and is composed of fibers from the perineal body, Denonvilliers' fascia, and the rectourethralis muscle.

The above-mentioned technique ensures accurate placement of the anastomotic sutures in the distal urethral segment and avoids damage to the neurovascular bundles (see Fig. 86–18). When placing the 6-o'clock suture in the urethral mucosa, the neurovascular bundles are protected from injury by the intact posterior layer of the striated sphincter complex. In the past, I placed this 6-o'clock suture through the striated sphincter "blindly" after the prostate was removed. I subsequently realized that many fewer patients were potent (Walsh, 1994) with this technique. **This observation highlights the fact that minor alterations in surgical technique can have a major impact on the recovery of sexual function following radical prostatectomy.** Using the technique described previously, postoperative potency rates have improved.

Identification and Preservation of Neurovascular Bundle

When releasing the neurovascular bundle, there should be no upward traction on the prostate. Rather, the prostate

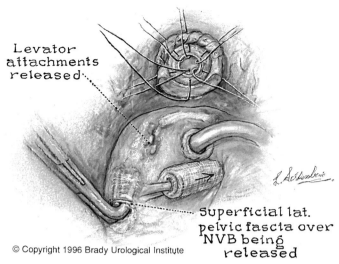

Levator attachments released

Superficial lat. pelvic fascia over NVB being released

© Copyright 1996 Brady Urological Institute

Figure 86–19. The lateral surface of the prostate is exposed to displacing the prostate on its side using a sponge stick. The site where the levator ani musculature was released from the apex of the prostate is seen. A right-angle clamp is inserted under the superficial layers of the lateral pelvic fascia. (Copyright 1996, Brady Urological Institute.)

should be rolled from side to side. This can be accomplished by removing the catheter during this portion of the dissection. Alternatively, some of the fluid in the No. 16 Fr Foley catheter balloon can be released, the end of the catheter can be ligated, and the catheter can be tucked against the pelvic sidewall on the contralateral side of the dissection. Without a catheter, or with a small soft No. 16 Fr Silastic catheter in place, the prostate is softer, and it appears easier to identify the correct plane for release of the neurovascular bundle.

Recall that the lateral pelvic fascia is composed of two layers, the levator fascia and the prostatic fascia. The

neurovascular bundle travels between these two layers (see Fig. 86–4). Using a right-angle clamp, the superficial layers of lateral pelvic fascia are released. This dissection should begin at the bladder neck where this fascia forms a thick band. When this band is divided, the prostate immediately becomes more mobile (Fig. 86–19). The superficial fascia should be released from the bladder neck to the apex (Fig. 86–20). This maneuver releases the bundle laterally, thus making it easier to perform the next step, where the bundle is released at the apex.

Once the superficial fascia has been released, the location of the neurovascular bundle can be identified by the presence of a subtle groove on the posterolateral edge of the prostate. **By tracing this groove to the apex of the prostate, one can determine where the neurovascular bundle begins to travel inferiorly away from the prostatic apex toward the urethra (see Fig. 86–20). Once the medial border of the neurovascular bundle has been identified at the apex, the dissection in the midline can be safely carried posteriorly toward the rectum** (Fig. 86–21). Having developed the plane between the rectum and prostate in the midline, it is now possible to release the neurovascular bundle from the prostate beginning at the apex and moving toward the base using the sponge stick to roll the prostate over on its side. **Beginning on the rectal surface, the bundle is released from the prostate by spreading a right-angle clamp gently. Once the dissection has been initiated at the apex, it should proceed to the midpoint of the prostate** (Fig. 86–22). Because the superficial layer of the lateral pelvic fascia has already been released, this dissection often proceeds quite easily. **Furthermore, in using this plane, Denonvilliers' fascia and the prostatic fascia remain on the prostate; only the residual fragments of the levator fascia are released from the prostate laterally.**

If the bundle does not fall off the prostate, there are

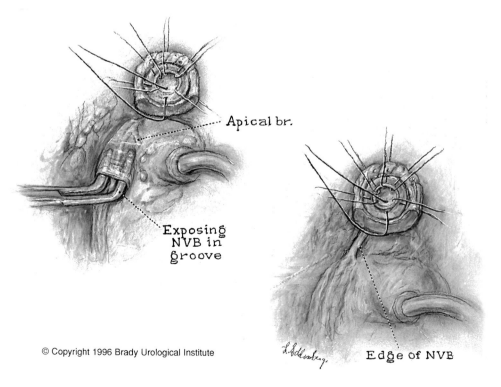

Apical br.

Exposing NVB in groove

Edge of NVB

© Copyright 1996 Brady Urological Institute

Figure 86–20. The superficial fascia is released all the way out to the apex. Once the superficial fascia has been released, the neurovascular bundle can be located by the presence of a subtle "groove" on the posterolateral edge of the prostate. By tracing this groove out to the apex of the prostate, one can determine where the neurovascular bundle begins to travel inferiorly away from the prostate toward the urethra. (Copyright 1996, Brady Urological Institute.)

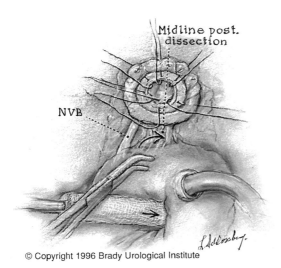

Midline post. dissection

NVB

© Copyright 1996 Brady Urological Institute

Figure 86–21. Once the medial border of the neurovascular bundle has been identified at the apex, the dissection in the midline can be safely pursued posteriorly down to the rectum. (Copyright 1996, Brady Urological Institute.)

likely to be small apical vessels tethering it in place. These are best controlled using small hemoclips placed parallel to the bundle (Fig. 86–23). **Electrocoagulation should never be used on the neurovascular bundle or its branches.** There is usually no need to clip the prostatic side of these tiny vessels; fine scissors should be used to divide them. The number of arterial and venous branches is extremely variable. By starting at the apex, however, one can easily identify them prospectively. **If the fixation of the bundle to the prostate cannot be explained by vascular branches, the neurovascular bundle should be excised** (see later). The surgeon should be aware that the bundle may travel more anteriorly in some patients. In these patients, one can confuse the groove with the potential space between the prostate and rectum. This is another good reason to release

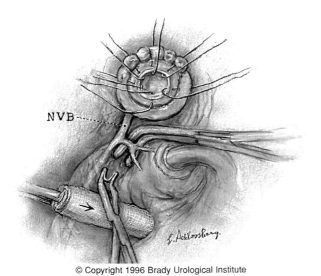

NVB

© Copyright 1996 Brady Urological Institute

Figure 86–22. Beginning posteriorly with a right angle, the neurovascular bundle is gently released from the prostate. Small arterial and venous branches are divided using clips. Because the superficial pelvic fascia was released previously, the neurovascular bundle usually falls off the prostate. (Copyright 1996, Brady Urological Institute.)

the bundle first at the apex. In addition, some patients have many veins on the lateral surface of the prostate, which anastomose between Santorini's plexus anteriorly and the neurovascular bundle posteriorly. The apical approach to the bundle facilitates management of this condition as well.

Some surgeons advocate releasing the neurovascular bundle before division of the dorsal vein complex or urethra. As is evident from the previous description, at the apex the neurovascular bundle is beneath the posterior striated urethral sphincter complex. Furthermore, it is often tethered in place by small apical vessels. Finally, to make certain that Denonvilliers' fascia is maintained on the prostate, the neurovascular bundles should be released by dissecting from the rectal surface anteriorly. **Using the principles described previously, I have not had positive surgical margins in men with organ-confined disease that were caused by inadvertently cutting into the prostate.**

Excision of Lateral Pelvic Fascia and Neurovascular Bundle

Under certain circumstances, it may be necessary to excise the lateral pelvic fascia and neurovascular bundles completely on one or both sides. **I do not believe that the bundle should "always" be excised on the side of the positive biopsy or palpable lesion. Rather, this decision should be based on the preoperative evaluation and the findings at surgery.**

1. **Surgery on an impotent patient.** If there is any question, the neurovascular bundles should be widely excised in impotent patients. If the neurovascular bundles "fall off" the prostate, however, I often preserve them because I believe that innervation from the neurovascular bundles may play a minor role in the recovery of urinary control.

2. **Induration involving the lateral sulcus found on preoperative physical examination.** It has always been obvious to me that the neurovascular bundle was closer to the apex of the prostate than the base (Walsh and Donker, 1982; Lepor et al, 1985; Schlegel and Walsh, 1987). For this reason, I more commonly excise the ipsilateral neurovascular bundle in patients with palpable apical lesions than in patients with lesions at the base.

3. **Estimation of pathologic stage based on preoperative prostate-specific antigen (PSA), Gleason score, and clinical stage.** Using nomograms, if the probability of capsular penetration is high, the surgeon should have a low threshold for excising the neurovascular bundle (Partin et al, 1993). Likewise, if perineural invasion is present in the biopsy specimen, there is a 95% chance that capsular penetration is present (Bastacki et al, 1995). Today, wide excision of the neurovascular bundle is performed less often than in the past because candidates are diagnosed earlier. For example, in the most recent 100 cases, one neurovascular bundle was excised widely in only 15% and partially in 11%. Of these 100 cases, 66% were T1c, in which the tumor is less often located in the peripheral zone. In those men, both bundles were preserved in 88%, one bundle was partially excised in 9%, and one bundle was widely excised in 3%; the surgical margins were negative in all of these cases.

4. **Induration in the lateral pelvic fascia found intraoperatively after the endopelvic fascia has been opened.**

5. **Fixation of the neurovascular bundle to the capsule**

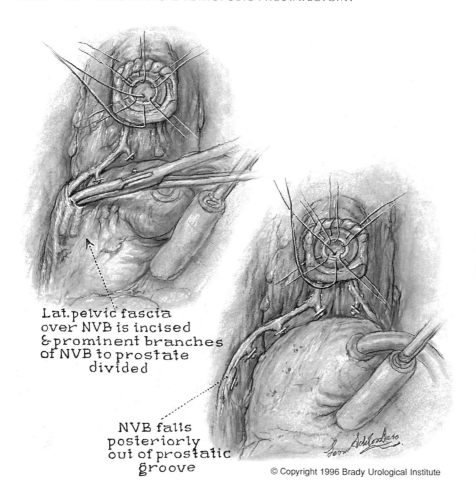

Lat. pelvic fascia
over NVB is incised
& prominent branches
of NVB to prostate
divided

NVB falls
posteriorly
out of prostatic
groove

Figure 86–23. Once the bundle has been identified and released at the apex, it should be released up to the midportion of the prostate. (Copyright 1996, Brady Urological Institute.)

© Copyright 1996 Brady Urological Institute

of the prostate detected once the lateral pelvic fascia has been divided. If the neurovascular bundle does not fall off the prostate easily and if there are no vascular branches that explain this fixation, the bundle should be widely excised.

Before excising the neurovascular bundle unilaterally, the contralateral neurovascular bundle should be freed from the prostate starting at the apex first. This avoids traction injury, which can occur during wide excision of the contralateral bundle. The neurovascular bundle to be excised is identified at the apex, and a right-angle clamp is passed from medial to lateral, immediately on the anterior surface of the rectum (Fig. 86–24). The bundle is divided without ligation in an effort to excise as much soft tissue as possible (Fig. 86–25). Later, if bleeding is troublesome, the distal end can be clipped. The dissection is continued by dividing the fascia on the lateral surface of the rectum from the apex to the base so that the neurovascular bundle and abundant fascial tissue are included in the specimen. This procedure is performed under direct vision with the dissection terminating at the tip of the seminal vesicle, where the neurovascular bundle is ligated and divided. In this way, the neurovascular bundle and the lateral pelvic fascia are excised under direct vision in a more complete way than previously possible.

Posterior Dissection and Division of Lateral Pedicles

Once the neurovascular bundles have been either preserved at the apex or widely excised and the prostate has been mobilized to its midpoint, the Foley catheter is replaced if it was removed. With light upward traction on the catheter, the rectum is separated from the prostate with finger dissection; next, the attachment between the rectum and Denonvilliers' fascia is divided in the midline posteriorly (Fig. 86–26). Because the neurovascular bundles have been freed, one may now apply traction to the catheter to gain exposure to the base of the prostate and seminal vesicles. In developing this plane, all layers of Denonvilliers' fascia should be left covering the seminal vesicles. Next, **the surgeon should look for a prominent arterial branch traveling from the neurovascular bundle over the seminal vesicles to supply the base of the prostate. This posterior vessel should be ligated on each side and divided** (see Fig. 86–26). **In doing so, the neurovascular bundles are no longer tethered to the prostate and fall posteriorly. This enables the lateral pedicle to be divided safely on the lateral surface of the seminal vesicles without injuring the neurovascular bundle** (Fig. 86–27).

At this point, the plane between the lateral edge of the seminal vesicles and the overlying lateral pelvic fascia should be developed. **The lateral pedicles are then divided without ligation. I usually divide the superficial portions of the lateral pedicle first, then divide the deeper portions** (see Fig. 86–27). Obvious arterial bleeders are simply controlled with hemoclips. With this approach, I am able to leave more soft tissue on the prostate and protect the neurovascular bundles from injury.

Before approaching the bladder neck, one should divide

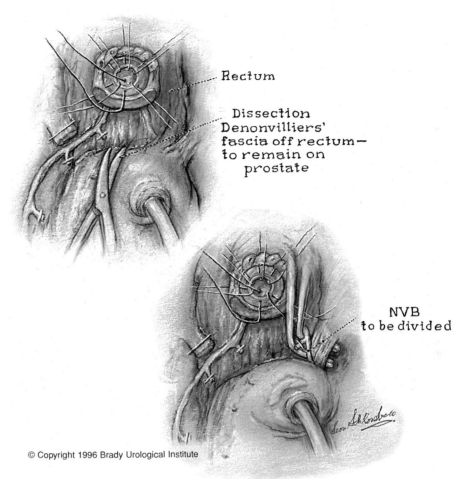

Rectum

Dissection
Denonvilliers'
fascia off rectum—
to remain on
prostate

NVB
to be divided

© Copyright 1996 Brady Urological Institute

Figure 86–24. Residual attachments of the apex of the prostate in the midline are released in preparation for wide excision of the right neurovascular bundle. A right-angle clamp is then passed directly on the anterior surface of the rectum from the midline laterally. If the right-angle clamp is passed from lateral to medial, a rectal injury is more likely to occur. (Copyright 1996, Brady Urological Institute.)

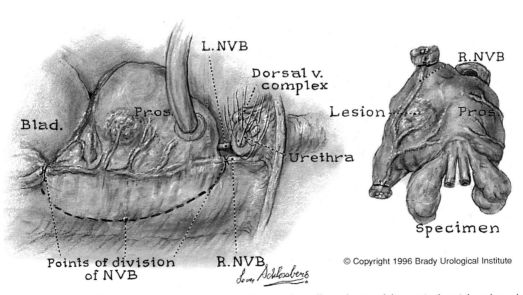

L. NVB

Dorsal v.
complex

Pros.

Blad.

Lesion

Pros.

R. NVB

Urethra

Points of division
of NVB

R. NVB

Specimen

© Copyright 1996 Brady Urological Institute

Figure 86–25. Extent of the division of the neurovascular bundle from the apex laterally to the tip of the seminal vesicle, where the neurovascular bundle is ligated. This provides extensive soft tissue covering the primary lesion. (Copyright 1996, Brady Urological Institute.)

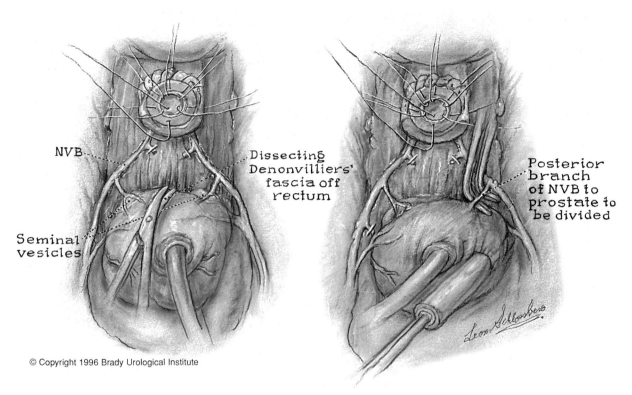

© Copyright 1996 Brady Urological Institute

Figure 86–26. Posterior dissection. The Foley catheter is replaced and used for traction. The attachment of Denonvilliers' fascia to the rectum is released maintaining all layers of Denonvilliers' fascia over the posterior surface of the seminal vesicles. Prominent branches from the neurovascular bundle to the posterior surface of the prostate are identified at the posterolateral angle of the rectum. By dividing these posterior branches, the neurovascular bundle is free to fall away from the prostate posteriorly. (Copyright 1996, Brady Urological Institute.)

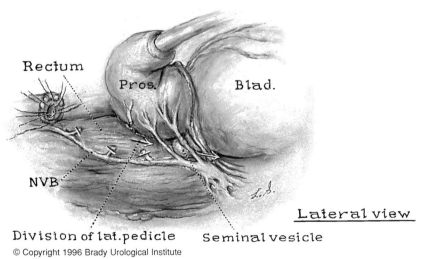

© Copyright 1996 Brady Urological Institute

Figure 86–27. Lateral view demonstrating location of the neurovascular bundle following ligation of the posterior branch to the prostate. The site for division of the lateral pedicle is indicated. An incision in this area should not damage the neurovascular bundle or pelvic plexus. (Copyright 1996, Brady Urological Institute.)

Denonvilliers' fascia near the tips of the seminal vesicles. This will make the dissection much easier. Some surgeons prefer to dissect the seminal vesicles at this stage for several reasons. They feel that visualization is better because there is less bleeding, and they are able to preserve more of the bladder neck musculature. To dissect the seminal vesicles, after dividing Denonvilliers' fascia over the seminal vesicles, one should proceed as described below to free the seminal vesicles and divide the vasa deferentia.

Division of Bladder Neck and Excision of Seminal Vesicles

The prostate has now been mobilized almost completely. The bladder neck is incised anteriorly at the prostatovesicular junction (Fig. 86–28). The incision is carried down to the mucosa, the mucosa is incised, the Foley balloon is deflated, and the two ends of the catheter are clamped together to provide traction. As the incision in the bladder neck is widened, branches running from the inferior vesical pedicle to the prostate are noted at 5-o'clock and 7-o'clock positions (Fig. 86–29). **After dividing these pedicles, it should be possible to visualize the plane between the anterior surface of the seminal vesicles and the posterior wall of the bladder. Using scissor dissection hugging the anterior surface of the seminal vesicles, the posterior bladder neck can be divided safely while observing the location of the ureteral orifices** (Fig. 86–30). After dividing the posterior bladder wall, the bladder neck is retracted with an Allis clamp and the vasa deferentia ligated with hemoclips and divided. The seminal vesicles are dissected free from surrounding structures (Fig. 86–31). Recall that the pelvic plexus is located on the lateral surface of the seminal vesicles. **To avoid injury to the pelvic plexus, the surgeon**

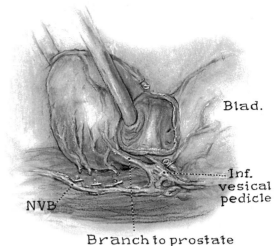

Figure 86–29. Branches from the inferior vesical pedicle to the prostate at 5- and 7-o'clock positions following division of the anterior bladder neck. Ligation of these branches exposes the angle between the bladder and seminal vesicles. (Copyright 1996, Brady Urological Institute.)

should perform this dissection with great care, especially laterally, and under direct vision should identify the small arterial branches that travel to the seminal vesicles and stay close to the seminal vesicles when ligating them with small clips. As the tips of the seminal vesicles are freed, small arterial branches at the tip of each seminal vesicle should be identified, ligated, and divided. Any residual attachments of Denonvilliers' fascia are then divided, and the specimen is removed. The specimen is inspected carefully to identify any areas where the margin of resection is uncertain. If there is any concern about the margin on the posterolateral surface of the prostate, the neurovascular bundle on that side should be excised.

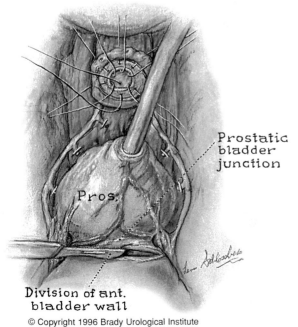

Figure 86–28. Division of the anterior bladder neck. (Copyright 1996, Brady Urological Institute.)

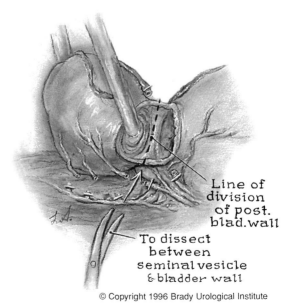

Figure 86–30. Plane between the anterior wall of the seminal vesicles and posterior wall of the bladder neck for division of the posterior bladder wall. (Copyright 1996, Brady Urological Institute.)

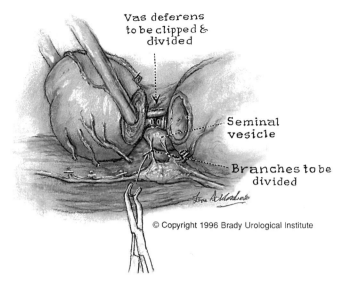

Vas deferens
to be clipped &
divided

Seminal
vesicle

Branches to be
divided

© Copyright 1996 Brady Urological Institute

Figure 86–31. Dissection of the vas deferens and seminal vesicle. The left vas deferens has been ligated and divided. The lateral wall of the seminal vesicle is carefully dissected free from the pelvic plexus with direct visualization and ligation of small arterial branches. (Copyright 1996, Brady Urological Institute.)

The bulldog clamps are removed, and the operative site is inspected carefully for bleeding. **To avoid injury to the fine nerve fibers, small bleeding vessels near the neurovascular bundle should not be cauterized.** Bleeding from these small vessels should be controlled with small hemoclips.

Bladder Neck Closure and Anastomosis

The bladder neck is reconstructed employing interrupted sutures of 2–0 chromic catgut to approximate full-thickness muscularis and mucosa forming a tennis racket closure (Fig. 86–32). The efflux of Indigo carmine from the ureteral orifices is noted while placing the sutures; ureteral catheters are not usually necessary. **By incorporating the mucosa in the closure, troublesome hematuria can be avoided.** The closure is initiated in the midline posteriorly and proceeds anteriorly until the bladder neck is narrowed to approximate the diameter of the index finger. Interrupted 4–0 chromic catgut sutures are used to advance the mucosa over the raw musculature of the bladder neck (see Fig. 86–32). In this way, a rosette of mucosa covers the bladder neck facilitating a mucosa-to-mucosa urethrovesical anastomosis. Finally, the bladder neck is narrowed to approximately No. 22 Fr with one or two additional chromic catgut sutures.

The operative site is inspected carefully for bleeding. A new silicone Foley catheter (No. 16 Fr, 5-ml balloon) is placed through the urethra into the pelvis. The six 3–0 Monocryl sutures that were previously placed in the distal urethra are now placed through the bladder neck in their corresponding positions from the inside to outside (Fig. 86–33). As mentioned previously, a French eye needle is used for placement of the 12-o'clock, 2-o'clock, and 5-o'clock sutures. The catheter is irrigated free of clots, the balloon is tested, and the catheter is placed through the bladder neck.

The anterior suture is tied initially because of the excellent tensile strength provided by the anterior dorsal vein complex. If there is any tension on the anastomosis, the table should be flattened and Balfour retractor released. After the first suture is tied, the balloon on the Foley catheter is inflated. After each suture is tied, the catheter is manipulated to make certain that the catheter is not caught in one of the sutures. The 2-o'clock, 5-o'clock, 10-o'clock, 7-o'clock, and 6-o'clock sutures are tied sequentially. The catheter is irrigated with saline to eliminate clots. After the

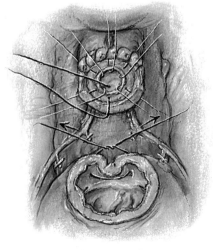

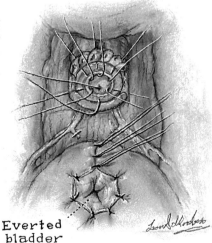

Everted
bladder
mucosa

Figure 86–32. Tennis racket closure of bladder neck using interrupted 2–0 chromic catgut suture incorporating all layers of the bladder wall. The bladder mucosa is then advanced over the raw bladder neck edges with interrupted 4–0 chromic catgut suture material to ensure a mucosa-to-mucosa anastomosis. (Copyright 1996, Brady Urological Institute.)

© Copyright 1996 Brady Urological Institute

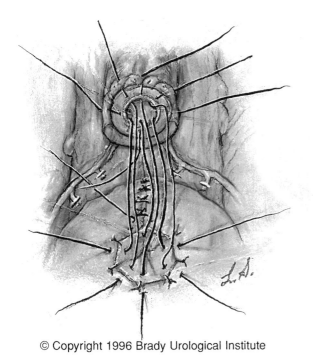

© Copyright 1996 Brady Urological Institute

Figure 86–33. Final anastomosis using six 3–0 Monocryl sutures at 12-, 2-, 5-, 6-, 7-, and 10-o'clock positions. (Copyright 1996, Brady Urological Institute.)

operative site is irrigated vigorously with saline, small suction drains are placed through the medial two thirds of the lower rectus muscles (Niesel et al, 1996). Placement of the drains in this location avoids injury to the intercostal nerves and inferior epigastric vessels and results in less pain at the drain site. The incision is closed with a running No. 2 nylon suture and skin clips. The catheter is carefully taped to the thigh.

POSTOPERATIVE MANAGEMENT

The postoperative recovery of men who undergo radical retropubic prostatectomy is usually uneventful. Patients ambulate the morning after their procedure. Pain control is achieved with intravenous patient-controlled analgesia using morphine. If pain control is not adequate, intravenous ketorolac tromethamine can also be used. **This combination of analgesic agents reduces postoperative ileus.** Patients are fed a clear liquid diet on the first postoperative day, a low-fat diet on the second postoperative day, and a regular diet on the third day. Closed suction drains are left in place until they cease to function. Patients are discharged from the hospital 3 to 5 days postoperatively with a Foley catheter in place. They return 3 weeks after the procedure for removal of the catheter.

COMPLICATIONS

Radical retropubic prostatectomy is well tolerated with minimal morbidity and a low mortality (0.2%). Complications can be divided into those occurring intraoperatively and those occurring postoperatively.

Intraoperative Complications

The most common intraoperative problem is hemorrhage, usually arising from venous structures. Hemorrhage may occur during the pelvic lymphadenectomy if one of the branches of the hypogastric vein is torn inadvertently. Venous injury such as this can often be controlled by temporary packing. If this is not successful, it can be repaired with fine cardiovascular sutures. Hemorrhage can also occur during incision in the endopelvic fascia if the incision is made too close to the prostate, during division of the puboprostatic ligaments if the ligaments are not dissected free from the superficial branch of the dorsal vein or anterior prostatic fascia, and during exposure of the apex of the prostate with transection of the dorsal vein complex. If one understands fully the anatomy of the dorsal vein complex, this bleeding is usually satisfactorily controlled once the dorsal vein has been divided and ligated. **Consequently, if there is troublesome bleeding from the dorsal vein complex at any point, the surgeon should completely divide the dorsal vein complex over the urethra and oversew the end. This is the single best means to control bleeding from the dorsal vein complex. Any maneuver short of this only worsens the bleeding.** To gain exposure for the prostatectomy, one must put traction on the prostate. If the dorsal vein is not completely divided, traction opens the partially transected veins and usually worsens the bleeding. It is imperative to obtain excellent hemostasis before the apex of the prostate is approached so that the anatomy can be viewed in a bloodless field. With careful technique and a thorough knowledge of anatomy, the average blood loss during radical prostatectomy is 1000 ml. Because substantial bleeding may occur unexpectedly, however, the surgeon should always be prepared by having adequate blood available from the blood bank.

Less common complications include obturator nerve injury during pelvic lymph node dissection, rectal injury, and ureteral injury. If the obturator nerve is inadvertently severed, an attempt should be made at reanastomosis using fine nonabsorbable sutures. Rectal injury is an infrequent but serious complication. In 1800 consecutive cases, we experienced 10 injuries to the rectum. They occur during apical dissection when attempting to develop the plane between the rectum and Denonvilliers' fascia. If a rectal injury occurs, the prostatectomy should be completed, the bladder neck should be reconstructed, and hemostasis should be excellent. The rectal injury should be repaired before placing the urethral sutures through the bladder neck. The edges of the wound are freshened and closed in two layers. It is wise to interpose omentum between the rectal closure and the vesicourethral anastomosis to reduce the possibility of a rectourethral fistula. This maneuver can be accomplished simply by making a small opening in the peritoneum, dividing the peritoneum in the rectovesical cul-de-sac, and feeding the end of an omental pedicle through this opening. The anal sphincter is dilated widely by an assistant. The wound should be copiously irrigated with antibiotic solution, and the patient should be maintained on broad-spectrum antibiotics for both aerobic and anaerobic bacteria. When this technique was used without a colostomy, all patients recovered without developing a wound infection, pelvic abscess, or rectourethral fistula (Borland and Walsh, 1992). If the patient has received prior radiotherapy, however, it is prudent to perform a diverting colostomy. Ureteral injury occurs secondary to inadvertent dissection within the layers of the trigone while attempting to identify the proper cleavage plane between the bladder and seminal vesicles. If this injury occurs, ureteral reimplantation should be undertaken.

Postoperative Complications

Postoperative complications are covered in depth in Chapter 87. Following is a review of my own institutional experience.

Delayed Bleeding

Bleeding after radical prostatectomy is defined as significant postoperative hemorrhage requiring acute blood transfusion to support blood pressure. In 1350 consecutive radical prostatectomies, seven cases (0.5%) met this criterion (Hedican and Walsh, 1994). Of these, four patients were explored for bleeding, and three were managed expectantly. The mean blood product requirements for explored patients was comparable to those managed conservatively, although total hospitalization was shorter in patients who underwent a secondary operation. In the three patients managed nonoperatively, the pelvic hematoma drained through the urethrovesical anastomosis resulting in symptomatic bladder neck contractures in all three and long-term problems with urinary control in two. Only one of four patients explored (25%) experienced prolonged mild incontinence. **These results suggest that patients requiring acute transfusions for hypotension after radical prostatectomy should be explored to evacuate the pelvic hematoma in an effort to decrease the likelihood of bladder neck contracture and incontinence.**

Incontinence

Incontinence after radical prostatectomy can be attributed to a variety of different mechanisms: damage to the distal sphincter mechanism, individual variation in the length of the distal urethral segment, bladder neck contracture, denervation, and bladder instability. By avoiding injury to the smooth muscle of the urethra by placing the sutures only on the edge of the mucosa and striated sphincter, continence has returned earlier. **The use of six sutures for the anastomosis has greatly reduced the frequency of bladder neck contractures.** Chao and Mayo (1995) suggest that detrusor abnormalities are rarely the sole cause of incontinence. **Thus, I believe that the major cause of incontinence is individual variability in the development of the distal urethral sphincter mechanism.**

Urinary continence was evaluated in the first 593 consecutive patients who underwent anatomic radical prostatectomy (Steiner et al, 1991). Complete urinary control was achieved in 92% of the patients, and stress incontinence was present in 8%. Six percent wore one pad per day, and stress incontinence was sufficient to require placement of an artificial sphincter in two men (0.3%). No patient was totally incontinent. Weight of the prostate, prior transurethral resection of the prostate, and pathologic stage had no significant influ-

ence on the preservation of urinary control. **In the patients older than 70 years, 86% were completely dry. This decrease in the continence rate did not reach statistical significance because of the small number of men older than 70 years in our series (4%). We believe, however, that this phenomenon is real. Continence was achieved in 94% of patients with preservation of both neurovascular bundles, 92% with preservation of only one neurovascular bundle, and 81% with excision of both neurovascular bundles. Although these differences did not reach statistical significance, they suggest that innervation from the pelvic plexus may have some influence on the urinary continence mechanism.** There was no correlation between postoperative potency and urinary continence; 94% of the potent patients and 90% of the impotent patients were dry. In the most recent 700 men, no one has experienced total urinary incontinence (Walsh et al, 1994). Eight men in this series who had the most severe incontinence (requiring more than one pad per day) were evaluated. Their average bladder capacity was 450 ml, and none exhibited uninhibited bladder contractions. In five men, leakage could not be demonstrated at full bladder capacity with Valsalva's maneuver, and in the remaining three the average leak point pressure was 65 cm H_2O. Pad weighing demonstrated that the average 24-hour urinary loss was 9% of the total urinary output.

During the recovery period, patients need constant encouragement and advice at regular intervals. The details of this program are reported elsewhere (Walsh and Worthington, 1995). **It is clear that the distal urethral sphincter mechanism is capable of maintaining passive urinary control in most but not all men. For the 8% of men in whom it is not sufficient, attempts at improving the surgical technique to provide an additional continence mechanism should be pursued.** Furthermore, because most of these patients have mild problems, postoperative injection of collagen into the submucosa adjacent to the bladder neck is helpful for many.

Impotence

Before the development of an anatomic approach to radical prostatectomy, virtually all patients were impotent. Recognizing that these patients had intact penile sensation and could achieve orgasm, it was clear that injury to the pudendal nerve was not responsible for impotence. Rather, impotence arose from damage to the autonomic innervation to the corpora cavernosa. **Before 1982, the exact anatomic location of the autonomic branches from the pelvic plexus to the corpora cavernosa was unknown.** In that year, Walsh and Donker described the anatomy of the pelvic plexus and the branches that innervate the corpora cavernosa and recommended minor modifications in the surgical procedure that could preserve potency. **It subsequently became clear that in older series, these nerves were not excised with the specimen but were merely cut and left in place** (Walsh et al, 1987). With further experience, we were able to demonstrate that it was possible to excise the nerves widely on one side without compromising sexual function in the majority of patients (Walsh et al, 1987).

A number of improvements in the surgical technique have continued to this date. We evaluated the recovery of sexual function in 600 consecutive men 34 to 72 years old who underwent an anatomic approach to radical prostatectomy between 1982 and 1988 (Quinlan et al, 1991a). Of the 503 patients who were potent preoperatively and followed for a minimum of 18 months, 68% were potent postoperatively. **Three factors were identified that correlated with the return of sexual function: age, clinical and pathologic stage, and surgical technique (preservation or excision of the neurovascular bundle).** Sexual function was preserved in 91% of men less than 50 years old, 75% of men 50 to 60 years old, 58% of men 60 to 70 years old, and 25% of men 70 years or older. Among men younger than 50 years, potency was similar in those who had both neurovascular bundles preserved and in patients who had one neurovascular bundle widely excised. With advancing age (>50 years), sexual function was better in patients in whom both neurovascular bundles were preserved than in those in whom one neurovascular bundle was excised (P <.05). When the relative risk of postoperative impotence was adjusted for age, the risk of postoperative impotence was twofold greater if there was capsular penetration or seminal vesicle invasion (P <.05). For example, 71% of patients 60 to 69 years old with organ-confined cancer and preservation of both neurovascular bundles were potent, compared with 44% with preservation of both neurovascular bundles but involvement of the seminal vesicles and only 17% with wide excision of one neurovascular bundle and seminal vesicle invasion. **Thus, patients who have the best recovery of sexual function are those who are young and have organ-confined disease. These patients also receive the most benefit from surgery.**

In this series, potency was defined as the ability to achieve an erection that was sufficient for intercourse. Patients who had full nocturnal erections but could not have intercourse were classified as impotent. Patients and their wives were sent an extensive questionnaire 18 months postoperatively inquiring about the recovery of sexual function (Walsh et al, 1994). This questionnaire was analyzed by an independent source and compared to the case records. In 90%, the results of the self-reported case record and the independent survey were identical. In 5%, however, the case record stated that the patient was impotent, yet the patient and his wife stated that he was potent. In another 5%, the case records stated that the patient was potent, yet the patient and his wife did not concur. When potent patients were asked to estimate the quality of erection compared to preoperative status, patients stated that it averaged 79% of preoperative status (range 60%–95%). Furthermore, they stated that the average duration of erection was 9 minutes. These data indicate that the return of sexual function postoperatively in men older than 50 years is quantitatively related to preservation of autonomic innervation, along with other factors (e.g., vascular). For men older than 50 in whom it is necessary to excise one neurovascular bundle, future consideration should be given to approaches that may restore autonomic function, for example, nerve regeneration, partial excision of the bundle, or cavernous nerve grafts (Burgers et al, 1991; Quinlan et al, 1991b). Until erections return, patients should be encouraged to resume sexual activity using vacuum erection devices or injection therapy. I believe that these measures encourage the earlier recovery of unassisted erections. Because erections may not recover for 24 to 48 months following surgery, patients require constant encouragement (Walsh and Worthington, 1995).

CANCER CONTROL

In 1994, we reviewed our 10-year experience with anatomic radical retropubic prostatectomy at The Johns Hopkins Hospital (Walsh et al, 1994). Between April 1982 and March 1991, 955 men with clinically localized prostate cancer (clinical stages T1 to T2) underwent staging pelvic lymphadenectomy and anatomic radical retropubic prostatectomy. **Using actuarial analysis, at 10 years the likelihood of an undetectable PSA level was 70%, isolated elevation of PSA 23%, distant metastases 7%, and local recurrence 4%. The actuarial likelihood of an elevated serum PSA increased with increasing pathologic stage: 10-year actuarial likelihood of freedom from PSA relapse was 85% for men with organ-confined disease, 82% with focal capsular penetration, 54% with established capsular penetration and Gleason score 2 to 6 disease, and 42% with established capsular penetration and Gleason 7 to 10 disease. These data indicate that radical prostatectomy cures the majority of men with organ-confined disease or with well-differentiated to moderately well-differentiated tumors that have penetrated the prostatic capsule to the extent where it is possible to obtain a clear surgical margin.** Fortunately, with the use of PSA in the early diagnosis and staging of prostate cancer, most men who undergo surgery fall into this favorable category. In a series of 200 consecutive cases, the tumor was organ confined in 43%; there was focal capsular penetration in 15%, established capsular penetration in 42%, positive surgical margins in 4.6%, seminal vesicle involvement in 2.4%, and lymph node involvement in 2.8%.

SUMMARY

During the last 15 years, there have been a number of advances in the diagnosis and treatment of localized prostate cancer. Today, more men are diagnosed with curable disease at a younger age. Men are also living longer; a man 65 to 70 years old has a 50% chance of living for another 15 years. Radical prostatectomy is an ideal form of treatment for patients who can be cured and who will live long enough to benefit from it. These patients also have the best quality of life postoperatively.

REFERENCES

Ansell JS: Radical transvesical prostatectomy: Preliminary report on an approach to surgical excision of localized prostate malignancy. J Urol 1959; 2:373.

Bastacki RN, Walsh PC, Epstein JI: Relationship between perineural tumor invasion on needle biopsy and radical prostatectomy: Capsular penetration in clinical stage B adenocarcinoma of the prostate. Am J Surg Pathol 1995; 17:336–341.

Borland RN, Walsh PC: The management of rectal injury during radical retropubic prostatectomy. J Urol 1992; 147:905–907.

Breza J, Abuseif SR, Orvis BR, et al: Detailed anatomy of penile neurovascular structures: Surgical significance. J Urol 1989; 41:437–443.

Burgers JK, Nelson RJ, Quinlan DM, Walsh PC: Nerve growth factor,

ANATOMIC RADICAL RETROPUBIC PROSTATECTOMY

nerve grafts, and amniotic membrane grafts restore erectile function in rats. J Urol 1991; 146:463–468.

Campbell EW: Total prostatectomy with preliminary ligation of the vascular pedicle. J Urol 1959; 81:464.

Chao R, Mayo ME: Incontinence after radical prostatectomy: Detrusor or sphincter causes. J Urol 1995; 154:16–18.

Chute R: Radical retropubic prostatectomy for cancer. J Urol 1954; 71:347.

Flocks RH: Arterial distribution within prostate gland: Its role in transurethral prostatic resection. J Urol 1937; 37:524–548.

Hedican SP, Walsh PC: Postoperative bleeding following radical retropubic prostatectomy. J Urol 1994; 152:1181–1183.

Jewett HJ, Eggleston JC, Yawn DH: Radical prostatectomy in the management of carcinoma of the prostate: Probable causes of some therapeutic failures. J Urol 1972; 107:1034.

Lepor H, Gregerman M, Crosby R, et al: Precise localization of the autonomic nerves from the pelvic plexus to the corpora cavernosa: A detailed anatomical study of the adult male pelvis. J Urol 1985; 133:207–212.

Lich R, Grant O, Maurer JE: Extravesical prostatectomy: A comparison of retropubic and perineal prostatectomy. J Urol 1949; 61:930.

Lue TF, Zeineh SJ, Schmidt RA, Tanagho EA: Neuroanatomy of penile erection: Its relevance to iatrogenic impotence. J Urol 1984; 131:273–280.

Memmelaar J: Total prostatovesiculectomy: Retropubic approach. J Urol 1949; 62:349.

Millin T: Retropubic Urinary Surgery. London, Livingstone, 1947.

Myers RP: Prostate shape, external striated urethral sphincter, and radical prostatectomy: The apical dissection. J Urol 1987; 138:543–550.

Myers RP: Male urethral sphincteric anatomy and radical prostatectomy. Urol Clin North Am 1991; 18:211–227.

Myers RP: Radical prostatectomy: Pertinent surgical anatomy. Atlas Urol Clin North Am 1994; 2:1–18.

Niesel T, Partin AW, Walsh PC: An anatomical approach for placement of surgical drains after radical retropubic prostatectomy: Long-term effects on post-operative pain. Urology 1996; 48:91–94.

Oelrich TM: The urethral sphincter muscle in the male. Am J Anat 1980; 158:229–296.

Partin AW, Yoo J, Carter HB, et al: The use of prostate specific antigen, clinical stage and Gleason score to predict pathologic stage in men with localized prostate cancer. J Urol 1993; 150:110.

Peters C, Walsh PC: Blood transfusion and anesthetic practices in radical retropubic prostatectomy. J Urol 1985; 134:81–83.

Polascik TJ, Walsh PC: Radical retropubic prostatectomy: The influence of accessory pudendal arteries on the recovery of sexual function. J Urol 1995; 153:150–152.

Quinlan DM, Epstein JI, Carter BS, Walsh PC: Sexual function following radical prostatectomy: Influence of preservation of neurovascular bundles. J Urol 1991a; 145:998–1002.

Quinlan DM, Nelson RS, Walsh PC: Cavernous nerve grafts restore erectile function in denervated rats. J Urol 1991b; 145:380–383.

Reiner WG, Walsh PC: An anatomical approach to the surgical management of the dorsal vein and Santorini's plexus during radical retropubic surgery. J Urol 1979; 121:198–200.

Schlegel P, Walsh PC: Neuroanatomical approach to radical cystoprostatectomy with preservation of sexual function. J Urol 1987; 138:1402–1406.

Sgrignoli AR, Walsh PC, Steinberg GD, et al: Prognostic factors in men with stage D1 prostate cancer: Identification of patients less likely to have prolonged survival after radical prostatectomy. J Urol 1994; 152:1077–1081.

Shir Y, Raja SN, Frank SM, Brendler CB: Intraoperative blood loss during radical retropubic prostatectomy: Epidural versus general anesthesia. Urology 1995; 45:993.

Steiner MS: The puboprostatic ligament and the male urethral suspensory mechanism: An anatomic study. Urology 1994; 44:530.

Steiner MS, Morton RA, Walsh PC: Impact of radical prostatectomy on urinary continence. J Urol 1991; 145:512–515.

Walsh PC: Technique of vesicourethral anastomosis may influence recovery of sexual function following radical prostatectomy. Atlas Urol Clin North Am 1994; 2:59–63.

Walsh PC: *Anatomic Radical Retropubic Prostatectomy: Surgical Technique After 20 Years of Refinement 1997 [videotape]*. Baltimore, James Buchanan Brady Urological Institute, 1997.

Walsh PC, Donker PJ: Impotence following radical prostatectomy: Insight into etiology and prevention. J Urol 1982; 128:492–497.

Walsh PC, Epstein JI, Lowe FC: Potency following radical prostatectomy with wide unilateral excision of the neurovascular bundle. J Urol 1987; 138:823–827.

Walsh PC, Lepor H, Eggleston JC: Radical prostatectomy with preservation of sexual function: Anatomical and pathological considerations. Prostate 1983; 4:473–485.

Walsh PC, Partin AW, Epstein JI: Cancer control and quality of life following anatomical radical retropubic prostatectomy: Results at 10 years. J Urol 1994; 152:1831–1836.

Walsh PC, Quinlan DM, Morton RA, Steiner MS: Radical retropubic prostatectomy: Improved anastomosis and urinary continence. Urol Clin North Am 1990; 17:679.

Walsh PC, Worthington JF: Treating prostate cancer: Radical prostatectomy. *In* The Prostate: A Guide for Men and the Women Who Love Them. Baltimore, Johns Hopkins University Press, 1995, pp 92–119.

Zvara P, Carrier S, Kour NW, Tanagho EA: The detailed neuroanatomy of the human striated urethral sphincter. Br J Urol 1994; 74:182–187.

87
RADICAL PERINEAL PROSTATECTOMY

Robert P. Gibbons, M.D.

Radical perineal prostatectomy was first described by Young more than 90 years ago. In the properly selected patient, this procedure provides disease-free survival rates comparable to the expected survival in similarly aged men for up to 30 years of observation (Young, 1905; Gibbons et al, 1989). Many urologists have not had the opportunity to learn this operation, however, and the procedure as described by Young and popularized by Belt usually resulted in erectile impotence (Belt et al, 1939). Despite these limitations, radical perineal prostatectomy remained the surgical treatment of choice for localized prostate cancer until the late 1970s. At that time, Walsh and associates described a series of technical modifications to the retropubic procedure that reduced the blood loss, incontinence, and erectile dysfunction associated with that technique and provided an anatomic approach that was more familiar to most urologists (Reiner and Walsh, 1979; Walsh and Donker, 1982; Walsh et al, 1983; Walsh et al, 1987). Weldon and colleagues described modifications to the perineal approach incorporating many of these observations so that the two procedures are virtually identical with regard to potency and pathologic outcomes (Weldon, 1988; Weldon and Tavel 1988; Weldon et al, 1995).

There has been a **renewed interest in learning the technique of radical perineal prostatectomy** for a variety of reasons. The long-term cancer control rates are well known. There is less patient discomfort following the perineal approach with more rapid postoperative return of appetite, bowel function, and resumption of activity, all of which shorten the length of hospitalization. With heightened patient and physician awareness of prostate cancer and more widespread utilization of prostate-specific antigen (PSA) and digital rectal exam (DRE), a **larger proportion of patients** with low-stage and low-grade cancers are being detected **in whom pelvic lymphadenectomy can be omitted. Technical advantages** include clear exposure and access to the apex of the prostate to optimize the complete removal of this critical margin and allow precise transection of the urethra; generally less blood loss because it is not necessary to transect the dorsal vein complex; and tying of the vesical-urethral anastomotic sutures under direct vision to perform a watertight closure that is without tension and dependent.

Disadvantages to the procedure exist, including the need for a preliminary approach to the pelvic lymph nodes in those patients at risk for nodal disease—assuming that frozen section examination of the lymph nodes is performed and the prostatectomy is not performed if the nodes are positive. Most patients who are candidates for radical prostatectomy (clinically organ-confined disease) have a low incidence of lymph node involvement. Several **guidelines have evolved employing clinical stage, grade, and PSA to use in selecting the majority of these patients who do not "routinely" need a preliminary pelvic lymph node dissection** (Partin et al, 1993; Bluestein et al, 1994; Epstein et al, 1994; Narayan et al, 1994; Bishoff et al, 1995). For example, none of the 100 Mayo Clinic patients with T1c cancer and a PSA 10 or less had a positive pelvic lymph node (Bluestein et al, 1994). Two large contemporary series of nearly 600 patients

2589

in whom cancer was detected using PSA for screening have found the incidence of positive lymph nodes 5% or less. Before PSA, their positive lymph node rate had been 20% (Petros and Catalona, 1992; Danella et al, 1993).

The exaggerated lithotomy position is infrequently a problem except for the rare patient with hip ankylosis or marked obesity. A **simple office test** is to have the patient lie supine on the examining table and bring his knees to his chest. The inability to do this is a contraindication to the procedure. Patients with gland weights exceeding 120 g can be difficult, especially if the pelvis is narrow. Removal can usually be accomplished by altering the sequence of the procedure to ligate and transect the lateral pedicles before dissection of the seminal vesicles and ampullae of the vasa deferentia, but in this setting a retropubic approach is probably technically easier. Radical perineal prostatectomy can be performed safely with acceptable morbidity within 4 weeks of transurethral prostatectomy. If not performed within this interval, it is advantageous to wait 4 months to lessen the risk of incontinence (Elder et al, 1984).

PATIENT SELECTION

Surgery is curative only if all of the tumor present is removed. Surgery is necessary only if the cancer will inflict morbidity or shorten the patient's expected survival. This is discussed in more detail in Chapter 84, but in summary, **the appropriate patient** should have disease that is confined to the prostate, an expected longevity longer than the natural history of the cancer, and no significant surgical risk factors present. This would include patients with clinical stage T1b, T1c, or T2 biopsy-proven tumors. There should be no area of extension beyond the capsule or fixation, ideally confirmed by two experienced urologists. The patient should have at least a 15-year life expectancy and, after discussion of the risks, quality of life, natural history, and options, a willingness to undergo surgery.

Surgery should be deferred for at least 2 weeks following transrectal prostate needle biopsy—longer if there was any associated bleeding or infection.

Preoperative Counseling

For the sexually active man, **whether to perform a nerve-sparing or extended wide-field dissection is an important decision.** Patients with positive surgical margins have recurrence rates (PSA failure) that are significantly higher than patients with specimen-confined disease (Epstein et al, 1993; Paulson, 1994; Weldon et al, 1995). Because the difference between specimen-confined or margin-positive status can be less than 1 mm, there have been concerns that sparing the neurovascular bundles might compromise the extent of the surgical margins obtained. Indeed, most surgeons perform a wide excision of the neurovascular bundle on the side of the tumor. In Weldon's pathologic analysis of 200 patients undergoing radical perineal prostatectomy, 15% had tumors completely penetrating the capsule but still specimen-confined because an extended dissection, including the adjacent posterolateral periprostatic fascia and enclosed neurovascular bundle, was performed. In addition, 7% of the

nerve-sparing dissections resulted in solitary, positive, posterolateral margins. Based on this experience, **Weldon and colleagues recommend an extended dissection sacrificing the neurovascular bundle on each side unless *all* of the following criteria are present:** good potency with a strong desire by the patient to preserve it, acceptance by the patient of the discretionary low risk of a positive margin, little or no clinically recognized adjacent tumor (and none with a Gleason score ≥7), and a neurovascular bundle that could be easily and cleanly dissected off the prostate. Patients are counseled that if impotence occurs after surgery, erectile function is lost, but **libido and the sensation of orgasm remain intact.** In these patients, mechanical (vacuum erection device or penile prosthesis) or pharmacologic-induced erections provide effective treatment (Carroll et al, 1989). **A bilateral extended dissection** sacrificing both neurovascular bundles is **advisable** for all impotent men, for those with marginal potency who are unlikely to retain it, and for those who do not wish to accept any increased risk of cancer recurrence to preserve erectile function.

Patients receive detailed postoperative instructions before admission to the hospital, including their anticipated postsurgical course. With preoperative discussion of these expectations, **most patients can be discharged on the second day after surgery.**

Autologous Blood

Patients have been encouraged to have autologous blood available, but when the surgeon's transfusion rate decreases to 5% to 10%, this becomes an unnecessary expense and causes a delay in surgery. The decision about need and type of blood products is an individual one that has to be based on the surgeon's transfusion rate, the availability of blood, and the patient desires.

PREHOSPITAL PREPARATION

Patients can have a regular diet up until midnight of the day before surgery. They take neomycin 1.0 g orally at 12:00 PM, 2:00 PM, 4:00 PM, 6:00 PM, 8:00 PM, and 10:00 PM on the day before surgery and give themselves a Fleet's enema at 9:00 PM. Patients are **admitted to the hospital on the morning of surgery** following the aforementioned at-home preparation and in the induction room receive gentamicin 80 mg intravenously and cefotetan 1.0 g intravenously. They are sent to the operating room with midthigh elastic antithromboembolic hose on both legs.

OPERATING ROOM PREPARATION

The small incision and the fact that much of the operation is performed bluntly make it necessary that one of the **two assistants** be familiar with both the perineal anatomy and the sequence of the procedure. Necessary **special instruments include a curved and straight Lowsley retractor.** A notched Young bulb retractor, short and deep lateral retractors, and lighted sucker are useful. Other standard instruments include four narrow Deavers, curved prostate scissors,

and a Heaney needle holder. A self-retaining retractor can relieve one of the assistants during the closure.

It is necessary that the operating room table not have a notch removed under the buttocks when the foot part of the table is lowered.

PROCEDURE

Anesthesia

This procedure lends itself well to an epidural or a spinal approach, but some anesthesiologists feel more comfortable with a general/endotracheal technique.

Position (Fig. 87–1)

It is important that the buttocks be brought down beyond the end of the table and that the end of the table be solid. If shoulder restraints are placed, pad them with 250-ml intravenous fluid containers wrapped in a towel and placed against the acromion process and not the soft trapezius muscle or side of the neck. Midthigh elastic antithromboembolic hose are placed (ideally by the patient before the anesthesia), and the lower legs, ankles, and feet are padded with egg crate sponge held in place with orthopedic stockinette. The ankles are then placed in the stirrups, and the foot section of the table is lowered. The patient is placed in the exaggerated lithotomy position by simultaneously rotating the stirrup poles cephalad. A bean bag is placed underneath the sacrum so that the perineum is almost parallel to the floor. Care is taken to ensure that any **pressure points are**

well padded. Three-inch tape stretching between the stirrups and posterior to the rectum secures the position. The arms should be abducted as little as possible and can be tucked next to the body if agreeable with the anesthesiologist. During the operation, **exposure is maintained as necessary by elevating the table and avoiding Trendelenburg's position,** which risks added pressure on the shoulders and loss of position.

Hair is shaved only in the perineum and posterior scrotum. Following standard preparation of the perineum and genitalia, a rectal sheath is placed and the perineum draped with TUR (transurethral resection of the prostate) drapes.

ANATOMIC CONSIDERATIONS

Figure 87–2 illustrates the relationship of the muscles of the perineum and the external rectal sphincter. The prostate can be approached by one of three routes through or around the fibers of the external rectal sphincter, which are retracted and not incised (Young, 1905; Belt et al, 1939; Hudson and Lilien, 1992).

The perineal route to the prostate is seen in Figure 87–3. Initially the apical region of the prostate serves as a palpable landmark. Following division of the rectourethralis muscle, Denonvilliers' fascia is encountered. This fascia is composed of an anterior and posterior layer. The fibrous membrane derived from the pelvic cul-de-sac of peritoneum and adjacent to the prostate capsule is designated the anterior layer, and the slightly thicker fascia around the rectal musculature is designated the posterior layer (Tobin and Benjamin, 1945). The posterior layer is also referred to as the *ventral-rectal fascia.* In the classic radical perineal prostatectomy, a

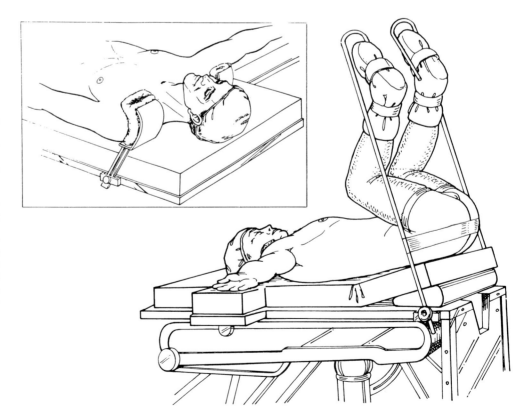

Figure 87–1. Exaggerated lithotomy position for radical perineal prostatectomy. If the end of the table under the buttocks is notched (as shown), it is important that this gap be bridged by a rigid support. Shoulder restraints are padded and placed against the acromion process. The upper extremity is not extended more than 45 degrees. (From Gibbons RP: Radical perineal prostatectomy: Definitive treatment for patients with localized prostate cancer. AUA Update Series, Volume 13, Lesson 5. AUA Office of Education, Houston, TX, 1994.)

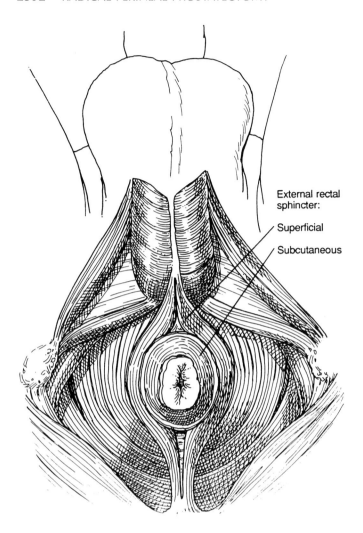

External rectal
sphincter:

Superficial

Subcutaneous

Figure 87–2. Muscles of perineum and external rectal sphincter. The dissection proceeds through the triangle formed by the subcutaneous and superficial fibers of the external rectal sphincter. The superficial fibers are retracted in a cephalad/lateral direction. None of these muscles are transected. (From Gibbons RP: Radical perineal prostatectomy: Definitive treatment for patients with localized prostate cancer. AUA Update Series, Volume 13, Lesson 5. AUA Office of Education, Houston, TX, 1994.)

plane is developed between the anterior and posterior layers of Denonvilliers' fascia. An extended wide-field radical dissection leaves both of Denonvilliers' layers attached to the prostate (Weldon, 1993). Invasion of Denonvilliers' fascia can lead to positive surgical margins if complete excision of this fascia is not performed (Villers et al, 1993).

INCISION

The incision is made from one ischial tuberosity to the other with the apex approximately 1.5 cm above the anus—just anterior to the mucocutaneous pigmentation line (Fig. 87–4). It is carried down to the fat, and the drape and rectal sheath are clipped to the lower skin edge. The ischiorectal fossa on each side of the rectum is bluntly developed with the index fingers directed toward the surgeon's toes (Fig. 87–5A). Fascia bands are sharply incised. By bringing the two index fingers together toward the midline, one can feel the rectal sheath and location of the rectum. An index finger is then bluntly tunneled beneath the superficial central tendon and above the ventral wall of the rectum, and the central tendon is transected (Fig. 87–5B). **A moist, folded sponge is placed over the exposed rectum for protection for the duration of the procedure.** If either the Belt or Hudson approach is used, fibers of the external rectal

sphincter are identified by their horizontal orientation. This part of the dissection is best performed bluntly using the finger or blunt end of a long knife handle to sweep the muscle fibers of the external rectal sphincter upward and lateral (Fig. 87–5C). These should not be incised. This exposes the longitudinal fibers of the ventral wall of the rectum, which are gently followed with finger dissection along this **avascular plane** to the rectourethralis muscle. Short, then long, lateral retractors are used to retract gently the levator ani muscles laterally. **At this point,** the curved Lowsley retractor is passed into the bladder and the wings are opened. By moving the handle of the Lowsley retractor cephalad, the prostate is rotated toward the incision, and the apex of the prostate can be palpated as well as the adjacent urethra. With the Lowsley retractor stabilizing the prostate, the rectourethralis muscle is transected with scissors to the apex of the prostate (Fig. 87–6). If the handle of the Lowsley retractor is pushed too firmly against the abdomen or in a caudad direction, it is possible to lift the ventral surface of the rectum into the line of incision, resulting in a **rectal injury.** If uncertain, double-glove one hand and insert a finger into the rectum to ascertain its location. **The rectourethralis muscle is usually thicker than one expects** (3–10 mm), and **sharp dissection** should continue toward the **apex** of the prostate until **Denonvilliers' fascia** is clearly identified by its more white and shiny appearance (Fig. 87–7).

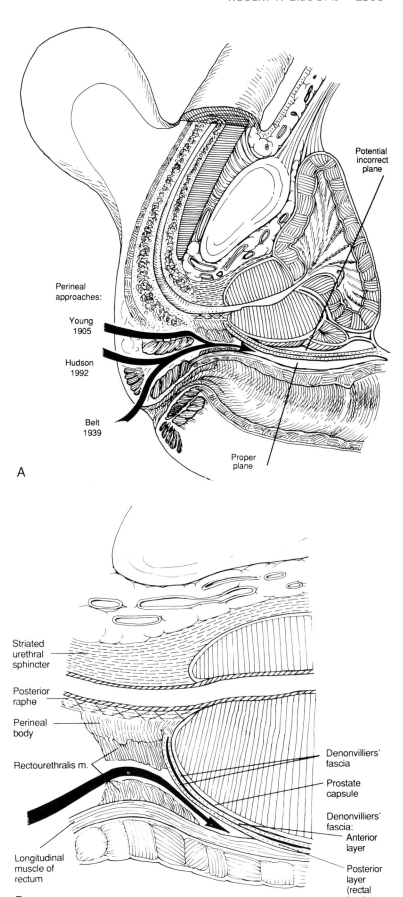

Figure 87–3. *A,* The three described perineal approaches to the prostate vary only in how they traverse the external rectal sphincter. The Young approach is the most direct route, but the Belt and Hudson approaches provide early visualization of the longitudinal fibers of the rectum, which are a useful landmark. *B,* Relationship of the rectum, rectourethralis muscle, striated urethral sphincter, Denonvilliers' fascia, and apex of the prostate.

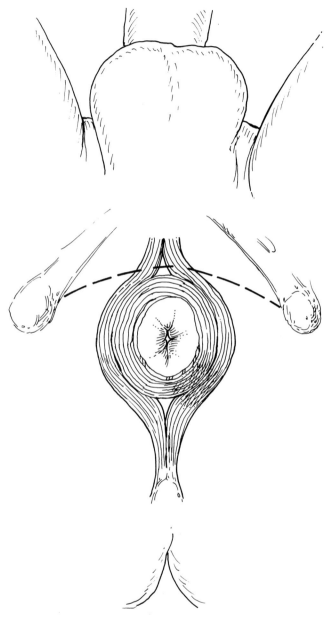

Figure 87–4. Incision. A gently curved incision is made between the ischial tuberosities with the apex just above the hyperpigmentation of the mucocutaneous junction. (From Gibbons RP: Radical perineal prostatectomy: Definitive treatment for patients with localized prostate cancer. AUA Update Series, Volume 13, Lesson 5. AUA Office of Education, Houston, TX, 1994.)

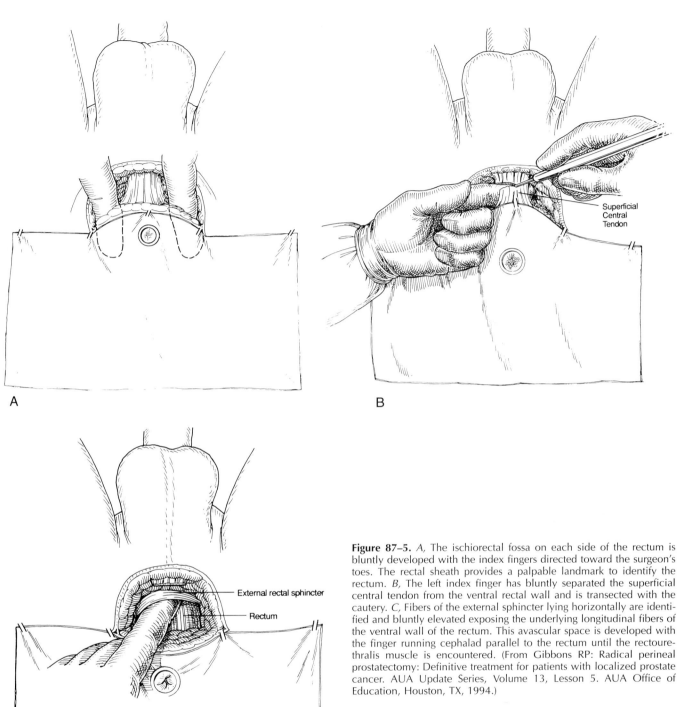

Figure 87–5. *A,* The ischiorectal fossa on each side of the rectum is bluntly developed with the index fingers directed toward the surgeon's toes. The rectal sheath provides a palpable landmark to identify the rectum. *B,* The left index finger has bluntly separated the superficial central tendon from the ventral rectal wall and is transected with the cautery. *C,* Fibers of the external sphincter lying horizontally are identified and bluntly elevated exposing the underlying longitudinal fibers of the ventral wall of the rectum. This avascular space is developed with the finger running cephalad parallel to the rectum until the rectourethralis muscle is encountered. (From Gibbons RP: Radical perineal prostatectomy: Definitive treatment for patients with localized prostate cancer. AUA Update Series, Volume 13, Lesson 5. AUA Office of Education, Houston, TX, 1994.)

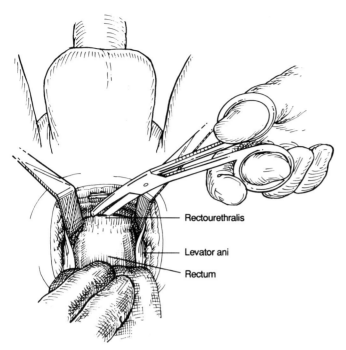

Figure 87–6. The curved Lowsley retractor has been placed so that the apex of the prostate is readily palpable on the opposite side of the rectourethralis muscle. The rectourethralis is sharply divided *(dotted line)* until the shiny, white Denonvilliers' fascia is clearly identified. Avoid forceful leverage on the Lowsley retractor, which would elevate the rectum into the line of incision. If there is doubt about the position of the rectum, double-glove one hand and insert a finger into the rectum to ascertain its location.

The rectal surface is bluntly and gently separated from the posterior layer of Denonvilliers' fascia. This separation is facilitated by gentle rocking of the curved Lowsley retractor, which provides countertraction. The rectum is usually attached at the base of the prostate/seminal vesicle junction (Fig. 87–8) and has to be sharply incised, following which it is possible to initiate a plane between the ventral surface

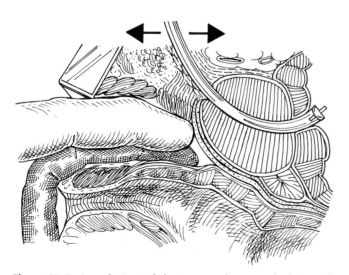

Figure 87–7. Lateral view of the transected rectourethralis muscle adjacent to the apex of the prostate. A moist, folded sponge is placed over the exposed rectum for protection for the duration of the procedure.

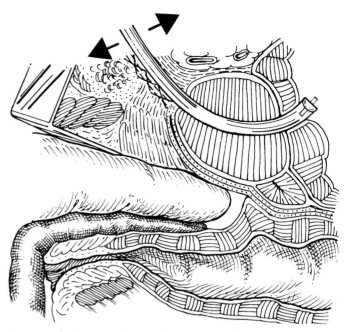

Figure 87–8. The space between the rectum and the posterior layer of Denonvilliers' fascia is bluntly developed with care to avoid entering the prostate capsule or rectal wall. The rectal wall is usually adherent at the base of the prostate/seminal vesicle junction.

of the rectum and dorsal surface of the seminal vesicles (Fig. 87–9). The use of three moist unfolded sponges placed into this space further exposes the dorsal surface of the surgical specimen and separates it further from the rectum (Fig. 87–10). Again, this space is more readily developed if the curved **Lowsley retractor is not pushed too firmly against the abdomen** and is alternately lifted toward the ceiling. The neurovascular bundles are located laterally between the two layers of Denonvilliers' fascia and can be damaged by excessive dissection or retraction.

The space between the lateral edge of the prostate and the adjacent fibers of the levator ani is now bluntly exposed as an avascular plane and developed to the junction of the apex of the prostate and urethra on both sides (Fig. 87–11). The **neurovascular bundles** are prominently seen at this point and are ligated and transected if this is an extended wide-field procedure. If this is a nerve-sparing procedure, the neurovascular bundles can be followed into the plane between the two layers of Denonvilliers' fascia, where they can be dissected out along their vertical course.

The apex of the prostate and adjacent urethra can be readily palpated by the presence of the Lowsley retractor. **Minimal dissection is performed,** and the urethra is not encircled to avoid injury to the striated urethral sphincter (Myers et al, 1987). The posterior membranous urethra is opened transversely, distal to the apex of the prostate, exposing the curved Lowsley retractor (Fig. 87–12A). If this is a nerve-sparing approach, care must be taken to keep the neurovascular bundles on the lateral side of this incision.

The curved Lowsley retractor is replaced with the straight Lowsley retractor, which is placed into the transected urethra and **rotated so that the bladder blades are in a vertical plane.** The anterior side of the urethra is now transected, completely separating the urethra from the prostate (Fig.

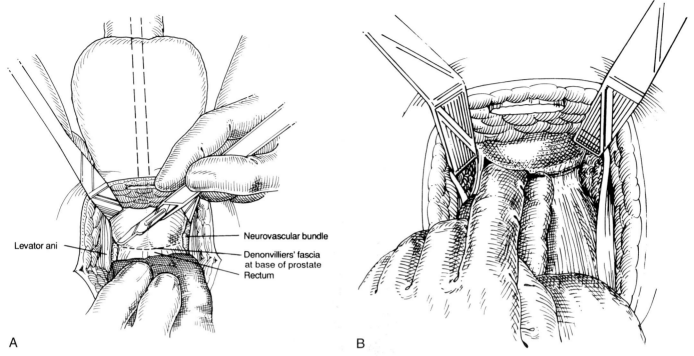

A   B

Figure 87–9. *A,* Sharply divide *(dotted line)* the adherent rectum from the base of the prostate/seminal vesicles. (From Gibbons RP: Radical perineal prostatectomy: Definitive treatment for patients with localized prostate cancer. AUA Update Series, Volume 13, Lesson 5. AUA Office of Education, Houston, TX, 1994.) *B,* The space between the rectum and the seminal vesicles can be bluntly developed with the finger and three open, moist sponges.

Figure 87–10. Lateral view detailing completed posterior dissection.

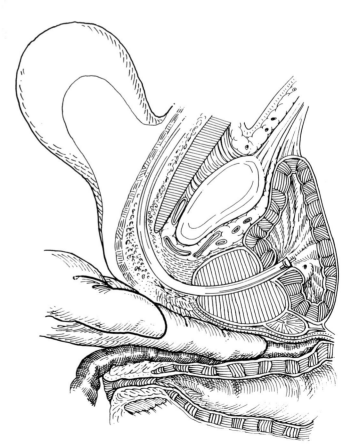

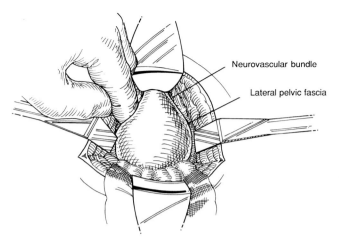

Figure 87–11. The space between the lateral lobe of the prostate and adjacent levator ani muscles is bluntly developed lateral to the neurovascular bundle in an extended wide field dissection. In a nerve-sparing modification, the neurovascular bundles can be followed into the plane between the two layers of Denonvilliers' fascia and dissected out along their vertical course.

87–12*B*). Care is taken to **minimize injury to the striated urethral sphincter** (Myers, 1991).

The prostate capsule is replaced at the apex and anterior surface with a merging of parenchyma of the prostate and striated muscle (Fig. 87–13). The anterior surface of the prostate is identified and **bluntly** followed in the midline to the anterior bladder neck, which is identified by the vertical blade of the Lowsley retractor (Fig. 87–14). **The dorsal vein complex lies anterior and is usually not encountered.** Both **puboprostatic ligaments** are felt on each side of the

finger where they fan out to insert on the prostate near the bladder neck. They should be **sharply transected** near their attachment to the prostate.

If the patient has had a **prior transurethral or open subtotal prostatectomy,** it is necessary to enter the space of Retzius bluntly or sharply at this time and mobilize the anterior bladder neck from any adherent scar tissue. Failure to do so makes it difficult to perform a tension-free vesicourethral anastomosis later.

The anterior bladder neck is sharply incised over the vertically placed blade of the straight Lowsley retractor, and the cystotomy is opened generously by spreading a right-angle clamp on each side of the exposed blade of the Lowsley retractor (Fig. 87–15*A*). A long right-angle clamp is now passed adjacent to the Lowsley retractor, and when the tip of the clamp is identified, the Lowsley retractor is removed and replaced with a No. 14 Fr red rubber catheter for future retraction (Fig. 87–15*B*).

The opening in the anterior bladder neck is widened sufficiently to accept the middle finger. Now the lateral attachments of the prostate with the bladder neck can be safely incised, either sharply or with cautery (Fig. 87–16). This ensures an **optimal surgical margin at the bladder neck.** The incision is carried three quarters of the way around the bladder neck on each side. Using narrow Deaver retractors placed into the open bladder, the trigone and ureteral orifices are identified. If symmetric, a No. 5 Fr olive-tipped catheter is placed into **one** ureter for future identification. Ureteral edema resulting in anuria can occur sometimes if catheters are placed bilaterally.

The trigone is transected 1 cm distal to the ureteral orifices (Fig. 87–17). This is best done with **right-angle scissors** so that the incision goes perpendicular to the floor and not up

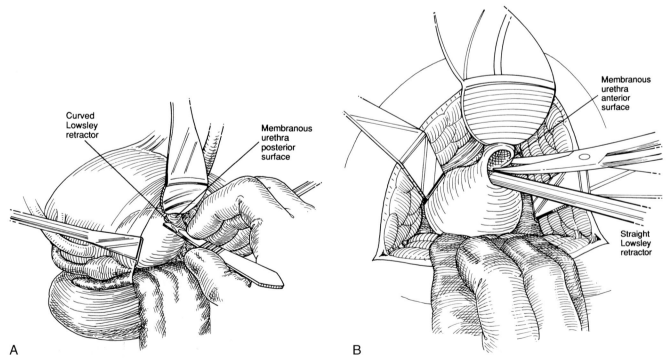

A   B

Figure 87–12. *A*, Transverse division of the posterior membranous urethra is performed distal to the apex of the prostate. Minimal lateral and anterior dissection is performed to avoid injury to the striated urethral sphincter. *B*, The anterior surface of the membranous urethra is visualized and transected following placement of the straight Lowsley retractor. (From Gibbons RP: Radical perineal prostatectomy: Definitive treatment for patients with localized prostate cancer. AUA Update Series, Volume 13, Lesson 5. AUA Office of Education, Houston, TX, 1994.)

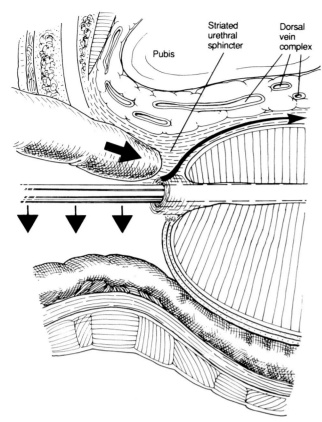

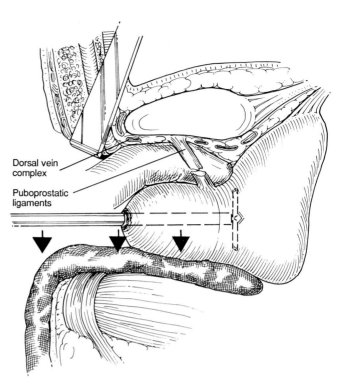

Figure 87–13. The anterior surface of the prostate is bluntly followed in the midline to the anterior bladder neck. This dissection is performed beneath the dorsal vein complex and is facilitated by applying downward pressure on the straight Lowsley retractor. If bleeding is encountered, secure with a 2–0 braided absorbable suture on a 5/8 circle needle passed toward the underside of the symphysis pubis.

Figure 87–14. The anterior bladder neck is identified by the vertically placed blade of the straight Lowsley retractor. The puboprostatic ligaments can be felt on each side of the finger where they fan out to insert on the prostate near the bladder neck and are sharply transected near their attachment to the prostate. (From Gibbons RP: Radical perineal prostatectomy: Definitive treatment for patients with localized prostate cancer. AUA Update Series, Volume 13, Lesson 5. AUA Office of Education, Houston, TX, 1994.)

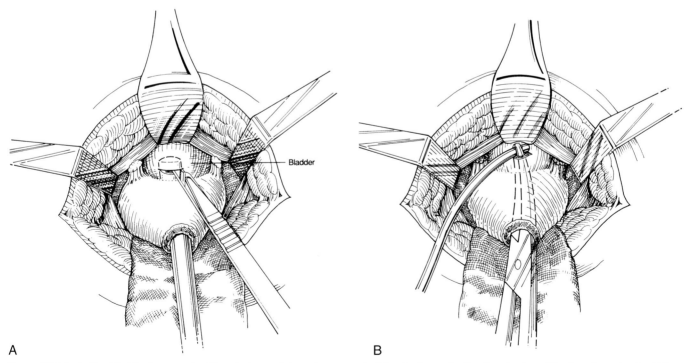

A

B

Figure 87–15. *A,* The bladder is opened at its anterior neck by a transverse incision to the vertically placed wing of the Lowsley retractor. When urine from the bladder is released, the cystotomy is bluntly expanded by spreading a right-angle clamp on each side of the exposed blade of the Lowsley retractor. *B,* A long right-angle clamp is now passed adjacent to the Lowsley retractor and grasps a No. 18 Fr red rubber catheter. Following removal of the Lowsley retractor, the red rubber catheter is brought through the prostatic urethra and used for future retraction. (From Gibbons RP: Radical perineal prostatectomy: Definitive treatment for patients with localized prostate cancer. AUA Update Series, Volume 13, Lesson 5. AUA Office of Education, Houston, TX, 1994.)

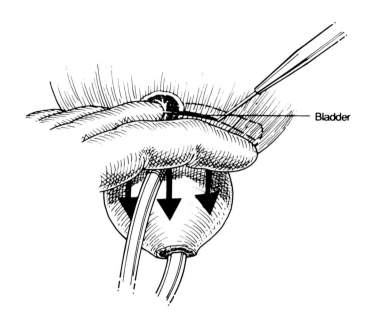

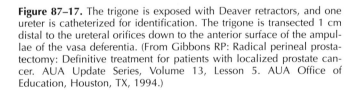

Figure 87–16. With the middle finger inside the bladder and the index-finger outside, the lateral attachments of the prostate are incised three quarters of the way around the bladder neck on both sides. (From Gibbons RP: Radical perineal prostatectomy: Definitive treatment for patients with localized prostate cancer. AUA Update Series, Volume 13, Lesson 5. AUA Office of Education, Houston, TX, 1994.)

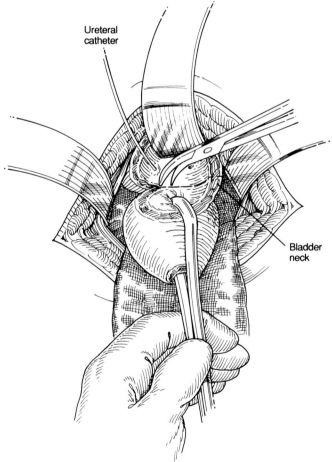

Figure 87–17. The trigone is exposed with Deaver retractors, and one ureter is catheterized for identification. The trigone is transected 1 cm distal to the ureteral orifices down to the anterior surface of the ampullae of the vasa deferentia. (From Gibbons RP: Radical perineal prostatectomy: Definitive treatment for patients with localized prostate cancer. AUA Update Series, Volume 13, Lesson 5. AUA Office of Education, Houston, TX, 1994.)

under the trigone. The incision is continued until the anterior surface of the ampullae of the vasa deferentia and seminal vesicles are identified (Fig. 87–18). These structures are bluntly separated from the overlying detrusor, and a **narrow Deaver retractor is placed beneath the trigone** to keep it elevated and provide exposure. The ampullae of the vasa are bluntly dissected with a right-angle clamp cephalad for a distance of several centimeters. This aids in the future identification and dissection of the tips of the seminal vesicles. The vasa are then transected with the cautery.

If the seminal vesicle is well visualized, it can be bluntly dissected free of its enveloping structures at this time using Russian forceps, the tip of the sucker, and cautery or small clips, as necessary. At other times, it is easier to ligate the lateral pedicles first before freeing up the seminal vesicles. This is particularly true with large prostates. Injury to the neurovascular bundles is minimized if the lateral pedicles are ligated adjacent to the prostate. However, shortening the length of the pedicle excised results in a potential risk of compromising the surgical margin (Weldon et al, 1995).

The **lateral pedicle** can be seen and palpated as a bundle of tissue lateral to the seminal vesicles. A right-angle clamp is passed beneath the pedicle lateral to the seminal vesicle. The clamp is spread to create a generous space and aid in the dissection of the seminal vesicle. A 2–0 braided absorbable ligature can then be placed in the clamp and the clamp removed (Fig. 87–19). Following ligation of the pedicle, it can be transected on the prostate side. It might take two or

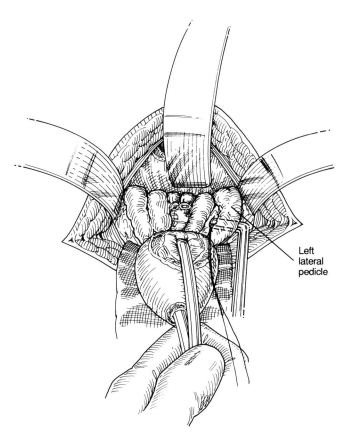

Figure 87–19. The lateral pedicles can be isolated with a right-angle clamp and ligated with 2–0 braided absorbable suture before they are incised. Injury to the neurovascular bundles is minimized if the pedicles are ligated adjacent to the prostate. The seminal vesicles can be bluntly dissected free of their enveloping structures using Russian forceps, tip of the sucker, and the cautery or small clips as necessary. If a nerve-sparing procedure is performed, the cautery is not used. (From Gibbons RP: Radical perineal prostatectomy: Definitive treatment for patients with localized prostate cancer. AUA Update Series, Volume 13, Lesson 5. AUA Office of Education, Houston, TX, 1994.)

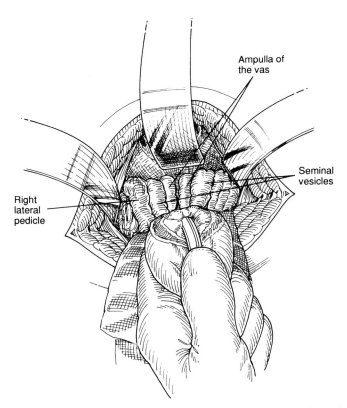

Figure 87–18. The space beneath the trigone and anterior surface of the ampullae of the vasa and seminal vesicles is bluntly developed. This is facilitated with a narrow Deaver retractor placed beneath the trigone. The vasa are bluntly dissected cephalad with a right-angle clamp to the tips of the seminal vesicles, where they are transected with the cautery. (From Gibbons RP: Radical perineal prostatectomy: Definitive treatment for patients with localized prostate cancer. AUA Update Series, Volume 13, Lesson 5. AUA Office of Education, Houston, TX, 1994.)

three such sutures to ligate completely all of the lateral pedicle tissue on each side. The specimen can be removed when the procedure has been performed bilaterally.

The operative site is inspected for any bleeding. In the unusual event that **bleeding from the dorsal vein complex** occurs, it can be controlled using 2–0 braided absorbable suture on a 5/8 circle needle passed toward the underside of the symphysis pubis.

The midline anterior and posterior walls of the bladder are identified with long Allis clamps. A No. 18 Fr urethral catheter is passed through the urethra to identify the urethral stump. The Allis clamp on the anterior bladder neck is removed, and the urethra is anastomosed to the anterior bladder neck at the 12-o'clock, 1-o'clock, and 11-o'clock positions with interrupted sutures of 2–0 braided absorbable suture with the knot tied on the outside of the lumen (Fig. 87–20A). Each suture placed should include a 3- to 4-mm portion of muscle and 1-mm segment of mucosa to reduce the formation of an anastomotic stricture. If a nerve-sparing procedure was performed, care must be exercised to avoid including the adjacent neurovascular bundle in the closing sutures.

The posterior bladder is closed with interrupted sutures of 2–0 braided absorbable suture material in a "tennis-racket"

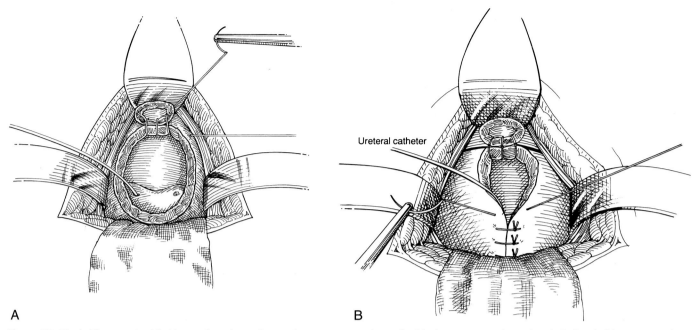

A   B

Figure 87–20. *A,* The anterior bladder neck and anterior urethra are reapproximated with three sutures of 2–0 braided absorbable suture at the 12-, 1-, and 11-o'clock positions with the knots tied outside the lumen. Each suture includes a generous portion of muscle and a 1-mm segment of mucosa. If a nerve-sparing procedure was performed, the suture must avoid the adjacent neurovascular bundle. *B,* The posterior bladder is closed in a "tennis-racquet" manner using interrupted sutures of 2–0 braided absorbable suture, avoiding the distal ureters. (From Gibbons RP: Radical perineal prostatectomy: Definitive treatment for patients with localized prostate cancer. AUA Update Series, Volume 13, Lesson 5. AUA Office of Education, Houston, TX, 1994.)

manner (Fig. 87–20*B*). During the closure of the bladder neck, the noncatheterized ureteral orifice should be observed for urine flow. Indigo carmine can be injected intravenously as an aid, if necessary. When clearly above the ureteral orifices, the ureteral catheter is removed to ensure that it has not been incorporated in a suture or the ureter otherwise damaged.

When the reanastomosis is nearly complete, a No. 20 Fr 5-ml Foley catheter is passed but not inflated. The bladder closure is completed, using a **figure-of-eight suture** placed in the manner of Jewett (Fig. 87–21) (Hodges, 1977). The 2–0 braided absorbable suture is first placed into the bladder (1) and crosses to the other side and up the urethra (2). The anterior bulb retractor is then repositioned so that the needle can incorporate tissue from the perineal membrane (3). The closure continues by reversing the course of the needle on the opposite side: perineal membrane (4), urethra (5), and bladder (6). A curved Heaney needle holder significantly aids in the placement of this suture. When the suture is tied, the urethra is broadly aligned with the adjacent bladder, with the tension on the perineal membrane fascia and bladder instead of the urethra (see Fig. 87–21—*inset*). The Foley catheter is inflated with 8 ml of saline and irrigated to ensure that there are no catheter problems, the anastomosis is watertight, and there is no significant hematuria. The wound is irrigated copiously with saline and reinspected for bleeding and rectal injury.

Two 1/4-inch Penrose drains are passed through a separate skin incision and placed on each side of the anastomosis. These are secured to the skin with 3–0 nylon sutures (Fig. 87–22*A*). The levator ani muscles are reapproximated with interrupted 2–0 braided absorbable suture. The central tendon is reapproximated with 2–0 braided absorbable suture with care taken to avoid the rectum (Fig. 87–22*B*). The dead

space is obliterated with interrupted 3–0 braided absorbable suture material, and the incision is closed with a running subcuticular 4–0 braided absorbable suture (Fig. 87–22*C*). Dressings are applied and held in place with fishnet shorts.

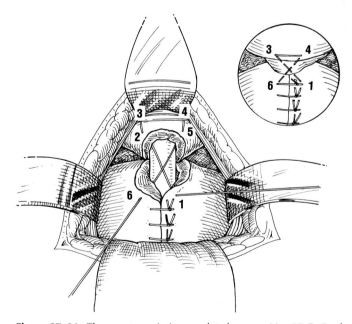

Figure 87–21. The anastomosis is completed over a No. 20 Fr 5-ml Foley catheter using a figure-of-eight suture placed in the order as diagrammed (see text). When tied, the posterior urethra is broadly coapted with the bladder with the tension away from the suture line *(inset).* (From Gibbons RP: Radical perineal prostatectomy: Definitive treatment for patients with localized prostate cancer. AUA Update Series, Volume 13, Lesson 5. AUA Office of Education, Houston, TX, 1994.)

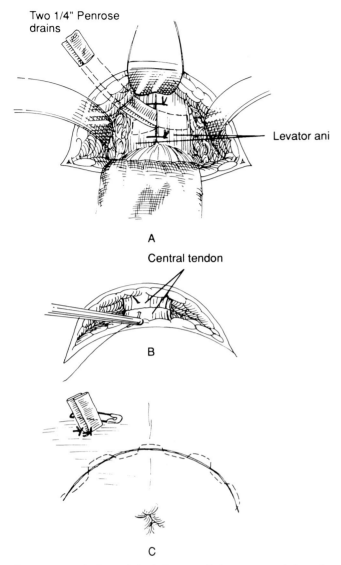

Two 1/4" Penrose drains

Levator ani

A

Central tendon

B

C

Figure 87–22. *A,* Two 1/4-inch Penrose drains are passed through a separate skin incision and levator ani muscles to the anastomosis. The levator ani muscles are reapproximated with interrupted 2–0 braided absorbable suture. *B,* The central tendon is reapproximated with care to avoid the rectum. *C,* Underlying dead space is obliterated, and the incision is closed with running subcuticular 4–0 braided absorbable suture. (From Gibbons RP: Radical perineal prostatectomy: Definitive treatment for patients with localized prostate cancer. AUA Update Series, Volume 13, Lesson 5. AUA Office of Education, Houston, TX, 1994.)

The Foley catheter is taped to the midline abdomen after shaving the hair in the appropriate location.

COMPLICATIONS

Most patients following radical perineal prostatectomy can be safely discharged on the second postoperative day. It is imperative that **patients be discharged with precise instructions** about activity, diet, pain control, bowel control, and, most important, **when to call the urologist** (e.g., if there is increased drainage, redness or swelling around the wound, chills or fever over 100°F, foul-smelling cloudy urine, increasing blood in the urine, inadequate bladder drainage, or loss of the catheter).

Rectal Injury

Rectal injuries are generally not a problem if the patient has been on a bowel preparation and the injury was noted and corrected intraoperatively (Lassen and Kearse, 1995). Injury is most likely to occur when dividing the rectourethralis muscle or establishing the plane between the rectum and prostate/seminal vesicles and **should be corrected at the time of injury** rather than delaying it to later in the procedure. The edges are freshened, and the mucosa is closed with a running suture of 4–0 braided absorbable suture turning the mucosa inward toward the lumen. A second layer of interrupted 4–0 monofilament absorbable sutures is placed in a Lembert's manner to invert the first layer. These sutures are placed approximately 4 mm apart. The proctotomy and operative site are copiously irrigated with 1 L of normal saline containing an antibiotic, such as 1 g of cefazolin sodium (Ancef). If a rectal injury has occurred, the patient is kept NPO (nothing by mouth) for 5 days following surgery and then given a soft diet for 2 days. The drain is left in for 5 days. The patient is given a stool softener but no mineral oil or other cathartic.

Inadvertent Removal of Catheter

If the catheter is inadvertently removed, a No. 18 Fr **coudé** catheter can be readily passed.

Fecal Fistula

A fecal fistula requires a diverting end-colostomy for 3 to 4 months, with careful study to be certain the fistula is closed before the colostomy is taken down. If a delayed fecal-urinary fistula occurs, this can be approached through the same perineal incision using a finger in the rectum for guidance. Both ends of the fistula are closed, and then the gracilis muscle is placed as a barrier (Ryan et al, 1985). A suprapubic tube is placed. A voiding cystourethrogram is performed via the suprapubic tube in 2 to 3 weeks, and the catheter is removed at that time if the fistula is closed.

Urinary Incontinence

Urinary incontinence can take 3 weeks to 3 months to resolve. Kegel exercises might be helpful. Some patients with a prolonged but small amount of stress urinary incontinence benefit from an alpha-adrenergic agonist, for example, pseudoephedrine hydrochloride (Sudafed) 60 mg every 4 to 6 hours, as necessary. Any type of penile clamp or condom catheter is to be avoided for the first 6 months. If the patient has significant incontinence after this interval, a penile clamp or artificial urinary sphincter should be considered. Incontinence of this severity was noted in 3% of patients surveyed by confidential third-party mail questionnaire.

Urinary Retention

If urinary retention occurs within a day or so of removal of the catheter, simply replace a No. 20 Fr coudé catheter for another week. If this is a delayed problem, the patient requires cystoscopy and probable urethral dilation of an anastomotic stricture. If this is a persistent problem, dilation under anesthesia followed by self-balloon dilation on a daily basis for 6 weeks should be considered. A direct vision internal urethrotomy often results in incontinence.

Impotence

These patients usually do not have an impaired sensation of orgasm. If erectile impotence is a problem beyond 3 months following surgery, the patient is started on a pharmacologic erection program or vacuum erection device. If this is a permanent problem, the patient can consider a penile prosthesis if he is not satisfied with the aforementioned treatments.

SUMMARY

"Because of the precision of approach, accuracy of hemostasis, visual control at all stages, ready adaptation to individual anatomic variations, large reduction in shock, rapidity of healing, and shortness of hospitalization," a radical perineal prostatectomy is an effective surgical procedure with many benefits. These advantages are as true today as when first written by Belt (Belt, 1939). The perineal approach represents another example of "minimal invasive surgery," and there is **an increasing number of patients with small, nonpalpable tumors detected only by a rising PSA in whom this is an appropriate treatment option.**

REFERENCES

Belt E, Ebert CE, Surber AC Jr: A new anatomic approach in perineal prostatectomy. J Urol 1939; 41:482–497.

Bishoff JT, Reyes A, Thompson IM, et al: Pelvic lymphadenectomy can be omitted in selected patients with carcinoma of the prostate: Development of a system of patient selection. Urology 1995; 45:270–274.

Bluestein DL, Bostwick DG, Bergstralh EJ, Oesterling JE: Eliminating the need for bilateral pelvic lymphadenectomy in select patients with prostate cancer. J Urol 1994; 151:1315–1320.

Carroll PR, Lue TF, Narayan P, Tanagho EA: Impotence and incontinence after radical prostatectomy: Pathophysiology and management. In DeVita VT, Hellman S, Rosenberg SA, eds: Important Advances in Oncology. Philadelphia, J.B. Lippincott, 1989, pp 161–180.

Danella JF, deKernion J, Smith RB, Steckel J: A contemporary incidence of lymph node metastases in prostate cancer: Implications for laparoscopic lymph node dissection. J Urol 1993; 149:1488–1491.

Elder JS, Gibbons RP, Correa RJ Jr, Brandon GE: Morbidity of radical perineal prostatectomy following transurethral resection of the prostate. J Urol 1984; 132:55–57.

Epstein JI, Pizov G, Walsh PC: Correlation of pathologic findings with progression after radical retropubic prostatectomy. Cancer 1993; 71: 3582–3593.

Epstein JI, Walsh PC, Carmichael M, Brendler CB: Pathologic and clinical findings to predict tumor extent of nonpalpable (stage T11c) prostate cancer. JAMA 1994; 271:368–374.

Gibbons RP, Correa RJ Jr, Brannon GE, Weissman RM: Total prostatectomy for clinically localized prostatic cancer: Long-term results. J Urol 1989; 141:564–566.

Hodges CV: Vesicourethral anastomosis after radical prostatectomy: Experience with the Jewett modification. J Urol 1977; 118:209–210.

Hudson PB, Lilien OM: Perineal surgery for benign conditions of the prostate. In Droller MJ, ed: Surgical Management of Urologic Disease. St. Louis, Mosby-Year Book, 1992, pp 713–719.

Lassen PM, Kearse WS Jr: Rectal injuries during radical perineal prostatectomy. Urology 1995; 45:266–279.

Myers RP: Male urethral sphincteric anatomy and radical prostatectomy. Urol Clin North Am 1991; 18:211–227.

Myers RP, Goellner JR, Cahill DR: Prostate shape, external striated urethral sphincter in radical prostatectomy: The apical dissection. J Urol 1987; 138:543–550.

Narayan P, Fournier G, Gajendran V, et al: Utility of preoperative serum prostate-specific antigen concentration and biopsy Gleason score in predicting risk of pelvic lymph node metastases in prostate cancer. Urology 1994; 44:519–524.

Partin AW, Yoo J, Carter HB, et al: The use of prostate-specific antigen, clinical stage and Gleason score to predict pathological stage in men with localized prostate cancer. J Urol 1993; 150:110–115.

Paulson DF: Impact of radical prostatectomy in the management of clinically localized disease. J Urol 1994; 152(suppl):1826–1830.

Petros JA, Catalona WJ: Lower incidence of unsuspected lymph node metastases in 521 consecutive patients with clinically localized prostate cancer. J Urol 1992; 147:1574–1575.

Reiner WJ, Walsh PC: An anatomical approach to the surgical management of the dorsal vein and Santorini's plexus during radical retropubic surgery. J Urol 1979; 121:198–200.

Ryan JA Jr, Gibbons RP, Correa RJ Jr: Urologic use of gracilis muscle flap for nonhealing perineal wounds and fistulas. Urology 1985; 26:456–459.

Tobin CE, Benjamin JA: Anatomical and surgical restudy of Denonvilliers' fascia. Surg Gynecol Obstet 1945; 80:373–388.

Villers A, McNeal JE, Freiha FS, et al: Invasion of Denonvilliers' fascia in radical prostatectomy specimens. J Urol 1993; 149:793–798.

Walsh PC, Donker PJ: Impotence following radical prostatectomy: Insight into etiology and prevention. J Urol 1982; 128:492–497.

Walsh PC, Epstein JI, Lowe FC: Potency following radical prostatectomy with wide excision of the neurovascular bundle. J Urol 1987; 138:823–827.

Walsh PC, Lepor H, Eggleston JC: Radical prostatectomy with preservation of sexual function: Anatomical and pathological considerations. Prostate 1983; 4:473–475.

Weldon VE: Extended radical perineal prostatectomy: An anatomical and surgical study (Abstract). J Urol 1988; 139:448a.

Weldon VE: Radical perineal prostatectomy. In Das S, Crawford ED, eds: Cancer of the Prostate. New York, Marcel Dekker, 1993, pp 225–266.

Weldon VE, Tavel FR: Potency-sparing radical perineal prostatectomy: Anatomy, surgical technique and initial results. J Urol 1988; 140:559–562.

Weldon VE, Tavel FR, Neuwirth H, Cohen R: Patterns of positive specimen margins and detectable prostate-specific antigen after radical perineal prostatectomy. J Urol 1995; 153:1565–1569.

Young HH: The early diagnosis and radical cure of carcinoma of the prostate: Being a study of 40 cases and presentation of a radical operation which was carried out in four cases. Johns Hopkins Hosp Bull 1905; 16:315–321.

88
RADIOTHERAPY AND CRYOTHERAPY FOR PROSTATE CANCER

Arthur T. Porter, M.D.
Peter Littrup, M.D.
David Grignon, M.D.
Jeffrey Forman, M.D.
James E. Montie, M.D.

RADIOTHERAPY FOR PROSTATE CANCER

History

Radiotherapy, or the use of ionizing radiation to destroy malignant tissue, has proved its usefulness in the treatment of many cancers and has a significant role to play in the management of genitourinary malignancies. In essence, radiation is effective at a cellular level by causing both single-strand and double-strand breaks within the DNA of a malignant cell. This leads to a loss of the reproductive integrity of the cell (i.e., it cannot divide and therefore ages naturally and dies).

Radiation can be naturally produced using gamma radiation of certain naturally occurring isotopes, such as cobalt 60, or it can be artificially produced. Artificially produced radiation includes the use of isotopes such as strontium 89, which is produced by bombarding inactive strontium with neutrons, and external radiation, which is generally produced using linear accelerators and represents the most common way radiation is delivered today. The linear accelerator is, in effect, a tube into which electrons are injected, are allowed to accelerate on a radiofrequency carrier wave, and then are forced to impact on a target, which converts their energy to x-rays or photons. The energy produced by the linear accelerator is variable and can be much higher than the energy (1.25 MeV) produced by cobalt 60 machines. **Energy is important in radiotherapy because the higher the energy, the deeper the penetration in tissue, allowing better beam characteristics for treating deep tumors such as prostate cancer.**

The second important physical requirement of the delivery of radiation involves treatment planning, or the arrangement of several beams of x-rays, to deliver as homogeneous a dose as achievable across the defined tumor volume with the lowest possible dose everywhere else, especially to those organs whose tolerance to radiation is low. Often computed tomography (CT) and the instillation of contrast materials into body cavities are used to help delineate the tumor and the surrounding normal tissues. Lead or lead substitute materials may be fabricated to allow the treatment-projected volume to conform to the volume of the tumor.

Other than the physics of getting radiation to the tumor with the least amount anywhere else, another important factor is the biology of the interaction of the radiation and different tissues. This underlies the reason for fractionation of radiation, in which the goal is to exploit differing repair characteristics of tumor and nontumor tissue. **Most external beam radiotherapy schedules employ doses of 180 to 200 cGy given daily. A dose between 4500 and 5000 cGy is generally thought to sterilize micrometastases, and doses of 6500 to 7500 cGy may be needed to treat bulky disease.**

Radiation Therapy—Treatment

Early-Stage Prostate Cancer

The overall goal of treatment for early-stage prostate cancer (stage T1-T2) is the attainment of cure of disease without the introduction of complications. The treatment of early-stage prostate cancer is controversial for several reasons. There are a wide variety of available therapies; there is a high incidence of comorbidity by virtue of age and overall general health of this population subgroup; and there is the recognition of substantial heterogeneity of disease evolution, progression, and impact within the spectrum of early-stage prostate cancer.

Since the 1960s, an accepted treatment for early-stage disease has been radiotherapy using the mechanism of ionizing radiation damage causing the loss of reproductive integrity of individual cells and tumor regression (Bagshaw et al, 1994). Many other treatment options have been explored. Radical prostatectomy has been increasingly offered as an option in patients with intracapsular tumor who are also surgical candidates (Epstein et al, 1993); however, as many have emphasized, truly valid comparisons of treatment options are lacking (Catalona, 1994).

The selection of treatment for patients with potentially curable prostate cancer is an exceedingly important health care issue. An estimated 240,000 new cases of prostate cancer were expected for 1995 (Boring et al, 1994), and the number of deaths expected are estimated at 40,000. Currently, more than 80% of cases are diagnosed in men over the age of 65. With improvements in early detection, younger men with clinically important cancer may be expected to be diagnosed in more curable stages.

Treatment decisions have become even more difficult because of the finding that in selected groups of patients all available treatment options, including no treatment, result in a survival rate that is comparable to that seen in the general population (Johansson et al, 1992; Adolfsson et al, 1994). The concept of "watchful waiting" appears to be an important option for many patients with prostate cancer and adds to the oncologic conundrum of determining which patients are best treated with more radical therapies and whether those therapies will result in desirable cure/complication probabilities.

RETROSPECTIVE DATABASE

The analysis of retrospective data for early-stage prostate cancer is fraught with difficulty. When patients are counseled that there is an equal chance of cure with radiation and surgery, a number of assumptions with regard to comparison of results are made. In fact, radiotherapy and surgical series are incomparable and cannot generally be matched in terms of prognostic indicators.

In surgical series, the patients have tended to be younger, be fitter, and have smaller tumors. In radiotherapy series, the patients have most often been "deselected" as noncandidates for surgery. Also, radiotherapy patients tend not to be surgically staged. Obviously an error would be made if one were to compare a group of pathologically staged T2aN0 patients with a clinically staged group of T2aNx radiation therapy patients. **If in a hypothetical series of patients, 50% of the clinical T2a patients may be expected to show capsular penetration (pathologic T3) after surgery, and a low local failure rate (say 5%) among those not upstaged must be understood in this context. An identical patient group receiving radiation treatment might exhibit a 30% positive postradiation biopsy rate. Among those achieving negative biopsy results, an additional 25% could ultimately fail. Considering the presence of positive margins, positive postradiation biopsy results, and frank local failure all to be iterations of overall treatment nonsuccess, there is substantial comparability between the outcomes resulting from radiotherapy and surgery.**

Numerous single-institution reports of radiotherapy series of early-stage prostate cancer have been published. Results from four centers are summarized in Table 88–1. The Stanford University experience was updated with 25 years' follow-up. Sufficient time has elapsed for these patients' failures to be documented clinically (i.e., without prostate-specific antigen [PSA]). The 773 patients with negative lymph nodes had a 15-year survival of 53%. Importantly, there was no evidence of any increased failure rate in the second decade of follow-up.

Long-term results from the M. D. Anderson Hospital (Zagars et al, 1988) and Washington University (Perez et al, 1988) are also available (see Table 88–1). The 5- and 10-year overall survivals and disease-free survivals from these centers are good and compare favorably with surgery. Even though these data sets were collected over lengthy periods of time, however, they suffer from not using PSA and other more modern technology in their assessment.

Table 88–1. RADIOTHERAPY FOR EARLY-STAGE PROSTATE CANCER: SINGLE INSTITUTION DATA

	SU	MDACC	MDACC	MIR	MIR	NTI
Number	773	114	82	41	185	197
Stage	T1-2N0	A-B	B	A2	B	T1-T2b
5-year*	85	89	93 (89)	(78)	(76)	(95)
10-year	65	68	70 (85)	(60)	(56)	
15-year	45					

*Overall survival is shown with disease-free survivals in parentheses.
SU, Stanford University; MDACC, M. D. Anderson Cancer Center; MIR, Mallinkrodt Institute of Radiology; NTI, Northwest Tumor Institute (^{125}I implant data).

PROSPECTIVE TRIALS AND DATABASES

Hanks and colleagues have re-examined the Patterns of Care Study (PCS), conducted by the American College of Radiology, and Radiation Therapy Oncology Group (RTOG) prostate cancer databases (Hanks et al, 1994). The RTOG has performed prospective, randomized studies of early prostate cancer, and the PCS patients are developed from a large survey using on-site chart review. For both PCS and RTOG patients with T1Nx (unknown nodal status) disease, there was no difference between treated patients and the expected survival for age-matched controls with 15 years' follow-up. Five- and 10-year survivals for T1Nx PCS patients (Table 88–2) were about 85% and 60%.

For patients with T2Nx disease in the 1973 and 1978 PCS studies, the 5- and 10-year survivals were 75% and 45% (see Table 88–2). For T1BN0 and T2N0 patients in RTOG 7706, the 5- and 10-year survivals were 87% and 63%, respectively (see Table 88–2), and greater than the expected survivals for age-matched patients (i.e., they were able to tolerate lymphadenectomy). This (select) group of patients is most comparable with prostatectomy candidates.

The only randomized trial comparing radiation with radical prostatectomy was done by the Veterans Administration Uro-Oncology Research Group (Paulson et al, 1982b). **This trial of 97 patients has been widely criticized. The randomization was flawed, many patients did not receive the treatment to which they were randomized, and the radiotherapy results were poor. Only 59% 5-year freedom from recurrence was found** (see Table 88–2). Although this study attempted to conclude that the case for the superiority of radical prostatectomy had been successfully developed, there was sufficient skepticism in the uro-oncologic community that the National Cancer Institute (NCI) sanctioned an intergroup study to compare radical surgery and radical radiotherapy. Statistical considerations required that more than 1000 patients be entered to answer the question. Unfortunately, this study closed prematurely because of inadequate patient entry.

Clinical end points considered previously (e.g., actuarial overall survival, disease-free survival) are straightforward and have been in use for many years. In general, they remain the most relevant clinical end points. Their weaknesses lie in the fact that many years must pass for results to mature, and in this situation these end points are confounded by the comorbidity that is prevalent in this cohort of patients. In the area of prostate cancer, clinicians are confronted with new end points, including biochemical (PSA) and histologic (margin positivity and postradiation biopsy positivity) indices. What implications does this shift in emphasis have?

From the work of Zietman and colleagues among others, it is becoming evident that initial PSA levels exceeding 15 ng/ml are associated with poor outcome and may not represent early-stage disease (Zietman et al, 1994). Thus, to compare treatment groups, it is necessary to stratify according to presenting PSA levels as well as tumor stage and histologic differentiation. Subsequently the results of treatment may be assessed biochemically. **Just as PSA should be undetectable after radical prostatectomy, patients with PSA nadir levels below 1.0 ng/ml after radiation therapy are considered to have a low probability of postradiation clinical failure.** The choice of end points may lead to selection bias and outcome bias.

EXTERNAL-BEAM RADIOTHERAPY TECHNIQUES

Although basic principles have not changed, the techniques of radiation treatment are rapidly evolving. The advantages of using multiple daily fields (or moving fields), adequate machine energy (>10 MV), and cast blocks are now well established. Proper simulation (including retrograde urethrogram) and assessment of day-to-day reproducibility (port films) have reduced the probability of marginal miss. Although most centers use conventional simulation, the recent literature supports reduced complications using three-dimensional conformal treatment planning (Mesina et al, 1994).

Debate continues with regard to the treatment or nontreatment of pelvic lymph nodes using radiotherapy. Either policy can be defended. Two randomized trials (RTOG 7506 and 7706) showed no difference with elective nodal radiation in stages A2, B, or C but did not prove or disprove the value of the treatment (Hanks et al, 1991). For example, in RTOG 7706, only 4% of patients could actually have been expected to harbor microscopic disease without distant metastasis (N + M0) and therefore benefit from nodal treatment. It may be possible to predict the approximate risk of pelvic lymph node involvement by using PSA, Gleason sum, and clinical stage (Roach et al, 1994) and then to omit pelvic irradiation in patients identified as low risk. At Wayne State University, greater than 95% of early-stage prostate treatments are designed using a CT image–based three-dimensional conformal planning system. Initially, beam apertures that include the

Table 88–2. PROSPECTIVE TRIALS OF RADIOTHERAPY FOR EARLY-STAGE PROSTATE CANCER

	PCS* 1973	PCS 1978	PCS 1973	PCS 1978	RTOG 7706† N0	RTOG 7706§ Nx	UOG XRT‡ N0
Number	60	312	115	381	104	40	56
Stage	T1Nx	T2Nx	T1Nx	T2Nx	T1b-T2	T1b-T2	A2-B
5-year* OS	84	75	85	74	87	76	594
10-year OS	54	46	63	43	63		
15-year OS	40	22					

*A national Patterns of Care Survey using on-site chart review and randomized selection of facilities and of patients within a facility.
†Data from RTOG 7706 for patients with pathologically negative lymph nodes (N0) or unknown lymph node status are shown.
‡Data from the Uro-Oncology Group trial radiotherapy arm.
§Five-year freedom from recurrence was reported.
 OS, Overall survival.

prostate and seminal vesicles (with a 1.5-cm margin) and four axial fields are treated using 15 MV photons, to a total dose of 4500 cGy at 180 cGy per day. The subsequent boost to the prostate is 2000 cGy to 2400 cGy in 200-cGy fractions. Either axial (four-field box) or nonaxial four-field techniques are used for the boost (Mesina et al, 1994).

TREATMENT-ASSOCIATED SEQUELAE

Acute effects of radiation to the pelvis are generally self-limiting and mainly include diarrhea, rectal irritation, dysuria, and frequency. An overall chronic complication rate of 5% or less can be expected with external beam radiation of the prostate. These late sequelae include chronic rectal and bladder injury, enteritis, impotence, urethral stricture, and incontinence. The PCS showed a 3.5% major complication rate at doses below 7000 cGy. A literature review of 2611 radiotherapy patients (all stages) showed 0.2% treatment-related mortality, 1.9% severe complications, and 0.9% incontinence (Shipley et al, 1994b). Thirty percent to 60% of patients maintained potency. Of 331 patients with stages T1-T2 tumors, 0% mortality, 0% severe complications, 0.4% incontinence, 5.4% strictures (1.2% persisting), 5.1% hematuria (0.9% persisting), and 5.4% rectal bleeding (0.6% persisting) were noted.

ROLE OF RADIOACTIVE ISOTOPE IMPLANTATION

Brachytherapy, or the implantation of radioactive isotopes, can theoretically deliver more radiation to the prostate with less dose to the surrounding normal organs than conventional radiation (Blasko et al, 1993). Higher intraprostatic dose may result in effective tumor sterilization with fewer complications. Permanent radioactive iodine (^{125}I) implants popularized in the 1970s were based on an open retropubic procedure with seeds placed after lymphadenectomy. The 5-year survival rates were encouraging, but the 10-year results were poor, most likely owing to inhomogeneous dose distributions and disadvantageous radiobiologic effects in treating higher-grade tumors (Fuks et al, 1991).

Improvements in methods (introduction of new radioisotopes, afterloading, computer dosimetry, and modern imaging) may enable brachytherapy to re-emerge as an effective modality. High clinical local control rates have been reported at the Northwest Tumor Institute (see Table 88–1) (Porter et al, 1995).

NEOADJUVANT HORMONES AND DOSE ESCALATION

Neoadjuvant hormonal cytoreduction is recommended for patients with large glands, because the volume of normal bladder and rectum irradiated decreases significantly with the downsizing of the prostate target volume (Forman et al, 1995). Hormonal therapy is also cytotoxic to prostate cancer cells, and neoadjuvant hormone treatment has been shown in RTOG 8610 to improve local control and disease-free survival in patients with locally advanced prostate cancer (Pilepich et al, 1993).

There is reason to believe that the advantages of cytoreduction of tumors may still be valid in early-stage disease. Current national protocols are ongoing. Interest in dose escalation is currently under investigation at several centers and

is based on the rationale that there appears to be a volume-dependent dose-response curve for prostate cancer above 7000 cGy (Hanks et al, 1988). Because a significant proportion of patients continue to have local recurrence after receiving standard radiation, doses of up to 8000 to 8100 cGy using three-dimensional conformal radiotherapy (3D-CRT) have been delivered at the Memorial Sloan-Kettering Cancer Center and at Wayne State University (Forman et al, 1993b).

Locally Advanced Prostate Cancer

The situation for locally advanced prostate cancer is somewhat different. **It is now recognized that the outcome after external beam radiotherapy using standard doses is low, with 10-year survivals ranging from 15% to 30%** (Cox and Stoffel, 1977; Harisiadis et al, 1978; Bruce et al, 1979; Rosen et al, 1985; Zagars et al, 1987; Perez et al, 1988; Crook et al, 1993). It is also recognized that there is a dose-response relationship between prostate tumor volume and radiation dose (Hanks, 1985). It has been further shown that as the volume of tumor increases, so does the probability of obtaining a positive biopsy result 18 to 24 months after therapy (Forman et al, 1993a; Freiha and Bagshaw, 1984). This probability, in some part, is related to the limitation of the radiation dose that can be achieved in the prostate without exceeding late-reacting normal tissue tolerance—for example, that of the rectal mucosa and the bladder. Therefore, the approach to the treatment of patients with stage T3-T4 prostate cancer must involve a knowledge of the natural history of the disease and of the potentials of the modality that is being used.

Two major concerns are present in the treatment of stage T3-T4 prostate cancer. The first is that of the bulk or volume of tumor present locally and the second, the propensity for occult metastatic disease as evidenced by pre-existing nodal involvement. Can radiation therapy be modified so as to attempt to tackle these two effects to the benefit of the patient? Concerning the bulk or volume of tumor, there is a second premise that has to be accepted: that improved local control ultimately results in improved survival (Kurth et al, 1977; Scardino et al, 1986; Kuban et al, 1987; Fuks et al, 1991; Kuban et al, 1992; Prestidge et al, 1992; Prestidge et al, 1994). What methods are therefore available for improving the effect of radiotherapy on bulky disease?

There are three major modifications that can be undertaken:

1. **Increasing the relative integral dose.**
2. **Decreasing the volume of tumor present.**
3. **Radiobiologic optimization.**

INCREASING THE RELATIVE INTEGRAL DOSE

One can increase the relative integral dose, or the dose that the tumor receives versus the dose received by the surrounding normal tissues, by using one of three means: conformal external beam radiotherapy, proton therapy, and brachytherapy.

Data in the literature now suggest that by conforming the beam shape to the tumor by the integration of complex three-dimensional treatment planning, it is possible to deliver

higher doses of radiation to the tumor without additional toxicity to the late-reacting normal tissues, and therefore, theoretically, the possibility exists to sterilize larger tumors (Sandler et al, 1991; Simpson et al, 1991; Forman et al, 1993b; Leibel et al, 1993). Forman and co-workers have demonstrated that doses of 7800 cGy can be effectively given, and early results suggest an improvement in histologic local control over historical values (Forman et al, 1993b; Leibel et al, 1993).

Proton radiotherapy, by virtue of the physics of dose distribution inherent in a proton beam, also allows the development of exceptionally conformed radiotherapy volumes, and a phase III trial is being undertaken in stage T3-T4 prostate cancer by the Massachusetts General Hospital Group (Shipley et al, 1994a).

The modality that has been most tested to achieve an enhanced relative integral dose in prostate cancer is brachytherapy, in which isotopes are placed directly into the prostate to achieve high doses (Porter and Forman, 1993). The results of brachytherapy have been confused because of the variability in the brachytherapy techniques and isotopes that have been employed (Porter, 1990). Isotopes such as ^{125}I used in a permanent implant situation, although having excellent radioprotection properties, have been associated, owing to their low energy and low dose rate, with poor efficacy in the treatment of rapidly dividing prostate cancer cells (Fuks et al, 1991). The best data in terms of sterilization of tumor have been those reported after temporary iridium 192 implant. Using these techniques, many workers have reported local control rates, confirmed by biopsy, of 70% to 90% in stage T3 prostate cancer (Martinez et al, 1985; Puthawala et al, 1985; Donnelly et al, 1991). Morbidity using these techniques, however, has been high, with damage to the rectal wall and to the bladder neck being common in early reported series.

HORMONAL CYTOREDUCTION

A further way of optimizing radiation therapy is to reduce the bulk of tumor present, using hormonal cytoreduction (Porter and Venner, 1990). **There have been several phase II studies that have suggested that hormonal cytoreduction before radiotherapy may improve local control. Two major phase III trials have been undertaken to validate these data. The Canadian Androcur Study (CDN/89/AND/1) has evaluated large-volume prostate cancer stratified by stage, grade, and surgical staging; randomized patients to receive immediate radiotherapy to a dose of 6500 cGy or to receive 12 weeks of cyproterone acetate 100 mg three times a day followed by radiotherapy; and then evaluated local control, PSA disease-free survival, and survival as end points. All patients entered in this study undergo a biopsy at 18 months to evaluate histologic control as an objective criterion. This study has not yet reported its findings** (Porter and Forman, 1994).

The RTOG has also reported a study (RTOG 86-10) in which patients with stage C (T3) prostate cancer were randomized to receive cytoreduction using goserelin 3.6 mg every 4 weeks and flutamide 250 mg three times a day for 3 months and then to receive radiation therapy to a dose of 6500 cGy or greater versus radical radiotherapy alone. A 3-

year interim analysis now demonstrates, with 255 patients eligible, a significant improvement in digitally evaluated local control in the group receiving the cytoreduction (84% versus 71%, P = .003) and significant improvements in the disease-free survival for patients again treated with the cytoreduction before radiotherapy. The disease-free survival rates without taking PSA into account were 61% and 43% (P = .0014), and when taking PSA into account and accepting a value of greater than 4.0 as being evidence of disease progression, disease-free survival rates of 46% and 26% (P = .0001) were identified (Pilepich et al, 1993; Porter and Forman, 1994).

Clearly, these data suggest that cytoreduction plus radiotherapy may be the preferential way to use radiation therapy in bulky prostate cancer disease, and, in fact, the RTOG has incorporated cytoreduction plus radiotherapy as the standard arm of their current study, RTOG 92-02, in which 2 years of adjuvant goserelin is being evaluated after optimal local therapy in a phase III study.

RADIOBIOLOGIC OPTIMIZATION

There are three major ways in which radiotherapy can be optimized by altering the radiobiologic parameters: altered fractionation, use of radiosensitizers, or neutron radiotherapy. There have now been two studies conducted using neutron therapy, taking advantage of the ability of neutrons to have an enhanced killing effect on hypoxic cells and a reduced variation in biologic effect across the cell cycle. **The RTOG and the Neutron Therapy Cooperative Working Group have now reported on a trial, 77-04, in which patients with bulky prostatic cancer were randomized to receive a mixed beam of photons and neutrons to a dose of 7000 cGy in 7 weeks or photons alone to 7000 cGy in 7 weeks. At 5 years, a significant difference in absolute survival of 70% versus 53% in favor of the mixed beam arm occurred, and this difference has been maintained at 10 years with survivals of 46% and 29% (P = .03). In terms of clinical, local, and regional control, there is a difference between the two groups in favor of the mixed beam arm of 85% and 62% at 5 years and of 70% and 56% at 10 years. This is one of the first phase III studies that have demonstrated a systemic survival effect on the basis of a change in local control in prostate cancer** (Griffin et al, 1988).

A second study has been performed using a pure neutron beam and comparing this to a photon beam. Patients were randomized to receive neutron therapy of 2040 cGy in 12 fractions over 4 weeks versus 7000-cGy photons in 35 fractions over 7 weeks. These data, which have been reported only at 3 years, do not yet show a significant difference in terms of survival but already show a difference in local regional tumor control in favor of the neutron-only arm that has reached statistical significance (Russell et al, 1993).

It is likely that many of these approaches to the treatment of large-volume disease may be used in conjunction with one another to optimize further the use of radiation in this disease. Forman and colleagues have demonstrated that neutrons can now be given using conformal techniques with three-dimensional treatment planning, which allows dose distributions of neutron- and photon-mixed beams to be

similar to those achieved with the best of photon planning (Forman et al, 1995). Of course, with larger-volume disease, there is also a greater probability of lymph node involvement and occult metastatic spread. Clearly, when treating this systemic disease, systemic remedies, such as adjuvant hormonal therapy, are needed.

Radiation Therapy—Pathology

Effects on Normal Prostate Tissue

The histologic changes induced in the normal tissues of the prostate gland by radiation therapy have been well described (Bostwick et al, 1982; Dhom and Degro, 1982; Siders and Lee, 1993). There is atrophy of normal glands with reduced numbers of acini and decreased gland diameters. The cytoplasm of the secretory epithelial cells is reduced in amount and stains more intensely amphophilic or basophilic. The nuclei generally are small and pyknotic; however, in some cells, they are enlarged and hyperchromatic with occasional nucleoli. The degree of cytologic atypia induced in normal glands is greater than in the neoplastic ones (Fig. 88–1) (Siders and Lee, 1993). Squamous metaplasia has been reported (Bostwick et al, 1982). The basal cells are typically small and shrunken, making their identification even more difficult than in normal tissues.

The fibromuscular stroma shows characteristic changes, including fibrosis with occasional atypical fibroblasts. There is intimal proliferation; luminal narrowing; and accumulation of foamy, lipid-laden macrophages in blood vessels (Bostwick et al, 1982).

The atypia in atrophic benign glands can result in major problems in differentiating benign glands from residual carcinoma. The application of basal cell–specific high-molecular-weight cytokeratin antibodies can be of great utility in this distinction (Brawer et al, 1989).

Effects on Prostate Cancer Tissue

Prostate cancer glands show highly variable treatment-related alterations between different patients and even within the same patient (Dhom and Degro, 1982). Typical changes

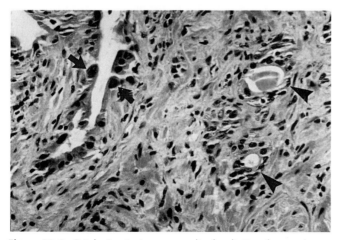

Figure 88–1. Cytologic atypia as a result of radiation therapy in normal glands.

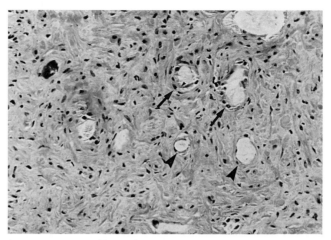

Figure 88–2. No visible nuclei are evident in prostate cancer glands as a result of radiation therapy.

include a decrease in the number and size of the malignant glands. Nuclei become irregular in size and shape with hyperchromasia; nucleoli may be absent or continue to be prominent. In the most severely affected yet still identifiable tumor cells, the cytoplasm is greatly increased in amount with or without vacuolization. This increase may result in the cells' appearing to have only cytoplasm without visible nuclei (Fig. 88–2). Paneth-like cells may also be prominent (Siders and Lee, 1993).

The net effect of these alterations can result in changes in the interpretation of histologic grade. Bostwick and associates reported a change in the Gleason score of 2 or greater in 7 of 26 biopsy specimens (27%) (Bostwick et al, 1982). **Siders and Lee (1993) found a significant increase in the Gleason score after radiation therapy. In the majority of instances, this increase reflects the application of Gleason scoring to treated cancer; a case with minimal residual tumor having marked therapy effects consists of isolated single cells, a Gleason grade 5 (score 10) pattern. It is unlikely that this reflects a dedifferentiation phenomenon but is more an artifact of grading** (Grignon and Sakr, 1995).

Patients with clinical local recurrence after radiation therapy frequently are of a much higher grade (Wheeler et al, 1993). In a study of 49 locally recurrent cancers (9–253 months after completion of radiation therapy), Wheeler and colleagues concluded that this was most consistent with progression through clonal evolution (Wheeler et al, 1993).

Clinical Significance of Positive Biopsy Results

There has been considerable controversy over the frequency and the significance of positive postradiation therapy biopsy results. Reported positive rates have ranged from 20% (Forman et al, 1993a) to 93% (Kabalin et al, 1989), with most series having numbers in the 50% to 60% range (Mollenkamp et al, 1975; Kurth et al, 1977; Kiesling et al, 1980). Several factors, including patient selection, biopsy strategy, time after radiation therapy, and type of radiation therapy, could influence the results obtained (Hanks, 1985). The potential for false-positive or false-negative results ow-

ing to pathologic interpretation has for the most part not been considered.

In some early reports, it was argued that biopsy results were not predictive of outcome (Cox and Stoffel, 1977). With the results of many more studies available, **it is now clear that the presence of tumor after completion of therapy correlates with an increased risk for local recurrence** (Scardino et al, 1986; Miller et al, 1993), **distant metastases** (Kurth et al, 1977; Kiesling et al, 1980; Miller et al, 1993; Freiha and Bagshaw, 1984), **and death from prostate cancer** (Scardino et al, 1986; Freiha and Bagshaw, 1984). A number of issues remain unresolved in the interpretation of postradiation therapy biopsy results. Early investigators observed a reduced frequency of positive biopsy results with increased time following completion of radiotherapy (Mollenkamp et al, 1975; Cox and Stoffel, 1977; Bostwick et al, 1982), although this was not universally found (Nachtsheim et al, 1978; Bruce et al, 1979). This observation was interpreted as indicating that tumors continued to regress for 6 to 12 months after the completion of treatment.

In a report on postradiation therapy biopsies in 100 consecutive patients, a group of 21 patients with initial positive biopsy results (Crook et al, 1993) subsequently had negative biopsy results. None of these patients had relapsed clinically or by serum PSA at the time of the report; this tends to support the earlier observation. It is also clear that there is a subset of patients with positive postradiation therapy biopsy results who do not show evidence of progression. In the report of Scardino and colleagues, 34% of patients with positive biopsy results showed no evidence of local progression (Scardino et al, 1986). Dhom and Degro (1982) and Schellhammer and co-workers (1980) have proposed systems to grade therapy effects. Patients treated by radiation therapy or with estrogens were followed by Dhom and Degro (1982) with repeat biopsies over time, and different patterns of therapy response were identified; to date, these changes have not been correlated with failure. In this regard, Crook and associates used antibody against proliferating cell nuclear antigen (PCNA) immunostaining to identify positive postradiation therapy biopsy results from 83 patients; PCNA-positive tumors had a significantly higher progression rate than those that were negative (53% [25 of 47] versus 22% [8 of 36]) (Crook et al, 1994).

The probability of obtaining a positive postradiation therapy biopsy result correlates with clinical stage (Nachtsheim et al, 1978; Scardino et al, 1986; Marinelli et al, 1992; Forman et al, 1993a; Freiha and Bagshaw, 1984), **pelvic lymph node status** (Scardino et al, 1986; Marinelli et al, 1992; Freiha and Bagshaw, 1984), **histologic grade** (Dugan et al, 1991; Marinelli et al, 1992; Freiha and Bagshaw, 1984), **and serum PSA** (Dugan et al, 1991; Forman et al, 1993a). Whether other biologic markers, such as indicators of cell proliferation or apoptosis, are also of value in this regard remains to be explored.

Practical Considerations Regarding Radiotherapy

Putting therapeutic benefits aside, how does the clinician discern if the treatment recommended for the patient is adequate, appropriate, and the best available at the present time? The following should serve as a rough guideline of the minimum and maximum expectations with the clinical setting that exists in the late 1990s. These considerations are based on the equipment available for the design and delivery of treatment as well as on the philosophy of the treating physician.

For patients with cancer limited to the prostate that would be classified as stages T1 and T2N0M0, typical fields of radiation should encompass the prostate and seminal vesicles with a margin of 1 to 2 cm. The use of elective nodal irradiation in this setting has not been demonstrated to lead to enhanced survival outcomes, and therefore the routine use of elective nodal irradiation for patients with early-stage disease is not warranted. In addition, the use of nodal irradiation increases the volume of normal tissue irradiation and may increase the morbidity of treatment (Porter and Daly, 1987).

The typical dosage range for treating patients with early-stage disease is between 6500 and 7000 cGy, in total, and typically is delivered at 180 to 200 cGy per day. Treatment planning should, at a minimum, consist of x-ray simulation. During this planning process, an attempt should be made to opacify and identify the small intestine as well as the bladder. Some attempt, through the use of barium in the rectum, during simulation, or by outlining the contour of the rectum on a treatment planning CT scan, should be made to identify the volume of the rectum. Finally, the use of urethrography at the time of simulation has been shown to aid more adequately in the identification of the inferior border of the field and thus may lead to a reduction in the volume of normal tissue irradiated and increased assurance of the inclusion of the prostate in the radiation field. The use of CT planning for patients with early-stage disease is also strongly recommended.

For patients with locally advanced disease, the recommendations for using x-ray simulation and CT scan–based treatment planning are similar to that described for early-stage prostate cancer. **The volume of radiation typically includes the prostate and seminal vesicle and often the periprostatic or pelvic lymph nodes. Again, in this setting, the use of elective nodal irradiation has not proven to be beneficial, although a stronger case can be made for the use of pelvic irradiation in this group because of the 30% to 50% probability of occult pelvic lymph node metastases.** If pelvic lymph node irradiation is used, a dose of around 4500 cGy delivered in 25 fractions is appropriate using a four-field orthogonal technique. The field is then reduced to include the prostate and seminal vesicles only to a total dose in the range of 7000 cGy. In patients with locally advanced disease, the use of neoadjuvant hormonal therapy has been demonstrated to improve the disease-free survival and delay recurrence significantly and should now be considered standard in the treatment of patients with locally advanced adenocarcinoma of the prostate with external beam therapy.

New strategies for the treatment of early-stage disease include the use of multiple nonaxial fields as well as some degree of dose intensification/dose escalation. These strategies are based on the fact that many patients with early-stage disease have evidence of recurrence based on biochemical failure with a rise in PSA, and up to 50% of patients may have residual local disease, including those patients with clinical local failure and histologic evidence of residual disease. Thus, these patients with localized disease are candidates for protocol therapy of dosage intensification, which includes neoadjuvant hormonal therapy, high-linear-energy transfer irradiation in the form of neutrons, proton boost, and even interstitial brachytherapy boost therapy. In addition, the use of nonaxial or nonplanar beam arrangements at standard doses has been shown to reduce the toxicity associated with the treatment of even early-stage patients. The use of multiple nonaxial fields by comparison to the standard four-field technique or to an arc rotational technique reduces the probability of complications by nearly a factor of 2.

For patients receiving postprostatectomy irradiation, recommendations on treatment design, field orientation, and total dose are somewhat more difficult to come by. There has been no standardization for the delivery of treatments in the postprostatectomy setting. **Typically, for patients with pathologic T3 disease who are being treated adjuvantly in the absence of pelvic lymph node irradiation, doses in the range of 6000 to 6400 cGy appear to be adequate in the majority of patients for controlling occult residual disease and preventing clinical and biochemical relapse.** Typically a four-field arrangement has been used with opposing anterior and posterior as well as right and left lateral fields. Shielding is designed to minimize the dose to the bladder and rectum. Knowledge of the region of positive margins can be helpful in designing the treatment fields so as to ensure inclusion of the perivesicular tissue, apical tissues, or posterior lateral tissues most commonly found to be involved at the time of surgery. It is important to delay the initiation of radiation therapy until adequate healing from surgery is evident and urinary continence restored. This is usually complete between 5 and 8 weeks after surgery.

For patients with biochemical relapse who have had evidence of extracapsular extension, field arrangements are basically the same. Because of the presence of an elevated PSA level, however, the dose of radiation should probably be higher to treat a larger tumor burden. The authors have typically used graded doses from 6400 to 7200 cGy depending on the degree of elevation of the PSA level. Typically, for patients with a serum PSA level at the time of relapse of 1.5 ng/ml or less, doses of 6800 cGy are used.

For patients with clinical local failure, doses are titrated according to the volume of residual disease. Often, patients with clinical local failure harbor a larger volume of residual disease than those patients with an intact prostate, and doses in excess of 7000 cGy may need to be used to ensure sterilization. With the advent of serum PSA observations in the postprostatectomy setting, however, the number of patients with clinical local relapse should be few. Finally, in the node-positive postprostatectomy setting, the utility of adjuvant radiation, even pelvic nodal irradiation, has yet to be proven, and cases need to be individualized with regard to the intent of treatment and the probability of success.

Radiotherapy for Palliation

Bone Metastases

In genitourinary cancers, bone metastases represent a common problem (Abrams et al, 1950; Gilbert and Dagan, 1976).

Many therapies are available for bone metastases, including surgery, medical management, and radiation. Radiation therapy can treat most patients with highly effective symptom relief.

The hallmark of osseous metastases is localized pain, which is frequently continuous and unrelenting regardless of the site. The pain caused by bone metastases is not well understood. Some investigators have hypothesized that irritation of the periosteal membrane or the release of biologic mediators is responsible for bone pain. The most serious complication of osseous metastases is spinal cord compression, which is discussed later.

Most bone metastases can be diagnosed by physical examination, plain radiographs, and a bone scan. Plain radiographs are highly accurate in detecting metastatic lesions, particularly when associated with pain; however, the sensitivity is poor. The radiographic pattern is typically blastic for prostate cancer. Bone scanning is a useful adjunct to plain films. Technetium 99m diphosphonate is taken up in areas of bone production and can be used for detection of bone metastases and to follow the response to therapy. Bone scintigraphy is approximately 50% to 80% more sensitive than plain radiographs (Pagani and Libshitz, 1982). It can frequently show metastatic lesions long before changes on plain films are appreciated. Several investigators have estimated that this may be 2 to 6 months (Wilner, 1982; Glasko, 1986). Plain films and bone scans are frequently used to plan radiation fields and define technique. CT and magnetic resonance imaging (MRI) are sometimes required if there is suspicion of bone involvement but x-ray and bone scan are negative or if there is soft tissue involvement.

Most clinical situations including pain management and preservation of bone integrity can be managed by the judicious use of radiation therapy. Planning radiation therapy requires a clear understanding of the patient's disease and the intent of treatment. Although radiation has been shown to be highly effective, actual treatment delivery, dose, fractionation, and volume can vary greatly from center to center without any apparent effect on efficacy. Therefore, treatment can be customized to the patient's needs. Certainly, a patient with a painful bone lesion and a poor prognosis is likely to have a different treatment regimen than a patient with a good prognosis. It is not unlikely for patients with bone metastases, especially from the prostate, to have many useful years of life.

The most widely quoted bone metastases study using radiation is the RTOG trial 74-02 reported by Tong and colleagues (1982). This study analyzed 1016 patients. All patients had at least one painful bone site, most required narcotic medications, and 56% described their pain as being constant and severe. These patients were randomized to receive several different radiation therapy regimens. Eighty-three percent of patients obtained a partial response, and 54% obtained a complete response usually within 2 to 4 weeks of treatment. Pain relief was influenced by the site and pain status before irradiation. More than 70% of patients who experienced some pain relief did not relapse before death. There were no significant differences in the frequency of pain relief among the various treatment arms. A reanalysis of this RTOG study by Blitzer (1985), however, concluded that the two high-dose protracted programs (270 cGy $\times$ 15 and 300 cGy $\times$ 10) had significantly better complete responses and decreased narcotic use, and patients treated to higher doses required fewer retreatments. Reviewing the data from currently available prospective studies has shown overall response rates ranging from 85% to 100% using various treatment schedules (Madsen, 1983; Price et al, 1988; Cole, 1989). Single-fraction regimens (800 cGy × 1) appear to be as effective as the other more protracted regimens but are also associated with increased acute morbidity, particularly to the abdominal organs. **A frequently used regimen in the United States is to give 3000 cGy in 10 divided fractions. This dosage is adequate for most osseous metastases.**

A metastasis to a weight-bearing region raises many concerns. A pathologic fracture can be painful and disabling both functionally and psychologically. Certain radiographic and clinical factors that warrant consideration of prophylactic surgical fixation include

1. An intramedullary lytic lesion equal to or greater than 50% of the cross-sectional diameter of the bone.

2. A lytic lesion involving a length of cortex equal to or greater than the cross-sectional diameter of the bone or greater than 2.5 cm in axial length (Lane et al, 1980).

These patients should be evaluated by an orthopedic surgeon. If a pathologic fracture has occurred in a weight-bearing region, surgical fixation is required for pain control and to promote adequate healing. In all situations, postoperative radiation is required. Because prostate cancer produces primarily blastic metastases, pathologic fracture is correspondingly infrequent.

Spinal Cord Compression

Spinal cord compression is a medical emergency. Failure to diagnose and treat promptly can lead to significant morbidity, including paraplegia and autonomic dysfunction. In a study by Bruckman and Bloomer (1978), genitourinary tumors, especially prostate and kidney, accounted for 13% of spinal cord compressions. Approximately 18,000 cases of spinal cord compression occur in the United States every year (Black, 1979).

The predominant symptom of cord compression is pain in about 95% of patients (Gilbert et al, 1978). **Pain usually precedes a diagnosis of spinal cord compression by about 4 months. Symptoms, however, can progress rapidly to neurologic dysfunction in a matter of hours to days. When a patient has progressed to paraplegia, return of function is infrequent. Therefore, early diagnosis and therapy are critical.**

Diagnostic tools include x-ray films, bone scan, CT, MRI, and myelogram (Rodichok et al, 1986). Plain films are positive in about 80% of patients with epidural compression but are neither specific nor sensitive. A major limitation of plain films is that the bone requires at least 50% decalcification before radiologic changes can be appreciated. Bone scans as mentioned earlier are more sensitive but are not specific. Plain films and bone scans with physical examination can detect most spinal cord compressions (85%–90%) (Portenoy et al, 1989). The gold standard for diagnosis has traditionally been the myelogram. The sensitivity and specificity are approximately 95% and 88%, respectively (Carmody et al, 1989). This test, however, is invasive, and several investiga-

tors have shown MRI to be of similar if not superior accuracy (Li and Poon, 1988; Sze et al, 1988). MRI has the added benefit of imaging the entire spine.

Once the diagnosis of spinal cord compression is made, the physician is left with the dilemma of how to treat. Effective regimens include surgery, radiation, hormonal therapy, or all of these. **Immediate androgen deprivation is required in these patients if previously untreated with hormones.** A luteinizing hormone–releasing hormone agonist alone is contraindicated because of the high potential of a tumor flare. **In most instances, radiation therapy and hormonal therapy suffice and obviate the need for surgery.** Several retrospective series have shown equivalent results between radiation alone and laminectomy, plus radiation in terms of pain control, and functional improvement. The most widely quoted study evaluating this issue is that of Gilbert and colleagues (1978). In general, despite the therapy instituted, if a patient is ambulatory, there is an 85% chance that the patient will remain ambulatory. If the patient is nonambulatory, there is a less than 50% chance of regaining ambulation, and if the patient is paraplegic, less than 5% of becoming ambulatory. Again, this emphasizes the need for early diagnosis and treatment. Improvement of pain is similar to those results obtained with radiotherapy for other bone metastases (Gilbert et al, 1978).

Radiation therapy can be instituted quickly and efficiently. Results of MRI or other diagnostic tests together with physical examination can help determine the appropriate treatment volume. Multiple epidural lesions can be treated in one continuous field or by multiple treatment fields. The volume treated is usually the level of cord involvement together with two vertebral bodies above and two below the epidural lesion. With the accuracy of MRI, however, many centers use one vertebral body above and one below the area of cord compression. The optimal radiation dose and fractionation scheme have not been firmly established. Different from the treatment of other bone metastases, however, the goal is not only pain relief, but also tumor reduction. It is for this reason that protracted fractionation for spinal cord compression is recommended.

Friedman and associates demonstrated a good response in 71% of patients who received more than 2500 cGy for epidural compression versus 34% for patients who received less than 2500 cGy (Friedman et al, 1976). The patients in this study had the diagnosis of lymphoma, which is usually more radiosensitive than other tumor histologies. Commonly employed dosages are 3000 to 4000 cGy over 2 to 4 weeks. In all cases, spinal cord tolerance to radiation should be respected. Often, initial doses of 300 to 500 cGy are given for the first two to three treatments to attempt quicker symptom palliation, but there are no firm data to support this.

There are a few instances in which surgery should be considered as an option before radiation, including pathologic fracture with spinal instability or compression of the spinal cord by bone, unknown tissue diagnosis, or a history of previous radiation to the same area.

Once the diagnosis of cord compression is made or even suspected, all patients should be placed on steroid therapy. Steroids can decrease vasogenic edema and provide striking analgesic benefit. The loading dose of dexamethasone (Decadron) is 4 to 100 mg followed by a maintenance dosage of 4 to 24 mg every 6 hours.

Palliative Systemic Radiotherapy

HEMIBODY IRRADIATION

The concept of palliative systemic radiation therapy has interested physicians since the 1950s. Over the years, the techniques and applications of this form of treatment have continued to progress. Before the 1970s, experience in systemic radiotherapy was primarily in the form of total body irradiation (TBI). Its use was mostly in the treatment of hematologic diseases. The main limitation of this form of treatment was bone marrow organ toxicity, which limited the maximal dose that can be given, 225 to 300 cGy.

Fitzpatrick and Rider (1976) began using hemibody irradiation (HBI) to circumvent the shortcomings associated with TBI in the early 1970s. In 1976, they published a landmark paper on their experiences with HBI (Fitzpatrick and Rider, 1976). Using single fractions of 500 to 1000 cGy, they treated 140 patients with symptomatic bone metastases and reported the results of 82 patients. HBI was tolerable and effective in achieving palliation of pain, many within 48 hours of treatment. Deaths from radiation pneumonitis and hematopoietic failure were few. The study also showed that systemic radiotherapy can be effective in treating solid tumors. Following this publication, several articles evaluating their retrospective data on HBI for palliation of bone metastases were reported (Salazar et al, 1978; Epstein et al, 1979). Results were encouraging and prompted the RTOG to evaluate this modality.

The final analysis of RTOG 78-10 was published in 1986 by Salazar and associates. The protocol explored increasing single doses of half-body irradiation in patients with multiple symptomatic osseous metastases. The doses used were 600 to 800 cGy in the upper hemibody and 800 to 1000 cGy in the lower or middle hemibody. The most common histologies treated were prostate (40%), breast (29%), and lung (18%). Pain relief was experienced in 73% of patients. Fifty percent of patients achieved pain relief within 48 hours and 80% within 1 week. There were no fatalities, and treatment was considered tolerable. Most effective and safest doses were 600 cGy for the upper hemibody and 800 cGy for the lower and middle hemibody. When compared to RTOG 74-02 (local irradiation for palliation of bone metastases), HBI achieved a similar number of patients experiencing pain relief; however, local irradiation achieved twice the number of complete responses. Another important finding was that recurrences of pain within irradiated fields were four times lower with HBI than with local irradiation. This indicated that prophylactic irradiation to bones can decrease the rate of disease involvement. Studies by Jacobsson and Naslund and Kaplan and associates showed that prostate cancer patients who received periaortic irradiation developed significantly fewer lumbar metastases than those who had whole-pelvis irradiation alone (Kaplan et al, 1990; Jacobsson and Naslund, 1991).

Based on the results of RTOG 78-10 and on the preliminary data on prophylactic irradiation, RTOG 82-06 was designed. This prospective, randomized study evaluated the effect of adjuvant systemic radiotherapy (HBI) in delaying the onset of bone metastases (Poulter et al, 1992). A total of 499 patients with painful bone metastases were randomized to either local radiation or local radiation and HBI 800 cGy. Those patients who received HBI had an increased progression-free survival, 12.6 months versus 6.3 months, and fewer retreatments. Overall the incidence of toxicities was 5% to 15%. There were no fatalities or radiating pneumonitis; lung shields were used. The authors of the study concluded that 800 cGy of HBI can cause micrometastases to regress and that HBI has the potential to be used to treat systemic and occult metastases and improve quality of life for these patients.

HBI is delivered by external beam irradiation. The typical dose is 600 cGy to upper hemibody and 800 cGy to the middle and lower hemibody given in a single fraction.

The major chronic toxicity associated with HBI is radiation pneumonitis. Without lung correction, the incidence of radiation pneumonitis is estimated to be 18% to 35% for doses of 600 to 1000 cGy and less than 10% if corrected for lung transmission (Rubin and Scarantino, 1994). Approximately 50% of patients have depression of the hematologic profile, and 10% of patients may require transient hematologic support. Irradiation of the head can cause xerostomia and cataract formation. If the head and brain has a low incidence of metastatic involvement, exclusion of the head from the upper hemibody is acceptable. The most troublesome acute complication is nausea and vomiting, which occurs in 80% of patients, particularly with upper and middle hemibody irradiation. With the use of premedication programs using prednisone, odansetron, and hydration, the incidence of emesis is less than 5% (Scarantino et al, 1994). **HBI should be considered in any patient with multiple bone disease sites that are not responsive to hormone or chemotherapy maneuvers and have adequate bone marrow function.**

SYSTEMIC RADIONUCLIDE THERAPY

The first report on the use of systemic radionuclides for the treatment of bone metastases was published by Pecher (1942) more than 50 years ago. Using this modality, all involved sites are addressed simultaneously with little toxicity. Selective absorption into bone metastases limits irradiation of normal tissues and increases the therapeutic ratio. Administration as a single intravenous injection in the outpatient clinic is a further advantage for many patients. Phosphorus 32 (^{32}P) and strontium 89 are the most studied radionuclides to date. Samarium 153 and rhenium 186 continue to be under clinical investigation. Tables 88–3 and 88–4 provide a summary of the physical characteristics and the clinical usefulness of the radionuclides discussed.

STRONTIUM 89

Physical Characteristics and Biokinetics. Strontium 89 decays by beta emission to yttrium 89 with a half-life of

Table 88–3. PHYSICAL CHARACTERISTICS OF RADIONUCLIDES REVIEWED

Radionuclide	Physical Half-life	Beta Energy (MeV)	Gamma Energy (KeV)	Chelate
^{32}P	14.3 days	1.71	0	Orthophosphate
^{89}Sr	50.6 days	1.46	0	Chloride
^{186}Re	90.6 hours	1.07	137	HEDP
^{153}Sm	46.3 hours	0.84	103	EDTMP

50.6 days. The average beta energy is 1.46 MeV. Chemically similar to calcium, strontium 89 is quickly taken up into the mineral matrix of bone. The fraction of strontium 89 retained is proportional to the metastatic tumor burden and varies between 20% and 80% of the administered dose (Blake et al, 1986). Preferential accumulation in and around metastatic deposits, where active bone formation takes place, has been demonstrated by bone scans with the gamma emitter strontium 85 (Blake et al, 1986; Breen et al, 1992) and by direct comparison of autoradiography and histologic sections of affected bone (Ben-Josef et al, 1995a). Once incorporated into the metastatic lesion, strontium 89 is not removed metabolically and remains deposited for as long as 100 days. Normal bone takes up only a small fraction of the injected dose and retains it for a much shorter period of time. **Elimination is through the kidneys, and careful disposal of urine is needed for 7 to 10 days after administration** (National Council on Radiation Protection and Measurements, 1978; Blake et al, 1988; Ben-Josef et al, 1995b). **Extra care in terms of urine handling and disposal is advised for incontinent patients. Because strontium 89 emits extremely little gamma radiation,** the patient is not a radiation hazard to family members or to hospital staff.

Clinical Experience with Strontium 89. The efficacy of strontium 89 has been demonstrated in multiple studies (Firusian et al, 1976; Correns et al, 1979; Silberstein and Williams, 1985; Robinson et al, 1987; Tennvall et al, 1988; Montebello and Hartson-Eaton, 1989; Williams and Dillehay, 1989; Laing et al, 1991). Most of these studies were conducted on patients with hormone-refractory prostate cancer. The limited experience in patients with metastatic breast cancer, however, suggests similar efficacy. In one retrospective review, 89% of 28 patients were reported to obtain moderate or good relief of pain (Robinson et al, 1992).

Lewington and co-workers, in a randomized, double-blind, cross-over study, demonstrated the superiority of strontium 89 over stable elemental strontium (Lewington et al, 1991). This study confirmed that the palliative effects of strontium 89 are due to its radioactive emission and not a pharmacologic inhibitory effect on osteoclast-mediated bone resorption.

In a multicenter trial, 22 patients with metastatic prostate cancer were treated with doses ranging from 0.7 to 3.0 MBq/kg. The optimal dose was found to be 1.5 MBq/kg with no appreciable increment in efficacy above this dose. Of 83 patients treated with at least 1.5 MBq/kg, 75% had partial relief of pain, and 22% were rendered pain-free. Pain relief began 10 to 20 days post-treatment and peaked at 6 weeks. Response was maintained for a median duration of 6 months (with a range of 4 to 15 months). RTOG has completed another phase I dose escalation study and concluded that

the maximum tolerated dose of strontium 89 is 6.5 mCi (approximately 3.4 MBq/kg) (Porter, 1994).

Toxicity of strontium 89 is mainly hematologic. Platelet depression is dose dependent. Most patients have a 20% to 50% drop in their counts following doses of 3 to 4 mCi (1.5 to 2 MBq/kg). Grade III toxicity is rare. Other adverse effects include a transient increase in bone pain in up to 10% of patients and rarely facial flushing. The pain flare occurs 1 to 2 weeks post-treatment, may last a few days, and usually heralds a favorable response.

The results of the Trans-Canada study have been reported by Porter and colleagues (1993). This prospectively randomized phase III trial was designed to evaluate the efficacy of strontium 89 adjuvant to local field external-beam radiotherapy. Patients were required to have multiple bone metastases secondary to hormone-refractory prostate cancer. Treatment consisted of local field radiotherapy (2000 cGy in 5 fractions or 3000 cGy in 10 fractions) and placebo or local field radiotherapy and strontium 89 (10.8 mCi).

A total of 126 patients were recruited to the study. Overall and complete responses (relief of pain at the index site) were higher in the treatment arm, but the differences did not reach statistical significance. Objectively measured responses (>50% reduction in serum PSA and alkaline phosphatase) were also significantly superior in the treatment arm. A significantly greater proportion of patients in the treatment arm had stopped taking analgesics and experienced an improvement in physical activity and quality of life. Strontium 89–treated patients had a significant delay in the appearance of new painful sites as well as prolongation in the time before further radiotherapy was required. At 3 months post-treatment, 58.7% and 34% of patients in the treatment and control arms, respectively, were free of new painful metastases. The median time to the requirement for further radiotherapy was 35.3 weeks and 20.3 weeks in the treatment and control arms, respectively. Hematologic toxicity was, as expected, higher in strontium 89–treated patients.

The UK Metastron Investigators' Group study (Bolger et al, 1993; Quilty et al, 1994) was designed to compare pain relief after strontium 89 with that after external-beam radiotherapy. Entry criteria were similar to those in the Trans-Canada study. Eligible patients were stratified as suitable for treatment with either local or hemibody radiotherapy. They were then randomized to treatment with that form of external-beam irradiation or strontium 89. Local field radiation schedules were usually 2000 cGy in 5 fractions, but a single 800-cGy fraction was occasionally used. Hemibody irradiation was given as a single fraction of 600 cGy (upper half) or 800 cGy (lower half). Strontium 89 was given at a dose of 200 MBq (5.4 mCi). Pain at each site was graded according to severity (mild to intractable) and type (intermittent or constant). Additional end points scored included analgesics usage, performance status, and mobility. Overall response was scored using a scale from "deterioration" to "dramatic improvement." A total of 284 patients were treated according to protocol. Overall and dramatic pain relief were similar with strontium 89 (61% and 44.1%), local radiotherapy (65.9% and 36.4%), or hemibody irradiation (63.6% and 43.2%). Patients receiving strontium 89 were significantly less likely to develop new sites of pain or require additional therapy than those treated with either form

Table 88–4. CLINICAL EFFICACY AND TOXICITY OF RADIONUCLIDES REVIEWED

Radionuclide	Response Rate (%)	Response Duration (months)	Toxicity
^{32}P	60–80	~5	+ +
^{89}Sr	60–90	~6	+
^{186}Re	75–80	1–2	+
^{153}Sm	75–90	2–3	+

of external-beam irradiation. The incidence of symptomatic side effects was markedly less after strontium 89.

The findings of the Trans-Canada trial and the UK trial are strikingly similar. Together, they have helped define a new paradigm for the treatment of osseous metastases: local field external-beam radiation directed at significant symptomatic disease interdigitated with systemic radiation targeting subclinical disease. This combination can be effectively used to increase the symptom-free interval (Friedell and Storaasli, 1950).

OTHER RADIONUCLIDES

Phosphorus 32. In 1950, Friedell and Storaasli reported on the successful use of ^{32}P for bone metastases. This radionuclide decays by beta emission to sulfur 32 with a half-life of 14.3 days. The maximum beta energy is 1.71 MeV. Following parenteral administration, ^{32}P skeletal uptake exceeds that of muscle, fat, or skin by a factor of 6 to 10. The results of 28 reported human studies have been reviewed by Silberstein (1993). Subjective decrease in pain occurs in 60% to 80% of patients. Although parathormone and testosterone can enhance ^{32}P uptake in bone, a clinically significant advantage is hard to prove. Pain relief is rapid, most often obtained within 14 days. The major toxicity reported is myelosuppression with pancytopenia. Nausea and vomiting are not uncommon. An increased incidence of acute leukemia has also been reported (Landaw, 1986).

Samarium 153. Samarium 153 is a man-made radionuclide that emits beta particles of 0.81 MeV (20%), 0.71 MeV (30%), and 0.64 MeV (50%) and gamma photons of 103 KeV (28%). It has a relatively short half-life of 46.3 hours and consequently a relatively high dose rate. Samarium 153 has been chelated to a phosphonate, ethylenediamine tetramethylene (EDTMP), to produce a bone-seeking complex. About 50% of an intravenously administered dose is retained in bone (Eary et al, 1993; Bayouth et al, 1994). Absorbed doses in bone and red marrow have been estimated at 2.5 cGy/MBq and 0.57 cGy/MBq (Eary et al, 1993). Clinical experience with samarium 153 is still limited. In a phase I/II clinical trial (Collins et al, 1993), the maximum tolerated dose was determined to be 2.5 mCi/kg. The principal toxicity observed was hematologic, with maximum myelosuppression occurring at 3 to 4 weeks. A flare of bone pain occurred in 12% of patients. The overall pain relief rate was 74% with a median duration of palliation of 2.6 months. In responders, relief was obtained promptly within 7 to 14 days of treatment. Response rates were significantly higher with 2.5 mCi/kg than with 1.0 mCi/kg.

Rhenium 186. Rhenium 186 emits beta particles of 1.07 MeV and a 137-KeV gamma ray and has a short half-life of 3.8 days. Similar to samarium 153, it has been complexed to a bone-seeking phosphonate, hydroxyethylenediphosphonic acid (HEDP). Retention in bone is about 50% of the injected dose, and the rest is excreted through the kidneys into the urine (Maxon et al, 1990). Rhenium 186 has been studied in a small number of patients with metastatic cancer of the prostate, breast, colon, and lung (Maxon et al, 1992). After administration of 33 to 35 mCi, 75% to 80% of patients experienced pain relief, most often within 2 weeks (Maxon et al, 1991). The average duration of palliation (5 weeks) appears shorter than that reported for strontium 89 or samar-

ium 153. The therapeutic efficacy of rhenium 186 has been confirmed in a double-blind, cross-over comparison with placebo (Porter and Forman, 1993). Myelosuppression begins 2 weeks after treatment, peaks at 4 to 6 weeks, and resolves by 8 weeks. A pain flare occurs in 10% of patients 2 to 3 days post-treatment and resolves within 1 week.

Future Directions

SURVIVAL

The UK Metastron study and the Trans-Canada study have not demonstrated a survival advantage to strontium 89–treated patients. In a much smaller study, however, Buchali and colleagues demonstrated a significant prolongation in survival for patients randomized to receive strontium 89 compared with those who received placebo (Buchali et al, 1988). Mertens and colleagues noted a median survival of greater than 8 months in patients treated with strontium 89 and low-dose *cis*-platin (Mertens et al, 1992). Correns and associates noted a significantly longer survival in patients who received 2.5 mCi/kg than in those who received 1.0 mCi/kg (median of 9 versus 6 months) (Correns et al, 1979). Although this was not a randomized study, there were no differences in either the extent of bone metastases or the performance status between the two groups. Larger controlled trials are required to determine whether systemic radionuclide therapy offers any survival advantage over supportive care.

ENHANCEMENT OF EFFICACY

The effectiveness of radionuclide therapy can potentially be enhanced by concomitant use of biphosphonates. These agents can inhibit osteoclast-mediated bone resorption and have been shown to reduce the frequency of pathologic fractures, bone pain, and hypercalcemia in patients with metastatic breast cancer (Van Holten-Verzantvoort et al, 1987). If given in combination with a radionuclide, they may enhance its effect. Similarly, chemotherapy can be administered to enhance tumor cell kill through radiosensitization. Concurrent administration of strontium 89 and low-dose *cis*-platin has resulted in complete and partial relief of pain in five (22%) and eight (52%) patients (Mertens et al, 1992). Duration of palliation ranged from 1 to 4 months.

In another study, 15 patients were treated with samarium 153–EDTMP in combination with bolus doxorubicin, mitomycin C, or 5-fluorouracil (Turner et al, 1992). Complete and partial responses have been obtained in four (7%) and eight (53%).

ADJUVANT TREATMENT

To date, all patients have been treated with systemic radionuclides at an advanced metastatic stage of disease. Better results might be expected if treatment were offered at an earlier stage when the overall tumor burden is smaller. It is not clear, however, if clinically occult micrometastases can trigger enough osteoblastic activity necessary for effective retention of strontium 89. Much basic and clinical research is needed to answer this question before strontium 89 can be used in a truly adjuvant setting.

CRYOTHERAPY FOR PROSTATE CANCER

Freezing Mechanisms, History, and Animal Models

The reintroduction of cytotoxic freezing temperatures to treat prostate cancer has been met with an emotional spectrum from enthusiasm to controversy. The biologic aspects of freezing have not significantly changed, but the technique and associated delivery mechanisms have markedly improved. The current technique is done through a percutaneous approach and as such is not adequately described as surgery. Likewise, prior and more recent data suggest that freezing may not produce complete ablation if specific technique considerations are not closely followed. Therefore, the term *cryotherapy* may best describe renewed attempts to use this modality for the treatment of prostate cancer. An overview of freezing mechanisms, history, current techniques, and results is presented with considerations for future research and development.

Cryotherapy is the destruction of tumor through the application of freezing temperatures. Mechanisms of in vivo tissue destruction include microvascular occlusion, evolution of intracellular toxic solutes via osmotic shifts during freeze-thaw cycles, and intracellular crystallization (Gill and Long, 1971; Mazur, 1977). An excellent summary of the thermodynamics of heat transfer, the freezing process, and new data concerning cryomicroscopy of human prostate has been published (Rubinski, 1995). As originally proposed by Mazur (1963, 1970), the cellular-level mechanisms of damage have two modes: **solute damage** at low cooling rates and **intracellular ice formulation** at high cooling rates. **Vascular damage,** however, caused by thrombosis of the vasculature, appears to be the dominant mechanism in living parenchymal tissue. The end result is coagulative or ischemic necrosis with minimal peripheral tissue damage, creating a relatively sharp line of demarcation between viable and ablated tissue. In vitro freezing experiments are thus insufficient to model the potentially dominant effects of tissue ischemia.

Initiation of tissue damage may correspond to the early coagulation of parenchymal capillaries and microvasculature. As the sink effect of flowing blood becomes limited or occluded, extracellular ice begins to form and creates a hypertonic environment, which dehydrates the regional cellular matrix. If adequate hypothermia continues, intracellular ice begins to form and is highly lethal to involved cells. Cellular rupture, however, also occurs in the thaw cycle owing to rehydration and rapid re-expansion of cells exposed only to extracellular ice. Cryoprotective mechanisms are needed to avoid these toxic mechanisms and dehydration before freezing is the primary treatment administered to (in vitro) cells for tissue banks (e.g., sperm samples). For cells surviving a limited freeze, ischemic cell death may occur from disrupted blood supply and inability to recanalize coagulated microvasculature.

The cytotoxic effects of severe hypothermia on parenchymal human prostate tissue has been best defined by Rubinski (1995). In his article, he presents data evaluating the effects of hypothermia to −40°C and −10°C, modeling intermediate cooling and slower cooling rates. This was done using cryomicroscopy, which clearly delineates major mechanisms of tissue damage. Beginning at −10°C, ice crystals begin to form within the capillaries and prostatic stroma, producing numerous tears (lacunae) in the tissue. This disrupts smooth muscle and the glandular epithelium with associated significant shrinkage and distortion of epithelial cells. Precryotherapy alteration of the in vivo extracellular fluid space is difficult to achieve because of its much smaller volume compared to in vitro experiments. At −40°C, the stromal disruption is more severe, with epithelial cells being severely dislodged from connective tissue with no evidence of intact cells. It would have taken two freezes at −10°C to produce a similar effect of a single −40°C freeze. For the in vivo model, cryotherapy appears to induce a more epithelial selective necrosis and may relate to these complex interactions of cellular and vascular effects. The formation of intracellular ice occurs somewhere beyond the −40°C level as it approaches the temperature of liquid nitrogen (−196°C). These findings are crucial to understanding inadequate freezing and cancer cell survival within the intact prostate and current human studies. Further subsequent vascular damage after a −40°C freeze (or double freeze at −10°C) helps explain the sharp delineation of viable and completely necrotic cells.

Prostate cryosurgery for the treatment of benign prostatic hyperplasia was first described in 1966 using a retrograde, transurethral approach (Gonder et al, 1966). Sloughing of the resultant necrotic tissue caused intermittent or prolonged obstruction, and the technique was abandoned. Application of cryosurgery for prostate cancer was then reported in 1968 using an open transperineal technique (Soanes and Gonder, 1968; Flocks et al, 1972). Monitoring of the cryosurgical procedure at that time was limited to palpation and direct visualization. One study of 229 patients with prostate cancer who underwent open perineal cryosurgery demonstrated equivalent, stage-for-stage, 10-year survival with radical prostatectomy and external-beam radiation therapy (Bonney et al, 1982). These encouraging long-term results are frequently quoted as justification for the current renewed interest in prostate cryotherapy. It should be emphasized, however, that these were nonrandomized, uncontrolled trials in which many of the patients had already received hormonal therapy.

Historical data analysis regarding the efficacy of prostate cryotherapy also suffers from uncertain comparisons of technique variation over time for radical prostatectomy and radiation therapy as well as improvements in cryotherapy. The older cryotherapy literature should therefore be viewed as historical data with no randomized data available for any current therapy of prostate cancer. Radical prostatectomy and radiation therapy have significantly longer and larger treatment trials showing excellent local control for clinically localized disease (Paulson et al, 1982a; Pilepich et al, 1987). PSA and postcryotherapy biopsy data may become adequate surrogates for long-term local control. Standardized cryotherapy techniques, however, need to be incorporated into current trials to ensure uniformity of any multicenter effort. Because diagnostic transrectal ultrasound (TRUS) and guidance are highly operator-dependent techniques, evaluation of current treatment and morbidity data requires assessment of technique variations.

The need for detailed cryotherapy treatment standards is reinforced by the complications noted in older literature that ultimately led to its prior discontinuation. Prostate cryotherapy, without the benefit of TRUS guidance, produced numerous complications (Ortved et al, 1967; O'Brien and Carswell, 1972; O'Donoghue et al, 1975; Loening et al, 1980, 1981; Bonney et al, 1982, 1983; Debruyne et al, 1984; Kunit, 1986), which are listed in Table 88–5 subdivided into immediate (or transient) and late (or persistent) sequelae. Perhaps the most significant complication of open cryosurgery was fistula formation, approaching 15% overall. Most of these were urethrocutaneous to the perineum and probably were related to the open approach (i.e., partially devitalized tissue) and the potential for backfreezing along shafts of the cryosurgical probes at that time. Impotence, however, was reported in only 7.4% of patients, and the overall morbidity was comparable to other radical treatment options.

The first description of TRUS-guided cryotherapy was reported by Ando in 1982 but still used an open perineal technique. Ultrasound characteristics of frozen and thawed canine prostate tissue were then defined in 1988 (Onik et al, 1988), but cryotherapy was performed with an open technique and did not attempt total gland destruction. The percutaneous technique of freezing the entire prostate in humans was instituted before any published results in an animal model. Despite the difficulties of canine morphologic differences, the authors attempted the first histologic documentation of whole-gland cryotherapy to address basic questions regarding TRUS guidance of cryoprobe placement and ice progression (Littrup et al, 1994b). Specifically the accuracy of TRUS in monitoring ice-ball extension through the posterior prostate while avoiding full-thickness rectal wall necrosis was addressed. This small feasibility study helped define the complete prostate cryodestruction, relationship to the adjacent rectal wall, and the potential effects of urethral and rectal warming.

Controversies still exist about the utility of urethral warming during cryotherapy. Sloughing of necrotic tissue in prior human studies of prostate cryotherapy induced the development of a closed-loop, double-lumen balloon catheter with a final inflation diameter of approximately 15 mm, circulating warm water at high flow rates. It was suggested that its use accounted for the minimal tissue sloughage in recent human reports (Onik et al, 1993); however, controlled comparisons and histologic documentation were lacking. The dog has an os penis, and the urethra makes a tight turn at the perineum, prohibiting the passage of this catheter. Other attempts to provide urethral warming appeared inadequate to prevent sloughage in the dog model (Littrup et al, 1994b). A limited attempt at continuous rectal warming during the height of freeze suggested some potential benefit in limiting ice-ball progression to the thin hypoechoic line in the rectal wall, the muscularis propria. The authors emphasized, however, the millimeter accuracy in monitoring ice-ball progression to the muscularis propria of the rectal wall rather than potential merits of rectal warming. Correlation of the progressing ice front with histologic damage was within 1 to 2 mm accuracy using TRUS, with irreversible necrosis occurring immediately behind the echogenic rim of an ice-ball maintained for at least 15 minutes (Littrup et al, 1994b). Any mild decrease in prostate echogenicity owing to hemorrhagic infarction or edema (or both) (Onik et al, 1988) was not readily discernible without adjacent residual normal parenchyma. Excellent correlation of TRUS ice-ball extent with complete infarction of the posterior prostate and only partial extension into the rectal wall was noted. This was achieved despite the thin posterior periprostatic region in dogs. In humans with thicker rectoprostatic tissues, this feasibility study should encourage thorough cryotherapy beyond the posterior margin of the prostate to ensure optimal potential clinical efficacy. These mechanisms of cryotherapy cytotoxicity, historical background, and animal model data all suggest the need for close evaluation of current human techniques.

Technique

The pivotal concern about modern, TRUS-guided cryotherapy should be the balance between a thorough, intensive freeze and resultant morbidity. Lee and colleagues detail the major anatomic and pathologic characteristics of cryotherapy, illustrating the greater technique flexibility in humans (Lee et al, 1994). More intensive freezes are possible with careful TRUS placement of five probes and controlling their ice formation. The following summary of technique details is suggested as the current state-of-the-art, producing optimal clinical results yet reducing the probabilities of infection or fistula formation:

1. For optimal prophylaxis, a volume cathartic bowel preparation is recommended (e.g., polyethylene glycol-electrolyte solution [GoLYTELY]). This also may delay any added stress on the rectal wall from immediate postoperative defecation. Intravenous antibiotics should be started immediately before the cryosurgery and continue through the first postoperative day. The patient may then be switched to oral antibiotics until catheter removal is appropriate.

2. Prostate volumes should be 40 to 50 ml to obtain adequate coverage of the entire prostate at optimal freezing intensity. Androgen deprivation therapy may significantly decrease prostate volume (i.e., 30%–50%), thereby simplifying the procedure and allowing for lower overall tissue temperatures.

Table 88–5. HISTORICAL COMPLICATIONS OF OPEN PERINEAL PROSTATE CRYOSURGERY*

Immediate Perioperative Complications(%)†	Delayed/Persistent Complications (%)†
Urethroperineal fistula (10.7)	Erectile impotence (7.4–38.5)
Urethrorectal fistula (1.4)	Stress incontinence (6.5)
Epididymitis (2.0)	Bladder neck
Obstruction by neoplasm (2.3)	Protracted severe urinary tract
Orchitis	infection
Acute pyelonephritis	Fibrosis of trigone and chronic renal
Periurethral abscess	failure
Incisional abscess	Urethral stricture
Urinary retention	Bladder calculi
Stress incontinence	Late hemorrhage
Acute renal failure	Osteitis pubis
Penile edema	Fecal incontinence

*Estimated rates of prostate cryosurgery complications using the open approach without TRUS guidance. Individual complications are not listed with percentages and are assumed to be infrequent or unusual. See text for references.
†Percents given when more than incidental.

3. A suprapubic tube is placed before the initiation of the procedure at most centers. Some investigators, however, have chosen to use standard Foley catheter drainage. During needle insertion, a urethral catheter allowing guide wire exchange is used to avoid inadvertent puncture of the subsequent urethral warming device. Following needle placement and guide wire exchange, the urethral integrity can be assessed by flexible cystoscopy. Urethral transgression or submucosal wire placement could lead to the subsequent cryoprobes overcoming the urethral warming device, causing greater urethral necrosis. At this step, it is much easier to reposition the needle and guide wire than after dilator and sheath exchange.

4. **Probe placement** should be well planned, considering cancer size and location in relation to the anticipated size of the eventual ice-ball. This requires optimized preoperative tumor mapping by directed TRUS biopsy of suspicious areas and complete sextant localization. Staging biopsies of seminal vesicles and adjacent neurovascular bundles should be considered, yet tailored to the relative risk for extracapsular extensions (e.g., PSA density >0.3 ng/ml/cc and adjacent TRUS lesion >1.5 cm) (Littrup and Sparashu, 1995). Initial probe tip location should be at the capsule in the base of the gland:

- **Confined cancer:** The anterior probes are placed 1.2 cm from the anterior gland margin, separated by approximately 1.8 cm and equidistant from the urethra. The relative pyramidal shape of most prostates suggests that posterior probe placements require more lateral anglation toward the base of the gland. The probes are spaced 1.2 cm from the posterior margin but less than 1 cm from the lateral aspect to allow better coverage of the neurovascular bundles. This may necessitate a free-hand approach rather than the straight parasagittal alignment achieved with needle guides or insertion templates.

- **Nonconfined cancer:** For larger-volume disease (i.e., greater than three of six positive cores or staging biopsy confirmation), several technique modifications may be applied. First, an asymmetric distribution toward the more involved side may be easily done without compromising coverage of the remaining gland if the prostate volume is less than 40 ml. Alternatively, documented or highly suspected lateral extensions may be first treated with a separate probe placement, followed by the standard five-probe coverage. Extension into the confluence of the seminal vesicles may be achieved by careful extension of the midline probe into this area, making sure the tip is 1.5 cm from the muscularis propria of the rectum. Bladder neck involvement may be treated by the anterior probes, but care is needed to prevent ice-ball extension into the bladder trigone.

5. Thermosensors produce assurance of adequate freezing temperatures (i.e., 5–40°C) in three crucial locations: the anterior margin just below the fibromuscular stroma, the superior neurovascular bundle(s), and the distal midline apex (Bahn et al, 1995). Once these thermosensors reach less than −40°C, probe flow rates should be decreased to help prevent excessive ice-ball extension and resultant complications. It should be noted that copper-constantan thermocouples are not approved for this use and should be cleared by institutional review board approval. Alternatively an 18-gauge needle has been suggested as a rough gauge of cytotoxic temperature when it becomes stuck within the advancing ice front (Bahn et al, 1995).

6. Following satisfactory guide wire localization, the 3-mm dilator and sheath are exchanged over the guide wires, and the dilator is removed. Visualization of the entire extent of the sheath is best done by filling the empty sheath with sterile water. Particular attention should be made to identify the cephalad extent of the sheath to prevent bladder damage from the eventual probes and ice-balls. The selected urethral warming device (Cohen and Miller, 1994) may now be carefully exchanged over the guide wire.

7. The best overall view of the freezing process is produced with a linear array TRUS probe to achieve better lateral visualization of the ice-ball shadow compared to sector array probes. Anterior probes are turned on first to allow accurate monitoring and prevent excessive anterior ice extension.

8. Next the ice-balls from the posterior probes should be monitored closely as they approach the rectum, requiring slower freezing rates. Freezing should be terminated just *before* the ice-ball reaches the thin hypoechoic layer of the rectum's muscularis propria because propagation of the ice-ball may occur after the probes are turned off.

9. The visualized thickness of the rectum can be significantly increased in most patients by more posterior placement of the entire transducer shaft or angulating the probe tip posterior. This allows detailed visualization of ice-ball progression and helps prevent rapid transmural freezing to the mucosal layer and potential urethorectal fistula.

10. In patients with a thin rectal wall or in whom the thickness cannot be increased by the above-mentioned maneuver, the rectoprostatic interspace may be injected with sterile saline via a 22-gauge needle. Care should be taken to inject the air from the needle's dead space in a region superior or inferior to the prostate. Even a tiny amount of air can produce shadowing and significantly degrade the TRUS image.

11. A 1- to 2-cm pull-back of the cryoprobes following the first complete freeze is recommended to better include the distal apex. As noted, the course of the probes near the external sphincter should be noted during initial needle placement so that they do not abut the urethral lumen. If the cryoprobes are too close to the urethra, they could overpower the heat-sink capacity of the urethral warmer and cause incontinence.

12. During the pull-back freeze, the superior ice margin from the first freeze should be continually monitored because freezing may be propagated through the initial ice-ball near the base of the gland. This could cause secondary transmural freezing of the rectum in a region that had been safe during the first freeze.

13. The flow through the urethral warming device should be continually checked throughout the procedure to confirm proper function.

14. Until a formally approved rectal warming (or circulation) device is developed, additional protection of the rectal mucosa may be achieved through direct flushing of the rectum with warm water via a 60-ml syringe. This has also been done through a water balloon at the tip of the TRUS probe (Littrup et al, 1994b).

15. At the conclusion of the procedure, the cryoprobes

are not removed until they are freely mobile within the residual ice because torque applied to the ice conglomerate may produce unnecessary bleeding.

Following these basic procedures, careful TRUS monitoring should minimize the complications encountered during the learning curve of this procedure. The reported complication rates for prostate cryotherapy in one series using these techniques are shown in Table 88–6 (Bahn et al, 1995). The complications of cryotherapy are much greater in patients who had prior radiation therapy, and these patients should be identified in current published series.

Two articles substantiate the need for detailed technique evaluation of cryotherapy (Cox and Crawford, 1995; Grampsas et al, 1995). Their marked complication rate of 54% (37 of 69) did not show improvement over time and was significantly (P = .0012) increased in their last 29 procedures, in which the urethral warming device could not be used (Cox and Crawford, 1995). This marked increase in overall complications is related to incontinence and urinary retention, corresponding to inadequate protection of the external sphincter and periurethral architectural matrix. Even before the discontinued use of the initial urethral warming catheter (Cryomedical Sciences, Inc., Rockville, MD), their urinary retention and incontinence rates (10% and 7.5%) were significantly higher than those reported in Table 88–6. This suggests significant differences in their cryotherapy technique (or reporting format) than with the detailed techniques described previously.

The histologic results of six patients having failed cryotherapy (Grampsas et al, 1995) also demonstrate the need for more technique detail. The previously discussed mechanisms of tissue damage (Rubinski, 1995) suggest that inadequate tissue temperatures were achieved (Grampsas et al, 1995) and seem to reflect prostate tissue temperatures of $-10°C$ or lower. It is difficult to assess the potential cooling rates experienced by these patients, because freezing times were noted to extend only from 5 to 15 minutes, and thermocouples were not used for documentation. Individual pretreatment volumes were also not specified. The TRUS image in the article by Grampsas and colleagues used a sector scan format, which produces significant lateral refraction artifact and incomplete visualization. They also describe the ice-ball as *hypoechoic*, which is a misnomer of the totally anechoic ultrasound absorption produced by ice. Therefore, the following cannot be determined from their study for comparison with the above-mentioned techniques: the temperature

of the visualized ice-ball, the completeness of sector scan visualization, or the utilization of a double freeze with pullback. Their results must be considered preliminary, yet they highlight the need for detailed technique specifications in current cryotherapy publications if one is to account for differences in treatment efficacy and complications.

Cryotherapy Following Radiation Therapy

Patients having persistent disease after radiation therapy pose a treatment dilemma in which few options exist for local control with low morbidity. The significance of reported high percentages of residual carcinoma on systematic biopsy (Kabalin et al, 1989) has been debated, yet persistent disease is consistent with significantly higher disease progression rates compared with those having negative biopsy results (Freiha and Bagshaw, 1984; Scardino et al, 1986). Salvage prostatectomy may be appropriate for younger patients with early rising PSA; however, it also has significantly higher morbidity rates than standard radical prostatectomy. For salvage prostatectomy, these include 30% urinary incontinence, 9% rectal injury, and 70% positive surgical margins (Pontes et al, 1993). Hormonal therapy has been the only other option for these patients, especially given the higher rates of systemic disease after recurrence. As suggested by salvage prostatectomy, if these patients are detected earlier by rising PSA, systemic therapy may be unnecessary if adequate local control could be achieved. TRUS-guided cryotherapy has therefore been investigated as a potential salvage therapy.

Given the current status of evolving expertise in cryotherapy, it is difficult to gain a reliable perspective for this most difficult group of patients. **As with salvage radical prostatectomy, it is recognized that postradiation patients have limited tissue reserves for healing and repair for any postoperative status.** Although several centers have reported initial results of cryotherapy in abstract format (Cohen et al, 1995; Miller et al, 1995; Schmidt et al, 1995; Shinohara and Carroll, 1995), only one published paper (Bahn et al, 1995) and one abstract (von Eschenbach et al, 1995) adequately separate the results of postradiation patients to assess treatment efficacy and morbidity. In the report by Bahn and colleagues, no significant difference in positive biopsy rate at 3 months was noted between radiation (3 of 27 = 11%) and nonradiation patients (7 of 103 = 6.7%) (Bahn et al, 1995). Both mean preoperative and postoperative PSA levels, however, were significantly higher than in the nonradiation patient group. This may indicate residual tumor burden (or systemic disease) and potential for delayed recurrence in postradiation patients. The M. D. Anderson experience confirms the low initial positive biopsy rate, and PSA levels decreased in 92% of patients, including 28% with an undetectable nadir (von Eschenbach et al, 1995). Interestingly, they also document the utility of the optimized techniques described previously, noting improvement in the 31% positive biopsy rate at 6 months to only 8% when they used a double freeze.

The complication rates encountered in postradiation patients have been the primary drawback to the otherwise promising local control data. The M. D. Anderson

Table 88–6. COMPLICATIONS OF TRUS-GUIDED RADICAL PROSTATE CRYOSURGERY*

Estimated Total Complications	Number (percent)
Death	0/210 (0%)
Urethrorectal fistula	5/210 (2.5%)
Urinary obstruction	6/210 (2.9%)
Total incontinence	3/130 (2.3%)
Stress incontinence	8/130 (6.2%)
Impotency in previously potent patients	11/47 (41%)
Penile and scrotal edema	Most patients: self-limited

*Estimated rates of various prostate cryosurgery complications using current techniques.
Data from Bahn et al, 1995, and Lee et al, 1994.

Table 88–7. RESIDUAL CANCER FOLLOWING PROSTATE CRYOSURGERY*

Bahn et al, 1995				
Biopsy Results	*3 months*	*6 months*	*12 months*	*Total*
Stage ≤T2	2/134 (1.5%)	1/78 (1.3%)	1/34 (3.9%)	4/134 (3.0%)
Stage T3	8/71 (11.3%)	2/39 (5.1%)	0/15 (0%)	10/71 (14.1%)

PSA Results	*Pretherapy*		*3 months*		*6 months*		*12 months*		
	N	PSA	N	PSA	N	PSA	N	PSA	
Total patients	130	12.6 ± 16.1	129	1.4 ± 8.1	91	1.0 ± 2.5	43	1.2 ± 5.0	
Negative biopsy	—	—	118	0.4 ± 0.8	88	0.5 ± 1.1	42	0.4 ± 0.8	

Miller et al, 1994				
Biopsy Results	*3 months* *(after first cryotherapy)*	*3 months†*	*12 months*	*24 months*
Stage T3	13/62 (21.0%)	3/58 (5.2%)	3/23 (13.0%)	1/4 (25.0%)

*Available treatment data from two cryotherapy trials that provided data in relation to patient stage.
†After one or two procedures.
PSA, Prostate-specific antigen.

group noted the highest incontinence rate of 50%, a third of which persisted for greater than 6 months (von Eschenbach et al, 1995). They also describe common immediate sequelae of perineal pain, temporary urinary obstruction, and hematuria. One episode of sepsis owing to prostatic abscess was also seen. Prolonged pelvic pain may relate in part to unmonitored anterior extension of the freeze to produce osteonecrosis of the symphysis pubis (Ortved et al, 1967), an early manifestation the authors noted when thermosensors or decreased freezing rates of the anterior probes were not used (Littrup et al, 1994a). This degree of pain was not demonstrated in the published series by Bahn and colleagues, and all of their patients with total incontinence (3 of 3) occurred in postradiation group, yielding only 11% (3 of 27) incontinence (Bahn et al, 1995). In patients who developed a urethrorectal fistula (2.4% = 5 of 210), 80% (4 of 5) occurred in postradiation patients for a rate of 15% (4 of 27). The greater fistula rate in their series may be due to the complete freeze attempted by pushing the ice-ball into the muscularis propria of the rectal wall, which may have already been partially compromised by prior radiation.

Cryotherapy of Clinically Confined Disease

The status of cryotherapy for stage T2 or lower prostate cancer is difficult to evaluate from available abstract data, in which patients are frequently grouped with more locally advanced disease (Cohen et al, 1995; Schmidt et al, 1995; Shinohara and Carroll, 1995). Some reports cannot be readily separated, whereas others merely suggest that only 40% of their cases are from clinically confined cancer patients (Shinohara and Carroll, 1995). The published series of more than 210 patients details the largest results from 130 patients having at least 3 months biopsy and PSA follow-up (Bahn et al, 1995). Of these 130 patients, 27 had prior radiation yet were included in stage separation of 82 patients with confined disease and 48 patients with histologic biopsy confirmation of extraprostatic disease. This was done because no significant differences in positive biopsy rates were

noted among those having received radiation. This presentation, however, makes the significantly higher postcryotherapy PSA results in radiation patients difficult to separate from those of patients receiving primary cryotherapy. Mean preoperative and postoperative PSA results were significantly higher in patients having a positive postcryotherapy biopsy result, regardless of radiation status. Further difficulties in data assessment arise from 88% (114 of 130) of patients having received neoadjuvant androgen deprivation therapy (Bahn et al, 1995). This may significantly skew the follow-up PSA for the first year, and the effect on biopsy status remains unknown.

The overall biopsy and PSA results for 130 patients are given in Table 88–7 (Littrup and Sparschu, 1995). **This clearly demonstrates lower positive biopsy rates for patients stage T2 or lower (4.9% = 4 of 82) compared to the 13% (10 of 78) positive biopsy rate for stage T3 patients.** Of the 14 patients with positive biopsy results, it can be presumed that the majority of the 10 patients having available PSA data with positive biopsy results were from the T3 group. A significant association between increasing positive biopsy rate was also noted with increasing Gleason score on precryotherapy biopsy specimens such that 29% (4 of 15) of Gleason 8–9 patients had positive biopsy results compared with 12.0% (7 of 58) and 5.2% (3 of 57) of Gleason 7 and Gleason 4–6. Owing to their initial experience of incomplete apical freeze, the majority of positive biopsy results occurred at the apex in the early phase of their study (Bahn et al, 1995). **These results suggest better performance of cryotherapy in lower-volume disease as evaluated by biopsy and PSA criteria. As with radical prostatectomy data, these initial encouraging results may be tempered over time by longer-term follow-up of these patients, particularly because of the lack of controls for neoadjuvant androgen deprivation.**

The complications in patients with clinically confined disease also show marked improvements, especially when compared with the previously described group of postradiation patients (Bahn et al, 1995). The overall complications for their published group of 210 patients are given in Table 88–6 and represent patient responses to self-administered questionnaires. Eliminating the radiation patients, the major complications of urethrorectal fistula and total incontinence are 0.5% (1 of 183) and 0%. Stress incontinence in 6.2% (8 of 130) of respondents was considered transient and markedly improved or absent at 3 months. Impotency was subjective and not clinically evaluated, thereby raising concerns of patient bias. Of available data on 36 patients at 1 year, however, 27 had been potent before cryotherapy. After cryotherapy, 33% (9 of 27) remained potent to achieve intercourse, 26% (7 of 27) described partial erectile function, and 41% (11 of 27) were impotent. Again, the use of neoadjuvant androgen deprivation clouds the significance and true course of potency response in the wide age group (i.e., 51–80, mean 67 years). The impotence rate in the first TRUS-guided cryotherapy series (Onik et al, 1993) was estimated to be 65% in those patients who were previously sexually active, suggesting a far more thorough or intensive freeze than in older series (Bonney et al, 1983; Kunit, 1986).

Cryotherapy of Bulky or Locally Advanced Disease

Cryotherapy for locally advanced disease should be further examined for improved local disease control compared to the standard external-beam radiation therapy (Miller et al, 1994; Cohen et al, 1995; Miller et al, 1995). Despite improvements in local control rates when neoadjuvant androgen deprivation is administered before external-beam radiation therapy, greater cancer ablation may be possible with TRUS-guided cryotherapy. The results from two published series (Miller et al, 1994; Bahn et al, 1995) that separated the data for stage T3 patients are also given in Table 88–7. The rates between these two series appear similar but are reported in slightly different formats. The abstracts by Cohen, Miller, and colleagues now have larger numbers and suggest only 5.6% (5 of 89) positive biopsy results in patients receiving one or two cryoprocedures (Cohen et al, 1995; Miller et al, 1995). They also report mean PSA of only 0.98 ng/ml at 3 months and only 13% (1 of 8) positive biopsy results at 2 years postcryotherapy. Relatively low-volume disease, however, may be present in T3 patients because the mean/median pretreatment PSA was only 13.4/9.1 ng/ml. The PSA data presented by Bahn and colleagues did not separate patients by stage and was reported only for the entire group and subdivided by postcryotherapy biopsy results (Bahn et al, 1995).

The complications of cryotherapy for stage T3 disease should not be significantly different from those previously detailed for confined disease. The technique may require more lateral or superior extension of the ice-ball but should not produce any greater threat of rectal damage if similar care is taken to monitor the entire course of the freeze and pull-back. The abstract by Miller and co-workers (1995) may suggest greater incontinence (3.1% = 3 of 96) than in the series by Bahn and colleagues (1995) but appears related to their initial experience (Miller et al, 1994) and probably not reflective of technique differences. Once again, most complications have been subjectively graded by the treating physicians and require further evaluation by standardized quality of life instruments completed by patients. Given the degree of early success in local control as defined by biopsy

and PSA data, the complications appear low when postradiation patients are excluded.

Discussion

Much has been learned about cryotherapy, and TRUS guidance produces superior results compared to older series using open technique. Canine feasibility studies demonstrated several important TRUS imaging characteristics with histopathologic correlation over time (Littrup et al, 1994b). Excellent correlation of TRUS ice-ball extent with complete infarction of the posterior prostate and only partial extension into the rectal wall was noted. In humans with thicker rectoprostatic tissues, the canine study should encourage thorough cryotherapy beyond the posterior margin of the prostate because of highly accurate visualization of the echogenic freeze front, ensuring optimal clinical efficacy.

TRUS appearance of the prostate after cryotherapy may be unremarkable. Postcryotherapy prostates appear diffusely isoechoic with some loss of anatomic boundaries between the transition and peripheral zones. In addition, any previously noted biopsy-proven, focal hypoechoic cancer may develop poorly visualized margins or become isoechoic to adjacent parenchyma. The demonstration of unremarkable TRUS appearance in early postcryotherapy dogs was in stark comparison to the total necrosis seen on pathology (Littrup et al, 1994b). The epithelial components of the prostate parenchyma appeared thoroughly necrotic on a background of a relatively preserved collagenous architecture. If the urethral warmer effectively prevented most tissue sloughage in humans, the homogeneous isoechoic appearance on long-term follow-up is easier to understand. The autodigestive mechanisms, inflammatory infiltrates, and fibrotic changes may actually fill in the epithelial "holes" of the remaining collagenous structural skeleton. In this manner, overall acoustic interfaces are minimally changed despite gross histologic alteration. Re-epithelialization of the urethra occurred as early as 3 days but appeared well established by day 20, showing epithelial-lined glands throughout the prostate (Littrup et al, 1994b). This raised the possibility of a transitional cell progenitor for the lining epithelium of at least some of the benign-appearing glands noted on human postcryotherapy biopsy specimens.

Cryotherapy for treatment of prostatic cancer has rapidly proceeded into clinical practice given its prior use. Better cryotherapy results are achieved in patients with lower-volume cancers and neoadjuvant hormones. Bahn and co-workers show a cumulative positive biopsy rate of only 4.9% in stage T2 patients (Bahn et al, 1995). The encouraging results also extend to stage T3 patients, and the 2-year data presented by Miller and associates suggest the longest local control to date (Miller et al, 1995). **Cryotherapy biopsy results, with or without neoadjuvant hormones, thus compare quite favorably with results for radiation therapy at their optimal biopsy time frame of 18 to 24 months (e.g., 30%–90% positive biopsy results).** The clinical significance of residual tumor on biopsy following either of these therapies remains controversial but should generally be considered an insufficient result, particularly in younger patients.

The potentially spared periurethral tissue following cryotherapy also has the possibility of producing PSA elevation after the initial PSA nadir. Differential rates of PSA nadir (or subsequent rises) may allow differentiation of those patients with residual tumor from those with residual spared periurethral tissue (Littrup et al, 1994a). Even if the rate of residual tumor after cryosurgery (with neoadjuvant hormonal therapy) is doubled with longer follow-up (e.g., 10% and 40% for T2 or T3 disease), it may still be comparable to the incidence of positive surgical margins after radical prostatectomy alone (e.g., 30%–50%). The positive surgical margins at prostatectomy may, in part, correspond to the greater than 40% rising PSA levels 2 years after surgery (Murphy, 1993). The operator-dependent nature of cryotherapy, however, also applies to radical prostatectomy and emphasizes the need for larger multicenter studies for cryotherapy using similar techniques at all institutions. Likewise, American College of Surgeons data reflect pooled results of many different surgeons with variable experience and skill. Herein lies the primary difficulty in evaluating the current efficacy of cryotherapy—the lack of long-term follow-up with PSA and continued aggressive biopsy. Perhaps biopsy may not be necessary in the presence of long-term stable PSA levels (i.e., <1 ng/ml), but investigators have noted persistent viable normal parenchyma in some biopsy specimens (Hanno et al, 1995) and radical prostate specimens (Grampsas et al, 1995) as a warning of possible future failure in more patients.

Varying cryotherapy techniques, therefore, become a primary consideration in the assessment of early data from various investigators. The most detailed accounts of TRUS-guided cryotherapy have been summarized to emphasize the operator-dependent nature of this procedure (Lee et al, 1994). Early experience of many investigators suggests severe potential complications of rectal damage with fistula formation and incontinence as the primary drawbacks to this promising technique. The low rates of severe complications by the two groups with the most experience (Onik et al, 1993; Miller et al, 1994; Bahn et al, 1995; Cohen et al, 1995; Miller et al, 1995), however, attest to the safety of cryotherapy if careful attention to good TRUS guidance and monitoring is achieved. The higher rates of complications in postradiation cryotherapy patients (von Eschenbach et al, 1995) may also be improved if more sophisticated monitoring techniques are applied (Bahn et al, 1995). Similarly, other institutions beginning cryotherapy may demonstrate fewer complications than currently reported (Cox and Crawford, 1995) if these detailed technique modifications are followed. The potentially compromised rectal wall and external sphincter in all postradiation patients, however, places them at inherently higher risk for any surgical procedure in this area.

Because no treatment for localized prostate cancer has ever been shown to decrease mortality in controlled trials, the morbidities of any therapy may have greater significance than slight differences in survival outcome. Quality-adjusted life years may become the most socially significant parameter for the evaluation of treatment choices for prostate cancer (Wasson et al, 1993; Krahn et al, 1994). If biochemical control or cure can be established by longer follow-up of the initial encouraging cryotherapy results, far more attention should be paid to quality of life parameters and judged by validated instruments. A large proportion of lost quality-

adjusted life years stems from potential impotence, and the authors proposed nerve-sparing modifications to current human cryotherapy techniques (Littrup et al, 1994a). Although still untested, the concept should not be considered completely theoretical because the medical and economic impetus already exists for limiting any treatment morbidity caused by the markedly increased detection of clinically localized prostate cancer (Catalona et al, 1993).

The future of clinical prostate cryotherapy research depends in large part on organized efforts to conduct appropriate trials that are accessible to many cancer patients. This requires some form of reimbursement for the procedure itself and may be justified if limited to specific centers documenting adherence to well-defined technique considerations. In its absence, the utility of cryotherapy may never be adequately evaluated and remain controversial because of the lack of multi-institutional, controlled data. Further investigations of thermosensors, urethral warmers, and rectal warmers may better define their role in decreasing incontinence or fistula formation. Tailored biopsy approaches directed at extensive sampling of any region considered for sparing (e.g., the distal apex in postradiation patients) may also improve the complication profile. Basic research on improved mechanisms to produce more thorough cytotoxicity (i.e., cryosensitizers) also needs to be balanced by concurrent efforts of morbidity reduction or prevention. As noted, the value of cryotherapy may be better judged in the future in relation to quality-adjusted life years and associated efficacy and morbidity comparisons to other treatments or observation alone.

REFERENCES

Abrams HL, Spiro R, Goldstein N: Metastases in carcinoma: Analysis of 1000 autopsied cases. Cancer 1950; 3:74–75.

Adolfsson J, Chisholm GD, Chodak GW, et al: Results of conservative management of clinically localized prostate cancer. N Engl J Med 1994; 330:242–248.

Ando K: Cryoprostatectomy under control of ultrasonotomography. Presented at the 14th Congress of the International Urologic Society, 1982.

Bagshaw MA, Cox RS, Hancock SL: Control of prostate cancer with radiotherapy: Long-term results. J Urol 1994; 152:1781–1785.

Bahn DK, Lee F, Solomon MH, et al: Prostate cancer: Ultrasound guided percutaneous cryoablation: Work in progress. Radiology 1995; 194:551–556.

Bayouth JE, Macey DJ, Kasi LP, Fossella FV: Dosimetry and toxicity of samarium-153-EDTMP administered for bone pain due to skeletal metastases. J Nucl Med 1994; 35:63–69.

Ben-Josef E, Lucas RD, Vasan S, Porter AT: Selective accumulation of strontium-89 in metastatic deposits in bone: Radio-histological correlation. Nucl Med Commun 1995a; 16:452–456.

Ben-Josef E, Maughan RL, Vasan S, Porter AT: A direct measurement of 89Sr activity in bone metastases. Nucl Med Commun 1995b; 16:457–463.

Black P: Spinal metastases: Current status and recommended guidelines for management. Neurosurgery 1979; 5:726–746.

Blake GM, Zivanovic MA, Blaquiere RM, et al: Strontium-89 therapy: Measurement of absorbed dose to skeletal metastases. J Nucl Med 1988; 29:549–557.

Blake GM, Zivanovic MA, McEwan AJ, et al: Sr-89 therapy: Strontium kinetics in disseminated carcinoma of the prostate. Eur J Nucl Med 1986; 12:447–454.

Blasko JC, Grimm PD, Ragde H: Brachytherapy and organ preservation in the management of carcinoma of the prostate. Semin Radiat Oncol 1993; 3:240–249.

Blitzer PH: Reanalysis of the RTOG study of the palliation of symptomatic osseous metastases. Cancer 1985; 55:1468–1472.

Bolger JJ, Dearnaley DP, Kirk D, et al: Strontium-89 (Metastron) versus external beam radiotherapy in patients with painful bone metastases secondary to prostatic cancer: Preliminary report of a multicenter trial: UK Metastron Investigators Group. Semin Oncol 1993; 20:32–33.

Bonney WW, Fallon B, Gerber WL, et al: Cryosurgery in prostatic cancer: Survival. Urology 1982; 19:37–42.

Bonney WW, Fallon B, Gerber WL, et al: Cryosurgery in prostatic cancer: Elimination of a local lesion. Urology 1983; 22:8–15.

Boring CC, Squires T, Tong T, Montgomery S: Cancer statistics, 1994. CA Cancer J Clin 1994; 44:7–26.

Bostwick DG, Egbert BM, Fajardo LF: Radiation injury of the normal and neoplastic prostate. Am J Surg Pathol 1982; 6:541–551.

Brawer MK, Nagle RB, Pitts W, et al: Keratin immunoreactivity as an aid to the diagnosis of persistent adenocarcinoma in irradiated human prostates. Cancer 1989; 63:454–460.

Breen SL, Powe JE, Porter AT: Dose estimation in strontium-89 radiotherapy of metastatic prostatic carcinoma. J Nucl Med 1992; 33:1316–1323.

Bruce AW, Mahan DE, Lott S: Radiation therapy for adenocarcinoma of the prostate. Can J Surg 1979; 22:424–427.

Bruckman JE, Bloomer WD: Management of spinal cord compression. Semin Oncol 1978; 5:135–140.

Buchali K, Correns HJ, Schuerer M, et al: Results of a double-blind study of 89-strontium therapy of skeletal metastases of prostatic carcinoma. Eur J Nucl Med 1988; 14:349–351.

Carmody RF, Yang PJ, Seely GW, et al: Spinal cord compression due to metastatic disease: Diagnosis with MR imaging versus myelography. Radiology 1989; 173:225–229.

Catalona WJ: Management of cancer of the prostate. N Engl J Med 1994; 331:996–1004.

Catalona WJ, Smith DS, Ratliff TL, Basler JW: Detection of organ-confined prostate cancer is increased through prostate-specific antigen-based screening. JAMA 1993; 270:948–954.

Cohen JK, Miller RJ: Thermal protection of urethra during cryosurgery of the prostate. Cryobiology 1994; 30:313–316.

Cohen JK, Miller RJ, Schumann BA: Cryosurgical ablation of the prostate: Patterns of failure and two year post treatment data as compared to external beam radiation therapy (Abstract 1098). J Urol 1995; 153(suppl):503A.

Cole DJ: A randomised trial of a single treatment versus conventional fractionation in the palliative radiotherapy of painful bone metastases. Clin Oncol 1989; 1:59–62.

Collins C, Eary JF, Donaldson G, et al: Samarium-153-EDTMP in bone metastases of hormone refractory prostate carcinoma: A phase I/II trial. J Nucl Med 1993; 34:1839–1844.

Correns HJ, Mebel M, Buchali K, et al: Strontium-89 therapy of bone metastases of carcinoma of the prostate gland. Eur J Nucl Med 1979; 4:33–35.

Cox JD, Stoffel TJ: The significance of needle biopsy after irradiation for stage C adenocarcinoma of the prostate. Cancer 1977; 40:156–160.

Cox RL, Crawford ED: Complications of cryosurgical ablation of the prostate to treat localized adenocarcinoma. Urology 1995; 45:932–935.

Crook J, Robertson S, Collin G, et al: Clinical relevance of trans-rectal ultrasound biopsy, and serum prostate-specific antigen following external beam radiotherapy for carcinoma of the prostate. Int J Radiat Oncol Biol Phys 1993; 27:31–37.

Crook J, Robertson S, Esche B: Proliferative cell nuclear antigen in postradiotherapy prostate biopsies. Int J Radiat Oncol Biol Phys 1994; 30:303–308.

Debruyne FMJ, Boerema JBJ, Kirkels WJ: Cryosurgery of prostatic cancer. Act Urol Belg 1984; 3:450–455.

Dhom G, Degro S: Therapy of prostatic cancer and histopathologic follow-up. Prostate 1982; 3:531–542.

Donnelly BJ, Pedersen J, Porter AT, McPhee M: Iridium-192 brachytherapy in the treatment of cancer of the prostate. Clin Urol 1991; 18:483–491.

Dugan TC, Shipley WU, Young RH, et al: Biopsy after external beam radiation therapy for adenocarcinoma of the prostate: Correlation with original histological grade and current prostate specific antigen levels. J Urol 1991; 146:1313–1316.

Eary JF, Collins C, Stabin M, et al: Samarium-153-EDTMP biodistribution and dosimetry estimation. J Nucl Med 1993; 34:1031–1036.

Epstein JI, Pizov G, Walsh PC: Correlation of pathologic findings with progression after radical retropubic prostatectomy. Cancer 1993; 71:3582–3593.

Epstein LM, Stewart BH, Antung AR, et al: Half and total body irradiation for carcinoma of the prostate. J Urol 1979; 12:330.

Firusian N, Mellin P, Schmidt CG: Results of strontium-89 therapy in patients with carcinoma of the prostate and incurable pain from bone metastases: A preliminary report. J Urol 1976; 116:764–798.

Fitzpatrick PJ, Rider WD: Halfbody radiotherapy. Int J Radiat Oncol Biol Phys 1976; 1:197.

Flocks RH, Neyon CMK, Boatman DL: Perineal cryosurgery for prostatic carcinoma. J Urol 1972; 108:933–935.

Forman JD, Kumar R, Haas G, et al: Neoadjuvant hormonal downsizing of localized carcinoma of the prostate: Effects on the volume of tissue irradiated. Cancer Invest 1995; 13:8–15.

Forman JD, Oppenheim T, Liu H, et al: Frequency of residual neoplasm in the prostate following three-dimensional conformal radiotherapy. Prostate 1993a; 23:235–243.

Forman JD, Orton C, Ezzell G, Porter AT: Preliminary results of a hyper-fractionated dose escalation study for locally advanced adenocarcinoma of the prostate. Radiother Oncol 1993b; 27:203–208.

Forman JD, Warmelink C, Devi S, et al: Alternating conformal neutron and photon irradiation for locally advanced adenocarcinoma of the prostate. Am J Clin Oncol 1995; 18(3):231–238.

Freiha FS, Bagshaw MA: Carcinoma of the prostate: Results of post-irradiation biopsy. Prostate 1984; 5:19–25.

Friedell HL, Storaasli JP: The use of radioactive phosphorus in the treatment of carcinoma of the breast with wide-spread metastases to bone. Am J Roentgenol Radiat Ther 1950; 64:559–575.

Friedman M, Kim TM, Panahon AM: Spinal cord compression in malignant lymphoma. Cancer 1976; 37:1485.

Fuks A, Leibel AA, Wallner KE, et al: The effect of local control on metastatic dissemination in carcinoma of the prostate: Long term results in patients treated with I-125 implantation. Int J Radiat Oncol Biol Phys 1991; 21:537–547.

Gilbert HA, Dagan AR: Metastases: Incidence, detection, and evaluation. In Weiss L, ed: Fundamental Aspects of Metastases. Amsterdam, Elsevier Excerpta Medica, 1976.

Gilbert RW, Kim JH, Posner JB: Epidural spinal cord compression from metastatic tumor: Diagnosis and treatment. Ann Neurol 1978; 3:40–51.

Gill W, Long WB: A critical look at cryosurgery. Int Surg 1971; 56:344–351.

Glasko CSB: Skeletal metastases. Clin Orthop 1986; 210:18–30.

Gonder MJ, Soanes W, Schulman S: Cryosurgical treatment of the prostate. Invest Urol 1966; 3:372–378.

Grampsas SA, Miller GJ, Crawford ED: Salvage prostatectomy after failed transperineal cryotherapy: Histologic findings from prostate whole-mount specimens correlated with intraoperative transrectal ultrasound images. Urology 1995; 45:936–941.

Griffin TW, Krall JM, Russell KJ, et al: Fast neutron irradiation of locally advanced prostate cancer. Semin Oncol 1988; 4:359–365.

Grignon DJ, Sakr WA: Histological effects of radiation therapy and total androgen blockade on prostate cancer. Cancer 1995; 75:1837–1841.

Hanks GE: Optimizing the radiation treatment and outcome of prostate cancer. Int J Radiat Oncol Biol Phys 1985; 11:1235–1245.

Hanks GE, Asbell S, Krall JM, et al: Outcome for lymph node dissection negative T-1b, T2 (A-2, B) prostate cancer treated with external beam radiation therapy in RTOG 7706. Int J Radiat Oncol Biol Phys 1991; 21:1099–1103.

Hanks GE, Hanlon A, Schultheiss T, et al: Early prostate cancer: The national results of radiation treatment from the Patterns of Care and Radiation Therapy Oncology Group studies with prospects for improvement with conformal radiation and adjuvant androgen deprivation. J Urol 1994; 152:1775–1780.

Hanks GE, Martz KL, Diamond JJ: The effect of dose on local control of prostate cancer. Int J Radiat Oncol Biol Phys 1988; 15:1299–1305.

Hanno P, Brandes S, Stern R, Seidmon EJ: Persistence of histologically viable appearing prostate tissue after cryosurgery (Abstract 1099). J Urol 1995; 153(suppl):503A.

Harisiadis L, Veenemar J, Senyzsyn JA, et al: Carcinoma of the prostate: Treatment with external radiotherapy. Cancer 1978; 41:2131–2142.

Jacobsson H, Naslund I: Reduced incidence of bone metastases in irradiated areas after external radiation therapy of prostatic carcinoma. Int J Radiat Oncol Biol Phys 1991; 20:1297–1303.

Johansson JE, Adami H-O, Andersson S-O, et al: High 10-year survival rate in patients with early, untreated prostatic cancer. JAMA 1992; 267:2191–2196.

Kabalin JN, Hodge KK, McNeal JE, et al: Identification of residual cancer in the prostate following radiation therapy: Role of transrectal ultrasound guided biopsy and prostate specific antigen. J Urol 1989; 142:326–331.

Kaplan ID, Valdagni R, Cox RS: Reduction of spinal metastases after preemptive irradiation in prostate cancer. Int J Radiat Oncol Biol Phys 1990; 18:1019.

Kiesling VJ, McAninch JW, Goebel JL, Agee RE: External beam radiotherapy for adenocarcinoma of the prostate: A clinical follow-up. J Urol 1980; 124:851–854.

Krahn MD, Mahoney JE, Eckman MH, et al: Screening for prostate cancer: A decision analytic view. JAMA 1994; 272:773–780.

Kuban DA, El-Mahdi AM, Schellhammer PF: Effective local tumor control on distant metastases and survival in prostate cancer. J Urol 1987; 30:420–426.

Kuban DA, El-Mahdi AM, Schellhammer P: The significance of post-irradiation prostate biopsy with long term follow-up. Int J Radiat Oncol Biol Phys 1992; 24:409–414.

Kunit G: Open perineal cryosurgery in carcinoma of the prostate—a possible curative alternative. Urol Res 1986; 14:3–7.

Kurth KH, Altwein JE, Skoluda D: Follow-up of irradiated prostatic carcinoma by aspiration biopsy. J Urol 1977; 117:615.

Laing AH, Ackery DM, Bayly RJ, et al: Strontium-89 chloride for pain palliation in prostatic skeletal malignancy. Br J Radiol 1991; 64:816–822.

Landaw SA: Acute leukemia in polycythemia vera. Semin Hematol 1986; 23:156–165.

Lane JM, Sculo TP, Zolan S: Treatment of pathologic fractures of the hip by endoprosthetic replacement. J Bone Joint Surg 1980; 62:954–959.

Lee F, Bahn DK, McHugh TA, et al: US-guided percutaneous cryoablation of prostate cancer. Radiology 1994; 192:769–776.

Leibel SA, Heimann R, Kutcher GJ, et al: Three-dimensional conformal radiation therapy in locally advanced carcinoma of prostate: Preliminary results of phase-I dose escalation study. Int J Radiat Oncol Biol Phys 1993; 28:55–65.

Lewington VJ, McEwan AJ, Ackery DM, et al: A prospective randomized double-blind crossover study to examine the efficacy of strontium-89 in pain palliation in patients with advanced prostate cancer metastatic to bone. Eur J Cancer 1991; 27:954–958.

Li KC, Poon PY: Sensitivity and specificity of MRI in detecting malignant spinal cord compression and in distinguishing malignant from benign compression fractures of vertebrae. MRI 1988; 6:547–556.

Littrup PJ, Mody A, Sparschu RA: Prostate cryosurgery complications. Semin Intervent Radiol 1994a; 11:226–230.

Littrup PJ, Mody A, Sparschu RA, Prchevski P, et al: Prostatic cryotherapy: Ultrasonographic and pathologic correlation in canine model. Urology 1994b; 44:175–184.

Littrup PJ, Sparschu RA: Transrectal ultrasound and prostate cancer risks: The "tailored" prostate biopsy. Cancer 1995; 75:1807–1813.

Loening S, Bonney WW, Fallon B, et al: Perineal cryosurgery of prostatic cancer. Urology 1981; 27(suppl):12–14.

Loening S, Hawtrey CE, Bonney WW, et al: Cryotherapy of prostate cancer. Prostate 1980; 1:279–286.

Loening S, Lubaroff D: Cryosurgery and immunotherapy for prostatic cancer. Urol Clin North Am 1984; 2:327–336.

Madsen EL: Painful bone metastases: Efficacy of radiotherapy assessed by the patient—a randomized trial comparing 4 Gy × 6 vs 10 Gy × 2. Int J Radiat Oncol Biol Phys 1983; 9:1775–1779.

Marinelli D, Shanberg AM, Tansey LA, et al: Follow-up prostate biopsy in patients with carcinoma of the prostate treated by 192-iridium template irradiation plus supplemental external beam radiation. J Urol 1992; 147:922–925.

Martinez A, Edmundsen JD, Cox RS, et al: A combination of external beam irradiation and multiple site perineal applicator for the treatment of locally advanced or recurrent prostate perineum and gynecological malignancies. Int J Radiat Oncol Biol Phys 1985; 11:391–398.

Maxon HR, Schroder LE, Hertzberg VA, et al: Re-186(Sn) HEDP for treatment of painful osseous metastases: Results of a double-blind cross-over comparison with placebo. J Nucl Med 1991; 32:1877–1881.

Maxon HR, Schroder LE, Thomas SR, et al: Re-186(Sn) HEDP for treatment of painful osseous metastases: Initial clinical experience in 20 patients with hormone-resistant prostate cancer. Radiology 1990; 176:155–159.

Maxon HR, Thomas SR, Hertzberg VA, et al: Rhenium-186 hydroxyethylidene diphosphonate for the treatment of painful osseous metastases. Semin Nucl Med 1992; 22:33–40.

Mazur P: Kinetics of water loss from cells at sub-zero temperatures and the likelihood of intracellular freezing. J Gen Physiol 1963: 47:347–369.

Mazur P: Cryobiology: The freezing of biological systems. Science 1970; 168:939–949.

Mazur P: The role of intracellular freezing in the death of cells cooled at supraoptimal rates. Cryobiology 1977; 14:251–272.

Mertens WC, Porter AT, Ried RH, Powe JE: Strontium-89 and low-dose cisplatinum for patients with hormone refractory prostate carcinoma metastatic to bone: A preliminary report. J Nucl Med 1992; 33:1437–1443.

Mesina CF, Sharma R, Rissman LS, et al: Comparison of a conformal nonaxial boost with a four-field boost technique in the treatment of adenocarcinoma of the prostate. Int J Radiat Oncol Biol Phys 1994; 30:427–430.

Miller EB, Ladaga LE, El-Mahdi AM, Schellhammer PF: Reevaluation of prostate biopsy after definitive radiation therapy. Urology 1993; 41:311–316.

Miller RJ, Cohen JK, Merlotti LA: Percutaneous transperineal cryosurgical ablation of the prostate for the primary treatment of clinical stage C adenocarcinoma of the prostate. Urology 1994; 44:170–174.

Miller RJ, Cohen JK, Schuman BA: Percutaneous transperineal cryosurgical ablation of the prostate as primary treatment for clinical stage C adenocarcinoma (Abstract 628). J Urol 1995; 153(suppl):385A.

Mollenkamp JS, Cooper JF, Kagan AR: Clinical experience with supervoltage radiotherapy in carcinoma of the prostate: A preliminary report. J Urol 1975; 113:374–377.

Montebello JF, Hartson-Eaton M: The palliation of osseous metastases with 32P or 89Sr compared with external beam and hemibody irradiation: A historical perspective. Cancer Invest 1989; 7:139–169.

Murphy GP: American College of Surgeons survey. Presented at the Detection and Treatment of Early Stage Prostate Cancer, Crystal City, VA, 1993.

Nachtsheim DA Jr, McAninch JW, Stutzman RE, Goebel JL: Latent residual tumor following external radiotherapy for prostate adenocarcinoma. J Urol 1978; 120:312–314.

National Council on Radiation Protection and Measurements: A Handbook of Radioactivity Measurements Procedure. Washington, D.C., 1978.

O'Brien J, Carswell GF: A complication of cryoprostatectomy. Br J Urol 1972; 44:713–715.

O'Donoghue EPN, Milleman LA, Flocks RH, et al: Cryosurgery for carcinoma of the prostate. Urology 1975; 5:308–316.

Onik G, Cobb C, Cohen J, et al: US characteristics of frozen prostate. Radiology 1988; 168:629–631.

Onik G, Cohen J, Reyes G, et al: Transrectal ultrasound percutaneous radical cryosurgical ablation of the prostate. Cancer 1993; 72:11291–11299.

Ortved WE, O'Kelly FM, Todd IAD, et al: Cryosurgical prostatectomy. Br J Urol 1967; 39:577–583.

Pagani JJ, Libshitz HI: Imaging in bone metastases. Radiol Clin North Am 1982; 20:545–560.

Paulson DF, Hodge GB, Hinshaw W, Stephani S: Radical surgery versus radiation therapy for adenocarcinoma of the prostate, J Urol 1982a; 128:502–504.

Paulson DF, Lin GH, Hinshaw W, Stephani S: The Uro-Oncology Research Group: Radical surgery versus radiotherapy for adenocarcinoma for the prostate. Urology 1982b; 128:502–504.

Pecher C: Biological investigations with radioactive calcium and strontium: Preliminary report on the use of radioactive strontium in treatment of metastatic bone cancer. University of California Publications Pharmacol 1942; 11:117–149.

Perez CA, Pilepich MV, Garcia D, et al: Definitive radiation therapy in carcinoma of the prostate localized to the pelvis: Experience at the Mallinckrodt Institute of Radiology. NCI Monogr 1988; 7:85–94.

Pilepich MV, Bagshaw M, Asbell SO, et al: Radical prostatectomy or radiotherapy in carcinoma of the prostate—the dilemma continues. Urology 1987; 30:18–21.

Pilepich MW, Krall J, Al-Sarraf M, et al: A phase-III trial of androgen suppression before and during radiation therapy for locally advanced prostatic carcinoma: Preliminary report RTOG Protocol 8610 (Abstract). Proceedings ASCO, 1993, p 703.

Pontes JE, Montie J, Klein E, Huben R: Salvage surgery for radiation failure in prostate cancer. Cancer 1993; 71:976–980.

Portenoy RK, Galer BS, Salamon O, et al: Identification of epidural neoplasm: Radiography and bone scintigraphy in the symptomatic and asymptomatic spine. Cancer 1989; 64:2207–2213.

Porter AT: Prostate brachytherapy. In Mould R, ed: Bachytherapy 1990. Amsterdam, Nucletron Inc, 1990, pp 165–171.

Porter AT: Use of strontium-89 in metastatic cancer: US and UK experience. Oncology 1994; 8(suppl):25–29.

Porter AT, Blasko JC, Grimm PD, et al: Brachytherapy for prostate cancer. CA Cancer J Clin 1995; 45:165–178.

Porter AT, Daly H: Retrograde urographic technique in the treatment planning of radiation therapy to prostate cancers. Med Dosim 1987; 12:29–30.

Porter AT, Fontanesi J: Palliative irradiation for bone metastases—a new paradigm. Int J Radiat Oncol Biol Phys 1994; 29:1199–1200.

Porter AT, Forman JD: Prostate brachytherapy: An overview. Cancer 1993; 71:950–958.

Porter AT, Forman JD: The role of radiotherapy in the management of locally advanced prostate cancer. Urology 1994; 44(suppl):43–46.

Porter AT, McEwan AJB, Powe JE, et al: Results of a randomized phase-III trial to evaluate the efficacy of strontium-89 adjuvant to local field external beam irradiation in the management of endocrine resistant metastatic prostate cancer. Int J Radiat Oncol Biol Phys 1993; 25:805–813.

Porter AT, Venner PM: The role of cytoreduction prior to definitive radiotherapy in locally advanced prostate cancer. Prog Clin Biol Res 1990; 359:231–239.

Poulter CA, Cosmatos D, Rubin P, et al: A report of RTOG 82-06: A Phase III study of the addition of single dose hemibody irradiation to standard fractionated local field irradiation alone in the treatment of symptomatic osseous metastases. Int J Radiat Oncol Biol Phys 1992; 23:207.

Prestidge BR, Kaplan I, Cox RS, Bagshaw MA: The clinical significance of a positive post-irradiation prostatic biopsy without metastases. Int J Radiat Oncol Biol Phys 1992; 24:403–408.

Prestidge BR, Kaplan I, Cox RS, Bagshaw MA: Predictors of survival after a positive post-irradiation prostate biopsy. Int J Radiat Oncol Biol Phys 1994; 28:17–22.

Price P, Hoskin PJ, Easton D, et al: Low dose single fraction radiotherapy in the treatment of metastatic bone pain: A pilot study. Radiother Oncol 1988; 12:297–300.

Puthawala A, Syed AMN, Tansey L: Temporary iridium-192 implant in the management of carcinoma of the prostate. Endocurietherapy/Hyperthermia Oncol 1985; 1:25–33.

Quilty PM, Kirk D, Bolger JJ, et al: A comparison of the palliative effects of strontium-89 and external beam radiotherapy in metastatic prostate cancer. Radiother Oncol 1994; 31:33–40.

Roach M III, Marquez C, Yuo H-S, et al: Predicting the risk of lymph node involvement using the pre-treatment prostate specific antigen and Gleason score in men with clinically localized prostate cancer. Int J Radiat Oncol Biol Phys 1994; 28:33–37.

Robinson RG, Preston DF, Baxter KG, et al: Clinical experience with strontium-89 in prostatic and breast cancer patients. Semin Oncol 1992; 20:44–48.

Robinson RG, Spicer JA, Preston DF, et al: Treatment of metastatic bone pain with strontium-89. Nucl Med Biol 1987; 14:219–222.

Rodichok RD, Ruckdeschel JC, Harper GR, et al: Early detection and treatment of spinal epidural metastases: The role of myelography. Ann Neurol 1986; 20:696–702.

Rosen E, Cassady JR, Connolly J, Chaffey JT: Radiotherapy for prostate carcinoma: The JCRT Experience: Factors related to tumor control and complications. Int J Radiat Oncol Biol Phys 1985; 11:726–730.

Rubin P, Scarantino CW: Hemibody irradiation. In Mauch PM, Loeffler JS, eds: Radiation Oncology: Technology and Biology. Philadelphia, W. B. Saunders, 1994.

Rubinski B: Percutaneous Prostate Cryoablation. St. Louis, MO, Quality Medical Publishing, Inc, 1995.

Russell KJ, Caplan RJ, Laramore GE, et al: Photon versus fast neutron external beam radiotherapy in the treatment of locally advanced prostate cancer: Results of a randomized prospective trial. Int J Radiat Oncol Biol Phys 1993; 28:47–54.

Salazar OM, Rubin P, Hendrickson FR, et al: Single-dose half-body irradiation for palliation of multiple bone metastases from solid tumors: Final Radiation Therapy Oncology Group Report. Cancer 1986; 58:29–36.

Salazar OM, Rubin P, Keller B, et al: Systemic (half-body) radiation therapy: Response and toxicity. Int J Radiat Oncol Biol Phys 1978; 4:937–950.

Sandler H, McShan D, Lichter AS: Potential improvement in the results of irradiation for prostate carcinoma using improved dose distribution. Int J Radiat Oncol Biol Phys 1991; 22:361–367.

Scarantino CW, Ornitz RD, Hoffman LG, et al: On the mechanism of radiation-induced emesis (RIE): The role of serotonin. Int J Radiat Oncol Biol Phys 1994; 30:825–830.

Scardino PT, Frankel JM, Wheeler TM, et al: The significance of post-irradiation biopsy results in patients with prostatic cancer. J Urol 1986; 135:510–516.

Schellhammer POF, Ladaga LE, El-Mahdi A: Histological characteristics of prostatic biopsies after iodine implantation. J Urol 1980; 123:700–705.

Schmidt JD, Parsons CL, Casola G, et al: Transperineal cryoablation for prostate cancer (Abstract 1096). J Urol 1995; 153(suppl):502A.

Shinohara K, Carroll PR: Improved results of cryosurgical ablation of the prostate (Abstract 627). J Urol 1995; 153(suppl):385A.

Shipley WU, Munzenrider JE, McManus PL, et al: Results of a randomized trial of total radiation dose for stage T3-T4 prostate cancer boosting with photons (to 67.2 cGe) or with conformal protons (to 75.6 cGe). Proceedings of the American Society of Therapeutic Radiation Oncology (ASTRO) 36th Annual Meeting. Int J Radiat Oncol Biol Phys 1994a; 30:211.

Shipley WU, Zietman AL, Hanks GE, et al: Treatment related sequelae following external beam radiation for prostate cancer: A review with an update in patients with stages T1 and T2 tumor. J Urol 1994b; 152:1799–1805.

Siders DB, Lee F: Histologic changes of irradiated prostatic carcinoma diagnosed by transrectal ultrasound. Hum Pathol 1993; 23:344–351.

Silberstein EB: The treatment of painful osseous metastases with phosphorus-32 labeled phosphates. Semin Oncol 1993; 20:10–21.

Silberstein EB, Williams C: Strontium-89 therapy for the pain of osseous metastases. J Nucl Med 1985; 26:345–348.

Simpson JR, Purdy JA, Manolis MV, et al: Three-dimensional treatment planning considerations for prostate cancer. Int J Radiat Oncol Biol Phys 1991; 21:243–252.

Soanes WA, Gonder MJ: Use of cryosurgery in prostatic cancer. J Urol 1968; 99:793–797.

Sze G, Krol G, Zimmerman RD: Malignant extradural spinal tumors: MR imaging with Gd-DTPA. Radiology 1988; 167:217–233.

Tennvall J, Darte L, Lindgren R, El Hassan AM: Palliation of multiple bony metastases from prostatic carcinoma with strontium-89. Acta Oncol 1988; 27:365–369.

Tong D, Gillick L, Hendrickson FR: The palliation of symptomatic osseous metastases: Final results of the Radiation Therapy Oncology Group. Cancer 1982; 50:893–899.

Turner JH, Claringbold PG, Martindale AA, et al: Samarium-153 EDTMP and radiosensitizing chemotherapy for treatment of disseminated skeletal metastases (Abstract). Eur J Nucl Med 1992; 16:S-125.

Van Holten-Verzantvoort AT, Bijvoet OLM, Cleton FJ, et al: Reduced morbidity from skeletal metastases in breast cancer patients during long-term bisphosphonate (APD) treatment. Lancet 1987; 2:983–985.

von Eschenbach AC, Pisters LL, Swanson DA, et al: Results of a phase I/II study of cryoablation for recurrent carcinoma of the prostate: The University of Texas M. D. Anderson Cancer Center experience (Abstract 1097). J Urol 1995; 153(suppl):503A.

Wasson J, Cushman CC, Bruskewitz RB, et al: A structured literature review of treatment for localized prostate cancer. Arch Fam Med 1993; 2:487–493.

Wheeler JA, Zagars GK, Ayala AG: Dedifferentiation of locally recurrent prostate cancer after radiation therapy. Cancer 1993; 71:3783–3787.

Williams JR, Dillehay LE: The radiobiology of exponentially decreasing dose rates in vitro and in vivo: Relevance to tumor therapy with radiolabeled antibodies (Abstract). Proceedings of the 37th Annual Meeting of the Radiation Research Society, Seattle, 1989, p 202.

Wilner D: Cancer metastases to bone. In Wilner D, ed: Radiology of Bone Tumors and Allied Disorders. Philadelphia, W. B. Saunders, 1982, pp 3641–3908.

Zagars GK, von Eschenbach AC, Johnson DE: Stage-C adenocarcinoma of the prostate: An analysis of 551 patients treated with external beam radiation. Cancer 1987; 60:1489–1499.

Zagars GK, von Eschenbach AC, Johnson DE, Oswald MJ: The role of radiation therapy in stages A2 and B adenocarcinoma of the prostate. Int J Radiat Oncol Biol Phys 1988; 14:701.

Zietman AL, Shipley WU, Coen JJ: Radical radiation therapy in the management of prostatic adenocarcinoma: The initial prostate specific antigen value as a predictor of treatment outcome. J Urol 1994; 151:640–645.

89
ENDOCRINE TREATMENT OF PROSTATE CANCER

Fritz H. Schröder, M.D.

ENDOCRINE DEPENDENCE OF PROSTATE CANCER

In patients suffering from prostate cancer, castration or the use of other mechanisms that lead to a decrease of testicular androgen production and of plasma testosterone levels usually results in a favorable response. Huggins and Hodges (1941) were the first to describe castration or treatment with diethylstilbestrol (DES) as effective. **They found that elevated levels of serum acid phosphatase decrease under endocrine treatment, and alkaline phosphatase initially shows a slow rise but then also decreases or normalizes. This response was associated with an improvement of symptoms related to prostate cancer.** The discovery, which was honored with the Nobel Prize, was the result of systematic research on the endocrine dependence of the dog prostate as well as of a carefully conducted morphologic study of the effect of castration on human benign prostatic hyperplasia (BPH) (Huggins et al, 1941). At this time, it was assumed that the impressive response of tumor-related parameters must be associated with a clinically important prolongation of life or even cure of some patients with prostate cancer. This assumption seemed to be confirmed when Nesbit and Baum (1950) published their results of a

large retrospective study in which the fate of 417 patients with metasases was compared, and 3-year survival showed a significant difference for those who had received endocrine treatment.

As is evident from this chapter, **endocrine treatment of prostate cancer is palliative.** Although intercurrent death of men suffering from this disease is common because of the natural occurrence of competing causes of death in the age group involved, convincing **evidence of cure of prostate cancer under endocrine treatment** has rarely been presented. Johansson and Ljunggren (1981) claimed cure of a nonmetastatic prostate carcinoma by estrogen treatment. The patient died of hemorrhage 14 years after the diagnosis was made: prostatic step sections showed no residual tumor. Some patients with metastatic prostate cancer lived for long periods of time under endocrine treatment. Reiner and colleagues reviewed a series of 56 patients with metastatic prostate cancer and a follow-up period of 10 to 15 years (Reiner et al, 1979). Five of these men lived longer than 10 years. One man died 15 years after initiation of treatment without clinical evidence of disease.

Endocrine treatment is commonly applied to either locally advanced or metastatic prostate cancer. In the still commonly used classification by Whitmore (1956), this disease is classified as stage C (locally extensive), stage

D1 (lymph node metastases), or stage D2 (other distant metastases). In the tumor, nodes, and metastases (TNM) system (Hermanek and Sobin, 1992), which is more commonly used by clinicians all over the world, locally extensive or metastatic disease falls within the T3, N0–3, and M1 categories (Table 89–1).

Exploitable Mechanisms in Endocrine Treatment

The full extent of the endocrine dependence of normal prostatic cells and prostate cancer cells is not known at this time, especially if the effect of cytokines and growth factors is included. Details can be found in Chapter 45. Within the context of this chapter, only those mechanisms that are of clinical importance at the time of writing are reviewed. This excludes the issue of suramin, a treatment that is specifically directed against growth factors, which may influence the growth of hormone-dependent and hormone-independent prostate cancer. Suramin is covered in Chapter 90.

Androgens and Androgen Withdrawal

The major source of androgens in males is the Leydig cells located in the testes. Testicular production of the main circulating androgen, testosterone, amounts to about 6.6 mg/day leading to serum concentrations of 5.72 ± 1.35 ng/ml (19.8 ± 4.7 nmol/l) in the adult. **After castration, serum testosterone decreases to 5% to 10% of the original values.** The remaining testosterone is derived from adrenal androgens, which may be metabolized to testosterone and **5-alpha-dihydrotestosterone (DHT), the most potent androgen at the level of the prostate,** which is derived from testosterone by 5-alpha reduction through the activity of the enzymes **5-alpha-reductase (5αR) type 1 and type 2.** The biologic activity of androgens is determined by their structure and by their affinity to the androgen receptor, which is about 7 times higher for DHT in comparison to testosterone. Adrenal androgens are rather weak but can be metabolized to DHT within the prostate and outside through the availability of the enzymes 17-beta-hydroxysteroid dehydrogenase and 5αR.

Adrenal androgens are produced in the zona fasciculata and reticularis of the adrenal cortex. The main adrenal androgens are androstenedione and dehydroepiandrosterone. Adrenal androgens in circulation are bound to albumin, whereas testosterone and DHT are bound to steroid hormone–binding globulin; only free androgens can exert androgenic actions.

Androgen production in the Leydig cells and the adrenals is under pituitary control through luteinizing hormone (LH) and adrenocorticotropic hormone (ACTH). Pituitary control mechanisms and hypothalamic control mechanisms of the pituitary are depicted in Figure 89–1.

The action of androgens at the target cell is mediated by the androgen receptor. The steroid androgen receptor complex binds to specific DNA sites and leads to the initiation of transcription. Without androgen receptor binding, steroid hormones cannot exert their biologic effects. Consequently, if androgen receptor binding is inhibited, biologic effects can be prevented. Antiandrogens interfere with the formation of the androgen receptor complex. There are several possible ways in which androgen deprivation can be achieved:

Surgical castration.
Medical castration: estrogens, luteinizing hormone–releasing hormone (LH-RH) agonists.
Androgen blockade at target cells: steroidal antiandrogens, pure antiandrogens.
Maximal androgen blockade.
5αR inhibition.

Other hormones have been found to have a stimulatory effect on animal and human prostates. These include prolactin (Grayhack et al, 1955) and growth hormone (Schally and Redding, 1987).

Growth Factors

The role of growth factors and their potential in prostatic growth control has been reviewed by Myers and colleagues (1993). There is interaction between steroid hormones; growth hormones; the natural growth hormone antagonist somatostatin; and growth factors that have been shown to be active on prostate and prostate cancer cells, including the epithelial growth factor family, the fibroblast growth factor family, insulin-like growth factors 1 and 2, and the transforming growth factor beta family, which plays an important physiologic role in suppressing the proliferation of prostatic epithelial cells. Growth factors act through membrane receptors and through binding to heparan sulfate, which is part of the extracellular matrix.

Effects of Androgen Depletion on Prostatic Tissues

Similar to the ventral prostate of the rat, which is one of the classic models for the study of endocrine dependence of prostatic tissue, **prostate cancer tissue shrinks if androgen is withdrawn.** Even normal androgen-dependent tissue, however, has the capability of regrowth if the androgenic stimulus is reactivated (Bruchovsky et al, 1987). That endo-

Table 89–1. TNM CLASSIFICATION OF LOCALLY ADVANCED OR METASTATIC PROSTATE CANCER

T3	Tumor extends through the prostate capsule
T3a	Unilateral extracapsular extension
T3b	Bilateral extracapsular extension
T3c	Tumor invades seminal vesicle(s)
T4	Tumor is fixed or invades adjacent structures other than seminal vesicles
T4a	Tumor invades the bladder neck, external sphincter, or rectum
T4b	Tumor invades the levator muscles and/or is fixed to the pelvic wall
N1–N3	Regional nodal metastases
M1	Distant metastases
M1a	Nonregional lymph nodes
M1b	Bone(s)
M1c	Other site(s)

Data from Hermanek P, Sobin LH, eds: UICC (Union International Contre le Cancer): TNM Classification of Malignant Tumors, 4th ed, 2nd rev. Berlin, Springer, 1992.

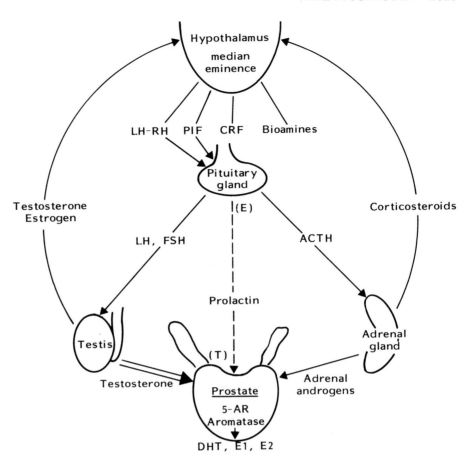

Figure 89–1. Endocrine factors regulating prostatic growth and function. LH-RH, luteinizing hormone–releasing hormones; PIF, pituitary factor for prolactin; E, estrogen; LH, luteinizing hormone; FSH, follicle-stimulating hormone; ACTH, adrenocorticotropic hormone; T, testosterone; DHT, 5-alpha-dihydrotestosterone; 5-AR, 5-alpha-reductase; CRF, corticotropin-releasing factor. (From Schröder FH, Röhrborn CG: Endocrine management of prostate cancer. *In* Lytton B, Catalona W, eds: Advances in Urology 4. St. Louis, Mosby-Year Book, 1991, pp 25–52.)

crine treatment of human prostate carcinoma leads to the shrinkage of cancerous tissue can best be shown by the decrease and disappearance of metastatic deposits. **The primary tumor volume decreases by an average of 30% to 40%** as shown in a longitudinal study by Sneller and associates (1992). The possibility of relapse of the primary tumor as well as of metastases under this treatment is best explained by the presence of hormone-resistant cell populations, which through clonal overgrowth eventually lead to the presence of a hormone-insensitive tumor, as has been shown for the Dunning rat prostatic carcinoma system by Isaacs and Coffey (1981).

What Can Be Expected from Endocrine Treatment

As mentioned earlier, cure of prostate cancer by means of endocrine treatment is highly unlikely. **Some men die of intercurrent deaths *with* prostate cancer rather than *of* prostate cancer.** Still these patients cannot be considered to be cured.

Rates of response of clinical prostate cancer under endocrine treatment strongly depend on the type of criteria used for the evaluation. **Objective and subjective response may vary between 40%,** as in most studies of the European Organization for Research and Treatment of Cancer (EORTC) as described by Newling (1988), **and 80%,** if the criteria of the National Prostatic Cancer Project (NPCP) as described by Murphy and Slack (1980) are applied. Re-

sponse to treatment is often associated with pain relief; improvement of symptoms of an obstructive micturition, which results from shrinkage of the primary tumor; and improvement of the performance status and of other tumor-related parameters, as was first quantitatively shown in the evaluation of the first prospective, randomized trial of the Veterans Administration Cooperative Urological Research Group (VACURG) in 1967 and in a later review by Byar and associates (1981). That the volume reduction of the primary tumor under endocrine treatment translates into an improvement of obstructive symptoms was shown in a study by Fleischmann and Catalona (1985), in which 69% of men responded with an objective improvement.

The duration of subjective and objective response is variable. **Time to clinical progression and death in studies varied between 18 to 24 and 30 to 36 months in patients with metastases** and may be substantially longer in those who have locally confined or extensive disease. Progression under endocrine treatment shows that endocrine-independent cell populations have achieved a sufficient tumor mass to determine the further clinical course. Progression to endocrine independence is poorly understood but is associated with increasing signs of genetic instability as shown by Isaacs and colleagues in the Dunning tumor model (Isaacs et al, 1982). Evidence of an increase of the proportions of poorly differentiated and aneuploid cells was presented by Adolfsson and Tribukait (1990), who carried out repeated cytologic biopsies in 84 patients over a 2-year period. The same authors have also shown that the proportion of aneuploid cells increases dramatically if primary tumors and metastatic disease are considered. Another possible marker for endocrine independence is E-cadherin, a cell adherence factor that has been shown to correlate with progression of locally confined disease. This marker is being developed by Umbas and co-workers (1994).

RESPONSE, PROGRESSION, AND SURVIVAL IN ADVANCED PROSTATE CANCER

A complete response consisting of a disappearance of all clinically identifiable disease and complete normalization of all markers is only rarely seen (5%–10%). Most responses are partial. Often enough, however, partial responses cannot be evaluated because the only clinically identifiable type of metastases, bone metastases, cannot be measured. Partial response requires a 50% decrease in size of such lesions. Lymph node metastases, which are probably the most common metastases in prostate cancer, are only rarely palpable and measurable or visible with imaging techniques (Murphy and Slack, 1980).

Progression, according to World Health Organization (WHO) standards, is defined as an increase in size of measurable lesions of 25% or more or as the appearance of new lesions. Disappearance of some lesions at one metastatic site and appearance of new lesions elsewhere (mixed response) is accounted for as progression. Markers such as prostate-specific antigen (PSA) and acid phosphatase are useful in some situations but not in others. Progression of disease under endocrine treatment without an elevation of markers is common and is discussed later in this section.

Acid phosphatase determined in the serum of patients with prostate cancer was the first useful tumor marker in human oncology and was introduced by Gutman and Gutman (1938). **Acid phosphatase in years of clinical practice was confirmed as what it was first described to be: a marker of metastatic disease, usually of bone metastases.** Acid phosphatase in itself is not an endocrine-dependent enzyme. With endocrine-induced regression of metastatic disease, however, acid phosphatase goes down. Alkaline phosphatase, which is often elevated in patients with bone metastases, is derived from increased metabolic activity in the area of bone metastases. Under successful endocrine treatment, alkaline phosphatase initially rises and then also shows a decrease paralleling acid phosphatase.

PSA was introduced into clinical medicine after Papsidero and co-workers developed the first assay allowing the determination of PSA in human serum (Papsidero et al, 1980). **PSA has turned out to be the most sensitive marker for human prostate cancer,** possibly the most sensitive marker available in human oncology at this time. PSA is widely used in the early detection of prostate cancer and in follow-up of patients after radical prostatectomy, in which an elevation of PSA above the lower limit of determination of the available routine assays of 0.1 ng/ml indicates residual disease and progression. **PSA is not a useful marker for the presence or absence of metastatic disease.** Its usefulness in studying response and progression under endocrine management of advanced disease is still under investigation. **A rise of PSA is indicative of progression.**

Theoretically the level of PSA at the time of diagnosis,

the nadir of PSA under treatment, and **the time necessary to reach a PSA nadir could be useful parameters for response to endocrine treatment.** Nadirs of 10 and 4 ng/ml were both found to correlate with longer times to progression and death under endocrine treatment (Mulders et al, 1992; Janknegt et al, 1993). Arai and colleagues reported on 50 patients who had frequent PSA determinations under endocrine treatment and found that those who reached the PSA nadir within 1 month had a significantly longer progression-free interval than those who reached a PSA nadir at 3 months or later (Arai et al, 1990). Thirteen percent to 25% of patients who suffer progression under endocrine treatment have been found to do so with normal PSA values, as described by Dupont and associates (1991) and Kadmon and associates (1991). Cooper and colleagues found that a rise of PSA under endocrine treatment precedes the demonstration of evidence of new metastases by bone scans or other clinical means by 6 to 12 months (Cooper et al, 1990).

Response criteria have to be repeatedly evaluable during the clinical course of a given disease. **Prognostic factors are usually evaluable only once.** The grade of the primary tumor, an important prognostic factor, is usually evaluated only at the time of biopsy or prostatic surgery. Prognostic factors in advanced prostate cancer are used to estimate the potential outcome for groups of patients or individuals under treatment. A wealth of literature on prognostic factors results from the evaluation of prospective phase III studies.

In an analysis of EORTC protocols 30761 and 30762, de Voogt and co-workers found that besides the presence or absence of pain and metastases, tumor-related prognostic factors showed a strong correlation with time to progression and survival (de Voogt et al, 1989). These were in sequence of the results of a multivariate analysis: **performance status, alkaline phosphatase, T category (T $\leq$ 3 versus T4), and chronic cardiovascular disease.** Grade, tumor size (by digital rectal examination), pain, and hemoglobin content were important factors in the monovariate analysis only. **The extent of metastatic disease** determined by numbers of metastases at the time of diagnosis was shown by Soloway and associates to have an impact on outcome; at least three prognostic categories, minimal, intermediate, and extensive, correlate significantly with time to progression and survival (Soloway et al, 1987).

Although **criteria for response are most important for phase II trials,** in which the effectiveness of a new treatment modality is evaluated, **the end points of phase III studies often include progression, disease-related mortality, and overall survival.** The importance of overall mortality survival as an end point, however, is adversely influenced by the relative frequency of intercurrent deaths in prostate cancer. The rate of progression and time to progression as an end point in phase III studies has the advantage of being tumor related but the disadvantage of being more difficult to determine. As already mentioned, time to progression evaluated by a rise of PSA may precede the occurrence of bone metastases by a year or even longer. For this reason, it has been suggested to evaluate progression separately according to each of the available subjective and objective parameters.

Overall Survival

The duration of overall survival is quite obviously the most important end point in the management of any malignancy. Unfortunately, overall survival has never been and probably never will be studied in a randomized fashion comparing endocrine treatment with no endocrine treatment. Because of its beneficial effect in symptomatic patients, endocrine treatment cannot be withheld once symptomatic progression occurs, as was demonstrated in the studies of VACURG (1967). Although several trials, mainly those comparing maximal androgen blockade to standard endocrine treatment, have shown small differences in overall survival, this is not confirmed in two meta-analyses, as is discussed further subsequently.

One phase III study of the EORTC GU Group compared castration to DES 1 mg/day, a regimen insufficient to suppress plasma testosterone to castrate levels and to a regimen of maximal androgen blockade (Robinson and Hetherington, 1986). Data from phase III studies show quite similar periods of overall survival: After 1 year, about 10% to 20% of men with metastatic prostate cancer die. This increases to 50%, 75%, and 90% after 3, 5, and 10 years. About 85% of patients with metastatic disease die of prostate cancer. Figure 89–2 shows the overall survival curves of the VACURG studies, as reported by Blackard and colleagues (1973); and an update of the Intergroup Study 0036 (maximal androgen blockade versus LH-RH analogue (2B) (Crawford, 1992). No differences in time to progression and overall survival are seen. **Recently available information does not reveal a clinically relevant advantage of any effective endocrine treatment regimen and of endocrine treatment in general in overall survival.**

Quality of Life

With the recognition of the purely palliative nature of endocrine treatment, subjective parameters related to the quality of life under endocrine treatment are more frequently and more seriously considered. Instruments for quality-of-life measurements specific to prostate cancer patients with and without metastases are being developed (Fossa, 1994)

and tested in prospective trials. The potential advantages and disadvantages of different types of endocrine treatment and of different regimens, such as early versus delayed and intermittent treatment, as well as minimally aggressive forms of treatment have to be re-evaluated. The key question: **Is it justified to maintain libido and potency at the price of accepting disease progression in the meantime?**

METHODS OF ENDOCRINE TREATMENT, RESULTS, AND SIDE EFFECTS

The methods of endocrine treatment are reviewed with concentration on those forms of management that are available at this time and that are in clinical use. Ongoing developments are discussed later.

Surgical Castration

History and General Remarks

Castration is still considered the gold standard of endocrine treatment of prostate cancer, even by investigators who are strong proponents of the simultaneous exclusion of testicular and adrenal androgens as initial forms of endocrine treatment of prostate cancer (Daneshgari and Crawford, 1993). **Bilateral orchiectomy was first used by Huggins and co-workers who demonstrated that 15 of 21 patients so treated (71%) had either subjective or objective improvement of pain or neurologic symptoms** resulting from metastatic prostate cancer (Huggins et al, 1941). In addition, there was a decrease in serum acid phosphatase in those patients who responded favorably. Although orchiectomy as a procedure may be unacceptable to some patients, the advantages are obvious: Orchiectomy can be carried out under local anesthesia in outpatient treatment, it is immediately effective, there is no compliance problem, and cost is

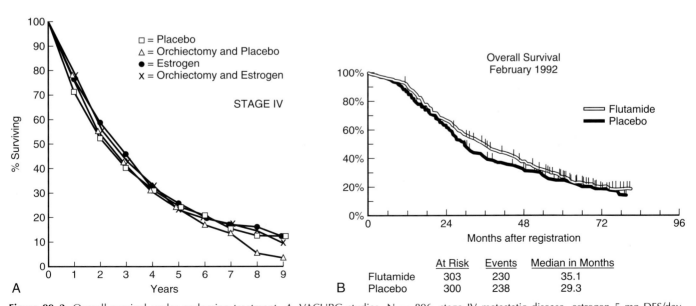

Figure 89–2. Overall survival under endocrine treatment. *A*, VACURG studies, N = 896, stage IV metastatic disease, estrogen 5 mg DES/day. *B*, NCI/Intergroup Study 0036, LH-RH analogue (Leupron) and placebo versus LH-RH and flutamide 3 × 250 mg (p-value not given).

contained. The cosmetic disadvantage can be eliminated by implanting a testicular prosthesis. **The frequent side effects of an almost immediate loss of libido and potency** are unavoidable and are inherent to any other treatment that eliminates the source or the effect of testicular androgens. It is unexplained why some patients remain potent under endocrine treatment. Ellis and Grayhack (1963) in a classic paper found that after castration, treatment with estrogens, or the combination of both, 16 of 38 previously potent patients remained potent. Greenstein and colleagues showed that 4 of 16 men could be stimulated to have functional erections by viewing an erotic tape (Greenstein et al, 1995). Other long-term side effects are hot flashes, osteoporosis, fatigue, loss of muscle mass, anemia, and weight gain. Endocrine treatment should be administered only on the basis of strict medical indications.

Technique

The technique of orchiectomy has been a subject of much debate since Riba (1942) introduced subcapsular orchiectomy. The advantage of this technique is that it does not leave behind an empty scrotum. Although it was initially doubted that subcapsular orchiectomy was complete and would lead to permanent castration values of plasma testosterone, ample evidence is now available in the literature that the source of testicular androgen can be removed effectively with the Riba technique. Bergman and associates studied plasma testosterone, follicle-stimulating hormone, LH, and prolactin over a 6-month period in a randomized study of total versus subcapsular orchiectomy in 22 men (Bergman et al, 1982). **With both techniques, the elimination of plasma testosterone was immediate and complete.** The results are reproduced in Figure 89–3. These findings were

confirmed by Clark and Houghton (1977) and by Senge and associates (1978). These authors also used a comparative group of 31 patients who were treated by 3 mg of DES orally and daily. Over a period of 2 to 3 years, plasma testosterone levels in 25 patients after bilateral subcapsular orchiectomy remained in the castration range, whereas patients treated with DES 3 mg/day had higher and more variable testosterone levels. Lin and co-workers pointed out that after bilateral orchiectomy, castration level of plasma testosterone is reached within 3 to 12 hours (mean 8.6 hours) (Lin et al, 1994). With DES treatment, 3 mg/day, castration levels were reached within 21 to 60 days with a mean of 38.3 days. An immediate effect certainly is desirable in patients who have cancer-related symptoms. The effects of different forms of endocrine treatment on plasma testosterone are summarized in Table 89–2. The most immediate way to achieve androgen deprivation is the use of an antiandrogen.

Results

The question whether castration is equally effective to other forms of management of prostate cancer has been subjected to a considerable number of prospective, randomized studies. One challenge comes from estrogen treatment. Study 1 of VACURG (1967) was a randomized study of patients with stage 3 (locally extensive) and stage 4 (metastatic) prostate cancer to determine the relative effectiveness of 5 mg of DES daily compared with orchiectomy, orchiectomy plus 5 mg of DES, and placebo. The first report on the study is by Mellinger and co-workers (1967). End points were progression to metastatic disease in the stage 3 group, overall survival, and prostate cancer mortality. The study is complicated by the fact that switchover from the placebo

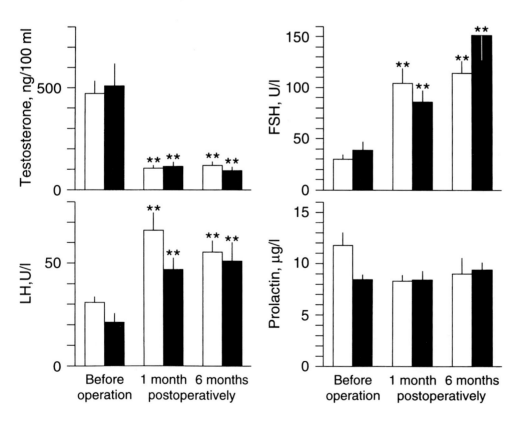

Figure 89–3. The mean serum concentrations of testosterone, follicle-stimulating hormone (FSH), luteinizing hormone (LH), and prolactin before and 1 and 6 months after orchiectomy. The shading in the histogram corresponds to subcapsular operations. SEM are indicated. *P < .05 and **P < .001, as compared to preoperative values. (From Bergman B, Damber JE, Tomic R: Urol Int 1982; 37:139–144. Basel, Karger.)

Table 89–2. EFFECT OF ENDOCRINE TREATMENT ON PLASMA TESTOSTERONE LEVELS

Treatment Modality	Plasma Testosterone (ng/ml)	Time to Nadir Level	References
Normal levels	6.11 ± 1.82 (2.12 ± 0.63 μmol/l)	—	Coffey, 1992
Surgical castration	0.2*	8.6 ± 3.2 hours†	Lin et al, 1994
Diethylstilbestrol 1 mg/day	0.8	Tested at 7 days	Mackler et al, 1972
	0.75	Tested at 1 month	Shearer et al, 1973
3 mg/day	0.2–0.5	38.3 ± 15.5 days	Lin et al, 1994
Polyestradiol phosphate, 80 mg	0.2–0.5	9 days	Lukkarinen et al, 1979
LH-RH	0.2–0.5	± 3 weeks	Fiet et al, 1993
Maximal androgen blockade (MAB)	0.2–0.5	± 2 weeks	Fiet et al, 1993

*Castration level, 5–10% of precastration levels.
†Half-life of circulating testosterone was 45 minutes.
LH-RH, Luteinizing hormone–releasing hormone.

arm to treatment arms was permitted. This option was used in 70% of stage 3 patients included in that arm; patients, however, were analyzed according to the original randomization. In the original analysis, no difference in survival was described (Blackard et al, 1973). **The most relevant finding was the discovery of the previously unknown toxic effects of DES, which led to a significant increase in cardiovascular mortality in the DES 5 mg arms.** Several independent analyses of these data are available. The overview by Byar (1973) seems to indicate that DES at a dosage of 5 mg/day prevents prostate cancer death more frequently than castration. Because most cardiovascular deaths occur during the first year of treatment, these patients died before prostate cancer could kill them; the lower rate of prostate cancer deaths in the DES arms must therefore be considered an artifact.

The EORTC GU Group conducted a study in newly diagnosed metastatic prostate cancer patients (protocol 30805) in which bilateral orchiectomy was compared with 1 mg of DES and orchiectomy plus cyproterone acetate (CPA). No difference in progression rates and survival were found in the final analysis by Robinson and colleagues (1995). This was the first randomized study of maximal androgen blockade ever conducted. As a result of the available information, clearly, bilateral orchiectomy produces results that are comparable to other standard methods of treatment. Maximal androgen blockade and castration are discussed later.

Medical Castration

A number of mechanisms are available and are used in the management of prostate cancer that suppress circulating testosterone to castration levels. Their effects and times to testosterone nadirs are summarized in Table 89–2.

Estrogens

The physiologic role of estrogens in the development of the male and of male reproductive organs is dealt with in Chapter 45. Estrogens are thought to interact with the prostatic stroma and to play a role in the development of BPH. Estrogen receptors are present in low concentrations in prostatic stroma. In physiologic concentrations, estrogens do not

seem to have a direct effect on prostatic cancer cells. They are effective in humans through their capability of exerting feedback control at the level of hypothalamus and in this way decreasing LH-RH and LH production (see Fig. 89–1).

DOSAGE. Synthetic estrogens are most commonly applied in the treatment of prostate cancer. DES has been used in clinical investigations at dosages of 0.2, 1.0, 3.0, and 5 mg/day. Dosages up to several hundred milligrams per day were common in clinical routine in the past. Some of these trials have already been discussed; some others are discussed later. Chlorotrianisene (TACE) is also a stilbene derivative of DES designed for oral use. This drug, however, has not been shown to lower plasma testosterone levels effectively and is therefore not in use. Polyestradiol phosphate is a drug that is frequently used as a parenteral depot injection at dosages of 80 or 160 mg per month in Northern European countries. **The advantage of the parenteral application may be a diminution of estrogenic side effects.** The effectiveness of polyestradiol phosphate at the indicated dosages is, however, still under investigation (Haapiainen et al, 1990). Another form of application of synthetic estrogens in a parenteral form is the treatment with high-dose DES diphosphate (Honvan). This drug is traditionally applied in some European countries at dosages around 1000 mg/day in hormone-refractory prostate cancer. This regimen has been insufficiently studied. Droz and colleagues have shown that DES diphosphate treatment lowers PSA in a substantial number of patients with progressive disease after castration or other forms of endocrine treatment (Droz et al, 1993). Table 89–2 summarizes the effects of common treatment regimens on plasma testosterone levels and the times until nadirs are reached.

With the description of severe cardiovascular side effects and a high rate of cardiovascular deaths within the VACURG studies (1967) and also with consideration of the high probability that there would be no exploitable direct effect of low-dose estrogen regimens on prostate cancer cells, the question of the lowest effective dosage of DES became relevant. Unfortunately, this question has never been answered. The second VACURG study was set up to investigate in a comparative fashion 0.2, 1.0, and 5.0 mg of DES. The results reported by Byar and Corle (1988) have shown clearly that the 0.2 mg/day regimen is less effective in preventing progression from stage 3 to stage 4 and death from prostate cancer than higher dosages. In a selected population derived from this trial, **Kent and associates studied plasma testosterone levels and found that neither 0.2 nor 1.0 mg suppresses plasma testosterone to castrate levels** (Kent et al, 1973). Interestingly, **the 1-mg dose was found to be equally effective as an anticancer agent as 5 mg of DES.** In their study, Kent and associates found that the level of plasma testosterone observed over 3- and 6-month periods remained in the range of two times those levels that were achievable with 5 mg of DES (Kent et al, 1973). This finding was supported by observations by Prout and co-workers (1976) and by Shearer and colleagues (1973), who found that DES 1 mg/day would not suppress the diurnal variations of plasma testosterone when compared with a 3 mg/day regimen. Beck and associates found that plasma testosterone is sufficiently suppressed by DES 1 mg/day (Fig. 89–4) (Beck et al, 1978). Probably as a result of this discussion and based on a number of subsequent studies in Europe and in the United States, **the dosage of 1 mg of DES orally three times a day has become standard treatment.** The dosage of 2 mg/day has not been explored in prospective studies.

In Scandinavian countries, parenteral estrogens, especially polyestradiol phosphate in depot preparation applied once a month in injections of 80 or 160 mg, are still commonly used. It is believed that the cardiovascular side effects seen with the oral application of DES can be avoided by eliminating the necessity of the initial passage through the portal system and through the liver (de Lignieres, 1993). Polyestradiol phosphate has been used in a number of studies in comparison to orchiectomy. The resulting data are at this time inconclusive (Haapiainen et al, 1990, 1991; Johansson et al, 1991).

SIDE EFFECTS. The severe cardiovascular side effects seen in men using the standard dosage of DES 5 mg/day were unknown before the report by Mellinger (1967) of the VACURG studies. **The key observation was a 36% in-**crease of non–cancer-related mortality in the estrogen groups, as compared to the non–estrogen-treated groups of males in these studies of more than 4000 patients. The majority of this excessive mortality was due to a large difference in cardiovascular mortality, which more than compensated for the small benefit in terms of prostate cancer mortality that was seen in the DES groups. DES-related cardiovascular mortality was usually seen during the first year of treatment; men died of DES before they could die of prostate cancer. Later on, the EORTC GU Group evaluated cardiovascular toxicity in their studies using DES 3 mg/day, DES 1 mg/day, estramustine phosphate 280 mg/day, medroxyprogesterone acetate (MPA) at standard dosage, and CPA at standard dosage. The risk of severe cardiovascular complications in the report by de Voogt and associates was highest in the DES 3 mg groups and was more pronounced during the first 6 months of treatment (de Voogt et al, 1986). Increasing age, body weight larger than 75 kg, and especially the presence of previous cardiovascular disease represented risk factors for the development of additional cardiovascular toxicity and death. Cardiovascular toxicity was lowest with CPA (steroidal antiandrogen) monotherapy. A full explanation of the mechanism of the side effects of oral application of estrogens is still lacking. Based on clinical data, it is likely that not only lipid metabolism, but also the blood coagulation system and fluid retention are directly influenced. Gynecomastia is seen with DES treatment in about 40% of cases (Smith et al, 1986); it can be prevented by low-dose irradiation to the mamillae before treatment with DES.

Luteinizing Hormone–Releasing Hormone

In 1971, Schally and co-workers isolated and described the structure of the gonadotropin-releasing hormone, which is active in stimulating the pituitary release of follicle-stimu-

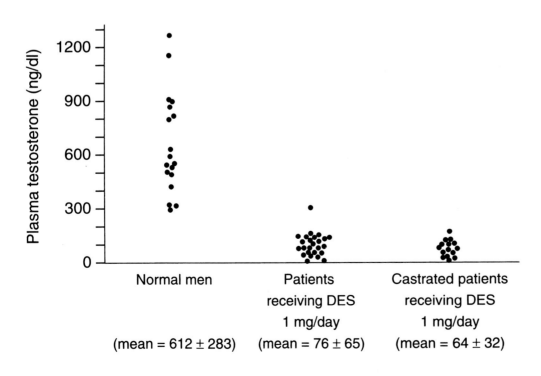

Figure 89–4. Plasma testosterone in normal men, in patients receiving diethylstilbestrol (DES), and in castrated patients receiving DES. (Reprinted by permission of the publisher from Beck PH, McAnich JW, Goebel JL, Stutman RE: Urology 1978; 11:157–160. Copyright 1978 by Elsevier Science Inc.)

lating hormone and LH. This discovery, which was honored by the Nobel Prize, opened the way to the development of a large number of peptides of which some have antagonist and some superagonist properties. It was found that synthetic LH-RH agonists with the substitution of glycine in position 6 by various D–amino acid residues (such as D-Trp[6] LH-RH) for glycine-6 are many times more powerful than the natural compounds. Although naturally occurring LH-RH stimulates LH release and supports its circadian rhythm, **it was soon found that superactive synthetic LH-RH agonists after an initial phase of stimulation lead to a suppression of LH and of testosterone production to castrate levels** (Auclair et al, 1977). Redding and Schally (1981) treated two sublines of the Dunning rat prostate carcinoma with the D-Trp[6] analogue of LH-RH and showed an inhibition of tumor growth that was similar to the growth suppression achieved by castration. Subsequently the same analogue was applied to ten patients who were observed during a 16-week period. A suppression of plasma testosterone, estradiol, and acid and alkaline phosphatase plasma levels was observed (Tolis et al, 1982). These findings opened the way to the broad clinical application of LH-RH agonists. LH-RH antagonists have also been developed. Despite a number of studies, these substances have not reached clinical application.

FORMS OF APPLICATION, DOSAGE, AND SIDE EFFECTS. The development of the clinical use of LH-RH agonists was hampered by difficulties in finding the proper ways of applying these drugs to patients. The short half-life initially necessitated either daily injections or, as in the case of D-Ser(TBU)[6]-EA[10] LH-RH (buserelin), several daily intranasal applications. The breakthrough came when monthly depot preparations were developed by coupling analogues to lactic acid polymers in the form of implants or microcapsules. This development allowed further progress in the establishment of an every-2-months injectable depot analogue; 3-month depots are being introduced at this time. **These depot LH-RH agonists allow the use of low dosages (e.g., 3.6 mg buserelin acetate, 3.75 mg leuprorelin, 3.6 mg goserelin, 3.75 mg triptorelin) and guarantee a sufficiently constant release over a 28- to 30-day period** to suppress plasma testosterone to castration levels in a reliable fashion. Depot preparations are available as subcutaneous rod implants or as microcapsule injections. LH-RH agonists have become standard forms of treatment of prostate cancer.

The **side effects of LH-RH agonists are compatible with those of castration.** Most of the large studies, which are reviewed later in this chapter, give a complete indication of the side effects encountered. In a carefully conducted phase II study of 56 patients with leuprolide depot 7.5 mg every 4 weeks, Sharifi and colleagues reported hot flashes in 57% and serious sweating in 10.7% of the patients together with loss of libido and potency and other probably not drug-related side effects (Sharifi et al, 1990).

FLARE PHENOMENON. Under treatment with LH-RH agonists, a stimulation of LH and testosterone secretion during the first 2 to 3 weeks occurs. This phenomenon may be associated with a rise in serum markers of prostate cancer, such as acid phosphatase and PSA. An early example is given in Figure 89–5. In this study of buserelin, it is shown that the initial rise in plasma testosterone is accompanied by a rise in acid phosphatase in this series of patients in which daily determinations of both parameters were carried out.

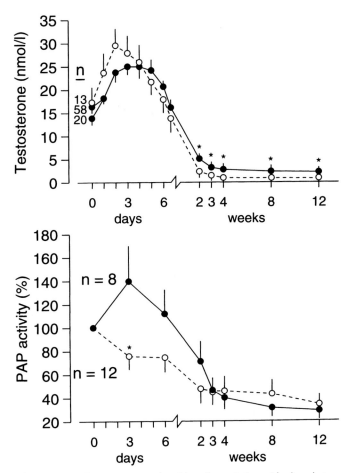

Figure 89–5. Testosterone and acid and prostatic acid phosphatase (PAP) levels in patients on buserelin only (●) or buserelin plus cyproterone acetate (CPA) (○). For plasma testosterone n = 58 for patients treated with buserelin alone (n = 20 for samples collected on days 1 through 6) and n = 13 for those on buserelin plus CPA. Results as mean and SEM. *P < 0.05. (From Klijn JGM, de Voogt HJ, Schröder FH, de Jong FH: Combined treatment with buserelin and cyproterone acetate in metastatic prostatic carcinoma (Letter). Lancet 1985; 2:493. © by The Lancet Ltd.)

This biochemical flare can be accompanied by clinical symptoms such as increase of bone pain. Radiologic evidence of acute progression has also been described. In patients who have a critical metastatic tumor mass, a marginal bone marrow reserve, or symptoms of spinal cord compression, the acute exacerbation can be detrimental and lead to acute situations, including paraplegia. Death from acute progression of prostate cancer has also been described. Thompson and associates, in a review retrieved from the literature of 765 patients with symptoms of flare noted that 15 died with the presence of acute symptoms of exacerbation (2%) (Thompson et al, 1990). Biochemical and clinical flare can be prevented by the use of a pure or steroidal antiandrogen either 1 week before the initiation of the LH-RH analogue treatment as proposed by Boccon-Gibod and colleagues (1986) or simultaneously with the initiation of LH-RH treatment (Schulze and Senge, 1990). In the first case, if a steroidal antiandrogen is used, the rise in plasma testosterone above pretreatment levels can be prevented together with the biochemical flare phenomenon. In the second case, the peak in plasma testosterone is still seen; however, biochemical flare is inhibited by the action of the antiandrogen as shown by Klijn and co-workers (1985). Most of the early large protocols, which were conducted to establish the clinical value of LH-RH agonists, could not take into account the possibility of clinical flare. It is remarkable that in the large study of the Leuprolide Study Group (1984), ten patients in the LH-RH group suffered early progression and were removed from the study for this reason, as opposed to only three in the DES group. A complete review of the flare issue has been given by Boccon-Gibod (1990). **A pure or steroidal antiandrogen in standard dosage should be given before or at the time of initiation of LH-RH analogue treatment, especially in patients with a large metastatic tumor mass.**

RESULTS OF RANDOMIZED STUDIES. A number of large studies were undertaken to establish the value of LH-RH agonists as standard treatment of prostate cancer after the endocrine effectiveness and mechanism have been established in phase I–II studies. The two approaches that were taken relate to comparisons with castration and with DES 3 mg/day. All these studies report a similar effect on rates of progression, time to progression, and overall survival. Large comparative studies of LH-RH analogues with castration have been reported by Parmar and colleagues (1987), Huben and associates (1988), Kaisary and associates (1991), Soloway and colleagues (1991), and de Voogt and colleagues (1990).

In the study by Huben and associates (National Prostatic Cancer Project Protocol 1700), a significant difference in the proportion of progression-free survival was found, to the detriment of the buserelin group, as compared to DES 3 mg/day or orchidectomy (Huben et al, 1988). The difference in progression-free survival occurs after 3 months. The authors speculate that this may be due to the flare phenomenon. Intranasal application of buserelin, however, was shown not to suppress plasma testosterone to castrate levels. In EORTC Study 30843 (de Voogt et al, 1990, 1995), the antiandrogen cyproterone acetate was used during the first 2 weeks of treatment, and clinical flare was not observed. Progression and survival curves for LH-RH and castration are superimposing. The largest studies comparing LH-RH analogues with DES 3 mg/day are those reported by the Leuprolide Study Group (1984) and by Waymont and colleagues (1992).

Androgen Blockade at Target Cells

Pure Antiandrogens

Antihormones are substances that counteract the effect of hormones at their target cell. Two types of antiandrogens are known: steroidal antiandrogens, which because of their progestational properties also act by suppressing gonadotropins and thereby lowering plasma testosterone (CPA, megestrol acetate), and so-called pure antiandrogens, which are nonsteroidal in structure and which do not have any antigonadotropic effects. All known antiandrogens interfere with androgen action by binding to the androgen receptor in a competitive fashion. In the case of CPA, this was established by Brinkman and co-workers (1995) and Huang and associates (1985). Because of their different mechanism of action, the biologic effects of antiandrogens and their impact on plasma hormones is quite different. A summary of these

effects is given in Table 89–3. **Pure antiandrogens obviously also block androgen receptors in the diencephalon,** the area that is crucial for LH-RH production and the feedback mechanism that regulates plasma testosterone levels through LH. This leads to an LH increase in endocrinologically intact males with the use of pure antiandrogens. This increase of LH and testosterone is inhibited by the antigonadotropic effect that is associated with the use of steroidal antiandrogens. For reasons that are not completely understood, with the use of pure antiandrogens the rise in plasma testosterone is temporary and self-limiting at a level of about 1.5 times the normal plasma testosterone levels in intact males. Obviously, at least in theory, steroidal and pure antiandrogens are useful to counteract androgenic activity from the adrenals, which is left over after castration or testicular suppression by interfering with the diencephalic, pituitary testicular feedback mechanisms. **In intact males, steroidal antiandrogens may be more useful if used in monotherapy because they do not lead to a rise of plasma testosterone and subsequently have to interfere with smaller amounts of androgens at the target cells.** The differential mechanism of pure and steroidal antiandrogens is depicted in Table 89–3. Another pure antiandrogen, Casodex, has recently been marketed in the U.S. and elsewhere. A review is given by Kaisary (1994).

In the subsequent sections, only the role of antiandrogens in monotherapy is reviewed. The structural formulas of the antiandrogens mentioned are indicated in Figure 89–6.

Steroidal Antiandrogens

In this section, mainly CPA is discussed. CPA is not available in the United States; it is, however, widely used in other parts of the world and in Europe. **Practical advantages are the oral use, the immediate effectiveness, and the lack of the cardiovascular side effects of estrogens.** The recommended dosage of CPA is 100 mg/day two to three times a day. Side effects include loss of libido and potency; gynecomastia is rarely a problem. Cardiovascular toxicity, although indicated as a possibility in the product informa-

Table 89–3. BIOLOGIC EFFECTS OF A STEROIDAL (CYPROTERONE ACETATE) AND A PURE ANTIANDROGEN (FLUTAMIDE) IN INTACT HUMAN MALES AND IN MALE RATS

	Cyproterone Acetate	Flutamide
Human		
Plasma		
Testosterone	Decrease	Increase
54-Dihydrotestosterone	Decrease	Increase
Estradiol	Decrease	Increase
Luteinizing hormone	Decrease	Increase
Volume BPH	Decrease	Decrease
Gynecomastia	–	+
Libido	Decrease	+
Potency	Decrease	+
Rat		
Accessory glands	Decrease	Decrease
Leydig cells	Atrophy	Hypertrophy

BPH, Benign prostatic hyperplasia.

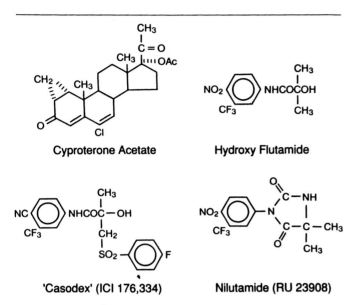

Figure 89–6. The structural formulas of currently used antiandrogens.

tion, has been shown in a retrospective analysis of EORTC studies by de Voogt and co-workers to be significantly less than with estrogens and is probably compatible with the prevalence of cardiovascular symptoms and death in the general population (de Voogt et al, 1986). This comparison has, however, not been made in any prospective protocol. Hepatic toxicity has been a subject of discussion. Elevations of liver function tests are rarely seen and are usually, but not always, reversible.

CPA in monotherapy has been compared to DES 3 mg/day by the EORTC GU Group (Pavone-Macaluso et al, 1986) and estradiol undecylate 100 mg/month intramuscularly (Jacobi et al, 1980). There were no differences in major end points, and these studies establish CPA as a standard form of treatment for prostate cancer. Unfortunately a direct comparison of CPA with castration has never been carried out.

CPA at dosages of 50 to 100 mg/day has been shown to be effective in preventing hot flashes, which occur under LH-RH agonist treatment or after castration. The mechanism of this has been described by Radlmaier and colleagues (1990). The effectiveness of CPA in preventing the flare phenomenon under LH-RH agonist treatment has already been described.

Pure Antiandrogens as Monotherapy

Flutamide, nilutamide and Casodex are discussed in this section.

A main clinical advantage of pure antiandrogen monotherapy is the maintenance of libido and potency. This phenomenon is most likely due to the maintenance of normal or elevated plasma testosterone levels. A number of unresolved questions are connected with this issue. Although it is well understood that there is a dissociation of the regulation of libido and potency, which is mainly governed by testosterone, with the regulation of growth and function of the prostate, which is mainly dependent on 5α-DHT, **it is poorly understood why the pure antiandrogen would**

not counteract testosterone at those cerebral androgen receptors that govern libido. Also, it has never been shown conclusively that the elevated androgen levels, which result under pure antiandrogen treatment, do not lead to a maintenance of androgen-induced proliferation of prostate cancer cell populations. As indicated in Table 89–3, a rise of plasma estradiol levels is also a result of monotherapy with pure antiandrogens. It could be that the elevation of estrogens, which probably is the reason for the high incidence of gynecomastia seen with flutamide monotherapy, also interferes with diencephalic feedback mechanisms leading to a stabilization of LH and testosterone production. The only conclusive way to exclude the possibility of stimulation of androgen-dependent cell populations by the elevated levels of testosterone seen with pure antiandrogen treatment would be a study of proliferation in human prostate cancer cell populations. Such a study, which obviously logistically poses great difficulties, has never been carried out.

DOSAGE AND SIDE EFFECTS. The recommended dosage of flutamide in monotherapy is 250 mg three times a day orally. Flutamide is metabolized in the liver to hydroxyflutamide, the active antiandrogen. Side effects of flutamide are probably best described by DeKernion and colleagues (1988). This paper presents the analysis of a prospective, randomized trial comparing flutamide to estramustine phosphate in hormone-refractory metastatic prostate cancer (NPCP Study 2400). Side effects included nausea and vomiting at various degrees in 46% and diarrhea in 21%. Gynecomastia is reported with an incidence of about 40%. Gynecomastia is probably due to the elevated circulating estrogen levels. A transient hepatitis-like syndrome occurs in about 3% of patients treated with flutamide either alone or in combination with other treatment regimens. For this reason, at least during the first months of therapy, liver enzymes should be monitored. Usually the hepatitis-like syndrome is reversible.

RESULTS OF PROSPECTIVE STUDIES. The first major report on flutamide monotherapy was by Sogani and colleagues (1984). The authors judge that there was a favorable response in 87.5% of 63 patients. The response criteria used were rather soft. Other studies, most of which are supportive of the use of flutamide, include those by MacFarlane and Tolley (1985), Lundgren and associates (1985), Delare and Thillo (1991), and Soloway and Matzkin (1993). Unfortunately a randomized study comparing flutamide to other standard forms of therapy is not yet available except for the small randomized comparative study of flutamide and DES of Lund and Rasmussen (1988), which was mainly designed to study the endocrine effects of both drugs and their side effects. Another randomized study, EORTC Protocol 30892, which compares CPA to flutamide at standard dosages in M1 disease, has recently been closed and evaluated. **Side effects, mainly painful gynecomastia, abnormal liver function, diarrhea, and gastrointestinal complaints, were significantly more frequent in the flutamide group** and led more frequently to discontinuation of flutamide treatment. Surprisingly, among those who were sexually active at entry, sexual activity decreased equally in both arms. About 30% of these men remained sexually active (Schröder et al, 1996). Unfortunately, at this time it remains uncertain whether monotherapy with pure and steroidal antiandrogens is equally effective. The higher incidence of bothersome side effects with pure antiandrogens of the flutamide type can be accepted only if a better outcome is shown.

NILUTAMIDE. Nilutamide is not recommended by its manufacturer for use in monotherapy. Results may be expected to be comparable to those of flutamide. Nilutamide may have the advantage of having a slightly longer half-life. Potential side effects are alcohol intolerance, a decrease in the speed of dark/light adaptation, and interstitial pneumonitis.

CASODEX. This drug has been studied in monotherapy in three different dosages (50 mg, 100 mg, 150 mg) in randomized comparison with castration. No recommendation for use in monotherapy has resulted so far (Kaisary, 1994). **The trials fail to show even equal effectiveness of Casodex monotherapy** (Iversen, 1996).

Maximal Androgen Blockade

Maximal androgen blockade, total androgen blockade, and total androgen suppression **are all terms that describe the initial, simultaneous exclusion of testicular and adrenal androgens as first-line endocrine treatment of prostate cancer.** The term *maximal androgen blockade* (as opposed to *total androgen blockade*), used by Labrie and colleagues, addresses the fact that commonly known antiandrogens are not capable of totally blocking receptor-mediated androgen action (Labrie et al, 1983, 1988). The exclusion of adrenal androgens as second-line endocrine treatment is discussed later. The first documented attempt to study first-line maximal androgen blockade in a phase III study is protocol 30805 of the EORTC GU Group. This protocol was designed in 1979 and used castration as the standard form of treatment. The two experimental arms were DES 1 mg/day and castration plus CPA 150 mg/day. The study compares standard treatment to a maximal form of endocrine ablation and to DES 1 mg, which was known at that time to be clinically equal to DES 5 mg/day but was also known at least in some studies not to suppress plasma testosterone to castration levels. The three-arm study recruited 335 patients with metastatic disease. No difference in progression rates, time to progression, and overall survival was found among the three treatment arms. The progression and survival curves are superimposing (Robinson et al, 1995).

In 1983, Labrie and coworkers published the results of a small phase II study in which response based on PSA and response criteria of the NPCP were related (Labrie et al, 1983). Thirty patients were treated with an LH-RH analogue and a pure antiandrogen. The results were interpreted as a dramatic improvement above standard treatment, especially based on the slopes of PSA decrease. Since then, the concept of maximal androgen blockade has been extensively studied internationally in at least 24 prospective, randomized trials. The overall results are reviewed subsequently.

Regimens, Dosages, and Side Effects

Maximal androgen blockade can be achieved in several different ways. **Castration or any other principle of treatment that excludes testicular androgen production is combined with the exclusion of adrenal androgens either at the production site or at the target cell.** The obvious

options are to combine castration, an LH-RH agonist, or estrogen treatment with an antiandrogen. Because the amount of androgen that remains after excluding testicular androgens is much smaller, an adaptation of the dosage of the antiandrogen in this situation could be considered. Still, in all studies concerned and in clinical practice, usually 250 mg flutamide three times is given.

Nilutamide, which has a considerably longer plasma elimination half-life (mean 56 hours), can be given in one daily dose of 300 mg for the first day to be followed by 150 mg/day orally. CPA, of which the recommended dosage in monotherapy is 200 to 300 mg, is usually reduced to 150 or 200 mg in the situation of maximal androgen blockade trials, and the same dosage reduction has been recommended for clinical use. The **side effects** of the three available antiandrogens have already been discussed. If pure antiandrogens are used in conjunction with castration or an LH-RH agonist, obviously those side effects that are due to increased levels of testosterone or estrogens are eliminated. The gastrointestinal and hepatic side effects, however, remain. Potency and libido are lost because of the elimination of testicular androgen production. In the case of nilutamide, delayed adaptation to darkness is seen in about 30%, and alcohol intolerance is seen in 20% of patients. Nilutamide is associated with a 2% incidence of interstitial lung disease, which may be higher in Japanese. Other side effects include mild hepatotoxicity and mild gastrointestinal adverse effects. These side effects as well as alcohol intolerance are rarely a reason for discontinuation of treatment. The literature on side effects has been reviewed by Harris and co-workers (1993).

Megesterol acetate has been proposed for the management of prostate cancer in combination with a low dose of 0.1 mg of DES. A phase I–II study has been reported by Geller and associates (1984). Megesterol acetate was applied at dosages between 40 and 160 mg/day. The regimen has never been studied in a phase III study. Similarly, Goldenberg and colleagues proposed the combination of CPA at a dosage of 200 mg daily with DES 0.1 mg/day (Goldenberg et al, 1988). The concept and rationale of maximal androgen blockade has been developed and presented by Labrie and associates on several occasions, including the publication in 1988 (Labrie et al, 1988).

Results of Prospective, Randomized Studies

An extensive literature search identified **24 studies using maximal androgen blockade** at least in one of the treatment arms that were initiated before 1989. The few studies that have been initiated after 1989 include one relevant one—the SWOG Intergroup Study 0105, which completed the recruitment of 1378 patients with distant metastatic disease during 1994. These patients were randomized in a double-blind, placebo-controlled fashion with regard to the antiandrogen into a group undergoing surgical castration and receiving a placebo and a group undergoing surgical castration and receiving flutamide. With a median follow-up of more than 3 years there was no difference in time to progression or in overall survival, neither in the whole population, nor in the subset of patients with favorable prognostic factors identified by up-front stratification.

In the meantime, it is difficult to judge whether there is a better treatment than the gold standard of orchiectomy or those forms of treatment that have been shown to be equivalent. It is impossible to review all of the available studies. This review is limited to those few protocols that have either shown significant differences with respect to their major end points or contributed in some other way to a better understanding of this complicated field of clinical research.

The largest positive study that has led to the widespread use of maximal androgen blockade as first-line endocrine treatment is **Protocol 0036 of the National Cancer Institute/Intergroup** (Crawford et al, 1989). In this protocol, the LH-RH agonist leuprolide given by daily injections without initial protection by an antiandrogen was compared with leuprolide plus flutamide. The study shows a significant difference in time to progression and in overall survival. Median times to progression and median survival times differed by 2.6 and 7.3 months in favor of the combination treatment arm. These differences were statistically significant. This study has been criticized because the possibility of flare in a considerable proportion of patients in the control arm (leuprolide unprotected) cannot be excluded. The progression curves are suggestive of such an effect. Furthermore, a subgroup analysis shows that the improvements are much more accentuated in patients with favorable prognostic factors, with minimal metastases limited to spine and pelvis, and without pain. The significance of this finding is poorly understood. In a more recent analysis reported by Crawford (1992), 5-year survival comparisons are shown that do not seem to differ (see Fig. 89–2B).

After completion of intergroup protocol 0036, the EORTC GU Group decided to do a similar study replacing the LH-RH agonist by castration. The results of Protocol 30853 were reported by Denis and colleagues (1993). This study recruited 327 patients. Castration was compared to the LH-RH agonist goserelin acetate (Zoladex) combined with flutamide 250 mg three times daily. This study also showed a significant difference in time to progression and overall survival in the same order of magnitude. The median duration of survival was 27.1 months in the orchiectomy and 34.4 months in the maximal androgen blockade arm. The same subgroup analysis was carried out. About 15% of the patients had favorable prognostic factors; the favorable effect seems to be limited to this particular group. The death hazard ratio for patients with poor prognostic factors (more than five bone metastases) was close to 1.0, which indicates no difference between the treatment arms.

Two other studies, both using nilutamide plus castration compared with castration alone (Béland, 1991; Janknegt et al, 1993), reported significant differences in either survival or progression-free survival rates. Interestingly, Béland and colleagues reported "no statistically significant difference between the two treatment groups for time to progression or survival" for the same study during the same year (1991) (Béland et al, 1991). These two studies were part of a group of seven randomized, double-blind trials that used the same protocol and recruited a total of 1191 patients. A total of 1056 patients were included in a meta-analysis that was reported by Bertagna and co-workers (1994). **This meta-analysis concluded that the combination of nilutamide and orchiectomy had a beneficial effect on pain of metastatic origin, levels of tumor markers, the objective re-sponse of disease, and the time to disease progression.** Cancer-specific and overall survival were not significantly improved. A more detailed analysis of the maximal androgen blockade issue is given by Schröder (1993) and from a medical statistical point of view by Blumenstein (1993).

An **overview analysis** goes back to the raw data collected from all available studies. In contrast to the technique of a meta-analysis, in which literature reports may be sufficient for a statistical reanalysis, an overview analysis has to use the original data of all patients gathered in identified protocols. It is essential for an overview analysis that all protocols during a clearly defined period of time are included without exception. Such an overview analysis has been undertaken by Dalesio and co-workers (1995). Data from 5600 patients randomized to 21 studies were collected. A total of 3212 patients had died at the time of this analysis. There was a 3% improvement of overall 5-year survival in favor of maximal androgen blockade; this result was not significantly different from castration or LH-RH agonist treatment. It was concluded that currently available **randomized evidence does not demonstrate that maximal androgen blockade results in longer survival than conventional treatment does.** The study showed also that at time periods earlier than 5 years there was no significant survival difference. Although there were differences in overall survival with respect to different antiandrogens, none produced a significant improvement.

At this time, the author agrees with Daneshgari and Crawford (1993) that castration remains the gold standard of endocrine treatment. The results of the overview analysis and the negative results of the largest study, SWOG Intergroup Study 0105, allow us to conclude that maximal androgen blockade has no additional value if time to progression and survival are considered. It remains poorly understood why some randomized studies are positive and others are negative.

Antiandrogen Withdrawal Syndrome

Scher and Kelly (1993) and Dupont and colleagues (1993) were first to observe that about 40% of patients who progress on maximal androgen blockade with the use of flutamide show a remission, biochemically or clinically, after discontinuation of flutamide. Such remissions may last more than 1 year. This phenomenon has been termed *antiandrogen withdrawal syndrome.* The mechanism of this paradoxical androgenic effect of flutamide is not understood at this time. The possibility of clonal proliferation of tumor cells with a mutated androgen receptor, however, cannot be excluded. One prostate cancer cell line (LNCaP) was shown to contain a mutation that leads to stimulation of growth by flutamide and other antiandrogens (Veldscholte et al, 1992). **If progression under maximal androgen blockade occurs, the antiandrogen, especially flutamide, should be discontinued.**

Second-Line Endocrine Treatment

Surgical hypophysectomy and adrenalectomy are historical. Several means exist to exclude adrenal androgens medically in second-line regimens: antiandrogens (at target cells); glucocorticoids, which indirectly suppress ACTH release and

in this way suppress adrenal cortical function; and drugs that interfere with cytochrome P-450–mediated hydroxylation reactions, such as aminoglutethimide, ketoconazole, and spironolactone. Moderate response rates have been reported for hypophysectomy and secondary adrenal suppression. These data are soft, and phase III studies are unavailable. For review, see Schröder (1985).

If progression under endocrine treatment occurs, this prostate cancer has become endocrine independent and cannot be controlled by endocrine means unless plasma testosterone is not at castrate level (compliance) or there is paradoxical stimulation by an antiandrogen. **In the first situation, previous treatment should be replaced by castration; in the second one, the antiandrogen should be discontinued.**

Prolactin Inhibition

Based on early observations, which indicate that the withdrawal of prolactin has an additional effect on the regression of the ventral prostate of the rat after castration, reported by Grayhack and colleagues (1955) and referred to earlier in this chapter, attempts to establish the clinical value of prolactin suppression in the management of prostate cancer have been made in the 1980s. Clinically, effectiveness was never conclusively established (Farnsworth et al, 1981; Jacobi, 1982).

5-Alpha-Reductase Inhibition

$5\alpha R$ inhibitors have been shown to decrease DHT in plasma and in prostatic tissue. A small study of patients with metastatic disease showed only slight effectiveness in lowering PSA levels in serum (finasteride). The same drug was used in comparison with placebo in men with a rising PSA after radical prostatectomy and showed a delay of PSA progression. The potential advantage of $5\alpha R$ inhibitors is preservation of libido and potency. Clinical effectiveness and its potential role, however, are limited at this time. Available data are reviewed by Gormley (1991).

ENDOCRINE TREATMENT, STAGE BY STAGE

In general, endocrine treatment is reserved for advanced stages of prostate cancer. **One of the important results of the studies of VACURG was that delay of endocrine treatment in stage III patients had no adverse influence on survival.** This finding has for some time determined clinical practice. The VACURG studies, however, were not set up to answer this question, and subsequently it has never been conclusively studied in a phase III situation.

Early Versus Delayed Endocrine Treatment in N+ (D1) Prostate Cancer

The question whether early or delayed endocrine treatment may be advantageous with relation to overall survival, unfor-

tunately, remains unanswered. Prospective, randomized studies on this issue must be considered one of the top priorities in clinical research in this field. Unfortunately the available information from retrospective studies is confusing and inconclusive. The side effects of endocrine treatment in asymptomatic patients are not negligible. The risk of loss of libido, impotence, and the other side effects, such as hot flashes, osteoporosis, loss of muscle mass, anemia, and gynecomastia, that may be inherent to the chosen endocrine treatment regimen is acceptable only in tradeoff with a survival benefit. If this is not the case, patients should be given a choice between early endocrine treatment and a long period until initial progression occurs, and delayed endocrine treatment with the advantage of maintenance of libido and potency, the lack of other side effects, and a shorter time to initial progression, with the potential for endocrine treatment. Unfortunately, all data that indicate that early endocrine treatment leads to better overall survival (Byar and Corle, 1988; review by Kozlowski et al, 1991) are severely flawed by methodologic problems (Walsh, 1989).

Much of the debate concerning early versus delayed treatment is taking place around those patients who are found at the time of evaluation for potentially curative treatment to have lymph node metastases (N+, D1 disease). **There is no question that early endocrine treatment delays progression.** Zagars and co-workers reported on long-term follow-up of 179 patients with N1–3 M0 disease who underwent pelvic lymphadenectomy without radical prostatectomy and immediate endocrine treatment (Zagars et al, 1994). The follow-up in this series is sufficiently long to calculate not only the median interval to disease progression, which was 67 months, but also the median survival after disease progression, which was 36 months. Van den Ouden and associates reported on untreated patients with N+ disease and found a median time to progression of 24 months (van den Ouden et al, 1993). Data presented by Sgrignoli and colleagues show that about 90% of 113 men with D1 disease after node dissection and radical prostatectomy show biochemical or clinical progression after 5 to 10 years (Sgrignoli et al, 1994). Median time to clinical progression without endocrine treatment, however, was more than 60 months.

Endocrine Treatment in Locally Extensive, Nonmetastatic Disease

Progression from locally extensive to metastatic disease can be delayed by early endocrine treatment. Patient choice and the specific medical and personal situation should play a decisive role in decision making. Locally extensive disease may be curable by radiotherapy or surgery. When the decision for early endocrine treatment is made, this possibility has to be considered.

Several reports in the literature confirm that **if urinary retention occurs in patients with large localized prostate carcinomas, endocrine treatment offers effective relief.** Hampson and associates described 31 patients in the situation, of which 21 were subsequently able to void without the need for surgical intervention (Hampson et al, 1993). Similar data are reported by Fleischmann and Catalona (1985).

Endocrine therapy in preparation for radiotherapy or

surgery is at this time an issue under discussion. Patients with large but localized lesions require a rather large field of radiotherapy. The volume reduction of prostate cancer 3 months after endocrine therapy averages more than 40%. The decrease in size of the radiotherapeutic field with a much smaller prostate may lead to a significant reduction of the risk of side effects. Again, retrospective, randomized studies on this issue are not available. The procedure described, however, has become common practice in many urologic centers. Preliminary data from a large American prospective study reported by Pilepich and colleagues does confirm a decrease of radiotherapeutic side effects (Pilepich et al, 1990). Up-front endocrine treatment before surgery is subject to prospective studies at the time of writing this chapter. Preliminary data on intermediate end points such as positive margins of resection do not allow an answer to the question whether the rate of curable patients can be increased. However, two of these studies were recently closed and analyzed; no difference was seen in the incidence of a rise of PSA with or without up-front endocrine treatment of 3 months' duration (Klotz et al, 1996; Soloway, 1996). This finding casts serious doubt on the effectiveness of this form of treatment.

UNRESOLVED ISSUES OF ENDOCRINE TREATMENT AND FUTURE DEVELOPMENTS

The field of prostate cancer is changing quickly. A number of important developments are at present occurring without having produced definitive results. Some of these issues are included in a brief review.

Quality of Life

Traditionally, in trials of prostate cancer, solid end points have been used in judging the effectiveness of treatment. In this respect, WHO recommendations were followed. Although the rather strict response criteria for phase II and phase III trials of the NPCP and of the EORTC GU Group have contributed much to a better understanding of endocrine therapy, softer end points related to quality-of-life issues may be warranted in a situation in which palliative treatment is evaluated. Instruments to measure quality of life are in the process of being developed. First steps have been described by Fossa (1994).

Intermittent Endocrine Treatment

Intermittent endocrine treatment is proposed by Akakura and co-workers (1993). A theoretical advantage of cyclic forms of endocrine treatment might be an increased quality of life during the nontreatment intervals and savings of expenses. The hypothesis that intermittent treatment may be equal to continuous treatment is at present being tested in a phase III trial.

Endocrine Prevention: Early Endocrine Treatment

There is strong evidence that prostate cancer with increase in size goes through a biologic development resulting in a decrease of endocrine dependence on androgens and in the development of less favorable prognostic factors. Larger lesions are more frequently poorly differentiated, show more frequently an aneuploid pattern, and seem to be less responsive to endocrine treatment. The possibility that small lesions are completely endocrine dependent and might even be curable by endocrine treatment cannot be excluded at this moment. With the availability of drugs that allow maintenance of libido and potency, the possibility of early endocrine treatment or even endocrine prevention exists. Substances that can potentially be used in this context are 5αR inhibitors and pure antiandrogens. At this moment, a large study of the Southwest Oncology Group/National Cancer Institute applies the 5αR inhibitor finasteride in a randomized endocrine prevention study.

Growth Factors and Growth Factor Inhibitors

Knowledge is increasing rapidly with respect to growth factors and growth factor inhibitors and their role in the progression and growth control of prostate cancer. A summary is given by Myers and associates (1993). Interference with growth factors and growth factor–related mechanisms will probably play an important role in phase I and phase II investigations in the near future.

REFERENCES

Adolfsson J, Tribukait B: Evaluation of tumor progression by repeated fine needle biopsies in prostate adenocarcinoma: Modal deoxyribonucleic acid value and cytological differentiation. J Urol 1990; 144:1408–1410.

Akakura K, Bruchovsky N, Goldenberg SL, et al: Effects of intermittent androgen suppression on androgen-dependent tumors. Cancer 1993; 71:2782–2790.

Arai Y, Yoshiki T, Yoshida O: Prognostic significance of prostate specific antigen in endocrine treatment for prostatic cancer. J Urol 1990; 144:1415–1419.

Auclair C, Kelly PA, Labrie F, et al: Inhibition of testicular luteinizing hormone receptor level by treatment with a potent LHRH agonist or human chorionic gonadotropin. Biochem Biophys Res Commun 1977; 76:855–862.

Barradell LB, Faulds D: Cyproterone: A review of its pharmacology and therapeutic efficacy in prostate cancer. Drugs Aging 1994; 5:59–80.

Beck PH, McAnich JW, Goebel JL, Stutman RE: Plasma testosterone in patients receiving DES. Urology 1978; 11:157–160.

Béland G: Combination of anandron with orchiectomy in treatment of metastatic prostate cancer: Results of a double-blind study. Urology 1991; 37(2 suppl):25–29.

Béland G, Elhilali M, Fradet Y, et al: Total androgen ablation: Canadian experience. Urol Clin North Am 1991; 18:75 82.

Bergman B, Damber JE, Tomic R: Effects of total and subcapsular orchidectomy on serum concentrations of testosterone and pituitary hormones in patients with carcinoma of the prostate. Urol Int 1982; 37:139–144.

Bertagna C, De Géry A, Hucher M, et al: Efficacy of the combination of nilutamide plus orchidectomy in patients with metastic prostatic cancer: A meta-analysis of seven randomized double-blind trials (1056 patients). Br J Urol 1994; 73:396–402.

Blackard CE, Byar DP, Jordan WP: Orchiectomy for advanced prostatic carcinoma. Urology 1973; 1:553–560.

Blumenstein BA: Some statistical considerations for the interpretation of trials of combined androgen therapy. Cancer 1993; 72:3834–3840.

Boccon-Gibod L: The prevention of LHRH induced disease flares in patients with metastatic carcinoma of the prostate. *In* Schröder FH, ed: EORTC Genitourinary Group Monograph 8: Treatment of Prostatic Cancer: Facts and Controversies. New York, Wiley-Liss, 1990, pp 125–129.

Boccon-Gibod L, Laudat MH, Dugue MA, Steg A: Cyproterone acetate lead-in prevents initial rise of serum testosterone induced by luteinizing hormone-releasing hormone analogs in the treatment of metastatic carcinoma of the prostate. Eur Urol 1986; 12:400–402.

Brinkman AO, Jenster G, Ris-Stalpers C, et al: Androgen receptor mutations. J Steroid Biochem Molec Biol 1995; 53:443–448.

Brogden RN, Crisp P: Flutamide: A review of its pharmacodynamic and pharmacokinetic properties, and therapeutic use in advanced prostatic cancer. Drugs Aging 1991; 1:104–115.

Bruchovsky N, Brown EM, Coppin CM, et al: The endocrinology and treatment of prostate tumor progression. *In* Bruchovsky N, Resnick MI, Karr JP, eds: Current Concepts and Approaches to the Study of Prostate Cancer. New York, Alan R. Liss, 1987, pp 347–387.

Byar DP: The Veterans Administration Cooperative Urological Research Group's study of cancer of the prostate. Cancer 1973; 32:1126–1130.

Byar DP, Corle DK: Veterans Administration Cooperative Urological Research Group: VACURG randomized trial of radical prostatectomy for stages I and II prostate cancer. Urology 1981; 17(4 suppl):7–11.

Byar DP, Corle DK: Hormone therapy for prostate cancer: Results of the Veterans Administration Cooperative Urological Research Group Studies. NCI Monogr 1988; 7:165–170.

Clark P, Houghton L: Subcapsular orchiectomy for carcinoma of the prostate. Br J Urol 1977; 49:419–425.

Coffey DS: The molecular biology, endocrinology and physiology of the prostate and seminal vesicles. *In* Walsh PC, Retik AB, Stamey TA, Vaugh ED, eds: Campbell's Urology, 6th ed. Philadelphia, WB Saunders, 1992, pp 221–266.

Cooper EH, Armitage TG, Robinson MRG, et al: Prostatic specific antigen and the prediction of prognosis in metastatic prostatic cancer. Cancer 1990; 66(suppl):19–22.

Crawford ED: Challenges in the management of prostate cancer. Br J Urol 1992; 70(suppl 1):33–38.

Crawford ED, Eisenberger MA, McLeod, et al: A controlled trial of Leuprolide with and without Flutamide in prostatic carcinoma. N Engl J Med 1989; 321:419–424.

Dalesio O, Schröder FH, Peto R (Writing Committee), and the Prostate Cancer Trialists' Collaborative Group: Maximal androgen blockade in advanced prostate cancer: an overview of 22 randomized trials with 3289 deaths in 5710 patients. Lancet 1995; 346:265–269.

Daneshgari F, Crawford ED: Endocrine therapy of advanced carcinoma of the prostate. Cancer 1993; 71:1089–1097.

DeKernion JN, Murphy GP, Priore R: Comparison of flutamide and emcyt in hormone-refractory metastatic prostatic cancer. Urology 1988; 31:312–317.

Delaere KPJ, van Thillo EL: Flutamide monotherapy as primary treatment in advanced prostatic carcinoma. Semin Oncol 1991; 18(suppl 6):13–18.

de Lignieres B: The case for a nonplasma lipoprotein etiology of reduced vascular risk in estrogen replacement therapy. Curr Opin Obstet Gynaec 1993; 5:389–395.

Denis LJ, Carneiro de Moura JL, Bono A, et al: Goserelin acetate and flutamide versus bilateral orchiectomy: A phase III EORTC trial (30853). Urology 1993; 42:119–130.

de Voogt HJ, Klijn JGM, Studer U, members of the EORTC GU Group: Orchidectomy versus buserelin in combination with cyproterone acetate, for 2 weeks or continuously, in the treatment of metastatic cancer: Preliminary results of EORTC trial 30843. J Steroid Biochem Molec Biol 1990; 37:965–969.

de Voogt HJ, Smith PhH, Pavone-Macaluso M, members of the EORTC GU Group: Cardiovascular side effects of diethylstilbestrol, cyproterone acetate, medroxyprogesterone acetate and estramustine phosphate used for the treatment of advanced prostatic cancer: Results from European Organization for Research on Treatment of Cancer trials 30761 and 30762. J Urol 1986; 135:303–307.

de Voogt HJ, Studer U, Schröder FH, members of the EORTC GU Group: Maximum androgen blockade (MAB) using LHR-agonist Buserelin in combination with short-term (2 weeks) or long-term (continuously) cyproterone-acetate (CPA), is not superior to standard androgen deprivation in the treatment of advanced prostate cancer: Final analysis of EORTC GU group trial 30843. Eur Urol 1995. In press.

de Voogt HJ, Suciu S, Sylvester R, members of the European Organization for Research on Treatment of Cancer Genitourinary Tract Cooperative Group: Multivariate analysis of prognostic factors in patients with advanced prostatic cancer: Results from 2 European Organization for Research on Treatment of Cancer trials. J Urol 1989; 141:883–888.

Droz J-P, Kattan J, Bonnay M, et al: High-dose continuous-infusion fosfestrol in hormone-resistant prostate cancer. Cancer 1993; 71:1123–1130.

Dupont A, Cusan L, Gomez J-L, et al: Prostate specific antigen and prostatic acid phosphatase for monitoring therapy of carcinoma of the prostate. J Urol 1991; 146:1064–1068.

Dupont A, Gomez J, Cusan L, et al: Response to flutamide withdrawal in advanced prostate cancer in progression under combination therapy. J Urol 1993; 150:908–913.

Ellis WJ, Grayhack JT: Sexual function in aging males after orchiectomy and estrogen therapy. J Urol 1963; 89:895–899.

Farnsworth WE, Slaunwhite WR, Sharma M, et al: Interaction of prolactin and testosterone in the human prostate. Urol Res 1981; 9:79–88.

Fiet J, Doré J-C, le Gô A, et al: Multivariate analysis of plasma hormones in patients with metastatic prostate cancer receiving combined LHRH-analog and antiandrogen therapy. Prostate 1993; 23:291–313.

Fleischmann JD, Catalona WJ: Endocrine therapy for bladder outlet obstruction from carcinoma of the prostate. J Urol 1985; 134:498–500.

Fossa SD: Quality of life after palliative radiotherapy in patients with hormone-resistant prostate cancer: Single institution experience. Br J Urol 1994; 74:345–351.

Geller J, Albert JD, Nachtsheim DA, Loza D: Comparison of prostatic cancer tissue dihydrotestosterone levels at the time of relapse following orchiectomy or estrogen therapy. J Urol 1984; 132:693–696.

Goldenberg SL, Bruchovsky N, Rennie PS, Coppin CM: The combination of cyproterone acetate and low dose diethylstilbestrol in the treatment of advanced prostatic carcinoma. J Urol 1988; 140:1460–1465.

Gormley GJ: Role of 5α-reductase inhibitors in the treatment of advanced prostatic carcinoma. Urol Clin North Am 1991; 18:93–98.

Grayhack JT, Bunce PL, Kearns JW, Scott WW: Influence of the pituitary on prostatic response to androgen in the rat. Bull Johns Hopkins Hosp 1955; 96:154–163.

Greenstein A, Plymate SR, Katz PG: Visually stimulated erection in castrated men. J Urol 1995; 153:650–652.

Gutman AB, Gutman EB: Acid phosphatase occurring in term of patients with metastasizing carcinoma of the prostate gland. J Clin Invest 1938; 17:473–481.

Haapiainen R, Rannikko S, Alfthan O, Finn Prostate Group: Comparison of primary orchiectomy and polyestradiol phosphatase in the treatment of advanced prostatic cancer. Br J Urol 1990; 66:94–97.

Haapiainen R, Rannikko S, Ruutu M, et al: Orchiectomy versus oestrogen in the treatment of advanced prostatic cancer. Br J Urol 1991; 67:184–187.

Hampson SJ, Davies JH, Charig CR, Shearer RJ: LHRH analogues as primary treatment for urinary retention in patients with prostatic carcinoma. Br J Urol 1993; 71:583–586.

Harris MG, Coleman SG, Faulds D, Crisp P: Nilutamide: A review of its pharmacodynamic and pharmacokinetic properties, and therapeutic efficacy in prostate cancer. Drugs Aging 1993; 3:9–25.

Hermanek P, Sobin LH, eds: UICC (Union International Contre le Cancer): TNM Classification of Malignant Tumors, 4th ed; 2nd rev. Berlin, Springer, 1992.

Huang JK, Bartsch W, Voigt KD: Interactions of antiandrogen (cyproterone acetate) with the androgen receptor system and its biological action in the rat ventral prostate. Acta Endocrinol 1985; 109:569–576.

Huben RP, Murphy GP, Investigators of the National Prostatic Cancer Project: A comparison of diethylstilbestrol or orchiectomy with buserelin and with methotrexate plus diethylstilbestrol or orchiectomy in newly diagnosed patients with clinical stage D2 cancer of the prostate. Cancer 1988; 62:1881–1887.

Huggins C, Hodges CV: Studies on prostate cancer: I. The effect of estrogen and of androgen injection on serum phosphatases in metastatic carcinoma of the prostate. Cancer Res 1941; 1:293–297.

Huggins C, Stevens RE, Hodges CV: Studies on prostatic cancer: II. The effects of castration on advanced carcinoma of the prostate gland. Arch Surg 1941; 43:209.

Isaacs JT, Coffey DS: Adaptation versus selection as the mechanism responsible for the relapse of prostatic cancer to androgen ablation therapy as studied in the Dunning R-3327-H adenocarcinoma. Cancer Res 1981; 41:5070–5075.

Isaacs JT, Wake N, Coffey DS, Sandberg AA: Genetic instability coupled to clonal selection as a mechanism for tumor progression in the Dunning

R-3327 rat prostatic adenocarcinoma system. Cancer Res 1982; 42:2353–2361.

Iversen P. Endocrine management of advanced prostate cancer—goals and limitations. *In* Schröder FH: Proceedings of the symposium on Progress and Controversies in Oncological Urology IV: Recent Advances in Prostate Cancer and BPH. Rotterdam, The Netherlands, April 11–13, 1996. Parthenon Publishing, Carnforth, United Kingdom, 1996. In press.

Jacobi GH: Intramuscular cyproterone acetate treatment for advanced prostatic carcinoma: Results of the first multicentric randomized trial. Proceedings Androgens and Antiandrogens, International Symposium, Utrecht, 1982, pp 161–169.

Jacobi GH, Altwein JE, Kurth KH, et al: Treatment of advanced prostatic cancer with parenteral cyproterone acetate: A phase III randomized trial. Br J Urol 1980; 52:208–215.

Janknegt RA, Abbou CC, Bartoletti R, et al: Orchiectomy and nilutamide or placebo as treatment of metastatic prostatic cancer in a multinational double-blind randomized trial. J Urol 1993; 149:77–83.

Johansson J-E, Andersson S-O, Holmberg L, Bergström R: Primary orchiectomy versus estrogen therapy in advanced prostatic cancer—a randomized study: Results after 7 to 10 years of follow-up. J Urol 1991; 145:519–523.

Johansson S, Ljunggren E: Prostatic carcinoma with hormonal treatment. Scand J Urol Nephrol 1981; 15:331–332.

Kadmon D, Thompson TC, Lynch GR, Scardino PT: Elevated plasma chromogranin-A concentrations in prostatic carcinoma. J Urol 1991; 146:358–361.

Kaisary AV: Current clinical studies with a new nonsteroidal antiandrogen, casodex. Prostate 1994; 5(Suppl):27–33.

Kaisary AV, Tyrrell CJ, Peeling WB, Griffiths K: Comparison of LHRH analogue (Zoladex) with orchiectomy in patients with metastatic prostatic carcinoma. Br J Urol 1991; 67:502–508.

Kent JR, Bischoff AJ, Arduino LJ, et al: Estrogen dosage and suppression of testosterone levels in patients with prostatic carcinoma. J Urol 1973; 109:858–860.

Klijn JGM, de Voogt HJ, Schröder FH, de Jong FH: Combined treatment with buserelin and cyproterone acetate in metastatic prostatic carcinoma (Letter). Lancet 1985; 2:493.

Klotz LH, Goldenberg LS, Bullock MJ, et al: Neoadjuvant cyproterone acetate (CPA) therapy prior to radical prostatectomy reduces tumour burden and margin positivity without altering 6- and 12-month post-treatment PSA. Results of a randomized trial (abstract 356). J Urol 1996; 155(Suppl):399A.

Kozlowski JM, Ellis WJ, Grayhack JT: Advanced prostatic carcinoma: Early versus late endocrine therapy. Urol Clin North Am 1991; 18:15–24.

Labrie F, Belanger A, Veilleux R, et al: Rationale for maximal androgen withdrawal in the therapy of prostate cancer. Bailliere's Clin Oncol 1988; 2:597–619.

Labrie F, Dupont A, Belanger A, et al: New approaches in the treatment of prostate cancer: Complete instead of partial withdrawal of androgens. Prostate 1983; 4:579–594.

Leuprolide Study Group: Leuprolide versus diethylstilbestrol for metastatic prostate cancer. N Engl J Med 1984; 311:1281–1286.

Lin BJT, Chen K-K, Chen M-T, Chang LS: The time for serum testosterone to reach castrate level after bilateral orchiectomy or oral estrogen in the management of metastatic prostatic cancer. Urology 1994; 43:834–837.

Lukkarinen O, Hammond GL, Kontturi M, Vihko R: Testicular steroid secretion and peripheral serum steroid concentrations in patients with prostatic carcinoma after short-term estrogen treatment. Invest Urol 1979; 16:453–456.

Lund F, Rasmussen F: Flutamide versus stilbestrol in the management of advanced prostatic cancer. Br J Urol 1988; 61:140–142.

MacFarland JR, Tolley DA: Flutamide therapy for advanced prostatic cancer; A Phase II study. Br J Urol 1985; 57:172–174.

Mackler MA, Liberti JP, Smith MJV, et al: The effect of orchiectomy and various doses of stilbestrol on plasma testosterone levels in patients with carcinoma of the prostate. Invest Urol 1972; 9:423–425.

McLeod DG, Crawford ED, Blumenstein BA, et al: Controversies in the treatment of metastatic prostate cancer. Cancer 1992; 7(Suppl):324–328.

Mellinger GT, as member of the Veterans Administration Co-operative Urological Research Group: Treatment and survival of patients with cancer of the prostate. Surg Gynecol Obstet 1967; 124:1011–1017.

Mulders PFA, Fernandez del Moral P, Theeuwes AGM, et al: Value of biochemical markers in the management of disseminated prostatic cancer. Eur Urol 1992; 21:2–5.

Murphy GP, Slack NH: Response criteria of the prostate of the USA National Prostatic Cancer Project. Prostate 1980; 1:375–382.

Myers C, Trepel J, Sartor O, et al: Antigrowth factor strategies. Cancer 1993; 71(3 suppl):1172–1178.

Myers RP, Larson-Keller JJ, Bergstralh EJ, et al: Hormonal treatment at time of radical retropubic prostatectomy for stage D1 prostate cancer: Results of long-term follow-up. J Urol 1992; 147:910–915.

Nesbit RM, Baum WC: Endocrine control of prostatic carcinoma. JAMA 1950; 143:1317–1320.

Papsidero LD, Wang MC, Valenzuela LA, et al: A prostate antigen in sera of prostatic cancer patients. Cancer Res 1980; 40:2428–2432.

Parmar H, Edwards L, Phillips RH, et al: Orchiectomy versus long-acting D-Trp-6-LHRH in advanced prostate cancer. Br J Urol 1987; 59:248–254.

Pavone-Macaluso M, de Voogt HJ, Viggiano G, et al: Comparison of diethylstilbestrol, cyproterone acetate and medroxyprogesterone acetate in the treatment of advanced prostatic cancer: Final analysis of a randomized phase III trial of the European Organization for Research on Treatment of Cancer Urological Group. J Urol 1986; 136:624–631.

Pilepich MV, John MJ, Krall JM, et al: Phase II Radiation Therapy Oncology Group study of hormonal cytoreduction with flutamide and zoladex in locally advanced carcinoma of the prostate treated with definite radiotherapy. Am J Clin Oncol 1990; 13:461–464.

Prostate Cancer Trialists' Collaborative Group: Maximum androgen blockade in advanced prostate cancer: An overview of 22 randomised trials with 3283 deaths in 5710 patients. Lancet 1995; 346:265–269.

Prout GR Jr, Kliman B, Daly JJ, et al: Endocrine changes after diethylstilbestrol therapy: Effects in prostatic neoplasm and pituitary gonadal axis. Urology 1976; 7:148–155.

Radlmaier A, Bormacher K, Neumann F: Hot flushes: Mechanism and prevention. EORTC Genitourinary Group Monograph 8: Treatment of Prostatic Cancer—Facts and Controversies. New York, Alan R. Liss, 1990, pp 131–140.

Redding TW, Schally AV: Inhibition of prostate tumor growth in two rat models by chronic administration of D-Trp^6 analogue of luteinizing hormone-releasing hormone. Proc Natl Acad Sci USA 1981; 78:6509–6512.

Reiner WG, Scott WW, Eggleston JC, Walsh PC: Long-term survival after hormonal therapy for stage D prostate cancer. J Urol 1979; 122:183–184.

Riba LW: Subcapsular castration for carcinoma of prostate. J Urol 1942; 48:384–387.

Robinson MRG, Hetherington J: The EORTC studies: Is there an optimal endocrine management for M1 prostatic cancer? World J Urol 1986; 4:171–175.

Robinson MRG, Smith PH, Richards B, et al: The final analysis of the EORTC Genito-Urinary Group Phase III clinical trial (Protocol 30805) comparing orchidectomy, orchidectomy plus cyproterone acetate and low dose stilboestrol in the management of metastatic carcinoma of the prostate. Eur Urol 1995; 28:273–283.

Schally AV, Arimura A, Baba Y, et al: Isolation and properties of the FSH and LH-releasing hormone. Biochem Biophys Res Commun 1971; 43:393–399.

Schally AV, Redding TW: Somatostatin analogs as adjuncts to agonists of luteinizing hormone–releasing hormone in the treatment of experimental prostate cancer. Proc Natl Acad Sci USA 1987; 84:7275–7279.

Scher HI, Kelly WK: The flutamide withdrawal syndrome: Its impact on clinical trials in hormone-refractory prostatic cancer. J Clin Oncol 1993; 11:1566–1572.

Schröder FH: Total androgen suppression in the management of prostatic cancer: A critical review. *In* Schröder FH, Richards B, eds: Progress in Clinical and Biological Research. EORTC GU Group Monograph 2, Part A: Therapeutic Principles in Metastatic Prostatic Cancer. New York, Alan R. Liss, 1985, pp 307–317.

Schröder FH: Prostate cancer: To screen or not to screen? BMJ 1993; 306:407–408.

Schröder FH, Röhrborn CG: Endocrine management of prostate cancer. *In* Lytton B, Catalona W, eds: Advances in Urology 4. St. Louis, Mosby-Year Book, 1991, pp 25–52.

Schröder FH, Whelan P, Kurth KH, et al: Antiandrogens as monotherapy for metastatic prostate cancer: a preliminary report on EORTC Protocol 30892. *In* Schröder FH: Proceedings of the symposium on Progress and Controversies in Oncological Urology IV: Recent Advances in Prostate Cancer and BPH. Rotterdam, The Netherlands, April 11–13, 1996. Parthenon Publishing, Carnforth, United Kingdom, 1996. In press.

Schulze H, Senge T: Influence of different types of antiandrogens on luteinizing hormone–releasing hormone analogue-induced testosterone surge in patients with metastatic carcinoma of the prostate. J Urol 1990; 144:934–941.

Senge T, Hulshoff T, Tunn U, et al: Testosteron Konzentration im Serum nach subkapsulaerer Orchiektomie. Urologe 1978; 17:382–384.

Sgrignoli AR, Walsh PC, Steinberg GD, et al: Prognostic factors in men with stage D1 prostate cancer: Identification of patients less likely to have prolonged survival after radical prostatectomy. J Urol 1994; 152:1077–1081.

Sharifi R, Soloway M, Leuprolide Study Group: Clinical study of leuprolide depot formulation in the treatment of advanced prostate cancer. J Urol 1990; 143:68–71.

Shearer RJ, Hendry WF, Sommerville IF, et al: Plasma testosterone an accurate monitor of hormone treatment in prostatic cancer. Br J Urol 1973; 45:668–677.

Smith PH, Suciu S, Robinson MRG, et al: A comparison of the effect of diethylstilbestrol with low dose estramustine phosphate in the treatment of advanced prostatic cancer: Final analysis of a phase III trial of the European Organization for Research on Treatment of Cancer. J Urol 1986; 136:619–623.

Sneller ZW, Hop WCJ, Carpentier PJ, Schröder FH: Prognosis and prostatic volume changes during endocrine management of prostate cancer: A longitudinal study. J Urol 1992; 147:962–966.

Sogani PC, Minoo R, Vagaiwala R, Whitmore WS: Experience with fluta-mide in patients with advanced prostatic cancer without prior endocrine therapy. Cancer 1984; 54:744–750.

Soloway MS: Randomized prospective study: Radical prostatectomy (RP) alone vs. RP preceded by androgen blockade in CT2b prostate cancer. Proceedings, American Association of Genitourinary Surgeons, Sea Is-land, GA, 1996, p 41.

Soloway MS, Chodak G, Vogelzang NJ, et al: Zoladex versus orchiectomy in treatment of advanced prostate cancer: A randomized trial: Zoladex Prostate Study Group. Urology 1991; 37:46–51.

Soloway MS, Hardeman SW, Hickey DP, et al: Simple grading system for bone scans correlates with survival for patients with stage D2 prostatic cancer (Abstract 1023). J Urol 1987; 137:359A.

Soloway MS, Matzkin H: Antiandrogenic agents as monotherapy in ad-vanced prostatic carcinoma. Cancer 1993; 71(3 suppl):1083–1088.

Thompson IM, Zeidman EJ, Rodriguez FR: Sudden death due to disease flare with luteinizing hormone–releasing agonist therapy for carcinoma of the prostate. J Urol 1990; 144:1479–1480.

Tolis G, Ackman D, Stellos A, et al: Tumor growth inhibition in patients with prostatic carcinoma treated with luteinizing hormone–releasing hor-mone agonists. Proc Natl Acad Sci USA 1982; 79:1658–1662.

Umbas R, Isaacs WB, Bringuier PP, et al: Decreased E-cadherine expression is associated with poor prognosis in patients with prostate cancer. Cancer Res 1994; 54:3929–3933.

van Aubel OGJM, Hoekstra WJ, Schröder FH: Early orchiectomy for patients with stage D1 prostatic carcinoma. J Urol 1985; 134:292–294.

van den Ouden D, Tribukait B, Blom JHM, et al, the European Organization for Research and Treatment of Cancer Genitourinary Group: Deoxyribo-nucleic acid ploidy of core biopsies and metastatic lymph nodes of prostate cancer patients: Impact on time to progression. J Urol 1993; 150:400–406.

Veldscholte J, Berrevoets CA, Brinkmann AO, et al: Anti-androgens and the mutated androgen receptor of LNCaP cells: Differential effects on binding affinity, heat-shock protein interaction, and transcription activa-tion. Biochemistry 1992; 31:2393–2399.

Veterans Administration Cooperative Urological Research Group (VA-CURG): Treatment and survival of patients with cancer of the prostate. Surg Gynecol Obstet 1967; 124:1011–1017.

Walsh PC: Benign and malignant neoplasms of the prostate (Editorial Comment). J Urol 1989; 141:1032–1033.

Waymont B, Lynch TH, Dunn JA, et al: Phase III randomised study of zoladex versus stilboestrol in the treatment of advanced prostate cancer. Br J Urol 1992; 69:614–620.

Whitmore WF Jr: Hormone therapy in prostatic cancer. Am J Med 1956; 21:697–701.

Zagars GK, Sands ME, Pollack A, von Eschenbach AC: Early androgen ablation for stage D1 (N1 to N3, M0) prostate cancer: Prognostic vari-ables and outcome. J Urol 1994; 151:1330–1333.

90
CHEMOTHERAPY FOR HORMONE-RESISTANT PROSTATE CANCER

Mario A. Eisenberger, M.D.

Clinical Considerations in the Management of Patients with Hormone-Resistant Prostate Cancer

Evaluation of Patients with Androgen-Resistant Prostate Cancer

Experience with Cytotoxic Chemotherapy

Palliative Management of Patients with Hormone-Refractory Prostate Cancer: Pain and Epidural Cord Compression

Future Directions with Chemotherapy

Prostate cancer represents a prime model of endocrine-dependent tumors in men. Although patients respond dramatically (subjectively and objectively) to a variety of androgen deprivation procedures, this effect is usually palliative and temporary. The development of a hormone-independent state is a categorical and irreversible phenomenon observed in the majority of patients and occurs within an almost predictable time frame after the initiation of androgen deprivation. Extensive data derived from large-scale, prospective studies involving patients with stage D_2 disease treated with virtually all combinations and permutations of androgen deprivation maneuvers indicate that the medians in time to progression and survival have ranged from 12 to 18 months and 2 to 3 years (Byar, 1980; The Leuprolide Study Group, 1984; Eisenberger et al, 1986; Turkes et al, 1987; Crawford et al, 1989; Denis et al, 1993; McLeod, 1995).

Many of the biologic events leading to a predominantly hormone-independent state remain undefined, although progress in cell and molecular biology over the past decade has enhanced understanding of the mechanisms involved in prostate cancer growth, differentiation, and metastasis. Although cancer cells demonstrating the androgen-independent phenotype can be identified during the early development of prostate cancer, as the tumor progresses and distant metastases become clinically evident, the pool of such hormone-independent cells reaches critical proportions. An increasing number of biologic events have been identified during the process of prostate cancer progression. Among these are a variety of phenotypic changes ranging from morphologic transformation, modification of cellular antigenic expression, changes in growth patterns, and differenti-

ation pathways. Similarly a number of other fundamental biologic events are likely to play a significant role in the complex pathogenesis of advanced prostate cancer. Among these are genetic alterations, such as mutations of tumor suppressor genes (Thompson et al, 1991), expression of various oncogenes affecting the control of cell growth, proliferation and cell death (Berges et al, 1993), enhanced tumor angiogenesis (Weidner et al, 1995), and gene mutations that result in a functionally altered expression of the androgen receptor (Taplin et al, 1995).

In the presence of androgens, prostatic cancer growth is based on a cell proliferation rate that exceeds that of cell death (Isaacs et al, 1992). Androgen ablation affects primarily the cell death rate by inducing a swift cascade of a self-destructive apoptosis (Isaacs et al, 1992). As the tumor progresses, the threshold of apoptosis progressively diminishes to a point that cell proliferation exceeds cell death (Berges et al, 1995). This increase in cell number is primarily due to the accumulation of endocrine-insensitive cells, which eventually dominate the biologic scenario of prostate cancer in late stages and result in a formidable array of clinical morbidity that eventually contributes to the demise of these patients.

The relatively low growth fraction expressed by adenocarcinoma of the prostate, compared with other common tumor types such as adenocarcinoma of the breast, is most likely an important factor to explain the differences in response rates observed with chemotherapy between these two, otherwise similar, tumor types. It should be pointed out, however, that the proliferation rate of prostate cancer, which is directly proportional to its growth fraction (Berges et al, 1995), appears to increase with tumor progression, especially after androgen ablation. The identification of proliferation antigens such as ki67, which can be demonstrated in paraffin-imbedded tissue (Cattoretti et al, 1992) and are expressed by cycling cells, may have important prognostic and therapeutic implications. This aspect is particularly important because most chemotherapeutic agents available are more effective in tumors with a high proliferative rate, such as lymphomas, small cell lung carcinomas, and germ cell tumors of the testis.

Changes in the differentiation pathway in prostate cancer have been increasingly demonstrated, particularly in the form of neuroendocrine cells (diSant'Agnese, 1995). Recognition of this important biologic feature is accomplished morphologically, immunohistochemically, molecularly, and clinically as well. Tumors with the neuroendocrine phenotype more often present in a hybrid manner characterized by poorly differentiated epithelial and neuroendocrine cells and demonstrate more aggressive clinical behavior. The evolving experience with cytotoxic chemotherapy suggests that this aggressive clinical entity is more responsive than the conventional differentiated adenocarcinoma type, although the prognosis remains poor (Logothetis et al, 1994).

The emphasis of a primary and direct effect of androgens on prostate cancer growth is being increasingly scrutinized. Evolving data suggest a prominent role of polypeptide growth factors in the pathogenesis of this disease (Eaton, 1982; Story, 1991). More knowledge on the precise function and significance of the effects of these proteins may add to the understanding of the biology of this disease and provide further support for developing therapeutic interventions specifically targeted at the growth factor–mediated tumor growth (Wilding, 1991; Eisenberger et al, 1995b).

CLINICAL CONSIDERATIONS IN THE MANAGEMENT OF PATIENTS WITH HORMONE-RESISTANT PROSTATE CANCER

Most patients with hormone-resistant prostate cancer demonstrate evidence of a rising prostate-specific antigen (PSA) level as the first manifestation of disease progression following androgen deprivation. Indeed, a prospective evaluation of PSA changes in 282 patients with stage D_2 disease treated with bilateral orchiectomy with or without the antiandrogen flutamide has shown that PSA progressions occur approximately 6 months before other clinical (radiologic, scintigraphic) evidence of disease progression (Eisenberger et al, 1995a).

Metastatic adenocarcinoma of the prostate has an overwhelming predilection to involve primarily bone. Although the explanation for this unique metastatic pattern has not been completely elucidated, it probably reflects a multistep combination of biologic factors starting at the time of metastatic spread. Circulating prostatic adenocarcinoma cells are arrested in the cortical and medullary bone spaces, where they subsequently adhere to bone surfaces via specific receptors for moieties such as integrins, collagens, laminin, and other bone-derived proteins. Cell growth is subsequently promoted by various factors, such as hormones, growth

factors, and various stromal epithelial biologic interactions of which most operate in the bone marrow. Expansion of tumor from the bone may cause pain, compression, or pathologic fractures, and extensive bone marrow replacement may cause a major impairment in hematologic function.

Typically, bone metastases in prostate cancer are osteoblastic in their appearance, which reflects an interaction between osteoclast/osteoblastic remodeling and tumor cells and an enhancement of the osteoblast-mediated bone repair mechanisms (Averbuch, 1993). **Mixed osteoblastic/osteolytic and pure osteolytic bone metastases are also seen less frequently. It is believed that osteolytic bone metastases in prostate cancer are usually a manifestation of tumors with more aggressive biologic behavior.**

Clinical involvement of visceral sites is relatively uncommon even in patients with widespread hormone-resistant disease. Table 90–1 illustrates the distribution of metastatic sites reported in different series included in chemotherapy phase II trials. These figures suggest that clinical evidence of visceral metastasis is observed in less than 10% of patients, whereas about 20% have demonstrable soft tissue nodal disease. Because patients with visceral involvement usually have a less satisfactory clinical outcome than those with soft tissue nodal disease, separation of these two groups (visceral versus nodal involvement) may be important for the evaluation of treatment responses in patients with measurable disease sites.

Patients with hormone-resistant prostatic carcinoma may present with a range of hematologic problems caused primarily by the disease or secondary to treatment. Anemia is the most common hematologic abnormality, which can be explained by a variety of factors such as anemia of chronic disease (Waterbury, 1979), bone marrow invasion (Berlin, 1974), and blood loss and in rare cases is secondary to a picture of microangiopathic hemolytic anemia that is commonly associated with a consumption coagulopathy (disseminated intravascular coagulation) (Antman et al, 1979; Coleman et al, 1979). A decrease in the red cell count of patients with advanced hormone-resistant prostate cancer is most commonly caused by a combination of prior treatment with local radiation to bone marrow harboring sites, systemic use of radiopharmaceuticals, and systemic chemotherapy as well as extensive bone marrow invasion by tumor resulting in substantial decrease in the bone marrow reserve. The only

Table 90–1. DISTRIBUTION OF METASTATIC SITES IN CHEMOTHERAPY TRIALS FOR PATIENTS WITH HORMONE-RESISTANT PROSTATE CANCER

Investigator	Total No.	Bone	Lung	Liver	Soft Tissue–Nodal
Pienta et al (1994)	42	42	3	5	13
Sella et al (1994)	39	36	3	3	9
Moore et al (1994)	27	22	2	2	10
Eisenberger et al (1995b)	109	108	6	4	15
Hudes et al (1992)	36	36	0	2	7
Total	253	244 (96%)	14 (5.5%)	16 (6.5%)	54 (21%)

effective approach in such cases is repeated support with blood transfusions, which is not devoid of complications such as allosensitization and an increased incidence of transfusion-related hepatitis. The use of erythropoietin in patients with transfusion-dependent anemia owing to decreased bone marrow reserve has not been successful (Miller et al, 1990), although this has not been tested specifically in prostate cancer. The use of iron preparations and vitamin supplementation provides unsatisfactory results. Granulocytopenia and thrombocytopenia are most commonly a complication of extensive radiation or systemic chemotherapy. Rarely, rapidly growing tumors with bone marrow involvement result in pancytopenia. Thrombocytosis is also a nonspecific manifestation associated with various neoplastic conditions including prostate cancer (Williams, 1977). Thrombotic complications associated with thrombocytosis are rarely seen in patients with prostate cancer, and treatment is not necessary.

Among the most important urologic complications in patients with advanced prostate cancer is the development of obstructive uropathy. This complication, related to the primary disease, can be devastating to the quality of life and can have major therapeutic implications. Besides an increased incidence of infection and pain, obstructed kidneys may critically impair the renal function to a degree that various chemotherapeutic agents, which depend largely on renal mechanisms for their clearance, cannot be safely employed. In general, patients who are otherwise candidates for treatment with cytotoxic drugs are best managed by relief of obstruction with placement of either internal stents or percutaneous nephrostomies.

Among the most important complications in oncology is the development of epidural cord compression (Sorensen et al, 1990) because of the frequent involvement of vertebral bodies by prostate cancer. The spectrum of clinical manifestations in epidural cord compression includes pain, sensory abnormalities, and progressive motor changes including the devastating development of loss of sphincter control of the bladder and bowel, which may result in stool and urinary incontinence. The presence of significant back pain in patients with extensive vertebral bone involvement is frequently the first sign. Early recognition and an aggressive therapeutic posture coupled with the widespread availability of noninvasive procedures such as magnetic resonance imaging provide the opportunity for more effective management of this potentially hazardous complication. The emergency management of these patients includes the administration of high-dose parenteral corticosteroids, external beam radiation, and surgical decompression with spinal stabilization (Sorensen et al, 1990).

EVALUATION OF PATIENTS WITH ANDROGEN-RESISTANT PROSTATE CANCER

Evolving data suggest that patients with hormone-refractory prostate cancer represent a heterogeneous group and that a complete characterization of response and type of prior endocrine treatment is a critical component in the management of these patients.

Usually the first manifestation of disease progression is a rising serum PSA level. This finding may precede other evidence of advancing disease by a period of about 6 months, and during this time patients may remain relatively asymptomatic (Eisenberger et al, 1995a). **Unless there are reasons to suspect treatment noncompliance or if the choice of prior treatment involved regimens known not to result in a sustained suppression of serum testosterone to the castrate range (such as monotherapy with nonsteroidal antiandrogens, low-dose estrogens, or 5-alpha-reductase inhibitors or with a combination thereof), routine evaluation of serum testosterone is unlikely to be cost-effective, especially if patients already demonstrate signs and symptoms of chronic hypogonadism.** A high rate of sequential responses, however, has been reported with the intermittent androgen deprivation approach reported by Goldenberg and colleagues (1995). Most patients who responded to subsequent reintroduction of treatment showed evidence of recovery of serum testosterone above the castrate range during the periods off treatment which suggests that evaluation of serum levels of testosterone may indeed be warranted in selected patients.

For several years, it has been postulated that discontinuation of androgen suppression in nonorchiectomized patients may influence the outcome of disease in terms of progression and survival (Taylor et al, 1993). Similarly, it has been shown that administration of exogenous testosterone and its derivatives may indeed produce a significant clinical flare, which results in severe pain, neurologic, urologic, and coagulation complications in a small proportion of patients (Fowler and Whitmore, 1981, 1982; Manni et al, 1988). In a retrospective analysis of 205 patients with hormone-refractory disease treated with chemotherapy, various prognostic variables, including orchiectomy, were evaluated by Hussain and colleagues (1994b). This multivariate analysis failed to indicate a significant correlation between prior orchiectomy and time to disease progression and survival. In Hussain and colleagues' patients, all medical forms of androgen deprivation were discontinued at least 4 weeks before initiation of chemotherapy, and contrary to that suggested by Taylor and co-workers (1995), discontinuation of treatment did not significantly affect outcome. **Until this issue is resolved, the author recommends that for clinical trials with chemotherapy, gonadal androgen suppression should be maintained during treatment, whereas in routine clinical practice if discontinuation of treatment is elected, intermittent monitoring of serum testosterone may provide potentially important information in the management of these patients.**

Another important management aspect discussed in more detail elsewhere in this chapter relates to antiandrogen withdrawal effects (Scher and Kelly, 1993). **Discontinuation of antiandrogens (both steroidal and nonsteroidal) can result in clinical responses expressed by decreases in PSA levels, symptomatic benefits, and less frequently objective improvements in soft tissue and bone metastasis. Because of this, the author recommends that in patients treated with antiandrogens in combination with other forms of androgen deprivation, the first step should involve the discontinuation of these agents and careful observation, including serial monitoring of PSA levels, for a period 4 to 8 weeks before embarking on the next therapeutic maneuver.**

The next step is to determine which modality of treatment

should be employed first: either administration of a relatively nontoxic treatment such as a second-line hormonal manipulation or cytotoxic chemotherapy. **Evolving data suggest that there might be a role for a second-line endocrine manipulation approach in selected patients** (Scher et al, 1995). Among agents that have been reported to produce some antitumor activity in this setting are aminoglutethimide (Sartor, 1995), ketoconazole (Wilding, 1991), and corticosteroids (Storlie et al, 1995) as well as the withdrawal of antiandrogens (Scher and Kelly, 1993; Small and Srinivas, 1995). An interesting observation is that previously reported experience with the same agents—aminoglutethimide (Drago, 1984), ketoconazole, and low-dose corticosteroids (Tannock et al, 1989)—was much less encouraging. The main difference between the current and old experience relates to patient selection factors and possible timing of initiation of therapies. It is possible that this relatively unexpected experience with these agents can be explained, at least partly, by the ability to recognize early progression with sequential PSA monitoring during hormonal therapy, thus allowing for changes in therapy at earlier points in time when the disease may still demonstrate some biologic dependence on hormones. More data about the clinical significance of these early observations are needed to define the relative impact of sequential endocrine approaches to patients with metastatic disease. It is possible that this may evolve in the same direction as in breast cancer, in which mostly short-lived responses can be seen in patients with tumors rich in estrogen and progesterone receptors. In view of the limited role of cytotoxic chemotherapy in advanced prostatic cancer and the frequent toxicity associated with this treatment modality, this sequential hormonal approach may be a reasonable alternative for those patients with relatively limited metastatic disease who remain asymptomatic at the time of disease progression.

Another important consideration is the initial assessment of the clinical behavior of these tumors, which is frequently alluded to as the metastatic phenotype. Poorly differentiated, anaplastic, or neuroendocrine tumors usually have a low likelihood of response and shorter duration of response to androgen deprivation. These patients frequently present with low or absent serum PSA levels, have a disproportionately high incidence of visceral involvement, and demonstrate an uncharacteristic bone involvement (lytic lesions). Recognition of these clinical characteristics may indeed play an important role in the selection of chemotherapeutic agents (see later). It has been suggested by some investigators (Logothetis et al, 1994) that systematic biopsies of visceral sites may elicit evidence of a small cell component in about 30% to 40% of patients; this, however, needs to be confirmed by other groups before one can recommend routine biopsies for this purpose only.

EXPERIENCE WITH CYTOTOXIC CHEMOTHERAPY

The conduct and evaluation of clinical trials in patients with metastatic prostate cancer is usually confounded by significant methodologic problems. Most of the difficulties are related to the pattern of predominant metastatic spread of the disease. As mentioned earlier, the most common metastatic site is bone, manifested by diffuse osteoblastic lesions, which cannot be measured reliably by current methods to allow for assessments of therapeutic benefits. The presence of soft tissue or visceral metastatic sites that allow for serial measurements is uncommon (see Table 90–1) and frequently associated with dominant bone disease that prevents a more global evaluation of these patients (Yagoda, 1984). Furthermore, the selection of patients with bidimensionally measurable disease for new drug development has been the subject of significant criticism. These patients are considered by many as a subgroup with distinct biologic features and not necessarily representative of the usual patients with prostate cancer who present with clinical evidence of bone metastasis only. In fact, much emphasis has been placed on defining the population of patients with hormone-resistant disease with regard to their prognostic variables. Table 90–2 summarizes the clinical and laboratory parameters known as important factors with regard to disease outcome measured by survival. Among those with consistent prognostic significance by most reports are baseline functional status (performance status) and pretreatment hemoglobin levels (above and below the median hemoglobin for the patient population evaluated). Other parameters likely to play a significant role with regard to disease outcome are baseline values of serum acid phosphatase, alkaline phosphatase, and lactic dehydrogenase. The data on the role of baseline PSA, extent of bone scan involvement (number of lesions or pattern of distribution of bone involvement), and maintenance of androgen suppression have been equivocal, and more study is needed at this time.

Despite the frequent finding of elevated PSA levels in patients with hormone-resistant disease, the usefulness of this test as a surrogate end point for clinical trials (i.e., relationship between changes in PSA and therapeutic benefits) remains to be determined. Although many series suggest that PSA changes with treatment indeed reflect a prognostically important finding, this observation requires

Table 90–2. COMMONLY DESCRIBED PROGNOSTIC FACTORS FOR SURVIVAL IN PATIENTS WITH HORMONE-RESISTANT CANCER OF THE PROSTATE

Prognostic Factor	Significance
Performance status	Definite—seen in all studies
Baseline hemoglobin	
Liver involvement	Possible—seen in some studies
Baseline acid phosphatase	
Alkaline phosphatase	
Lactic dehydrogenase	
Time from initiation of androgen deprivation to initiation of chemotherapy	
Response to therapy (measurable)	
≥50% decline in PSA (1 or ≥4 weeks)	
Baseline PSA	Equivocal—more data needed
Extent of disease on bone scan	
Permanent androgen deprivation	

PSA, Prostate-specific antigen.
Based on Petrylak et al, 1992; Kelly, 1993; Taylor, 1993; Hussain et al, 1994b; Sridhara et al, 1995.

proper evaluation in specifically designed phase III trials. Despite this, current clinical trials involving patients with hormone-resistant disease frequently refer to a 50% or greater decline in PSA from the baseline values for a period of 4 weeks or longer as evidence of therapeutic benefits (Kelly, 1993). More recently, another detailed analysis of PSA changes in patients with hormone-resistant prostate cancer supported the prognostic significance of PSA changes with treatment; however, it failed to define a measure of decline that demonstrated sufficient specificity to be used as a reasonable end point in uncontrolled new drug trials (Sridhara et al, 1995). Sridhara and colleagues have argued against the routine use of this parameter as the sole indication of therapeutic efficacy in the process of clinical screening for new drug activity (Sridhara et al, 1995). Furthermore, the interpretation of therapeutic results on the basis on PSA declines needs to be cautiously undertaken because various drugs have been shown to reduce PSA secretion without changing tumor growth (Larocca et al 1191, Steiner et al, 1995). The use of other tests such as serum acid phosphatase (by any method of measurement) and alkaline phosphatase has not been proven beneficial (Yagoda, 1984).

Most of the single chemotherapeutic agents available in practice have been employed in patients with hormone-resistant prostate cancer (Eisenberger et al, 1985; Eisenberger, 1988). The data reported in the literature should be evaluated with regard to the time of their report. Clinical trials reported before the late 1980s should be evaluated separately from those reported subsequently. The main issue relates to the availability of serum PSA and the development of instruments to evaluate and measure quality of life end points. Although PSA and quality of life still need to be better evaluated with regard to their utility as surrogate end points, it has become clear that higher response rates using these two parameters have been reported in contemporary studies (see Table 90–6). It is possible that some of the patients included in the previously described stable disease category (Schmidt et al, 1976; Slack et al, 1980) may indeed be further characterized as responders with the demonstration of significant PSA declines. Furthermore, it is likely that patients currently referred to medical oncologists and entered into clinical trials have less advanced and symptomatic disease than those treated before the availability of PSA. This lead-time factor is also important when survival is assessed in this patient population. **The evolving data with chemotherapy during this decade suggest that the survival of patients with hormone-resistant prostate cancer is most likely between 12 and 18 months** (Eisenberger et al, 1995a) **as opposed to between 6 and 12 months as previously described** (Eisenberger et al, 1985; Eisenberger, 1988), **and this may simply be a reflection of a lead-time bias rather then therapeutic effects.**

The studies conducted before the late 1980s should be carefully scrutinized because of their differences in criteria for evaluation, in addition to patient selection factors, as well as the above-mentioned inherent difficulties in the evaluation of response in patients with advanced prostate cancer. Undoubtedly, these methodologic issues account for the variability in responses reported with the same agent by different investigators. Table 90–3 describes the selected experience with commonly used single agents in this disease before availability of PSA, and Table 90–4 illustrates more recent

experience using PSA assessments. The same data regarding combinations of drugs are shown in Tables 90–5 and 90–6.

The interpretation of some studies is also confounded by the previously unrecognized flutamide withdrawal syndrome (Scher and Kelly, 1993). **This syndrome is characterized by a decrease in PSA and less frequently by objective reductions of measurable tumors following the discontinuation of the nonsteroidal antiandrogen flutamide, and this may have contributed to some of the clinical responses reported with chemotherapy. Typically, following discontinuation of flutamide, the manifestations of tumor response have a short median duration (approximately 3 months). Although it may confound the evaluation of subsequent treatment, the actual therapeutic value of the flutamide withdrawal effect is probably quite limited and palliative. A prospective evaluation of patients with stage D₂ disease treated with flutamide suggests that the actual incidence of a meaningful flutamide withdrawal response is uncommon (15%)** (Small and Srinivas, 1995) **and that this may be enhanced by the use of corticosteroids** (Sartor and Myers, 1995).

The data in Tables 90–3 through 90–6 suggest that among the single agents with modest activity are the bifunctional alkylating drug cyclophosphamide, which has shown modest antitumor effects in about 10% to 20% based on the older literature. Interestingly, in contemporary trials, cyclophosphamide given in standard oral doses or high intravenous doses with hematopoietic growth factor support has been reported to have a higher order of activity (Von Roemeling et al, 1992; Smith D et al, 1992; Abell et al, 1995). Doxorubicin, 5-fluorouracil, and cisplatin, agents with significant activity in various tumor types, have demonstrated only modest single-agent benefits in patients with hormone-resistant prostate cancer. Mitroxantrone, a semisynthetic anthracenedione derivative, has shown modest subjective benefits with otherwise minimal evidence of objective antitumor activity (Osborne et al, 1983; Raghavan et al, 1986; Rearden et al, 1995). This agent was evaluated in combination with low-dose prednisone (10 mg/day orally) and resulted in significant palliative benefits, which could, however, be attributed to the corticosteroid alone (Moore et al, 1994). In a prospective, randomized comparison of mitoxantrone plus prednisone versus prednisone alone, however, the combination resulted in significant improvements of various quality of life issues (Tannock et al, 1995). Interestingly, other objective measures of therapeutic efficacy, such as time to disease progression, decline in PSA levels, and survival, were not significantly different between the treatment arms. This study represents the first randomized comparison designed specifically to evaluate an end point that has been a major focus of attention over the past decade; however, the significance and impact of such assessments obviously require additional scrutiny in carefully designed clinical trials.

Estramustine phosphate is a nitrogen mustard derivative of estradiol-17β phosphate that has demonstrated limited single-agent activity in prostate cancer (see Tables 90–3 and 90–4). In fact, in a prospective, randomized study in patients with hormone-refractory disease, estramustine phosphate given in a dose of 560 mg/day orally was not shown to be superior to a placebo in terms of both palliative effects and survival (Iversen and Rasmussen, 1995) (Table 90–7). This drug has been shown in more recent preclinical evaluation

Table 90–3. REPRESENTATIVE EXPERIENCE REPORTED WITH SINGLE AGENTS BEFORE THE AVAILABILITY OF SERUM PROSTATE-SPECIFIC ANTIGEN

Drug	Reference	Dosage/Schedule	Overall Responses	Common Toxicities	Response Criteria
Cyclophosphamide	Review by Carter and Wasserman, 1975	Multiple oral and IV	8/57 (14%)	N + V, heme	Not specified
Doxorubicin	O'Bryan et al, 1973	30–60 mg/m² IV every 3 weeks	13/88 (14.5%)	N + V, heme, cardiac	Not specified
	O'Bryan et al, 1977 Scher et al, 1984 Torti et al, 1983	10–20 mg/m² IV weekly			MSKCC (Yagoda, 1984) NPCP (Schmidt et al, 1976)
Estramustine phosphate	Mittleman et al, 1976	Multiple	15/86 (17%)	N + V, heme, edema, thromboembolic, gynecomastia	Multiple response criteria
	Kuss et al, 1980 Veronesi et al, 1982	Oral and IV			
Cis-platin	Yagoda et al, 1979	50–80 mg/m² IV every 3 weeks with hydration before and after	24/146 (13.5%)	N + V, renal heme	MSKCC (Yagoda, 1984) NPCP (Schmidt et al, 1976) or not specified
	Merrin, 1979 Rossof et al, 1979 Qazi and Khandekar, 1983 Moore et al, 1986				
Mitoxantrone	Osborne et al, 1983 Raghavan et al, 1986	12–14 mg/m² IV every 3 weeks	3/64 (5%)	N + V, heme	Southwest Oncology Group (Osborn et al, 1983) and World Health Organization (Raghavan et al, 1986). 13 additional patients had improvements of one or more quality of life end points
Vinblastine	Review by Yagoda, 1993	Multiple doses IV bolus and by continuous infusion × 5 days	Total number unclear (8%), 8/39 (21%)	Neuro, heme	Various response criteria M. D. Anderson (Logothetis, 1983) were used in the continuous infusion study.
5-Fluorouracil	Review by Eisenberger, 1988	Multiple doses orally and IV bolus	Unclear	Heme, mucositis	Unclear response criteria—however, overall response rates probably <20%

IV, Intravenous; N + V, nausea and vomiting; heme, hematologic (myelosuppression); neuro, neurotoxicity; NPCP, National Prostatic Cancer Project; MSKCC, Memorial–Sloan Kettering Cancer Center.
Modified from Eisenberger MA, Simon R, O'Dwyer P, et al: J Clin Oncol 1985; 3:827–841; and Eisenberger MA: NCI Monogr 1988; 7:151–163.

to exert its cytotoxic activity through microtubular inhibition (Hudes et al, 1992) and binding to nuclear matrix (Hartley-Asp and Kruse, 1986). In an attempt to enhance the cytotoxicity of estramustine phosphate, investigators combined this agent with other drugs that also exert cytotoxic effects at the level of the microtubule, such as vinblastine and taxol (Seidman et al, 1992; Hudes et al, 1992, 1995). Similarly, it has been shown that etoposide acts synergistically with estramustine phosphate by affecting the nuclear matrix (Pienta et al, 1994). Indeed, clinical trials testing the combination of estramustine plus vinblastine or etoposide or taxol have resulted in promising preliminary evidence of antitumor activity (see Table 90–5). As with estramustine phosphate, etoposide, vinblastine, and taxol have minimal activity in patients with hormone-resistant prostate cancer (see Tables 90–3 and 90–4), which suggests that the mechanistic preclinical observations may be clinically pertinent.

The importance of autocrine growth factors in the control of prostate cancer growth has been emphasized (Story, 1991; Wilding, 1991). Suramin is an old compound that was used for the treatment of parasitic disorders during the early 1900s; it resurfaced in the mid-1980s when it was evaluated for the treatment of patients with acquired immunodeficiency syndrome (AIDS). Suramin is a polysulfonated naphtylurea with multiple biologic functions, including inhibition of binding of various autocrine growth factors to their cellular receptors (Myers et al; 1992; Eisenberger et al, 1995b). Suramin has complex pharmacologic properties (tight protein binding with slow release, long terminal half-life) and an unusual toxicity pattern (neurotoxicity and renal toxicity and a syndrome of malaise fatigue and anorexia), which have now been appropriately characterized. This knowledge and experience about the pharmacology and toxicity pattern of this interesting agent have allowed the development of safe,

Table 90–4. SINGLE AGENT EXPERIENCE WITH THE USE OF PROSTATE-SPECIFIC ANTIGEN

Drug	Reference	Dosage/Schedule	Overall Responses	Common Toxicities	Response Criteria
Cyclophosphamide	Von Roemeling et al, 1992	75–150 mg/day orally	4/13 (30%)	Nausea, heme	Primarily ≥50% PSA decline but measurable responses also seen
	Abell et al, 1995	100 mg/m² /day orally × 14 days every 2 weeks × 3 cycles	6/20 (30%)	Nausea, heme	
	Smith et al, 1992	1.5–4.5 g/m² + GM-CSF + mesna	6/10	Nausea, heme	
Taxol	Roth et al, 1992	135–170 mg/m² IV in 24 hours	1/23	Heme, cardiovascular, anaphylaxis reactions	Measurable criteria and PSA responses (≥50%)
Mitoxantrone	Rearden et al, 1995	3–4 mg/m² IV weekly	0/14	Heme	One measurable response and three subjective improvements 0/14 ≥50% decline in PSA
Estramustine phosphate	Yagoda et al, 1991	14 mg/kg/day orally 3 × daily	9/42 (21%)	Nausea, heme thromboembolic, gynecomastia	≥50% decline in PSA
5-Fluorouracil	Kuzel et al, 1993	1000 mg/m² /day × 5 days by continuous IV infusion every 28 days	0/18	Heme, mucositis	No objective measurable responses or ≥50% PSA decline
Etoposide	Hussain et al, 1994	50 mg/m² /day orally × 21 days, monthly	2/24 (8%)	Heme	One patient had ≥50% decline in PSA, and one had a measurable response
Carboplatin	Canobbio et al, 1993	150 mg/m² IV weekly	3(2)/25 (12%)	Heme	Three had ≥50% PSA declines, and two had measurable responses
Losoxantrone	Huan et al, 1995	50 mg/m² IV every 21 days	5/29 (25%)	Heme	60% had subjective improvements

Heme, Hematologic (myelosuppression); GM-CSF, granulocyte macrophage colony-stimulating factor; IV, intravenous; PSA, prostate-specific antigen.

effective schedules currently undergoing extensive clinical testing in prostate cancer as well as other tumor types. Prospective, randomized trials in patients with hormone-resistant disease and in patients with hormone-naive, stage D₂ prostate cancer should provide more definitive evidence with regard to the role of this new agent in this disease. If proven effective, it will introduce the first clinical evidence that interference with the function of autocrine growth factors may indeed reflect an effective and therapeutic tool for prostate cancer and thus create new opportunities for developing other effective agents targeting this mechanism.

Randomized studies provide the opportunity to evaluate survival, which indeed is the fundamental end point for the evaluation of therapeutic efficacy in this disease. Table 90–7 illustrates selected phase III trials reported in patients with hormone-resistant disease. **The data in Table 90–7 demonstrate that none of the chemotherapeutic regimens tested in these trials was shown to be superior to another with regard to survival. It also points out that the survival of these patients was invariably limited to less than 1 year.**

Laboratory and clinical evidence indicates that major alterations in the differentiation pathway (neuroendocrine transformation) of prostate cancer can be seen in a variable proportion of patients with primarily advanced disease (Lo-

gothetis et al, 1994; diSant'Agnese, 1995). The therapeutic implications of this finding are of significance because tumors demonstrating the neuroendocrine phenotype usually represent an inherently endocrine-resistant disease. These tumors express a number of biologic characteristics unique to neuroendocrine tumors that also occur in other organs, such as lung. Among these are the expression of receptors to various neuroendocrine peptide growth factor, such as bombesin/gastrin-releasing-peptide antagonist, somatostatin, chromogranin-A, and serotonin as well as parathyroid hormone–related protein and p53 mutations. These tumors have rather uncharacteristic clinical behavior reflected by frequent visceral involvement and rapidly growing soft tissue metastasis. Appropriate diagnosis is accomplished clinically and histologically (with demonstration of a small cell variant in the biopsy tissue) and in the laboratory with the demonstration of neuroendocrine markers in the urine (diSant'Agnese, 1995). Treatment is usually similar to that in patients with other neuroendocrine tumors (e.g., small cell carcinoma of the lung) and include combinations of *cis*-platin and etoposide (Frank et al, 1995), although doxorubicin-containing combinations have also been shown to be moderately effective (Logothetis et al, 1994). Despite obvious responses, the prognosis of these patients remains limited and is dependent

Table 90–5. OVERALL EXPERIENCE WITH SELECTED COMBINATION REGIMENS IN PHASE II TRIALS WITHOUT PROSTATE-SPECIFIC ANTIGEN ASSESSMENTS

Regimen	Response	Toxicity
Cyclophosphamide + doxorubicin	12/93 (13%)	N + V, heme
Estramustine + 5-fluorouracil	3/25 (12%)	Gynecomastia, nausea, thromboembolism, mucositis, heme
Carmustine + cyclophosphamide + doxorubicin	7/27 (25%)	Heme, N + V
Cyclophosphamide + prednisolone	7/83 (8%)	Heme, N + V
Doxorubicin + 5-fluorouracil	31*/92 (34%)	Heme, N + V, mucositis
Melphalan + methotrexate + 5-fluorouracil + vincristine + prednisone	27†/84 (32%)	Heme, N + V, mucositis

*30 patients responded according to M. D. Anderson response criteria (Logothetis, 1983); otherwise, responses are unclearly defined.
†24 patients had a ≥50% decrease in acid phosphatase, and 3 of 7 had measurable responses.
N + V, Nausea and vomiting; heme, hematologic (myelosuppression).
Modified from Eisenberger MA, Simon R, O'Dwyer P, et al: J Clin Oncol 1985; 3:827–841; and Eisenberger MA: NCI Monogr 1988; 7:151–163.

on various factors, including extent of disease at the time of presentation.

The extensive experience with chemotherapy for patients with hormone-resistant prostate cancer has been described and discussed here. Some of the complex clinical characteristics of this unique disease in the context of therapeutic interventions have also been illustrated. Despite the relatively small, primarily palliative advances accomplished thus far with nonhormonal chemotherapy, it is clear that the identification of active chemotherapeutic agents and other nonhormonal modalities to treat this disease is critical for the accomplishment of meaningful results in patients who are not cured by local treatment modalities. Undoubtedly, during the last decade, advances in tumor biology in the laboratory as well as a systematic prospective evaluation of the clinical behavior of prostate cancer within the organized environment of clinical trials have enhanced understanding of this prevalent disease and created more plausible opportunities for a rational and tumor-specific design of systemic treatment regimens.

PALLIATIVE MANAGEMENT OF PATIENTS WITH HORMONE-REFRACTORY PROSTATE CANCER: PAIN AND EPIDURAL CORD COMPRESSION

As in other disseminated malignant neoplasms, palliation of symptoms and maintenance of adequate levels of quality of life represent the most important objectives in the management of advanced prostate cancer. **Cancer-related pain is undoubtedly the most debilitating symptom associated with metastatic prostatic carcinoma. Prompt recognition** of the various pain syndromes associated with this disease is critical to accomplish effective control of this devastating symptom. Table 90–8 describes the most common pain syndromes and their respective therapeutic considerations.

Despite extensive efforts, the pathogenesis of bone metastases and pain in prostate cancer remains poorly understood. Alteration in the normal process of bone absorption and formation, which usually follows in an orderly and sequential basis, appears to be a key determining factor (Galasko, 1986) in the development of bone metastasis associated with most malignant neoplasms. Under normal physiologic conditions, the process of bone remodeling is initiated by an increase in osteoclastic activity followed by an increase in osteoblastic differentiation and maturation, which results in the formation of new bone and repair of the initial absorption caused by osteoblasts. Bone loss associated with metastatic cancer can result from enhanced osteoclastic activity, which, in turn, causes excessive resorption of bone mineral and organic matrix. Tumor cells may also cause mineral release and matrix resorption in the areas involved by metastatic disease (Galasko, 1986). In addition to various cytokines, growth factors, tumor necrosis factors, and bone morphogenic proteins have been shown in preclinical studies to play a major role in the induction of both osteoclastic and osteoblastic activity (Galasko, 1986; Reddi and Cunningham, 1990). In prostate cancer, bone metastases are predominantly blastic which reflects a predominance of osteoblast activity in the process of bone remodeling (Averbuch, 1993). This phenomenon may be due to secretion of a specific growth factor that is responsible for the induction of osteoblastic activity (Jacobs et al, 1979). Similarly, there is lack of significant osteoclastic activity, which may explain the relative rarity of hypercalcemia in metastatic prostate cancer (Jacobs et al, 1979; Story, 1991); in fact, significantly elevated serum Ca^{++} levels are most frequently (although the actual incidence is rare) due to the neuroendocrine prostate cancer phenotype discussed previously (deSant'Agnese, 1995).

Focal bone pain in patients with hormone-refractory disease can be well controlled by external localized radiotherapy. **In general, the author also recommends that painful areas known to be positive on bone scan should be evaluated with plain radiographs to exclude the presence of lytic lesions or pathologic fractures.** Such considerations become even more important when the painful area(s) affects extremities and weight-bearing sites. **Sizable lytic bone metastasis, especially in weight-bearing areas, should be routinely irradiated, regardless of pain status, and surgical stabilization should be considered when there is evidence of cortical bone destruction or pathologic fractures.**

The management of diffuse bone pain is an even more challenging problem. **Aggressive administration of narcotic analgesics should be employed because this has shown unequivocal improvement of quality of life** (Foley, 1993; U.S. DHHS, 1994). Other adjuvant pharmacologic approaches include corticosteroids (Tannock et al, 1989, Storlie et al, 1995), biphosphonates (Averbuch, 1993), and nonsteroidal anti-inflammatory drugs (U.S. DHHS, 1994). The introduction of bone-seeking radiopharmaceuticals has

Table 90–6. EXPERIENCE WITH NEWER COMBINATIONS USING PROSTATE-SPECIFIC ANTIGEN ASSESSMENTS

Regimen	Reference	Responses		Toxicity	Comments
		≥50% Decline in PSA	Measurable Responses		
Estramustine phosphate (10 mg/kg/day orally in 3 divided doses × 6–7 weeks) + Vinblastine (4 mg/m²/ IV/weekly)	Seidman et al, 1992 Hudes et al, 1992	13/24 22/36	2/5 1/7	Heme, N + V, gynecomastia, thromboembolism	No information on prior flutamide treatment
Estramustine phosphate (15 mg/kg/day orally × 3 weeks) + Etoposide (50 mg/m²/ day orally × 3 weeks)	Pienta et al, 1994	29/42 (69%)	9/18 (50%)	As above; 25% had severe heme	Prior flutamide treatment effects unclear. Responses seen in patients with no prior antiandrogen treatment
Estramustine phosphate (600 mg/m² orally/ day) + Taxol (120–140 mg/m² × 96 hours infusion)	Hudes et al, 1995	10/17 (59%)	3/6	Heme, mucositis, N + V, edema	All patients with prior flutamide had objective progression before study entry
Doxorubicin (40 mg/ m² IV) + Cyclophosphamide (800–2000 mg/m²) + G-CSF (5 mg/kg/day)	Small et al, 1995	12/29	4/12	Heme, N + V	As above
Suramin (various dosages/schedules) + Hydrocortisone (30–40 mg/day orally)	Review by Eisenberger et al, 1995b; 9 studies	128/338 (38%)	25/85 (29.5)	Malaise, anorexia, renal, neuro, adrenal insufficiency	This is a review of nine studies. Individual responses have ranged from 20–65%
Mitoxantrone (12 mg/ m² IV every 3 weeks) + Prednisone (10 mg orally daily)	Moore et al, 1994	5/23 (21.5%)	1/7	Heme	Nine of 25 were reported to have good palliative responses
Ketoconazole (1200 mg orally daily) + Doxorubicin (20 mg/ m² × 24 hours; infusion weekly) + Hydrocortisone (30 mg/day) (to most patients)	Sella et al, 1994	21/39 (55%)	7/12	Heme, mucositis, adrenal insufficiency	Flutamide withdrawal possible in some, but responses seen in patients with no prior antiandrogen treatment

PSA, Prostate-specific antigen; IV, intravenous; heme, hematologic (myelosuppression); N + V, nausea and vomiting.

provided a useful resource for the management of diffuse bone pain. Among the most commonly used compounds are radioactive phosphorus (P³²) (Silberstein and Williams, 1985; Silberstein, 1993) and strontium 89 (Sr 89) (Porter et al, 1993; Porter and Davis, 1994). This latter compound has been shown to palliate pain to various degrees in 25% to 65% of patients with hormone-refractory disease with diffuse pain (Porter et al, 1993; Porter and Davis, 1994), and in one clinical trial it resulted in more durable pain control when combined with local external beam radiotherapy for localized bone pain (Porter and Davis, 1994). The pharmacokinetics of Sr 89 vary considerably according to the extent of bony involvement. The retention of the isotope is signifi-

cantly longer in patients with diffuse osteoblastic metastasis than in those with relatively limited bone involvement (Robinson et al, 1989). This factor is important to recognize because it undoubtedly affects the degree and duration of myelotoxicity associated with this radioactive compound. A study reported encouraging synergism with Sr 89 and doxorubicin, a known and well-studied radiosensitizer (Tu et al, 1995), and additional studies evaluating the same or other drugs with Sr 89 are under way.

Epidural metastases are a common and potentially devastating complication of systemic cancer. In view of the propensity of prostate cancer to metastasize to the vertebrae and paravertebral region, the incidence of epi-

Table 90–7. SURVIVAL COMPARISONS IN PROSPECTIVE RANDOMIZED TRIALS*

Drug/Regimen	Median Survival (Weeks)	Comments
Cyclophosphamide	47	More patients on the chemotherapy arms had stable disease. Difference in survival not significant statistically
5-Fluorouracil	44	
No chemotherapy†	38	
Estramustine phosphate	26	
Streptozotocin	25	As above
No chemotherapy†	24	
Cyclophosphamide	27	Survival difference not significant
Dacarbazine	40	
Procarbazine	31	
Estramustine + prednimustine	37	As above
Prednimustine	36	
Cyclophosphamide	41	High inevaluability rate. Survival differences not statistically significant
Semustine	22	
Hydroxyurea	19	
Estramustine (E)	26	As above
Vincristine (V)	27	
E + V	32	
Estramustine	43	As above
Methotrexate	37	
Cis-platin	33	
Estramustine (E)	38	As above
Cis-platin (C)	28	
E + C	40	
Doxorubin	29	Survival differences not statistically significant
5-Fluorouracil	24	
CAF	25	As above
5-Fluorouracil	34	
CA	27	No difference in survival
Hydroxyurea	28	
Estramustine§	34	Survival differences not statistically significant
Placebo	24	

*This includes only trials with at least 20 evaluable patients per treatment arm.
†No chemotherapy: palliative treatment with radiation, corticosteroids, and other hormones or analgesics only.
§Iversen and Rasmussen, 1995.
CA, Cyclophosphamide + doxorubicin (Adriamycin); CAF, cyclophosphamide + doxorubicin (Adriamycin) + 5-fluorouracil.
Modified from Eisenberger MA, Simon R, O'Dwyer P, et al: J Clin Oncol 1985; 3:827–841; and Eisenberger MA: NCI Monogr 1988; 7:151–163.

dural cord compression is particularly high. **Early diagnosis and treatment of epidural metastasis are critical in preserving ambulation and bowel and bladder function and aid in the management of back pain** (Rodichok et al, 1981, 1986; Grossman and Lossignol, 1990). Epidural cord compressions arising from vertebral bodies account for the vast majority of all spinal cord compressions, whereas only less than 10% result from tumors involving the paravertebral region. The vast majority of patients have positive bone scans and abnormal x-ray studies at the time of diagnosis; however, an abnormal neurologic examination may be the only finding in patients who have epidural metastasis from a paravertebral region (Wright, 1963).

The diagnosis of epidural cord compression is accomplished by clinical and radiologic evaluation. **All patients with persistent back pain and known skeletal involve-**ment on bone scans with or without abnormal neurologic findings are at high risk for epidural involvement of tumor and should be evaluated radiologically.** Spinal magnetic resonance imaging is a noninvasive technique routinely used to exclude the possibility of significant epidural disease, and it has almost entirely replaced other methodology such as computed tomography myelography and conventional myelography. Recognition of the risks and complications of epidural metastasis as well as widespread emphasis on magnetic resonance imaging is essential for early diagnosis and effective treatment of this complication; however, a high index of suspicion is always required to achieve the optimum outcome. The most common symptom is radicular back pain, sensory levels and motor weakness on neurologic examination, and bladder and bowel dysfunction in advanced cases. In addition to confirming a clinical diagnosis, magnetic resonance imaging also provides important diagnostic information about localization, extent, and delineation of disease for radiation planning. About 20% of patients with epidural cancer have multiple tumor deposits (Grossman and Lossignol, 1990). The use of gadolinium may enhance the ability to image the meninges, especially when direct meningeal extension is suspected in addition to evaluating for intramedullary disease. **The two most important prognostic indicators for outcome are the presence and severity of abnormal neurologic findings and radiation sensitivity of the tumor** (Grossman and Lossignol, 1990). **The first therapeutic intervention should include the administration of high doses of intravenous glucocorticoids.** Dexamethasone at doses ranging from 16 to 100 mg daily is most commonly employed. Although most frequently patients are given an intravenous loading dose of 10 mg of dexamethasone followed by 4 mg every 6 hours, the optimal dose of treatment remains relatively undefined. On improvement of symptoms, which can be accomplished promptly with steroids, the treatment dose may be tapered over a 2- to 3-week period (Greenberg et al, 1980).

Radiation therapy is often the main modality of treatment except when patients present with evidence of progression of signs and symptoms during radiotherapy, develop or present with unstable pathologic fractures, or have recurrence after radiotherapy, at which point surgery is recommended. Chemotherapy is rarely used to treat epidural cord compressions. In view of the limited relative value of chemotherapy in this disease and the potential for toxicity, this modality should not be employed as the primary treatment of this complication at this time.

FUTURE DIRECTIONS WITH CHEMOTHERAPY

Several new classes of compounds, designed to target various important steps in tumor biology, are now being developed. These newer compounds, some of which have unique mechanisms of action, are undoubtedly the forefront of new drug development. It is possible that a combination of strategies, aiming at different targets in the process of development of neoplasia, may indeed offer optimal chances for more meaningful clinical benefits in this disease.

Among some of the most promising anticancer compounds are those designed to target topoisomerase I inhibi-

Table 90–8. COMMON PAIN SYNDROMES IN METASTATIC HORMONE-REFRACTORY PROSTATE CANCER*

Pain Syndrome	Initial Management	Other Therapeutic Alternatives
Focal bone pain	Pharmacologic pain management Localized radiotherapy (special attention to weight-bearing areas, lytic metastasis, and extremities	Surgical stabilization of pathologic fractures or extensive bone erosions Epidural metastasis and cord compression should be evaluated in patients with focal back pain Radiopharmaceuticals should be considered if local radiation fails
Diffuse bone pain	Pharmacologic pain management "Multispot" or wide field radiotherapy Radiopharmaceuticals	Corticosteroids Biphosphonates Calcitonin Chemotherapy Pharmacologic pain management
Epidural metastasis and cord compression	High-dose corticosteroids Radiotherapy Surgical decompression and stabilization should be indicated in high-grade epidural blocks, extensive bone involvement, or recurrence postradiation	
Plexopathies—caused by direct tumor extension or prior therapy (rare)	Pharmacologic pain management Radiation therapy (if not previously employed) Neurolytic procedures (nerve blocks)	Tricyclics (amitriptyline) Anticonvulsants
Miscellaneous neurogenic causes: Postherpetic neuralgia, peripheral neuropathies	Careful neurologic evaluation Pharmacologic pain management Discontinuation of neurotoxic drug(s): taxol, vinca alkaloids, platinum compounds, suramin	Tricyclics (amitriptyline) Anticonvulsants
Other uncommon pain syndromes: extensive skull metastasis with cranial nerve involvement; extensive painful liver metastasis or pelvic masses	Radiotherapy Pharmacologic pain management Corticosteroids (cranial nerves involvement)	Intrathecal chemotherapy may ameliorate symptoms of meningeal involvement; regional infusions may be considered

*Recommended reference U.S. DHHS, 1994.

tion (TOPO-I). TOPO-I is a ubiquitous nuclear enzyme involved in RNA transcription, DNA replication, and possibly DNA repair and genetic rearrangements (Vosberg, 1985). Although initial clinical trials with the prototypic TOPO-I inhibitor, camptothecin, resulted in significant toxicity and thus delayed for more than two decades further development of this compound, newer analogues to the parent drug have demonstrated reasonable tolerance and activity (Slichenmyer et al, 1993). Camptothecin represents one of the most active compounds against prostate cancer cell lines; its cytotoxic effect, however, is cell cycle dependent. In view of the relatively low growth fraction in prostate cancer, in vivo it is likely that optimal administration of TOPO-I inhibitors requires long-term drug exposure. Oral forms of campto-thecin analogues are being developed, and this clearly facilitates drug development of protracted schedules of administration.

Better understanding of the molecular mechanisms of cancer invasion and metastasis has also provided the opportunity for developing agents and strategies to treat human cancer. The expression of the metastatic phenotype has been shown to depend on a balance between positive and negative gene products. Metalloproteinases represent various enzymes that have been shown to operate prominently in the process of tumor invasion (Alvarez et al, 1990). Tissue inhibitors of metalloproteases, known as TIMPs, are currently being evaluated in prostate cancer at various stages. The toxicity of these compounds is likely to be low because appropriate biologic effects can be seen at lower, nontoxic doses (Brown, 1993). Furthermore, the availability of oral forms makes it especially suitable for long-term outpatient administration. It is likely that TIMPs will be especially targeted for earlier stages of the disease because their effects are primarily aimed at the delay of tumor progression (Brown, 1993).

Imbalanced calcium homeostasis and aberrant calcium regulation may play important roles in the malignant process. Carboxyamidotriazole (CAI) offers a novel approach to target at calcium-mediated signal transduction in the regulation of tumor growth and metastasis. Furthermore, it may also affect ras oncogene signal transduction. CAI has shown encouraging effects in preclinical models evaluating both primary and metastatic tumor growth (Feldman, 1992).

It has been established that solid tumors require capillary proliferation to maintain growth, suggesting that inhibition of tumor angiogenesis could be a reasonable therapeutic strategy (Weidner et al, 1991). The process of tumor angiogenesis may be inhibited by various mechanisms, and some compounds are actually in active stages of development, including TNP-470, which is an analogue of fumagillin, an antibiotic derived from the fungus *Aspergillus fumigatus* that exerts potent angiogenesis activity in various systems and inhibits tumor growth of various cell lines, including prostate carcinoma lines (Yamaoka et al, 1993). Various compounds have demonstrated significant angiogenesis inhibition and are in active process of development, including CM-101, which is a polysaccharide endotoxin (Hellerqvist et al, 1993), and tecogalan, a sulfated polysaccharide isolated from arthrobacter species AT-25 (Tulpule et al, 1995), among others.

Differentiation-inducing agents have demonstrated significant activity in various preclinical and clinical trials.

Among agents with demonstrable activity are the retinoids (Smith M et al, 1992), vitamin D derivatives (Colston et al, 1992), and butyrates (phenylbutyrate, phenylacetate, and tributyrin), which have shown a variety of biologic effects including induction of terminal differentiation (Prasad, 1980; Samid et al, 1992). Current data in phase I trials indicate that these compounds are likely to be associated with modest toxicity. Other promising and evolving strategies include the development of a gene-modified prostate cancer cell vaccine (genetherapy) that involves the transfer of known genes into the cancer and elicits a number of biologic responses (Sanda et al, 1994), combined systemic use of radiopharmaceuticals and radiosensitizing chemotherapy (Tu et al, 1995), and other growth factor antagonists similar to suramin in structure and biologic properties but possibly with less toxicity (Eisenberger et al, 1995b).

Finally, a resurgence in the interest in monoclonal antibodies as a therapeutic tool has taken place in view of the identification of what may be perceived as feasible targets that mimic human conditions (Trail et al, 1993). In view of the radiosensitivity of prostate cancer, these compounds are conjugated with various sources of systemic radiation and used for therapy (Bander, 1994). Furthermore, the widespread use of effective supportive measures may add to the relative benefit of established compounds by improving the therapeutic index. A more effective control of chemotherapy-induced emesis with the newer compounds with great affinity and specificity to 5-HT3 (sterotonin) receptors (Gralla, 1993); reduction in the incidence, degree, and especially duration of chemotherapy-induced myelosuppression with hematopoietic growth factors (Sieff, 1987), erythropoietin (Miller et al, 1990), and possibly platelet growth factors in development; evolving experience with new neuroprotective compounds; and appropriate management of other toxicities are among examples available for clinical use or in active stages of clinical development.

REFERENCES

Abell F, Wilkes J, Divers L, et al: Oral cyclophosphamide for hormone-refractory prostate cancer (Abtract 646). Proc Am Soc Clin Oncol 1995; 14:213.
Alvarez O, Carmichael D, DeClerck Y: Inhibition of collagenolytic activity and metastasis of tumor cells by a recombinant human tissue inhibitor of metalloproteinases. J Natl Cancer Inst 1990; 82:589–595.
Antman K, Skarin A, Mayer R; Microangiopathic anemia and cancer: Review. Medicine (Baltimore) 1979; 58:377–384.
Atkins J, Muss H, Case D: High dose 24 hour infusion of 5-fluorouracil in metastatic prostate cancer. Am J Clin Oncol 1991; 14:526–529.
Averbuch SD: New bisphosphonates in the treatment of bone metastases. Cancer 1993; 72(11suppl):3443–3452.
Bander N: Current status of monoclonal antibodies for imaging and therapy of prostate cancer. Semin Oncol 1994; 21:607–612.
Berges R, Furuya Y, Remington L, et al: Cell proliferation, DNA repair and p-53 are not required for programmed cell death of prostatic glandular cells induced by androgen ablation. Proc Natl Acad Sci USA 1993; 90:8910–8914.
Berges R, Vukanovic J, Epstein J, et al: Implications of cell kinetic changes during the progression of human prostatic cancer. Clin Cancer Res 1995; 1:473–480.
Berlin N: Anemia of cancer. Ann NY Acad Sci 1974; 230:209–211.
Brown P: Proteinase inhibition: A new approach to cancer therapy. Cancer Topics Nov/Dec 1993.
Byar D: Review of the Veterans Administration studies of cancer of the prostate and new results concerning treatment of stage I and II tumors. In Pavone-Malacuso M, Smith P, Edsmyr F, eds: Bladder Tumors and Other Topics in Urological Oncology. New York; Plenum-Press, 1980, pp 471–492.
Canobbio L, Guarneri D, Miglietta L, et al: Carboplatin in advanced hormone-refractory prostatic cancer patients. Eur J Cancer 1993; 29A:2094–2096.
Carter SK, Wasserman TH: The chemotherapy of urologic cancer. Cancer 1975; 36:729–747.
Cattoretti G, Becker M, Key G, et al: Monoclonal antibodies against recombinant parts of the Ki-67 antigen (MIBI) and (MIB3) detect proliferating cells in microwave processed formulation-fixed paraffin sections. J Pathol 1992; 168:357–363.
Coleman R, Robboy S, Minna J: Disseminated intravascular coagulation: A reappraisal. Ann Rev Med 1979; 30:359–374.
Colston K, Mackay A, James S: EB1089: A new vitamin D analogue that inhibits the growth of breast cancer cells in vivo and in vitro. Biochem Pharmacol 1992; 44:2273–2280.
Crawford E, Eisenberger M, McLeod D, et al: A controlled randomized trial of leuprolide with and without flutamide in prostatic cancer. N Engl J Med 1989; 321:419–424.
Denis L, Whetan P, Carneiro DE, et al: Goserelin acetate and flutamide versus bilateral orchiectomy: A phase III EORTC study (30853). Urology 1993; 42:119–130.
diSant'Agnese P: Neuroendocrine differentiation in prostatic carcinoma: Recent findings and new concepts. Cancer 1995; 75(suppl):1850–1859.
Eaton C: Growth factors, oncogenes and prostate cancer. Rev Endocr Rel Cancer 1982; 40:5–12.
Eisenberger MA: Chemotherapy for prostate carcinoma. NCI Monogr 1988; 7:151–163.
Eisenberger M, Crawford E, McLeod D, et al: The prognostic significance of prostate specific antigen in stage D2 prostate cancer: Interim evaluation of intergroup 0105 [Abstract 613]. Proc Am Soc Clin Oncol 1995a; 14:236.
Eisenberger MA, O'Dwyer PJ, Friedman MA: Gonadotropin hormone releasing analogues: A new therapeutic approach for prostate cancer. J Clin Oncol 1986; 4:414–419.
Eisenberger M, Reyno L, Sinibaldi V, et al: The experience with suramin in advanced prostate cancer. Cancer 1995b; 75(suppl):1927–1934.
Eisenberger MA, Simon R, O'Dwyer P, et al: A reevaluation of non-hormonal cytotoxic chemotherapy in the treatment of prostate cancer. J Clin Oncol 1985; 3:827–841.
Felder C: The activity of oral CAI in tumor xenografts. J Pharmacol Exp Ther 1992; 257:967–971.
Foley K: Changing concepts of tolerance to opioids: What the cancer patient has taught us. In Chapman CR, Foley KM, eds: Current and Emerging Issues in Cancer Pain: Research and Practice. New York, Raven Press, 1993; pp 331–350.
Fowler J Jr, Whitmore W Jr: The response of metastatic adenocarcinoma of the prostate to exogenous testosterone. J Urol 1981; 126:372–375.
Fowler J Jr, Whitmore W Jr: Consideration for the use of testosterone with systemic chemotherapy in prostate cancer. Cancer 1982; 49:1373–1377.
Frank S, Amsterdam A, Kelly W, et al: Platinum-based chemotherapy for patients with poorly differentiated hormone-refractory prostate cancer: Response and pathologic considerations (Abstract 601). Proc Am Soc Clin Oncol 1995; 14:232.
Galasko C: Mechanisms of bone destruction in the development of skeletal metastasis. Nature 1986; 263:507–508.
Goldenberg S, Bruchovsky N, Gleave M, Sullivan L: Intermittent androgen suppression in the treatment of prostate cancer (Abstract 880). Proc Am Urol Assoc 1995; 153:448.
Gralla R: Antiemetic therapy. In DeVita V, Hellman S, Rosenberg S, eds:. Principles and Practice of Oncology, 4th ed. Philadelphia, J. B. Lippincott, 1993, pp 2338–2348.
Greenberg H, Kim J, Posner J: Epidural spinal cord compression from metastatic tumor: Results with a new protocol. Ann Neurol 1980; 8:361–366.
Grossman S, Lossignol D: Diagnosis and treatment of epidural metastasis. Oncology 1990; 4:47–54.
Hartley-Asp B, Kruse E: Nuclear protein matrix as a target for estramustine-induced cell death. Prostate 1986; 9:387–395.
Hellerqvist C, Thurman G, Page D, et al: Antitumor effects of GBS toxin: A polysaccharide exotoxin from group B β-hemolytic streptococcus. J Cancer Res Clin Oncol 1993; 120:63–70.
Huan S, Natale R, Stewart D, et al: A phase II multicenter trial of losoxantrone (DUP-941) in patients with metastatic hormone-refractory prostate cancer (Abstract 626). Proc Am Soc Clin Oncol 1995; 14:238.

Hudes G, Greenberg R, Krigel R: Phase-II study of estramustine and vinblastine, two microtubule inhibitors, in hormone-refractory prostate cancer. J Clin Oncol 1992; 10:1754–1761.

Hudes G, Nathan F, Chapman A, et al: Combined antimicrotubule therapy of metastatic prostate cancer with 96-hr paclitaxel and estramustine: Activity in hormone-refractory disease (Abstract). Proc Am Soc Clin Oncol 1995; 14:236.

Hussain M, Pienta K, Redman B, et al: Oral etoposide in the treatment of hormone refractory prostate cancer. Cancer 1994a; 74:100–103.

Hussain M, Wolf M, Marshall E, et al: Effects of continued androgen deprivation therapy and other prognostic factors on response and survival in phase-II chemotherapy trials for hormone-refractory prostate cancer: A Southwest Oncology Group report. J Clin Oncol 1994b; 12:1868–1875.

Isaacs JT, Lundmo PI, Berges R, et al: Androgen regulation of programmed cell death of normal and malignant prostatic cells. J Androl 1992; 13:457–464.

Iversen P, Rasmussen F: Estramustine phosphate versus placebo in hormone-refractory prostate cancer: Danish prostate cancer group study 9002 (Abstract 41). Proc Am Urol Assoc 1995; 153:239A.

Jacobs S, Pikna D, Lawson R: Prostatic osteoblastic factor. Invest Urol 1979; 17:195–198.

Kelly WK, Scher HI, Mazumdar M, et al: Prostate-specific antigen as a measure of disease outcome in metastatic hormone-refractory prostate cancer. J Clin Oncol 1993; 11:607–615.

Kuss R, Khoury S, Richard F, et al: Estramustine phosphate in the treatment of advanced prostatic cancer. Br J Urol 1980; 52:29–33.

Kuzel T, Tallman M, Shevrin D, et al: A phase-II of continuous infusion 5-flourouracil in advanced hormone refractory prostate cancer. Cancer 1993; 72:1965–1968.

Larocca RV, Danesi R, Cooper MR, Myers C: Effect of suramin on human prostate cancer cells in vitro. J Urol 1991; 145:393–398.

Logothetis C, Joosein N, Hsieh J: The clinical and biological study of androgen independent prostate cancer. Semin Oncol 1994; 21:620–629.

Logothetis CJ, Samuels ML, von Echenback AC: Doxorubicin, mitomycin-C, and 5-fluorouracil (DMF) in the treatment of metastatic hormone-refractory adenocarcinoma of the prostate, with a note on the staging of metastatic prostate cancer. J Clin Oncol 1983; 1:368–378.

Manni A, Bartholomew M, Chaplain R: Androgen priming and chemotherapy in advanced prostate cancer: Evaluation of determinants of clinical outcome. J Clin Oncol 1988; 6:1456–1466.

McLeod D: Hormonal therapy in the treatment of carcinoma of the prostate. Cancer 1995; 75:1914–1919.

Merrin C: Treatment of genitourinary tumors with cis-dichlorodiammineplatinum (II): Experience in 250 patients. Cancer Treat Rep 1979; 63:1579–1589.

Miller CB, Jones RJ, Piantadosi S: Decreased erythropoietin response in patients with the anemia of cancer. N Engl J Med 1990; 322:1689–1992.

Mittleman A, Shukla SK, Murphy GP: Extended therapy of stage D carcinoma of the prostate with oral estramustine phosphate. J Urol 1976; 115:403–412.

Moore M, Osoba D, Murphy K, et al: Use of palliative endpoints to evaluate the effects of mitoxantrone and low-dose prednisone in patients with hormonally resistant prostate cancer. J Clin Oncol 1994; 12:689–694.

Moore M, Troner M, DeSimone P, et al: Phase II evaluation of weekly cisplatin in metastatic hormone-resistant prostate cancer: A Southeastern Cancer Study Group trial. Cancer Treat Rep 1986; 70:541–542.

Myers C, Cooper M, Stein C, LaRocca R: Suramin: A novel growth factor antagonist with activity in hormone refractory prostate cancer. J Clin Oncol 1992; 10:881–889.

O'Bryan R, Baker L, Gottlieb J, et al: Dose-response evaluation of adriamycin in human neoplasia. Cancer 1977; 39:1940–1948.

O'Bryan R, Luce J, Talley RW, et al: Phase II evaluation of adriamycin in human neoplasia. Cancer 1973; 32:1–8.

Osborne C, Drelichman A, VonHotoll D: Mitoxantrone: Modest activity in a phase-II trial in advanced prostate cancer. Cancer Treat Rep 1983; 67:1133–1135.

Petrylak D, Scher H, Zhaohai L, et al: Prognostic factors for survival of patients with bidimensionally measurable metastatic hormone refractory prostatic cancer treated with single agent chemotherapy. Cancer 1992; 70:2870–2878.

Pienta K, Redman B, Hussain M: Phase-II study of estramustine and oral etoposide in hormone-refractory adenocarcinoma of the prostate. J Clin Oncol 1994; 12:2005–2012.

Porter A, Davis L: Systemic radionuclide therapy of bone metastases with strontium-89. Oncology 1994; Feb:173–177.

Porter A, McEwan A, Powe J, et al: Results of a randomized phase-III trial to evaluate the efficacy of strontium-89 adjuvant to local field external beam irradiation in the management of endocrine resistant prostate cancer. Int J Radiat Oncol Biol Phys 1993; 25:805–813.

Prasad K: Butyrates as differentiating agents. Life Sci 1980; 27:1351–1358.

Qazi R, Khandekar J: Phase II study of cisplatin for metastatic prostatic carcinoma: An Eastern Cooperative Oncology Group study. Am J Clin Oncol 1983; 6:203–205.

Raghavan D, Bishop J, Woods J: Mitoxantrone, a non-toxic, moderately active agent for hormone resistant prostate cancer (Abstract 395). Proc Am Soc Clin Oncol 1986; 5:102.

Rearden T, Small E, Valone F, et al: Phase II study of mitoxantrone for hormone refractory prostate cancer (Abstract 688). Proc Am Soc Clin Oncol 1995; 14: 218.

Reddi A, Cunningham N: Bone induction by osteogenic and bone morphogenic proteins. Biomaterials 1990; 11:33–34.

Robinson R, Blake G, Preston D, et al: Strontium-89: Treatment results and kinetics in patients with painful metastatic prostate and breast cancer in bone. Radiographics 1989; 9:271–281.

Rodichok L, Harper G, Ruckdeschel J: Early diagnosis of spinal epidural metastasis. Am J Med 1981; 70:1187–1188.

Rodichok L, Ruckdeschel J, Harper J: Early detection and treatment of spinal epidural metastasis: The role of myelography. Ann Neurol 1986; 20:696–702.

Rossof A, Talley R, Stephens R, et al: Phase-II evaluation of cis-dichlorodiammineplatinum (II) in advanced malignancies of the genitourinary and gynecologic organs: A Southwest Oncology Group study. Cancer Treat Rep 1979; 63:1557–1564.

Roth B, Yeap B, Wilding G, et al: Taxol (NSC 125973) in advanced hormone-refractory prostate cancer: An ECOG phase-II trial (Abstract 598). Proc Am Soc Clin Oncol 1992; 11:196.

Sack GH, Levin J, Bell WR: Trousseau's syndrome and other manifestations in chronic disseminated coagulopathy in patients with cancer. Medicine (Baltimore) 1977; 56:1–37.

Samid D, Shack S, Sherman L: Phenylacetate: A novel non toxic inducer of tumor cell differentiation. Cancer Res 1992; 52:1988–1992.

Sanda M, Ayxagari S, Jaffee E, et al: Demonstration of a rational strategy for human prostate cancer gene therapy. J Urol 1994; 151:622–628.

Sartor O, Myers C: The influence of aminoglutethimide and corticosteroids on the therapeutic benefits of flutamide withdrawal. Proc Am Soc Clin Oncol 1995; 14:245.

Scher H, Kelly KW: Flutamide withdrawal syndrome: Its impact on clinical trials in hormone refractory prostate cancer. J Clin Oncol 1993; 11:1566–1572.

Scher H, Steineck G, Kelly W: Hormone-refractory (D₃) prostate cancer: Refining the concept. Urology 1995; 46:142–148.

Scher H, Yagoda A, Watson R, et al: Phase II trial of doxorubicin in bidimensionally measurable prostatic adenocarcinoma. J Urol 1984; 13:1099–1102.

Schmidt JD, Gibbons RP, Johnson DE, Murphy GP: Chemotherapy of advanced prostate cancer: Evaluation of response parameters. Urology 1976; 7:607–610.

Seidman AD, Scher HI, Petrylak D, et al: Estramustine and vinblastine: Use of prostatic specific antigen as a clinical trial endpoint for hormone refractory prostatic cancer. J Urol 1992; 147:931–934.

Sella A, Kilbourn R, Amato R, et al: Phase-II study of ketoconazole combined with weekly doxorubicin in patients with androgen-independent prostate cancer. J Clin Oncol 1994; 4:683–688.

Sieff C: Hematopoietic growth-factors. J Clin Invest 1987; 79:1549–1557.

Silberstein E: The treatment of painful osseous metastasis with phosphorus-32-labeled phosphates. Semin Oncol 1993; 20(suppl 2):10–21.

Silberstein E, Williams C: Strontium-89 therapy for the pain of osseous metastasis. J Nucl Med 1985; 26:345–348.

Slack N, Mittleman A, Brady MF, Murphy GP: The importance of the stable category for chemotherapy treated patients with advanced and relapsed prostate cancer. Cancer 1980; 46:2393–2402.

Slichenmyer W, Rowinsky E, Donehower R, et al: The current status of camptothecin analogues as antitumor agents. J Natl Cancer Inst 1993; 85:271–291.

Small E, Srinivas S: The antiandrogen withdrawal syndrome: Experience in a large cohort of unselected advanced prostate cancer patients (Abstract 878). Proc Am Urol Assoc 1995; 153:448.

Small E, Srinivas S, Madhavan S, Rearden T: Use of doxorubicin and dose-escalated cyclophosphamide with granulocyte colony stimulating factor in the treatment of hormone refractory prostate cancer (Abstract 648). Proc Am Soc Clin Oncol 1995; 14:243.

Smith D, Vogelzang N, Goldberg H, et al: High-dose cyclophosphamide with granulocyte-macrophage colony stimulating factor in hormone-refractory prostate cancer (Abstract 666). Proc Am Soc Clin Oncol 1992; 11:213.

Smith E, Hampel N, Ruff R, et al: Spinal cord compression secondary to prostate cancer: Treatment and prognosis. J Urol 1993; 149:330–333.

Smith M, Parkinson D, Cheson B, Friedman M: Retinoids in cancer therapy. J Clin Oncol 1992; 10:839–864.

Sorensen PS, Borgensen SE, Rohde K: Metastatic epidural spinal cord compression: Results of treatment and survival. Cancer 1990; 65:1502–1510.

Sridhara R, Eisenberger M, Sinibaldi V, et al: Evaluation of prostate specific antigen as a surrogate marker for response of hormone refractory prostate cancer to suramin therapy. J Clin Oncol 1995; 13:2687–2692.

Steiner MS, Seckin B, Anthony CT, Murphy B: Can prostate specific antigen be used as a valid endpoint for chemotherapy efficacy in advanced prostate cancer (Abstract 1245). Proc AACR 1995; 36:209.

Storlie J, Buckner J, Wiseman G, et al: Prostate specific antigen levels and clinical response to low dose dexamethasone for hormone-refractory metastatic prostate carcinoma. Cancer 1995; 76:96–100.

Story MT: Polypeptide modulators of prostatic growth and development. In Isaacs JT, ed: Prostate Cancer: Cell and Molecular Mechanisms in Diagnosis and Treatment. New York, Cold Spring Harbor Laboratory Press, 1991, pp. 123–146.

Tannock I, Gospodarowicz M, Meakin W, et al: Treatment of metastatic prostate cancer with low-dose prednisone: Evaluation of pain and quality of life as pragmatic indices of response. J Clin Oncol 1989; 7:790–797.

Tannock I, Osoba D, Ernst S, et al: Chemotherapy with mitoxantrone palliates patients with hormone-resistant prostate cancer: Results of a Canadian randomized trial (Abstract 353). Proc Am Soc Clin Oncol 1995; 14:245.

Taplin ME, Bubley GJ, Shuster TD, et al: Mutation of the androgen-receptor gene in metastatic androgen-independent prostate cancer. N Engl J Med 1995; 332:1393–1398.

Taylor CD, Elson P, Trump DL: Importance of continued testicular suppression in hormone-refractory prostate cancer. J Clin Oncol 1993; 11:2167–2172.

The Leuprolide Study Group: Leuprolide versus diethylstilbestrol for metastatic prostate cancer. N Engl J Med 1984; 311:1281–1289.

Thompson T, Kadmon D, Timme T, et al: Experimental oncogene induced prostate cancer. In Isaacs JT, ed: Prostate Cancer: Cell and Molecular Mechanisms in Diagnosis and Treatment. New York, Cold Spring Harbor Laboratory Press, 1991; pp 55–71.

Torti F, Aston D, Lum BL, et al: Weekly doxorubicin in endocrine refractory carcinoma of the prostate. J Clin Oncol 1983; 1:477–482.

Trail P, Willner D, Lash S: Cure of xenographed human carcinomas by Br-96-doxorubicin immunoconjugates. Science 1993; 261:212–215.

Tu S, Jones D, Finn L: Strontium-89 combined with adriamycin in the treatment of patients with androgen independent prostate carcinoma (Abstract 608). Proc Am Soc Clin Oncol 1995; 14:233.

Tulpule A, Espina B, Higashi L, et al: A phase-I study of tecogalan, a novel angiogenesis inhibitor in the treatment of AIDS-related Kaposi's sarcoma and solid tumors. Proceedings New Cancer Strategies: Angiogenesis Inhibitors, Washington, DC, 1995.

Turkes A, Peeling W, Griffith H: Treatment of patients with advanced cancer of the prostate: Phase III trial, zoladex against castration: A study of the British prostate group. J Steroid Biochem 1987; 27:543–549.

U.S. Department of Health and Human Services (U.S. DHHS): Management of cancer pain. Clinical Practice CE Guideline 1994; 9:23–38.

Veronesi A, Zattoni F, Frustacci S, et al: Estramustine phosphate (Estracyt) treatment of T3-T4 prostatic carcinoma. Prostate 1982; 3:159–164.

Von Roemeling R, Fisher HAG, Horton J: Daily oral cyclophosphamide is effective in hormone-refractory prostate cancer: A phase-I/II pilot study (Abstract 665). Proc Am Soc Clin Oncol 1992; 11:213.

Vosberg H: DNA topoisomerase: Enzymes that control DNA conformation. Curr Top Microbiol Immunol 1985; 114:91–102.

Waterbury L: Hematologic problems. In Abeloff MD, ed: Complications of Cancer: Diagnosis and Management. Baltimore, Johns Hopkins Press, 1979, pp 121–145.

Weidner N, Carroll PR, Faux J, et al: Tumor angiogenesis correlates with metastasis in invasive prostate cancer. Am J Pathol 1993; 143:401–409.

Weidner N, Sample J, Welch W, Folkman J: Tumor angiogenesis and metastasis correlation in invasive breast cancer. N Engl J Med 1991; 324:1–8.

Wilding G: Response of prostate cancer cells to peptide growth factors: Transforming growth factor–β. In Isaacs JT, ed: Prostate Cancer: Cell and Molecular Mechanisms in Diagnosis and Treatment. New York, Cold Spring Harbor Laboratory Press, 1991, pp 123–146.

Williams W: Thrombocytosis. In Williams W, Beutler E, Erslew A, Rundles R, eds: Hematology, 2nd ed. New York: McGraw-Hill, 1977, pp 1364–1367.

Wright R: Malignant tumors in the spinal extradural space: Results of surgical treatment. Ann Surg 1963; 157:227–231.

Yagoda A, Petrylak D: Cytotoxic chemotherapy for advanced hormone-resistant prostate cancer. Cancer (suppl) 1993; 71:1098–1109.

Yagoda A, Smith JA, Soloway M: Phase II study of estramustine phosphate in advanced hormone-refractory prostate cancer with increasing prostate specific antigen. J Urol 1991; 145:384A.

Yagoda A, Watson RC, Natale RB, et al: A critical analysis of response criteria in patients with prostatic cancer treated with cis-diamminedichloride platinum II. Cancer 1979; 44:1553–1562.

Yagoda A: Response in prostate cancer: An enigma. Semin Urol 1984; 1:311–319.

Yamaoka M, Yamamoto T, Ikeyama S: Angiogenesis inhibitor TNP-470 inhibits the tumor growth of hormone-independent breast and prostate cancer cell lines. Cancer Res 1993; 53:5233–5236.

XII
URINARY
LITHIASIS

91
URINARY LITHIASIS: ETIOLOGY, DIAGNOSIS, AND MEDICAL MANAGEMENT

Mani Menon, M.D.
Bhalchondra G. Parulkar, M.D.
George W. Drach, M.D.

Urinary stones have afflicted humankind since antiquity, with the earliest recorded example being bladder and kidney stones detected in Egyptian mummies dated to 4800 B.C. (Table 91–1). The specialty of urologic surgery was recognized even by Hippocrates, who wrote, in his famous oath for the physician, "I will not cut, even for the stone, but leave such procedures to the practitioners of the craft" (Clendening, 1942). The prevalence of urinary tract stone disease is estimated to be 2% to 3%, and the likelihood that a white man will develop stone disease by age 70 is about 1 in 8. The recurrence rate without treatment for calcium oxalate renal stones is about 10% at 1 year, 35% at 5 years, and 50% at 10 years (Uribarri et al, 1989).

Until the 1980s, urinary stones were a major health problem, with a significant proportion of patients requiring extensive surgical procedures and a sizable minority losing their kidney. One study showed that about 20% of patients with recurrent stone disease who underwent surgery for obstruction and infection went on to develop mild renal insufficiency (Menon and Koul, 1992). The advent of extracorporeal techniques for stone destruction and refinements in endoscopic surgery, however, have greatly decreased the morbidity associated with stone surgery, and it is possible that the disorder is changing from a major health problem to a major inconvenience. These procedures treat stones but do not prevent them, and it is too early to see if the treatment is associated with long-term morbidity.

The management of urinary lithiasis requires cooperation between the urologist and his or her medical colleagues. Critical to the selection of proper therapy is knowledge of both medical and surgical methods of treating urinary stone disease. Urologists must, therefore, understand all aspects of the etiology, diagnosis, and medical and surgical treatment of urinary lithiasis. This chapter expands on the excellent chapters by Drach, who authored this topic in the previous three editions of *Campbell's Urology*, and adds information gleaned over the last 5 years.

EPIDEMIOLOGIC ASPECTS

Intrinsic Factors

Heredity

Numerous workers have noted that urinary calculi are relatively rare in Native Americans, blacks of Africa and America, and native-born Israelis. Conversely, the incidence of stone disease is highest in some of the colder temperate areas of the world populated primarily by Asians and whites. Although the incidence of bladder stones seems to be related primarily to dietary habits and malnutrition in underdeveloped and primitive countries, dietary improvement over the years has probably resulted only in a change of the site of occurrence of urinary calculi from bladder to kidney (Sutor, 1972).

Genetic studies performed by Resnick and co-workers (1968) and by McGeown (1960) have concluded that urolithiasis is associated with a polygenic defect and partial penetrance. White (1969), however, cautions against accepting familial or hereditary theories of stone formation too readily. White noted that urinary calcium excretion was significantly higher in spouses of patients who were stone formers than in the control persons of the same sex in households of persons who did not form stones. Hence, household diet as well as familial tendencies must be considered in theories of etiology of urinary lithiasis.

Several disorders that cause renal stones are hereditary. Familial renal tubular acidosis (RTA) is associated with nephrolithiasis and nephrocalcinosis in almost 70% of patients (Dretler et al, 1969). Cystinuria is a homozygous recessive disease. Similarly, hereditary xanthinuria and dehydroxyadeninuria are disorders that cause renal stones.

Age and Sex

The peak incidence of urinary calculi occurs in the twenties to forties (Fetter and Zimskind, 1961; Blacklock, 1969; Pak, 1987a,b). The majority of patients, however, report onset of disease in their teens. About three males are afflicted for every female. A relatively greater proportion of upper urinary tract calculus disease is caused by chronic urinary tract infections or defects, such as cystinuria or hyperparathyroidism, in women than in men (Baker et al, 1993). Several investigators have commented on the apparently equal tendency toward urinary lithiasis in males and females during childhood (Prince and Scardino, 1960; Malek and Kelalis, 1975). This observation, coupled with reports that increased serum testosterone levels resulted in increased endogenous oxalate production by the liver (Liao and Richardson, 1972), led Finlayson (1974) to postulate that lower serum testosterone levels may contribute to some of the protection women and children have against oxalate stone disease. Yet, Van Aswegen and associates found that the urinary testosterone concentration of patients who were stone formers was lower than that of controls (Van Aswegen et al, 1989). Welshman and McGeown (1975) have demonstrated increased urinary citrate concentrations in the urine of women. They postulate that this finding may aid in protecting females from calcium urolithiasis.

Extrinsic Factors

Geography

The prevalence of urinary calculi is higher in those who live in mountainous, desert, and tropical areas. Finlayson (1974) reviewed several worldwide geographic surveys and stated that the United States is relatively high in the incidence of urinary calculus disease for its population. Other high-incidence areas are the British Isles, Scandinavian countries, Mediterranean countries, northern India and Pakistan, northern Australia, Central Europe, portions of the Malayan peninsula, and China. Low-incidence areas include Central and South America, most of Africa, and those areas of Australia populated by aborigines. Lonsdale (1968a,b) and Sutor and Wooley (1970, 1971, 1974a; Sutor et al, 1974) have noted that stones from Great Britain, Scotland, and Sudan are composed primarily of mixed calcium oxalate and calcium phosphate. Upper urinary tract calculi composed of uric acid tend to be more common in Israel (Herbstein et al, 1974). Table 91–2 shows the crystalline constituents and mineralogic names of common urinary calculi.

Table 91–1. MILESTONES IN URINARY STONE DISEASE

4800 B.C.	First urinary stones discovered at El Amrah, Egypt
12th century B.C.	Susruta performs perineal lithotomy
4th century B.C.	Hippocrates notes the presence of renal stones together with a renal abscess, describes gout, writes Hippocratic oath: "I will not cut, even for the stone." (Obviously, Hippocrates was not a urologist)
1668	Duclos isolates oxalate from sorrel
1683	Sydenham characterizes gout
17th and 18th centuries	Itinerant lithotomists including Frere Jacques
1776	Scheele isolates uric acid from kidney stones
1797	Wollaston identifies calcium oxalate in kidney stones
1810	Wollaston describes "cystic oxide" bladder stones
1824	Stromeyer notes hexagonal crystals in the urine
1833	Berzelius coins the word cystine
1840	Brooke identifies calcium oxalate monohydrate in rocks
1863	Garrod suggests that serum uric acid is increased in gouty patients
1871	Simon performs nephrectomy for stone disease
1879	Heinecke performs pyelolithotomy
1908	Garrod calls cystinuria an inborn error of metabolism. He describes other inborn errors of metabolism. He is right about the rest, but wrong about cystinuria
1912	Hugh Hampton Young examines a massively dilated ureter in a child using a cystoscope
1926	Sumner isolates the first enzyme, urease. He later wins the Nobel Prize for this
1936	Bannister and Hey identify calcium oxalate dihydrate at the bottom of the Weddell Sea
1939	Flocks describes the association between hypercalciuria and kidney stones
1940	Albright describes citrate therapy of renal tubular acidosis
1941	Kissin and Locks observe decreased urinary citrate in kidney stone formers
1941	Rupel and Brown remove a kidney stone through an established nephrostomy tract
1951	Dent and Rose propose that cystinuria is a transport defect
1953	Albright coins the term *idiopathic hypercalciuria*
1957	Watts describes primary hyperoxaluria
1957	Yendt uses thiazides for the treatment of hypercalciuria
1962	McGovern and Walzak perform flexible ureteroscopy for stone
1967	Lloyd Smith and Hibbard Williams identify enzymatic defect in primary hyperoxaluria type I; 28 years later, they are proved wrong
1968	Vernon Smith and Boyce perform anatrophic nephrolithotomy
1968	Williams and Smith describe primary hyperoxaluria type II
1968	Prien and Gutman report that patients with gout form calcium oxalate kidney stones also
1969	Dornier GMBH starts studies on the effects of shock waves on tissues
1969	Vernon Smith uses allopurinol for recurrent calcium oxalate stones
1971	Robertson and Nordin start studies on the role of oxalate in kidney stone formation
1972	Dornier and the Urology Department at the University of Munich start work on shock waves and kidney stones
1972	Nordin describes *absorptive hypercalciuria*
1973	Griffith and Musher show that urease is the principal cause of infection stones and that acetohydroxyamic acid inhibits struvite calculation
1973	Coe describes renal leak hypercalciuria
1973	Coe and Raisen describe hyperuricosuric calcium oxalate nephrolithiasis
1973	Ettinger and Kolb report randomized trial on medical therapy of nephrolithiasis: acid phosphates do not work
1974	Pak classifies the hypercalciurias; suggests that absorptive hypercalciuria is the most common
1976	Fernstrom and Johansson describe planned percutaneous nephrolithotomy
1978	Lynwood Smith describes enteric hyperoxaluria
1978	Lyon uses pediatric cystoscope to examine the lower ureter in an adult
1979	Coe describes familial hypercalciuria
1979	Arthur Smith et al coin the term *endourology*
1980	Chaussy first uses ESWL for the treatment of patient with renal stone
1980	Perez-Castro examines renal pelvis through ureteroscope
1981	Alken et al describe percutaneous ultrasonic kidney stone fragmentation
1981	Das reports ureteroscopic stone manipulation
1982	Marberger et al develop nephroscope designed for percutaneous use
1983	Menon and Pak simultaneously show that hypocitraturia is a common abnormality in kidney stone patients
1984	Williams publishes randomized trial of acetohydroxyamic acid in struvite stones
1984	Baggio reports that oxalate transport is increased in the red blood cells of patients with calcium oxalate stones, raising the possibility that calcium oxalate nephrolithiasis is a cellular disease
1984	FDA approves ESWL for the treatment of urinary stones
1985	FDA approves potassium citrate for the treatment of nephrolithiasis, based primarily on Pak's studies
1986	Ettinger publishes randomized trial of allopurinol in calcium oxalate stone disease—allopurinol works
1986	Danpure and Jennings identify AGT deficiency as the cause of primary hyperoxaluria type I
1990	Danpure sequences human AGT gene

ESWL, Extracorporeal shock wave lithotripsy; FDA, Food and Drug Administration; AGT, alanine-glyoxylate aminotransferase.

Table 91–2. CRYSTALLINE CONSTITUENTS OF URINARY CALCULI

Substance	Mineralogic Name	Formula
Oxalate		
Calcium oxalate monohydrate	Whewellite	$CaC_2O_4 \cdot H_2O$
Calcium oxalate dihydrate	Weddellite	$CaC_2O_4 \cdot 2H_2O$
Phosphates		
Hydroxyapatite	Hydroxyapatite	$Ca_{10}(PO_4)_6(OH)_2$
Carbonate-apatite	Carbonate-apatite	$Ca_{10}(PO_4, CO_3, OH)_6(OH)_2$
Calcium hydrogen phosphate dihydrate	Brushite	$CaHPO_4 \cdot 2H_2O$
Tricalcium phosphate	Whitlockite	$Ca_3(PO_4)_2$
Octacalcium phosphate	—	$Ca_4H(PO_4)_3 \cdot 2 \cdot 5H_2O$
Magnesium ammonium phosphate hexahydrate	Struvite	$MgNH_4PO_4 \cdot 6H_2O$
Magnesium hydrogen phosphate trihydrate	Newberyite	$MgHPO_4 \cdot 3H_2O$
Uric acids		
Anhydrous uric acid	—	$C_5H_4N_4O_3$
Uric acid dihydrate	—	$C_5H_4N_4O_3 \cdot 2H_2O$
Urates		
Ammonium acid urate	—	$C_5H_3N_4O_3NH_4$
Sodium acid urate monohydrate	—	$C_5H_3N_4O_3Na \cdot H_2O$

Boyce and co-workers (1956) and Sierakowski and associates (1978) performed an extensive study of the incidence of calculus disease in the United States. Mandel and Mandel (1989a,b) reviewed hospital discharge data for urinary tract stone disease in the Veteran patient population of the entire United States between 1983 and 1986. Southeastern United States showed an increased discharge rate but only for calcium oxalate stones (Mandel and Mandel, 1989a) (Fig. 91–1). The Eastern seaboard had a higher rate of uric acid lithiasis (Mandel and Mandel, 1989a). Mandel and Mandel (1989b) observed that the stone discharge rate had not changed significantly in the last three decades despite advances in urolithiasis research.

Geography influences the incidence of urinary calculi and the types of calculi that occur within a given area. The capability of individuals to transport intrinsic genetic tendencies of urinary stone formation from area to area, however, makes it likely that the major tendencies contributing to urinary lithiasis reside in the individual. Geography represents just one aspect of environmental factors, such as dietary habits, temperature, and humidity, superimposed on intrinsic factors that predispose to stone formation.

Climatic and Seasonal Factors

The effect of geography on the prevalence of stone disease may be indirect, through its effect on temperature. Several workers show a relationship between higher environmental temperature and higher seasonal incidence of urinary stone disease. Prince and associates found that the incidence of urinary calculi was higher during the summer months (Prince et al, 1956). Prince and Scardino (1960) followed this study with a prospective analysis of 922 occurrences of ureteral stones. Once again, the peak incidence occurred in July,

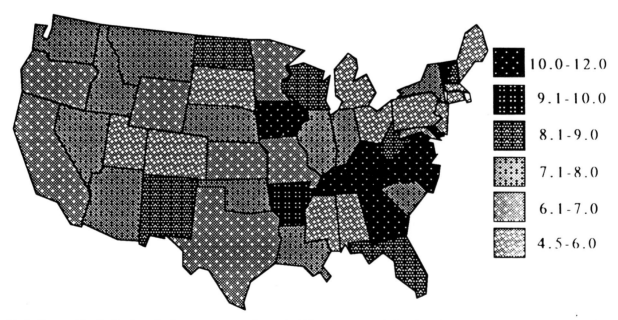

Figure 91–1. Geographic distribution of urinary tract stone disease in U.S. veteran population from 1983 to 1986. Data are expressed as urinary tract stone patients per 1000 hospital discharges. (From Mandel NS, Mandel GS: J Urol 1989; 142:1516.)

August, and September. The highest incidence of urinary calculi appears to occur 1 to 2 months following the achievement of the maximum mean annual temperature in the study area.

Bateson (1973) reported on the incidence of upper urinary tract calculi in the area surrounding Perth in Western Australia. The peak incidence of urinary calculi occurs in December through March. This finding coincides with the peak maximum summer temperatures in that geographic area. Baker and colleagues investigated the trends in renal stone formation in residents of South Australia between 1977 and 1991 (Baker et al, 1993). They observed no significant seasonal variation with calcium oxalate or calcium phosphate stones. The incidence of uric acid stones increased significantly during summer and autumn, and that of infectious stones decreased significantly during spring and summer.

High temperatures increase perspiration, which may result in concentrated urine. This promotes increased urinary crystallization. Hallson and Rose (1977) have shown increased crystalluria during summer months in patients who form stones. Patients with a tendency toward formation of uric acid or cystine calculi have an additional risk. Concentrated urine tends to be acidic, and acid urine holds much less uric acid or cystine in solution.

Parry and Lister (1975) present an alternative viewpoint. They suggest that increased exposure to sunlight causes increased production of 1,25-dihydroxyvitamin D_3 and increased urinary calcium excretion (see section on hypercalciuria). This may cause the higher incidence of urolithiasis during the summer months.

Water Intake

One of the prevailing assumptions in the literature on urolithiasis is that increased water intake and increased urinary output decrease the incidence of urinary calculi in those patients who are predisposed to the disease. Two factors involved in the relationship between water intake and urolithiasis are (1) the volume of water ingested as opposed to that lost by perspiration and respiration and (2) the mineral or trace element content of the water supply of the region.

In their survey of urolithiasis in the United States, Burkland and Rosenberg (1955) questioned urologists about their opinions of methods of preventing recurrence of urinary stone disease. "Forcing water" received the highest total number of positive responses, along with elimination of infection and elimination of urinary obstruction. This opinion is reaffirmed in reviews by Finlayson (1974) and Thomas (1975). Although urine dilution by increased water intake may increase ion activity coefficients and, hence, urinary crystallization, water diuresis reduces the average time of residence of free crystal particles in urine and dilutes the components of urine that may crystallize. Finlayson concluded that the dilutional effects of water diuresis outweigh the changes in ion activity and, therefore, do help to prevent stone formation.

Frank and de Vries first investigated the epidemiologic aspects of occurrence of urinary lithiasis in native and immigrant groups populating Israeli communities (Drach, 1992). They noted that the areas of highest incidence of urolithiasis were the warmer desert regions as opposed to the cooler mountain regions. Within desert areas, the incidence of cal-

culi formation was highest in immigrants from Europe, lower in those from East and North Africa, and lowest in the native-born population of Israel.

The mineral content of water also may contribute to the causation of stone disease. Some state that excessive water hardness (e.g., sodium carbonate) causes a greater incidence of stone disease (Sierakowski et al, 1978). Data, however, are conflicting (Churchill et al, 1980; Shuster et al, 1982).

The presence or absence of certain trace elements in water has been implicated in the formation of urinary calculi. For example, zinc is an inhibitor of calcium crystallization (Elliot and Eusebio, 1967). Low urinary levels of zinc, therefore, may increase the tendency toward stone formation. Yet, Yendt and Cohanim (1973) reported that thiazide treatment decreased stone recurrences in their patients, even though urinary zinc concentrations declined in most of them.

Diet

Dietary intake of various foods and fluids that result in greater urinary excretion of substances that produce stones has a significant effect on the incidence of urinary calculi. Ingestion of excessive amounts of purines (Hodgkinson, 1976), oxalates (Thomas, 1975), calcium, phosphate, and other elements often results in excessive excretion of these components in urine. The effects of diet in relation to specific types of urinary calculi are reviewed in later sections.

Lonsdale (1968b) points out that patients who form stones may have exceptional dietary patterns. Peculiar dietary excesses may also occur, such as the following: use of large amounts of Worcestershire sauce with its high oxalate content (Holmes, 1971), a vegetarian diet associated with childhood urolithiasis, and habitual excessive ingestion of milk products in the form of cheese or ice cream. In contrast, in a study of more than 45,000 men, Curhan and associates found that the prevalence of stone disease was lowest in patients on a high-calcium diet (Curhan et al, 1994).

Not only the diet, but also its source may be important. Identical vegetables grown in various parts of Thailand contain amounts of oxalate that differ by 50% or more (Suvachittanont et al, 1973). A careful dietary history is critical to the evaluation of every individual who forms stones.

Occupation

Lonsdale (1968b) indicated that urinary calculi are much more likely to be found in individuals who have sedentary occupations. Blacklock (1969) reported that the incidence of urinary calculi was higher in administrative and sedentary personnel of the royal Navy than in manual workers. The highest incidences were found in cooks and engineering room personnel.

Sutor and Wooley (1974a) correlated occupation with incidence of urinary calculi in 856 patients. Professional and managerial groups had a much higher than expected incidence. Manual workers had a much lower than expected frequency of urinary calculi. Whitson and colleagues examined the physiologic changes of metabolic and environmental origin in astronauts spending time in the microgravity environment of space (Whitson et al, 1993). The risk of calcium oxalate and uric acid stone formation increases after a space flight because of hypercalciuria, hypocitraturia, decreased pH, and lower urine volumes.

Robertson and colleagues performed extensive studies of the relationships between occupation, social class, and risk of stone formation (Robertson et al, 1980). They confirmed that the risk of formation of calcareous urinary calculi was increased in the most affluent countries, regions, societies, and individuals. These persons have more disposable income to spend on animal protein, which leads to increased urinary concentrations of calcium, oxalate, and uric acid. In fact, these investigators have gone so far as to suggest that recurrent calcium oxalate stone formers should become vegetarians (Robertson et al, 1979b). It becomes difficult to assess whether occupation is a primary factor in stone disease or whether it merely establishes other aspects of environment, such as diet, heat exposure, and water drinking. Alterations in these factors may be the actual instigators of urolithiasis.

PHYSICAL CHEMISTRY

Thermodynamic Solubility Product, Saturation, and Supersaturation

The central event in stone formation is supersaturation. Picture a glass of water containing salt or sodium chloride crystals in it. If there is little salt, it dissolves. As more salt is added, a point is reached at which the concentration of sodium chloride in the water is just high enough to prevent the crystals from dissolving. At this concentration, the solution is said to be saturated. If more crystals are added, the crystals precipitate, unless the temperature or pH is changed or another chemical that allows the salt to dissolve is added. The point at which saturation is reached and crystallization begins is referred to as the *thermodynamic solubility product* (K_{sp}). This is a constant, equal to the product of the concentration of the pure chemical components at which the solid and solvent stages are in equilibrium. For calcium oxalate monohydrate, the K_{sp} in distilled water at 37°C is 2.34×10^{-9} (Fig. 91–2).

Imagine now what happens in urine. If the product of calcium and oxalate concentrations in urine exceeds its thermodynamic solubility product in water, calcium oxalate crystals should precipitate. Urine, however, contains inhibitors and other molecules that allow higher concentrations of calcium oxalate to be held in solution. Thus, urine is said to be *metastable* with respect to calcium oxalate. As calcium oxalate concentrations are increased further, a point is reached at which it can no longer be held in solution. This concentration or K_F is the formation product of calcium oxalate in urine (see Fig. 91–2). The concentrations of most stone components in urine are in the metastable range between K_{sp} and K_F. Thus, the question really is not why some people form stones, but why most do not.

It is possible to estimate the state of saturation for a specific crystal system in urine. Pak and co-workers have developed a relatively simple method of estimating calcium oxalate and calcium phosphate saturation (Pak et al, 1977a).

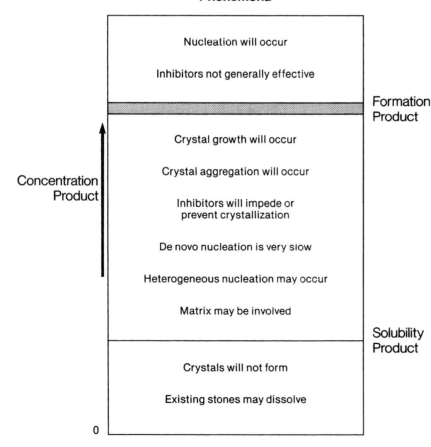

Phenomena

Figure 91–2. States of saturation. Listed are solid-solution phenomena that are likely to occur at a given range of concentration products. Three general situations are considered: (1) concentrations less than the solubility product (undersaturation), (2) concentrations that are metastable with respect to de novo precipitation (between the solubility product and the formation product), and (3) concentrations that are greater than the formation product (unstable). (From Meye JL: Physicochemistry of stone formation. *In* Resnick MI, Pak CYC, eds: Urolithiasis: A Medical and Surgical Reference, Philadelphia, W. B. Saunders, 1990, pp 11–34.)

They term it the *activity product ratio*. A second technique uses a computer program (EQUIL 93) to measure the state of saturation (Brown et al, 1994). One needs to measure the urine pH and the concentration of the major urinary ions. This program has been used by many prominent investigators in urolithiasis to monitor the results of therapy on urinary supersaturation. Temperature and pH are always specified for any crystallization process. Alteration in either factor may greatly change the amount of solute that may be held in solution. Perhaps the best-known illustration of the effects of temperature on solubility is the increased solubility of sugar as water is heated. For practical purposes, there need be no concern about temperature in this discussion of urolithiasis because it must occur at body temperature, near 37°C. One must be cautious in analyzing the results of crystallization studies performed at room temperature rather than at body temperature (Finlayson and Smith, 1974). Because urine varies widely in pH, this factor must be considered in any in vitro study of crystallization.

Saturation and solubility product in water are simple to define, but urine is a much more complex solution. In urine, when the concentration of a substance reaches the point at which saturation would occur in water, crystallization does not occur as expected. Urine has the ability to hold more solute in solution than does pure water. Although all elements and molecules in urine are suspended in water, the mixture of many electrically active ions in urine causes interactions that change the solubility of their elements. In addition, many organic molecules, such as urea, uric acid, citrate, and complex mucoproteins of urine, mutually affect the solubility of other substances. For example, citrate is known to combine with calcium to form a soluble complex. It therefore prevents some calcium from combining with oxalate or phosphate and becoming crystalline. As a corollary to this statement, Welshman and McGeown (1975), Menon and Mahle (1983c), Nicar and co-workers (1983), and Schwille and co-workers (1982) have reported that deficiency in urinary citrate is an important risk factor for calcium oxalate stone formation.

Nucleation, Crystal Growth, and Aggregation

In normal urine, the concentration of calcium oxalate is four times higher than its solubility (Coe and Parks, 1988a). Low urinary volumes; high rates of calcium, oxalate, phosphate, or urate excretion; and low citrate and magnesium excretion all increase calcium oxalate supersaturation. Once calcium oxalate concentration exceeds its K_{sp}, crystallization can occur. Because of inhibitors and other molecules, however, calcium oxalate precipitation in urine occurs only when its supersaturation is 7 to 11 times its solubility. The process by which nuclei form in pure solutions is called *homogeneous nucleation*. These nuclei form the earliest crystal structure that will not dissolve and have the form of a lattice that is characteristic of that crystal. In urine, however, crystal nuclei usually form on existing surfaces (heterogeneous nucleation). Epithelial cells, cell debris, urinary casts, other crystals, and red blood cells can all act as heterogeneous nuclei (Brown and Purich, 1992). Epithelial cell injury can lower the concentration at which crystals form. Biologic processes can create nucleation sites (Randall, 1937; Carr, 1969; Drach and Boyce, 1972). Stones then grow on these preformed nuclei.

Another concept necessary to promote understanding of the genesis of urinary calculi is that of aggregation. Crystal nuclei cannot grow large enough to attach to and occlude renal tubular lumens within the 5 to 7 minutes that it takes them to pass through tubules and enter the renal pelvis. They can, however, aggregate into large clumps within a minute (Kok et al, 1990). Thus, although crystal growth alone cannot explain clinical stone disease, a combination of growth and aggregation can. Magnesium and citrate inhibit crystal aggregation. Nephrocalcin, an acidic glycoprotein of renal origin, inhibits calcium oxalate nucleation, growth, and aggregation (Nakagawa et al, 1987; Asplin et al, 1991). Tamm-Horsfall mucoprotein, the most abundant protein in urine, inhibits aggregation (Hess et al, 1991), whereas uropontin inhibits crystal growth (Shiraga et al, 1992). Interference with crystal growth and aggregation is a possible therapeutic strategy for the prevention of recurrent stone disease.

Free Particle Nucleation and Fixed Nucleation or Crystal Retention

The standard laws of the physical chemistry of crystallization can explain the occurrence of crystals in a static solution. Normal urine, however, is not a static solution. It flows continuously, and new solutes are added and subtracted from the solution. Urine moves from the glomerulus through the nephron into the collecting system within 2 to 5 minutes. The point of greatest supersaturation of the urine is usually the renal papilla (Vermeulen and Lyon, 1968; Jordan et al, 1978; Hautmann et al, 1980). The lumen of the nephron at the level of the collecting duct is 50 to 200 μm. A newly formed crystal within the nephron requires anywhere from 90 to 1500 minutes to grow to a diameter of 200 μm at levels of conventional urinary supersaturation (Finlayson B, personal communication, 1980). Although crystal aggregation can result in urinary microliths large enough to occlude collecting ducts, in most instances, this mechanism is simply not enough to explain the genesis of renal calculi. Thus, factors must exist that cause the crystals to be retained within the kidney. If a crystal mass becomes lodged in the renal papilla or tubule, it is no longer able to move through the system (Fig. 91–3). If a crystal is retained in the kidney, growth can occur for long periods of time whenever urinary supersaturation or aggregation of new crystals occurs. Many kidney stones have a layered structure, suggesting intermittent growth during periods of supersaturation. Anatomic abnormalities, such as medullary sponge kidney or ureteropelvic junction obstruction, can predispose to increased crystal retention. Increased stickiness of the tubular epithelium can cause crystal retention. Finally, abnormalities in renal cellular calcium or oxalate transport may result in intracellular or interstitial crystal deposition and stone formation (Kumar et al, 1991; Menon and Koul, 1992; Scheid et al, 1996).

Modifiers of Crystal Formation: Inhibitors, Complexors, and Promoters

Urine contains substances that alter or modify crystal formation (Drach and Boyce, 1972; Fleisch, 1978; Coe et al,

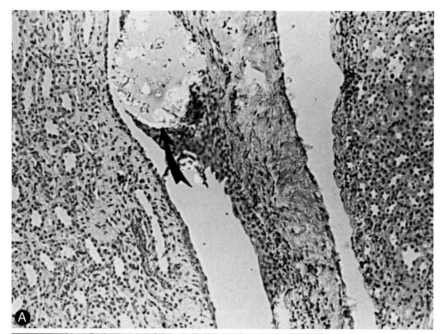

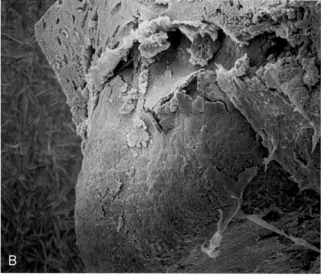

Figure 91–3. Randall's plaque. *A,* A subepithelial collection of calcified material has acquired additional calcium oxalate crystals and has begun to erupt through the epithelium (100 × partly crossed polars). *B,* Scanning electron micrograph of calcium oxalate stone at the tip of human papilla. (*B* courtesy of Dr. S. R. Khan, University of Florida, Gainesville, FL.)

1980a; Garside, 1982). These can be divided into inhibitors, complexors, and promoters. Robertson and Peacock (1972) showed that patients who formed calcium stones excrete considerably more oxalate and calcium than normal patients do. There was overlap, however, in the degree of saturation between normal subjects and patients with stone formation. This suggests that a certain percentage of normal subjects are indistinguishable biochemically from patients with stones, yet they do not form stones. Although all patients with cystinuria have an excessive amount of cystine in the urine, many of them do not form calculi. Many investigators believe that the reason some individuals with supersaturated urine are able to prevent crystallization in the urine is because they possess inhibitors of crystallization in the urine.

Robertson and colleagues have derived a saturation-inhibition index that differentiates stone formers from controls with a high degree of accuracy (Robertson et al, 1976). Urinary inhibitors attach to growth sites on crystals, retarding further growth and aggregation. Urinary inhibitors

may be organic or inorganic. The earliest investigation into inhibitors was performed by Howard and colleagues (1967). They showed that urine from normal subjects prevented the setting of Portland cement, whereas urine of stone formers did not. They postulated that the urine of normal subjects contains a chemical that prevents precipitation of Portland cement. Initially, this inhibitor was thought to be a peptide, and it has been studied extensively by Howard and colleagues (1967) and subsequently by Robertson and colleagues (1969) and Smith (1989). This substance was subsequently identified as phosphocitrate (Tew et al, 1981).

In urine, inhibitors have been identified for the calcium phosphate and the calcium oxalate crystal systems but not the urate system. Magnesium, citrate, pyrophosphate, and nephrocalcin make up most of the inhibition present for the calcium phosphate crystal system (Ito and Coe, 1977). Inhibitors of calcium oxalate crystal formation present in urine include citrate, pyrophosphate, glycosaminoglycans, RNA fragments, and nephrocalcin, with much of the inhibition coming from large-molecular-weight compounds (Garside, 1982; Khan et al, 1988). Two urinary glycoproteins—nephrocalcin and Tamm-Horsfall glycoprotein—are potent inhibitors of calcium oxalate monohydrate crystal aggregation (Nakagawa et al, 1987). Nephrocalcin is synthesized by the proximal tubules and the thick ascending limb and is the most potent inhibitor of calcium oxalate monohydrate crystal growth in simple solutions. Urinary nephrocalcin from calcium oxalate stone formers inhibits calcium oxalate monohydrate crystal aggregation tenfold less than nephrocalcin from normal urine. This nephrocalcin lacks gamma-carboxyglutamic acid, which normally is present at two to three residues per molecule. A second protein, lithostatine, colocalizes with nephrocalcin in the kidney but appears to be immunologically different (Verdier et al, 1992). Tamm-Horsfall mucoprotein, synthesized in renal thick ascending limb and the distal tubule, does not inhibit calcium oxalate crystal growth but does inhibit crystal aggregation. Tamm-Horsfall protein is the most potent aggregation inhibitor as yet identified. At physiologic concentrations of 0.5 mmol, Tamm-Horsfall protein is as potent an inhibitor of aggregation as nephrocalcin, whereas at lower concentrations, Tamm-Horsfall protein is ten times as potent as equimolar concentrations of nephrocalcin (Grover et al, 1994). The effectiveness of Tamm-Horsfall protein as an inhibitor is reduced by self-aggregation. Although there is no difference in the urinary excretion of Tamm-Horsfall protein between stone formers and normal subjects, Tamm-Horsfall protein in stone formers exists in the predominantly self-aggregated form, reducing its effectiveness as an aggregation inhibitor.

Even though nephrocalcin and Tamm-Horsfall protein are excellent inhibitors of aggregation at urinary concentration, the aggregation assays showing this were performed in simple solutions and not in urine. Ryall and colleagues have pointed out that when inhibition is measured in normal urine, urinary prothrombin fragment 1 is the most potent inhibitor studied (Ryall et al, 1995). These studies are still preliminary, and the exact role of urinary prothrombin fragment 1 in crystal inhibition is yet to be determined (Stapleton and Ryall, 1995).

Another important inhibitor of calcium oxalate crystal growth present in urine is uropontin (Shiraga et al, 1992). This aspartic acid-rich protein shares N-terminal amino acid sequences with human osteopontin. Indeed, osteopontin is produced by mouse kidney cortical cells in culture (Worcester et al, 1992) and is present in the distal tubules of stone-forming rats (Kohri et al, 1993). Both uropontin and osteopontin are major components of the matrix of calcium oxalate monohydrate stones. They contain functional Arg-Gly-Asp–cell-binding sequences that may facilitate interactions between cells and mineralizable matrix. Thus, these proteins, under certain conditions, may promote crystal adherence to renal epithelial cells (Oldberg et al, 1986; Reinholt et al, 1990). Another protein present in renal stones is alpha$_1$-antitrypsin or a related molecule (Umekawa et al, 1993). This protein does not bind calcium, but it has an important role in inflammation. The presence of this protein in renal stones suggests that stone crystals may have been in contact with blood cells during their formation or growth. The reaction between crystals and blood cells may cause crystal adherence (Umekawa et al, 1993).

Substances that form soluble complexes with the lattice ions for specific crystals, such as calcium oxalate, decrease the free ion activity of that ion and effectively decrease the state of saturation for that ion system. Citrate is the most potent complexer of calcium and exerts its maximum effect at a pH of 6.5. In the calcium oxalate system, magnesium forms soluble complexes with oxalate by complexation. Thus, both citrate and magnesium act not only as inhibitors, but also as complexors (Malek and Boyce, 1973; Malagodi and Moye, 1981).

A third group of substances acts as promoters of crystal formation. A substance may promote one stage of crystal formation such as growth and inhibit another stage such as aggregation. For instance, glycosaminoglycans promote crystal nucleation but inhibit crystal aggregation and growth (Malek and Boyce, 1977). Tamm-Horsfall protein, depending on its molecular size and state of self-aggregation, may act either as an inhibitor or as a promoter of crystal formation (Meyer, 1981).

Role of Matrix

A noncrystalline protein-like matrix of urinary calculi was first described by Anton Von Heyde in 1684 (King, 1967). Boyce (1969) pursued the role of matrix in stone formation since his earliest report in 1954. Extensive investigations have characterized matrix as a derivative of several of the mucoproteins of urine and serum (Sugimoto et al, 1985; Rahman et al, 1986). The matrix content varies from stone to stone, but most solid urinary calculi have a matrix content of about 3% by weight (Boyce and King, 1959). Alternatively, matrix calculi, composed of an average of 65% of matrix by weight, may occur, especially in association with urinary infection (Allen and Spence, 1966; Mall et al, 1975).

Chemical analysis of stone matrix reveals it to be about 65% hexosamine and 10% bound water (Boyce, 1968). Uromucoid, the major component of urine, is similar in composition to matrix except that it contains about 3.5% sialic acid, whereas matrix has none. Malek and Boyce (1973) have postulated that this distinctive lack of sialic acid may be due to cleavage of the acid from uromucoid molecules by the renal enzyme sialidase.

Finlayson and associates (1961) and Vermeulen and Lyon (1968) have indicated that matrix may be only an adventitious precipitate with the crystals that form stones. Polymerization of matrix must occur to form the matrix stone. Watanabe (1972) and Lanzalaco and co-workers (1988) believe that matrix participates in the formation of stone crystals. Matrix must originate in the renal tubules, probably in the proximal tubule (Malek and Boyce, 1973). Malek and Boyce (1973) demonstrated intranephronic calculi in the renal tubules in patients with idiopathic calcium lithiasis. These microliths are laminated structures of matrix and crystals that mimic the structures of larger stones. Such microliths were not found in kidneys of patients who formed struvite, uric acid, or cystine stones.

Boyce and associates described one component that is immunologically unique to stone matrix and is different from any of the other mucoids of urine (Boyce et al, 1962). This *substance A* was found on the matrix of all calciferous stones, in the kidneys of patients who had stone disease, and in the urine of patients who formed calcium stones. It was also found in the urine of patients who had renal inflammation because of infection, infarction, or cancer (Keutel and King, 1964). Substance A was detected not as a single protein but as three or four antigens unique to stones (Moore and Gowland, 1975). They detected these "stone-specific antigens" in the urine of 85% of patients who formed stones but in no urine of normal individuals.

Dutoit and colleagues have hypothesized that a factor in the pathogenesis of renal stones is the alteration of excretion of the urinary enzymes urokinase and sialidase (Dutoit et al, 1992). According to their theory, patients with stones have decreased urokinase and increased sialidase activity in the urine, which leads to the formation of a mineralizable stone matrix. The authors found that *Proteus mirabilis* and *Escherichia coli* decrease urokinase and increase sialidase activity. Up to one third of patients with calcium stones have a history of urinary tract infection, usually due to *E. coli* (Holmgren et al, 1989). A non–urease-producing bacterium such as *E. coli* may play a role in stone formation by increasing the production of urinary matrix substances, thereby increasing crystal adherence to the renal epithelium.

Matrix undoubtedly plays some role in stone formation. Whether it is active or passive, qualitative or quantitative, enhancing or inhibitory remains to be decided.

Summary

Urinary stones do not occur unless crystals of the offending substance form in urine. For crystals to occur, the urine should be supersaturated with the salt in consideration. An increase in the urinary excretion of the chemicals that constitute the crystals results in an increase in the potential for crystallization. Urine does not need to be continuously supersaturated for crystals to form or grow: Intermittent supersaturation, as is seen during periods of dehydration or after meals, is sufficient. Because urine is a complex solution, several factors affect the availability of ions required for crystallization. Thus, the crystallizing potential for calcium oxalate is related not so much to the total concentration of calcium or oxalate in urine but to the chemical activity of the ions in solution. Compounds such as citrate and phosphate form complexes with calcium, and elements such as magnesium and sodium form complexes with oxalate, effectively reducing the free ionic concentrations of each.

Urinary supersaturation alone does not explain the formation of urinary stones. Urinary crystals can be seen in most urine specimens, particularly after storage, yet most individuals do not form stones. Stone formers as a group excrete larger crystals and crystal aggregates than healthy individuals. Normal subjects have inhibitors of crystal formation, growth, and aggregation in their urine. These include low-molecular-weight compounds such as citrate and pyrophosphate and larger molecules, such as glycosaminoglycans, nephrocalcin, and Tamm-Horsfall protein. Urine from patients with recurrent calcium oxalate stones tends to have higher calcium and oxalate saturation and lower inhibitors than urine from patients without stones, and a mathematically derived saturation-inhibition index has been reported to discriminate between the groups with better than 90% accuracy.

Free crystals formed within the kidney do not have the ability to grow to a size large enough to occlude a collecting duct and form a stone in a free-flowing urinary system. Crystal aggregation and retention within the kidney are prerequisites for urinary crystals to be converted to urinary calculi. Crystal aggregation is enhanced in individuals who lack inhibitors of aggregation. The urinary glycoproteins nephrocalcin and Tamm-Horsfall protein are potent inhibitors of crystal aggregation in simple solutions, whereas citrate and magnesium are inhibitors of crystal growth.

Anatomic abnormalities, such as medullary sponge kidney or ureteropelvic junction obstruction, or increased "stickiness" of the tubular epithelium can predispose to increased crystal retention. Urate and calcium oxalate crystals anchor to surfaces of cultured renal epithelial cells and may adhere in vivo to tubular cells or urothelium. Although not proven, bacterial infection may promote calcium oxalate stone formation by increasing urinary matrix, which, in turn, promotes crystal adherence. Finally, altered transport of calcium and oxalate by renal epithelial cells may result in intracellular or interstitial crystallization. These crystals are retained in the kidney and can become the nidus for stone formation (see Fig. 91–3).

MINERAL METABOLISM

The following is a brief description of mineral metabolism for the clinical urologist. In-depth reviews are available (Coe and Favus, 1992).

Calcium, Magnesium, Phosphorus, Vitamin D, and Parathyroid Hormone

The calcium content of the average Western adult diet ranges from 600 to 1200 mg, or about 15 mg per kg body weight (Pak et al, 1981c). Of this, about 30% to 45% (300–400 mg) is absorbed. The intestinal absorption of calcium changes inversely to dietary calcium intake. Thus, absorption of calcium is greater on low-calcium diets than on high-calcium diets. About 100 to 200 mg of the absorbed calcium is secreted into the bowel; **the net absorption of calcium is, thus, 100 to 300 mg** (Fig. 91–4). **Intestinal calcium absorption is mediated via cellular and pericellular pathways** (Favus, 1992). At high luminal concentrations, absorption is primarily through diffusion along pericellular pathways, whereas at low concentrations (<10 mmol), cellular pathways become more important. Calcium is absorbed in the ionic state: Therefore, substances that complex calcium, such as phosphate, citrate, sulfate, oxalate, and fatty acids, decrease the calcium available for absorption (Menon, 1986). Because calcium oxalate complexation is low below a pH of 6.1, calcium is probably maximally absorbed in the jejunum and the proximal portion of the ileum, where the luminal pH is usually below 6. Some calcium, however, is absorbed along the length of the entire gastrointestinal tract (Menon, 1986; Favus, 1992). The most important factor that mediates active or transcellular calcium absorption is 1,25-dihydroxyvitamin D_3, or calcitriol. 1,25-Dihydroxyvitamin

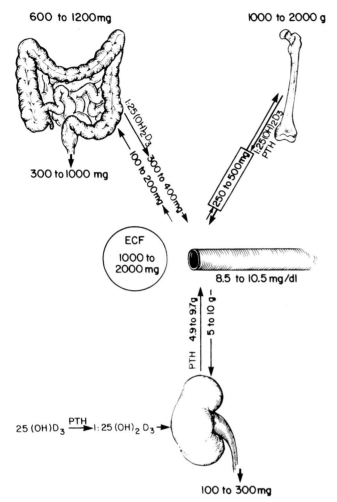

600 to 1200mg

1000 to 2000 g

1,25(OH)2D3
300 to 400 mg
100 to 200 mg

250 to 500 mg
1,25(OH)2D3
PTH

ECF
1000 to
2000 mg

300 to 1000 mg

8.5 to 10.5 mg/dl

PTH 4.9 to 9.7g
5 to 10 g

25 (OH)D₃ →PTH→ 1: 25 (OH)₂ D₃

100 to 300mg

Figure 91–4. The absorption and excretion of calcium. Ranges of values shown are approximate. Intestinal calcium absorption varies inversely with dietary calcium content. Under conditions of normal metabolic balance, rates of calcium uptake from and release into bone are equal. ECF, extracellular fluid; PTH, parathyroid hormone. (From Menon M: Calcium oxalate renal lithiasis: Endocrinology and metabolism. *In* Rajfer J, ed: Urological Endocrinology. Philadelphia, W. B. Saunders, 1986, p 387.)

D_3 increases calcium absorption by the brush border membranes of intestinal mucosa. It may alter membrane lipid concentration, allowing for a rapid increase in membrane permeability to calcium (Rasmussen et al, 1979; Matsumoto et al, 1981). When the amount of dietary calcium is low, production and serum levels of 1,25-dihydroxyvitamin D_3 are high—calcium is absorbed through the duodenum, jejunum, ileum, and colon.

Although about 37 metabolites of vitamin D have been characterized, it is generally accepted that **1,25-dihydroxyvitamin D_3 is the vitamin D metabolite that is the most potent stimulator of intestinal calcium absorption** (De Luca, 1980; Favus, 1981; Henry and Norman, 1992). Sunlight results in the conversion of 7-dehydrocholesterol in the malpighian layer of the skin to previtamin D_3. This is then transported to the liver, where it is hydroxylated to 25-hydroxyvitamin D_3. This metabolite is hydroxylated in the proximal renal tubules to 1,25-dihydroxyvitamin D_3. The conversion of 25-hydroxyvitamin D_3 to 1,25-dihydroxyvita-

min D_3 is stimulated by parathyroid hormone (PTH) and by hypophosphatemia. **PTH stimulates the enzyme 1α-hydroxylase located in the mitochondria of the proximal tubules.** Calcitriol is then secreted into the blood and transported to the intestine, where it binds to receptors in the brush border membrane epithelial cells. Although the kidney is the most important producer of calcitriol, activated macrophages and other cells also probably contribute to its production (Henry and Norman, 1992).

In addition to promoting intestinal calcium absorption, 1,25-dihydroxyvitamin D_3 has important, albeit perhaps indirect, effects on bone and kidney (see Fig. 91–4). In bone, 1,25-dihydroxyvitamin D_3 stimulates bone resorption by increasing osteoclast activity, probably in concert with PTH (Raisz et al, 1972; Menon, 1986). Consequently the amount of calcium and phosphate presented to the kidney increases, but PTH promotes renal calcium resorption and phosphate excretion. The net result is a rise in the serum calcium, suppressing PTH secretion and the production of 1,25-dihydroxyvitamin D_3.

Another factor important in normal mineral metabolism is PTH. **Human PTH is an 84–amino acid, single-chain polypeptide secreted by the parathyroid gland.** All known biologic activity resides in the amino terminal fragment, containing the 1-to-34 sequence. The most potent stimulus for the secretion of PTH is a decrease in serum calcium, in particular, the ionized fraction. **PTH stimulates osteoclasts to demineralize bone, by breaking down the bone crystal, apatite.** The dissolution of apatite results in the release of calcium and phosphate (PO_4^{3-}) into the blood stream. PTH stimulates renal adenylate cyclase. Within minutes, an increase in urinary cyclic adenosine monophosphate (cAMP) can be detected. **PTH increases renal calcium resorption of calcium and decreases the renal tubular resorption of phosphate.** As discussed earlier, PTH stimulates 1,25-dihydroxyvitamin D_3 production in the kidney and increases calcium and phosphate absorption in the intestine. In turn, 1,25-dihydroxyvitamin D_3 lowers PTH production. PTH does not appear to have a direct action on intestinal calcium absorption (Bushinsky and Krieger, 1992).

Similar to calcium, inorganic phosphorus is transported across the intestine through active and passive mechanisms. **Approximately 60% of the dietary intake of phosphate is absorbed by the intestine** (Yanagawa and Lee, 1992). 1,25-Dihydroxyvitamin D_3 stimulates phosphorus absorption in the duodenum and jejunum through a sodium-dependent active transport process (Kowarski and Schachter, 1969; Chen et al, 1974). The transport of phosphate is pH dependent: A decrease in luminal pH inhibits phosphate transport, and an increase in pH stimulates phosphate transport. At concentrations of greater than 3 mmol, intestinal absorption of phosphorus is mediated via passive diffusion. In contrast to calcium, inorganic phosphorus is secreted by the ileum and colon.

About 65% of the absorbed phosphate is excreted by the kidney, the remainder by the intestine. Under normal conditions, approximately 20% of the filtered load is excreted, the other 80% being absorbed by the proximal tubule. It is not clear whether the distal nephron possesses the ability to resorb phosphorus. PTH is the major hormonal regulator of renal phosphate resorption. Daily, about 150 to 200 mmol of calcium and about 100 mmol of phosphorus are filtered:

Only 5 mmol of calcium and 10 mmol of phosphorus are excreted in the urine. Thus, 97% to 99% of calcium and 85% to 90% of phosphorus are resorbed by the kidney.

Magnesium also is absorbed via active and passive mechanisms by the intestine. Under basal conditions, absorption is predominantly through passive diffusion. About 35% to 40% of ingested magnesium is absorbed (King and Stanbury, 1970). Although magnesium is absorbed mostly in the small intestine, some is absorbed by the large bowel also. Both vitamin D and PTH increase magnesium absorption.

Magnesium inhibits PTH excretion, perhaps by increasing calcium within parathyroid cells (Arnaud and Pun, 1992). About 95% of filtered magnesium is resorbed by the kidney, mostly by the loop of Henle (Rouffignac, 1992). A small portion is resorbed by the proximal and distal tubules.

Oxalate Metabolism

Oxalic acid is present in many foods and beverages. Its content is highest in leaf tea and powdered coffee, when expressed as percent content. Spinach and rhubarb, however, are the foods that are highest in oxalate per average serving. **In normal subjects, oxalate is absorbed poorly from the intestine, and urinary oxalate levels increase by only 3% after the ingestion of synthetic oxalate. In contrast, oxalate absorption is markedly increased in patients with small bowel resection or inflammatory bowel disease in whom the colon is present.** Although the entire intestinal tract is capable of absorbing oxalate, the stomach and distal bowel may be the primary sites for oxalate absorption (Menon and Mahle, 1982; Hautmann, 1993). Oxalate absorption is increased in patients with increased intestinal calcium absorption: In normal subjects, it is inversely related to dietary intake of calcium (Earnest et al, 1974; Barilla et al, 1978a). Although most of the oxalate is absorbed by passive diffusion, facilitated diffusion has been demonstrated across brush border membrane vesicles of ileum (Knickelbein et al, 1986). Approximately half of the ingested oxalate is destroyed by bacterial action, and about 25% is excreted unchanged in the feces (Menon and Mahle, 1983b; Williams and Smith, 1983). Two bacteria, *Oxalobacter formigenes* and *Pseudomonas oxalitcus*, contain enzymes that degrade oxalate within the physiologic pH range (Allison et al, 1986; Dawson et al, 1988). Some patients with nephrolithiasis may have a paucity of intestinal *O. formigenes* (Kleinschmidt et al, 1995). About 25% of the oxalate is excreted unchanged in the feces and the remainder in the urine. **Eighty percent of the oxalate found in urine comes from endogenous production in the liver (40% from ascorbic acid, 40% from glycine), and 10% comes from dietary sources** (see section on primary hyperoxaluria). Ascorbic acid undergoes enzymatic and nonenzymatic conversion to oxalate. Although less than 15% of administered glycine appears as urinary oxalate, its ubiquity in the diet causes it to be an important precursor of oxalate (Fig. 91–5).

Oxalate is freely filtered at the glomerulus and is secreted along the entire length of the proximal tubule (Greger et al, 1978; Weinman et al, 1978). Despite its importance, understanding of renal handling of oxalate is far from complete. In human kidney, oxalate undergoes bidirectional transport in the renal tubules. Micropuncture studies demon-

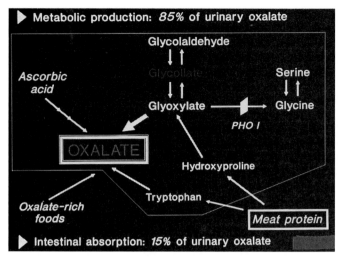

Figure 91–5. Oxalate metabolism. Role of dietary intake and metabolic production. (Courtesy of B. Hess, University Hospital, Berne.)

strated net secretion of oxalate in the kidney and showed that this secretory flux is predominantly located in proximal tubule (Senekjian and Weinman, 1982). It is estimated that 10% to 30% of urinary oxalate derives from net tubular secretion in normal conditions. Active secretion of oxalate in the proximal tubule requires oxalate uptake from the basolateral cell surface into the cell and luminal secretion through apical membrane. This notion is supported by direct demonstration of oxalate:chloride exchange process in apical membrane vesicles and oxalate:sulfate (bicarbonate) exchange in the basolateral membrane vesicles (Kuo and Aronson, 1980; Karniski and Aronson, 1987). The authors' studies using monolayers of renal proximal tubular epithelial cells (LLC-PK1 cells) in tissue culture system demonstrated polarized distribution of these functionally distinct oxalate transport systems in the intact living epithelial cells, with the oxalate:chloride exchange system being localized to the apical membrane domain and the oxalate:sulfate (bicarbonate) to the basolateral domain of these cells (Koul et al, 1994).

Baggio and colleagues (1986) measured the rate of oxalate flux across erythrocyte membranes in 114 patients with a history of calcium oxalate kidney stones and in 25 controls. An increased flux rate was seen in 70% to 80% of the patients studied. Intestinal oxalate absorption was increased in the five patients in whom it was determined. Others (Jenkins et al, 1988; Narula et al, 1988) have confirmed this observation.

Hydrogen Ion or Acid

The metabolic degradation of ingested carbohydrates, fats, and particularly proteins accounts for the production of 40 to 60 mmol (0.8–1.0 mg/kg) of acid per day (Davidman and Schmitz, 1988). In addition, about 20 to 40 mmol of bicarbonate are lost daily in the feces, which results in the addition of hydrogen ion (H^+) to the body (Gennari, 1989). This entire H^+ load must be excreted in the urine. In addition, the kidneys filter 180 L of plasma daily, containing about 4500 mmol of bicarbonate. This must be reabsorbed or regenerated. **Thus, the kidney must excrete the entire H^+ load produced by the body and reclaim all the bicarbonate that is filtered.** A defect in either acid excretion or bicarbonate resorption can lead to metabolic acidosis (Fig. 91–6).

The proximal nephron resorbs bicarbonate through coupled secretion of H^+ into the tubular lumen. The driving force for this reaction is sodium potassium ATPase (Na^+-K^+-ATPase) located on the basolateral membrane of the tubular cells. Sodium is pumped out of the cell and into the circulation in exchange for potassium. This results in a decrease in intracellular sodium, setting up an electrochemical gradient that drives a Na^+:H^+ exchanger located on the brush border. This exchanger maintains electrical neutrality by excreting protons into the tubular lumen in exchange for sodium resorbed from the tubule. Protons are produced in the tubular cell by the action of carbonic anhydrase (Kinkead and Menon, 1995). This enzyme is located on the brush border membranes and within the cell and catalyzes both the synthesis and the degradation of carbonic acid. Carbonic acid disassociates readily into bicarbonate and protons. The bicarbonate diffuses freely across the basal lateral membrane and into the circulation in exchange for chloride and represents reclaimed bicarbonate: H^+ is free to exchange with sodium at the brush border to maintain the cycle. **The proximal nephron is a high-capacity, low-gradient transport system with regards to H^+ secretion. It can secrete large quantities of protons but cannot generate a proton gradient between blood and urine steep enough to lower urinary pH significantly** (Rocher and Tannon, 1986).

About 80% of the filtered bicarbonate is resorbed by the proximal nephron; the remainder is reclaimed by the distal nephron through a mechanism similar to that described. The process of H^+ secretion in the distal nephron, however, differs in several ways from the process in the proximal nephron. In the distal nephron, H^+ secretion occurs by means of an active H^+ transporting ATPase or proton pump, located on the brush border. H^+ in the distal tubular lumen combines with urinary buffers such as phosphate and ammonia, rather than with bicarbonate. Divalent phosphate is minimally permeable and accounts for the vast majority of titratable acid, measured as the amount of acid required to restore the pH to neutrality. Ammonia, generated in the tubular cell from glutamine metabolism, diffuses readily into the tubular lumen and binds with protons to form the poorly diffusible NH_4^+ ion. The amount of NH_4^+ and HPO_4^{2-} in the final urine minus the excretion of bicarbonate—normally negligible—is termed *net acid excretion* (Morris and Sebastian, 1983). Carbonic anhydrase is absent in the lumen of the collecting ducts; aldosterone stimulates proton pumps, sodium resorption, and ammonia production and increases the electrical gradient. As a result of all these mechanisms, **the distal nephron can generate a 1000 to 1 H^+ gradient between the cell and tubular lumen, allowing the production of urine with a pH of 4.5 to 5.0 during periods of systemic acidosis. The distal nephron is a low-capacity, high-gradient proton pump** (see Fig. 91–6).

Citrate

Citrate is the most important complexor of calcium in urine and reduces ionic calcium concentration (Meyer and Smith, 1975; Pak, 1982a). It inhibits both spontaneous and heterogeneous nucleation of calcium oxalate crystals

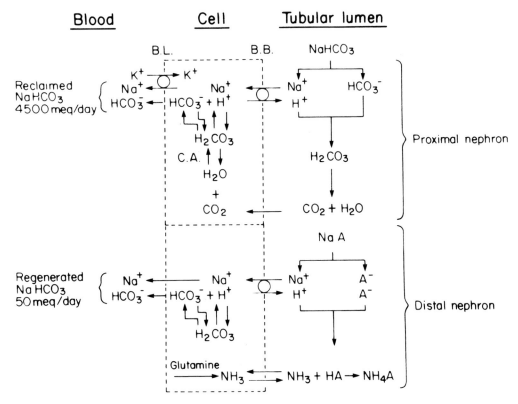

Figure 91–6. Mechanism of renal acidification, modified from that of Morris and Sebastian (1983). Bicarbonate ($NaHCO_3$) resorption occurs mainly in the proximal tubule and regeneration in the distal tubule. Sodium (Na^+) and potassium (K^+) exchange in proximal tubule is catalyzed by sodium-potassium adenosine triphosphatase. Dehydration of carbonic acid (H_2CO_3) is catalyzed by carbonic anhydrase (C.A.) in proximal tubule but not in distal nephron. Net acid excretion is 1 to 3 mEq/kg/day. B.L., basolateral membrane; B.B., brush border membrane; HCO_3, bicarbonate ion; NH_3, ammonia; HA, acid; A^-, base; Na A, sodium sulfate; NH_4A, ammonium acid (ammonium salt of nonvolatile acid). (From Pohlman T, Hruska KA, Menon M: J Urol 1984; 132:432.)

(Meyer and Smith, 1975; Kok et al, 1986; Nicar et al, 1987). Although on a molar basis its inhibitory activity is much less than that of other substances, urinary concentrations of citrate are so much higher than those of other inhibitors that at physiologic concentrations it is a potent inhibitory agent.

Citrate is widely distributed in the body and is an important energy source. Less than 1% of the citrate present in food appears unaltered as citrate in the urine. Absorbed citrate is oxidized, yielding an alkali load. This alkali raises the pH and bicarbonate concentration within the renal tubular cell and inhibits tubular resorption by decreasing citrate transport into renal cortical mitochondria (Simpson, 1963; Adler et al, 1971; Simpson and Hager, 1979). In normal subjects, orally administered potassium bicarbonate or potassium citrate increases urinary pH and citrate excretion to an equivalent degree (Sakhaee et al, 1991). Sakhaee and colleagues found a positive correlation between urinary citrate excretion and net alkali absorption with no difference between normal subjects and stone formers (Sakhaee et al, 1991).

In the circulation, citrate is present at a concentration of about 0.14 mmol, mostly as a free trivalent anion (Pak, 1990). Of the citrate filtered by the kidney, 75% is resorbed, mostly in the proximal tubule; the rest is excreted. Citrate concentration in the renal cortex often exceeds that of the peripheral blood. Citrate resorbed by the proximal tubule cell is transported into mitochondria, where it is oxidized into carbon dioxide and water via the citric acid cycle. **The major determinant of renal citrate handling is the acid-base status of the body. Metabolic acidosis facilitates the influx and inhibits the efflux of citrate from renal cortical mitochondria.** The metabolism of citrate by mitochondria is stimulated, resulting in a fall in cytosolic citrate concentration. This, in turn, increases citrate uptake by the sodium-citrate cotransporter in the brush border membrane (Jenkins et al, 1985). **Thus, metabolic acidosis reduces citrate excretion by augmenting citrate resorption and mitochondrial oxidation.** Metabolic alkalosis decreases mitochondrial uptake of citrate and increases urinary citrate excretion. Conditions that predispose to intracellular acidosis, such as hypokalemia (Fourman and Robinson, 1953), a high-protein diet with its acid load, and exercise, decrease citrate excretion. In contrast, organic acids such as malate, fumarate, succinate, and tartrate (Baruch et al, 1975; Down et al, 1977) enhance citrate excretion by providing an alkali load and increased substrate for intrarenal citrate synthesis. Urinary citrate excretion increases during pregnancy, perhaps as a consequence of the action of estrogen or progesterone (Shorr et al, 1942a,b). It is suggested that PTH, calcitonin, and vitamin D increase citrate secretion, and androgens reduce citrate secretion (Costello et al, 1970).

Cystine

Cystine is a dibasic amino acid. **It is absorbed by the intestine from dietary sources and also converted from methionine. In normal individuals, filtered cystine is almost completely resorbed in the proximal nephron: Urinary cystine excretion is less than 20 mg/day.** The details of cystine transport by the kidney are not completely detailed in humans; the following is probably what happens. Cystine

is transported by the proximal tubular cell from peritubular blood, through transporters located at the basolateral membrane. It is both secreted and resorbed across the brush border membrane of the proximal nephron. The gene for cystine transport has been mapped to chromosome 2, and at least four mutations responsible for cystinuria have been identified (Pras et al, 1994). The mutant gene in cystinuria codes for an abnormal transport system involving cystine, ornithine, lysine, and arginine. **The secretion and paracellular leakage of cystine are apparently normal in patients with cystinuria; however, there is impaired resorption of cystine across the brush border membrane.** Increased urinary sodium stimulates cystine excretion to a modest degree. Patients with cystinuria often excrete twice as much lysine than cystine in the urine. Because lysine, arginine, and ornithine are freely soluble, however, they do not form renal stones. The intestinal transport of cystine has been measured from the in vitro uptake of radiolabeled cystine by biopsy specimens of the jejunal mucosa and from measuring plasma cystine levels following an oral cystine load. Three defects in intestinal transport have been described in cystinuria. In type 1 cystinuria, there is total loss of intestinal transport of cystine, lysine, and arginine. In type 2, some cystine uptake is detected in the jejunal mucosa. In type 3, there is reduced uptake by jejunal mucosa as well as following an oral cystine load.

PATHOPHYSIOLOGY OF STONE FORMATION

Calcium Oxalate Stones

Hypercalciuria

The association between increased urinary calcium excretion and calcium oxalate renal stones was initially reported by Flocks (1939) and subsequently by Albright and colleagues (1948). **Between 30% and 60% of all patients with calcium oxalate kidney stones have increased urinary calcium excretion in the absence of raised serum calcium levels.** This condition—idiopathic hypercalciuria—has received much attention from researchers of urolithiasis. There are several different definitions of *hypercalciuria*. Urinary calcium excretion largely depends on dietary calcium intake, which varies between 400 and 2000 mg per day in Western countries. The most stringent definition of hypercalciuria is that of Pak (1987b), who defined it as the excretion of greater than 200 mg of calcium per 24 hours after 1 week's adherence to a 400-mg calcium, 100-mEq sodium diet. Alternatively, hypercalciuria has been defined as the excretion of greater than 4 mg calcium per kg body weight per day or greater than 7 mmol in men and 6 mmol in women (Parks and Coe, 1986). A final definition is the excretion of urinary calcium of greater than 0.11 mg/100 ml of glomerular filtrate (Broadus et al, 1978). Hypercalciuria contributes to calcium stone formation by increasing the relative supersaturation of urine and by creating a complex with anionic inhibitors of stone formation, such as citrate and glycosaminoglycans. It has also been suggested, however, that it may paradoxically increase the inhibitor activity of nephrocalcin.

Two broad concepts exist about the pathogenesis of hypercalciuria. In 1974, Pak and associates suggested that hypercalciuria was heterogeneous in origin and that three types existed: **(1) absorptive hypercalciuria, in which the primary abnormality was an increased intestinal absorption of calcium; (2) renal hypercalciuria, characterized by a primary renal leak of calcium; and (3) resorptive hypercalciuria, characterized by increased bone demineralization. Coe and associates, however, eschew such a distinction and maintain that patients with hypercalciuric nephrolithiasis suffer from multiple disturbances in renal tubular function, a disturbance in phosphate transport, and accelerated 1,25-dihydroxyvitamin D$_3$ synthesis, resulting in increased intestinal calcium absorption** (Coe et al, 1992). Supporters of the theory that there are several forms of hypercalciuria point out that therapy designed to correct specific metabolic abnormalities is associated with high success rates. Proponents of the unifying hypothesis point out that bone mineral density is reduced to an equivalent extent in hypercalciuric stone formers regardless of dietary calcium restriction, suggesting that an element of bone demineralization is present in all patients. There is currently no controlled investigation that demonstrates that therapy designed specifically to correct absorptive, renal, or resorptive hypercalciuria is more successful in preventing stone recurrences than nonspecific methods of lowering urinary calcium. Nonetheless, subclassification of hypercalciurias helps to understand why many patients with kidney stones have increased urinary calcium excretion, and therefore the subclassifications proposed by Pak et al (1974) are described.

Absorptive Hypercalciuria

In absorptive hypercalciuria, the primary abnormality is increased intestinal calcium absorption. Some investigators restrict this term to patients in whom the hyperabsorption of calcium is primary, whereas others use it to encompass patients in whom the increase in intestinal calcium absorption is secondary to increases in 1,25-dihydroxyvitamin D$_3$ production or mild hypophosphatemia. In absorptive hypercalciuria type 1, intestinal hyperabsorption of calcium exists, whether or not the patient is on a calcium-restricted diet. Intestinal perfusion studies have demonstrated selective hyperabsorption of calcium in the jejunum but not in the ileum. Intestinal magnesium absorption is normal in patients with absorptive hypercalciuria, but oxalate absorption is increased (Menon and Koul, 1992). Two observations suggest that increased absorption of calcium detected is independent of vitamin D. Classically, vitamin D increases calcium and magnesium, but not oxalate, absorption in both the jejunum and the ileum. In addition, intestinal calcium absorption remains elevated in many patients with hypercalciuria, despite treatment with corticosteroids or orthophosphates, agents that decrease vitamin D–mediated calcium absorption. Nonetheless, **1,25-dihydroxyvitamin D$_3$ levels are elevated in up to 50% of patients with absorptive hypercalciuria, suggesting that, at least in some individuals, this condition is secondary to increased production of or increased sensitivity to vitamin D metabolites.** Absorptive hypercalciuria type 2 is a variant of this disorder wherein patients exhibit increased urinary calcium excretion while on their normal diet but normal calcium excretion on a low-calcium, low-sodium diet. In the final subcategory, absorptive hypercalciuria type 3, the serum phosphate is low, suggesting that the increased intestinal calcium absorption is the result of a stimulation in vitamin D production as the result of the lowered serum phosphate.

The mechanism by which increased absorption of calcium leads to hypercalciuria is shown in Figure 91–7. As calcium absorption is exaggerated in the intestine, serum calcium levels tend to rise yet remain within the normal range. The filtered load of calcium increases, whereas PTH secretion is suppressed. The relative deficiency of PTH decreases renal tubular resorption of calcium, and consequently 1,25-dihydroxyvitamin D$_3$ production is suppressed. The combination of increased filtration and decreased resorption leads to hypercalciuria. A new steady state with respect to serum calcium is established, albeit with suppressed parathyroid function and hypercalciuria.

Renal Hypercalciuria

In this condition, the underlying abnormality is a primary renal wasting of calcium. The consequent reduction

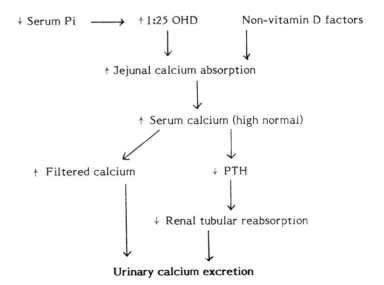

Figure 91–7. Mechanisms of absorptive hypercalciuria. (From Menon M, and Krishnan CS: Urol Clin North Am 1983; 10:596.)

in circulating serum calcium stimulates PTH production (Fig. 91–8). This results in the hydroxylation of 25-hydroxy-vitamin D to 1,25-dihydroxyvitamin D₃, thus increasing intestinal calcium absorption. These effects restore the serum calcium to normal (in contrast to in primary hyperparathyroidism) but at the expense of increased PTH and 1,25-dihydroxyvitamin D₃. Two facts must be stressed: First, intestinal absorption of calcium is increased in both absorptive and renal hypercalciuria; second, parathyroid function is suppressed in absorptive hypercalciuria but stimulated in renal hypercalciuria. Fasting urinary calcium levels are normal in patients with absorptive hypercalciuria, provided that they have fasted long enough to excrete the excessively absorbed calcium. They remain **elevated, however, in renal hypercalciuria. These two criteria—elevated fasting urinary calcium levels and stimulated parathyroid function—serve to distinguish renal from absorptive hypercalciuria.**

The cause of renal calcium leak remains to be clarified. A high serum osteocalcin level has been reported in some patients with renal hypercalciuria but not in patients with absorptive hypercalciuria (Menon and Kaul, 1992). Up to one third of patients with renal hypercalciuria have an antecedent history of urinary tract infection, but it is not clear whether the infection is a renal infection. Many also have low urinary citrate excretion (Nicar et al, 1983). In one study, subtle radiologic signs of tubular ectasia were present in some patients with renal hypercalciuria, suggesting that primary structural abnormalities in the tubule may be responsible for the condition (Yendt et al, 1981). In another study, a functional defect in the proximal tubule with impaired resorption of sodium, calcium, phosphorus, and magnesium was detected (Sutton and Walker, 1980). Patients with renal hypercalciuria sometimes exhibit an exaggerated calciuric response to an oral glucose load (Barilla et al, 1978b). These studies suggest that tubular function may be abnormal in patients with renal hypercalciuria. Muldowney and colleagues have suggested that renal hypercalciuria is secondary to excessive dietary intake of sodium (Muldowney et al, 1982). In normal subjects on controlled diets, a sodium chloride load of 240 mEq/day induces all the biochemical changes of renal hypercalciuria, including an elevation in serum PTH, 1,25-dihydroxyvitamin D₃, and intestinal calcium absorption (Breslau et al, 1982a). Similar changes can be seen as a result of furosemide-induced natriuresis (Bushinsky et al, 1986). Restricting sodium intake, however, does not normalize the biochemical changes seen in patients with renal hypercalciuria (Pak, 1990).

Prostaglandins can increase glomerular filtration rates and renal calcium excretion. Buck and associates initially demonstrated that urinary prostaglandin (prostaglandin E₂) levels were increased in hypercalciuric recurrent stone formers and that nonsteroidal anti-inflammatory agents reduced urinary calcium excretion in them (Buck et al, 1981, 1983). Other investigators (Houser et al, 1984; Calo et al, 1990; Henriquez-LaRoche et al, 1992) have confirmed this observation. Prostaglandin synthetase inhibitors lower urinary calcium levels in patients with hypercalciuria and stones (Sharma et al, 1992). In a double-blind study, Buck and colleagues found that the administration of fish oil or evening primrose oil, agents that inhibit conversion of arachidonic acid to prostaglandins, reduced urinary calcium excretion in stone formers with idiopathic hypercalciuria, although they increased intestinal calcium absorption (Buck et al, 1992).

Resorptive Hypercalciuria

This syndrome is synonymous with subtle hyperparathyroidism. **Hypercalciuria results from excessive PTH-dependent bone resorption as well as enhanced intestinal absorption of calcium** caused by PTH itself or by a PTH-dependent synthesis of 1,25-dihydroxyvitamin D₃. Although PTH causes increased tubular resorption of calcium, the increase in the filtered load of calcium overwhelms this and results in excessive urinary calcium excretion.

Idiopathic Hypercalciuria

Idiopathic hypercalciuria occurs in 5% to 10% of normal people (Coe et al, 1979; Coe and Bushinsky, 1984) and in about half the patients with calcium nephrolithiasis. Familial clustering of hypercalciuria has been reported by several investigators (Coe et al, 1979; Mehes and Szelid, 1980; Pak et al, 1981a). In an early study, Coe and associates determined the frequency of hypercalciuria in the families of nine patients with idiopathic hypercalciuria and recurrent calcium oxalate nephrolithiasis (Coe et al, 1979). Hypercalciuria occurred in 26 of 73 relatives over multiple generations. Nineteen of the 44 first-degree relatives had idiopathic hypercalciuria, and a similar number formed stones. The syndrome of

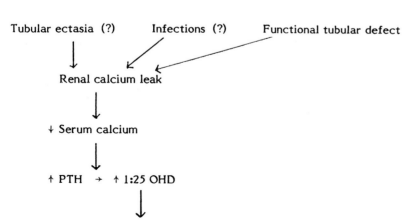

Tubular ectasia (?)   Infections (?)   Functional tubular defect

Renal calcium leak

↓ Serum calcium

↑ PTH → ↑ 1:25 OHD

↑ **Intestinal calcium absorption**

Figure 91–8. Mechanism of renal hypercalciuria. This represents an idealized version of the pathophysiologic processes involved in renal hypercalciuria. Increased levels of parathyroid hormone (PTH) have not been reported by some investigators. (From Menon M, Krishnan CS: Urol Clin North Am 1983; 10:597.)

renal phosphate leak, elevated 1,25-dihydroxyvitamin D_3, and absorptive hypercalciuria has been demonstrated in members of a Bedouin tribe in which intermarriage is common (Tieder et al, 1985, 1987). Animal models of renal and absorptive hypercalciuria exist (Favus and Coe, 1979; Lau and Ebny, 1982). Hypercalciuria is seen in some patients with pseudoxanthoma elasticum or cystic fibrosis (Mallette and Mechanick, 1987; Katz et al, 1988). In one study by Bianchi and colleagues, erythrocyte membrane calcium-magnesium-ATPase was increased in patients with hypercalciuria and correlated with 24-hour urinary calcium excretion (Bianchi et al, 1988). **These studies suggest that idiopathic hypercalciuria may be inherited as an autosomal dominant trait, although the pattern can reflect polygenic control of calcium excretion as well** (Holmes et al, 1995).

A contradictory opinion has been raised by Pak (1990). Among 3473 stone-forming patients who had 24-hour urine measurements, hypercalciuria was seen in 40%. Among these hypercalciuria patients, 25% had hyperuricosuria, 23% had hyperoxaluria, 17% had hypocitraturia, 17% had low urinary pH, 69% had low urinary volume, 38% had high urinary sodium, and 3% had low urinary magnesium. The coexistence of these abnormalities suggested to Pak that they may be environmental or nutritional in origin because a genetic defect is more likely to cause a single metabolic abnormality. The co-occurrence of multiple derangements, however, can also result from the superimposition of dietary and environmental factors on an underlying genetic defect.

Differential Diagnosis of Idiopathic Hypercalciuria: Calcium Load Test. After 7 days of a low-calcium, low-sodium diet, patients fast for 12 hours from 9 PM. Distilled water is provided at 9 PM and midnight. At 7 AM the next day, patients completely empty their bladder and discard the urine. They drink an additional 600 ml of distilled water. Urine is collected from 7 to 9 AM. This is the fasting sample. At 9 AM, 1 g of calcium mixed in a liquid synthetic meal is given orally. A urine sample is collected from 9 AM to 1 PM. This is the postload sample. Both urine samples are analyzed for calcium, creatinine, and cAMP (Table 91–3). cAMP measurements are used as an indirect estimate of parathyroid function because most PTH assays are insensitive to rapid changes in serum calcium.

The conditions of this test are fairly rigorous, and the values are valid only if conditions have been followed strictly. Absorptive hypercalciuria is diagnosed by a fasting urinary calcium of less than 0.11 mg per 100 ml of glomerular filtrate, increasing to greater than 0.20 mg per 100 ml following the calcium load. cAMP is less than 6.85 nmol/

100 ml of glomerular filtrate while fasting and remains suppressed after the calcium load. Renal hypercalciuria has a fasting urinary calcium excretion of greater than 0.11 mg/100 ml glomerular filtrate and cAMP levels greater than 6.85 nmol/100 ml filtrate. Following the calcium load, urinary calcium levels increase to greater than 0.20 mg/dl, whereas cAMP levels fall to normal. In patients with resorptive hypercalciuria or normocalcemic primary hyperparathyroidism, urinary calcium and cAMP levels remain elevated both in the fasting and in the postload situations, indicating nonsuppressibility of parathyroid function (see Table 91–3).

Hypercalcemic Nephrolithiasis

Primary Hyperparathyroidism

The association between primary hyperparathyroidism and renal calculus disease has been known since the 1920s. Indeed, the first patient undergoing parathyroidectomy in the United States died as a result of complications from kidney stone formation (Barzel, 1977). Routine screening measurements of serum calcium have resulted in hyperparathyroidism being detected when it is relatively asymptomatic. Thus, although between 39% and 78% of patients in many early series presented with renal calculi (Cope, 1966; Yendt and Gagne, 1968; Heath et al, 1980), more recent series have indicated that the prevalence of stone disease in hyperparathyroidism is only about 1%, a figure not much different from the prevalence of stone disease among general hospital admissions (Heath et al, 1980).

DIAGNOSIS

The diagnosis of primary hyperparathyroidism can sometimes be difficult. Classically, **it requires a demonstration of hypercalcemia in the absence of any other disorder that elevates serum calcium** (Breslau and Pak, 1982). Serum calcium determinations are often inaccurate by about 5%, and elevations in serum calcium seen in patients with mild hyperparathyroidism may be much less than 5% (Yendt and Gagne, 1968). Thus, multiple determinations of serum calcium may be required for the diagnosis of primary hyperparathyroidism. **Hyperparathyroidism should be suspected in patients with renal stones who have a serum calcium close to the upper limit of normal, or over 10.1 mg/dl** (Menon, 1986). In some patients with normal total serum calcium, ionized serum calcium is elevated (Muldow-

Table 91–3. DIFFERENTIAL DIAGNOSIS OF THE HYPERCALCIURIAS*

	Fast		Load	
	UCa (mg/mg cr)	UcAMP (mg/100 ml GF)	UCa (mg/mg cr)	UcAMP (mg/100 ml GF)
AH	<0.11	<6.85	>0.20	<4.6
RH	>0.11	>6.85	>0.20	<6.85
PHPT	>0.11	>6.85	>0.20	<6.85

*The conditions of the test are as described by Pak (1982a). Patients are maintained on a 100-mg calcium, 100-mEq sodium diet for 1 week. They fast overnight before the test except for tap water as desired. The first morning voided urine is discarded, and a 2-hour fasting urine specimen is obtained. A test meal containing 1 g of Neo-calglucon in 240 ml of Calci-test is then given, and urine is collected after 4 hours.
AH, Absorptive hypercalciuria; RH, renal hypercalciuria; PHPT, primary hyperparathyroidism; UCa, urinary calcium; UcAMP, urinary cAMP.
From Menon M, Krishnan CS: Urol Clin North Am 1983; 10:598.

ney et al, 1976; Yendt and Gagne, 1968). Bilezikian (1992) believes that the most useful test for primary hyperparathyroidism is the measurement of PTH. **Assays that measure the intact hormone, the midmolecule, or the carboxy-terminal regions of PTH are elevated in more than 90% of patients with surgically proven primary hyperparathyroidism.** These assays are more sensitive than assays directed against the N-terminal fragment.

PTH acts on the kidney and causes the release of cAMP (Broadus, 1980). Thus, urinary cAMP is elevated in patients with primary hyperparathyroidism. PTH-mediated changes in cAMP are rapid, and urinary cAMP can be used as an indicator of the response of the parathyroid gland to oral calcium loading. PTH promotes proximal tubular excretion of bicarbonate and phosphorus, resulting in phosphaturia and mild hyperchloremic acidosis. Some authors have used the serum chloride-to-phosphate ratio as a diagnostic parameter. If the ratio is above 33, and the serum phosphorus is below 2.5 mg/dl, hyperparathyroidism can be strongly suspected (Aro et al, 1977). A better indicator may be the determination of the renal phosphate threshold (Bijvoet, 1977). Determination of this ratio requires analysis of spot urine and serum specimens for phosphate and creatinine content. The tubular resorption of phosphate is calculated, and the renal phosphate threshold is derived from a nomogram. This test is extremely reliable in patients with normal renal function suspected to have primary hyperparathyroidism.

TREATMENT

The treatment of patients with primary hyperparathyroidism who form stones is surgical removal of the adenoma, with success rates of greater than 90% (Coe and Parks, 1988a). The treatment of asymptomatic hyperparathyroidism, usually seen in postmenopausal women, is much more controversial. Many authorities do not recommend parathyroidectomy in postmenopausal women with mild symptoms. In these patients, no treatment or estrogens, which inhibit the action of PTH on bone, may be used (Coe and Parks, 1988a). In one study (Thomas et al, 1985), however, most patients with "asymptomatic" hyperparathyroidism, picked up on routine serum calcium measurements, admitted to nonspecific symptoms such as malaise, fatigue, abdominal pain, bone pain, constipation, or depression. Seventy-five percent of the symptoms improved after removal of the parathyroid gland. In contrast, a similar group of patients undergoing operations for thyroid nodules had only a 9% improvement in elicited symptoms.

If a patient with primary hyperparathyroidism presents with symptomatic hypercalcemia and asymptomatic renal calculi, the first approach to therapy involves surgical removal of the parathyroid gland. If the patient presents with symptomatic or obstructive renal calculi, the stones should be treated initially, if the patient is not in hypercalcemic crisis (Sonda et al, 1982).

MECHANISM OF STONE FORMATION

Some patients with primary hyperparathyroidism present with bone disease and some with stone disease (Albright and Reifenstein, 1948). Absolute levels of serum or urinary calcium, PTH measurements, alkaline phosphates, and a variety of other parameters do not allow distinction between the two groups. Patients with bone disease may have larger adenomas than patients with stones (Bilezikian, 1992). When patients with hyperparathyroidism are analyzed on the basis of calcium absorption, those with higher levels of 1,25-dihydroxyvitamin D_3 and greater calcium absorption tend to have renal stones (Broadus et al, 1980). When patients are analyzed according to whether they have stones or do not, however, no differences in calcium absorption or vitamin D levels are detected between stone formers and non–stone formers (Pak et al, 1981b). In a study in Pak's laboratory (Pak et al, 1981b), the concentration at which spontaneous crystallization of calcium oxalate occurs was lower in patients with stones. Because all other parameters were similar whether or not patients had stones, Pak and co-workers concluded that this increase in crystallization was the result of either decreased inhibitors or increased promoters in the urine (Pak et al, 1981b). Jenkins and colleagues demonstrated that urinary citrate levels were decreased in hyperparathyroid patients with renal calculi (Jenkins et al, 1982).

Malignancy-Associated Hypercalcemia

Although primary hyperparathyroidism is the most prevalent cause of hypercalcemia in an outpatient setting (Rizzoli and Bonjour, 1992)**, in an inpatient setting, the most common cause of hypercalcemia is a malignancy.** In the past, the detection of hypercalcemia in the hospital setting often prompted an energetic work-up for occult cancer. **Assays for intact PTH now completely separate individuals with hyperparathyroidism from those with other causes of hypercalcemia** (Table 91–4).

Lung and breast cancers account for 60% of malignancy-associated hypercalcemia, renal cell cancer for 10% to 15%, head and neck cancer for 10%, and hematologic malignancies such as lymphoma and myeloma for another 10%. Hypercalcemia is rarely seen in prostate cancer (Nussbaum, 1993). Malignancy-associated hypercalcemia is an exceedingly rare cause of renal stones. In the report from Parks and associates, 1 out of 1132 consecutive patients with nephrolithiasis had a malignancy—multiple myeloma (Parks et al, 1980). Neither Pak nor the authors (Menon, 1986) have seen a single patient with an undiagnosed malignancy who presented with nephrolithiasis as the primary symptom.

It was originally thought that direct mechanical destruction of bone by malignant cells was the cause of tumor hypercalcemia. Hypercalcemia, however, does not occur in all patients with extensive metastases. Malignancies, in particular multiple myeloma, secrete a number of cytokines that act locally in the bone marrow to stimulate osteoclastic bone resorption (Eilon and Mundy, 1978; Ralston et al, 1982). These cytokines are called *osteoclast-activating factors* and consist of prostaglandin E, tumor necrosis factors alpha and beta, interleukin-1 alpha and beta, and transforming growth factors alpha and beta (Mundy, 1989; Orloff and Stewart, 1992). These factors stimulate the osteoclast to release the necessary hydrolysates required to dissolve bone.

The most common cause of malignancy-associated hypercalcemia, even in patients with skeletal metastasis, is the production by the tumor of a bone-resorbing substance called *PTH-related polypeptide* (Edelson and Kleere-koper, 1995). This clinical syndrome is now called *humoral*

Table 91–4. HYPERCALCEMIC STATES

Condition	Parathyroid Hormone	Phosphorus	Urine Calcium	Glomerular Filtration Rate	Other
Thiazide	N	N	L	N	Low K^+
Malignant tumors	NLH	L/N	H	N/L	Osteolytic or sclerotic bone lesions
Vitamin D excess	L	N/H	H	N/L	High $1,25(OH)_2D_3$
Sarcoidosis	L	N	H	N/L	High $1,25(OH)_2D_3$
Coccidioidomycosis	L	N	H	N/L	High $1,25(OH)_2D_3$
Silicosis	L	N	H	N/L	High $1,25(OH)_2D_3$
Plasma cell granuloma	N	N	—	L	High $1,25(OH)_2D_3$
Leprosy	N	N	H	L	High $1,25(OH)_2D_3$
Hypothyroidism	H	L	L	N	High $1,25(OH)_2D_3$
Primary increase in $1,25(OH)_2D_3$	L	N	H	N	High $1,25(OH)_2D_3$
Pheochromocytoma	L/N	N	H	N	High calcitonin has been reported
Hyperthyroidism	N	N	H	N	
Tuberculosis	L	H	H	L	
Addison's disease					
Familial hypocalciuric hypercalcemia	N	N	L/N	N	Asymptomatic
Lithium	H	N	N	N	
Theophylline	N	—	—	—	
Paget's disease	L	N	H	N	
Immobilization	L	N	H	N	Usually only hypercalciuric
Acquired immunodeficiency syndrome	L	L/N	—	—	Low $1,25(OH)_2D_3$

N, Normal; L, low; H, high; $1,25(OH)_2D_3$, 1,25-dihydroxyvitamin D_3.
From Coe FL, Parks JH, eds: Nephrolithiasis: Pathogenesis and Treatment. Chicago, Year Book Medical Publishers, 1988, p 85.

hypercalcemia of malignancy (Orloff and Stewart, 1992). PTH-related polypeptide has 146 amino acids, whereas PTH has only 84 (Krane and Potts, 1990). Both peptides exhibit full biologic activity on mineral ion homeostasis (Horiuchi et al, 1988), and both hormones bind to an identical receptor on bone and kidney target tissue (Juppner et al, 1991). Approximately 80% of patients with malignancy-associated hypercalcemia have humoral hypercalcemia of malignancy, mediated by the PTH-related peptide.

Hypercalcemia occurs in up to 5% of patients with lymphoma (Cannellos, 1974). Almost all patients with HTLV-1 lymphomas or leukemias develop hypercalcemia in the absence of skeletal metastasis. These patients secrete the hormone responsible for humoral hypercalcemia of malignancy. Other tumors may cause hypercalcemia by secreting prostaglandin E_2 (Metz et al, 1981) or a novel and as yet uncharacterized factor (Bringhurst et al, 1986). Prostaglandin E_2 stimulates osteoclastic bone resorption in tissue cultures. This prostaglandin may be produced by the tumor or by monocytes and macrophages recruited by the immune response to the tumor.

Sarcoidosis and Other Granulomatous Diseases

Many granulomatous diseases, including sarcoidosis, tuberculosis, histoplasmosis, coccidioidomycosis, leprosy, and silicosis, have been reported to produce hypercalcemia (see Table 91–4). The most common cause of hypercalcemic nephrolithiasis among these disorders is sarcoidosis. Sarcoidosis is a multisystem granulomatous disorder of unknown etiology most commonly affecting young adults and presenting with bilateral lymphadenopathy, pulmonary infiltration, and skin and eye lesions (Johns, 1980). **The sarcoid granuloma produces 1,25-dihydroxyvitamin D_3, causing increased intestinal calcium absorption, hypercalcemia, and hypercalciuria** (Hendrix, 1966; Bell et al, 1979). Al-

though hydroxylation of 25-hydroxyvitamin D_3 to 1,25-dihydroxyvitamin D_3 occurs under normal circumstances only in the kidney, pulmonary alveolar macrophages and lymph node homogenates from patients with sarcoidosis are capable of synthesizing the hormone. The differentiation between sarcoidosis and other hypercalcemic conditions is not difficult when classic manifestations of the disease are present; however, it can be troublesome when the only clinical manifestation is renal stones. The distinction between sarcoidosis and intermittent hypercalcemic hyperparathyroidism may be particularly elusive, but refinements in PTH assays have made the distinction easier. **Most patients with sarcoidosis have low or unmeasurable levels of PTH** (Cushard et al, 1972). From a practical standpoint, an important diagnostic factor is the response of hypercalcemia to steroid therapy. Breslau and associates found that serum calcium levels fell in response to short-term glucocorticoid administration in all patients with sarcoidosis, whereas they rose in patients with primary hyperparathyroidism (Breslau et al, 1982b). Breslau and associates believed that steroids act primarily on the intestinal mucosa in patients with sarcoidosis, decreasing intestinal calcium absorption (Breslau et al, 1982b). In patients with primary hyperparathyroidism, the steroids act primarily on the bone and stimulate bone resorption.

Hyperthyroidism

About 5% to 10% of patients with hyperthyroidism develop hypercalcemia. Because mean serum albumin level is low in these patients, the incidence of hypercalcemia may be underestimated. Indeed, when serum ionized calcium is measured, about 50% of patients with thyrotoxicosis have been demonstrated to have mild hypercalcemia (Burman et al, 1976; Mosekilde and Christiansen, 1977).

Thyrotoxicosis is readily apparent in most patients by the history and the physical examination. The hypercalcemia is usually mild, rarely exceeding 11.5 mg/dl. When severe hypercalcemia occurs in a thyrotoxic patient, the existence of a parathyroid adenoma must be considered (Menon, 1986). **Hypercalcemia and hypercalciuria result from a stimulation of bone resorption mediated by thyroxine and triiodothyronine** and are reflected by an increase in serum alkaline phosphatase and urinary hydroxyproline excretion. PTH levels are low in hypercalcemic patients with hyperthyroidism (Menon, 1986). Renal calculi are distinctly uncommon in the thyrotoxic patient.

Glucocorticoid-Induced Hypercalcemia

Glucocorticoids affect calcium metabolism through three mechanisms—their action on bone, intestine, and the parathyroid glands. Of these, their action on bone is the most important. **Glucocorticoid excess leads to increased bone resorption, decreased bone formation, and osteopenia.** Prednisone inhibits intestinal absorption; this effect favors a reduction in serum calcium and urinary calcium excretion. It is this action of glucocorticoids that has resulted in its being used to treat hypercalcemia associated with sarcoidosis. Glucocorticoids also have a direct stimulatory effect on the parathyroid gland. Cortisol has been shown to stimulate the release of PTH from cultured rat parathyroid glands. The acute infusion of cortisol to normal subjects causes an immediate increase in PTH levels, without altering serum calcium (Fucik et al, 1975). Renal calculi are not rare in Cushing's syndrome, and Cushing's original patient had renal stones (Cushing, 1932). Between 4% and 65% of patients with Cushing's syndrome have renal stones (Pyrah, 1979). The incidence of asymptomatic renal calcification is even higher (Scholz et al, 1957).

Pheochromocytoma

Hypercalcemia, when seen in patients with pheochromocytoma, occurs most often in patients with multiple endocrine neoplasia type 2, in which primary hyperparathyroidism, medullary carcinoma of the thyroid, and adrenal gland tumor coexist (Samaan et al, 1976; Drezner and Lebovitz, 1978). Catecholamines are known to stimulate secretion of PTH in vitro (Sackner et al, 1960) and may also stimulate osteoclast-activated bone resorption. Islet cell tumors of the pancreas secrete vasoactive intestinal polypeptide (VIP), which can also cause hypercalcemia.

Familial Hypocalciuric Hypocalcemia

Familial hypocalciuric hypocalcemia is an autosomal dominant and apparently benign disorder that is characterized by hypercalcemia presenting in childhood (Law and Heath, 1985). Patients tend to be asymptomatic and lack the characteristic manifestations of primary hyperparathyroidism. It is diagnosed by documenting hypercalcemia in blood relatives and is best left untreated.

Immobilization

Prolonged bed rest can lead to hypercalcemia, as the result of increased bone turnover. Hypercalcemia caused exclusively by immobilization, however, is rare in patients whose underlying bone metabolism is normal. Hypercalcemia is seen most often when another condition, such as Paget's disease—with accelerated bone turnover—primary hyperparathyroidism, or malignancy, coexists in an immobilized patient.

Iatrogenic Hypercalcemia

Thiazide diuretics may cause hypercalcemia by increasing proximal tubular resorption of calcium, reducing plasma volume, and enhancing sensitivity of target tissues to PTH (Orloff and Stewart, 1992). In some patients, **thiazide-induced hypercalcemia leads to the unmasking of subtle primary hyperparathyroidism**. Similarly, lithium may induce a condition that mimics primary hyperparathyroidism. Mallette and co-workers found that serum ionized calcium increased in patients treated with lithium without any change in PTH levels initially (Mallette et al, 1989). With long-term treatment, circulating PTH levels also significantly increased.

Hypercalcemia has been reported in patients with extensive skeletal metastasis from breast cancer who have been treated with estrogens and antiestrogen (tamoxifen) (Legha et al, 1981). This is probably the result of the cytotoxic effects of therapy on skeletal metastasis. Patients who ingested large amounts of milk and absorbable alkali for the treatment of peptic ulcer disease rarely develop a syndrome called the milk-alkali syndrome. These patients usually ingest up to 10 g of calcium, together with large amounts of alkaline. The patients develop metabolic alkalosis, hypercalcemia, a tendency toward hyperphosphatemia, nephrocalcinosis, and renal insufficiency (Orwoll, 1982) but typically do not have hypercalciuria. Excessive vitamin D ingestion can cause severe hypercalcemia. Although this can happen in patients with food fads, it most commonly occurs during the course of treatment for hypoparathyroidism. Vitamin A toxicity, by causing increased bone resorption, may rarely cause hypercalcemia.

Treatment of Hypercalcemia

The treatment of hypercalcemia is best accomplished by treating the underlying cause. Emergency treatment is required when a hypercalcemic crisis exists. The clinical findings include dehydration, metabolic encephalopathy, gastrointestinal symptoms, and a serum calcium usually greater than 14 mg/dl (Nussbaum, 1993; Edelson and Kleerekoper, 1995). The most common cause of a hypercalcemic crisis is an underlying malignancy, usually occurring in a patient in whom the primary diagnosis is well established. Therapy must be directed toward decreasing bone resorption and increasing the urinary excretion of calcium. **Initial therapy should include volume expansion as rapidly and completely as possible. Normal saline expands the volume and induces urinary calcium excretion.** Patients may need up to 4 L a day for the first 48 hours. Thiazide therapy should be discontinued because of its effect on increasing renal tubular resorption of calcium. A loop diuretic such as furosemide promotes urinary excretion of calcium. **Bisphosphonates are one of the mainstays for the therapy of severe hypercalcemia** (Bilezikian, 1992). These drugs effectively inhibit osteoclast activity and decrease bone resorption. Pamidronate (30–90 mg) is the preferred agent because of its potency and its ability to be infused intravenously (Garabedian et al, 1972).

Similar to the bisphosphonates, calcitonin inhibits osteoclast-induced bone resorption. It is administered subcutaneously or intramuscularly and acts rapidly, lowering serum calcium within a few hours of administration. Mithramycin, which used to be one of the first-line drugs for the treatment of hypercalcemia, has been replaced by the bisphosphonates or calcitonin because of its potential side effects. These include soft tissue irritation if extravasation occurs, alteration in liver enzymes, nephrotoxicity, and thrombocytopenia. Glucocorticoids are effective in patients with hematologic malignancies and in hypercalcemia associated with sarcoidosis. Gallium nitrate has been approved for the treatment of severe hypercalcemia. It inhibits bone resorption, although the precise mechanism is not clear (Edelson and Kleerekoper, 1995). It can cause nephrotoxicity and generally should not be administered to patients with serum creatinine levels greater than 2.5 mg/dl. Intravenous phosphate is not used commonly for hypercalcemia because of the potential for intravascular and ectopic soft tissue calcifications.

Summary

Almost all patients with hypercalcemia who form stones have primary hyperparathyroidism. In the series from Chicago, 56 of 66 hypercalcemic stone formers had primary hyperparathyroidism; 7 were undiagnosed; and 1 each had hyperthyroidism, sarcoidosis, and multiple myeloma (Parks et al, 1980).

Hyperoxaluria

Hyperoxaluria is associated with calcium oxalate nephrolithiasis in three different clinical scenarios (Table 91–5). **Primary hyperoxaluria is a rare genetic disorder resulting from increased hepatic production of oxalate. Enteric hyperoxaluria occurs in patients with short bowel syndrome or malabsorption. Finally, a group of patients with recurrent idiopathic calcium oxalate lithiasis exhibits mild hyperoxaluria or increased transport of oxalate by red blood cells.**

Increased Oxalate Production

PRIMARY HYPEROXALURIA

Two types of primary hyperoxaluria exist. Primary hyperoxaluria type I (MIM, #25990) is an autosomal recessive inborn error of metabolism characterized by nephrocalcinosis, tissue deposition of oxalate (oxalosis), and death from renal failure before the age of 20 in untreated patients (Williams and Smith, 1978). The disease is characterized by

Table 91–5. TYPES OF HYPEROXALURIA

I   Increased oxalate production
Primary hyperoxaluria
Increased hepatic conversion
II Increased oxalate absorption
III Hyperoxaluria in idiopathic calcium oxalate stone disease

increased urinary excretion of oxalic, glycolic, and glyoxylic acids (Menon and Mahle, 1982). It was originally thought that the underlying biochemical abnormality was a deficiency in the activity of the enzyme α-ketoglutarate–glyoxylate carboligase (Williams and Smith, 1978). In 1986, however, Danpure and Jennings demonstrated conclusively that **primary hyperoxaluria type I is due to a defect of the enzyme alanine–glyoxylate aminotransferase (AGT) in the liver.** In humans, AGT is normally located in hepatic peroxisomes. Primary hyperoxaluria type I may be the result of either a complete deficiency of peroxisomal AGT or altered trafficking of AGT wherein it is displaced into mitochondria (Danpure et al, 1989). Liver biopsy specimens in patients with primary hyperoxaluria type I have shown that two thirds of patients have undetectable AGT activity, whereas one third have significant activity, albeit in the mitochondria (Danpure and Jennings, 1988). Heterozygotes have diminished enzyme activity in the peroxisome, sufficient to allow normal detoxification of glyoxylate.

In normal human liver, AGT catalyzes the transamination or detoxification of glyoxylate to glycine, a function that it can perform only if it is located in the peroxisome (Fig. 91–9). Its deficiency in primary hyperoxaluria results in glyoxylate's being oxidized to oxalate (Danpure, 1994). The human AGT gene has been cloned and sequenced, and the mutations responsible for abnormal trafficking have been identified. Primary hyperoxaluria type I can be definitively diagnosed even in patients who present in end-stage renal failure by assaying the amount and subcellular distribution of AGT in percutaneous needle biopsy specimens of the liver. Prenatal diagnosis of primary hyperoxaluria type I can be achieved either by measuring AGT in fetal liver biopsy specimens or by DNA analysis of chorionic villus (Danpure et al, 1994).

Primary hyperoxaluria type II or L-glyceric aciduria (MIM #26000) is a much rarer variant of the disease (Williams and Smith, 1968). **Deficiencies of the hepatic enzymes D-glycerate dehydrogenase and glyoxylate reductase lead to increases in urinary oxalate and glycerate excretion.** To date, only 21 cases have been reported with limited long-term follow-up (Chlebeck et al, 1994).

Both forms of primary hyperoxaluria cause a high level of oxalate production and urinary excretion of oxalate of 1.5 to 3 mmol daily (Itami et al, 1990; Scheinman, 1991). Stone formation often begins in childhood. Nephrocalcinosis, tubulointerstitial nephropathy, and chronic renal failure often result (Yendt and Cohanim, 1985; Watts et al, 1991). About one third of the patients present with completely silent renal failure (Scheinman, 1991). Serum oxalate levels are elevated (Worcester et al, 1986), and oxalate deposition in the heart, bone, joints, eyes, and other tissues occurs (oxalosis). Some patients with primary hyperoxaluria type II have a more indolent illness, with one patient, detected through screening, having had no evidence of renal stones over 21 years of follow-up (Chlebeck et al, 1994).

Primary hyperoxaluria is treated with pyridoxine supplements (200–400 mg/day), which lower oxalate production in some patients. Pyridoxine acts as a cofactor in the transamination of glyoxylate to glycine and lowers urinary oxalate excretion in some patients with primary hyperoxaluria. The treatment of pyridoxine-resistant hyperoxaluria requires increasing urinary volume to 3.5 L/day and adding

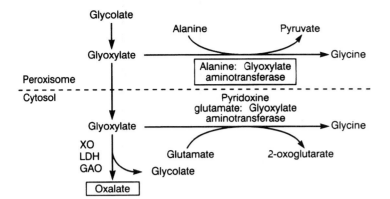

Figure 91–9. Glyoxylate metabolism within the peroxisome and the cytosol. Alanine: glyoxylate aminotransferase deficiency increases cytosolic glyoxylate and causes increased production of oxalate. XO, xanthineoxidase; LDH, lactate dehydrogenase; GAO, glycolic acid oxidase. (From Smith LH: Hyperoxaluric states. *In* Coe FL, Favus MJ, eds: Disorders of Bone and Mineral Metabolism. Philadelphia, Lippincott-Raven, 1992, p 721.)

supplemental oral citrate, thiazides, neutral phosphates, or magnesium gluconate (Thomas et al, 1979; Scheinman, 1991). Patients who progress to renal failure and are treated with long-term dialysis die from effects of systemic oxalosis because treatment regimens that control uremia are not sufficient to eliminate the oxalate overload (Watts et al, 1984). Isolated renal transplantation is often unsuccessful because of recurrent stone formation and nephrocalcinosis. Watts and co-workers have suggested that hepatic transplantation, which corrects the underlying metabolic abnormality, should be performed before end-stage renal failure develops (Watts et al, 1991). When necessary, this should be supplemented with renal transplantation and vigorous dialysis to deplete the body stores of oxalate. What is needed, however, is replacement of the defective AGT gene in the liver.

INCREASED HEPATIC CONVERSION

Three other conditions result in oxalate overproduction—pyridoxine deficiency, ethylene glycol ingestion, and methoxyflurane anesthesia. Ethylene glycol is readily converted to glycolaldehyde and to glycolic acid. The anesthetic drug methoxyflurane is also converted to oxalate. Intratubular oxalate precipitates and interstitial oxalosis have been described as a consequence of its use (Williams and Smith, 1983).

Enteric Hyperoxaluria

Ingested oxalate is absorbed through the stomach (Hautmann, 1993) and the colon (Madorsky and Finlayson, 1977; Menon and Mahle, 1982). **Malabsorption from any cause, including small bowel resection** (Smith et al, 1972), **intrinsic disease, or jejunoileal bypass** (Cryer et al, 1975; Vainder and Kelly, 1976), **increases the colonic permeability of oxalate as the result of exposure of the colonic epithelium to bile salts. Furthermore, loss of calcium in the feces results in the presence of less calcium in the intestinal lumen, allowing oxalate to exist in a soluble form.** Earnest and colleagues demonstrated that 30% of ingested oxalate in a 100-mg spinach meal was absorbed by patients with extensive ileal resection, in contrast to 6% absorbed by normal subjects or patients with ileostomy (Earnest et al, 1974). The hyperoxaluria from small bowel malabsorption often exceeds 1 mmol/day and causes recurrent nephrolithiasis, nephrocalcinosis, and renal oxalate deposition.

The treatment of enteric hyperoxaluria is unsatisfactory.

Often, a combination of treatment modalities needs to be used. General methods of treatment include oral hydration and a low-oxalate and low-fat diet. These measures are difficult to achieve, however, in an individual with malabsorption. Calcium carbonate by mouth, 1 to 4 g with each meal, binds oxalate in the gut so that it cannot be absorbed (Andersson and Jagenburg, 1974; Smith, 1992). Some studies, however, have suggested that the urinary saturation with calcium oxalate is not altered with calcium supplementation because the increase in the urinary calcium balances the decrease in urinary oxalate. Cholestyramine, a nonabsorbable resin that binds fatty acids, bile salts, and oxalate, can be used at doses at 1 to 4 g with each meal and at bedtime. It is tolerated poorly, however, by many patients. Lindsjo (1989) has used an organic marine hydrocolloid charged with calcium in 10 patients with enteric hyperoxaluria treated for 6 months to 3 years. Urinary oxalate decreased by 20%, and clinical improvement was seen in some patients. Many clinicians (Coe et al, 1992; Smith, 1992) prefer to use all treatments together and increased one by one until urinary oxalate level reaches a nadir. In patients with jejunoileal bypass, reversion of the bypass restores urinary oxalate levels to normal. This needs to be done only rarely. Kleinschmidt and colleagues have shown that patients with recurrent calcium oxalate stone disease have a decrease in intestinal *O. formigenes* and thus have a decrease in oxalate degradation in the intestine (Kleinschmidt et al, 1995).

Mild Metabolic Hyperoxaluria

Several studies suggest that **mild hyperoxaluria is as least as important a factor in the pathogenesis of idiopathic calcium oxalate stones as hypercalciuria** (Menon, 1986; Robertson and Hughes, 1993). Increased urinary oxalate excretion can be detected in 0.3% to 50% of patients with calcium stones (Menon and Mahle, 1983a). In general, investigators using imprecise assays and stringent definitions of hyperoxaluria find a lower prevalence of the disorder, whereas investigators who use more precise assays and a less precise definition of hyperoxaluria show higher preponderance of the disorder. When excretion greater than the 90th percentile of control was used to define hyperoxaluria, 37% of patients with stone disease proved to have the entity (Wallace et al, 1981). A detailed risk factor analysis comparing patients with renal stones and normal controls suggested that the probability of new stone formation correlated best with the decrease in urinary volume and an increase in urinary oxalate (Robertson et al, 1978). In several series, the activity of stone disease correlates better with absolute levels of urinary oxalate than with levels of urinary calcium (Robertson et al, 1978; Thomas et al, 1979; Lindsjo, 1989).

The most compelling evidence indicating that an abnormality in the way the body handles oxalate is responsible for calcium oxalate nephrolithiasis comes from the work of Baggio and colleagues (1986). **They found an increase in oxalate self-exchange across the red blood cell membrane in 79% of patients with idiopathic calcium oxalate nephrolithiasis.** Others (Jenkins et al, 1988; Narula et al, 1988; Motola et al, 1992) have confirmed this finding. Because less than 50% of the patients with the red cell anomaly exhibited hyperoxaluria, one can say that altered membrane transport of oxalate (hyperoxaluria sans oxalate) may be the most common defect involved in idiopathic calcium oxalate nephrolithiasis. Many of Baggio's patients had associated abnormalities in distal acidification (Gambaro et al, 1988).

The exact etiology of increased urinary oxalate excretion remains to be elucidated. Increased dietary protein intake and altered renal excretion of oxalate have been postulated as causes by some investigators (Pinto et al, 1974; Robertson et al, 1979a). Rose (1988a) has suggested that some patients with renal stones may have a mild metabolic hyperoxaluria, a condition characterized by increased urinary glycolate and oxalate excretion. Wilson and colleagues have suggested that such patients have an abnormality of renal tubular excretion of oxalate characterized by an increase in the fractional excretion of oxalate (Wilson et al, 1984). Others believe, however, that increased intestinal absorption is the cause for hyperoxaluria in patients with stones (Marangella et al, 1982; Lindsjo, 1989). Hodgkinson (1978) found that urinary oxalate excretion normalized when patients fasted. Marangella and associates and Lindsjo found that patients with hyperoxaluria also had hypercalciuria. The absorption of ^{14}C oxalate was increased in hypercalciuric patients. When dietary calcium was restricted but oxalate remained constant, urinary oxalate excretion increased further. These observations led these investigators to conclude that oxalate absorption was increased in patients with increased calcium absorption (Marangella et al, 1982).

The treatment of mild hyperoxaluria is difficult. Dietary restriction of oxalate results in decreased oxalate excretion, but the decrease may not be significant. A no-oxalate diet is difficult if not impossible to adhere to (Gregory et al, 1977). **Dietary calcium restriction is counterproductive because urinary oxalate excretion rises. Pyridoxine decreases urinary oxalate excretion in 50% of patients with mild metabolic hyperoxaluria** (Rose, 1988b). **Administration of thiazides causes a decrease in urinary oxalate excretion and normalizes erythrocyte oxalate fluxes** (Yendt and Cohanim, 1978; Baggio et al, 1986). Tyrosine, by inhibiting the conversion of hydroxyproline to oxalate, may reduce urinary oxalate excretion (Zinsser and Karp, 1973). The administration of calcium decreases urinary oxalate excretion, but because urinary calcium levels rise, the relative urinary supersaturation of calcium oxalate is affected little. The administration of nonabsorbable cations such as aluminum may decrease calcium absorption without increasing oxalate absorption, but clinical studies are not available. Finally, an oral mixture of glycosaminoglycans has inhibited

erythrocyte oxalate fluxes and decreased urinary oxalate excretion (Baggio et al, 1991a,b).

Hyperuricosuria

In 1968, Gutman and Yu as well as Prien and Prien observed that patients with gout or hypouricemia formed not only uric acid, but also calcium oxalate stones. Smith and associates noted that serum urate concentration was higher in patients with idiopathic calcium oxalate nephrolithiasis than in normal subjects (Smith et al, 1969). Much of the work linking hyperuricosuria and calcium oxalate stones, however, has come from Coe's laboratories (Coe and Raisen, 1973; Coe and Kavalich, 1974).

Physical Chemistry

Uric acid promotes calcium oxalate crystallization by facilitating the formation of nuclei. Addition of crystals of uric acid to supersaturated calcium oxalate solutions (Deganello and Chou, 1984) induces the deposition of well-oriented crystals of calcium oxalate over the uric acid. Both sodium hydrogen urate and uric acid crystals can initiate calcium oxalate crystal growth in a seeded solution. Sodium hydrogen urate crystals, however, are not seen in fresh human urine or kidney stones.

Robertson (1976) has suggested that **sodium acid urate may produce calcium oxalate stone disease by nullifying the effectiveness of naturally occurring inhibitors of calcium oxalate crystal growth.** Monosodium urate can absorb glycosaminoglycans such as heparin (Finlayson and Dubois, 1978; Pak et al, 1979) and other naturally occurring urinary macromolecules such as glycopeptide, reducing the inhibitory activity of these macromolecules against crystal growth of calcium oxalate.

Hyperuricosuria was seen in 277 out of 1117 (24%) calcium stone formers evaluated by Coe and Parks (1988) **and in 10% of patients seen in Dallas (Pak, 1990). In Dallas, it coexisted with other abnormalities in 40% of patients. Of the stones analyzed by the Coe group, 12% contained a mixture of calcium oxalate and uric acid.**

Mechanisms of Hyperuricosuria

Excessive dietary purine intake is the main cause of hyperuricosuria (Coe and Kavalich, 1974). In addition, some patients appear to overproduce uric acid. These patients excrete more uric acid in the urine than do normal subjects, even on a purine-free diet. This may be the result of increased uric acid production from endogenous purine metabolism.

The majority of hyperuricosuric calcium oxalate stone formers have normal serum uric acid concentrations. Increased purine intake tends to increase serum uric acid levels in normal people to high normal or abnormal levels over a short time (Steele and Reiselbach, 1967). The fact that serum uric acid is almost always normal despite dietary purine gluttony indicates that patients with hyperuricosuric nephrolithiasis may have an alteration in the tubular handling of urate. **Between 80% and 90% of patients with hyperuricosuric nephrolithiasis are men,** opposed to about 70% of calcium stone patients without hyperuricosuria. Coe (1978) and Fellstrom and colleagues (1982) have found that patients with hyperuricosuria have higher rates of stone formation than patients with hypercalciuric calcium nephrolithiasis. **Patients with hyperuricosuria tend to have more severe symptoms, as evidenced by the number of procedures that they undergo, in comparison to those without hyperuricosuria** (Coe, 1978). Patients with mixed uric acid and calcium oxalate stones have lower urinary pH than patients with pure calcium oxalate stones.

Management of Hyperuricosuric Calcium Nephrolithiasis

Dietary purine restriction, in theory, should prevent hyperuricosuria and nephrolithiasis (Appendix A). This requires limiting red meat, poultry, and fish. Both Coe and Pak, however, have had difficulty in obtaining patient compliance with this diet. Therefore, Coe "like cowards, gives **allopurinol**" (Coe and Parks, 1988). Allopurinol inactivates xanthine oxidase and decreases uric acid synthesis. Allopurinol is well tolerated, the principal side effects being a rare skin rash and hepatic enzyme abnormalities.

Hypocitraturia

This chapter in the 6th edition of *Campbell's Urology* did not feature hypocitraturia as a cause of calcium oxalate stone disease; yet, today, hypocitraturia is considered to be a major, correctable cause of calcium oxalate nephrolithiasis. A role for decreased urinary citrate excretion in the pathogenesis of calcareous calculi has been postulated since the 1930s, when Sabatini demonstrated the ability of citric acid to complex with calcium (Scott et al, 1943). In 1934, Boothby and Adams showed that urinary excretion of citrate was decreased in two patients with renal calculi. These findings were largely ignored, however, when it was shown that urinary citrate excretion was decreased only in patients with a urinary tract infection, the assumption being that hypocitraturia was the result of bacterial infection (Conway et al, 1979). Rudman and colleagues (1980), Menon and Mahle (1983c), and Nicar and colleagues (1983) rediscovered that urinary citrate excretion was decreased in patients with renal calculi. **Hypocitraturia has been reported in 15% to 63% of patients with nephrolithiasis** (Menon and Mahle, 1983a; Pak, 1987a). **In about 10% of patients, hypocitraturia exists as an isolated anomaly; in the rest, it coexists with other metabolic abnormalities** (Menon and Mahle, 1983a; Pak et al, 1985a). Urinary citrate is normally greater in women than in men and in premenopausal than in postmenopausal women (Pak, 1990). Because of this, different normal ranges for urinary citrate have been established by different laboratories. Hypocitraturia is more common in stone-forming women than in men (Parks and Coe, 1986; Pak, 1990).

Much of the understanding about hypocitraturic calcium nephrolithiasis comes from the work of Pak and colleagues (Pak et al, 1986b; Nicar et al, 1987; Pak, 1987a). The Dallas group defines the low normal limit for citrate as 220 mg/day for both men and women, regardless of age, whereas Menon and Mahle (1983c) define hypocitraturia as citrate excretion

of less than 0.60 mmol (115 mg) in men and 1.03 mmol (200 mg) in women. Causes of hypocitraturic calcium nephrolithiasis are outlined in Table 91–6 (Pak, 1990). **Acidosis is probably the most important etiologic factor in hypocitraturia.** In patients with inflammatory bowel disease and chronic diarrhea, intestinal alkali loss results in metabolic acidosis (Rudman et al, 1980). A decrease in urinary magnesium excretion results in a decreased complexation of citrate in the urine and increased absorption of citrate in the proximal tubule. Thiazide-induced hypokalemia and intracellular acidosis are other causes of decreased urinary citrate excretion (Morris, 1985; Pak et al, 1985b; Preminger et al, 1985). A diet rich in animal protein may produce an acid load (Breslau et al, 1988). Strenuous physical exercise and increased sodium intake can likewise produce hypocitraturia. Urinary tract infection with bacteria degrading citrate lowers urinary citrate excretion.

The primary mechanism of action of citrate is as a complexing agent for calcium. Calcium citrate complexes are considerably more soluble than calcium oxalate. In addition, citrate inhibits the spontaneous nucleation of calcium oxalate, the crystal growth of calcium oxalate and phosphate, and the aggregation of calcium oxalate or calcium phosphate (Tiselius et al, 1993b). Tiselius and colleagues demonstrated that physiologic concentrations of citrate inhibited calcium oxalate monohydrate sedimentation and aggregation (Tiselius et al, 1993a). Hess and colleagues (1993) demonstrated that citrate restored the inhibitory reactivity of Tamm-Horsfall protein in stone formers.

Fegan and colleagues measured the gastrointestinal absorption of citrate in patients with idiopathic hypocitraturia and in control subjects (Fegan et al, 1992). They found no difference in citrate absorption between the two groups. Greater than 90% of administered citrate was absorbed, suggesting that impaired gastrointestinal absorption of citrate is unlikely to be the cause of hypocitraturia in recurrent calcium oxalate stone disease.

Minisola and colleagues examined the renal handling of citrate in normal controls and patients with kidney stones (Minisola et al, 1989). Serum citrate levels were similar in the two groups, but 24-hour urinary citrate and the fasting citrate-to-creatinine ratio was significantly reduced in stone formers. **The tubular resorption of citrate was increased in kidney stone patients, suggesting that this, and not decreased intestinal absorption of citrate, may be the cause of hypocitraturia in patients with renal calculi.**

Table 91–6. CAUSES OF HYPOCITRATURIC CALCIUM NEPHROLITHIASIS

Distal renal tubular acidosis
  Complete
  Incomplete
Chronic diarrheal syndrome
Thiazide-induced hypocitraturia
Idiopathic
  Diet high in animal protein
  Strenuous physical exercise
  High sodium intake
  Active urinary tract infection
  Intestinal malabsorption of citrate

From Pak CYC: *In* Resnick MI, Pak CYC, eds: Urolithiasis: A Medical and Surgical Reference. Philadelphia, W. B. Saunders, 1990, p 94.

Hypomagnesuria

Many experimental studies have suggested that administration of magnesium salts prevents stone disease. Rats fed a pyridoxine-deficient diet tend to form stones, prevented by the addition of magnesium (Andrus et al, 1960). Melnick and associates reported that the stone belt in the southeastern United States roughly corresponds to a region with magnesium-deficient soil (Melnick et al, 1971). King and co-workers found that a low urinary magnesium-to-calcium ratio was present in many patients with stones (King et al, 1968). Some reports show decreased urinary magnesium excretion in patients with stone disease, whereas others do not. In the large series from Dallas (Preminger et al, 1989), hypomagnesuria with calcium stones was detected in 4.3% of patients. Johansson and colleagues compared the metabolism of magnesium in 70 patients who formed stones and 58 matched controls (Johansson et al, 1980). The intestinal absorption of magnesium was similar in both groups. Serum and urinary magnesium levels were not different in the two groups. The muscular content of magnesium and the retention of an intravenously administered magnesium load were also identical, indicating that stone formers did not have magnesium deficiency. Patients who formed stones excreted more calcium in their urine than controls. These observations led to the conclusion that dietary deficiency and negative magnesium balance are not found in patients who formed stones. The low urinary magnesium-to-calcium ratio in Johansson's patients appeared to be related more to hypercalciuria than hypomagnesuria. King and co-workers believe, however, that the magnesium-to-calcium ratio is an independent risk factor in stone formation, even when corrected for urinary calcium levels (King et al, 1968).

By far, **the most common cause of overt hypomagnesuria is inflammatory bowel disease associated with malabsorption.** Most patients with hypomagnesuria also have hypocitraturia (Preminger et al, 1989). This loss of inhibitory or complexing activity of magnesium or citrate (or both) is responsible for calcium oxalate crystallization in these individuals. Several clinical trials have examined the efficacy of magnesium therapy for the prevention of stone recurrences. Gershoff and Prien (1967) showed a remission rate of 89% and a decrease in stone episode rate from 1.3 to 0.1 per patient per year during treatment with magnesium oxide and pyridoxine. Melnick and associates reported a decrease in stone rate from 1.45 to 0.31 during the first 2 years of magnesium oxide therapy and to 0.11 during the second 2 years (Melnick et al, 1971). Patients who were not treated with magnesium had rates of 1.52, 0.86, and 0.64 over 4 years. Johansson and colleagues found that stones recurred in 12% of treated and 44% of control subjects at 2 years of follow-up (Johansson et al, 1980). A randomized clinical trial by Ettinger and co-workers showed no differences in recurrence rates between treated and untreated patients (Ettinger et al, 1985). Details of randomization were not given, however, and the patients were not described in detail. Lindberg and associates suggested that the beneficial effects of magnesium on urinary biochemistry occur only when magnesium salts were provided with meals and not on an empty stomach (Lindberg et al, 1990a). In none of the studies is it clear that this was emphasized. They suggest that **magnesium citrate may be the ideal agent for the** treatment of hypomagnesuric calcium nephrolithiasis (Lindberg et al, 1990b; Pak, 1990).

Multiple Metabolic Abnormalities

Although the derangements presented here have been discussed as separate and distinct, in many patients these abnormalities coexist with one another. Menon and Mahle (1983a) originally reported that 26 of 52 consecutive patients with calcium oxalate renal lithiasis seen over a 1-year period had hyperoxaluria. Of the patients with hyperoxaluria, 48% had hypercalciuria, 38% had hyperuricosuria, and 21% had hypocitraturia. Hyperoxaluria occurred as an isolated abnormality in only 12% of patients. Laminski and associates found associated metabolic abnormalities in three fourths of their patients with mild hyperoxaluria (Laminski et al, 1991). Pak (1990) reported that analysis of urine samples from 3473 stone-forming patients revealed hypercalciuria in 41%. Among these, 25% had hyperuricosuria, 23% had hyperoxaluria, and 17% had hypocitraturia. These data suggest that patients with nephrolithiasis may have a nonspecific abnormality in intestinal or renal handling of the metabolites involved in stone formation.

Sex Hormones and Renal Stones

Calcium oxalate renal stones occur much more frequently in men than in women. Even when a disease such as hyperparathyroidism, which has a distinct female preponderance, is considered, the proportion of male stone formers is greater than that of female stone formers (Robertson et al, 1978; Wikstrom et al, 1983). Similarly, hyperoxaluria is present in all patients following jejunoileal bypass; yet, only 8 of 84 women (10%) as opposed to 6 of 14 men (42%) seen by the authors developed calcium oxalate stones (unpublished observations).

Several observations suggest that sex hormones play a role in the pathogenesis of renal stones. Estrogen, progesterone, and testosterone modulate the synthesis of 1,25-dihydroxyvitamin D_3 and the intestinal absorption of calcium by stimulating 1α-hydroxylase in the kidney (De Luca, 1980). Some investigators have found that urinary citrate excretion is greater in normal women than in men but drops to a greater extent in women with stones than in men with stones (Ljunghall and Hedstrand, 1978; Menon and Mahle, 1983c). Testosterone increases renal oxalate deposition and urinary oxalate excretion in castrated rats fed diets supplemented with glycolate (Bell et al, 1979). In one study, the administration of estrogens decreased urinary oxalate excretion in patients with primary hyperoxaluria (Tiselius et al, 1980). Tiselius and colleagues (1980) and Zarembski and Hodgkinson (1969) found that urinary oxalate excretion did not change significantly in patients with metastatic prostate cancer undergoing castration. Similarly, Drach (1976) was unable to detect any correlation between plasma testosterone concentrations and urinary oxalate excretion. Van Aswegen and colleagues found that urinary testosterone levels were *lower* in young stone patients than in matched controls (Van Aswegen et al, 1989). They suggested that low testosterone results in low urokinase, which, in turn, leads to high uromucoid concentrations. They postulate that the elevation of uromucoid may predispose to calcium oxalate crystal aggregation and stone formation. Although there is a distinct male preponderance to calcium oxalate nephrolithiasis and although sex steroid hormones may influence the metabolism of factors involved in stone formation, their role in the pathogenesis of stone formation remains to be defined.

Calcium Phosphate Stones and Renal Tubular Acidosis

Stones composed predominantly of calcium phosphate average around 10% of stones of renal origin (Gault et al, 1988, 1991). Although some amount of calcium phosphate is often found in calcium oxalate calculi, pure calcium phosphate stones are quite rare. Such stones are more common in women and are often associated with tubular acidification defects (Gault et al, 1988, 1989, 1991) **Calcium phosphate stones occur only when the chemical pressure for crystallization is quite high and, thus, are usually seen in active stone disease** (Tiselius and Larson, 1993). **If a stone analysis comes back showing pure calcium phosphate, a search for distal renal tubular acidosis is mandated; rarely, the authors have seen such stones in primary hyperparathyroidism and sarcoidosis.**

Renal Tubular Acidosis

Renal tubular acidosis (RTA) (MIM #17980) is a clinical syndrome that results from specific defects in renal tubular H^+ secretion and urinary acidification. If the kidneys lose some of their ability to lower urinary pH, the resulting higher pH increases the divalent and trivalent forms of phosphate, which raises calcium phosphate supersaturation (Coe et al, 1992b). Three major types of RTA—I, II, and IV—are currently recognized.

Type I (Distal) Renal Tubular Acidosis

Distal RTA is characterized by hypokalemic, hyperchloremic, non–anion gap metabolic acidosis and a urinary pH consistently above 6.0. The primary abnormality is the inability of the distal nephron to establish and maintain a proton gradient between tubular fluid and the blood. At least four major pathogenic mechanisms have been identified: a permeability defect, a proton pump secretory defect, a voltage-dependent defect, and carbonic anhydrase deficiency (Pohlman et al, 1984).

Distal RTA may present as an isolated entity or may be the secondary manifestation of a variety of systemic and renal disorders. More than two thirds of patients with distal RTA are adults, and one third are children, mostly infants. Infants generally present with vomiting or diarrhea, failure to thrive, and growth retardation. Children present with metabolic bone disease and renal stones. Adults present with symptoms referable to nephrolithiasis and nephrocalcinosis.

Up to 70% of adults with distal RTA have kidney stones (Caruana and Buckalew, 1988). Symptoms referable to nephrolithiasis were the presenting manifestation in about 50% of patients with RTA seen in the Mayo Clinic (Van Den Berg, 1987). Stone disease in RTA is often severe enough to cause considerable morbidity and even mortality.

RTA is endemic in the northeast plateau of Thailand, where it can present with hypokalemic periodic paralysis and sudden unexplained nocturnal death (Nimmannit et al, 1991). Primary distal RTA is usually sporadic in occurrence; however, a hereditary form with an autosomal dominant mode of inheritance has been reported (Pohlman et al, 1984; Buckalew and Caruana, 1985). Patients with familial RTA usually present in childhood. Secondary and sporadic forms may present at any age; **up to 80% of the patients are women.** Urologists need to be aware that obstructive uropathy, pyelonephritis, acute tubular necrosis, renal transplantation, analgesic nephropathy, sarcoidosis, idiopathic hypercalciuria, and primary hyperparathyroidism can lead to secondary RTA (Buckalew, 1989).

The stones of distal RTA are calcium phosphate (brushite), although oxalate and struvite stones may be seen also. Stone formation typically occurs in the papillary tips and in the medulla. Cortical nephrolithiasis and nephrocalcinosis are unusual. Typical plain radiographic and ultrasonic presentations of type I RTA are shown in Figure 91–10. In one study, all patients with distal RTA followed 6 to 18 years developed renal cysts, usually multiple and bilateral. These cysts may arise from dilation of the distal tubules caused by hypokalemia.

Figure 91–11 shows the physiologic basis for the clinical features seen in patients with distal RTA. **Stone formation is the result of hypercalciuria, hypocitraturia, and increased urinary pH.** Hypercalciuria is the result of the effects of systemic acidosis on bone demineralization and secondary hyperparathyroidism as the result of decreased production of 1,25-dihydroxyvitamin D_3. Hypocitraturia results from a primary defect in renal tubular citrate transport, again, the result of metabolic acidosis. Urinary citrate levels may be less than 50 mg per 24 hours in the presence of systemic acidosis (Smith, 1986). Systemic acidosis increases transmitochondrial citrate transport and mitochondrial citrate metabolism (Osther et al, 1989). **Hypocitraturia is probably the most important metabolic factor for stone formation in patients with type I RTA.**

Type II (Proximal) Renal Tubular Acidosis

As in type I RTA, hypokalemic, hyperchloremic non–anion gap metabolic acidosis also occurs in type II RTA. Because distal tubular function is intact, however, the kidney is able to create a proton gradient and acidify urine appropriately. **The primary defect here is a failure of bicarbonate resorption in the proximal tubule leading to urinary bicarbonate excretion.** At normal serum bicarbonate levels, greater than 15% of the filtered load of bicarbonate is lost. Type II RTA is usually associated with a disorder of proximal tubular dysfunction known as Fanconi's syndrome, manifested by increased urinary excretion of glucose, amino acids, uric acid, and phosphate in addition to bicarbonate (Rocher and Tannon, 1986). The defect in proximal tubular bicarbonate absorption is associated with increased urinary citrate excretion. **Thus, most individuals believe that nephrolithiasis and nephrocalcinosis do not occur in patients with classic proximal RTA.** Three reports (Backman et al, 1980b; Tessitore et al, 1985; Jaeger et al, 1986a) go against conventional wisdom and suggest that nephrolithiasis can

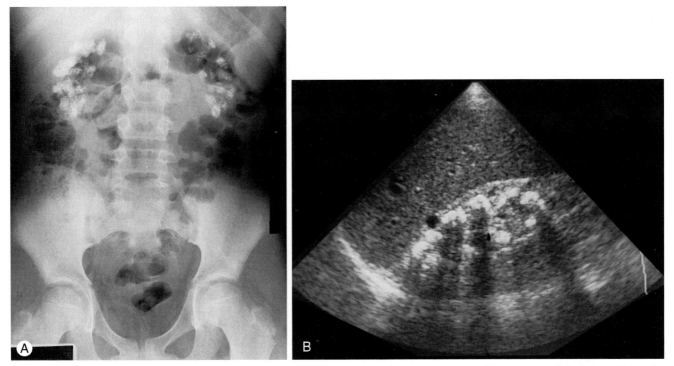

Figure 91–10. Plain radiographic *(A)* and ultrasonic *(B)* presentations of nephrocalcinosis. (Courtesy of Department of Radiology, University of Massachusetts, Worcester, MA.)

occur in patients with type II RTA. Buckalew and Caruana (1985) have suggested, however, that these patients may be better characterized as having incomplete type I RTA. Tesitore and colleagues found that 8 of 28 stone formers with renal hypercalciuria had reduced bicarbonate resorption, indicating the presence of type II RTA (Tesitore et al, 1985). Jaeger and associates demonstrated many defects in tubular function in patients with stone disease, including increased fractional excretion of glucose, insulin, phosphate, and uri-

nary lysozyme (Jaeger et al, 1986). In their study, 35% of stone formers had an increased fractional excretion of bicarbonate.

Type III Renal Tubular Acidosis

This syndrome is a hybrid of types I and II and was formerly used to describe infants who manifested both renal bicarbonate wasting and a disorder of distal renal acidifica-

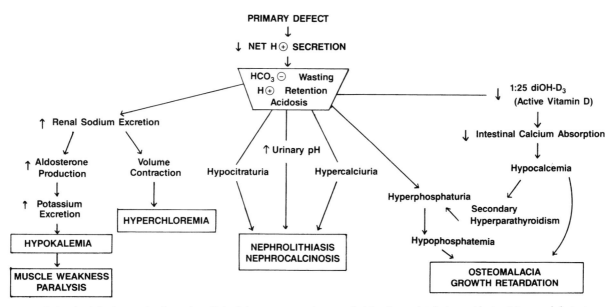

Figure 91–11. Pathophysiologic mechanisms for clinical features seen in type 1 (distal) renal tubular acidosis. Primary defects in renal acid excretion lead directly and through hormonally mediated pathways to metabolic abnormalities that produce the clinical syndromes seen in renal tubular acidosis. (From Kinkead TM, Menon M: AUA Update 1995; 14:54.)

tion. This syndrome is now considered a variant of distal RTA (Kinkead and Menon, 1995).

Type IV Renal Tubular Acidosis

Nephrolithiasis and nephrocalcinosis are uncommon in type IV renal tubular acidosis, a disorder commonly seen in patients with diabetic nephropathy and interstitial renal disease. Chronic renal parenchymal damage results in moderate reductions in glomerular filtration rate, hyperkalemia, and hyperchloremic metabolic acidosis with reduced net acid excretion (Pohlman et al, 1984). Uriberri and colleagues examined urinary biochemistry in 12 patients with type IV RTA and matched controls with a similar degree of kidney impairment (Uriberri et al, 1994). Urinary citrate was low but not as low as in patients with type I RTA. Urinary pH, calcium, and uric acid were lower in patients with type IV RTA than in matched controls. **Thus, patients with type IV RTA do not make uric acid stones because their uric acid excretion is low, and they do not make calcium stones because their calcium excretion is low.**

Diagnosis

Table 91–7 indicates clinical circumstances under which an evaluation for RTA is indicated. The diagnosis of complete distal RTA is not difficult. **The patient has hypokalemia, hyperchloremia, metabolic acidosis, and a urine pH of 5.5 or greater.** The urine pH should be measured with a pH meter, in a specimen free of bacterial infection. **Urinary citrate is low, usually less than 50 mg per 24 hours.** Hypercalciuria is often seen.

If the urinary pH is greater than 5.5 but acidosis is mild or absent, the patient may have incomplete distal RTA or may be normal. Metabolic acidosis must then be induced, usually by means of oral ammonium chloride loading. The fasting patient is given 0.1 g of ammonium chloride per kg body weight in crushed granules mixed with a soft drink. Subsequently, hourly measurements of urinary pH and 2-hourly measurements of serum pH or bicarbonate are taken over 4 to 6 hours (Pohlman et al, 1984; Smith, 1986). If the serum pH falls below 7.32, or the bicarbonate falls below 16 mmol/L but urinary pH remains at or above 5.5, the diagnosis of incomplete distal RTA is confirmed. If at any time the urinary pH falls below 5.5, the diagnosis of incomplete distal RTA is excluded. Chafe and Gault (1994) found that 9 of 10 patients who had incomplete RTA diagnosed from the ammonium chloride load also had a first and second

Table 91–7. CLINICAL SITUATIONS IN WHICH AN EVALUATION FOR RENAL TUBULAR ACIDOSIS IS INDICATED

Calcium phosphate stones
Recurrent stones >2/year
Bilateral stones
Medullary nephrocalcinosis
Medullary sponge kidney
Hypocitraturia <0.5 mmol/24 hours
Hypokalemia
Chronic pyelonephritis
Azotemia

1) Obtain serum electrolytes and arterial blood gas— hypokalemic, hyperchloremic, non-anion gap metabolic acidosis

2) Rule out other causes of acidosis by history and physical exam

3) Obtain urinary pH (fasting morning specimen, under oil, pH meter)—If pH >5.5, diagnosis is complete distal RTA (Type 1)

4) If urinary pH >5.5, but systemic acidosis mild or absent, perform ammonium chloride loading test and measure urinary bicarbonate—if urine pH does not decrease to <5.5 after acid loading, diagnosis is incomplete distal RTA (iRTA)

5) If bicarbonaturia present, perform bicarbonate loading test—If fractional excretion of bicarbonate >15 percent at normal serum bicarbonate levels, diagnosis is proximal RTA (Type 2)

6) If hyperkalemia present, diagnosis is Type 4 RTA.

Figure 91–12. Diagnostic evaluation of renal tubular acidosis (RTA). (From Kinkead TM, Menon M: AUA Update 1995; 14:54.)

morning urine pH above 6.0. In contrast, only 4 of 100 individuals without incomplete RTA had a first and second morning urine pH at or above 6.0. **Thus, a first and second morning urine pH is a good screening test for the detection of incomplete RTA.** Alternatively the measurement of urinary pH following an oral dose of 40 mg of furosemide can be used as a screening test for the detection of renal tubular acidification defect (Reynolds et al, 1993).

Figure 91–12 gives a simplified approach to the diagnosis of RTA. This is a practical algorithm for the urologist to formulate guidelines for the treatment of patients with renal stones and RTA (Kinkead and Menon, 1995).

Therapy

Alkali therapy decreases stone growth and new stone formation, delays the development of nephrocalcinosis, normalizes retarded growth in children, and corrects the metabolic changes of hypokalemia (Rocher and Tannon, 1986). **Potassium bicarbonate or citrate (1–2 mmol/kg daily in two to three divided doses) corrects systemic acidosis and normalizes urinary citrate. The goal of treatment is to restore urinary citrate to high normal levels and not simply to correct metabolic acidosis.** Patients can continue to form stones in the absence of metabolic acidosis if urinary citrate remains low. Spot urine testing for *N*-acetylglucosaminidase, which is elevated with hypercalciuric renal tubular cell damage, has been recommended for monitoring therapy, eliminating the need of 24-hour urine collections, particularly in children (Sinaniotis et al, 1989). **If hypercalciuria persists on alkali therapy, a thiazide diuretic is added to the therapeutic regimen** (Coe et al, 1992).

Uric Acid Stones

Humans do not have the ability to convert the uric acid by-products of purine metabolism into the substance allantoin, which is freely water soluble (Yu, 1981). Therefore, humans have a level of uric acid in their system that is ten times greater than those of other mammals (Watts, 1976; Fanelli, 1977; Yu 1981). Humans not only produce excessive, relatively insoluble uric acid but also excrete urine that is predominantly acid because of the acid end products of metabolism. When uric acid enters human urine, it exists in two forms: free uric acid and urate salt, which forms a complex mostly with sodium. Sodium urate is approximately 20 times more soluble in water than free uric acid and does not crystallize under normal conditions.

Factors That Control Uric Acid Crystallization

The principal cause of uric acid crystallization is the supersaturation of urine with respect to undissociated uric acid (Finlayson and Smith, 1974a; Pak et al, 1977b). There is no known inhibitor of uric acid crystallization. Thus, if urine becomes supersaturated with uric acid, crystals precipitate. The solubility of undissociated uric acid in urine at a temperature of 37°C is about 100 mg/L (Coe et al, 1980b). The dissociation constant for the first proton of uric acid is near 5.35: At that pH, one half of the uric acid is ionized as urate salt, and the other half exists as free uric acid. Because normal 24-hour urinary uric acid excretion is between 500 and 600 mg per L of urine, urine is invariably supersaturated at a pH below 6. At a pH of 5, 1 L of urine can hold about 100 mg of uric acid in solution, whereas at a pH of 6, it can dissolve 500 mg of uric acid. Figure 91–13*A* shows the relationship between pH and the dissociation of uric acid. The curve is sigmoidal, and greater than 90% of uric acid is soluble at a pH of about 6.5.

Patients with uric acid stones often have prolonged periods of acidity in the urine. Normal individuals have variation in the pH of urine resulting from postprandial alkaline tides that take the pH well above 6.5. Millman and colleagues found that the mean pH of urine in patients with uric acid stones was 5.5 ± 0.4 (SEM) as compared with 6.0 ± 0.4 in patients who form calcium oxalate stones (Millman et al, 1982). Exogenous purines ingested with the evening meal result in the production of fixed acid, which further lowers urinary pH. In one study, the first morning urinary acid pH was greater than 5.7 in more than 26% of normal people, whereas only 10% of urine samples from patients

with gout or uric acid stones had a pH of 5.7 (Gutman and Yu, 1968).

Patients with gout excrete relatively less ammonium and more titratable acid than do normal subjects (Gutman and Yu, 1961). The exact mechanism for the low urinary ammonium level has not been worked out. Ammonia is produced in the tubular cell by the deamidization or deaminization of glutamine. It then diffuses into the tubular lumen, where it combines with a free proton, forming a nondiffusible NH^4 ion. The net result is buffering of urine to a more alkaline pH. This results in a decrease in the titratable acidity. A defect in glutamine deamination results in deficient renal NH_3 production and a more acid urine. The pKa of NH^{4+} is 9, so NH_3 can accept protons in the tubule where the pH is below 7 without lowering the pH. Urine NH^{4+} accounts normally for approximately 60% to 70% of acid excretion. Thus, a decrease in ammonia production can affect urinary pH profoundly.

Patients with gout or uric acid stones exhibit two other metabolic defects—overproduction of uric acid and an impaired renal uric acid excretion (Seegmiller et al, 1968; Wyngaarden and Kelley, 1972). The exact cause of uric acid overproduction in primary gout is unknown, it is not due to an enzymatic defect in uric acid biosynthesis (Benedict et al, 1952). It may be that many patients with uric acid stones or gout ingest more purines than people without these disorders. Patients with gout have a slight diminution of urate clearance also (Wyngaarden and Kelley, 1972). The ratio of urate to insulin clearance is lower in patients with gout than in normal subjects at any serum urate concentration. Finally, patients with uric acid urolithiasis often excrete a reduced volume of urine (Atsmon et al, 1963; Toor et al, 1964; Sakhaee et al, 1987). These patients may live in hot climates, work in hot places, be dehydrated because of diarrhea, or simply not like to drink much water. Coe and Parks (1988) suggest that certain occupations, such as bus drivers, surgeons, or investment bankers (long meetings), may predispose to uric acid stone formation.

Three factors are involved in uric acid urolithiasis. First, patients tend to excrete excessively acid urine at relatively fixed, low urinary pH. Second, they may absorb, produce, or excrete more uric acid than patients

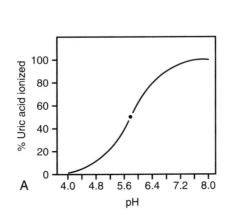
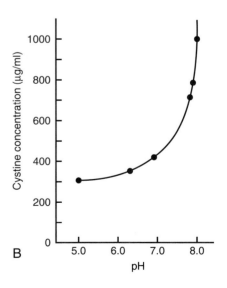

Figure 91–13. *A,* Dissociation of uric acid. At pH of 5.75, one half of uric acid is ionized as urate salts and is therefore soluble. As pH increases, more becomes ionized and soluble. *B,* Solubility of cystine in relation to urinary pH. (*A* from Gutman AB, Yu TF: Am J Med 1968; 45:756. *B* from Dent CE, Senior B: Studies on the treatment of cystinuria. Br J Urol 1955; 27:317. Blackwell Scientific Publications, Ltd.)

without gout or uric acid stones. Third, urinary volume is diminished in these patients. The combination of these factors is ideal for the crystallization of uric acid in the urine.

Clinical Picture

Uric acid stones are seen in 1 in 1000 adults in the United States, accounting for 5% to 10% of all renal stones. Between 75% and 80% of uric acid stones are composed of pure uric acid; the rest contain calcium oxalate (Uhlman, 1972; Pak and Holt, 1976). In Israel, Atsmon and colleagues have reported that 75% of stones are composed of uric acid (Atsmon et al, 1963).

This condition exists in both a sporadic and a familial form (Gutman and Yu, 1968). Women and men are affected equally, and an ethnic predilection for Jews and Italians has been seen (Melick and Henneman, 1958). The familial variety is transmitted as an autosomal dominant trait. In the absence of treatment, recurrence is the rule.

Secondary Uric Acid Stones

The frequency of uric acid stones in gout is about 20%. Hall and co-workers found that 12% of men with uric acid levels between 7 and 8 mg/dl, 22% of men with levels between 8 and 9 mg/dl, and 40% of men with levels greater than 9 mg/dl had renal stones (Hall et al, 1967). Eleven percent of patients with urinary uric acid excretion less than 300, 21% of patients between 300 and 699, 35% of patients between 700 and 1100, and 50% of patients more than 1100 mg per 24 hours developed uric acid stones (Yu and Gutman, 1967). In another study, the risk of stones in gout was roughly 1% per year after the first attack of gout (Fessel, 1979). Occasionally individuals have specific enzyme defects, such as increased activity of 5-phosphoribosyl-1-pyrophosphate synthetase, the enzyme that initiates purine metabolism. High levels of serum uric acid are seen in patients with the Lesch-Nyhan syndrome, who have a deficiency or complete lack of the enzyme hypoxanthine-guanine phosphoribosyl transferase. This results in a shunting of hypoxanthine to the xanthine/uric acid pathway with resultant hyperuricemia and extreme hyperuricosuria.

Myeloproliferative disorders such as acute leukemia are an important cause of severe hyperuricosuria, particularly in childhood. Patients should be placed on allopurinol before the time they are treated to avoid this problem. Cytotoxic chemotherapy results in cell necrosis, liberating large amounts of nucleic acids, which are converted to uric acid. Massive hyperuricosuria may result, the crystals plugging the intrarenal collecting system and both ureters. This can occur in the absence of ureteric colic and result in oliguria or anuria (Kjellstrand et al, 1974; Conger, 1981).

Evaluation

Evaluation of patients with uric acid lithiasis requires observation of daily urinary pH, by measuring and recording the pH of every voiding with Nitrazine or other pH paper, determining the serum and urinary uric acid levels, assessing the degree of ingestion of dietary purines, and analyzing the work and play conditions for dehydration. If the patient has

evidence of hyperuricemia, evaluation should include a brief survey to rule out myeloproliferative or neoplastic disease (Seftel and Resnick, 1990).

Uric acid stones are the most common radiolucent urinary calculus and may form staghorn stones (Fig. 91–14). Uric acid lithiasis may be associated with urinary obstruction through showers of small crystals rather than a single large stone. For this reason, microscopic examination of the urine can be helpful both in diagnosing uric acid urolithiasis and in determining therapy success. Patients under medical control should not have evidence of uric acid crystals in the urine at any time.

Therapy

Hydration, alkali, allopurinol, and diet are the cornerstones for the treatment for uric acid stones. The goal of therapy is to make urine undersaturated with uric acid. Any combination of therapeutic modalities that achieves this goal is effective.

Initial and immediate therapy involves instructing the patient to drink enough fluids to ensure urinary output in excess of 1500 to 2000 ml/day and verifying that the instructions are followed. The urine should be alkalinized to a level between 6.5 and 7.0. It is not necessary to raise the pH above 7.0: This may actually be detrimental, allowing precipitation of monosodium urate or apatite. The form of the alkali may be sodium bicarbonate 650 mg or more every 6 to 8 hours or balanced citrate solutions at doses of 15 to 30 ml three to four times a day (Thomas, 1975; Drach, 1976). Sakhaee and co-workers suggest that potassium citrate is the treatment of choice (Sakhaee et al, 1983). At a dose of 30 to 60 mEq/day, potassium citrate increased urinary pH from a mean of 5.3 to above 6.2 but less than 7.0. Sodium citrate may be as effective as potassium citrate in preventing uric acid nephrolithiasis; however, it may increase urinary calcium excretion and promote urate-induced crystallization of calcium oxalate (Pak et al, 1983; Sakhaee et al, 1983). Coe and Parks (1988) suggest that the last dose of alkali be given at bedtime and nocturnal urinary pH be checked with a pH paper to make sure that the pH remains above 6.5 at night. If the pH falls below 6.5, they suggest a single dose of 250 mg of acetazolamide, a carbonic anhydrase inhibitor (Coe and Parks, 1988). **If the patient has hyperuricemia or if urinary uric acid excretion is greater than 1200 mg/day, the patient should be treated with allopurinol, 300 to 600 mg/day in addition.** This drug inhibits the conversion of hypoxanthine and xanthine to uric acid. Complications of allopurinol include skin rash, drug fever, or an attack of acute gout. Rarely an exfoliative skin reaction with hemorrhagic skin lesions and systemic vasculitis can occur (Young et al, 1974; Ellman et al, 1975). Skin reactions are preceded by itching, which is an indication for stopping the drug treatment. The major side effect of sodium bicarbonate is excessive flatulence. This is one condition in which medical therapy is successful in dissolving pre-existing renal stones. The authors have seen partial and near-complete staghorn calculi of uric acid stones dissolving within a matter of a few days with alkalinization and hydration.

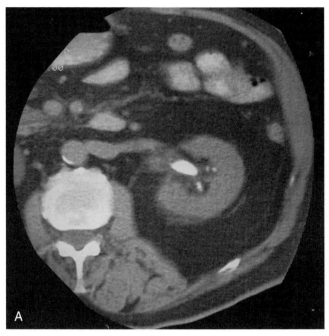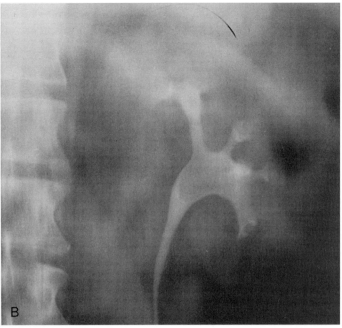

Figure 91–14. *A,* Nonenhanced computed tomography scan of uric acid calculus in the left renal pelvis. *B,* Intravenous pyelogram shows a negative well-demarcated shadow of uric acid calculus in renal pelvis. (Courtesy of Department of Radiology, University of Massachusetts, Worcester, MA.)

Struvite Stones (Infection Stones)

The earliest type of stone known to afflict humankind was the struvite stone. The mineral magnesium phosphate hexahydrate was identified in part by the Swedish geologist Ulex who named it *struvite* in honor of the Russian diplomat and naturalist H. C. G. Von-struve (Dana, 1920). **The stone is composed of magnesium, ammonium, and phosphate, mixed with carbonate.** Struvite calculi have also been commonly referred to as *infection* or *triple-phosphate* stones and account for 2% to 20% of all stones (Herring, 1962; Sharma et al, 1989).

Pathogenesis

Much of the understanding about the pathogenesis of struvite stones comes from the work of Griffith and colleagues (Griffith and Musher, 1973; Griffith and Obsorn, 1987). **Two conditions must coexist for the crystallization of struvite—a urine pH of 7.2 or above and the presence of ammonia in the urine** (Nemoy and Stamey, 1971). **The driving force behind struvite stones is infection of the urine with urease-producing bacteria.** In 1901, Brown proposed that the splitting of urea by bacteria results in ammoniacal urine, alkalinity, and stone formation. It was suggested that a bacterial enzyme, urease, was responsible for the hydrolysis of urea (Hagar and Magath, 1925).

Urease-producing bacteria hydrolyze urea to carbon dioxide and ammonium molecules:

$$NH_2-CO-NH_2 + H_2O \xrightarrow{\text{urease}} 2NH_3 + CO_2$$

The pK of ammonia is 9; thus, they take up hydrogen ions from water to become ammonium:

$$NH_3 + H_2O \rightarrow NH_4^+ + OH^-$$

Carbon dioxide is hydrated to carbonic acid (pK = 4.5), which dissociates to bicarbonate (pK = 6.33) and proton:

$$CO_2 + H_2O \rightarrow H_2CO_3$$

Further breakdown of bicarbonate results in the production of two hydrogen ions and one carbonate ion (pK = 10.1):

$$H_2CO_3 \rightarrow H^+ + HCO_3^- \rightarrow 2H^+ + CO_3^{2-}$$

Thus, the hydrolysis of urea releases both an acid (carbonic acid) and a base (ammonia). Because two molecules of ammonia are produced from one molecule of urea, neutralization of the base is incomplete. As a result of this, the urinary pH rises.

Bacteriology

Table 91–8 lists bacteria that produce urease. By far, the most common organism associated with struvite calculi is *P. mirabilis* (Silverman and Stamcy, 1983). It should be noted that *E. coli*, although associated with kidney stones, does not produce urease. *Ureaplasma urealyticum* produces urease that may hydrolyze urea at low urinary pH (Hedelin et al, 1984).

A second mechanism by which bacterial infection may induce stone formation is by increasing crystal adherence. Parsons and colleagues demonstrated that ammonium damages the glycosaminoglycan layer that covers normal bladder mucosa and allows bacterial adherence to the mucosal surface (Parsons et al, 1984). The removal of this layer from rat bladder increases the adherence of struvite crystals to the bladder (Grenabo et al, 1988.) Griffith and Osborne

Table 91–8. ORGANISMS THAT MAY PRODUCE UREASE

Organisms	Usually (>90% of Isolates)	Occasionally (5%–30% of Isolates)
Bacteria		
Gram-negative	*Proteus rettgeri*	*Klebsiella pneumoniae*
	Proteus vulgaris	*Klebsiella oxytoca*
	Proteus mirabilis	*Serratia marcescens*
	Proteus morganii	*Haemophilus parainfluenzae*
	Providencia stuartii	*Bordetella bronchiseptica*
	Haemophilus influenzae	*Aeromonas hydrophila*
	Bordetella pertussis	*Pseudomonas aeruginosa*
	Bacteroides corrodens	*Pasteurella* spp.
	Yersinia enterocolitica	
	Brucella spp.	
	Flavobacterium spp.	
Gram-positive	*Staphylococcus aureus*	*Staphylococcus epidermidis*
	Micrococcus varions	*Bacillus* spp.
	Corynebacterium ulcerans	*Corynebacterium murium*
	Corynebacterium renale	*Corynebacterium equi*
	Corynebacterium ovis	*Peptococcus asaccharolyticus*
	Corynebacterium hofmannii	*Clostridium tetani*
		Mycobacterium rhodochrous group
Mycoplasma	T-strain *Mycoplasma*	
	Ureaplasma urealyticum	
Yeasts	*Cryptococcus*	
	Rhodotorula	
	Sporobolmyces	
	Candida humicola	
	Trichosporon cutaneum	

From Gleeson MJ, Griffith DP: Infection stones. *In* Resnick MI, Pak CYC, eds: Urolithiasis: A Medical and Surgical Reference. Philadelphia, W. B. Saunders, 1990, p 115.

(1987) have proposed that bacterial infection may in a similar manner damage the glycosaminoglycan layer within the renal collecting system. This facilitates bacterial adherence, tissue inflammation, production of an organic matrix, and crystal matrix interaction.

Although it is accepted that urease-producing bacteria cause struvite stones, the role of non–urease-producing bacteria in stone disease is less clear. In one study (Holmgren et al, 1989), 371 of 1325 patients hospitalized with stone disease had positive cultures at some time during follow-up. Surprisingly, *E. coli* was the most common microorganism identified on urine culture, the prevalence being even higher than that of *Proteus*. Of the patients with an *E. coli* infection, 13% had struvite calculi. Dutoit and colleagues demonstrated that *E. coli* decreases urokinase and increases sialidase activity (Dutoit et al, 1989). This may lead to the production of urinary matrix substances, increasing crystal adherence to the renal epithelium. This altered enzymatic activity may explain the association between non–urease-producing bacteria and struvite stones.

Clinical Presentation

Struvite calculi account for the majority of staghorn stones observed in most countries (Fig. 91–15). They can grow quite large and may fill the collecting system. Struvite stones can form on a nidus of calcium oxalate stones and can grow quite rapidly. Most infection stones are radiopaque, but poorly mineralized matrix stones are faintly radiopaque or radiolucent. Women, perhaps because of their increased susceptibility to urinary tract infections, are more commonly affected than men (Resnick, 1981; Silverman and Stamey, 1983). Two other urologic conditions contribute to the ten-

dency to form struvite calculi—the presence of a foreign body in the urinary tract and neurogenic bladder. Comarr and associates found that 8% of patients with spinal cord injury developed infection stones (Comarr et al, 1962). Patients with indwelling Foley catheters, urinary diversion, or lower tract voiding dysfunction are prone to develop these stones (Comarr et al, 1962; Koff and Lapides, 1977).

Struvite calculi harbor infective bacteria within their interstices (Nemoy and Stamey, 1971; Thompson and Stamey, 1973). Indeed, bacteria have been cultured from the cores of stones that have been stored in formalin for several years. The penetration of antibiotics into these stones is inadequate for cure; therefore, the presence of an infected urinary calculus acts as a source for continued urinary infection. As long as infected urinary stones exist anywhere in the urinary tract, it is unlikely that the urinary system can be sterilized.

Patients with struvite stones may present acutely with fever, loin pain, dysuria, frequency, and hematuria. The combination of urinary tract obstruction plus fever can mimic an acute abdomen, and patients have been misdiagnosed as having appendicitis or generalized peritonitis. **A substantial proportion of patients present with symptoms of malaise, weakness, and loss of appetite.** Occasionally, patients develop xanthogranulomatous pyelonephritis, characterized by a nonfunctioning kidney or a portion of it and a mass lesion. The distinction between xanthogranulomatous pyelonephritis and a renal cell carcinoma may be difficult, particularly when the stone is small and the mass is large. Xanthogranulomatous pyelonephritis and carcinoma can coexist in the same kidney.

It is not clear whether patients with struvite stones also have associated metabolic abnormalities that predispose to

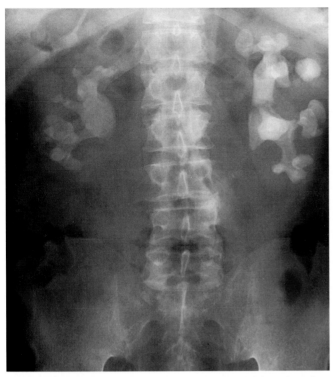

Figure 91–15. Kidney, ureter, bladder radiograph of bilateral staghorn stones. (Courtesy of Department of Radiology, University of Massachusetts, Worcester, MA.)

stone formation. Kristensen and co-workers demonstrated that such patients had a slightly reduced glomerular filtration rate compared with normal subjects, perhaps related to the size of the stones (Kristensen et al, 1987). They also found that urinary calcium excretion was increased in patients with struvite stones. Resnick (1981) has found that metabolic disorders are present in a substantial proportion of patients with infection stones. Other investigators, however, have not found this to be the case. Lingeman and colleagues have reviewed the literature and concluded that **metabolic abnormalities are present in patients with mixed calcium oxalate and struvite stones but not in patients with pure struvite stones** (Lingeman et al, 1995).

Treatment

Although it is widely accepted that patients presenting with acute symptoms should be treated, the authors have seen many patients with mildly symptomatic calculi being followed conservatively by internists and nephrologists in the prelithotripsy era. Blandy and Singh (1976) reported a 28% mortality within 20 years of follow-up in patients with staghorn calculi who were followed nonoperatively. All survivors had persistent pain and urinary tract infection. Vargas and colleagues demonstrated that only 1 of 22 staghorn calculi managed nonsurgically remained truly asymptomatic (Vargas et al, 1982). Seventeen (77%) had significant complications, two of which resulted in death within a follow-up period of 1 to 6 years. Thus, **patients with staghorn calculi should not be followed without treatment. The initial treatment is procedural to render the patient** stone-free, followed by supportive medical therapy to prevent recurrent urinary tract infection.

PROCEDURAL THERAPY

To cure infection stones, one needs to remove them completely. Open surgical procedures were the cornerstone of treatment for infection stones until the early 1980s (Table 91–9). In many patients, renal function improved with relief of intrarenal obstruction. The overall stone recurrence rate was 30%, and the risk of recurrent urinary tract infections was 40% (Griffith, 1978). **Percutaneous nephrolithotomy has been used increasingly for the treatment of staghorn calculi and has replaced open stone surgery in all but the rarest of instances.** At this point, anatrophic nephrolithotomy is relegated to the few patients who have a complete staghorn calculus associated with infundibular stenosis or distortion of intrarenal anatomy. Stone-free rates at 3 months with percutaneous approaches average about 60%. It is to be expected that with longer follow-up, the percentage of kidneys that are stone-free will drop. Percutaneous nephrolithotomy may be less expensive than anatrophic nephrolithotomy, require a shorter hospital stay, and allow a more rapid return to work (Charig et al, 1986; Lingeman et al, 1986; Snyder and Smith, 1986).

Extracorporeal shock wave lithotripsy (ESWL) is a less invasive procedure than percutaneous nephrolithotomy. When used as an isolated modality for the treatment of infection stones, stone-free results ranging from 30% to 66% have been achieved (see Table 91–9). Although most patients have residual stones at the time of discharge from the hospital, the stone-free rate increases over time as spontaneous passage of the stones occurs. The use of in situ irrigation increases the percentage of patients who are rendered stone-free (Rocco et al, 1988). Stone-free rates are greater in patients with smaller stones, particularly if they are not located in the lower pole of the kidney (Harada et al, 1988). In a large series, Wirth and Frohnmuller (1988) reported that 29% of patients with partial staghorn calculi and 48% of patients with complete staghorn calculi required multiple lithotripsies.

Most clinicians use a combination of percutaneous nephrolithotomy and ESWL for the treatment of patients with large staghorn calculi, particularly if many branches of the collecting system are involved. In a multicenter prospective, randomized study comparing ESWL monotherapy with combination therapy, Sohn and co-workers reported that only 30% of patients treated with ESWL monotherapy became stone-free compared with 54% of patients treated with a combination (Sohn et al, 1988). Lingeman and colleagues have reported that 92% of kidneys with partial staghorn calculi and 91% with complete staghorn calculi became stone-free after a three-stage procedure consisting of initial percutaneous nephrolithotomy, secondary ESWL, and repeat percutaneous nephrolithotomy with flushing out of residual stone debris (Lingeman et al, 1988).

MEDICAL TREATMENT

Antibiotics. Antibiotic therapy can sterilize the urine, reduce urinary pH, and thus render urine undersaturated with respect to struvite. This can result in complete or partial

Table 91–9. DIFFERENT METHODS OF TREATMENT OF STRUVITE CALCULI

Author	Year	No.	Technique	Residual/Recurrent Stones (%)
Smith & Boyce	1968	129	Open lithotomy	11
Wickham et al	1974	74	Open lithotomy	0
Boyce & Elkins	1974	60	Open lithotomy	18
Silverman & Stamey	1983	46	Open lithotomy and irrigation	20
Kerlan et al	1985	20	PCNL monotherapy	10
Snyder & Smith	1986	75	PCNL monotherapy	15
Lee et al	1986	124	PCNL monotherapy	15
Eisenberger et al	1987	42	PCNL monotherapy	31
Eisenberger et al	1987	31	ESWL monotherapy	50
Rocco et al	1988	84	ESWL monotherapy	47
Wirth & Frohnmuller	1988	174	ESWL monotherapy	46
Harada et al	1988	47	ESWL monotherapy	49
Pode et al	1988	41	ESWL monotherapy	56
Schulze et al	1986	87	PCNL + ESWL	42
Kahnoski et al	1986	36	PCNL + ESWL	15
Eisenberger et al	1987	78	PCNL + ESWL	40
Lingeman	1988	313	PCNL + ESWL	8

PCNL, Percutaneous nephrolithotomy; ESWL, extracorporeal shock wave lithotripsy.
Data from Coe and Parks, 1988; Gleeson and Griffith, 1990.

dissolution of the stone. **Long-term, culture-specific antimicrobials often reduce the bacterial burden, even if they do not completely sterilize the urine.** The reduction of bacterial colony count from 10^7 to 10^5 ml reduces urease production by 99% (Griffith and Osborne, 1987). **Bacteria are still located on the surface or within the lattice of the stones, however, and thus reinfection is common with cessation of antibiotic therapy.** The majority of urease-producing infections are caused by *P. mirabilis*, greater than 90% of which are sensitive to penicillin or ampicillin (Feit and Fair, 1979). Tetracyclines or fluoroquinolones such as ciprofloxacin or norfloxacin can be used for the treatment of patients with *Pseudomonas* or *Ureaplasma* urinary tract infections (Musher et al, 1975; Hedelin et al, 1984). Long-term antibiotic therapy is not recommended as prima facie treatment for patients with infection stones. **Antibiotics are an adjunct to procedural therapy and should be used to prevent stone recurrences or growth after operative procedures.**

Acetohydroxamic Acid. Acetohydroxamic acid, a chemical that has structural similarity to urea, is a potent, irreversible inhibitor of urease (Fishbein and Carbone, 1965). In 1973, Griffith and Musher showed that acetohydroxamic acid prevented the crystallization of struvite and carbonate apatite in vitro and in a rat model. Acetohydroxamic acid is rapidly absorbed from the gastrointestinal tract and reaches peak plasma levels after about 1 hour (Putcha et al, 1985). The half-life is 3.5 to 10 hours in normal subjects and 15 to 24 hours in patients with diminished renal function (Summerskill et al, 1967; Feldman et al, 1978).

The effectiveness of acetohydroxamic acid depends on its concentration in the urine. At doses of 250 mg every 8 hours, urinary concentrations of 15 to 30 mg/dl are usually achieved in patients with normal serum creatinine (Griffith et al, 1988b). When the serum creatinine exceeds 2.0 mg/dl, therapeutic concentrations of acetohydroxamic acid are usually not achievable.

There have been three double-blind, placebo-controlled trials of acetohydroxamic acid in patients with infection

stones, involving a total of 341 patients (Williams et al, 1984; Griffith et al, 1988b; Gleeson and Griffith, 1990). In each study, antibiotics were given concurrently. The side effects of therapy included deep vein thrombosis, tremor, headache, palpitations, edema, nausea, vomiting, diarrhea, loss of taste, hallucinations, rash, alopecia, abdominal pain, and anemia. Forty-five percent of Williams's patients, 68% of Griffith's patients, and 22% of Gleeson's patients had significant side effects, often resulting in withdrawal from the study. Of the placebo-treated patients, 46% to 60% had stone growth or recurrence within 24 months. In contrast, although sterile urine was not achieved in any patient, those treated with acetohydroxamic acid had only a 17% to 42% stone growth or recurrence rate. Griffith recommends that **acetohydroxamic acid be used in conjunction with antibiotic therapy in patients with infection stones in whom surgical intervention is contraindicated** (Griffith et al, 1988b).

Other inhibitors of urease include hydroxyurea, propionohydroxamic acid, chlorobenzamidoacetohydroxamic acid, hydroxycarbamide, nicotinohydroxamic acid, and flurofamide. These agents have not been studied extensively in humans. Details of their usage are given by Gleeson and Griffith (1990).

DIET

One of the earliest methods of treatment of struvite stones was alteration of diet (Shorr, 1945; Shorr and Carter, 1950) (Appendix B). A low-calcium, low-phosphorus diet with aluminum gels was recommended. Aluminum hydroxide or aluminum carbonate (basal gel) binds phosphate in the intestinal lumen to form insoluble aluminum phosphate. This decreases urinary phosphate excretion. In an early study, Lavengood and Marshall (1972) found that stones recurred in 19.8% of infected patients on the Shorr regimen compared with 30% of patients not on the regimen. In patients free of urinary tract infection, stone recurrences were 0% with the Shorr diet compared with 22% in patients not on the diet. Dietary compliance, however, was difficult.

IRRIGATION AND CHEMOLYSIS

One important aspect of medical treatment is the dissolution of calculi with irrigation. In 1938, Hellstrom used a combination of urinary antiseptic and acidifying agents for the dissolution of struvite calculi. Acidic solutions were also used by Suby and associates (1942) and Suby and Albright (1943). Mulvaney (1960) and Mulvaney and Hennings (1962) reported on hemiacidrin for dissolution of urinary calculi of struvite.

Nemoy and Stamey (1971), Blaivas and co-workers (1975), Jacobs and Gittes (1976), and Dretler and Pfister (1984) reviewed the development of hemiacidrin irrigation and the problems associated with it. For many years, reports in the literature indicated that this agent was extremely toxic and may have caused death. These investigators, however, state that in reviewing the literature they believed that the majority of patients who had toxicity with this irrigation technique were actually afflicted with severe urinary infection and sepsis. **All groups therefore now strongly recommend that the irrigation-dissolution technique be used only in a patient in whom the urinary tract infection is completely under control.** Hypermagnesemia must also be avoided (Cato and Tulloch, 1974).

Albright and co-workers observed that citric acid solutions would disintegrate predominantly calcium (apatite) stones not only because of the acid pH of the solutions, but also because of the formation of a calcium and citrate ion complex (Albright et al, 1948). Subsequent to the introduction of the "buffered" citrate solution by Albright, solutions G and M were developed by Suby.

These solutions have not always been effective in dissolving phosphate calculi. Mulvaney (1960), as noted, reported his experience with a new solvent designed especially for struvite and apatite calculi. This solution was called hemiacidrin (Renacidin). He stated that calcium phosphate, ammonium phosphate, and magnesium phosphate stones were soluble. The solvent appeared to have little effect on calcium oxalate and uric acid calculi. The technique for management of irrigation in suitable patients is thoroughly outlined in the article by Nemoy and Stamey (1971) and in Stamey's text (1972).

It is absolutely necessary that **no irrigation be attempted until the urine is completely sterile.** If surgery has been performed, a nephrostomy tube is left in place postoperatively. If the patient is in poor clinical condition and surgery is contraindicated, a percutaneous nephrostomy catheter may be inserted.

With either method, **the renal pelvis is first irrigated with a sterile saline solution at a rate of 120 ml/hour for 24 to 48 hours, beginning on the fourth or fifth postoperative day.** The height of irrigation is adjusted to the lowest level necessary to maintain the flow rate at 120 ml/hour. If there is leakage around a surgical drain or through the incision, irrigation is stopped until additional healing occurs. The patient is observed carefully for development of fever or any flank discomfort and for elevation of serum creatinine, magnesium, or phosphate levels (Dretler and Pfister, 1984). Occurrence of any of these conditions requires immediate cessation of irrigation.

If after 48 hours the patient's condition remains satisfactory and if there is no infection, no leakage, and no fever or flank discomfort, irrigation with an appropriate solution is begun. Flow rate is continued at 120 ml/hour through the irrigation tube or catheter. Nemoy and Stamey (1971), Jacobs and Gittes (1976), and Palmer and colleagues (1987) instruct their patients to stop the irrigation themselves if there is evidence of flank pain at any time.

The progress of irrigation is followed by obtaining radiographic tomographs of the calculi at intervals. Irrigation is continued for 24 to 48 hours after the last radiographically visible fragments have disappeared. In some instances, the rate of irrigation may be reduced to prevent irritation of the kidney or bladder, or sterile saline solutions may be alternated with irrigating solutions. Palmer and colleagues applied these concepts of treatment to outpatients (Palmer et al, 1987).

A cost/benefit analysis (Helal et al, 1995) has shown that a combination of percutaneous nephrolithotomy and ESWL is the most cost-effective treatment for patients with large struvite stones. Up to 50% of these patients, however, have stone recurrences or urinary tract infection (or both) over a 10-year follow-up. In contrast, Silverman and Stamey (1983) found only one stone recurrence in 46 kidneys treated with a combination of open surgery and chemolytic irrigation, after a mean follow-up of 7 years. Thus, it may be that traditional (i.e., outdated) surgical approaches provide the best therapeutic outcomes over the long term for patients with complex struvite stones.

Cystine Stones

Cystine stones account for about 1% of all urinary calculi in the United States and occur only in patients who have cystinuria (MIM 22010). Cystinuria is an autosomal recessive disorder of transmembrane cystine transport manifested in the intestine and in the kidney (Thier and Segal, 1972). In 1908, Garrod called cystinuria an inborn error of metabolism, but it is not. Cystinuria is a transepithelial transport defect, resulting in a decrease in cystine absorption in the intestine and of cystine resorption in the proximal renal tubule. Heterozygous cystinuria occurs in 1 out of 20 to 1 out of 200 individuals, whereas the homozygous cystinuria occurs in about 1 per 20,000 persons in the United States (Pak, 1990; Gleeson et al, 1992). Only homozygotes form cystine stones.

Cystine stones are radiopaque, although less so than calcium oxalate stones. The radiopacity is the result of the disulfide bond in cystine. **The stones are yellowish and have a waxy appearance. They are often multiple, are large, and may form staghorns. Cystinuria can cause renal stones in childhood, but the peak of clinical expression is in the second and third decades** (Thier, 1985). Two thirds of patients with homozygous cystinuria form pure cystine stones, and one third form stones that contain a mixture of calcium oxalate and cystine. Sakhaee and colleagues found that hypercalciuria was present in 18.5%, hyperuricosuria in 22.2%, and hypocitraturia in 44.4% of patients with cystinuria (Sakhaee et al, 1989). **Cystine stones form because cystine is poorly soluble within the range of normal urinary pH.** At a pH of 5, the solubility of cystine is 300 mg/L; at a pH of 7, it is 400 mg/L; at the physiologically unreachable pH of 9, it is greater than 1000 mg/L (Dent and Senior, 1955) (see Fig. 91–13).

Diagnosis

The first morning urine specimen should be examined for the presence of typical benzene ring or hexagonal cystine crystals. The cyanide-nitroprusside calorimetric test gives a magenta ring at urinary cystine levels of greater than 75 mg/L (Brand et al, 1930). If the screening test is positive, urinary cystine excretion should be quantitated with amino acid chromatography. A level of greater than 250 mg per 24 hours is usually diagnostic of cystinuria.

Treatment

The goal of therapy is to lower cystine concentration in urine below 200 mg/L.

DIET

Cystine is produced from the essential amino acid methionine, which is abundant in meat, poultry, fish, and dairy products. Thus, a low-methionine diet decreases urinary cystine excretion. Such a diet is unpalatable, however, and patient compliance is poor. Cystine excretion increases with sodium excretion, perhaps because amino acid transport across renal and intestinal brush borders is partially sodium dependent. Although long-term studies have not been performed, rigid dietary sodium restriction may result in a modest decrease in urinary citrate excretion.

ORAL HYDRATION AND ALKALINIZATION

Roughly 250 mg of cystine can dissolve in 1 L of saline and, presumably, urine. Thus, increasing the urinary output to 3 L/day allows dissolution of existing stones and prevention of new cystine stones at urinary cystine excretion of up to 750 mg/day. In this regard, fruit juices may have a dual benefit because they provide not only water, but also alkali.

Because the pKa of cystine is 8.3, alkalinization above 7.5 is necessary for the dissolution of cystine crystals. Such a high pH is difficult to achieve with oral medications. Sodium bicarbonate (15–25 g/day) and potassium citrate (15–20 mmol two to three times a day) are commonly used for alkalinizing urine. Acetazolamide (250 mg three times a day) increases urinary bicarbonate excretion by inhibiting carbonic anhydrase. It can be used to augment the alkalinization achieved with bicarbonate or citrate (Freed, 1975).

Urinary cystine excretion can be reduced by the administration of glutamine (2 g/day in three divided doses) (Jaeger et al, 1986b). This occurs, however, only when the sodium intake is high. The effect of glutamine in lowering urinary cystine is equivalent to that produced by dietary sodium restriction—modest.

PHARMACOLOGIC AGENTS

If hydration and alkalinization are ineffective in reducing the total cystine excretion or preventing stone formation, a cystine complexing agent should be added to the therapeutic regimen. Two agents can be used—D-penicillamine or α-mercaptopropionylglycine (MPG) (or tiopronin). Both agents bind cystine, forming a complex that is soluble in urine. D-penicillamine is a tried and proven agent; MPG is a new agent. The dose of either agent should be titrated to lower urinary cystine concentrations to below 200 mg/L.

A substantial number of patients develop adverse reactions to D-penicillamine. Side effects include gastrointestinal complications, such as nausea, vomiting, diarrhea, and impairment in taste and smell; dermatologic complications, such as urticaria and pemphigus; hypersensitivity reactions; fevers; chills; and arthralgia. Each increase in D-penicillamine dosage of 250 mg/day lowers urinary cystine by 75 to 100 mg/day. **In up to 50% of patients, the dose of penicillamine required to lower cystine levels to the acceptable range results in side effects that are so marked that therapy has to be discontinued.**

Available data from Japan and Europe suggest that MPG is as effective as D-penicillamine in inhibiting cystine stone formation. Its major advantage is its reduced toxicity. Pak and colleagues reported that side effects occurred in 35 out of 120 cystinuria patients being treated with MPG (Pak et al, 1986a). The adverse reactions were generally less serious than those with D-penicillamine; only two patients had to stop taking the medication because of adverse reactions. In a study from Dallas (Pak et al, 1986a), MPG was used in patients with known toxicity to D-penicillamine. Among 34 patients who could not tolerate D-penicillamine, only 10 had a similar reaction to MPG. Finally, two reports indicate that captopril reduces urinary cystine excretion by forming a captopril–cystine disulfide complex, which is 200 times more soluble than cystine (Sloand and Izzo, 1987).

In many patients, cystine stones are so large and so obstructive that procedural therapy should be used initially to debulk or remove the stone. Percutaneous chemolysis with N-acetylcysteine, tromethamine (Tham-E), sodium bicarbonate, or D-penicillamine has been used as an adjunct to stone removal (Smith et al, 1979; Stark and Savir, 1980). N-acetylcysteine, when applied as a topical solution, forms a soluble complex with cystine. Tham-E has a pH of 10.2 and thus increases the solubility of cystine. Finally, in patients with end-stage renal disease and cystinuria, renal transplantation corrects the defect in renal tubular resorption and thus cures cystinuria (Kelly and Nolan, 1980).

Miscellaneous Stones

Dihydroxyadenine Stones

Patients with dihydroxyadenine stone have a deficiency in the enzyme adenine phosphoribosyltransferase (Simmonds et al, 1976, 1978; Barratt et al, 1979). This results in an interference in the normal metabolism of dietary adenine. With the normal pathway blocked, adenine is oxidized by xanthine oxidase to 8-hydroxyadenine and 2,8-dihydroxyadenine. Because dihydroxyadenine is not soluble, it precipitates, forming a calculus. The condition of 2,8-dihydroxyadeninuria is extremely rare, with the incidence of heterozygosity being less than 1%. Dihydroxyadenine stones are radiolucent and thus resemble uric acid stones. They are not soluble, however, within the physiologic range of urinary

pH. Thus, alkalinization may actually cause stone growth. Uric acid stones are smooth and pale yellow, and stones of 2,8-dihydroxyadenine are rough and pale gray in appearance. Infrared spectroscopy distinguishes between uric acid and 2,8-dihydroxyadenine; however, a colorimetric assay cannot distinguish between the two. This condition, although rare, should be suspected in any child with radiolucent stones.

Diagnosis can be confirmed by the assay of adenine phosphoribosyl transferase activity in erythrocytes. Simmonds and colleagues demonstrated dihydroxyadenine in 14 of 10,000 stones analyzed, including 7 of 700 in children (Simmonds et al, 1992). They suggest that dihydroxyadenine urolithiasis may be underdiagnosed because patients with suspected uric acid lithiasis are treated successfully with allopurinol without a correct diagnosis. Finally, Maddocks (1992) states that dihydroxyadenine dipped into liquid nitrogen and exposed to ultraviolet light demonstrates an intense blue phosphorescence, whereas uric acid does not.

Xanthine Stones

Hereditary xanthinuria (MIM #27830) causes the formation of xanthine stones, also radiolucent and also confused with uric acid stones. **Xanthinuria is an inborn error of metabolism, inherited as an autosomal recessive trait and characterized by a deficiency of xanthine oxidase** (Wyngaarden, 1972). The oxidation of hypoxanthine to xanthine and then to uric acid is blocked. Serum uric acid levels are low, averaging less than 1.5 mg/dl. Serum and urine levels of xanthine and hypoxanthine are significantly increased. Because xanthine is less soluble than hypoxanthine, xanthine stones develop. Rarely, crystals of xanthine and hypoxanthine may be deposited in muscle.

Occasionally, patients who are given allopurinol treatment of uric acid urolithiasis or gout form xanthine calculi (Seegmiller et al, 1968). Allopurinol inhibits xanthine oxidase activity only partially, however, and rarely reduces serum uric acid below 3 mg/dl; thus, this is a rare occurrence.

The most effective therapy for xanthine stones is a high fluid intake. Paradoxically, allopurinol, by inhibiting residual xanthine oxidase, may inhibit the oxidation of hypoxanthine to xanthine, resulting in decreased crystallization.

Xanthine stones can occur in patients with the Lesch-Nyhan syndrome who are treated with large doses of allopurinol (Sperling et al, 1978; Loris et al, 1983). In this syndrome, a deficiency of the enzyme hypoxanthine guanine phosphoribosyltransferase leads to the accumulation of hypoxanthine. Hypoxanthine is oxidized by xanthine oxidase to xanthine and subsequently to uric acid. Serum uric acid tends to be high in patients with this syndrome, and massive amounts of allopurinol are sometimes necessary to lower the serum uric acid. Such large doses of allopurinol allow the buildup of large amounts of xanthine in the urine, and xanthine stones form.

Iatrogenic Stones

Iatrogenic stones composed primarily of proteinaceous material and fungus balls are sometimes seen in patients treated with prolonged courses of antibiotic therapy.

Triamterene Stones

Triamterene is a potassium-sparing diuretic that is often given singly or in combination with hydrochlorothiazide in the treatment of hypertension. This combination tends to avoid the potassium depletion that oral hydrochlorothiazide alone causes and has also been used for the treatment of fluid retention and hypercalciuric calcium nephrolithiasis. Up to 70% of orally administered triamterene appears in urine, and a few patients have developed either pure or mixed triamterene stones. Ettinger and co-workers found triamterene in 181 of 50,000 stones analyzed (Ettinger et al, 1980). Triamterene was the sole component in 36% of stones, or 0.13% of the total stone population. In the remaining stones, it occurred as a mixture with calcium oxalate or uric acid, most often in the nucleus. Patients with triamterene stones almost always have a history of nephrolithiasis.

In a study of patients enrolled in a prepaid health maintenance organization, the incidence of hospitalization for renal stones in patients treated with triamterene was not different from those treated with hydrochlorothiazide alone or in the general population (Jick et el, 1982). Nonetheless, with the advent of other potassium-sparing diuretics such as amiloride, which may directly lower urinary calcium, it appears prudent not to use triamterene in patients with a history of nephrolithiasis.

Silicate Calculi

Silicate urinary calculi occur in domestic cattle grazing in sandy areas (Joekes et al, 1973; Levison et al, 1982), but they are extremely rare in humans, occurring only in patients taking large amounts of antacids containing silicates (e.g., magnesium trisilicate) (Joekes et al, 1973; Levison et al, 1982; Haddad and Kouyoumdjian, 1986). The urinary excretion of silicate is normally less than 10 mg/day but approaches 500 mg/day in patients taking magnesium trisilicate. Trisilicate is converted to silica or silicon dioxide by gastric acid. Silicate calculi are radiolucent but have a spiky appearance. Treatment is stopping silicate therapy.

Matrix Calculi

Matrix calculi are found predominantly in individuals with infections caused by urease-producing organisms. *Proteus* species are especially likely to be associated with matrix calculi. Boyce (1968) has defined matrix calculi as those stones composed of coagulated mucoids with little crystalline component. Several clinical reports of these stones have appeared (Allen and Spence, 1966; Mall et al, 1975). They are radiolucent and may be confused with uric acid calculi. Their association with alkaline urinary tract infection, however, usually assists in making a presumptive diagnosis because uric acid calculi are usually formed in acidic, sterile urine. In most instances, surgical manipulation is required for their removal because they are not dissolved by any means yet known. Stones composed of β2-microglobulin, a protein that is filtered and appears in the urine, may form in the kidneys of uremic patients (Linke et al, 1986).

Ammonium Acid Urate Calculi

Three conditions predispose to this rare type of stone, which accounts for about 0.2% of all stones. The first is urealytic infection in the presence of excessive uric acid excretion; the second is urinary phosphate deficiency; and the third is the low fluid intake found in children of developing countries (Hsu, 1966; Klohn et al, 1986). Treatment involves eradication of infection and clearance of infected stone or restoration of normal phosphate metabolism (Klohn et al, 1986). Ammonium acid urate renal calculi have been detected in women with a history of laxative abuse (Dick et al, 1990). These women put out small volumes of concentrated urine, low in sodium, citrate, and potassium. Chronic extracellular volume depletion together with intracellular acidosis create a urinary environment conducive to the crystallization of ammonium acid urate.

Spurious Calculi

Spurious or fake urinary calculi are not at all unusual. Most laboratories report that approximately 1% to 2% of all calculi submitted are produced outside the human body. Sutor and O'Flynn (1973) reported one patient who inserted boiler scale into her bladder to mimic the production of urinary calculi. Drach (1992) reported on a patient whose wife stated that she had extracted urinary calculi from his urethra, and the patient was thus convinced that he had calculi. It was only after confrontation with the fact that the calculi were composed of standard creek-bed stones that the wife admitted that she had palmed the calculi, placed them in his urethra, and subsequently expelled them under the eyes of her husband.

The emergency departments of North America's hospitals are occasionally visited by individuals who fake urinary calculus disease (usually due to "uric acid stones") for secondary gain to obtain drugs (Sharon and Diamond, 1974). The standard story of these individuals is that they know they have uric acid stone disease and they are allergic to intravenous contrast material.

A high degree of suspicion is in order when an individual from out of town arrives in the emergency department with this story, has a severe degree of pain, and dramatizes this pain to an excessive degree. Several foreign patients have developed a true Munchausen's syndrome and have traveled the United States with supposed stone disease (Atkinson and Earll, 1974). It is better for the physician, however, to give an addict meperidine than to withhold it mistakenly from a true sufferer of ureteral colic.

CLINICAL PRESENTATION

Acute Stone Episode

General Observations

A urinary calculus usually presents with an acute episode of renal or ureteral colic as the result of a stone obstructing the urinary tract. There are five locations where stones can be infected in the urinary tract. First, stones may become impacted in a calyx of the upper urinary tract. Individual calyces may, therefore, become distended and painful and

create hematuria. The second area in which a calculus may become impacted is the ureteropelvic junction. It is here that the relatively large diameter of the renal pelvis (1 cm) abruptly decreases to that of the ureter (2–3 mm). A third area of impaction is at or near the pelvic brim, where the ureter begins to arch over the iliac vessels posteriorly into the true pelvis. The fourth area, especially in females, is the posterior pelvis, where the ureter is crossed anteriorly by the pelvic blood vessels and by the broad ligament. Finally, the most constricted area through which the urinary calculus must pass is the ureterovesical junction, which is the most common site of impaction. The majority of impacted ureteral stones are found in the pelvic portion of the ureter. To become impacted, calculi usually must have one diameter in excess of 2 mm. If the smaller diameter is less than 4 mm, spontaneous stone passage is likely (Fig. 91–16) (Prince and Scardino, 1960; Drach, 1983).

Renal Colic

Renal or ureteric colic is a symptom complex that is characteristic for the presence of obstructing urinary tract calculi. A typical episode occurs during the night or early morning hours, is abrupt in onset, and usually affects the patient while sedentary or at rest. The partially obstructing, continuously moving calculus appears to create the greatest amount of colic. The extreme crescendo of pain begins in the area of the flank, courses laterally around the abdomen, and generally radiates to the area of the groin and testicle in the male or to the labia majora and round ligament in the female. This radiation of pain may be related to the blood supply of the cord and testicular or ovarian vessels. Patients with renal colic find it impossible to be still and toss about writhing in pain. As the stone moves to the midureter, pain generally tends to radiate to the lateral flank and abdominal area. When ureteral stones are near the bladder, patients often develop the symptoms of urinary frequency and urgency. Because the autonomic nervous system transmits visceral pain, confusion about the source of the pain is not uncommon. The celiac ganglion serves both kidneys and stomach; therefore, nausea and vomiting are commonly associated with renal colic. In addition, ileus, intestinal stasis, or diarrhea associated with local irritation is not infrequent. The similarity of these symptoms to those arising from the gastrointestinal tract causes renal colic to be confused with a number of abdominal diseases, including gastroenteritis, acute appendicitis, colitis, and salpingitis.

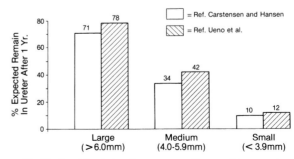

Figure 91–16. Combined data from two studies provide an estimate of percentages of stones first seen in the pelvic ureter and their likelihood of retention for 1 year. (From Drach GW: Urol Clin North Am 1983; 10:709.)

Physical Signs

Individuals with urinary lithiasis rarely can find comfort in any position. They sit, stand, pace, recline, and move continuously in an attempt to "shake off" whatever it is that is creating discomfort. Fever is not present unless urinary infection occurs along with the calculus. Pulse rate and blood pressure may be elevated because of pain and agitation. Examination of the abdomen reveals moderate deep tenderness on palpation over the location of the calculus and the area of the loin.

Urinalysis

Urinalysis in most patients with urinary lithiasis reveals the presence of microscopic or gross hematuria. Press and Smith (1995), however, reported that 15% of a series of 140 patients had no hematuria. In some instances, gross hematuria may be the only presenting complaint. Moderate pyuria may occur even in patients with uninfected urinary lithiasis. When significant numbers of pus cells are present in the urine, however, a thorough search for infection should be made, particularly in women, in whom urinary infection is likely to be a common cause of urinary lithiasis.

On occasion, a patient who is in an active phase of urinary lithiasis has the urine crystals of the same type that are creating the calculus. The observation of cystine, uric acid, or struvite crystals in the urine may be an indication of the type of calculus ultimately found. Calcium oxalate crystalluria may be absent, however, in patients with calcium oxalate stones, especially if urine samples are examined when fresh, and may be present in patients without stones, if the urine has been allowed to sit (Table 91–10; Fig. 91–17).

Radiographic Examination

PLAIN ABDOMINAL FILMS

In the initial evaluation, the first routine radiographs ordered are plain kidney-ureter-bladder (KUB) radiographs. Plain films of the abdomen often show densities such as pelvic phleboliths. A ureteric stone often looks like the root of a tooth, whereas pelvic phleboliths are usually round (Bloom et al, 1988). Renal tomography without contrast material can also be helpful. Calculi that contain calcium are radiodense (Lalli, 1974). Roth and Finlayson (1973) have shown that calcium phosphate (apatite) stones are the most radiopaque and have a density similar to that of bone. Cal-

Table 91–10. APPEARANCE OF URINARY CRYSTALS UNDER THE MICROSCOPE

Crystal	Shape Under Optical Microscope
Calcium oxalate monohydrate	Dumbbell or hourglass
Calcium oxalate dihydrate	Envelope or bipyramidal
Calcium phosphate-apatite	Amorphous
Brushite	Needle-shaped
Cystine	Hexagonal or benzene ring
Struvite	Coffin lid
Uric acid	Irregular plates or rosettes Amorphous

cium oxalate calculi are almost as opaque. Magnesium ammonium phosphate (struvite) calculi are somewhat less radiopaque than calcium calculi and have a laminated, rough character. Cystine calculi are slightly radiodense because of their sulfur content (Figs. 91–18 and 91–19). Coe and Parks (1988) have likened nephrocalcinosis to "stars on a dark night sky" (see Fig. 91–10). Nephrocalcinosis is common in medullary sponge kidney because crystals accumulate in dilated collecting ducts.

The degree of radiodensity is one factor in visualization of the calculus on the plain film, but the structure and configuration of the calculus also contribute. Calcium oxalate calculi must be at least 2 mm thick to appear on most radiographs. For cystine calculi, a degree of thickness approximating 3 to 4 mm is necessary for the stone to be visualized at all. Staghorns are large stones that replicate pelvicalyceal anatomy. They are usually made of struvite, cystine, or uric acid. Only calculi of pure uric acid, xanthine, dehydrohydroxyadenine, or triamterene or of matrix can be considered truly radiolucent. They too appear radiopaque, however, on nonenhanced computed tomography (CT) (Stoller et al, 1994).

INTRAVENOUS UROGRAM

The diagnosis of an obstructing urinary tract stone is confirmed by the demonstration of delay in the appearance of the contrast medium in the kidney after intravenous injection. Lalli (1974) and Van Arsdalen and colleagues (1990) point out that presence of such a delay indicates that the usual 5-, 10-, and 20-minute urographic films are not likely to be useful in defining the location and presence of the calculus. Therefore, it is better to extend the period of observation and obtain films at perhaps 20, 30, and 60 minutes. Delayed films may be obtained several hours or even 1 day after the injection of contrast material.

Some physicians prefer infusion urography for detection of renal calculi. Several authors report spontaneous urinary extravasation after infusion urography (Silver et al, 1973; Borkowski and Czapliczki, 1974). This is the result of extravasation of urine through renal fornices (Fig. 91–20). In patients with uninfected urine, this radiologic sign has no clinical importance.

Elton and colleagues wondered whether an intravenous urogram was necessary for the diagnosis of ureteral calculi in an emergency setting (Elton et al, 1993). In a series of 203 patients with renal colic and hematuria, they compared the accuracy of diagnosis comparing the plain abdominal film alone to the plain film and an intravenous urogram. In a patient with acute onset of flank pain and hematuria, a positive plain abdominal film diagnosed the presence of ureteral calculi with 96% accuracy. If the abdominal film was negative or equivocal, the diagnostic accuracy was much less. Based on this study, it appears that an intravenous urogram may not be necessary for the *diagnosis* of a ureteric calculus in the emergency setting, provided that the patient has acute flank pain, hematuria, and a positive abdominal film. An intravenous urogram may be necessary in some instances to decide whether the patient needs procedural therapy.

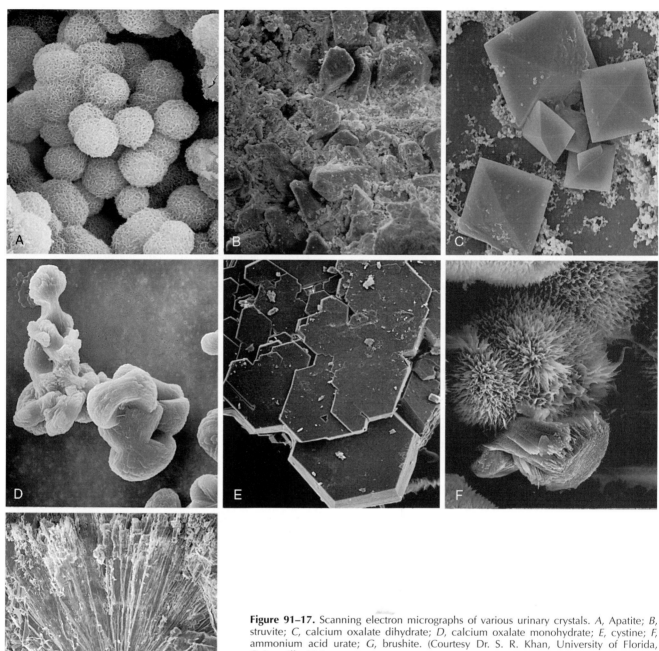

Figure 91–17. Scanning electron micrographs of various urinary crystals. *A*, Apatite; *B*, struvite; *C*, calcium oxalate dihydrate; *D*, calcium oxalate monohydrate; *E*, cystine; *F*, ammonium acid urate; *G*, brushite. (Courtesy Dr. S. R. Khan, University of Florida, Gainesville, FL.)

COMPUTED TOMOGRAPHY

This technique is especially useful in defining classically "radiolucent" uric acid calculi (Resnick et al, 1984). Studies without contrast material precede those with contrast material. Some investigators have attempted to use CT scanning to define the composition of stones, but this technique has been questioned (Van Arsdalen et al, 1990).

A modified spiral CT technique has supplanted intravenous urography for the evaluation of ureteric colic in some institutions.

ULTRASONOGRAPHY

Ultrasound is a noninvasive method of demonstrating both the urinary stone and the consequent hydronephrosis. Color

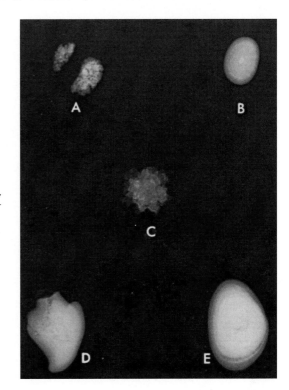

Figure 91–18. Radiodensities in air (to improve contrast) of five human calculi. A, Calcium oxalate; B, calcium phosphate; C, uric acid; D, cystine; E, magnesium ammonium phosphate. Note that only the uric acid calculus is truly radiolucent.

Doppler ultrasound examination may demonstrate an increased resistive index in the obstructed kidney and asymmetry or absence of ureteral jets in the urinary bladder, thereby reducing the number of false-negative results. In several institutions, it has supplanted intravenous urography as the diagnostic test of choice for the detection of renal stones and is reported to have a sensitivity of about 95% (Haddad et al, 1992). It may be falsely normal, however, in patients with small stones who have forniceal disruption and no hydronephrosis, and thus up to one fourth of patients with normal ultrasound studies have ureteric stones detected on urography (Menon, 1993).

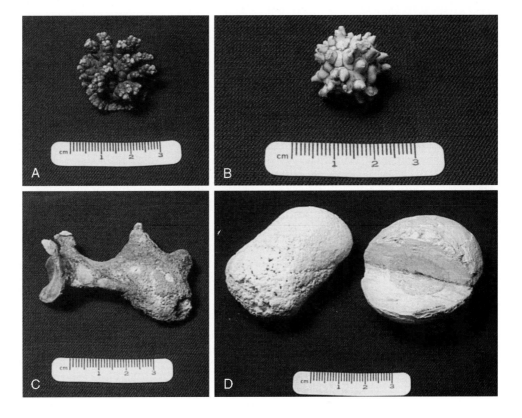

Figure 91–19. Examples of urinary calculi. *A,* Calcium oxalate monohydrate (whewellite)—also called "mulberry stone." *B,* Uric acid calculus—also called "Jackstone." *C,* Staghorn calculus—magnesium ammonium phosphate "struvite." *D,* Concentric character of magnesium ammonium phosphate "struvite." (Courtesy of Worcester District Medical Society, Worcester, MA.)

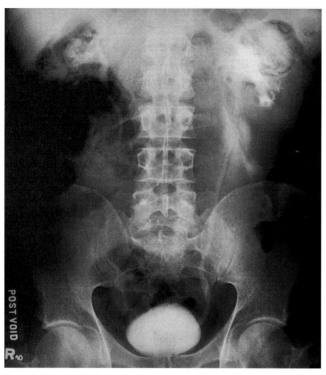

POST VOID
R

Figure 91–20. Infusion pyelography showing spontaneous extravasation on left side secondary to a left lower third ureteric calculus. (Courtesy of Department of Radiology, University of Massachusetts, Worcester, MA.)

RETROGRADE PYELOGRAPHY

Retrograde pyelography is necessary only rarely, perhaps in cases of relatively radiolucent calculi that are difficult to locate by other techniques.

Diagnostic and Treatment Decision Process

After a urolith is diagnosed, the first assessment is the degree of seriousness of the disease process. Coe and Parks (1988) report that 20% to 40% of patients with stone attacks may need hospital admission; however, the authors' experience is that less than 10% of patients need hospitalization. Bypassing obstruction or extraction of a stone is necessary when there is evidence of significant obstruction, progressive renal deterioration, refractory pyelonephritis, or unremitting pain. An obstructed and infected kidney should be drained expeditiously or as soon as the patient is stable.

The majority of patients with renal colic require prompt therapy for pain relief. Most patients gain relief from the intramuscular injection of 50 to 100 mg of meperidine or 10 to 15 mg of morphine, depending on body size and severity of pain. One study, however, showed that even with intravenous morphine, pain relief averaged only 36% at 30 minutes when measured on a visual analogue scale (Cordell et al, 1994). Liberal use of narcotics to treat the pain of urolithiasis has resulted in some addicted patients who feign symptoms. Drug addicts most frequently relate they are "allergic" to intravenous contrast material and relay information that may indicate that previous stones are known to be radiolucent. The absence of uric acid crystals or infection in the urine

helps confirm one's suspicion of drug dependency (see section on spurious calculi).

Hospitalization for renal stones is mandatory under three clinical circumstances: in patients with symptoms not controlled with oral medications; in the presence of calculus anuria, seen usually in patients with a solitary kidney; or in patients with an obstructing stone and an infected urine or fever. Finally, patients with obstructing ureteric stones greater than 6 mm are seldom likely to pass their stone spontaneously, and early admission for procedural therapy may be prudent. All other patients can be safely managed on an ambulatory basis.

It is almost a universal adage that fluids must be forced on patients with stones. An increase in diuresis, however, may reduce the rate of ureteral peristalsis. If so, forced water drinking may inhibit the ability to pass the stone spontaneously.

Some workers have advised antispasmodic or anti-inflammatory agents in the treatment of urinary calculus disease (Peters and Eckstein, 1975; Flannigan et al, 1983). In one study, acupuncture was demonstrated to have a more rapid analgesic onset and fewer side effects than narcotic analgesic analogue in the treatment of renal colic (Lee et al, 1992).

The majority of calculi less than 4 to 5 mm in size pass spontaneously. The patient must understand that it is critical to recover any calculus or gravel that is passed. One of several commercially available funnel-like straining devices can be provided. The simplest way for the patient to observe passage of a calculus, however, is to urinate into a clear glass jar. The density of the calculus causes it to fall to the bottom. Stone analysis is performed on any calculus that is recovered. Stone analysis provides information about composition and allows planning of future therapy for the majority of patients with urinary calculus disease.

Effects of Ureteral Obstruction on Renal Function

Ureteral obstruction, whether partial or complete, produces a progressive decrease in renal excretory function. After obstruction, a rapid redistribution of renal blood flow from medullary to cortical nephrons occurs. This redistribution results in a decrease in glomerular filtration rate and renal plasma flow, reflecting a decrease in both glomerular and tubular function (Lackner and Barton, 1970; Jones et al, 1989). Finkle and Smith (1970) and Vaughan and associates (1971) observed that these decreases resulted from reduced renal blood flow. Stecker and Gillenwater (1971) observed a significant concentration defect and reduced urinary acid excretion following partial ureteral obstruction.

Moody and co-workers divided renal response to ureteral occlusion into three phases: At 0 to 12 hours, ipsilateral renal blood flow and ureteral pressures rose; at 5 to 12 hours, renal blood flow fell, while ureteral pressures continued to rise; and at 5 to 18 hours, both renal blood flow and ureteral pressures fell (Moody et al, 1975). Vaughan and associates showed further that contralateral renal blood flow increased as function and renal blood flow of the obstructed kidney decreased (Vaughan et al, 1970).

Obstruction results not only in decreased renal function

but also in fairly rapid changes in ureteral peristaltic function. Gee and Kiviat (1975) observed hypertrophy of rapid ureteral musculature after only 3 days of obstruction. If obstruction continued for 2 weeks, connective tissue deposits (scar) occurred between muscle bundles. Such changes were considered as marked at 8 weeks. Chronic ureteral obstruction results in decreased peristalsis and decreased pressure. The presence of urinary infection totally impaired ureteral function. Perhaps this is why fewer stones pass spontaneously in patients with infection (Westbury, 1974).

Relief of obstruction after 8 weeks results in a rapid increase in ipsilateral renal blood flow and partial reversal of functional defects in the dog (Vaughan et al, 1970). Finkle and Smith (1970) believe that the major effects of obstruction are on the tubules. Stecker and Gillenwater (1971) and Jones and associates (1989) state, however, that the glomerulotubular balance is maintained in the obstructed kidney and that relief of obstruction results in improvement of both glomerular filtration rate and renal plasma flow.

How long can one wait before treating the stone? If infection exists behind the obstruction, the answer is clear: Relieve the obstruction as quickly as possible. In the absence of infection and with complete obstruction, renal deterioration begins within 18 to 24 hours in the dog. Some irreversible renal functional loss occurs within 5 to 14 days. After 16 weeks of obstruction, only "slight recovery" can be expected (Stecker and Gillenwater, 1971). Partial obstruction is less damaging but may still result in some irreversible functional damage. Schweitzer (1973) studied chronic partial obstruction in animals and concluded that renal damage occurs early. He suggested that intervention of some kind may well be necessary earlier than is usually practiced, if renal damage is to be avoided completely. **In the authors' opinion, detectable renal damage does not occur in previously normal kidneys until complete obstruction has been present for 4 weeks, and so one can give the patient up to 4 weeks to pass the stone spontaneously.**

Analysis of Uroliths

Most medical therapy for stone disease is now based on analysis of calculi, and decisions about proper procedures for treatment require knowledge of stone composition (Dretler, 1990). Table 91–11 shows the types of stones seen in the United States.

Chemical analysis of renal calculi has been all but abandoned. Significant error may occur because qualitative and semiquantitative chemical analysis methods are not accurate (Vergauwe et al, 1994). Schneider and co-workers compared chemical, x-ray diffraction, infrared spectroscopy, and thermoanalytic procedures in analysis of urinary calculi (Schneider et al, 1973). They found all of these methods accurate in detecting the components of urinary calculi.

Prien and Frondel (1947) emphasized the greater accuracy of optical crystallography and x-ray crystallography. Physical methods can distinguish between the different minerals in the stones, and they need a smaller sample. Thermal analysis needs relatively more sample but can give quantitative results. Optical methods give only qualitative results but can analyze small samples. Prien (1963, 1974) and colleagues (Sutor, 1968; Sutor and Scheidt, 1968) point out that the x-ray diffraction technique allows some minor components of mixed urinary calculi to go undetected in as many as 20% to 30% of stones.

Elliot (1973) recommended optical crystallographic examination combined with initial careful dissection of the stone, under a binocular stereoscopic microscope. In this way, separate layers and segments of the stone may be analyzed. In calcium oxalate calculi, Elliot found that calcium oxalate monohydrate (whewellite) formed the nucleus or initiating crystal of two thirds of all stones. The majority of surface deposits were composed of calcium oxalate dihydrate (weddellite).

Infrared spectroscopic analysis of urinary calculi can detect crystalline and amorphous minerals. It has been reported by Hazarika and Rao (1974) and Takasaki (1975). It can perform semiquantitative analysis on a small volume of stones (Vergauwe et al, 1994). It can identify "unexpected" stone constituents (Vergauwe et al, 1994). Volmer and co-workers have used partial least squares analysis employing infrared spectra of several urinary stones and artificial mixtures (Volmer et al, 1993). They found that partial least squares analysis was superior with respect to accuracy and necessity of expert knowledge.

Peuchant and associates have compared near infrared re-

Table 91–11. URINARY STONE ANALYSIS

	% Stones Analyzed				
	Prien and Frondel (1947)	*Prien (1963)*	*Herring (1962)*	*Smith (1988)*	*Mandel and Mandel (1989)*
No. stones	600	24,000	10,000	4525	10,163
Major crystal					
Calcium oxalate	36.1	—	—	58.8	—
Calcium oxalate monohydrate	—	—	31.4	—	55.4
Calcium oxalate dihydrate	—	71–84	40.9	—	34.6
Calcium oxalate/calcium phosphate	31	—	—	11.4	—
Calcium phosphate	—	—	17.3	8.9	28.9
Magnesium ammonium phosphate	21.5	6–14	15.7	9.3	12.6
Uric acid	6.1	6–10	7.4	10.1	16.7
Urates	—	—	0.87	—	—
Cystine	3.8	1–2	0.89	0.7	0.5
Miscellaneous	1.6	0.5–1.5	3.6	0.8	1.8

From Smith LH: J Urol 1989; 141:709.

flectance analysis to infrared spectroscopy (Peuchant et al, 1992). Infrared reflectance analysis is fast (takes <1 minute), requires small amounts of calculus in powder form (<100 μg), needs no reagents, and permits accurate semiquantitative analysis (Peuchant et al, 1992). Artificial neural network has been used in conjunction with infrared spectroscopy to detect the most frequently occurring compositions of urinary calculi (Volmer et al, 1994). Neural network analysis is more accurate than the library search and requires less expert knowledge (Volmer et al, 1994). Thin-section transmission electron microscopic analysis of calculi has been reported by Meyer and co-workers (1971). Their analyses of uric acid, oxalate, and phosphate stones reveal that stone material is finely divided and highly aggregated. A combination of refined morphologic and structural examination of stone with optical microscopy and compositional analysis using infrared spectroscopy of the core has been shown to provide a cost-effective, precise, and reliable analysis of the stone (Daudon et al, 1993).

With the widespread use of ESWL, fewer stones are being analyzed because of difficulties in collecting stone samples. Bowsher and colleagues analyzed urine samples immediately following lithotripsy using a combination of electron microscopy and x-ray spectroscopy (Bowsher et al, 1990). The results correlated well with analysis of voided stone fragments.

For the practicing urologist without in-house analytic laboratories, facilities for stone analysis are available by mail and certified by national agencies. Polarizing microscopy, x-ray diffraction, and infrared spectroscopy all are acceptable techniques for analyzing renal stones.

MEDICAL EVALUATION

The following discussion is based on the rationale just described. The authors' approach to evaluating patients is simply one method of doing this, not the only method. An expanded step-by-step version of this approach has been published (Pak et al, 1993). The authors' approach follows the guidelines suggested by the Concensus Conference on the prevention and treatment of kidney stones (1988).

History

The etiology of urinary calculi is multifactorial in the majority of cases, and rarely can a single factor in the patient's history account for the presence of the stone. For this reason, a detailed history should be taken, emphasizing the following areas:

1. *Diet and fluid intake.* Several investigators request every patient to keep a dietary diary for 1 week. A high meat intake increases the urinary restriction of calcium, oxalate, and uric acid and decreases urinary pH and citric excretion. Burns and Finlayson (1981) have shown that the effect of dietary protein on urinary calcium excretion follows the equation:

$$y = 6.8\beta^{0.4}$$

where *y* equals the increase in percent of urinary calcium caused by protein ingestion, and β is dietary protein nitrogen in grams. Using this formula, it can be shown that 10 ounces of meat ingested daily causes a 156% increase in urinary calcium excretion. The other effects of meat intake are believed to be the result of the high content of sulfur-containing amino acids found in animal protein. Increased acidity of the urine may diminish the inhibitory action of urinary glycosaminoglycans, potent inhibitors of calcium oxalate crystal growth and aggregation. It has been estimated that roughly half the increased levels of urinary calcium, oxalate, and uric acid seen in stone-forming patients may be attributed to a diet rich in animal protein.

Milk ingestion can cause hypercalciuria both because of increased calcium intake and because of the high lactose content of milk, lactose being a potent stimulator of intestinal calcium absorption. Milk or multivitamin tablets also contain vitamin D, which can increase intestinal absorption of calcium. Megadoses of ascorbic acid (>10 g) may predispose to hyperoxaluria.

2. *Medications.* Corticosteroids can increase enteric absorption of calcium leading to hypercalciuria. Hypercalciuria can also be seen with the ingestion of aluminum-containing antacids (which bind phosphate), loop diuretics, and vitamin D. Chemotherapeutic agents lead to cell breakdown and can cause uric acid stones. Uricosuric agents such as colchicine or probenecid also cause hyperuricosuria. The triamterene-containing antihypertensive Dyazide has been associated with triamterene stones.

3. *Infection.* Urinary tract infection, particularly with urease-producing bacteria such as *Proteus*, *Klebsiella*, *Serratia*, and *Enterobacter* species, may lead to struvite stones. Up to 30% of patients with calcium oxalate stones have a history of an *E. coli* infection, presumably causing stones by an alteration in matrix production.

4. *Activity level.* Periods of immobilization secondary to illness or injury may lead to bone demineralization and hypercalciuria. This is known to exacerbate stone formation in patients with a pre-existing tendency.

5. *Systemic disease.* Diseases such as primary hyperparathyroidism, RTA, gout, and sarcoidosis can cause urolithiasis.

6. *Genetics.* A family history of stones may suggest certain causes such as RTA, cystinuria, or absorptive hypercalciuria. The history of a family member having stone disease increases the likelihood of recurrences fourfold.

7. *Anatomy.* Urinary tract obstruction, congenital (ureteropelvic junction obstruction or horseshoe kidney) or acquired (benign prostatic hypertrophy, urethral stricture), leads to urinary stasis and stone formation. Medullary sponge kidney is the most common renal structural abnormality seen in patients with calcium-containing stones; up to 2% of patients have this. Schulz and colleagues have found good correlation between caliceal anatomy and stone formation, even in patients with normal upper tracts (Schulz et al, 1989). Review of excretory urograms from patients with kidney stones indicated that an equation taking into consideration the total area of the collecting system (A_t), caliceal angle (Σ_{ai}), and angle between the pelvis and the ureter (β) was able to discriminate between stone formers and normal controls with 80% accuracy (Schulz et al, 1989):

$$X = 3 \cdot 672 \times 10^{-1} \ A_t/mm^2 - 1 \cdot 839 \times 10^{-2} \ \Sigma_{ai}/degree - 2 \cdot 137 \times 10^{-2} \ \beta/degree$$

A value for X of -0.5 or less indicated the absence of stones, whereas a value of more than -0.5 indicated the presence of stones.

8. *Previous surgery.* A history of previous abdominal surgery with bowel resection resulting in diarrhea should initiate a search for hyperoxaluria or hypocitraturia.

Evaluation of the Patient with the First Stone

The first step in the evaluation is to assess the link of stone recurrences. Although imperfect, Figure 91–21 offers some guidelines as to which patients are at greater risk. In patients who are not at risk, a simplified metabolic evaluation is done (Fig. 91–22). All patients should have excretory urography, urinalysis, urine culture, a complete blood count, and a SMA-20. All stones should be analyzed. If the stone cannot be recovered, a urine cystine screen should be performed (Fig. 91–23), as outlined in the laboratory study protocol.

The presence of multiple stones or nephrocalcinosis on intravenous urography indicates a need for a more detailed metabolic work-up and aggressive medical therapy. A urinary pH of below 6 in a patient with radiolucent stones suggests that persistently acid urines may be the cause of uric acid crystallization. The presence of benzene crystals strongly suggests cystinuria; the presence of coffin lid crystals suggests struvite stones; and the presence of uric acid crystals suggests uric acid lithiasis. A urine culture that grows urease-splitting organisms indicates the presence of an infection stone, requiring aggressive treatment of the infection. The complete blood count may reveal unsuspected hematologic malignancy. Serum chemistries may suggest the

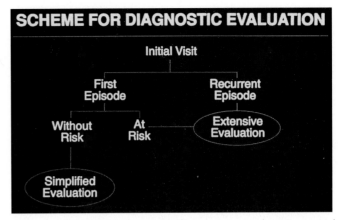

Figure 91–22. Selection of simplified or extensive evaluation at initial visit. Apply a simplified evaluation in a patient with a single stone episode without risk. Consider an extensive evaluation in patients with recurrent episode or first episode at risk. (Courtesy of Mission Pharmacal Co., San Antonio, TX.)

presence of metabolic acidosis. Together with the urine pH of greater than 5.4, this confirms the diagnosis of complete distal RTA. An elevated serum calcium suggests hyperparathyroidism or, more rarely, sarcoidosis. A decrease in serum phosphate is seen in absorptive hypercalciuria type III. An increase in uric acid is seen in gouty diatheses (Fig. 91–24).

Evaluation of the Patient with Multiple or Recurrent Stones

An ambulatory evaluation of stone disease is as efficient as an inpatient evaluation in detecting metabolic abnormalities. Figures 91–25 and 91–26 detail the authors' approach

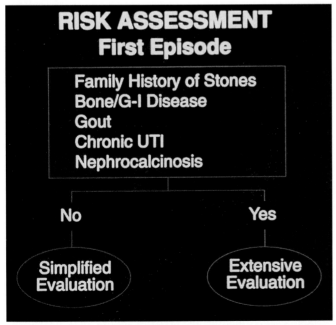

Figure 91–21. History constituting increased risk for stone development. If present in patients with first episode, an extensive evaluation is advised. If absent, a simplified evaluation may be applied. G-I, gastrointestinal; UTI, urinary tract infection. (Courtesy of Mission Pharmacal Co., San Antonio, TX.)

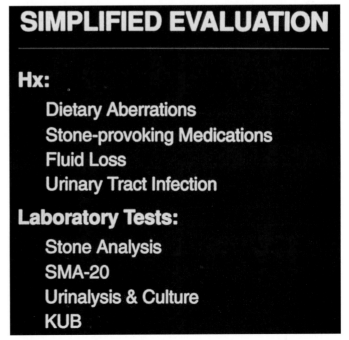

Figure 91–23. Recommended history (Hx) and laboratory tests to be obtained during simplified evaluation. KUB, kidney, ureter, bladder. (Courtesy of Mission Pharmacal Co., San Antonio, TX.)

SMA-20

↑ Ca, ↓ P	:	Primary Hyperparathyroidism
↓ K, ↓ CO_2	:	RTA
↑ Uric Acid	:	Gouty Diathesis
↓ P	:	Hypophosphatemic AH

If present, extensive evaluation

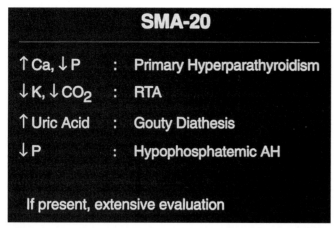

Figure 91–24. During simplified evaluation, diagnostic utility of SMA-20. Ca, calcium; P, phosphorus; K, potassium; CO_2, carbon dioxide; RTA, renal tubular acidosis; AH, absorptive hypercalciuria. (Courtesy of Mission Pharmacal Co., San Antonio, TX.)

to the evaluation of patients at risk for stone recurrence. Two evaluations—for a clinical and for a research setting—are given.

The analysis of urinary metabolites in 24-hour urine collections requires proper sample collection and processing techniques (Ng et al, 1984). A system of sequential acidification to pH 1.5 and alkalinization to pH 9 followed by heating at 56°C for 10 minutes allows accurate analysis of all urinary metabolites needed for the differential diagnosis for patients with renal calculi. Calcium, oxalate, magnesium, and phosphorus should be analyzed in the acidified sample; uric acid in the alkaline sample; and creatinine in untreated aliquots (Ng et al, 1984).

A commercial service, the Stone Risk Profile, is available in the United States (Pak et al, 1985c). The kit contains a container for collecting a 24-hour urine sample, a volume marker, and appropriate preservatives. After collection of the 24-hour sample, two 30-ml aliquots are sent to a central laboratory. This center then calculates the total volume from the dilution of the volume marker and analyzes metabolic risk factors (calcium, oxalate, uric acid, citrate, and pH) as well as total volume, sodium, sulfate, phosphorus, and magnesium. Each risk factor is visually displayed on a vertical line with linear or logarithmic scales. The ratios of supersaturation for calcium oxalate, brushite, sodium rate, struvite, and uric acid are calculated, and the relative risk is graphically displayed.

1. Automated Stone Risk Analysis (eg StoneRisk® Profile)
2. Dietary Modification pending results of 1
3. Abbreviated Stone Risk Analysis (eg StoneTrack®) plus SMA-20 & PTH following dietary modification
4. Bone Density in Hypercalcemia or Marked Hypercalciuria

Figure 91–25. Simplified ambulatory evaluation representing an extensive evaluation designed for a private practice setting. PTH, parathyroid hormone. (Courtesy of Mission Pharmacal Co., San Antonio, TX.)

Visit 1 : Random diet
History
Sequential multichannel analysis (SMA)-20
24-hr urine for stone risk factors

Visit 2 : Random diet
Repeat 24-hr urine for stone risk factors
Instruction on a diet restricted in calcium, sodium, oxalate

Visit 3 : Restricted diet
SMA-20 and PTH
24-hr urine for stone risk factors
Fast and calcium load test

Visit 1 & 2 - one week apart if possible
Bone density if available

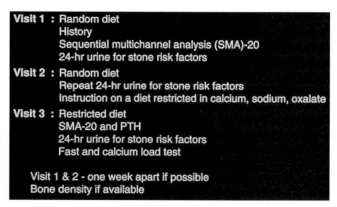

Figure 91–26. Full ambulatory protocol representing an extensive evaluation useful in a research setting. PTH, parathyroid hormone. (Courtesy of Mission Pharmacal Co., San Antonio, TX.)

PRINCIPLES OF MEDICAL THERAPY

Medical therapy for stone disease serves two purposes: treatment of the acute episode and prevention of stone recurrences or new stone formation. The treatment of the acute stone episode has been discussed earlier in this chapter. Only rarely is medical treatment useful for the treatment of the patient with existing stones—in the vast majority of instances, procedural or surgical therapy is indicated. The primary exception is the patient with uric acid stones, in whom medical therapy is extremely successful in causing stone dissolution. It is less successful in dissolving cystine stones or struvite stones. These issues are discussed in the relevant sections of this chapter. This section discusses the role of medical therapy in the prevention of recurrences of calcium oxalate renal stones.

Who Needs Medical Therapy

Between 25% and 75% of all patients who present with an initial stone develop a recurrent stone over prolonged follow-up, lasting from 10 to 20 years (Ljunghall et al, 1975; Marshall et al, 1975; Johnson et al, 1979; Strauss, et al, 1982; Sutherland et al, 1985). The recurrence rate was 5% per year in patients attending a urologic stone clinic (Marshall et al, 1975) and 10% to 23% in patients who formed a control group for randomized clinical trials (Ettinger, 1976; Brocks et al, 1981; Scholz et al, 1982; Laerum and Larsen, 1984; Ettinger et al, 1985). In a community urologic practice, the median time to recurrence, or the time by which 50% of patients had developed a second stone, was 8.8 ± 1.2 (SEM) years (Sutherland et al, 1985). Thus, **it can be predicted that the recurrence rate will be about 7% per year, with 50% of patients having recurrences within 10 years, in an unselected urologic practice.**

If only 50% of patients develop a stone recurrence over 10 years of follow-up, how can it be determined which patients will develop recurrence? This would be simple if metabolic abnormalities occurred mostly or only in patients with recurrent stones. This is not the case, however. **Patients who present after the first stone have the same pattern of metabolic disorders as patients with multiple stones** (Pak, 1982b; Strauss et al, 1982). Patients with more than

10 stones have metabolic disorders similar to those of all patients (Coe, 1977). Thus, metabolic testing does not allow the prediction of which patients will develop stone recurrence or will need long-term medical treatment.

Most patients who present with a stone are encouraged to drink more fluid and avoid dietary excesses after resolution of the acute stone episode. Hosking and colleagues reviewed the clinical course of 108 patients with idiopathic calcium urolithiasis who were given such advice (Hosking et al, 1983). After a mean follow-up of more than 5 years, 58% of the patients showed no evidence of stone growth or new stone formation (Hosking et al, 1983). This has been termed the **stone clinic effect**. Other investigators have noted similar recurrence rates over long-term follow-up. **If only 50% of patients develop a stone recurrence over 10 years of follow-up, the rationale for an extensive metabolic work-up and compulsory follow-up becomes less compelling for the patient with a first stone**.

A contrasting opinion has been raised. Parks and Coe (1994) analyzed stone recurrences in 370 men with calcium oxalate stone disease evaluated in their nephrolithiasis unit. **Men with increasing number of stones had more recurrences, whether they were treated or not.** Urinary risk factors such as calcium, oxalate, and citrate did not predict differences in stone-forming rate, whereas age and pretreatment urine volume did. Patients who entered the metabolic treatment program after their first stone episode had a 15% relapse rate at 10 years, those with two stone events had a 30% relapse rate, and those with three or more stone events before starting treatment had a 55% relapse rate at 10 years. These authors found that the number of stone episodes and the total number of stones were independent correlates of relapses, suggesting that patients who passed multiple stones during a stone episode were at a greater risk for stone recurrence than a patient with only a single stone during a stone event. **The authors concluded that increasing time of observation pretreatment correlated with the relapse rates. If such is the case, early intervention after the first stone event may be a better prevention strategy than allowing patients to form more stones.**

The best study directly examining the effect of pharmacologic therapy on stone recurrences in the first-time stone former was performed by Scott and Lewi (1989). They studied 301 patients presenting to a urologic practice with their first stone episode—a population similar to what a urologist in practice may see. Of these, 129 were treated with dietary modification and hydration; the rest were treated with thiazides if hypercalciuric, and allopurinol if not. The stone recurrence rate was 34% in patients treated with drugs regardless of the drug used and 61% in patients on conservative treatment.

Admitting that this approach may be biased, or even wrong, the authors elect to treat initial stone formers with hydration and avoidance of dietary excesses. The authors follow the recommendations of the Consensus Conference on nephrolithiasis (1988) and suggest that patients increase their urinary output to greater than 2 L/day. **Patients who have had only their first stone episode do not undergo a formal metabolic evaluation but rather have a urinalysis, a urine culture, and a blood chemical profile, including calcium, uric acid, electrolytes, and creatinine concentration.** Patients in whom the initial episode involves multiple stones, who have had a stone recurrence within 1 year of follow-up, or who have risk factors for recurrence have a more complete metabolic evaluation and specific medical therapy.

Patients with Asymptomatic Kidney Stones

Glowacki and associates evaluated the natural history of asymptomatic urolithiasis in 107 patients who were identified by radiographic or ultrasonographic techniques as having renal stones (Glowacki et al, 1992). In each patient, the stone was asymptomatic for at least 6 months after identification. Over a 32-month follow-up, 68% of the patients continued to be asymptomatic. Of the 32% who developed symptoms, half passed the stone spontaneously, whereas half required urologic procedures. The cumulative 5-year probability of a symptomatic event was close to 50% and correlated with the number of previous stones as well as the number of stones at identification.

General Measures of Prevention

Hydration

Although, to the authors' knowledge, the effect of increasing urinary output on stone recurrences has not been studied in a prospective, randomized fashion, historical data strongly suggest that hydration is effective in preventing stone formation. The incidence of stones is higher in hot climates, where extrarenal fluid losses result in a low urine output. Blacklock (1969) reported that stone formation rates dropped by 86% in the British Navy when the average urinary output was increased from 800 to 1200 ml/day. Experimental evidence (Pak et al, 1980) indicates that high fluid intake results in the reduction of the saturation of calcium phosphate, calcium oxalate, and monosodium urate and increases the threshold at which calcium oxalate crystallizes. In a stepwise discriminant analysis of patients attending a stone clinic, the Coe group identified a failure to increase urinary output as the most important factor that predicted stone recurrence (Strauss et al, 1982). The authors calculated a discriminant score that correlated strongly with recurrence:

$$\text{Discriminant score} = 0 \cdot 2373t - 0 \cdot 4623\,Ca + 1 \cdot 113\,\Lambda V + 0 \cdot 9509$$

where t = time in years since last stone; Ca = 24-hour urine calcium in mg/kg on treatment; and Λ = treatment—pretreatment urine volume in liters.

A patient with a positive score had a 90% chance of not relapsing, whereas a patient with a negative score had a 37% chance of relapsing. This score can be calculated quite easily and may be used prospectively to monitor therapy.

There is some association between the mineral content of the drinking water and the incidence of stones. In a study of 2400 patients, those who formed calcium stones were found to be twice as likely to be drinking water from a private well than those who did not. Some investigators have found a direct relationship between water hardness and stone disease (Rose and Westbury, 1975); others have found an inverse correlation (Sierakowski et al, 1976).

Because hydration has been for so long the mainstay of any treatment program aimed to prevent stone recurrences, it is hard to find a study in which hydration was not used. There is also no study that evaluates the timing or the absolute level of hydration that is required to prevent stone recurrence. Stone growth probably does not occur throughout the entire day but rather during certain critical periods when the urine becomes supersaturated, such as overnight, several hours after a meal, and during periods of extrarenal fluid loss. Thus, maximum intake of fluid should occur within 3 hours after meals, during periods of strenuous physical activity, at bedtime, and once in the middle of the night. Patients can set an alarm clock to wake up in the middle of the night to drink water. Patients should measure their 24-hour urinary output once a week and adjust the fluid intake to maintain an output of 3 L/day or more. Alternatively, the Hydrate 1 (Gyrus Medical Ltd., UK) system can be used to monitor urine osmolarity with a simple calorimetric method (Dilworth and Segura, 1993). Compliance with a strict regimen of hydration is sporadic, however, and determined primarily by occupational and lifestyle factors or by the frequency of pretreatment stone formation. Burns and Finlayson (1981) have been more optimistic about the likelihood of long-term compliance. They believe that within a short period of time, the decrease in urinary concentrating capacity induced by diuresis stimulates thirst mechanisms so that fluid intake becomes automatic.

Diet

If one assumes that the constituents of renal stones come from ingested food, dietary restriction becomes one of the most important strategies for therapy. In several reviews of the putative role of dietary factors in the pathogenesis of calcium oxalate stone disease, Goldfarb (1994) states that three criteria must be fulfilled for a dietary factor to be implicated in stone formation: (1) Intake of the dietary constituent should be increased in stone patients compared to controls, (2) restriction of the factor should decrease stone formation, and (3) the reason why the dietary factor causes stones should be identified. Although definitive proof according to these criteria does not exist, substantial indirect evidence suggests that dietary factors have a significant role in recurrent nephrolithiasis.

DIETARY PROTEIN

Epidemiologic studies from a number of countries have shown that the incidence of renal stones is higher in populations in which protein intake is greater. For example, in northern and western regions of India, animal protein intake is approximately 100% greater than in the southern and eastern regions, and the rate of kidney stones is four times greater. In the United Kingdom, the frequency of upper tract stone disease correlates with the per capita expenditure on foodstuffs (Robertson et al, 1979c, 1982). This effect may be partly because protein intake is higher in affluent people, and stone formation, for some reason, seems to be higher in the economically advantaged. When populations are matched

for economic status, the intake of protein and other dietary constituents does not differ in recurrent stone patients and controls. Even in subjects thus matched, however, stone patients secrete greater quantities of calcium in the urine than controls for a given intake of protein (Wasserstein et al, 1987). Thus, stone patients may be more sensitive to dietary protein loading than normal subjects. **Proteins increase urinary calcium, oxalate, and uric acid excretion and the mathematically calculated probability of stone formation even in normal subjects.** Indeed, according to Burns and Finlayson (1981), ingestion of protein is second only to ingestion of vitamin D in enhancing intestinal absorption of calcium. Stone patients also exhibit inappropriate hypercalciuria in response to carbohydrate, sodium, and oxalate intake.

Protein ingestion increases endogenous acid production and secretion. Acidosis inhibits calcium resorption in the distal nephron, thereby increasing urinary calcium excretion. Metabolism of dietary methionine results in sulfate formation, which may cause the formation of calcium-sulfate complexes in the tubular lumen and result in hypercalciuria. Acidosis also decreases urinary citrate excretion and, indirectly, the potential for calcium oxalate crystallization. An increase in dietary protein or purine results in an increase in uric acid excretion. Hyperuricosuric stone formers eat more purine-rich foods than normal subjects (Kavalich et al, 1976).

Not all investigators have noticed the relationship between the intake of meat and hypercalciuria. Brockis and colleagues demonstrated that mean urinary excretion of calcium and oxalate were similar in matched groups of Seventh Day Adventists (vegetarians) and Mormons (nonvegetarians) (Brockis et al, 1982). In a detailed epidemiologic study, Power (1983) found no differences in dietary meat intake between stone formers and controls, when matched for economic status. A large study at the University of Pennsylvania found that patients with recurrent nephrolithiasis consumed a diet similar in composition to that of case controls (Goldfarb, 1994). Therefore, intake of meat may not lead directly to calcium oxalate stone disease. It may be that intake of meat acts indirectly by causing obesity. Obesity has been associated with impaired carbohydrate tolerance and an inappropriate calcium response to glucose ingestion. Thus, the hypercalciuria seen in meat eaters may be a function of increased body weight (Menon and Krishnan, 1983).

DIETARY CALCIUM

Increased gastrointestinal calcium absorption occurs in many patients with renal stones; however, less than 10% of an oral calcium load is excreted in the urine by normal individuals (Sutton and Walker, 1981). Dietary calcium restriction can decrease urinary calcium excretion, especially in patients with hypercalciuria. Thus, restriction of dietary calcium intake has been a mainstay for the prevention of recurrent nephrolithiasis.

Little is known about the effect of dietary calcium restriction on the rate of kidney stone recurrence. In a landmark study, Curhan and associates examined the association between the intake of calcium and other nutrients and the incidence of kidney stones in a cohort of 45,619 men with no history of renal calculi (Curhan et al, 1993). Patients were followed with questionnaires on diet sent at 2 and 4 years. The validity of the questionnaire was verified by weighing all foods and beverages consumed by 127 men during 2-week periods 6 to 8 months apart. Total follow-up was more than 165,000 person-years, during which 505 symptomatic kidney stones were reported.

In Curhan's study (1993), mean calcium intake was significantly **lower** in men who developed kidney stones compared with those who did not. After correcting for age and energy intake, **a higher intake of dietary calcium was strongly associated with a** decreased **risk of kidney stones.** The incidence of symptomatic kidney stones was lower by almost 50% in men with the highest calcium intake (1326 mg/day) compared with those whose intake was the lowest (516 mg/day) (Fig. 91–27). Men who drank two or more glasses of milk per day had a relative risk of kidney stones approximately one half of those who drank less than one glass per month. Inverse relationships were also found for cottage cheese, ricotta cheese, yogurt, sherbet, and nondairy sources of calcium such as oranges and broccoli. Dietary calcium supplementation, however, did not protect against renal calculi. This study strongly suggests that dietary calcium restriction is inappropriate in patients with recurrent calcium nephrolithiasis. It may even be potentially dangerous: Severe dietary calcium restriction results in a markedly negative calcium balance as a result of continued gastrointestinal calcium losses and increased bone resorption (Coe et al, 1982; Maierhofer et al, 1983). This loss of bone calcium may lead to osteoporosis, particularly in older women.

DIETARY SODIUM

Increased dietary sodium results in natriuresis. Sodium and calcium are resorbed at common sites along the distal tubule—the proximal nephron, thick ascending limb, and distal nephron. Thus, there is good correlation between urinary sodium excretion and calcium excretion. **Natriuresis causes hypercalciuria. Patients with recurrent nephrolithiasis do not ingest greater amounts of sodium than controls; however, they are more sensitive to sodium than normal subjects. Thus, avoiding excessive sodium is a reasonable strategy for the prevention of recurrent calcium stone formation.** Nonetheless, it should be noted that sodium consumption was not associated with stone risk in Curhan's study (Curhan et al, 1993). Dietary sodium restriction causes a modest reduction of urinary cystine excretion in patients with cystinuria and stones.

In one study (Sakhaee et al, 1993) of normal subjects, supplementation of the diet with 250 mmol sodium chloride per day significantly decreased urinary citrate and increased urinary pH, in addition to its effect on sodium and calcium. The urinary saturation of calcium phosphate and monosodium urate increased, and the inhibitory activity against calcium oxalate decreased, creating an environment conducive to calcium oxalate crystallization.

DIETARY OXALATE

A small increase in urinary oxalate excretion affects calcium oxalate supersaturation as much as a much larger increase in urinary calcium excretion. About 40% of the oxalate present in urine comes from metabolic production in the liver, 40% comes from the conversion of ascorbate, and less than 10% comes from dietary sources. Under normal circumstances, ingestion of rather high doses of ascorbic acid does not result in an increase in urinary oxalate excretion (Tiselius and Almgard, 1977); however, some individuals may exhibit increased conversion of ascorbate to oxalate. **Thus, it appears prudent to avoid excesses of vitamin C in patients with recurrent calcium oxalate stone formation, especially if urinary oxalate is elevated.** A low-oxalate diet (Appendix C) may result in a decrease in urinary

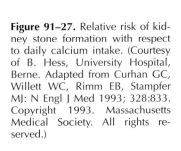

Figure 91–27. Relative risk of kidney stone formation with respect to daily calcium intake. (Courtesy of B. Hess, University Hospital, Berne. Adapted from Curhan GC, Willett WC, Rimm EB, Stampfer MJ: N Engl J Med 1993; 328:833. Copyright 1993. Massachusetts Medical Society. All rights reserved.)

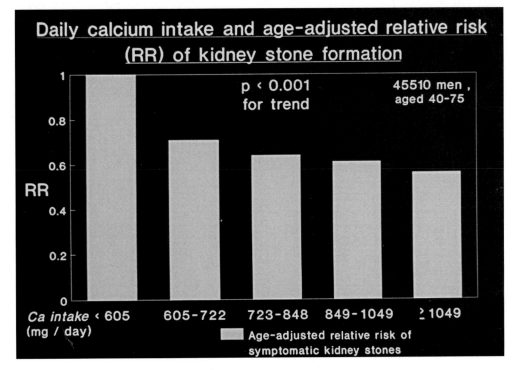

oxalate excretion; however, it tends to be quite unpalatable, and it is the rare patient who can stick to this diet over a prolonged period of time.

DIETARY PHOSPHATE

A low-phosphate diet has been used for the prevention of struvite stones because it in theory lowers the urinary supersaturation of magnesium ammonium phosphate (Shorr and Carter, 1950; Lavengood and Marshall, 1972). Such dietary restriction does not strike at the core of the problem—urinary infection with urease-splitting organisms. A low-phosphate diet results in increased production of 1,25-dihydroxyvitamin D3, increased calcium absorption, and hypercalciuria. If dietary modification is sufficiently severe, myopathy and osteomalacia may occur (Martin et al, 1975).

DIETARY FIBER

Patients with calcium oxalate stones eat less dietary fiber than healthy subjects. Fiber, or its phytic acid component, binds intestinal calcium and decreases calcium absorption. Fiber may also decrease intestinal transit time (Shah et al, 1980; Tizzani et al, 1989). Phytate-free bran is less effective than regular bran in reducing the rate of calcium excretion (Ohkawa et al, 1983). Supplementation of diet with wheat, soya, or rice bran decreases stone recurrences (Ebisuno et al, 1986; Robertson, 1987; Gleeson et al, 1990).

A decrease in intestinal calcium absorption may be expected to result in an increase in oxalate absorption and urinary oxalate excretion. Indeed, several studies (Ebisuno et al, 1986; Gleeson et al, 1990) have shown that patients ingesting bran supplements do exhibit a modest increase in urinary oxalate excretion. This effect, however, decreases with time.

Summary

The authors advise patients to drink sufficient water to keep the urine volume above 3 L/day, hoping that they will accomplish at least 2 L/day. Patients are instructed to limit their daily meat intake to 8 ounces or less, to substitute whole wheat bread for white bread, and to eat natural fiber cereals. The authors suggest that patients limit their intake of oxalate-rich foods and that they do not add salt at the table. Patients are told not to restrict dairy products but to avoid overindulgence—no more than three glasses of milk a day. Patients are advised that such a diet will not only decrease their likelihood of stone recurrences but also benefit their general health overall, by reducing the risk of hypertension, heart disease, and colon disease. The authors suggest that the entire family follow a similar diet (Fig. 91–28).

Specific Measures

Thiazides

Thiazides were originally used by Yendt and associates for the treatment of patients with idiopathic hypercalciuria in 1966. Over the last 30 years, this is the group of drugs

High Fluid Intake
Sodium Restriction
Oxalate Restriction
Avoidance of Purine Gluttony if possible
Increased Citrus Fruit Intake
Calcium Restriction (moderate) in Hypercalciuria
Only in the presence of normal bone density

Figure 91–28. Dietary modifications (for long-term treatment) apply to all patients with recurrent episode or first episode at risk (whether or not metabolic abnormalities are present). (Courtesy of Mission Pharmacal Co., San Antonio, TX.)

that has been used most extensively in the medical management of recurrent calcium oxalate stone disease. **Thiazides directly stimulate calcium resorption in the distal nephron while promoting excretion of sodium. Long-term thiazide therapy results in volume depletion, extracellular volume contraction, and proximal tubular resorption of sodium and calcium.** Thiazides also stimulate the effect of PTH in augmenting the renal resorption of calcium. Thiazides do not affect intestinal calcium absorption in normal subjects (Earnest et al, 1974) or in patients with absorptive hypercalciuria (Zerwekh and Pak, 1980; Preminger and Pak, 1987) but decrease it in patients with renal hypercalciuria. Chlorthalidone improves calcium balance in severe idiopathic hypercalciuria by lowering urinary calcium excretion more than it lowers intestinal calcium absorption (Coe et al, 1988). Thus, bone density may increase during thiazide treatment of absorptive hypercalciuria (Preminger, 1995). Prolonged treatment, however, stabilizes the bone density and attenuates the hypocalciuric effect of thiazides. **At doses of 50 mg twice daily, hydrochlorothiazide causes mean reduction of urinary calcium of 150 mg/day in normocalciuric patients and 400 mg/day in hypercalciuric patients** (Yendt and Cohanim, 1978).

Thiazides may increase urinary excretion of magnesium and zinc, but these responses are not consistent. Potassium losses from thiazide therapy can cause hypocitraturia. The urinary excretion of oxalate increases initially but decreases with longer treatment (Yendt and Cohanim, 1978).

Table 91–12 gives a summary of the results of randomized trials that compare thiazides and one study that uses a nonthiazide diuretic, indapamide, with placebo in the treatment of calcium oxalate stone disease. **Although the results of therapy are impressive when recurrence rates after treatment are compared with recurrence rates before treatment, equally impressive decreases in recurrence rates are obtained in placebo-treated patients.** Overall, 73% of placebo-treated patients remained in remission, as compared to 85% of patients treated with thiazides. **Any beneficial effect of thiazides is seen only in studies that have follow-ups of more than 2 years.** Thiazides may be specifically indicated in patients with renal hypercalciuria. When used in this condition, stone formation rates drop by about 90%, compared to pretreatment stone rates but not to placebo treatment (Pak et al, 1981c; Pak, 1982a).

The standard dose of hydrochlorothiazide for the treatment of calcium oxalate stone disease is 25 to 50 mg twice

Table 91–12. RANDOMIZED TRIALS OF DIURETIC THERAPY FOR THE PREVENTION OF CALCIUM OXALATE STONES

Year	Author	Diagnosis	Agent	Patients	Controls	Efficacy	Follow-Up	Comments
1981	Brocks et al	Recurrent calcium stones	Bendroflumethiazide 2.5 mg tid	29	33	83% remission in controls, 85% in treated: not significant	1.6 years	Not all patients were hypercalciuric. Only 16% of expected stones formed in controls, 24% in treated
1982	Scholz et al	Recurrent calcium stones	Hydrochlorothiazide 25 mg bid	25	26	77% remission in controls, 76% in thiazide: not significant	1 year	Fasting urinary calcium increased before treatment, decreased with thiazides, but not in controls. Urine output increased in both groups, indicating that hydration was sufficient
1984	Laerum and Larsen	Recurrent stone formers	Hydrochlorothiazide 25 mg bid	25	25	45% remission in controls, 75% in thiazides: significant difference. Controls formed 21 stones. Treated formed 20 stones: not significant	3 years	General practice study. 75% of patients did not have hypercalciuria. Differences seen only after 18 months
1988	Ettinger et al	Recurrent calcium stones	Chlorthalidone 25 or 50 mg/day	42	31	55% remission in controls, 86% in treated: significant	3 years	Only 15% of patients had hypercalciuria. Compliance to diet not encouraged or assessed; to drugs, assessed. Urine output not measured. 16% dropout rate in controls, 35–40% drop out rate with chlorothalidone
1984	Wilson et al	Recurrent calcium stones	Hydrochlorothiazide 100 mg/day	21	23	65% remission in controls, 70% in treated: not significant. 0.32 stones per year in controls, 0.15 stones per year in treated: significant	2.8 years	All patients not hypercalciuric. Other treatments—phosphates, magnesium, allopurinol—were ineffective
1992	Ohkawa et al	Idiopathic hypercalciuria	Trichlormethiazide 4 mg/day	82	93	86% remission in controls, 92% in thiazides: not significant. Stone formation rate significantly lowered in treated patients	<3 years	Multi-institution study. All patients had hypercalciuria. Many were single stone formers
1993	Borghi et al	Idiopathic hypercalciuria	Indapamide 2.5 mg/day or indapamide plus allopurinol 300 mg/day	25	25	65% remission in controls, 95% in treated: significant	3 years	Urinary output did not rise in either group, thus hydration may not have been effective
Total				253	252	73% remission in controls, 85% in treated patients		Beneficial effects with treatment seen only in trials with follow-up of ≥2 years

daily. Alternatively, trichlormethiazide 2 mg twice a day or bendroflumethiazide 2.5 mg two to three times a day may be used. Side effects may be minimized by starting with a small dose and escalating it over a period of 1 to 3 weeks. **Although side effects are generally mild, they occur in about 30% to 35% of treated patients, most of whom drop out of treatment. Side effects usually are seen on initiation of treatment, disappearing with continued treatment.** Lassitude and sleepiness are the most common symptoms and can occur in the absence of hypokalemia. Potassium supplementation need not be given routinely, but patients with evident potassium deficiency, patients on digitalis therapy, and patients who develop hypocitraturia need potassium supplementation. Rarely, thiazides unmask or induce primary hyperparathyroidism. They may also cause impaired carbohydrate tolerance and hyperuricemia. A more distressing complication is the occurrence of decreased libido or sexual dysfunction. Such a side effect is alarming to the typical patient with calcium oxalate stone disease—the young man.

Orthophosphates

Orthophosphate salts have been used for a number of years in the management of calcium urolithiasis but are currently waning in popularity, perhaps because of the lack of randomized trials showing efficacy and the occurrence of side effects. Initially, phosphates were used in the hope of binding dietary calcium in the intestine and thus reducing its absorption. The fractional absorption of calcium, however, appears to be unaffected in subjects who are administered orthophosphates (Thomas, 1976). Orthophosphates, however, decrease the production of 1,25-dihydroxyvitamin D3 without affecting parathyroid function (Van Den Berg et al, 1980; Insogna et al, 1989). **Clinically, urinary excretion of calcium decreases by about 50% in patients with absorptive hypercalciuria and by about 25% in patients without this disorder.** Orthophosphates may augment the renal tubular resorption of calcium.

Uncontrolled studies have reported remission rates of 75% to 91% in recurrent stone formers treated with orthophosphates (Smith et al, 1973; Pak et al, 1981c). In a double-blind, prospective study, Ettinger (1976) evaluated 71 patients with recurrent calcium oxalate stones treated with an inert placebo, a low-calcium diet, or potassium acid phosphate. With a follow-up of close to 3 years, mean urinary calcium levels dropped in patients on phosphate therapy by 33%; however, there was no appreciable decrease in renal stone formation. After 3 years of follow-up, 73% of patients treated with placebo, 47% of patients treated with a low-calcium diet, and 50% of patients treated with potassium acid phosphate developed recurrences. Examination of the pattern of recurrences, however, indicates that, as opposed to thiazides, phosphates may decrease stone recurrences within the first 2 years of follow-up but lose their effectiveness with longer treatment. This study has been criticized because an acid rather than a neutral form of phosphate was used; nonetheless, it represents a rare, prospective, randomized study of orthophosphates in the prevention of calcium oxalate stone disease.

Urinary phosphorus excretion is markedly increased during therapy with neutral or alkaline phosphate, which results in an increase in the inhibitor activity of urine, perhaps because of increased renal excretion of pyrophosphate and citrate (Preminger, 1995). Thus, the urinary saturation of calcium oxalate is lowered, whereas that of calcium phosphate is increased. This treatment has been reported to cause soft tissue calcification in patients with renal insufficiency. It is contraindicated in patients with magnesium ammonium phosphate stone disease. Orthophosphates can cause gastrointestinal disturbances and diarrhea.

Sodium Cellulose Phosphate

Sodium cellulose phosphate is a nonabsorbable resin that binds calcium and inhibits intestinal calcium absorption. In one series, sodium cellulose phosphate decreased intestinal calcium absorption by 85% in patients with absorptive hypercalciuria and recurrent nephrolithiasis (Blacklock and MacLeod, 1974). Acute treatment with cellulose phosphate decreases urinary calcium excretion by 50% to 70%; however, it increases urinary oxalate excretion (Hayashi et al, 1975). The rate of saturation of urine with respect to calcium oxalate is affected inconsistently. Uncontrolled studies have shown a decrease in stone formation in patients being treated with sodium cellulose phosphate (Blacklock and MacLeod, 1974; Pak et al, 1981c). In Pak's study, 18 patients with absorptive hypercalciuria type I were treated with sodium cellulose phosphate at 10 to 15 g/day in divided doses. Oral magnesium supplementation and moderate dietary restriction of calcium and oxalate were also used. At a mean follow-up of 2.4 years, 78% of the patients were in remission, and the rest showed reduced stone formation. In another study, Backman and colleagues compared the effects of cellulose phosphate with those of diet and hydration (Backman et al, 1980a). Although this study was not randomized, 47% of the renal stone formers treated with cellulose phosphate developed a stone recurrence within 2 years of follow-up, not much different from control subjects.

Sodium cellulose phosphate is poorly tolerated by some individuals, giving rise to nausea and diarrhea. When used in patients with normal intestinal calcium absorption, it may cause negative calcium balance and parathyroid stimulation. The resin also binds magnesium, resulting in hypomagnesuria. Finally, it binds calcium of the gut, making more oxalate available for absorption. Thus, it may increase urinary oxalate excretion. For these reasons, **sodium cellulose phosphate should be used only in documented cases of absorptive hypercalciuria. Oral magnesium supplementation and a moderate dietary restriction of oxalate should be used simultaneously.** Under these conditions, sodium cellulose phosphate reduces urinary calcium, reduces crystallization of calcium salts, maintains bone density, and is clinically effective (Preminger, 1995). Rice bran (Ebisuno

et al, 1991) also binds intestinal calcium and increases urinary pyrophosphate. In an uncontrolled long-term study, rice bran reduced stone recurrences. In another study, 73 patients with recurrent urinary stone formation were treated with 40 g of unprocessed bran daily. Hydrochlorothiazide was added during the summer months. Over a 2-year follow-up, three fourths of the patients were free of stones. The combination of thiazide and bran was superior to bran alone in preventing stone formation (Ala-opas et al, 1987)

Allopurinol

Allopurinol inhibits xanthine oxidase and decreases the production of uric acid. It has been used at doses of 100 mg three times a day for the treatment of hyperuricosuric calcium oxalate and uric acid nephrolithiasis. In several studies, allopurinol has been used in patients with recurrent calcium stones, not all of whom having hyperuricosuria (Smith, 1977; Scott et al, 1979; Wilson et al, 1984; Fellstrom et al, 1985; Marangella et al, 1985; Miano et al, 1985; Robertson et al, 1985). In these studies, although there has been a decrease in calculus events, the decrease is no greater than would be expected with hydration and avoidance of dietary excesses. In contrast, Coe (1977) found that allopurinol, when used in patients with hyperuricosuria and normocalciuria, resulted in post-treatment calculus rates of 0.08 and 0.04 per patient per year, less than one would expect with placebo alone. In a double-blind, prospective, randomized study, Ettinger and associates administered allopurinol to 60 patients with hyperuricosuria and normocalciuria and recurrent calcium oxalate stones (Ettinger et al, 1986). A 6-month "grace period" was established, during which time any new calculus that was passed was not considered to represent failure of therapy. With a follow-up of up to 39 months, new stone events (stone growth or recurrence) occurred in 58% of the patients on placebo and in 31% of the patients on allopurinol. The placebo group had 63.4% fewer calculi, whereas the allopurinol group had 81.2% fewer calculi. The mean rate of calculus events was 0.26 per patient per year in the placebo group and 0.12 in the allopurinol group. The allopurinol group was found to have a significantly longer time before the recurrence of stones. The Ettinger study offers the most compelling proof that allopurinol is effective in the treatment of hyperuricosuric nephrolithiasis (Fig. 91–29).

The side effects of allopurinol are mainly drug reactions. Severe allopurinol hypersensitivity has been seen in association with thiazides in patients with prior renal compromise (Young et al, 1974).

Citrates

Two agents have been used for the treatment of hypocitraturia: sodium potassium citrate, commonly used in Europe, and potassium citrate—in liquid form or as a wax matrix tablet—used in the United States. The usual therapeutic dose is 30 to 60 mEq/day given in three divided doses (Pak et al, 1985a; Sakhaee et al, 1991) or as a single evening dose (Berg et al, 1992). In Europe, sodium potassium citrate is favored because of the relative unpalatability of potassium citrate (Hermann et al, 1992). This problem has not been reported in the United States. Pak prefers potassium citrate

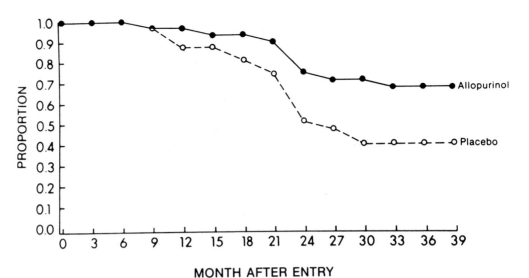

Figure 91–29. Life table plot showing proportion of patients without calculus events during treatment with allopurinol or placebo. (From Ettinger B, Tang A, Citron JT, et al: N Engl J Med 1986; 315:1388. Copyright 1986; Massachusetts Medical Society. Reprinted by permission of *The New England Journal of Medicine*.)

because it appears to decrease urinary calcium excretion, at least transiently (Pak, 1987a). Sodium citrate does not lower urinary calcium excretion, perhaps as the result of the increased sodium load associated with therapy (Sakhaee et al, 1983).

There are conflicting reports about the efficacy of citrate in preventing stone recurrences. Pak and colleagues initially used potassium citrate to treat 13 patients with hypercalciuria who failed thiazide therapy (Pak et al, 1985a). Over a 1- to 2-year follow-up, all patients had reduced stone formation, and 10 out of 13 patients (77%) stopped forming stones altogether. Pak (1987a) subsequently reported on the use of potassium citrate in 35 patients with hypocitraturia. Over a 1.7-year follow-up, 88% of patients were free of recurrences. In contrast, Berg and colleagues (1992) found a 28% recurrence rate in 72 patients treated with sodium potassium citrate, although only half of these patients had hypocitraturia.

Two small randomized studies have compared citrate therapy with oral hydration in the treatment of patients with calcium stone disease. Hofbauer and colleagues compared sodium potassium citrate to general prophylaxis in 50 patients with a follow-up of 3 years (Hofbauer et al, 1994). Sixty-five percent of the control subjects and 72% of the treated group had hypocitraturia. Sixty-nine percent of the patients in the treatment group and 73% of the patients in the control group continued to form stones. The rate of stone recurrence dropped from 2.1 to 0.9 stones per patient per year with treatment. In the control group, the corresponding numbers were 1.8 and 0.7. This study has been criticized because sodium potassium citrate was used, which may have caused hypercalciuria. Of the treated patients, however, 48% had hypercalciuria before therapy, whereas only 25% had hypercalciuria during therapy. Thus, it appears that alkali citrate did lower urinary calcium excretion in some of these patients. Furthermore, no prospective, randomized study has confirmed the superiority of potassium citrate over sodium potassium citrate in the prevention of stone recurrences. In another study, Abdulhadi and colleagues (1993) reported on the results of long-term potassium citrate therapy in 10 patients with hypocitraturia and recurrent calcium nephrolithiasis compared to 13 controls with stone disease who were treated with hydration alone. New stone formation rate decreased 62% in the citrate group and 70% in the controls. Twenty percent of the treated patients and 31% of the controls continued to form stones. Patients in this study were frankly hypercalciuric, and urinary citrate excretion averaged 69 mg per 24 hours. Thus, some of these patients may have had RTA, a condition that is notoriously difficult to treat.

Thus, **citrate therapy is a new and promising method for the prevention of recurrent calcium oxalate stone disease. Its efficacy needs to be verified, however, in long-term, prospective trials.** Even in the negative trials, investigators have believed that stones passed with less severe colic (Hofbauer et al, 1994). If this is the case, citrate therapy will be a boon to the average patient, even if it does not decrease stone recurrence.

Magnesium

The administration of magnesium salts was first advocated on the ground that it reduced urinary excretion of oxalate. **Some magnesium salts increase urinary magnesium excretion and thus produce a more favorable magnesium-to-calcium ratio in the urine, a condition that offers relative protection against stone formation. Magnesium decreases renal tubular citrate resorption through the chelation of citrate and thus increases urinary citrate excretion.** Melnick and co-workers found that stone recurrence dropped from 6 stones per year to 0.073 stone per year in a group of 149 recurrent calcium oxalate stone formers treated with magnesium oxide (Melnick et al, 1971). Prien and Greshoff (1974) reported that about 70% of patients administered 300 mg of magnesium oxide and 100 mg of pyridoxine demonstrated a complete cessation of stone formation. Johansson and associates treated 56 patients with 400 to 500 mg of magnesium hydroxide (Johansson et al, 1980). Eighty percent of the treated patients were free of stones, in comparison to 50% who did not receive magnesium supplementation. The rate of stone formation dropped from 0.80 stone per year to 0.03 stone per year in the treated patients and from 0.50 stone per year to 0.22 stone per year in the control subjects. Two randomized trials (Wilson et al, 1984; Ettinger et al, 1988) showed no difference in recurrence rates between treated and untreated patients. In these studies, details of randomization were not given, and the biochemical abnormalities were not described in detail.

Several magnesium salts have been used for the treatment of stone disease. Magnesium oxide and magnesium hydroxide are poorly absorbed and produce only a slight decrease in urinary oxalate and a modest increase in urinary magnesium (Barilla et al, 1978a; Johansson et al, 1980; Ahlstrand and Tiselius, 1984). Urinary calcium levels are increased during magnesium oxide supplementation (Melnick et al, 1971; Fetner et al, 1978; Tiselius et al, 1980), and thus urinary saturation of calcium oxalate is not significantly lowered with magnesium oxide. Lindberg and colleagues found that either magnesium citrate or magnesium oxide induced only modest beneficial changes in urinary biochemistry when administered on an empty stomach (Lindberg et al, 1990a). **When the magnesium salts were provided with meals, however, they caused more prominent changes in urinary biochemistry** and lowered the relative saturation of urine with calcium oxalate or brushite.

Gastrointestinal intolerance is the major side effect of magnesium therapy. At this time, magnesium supplementation is not widely used. It may be indicated in patients with hypomagnesuric calcium oxalate nephrolithiasis, seen in less than 5% of patients with recurrent calcium stones. Magnesium supplementation may be used together with sodium cellulose phosphate in the treatment of patients with absorptive hypercalciuria type I and with potassium citrate in patients with chronic diarrheal syndromes.

Selective Versus Nonselective Therapy

The rationale for using selective therapy for nephrolithiasis based on urinary biochemistry is the assumption that normalization of urinary parameters prevents stone recurrences and that selective therapy is more effective and safer than random therapy in accomplishing this goal. In the first study examining this concept, Pak and colleagues found that selective therapy induced a remission rate of between 70% and 91% and reduced stone formation in 88% to 100% of patients so treated (Pak et al, 1981c). Each treatment program produced a significant decline in stone formation in the targeted population. In other studies, Ettinger and colleagues (1986) found that allopurinol was more effective in patients with pure hyperuricosuria than in patients with hypercalciuria. In a study at Dallas (Pak et al, 1985a), potassium citrate was more effective in patients with hypocitraturia than in patients with normal urinary citrate.

Pak worries about the side effects of nonselective therapy (Pak, 1990). Treatment of renal hypercalciuria with sodium cellulose phosphate, an agent that reduces calcium absorption from the intestine while allowing continued renal losses of calcium, may exaggerate secondary hyperparathyroidism and promote bone demineralization. Thiazides may cause calcium deposition in the bones of patients with absorptive hypercalciuria, and hypercalcemia in patients with resorptive hypercalciuria. Orthophosphates may also cause calcium retention in patients with normophosphatemic absorptive hypercalciuria. Potassium citrate, used in the presence of urinary tract infection, may increase urinary pH and promote stone growth. Sodium citrate may increase urinary calcium

excretion, increasing the saturation of calcium salts and promoting urate-induced crystallization.

It is intellectually appealing to categorize stone disease on the basis of urinary metabolites and to use selective therapy. There is no proof, however, that selective therapy is more efficacious than nonselective therapy. One advantage of using nonselective therapy is that it avoids the expense and work involved in categorizing calcium oxalate stone disease. It is also sobering to note that in three of the four randomized trials in which thiazides were found to be effective, the agent was used on a nonselective basis, and only a minority of patients had hypercalciuria (Laerum and Larsen, 1984; Wilson et al, 1984; Ettinger et al, 1988). It is also true that most patients do not have an isolated metabolic abnormality but rather a combination of abnormalities, and thus selective treatment may be too precise. Finally, Coe and co-workers have questioned the subcategorization of idiopathic hypercalciuria into tight compartments of absorptive, renal, and resorptive hypercalciuria (Coe et al, 1992). They have suggested that hypercalciuria represents a continuum of disorders, with varying elements of absorptive, renal, and resorptive disturbance.

Although the authors prefer to use selective therapy, in the absence of conclusive proof that this is better and safer than nonselective therapy, they have no quarrel with those who prefer a simpler approach. Table 91–13 shows currently accepted methods for selective medical therapy of patients with renal stones.

Problems in the Literature Dealing with Prevention of Recurrences

The literature that deals with the prevention of stone recurrences can broadly be divided into two categories: studies in which clinical outcomes are measured before and during intervention, and randomized clinical trials (Churchill, 1987). The vast majority of clinical studies have employed the former strategy. Because calcium oxalate stone disease has a quixotic and unpredictable recurrence pattern, such studies are flawed in concept. Patients generally come to a specialized center or stone clinic when they have a flare-up of stone disease; any remission of their symptoms may be the result of variable natural history, rather than a benefit of intervention. It is difficult to do prospective, randomized clinical trials in stone disease, and thus few have been done: six with thiazides (Ettinger, 1976; Brockis et al, 1981; Scholz et al, 1982; Laerum and Larsen, 1984; Wilson et al, 1984; Robertson et al, 1985), three with orthophosphates (Ettinger, 1976; Wilson et al, 1984; Robertson et al, 1985), none with sodium cellulose phosphate, five with allopurinol (Smith, 1977; Wilson et al, 1984; Ettinger et al, 1985; Miano et al, 1985; Robertson et al, 1985), one with magnesium hydroxide (Ettinger et al, 1985), and two with citrate (Abdulhadi et al, 1993; Hofbauer et al, 1994). **These studies suggest that thiazides are efficacious in preventing stone recurrence, if the follow-up is greater than 2 years. Allopurinol is efficacious in patients with hyperuricosuria without hypercalciuria. The effectiveness of magnesium, sodium cellulose phosphate, orthophosphates, and citrate remains to be proven in randomized clinical trials.**

Table 91–13. SELECTIVE TREATMENT OF RECURRENT STONES

Disorder	Treatment	Mechanism of Action	Side Effects
Low urine volume	High fluid intake	Increases urinary volume, decreases urinary saturation	None
Absorptive hypercalciuria, type I	Sodium cellulose phosphate	Decreases intestinal calcium absorption	Mild gastrointestinal discomfort, unpleasant taste, arthritis
	Thiazides and other hypocalciuric diuretics	Decreases urinary calcium excretion	Lassitude, sleepiness, weakness, sexual dysfunction, impaired glucose tolerance, hypokalemia, increased serum cholesterol, increased calcium deposition in bone (?)
Absorptive hypercalciuria, type II	Low-calcium diet, sodium cellulose phosphate	Decreases intestinal calcium absorption	Bone mineral loss
Absorptive hypercalciuria, type III	Orthophosphates	Decreases 1,25-dihydroxyvitamin D_3 and urinary calcium, increases urinary citrate and pyrophosphate	Diarrhea, bloating, arthralgia (?)
Hypocitraturia, including renal tubular acidosis	Potassium citrate	Increases urinary citrate, increases urinary pH	Gastrointestinal intolerance
Hypomagnesiuria	Magnesium citrate	Increases urinary magnesium and citrate	Gastrointestinal intolerance
Hyperuricosuria with calcium oxalate stones	Allopurinol Potassium alkali salts Reduced urine intake	Decreases urinary uric acid, increases urinary citrate and pH, decreases urinary uric acid	Drug reactions, especially in patients on thiazides; gastrointestinal intolerance; lack of compliance
Uric acid stones	Potassium alkali salts	Increases urinary citrate, increases urinary pH	Gastrointestinal intolerance
	Allopurinol	Decreases urinary uric acid	Drug reactions
Enteric hyperoxaluria	Pyridoxine Oral calcium supplementation	Decreases urinary oxalate, increases oxalate binding in the intestine	
Chronic diarrheal syndromes	Cholestyramine	Decreases oxalate absorption	Worsening diarrhea, vitamin K depletion, drug interactions
	Potassium alkali salts	Increases urinary citrate	Gastrointestinal intolerance
Infection stones	Acetohydroxamic acid	Decreases urease, ammonium, and pH	Headaches, tremor, deep vein thrombosis
Cystinuria	D-penicillamine or tiopronin (MPG)	Increases solubility of cystine	Impaired taste and smell, proteinuria, serum sickness, anemia

Modified from Pak CYC: General guidelines in management. *In* Resnick MI, Pak CYC, eds: Urolithiasis: A Medical and Surgical Reference. Philadelphia, W. B. Saunders, 1990, p 17; and modified from Coe FL, Parks JH, Asplin JR: N Engl J Med 1992; 327:1141. Copyright 1992. Massachusetts Medical Society. All rights reserved.

The dramatic therapeutic success that is reported in studies that compare clinical outcomes before and during intervention are not borne out in randomized clinical trials. Even in the trials that show a putative benefit, there are methodologic flaws, such as patients lost to follow-up; grace periods; or demonstration that hydration, the placebo treatment, really has been implemented. The longest trials have a follow-up of about 3 years—hardly long enough for a disease with a variable and lifelong recurrence pattern.

In the absence of randomized trials, the authors suggest the following criteria be used in interpreting results of trials with historical controls. Bek-Jensen and Tiselius (1989) have suggested that the bias that is introduced when stone recurrences immediately before intervention are compared to those during intervention can be avoided by using the stone recurrence pattern at initiation of disease—rather than immediately before treatment—as the control period. The authors agree. **Alternatively, stone recurrence rate without treatment averages between 5% and 10% per year. Thus, any treatment that does not induce a stone remission of greater than 70% at 3 years should be considered ineffective.**

OTHER ANATOMIC LOCATIONS
Vesical Calculi

In certain parts of the world, the incidence of vesical calculi is high. In other areas, a steady, pronounced decrease in incidence of stones in the bladder has occurred since the 19th century. This decrease has been attributed to dietary and nutritional progress. In England and France during the 19th century, calculus disease was largely limited to children. Now, it is a disease of adults (Hodgkinson and Marshall, 1975). The decrease in vesical calculi in childhood is probably due to improvement in nutrition. In some areas of the world, such as Thailand and Indonesia, bladder calculi continue to occur in children. A symposium on idiopathic urinary bladder stone disease has been published (Van Reen, 1977).

Vesical calculus is predominantly a disease of men. In the United States, vesical calculi occur usually in men over 50 years old and are associated with bladder outlet obstruction. The diagnosis of a bladder stone should result in a complete urologic evaluation for factors that give rise to retention of urine, such as stricture of the urethra, prostatic hypertrophy, diverticulum of the bladder, and neurogenic bladder.

In contrast to renal stones, bladder stones are usually composed of uric acid (in noninfected urine) or struvite (in infected urine). Reports from the United States have revealed uric acid stones in nearly 50% of patients with bladder stones (Douenias et al, 1991). Such patients often have bladder outlet obstruction, causing them to decrease fluid intake, with the resultant production of concentrated, acid urine. The occurrence of calcium oxalate or cystine stones in the bladder suggests the presence of calculi in the kidney.

Usually a single stone is observed in the bladder, but in the presence of retained urine, multiple stones may be present (Sarica et al, 1994). Multiple stones are formed more frequently when there is a diverticulum of the bladder. Multiple stones may become faceted and vary in size (Fig. 91–30).

Symptoms

In patients with prostatic enlargement and residual urine, the complaints may be those of prostatic obstruction, with the calculus being found incidentally. Typical symptoms of vesical stone are intermittent, painful voiding with terminal hematuria. Discomfort may be dull, aching, or sharp suprapubic pain, which is aggravated by exercise and sudden movement. Severe pain usually occurs near the end of micturition, as the stone impacts at the bladder neck. Relief may be afforded by assuming a recumbent position. The pain may be referred to the tip of the penis, scrotum, or the perineum and on occasion to the back, the hip, or even the heel or sole of the foot. Besides pain, there may be an interruption of the urinary stream from impaction of the stone at the bladder neck or urethra. Priapism and nocturnal enuresis may occur in children.

Diagnosis

Often evidence of vesical calculi is not seen in plain films because of the presence of uric acid in many of the calculi and because of overlying prostatic tissue. Such stones form negative shadows in the cystogram phase of an intravenous urogram. Ultrasonography is useful for detecting radiolucent calculi. Cystoscopic examination is the surest method for detecting vesical calculi.

Treatment

Eradication of obstruction, correction of bladder stasis, and removal of foreign bodies minimize recurrence. Stone dissolution with the use of Suby's G or M solution is protracted and is now rarely employed. Renacidin may be employed to dissolve struvite or phosphate calculi and may prove beneficial in irrigating indwelling suprapubic or ure-

thral catheters to prevent formation of calculus. Twice-daily or thrice-daily irrigations with 0.25% or 0.5% acetic acid solution also serve as beneficial prophylaxis against recurrent struvite calculi when catheters must be left indwelling for long periods. Uric acid calculi may be dissolved by irrigation with alkaline solutions. The basis of treatment, however, is interventional (Drach, 1979).

Calculi of the Prostate and Seminal Vesicles

Classification

True prostatic calculi are those that develop in the tissues or acini of the gland and are not to be confused with urinary calculi lodged in a dilated prostatic urethra or in a pouch of the urethra. True prostatic calculi are formed by the deposition of calcareous material on corpora amylacea. These are 2- to 5-mm, round or ovoid bodies present in the alveoli of the prostate gland. They are rare in boys but frequent in men over 50 years old. Corpora amylacea have a laminated structure composed of lecithin and a nitrogenous substance of an albuminous nature, which is apparently formed around desquamated epithelial cells. Inorganic salts (calcium phosphate and calcium carbonate) impregnate the corpora amylacea, converting them into calculi. Sutor and Wooley (1974b) observed that "false" prostatic calculi probably arise from the precipitation of salts found in normal prostatic fluid, that is, calcium and magnesium phosphates. Infection also contributes to formation of some prostatic calculi. Ochronosis, associated with alkaptonuria and precipitation of homogentisic acid, has been rarely associated with prostatic calculi (Douenias et al, 1991).

Incidence

The prevalence of symptomatic prostatic calculi is not known because, in many instances, they are noted incidentally during a routine roentgenographic or ultrasonic survey.

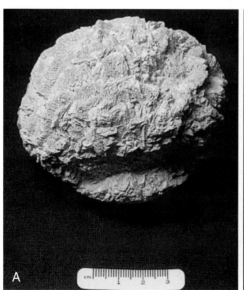
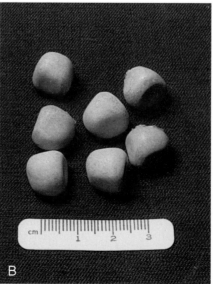

Figure 91–30. Vesical calculus: *A*, Solitary struvite. *B*, Multiple faceted stones. (Courtesy of Worcester District Medical Society, Worcester, MA.)

Joly (1931) observed 34 cases of prostatic calculi in a series of 636 cases of urinary calculi, an incidence of 5.3%.

Stones in the seminal vesicles are an extremely rare condition (White, 1928). The nucleus is composed of epithelial cells and a mucoid substance that is covered with lime salts. The stones are smooth and hard and range in size from 1 mm to 1 cm in diameter.

Composition

Generally, stones in the prostate are composed of calcium phosphate. Huggins and Bear (1944) observed that the organic components proteins, cholesterol, and citrate composed about 20% of the calculus. True prostatic calculi are composed solely of calcium phosphate trihydrate (whitlockite) and carbonate (Sutor and Wooley, 1974b).

Symptoms

No symptoms are pathognomonic of calculus disease of the prostate gland. Symptoms, when present, may be due to prostatic hypertrophy, stricture of the urethra, or chronic prostatitis. Terminal urinary bleeding may be present. A stone in the seminal vesicle may be silent and produce no symptoms. In some cases, hematospermia, painful erections, and perineal discomfort at the time of ejaculation have occurred (Drach, 1975).

Diagnosis

Panendoscopic examination usually reveals only prostatic enlargement. Stones are seldom seen endoscopically in patients with prostatic calculi. Occasionally, grating is felt on passing the urethroscope. A calculus sometimes protrudes into and obstructs the urethra. Roentgenographic or ultrasonic study usually confirms diagnosis of prostatic calculi (Fig. 91–31). Diffuse shadows may be generally distributed throughout the gland and are more likely to be related to chronic inflammatory processes, such as tuberculosis. In other, more frequently observed types, there are so-called horseshoe or ring arrangements. The shadows surround a clear central portion formed by the central prostate (the adenoma of the urethra). In the horseshoe type, the stones

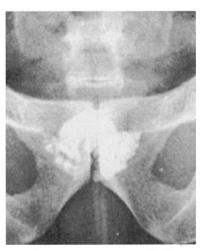

Figure 91–31. Prostatic calculi.

are present laterally on both sides of the gland but are absent anterior to the urethra, as evidenced by the clear space that is the opening of the horseshoe. In other instances, a large solitary calculus is observed.

Treatment

No treatment is indicated for patients with asymptomatic prostatic calculi. In patients with significant symptoms, a transurethral or suprapubic prostatectomy may be contemplated. In the presence of multiple symptomatic calculi and intractable infection, total prostatectomy and bilateral seminal vesiculectomy, although drastic, usually affords a cure (Drach, 1992).

Urethral Calculi

The majority of urethral calculi in the male consist of stones expelled from the bladder into the urethra. Rarely a calculus may form primarily in the urethra when stricture is present, or it may form in a pouch or diverticulum that opens into the urethra. Among the natives of developing countries, urethral calculi are common in children because stones of the bladder are also frequent. Otherwise, urethral calculi represent less than 1% of all urinary stone disease. Calculi that migrate to the urethra obviously have the same constituents as bladder or upper urinary tract calculi. If there is associated infection, a primary urethral calculus is composed of struvite. Usually only a single stone is encountered.

Symptoms

While urinating, the patient with a urethral calculus may experience a sudden stoppage and be therefore unable to empty the bladder. Dribbling also occurs. A patient may be able to palpate the stone within the scrotal or penile urethra. Pain occasioned by the stone may be rather severe and may radiate to the head of the penis. When the calculus is lodged in the posterior urethra, the pain is referred to the perineum or the rectum. When the stone is lodged in the anterior urethra, the pain should be localized at the site of impaction. A stone may be present in a diverticulum of the urethra for an extended period without producing symptoms. Urethral discharge may be observed—the result of the infection in the diverticulum. The patient may be aware of a painful lump that has gradually increased in size and hardness on the undersurface of the penis. Usually, no change occurs in the caliber of the stream or urine, and no dribbling occurs.

Treatment

Treatment is influenced by the size, shape, and position of the calculus and by the status of the urethra. At times, a stone in the anterior urethra may be grasped and removed with forceps. Pressure is exerted simultaneously on the urethra proximal to the stone so that it is not forced into the bladder. A small stone may sometimes be gently massaged or milked outward, so that it can be expelled. A novel noninvasive procedure uses intraurethral instillation of 2% lidocaine jelly for spontaneous expulsion of impacted urethral stones. El-Sherif and El-Hafi (1991) reported spontaneous expulsion of the stone in 14 of 18 patients treated in this manner. Lithotripsy and removal of a stone via the urethroscope may be advisable. When a stricture obstructs passage of the stone, a preliminary internal urethrotomy may be performed. When a large stone has been impacted for some time in the urethra, an external urethrotomy may be required. A calculus lodged in the navicular fossa often can be removed by meatotomy. A calculus recently impacted in the posterior urethra frequently can be pushed back into the bladder and then crushed (Sharfi, 1991). If the stone is large and immovable, it may be removed through the perineal or suprapubic route. When the calculus occupies a urethral diverticulum, diverticulectomy and repair should be performed.

Urethral Calculi in Women

The occurrence of urethral calculi in women is infrequent in comparison with that in men. This may be attributed to two factors — the short urethra in women and the infrequency of vesical calculi in women. Calculi in the female urethra are usually associated with a urethral diverticulum or a urethrocele.

Symptoms and Diagnosis

The symptoms of urethral diverticulum, with or without calculus, are those of infection of the lower urinary tract. Pain during coitus is a prominent symptom. Occasional discharge of pus may occur, giving the patient only temporary relief. Examination discloses a hard mass in the anterior vaginal wall in the area of the urethra.

Treatment

The treatment of a urethrocele or diverticulum containing a calculus is surgical, with excision of the sac containing the calculus. The technique varies according to the preference of the operating surgeon.

Preputial Calculi

Preputial calculi usually form when phimosis is present. Three types of preputial calculi are noted. First are calculi arising from inspissated smegma that becomes impregnated with lime salts. The second type includes calculi that form in stagnant urine retained in the sac because of phimosis. They are composed of magnesium ammonium phosphate or calcium phosphate. Third are calculi that have been expelled from the bladder into the urethra and have gained entrance into the preputial sac by way of the urethral meatus or by ulceration through the navicular fossa.

In the United States, these calculi are rare. It is primarily a disease of adults. There may be no symptoms referable to the calculus. The usual symptoms are those of balanoposthitis. Carcinoma may also coexist when the calculus has been present for a long time. The diagnosis is established by palpation of the stone.

When an acute infection is present, a dorsal slit should be performed to establish drainage. The ultimate treatment consists of circumcision.

PEDIATRIC UROLITHIASIS

Urinary stones in children fall into three broad epidemiologic patterns: renal stones seen in premature infants of very low birth weight, upper tract stones seen in children and adolescents, and endemic bladder stones.

Stone Disease in Very-Low-Birth-Weight Infants

Nephrocalcinosis occurs in a significant proportion of infants with birth weight less than 1500 g. Between 30% and 90% of very-low-birth-weight infants treated with furosemide have renal calcifications on ultrasonography (Adams and Rowe, 1992). These children are usually very ill and require respiratory and nutritional support. **Initially, stone formation was attributed exclusively to furosemide-induced hypercalciuria; however, it has become apparent that renal calcifications can occur in infants who have not received furosemide** (Polinsky et al, 1993; Campfield et al, 1994). Other factors that may contribute to the development of urolithiasis and nephrocalcinosis in these infants include dietary sodium, calcium, and vitamin D supplementation or the administration of parenteral hyperalimentation solutions. Hypercalciuria may be caused by the administration of steroids or theophylline. Many premature infants have metabolic or respiratory acidosis, leading to hypocitraturia.

Urinary oxalate excretion is increased in very-low-birth-weight infants receiving hyperalimentation, perhaps as a result of the conversion of ascorbate and glycine present in these solutions to oxalate (Polinsky et al, 1993; Campfield et al, 1994). Campfield and colleagues examined urinary oxalate excretion in calcium oxalate and phosphate saturation in premature and term infants fed with formula or human milk. Calcium oxalate supersaturation was markedly higher in preterm infants when compared to term infants or adult controls, regardless of the method of nutrition. The highest oxalate excretion occurred in formula-fed preterm infants. Multiple factors contribute to increased urinary oxalate excretion in very-low-birth-weight infants, including abnormal fat absorption, increased intake of ascorbic acid, and alternative pathways of oxalate metabolism. In many infants with hypercalciuria, and some without hypercalciuria, reduction of furosemide and addition of thiazide diuretics causes halting or even reversal of nephrocalcinosis or urolithiasis.

Nephrolithiasis in Children and Adolescents

Renal calculi occurring in children or adolescents can be divided into two broad categories: those with an underlying urologic cause and those without such a cause (Table 91–14). In general, reports from centers of pediatric urology find the occurrence of anatomic abnormalities in between 10% and 40% of patients. **In those series that**

Table 91–14. PREVALENCE OF METABOLIC STONE DISEASE IN CHILDREN WITH RENAL STONES

Author	Year	Metabolic (%)	Structural (%)
Choi et al	1987	55	35*
Diamond et al	1994	30	33*
Malek & Kelalis	1975	68	32*
Cheah et al	1994	Not done	9
Noe et al	1983	63	19
Perrone et al	1992	80	4

*Report from pediatric urology centers.

provide breakdown of anatomic lesions responsible for stone formation, ureteropelvic junction obstruction is the most common lesion. These series also note a high prevalence of urinary tract infection: up to 75% (Diamond and Menon, 1991). Many series, however, do not clearly distinguish between stones caused by infection (struvite stones) or stones associated with infection (usually calcium oxalate stones). **Diseases such as meningomyelocele or neurogenic bladder are prime causes of struvite stones, particularly if associated with urologic intervention.**

In the absence of anatomic disorders or urologic intervention, stone disease seen in children parallels that seen in adults. Such patient series are usually reported in collaboration with or exclusively by nephrologists. For instance, Noe and colleagues and Perrone and colleagues reported that 63% to 86% of their patients had underlying metabolic abnormalities (Noe et al, 1983; Perrone et al, 1992). Such metabolic abnormalities are often under-reported because they have not been sought out in many instances. In these series, the prevalence of anatomic abnormalities was less than 20%.

Children with renal stones seldom present with typical ureteric colic. In most series, about 70% of patients are diagnosed during work-up of a urinary tract infection. Hematuria and abdominal pain are other presenting symptoms, with typical ureteric colic occurring in less than 15% of individuals (Diamond and Menon, 1991). Indeed, some children with unexplained hematuria and hypercalciuria develop renal stones on follow-up (Stapleton et al, 1984). The distribution of metabolic stone disease parallels that of adults, with calcium oxalate and phosphate stones being predominant and uric acid stones accounting for between 5% and 10% of all stones. Cystinuria and primary hyperoxaluria are seen in 1% to 2% of patients. Distal RTA, sometimes associated with type I glycogen storage disease, is a rare cause of pediatric nephrolithiasis (Restaino et al, 1993).

The average age at presentation of children with renal stones is between 8 and 10 years. The male-to-female ratio is around 1.5:1, lower than the 3:1 ratio seen in adults (Diamond and Menon, 1991). Hypercalciuria is the most common metabolic abnormality seen in patients with noninfected, nonanatomic renal stones. The excretion of urinary metabolites is usually indexed to $1 \cdot 73 \text{ m}^2$ of body surface area, to conform with values obtained in adults. Absorptive hypercalciuria is diagnosed if fasting urinary calcium/urinary creatinine is below 0.21 and post–calcium load urinary calcium/urinary creatinine exceeds this level. Renal hypercalciuria is diagnosed if fasting urinary calcium/urinary creatinine is greater than 0.21. In most series, hypercalciuria accounts for 75% to 80% of metabolic causes, with renal hypercalci-

uria occurring at a higher rate than in adults. Between 20% and 25% of patients demonstrate uric acid hyperexcretion. **When metabolic abnormalities are diligently searched for, about 90% of patients with nonanatomic renal stones prove to have underlying metabolic abnormalities.** This number may actually be low because detailed evaluations of acid, citrate, and oxalate handling have not been uniformly performed in the pediatric population.

The radiologic diagnosis of calculi in children is similar to that in adults. One significant radiologic difference between children and adults with stones has been reported by Breatnach and Smith (1983). In a group of 50 children who had intravenous urography for calculi, increased nephrographic density or the adult intravenous urogram pattern of acute ureteric obstruction was not seen. Because 80% of these children had associated urinary infections, generalized ureteral dilation and calicectasis were quite common and may have masked the typical radiologic signs of stone obstruction. The occurrence of lucent calculi (uric acid and, to some degree, cystine) requires urography. About 3% to 10% of calculi are radiolucent (Rambar and MacKenzie, 1978; Borgmann and Nagel, 1982; Steele et al, 1983).

Some physicians tend to avoid intravenous urography in younger children because of excessive radiation exposure. Certainly, genitalia and gonads should be shielded whenever possible. Higher degrees of radiation can be avoided by the performance of a tailored urogram. Imaging by ultrasound methods can illustrate stone effectively. Often a KUB accompanied by ultrasound of the kidneys, ureters, and bladder is sufficient. Urethral stones often present with hematuria accompanied by dysuria. Sonographic evaluation of the urethra may be carried out via a scan of the penis for anterior urethra and via the abdomen (using the bladder as an acoustic window) or perineum for the posterior urethra (Kessler et al, 1992).

Because children with stone disease are at risk for a longer period than adults, the cumulative likelihood of stone recurrences may be higher in children. Thus, most authorities agree that a thorough metabolic evaluation is mandatory in children with nephrolithiasis. **In most series, about two thirds of patients require procedural therapy to remove the stone.** This is much higher than in the adult population. Interestingly, once surgical correction has been performed, the recurrence rates for stones of the pediatric age group seems to be lower, or at least no greater, than for adults (Steele et al, 1983; Diamond et al, 1989). Thereafter, appropriate therapy can be assigned. The usual admonitions to increase fluid intake and output seem universally accepted. Primary hyperoxaluria or hypercalciuria has been treated by dietary limitation of oxalate or calcium with or without neutral orthophosphates (Noe et al, 1983). Hypercalciuric children may be treated with thiazides (1 mg/kg/day). Urinary calcium excretion reaches its lowest value after 2 weeks and continues to be below the initial value at the end of 3 months of treatment (Reusz et al, 1993). A significant rise in the total cholesterol and low-density lipoproteins is observed at the end of 3 months (Reusz et al, 1993). Other side effects, such as potassium wasting, uric acid retention, and elevated blood glucose, have been reported by Reusz and colleagues (1993). Long-term observation of children for side effects of therapy becomes as important as that of adults.

Endemic Bladder Calculi

Before the 20th century, the major incidence of urinary lithiasis was bladder stones in children. As nations increased productivity and moved into the industrial age, average income and food quality improved. These events resulted in the gradual disappearance of endemic bladder stone disease from previously afflicted populations. Such stones are now found mostly in North Africa, the Middle and Near East, Burma, Thailand, and Indonesia (Van Reen, 1977). Most pediatric bladder calculi in endemic areas are composed of ammonium acid urate (Brockis et al, 1981), calcium oxalate, or mixtures thereof. **The occurrence of such stones may be traced to the common practice in endemic areas of feeding infants human breast milk and cereal foods, such as polished rice or millet.** Human breast milk, in contrast to cow's milk, is low in phosphorus, as is polished rice (Anderson, 1962; Thalut et al, 1976). Such low-phosphate diets result in high peaks of urinary ammonia excretion (Brockis et al, 1981). Also, ingestion of oxalate-rich vegetables contributes to the high degree of crystalluria often seen in these children (Valyasevi and Dhanamitta, 1974). Consumption of diets rich in acid ash (animal protein) is known to lower urinary citrate excretion (Pak, 1988; Lerner et al, 1989). Anatomic urologic disease may coexist with bladder stones of nutritional etiology. Neurogenic bladders, which often require catheterization or augmentation cystoplasty (Palmer et al, 1993), are significant risk factors for the development of recurrent urolithiasis. The use of staples and intestinal mucus have been implicated as causes (Palmer et al, 1993).

STONES IN PREGNANCY

The incidence of symptomatic urinary calculi in pregnancy is reported to be anywhere from 1:1500 (Rodriguez and Klein, 1988) to 1:2500 (O'Reagan et al, 1984) depending on location and referral status (high-risk pregnancy centers). The incidences and rates of recurrence are similar to an age-matched population (Kroovand, 1992). Although some series have shown a predisposition for right side over left (Cumming and Taylor, 1979), generally calculi occur with equal frequency on both sides (Lattanzi and Cook, 1980; Kroovand, 1992).

Multiparous women tend to be more commonly predisposed to urinary stones than primiparae (Stothers and Lee, 1992). Most patients present in the second or third trimester

(Denstedt and Razvi, 1992). **Although pregnancy by itself does not predispose to calculi, the physiologic dilatation of the ureters and back pressure changes because of the gravid uterus allow preformed calculi more room for movement, resulting in renal colic and hematuria.**

Most pregnant women have absorptive hypercalciuria (Gertner et al, 1986) and hyperuricosuria (Swanson et al, 1995). Hypercalciuria is the result of an elevation of 1,25-dihydroxyvitamin D_3 manufactured in placenta and consequent suppression of PTH secretion (Gertner et al, 1986). Dietary supplementation with calcium further augments urinary calcium excretion. The increased quantities of inhibitors present in urine during gestation (Maikranz et al, 1987) and increased urine output, however, may counter the risk imposed by hypercalciuria. In fact, in one series of 78 women with a history of urolithiasis, no increase in symptomatic urolithiasis occurred with pregnancy (Coe et al, 1978b).

The diagnosis and treatment of urolithiasis in pregnancy is difficult. Pregnancy masks the symptoms and signs of renal colic. Although typical renal colic is the most common presentation, patients may present with vague abdominal pain. Unexplained fever, unresolved bacteriuria, and microscopic hematuria also should tip the clinician off about the presence of renal stones. A high index of suspicion is necessary in evaluating pregnant women with the aforementioned clinical features. It is critical to establish the diagnosis of urolithiasis in pregnancy.

The plain abdominal film and ultrasound have become the cornerstone of evaluation of suspected renal colic in pregnancy. Physiologic dilatation of pelvicalyceal system in pregnancy, especially on the right side, lowers the sensitivity of ultrasound screening, unless the sonographer is skilled enough to demonstrate the actual stone. When ultrasonography is inconclusive, appropriate radiographic evaluation should be performed. The overlapping fetal skeleton may compromise the ability of the plain abdominal film to detect calculi. Swartz and Reichling (1978) have identified **the first trimester as the most significant risk period for fetal malformation and spontaneous abortion following radiation exposure** (Swartz and Reichling, 1978). They estimated that exposure to 25 to 80 rad of radiation doubles the risk of teratogenesis in the fetus; however, the exposure to radiation after a single x-ray film is 20 mrad, or less than 1% of the critical dose. Proper shielding of the asymptomatic side may further reduce the risk of radiation exposure. A tailored intravenous pyelogram, consisting of a scout, 30-second nephrogram, and a 20-minute film, has minimal risk in the second and third trimester; however, fluoroscopy should be avoided.

Approximately 66% to 85% of pregnant women with ureteric colic spontaneously pass the calculi when treated conservatively with hydration, analgesics, and, if infected, with antibiotics (Jones et al, 1979; Stothers and Lee, 1992). The goal of therapy for the remaining patients is to do the least required to keep the kidney functioning, the patient free from symptoms, and the urine uninfected. **Stents should be placed cystoscopically with minimal radiographic or sonographic monitoring** (Loughlin and Bailey, 1986; Jarrard et al, 1993). Some studies have shown increased encrustation of stents requiring frequent change over a guide wire. In some instances, the stents migrate down the ureter because of the physiologic dilatation (Stothers and Lee,

1992). Stents should be changed at least every 6 to 8 weeks (Kavoussi et al, 1992). They recommend stent placement preferably in the late second or third trimesters only. Some patients may continue to have significant lower urinary discomfort (Denstedt and Razvi, 1992) and flank pain (during voiding) because of vesicoureteral reflux after stent placement. If the symptoms do not resolve with appropriate treatment, alternative therapy such as percutaneous nephrostomy should be considered. It is particularly risky to attempt ureteroscopy and basketing in pregnant patients (Rittenberg and Bagley, 1988). Ultrasound-guided percutaneous nephrostomy drainage under local anesthesia is an effective temporizing option (Kavoussi et al, 1992), especially in the first and second trimester. The procedure can be performed without fluoroscopy. Definitive procedures such as ultrasonic/electrohydraulic lithotripsy should be avoided until after delivery because there are no studies detailing the risk of these energy sources on the fetus and mother, and there are documented episodes of anesthesia-related premature labor, spontaneous abortion, and intrauterine growth retardation (Duncan et al, 1986). **Thus, pregnancy is an absolute contraindication for the use of lithotripsy in any form** (Denstedt and Razvi, 1992; Kroovand, 1992). In exceptional circumstances in which persistent pain, sepsis, or recurrent obstruction demands an intervention, percutaneous stone removal under carefully monitored anesthesia and suitable radiation shielding has been advocated by some (Kavoussi et al, 1992).

REFERENCES

Abdulhadi MH, Hall PM, Streem SB: Can citrate therapy prevent nephrolithiasis? Urology 1993; 41:221–224.

Adams ND, Rowe JC: Nephrocalcinosis. Clin Perinatol 1992; 19:179–195.

Adler S, Anderson B, Zemotel L: Metabolic acid-base effects on tissue citrate content and metabolism in the rat. Am J Physiol 1971; 220:986–992.

Ahlstrand C, Tiselius HG: Biochemical effects in patients with calcium oxalate stone disease during combined treatment with bendroflumethiazide and magnesium oxide. Br J Urol 1984; 56:125–130.

Ala-opas M, Elomaa I, Prokka L, Alfthan O: Unprocessed bran and intermittent thiazide therapy in prevention of recurrent urinary calcium stones. Scand J Urol Nephrol 1987; 21:311–314.

Albright F, Reifenstein EC: The Parathyroid Glands and Metabolic Bone Disease. Baltimore, Williams & Wilkins, 1948a.

Albright F, Suby H, Sulcowitch HE: In Albright F, Reifenstein EC Jr, eds: The Parathyroid Glands and Metabolic Bone Disease. Baltimore, Williams & Wilkins, 1948b.

Allen TD, Spence HM: Matrix stone. J Urol 1966; 95:284–290.

Allison MG, Cook HM, Milne DB, et al: Oxalate degradation by gastrointestinal bacteria from humans. J Nutr 1986; 116:455–460.

Anderson DA: The nutritional significance of primary bladder stone. Br J Urol 1962; 34:160.

Andersson H, Jagenburg R: Fat reduced diet in the treatment of hyperoxaluria in patients with ileophathy. Gut 1974; 15:360–366.

Andrus SB, Gerhoff SN, Faragolla FF: Production of calcium oxalate renal calculi in vitamin B₆ deficient rats: Study of the influence of urine pH. Lab Invest 1960; 9:7.

Arnaud CD, Pun K: Metabolism and assay of parathyroid hormone. In Coe FL, Favus MJ, eds: Disorders of Bone and Mineral Metabolism. New York, Raven Press, 1992, pp 107–122.

Aro A, Pelkonen R, Sivula A: Hypercalcemia: Serum chloride and phosphate (Letter). Ann Intern Med 1977; 86:664.

Asplin J, DeGannelli S, Nakagawa Y, Coe FL: Evidence that nephrocalcin and urine inhibit nucleation of calcium oxalate nephrolithiasis. Am J Physiol 1991; 260:F569–578.

Atkinson RL Jr, Earll JM: Munchausen syndrome with renal stones. JAMA 1974; 230:89.

Atsmon A, DeVries A, Frank M: Uric Acid Lithiasis. Amsterdam, Elsevier Publishing, 1963; pp 1–13.

Au WY: Cortisol stimulation of parathyroid hormone secretion by rat parathyroid glands in organ cultures. Science 1976; 193:1015–1017.

Aub JC, Brauer W, Heath CH: Studies of calcium and phosphorus metabolism: III. The effects of the thyroid hormone in thyroid disease. J Clin Invest 1929; 7:97.

Backman U, Danielson BG, Johansson G, et al: Treatment of recurrent calcium stone formation with cellulose phosphate. J Urol 1980a; 123:9–13

Backman U, Danielson BG, Johanson G, et al: Incidence and clinical importance of renal tubular defects in recurrent renal stone formers. Nephron 1980b; 25:96–101.

Baggio B, Gambaro G, Marchini F, et al: An inheritable anomaly of red cell oxalate transport in "primary" calcium nephrolithiasis correctable with diuretics. N Engl J Med 1986; 314:599–604.

Baggio B, Gambaro G, Marchini F, et al: Correction of erythrocyte abnormalities in idiopathic calcium oxalate nephrolithiasis and reduction of urinary oxalate by oral glycosaminoglycans. Lancet 1991a; 338:403–404.

Baggio B, Gambaro G, Marzaro G, et al: Effects of the oral administration of glycosaminoglycans on cellular abnormalities associated with idiopathic calcium oxalate nephrolithiasis. Eur J Clin Pharmacol 1991b; 40:237–240.

Baker PW, Coyle P, Bais R, Rofe AM: Influence of season, age and sex on renal stone formation in South Australia. Med J Aust 1993; 159:390–392.

Barilla DE, Townsend J, Pak CY: Renal oxalate excretion following oral oxalate loads in patients with ileal disease and with renal and absorptive hypercalciurias: Effect of calcium and magnesium. Am J Med 1978a; 64:579–585.

Barilla DE, Townsend J, Pak CYC: An exaggerated augmentation of renal calcium excretion after oral glucose ingestion in patients with renal hypercalciuria. Invest Urol 1978b; 15:486–488.

Barratt TM, Simmonds HA, Cemeron JS, et al: Complete deficiency of adenine phosphoribosyl transferase. Arch Dis Child 1979; 54:25–31.

Baruch SB, Burich RL, Eun CK, King VF: Renal metabolism of citrate. Med Clin North Am 1975; 59:569–582.

Barzel US: The changing face of hyperparathyroidism. Hosp Pract 1977; 12:89–94.

Bateson EM: Renal tract calculi and climate. Med J Aust 1973; 2:111–113.

Bek-Jensen H, Tiselius HG: Stone formation and urine composition in calcium stone formers without medical treatment. Eur Urol 1989; 16:144–150.

Bell NH, Stern PH, Pantzer E, et al: Evidence that increased circulating 1 alpha 25-dihydroxy vitamin D is the probable cause for abnormal calcium metabolism in sarcoidosis. J Clin Invest 1979; 64:218–225.

Benedict JD, Roche M, Yu TF: Incorporation of glycine nitrogen into uric acid in normal and gouty man. Metabolism 1952; 1:3–12.

Berg C, Larsson L, Tiselius HG: The effects of a single evening dose of alkaline citrate on urine composition and calcium stone formation. J Urol 1992; 148:979–985.

Bianchi G, Vezzoli G, Cusi D, et al: Abnormal red cell calcium pump in patients with idiopathic hypercalciuria. N Engl J Med 1988; 319:897–901.

Bijovet OLM: Kidney function and calcium phosphate metabolism. In Avioli LV, Krane SM, eds: Metabolic Bone Disease, Vol 1. New York, Academic Press, 1977, pp 49–140.

Bilezikian JP: Hypercalcemic states. In Coe FL, Favus MJ, eds: Disorders of Bone and Mineral Metabolism. New York, Raven Press, 1992, pp 493–521.

Black KS, Mundy GR, Garrett IR: Interleukin-6 causes hypercalcemia in vivo and enhances the bone resorbing potency of interleukin-1 and tumor necrosis factor by two orders of magnitude in vitro. J Bone Miner Res 1990; 5:S271.

Blacklock NJ: The pattern of urolithiasis in the Royal Navy. In Hodgkinson A, Nordin BEC, eds: Renal Stone Research Symposium. London, J & A Churchill Ltd, 1969, pp 33–47.

Blacklock NJ, MacLeod MA: The effect of cellulose phosphate on intestinal absorption and urinary excretion of calcium. Br J Urol 1974; 46:385–392.

Blaivas JG, Pais VM, Spellman RM: Chemolysis of residual stone fragments after extensive surgery for staghorn calculi. Urology 1975; 6:680–686.

Blandy JP, Singh M: The case for a more aggressive approach to staghorn stones. J Urol 1976; 115:505–506.

Bloom A, Libson E, Verstandig A, Rackow M: The tooth-root sign: A characteristic appearance of distal ureteral calculi. Acta Radiol 1988; 39:212–213.

Boothby WM, Adams M: The occurrence of citric acid in urine and body fluids. Am J Physiol 1934; 107:47.

Borghi L, Meschi T, Guerra A, Novarini A: Randomized prospective study of a nonthiazide diuretic, Indapamide, in preventing calcium stone recurrences. J Cardiovasc Pharmacol 1993; 22(suppl):578–586.

Borgmann V, Nagel R: Urolithiasis in childhood—a study of 181 cases. Urol Int 1982; 37:198–204.

Borkowski A, Czapliczki M: Nontraumatic extravasation from the ureter. Int Urol Nephrol 1974; 5:271–275.

Bors E: Neurogenic bladder. Urol Surv 1957; 7:177.

Bowsher WG, Crocker P, Ramsay JW, Whitfield HN: Single urine sample diagnosis: A new concept in stone analysis. Br J Urol 1990; 65:236–239.

Boyce WH: Organic matrix of human urinary concretions. Am J Med 1968; 45:673–683.

Boyce WH: Organic matrix of native human urinary concretions. In Hodgkinson A, Nordin BEC, eds: Renal Stone Research Symposium. London, J & A Churchill Ltd, 1969, p 93.

Boyce WH, Elkins IB: Reconstructive renal surgery following anatrophic nephrolithotomy: Follow-up of 100 consecutive cases. J Urol 1974; 11:307–312.

Boyce WH, Garvey FK, Strawcutter HE: Incidence of urinary calculi among patients in general hospital: 1948–1952. JAMA 1956; 161:1437.

Boyce WH, King JS Jr: Crystal-matrix interrelations in calculi. J Urol 1959; 81:351.

Boyce WH, King JS, Fielden ML: Total non-dialyzable solids (TNDS) of human urine: XIII. Immunological detection of a component peculiar to renal calculous matrix and to urine of calculous patients. J Clin Invest 1962; 41:1180.

Brand E, Harris MM, Biloon S: Cystinuria, excretion of a cystine complex which decomposes in the urine with the liberation of free cystine. J Biol Chem 1930; 86:315.

Breatnach E, Smith SEW: The radiology of renal stones in children. Clin Radiol 1983; 34:59–64.

Breslau NA, Brinkley L, Hill RD, Pak CYC: Relationship role of animal protein-rich diet to kidney stone formation and calcium metabolism. Med J Clin Endocrinol Metab 1988; 66:140–146.

Breslau NA, McGuire JL, Zerwekh JE, Pak CY: The role of dietary sodium on renal excretion and intestinal absorption of calcium and on vitamin D metabolism. J Clin Endocrinol Metab 1982a; 55:369–373.

Breslau NA, Pak CY: Endocrine aspects of nephrolithiasis. In Cohen P, Foa P, eds: Special Topics in Endocrinology and Metabolism, Vol III. New York, Allan R. Liss, 1982, pp 57–86.

Breslau NA, Zerwekh JE, Nicar MJ, Pak CY: Effects of short-term glucocorticoid administration in primary hyperparathyroidism: Comparison to sarcoidosis. J Clin Endocrinol Metab 1982b; 54:824–830.

Bringhurst FR, Bierer BE, Godeau F, et al: Humoral hypercalcemia of malignancy: Release of a prostaglandin-stimulating bone resorbing factor in vitro by human transitional-cell carcinoma cells. J Clin Invest 1986; 77:456–464.

Broadus A: Nephrolithiasis in primary hyperparathyroidism. In Coe F, Brenner B, Stein J, eds: Nephrolithiasis, New York, Churchill Livingstone, 1980, pp 59–85.

Broadus AE, Domingues M, Bartter FC: Pathophysiological studies in idiopathic hypercalciuria: Use of an oral calcium tolerance test to characterize distinctive hypercalciuric subgroups. J Clin Endocrinol Metab 1978; 47:751–760.

Broadus AE, Horst RL, Lang R, et al: The importance of circulating 1,25-dihydroxyvitamin D in the pathogenesis of hypercalciuria and renal stone formation in primary hyperparathyroidism. N Engl J Med 1980; 302:421–426.

Brockis JG, Bowyer RC, McCulloch RK, et al: Pathophysiology of endemic bladder stones. In Brockis JG, Finlayson B, eds: Urinary Calculus. Littleton, MA, PGS Publishing, 1981.

Brockis JG, Levitt AJ, Cruther SM: The effects of vegetables and animal protein diets on calcium, urate and oxalate excretion. Br J Urol 1982; 54:590–593.

Brocks P, Dahl C, Wolf H, Transbol I: Do thiazides prevent recurrent idiopathic renal calcium stones? Lancet 1981; 2:124–125.

Brown CM, Ackermann DK, Purich DL: Equil 93: A tool for experimental and clinical urolithiasis. Urol Res 1994; 22:119–126.

Brown CM, Purich DL: Physical chemical processes in kidney stone formation. In Coe FL, Flavus MJ, eds: Disorders of Bone and Mineral Metabolism. New York, Raven Press, 1992, pp 613–624.

Buck AC, Lote CJ, Sampson WF: The influence of renal prostaglandins on urinary calcium excretion in idiopathic urolithiasis. J Urol 1983; 129:421–426.

Buck AC, Sampson WF, Lote CJ, Blacklock NJ: The influence of renal prostaglandins on glomerular filtration rate (GFR) and calcium excretion in urolithiasis. Br J Urol 1981; 53:485–491.

Buck AC, Smellie WS, Jenkins A, et al: The treatment of idiopathic recurrent urolithiasis with fish oil and evening primrose oil—a double blind study. In Ryall R, Bais R, Marshall VR, et al, eds: Urolithiasis 2. New York, Plenum Press, 1992, pp 575–580.

Buckalew VM Jr: Nephrolithiasis in RTA. J Urol 1989; 141:731–737.

Buckalew VM Jr, Caruana RJ: The syndrome of distal (type 1) renal tubular acidosis. In Gonick HC, Buckalew VM Jr, eds: Renal Tubular Disorders: Pathophysiology, Diagnosis and Management. New York, Marcel Dekker, 1985, pp 357–386.

Burkland CE, Rosenberg M: Survey of urolithiasis in the United States. J Urol 1955; 73:198.

Burman KD, Monchik JM, Earl JM, Wartofsky L: Ionized and total serum calcium and parathyroid hormone in hyperthyroidism. Ann Intern Med 1976; 84:668–671.

Burns JR, Finlayson B: Strategies for the medical management of patients with urinary stone disease. Monogr Urol 1981; 2:106–125.

Bushinsky DA, Favus MJ, Langman CB, Coe FL: Mechanism of chronic hypercalciuria with furosemide: Increased calcium absorption. Am J Physiol 1986; 251(Renal Fluid Electrol Physiol 20):F17–F24.

Bushinsky DA, Krieger NS: Integration of calcium metabolism in the adult. In Coe FL, Favus MJ, eds: Disorders of Bone and Mineral Metabolism. New York, Raven Press, 1992.

Calo L, Cantaro S, Marchini F, et al: Is hydrochlorothiazide-induced hypocalciuria due to inhibition of prostaglandin E_2 synthesis? Clin Sci 1990; 78:321–325.

Campfield T, Braden G, Flynn-Valone P, Clark N: Urinary oxalate excretion in premature infants: Effect of human milk versus formula feeding. Pediatrics 1994; 94:674–678.

Cannellos GP: Hypercalcemia in malignant lymphoma and leukemia. Ann NY Acad Sci 1974; 230:240–250.

Carr RJ: Aetiology of renal calculi: Micro-radiographic studies. In Hodgkinson A, Nordin BEC, eds: Renal Stone Research Symposium. London, J & A Churchill, Ltd, 1969, p 123.

Caruana RJ, Buckalew VM Jr: The syndrome of distal (type 1) renal tubular acidosis: Clinical and laboratory findings in 58 cases. Medicine 1988; 67:84–89.

Cato AR, Tulloch AGS: Hypermagnesemia in a uremic patient during renal pelvic irrigation with Renacidin. J Urol 1974; 111:313–314.

Chafe L, Gault MH: First morning urine pH in the diagnosis of renal tubular acidosis with nephrolithiasis. Clin Nephrol 1994; 41:159–162.

Charig CT, Webb DR, Payne Sr, Wickham JEA: Comparison of treatment of renal calculi by open surgery, percutaneous nephrolithotomy and extra corporeal shock-wave lithotripsy. Br Med J 1986; 292:879–882.

Cheah WK, King PA, Tan HL: A review of pediatric cases of urinary tract calculi. J Pediatr Surg 1994; 29:701–705.

Chen TC, Castillo L, Korychka-Dahl M, Deluca HF: Role of vitamin D metabolites in phosphate transport of rat intestine. J Nutr 1974; 104:1056–1060.

Chlebeck PT, Milliner DS, Smith LH: Long term prognosis in primary hyperoxaluria type II (L-glyceric aciduria). Am J Kidney Dis 1994; 23:255–259.

Choi H, Snyder HM 3d, Duckett JW: Urolithiasis in childhood: Current management. J Pediatr Surg 1987; 22:158–164.

Choyke PL: The urogram: Are rumors of its death premature? Radiology 1992; 184:33–36.

Churchill DN: Medical treatment to prevent recurrent calcium urolithiasis—a guide to critical appaaisal. Miner Electr Metab 1987; 13:294–304.

Churchill DN, Maloney CM, Bear J, et al: Urolithiasis: a study of drinking water hardness and genetic factors. J Chronic Dis 1980; 33:727–731.

Clendening L: Source Book of Medical History. New York, Dove Publications, 1942, p 14.

Coe FL: Treated and untreated recurrent calcium nephrolithiasis in patients with idiopathic hypercalciuria, hyperuricosuria or no metabolic disorders. Ann Intern Med 1977; 87:404–410.

Coe FL: Hyperuricosuric calcium oxalate nephrolithiasis. Kidney Int 1978; 13:418–426.

Coe FL, Bushinsky DA: Pathophysiology of hypercalciuria (Review). Am J Physiol 1984; 247:F1–F13.

Coe FL, Favus MJ, eds: Disorders of Bone and Mineral Metabolism. New York, Raven Press, 1992.

Coe FL, Favus MJ, Crocket T: Effects of low-calcium diet on urine calcium excretion, parathyroid functional serum 1, 25(DH)—2D-3 levels in patients with idiopathic hypercalciuria and in normal subjects. Am J Med 1982; 72:25–32.

Coe FL, Kavalich AG: Hypercalciuria and hyperuricosuria in patients with calcium nephrolithiasis. N Engl J Med 1974; 291:1344–1350.

Coe FL, Margolis HC, Deutsch LH: Urinary macromolecular crystal growth inhibitors in calcium nephrolithiasis. Miner Electr Metab 1980a;3:268.

Coe FL, Moran E, Kavalich AG: The contribution of dietary purine over consumption to hyperuricosuria in calcium oxalate stone formers. J Chronic Dis 1976; 29:793–800.

Coe FL, Parks JH: Nephrolithiasis: Pathogenesis and Treatment, 2nd ed. Chicago, Year Book Medical Publishers, 1988.

Coe FL, Parks JH, Asplin Jr: The pathogenesis and treatment of kidney stones. N Engl J Med 1992; 327:1141–1152.

Coe FL, Parks JH, Bushinsky DA, et al: Chlorthalidone promotes mineral retention in patients with idiopathic hypercalciuria. Kidney Int 1988; 33:1140–1146.

Coe FL, Parks JH, Lindheimer MD: Nephrolithiasis associated with pregnancy. N Engl J Med 1978; 298:324–326.

Coe FL, Parks JH, Moore ES: Familial idiopathic hypercalciuria. N Engl J Med 1979; 300:337–340.

Coe FL, Parks JH, Nakagawa Y: Inhibitors and promoters of calcium oxalate crystallization. In Coe FL, Favus MJ, eds: Disorder of Bone and Mineral Metabolism. New York, Raven Press, 1992, pp 757–780.

Coe FL, Raisen L: Allopurinol treatment of uric-acid disorders in calcium stone formers. Lancet 1973; 1:129–131.

Coe FL, Strauss AL, Tembe V, LeDun S. Uric acid saturation in calcium nephrolithiasis. Kidney Int 1980b; 17:662–668.

Comarr AE, Kawaichi GR, Bors E: Renal calculosis in patients with traumatic cord lesions. J Urol 1962; 85:647–656.

Conger JD: Acute uric acid nephropathy. Semin Nephrol 1981; 1:69–74.

Consensus Conference: Prevention and treatment of kidney stones. JAMA 1988; 260: 977–981.

Conway NW, Maitland ATK, Rennie JB: The urinary citrate excretion in patients with renal caculi. Br J Urol 1979; 21:30.

Cope O: The story of hyperparathyroidism at the Massachusetts General Hospital. N Engl J Med 1966; 274:1174–1182.

Cordell WH, Larson TA, Lingeman JE, et al: Indomethacin suppositories versus intravenous titrated morphine for the treatment of ureteral colic. Ann Emerg Med 1994; 23:262–269.

Costello LC, Stacey R, Franklin R: Parathyroid hormone effects on soft tissue citrate levels. Horm Metab Res 1970; 2:242–245.

Cryer PE, Garber AJ, Joffsten P, et al: Renal failure after small intestinal bypass for obesity. Arch Intern Med 1975; 135:1610–1612.

Cumming DC, Taylor PJ: Urologic and obstetric significance of urinary calculi in pregnancy. Obstet & Gyn 1979; 53:505–508.

Curhan GC, Rimm EB, Willett WC, Stampfer MJ: Regional variation in nephrolithiasis incidence and prevalence among United States men. J Urol 1994; 151:838–841.

Curhan GC, Willett WC, Rimm EB, Stampfer MJ: A prospective study of dietary calcium and other nutrients and the risk of symptomatic kidney stones. N Engl J Med 1993; 328:833–838.

Cushard WG, Simon AB, Canterbury JM, Reiss E: Parathyroid function in sarcoidosis. N Engl J Med 1972; 286:395–398.

Cushing M: Basophil adenomas of pituitary body and their clinical manifestations (pituitary basophilism). Bull Johns Hopkins Hosp 1932; 50:137.

Dana ES: Descriptive Mineralogy. New York, John Wiley & Sons, 1920.

Danpure CJ: Molecular and cell biology of primary hyperoxaluria type 1. Clin Invest Med 1994; 72:725–727.

Danpure CJ, Birdsey GM, Rumsby G, et al: Molecular characterization and clinical use of a polymorphic tandem repeat in an intron of the human alanine: glyoxylated aminotransferase gene. Hum Genet 1994; 94:55–64.

Danpure CJ, Cooper PJ, Wise PJ, Jennings PR: An enzyme trafficking defect in two patients with primary hyperoxaluria type 1: Peroxisomal alanine/glyoxalate aminotransferase rerouted to mitochondria. J Cell Biol 1989; 108:1345–1352.

Danpure CJ, Jennings PR: Peroxisomal alanine: Glyoxylate aminotransferase deficiency in primary hyperoxaluria type I. FEBS Letters 1986; 201:20–24.

Danpure CJ, Jennings PR: Further studies on the activity and subcellular distribution of alanine: Glyoxylate aminotransferase in the livers of patients with hyperoxaluria type 1. Clin Sci 1988; 75:315–322.

Daudon M, Bader CA, Jungers P: Urinary calculi: Review of classification methods and correlations with etiology. Scann Microsc 1993; 7:1081–1106.

Davidman M, Schmitz P: Renal tubular acidosis—a pathophysiologic approach. Hosp Pract 1988; 23:77–81.

Dawson KA, Allison MJ, Hartman PA: Isolation and some characteristics of anerobic oxalate degrading bacteria from the Rumen. Appl Environ Microbiol 1988; 40:833–839.

Deganello S, Chou C: The uric acid-whewellite association in human kidney stones. Scan Electron Microsc (pt 2) 1984; 927–933.

De Luca HF: The vitamin D hormonal system: Implications for bone disease. Hosp Pract 1980; 15:57–63.

Denstedt JD, Razvi H: Management of urinary calculi during pregnancy. J Urol 1992; 108:1072–1075.

Dent CE, Senior B: Studies on the treatment of cystinuria. Br J Urol 1955; 27:317–332.

Diamond DA, Menon M: Pediatric urolithiasis. AUA Update Series 1991; 40:314–320.

Diamond DA, Menon M, Lee PH, et al: Etiological factors in pediatric stone recurrence. J Urol 1989; 142:606–608.

Diamond DA, Rickwood AM, Lee PH, Johnston JH: Infection stones in children: A twenty-seven year review. Urology 1994; 43:525–527.

Dick WH, Lingeman JE, Preminger GM, et al: Laxative abuse as a cause of ammonium-urate renal calculi. J Urol 1990; 143:244–247.

Dilworth JP, Segura JW: Compliance with use of the hydrate 1 system by patients with treated urolithiasis. J Endourol 1993; 7:197–199.

Douenias R, Rich M, Badlani G, et al: Predisposing factors in bladder calculi: Review of 100 cases. Urology 1991; 37:240–243.

Down WH, Sacharin RN, Chasseaud LF, et al: Renal and bone uptake of tartaric acid in rats: Comparison of L+ and DL-forms. Toxicology 1977; 8:333–334.

Drach GW: Prostatitis: Man's hidden infection. Urol Clin North Am 1975; 2:499–520.

Drach GW: Urolithiasis. In Conn HG, ed: Current Therapy. Philadelphia, W. B. Saunders, 1976, p 552.

Drach GW: Urinary lithiasis. In Harrison JH, Gittes RF, Perlmutter AD, et al, eds: Campbell's Urology, 4th ed. Philadelphia, W. B. Saunders, 1979, pp 779–880.

Drach GW: Transurethral ureteral stone manipulation. Urol Clin North Am 1983; 10:709–717.

Drach GW: Urinary lithiasis: Etiology, diagnosis, and medical management. In Walsh PC, Retick AB, Stamey TA, Vaughan ED, eds: Campbell's Urology, 6th ed. Philadelphia, W. B. Saunders, 1992, pp 2085–2156.

Drach GW, Boyce WH: Nephrocalcinosis as a source for renal stone nuclei: Observations on humans and squirrel monkeys and on hyperparathyroidism in the squirrel monkey. J Urol 1972; 107:897–904.

Dretler SP: Ureteral stone disease: Options for management. Urol Clin North Am 1990; 17:217–230.

Dretler SP, Coggins CH, McIver MA, Their SO: The physiologic approach to renal tubular acidosis. J Urol 1969; 102:665–669.

Dretler SP, Pfister RC: Primary dissolution therapy of struvite calculi. J Urol 1984; 131:861–863.

Drezner MK, Lebovitz HE: Primary hyperparathyroidism in paraneoplasic hypercalcemia. Lancet 1978; 1:1004–1006.

Duncan PG, Pope WD, Cohen MM, Green N: Fetal risk of anesthesia and surgery during pregnancy. Anesthesiology 1986; 64:790–794.

Dutoit PJ, Van Aswegen CH, Steyn PL, et al: Effects of bacteria involved with the pathogenesis of infection induced urolithiasis on the urokinase and sialidase (neuraminidase) activity. Urol Res 1992; 20:393–397.

Earnest DL, Johnson G, Williams HE, Admirand WM: Hyperoxaluria in patients with ileal resection: An abnormality in dietary oxalate absorption. Gastroenterology 1974; 66:1114–1122.

Ebisuno S, Morimoto S, Yasukawa S, Ohkawa T: Results of long term rice bran treatment on stone recurrence and hypercalciuric patients. Br J Urol 1991; 67:237–249.

Ebisuno S, Morimota S, Yoshida T, et al: Rice-bran treatment for calcium stone formers with idiopathic hypercalciuria. Br J Urol 1986; 58:592–595.

Edelson GW, Kleerekoper M: Hypercalcemic crisis. Med Clin North Am 1995; 79:79–92.

Eilon G, Mundy GR: Direct resorption of bone by human breast cancer cells in vitro. Nature 1978; 276:726–728.

Eisenberger F, Rassweiler J, Bub P: Differentiated approach to staghorn calculi using extracorporeal shock-wave lithotripsy and percutaneous nephrolithotomy: An analysis of 151 consecutive cases. World J Urol 1987; 5:248–254.

Elliot JS: Structure and composition of urinary calculi. J Urol 1973; 109:82–83.

Elliot JS, Eusebio E: Calcium oxalate solubility: The effects of trace metals. Invest Urol 1967; 4:428–430.

Ellman MH, Fretzin DF, Olson W: Toxic epidermal neurolysis associated with allopurinol administration. Arch Dermatol 1975; 111:986–990.

El-Sherif AC, El-Hafi R: Proposed new method for non-operative treatment of urethral stones. J Urol 1991; 146:1546–1547.

Elton TJ, Roth CS, Berquist TH, Silverstein MD: A clinical prediction rule for the diagnosis of ureteral calculi in emergency departments. J Gen Intern Med 1993; 8:57–62.

Erkyn S, Bultitude MI, Mayo ME, Lloyd-Davies RW: Prostatic calculi as a source of recurrent bacteriuria in the male. Br J Urol 1974; 46:527–532.

Ettinger B: Recurrent nephrolithiasis: Natural history and effect of phosphate therapy—a double blind controlled study. Am J Med 1976; 61:200–206.

Ettinger B, Citron JR, Livermore B, Dolman LI: Chlorthalidone reduces calcium oxalate calculus recurrence but magnesium hydroxide does not. J Urol 1988; 139:679–684.

Ettinger B, Citron JT, Tang A, Livermore B: Prophylaxis of calcium oxalate stones: Clinical trials of allopurinol, magnesium hydroxide and chlorthalidone. In Schwille PO, Smith LH, Robertson WG, Vahlensieck EW, eds: Urolithiasis and Related Clinical Research. New York, Plenum Press, 1985, pp 549–552.

Ettinger B, Oldroyd NO, Sorgel F: Triamterene nephrolithiasis. JAMA 1980; 244:2443–2446.

Ettinger B, Tang A, Citron JT, et al: Randomized trial of allopurinol in the prevention of calcium oxalate calculi. N Engl J Med 1986; 315:1386–1389.

Fanelli GM Jr: Urate excretion. Ann Rev Med 1977; 28:349–354.

Favus MJ: Factors affecting calcium metabolism in disorders of the kidney. Ann Clin Lab Sci 1981; 11:327–332.

Favus MJ: Intestinal absorption of calcium, magnesium and phosphorus. In Coe FL, Favus MJ, eds: Disorders of Bone and Mineral Metabolism. New York, Raven Press, 1992, pp 57–82.

Favus MJ, Coe FL: Evidence for spontaneous hypercalciuria in the rat. Miner Electrol Metab 1979; 2:150–154.

Fegan J, Khan P, Poindexter J, Pak CYC: Gastrointestinal citrate absorption in nephrolithiasis. J Urol 1992; 147:1212–1214.

Feit RM, Fair WR: The treatment of infection stones with penicillin. J Urol 1979; 122:592–594.

Feldman S, Putcha L, Griffith DP: Pharmacokinetics of acetohydroxamic acid-preliminary investigations. Invest Urol 1978; 15:498–501.

Fellstrom B, Backman U, Danielson BG, et al: Urinary excretion of urate in renal calcium stone disease and in renal tubular acidification disturbances. J Urol 1982; 127:589–592.

Fellstrom B, Backman U, Danielson BG, et al: Allopurinol treatment of renal calcium stone disease. Br J Urol 1985; 57:375–379.

Fessel WJ: Renal outcomes of gout and hyperuricemia. Am J Med 1979; 67:74–82.

Fetner CD, Barilla DE, Townsend J, Pak CYC: Effects of magnesium oxide on the crystallization of calcium salts in urine in patients with recurrent nephrolithiasis. J Urol 1978; 120: 399–401.

Fetter TL, Zimskind PD: Statistical analysis of patients with urinary calculi. JAMA 1961; 186:21.

Finkle AL, Smith DR: Parameters of renal functional capacity in reversible hydroureteronephrosis in dogs: V. Effects of 7 to 10 days of ureteral construction on RBF-Kr, C-In, Tc-H, O, C-PAH, osmolality, and sodium reabsorption. Invest Urol 1970; 8:299–310.

Finlayson B: Renal lithiasis in review. Urol Clin North Am 1974; 1:181–212.

Finlayson B, Dubois L: Absorption of heparin on sodium acid urate. Clin Chim Acta 1978; 84:203–206.

Finlayson B, Smith A: Stability of first dissociable proton of uric acid. J Chem Eng Data 1974; 19:94–97.

Finlayson B, Vermeulen W, Stewart RJ: Stone matrix and mucoprotein from urine. J Urol 1961; 86:355.

Fishbein WN, Carbone PO: Urease catalysis: II. Inhibition of the enzyme by hydroxyurea, hydroxylamine and acetohydroxamic acid. J Biol Chem 1965; 240:2407–2414.

Flannigan GM, Clifford RPC, Carver RA, et al: Indomethacin—an alternative to pethidine in ureteric colic. Br J Urol 1983; 55:6–9.

Fleisch H: Inhibitors and promoters of stone formation. Kidney Int 1978; 13:361–371.

Flocks RH: Calcium and phosphorus excretion in the urine of patients with renal or ureteric calculi. JAMA 1939; 113:1466.

Fourman P, Robinson JR: Diminished urinary excretion of citrated ring deficiencies of potassium in man. Lancet 1953; 2:656–657.

Freed SZ: The alternating use of an alkaline salt and acetazolamide in the management of cystine and uric acid stones. J Urol 1975; 113:96–99.

Fucik RF, Kukreja SC, Hargis GR, et al: Effects of glucocorticoids on function of the parathyroid glands in man. J Clin Endocrinol Metab 1975; 40:152–155.

Gambaro G, Marchini F, Bevilacgan M, et al: Red blood cell anomaly of oxalate transport and urinary acidification in idiopathic calcium oxalate mephrolithiasis. Kidney Int 1988; 35:754.

Garabedian M, Holick MF, DeLuca HF, Boyle IT: Control of 25-hydroxy-cholecalciferol metabolism by parathyroid glands. Proc Natl Acad Sci USA 1972; 69:1973–1976.

Garside J: Nucleation. In Nancollas GH, ed: Biological mineralization and demineralization. New York, Springer-Verlag, 1982, pp 23–25.

Gault MH, Chafe L, Morgan JM, et al: Comparison of patients with idiopathic calcium phosphate and calcium oxalate stones. Medicine 1991; 70:345–359.

Gault MH, Chafe L, Parfrey P, Robertson WG: The kidney-ureter stone sexual paradox: A possible explanation. J Urol 1989; 141:1104–1106.

Gault MH, Parfrey PS, Robertson WG: Idiopathic calcium phosphate nephrolithiasis (Editorial). Nephron 1988; 48:265–273.

Gee WF, Kiviat MD: Ureteral response to partial obstruction: Smooth muscle hyperplasia and connective tissue proliferation. Invest Urol 1975; 12:309–316.

Gennari FJ: Normal chemistry and physiology of acid-base homeostasis. In Massary SG, Glasscock RJ, eds: Textbook of Nephrology, 2nd ed. Baltimore, Williams & Wilkins, 1989, pp 357–365.

Gershoff SN, Prien EL: Effects of daily Mg and vitamin B6 administration to patients with recurring calcium oxalate kidney stones. Am J Clin Nutr 1967; 20:393–399.

Gertner JM, Coutan DR, Liger AS, et al: Pregnancy as state of physiologic absorptive hypercalciuria. Am J Med 1986; 81:451–456.

Gleeson MJ, Griffith DP: Infection stones. In Resnick MI, Pak CYC, eds: Urolithiasis: A Medical and Surgical Reference. Philadelphia, W. B. Saunders, 1990, pp 113–132.

Gleeson MJ, Kobashi K, Griffith DP: Non calcium nephrolithiasis. In Coe FL, Favus MJ, eds: Disorders of Bone and Mineral Metabolism. New York, Raven Press, 1992, pp 801–830.

Gleeson MJ, Thompson AS, Mehta S: Effect of unprocessed wheat bran on calciuria and oxaluria in patients with urolithiasis. Urology 1990; 35:231–234.

Glowacki LS, Beecroft ML, Cook RJ, et al: The natural history of a symptomatic urolithiasis. J Urol 1992; 147:319–321.

Goldfarb S: Diet and nephrolithiasis. Endocrinol Metab Clin North Am 1994; 45:235–243.

Greger R, Lang F, Oberleithner H, Deetjen P: Handling of oxalate by the rat kidney. Pflugers Arch 1978; 374:243–248.

Gregory JG, Park KY, Schoenberg HW: Oxalate stone disease after intestinal resection. J Urol 1977; 117:631–634.

Grenabo L, Hedelin H, Pettersson S: Adherence of urease induced crystals to rat bladder epithelium. Urol Res 1988; 16:49–52.

Griffith DP: Struvite stones. Kidney Int 1978; 13:372–382.

Griffith DP, Khonsari F, Skurnick JH: Experimental and clinical trials of lithostat (acetohydroxamic acid-AHA). In Martelli A, Buli P, Marchesini B, eds: Inhibitors of Crystallization in Renal Lithiasis and Their Clinical Application. Bologna, Italy, Acta Medica, 1988a, pp 228–235.

Griffith DP, Khonsari F, Skurnick JH, James KE: VA cooperative study group: A randomized trial of acetohydroxamic acid for the treatment and prevention of infection induced urinary stones in spinal cord injury patients. J Urol 1988b; 140:318–324.

Griffith DP, Musher DM: Prevention of infected urinary stones by urease inhibition. Invest Urol 1973; 11:228–233.

Griffith DP, Osborne CA: Infection (urease) stones. Miner Electrol Metab 1987; 13:278–285.

Grover PK, Marshall VR, Ryall RL: Tamm-Horsfall mucoprotein reduces promotion of calcium oxalate crystal aggregation induced by urate in human urine in vitro. Clin Sci 1994; 87:137–142.

Gutman AB, Yu TF: A three component system for regulation of renal excretion of uric acid in man. Trans Assoc Am Phys 1961; 74:353–363.

Gutman AB, Yu TF: Uric acid nephrolithiasis. Am J Med 1968; 45:756–779.

Haddad FS, Kouyoumdjian A: Silica stones in humans. Urol Int 1986; 41:70–76.

Haddad MC, Sharif HS, Abomelha MS, et al: Management of renal colic: Redefining the role of the urogram. Radiology 1992; 184:35–36.

Hagar BH, Magath TB: The etiology of incrusted cystitis with alkaline urine. JAMA 1925; 85:1352–1355.

Hall AP, Barry PE, Dawber TR, McNamara PM: Epidemiology of gout and hyperuricemia: A long term population study. Am J Med 1967; 42:27–37.

Hallson PC, Rose GA: Seasonal variations in urinary crystals. Br J Urol 1977; 49:227–284.

Harada M, Okuda Y, Maeda H: ESWL treatment of staghorn calculi and large stones. Presented at 4th Symposium on Shock Wave Lithotripsy: State of the Art, Indianapolis, 1988.

Hautmann RE: The stomach: A new and powerful oxalate absorption site in man. J Urol 1993; 149:1401–1404.

Hautmann R, Lehmann A, Kumar S: Calcium and oxalate concentrations in human and renal tissue: The key to the pathogenesis of stone formation. J Urol 1980; 123:317–319.

Hayashi Y, Kaplan RA, Pak CYC: Effect of cellulose phosphate therapy on crystallization of calcium oxalate in urine. Metabolism 1975; 24:1273–1278.

Hazarika EZ, Rao BN: Spectrochemical analysis of urinary tract calculi. Ind J Med Res 1974; 62:776–780.

Heath H 3d, Hodgson SF, Kennedy MA: Primary hyperparathyroidism: Influence, morbidity and potential economic impact in the community. N Engl J Med 1980; 302:189–193.

Hedelin H, Brorson JE, Grenabo L, Pettersson S: Ureaplasma urealyticum and upper urinary tract stones. Br J Urol 1984; 56:244–249.

Helal M, Mastandrea F, Black T, Lockhart J: Cost comparison and effectiveness between ESWL and percutaneous nephrolithotripsy in the management of staghorn calculi (Abstract 223). J Urol 1995; 153:284a.

Hellstrom J: The significance of staphylococci in the development and treatment of renal and ureteric stones. Br J Urol 1938; 10:348–378.

Hendrix JZ: Abnormal skeletal mineral metabolism in sarcoidosis. Ann Intern Med 1966; 64:797–805.

Henriquez-La Roche C, Rodriguez-Iturbe B, Parra G: Increased urinary excretion of prostaglandin E_2 in patients with idiopathic hypercalciuria is a primary phenomenon. Clin Sci 1992; 83:75–80.

Henry HL, Norman AW: Metabolism of vitamin D. In Coe FL, Favus MJ, eds: Disorders of Bone and Mineral Metabolism. New York, Raven Press, 1992, pp 149–162.

Herbstein FH, Kleeberg J, Shalitin Y, et al: Chemical and x-ray diffraction analysis of urinary stones in Israel. Isr J Med Sci 1974; 10:1493–1449.

Hermann U, Schwille PO, Schwarxalaender H, et al: Citrate and recurrent idiopathic calcium urolithiasis. Urol Res 1992; 20:347–353.

Herring LC: Observations of 10,000 urinary calculi. J Urol 1962; 88:545.

Hess B, Nakagawa Y, Parks JH, Coe FL: Molecular abnormality of Tamm-Horsfall glycoprotein in calcium oxalate nephrolithiasis. Am J Physiol 1991; 260:F569–578.

Hess B, Zipperle L, Jaeger P: Citrate and calcium effects on Tamm-Horsfall glycoprotein as a modifier of calcium oxalate crystal aggregation. Am J Physiol 1993; 265:F784–F791.

Hodgkinson A: Uric acid disorders in patients with calcium stones. Br J Urol 1976; 48:1–5.

Hodgkinson A: Evidence of increased oxalate absorption in patients with calcium oxalate kidney stones. Clin Sci Mol Med 1978; 54:291–294.

Hodgkinson A, Marshall RW: Changes in the composition of urinary tract stones. Invest Urol 1975; 13:131–135.

Hofbauer J, Hobarth R, Szabo N, Marberger M: Alkali citrate prophylaxis in idiopathic recurrent calcium oxalate urolithiasis—a prospective randomized study. Br J Urol 1994; 73:362–365.

Holmes G: Worcestershire sauce and the kidneys. Br Med J 1971; 3:252.

Holmes RP, Goodman HD, Assimos DG: The distribution of urinary calcium excretion in individuals on controlled diets (Abstract 488). J Urol 1995; 153:350A.

Holmgren K, Danielson BG, Fellstrom B, et al: The relation between urinary tract infections and stone composition in renal stone formers. Scand J Urol Nephrol 1989; 23:131–136.

Horiuchi N, Caulfield MD, Fisher JE: Similarity of synthetic peptide from human tumor to PARATHYROID HORMONE in vivo and in vitro. Science 1988; 138:1566–1568.

Hosking DH, Erickson SB, Van Den Berg CJ, et al: The stone clinic effect in patients with idiopathic calcium urolithiasis. J Urol 1983; 130:1115–1118.

Houser M, Zimmerman B, Davidson M, et al: Idiopathic hypercalciuria associated with hyperreninemia and high urinary prostaglandin E. Kidney Int 1984; 26:176–182.

Howard JE, Thomas WC, Barker LM, et al: The recognition and isolation from urine and serum of a peptide inhibitor to calcification. Johns Hopkins Med J 1967; 120:119–136.

Hsu TG: Ammonium acid urate lithiasis, experimental observations. J Urol 1966; 96:88–94.

Huggins C, Bear RS: Course of prostatic ducts and anatomy: Chemical and x-ray diffraction analysis of prostatic calculi. J Urol 1944; 51:37.

Insogna KL, Ellison AS, Burtis WJ, et al: Trichlormethiazide and oral phosphate therapy in patients with absorptive hypercalciuria. J Urol 1989; 141:269–274.

Itami N, Yasoshima K, Akutsu Y, Nonomura K: Spot urine screening for primary hyperoxaluria. Nephron 1990; 56:337–338.

Ito H, Coe FL: Acidic peptide and polyribonucleotide crystal growth inhibitors in human urine. Am J Physiol 1977; 233:F455–463.

Jacobs SC, Gittes RF: Dissolution of residual renal calculi with hemiacidrin. J Urol 1976; 115:2–4.

Jaeger P, Portmann L, Ginalski JM, et al: Tubulopathy in nephrolithiasis: Consequence rather than cause. Kidney Int 1986a; 29:563–571.

Jaeger P, Portmann L, Saunders A, et al: Anticystinuric effects of glutamine and of dietary sodium restriction. N Engl J Med 1986b; 315:1120–1123.

Jarrard DJ, Gerber GS, Lyon ES: Management of acute ureteral obstruction in pregnancy utilizing ultrasound guided placement of ureteral stents. Urology 1993; 42:263–268.

Jenkins AD, Dousa TP, Smith LH: Transport of citrate across renal brush border membrane, effects of dietary acid and alkali loading. Am J Physiol 1985; 249(Renal Fluid Electrol Physiol 18):F590–F595.

Jenkins AD, Langley MJ, Bobbitt MW: Red blood cell oxalate flux in patients with calcium urinary lithiasis. Urol Res 1988; 16:209.

Jenkins AD, Purnell DC, Scholz DA: Urolithiasis in primary hyperparathyroidism (Abstract #366). Presented at American Urological Association Meeting, Kansas City, MO, 1982.

Jick H, Dinan BJ, Hunter JR: Triamterene and renal stones. J Urol 1982; 127:224–225.

Joekes AM, Rose GA, Sutor J: Multiple renal silica calculi. Br Med J 1973; 1:146–147.

Johansson G, Backman U, Danielson BG, et al: Biochemical and clinical effects of the prophylactic treatment of renal calcium stones with magnesium hydroxide. J Urol 1980; 124:770–774.

Johns CJ: Sarcoidosis. In Isselbacher KJ, Sinba TK, DeLuca HF, eds: Harrison's Principles of Internal Medicine. New York, McGraw-Hill, 1980, p 928.

Johnson CM, Wilson DM, O'Fallon WM, et al: Renal stone epidemiology: A 25 year study in Rochester, Minnesota. Kindey Int 1979; 16:624–631.

Joly JS: Stone and Calculous Disease of the Urinary Organs. St. Louis, C. V. Mosby, 1931.

Jones DA, Atherton JC, O'Reilly PH Jr, et al: Assessment of the nephron segments involved in post-obstructive diuresis in man, using lithium clearance. Br J Urol 1989; 64:559–563.

Jones WA, Correa RJ Jr, Ansell JS: Urolithiasis associated with pregnancy. J Urol 1979; 122:333–335.

Jordan WR, Finlayson B, Luxenberg M: Kinetics of early time calcium oxalate nephrolithiasis. Invest Urol 1978; 15:465–468.

Juppner H, Abou-Samra AB, Freeman M, et al: A G-protein linked receptor for parathyroid hormone and parathyroid hormone related peptide. Science 1991; 254:1024–1026.

Kahnoski RJ, Lingeman JE, Coury TA: Combined percutaneous and extracorporeal shock wave lithotripsy for staghorn calculi: An alternative to anatrophic nephrolithotomy. J Urol 1986; 135:679–681.

Karniski LP, Aronson PS: Anion exchange pathways for chloride transport in rabbit renal microvilli membranes. Am J Physiol 1987; 253:F513–F521.

Katz SM, Krueger LJ, Falkner B: Microscopic nephrocalcinosis in cystic fibrosis. N Engl J Med 1988; 319:263–266.

Kavalich AG, Moran E, Coe FL: Dietary purine over consumption to hyperuricosuria in calcium oxalate kidney stone formers and normal subjects. J Chronic Dis 1976; 29:793–800.

Kavoussi LR, Albala DM, Basler JW, et al: Percutaneous management of urolithiasis during pregnancy. J Urol 1992; 148:1069–1071.

Kelly S, Nolan EP: Postscript on excretion rates in posttransplant cystinuric patient (letter). JAMA 1980; 243:1897.

Kerlan RK, Kahn RK, Laberge JM: Percutaneous removal of renal staghorn calculi. AJR 1985; 145:797–801.

Kessler A, Rosenberg HK, Smoyer WE, Blyth B: Urethral stones: US for identification of boys with hematuria and dysuria. Radiology 1992; 185:767–768.

Keutel HJ, King JS Jr: Further studies of matrix substance. Invest Urol 1964; 2:115.

Khan SR, Shevock PN, Hackett RL: In vitro precipitation of calcium oxalate in the presence of whole matrix or lipid components of the urinary stones. J Urol 1988; 139:418–422.

King JS, O'Connor FJ, Smith MJV: The urinary calcium/magnesium ratio in calcigerous stone formers. Invest Urol 1968; 6:60–65.

King JS Jr: Etiologic factors involved in urolithiasis: A review of recent research. J Urol 1967; 97:583–591.

King RG, Stanbury SW: Magnesium metabolism in primary hyperparathyroidism. Clin Sci 1970; 39:281–303.

Kinkead TM, Menon M: RTA. AUA Update Series 1995; 7:54–60.

Kjellstrand CM, Campbell DC, Von Hartitzsch B, Buselmeier TJ: Hyperuricemic acute renal failure. Arch Intern Med 1974; 133:349–359.

Kleinschmidt K, Mahlmann A, Hautmann RE: Intestinal oxalate degrading bacteria decrease urinary oxalate in stone formers: Proceedings of AUA (Abstract 791). J Urol 1995; 151:425a.

Klohn M, Bolle JF, Reverdin NP, et al: Ammonium urate urinary stones. Urol Res 1986; 14:315–318.

Knickelbein RG, Aronson PS, Dobbins JW: Oxalate transport by anion exchange across rabbit ileal brush border. J Clin Invest 1986; 77:170–175.

Koff SA, Lapides J: Altered bladder function in staghorn calculous disease. J Urol 1977; 117:577–580.

Kohri K, Nomura S, Kelamura Y, et al: Structure and expression of the m RNA encoding urinary stone protein (osteopontin). J Biol Chem 1993; 268:15180–15184.

Kok DJ, Papapoulos SE, Bijovet OL: Crystal agglomeration is a major element in calcium oxalate urinary stone formation. Kidney Int 1990; 37:51–56.

Kok DJ, Papapoulos SE, Bijovet OLM: Excessive crystal agglomeration with low citrate excretion in recurrent stone-formers. Lancet 1986; 10:1056–1058.

Koul H, Renzulli L, Yanagawa M, et al: Polarized distribution of oxalate transport systems in LLC-PK$_1$ cells, a line of renal epithelial cells. Am J Physiol 1994; 266:F266–F274.

Kowarski S, Schachter D: Effects of vitamin D on phosphate transport and incorporation into mucosal constituents of rat intestinal mucosa. J Biol Chem 1969; 244:211–217.

Krane S, Potts JT Jr: Skeletal remodeling and factors in influencing bone and mineral metabolism. In Isselbacher KJ, Sinba TK, DeLuca HF, eds: Harrison's Principles of Internal Medicine. New York, McGraw-Hill, 1990, p 1824.

Kristensen C, Parks JH, Lindheimer M, Coe FL: Reduced glomerular filtration rate and hypercalciuria in primary struvite nephrolithiasis. Kidney Int 1987; 32:749–753.

Kroovand RL: Stones in pregnancy and in children (Editorial). J Urol 1992; 148:1076–1078.

Kumar S, Sigmon D, Miller T, et al: A new model of nephrolithiasis involving tubular dysfunction/injury. J Urol 1991; 146:1384–1389.

Kuo SM, Aronson PS: Oxalate transport via the sulphate/HCO$_3$ exchanger in rabbit renal basolateral membrane vesicles. J Biol Chem 1980; 263:9710–9717.

Lackner H, Barton LJ: Cortical blood flow in ureteral obstruction. Invest Urol 1970; 8:319–323.

Laerum E, Larsen S: Thiazide prophylaxis of urolithiasis: A double blind study in general practice. Acta Med Scand 1984; 215:383–389.

Lafferty FW: Pseudohyperparathyroidism. Medicine 1966; 45:247–260.

Lalli AF: Roentgen aspects of renal calculous disease. Urol Clin North Am 1974; 1:213–227.

Laminski NA, Meyers AM, Kruger M, et al: Hyperoxaluria in patients with recurrent calcium oxalate calculi: Dietary and other risk factors. Br J Urol 1991; 68:454–458.

Lanzalaco AC, Singh RP, Smesko SA, et al: The influence of urinary macromolecules on calcium oxalate monohydrate crystal growth. J Urol 1988; 139:190–195.

Lattanzi DR, Cook WA: Urinary calculi in pregnancy. Obstet Gynecol NY 1980; 56:462–466.

Lau K, Ebny BK: Tubular mechanism for the spontaneous hypercalciuria in laboratory rats. J Clin Invest 1982; 70:835–844.

Lavengood RW Jr, Marshall VF: The prevention of renal phosphatic calcium in the presence of infection by the Shorr regimen. J Urol 1972; 108:368–371.

Law WM Jr, Heath H III: Familial benign hypercalcemia (hypocalciuric hypercalcemia): Clinical and pathogenetic studies in 21 families. Ann Intern Med 1985; 102:511–519.

Lee WJ, Smith AD, Cubelli V, Vernace FM: Percutaneous nephrolithotomy: Analysis of 500 consecutive cases. Urol Radiol 1986; 8:61–66.

Lee YH, Lee WC, Chen MT, et al: Acupuncture in the treatment of renal colic. J Urol 1992; 147:16–18.

Legha SS, Powell K, Buzdar AU, Blumenschein GR: Tamoxifen induced hypercalcemia in breast cancer. Cancer 1981; 47:2803–2806.

Lerner SP, Gleeson MJ, Griffith DP: Infection stones. J Urol 1989; 141:753–758.

Levison DA, Banim S, Crocker PR, Wallace DMA: Silica stones in the urinary bladder. Lancet 1982; 1:704–705.

Liao LL, Richardson KE: The metabolism of oxalate precursors in isolated perfused rat livers. Arch Biochem Biophys 1972; 153:438–448.

Lindberg J, Harvey J, Pak CY: Effect of magnesium citrate and magnesium oxide on the crystallization of calcium salts in urine: Changes produced by food-magnesium interaction. J Urol 1990a; 143:248–251.

Lindberg JS, Zobitz MM, Poindexter JR, Pak CYC: Magnesium bioavailability from magnesium citrate and magnesium oxide. J Am Coll Nutr 1990b;9:48–55.

Lindsjo M: Oxalate metabolism in renal stone disease with specific reference to calcium metabolism and intestinal absorption. Scand J Urol Nehrol 1989; 119(suppl):1–53.

Lingeman JE: Results of 313 staghorn treatments. Presented at 4th Symposium on Shock Wave Lithotripsy: State-of-the-Art, Indianapolis, 1988.

Lingeman JE, Saywell RM Jr, Woods JR, Newman DM: Cost analysis of extracorporeal shock wave lithotripsy relative to other surgical and non surgical treatment alternatives for urolithiasis. Med Care 1986; 24:1151–1160.

Lingeman JE, Siegel YL, Steele B: Metabolic evaluation of infected renal lithiasis—clinical relevance. J Endourol 1995; 9:51–54.

Linke RP, Bommer J, Ritz E, et al: Amyloid kidney stones of uremic patients consist of beta 2 microglobulin fragments. Biochem Biophys Res Commun 1986; 136:665–671.

Ljunghall S, Backman U, Danielson BG, et al: Epidemiology of renal stones in Sweden in a middle aged male population. Acta Med Scand 1975; 197:439–445.

Ljunghall S, Hedstrand H: Glucose metabolism in stone-formers. Urol Int 1978; 3:417–421.

Lloyd LM: Primary hyperparathyroidism: An analysis of the role of the parathyroid tumor. Medicine 1968; 47:53–71.

Lonsdale K: Epitaxy as on growth factor in urinary calculi and gallstones. Nature 1968a; 217:56–58.

Lonsdale K: Human stones. Science 1968b; 159:1199–1207.

Loris PC, Oliver-del-Cacho MJ, Heras GM, et al: Xanthine lithiasis in a case of Lesch-Nyhan syndrome treated with allopurinol. An ESP de Pediatria 1983; 19:401–404.

Loughlin KR, Bailey BBJ: Internal ureteral stents for conservative management of ureteral calculi during pregnancy. N Engl J Med 1986; 315:1647–1649.

Maddocks JL: 2–8 dihydroxyadenine urolithiasis (Letter to editor). Lancet 1992; 339:1050–1051.

Madorsky ML, Finlayson B: Oxalate absorption from intestinal segments of rats. Invest Urol 1977; 14:274–277.

Maierhofer WJ, Gray RW, Cheung HS, LeMann J Jr: Bone resorption stimulated by elevated serum 1, 25-(OH) 2 vitamin D concentrations in healthy men. Kidney Int 1983; 72:25–32.

Maikranz P, Coe FL, Parks J, Lindheimer MD: Nephrolithiasis in pregnancy. Am J Kidney Dis 1987; 9:354–358.

Malagodi MH, Moye HA: Physical and chemical characteristics of renal stone matrix. Urol Surv 1981; 31:81–87.

Malek RS, Boyce WH: Intranephronic calculosis: Its significance and relationships to matrix in nephrolithiasis. J Urol 1973; 109:551–555.

Malek RS, Boyce WH: Observations on the ultrastructure and genesis of urinary calculi. J Urol 1977; 117:336–341.

Malek RS, Kelalis PP: Pediatric nephrolithiasis. J Urol 1975; 113:545–551.

Mall JC, Collins PA, Lyon ES: Matrix calculi. Br J Radiol 1975; 48:807–810.

Mallette LE, Khouri K, Zengotita H, et al: Lithium treatment increases intact and midregion parathyroid hormone and parathyroid volume. J Clin Endocrinol Metab 1989; 68:654–660.

Mallette LE, Mechanick JI: Heritable syndrome of pseudoxanthoma elasticum with abnormal phosphorous and vitamin D metabolism. Am J Med 1987; 83:1157–1162.

Mandel NS, Mandel GS: Urinary tract stone disease in the United States veteran population: I. Geographical frequency of occurrence. J Urol 1989a; 142:1513–1515.

Mandel NS, Mandel GS: Urinary tract stone disease in the United States veteran population: II. Geographical analysis of variations in composition. J Urol 1989b; 142:1516–1520.

Marangella M, Futtero B, Bruno M, Linari F: Hyperoxaluria in idiopathic calcium oxalate stone disease: Further evidence of intestinal hyperabsorption of oxalate. Clin Sci 1982; 63:381–385.

Marangella M, Tricerri A, Rouzani M: The relationship between clinical outcome and urine biochemistry during various forms of therapy for idiopathic calcium stone disease. *In* Schwille P, Smith LH, Robertson WG, Vahlensieck W, eds: Urolithiasis and Related Clinical Research. New York, Plenum Press, 1985, pp 561–564.

Marshall V, White RH, DeSaintonge MC, et al: The natural history of renal and ureteric calculi. Br J Urol 1975; 47:117–124.

Martin DW Jr, Watts HD, Smith LH Jr: Hyperphosphatemia—medical staff conference, University of California, San Francisco. West J Med 1975; 122:482.

Matsumoto T, Fontaine O, Rasmussen H: Effect of 1,25 dihydroxyvitamin D₃ on phospholipid metabolism in chick duodenal mucosal cell. J Biol Chem 1981; 256:3354–3360.

McGeown MG: Heredity in renal stone disease. Clin Sci 1960; 19:465.

Mehes K, Szelid Z: Autosomal dominant inheritance of hypercalciuria. Eur J Pediatr 1980; 133:239–242.

Melick RA, Henneman PH: Clinical and laboratory studies of 207 consecutive patients in a kidney stone clinic. N Engl J Med 1958; 259:307–314.

Melnick I, Landes RR, Hoffman AA: Magnesium oxide therapy for recurrent calcium oxalate urolithiasis. Proceedings of First Symposium on Magnesium Deficiency in Human Pathology, 1973.

Melnick I, Landes RR, Hoffman AA, Burch JF: Magnesium therapy for recurring calcium oxalate urinary calculi. J Urol 1971; 105:119–122.

Menon M: Calcium oxalate renal lithiasis: Endocrinology and metabolism. *In* Rajfer J, ed: Urologic Endocrinology. Philadelphia, W. B. Saunders, 1986, pp 386–407.

Menon M: 2–8 Dihydroxyadenine urolithiasis (Editorial). J Urol 1992; 148:1632.

Menon M: Editorial comment to Choyke PL: Urogram: Are rumors of its death premature? J Urol 1993; 149:431.

Menon M, Koul H: Clinical review 32: Calcium oxalate nephrolithiasis. J Clin Endocrinol Metab 1992; 74:703–707.

Menon M, Krishnan CS: Evaluation and medical management of the patient with calcium stone disease. Urol Clin North Am 1983; 10:595–615.

Menon M, Mahle CJ: Oxalate metabolism and renal calculi. J Urol 1982; 127:148–151.

Menon M, Mahle CJ: Prevalence of hyperoxaluria in "idiopathic" calcium oxalate urolithiasis: Relationship to other metabolic abnormalities (Abstract 458). Presented at American Urological Association, Las Vegas, 1983a.

Menon M, Mahle CJ: Oxalate transport by intestinal brush border membrane vesicles. West J Urol 1983b; 1:163–169.

Menon M, Mahle CJ: Urinary citrate excretion in patients with renal calculi. J Urol 1983c; 129:1158–1160.

Metz SA, McRae JR, Robertson RP: Prostaglandins as mediators of paraneoplastic syndromes: Review and update. Metabolism 1981; 30:299–316.

Meyer AS, Finlayson B, Dubois L: Direct observation of urinary stone ultrastructure. Br J Urol 1971; 43:154–163.

Meyer JL: Nucleation kinetics in the calcium oxalate sodium urate monohydrate system. Invest Urol 1981; 19:197–201.

Meyer JL, Smith LH: Growth of calcium oxalate crystals. Invest Urol 1975; 13:36–39.

Miano L, Petta S, Paradiso GG, et al: A placebo controlled double-blind study of allopurinol in severe recurrent idiopathic renal lithiasis: Preliminary results. *In* Schwille PO, Smith LH, Robertson WG, Vahlensieck W, eds: Urolithiasis and Related Clinical Research. New York, Plenum Press, 1985, pp 521–524.

Millman S, Strans AA, Parks JH, Coe FL: Pathogenesis and clinical course of mixed calcium oxalate and uric acid nephrolithiasis. Kidney Int 1982; 22:366–370.

Minisola S, Rossi W, Pacitti MI, et al: Studies on citrate metabolism in normal subjects and kidney stone patients. Miner Electrol Metab 1989; 15:303–308.

Moody TE, Vaughan ED Jr, Gillenwater JY: Relationship between renal blood flow and ureteral pressure during 18 hours of total unilateral occlusion. Invest Urol 1975; 13:246–251.

Moore S, Gowland G: The immunological integrity of matrix substance A and its possible detection and quantitation in urine. Br J Urol 1975; 47:489–494.

Morris RC Jr: Relation of stone formation to renal tubular acidosis. Presented at the VIth International Symposium on Urolithiasis, Vancouver, 1995.

Morris RC Jr, Sebastian AA: Renal tubular acidosis and Fanconi syndrome. *In* Stanbury JB, Wyngaarden JB, Fredrickson DS, et al, eds: The Metabolic Basis of Inherited Disease, 5th ed. New York, McGraw-Hill, 1983, pp 1808–1843.

Mosekilde L, Christiansen MS: Decreased parathyroid function in hyperthyroidism: Relationship between serum parathyroid hormone, calcium phosphorous metabolism and thyroid functions. Acta Endocrinol (Copenh) 1977; 84:566–575.

Motola JA, Urivetsky M, Molia L, Smith AD: Transmembrane oxalate exchange: Its relationship to idiopathic calcium oxalate nephrolithiasis. J Urol 1992; 147:549–552.

Muldowney FP, Freaney R, McMullin JP: Serum ionized calcium and parathyroid hormone in renal stone disease. Q J Med 1976; 45:75–86.

Muldowney FP, Freaney R, Moloney MF: Importance of dietary sodium in the hypercalciuria syndrome. Kidney Int 1982; 22:292–296.

Mulvaney WP: The clinical use of Renacidin in urinary calcifications. J Urol 1960; 84:206.

Mulvaney WP, Hennings DC: Solvent treatment of urinary calculi: Refinements in technique. J Urol 1962; 88:145.

Mundy GR: Hypercalcemic factors other than parathyroid hormone related protein. Endocrinol Metab Clin North Am 1989; 18:741–752.

Musher D, Minuth J, Thorsteinsson SB, Holmes T: Effectiveness of achievable urinary concentrations of tetracycline against "tetracycline resistant" pathogenic bacteria. J Infect Dis 1975; 31(suppl):40–44.

Nakagawa Y, Ahmed M, Hall SL, et al: Isolation from human calcium oxalate renal stones of nephrocalcin, a glycoprotein inhibitor of calcium oxalate crystal growth: Evidence that nephrocalcin from patients with calcium oxalate nephrolithiasis is deficient in gamma carboxy glucotamic acid. J Clin Invest 1987; 79:1782–1787.

Narula R, Sharma SH, Sidhu H, et al: Transport of oxalate in intact red blood cell can identify potential stone-formers. Urol Res 1988; 16:193.

Nemoy NJ, Stamey TA: Surgical, bacteriological and biochemical management of "infection stones." JAMA 1971; 215:1470–1476.

Ng RH, Menon M, Landenson JH: Collection and handling of 24 hour urine specimens for measurement of analytes related to renal calculi. Clin Chem 1984; 30:467–471.

Nicar MJ, Hill K, Pak CY: Inhibition by citrate of spontaneous precipitation of calcium oxalate, in vitro. J Bone Miner Res 1987; 2:215–220.

Nicar MJ, Skurla C, Sakhaee K, Pak CY: Low urinary citrate excretion in nephrolithiasis. Urology 1983; 21:8–14.

Nickel JC, Eintage J, Costerton JW: Ultrastructural microbial ecology of infection-induced urinary stones. J Urol 1985; 133:622–627.

Nimmannit S, Malasit P, Chaovakul V, et al: Pathogenesis of sudden unexplained nocturnal death (Lai tai) and endemic distal renal tubular acidosis. Lancet 1991; 338:930–932.

Noe HN, Stapleton FB, Jerkins GR, Roy S 3d: Clinical experience with pediatric urolithiasis. J Urol 1983; 129:1166–1168.

Nussbaum SR: Pathophysiology and management of severe hypercalcemia. Endocrinol Metab Clin North Am 1993; 22:343–362.

Ohkawa T, Ebisuno S, Kitagenia M, et al: Rice bran treatment for hypercalciuric patients with urinary calculus disease. J Urol 1983; 129:1009–1011.

Ohkawa T, Tokunaga S, Nakashima T, et al: Thiazide treatment for calcium urolithiasis in patients with idiopathic hypercalciuria. Br J Urol 1992; 69:571–576.

Oldberg A, Franzen A, Heinengard D: Cloning and sequence analysis of rat bone sialoprotein (osteopontin) c-DNA reveals an Arg-Gly-Asp cell binding sequence. Proc Natl Acad Sci USA 1986; 83:8819–8823.

O'Reagan S, Laberge I, Homsy Y: Urolithiasis in pregnancy. Eur Urol 1984; 10:40–42.

Orloff NA, Stewart AF: Disorders of serum minerals caused by cancer. *In* Coe FL, Favus MJ, eds: Disorders of Bone and Mineral Metabolism. New York, Raven Press, 1992, pp 539–562.

Orwoll ES: The milk-alkali syndrome: Current concepts. Ann Intern Med 1982; 97:242–248.

Osther PJ, Hansen AB, Rohl HF: Screening renal stone formers for distal renal tubular acidosis. Br J Urol 1989; 63:581–583.

Pak CYC: Medical management of nephrolithiasis. J Urol 1982a; 128:1157–1164.

Pak CYC: Should patients with single renal stone occurrence undergo diagnostic evaluation. J Urol 1982b; 127:854–858.

Pak CYC: Citrate and renal calculi. Miner Electrol Metab 1987a; 13:257–266.

Pak CYC: Renal Stone Disease. Boston, Martinus Nijhoff Publishing, 1987b.

Pak CYC: Medical management of nephrolithiasis in Dallas: Update 1987. J Urol 1988; 140:461–467.

Pak CYC: Hypercalciuric calcium nephrolithiasis. *In* Resnick MI, Pak CYC, eds: Urolithiasis: A Medical and Surgical Reference. Philadelphia, W. B. Saunders, 1990, pp 79–88.

Pak CYC, Fuller C, Sakhaee K, et al: Long-term treatment of calcium nephrolithiasis with potassium citrate. J Urol 1985a; 134:11–19.

Pak CYC, Fuller C, Sakhaee K, et al: Management of cystine nephrolithiasis with alphamercaptopropionylglycine. J Urol 1986a; 136:1003–1008.

Pak CYC, Griffith DP, Menon M, et al: ABC's of medical management of stones. Educational monogram, Mission Pharmacal, San Antonio, 1993.

Pak CYC, Hayashi Y, Finlayson B, Chu S: Estimation of the state of saturation of brushite and calcium oxalate in urine: A comparison of three methods. J Lab Clin Med 1977a; 89:891–901.

Pak CYC, Holt K: Nucleation and growth of brushite and calcium oxalate in urine of stone formers. Metabolism 1976; 25:665–673.

Pak CYC, Holt K, Zerewekh JE: Attenuation by monosodium urate of the inhibitory effect glycosaminoglycans on calcium oxalate nucleation. Invest Urol 1979; 17:138–140.

Pak CYC, McGuire J, Peterson R, et al: Familial absorptive hypercalciuria in a large kindred. J Urol 1981a; 126:717–719.

Pak CYC, Nicar MJ, Peterson R, et al: A lack of unique pathophysiological background for nephrolithiasis of primary hyperparathyroidism. J Clin Endocrinol Metab 1981b; 53:536–542.

Pak CYC, Ohata M, Lawrence EC, Snyder W: The hypercalciurias: Courses, parathyroid functions and idiopathic criteria. J Clin Invest 1974; 54:387–400.

Pak CYC, Peters P, Hurt G, et al: Is selective therapy of recurrent nephrolithiasis possible? Am J Med 1981c; 71:615–622.

Pak CYC, Peterson R, Sakhaee K, et al: Correction of hypocitraturia and prevention of stone formation by combined thiazide and potassium citrate therapy in thiazide-unresponsive hypercalciuric nephrolithiasis. Am J Med 1985b; 79:284–288.

Pak CYC, Sakhaee K, Crowther C, Brinkley L: Evidence justifying a high fluid intake in treatment of nephrolithiasis. Intern Med 1980; 93:36–39.

Pak CYC, Sakhaee K, Fuller CJ: Physiological and physicochemical prevention of calcium-stone formation by potassium citrate therapy. Trans Assoc Am Phys 1983; 96:294–305.

Pak CY, Sakhaee K, Fuller C: Successful management of uric acid nephrolithiasis with potassium citrate. Kidney Int 1986b; 30:422–428.

Pak CYC, Skurla C, Harvey J: Graphic display of urinary risk factors for renal stone formation. J Urol 1985c; 134:867–870.

Pak CYC, Waters O, Arnold L, et al: Mechanism for calcium nephrolithiasis among patients with hyperuricosuria—supersaturation of urine with respect to monosodium urate. J Clin Invest 1977b; 59:426–431.

Palmer JM, Bishai MB, Mallon DS: Outpatient irrigation of the renal collecting system with 10% hemiacidrin: Cumulative experience of 365 days in thirteen patients. J Urol 1987; 138:262–265.

Palmer LS, Franco I, Kogan SJ, et al: Urolithiasis in children following augmentation cystoplasty. J Urol 1993; 150:726–729.

Parks JH, Coe FL: A urinary calcium-citrate index for the evaluation of nephrolithiasis. Kidney Int 1986; 30:85–90.

Parks JH, Coe FL: An increasing number of calcium oxalate stone events worsens treatment outcome. Kidney Int 1994; 45:1722–1730.

Parks JH, Coe FL, Favus M: Hyperparathyroidism in nephrolithiasis. Arch Intern Med 1980; 140:1479–1481.

Parks JH, Coe FL, Strauss AL: Calcium nephrolithiasis and medullary sponge kidney in women. N Engl J Med 1982; 306:1088–1091.

Parry ES, Lister IS: Sunlight and hypercalciuria. Lancet 1975; 1:1063–1065.

Parsons CL, Stauffer C, Mulholland SG, Griffith DP: The effect of ammonium on bacteria adherence to bladder transitional epithelium. J Urol 1984; 132:365–366.

Perrone HC, Santos DDR, Santos MV, et al: Urolithiasis in childhood metabolic evaluation. Pediatr Nephrol 1992; 6:54–56.

Peters HJ, Eckstein W: Possible pharmacological means of treating renal colic. Urol Res 1975; 3:55–59.

Peuchant E, Heches X, Sess D, Clerc M: Discriminant analysis of urinary calculi by near infra-red reflectance spectroscopy. Clin Chim Acta 1992; 205:19–30.

Pinto B, Crespi G, Sole Balcells F, Barcelo P: Patterns of oxalate metabolism in recurrent oxalate stone formers. Kidney Int 1974; 5:285–291.

Pode D, Verstandig A, Shapiro A: Treatment of complete staghorn calculi by extracorporeal shock wave lithotripsy monotherapy with special reference to internal stenting. J Urol 1988; 140:260–265.

Pohlman T, Hruska KA, Menon M: Renal tubular acidosis. J Urol 1984; 132:431–436.

Polinsky MS, Kaiser BA, Baluarte HJ, Gruskin AB: Renal stones and hypercalciuria. Adv Pediatr 1993; 40:353–384.

Power C: Diet and renal stones: A case-control study. Presented at Second International Urinary Stone Conference, Singapore, 1983.

Pras E, Arber N, Aksentijevich I, et al: Localization of a gene causing cystinuria to chromosome 2p. Nature Genet 1994; 6:415–419.

Preminger GM: Medical management of urinary calculus disease: Part II. Classification of metabolic disorders and selective medical management. AUA Update Series 1995; 14:1–8.

Preminger GM, Baker S, Peterson R: Hypomagnesiuric hypocitraturia: An apparent new entity for calcium nephrolithiasis. J Lith Stone Dis 1989; 1:22–25.

Preminger GM, Pak CY: Eventual attenuation of hypocalciuric response to hydrochlorothiazide in absorptive hypercalciuria. J Urol 1987; 137:1104–1109.

Preminger GM, Sakhaee K, Skurla C, Pak CYC: Prevention of recurrent calcium stone formation with potassium citrate therapy in patients with distal renal tubular acidosis. J Urol 1985; 134:20–23.

Press SM, Smith AD: Incidence of negative hematuria in a patient with acute urinary lithiasis presenting to the emergency room with flank pain. Urology 1995; 45:753–757.

Prien EL, Frondel C: Studies in urolithiasis: The composition of urinary calculi. J Urol 1947; 57:949.

Prien EL, Prien EL Jr: Composition and structure of urinary stones. Am J Med 1968; 45:654–672.

Prien EL Sr: Crystallographic analysis of urinary calculi: 23-year survey study. J Urol 1963; 89:917.

Prien EL Sr: Symposium on renal lithiasis: The analysis of urinary calculi. Urol Clin North Am 1974; 1:229–240.

Prien EL Sr, Gershoff SF: Magnesium oxide–pyridoxine therapy for recurrent calcium oxalate calculi. J Urol 1974; 112:509–512.

Prince CL, Scardino PL: A statistical analysis of ureteral calculi. J Urol 1960; 83:561.

Prince CL, Scardino PL, Wolan TC: The effect of temperature, humidity, and dehydration on the formation of renal calculi. J Urol 1956; 75:209.

Putcha L, Griffith DP, Feldman S: Pharmacokinetics of acetohydroxamic acid in patients with staghorn renal calculi. Eur J Clin Pharmacol 1985; 28:439–445.

Pyrah LH: Renal Calculus. New York, Springer Verlag, 1979, pp 84–85.

Rahman MA, Rahman B, Perveen S: Studies on serum mucoproteins in patients with urinary calculi. Biomed Pharmacother 1986; 40:311–313.

Raisz LG, Trummel CL, Holick MF, Deluca HF: 1,25-Dihydroxycholecalciferol: A potent stimulator of bone resorption in tissue culture. Science 1972; 175:768–769.

Ralston S, Fogelman I, Gardner MD: Hypercalcemia and metastatic bone disease: Is there a causal link? Lancet 1982; 2:903–905.

Rambar AC, MacKenzie RG: Urolithiasis in adolescents. Am J Dis Child 1978; 132:1117–1120.

Randall A: The origin and growth of renal calculi. Ann Surg 1937; 105:1009.

Rapado A, Traba ML, Castrillo JM: Incidence of hyperoxaluria in renal lithiaisis. In Rose GA, Robertson WG, Watts RWE, eds: Oxalate in Human Biochemistry and Clinical Pathology. London, The Wellcome Foundation, 1979, p 168.

Rasmussen H, Fontaine O, Max E, Goodman DBP: The effect of 1-hydroxyvitamin D_3 administration on calcium transport in chick intestine brush border membrane vesicles. J Biol Chem 1979; 254:2993–2999.

Reinholt FP, Hultenby K, Oldberg A, Heinegard D: Osteopontin—a possible anchor or osteoclasts to bone. Proc Natl Acad Sci USA 1990; 87:4473–4475.

Resnick MI: Evaluation and management of infection stones. Urol Clin North Am 1981; 8:265–276.

Resnick MI, Kursh ED, Cohen AM: Use of computerized tomography in the delineation of uric acid calculi. J Urol 1984; 131:9–10.

Resnick MI, Pridgen DB, Goodman HO: Genetic predisposition to formation of calcium oxalate renal calculi. N Engl J Med 1968; 278:1313.

Restaino I, Kaplan BS, Stanely C, Baker L: Nephrolithiasis, hypocitraturia and a distal renal tubular acidification defect in type 1 glycogen storage disease. J Pediatr 1993; 122:392–395.

Reusz GS, Dobos M, Tulassay T, Miltenyi M: Hydrochlorothiazide treatment of children with hypercalciuria: Effects and side effects. Pediatr Nephrol 1993; 7:669–702.

Reynolds TM, Burgess N, Matanhelia S, et al: The furosemide test: Simple screening test for renal acidification defect in urolithiasis. Br J Urol 1993; 72:153–156.

Rittenberg MN, Bagley DH: Ureteroscopic diagnosis and treatment of urinary calculi during pregnancy. Urology 1988; 32:427–428.

Rizzoli R, Bonjour JP: Management of disorders of calcium homeostasis. Baillieres Clin Endocrinol Metab 1992; 6:129–142.

Robertson WG: Physical chemical aspects of calcium stone formation in the urinary tract. *In* Fleisch H, Robertson WG, Smith LH, eds: Urolithiasis Research. New York, Plenum Publishing, 1976, pp 25–42.

Robertson WG: Diet and calcium stones. Miner Electrol Metab 1987; 13:228–234.

Robertson WG, Hambleton J, Hodgkinson A: Peptide inhibitors of calcium phosphate precipitation in the urine of normal and stone-forming men. Clin Chim Acta 1969; 25:247–253.

Robertson WG, Heyburn PJ, Peacock M, et al: The effect of high animal protein intake on the risk of calcium stone-formation in the urinary tract. Clin Sci 1979a; 57:285–288.

Robertson WG, Hughes H: Importance of mild hyperoxaluria in the pathogenesis of urolithiasis: New evidence from studies in the Arabian Peninsula. Scann Microsc 1993; 7:391–402.

Robertson WG, Peacock M: Calcium oxalate crystalluria and inhibitors of crystallization in recurrent renal stone formers. Clin Sci 1972; 43:499–506.

Robertson WG, Peacock M: The pattern of urinary stone disease in the United Kingdom in relation to animal protein intake during the period 1960–1980. Urol Int 1982; 37:394–399.

Robertson WG, Peacock M, Heyburn PJ, et al: Risk factors in calcium stone disease of the urinary tract. Br J Urol 1978; 50:449–454.

Robertson WG, Peacock M, Heyburn PJ, et al: Should recurrent calcium oxalate stone-formers become vegetarians? Br J Urol 1979b; 51:427–431.

Robertson WG, Peacock M, Heyburn PJ, Hanes FA: Epidemiological risk-factors in calcium stone formation. Scand J Urol Nephrol 1980; 53:15–30.

Robertson WG, Peacock M, Hodgkinson A: Dietary changes and the incidence of urinary calculi in the UK between 1958 and 1976. J Chron Dis 1979c; 37:394–399.

Robertson WG, Peacock M, Marshall RW, et al: Saturation inhibition index as a measure of the risk of calcium oxalate stone formation in the urinary tract. N Engl J Med 1976; 294:249–252.

Robertson WG, Peacock M, Selby PL: A multicenter trial to evaluate three treatments for recurrent idiopathic calcium stone disease: a preliminary report. *In* Schwille PO, Smith LH, Robertson WG, Vahlensieck W, eds: Urolithiasis and Related Clinical Research. New York, Plenum Press, 1985, pp 545–548.

Rocco F, Larcher P, Caimi D, Decobelli O: Treatment of renal staghorn calculi with ESWL monotherapy using the Rocco EXL catheter. Presented at 4th Symposium on Shock Wave Lithotripsy: State of the Art, Indianapolis, 1988.

Rocher LL, Tannon RL: The clinical spectrum of renal tubular acidosis. Ann Rev Med 1986; 37:319–331.

Rodriquez PN, Klein AS: Management of urolithiasis during pregnancy. Surg Obstet Gynecol 1988; 166:103–106.

Rose GA: Mild metabolic hyperoxaluria: A new syndrome. *In* Rose GA, ed: Oxalate Metabolism in Relation to Urinary Stones. London, Springer-Verlag, 1988; pp 121–130.

Rose GA, Westbury EJ: The influence of calcium content of water intake of vegetables, fruit and of other food factors upon the incidence of renal calculi. Urol Res 1975; 3:61–66.

Roth R, Finlayson B: Observations on the radiopacity of stone substances with special reference to cystine. Invest Urol 1973; 11:186–189.

Rouffignac CD: Regulation of magnesium excretion. *In* Coe FL, Favus MJ, eds: Disorders of Bone and Mineral Metabolism. New York, Raven Press, 1992, pp 41–56.

Rudman D, Dedonis JL, Fountain MT, et al: Hypocitraturia in patients with gastrointestinal mal absorption. N Engl J Med 1980; 303:657–661.

Ryall RL, Grover PK, Stapleton AMF, Tang Y: Effect of urinary prothrombin fragment 1 on calcium oxalate crystallization in undiluted human urine: Proceedings of AUA (Abstract 483). J Urol 1995; 153:349a.

Sackner MA, Spirak AP, Balia LJ: Hypercalcemia in the presence of osteoblastic metastases. N Engl J Med 1960; 262:173–176.

Sakhaee K, Alpern R, Jacobson HR, Pak CY: Contrasting effects of various potassium salts on renal citrate excretion. J Clin Endocrinol Metabol 1991; 72:396–400.

Sakhaee K, Harvey JA, Padalino PK, et al: The potential role of salt advice on the risk of kidney stone formation. J Urol 1993; 150:310–312.

Sakhaee K, Nicar M, Hill K, Pak CYC: Contrasting effects of potassium citrate and sodium citrate therapies on urinary chemistries and crystallization of stone-forming salts. Kidney Int 1983; 24:348–352.

Sakhaee K, Nigam S, Snell P, et al: Assessment of the pathogenetic role of physical exercise in renal stone formation. J Clin Endocrinol Metab 1987; 65:974–979.

Sakhaee K, Poindexter JR, Pak CY: The spectrum of metabolic abnormalities in patients with cystine nephrolithiasis. J Urol 1989; 141:819–821.

Samaan NA, Hickey RC, Sethi MR, et al: Hypercalcemia in patients with known malignant disease. Surgery 1976; 80:382–389.

Sarica K, Baltaci S, Kilic S, et al: 371 bladder calculi in a benign prostatic hyperplasia patient. Int Urol Nephrol 1994; 26:23–25.

Scheid CR, Koul H, Adam W, et al: Oxalate ion and calcium oxalate crystal interaction with renal epithelial cells. *In* Coe FL, Favus MJ, Pak CY, et al, eds: Kidney Stones: Medical and Surgical Management. Philadelphia, Lippincott–Raven Press, 1996, p 129.

Scheinman JI: Primary hyperoxaluria: Therapeutic strategies for the 90's. Kidney Int 1991; 40:389–399.

Schneider HJ, Berenyi M, Hesse A, Tscharnke J: Comparative urinary stone analyses: Quantitative chemical, x-ray diffraction, infrared spectroscopy and thermoanalytical procedures. Int Urol Nephrol 1973; 5:9–17.

Scholz D, Schwille PO, Sigel A: Double blind study with thiazide in recurrent calcium lithiasis. J Urol 1982; 128:903–907.

Scholz DA, Sprague RG, Kernohan JW: Cardiovascular and renal complications of Cushing's syndrome. A clinical and pathological study of 17 cases. N Engl J Med 1957; 256:833.

Schulz E, Borner R, Brundig P, Maurer F: Influence of different factors on the formation of calcium oxalate stones: II. Discriminant analytical computations of morphological parameters of pelvic-calyceal systems and clinicochemical urine parameters of controls and calcium oxalate stone formers. Eur Urol 1989; 16:218–222.

Schulze H, Hertle L, Graff J: Combined treatment of branched calculi by percutaneous nephrolithotomy and extracorporeal shock-wave lithotripsy. J Urol 1986; 135:1138–1141.

Schweitzer FA: Intra-pelvic pressure and renal function studies in experimental chronic partial ureteric obstruction. Br J Urol 1973; 45:2–7.

Schwille PO, Scholz D, Schwille K, et al: Citrate in urine and serum and associated variables in subgroup of urolithiasis. Nephron 1982; 31:194–202.

Scott R, Lewi H: Therapeutic management of upper urinary tract stone disease in 172 subjects. Urology 1989; 33:277–281.

Scott R, Mathieson A, McLelland A: The reduction in stone recurrence and oxalate excretion by allopurinol. *In* Rose GA, Robertson WG, Watts RWE, eds: Oxalate in Human Biochemistry and Clinical Pathology: Proceedings of an International Meeting in London, 1979. London, Wellcome Foundation, 1979, pp 191–197.

Scott WW, Huggins C, Selman BC: Metabolism of citric acid in urolithiasis. J Urol 1943; 50:202.

Seegmiller JE, Laster L, Howell RR: Biochemistry of uric acid and its relation to gout. N Engl J Med 1968; 268:712.

Seftel A, Resnick MI: Metabolic evaluation of urolithiasis. Urol Clin North Am 1990; 17:159–169.

Senekjian HO, Weinman EJ: Oxalate transport by proximal tubule of rabbit kidney. Am J Physiol 1982; 243:F271–F275.

Shah PJ, Green NA, Williams G: Unprocessed bran and its side effect on urinary calcium excretion in idiopathic hypercalcuria. Br Med J 1980; 281:426.

Sharfi AR: Presentation and management of urethral calculi. Br J Urol 1991; 68:271–272.

Sharma RN, Shah I, Gupta S, et al: Thermogravimetric analysis of urinary stones. Br J Urol 1989; 64:564–566.

Sharma S, Vaidyanathan S, Thind SK, Nath R: Therapeutic role of diclofenac sodium in management of hypocitraturia and hypophosphaturia in idiopathic stone formers. *In* Ryall R, Bais R, Marshall VR, et al, eds: Urolithiasis 2. New York, Plenum Press, 1992, p 666.

Sharon E, Diamond HS: Factitious uric acid urolithiasis as a feature of Munchausen syndrome. Mt Sinai J Med 1974; 41:698–699.

Shiraga H, Min W, Van Dusen WJ: Inhibition of calcium oxalate crystal growth in vitro by uropontin: Another member of the aspartic acid rich protein super family. Proc Natl Acad Sci USA 1992; 89:426–430.

Shorr E: The possible usefulness of estrogen and aluminum hydroxide gels in the management of renal stone. J Urol 1945; 53:507–520.

Shorr E, Almy TP, Sloan MH, et al: The relation between the urinary excretion of citric acid and calcium: Its implications for urinary calcium stone formation. Science 1942a; 96:587.

Shorr E, Bernheim AR, Taussky H: The relation of urinary citric acid excretion to the menstrual cycle and the steroidal reproductive hormones. Science 1942b; 95:606–607.

Shorr E, Carter AC: Aluminum gels in the management of renal phosphatic calculi. JAMA 1950; 144:1549–1556.

Shuster J, Finlayson B, Schaeffer R, et al: Water hardness and urinary stone disease. J Urol 1982; 128:422–425.

Sierakowski R, Finlayson B, Landes R: Stone incidence as related to water hardness in different geographical regions of the United States. Urol Res 1978; 7:157–160.

Sierakowski R, Hemp B, Finlayson B: Water hardness and the incidence of urinary calculi. *In* Finlayson B, Thomas WC, eds: Colloquium on Renal Lithiasis. Gainesville, University Presses of Florida, 1976.

Silver TM, Koff SA, Thornbury J: An unusual pathway of urine extravasation associated with renal colic. Radiology 1973; 109:537–538.

Silverman DE, Stamey TA: Management of infection stones: The Stanford experience. Medicine 1983; 62:44–51.

Simmonds HA, Potter CF, Sahota A, et al: Adenine phosphoribosyl deficiency presenting with supposed "uric acid" stones: Pitfalls and diagnosis. Jr Soc Med 1978; 71:791–795.

Simmonds HA, Van Acker KJ, Cameron JS, Snedden W: The identification of 2, 8-dihydroxy adenine, a new component of urinary stones. Biochem J 1976; 157:485–487.

Simmonds HA, Van Acker RJ, Sahota A: S, 2–8 dihydroxyadenine urolithiasis (Letter to editor). Lancet 1992; 339:1295–1296.

Simpson D, Hager SR: pH and bicarbonate effects on mitochondrial anion accumulation. J Clin Invest 1979; 63:704–712.

Simpson DP: Tissue citrate levels and citrate utilization after sodium bicarbonate administration. Proc Soc Exp Biol Med 1963; 114:263–265.

Sinaniotis CA, Koukoutsakis P, Spyridis P: Estimation of urinary N-acetyl-B-D: Glucosaminidase activity for monitoring therapy of distal renal tubular acidosis. Acta Paediatr Scand 1989; 78:453–456.

Sloand JA, Izzo JL: Captopril reduces urinary cystine excretion in cystinuria. Arch Intern Med 1987; 147:1409–1412.

Smith A, Lange P, Miller R: Dissolution of cystine calculi by irrigation E acetylcysteine through percutaneous nephrostomy. Urology 1979; 13:422–423.

Smith LH: Renal tubular acidosis. Update, Boston AUA Office of Education, 1986.

Smith LH: Urolithiasis. *In* Schrier RW, Gottschalk CW, eds: Diseases of the Kidney, 4th ed. Boston, Little, Brown, 1988, pp 785–813.

Smith LH: Medical aspects of urolithiasis: An overview. J Urol 1989; 141:707–710.

Smith LH: Hyperoxaluric states. *In* Coe FL, Favus MI, eds: Disorders of Bone and Mineral Metabolism. New York, Raven Press, 1992, pp 707–728.

Smith LH, Thomas WC Jr, Arnand CD: Orthophosphate therapy in calcium renal lithiasis. *In* Urinary Calculi—Proceedings of the International Symposium on Renal Stone Research, Madrid, 1972. Basel, Karger, 1973, pp 188–197.

Smith MJV: Placebo vs. allopurinol for renal calculi. J Urol 1977; 117:690–692.

Smith MJV, Boyce WH: Anatrophic nephrotomy and plastic calyrhaphy. J Urol 1968; 99:521–527.

Smith MJV, Hunt LD, King JS Jr, Boyce WH: Uricemia and urolithiasis. J Urol 1969; 101:637–642.

Snyder JA, Smith AD: Staghorn calculi: Percutaneous extraction versus anatrophic nephrolithotomy. J Urol 1986; 136:351–354.

Sohn M, Deutz FJ, Rohrmann D: Anesthesia-free ESWL monotherapy with double J stents versus PCNL/ESWL combined approach in staghorn disease: A prospective randomized study. Presented at 4th Symposium on Shock Wave Lithotripsy: State-of-the-Art, Indianapolis, 1988.

Sonda LP III, Thompson NW, Fischer CP: Simultaneous presentation of untreated hyperparathyroidism and obstructing ureteral calculi: Surgical considerations. J Urol 1982; 127:26–28.

Sperling O, Brosh S, Boer P, et al: Urinary xanthine stones in an allopurinol treated gouty patient with partial deficiency of hypoxanthine-guanine phosphoribosylltransferase. Isr J Med Sci 1978; 14:288–292.

Stamey TA: Urinary Infections. Baltimore, Williams & Wilkins, 1972.

Stapleton AMF, Ryall RL: The development of a specific antibody to prothrombin fragment 1 and its potential role in urolithiasis: Proceedings of AUA (Abstract 482). J Urol 1995; 153:349a.

Stapleton FB, Roy S 3d, Noe HN, Jerkins G: Hypercalciuria in children with hematuria. N Engl J Med 1984; 310:1345–1348.

Stark H, Savir A: Dissolution of cystine calculi by pelviocaliccal irrigation with D-penicillamine. J Urol 1980; 124:895–898.

Stauss AL, Coe FL, Parks JH: Formation of a single calcium stone of renal origin. Arch Intern Med 1982; 142:504–507.

Stecker JF Jr, Gillenwater JY: Experimental partial ureteral obstruction: I. Alteration in renal function. Invest Urol 1971; 8:377–385.

Steele BT, Lowe P, Rance CP, et al: Urinary tract calculi in children. Int J Pediatr Nephrol 1983; 4:47–52.

Steele TH, Reiselbach RE: The renal mechanism for urate homeostasis in normal man. Am J Med 1967; 43:876–886.

Stewart AF, Horst R, Deftos LJ, et al: Biochemical evaluation of patients with cancer associated hypercalcemia: Evidence for humoral and nonhumoral groups. N Engl J Med 1980; 303:1377–1383.

Stoller ML, Gupta M, Bolton D, Irby PB 3d: Clinical correlates of the gross radiographic and histologic features of urinary matrix calculi. J Endourol 1994; 8:335–340.

Stothers L, Lee LM: Renal colic in pregnancy. J Urol 1992; 148:1383–1387.

Strauss A, Coe FL, Deutsch L, Parks JH: Factors that predict relapse of calcium nephrolithiasis during treatment: A prospective study. Am J Med 1982; 72:17–24.

Suby HI, Albright F: Dissolutions of phosphatic urinary calculi by retrograde introduction of a citrate solution containing magnesium. N Engl J Med 1943; 228:81.

Suby HI, Suby RM, Albright F: Properties of organic solutions which determine their irritability to the bladder mucosa and the effect of magnesium ions in overcoming this irritability. J Urol 1942; 48:549.

Sugimoto T, Funae Y, Rhbben H, et al: Resolution of proteins in the kidney stone matrix using high-performance liquid chromatography. Eur Urol 1985; 11:334–340.

Summerskill WHJ, Thorsell F, Feinberg HJ, Aldrete JS: Effects of urease inhibition in hyperammonemia—clinical and experimental studies with acetohydroxamic acid. Gastroenterology 1967; 54:20–26.

Sutherland JW, Parks JH, Coe FL: Recurrence after a single renal stone in a community practice. Miner Electrol Metab 1985; 11:267–269.

Sutor DJ: Difficulties in the identification of components of mixed urinary calculi using the ray method. Br J Urol 1968; 40:29–32.

Sutor DJ: The nature of urinary stones. *In* Finlayson B, ed: Urolithiasis: Physical Aspects. Washington, D.C., National Academy of Sciences, 1972, p 43.

Sutor DJ, O'Flynn JD: Matrix formation in crystalline material in vivo. *In* Cifuentes L, Rapado A, Hodgkinson A, eds: Urinary Calculi: International Symposium on Renal Stone Research. Basel, S. Karger, 1973, p 280.

Sutor DJ, Scheidt S: Identification standards for human urinary calculus components using crystallographic methods. Br J Urol 1968; 40:22–28.

Sutor DJ, Wooley SE: Composition of urinary calculi by x-ray diffraction: Collected data from various localities: VIII. Leeds, England. Br J Urol 1970; 42:302–305.

Sutor DJ, Wooley SE: Composition of urinary calculi by x-ray diffraction: Collected data from various localities: IX–XI. Glasgow, Scotland; United States of America; and Sudan. Br J Urol 1971; 43:268–272.

Sutor DJ, Wooley SE: Composition of urinary calculi by x-ray diffraction: Collected data from various localities: XV–XVIII. Royal Navy; Bristol, England; and Dundee, Scotland. Br J Urol 1974a; 46:229–232.

Sutor DJ, Wooley SE: The crystalline composition of prostatic calculi. Br J Urol 1974b; 46:533–535.

Sutor DJ, Wooley SE, Illingworth JJ: Some aspects of the adult urinary stone problem in Great Britain and Northern Ireland. Br J Urol 1974; 46:275–288.

Sutton RAL, Walker VR: Responses to hydrochlorothiazide and acetazolamide in patients with calcium stones: Evidence suggesting a defect in renal tubular function. N Engl J Med 1980; 302:709–713.

Sutton RAL, Walker VR: Relationship of urinary calcium to sodium excretion in calcaneous renal stone formers: Effects of furosemide. *In* Schwille PO, Smith LH, Robertson WG, Vahlensieck W, eds: Urolithiasis and Related Clinical Research. New York, Plenum Press, 1981, pp 61–66.

Suvachittanont O, Mersongsee LA, Dhanamitta S, Valyasevi A: The oxalic acid content of some vegetables in Thailand, its possible relationships with the bladder stone disease. J Med Assoc Thailand 1973; 6:645–653.

Swanson SK, Heilman RI, Eversman WG: Urinary tract stones in pregnancy. Surg Clin North Am 1995; 75:123–142.

Swartz HM, Reichling BA: Hazards of radiation exposure for pregnant women. JAMA 1978; 239:1907–1908.

Takasaki E: An observation on the composition and recurrence of urinary calculi. Urol Int 1975; 30:228–236.

Tessitore N, Ortalda V, Fabris A, et al: Renal acidification defects in patients with recurrent calcium nephrolithiasis. Nephron 1985; 41:325–332.

Tew WP, Malis CD, Howard JE, Lehninger AL: Phosphocitrate inhibits mitochondrial and cytosolic accumulation of calcium in kidney cells in vivo. Proceedings of the National Academy of Sciences of the United States of America 1981; 78:5528–5532.

Thalut K, Rizal A, Brockis JG, et al: The endemic bladder stones of Indonesia—epidemiology and clinical features. Br J Urol 1976; 48:617–621.

Thier SO: Cystinuria. *In* Wyngaarden JB, Smith LH, eds: Cecil Textbook of Medicine, Vol. 1. Philadelphia, W. B. Saunders, 1985, p 611.

Thier SO, Segal S: Cystinuria. *In* Stanbury JB, Wyngaarden JB, Fredrickson DS, eds: The Metabolic Basis of Inherited Disease. New York, McGraw-Hill, 1972, pp 504–1519.

Thomas J, Champagnac A, Thomas E: Urinary oxalate and its relationship to calcium oxalate lithiasis. *In* Rose GA, Robertson WG, Watts RWE, eds: Urinary Oxalate in Human Biochemistry and Clinical Pathology. London, Wellcome Foundation, 1979, p 186.

Thomas JM, Cranston D, Knox AJ: Hyperparathyroidism: Patterns of presentation, symptoms and response to operation. Ann R Coll Surg Engl 1985; 67:79–82.

Thomas WC Jr: Clinical concepts of renal calculus disease. J Urol 1975; 113:423–432.

Thomas WC Jr: Renal Calculi: A Guide to Management. Springfield, IL, Charles C. Thomas, 1976.

Thompson RB, Stamey TA: Bacteriology of infected stones. Urology 1973; 2:627–633.

Tieder M, Modai D, Samuel R, et al: Hereditary hypophosphatemic rickets with hypercalciuria. N Engl J Med 1985; 312:611–617.

Tieder M, Modai D, Shaked U, et al: Idiopathic hypercalciuria and hereditary hypophosphatemic rickets: Two phenotypical expressions of a common genetic defect. N Engl J Med 1987; 316:125–129.

Tiselius HG, Ahlstrand C, Larsson L: Urine composition in patients with urolithiasis during treatment with magnesium oxide. Urol Res 1980; 8:197–206.

Tiselius HG, Almgard LE. The diurnal excretion of oxalate and the effect of pyridoxine and ascorbate on oxalate excretion. Eur Urol 1977; 3:41–46.

Tiselius HG, Berg C, Fornander AM, Nilsson MA: Effects of citrate on the different phases of calcium oxalate crystallization. Scann Microsc 1993a; 7:381–390.

Tiselius HG, Fornander AM, Nilsson MA: The effects of citrate and urine on calcium oxalate crystal aggregation. Urol Res 1993b; 21:363–366.

Tiselius HG, Larsson L: Calcium phosphate: An important crystal phase in patients with recurrent calcium stone formation? Urol Res 1993; 21:175–180.

Tiselius HG, Varenhorst E, Carlstrom K, Larrson L: Urinary oxalate excretion during antiandrogenic therapy. Invest Urol 1980; 18:110–111.

Tizzani A, Casetta G, Piana P, Vercelli D: Wheat bran in the selective therapy of absorptive hypercalciuria: A study performed on 18 lithiasis patients. J Urol 1989; 142:1018–1020.

Toor M, Massry S, Katz AI, Agmon J: The effect of fluid intake on the acidification of urine. Clin Sci 1964; 27:259.

Uhlman DR: Crystal growth from solutions: Interface structure and interface kinetics. *In* Finlayson B, ed: Urolithiasis: Physical Aspects. Washington, D.C., National Academy of Science, 1972, pp 169–176.

Umekawa T, Kohri KL, Amasaki N, et al: Sequencing of urinary stone protein, identical to alpha-one antitrypsin, which lacks 22 amino acids. Biochem Biophys Res Commun 1993; 193:1049–1053.

Uribarri J, Man S, Carroll JH: The first kidney stone. Ann Intern Med 1989; 111:1006–1009.

Uribarri J, Oh MS, Pak CYC: Renal stone risk factors in patients with type IV renal tubular acidosis. Am J Kidney Dis 1994; 23:784–787.

Vainder M, Kelly J: Renal tubular dysfunction secondary to jejunoileal bypass. JAMA 1976; 235:1257–1258.

Valyasevi A, Dhanamitta S: Studies of bladder stone disease in Thailand: XVII. Effect of exogenous source of oxalate on crystalluria. Am J Clin Nutr 1974; 27:877–882.

Van Arsdalen KN, Banner MP, Pollack HM: Radiographic imaging and urologic decision making in the management of renal and ureteral calculi. Urol Clin North Am 1990; 17:171–190.

Van Aswegen CH, Hurter P, Van Der Merwe CA, Du Plessis DJ: The relationship between total urinary testosterone and renal calculi. Urol Res 1989; 17:181–183.

Van Den Berg CJ: Renal tubular acidosis and urolithiasis. *In* Rous SN, ed: Stone Disease Diagnosis and Management. Orlando, Grune & Stratton, 1987, pp 131–134.

Van Den Berg CJ, Kumar R, Wilson DN: Orthophosphate therapy decreases urinary calcium excretion and serum 1,25 dihydroxyvitamin D concentration in idiopathic hypercalciuria. J Clin Endocrinol Metab 1980; 51:998–1001.

Van Reen R, ed: Idiopathic urinary bladder stone disease. Fogarty International Center Proceedings, no. 37, 1977.

Van Reen R: Geographical and nutritional aspects of endemic stones. *In* Brockis JG, Finlayson B, eds: Urinary Calculus. Littleton, MA, PSG Publishing Company, 1981.

Vargas AD, Bragin SD, Mendez R: Staghorn calculus: Its clinical presentation, complications and management. J Urol 1982; 127:860–862.

Vaughan ED Jr, Shenasky JH II, Gillenwater JY: Mechanism of acute hemodynamic response to ureteral occlusion. Invest Urol 1971; 9:109–118.

Vaughan ED Jr, Sorenson EJ, Gillenwater JY: The renal hemodynamic response to chronic unilateral complete ureteral occlusion. Invest Urol 1970; 8:78–90.

Verdier M, Dussol B, Casanova P, et al: Evidence that human kidney produces a protein similar to lithostatine, the pancreatic inhibitor of $CaCO_3$ crystal growth. Eur J Clin Invest 1992; 22:469–474.

Vergauwe DA, Verbeeck RM, Oosterlinck W: Analysis of urinary calculi. Acta Urol Belg 1994; 62:5–13.

Vermeulen CW, Lyon ES: Mechanism of genesis and growth of calculi. Am J Med 1968; 45:684–692.

Volmer M, Bolck A, Wolthers BG, et al: Partial least squares regression for routine analysis of urinary calculus composition with Fourier transform infrared analysis. Clin Chem 1993; 39:948–954.

Volmer M, Wolthers BG, Metting HJ, et al: Artificial neural network predictions of urinary calculus compositions analyzed with infrared spectroscopy. Clin Chem 1994; 40:1692–1697.

Wallace MR, Mason K, Gray J: Urine oxalate and calcium in idiopathic stone formers. N Z Med J 1981; 94:87–89.

Wasserstein AG, Stolley PD, Soper KA: Case control study of risk factors for idiopathic calcium nephrolithiasis. Miner Electrol Metab 1987; 13:85–95.

Watanabe T: Histochemical studies on mucosubstances in urinary stones. Tohoku J Exp Med 1972; 107:345–357.

Watts RW: Uric acid biosynthesis and its disorders. J R Coll Phys Lond 1976; 11:91–106.

Watts RWE, Morgan SH, Danpure CJ, et al: Combined hepatic and renal transplantation in primary hyperoxaluria type I: Clinical report of nine cases. Am J Med 1991; 90:179–188.

Watts RWE, Veall N, Purkiss P: Oxalate dynamics and removal rates during hemodialysis and peritoneal dialysis in patients with primary hyperoxaluria and severe renal failure. Clin Sci 1984; 66:591–597.

Weinman EJ, Frankfurt SJ, Ince A, Sansom S: Renal tubular transport of organic acids: Studies with oxalate and paraaminohippurate in the rat. J Clin Invest 1978; 61:801–806.

Welshman SG, McGeown MG: The relationship of the urinary cations calcium, magnesium, sodium and potassium in patients with renal calculi. Br J Urol 1975; 47:237–242.

Westbury EJ: Some observations on the quantitative analysis of over 1,000 urinary calculi. Br J Urol 1974; 46:215.

White JL: Stones in the prostate and seminal vesicles. Texas J Med 1928; 23:581.

White RW: Minerals in the urine of stone formers and their spouses. *In* Hodgkinson A, Nordin BEC, eds: Proceedings of the Renal Stone Research Symposium. London, J & A Churchill Ltd, 1969.

Whitson PA, Pietrzyk RA, Pak CY, Cintron NM: Alterations in renal stone risk factors after space flight. J Urol 1993; 150:803–807.

Wickham JEA, Coe N, Ward JP: One hundred cases of nephrolithotomy under hypothermia. J Urol 1974; 112:702–705.

Wikstrom B, Backman U, Danielson BG, et al: Ambulatory diagnostic evaluation of 389 recurrent renal stone formers. Klin Wochenschr 1983; 61:85–90.

Williams HE, Smith LH Jr: Disorders of oxalate metabolism. Am J Med 1968; 45:715–735.

Williams HE, Smith LH Jr: L-Glyceric aciduria: A new genetic variant of primary hyperoxaluria. N Engl J Med 1978; 278:233–328.

Williams HE, Smith LH Jr: Primary hyperoxaluria. *In* Stanbury JB, Wyngaarden JB, Fredrickson DS, eds: The Metabolic Basis of Inherited Disease, 5th ed. New York, McGraw-Hill, 1983, pp 204–228.

Williams JJ, Rodman JS, Peterson CM: A randomized double-blind study of acetohydroxamic acid in struvite nephrolithiasis. N Engl J Med 1984; 311:760–764.

Wilson DR, Strauss AL, Manuel MA: Comparison of medical treatments for the prevention of recurrent calcium nephrolithiasis (Abstract). Urol Res 1984; 12:39–40.

Wirth MP, Frohnmuller HGW: Results of primary treatment of staghorn calculi with extracorporeal shock wave lithotripsy. Presented at 4th Symposium on Shock Wave Lithotripsy: State-of-the-Art, Indianapolis, 1988.

Worcester EM, Blumenthal SS, Bershensky AM, Leward DL: Calcium oxalate crystal growth inhibitor produced by mouse kidney cortical cells in culture is osteopontin. J Bone Miner Res 1992; 71029–1036.

Worcester EM, Nakagawa Y, Bushinsky DA, Coe FL: Evidence that serum calcium oxalate supersaturation is consequence of oxalate retention in patients with chronic renal failure. J Clin Invest 1986; 77:1888–1896.

Wyngaarden JB: Xanthinuria. *In* Stanbury JB, Wyngaarden JB, Fredrickson DS, eds: The Metabolic Basis of Inherited Disease, 3rd ed. New York, McGraw-Hill, 1972, pp 992–1002.

Wyngaarden JB, Kelley WN: Gout. *In* Stanbury JB, Wyngaarden JB, Fredrickson DS, eds. The Metabolic Basis of Inherited Disease. New York, McGraw-Hill, 1972, pp 889–968.

Yanagawa N, Lee DBN: Renal handling of calcium and phosphorus. *In* Coe FL, Favus MJ, eds: Disorders of Bone and Mineral Metabolism. New York, Raven Press, 1992, pp 3–40.

Yendt ER, Cohanim M: Ten years experience with the use of thiazides in the prevention of kidney stones. Trans Am Clin Climat Assoc 1973; 85:65–75.

Yendt ER, Cohanim M: Prevention of calcium stones with thiazides. Kidney Int 1978; 13:397–409.

Yendt ER, Cohanim M: Response to a physiologic dose of pyridoxine in type I primary hyperoxaluria. N Engl J Med 1985; 312:953–957.

Yendt ER, Gagne RJA: Detection of primary hyperparathyroidism with special reference to its occurrence in hypercalciuric females with "normal" or borderline serum calcium. Can Med Assoc J 1968; 98:331–336.

Yendt ER, Gagne RJ, Cohanim M: The effects of thiazides in idiopathic hypercalciuria. Am Med Sci 1966; 251:409–416.

Yendt ER, Jarzylo S, Finnis WA: Medullary sponge kidney (tubular ectasia) in calcium urolithiasis. *In* Smith LH, Robertson WG, Finlayson B, eds: Urolithiasis Clinical and Basic Research. New York, Plenum Press, 1981, pp 105–112.

Young JL Jr, Boswell RB, Nies AS: Severe allopurinol hypersensitivity association with thiazides and prior renal compromise. Arch Intern Med 1974; 134:553–558.

Yu TF: Urolithiasis in hyperuricemia and gout. J Urol 1981; 126:424–430.

Yu TF, Gutman AB: Uric acid nephrolithiasis in gout: Predisposing factors. Ann Intern Med 1967; 67:1133–1148.

Zarembski PM, Hodgkinson A: Some factors influencing the urinary excretion of oxalic acid in man. Clin Chim Acta 1969; 25:1–10.

Zerwekh HE, Pak CY: Selective effects of thiazide therapy on serum alpha 2–5-dihydroxyvitamin D and intestinal calcium absorption in renal and absorptive hypercalciuria. Metab Clin Exp 1980: 29:13–17.

Zinsser H, Karp F: How to diminish endogenous oxalate excretion by L-tyrosine administration. Invest Urol 1973; 10:249–252.

Appendix A. LOW-PURINE DIET*

Breakfast

Fruit	1 serving
Cereal (no oatmeal)	1 serving
Eggs	2
Toast	1 slice
Butter or margarine	As desired
Beverage	Sanka, Kaffee Hag, or Postum
Milk	As desired
Cream	As desired
Sugar	As desired

Lunch

Soup	1 serving (see list)
Cheese	2 ounces
Vegetable (cooked)	1 serving
Vegetable (raw)	1 serving
Bread	1 slice
Butter or margarine	As desired
Dessert	1 serving (see list)
Milk	1 glassful

Dinner

Allowed soup	If desired
Meat, fish, fowl	2 ounces (twice weekly)
Potato	1 serving
Vegetable (cooked or raw)	1 serving
Bread	1 slice
Butter or margarine	As desired
Dessert	1 serving (see list)
Milk	1 glassful

Special Instructions

1. Avoid liver, sweetbreads, brains, and kidney. A 2-ounce portion of any other meat, fish, or fowl may be served twice weekly.
2. Serve cheese and eggs as meat substitutes. Fish roe and caviar may be used as desired.
3. Use 1–2 pints of milk daily.
4. Omit all meat extracts, broth soups, and gravies.
5. Omit the following vegetables entirely from the diet: Dried beans, lentils, dried peas, spinach.
6. Avoid coffee, tea, chocolate, and cocoa.
7. Omit alcoholic beverages of all kinds.
8. Use fruits of all kinds—fresh, canned, and dried.
9. Allow cereals of all kinds except oatmeal.
10. Soups allowed are milk soups made with any vegetables except those forbidden.
11. Desserts allowed are fruit, puddings, cake, ice cream, gelatin desserts, or pie.
12. Beverages allowed are milk or buttermilk and any decaffeinated coffee or cereal coffee.

*Carbohydrate—223, Protein—89, Fat—115: Cal. 2283.

Appendix B. LOW-CALCIUM, LOW-OXALATE DIET (300 mg calcium)

Food Groups	Foods Allowed	Foods to Avoid
Beverage	Carbonated beverages, cereal beverages; limit tea and coffee to 3 cups daily of either	Malted beverages, milk, milk drinks, chocolate beverages
Breads and cereals	White and wheat bread, refined cereals, crackers, rye or variety breads, donuts, pastries, sweet rolls	Any cereal enriched with calcium, such as instant-type hot cereals; cereals containing bran, such as All-Bran or Granola; pancakes, waffles, and other "quick breads"; breads containing bran; 100% whole wheat bread
Desserts	Gelatin desserts made of allowed foods, fruit ices, sherbets. Cakes, cookies, or other products not made from milk	Desserts made with milk, such as custard, pudding, ice cream, ice milk; cream pies and cream-filled baked products
Fats	Butter or margarine, cream (up to 1/3 cup daily), salad oils, cooking fat, nondairy creamer, cream cheese (up to 2 ounces per day)	Half-and-half, sour cream (can be included in 1/3 cup allowance)
Fruit	Canned, cooked, or fresh fruit except those excluded, dried fruit (up to 1/2 cup daily)	Rhubarb,* cranberries,* plums,* gooseberries,* and raspberries*
Meat and meat substitutes	Meat, fish, and fowl except those excluded. Not more than 2 eggs daily, including those used in cooking†	Sardines, shrimp, and oysters; cheese—yellow, natural, and processed; white cheese, including cottage cheese and Parmesan cheese; yogurt
Potato or substitute	Potato, macaroni, noodles, spaghetti, refined rice	Whole grain rices
Soups	Broth, vegetable, or meat soup made from allowed foods	Bean or pea soup; cream or milk-based soups
Sweets and nuts	Candy without chocolate, almonds, or peanuts; honey, jam, jelly, syrups, and sugar; other nuts	Chocolate,* molasses, cocoa,* almonds, peanuts
Vegetables	Canned, cooked, or fresh vegetables or vegetable juice except those excluded	Asparagus,* dried beans and peas, broccoli, beet greens, swiss chard, collards, mustard greens, turnip greens, kale, spinach*
Miscellaneous	Salt, spices, and pepper (in moderation), vinegar	Cream sauce, milk gravy, peanut butter, ripe olives

*Foods high in oxalate.
†Robertson et al (1979b) believe that limited animal protein intake also benefits calcium stone formers.

Appendix C. LOW-PHOSPHATE DIET REGIMEN
(SHORR REGIMEN)*

1. Daily dietary intake of phosphorus restricted to less than 300 mg/day; calcium restricted to less than 700 mg/day.
2. Patient takes 40 ml of basic aluminum carbonate gel four times daily.
3. Fluid intake of at least 3000 ml/day and more as needed to keep urinary output at 2000 ml/day.
4. Analysis of urinary phosphorus excretion, which should be less than 250 mg/day, is done at intervals.

*Modified from Marshall VF, Lavengood RW, Jr, and Kelly D.: Ann Surg 1965; 162:366.

92
SHOCK-WAVE LITHOTRIPSY

Thomas V. Martin, M.D.
R. Ernest Sosa, M.D.

Throughout the history of medicine, perhaps no technologic advance has exerted a more revolutionary effect than shock-wave lithotripsy (SWL). Twenty-five years ago, open surgery was the sole form of therapy for urinary calculous disease. Noninvasive therapies that would replace surgical interventions were little more than the subject of science fiction. The development of SWL provided a truly noninvasive therapy for urinary calculi. SWL displayed good success rates in treating urinary calculi while decreasing morbidity, length of hospitalization, and anesthesia requirements. Over the past decade, SWL has maintained a leading role in the management of urinary calculi.

Although the development of SWL has proceeded at a breathtaking pace since initial descriptions of its clinical use in 1982 (Chaussy et al, 1982), significant challenges remain. Large efforts have been directed at improving lithotriptor technology to increase treatment efficacy and to eliminate the need for anesthesia. At the same time, examination of the clinical uses of SWL continues in hopes of better defining criteria that allow for the selection of patients most likely to benefit from this therapy, while identifying those patients who would be best managed with other modalities.

Each lithotriptor requires the coordination of several different functions for effective operation. Shock wave generation, focusing, coupling, and stone localization are coordinated by a computer.

Lithotriptors are commonly characterized by the type of **shock wave generator** they employ. Commercially available lithotriptors use electrohydraulic, electromagnetic, or piezoelectric generators.

Shock wave focusing allows for the concentration of shock wave energy at a focal point. Unfocused shock waves can effect stone fragmentation only at extremely high power. At high power, shock waves are more likely to injure surrounding tissues. Shock waves may be focused by several different methods. Each method relies on the ability to alter the direction of shock waves with reflectors or lenses. Two important variables to be considered in shock wave focusing are the shock wave aperture and the focal area. The shock wave aperture refers to the width of the hemiellipsoid reflector, shock tube, or reflector dish. The size of the aperture corresponds to the body surface area that the shock waves traverse to enter the body. In general, lithotriptors with larger apertures, such as piezoelectric lithotriptors, are associated with less pain during treatment. The focal area refers to the volume within which the shock waves are concentrated. Within the focal area, effective stone fragmentation generally takes place. Lithotriptors with large focal areas, such as the Dornier HM-3, require less precise stone localization but require greater anesthesia. Lithotriptors with smaller focal volumes may require more precise stone localization and a lesser degree of anesthesia.

Shock wave coupling allows for the propagation of shock waves through the medium within which they are generated and into the patient without significant loss of energy. Initial lithotriptors used a large water bath to provide coupling, whereas newer machines use a smaller water pool or an enclosed water cushion and acoustic gel.

Stone localization allows for the precise placement of a stone within the focal area of a shock wave generator. This requires imaging by way of radiography (real-time fluoroscopy or hard copy radiograph) or ultrasonography. Patient positioning is accomplished by a remote-controlled mobile gantry or tabletop.

METHODS OF SHOCK WAVE GENERATION

Commercially available lithotriptors use electrohydraulic, electromagnetic, or piezoelectric shock wave generators. Other methods of shock wave generation include laser-induced shock wave generation and microexplosive shock wave generation. These methods, however, have not been applied in commonly available lithotriptors. Spark-gap, microexplosive, and laser shock wave generators are referred to as point source generators because the shock wave energy originates from a single point and then diverges before being refocused at a distant point. In contrast, extended source generators, such as electromagnetic and piezoelectric devices, are characterized by shock waves that are generated along a broad front and are then focused at a distant point. Differences in treatment efficiency, anesthesia requirements, and the nature of stone fragmentation may exist among generators (Table 92–1) (Zhong and Preminger, 1994).

Table 92–1. ADVANTAGES AND DISADVANTAGES OF DIFFERENT SHOCK WAVE GENERATORS

Shock Wave Generator	Advantages	Disadvantages
Spark-gap electrode	Wide range of energy Flexible aperture	Short life span (2000–4000 shock waves)
Piezoelectric	Long life span Variable shock wave frequency	Limited energy range Large aperture
Electromagnetic	Wide range and continuous graduation of energy Long life span	Metallic membrane must be periodically replaced

Electrohydraulic (Spark Gap) Generators

Electrohydraulic lithotriptors use shock waves produced by a spark gap electrode situated in a water medium (Fig. 92–1). A high-voltage spark discharge causes the explosive vaporization of water at the electrode tip, the first focal point (F_1). This sudden expansion generates shock waves through the surrounding medium (Chaussy et al, 1982). When the spark electrode is located within a hemiellipsoidal reflector, shock waves are reflected by the ellipsoid to a second focal point (F_2), where they are concentrated. This arrangement allows for the projection of the majority of the original shock wave energy from the electrode tip (F_1) to a distant point at which a stone is located (F_2). Because the shock waves have not converged proximal to this point, however, the effect on intervening tissues is minimized.

Electromagnetic Generators

Electromagnetic lithotriptors use a water-filled *shock tube* containing a thin metallic membrane that is associated with an electromagnetic coil (Fig. 92–2). When electric current is applied to the coil, the membrane is repelled owing to the opposing magnetic fields. This results in the development of shock waves, which then exit the shock tube and are focused by either an acoustic lens or a parabolic reflector. These

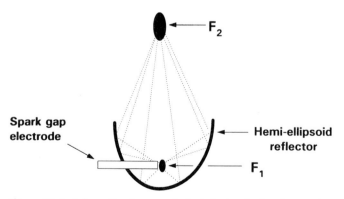

Figure 92–1. Schematic diagram of electrohydraulic (spark gap electrode) shock wave generation. Shock waves generated by a spark gap electrode are focused by a hemiellipsoid reflector at the second focal point (F_2).

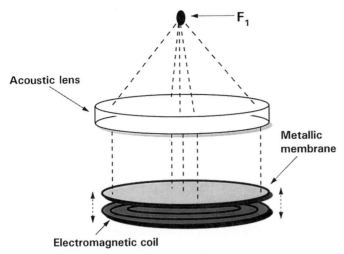

Figure 92–2. Schematic diagram of electromagnetic shock wave generation. When electrical current is applied to an electromagnetic coil, the coil repels a metallic membrane, resulting in the generation of shock waves. Shock waves are focused by an acoustic lens of parabolic reflector.

shock waves originate from the broad surface of the membrane rather than from a single point as in the electrohydraulic generator. Therefore, when focused for treatment, they converge at the electromagnetic lithotriptor's first focal point (F_1).

Piezoelectric Generators

Piezoelectric lithotriptors use a series of ceramic elements that line a reflector dish (Fig. 92–3). When such elements are activated with a high-voltage electric current, they rapidly expand. When simultaneously activated, the series of elements is capable of generating shock waves in a surrounding fluid medium. The reflector dish is configured so that shock waves generated by each ceramic element converge at a distant focal point (F_1) without the use of additional focusing mechanisms.

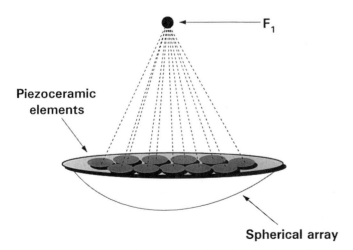

Figure 92–3. Schematic diagram depicting piezoelectric shock wave generation. Piezoceramic elements arranged in series line the surface of a spherical dish. Electrical current application results in the creation of a focused shock wave.

Microexplosive Generators

The Yachiyoda SZ-1 lithotriptor uses shock waves generated by exploding a small lead azide pellet within an ellipsoid reflector (Kuwahara et al, 1986, 1987a, 1987b). Lead azide is a potent explosive, and the difficulties with its safe usage and storage are drawbacks of this technique.

IMAGING SYSTEMS

See Table 92–2 for a comparison of imaging systems.

Radiography

The majority of commercially available lithotriptors use real-time fluoroscopy for stone imaging. Early lithotriptors employed two fluoroscopes arrayed at oblique angles to the patient and 90 degrees from each other to localize the stone at the F_2 focal point. Later models use anteroposterior and craniocaudal fluoroscopy for the same function to limit interference from the spine. The advantages of fluoroscopy include familiarity to urologists, ability to visualize radiopaque calculi throughout the urinary tract (including the ureter), and ability to use iodinated contrast material to aid stone localization and anatomic definition. The disadvantages include inability to visualize radiolucent calculi without the use of radiographic contrast material, the exposure of both patient and staff to ionizing radiation, and high maintenance requirements (Bush et al, 1987; Pollock, 1987; Van Swearingen et al, 1987).

Hard copy radiographs have been used as both an aid and an alternative to real-time fluoroscopy. Short-exposure, high-intensity radiographs or spot films may provide additional resolution of calculi that are difficult to visualize with fluoroscopy alone (Jenkins, 1988). Alternatively, hard copy radiographs may be used for stone positioning when combined with a computer-integrated system that places the stone at the shock wave focal point (Saltzman, 1988).

Ultrasonography

The use of ultrasonography for lithotriptor imaging was triggered by the development of multifunctional lithotriptors

Table 92–2. COMPARISON OF IMAGING MODALITIES FOR SHOCK-WAVE LITHOTRIPSY

Modality	Advantages	Disadvantages
Fluoroscopy	Familiarity to urologists Radiopaque stones visible throughout urinary tract Radiographic contrast material may be used to aid visualization	Inability to visualize radiolucent stones without contrast material Radiation exposure Higher maintenance costs
Ultrasound	Continuous real-time monitoring of treatment Visualization of radiolucent stones Lower maintenance cost	Steeper learning curve Inability to visualize most ureteral stones

2738 SHOCK-WAVE LITHOTRIPSY

designed for the treatment of both urinary and biliary calculi (Rassweiler et al, 1990). Because most biliary calculi are radiolucent, ultrasound imaging was necessary for such lithotriptors. Ultrasound, however, provides several advantages to the urologist as well, including the visualization of radiolucent urinary calculi, continuous real-time monitoring of treatment without radiation exposure, lower maintenance requirements, and lower cost (Preminger, 1989). Disadvantages include difficulty in localizing ureteral calculi because of overlying bowel and the relative unfamiliarity of performing abdominal ultrasonography to most urologists. The replacement of biliary lithotripsy by laparoscopic cholecystectomy as primary therapy for biliary calculi combined with the increasing interest in treating ureteral calculi by SWL has caused most manufacturers to use radiographic imaging systems primarily at this time, although some units may include ultrasonic capability as well.

MECHANISMS OF STONE FRAGMENTATION

Objects such as calculi maintain their form because of innate comprehensive forces. Fragmentation occurs when the

tensile strength of a calculus is overcome by opposing forces created by shock waves (Forssmann et al, 1977).

Shock waves may accomplish stone fragmentation by three mechanisms. First, as a shock wave strikes the anterior surface of a stone, it is divided into two components (Fig. 92–4A through C). One component is reflected backward toward the shock wave source. This component is referred to as the tensile component. The remaining portion of the shock wave proceeds forward through the stone and is referred to as the compressive component. These opposing forces create a pressure gradient across the anterior surface of the stone producing fragmentation and erosion (Chaussy and Fuchs, 1987a).

Second, as the compressive component strikes the posterior stone surface, a similar phenomenon occurs. Newly generated opposing forces act on the posterior surface, characteristically resulting in the separation of a spherical cap from the posterior stone surface. This process is referred to as *spalling* (Chuong et al, 1992).

Third, cavitation (Fig. 92–4D through F) is believed to play a role in SWL-induced stone fragmentation. This is an acoustic phenomenon in which pressure changes cause the rapid expansion of gaseous bubbles in a liquid medium. These bubbles are extremely unstable and collapse explo-

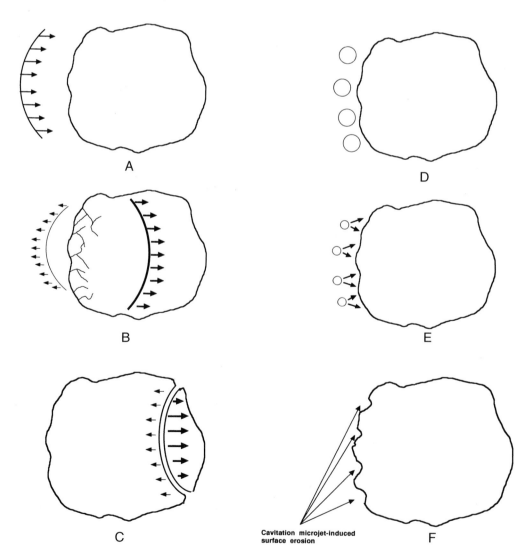

Cavitation microjet-induced surface erosion

Figure 92–4. *A,* Shock wave approaches the anterior surface of a stone. *B,* A shock wave strikes the anterior surface of stone; it is divided into tensile *(small arrows)* and compressive *(large arrows)* components. This results in fragmentation at the anterior stone surface. *C,* As original compressive component proceeds through the stone, it is similarly divided into opposing components, resulting in the separation of a spherical cap from the posterior stone surface. This process is referred to as "spalling." *D,* Cavitation occurs when unstable gas bubbles form at the stone surface after shock wave administration. *E,* When unstable bubbles collapse, cavitation microjets may be directed toward the stone surface *(arrows).* *F,* Microjets result in erosion and small fractures at the stone surface.

sively when struck by ensuing shock waves. This leads to the formation of microjets, which strike the stone surface at high velocities causing erosion and microscopic fractures (Crum, 1988; Delius et al, 1988). The importance of this effect has been likened to the small taps of the stonemason's hammer along a desired line of fracture. This induces a small fissure, and a forceful blow, similar to subsequent shock waves, then fractures the stone cleanly.

BIOEFFECTS OF SHOCK WAVES

Ideally the effect of shock waves is limited exclusively to the targeted calculus. Surrounding tissues, however, may be affected by the shock waves as well (Delius et al, 1987). Experimental studies have examined these effects and have aided in the development of safe treatment parameters.

Renal Effects

A variety of animal models have examined the impact of SWL on the kidney. Although initial studies by Chaussy and associates revealed the absence of pathologic changes in the canine kidney after SWL, subsequently more extensive studies have demonstrated that a variety of changes may occur (Chaussy et al, 1982). The most frequently reported effect is renal hemorrhage, which has been described in perinephric, subcapsular, and intraparenchymal locations (Brendel, 1986; Newman et al, 1987; Abrahams et al, 1988; Delius, 1988; Delius et al, 1988; Donovan et al, 1989; Morris et al, 1989). Thin-walled veins appear to be especially susceptible to shock wave damage. Importantly, the extent of hemorrhage correlates directly with the kilovoltage used and number of shock waves administered (Newman et al, 1987; Delius et al, 1988).

Additional pathologic findings in animal models have included chronic renal fibrosis (Abrahams et al, 1988; Recker et al, 1989). Such changes have raised concern about the development of SWL-induced hypertension (see later). The rationale for this concern is that fibrotic changes are also seen in the kidney after renal trauma, which is also associated with the development of hypertension.

Numerous studies have examined the effects of SWL on renal tubular and glomerular cells. Gilbert and associates demonstrated reversible, nephrotic-range proteinuria in patients after electrohydraulic shock-wave lithotripsy (ESWL) (Gilbert et al, 1988). Similarly, reversible changes in urinary levels of substances such as N-β-acetylglucosamidase, beta-galactosidase, gamma-glutamyl/transferase, creatine phosphokinase, lactate dehydrogenase, and alpha$_2$ macroglobulin have also been demonstrated in both animal and human studies (Assimos et al, 1989; Jaegar and Constantinides, 1989; Lingeman et al, 1986a, 1989). Such substances may eventually serve as markers, which allow for the determination of optimal treatment parameters to minimize the possibility of renal damage after ESWL.

Effects on Other Tissues

The effect of SWL on other tissues has also been evaluated. Pulmonary hemorrhage and contusion have been in-

duced in animal models. Pulmonary injury appears to be reversible (Kroovand et al, 1987) and, more importantly, may be prevented by shielding the lung fields with styrofoam (Chaussy et al, 1982; Newman and Riehle, 1987). Because of their proximity to the kidney, gastrointestinal structures are also subjected to shock waves. Minor submucosal bowel hematomas and liver petechiae have been demonstrated (Chaussy et al, 1982; Abrahams et al, 1988). Fortunately, however, these findings appear to be of little clinical significance. McCullough and colleagues reported that ESWL caused no undue effects to the rat ovary but urged caution in extrapolating these findings to humans (McCullough et al, 1989). It is therefore prudent to avoid SWL of lower ureteral calculi in women of reproductive age. Moran and co-workers described the disastrous effects of shock waves on chick embryos, and this work has served as the basis for the contraindication of ESWL during pregnancy (Moran et al, 1990).

Chaussy and associates examined the effect of ESWL on circulating blood cell elements, an important consideration given the highly vascular nature of the kidney (Chaussy et al, 1982). Although in vitro studies of red blood cell samples placed at the shock wave focal point revealed extensive hemolysis, these results were not reproduced in a live canine model because free hemoglobin levels were only slightly elevated. This was believed to be due to the relatively small amount of circulating blood within the focal area at any particular time. Similarly, lymphocyte activity was not affected.

CONTRAINDICATIONS TO SHOCK-WAVE LITHOTRIPSY

The previously noted bioeffects have helped delineate potential complications of SWL. Consideration of these tissue effects should help prevent the development of untoward complications.

Pregnancy is an absolute contraindication to SWL. Concern regarding miscarriage and birth defects after SWL prohibits treatment of gravid patients.

Uncontrolled coagulopathy also remains an absolute contraindication. The occurrence of perinephric, subcapsular, and intraparenchymal hemorrhage observed both in the previously noted animal studies and after treatment of humans with normal coagulation profiles (Kaude et al, 1985; Rubin et al, 1987) prohibits treatment in the presence of uncorrected coagulopathy. Patients with coagulopathies should undergo hematologic evaluation with the administration of supplemental platelets and clotting factors as necessary before SWL. Alternative therapies should be considered for patients in whom a coagulopathy cannot be corrected. In addition, patients taking anticoagulants such as warfarin (Coumadin), aspirin, and nonsteroidal anti-inflammatory drugs (NSAIDs) are at an increased risk to suffer hemorrhagic complications. These patients should discontinue the above-listed medications for an appropriate interval before SWL.

Hemorrhagic complications are also more likely to occur in those with uncontrolled hypertension (Knapp et al, 1988). Therefore, uncontrolled hypertension is a contraindication to

SWL. Appropriate diagnostic evaluation and management should be instituted before initiating ESWL.

Urinary tract obstruction distal to a calculus is a contraindication to SWL because the passage of resulting fragments cannot be ensured. Such obstruction may be due to a variety of causes including infundibular stenosis, ureteropelvic junction obstruction, and ureteral stricture. Patients with urinary obstruction are best managed either by an endoscopic approach, which allows simultaneous management of both the calculus and the cause of obstruction, or by correction of the obstruction followed by ESWL.

Urine cultures should be obtained before SWL. If urinary tract infection is present, appropriate antibiotic therapy should be instituted. Preferably, clearance of infection should be documented before SWL. It may be impossible, however, to clear some urinary infections before SWL, such as in patients with struvite stones. In these cases, it may be necessary to administer oral antibiotics before and after treatment and intravenous antibiotics at the time of treatment. In addition, urinary tract obstruction may be associated with persistent infections. Decompression of the obstructed system should be carried out. The presence of febrile urinary tract infection is a contraindication to SWL. Urinary tract drainage and antibiotic therapy should be instituted in these patients before proceeding with SWL.

Most centers have avoided SWL of distal ureteral calculi in women of childbearing age because of the uncertain effects of SWL on the ovary and uterus. Although McCullough and colleagues demonstrated the absence of deleterious effects of shock waves on the rat ovary, the applicability of these results to other species is uncertain (McCullough et al, 1989). Vieweg and associates reported a series of 84 women of reproductive age treated with SWL (Vieweg et al, 1992). Six patients subsequently delivered seven normal infants. Three patients suffered miscarriages, but all occurred more than 1 year after ESWL. Although suggestive of the safety of SWL in this population, this study's small size prohibits general conclusions. Because the safety of SWL of distal ureteral stones in this population remains unclear, the authors continue to recommend other therapies to these patients.

CLINICAL USE

Stone Composition

Calculi with different compositions may fragment with differing degrees of success (Table 92–3). Pure cystine stones tend to resist fragmentation by SWL. Therefore, cystine stones are best treated by percutaneous nephrostolithotomy (PNL) (Katz et al, 1990). Calcium oxalate monohydrate calculi also fragment poorly. They tend to fragment

Table 92–3. EASE OF FRAGMENTATION OF VARIOUS URINARY CALCULI

Easy to Fragment	Difficult to Fragment
Uric acid	Calcium oxalate monohydrate
Struvite	Calcium phosphate (apatite)
Calcium oxalate dihydrate	Cystine

into larger pieces than other varieties of stones. In contrast, calcium oxalate dihydrate calculi are much more fragile and form sand-like fragments. Of the remaining common urinary stones, struvite calculi tend to be susceptible to shock waves, as are uric acid calculi, although the radiolucent nature of the latter may pose problems in stone visualization (Newman et al, 1988).

Stone Size

It has become apparent that stone-free rates after SWL decrease as stone size increases. This appears to hold true for stones in all locations, including the calyces, renal pelvis, and the ureter (Chaussy et al, 1982, Drach et al, 1986, Lingeman et al, 1987, Riehle and Naslund, 1987a; Bierkens et al, 1992; Ehreth et al, 1994; Cass, 1995). Similarly, the need for additional treatments, either repeat ESWL or endoscopic stone extraction, appears to increase with increasing stone size. A cut-off point that distinguishes between a stone size appropriate for primary SWL and a size that calls for an alternative therapy is controversial. In the United States, cost efficiency has assumed an important role in this decision-making process, with third-party payers increasingly unwilling to pay for multiple expensive procedures. Currently the authors manage renal calculi that are 2 cm or less in diameter with SWL. Larger renal stones, which are unlikely to clear with SWL, are managed primarily with PNL, with follow-up SWL if needed for the management of residual fragments. Ureteral calculi 1 cm or less may likewise be managed with ESWL, but larger calculi appear to be best managed endoscopically.

Renal Calculi

Calyceal Calculi

The renal calyces are the most common location for asymptomatic or incidentally discovered urinary calculi. Such stones may also be diagnosed during the evaluation of flank pain, microscopic hematuria, and urinary infection. Upper-pole and midpole calyceal stones that are 2 cm or less in diameter have been treated with ESWL with stone-free rates of up to 90% (Chaussy et al, 1982; Lingeman et al, 1986a; Graff et al, 1988). PNL appears to provide superior results for upper-pole and midpole stones greater than 2 cm in diameter (Lingeman et al, 1987).

The management of lower-pole calculi is more controversial. Stone-free rates after ESWL range from 41% to 79%, lower than those reported for upper-pole and midpole stones (Drach et al, 1986; Graff et al, 1988, 1989; McCullough, 1989; McDougall et al, 1989; Netto et al, 1991b; Lingeman et al, 1994). Persistent stone fragments are likely due to the dependent position and poor drainage of the lower pole (Sampaio and Arago, 1992). PNL for lower-pole calculi appears more efficacious, with stone-free rates approaching 100% (McDougall et al, 1989; Netto et al, 1991b; Lingeman et al, 1987, 1994). Inversion therapy, in which a patient is suspended in a head-down position, has been attempted as a means to facilitate lower-pole drainage after ESWL (McCullough et al, 1989; Brownlee et al, 1990). This technique does not appear to provide significant benefit. Although the noninvasive nature of ESWL is attractive to both patient and urologist, the greater efficacy of PNL, especially for larger lower-pole calculi, should be considered before selecting a course of ESWL, which may entail multiple costly treatments with no guarantee of success.

Calculi in Calyceal Diverticula

Calyceal diverticula are congenital anomalies found on less than 0.5% of all intravenous pyelograms (Middleton and Pfister, 1974). They are usually drained by a narrow connection to the collecting system. This may predispose to stone formation and hinder the passage of stone fragments. Approximately 10% of such diverticula contain calculi, with presenting symptoms including hematuria, flank pain, and urinary infection (Wulfsohn, 1980). The use of ESWL for treatment of such calculi has been investigated. Stone-free rates have been quite low ($\leq$20%). Relief of symptoms, however, has been achieved in up to 70%, at least temporarily (Psirhamis and Dretler, 1987; Hendrikx et al, 1992). Other investigators have advocated SWL for carefully selected patients with small calculi and demonstrably patent diverticular necks. Streem and Yost (1992) reported that 50% of such patients were rendered stone-free, whereas 83% were relieved of symptoms, again suggesting that symptom relief is independent of the achievement of a stone-free state. The durability of such symptom relief in the presence of residual stone fragments and the persistence of the diverticulum is doubtful. Percutaneous techniques may be applied to the treatment of stones in diverticula. Simultaneous stone removal and definitive management of the diverticulum may be accomplished with stone-free rates ranging from 71% to 100% (Hulbert et al, 1986; Jones et al, 1991). Again, although the less invasive nature of ESWL is attractive, the superior efficacy of percutaneous techniques must be emphasized.

Renal Pelvic Calculi

Uncomplicated calculi within the renal pelvis that are 2 cm or less in diameter may be managed with SWL. Stone-free rates of 66% to 99% have been reported (Drach et al, 1986; Lingeman et al, 1986b; Bierkens et al, 1992; Grabe et al, 1992; Ehreth et al, 1994; Cass, 1995). Calculi that are greater than 2 cm often require multiple SWL treatments (Guzina et al, 1992) and are more effectively managed with PNL.

Staghorn Calculi

The concept of primary SWL treatment (SWL monotherapy) of staghorn calculi has been extensively evaluated (Pode et al, 1988; Winfield et al, 1988; Constantinides et al, 1989; Gleeson and Griffith, 1989; Schulze et al, 1989; Vandeursen and Baert, 1990; Michaels and Fowler, 1991). Examination of these reports reveals several important findings. First, stone-free rates are disappointingly low, with a median value of 50% (Segura et al, 1994). Residual fragments are associated with persistent urinary infection and stone regrowth. Second, patients frequently required additional procedures, including pretreatment ureteral stent placement to prevent obstruction. Third, repeat SWL or PNL was frequently indicated for treatment failures, and ureteroscopic intervention is often necessary for extraction of obstructing ureteral fragments. PNL has also been evaluated in the treatment of staghorn calculi (Clayman et al, 1983; Winfield et al, 1988; Schulze et al, 1989) and has been found to have superior stone-free rates and less need for additional procedures (Segura et al, 1994). After considering these findings, the American Urological Association Clinical Guidelines Panel on the Management of Staghorn Calculi established that "percutaneous stone removal, followed by ESWL and/or repeat percutaneous procedures as warranted should be used for most standard patients with struvite staghorn calculi.... ESWL may be considered as primary therapy for carefully selected small volume calculi in normal collecting systems" (Segura et al, 1994).

Ureteral Calculi

ESWL and ureteroscopy are currently the principal interventional options in the management of ureteral calculi. Stone location is again the critical factor in selecting optimal therapy for each calculus. In addition, because of the ureter's relatively small size and its role as an active conduit, stone size and composition and the degree of accompanying obstruction must be seriously considered.

Proximal Ureteral Calculi

Ureteral calculi that are located between the ureteropelvic junction and the superior border of the bony pelvis have been treated with ESWL with stone-free rates ranging from 80% to 99% (Drach et al, 1986; Danuser et al, 1993; Ehreth et al, 1994; Mobley et al, 1994; Cass, 1995). Factors contributing to these favorable results include the higher treatment power and number of shocks used and the relative ease of imaging calculi in the proximal ureter.

Initially, it was thought that the efficacy of SWL of proximal ureteral calculi could be enhanced by bypassing the stone with a ureteral stent or by manipulating the stone back into the kidney (Dretler et al, 1986; Lingeman et al, 1986a; Riehle and Naslund, 1987a). More recent studies have found little advantage to these additional procedures (Cass, 1992; Danuser et al, 1993; Cass, 1994a; Kumar et al, 1994; Mobley et al, 1994). The current recommendation for smaller ($\leq$1 cm), nonobstructing ureteral stones is to proceed with in situ ESWL. Stenting and stone manipulation are reserved for larger stones, stones that are difficult to visualize, and stones associated with significant obstruction. In addition, multiple, large, hard (cystine), or impacted stones and stones associated with obstruction are best managed by way of endoscopic approaches.

Midureteral Calculi

Ureteral calculi located between the superior and inferior borders of the sacroiliac joint may present a difficult management problem. SWL must be performed with the patient in the prone position. The pelvic bones interfere with the transmission of shock waves if the patient is maintained in the prone position. With some lithotriptors, the prone position may be difficult to obtain. In addition, some patients, especially those with cardiac or pulmonary disease, may not be able to tolerate this position. Radiographic visualization of midureteral calculi may be difficult because of the underlying pelvic bones, and ultrasound visualization is generally impossible. Ureteroscopic stone fragmentation and extraction may be equally difficult in this portion of the ureter because of its tortuous course over the iliac vessels. Flexible ureteroscopy may be helpful in accessing stones in this region (Bagley, 1990, 1994). Nevertheless, satisfactory results in terms of stone-free (up to 80%) and re-treatment rates (as low as 6%) are possible with SWL if prone positioning can be obtained and stone visualization is achieved (Drach et al, 1986; Tiselius et al, 1989; Ahlawat et al, 1991; Cass, 1994b; Ehreth et al, 1994).

Distal Ureteral Calculi

The optimal management of ureteral calculi located between the inferior border of the sacroiliac joint and the ureterovesical junction remains controversial (Chaussy and Fuchs, 1987b). Convincing arguments in favor of both ureteroscopy and SWL have been advanced.

Proponents of SWL have cited good success rates, decreased operating time, and minimal anesthetic requirements and hospital stays. Opponents of SWL emphasize the frequent difficulty of imaging distal ureteral calculi, the need for prone patient positioning, the periodic need for re-treatment, and the higher cost of SWL. Stone-free rates reported after SWL of distal ureteral stones have ranged from 78% to 97% (Kirkali et al, 1992; Landau et al, 1992; Erturk et al, 1993; Hofbauer et al, 1993; Thomas et al, 1993, Anderson et al, 1994). Stone-free rates may vary depending on the type of lithotriptor used, with lower-power second-generation and third-generation lithotriptors being less effective. The vast majority of these patients were treated on an outpatient basis with intravenous sedation anesthesia. Re-treatment rates have ranged up to 14%, and complication rates were low. Proponents of ureteroscopic management of ureteral calculi cite superior success rates with single treatments and lower costs as strengths of this approach (El-Faqih et al, 1988; Dretler, 1989; Chang et al, 1993). Ureteroscopy, however, has been associated with the need for general anesthesia, hospital admission, and ureteral stent placement more frequently than SWL (Netto et al, 1991a; Anderson et al, 1994), although these studies may not reflect more recent trends toward outpatient ureteroscopy with intravenous sedation anesthesia (Grasso et al, 1995). In addition, the inclusion of "dangler" strings at the distal end of ureteral stents has eliminated the need for an additional cystoscopy for stent removal.

It is apparent that both SWL and ureteroscopy retain roles in the management of distal ureteral calculi. For the urologist who has ready access to SWL facilities, SWL is a reasonable first-line treatment option for patients with single, small (≤1 cm) calculi that are not impacted and that are not composed of calcium oxalate monohydrate or cystine. Patients must be willing to accept a longer time interval to achieve a stone-free state while fragments pass. Patients who desire the quickest route to a stone-free state or who desire the single treatment with the greatest chance for success should be managed with ureteroscopy. Patients living in

Table 92–4. INDICATIONS FOR ENDOSCOPIC MANAGEMENT OF URINARY CALCULI

Renal Calculi	Ureteral Calculi
Stone size >2 cm diameter	Stone size >1 cm diameter
Stones located in lower-pole calyces and calyceal diverticula	Stones associated with distal obstruction (e.g., owing to ureteral stricture, extrinsic compression)
Staghorn calculi	Distal ureteral stones in women of childbearing age
Stones associated with distal obstruction	Multiple stones
Cystine stones	Impacted stones
	Extracorporeal shock-wave lithotripsy failures

areas without ready access to ESWL facilities may also be managed successfully with ureteroscopy. In addition, ureteroscopy is first-line therapy for larger (>10 mm) calculi, impacted calculi, multiple calculi, monohydrate or cystine calculi, and female patients of childbearing age (Table 92–4).

Bladder Calculi

Bladder calculi have been managed successfully with SWL. This approach requires prone positioning. Stones are generally well visualized, especially with ultrasound (Dawson and Whitfield, 1994). Advantages of this technique include the avoidance of urethral instrumentation and general or regional anesthesia, which are associated with cystolitholapaxy. Disadvantages include the cost and the inability to address associated bladder outlet obstruction, which is frequently the cause of bladder calculi, especially in the Western world.

COMPLICATIONS

Steinstrasse

The development of SWL was associated with the simultaneous development of a new condition termed *steinstrasse,* German for "street of stone." Steinstrasse is the result of the accumulation of multiple stone fragments within the ureter. Such accumulations are associated with SWL of larger stone burdens and may be prevented in some cases by pre-SWL stent placement. Patients with steinstrasse may be asymptomatic or may present with any of the symptoms characteristic of ureteral calculi. Management depends on the clinical situation. Asymptomatic patients may be observed initially to allow for spontaneous stone passage. Patients with significant obstruction or infection should be managed with prompt urinary tract decompression by nephrostomy tube placement. Coptcoat (1987) reported that this measure alone permitted passage of all fragments in 72% of cases. Primary ureteral stent placement is discouraged because an inflamed, stone-packed ureter may be more susceptible to perforation. Fragments that do not pass, especially if a large leading fragment is present, may be managed with ureteroscopic fragmentation and retrieval or alternatively with SWL.

Bleeding Complications

A spectrum of bleeding complications may occur after SWL. Hematuria occurs in most patients and is generally self-limited, lasting less than 24 hours, and is of little clinical consequence. Perinephric and renal hematomas have been reported in 0.2% to 0.66% of patients undergoing SWL (Drach et al, 1986; Knapp et al, 1988; Ehreth et al, 1994). These hematomas are usually associated with increasing pain after treatment but also may be associated with abdominal pain, ileus, hypotension, and decreased hematocrit. When such symptoms are present, an imaging study should be performed to evaluate for the presence of significant bleeding. Most hematomas may be managed conservatively and do not require transfusion. Cases requiring angiography, embolization, and even nephrectomy, however, have been reported (Donohue et al, 1989). Significant hemorrhagic complications have occurred after treatment of patients taking anticoagulant medications such as warfarin (Coumadin) and aspirin and in patients with abnormal clotting parameters (Pliskin et al, 1989; Rius and Saltzman, 1990).

Gastrointestinal Side Effects

A variety of gastrointestinal side effects have been reported following SWL, including pancreatitis, elevations of hepatic enzymes, incidental fragmentation of gallbladder calculi with resulting biliary colic, and mucosal erosions and submucosal hematomas of the colon (Drach et al, 1986; Lingeman et al, 1986a; Karawi et al, 1987; Michaels and Fowler, 1989). These complications are infrequent and are generally self-limited.

Mortality

The American Urological Association (AUA) Ad Hoc Lithotripsy Committee (McCullough, 1987) reported that SWL was associated with a mortality rate of 0.02% in a series of more than 62,000 patients. That many of these deaths occurred weeks after treatment and that some of the included deaths were due to unrelated causes, such as suicide and previously unrecognized cancer, underscores the relative safety of SWL.

SHOCK-WAVE LITHOTRIPSY AND HYPERTENSION

The existence of a cause-and-effect relationship between SWL and hypertension has been a hotly debated topic for more than 10 years. SWL represents a controlled form of blunt renal trauma, and renal trauma has been associated with the development of hypertension (Spark and Berg, 1976; Jakse et al, 1984). Arguments for and against the relationship between SWL and hypertension are rendered difficult because of the prevalence of hypertension in the general population and among patients with urolithiasis.

A variety of animal models have been equivocal in defining the effects of shock waves on blood pressure (Gunasek-

aran et al, 1990; Karlsen et al, 1990; Neal et al, 1991; Weber et al, 1995). This may be due to differences in kidney size and susceptibility to shock waves, the number and strength of shock waves administered, and the thickness of intervening tissues among species.

Clinical studies examining the relationship between SWL and hypertension have also been inconsistent. Early studies noted up to an 8.2% rate of new-onset hypertension among SWL patients (Lingeman and Kulb, 1987). Similar results have been reported in other series (Montgomery et al, 1989; Yokoyama et al, 1992; Claro et al, 1993). Still other studies have failed to demonstrate such an association (Puppo et al, 1989). The significance of each of these studies, however, has been limited by the absence of matched control groups of stone patients managed with alternative therapies, by the absence of standardized blood pressure measurement, and by the failure to exclude patients with underlying renal disease and pre-existing hypertension. The National Electrical Manufacturers Association Kidney Stone Blood Pressure Study Group initiated a prospective, controlled study to evaluate the effects of SWL on patients with normal blood pressure and renal function. These effects were compared to a matched control group of stone patients undergoing alternative treatments. At 2-year follow-up, there was no difference in average renal function or blood pressure between groups. In addition, there was no difference in the rate of new-onset hypertension among groups (Vaughan et al, 1996).

PATIENT PREPARATION FOR SHOCK-WAVE LITHOTRIPSY

In preparation for ESWL, patients routinely undergo radiologic evaluation in the form of intravenous urography, ultrasonography, or computed tomography scan to delineate the size and position of calculi, to define renal and collecting system anatomy and function, and to evaluate the presence of urinary tract obstruction (Table 92–5). In addition, patients undergo preoperative complete blood count; prothrombin and partial thromboplastin times; and serum electrolyte, blood urea nitrogen, and creatinine determinations. Urinalysis and culture are obtained. If infection is present, antibiot-

Table 92–5. PATIENT PREPARATION FOR
SHOCK-WAVE LITHOTRIPSY

History and physical examination
Medication history
   Patients must stop anticoagulants and NSAIDs at appropriate
     intervals before treatment
Urine culture
   Patients with acute infection should be treated with appropriate
     antibiotic therapy before treatment
Blood tests
   Complete blood count including platelets
   Serum blood urea nitrogen, creatinine, and electrolytes
   Prothrombin time and partial thromboplastin time
IVP/CT scan/retrograde pyelogram
   Determine size and location of stone and presence of urinary tract
     obstruction
Pre-SWL ureteral stent placement
   For patients with large stone burdens or difficult-to-visualize stones

NSAIDs, Nonsteroidal anti-inflammatory drugs; IVP, intravenous pyelogram; CT, computed tomography; SWL, shock-wave lithotripsy.

ics are administered. Repeat urine culture is obtained after antibiotic therapy is complete. Because shock wave delivery is controlled by the patient's electrocardiogram (ECG), a preoperative ECG should be obtained to exclude the presence of abnormalities of cardiac rate or rhythm. A chest x-ray may also be indicated based on the patient's age and medical condition. Patients are instructed to discontinue anticoagulants, such as warfarin (Coumadin), aspirin, and NSAIDs, at appropriate intervals before treatment and are instructed to take nothing by mouth after midnight the night before the procedure.

On the day of the procedure, patients undergo a plain abdominal radiograph to confirm stone position. Routine intravenous antibiotics need not be administered in the absence of documented infection or infection-related stone. Anesthetic requirements for ESWL depend on the lithotriptor being used, but even patients treated with the Dornier HM-3 may be managed with intravenous sedatives and analgesics. In addition, piezoelectric lithotriptors may offer treatment with minimal or no anesthesia.

TREATMENT PRINCIPLES

To ensure optimal treatment outcomes, each urologist must master patient positioning, imaging, and shock wave administration for the particular lithotriptor in use. Although there are differences in how these functions are accomplished by various lithotriptors, certain uniform principles exist for all devices.

Patient Positioning

Two important goals must be kept in mind during patient positioning. The first is placement of the patient on the lithotriptor so that the stone can be imaged and placed within the shock wave focal area. The second goal is the assurance of patient safety during treatment.

The patient is positioned on the lithotriptor so that the targeted stone can be imaged. Factors that may make stone visualization difficult include obesity, skeletal abnormalities, radiolucent stones, osseous structures, bowel gas, stool, and the presence of ectopic or horseshoe kidneys. If it is anticipated that a particular stone will be difficult to visualize or place in the F_2 focus, a simulation may be performed. Renal and proximal ureteral stones may be treated with the patient in the supine position, whereas midureteral and distal ureteral stones require prone positioning to prevent the obstruction of shock waves by the pelvic bones.

Once a stone has been localized and treatment has begun, maintenance of position should be confirmed by imaging periodically. The authors confirm positioning and monitor the progress of fragmentation by imaging at intervals of approximately 300 to 500 shocks depending on patient cooperation and movement.

The urologist must ensure patient safety during positioning because patients are frequently under anesthesia or heavily sedated and are incapable of protecting themselves. Weight-bearing surfaces such as heels, knees, and elbows should be padded. The head and extremities must be kept clear of moving machinery to prevent inadvertent injury.

Prone positioning may be dangerous for patients with cardiac or pulmonary disease or spinal problems.

Imaging

Lithotriptors may use fluoroscopy, ultrasonography, or hard copy x-rays for imaging. Fluoroscopy and hard copy radiography are imaging modalities familiar to most urologists. They provide adequate imaging for radiopaque calculi and allow for visualization of radiolucent calculi if radiographic contrast material is administered. Each urologist must be familiar with the imaging system employed on the lithotriptor to be used. It is important to understand the orientation of the fluoroscopy images generated by a given system, whether craniocaudad images or oblique images. This avoids excessive fluoroscopy use and patient repositioning to find the stone. It is similarly important that the urologist understand how to adjust the penetration power and exposure time of the unit to optimize imaging for each patient. Finally, during a urologist's initial use of a lithotriptor, it may be necessary to image continuously during stone localization, but with experience the amount of movement obtained when pressing a directional button may be anticipated without continuous monitoring.

Because of the risks of exposure of the patient and staff to ionizing radiation, the following precautions should be noted. Fluoroscopy and hard copy radiography should be used judiciously and efficiently. The lithotripsy console and anesthesia station should be protected by leaded glass shields, and personnel leaving these protected areas should wear leaded body and thyroid shields.

Ultrasonography may be used for imaging with some lithotriptors. Real-time ultrasonography remains an acquired skill that appears to have a longer learning curve. There are several advantages to ultrasonography, including the ability to visualize radiolucent stones and the avoidance of exposure to ionizing radiation. Moreover, because there is no radiation exposure, ultrasound imaging can be activated throughout the case, which may allow for more effective shock wave targeting and monitoring of stone fragmentation.

Shock Wave Administration

Familiarity with the control console of the lithotriptor to be used is important in effective shock wave administration. Monitors that display the kilovoltage in use, the number of shocks administered, and the degree of electrode consumption should be consulted frequently throughout the case. The maximum allowable kilovoltage and the number of shocks vary depending on the lithotriptor in use and on the location of the stone. Generally, ureteral stones may be treated at a higher kilovoltage and for a greater number of shocks than renal stones. Regardless of the lithotriptor or stone location, it is helpful to begin treatment at low power to minimize the "startle" response from the patient when the first shocks are administered. This may prevent movement of the stone away from the shock wave focal area. The authors follow a similar procedure when resuming treatment after pausing for imaging and have found it helpful in maintaining patient comfort and immobility.

POST–SHOCK-WAVE LITHOTRIPSY PATIENT CARE

Nearly all SWL is performed on an outpatient basis. After treatment, patients are encouraged to maintain an adequate oral fluid intake and to strain their urine for fragments. Oral narcotics are prescribed as needed for pain relief. Pain that is increasing in severity or that is out of proportion to that normally encountered after SWL mandates careful evaluation: Temperature and vital signs should be closely monitored and a complete blood count obtained. If urinary obstruction or renal hemorrhage is suspected, a renal imaging study is performed. Renal ultrasonography may provide the most rapid examination for these complications. If complications are found to be present, corrective measures should be instituted promptly.

Patients generally undergo a plain abdominal radiograph before discharge home to assess the extent of stone fragmentation (Riehle and Naslund, 1987b). An additional film should be obtained 1 to 2 weeks after treatment to assess the size and location of any residual fragments. In patients with radiolucent stones, ultrasonography or noncontrast CT may be necessary to exclude the presence of residual fragments. If stone-free, the patient should be followed up at 3 months postprocedure for repeat plain film and metabolic evaluation if indicated. If not stone-free, plain films should be assessed for the degree of fragmentation after ESWL, and, depending on the location of such fragments, intravenous pyelogram or renal ultrasound should be obtained to evaluate for the presence of obstruction. Patients should then be reassessed at approximately 2-week intervals. If residual fragments are large and unlikely to pass spontaneously or if they do not pass over a reasonable interval, additional interventions may be indicated.

TREATMENT OF SPECIAL CASES

Children

The use of SWL in the pediatric population has become relatively routine (Kroovand et al, 1987; Newman et al, 1986, 1988; Nijman et al, 1989; Abara et al, 1990). Shielding of the lung fields with lead or styrofoam has been recommended (Chaussy et al, 1982). Newer lithotriptors with smaller focal volumes and less powerful shock waves, however, may decrease the risk of pulmonary injury and render shielding unnecessary, especially in larger children (Rassweiler et al, 1992). Anesthetic requirements may vary as well, depending on the type of lithotriptor in use as well as the ability of the child to cooperate. Abara and colleagues stressed the importance of ensuring adequate shock wave coupling, which may be difficult given a child's bony body habitus (Abara et al, 1990). They also note that patient positioning may be facilitated by newer, water bath–less lithotriptors, which in contrast to older models do not require modifications of the patient gantry for pediatric use. Tiselius and co-workers have cautioned against treating stones overlying the sacroiliac joint because this may place the epiphyseal plates in the blast path, with skeletal growth disturbances as a possible result (Tiselius et al, 1989).

Anomalous Kidneys

Solitary, pelvic, and horseshoe kidneys may be safely treated with SWL. Previously described principles regarding stone location, size, and composition are equally applicable to these cases. SWL of calculi in solitary kidneys results in success rates comparable to those found in patients with two kidneys. In addition, complication rates do not differ (Cohen and Schmidt, 1990; Zanetti et al, 1992; Chandhoke et al, 1992). Regardless of the size of the stone burden, ureteral stent placement before SWL is recommended in these patients to prevent obstruction of the solitary renal unit by fragments.

Stones located in pelvic kidneys may be treated with SWL (Jenkins and Gillenwater, 1988; Bush and Brannen, 1987; Baltaci et al, 1994). Prone positioning may be required for effective treatment. In addition, stone localization may be challenging because of the underlying bony pelvis.

Stone localization and patient positioning may be similarly difficult in the case of stones located in horseshoe kidneys. The characteristic medial displacement of the calyces and pelvis may make stone visualization difficult because of interference from the spine and bony pelvis. Prone positioning may be necessary for horseshoe kidneys that are low in the abdomen. In addition, the characteristic high insertion of the ureter into the renal pelvis may hinder fragment passage. Nevertheless, stone-free rates of up to 79% have been reported (Jenkins and Gillenwater, 1988; Smith et al, 1989; Locke et al, 1990; Lampel et al, 1991; Vera-Denoso et al, 1991).

Abdominal Aortic and Renal Artery Aneurysms

Calcified abdominal aortic and renal artery aneurysms have been thought to represent contraindications to SWL. Research has suggested, however, that these conditions are not absolute contraindications to ESWL. Winfield and colleagues reported that shock waves administered to rabbit abdominal aorta resulted in no significant structural damage (Winfield et al, 1990). Vasavada and associates administered shock waves to calcified aneurysmal tissue placed at F_2 and reported no pathologic damage to this tissue (Vasavada et al, 1994). Carey and Streem (1992) have safely treated a small series of aneurysm patients with no ill effects, including rupture or distal thrombosis. All patients in this series had small (<5 cm in diameter), asymptomatic aneurysms that were located at least 5 cm away from the targeted calculus. Multiple associated medical problems often make these patients difficult management problems, and the risks of more invasive therapies must be balanced against those of SWL. Even if SWL provides the best option to carefully selected patients, aggressive intraoperative hemodynamic monitoring and blood pressure control are recommended.

Cardiac Pacemakers

Because of the electrical discharge that is required for shock wave generation, patients with cardiac pacemakers were initially considered unsuitable for SWL. There was fear of pacemaker malfunction with resulting arrhythmia. Multiple studies, however, have subsequently demonstrated that SWL may be performed safely in patients with pacemakers (Abber et al, 1988; Cooper et al, 1988; Theiss et al, 1990). Cooper and associates have suggested a series of guidelines for the safe treatment of patients with pacemakers (Cooper et al, 1988). In addition, Drach and co-workers have recommended that SWL not be performed unless a cardiologist or other physician with experience with pacemakers is available in case of malfunction (Drach et al, 1990).

Obesity

Some centers consider obesity a contraindication to SWL. Obesity may cause difficulty in imaging, in placement of the calculus at the shock wave focal point, and in patient positioning owing to equipment limits on patient weight. SWL is a desirable alternative for obese patients, however, who are at significantly increased risk for complications after more invasive procedures (Strauss and Wise, 1978). Thomas and Cass (1993) used several modifications to treat successfully a series of 81 patients with a mean weight of 326 pounds and renal and upper ureteral stones on a second-generation tubless lithotriptor. Radiologic techniques were modified to obtain adequate imaging, and abdominal compression was used to assist in positioning the stone at the focal point. Also, stones were treated in the extended blast path if they could not be localized to the focal point. These modifications allowed for treatment efficacy comparable to that seen in the general population. SWL should therefore be considered for renal and upper ureteral stones in obese patients, although the type of lithotriptor available as well as pertinent maintenance and warranty agreements must be taken into account before proceeding.

OVERVIEW OF LITHOTRIPTORS

Table 92–6 lists characteristics of lithotriptors in use.

Electrohydraulic Lithotriptors

Dornier HM-3

The Dornier HM-3 (Fig. 92–5) was the first commercially available lithotriptor. Although still in use at many centers, it is no longer manufactured. It does remain the gold standard, however, to which later-generation lithotriptors are compared. The HM-3 uses a water bath in which the patient is immersed for shock wave coupling. Stone localization is accomplished by way of biplanar fluoroscopy. Spark gap, electrohydraulic shock wave generation is used and is characterized by a narrow aperture and a large focal volume. As previously mentioned, these characteristics may be associated with an increased level of discomfort and increased anesthetic requirements but increased treatment efficacy. In addition to the anesthetic requirements, other disadvantages of this device include the cumbersome water bath and the difficulty in treating patients with distal ureteral calculi in the prone position (Jenkins, 1988).

Dornier HM-4

The HM-4 addressed several of the shortcomings of the HM-3. First, the water bath was replaced by a water cushion, which alleviated the need for water drainage and degassification after each treatment. In addition, the shock wave aperture was decreased from 9 × 1.5 cm for the HM-3 to 5 × 1.3 cm for the HM-4 (Eisenberger et al, 1989). This allowed for decreased anesthetic requirements, albeit at the expense of slightly decreased efficacy, especially in terms of re-treatment rates (Tailly and Gillis, 1988; Maggio et al, 1992).

Table 92–6. CHARACTERISTICS OF COMMONLY USED LITHOTRIPTORS

Device	Shock Wave Generation	Focusing	Coupling	Imaging Modality	Date Introduced
Dornier					
HM-3	Electrohydraulic	Hemiellipsoid	Water bath	Fluoroscopy (2 under-couch x-ray tubes)	1980
HM-4	Electrohydraulic	Hemiellipsoid	Water cushion	Fluoroscopy (2 under-couch x-ray tubes)	1980
MPL-9000/9000X	Electrohydraulic	Hemiellipsoid	Water cushion	Ultrasound (9000X adaptable to C-arm fluoroscopy)	1987/1989
MFL-5000	Electrohydraulic	Hemiellipsoid	Water cushion	Fluoroscopy (1 rotating x-ray tube)	1990
Technomed					
Sonolith 3000	Electrohydraulic	Hemiellipsoid	Partial water bath	Lateral/coaxial ultrasound	1985
Medstone STS	Electrohydraulic	Hemiellipsoid	Water cushion	Hard copy radiographs	
Siemens					
Lithostar	Electromagnetic (flat coil)	Acoustic lens	Water cushion	Fluoroscopy (2 over-couch x-ray tubes)	1986
Lithostar Plus	Electromagnetic (flat coil)	Acoustic lens	Water cushion	Coaxial ultrasound	1989
Storz					
Modulith SL-10	Electromagnetic (cylindrical coil)	Acoustic lens	Water cushion	Coaxial ultrasound/adaptable to external C-arm fluoroscopy	1991
Modulith SL-20	Electromagnetic (cylindrical coil)	Acoustic lens	Water cushion	Fluoroscopy	1989
Wolf Piezolith 2500	Piezoelectric	Spherical array	Water cushion	Dual ultrasound/fluoroscopy	1989
EDAP LT-02	Piezoelectric	Spherical array	Water cushion	Coaxial ultrasound/fluoroscopy	1991

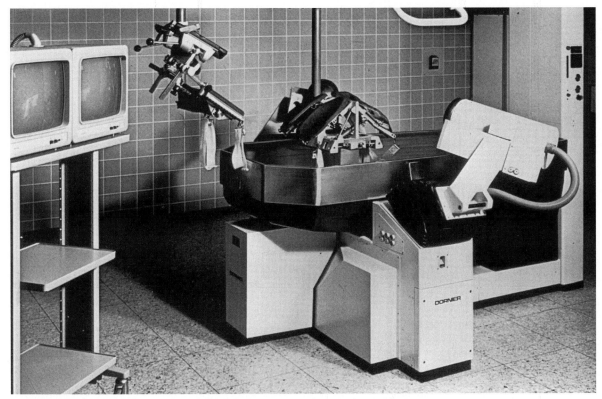

Figure 92–5. The Dornier HM-3, the first commercially available lithotriptor (Dornier Medical Systems, Kennesaw, GA).

Dornier MPL-9000

The Dornier MPL-9000 was initially developed for the treatment of biliary calculi and was subsequently applied to the treatment of urinary calculi. It uses a treatment table that allows easy patient positioning in both the supine and the prone positions. It has a wide shock wave aperture (21 cm) and a small focal area (0.34 cm $\times$ 4.2 cm), allowing for treatments with minimal anesthesia. Because of its intended use for gallstones, ultrasound stone localization is used. This allows for the visualization of radiolucent urinary calculi but makes the treatment of most ureteral calculi difficult, if not impossible (Tailly, 1992). In addition, the learning curve for ultrasound localization of urinary calculi has been described as steep (Keeler et al, 1991). To address these concerns, an accessory fluoroscopy unit has been developed (Rauchenwald et al, 1992). It requires the use of a different treatment electrode, however, which, in turn, increases the shock wave focal length and decreases the pressure at F_2. This may have an adverse effect on efficacy.

Dornier MFL-5000

The Dornier MFL-5000 (Fig. 92–6) is a multifunctional lithotriptor that may be used for (1) diagnostic x-ray procedures, (2) endoscopic and endourologic procedures, and (3) renal and ureteral ESWL (Lingeman and Newman, 1991). It includes a treatment table that is easily adaptable to supine, prone, flank, and lithotomy positioning. A C-arm fluoroscopy unit provides anteroposterior and craniocaudad imaging for SWL stone localization. An automated positioning system then places the stone at F_2. An electrohydraulic shock wave

generator is used with a wider aperture and smaller focal volume than the HM-3, again allowing for treatment with intravenous sedation. A water cushion is used for easy shock wave coupling.

Medstone STS

The Medstone Shockwave Therapy System (STS) also uses an electrohydraulic shock wave generator. Imaging is accomplished by way of a dual system of ultrasound and high-resolution x-rays. High-resolution anteroposterior and oblique hard copy radiographs are digitized, and a computer system positions the stone at F_2. Stone fragmentation may be monitored by ultrasound or by a supplemental fluoroscopy unit. This device is also adaptable to the performance of endoscopic procedures (Hammond et al, 1991).

Technomed Sonolith 3000

The Sonolith 3000 uses a unique electrohydraulic shock wave generator. Rather than the traditional spark plug, this device uses a pair of positive and negative electrodes that are continuously maintained in proper position relative to each other and to a hemiellipsoid reflector by a computer-controlled system. Its designers believed that this is a preferable design because it maintains even shock wave pressures and consistent focusing better than the spark gap design, which has been demonstrated to produce shock waves that vary in intensity by up to 50% (Hunter et al, 1980). Surges in shock wave intensity may increase the perception of pain. In addition, the Sonolith 3000 makes use of a wide shock wave aperture (22 cm) to decrease pain further during treat-

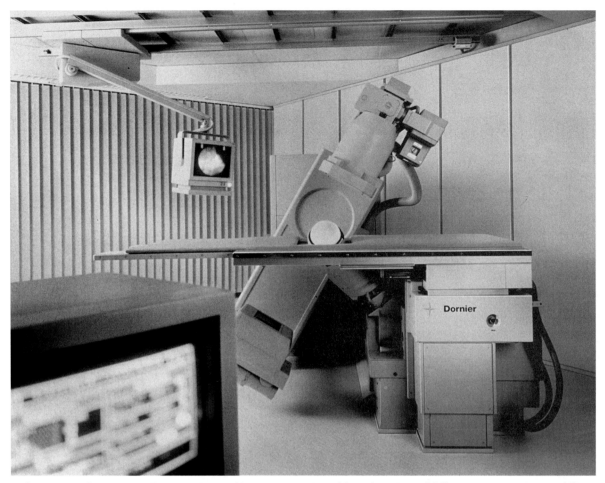

Figure 92–6. The Dornier MFL-5000. Note multipurpose operating table and craniocaudal fluoroscopic imaging capability.

ment. The Sonolith 3000 is further distinguished by the use of a small water pool (10 gallons) rather than an enclosed water cushion for shock wave coupling. Stone localization is by way of ultrasound. Fragmentation may be monitored by ultrasound or by portable x-ray (Tomera and Hellerstein, 1991).

Northgate SD-3

The Northgate SD-3 is a bathless electrohydraulic lithotriptor that is distinguished by its portability; its ability to use standard 110-volt, 15-amp electrical outlets; and its relative inexpense (Swanson et al, 1991). Stone localization is by way of ultrasound, although radiographic systems are under development.

B and L Technologies DP-1

The DP-1 is also a portable, bathless, and relatively inexpensive lithotriptor. It is compact and is roughly the size of a portable x-ray unit. Ultrasound stone localization is used, and minimal anesthesia is required (Begun, 1991).

Direx Tripter X-1

The Direx Tripter X-1 is also a portable, bathless device that is the least expensive of all lithotriptors because an

imaging system is not included. Users provide their own C-arm fluoroscopy unit. The C-arm and lithotriptor are attached to the treatment table so that the C-arm rotates around F_2 (Saltzman, 1991). This unit allows for centers to obtain lithotriptor technology inexpensively and to maximize the use of radiography equipment that is usually already in place.

Electromagnetic Lithotriptors

Siemens Lithostar and Lithostar Plus

The Siemens Lithostar was the first electromagnetic lithotriptor. It is a widely used device; it uses a flat electromagnetic coil and thin metallic membrane for shock wave generation and a water cushion for coupling. Stone localization is by way of biplanar fluoroscopy (anteroposterior and craniocaudad) or ultrasound (in the Lithostar Plus). Unique features of the Lithostar lithotriptors include (1) the presence of right-sided and left-sided shock wave generators, which allow for bilateral treatments without repositioning; (2) the inclusion of the lithotriptor in a multipurpose urology table; and (3) the durability of the shock wave generators, which have a life span of 600,000 to 1 million shocks before replacement is necessary. Although electromagnetic shock wave generator replacement is not as simple as spark plug replacement, generator failure during treatment may be addressed by flipping the patient to the prone position and continuing treatment with the contralateral generator (Psirhamis and Jewett, 1991).

Storz Modulith SL-10 and SL-20

The Modulith is an electromagnetic lithotriptor that uses a cylindrical coil and membrane rather than the flat coil and membrane found in the Lithostar. Only ultrasound imaging was available with the Modulith SL-10, but fixed x-ray with fluoroscopy has been included in the SL-20 (Klein, 1991).

Piezoelectric Lithotriptors

EDAP LT-01 and LT-02

The EDAP LT-01 was the first piezoelectric lithotriptor. This device is a bathless design that uses ultrasound for stone localization. The distinguishing characteristic of these and other piezoelectric lithotriptors is that treatment may be carried out without anesthesia in some patients (Miller, 1991). This is because of the wide aperture and small focal area that is characteristic of such lithotriptors.

Richard Wolf Piezolith 2300 and 2500

The Piezolith lithotriptors have been most frequently associated with true anesthesia-free treatment (Preminger, 1991). This comes at the expense of lower efficacy, however, especially as measured by re-treatment rates. Bierkens and co-workers reported a re-treatment rate of more than 30%, which was higher than all other devices examined (Bierkens et al, 1992).

Therasonics Lithotripsy System

The Therasonics Lithotripsy System is distinguished from other piezoelectric devices by its use of a single sheet of piezoceramic material for shock wave generation rather than a series of smaller individual elements. This device also has addressed some of the weaknesses of an ultrasound stone localization system by including an x-ray prelocalization system.

Comparison of Lithotriptors

The comparison of lithotriptors may be quite difficult. A plethora of variables must be considered, ranging from lithotriptor characteristics (methods of shock wave generation, power levels, imaging systems, focal area size) to efficacy (stone-free rates and re-treatment and auxiliary procedure rates) to practical considerations (anesthesia requirements, cost, portability, durability, size, and multifunctionality). Denstedt and colleagues (1990) proposed the efficiency quotient as a means of making more valid comparisons between different lithotriptors. The efficiency quotient is defined as

$$\frac{100\% \times \% \text{ stone-free}}{100\% \text{ first treatment} + \% \text{ re-treatment} + \% \text{ auxiliary procedures}}$$

This may be helpful in comparing the efficacy of different generators (Table 92–7), but it is difficult to attach a value to factors such as cost, portability, and multifunctionality. In addition, with trends toward the treatment of ureteral calculi with SWL, the disadvantage of ultrasound stone localization in a given lithotriptor might offset the benefit of a high efficiency quotient, thereby making a less efficient but fluoroscopy-equipped device preferable. Each stone center must therefore consider carefully its own needs and treatment goals in selecting a lithotriptor.

SUMMARY AND FUTURE PERSPECTIVES

After a period of explosive and revolutionary growth, it now appears that SWL is entering an era of fine-tuning, which, although less dramatic, will be no less important. Clinically the identification of patients who can expect to receive the best results in the fewest number of treatments is an important goal. Initially, any renal stone was "fair game" for SWL, but clinical research thus far has identified staghorn and calyceal diverticular calculi as stones that are more effectively and efficiently treated by other methods. Conversely, initial investigators were slow to treat ureteral calculi with SWL. It is now clear that many of these patients may be managed successfully with SWL. Future clinical research can only serve to make the use of SWL more efficient and cost-effective. In addition, continued efforts to understand better the effects of shock waves on living tissue remain important to continue to develop optimal parameters for safe treatment. Renal injury and hypertension are areas that need to be examined further.

In terms of technology, the search for the ideal shock wave will continue in hopes of developing increasingly efficient, yet anesthesia-free treatment. The examination of shock wave characteristics such as intensity, number, and rate of delivery and how these affect the mechanisms of stone fragmentation and tissue injury is an area that may allow for the development of more effective and safe treatment parameters.

Table 92–7. COMPARISON OF DIFFERENT LITHOTRIPTORS USING THE EFFICIENCY QUOTIENT

Lithotriptor	% Stone-free	% Re-SWL	% Auxiliary Procedures	EQ
For Stones <1 cm				
Dornier HM-3	77	5	12	0.66
EDAP LT-01	72	29	2	0.55
Siemens Lithostar	74	7	16	0.60
Piezolith 2300	86	16	4	0.72
For Stones 1–2 cm				
Dornier HM-3	75	10	11	0.62
EDAP LT-01	64	68	6	0.37
Siemens Lithostar	65	12	12	0.52
Piezolith 2300	69	27	2	0.53

SWL, Shock-wave lithotripsy; EQ, efficiency quotient.

REFERENCES

Abara E, Merguerian PA, McLorie GA, et al: Lithostar extracorporeal shock wave lithotripsy in children. J Urol 1990;144:489.

Abber JD, Langberg J, Muller SC, et al: Cardiovascular pathology and extracorporeal shock wave lithotripsy. J Urol 1988;140:408.

Abrahams C, Lipson S, Ross L: Pathologic changes in the kidneys and other organs of dogs undergoing extracorporeal shock wave lithotripsy with a tubless lithotripter. J Urol 1988;140:391.

Ahlawat RK, Bhandari M, Kumar A, et al: Treatment of ureteral calculi with extracorporeal shock wave lithotripsy using the Lithostar device. J Urol 1991;146:737.

Anderson KR, Keetch DW, Albala DM, et al: Optimal therapy for the distal ureteral stone: Extracorporeal shock wave lithotripsy versus ureteroscopy. J Urol 1994;152:62.

Assimos DG, Boyce WH, Farr EG, et al: Selective elevation of urinary enzyme levels after extracorporeal shock wave lithotripsy. J Urol 1989;142:687.

Bagley DH: Removal of upper tract urinary calculi with flexible ureteropyeloscopy. Urology 1990;35:412.

Bagley DH: Ureteroscopic stone retrieval: Rigid versus flexible endoscopes. Semin Urol 1994;12:32.

Baltaci S, Sarica K, Ozdiler E, et al: Extracorporeal shockwave lithotripsy in anomalous kidneys. J Endourol 1994;8:179.

Begun FP: B&L Technologies DP-1 lithotripter: The third generation. Semin Urol 1991;9:217.

Bierkens AF, Hendrikx AJM, de Kort VJW, et al: Efficacy of second generation lithotriptors: A multicenter comparative study of 2,206 extracorporeal shock wave lithotripsy treatments with the Siemens Lithostar, Dornier HM4, Wolf Piezolith 2300, Direx Tripter X-1, and Breakstone lithotriptors. J Urol 1992;148:1052.

Brendel W: Effect of shock waves on canine kidney. In Gravenstein JS, Peter K, eds: Extracorporeal Shock Wave of Renal Stone Disease: Technical and Clinical Aspects. Stoneham, MA, Butterworths, 1986, p 141.

Brownlee N, Foster M, Griffith DP, et al: Controlled inversion therapy: An adjunct to the elimination of gravity dependent fragments following extracorporeal shock wave lithotripsy. J Urol 1990;143:1096.

Bush WH, Brannen GE: Extracorporeal shock wave lithotripsy (ESWL) of pelvic kidney calculus: Use of C-arm fluoroscopy for correct patient positioning. Urology 1987;29:357.

Bush WH, Jones D, Gibbons RP: Radiation dose to patient and personnel during extracorporeal shock wave lithotripsy. J Urol 1987;138:716.

Carey SW, Streem SB: Extracorporeal shock wave lithotripsy for patients with calcified ipsilateral renal arterial or abdominal aortic aneurysms. J Urol 1992;148:18.

Cass AS: Do upper ureteral stones need to be manipulated (push back) into the kidneys before extracorporeal shock wave lithotripsy? J Urol 1992;147:349.

Cass AS: Nonstent or noncatheter extracorporeal shock wave lithotripsy for ureteral stones. Urology 1994a;43:178.

Cass AS: Extracorporeal shock wave lithotripsy for stones in the middle third of ureter (overlying pelvic bone). Urology 1994b;43:182.

Cass AS: Comparison of first generation (Dornier HM3) and second generation (Medstone STS) lithotriptors: Treatment results with 13,864 renal and ureteral calculi. J Urol 1995;153:588.

Chandhoke PS, Albala DM, Claymenn RV: Long-term comparison of renal function in patients with solitary kidneys and/or moderate renal insufficiency undergoing extracorporeal shock wave lithotripsy or percutaneous hephrolithotomy. J Urol 1992;147:1226.

Chang SC, Ho CM, Kuo HC: Ureteroscopic treatment of lower ureteral calculi in the era of extracorporeal shock wave lithotripsy: From a developing country point of view. J Urol 1993;150:1395.

Chaussy C, Schmeidt E, Jochman D, et al: First clinical experience with extracorporeally induced destruction of kidney stones by shock waves. J Urol 1982;131:417.

Chaussy CG, Fuchs GJ: Extracorporeal shock wave lithotripsy. Monogr Urol 1987a;4:80.

Chaussy CG, Fuchs GJ: Extracorporeal shock wave lithotripsy of distal ureteral calculi: Is it worthwhile? J Endourol 1987b;1:1–8.

Chaussy CG, Schmiedt E, Jochman D, et al: Extracorporeal shock wave lithotripsy: New aspects in the treatment of kidney stone disease. In Chaussy C, ed: Extracorporeal Shock Wave Lithotripsy. Munich, Karger Verlag, 1982, pp 22–35.

Chuong CJ, Zhong P, Preminger GM: A comparison of stone damage caused by different modes of shock wave generation. J Urol 1992;148:200.

Claro A, Lima ML, Ferreira U, et al: Blood pressure changes after extracorporeal shock wave lithotripsy in normotensive patients. J Urol 1993;150:1765.

Clayman RV, Surya V, Miller RP, et al: Percutaneous nephrolithotomy: An approach to branched and staghorn renal calculi. JAMA 1983;250:73.

Cohen ES, Schmidt JD: Extracorporeal shock wave lithotripsy for stones in solitary kidney. Urology 1990;36:52.

Constantinides C, Recker F, Jaeger P, et al: Extracorporeal shock wave lithotripsy as monotherapy of staghorn calculi. J Urol 1989;142:1415.

Cooper D, Wilkoff B, Masterson M, et al: Effects of extracorporeal shock wave lithotripsy on cardiac pacemakers and its safety in patients with implanted cardiac pacemakers. PACE 1988;11:1607.

Coptcoat MJ, Webb DR, Kellet MJ, et al: The steinstrasse: A legacy of extracorporeal shock wave lithotripsy? Eur Urol 1988;14(2):93–95.

Crum LA: Cavitation microjets as a contributory mechanism for renal calculi disintegration in ESWL. J Urol 1988;140:1587.

Danuser H, Ackerman DK, Marth DC, et al: Extracorporeal shock wave lithotripsy in situ or after push up for upper ureteral calculi: A prospective randomized trial. J Urol 1993;150:824.

Dawson C, Whitfield HN: The long-term results of treatment of urinary stones. Br J Urol 1994;74:397.

Delius M: Effect of extracorporeal shock waves on the kidney. J Urol 1988;140:390.

Delius M, Eizenhoefer H, Denk R, et al: Biological effects of shock waves. Proceedings IEEE Symposium on Sonics and Ultrasonics, Denver, 1987.

Delius M, Jordan M, Eizenhoefer H, et al: Biological effects of shock waves in dogs—administration rate dependence. Ultrasound Med Biol 1988;14:689.

Denstedt JD, Clayman RV, Preminger GM: Efficiency quotient as a means of comparing lithotripters. J Endourol 1990;4(Suppl):100.

Donohue AL, Linke CA, Rowe JM: Renal loss following extracorporeal shock wave lithotripsy. J Urol 1989;142:809.

Donovan JM, Weber C, Farjardo LL, et al: The effects of ESWL on the rabbit kidney and microvasculature. J Urol 1989;141:227A.

Drach GW, Dretler S, Fair W, et al: Report of the United States Cooperative Study of Extracorporeal Shock Wave Lithotripsy. J Urol 1986;135:1127.

Drach GW, Weber C, Donovan JM: Treatment of pacemaker patients with extracorporeal shock wave lithotripsy: Experience from 2 continents. J Urol 1990;143:895.

Dretler SP: In situ ESWL v ureteroscopy: The case for ureteroscopy. J Endourol 1989;3:301.

Dretler SP, Keating MA, Riley J: An algorithm for the management of ureteral calculi. J Urol 1986;136:1190.

Ehreth JT, Drach GW, Arnett ML, et al: Extracorporeal shock wave lithotripsy: Multicenter study of kidney and upper ureter versus middle and lower ureter treatments. J Urol 1994;152:1379.

Eisenberger F, Rassweiler J, Bub P: Second generation lithotripters in urology: In vitro efficacy, pain, and handling in a comparative study. AUA Update Series, Vol VIII, Lesson 35, 1989.

El-Faqih SR, Husain I, Ekman PE, et al: Primary choice of intervention for distal ureteric stone: Ureteroscopy or ESWL? Br J Urol 1988;62:13.

Erturk E, Herrman E, Cockett ATK, et al: Extracorporeal shock wave lithotripsy for distal ureteral stones. J Urol 1993;149:1425.

Forssmann B, Hepp W, Chaussy CG, et al: Eine Methode Zeer Behruhrungfreien zertrummerung von nieren-steinen durch stosswellen. Biomed Tech (Berlin) 1977;22:164.

Gilbert BR, Riehle RA Jr, Vaughan ED Jr: Extracorporeal shock wave lithotripsy and its effect on renal function. J Urol 1988;139:482.

Gleeson MJ, Griffith DP: Extracorporeal shock wave lithotripsy monotherapy for large renal calculi. Br J Urol 1989;64:329.

Grabe T, Kinn AC, Ahlgren G, et al: Treatment of renal and ureteric stones with the Lithocut C-3000 lithotriptor. J Endourol 1992;6:403–406.

Graff J, Benkert S, Pastor J, et al: Experience with a new multifunctional lithotriptor, the Dornier MFL-5000: Results of 415 treatments. J Endourol 1989;3:315.

Graff J, Schmidt A, Pastor J, et al: New generator for low pressure lithotripsy with the Dornier HM3: Preliminary experience of 2 centers. J Urol 1988;139:904.

Grasso M, Beaghler M, Loisides P: The case for primary endoscopic management of upper urinary tract calculi: II. Cost and outcome assessment of 112 primary ureteral calculi. Urology 1995;45:372.

Gunasekaran S, Donovan JM, Chvapil M, et al: Effects of extracorporeal shock wave lithotripsy on the structure and function of the rabbit kidney. J Urol 1990;141:1250.

Guzina T, Babic M, Alagic MD, et al: Extracorporeal shock wave lithotripsy with Dornier MPL-9000 in 2005 patients. J Endourol 1992;6:393–402.

Hammond GW Jr, Bass RB Jr, Cass AS: The Medstone STS: A technical review. Semin Urol 1991;9:239.

Hendrikx AJM, Bierkens AF, Bos R, et al: Treatment of stones in calyceal diverticula: Extracorporeal shock wave lithotripsy vs. percutaneous neph-rolithalopaxy. Br J Urol 1992;70:478.

Hofbauer J, Tuerk C, Hasun R, et al: ESWL in situ or ureteroscopy for ureteric stones? World J Urol 1993;11:54–58.

Hulbert JC, Reddy PK, Hunter DW, et al: Percutaneous techniques for the management of calyceal diverticula containing calculi. J Urol 1986;135:225.

Hunter P, Finlayson B, Hirko R, et al: Measurement of shock wave pressures used for lithotripsy. J Urol 1980;136:733.

Jaegar P, Constantinides C: Canine kidneys: Changes in blood and urine chemistry after exposure to extracorporeal shock waves. In Lingeman JE, Newman DM, eds: Shock Wave Lithotripsy 2. New York, Plenum Press, 1989, p 7.

Jakse G, Putz A, Gassner I, et al: Early surgery in the management of pediatric blunt renal trauma. J Urol 1984;131:920.

Jenkins AD: Dornier extracorporeal shock wave lithotripsy for ureteral stones. Urol Clin North Am 1988;15:377.

Jenkins AD, Gillenwater JY: Extracorporeal shock wave lithotripsy in the prone position: Treatment of stones in the distal ureter and the anomalous kidney. J Urol 1988;135:679.

Jones JA, Lingeman JE, Steidle CP: The roles of extracorporeal shock wave lithotripsy and percutaneous nephrostolithomy in the management of pyelocaliceal diverticula. J Urol 1991;146:724.

Karawi MA, Mohamed AR, El-Etaibi KE: Extracorporeal shock wave lithotripsy (ESWL) induced erosions in upper gastrointestinal tract. Urol-ogy 1987;30:224.

Karlsen SJ, Smevik B, Stenstroem J, et al: Acute physiological changes in canine kidneys following exposure to extracorporeal shock waves. J Urol 1990;143:1280.

Katz G, Lencorsky A, Pide D, et al: Place of extracorporeal shock wave lithotripsy (ESWL) in the management of cystine calculi. Urology 1990;36:124.

Kaude J, Williams C, Millner M, et al: Renal morphology and physiology immediately after extracorporeal shock wave lithotripsy. AJR 1985; 145:305.

Keeler LL, McNamara TC, Dorey FO, et al: The MPL-9000. Semin Urol 1991;9:230.

Kirkali Z, Mungan U, Sade M: Extracorporeal electromagnetic shock wave lithotripsy of ureteral stones. J Endourol 1992;6:411.

Klein FA: Storz Modulith SL-200: The new optimal acoustic source for extracorporeal lithotripsy. Semin Urol 1991;9:269.

Koch MO: Therasonics lithotripsy system. Semin Urol 1991;9:275.

Knapp PM, Kulb TB, Lingeman JE, et al: Extracorporeal shock wave lithotripsy-induced perirenal hematomas. J Urol 1988;139:700.

Kroovand RL, Harrison LH, McCullough DL: Extracorporeal shock wave lithotripsy in children. J Urol 1987;138(part 2):1106.

Kumar A, Kumar RV, Mishra VK, et al: Should upper ureteral calculi be manipulated before extracorporeal shock wave lithotripsy? A prospective controlled trial. J Urol 1994;152:320.

Kuwahara M, Kambe K, Kurosu S, et al: Extracorporeal stone disintegration using chemical microexplosive pellets as an energy source of underwater shock waves. J Urol 1986;135:814.

Kuwahara M, Orikesa S: Clinical application of extracorporeal shock wave lithotripsy using microexplosives. J Urol 1987b;137:837.

Kuwahara M, Takayama K: Extracorporeal microexplosive lithotripter. In Kandel LB, Harrison LH, McCullough DL, eds: State of the Art Extracor-poreal Shock Wave Lithotripsy. Mt. Kisco, NY, Futura Publishing, 1987a.

Lampel A, Hohenfellner M, Schultz-Lampel D, et al: ESWL in horseshoe kidneys. J Endourol 1991;5(suppl):73.

Landau EH, Pode D, Lencovsky Z, et al: Extracorporeal shock wave lithotripsy (ESWL) monotherapy for stones in lower ureter. Urology 1992;40:132.

Lingeman JE, Coury TA, Newman DM, et al: Comparison of results of percutaneous nephrostolithotomy and extracorporeal shock wave litho-tripsy. J Urol 1987;138:485.

Lingeman JE, Kulb TB: Hypertension following extracorporeal shock wave lithotripsy. J Urol 1987;137:142A.

Lingeman JE, Newman DM: Dornier MFL 5000 and Compact lithotriptors. Semin Urol 1991;9:225.

Lingeman JE, Newman DM, Mertz JHO, et al: Extracorporeal shock wave lithotripsy: The Methodist Hospital of Indiana experience. J Urol 1986a;135:1134.

Lingeman JE, Siegel YI, Steele B, et al: Management of lower pole nephrolithiasis: A critical review. J Urol 1994;151:663.

Lingeman JE, Sonda LP, Kahnoski J, et al: Ureteral stone management: Emerging concepts. J Urol 1986b;135:1172.

Lingeman JE, Woods J, Toth PO, et al: The role of lithotripsy and its side effects. J Urol 1989;141:793.

Locke DR, Newman RC, Steinbock GS, et al: Extracorporeal shock wave lithotripsy in horseshoe kidneys. Urology 1990;35:407.

Maggio MI, Nicely ER, Peppas DS, et al: An evaluation of 646 stone patients treated on the Dornier HM4 extracorporeal shock wave lithotrip-tor. J Urol 1992;148:1114.

McCullough DL, chairman: American Urological Association Ad Hoc Lithotripsy Committee Report, Baltimore, 1987.

McCullough DL: Extracorporeal shock wave lithotripsy and residual stone fragments in lower calices. J Urol 1989;141:140.

McCullough DL, Yeaman LD, Bo W, et al: Effects of shock waves on the rat ovary. J Urol 1989;141:666.

McDougall EM, Denstedt JD, Brown RD, et al: Comparison of extracorpo-real shock wave lithotripsy and percutaneous nephrostolithotomy for the treatment of renal calculi in lower pole calices. J Endourol 1989;3:265.

Michaels EK, Fowler JE Jr: Extracorporeal shock wave lithotripsy for struvite calculi: Prospective study with extended followup. J Urol 1991;146:728.

Middleton AW Jr, Pfister RC: Stone-containing pyelocaliceal diverticulum: Embryogenic, anatomic, radiologic, and clinical characteristics. J Urol 1974;111:2.

Miller HC: EDAP LT-01 piezoelectric lithotriptor. Semin Urol 1991;9:279.

Mobley TB, Myers DA, Jenkins JM, et al: Effects of stents on lithotripsy of ureteral calculi: Treatment results with 18,825 calculi using the Lithostar lithotriptor. J Urol 1994;152:53.

Montgomery BSI, Cole RS, Palfrey ELH, et al: Does extracorporeal shock wave lithotripsy cause hypertension? Br J Urol 1989;64:567.

Moran ME, Sandock D, Bottacini MR, et al: Chick embryo model to study effects of high energy shock waves on rapidly proliferating tissues. J Endourol 1990;4:315.

Morris JS, Husmann DA, Wilson WT, et al: Piezoelectric versus spark gap lithotripsy: A comparison of morphologic and functional alterations. J Urol 1989;141:228A.

Neal DE, Kaack MB, Harmon EP, et al: Renin production after experimental extracorporeal shock wave lithotripsy: A primate model. J Urol 1991;146:548.

Netto NR Jr, Claro JF, Ferreira U, et al: Lumbar ureteric stones: Which is the best treatment? Urology 1991a;38:443.

Netto NR Jr, Claro JF, Lemos GC, et al: Renal calculi in lower pole calices: What is the best method of treatment? J Urol 1991b;146:721.

Newman DM, Coury T, Lingeman JE, et al: Extracorporeal shock wave lithotripsy experience in children. J Urol 1986;136:238.

Newman DM, Scott JW, Lingeman JE: Two year followup of patients treated with extracorporeal shock wave lithotripsy. In Lingeman JE, Newman DM, eds: Shock Wave Lithotripsy. New York, Plenum Press, 1988, p 159.

Newman R, Hackett R, Senior D, et al: Pathologic effects of ESWL on canine renal tissue. Urology 1987;29:194.

Newman RC, Riehle RA Jr: Principles of treatment. In Riehle RA Jr, ed: Principles of Extracorporeal Shock Wave Lithotripsy. New York, Churchill Livingstone, 1987, p 82.

Nijman RJM, Ackaert K, Scholtmeijer RJ, et al: Long-term results of extracorporeal shock wave lithotripsy in children. J Urol 1989;142:609.

Pliskin MJ, Wikert GA, Dresner ML: Hemorrhagic complication of extra-corporeal shock wave lithotripsy in an anti-coagulated patient. J Endourol 1989;3:405.

Pode D, Verstandig A, Shapiro A, et al: Treatment of complete staghorn calculi by ESWL monotherapy with special reference to internal stenting. J Urol 1988;140:260.

Pollock HM: Radiation exposure and extracorporeal shock wave lithotripsy. J Urol 1987;138:850.

Preminger G: Sonographic piezolithotripsy: More bang for your buck. J Endourol 1989;3:321.

Preminger GM: Richard Wolf piezoelectric lithotripters: Piezolith 2300 and 2500. Semin Urol 1991;9:288.

Psirhamis KE, Dretler SP: Extracorporeal shock wave lithotripsy of caliceal diverticula calculi. J Urol 1987;138:707.

Psirhamis KE, Jewett MAS: Extracorporeal shock wave lithotripsy with the Siemens Lithostar lithotriptor. Semin Urol 1991;9:260.

Puppo P, Germinale T, Ricciotti G, et al: Hypertension after extracorporeal shock wave lithotripsy: A false alarm. J Endourol 1989;3:401.

Rassweiler J, Kohrmann KU, Alken P: ESWL, including imaging. Curr Opin Urol 1992;2:291.

Rassweiler J, Kohrmann KU, Heine G, et al: Experimental introduction and first clinical experience with a new disciplinary lithotripter. Eur Urol 1990;18:237.

Rauchenwald M, Colombo T, Petritsch PH, et al: In situ extracorporeal shock wave lithotripsy of ureteral calculi with the MPL-9000X lithotriptor. J Urol 1992;148:1097.

Recker F, Rubben H, Bex H, et al: Morphological changes following ESWL in the rat kidney. Urol Res 1989;17:229.

Riehle RA Jr, Naslund EB: Treatment of calculi in the upper ureter with extracorporeal shock wave lithotripsy. Surg Gynecol Obstet 1987a;164:1.

Riehle RA Jr, Naslund EB: Patient management and results after ESL. In Riehle RA Jr, ed: Principles of Extracorporeal Shock Wave Lithotripsy. New York, Churchill Livingstone, 1987b, p 121.

Rius H, Saltzman B: Aspirin induced bilateral renal hemorrhage after extracorporeal shock wave lithotripsy: Implications and conclusions. J Urol 1990;143:791.

Rubin J, Arger P, Pollack H, et al: Kidney changes after extracorporeal shock wave lithotripsy: CT evaluation. Radiology 1987;162:21.

Saltzman B: Second generation shock wave lithotripters. Urol Clin North Am 1988;15:385.

Saltzman B: Direx Tripter X-1. Semin Urol 1991;9:222.

Sampaio FJB, Arago AHM: Inferior pole collecting system anatomy: Its probable role in extracorporeal shock wave lithotripsy. J Urol 1992;147:322.

Schulze H, Hertle L, Kutta A, et al: Critical evaluation of treatment of staghorn calculi by percutaneous nephrolithotomy and extracorporeal shock wave lithotripsy. J Urol 1989;141:822.

Segura JW, Preminger GM, Assimos DG, et al: Nephrolithiasis clinical guidelines panel summary report on the management of staghorn calculi. J Urol 1994;151:1648.

Smith JE, Van Arsdalen KN, Hanno PM, et al: Extracorporeal shock wave lithotripsy treatment of calculi in horseshoe kidneys. J Urol 1989;142:683.

Spark RF, Berg S: Renal trauma and hypertension: The role of renin. Arch Intern Med 1976;136:1097.

Strauss RJ, Wise L: Operative risks of obesity. Surg Gynecol Obstet 1978;146:286.

Streem SB, Yost A: Treatment of caliceal diverticular calculi with extracorporeal shock wave lithotripsy: Patient selection and extended followup. J Urol 1992;148:1043.

Swanson SK, Larson TR, Boyle ET Jr: The Northgate SD-3 dual purpose lithotriptor. Semin Urol 1991;9:247.

Tailly G: Experience with the Dornier HM4 and MPL-9000 lithotriptors in urinary stone management. J Urol 1992;144:622.

Tailly G, Gillis J: Painless extracorporeal shock wave lithotripsy on the HM4: Preliminary results. Acta Urol Belg 1988;56(3):420.

Theiss M, Wirth MP, Frohmuller HGW: Extracorporeal shock wave lithotripsy in patients with cardiac pacemakers. J Urol 1990;143:479.

Thomas R, Cass AS: Extracorporeal shock wave lithotripsy in morbidly obese patients. J Urol 1993;150:30.

Thomas R, Macaluso JN, Vandenberg T, et al: An innovative approach to management of lower third ureteral calculi. J Urol 1993;149:1427.

Tiselius HG, Petterson B, Andersson A: Extracorporeal shock wave lithotripsy of stones in the mid-ureter. J Urol 1989;141:280.

Tomera KM, Hellerstein DK: The Sonolith 3000. Semin Urol 1991;9:253.

Vandeursen H, Baert L: Extracorporeal shock wave lithotripsy for staghorn calculi with the second generation lithotriptors. J Urol 1990;143:252.

Van Swearingen FL, McCullough DL, Dyer R, et al: Radiation exposure to patients during extracorporeal shock wave lithotripsy. J Urol 1987;138:18.

Vasavada SP, Streem SB, Kottke-Marchant K, et al: Pathological effects of extracorporeally generated shock waves on calcified aortic aneurysm tissue. J Urol 1994;152:45.

Vaughan ED Jr, Tobin JN, Alderman MH, et al: Extracorporeal shock wave monotherapy does not cause renal dysfunction or elevated blood pressure. J Urol 1996;155(5) Abs #915.

Vera-Denoso CD, Ruiz E, Broseta F, et al: ESWL in patients with congenital renal anomalies. J Endourol 1991;5(suppl):73.

Vieweg J, Weber HM, Miller K, et al: Female fertility following extracorporeal shock wave lithotripsy of distal ureteral calculi. J Urol 1992;148:1007.

Weber C, Gluck U, Staehler G, et al: Extracorporeal shock wave treatment raises blood pressure in borderline hypertensive rats. J Urol 1995;154:232.

Winfield HN, Clayman RV, Chaussy CG, et al: Monotherapy of staghorn renal calculi: A comparative study between percutaneous nephrostolithotomy and extracorporeal shock wave lithotripsy. J Urol 1988;146:728.

Winfield HN, Loening SA, Heidger PM: Effect of extracorporeal shock waves on rabbit abdominal aorta. J Endourol 1990;4:S56.

Wulfsohn MA: Pyelocaliceal diverticula. J Urol 1980;123:1.

Yokoyama M, Shoji F, Yanagizawa R, et al: Blood pressure changes following extracorporeal shock wave lithotripsy for urolithiasis. J Urol 1992;147:553.

Zanetti GR, Montanari E, Guarneri A, et al: Long-term followup after extracorporeal shock wave lithotripsy treatment of kidney stones in solitary kidneys. J Urol 1992;143:1011.

Zhong P, Preminger G: Differing modes of shock wave generation. Semin Urol 1994;12:2.

XIII

ENDOUROLOGY
AND LAPAROSCOPY

93
URETEROSCOPY

Jeffry L. Huffman, M.D., M.H.A.

The trend in medicine continues to be toward nonoperative or *minimally invasive* surgical procedures. This has been apparent in gastrointestinal surgery, orthopedics, otolaryngology, and urology. Often, minimally invasive endoscopic procedures replace open surgical procedures. As part of this increasing trend toward nonoperative therapy, there has been a steady increase in the number of endoscopic procedures performed within the upper urinary tract, including transurethral ureteroscopy, percutaneous nephroscopy, and antegrade ureteroscopy. This chapter discusses transurethral ureteroscopy and nephroscopy using both rigid and flexible instrumentation. Ureteroscopy is an extension of cystoscopic tech-

Some passages in this chapter are reproduced with permission from Huffman JL, Bagley DH, Lyon ES: Ureteroscopy. Philadelphia, W. B. Saunders, 1988.

niques used in the bladder and involves similar indications. The main differences relate to the anatomy of the ureter and kidney compared with the lower tract, the smaller size of instrumentation, and the narrower safety margin for the prevention of complications. The major components of transurethral ureteroscopy that have contributed most to the success and safety of this procedure are as follows:

- Understanding of upper urinary tract anatomy as it relates to endoscopy of the ureter and kidney has improved.
- The indications for rigid and flexible ureteroscopy have been clarified. This subject is changing constantly relative to stone disease treatment, with noninvasive shock-wave lithotripsy devices used more frequently for stones in the ureter.
- Rigid and flexible instruments continue to be improved and refined. Miniaturization of instruments and accessory devices has been a major step toward making the procedure more successful and safer.
- Methods of intraureteral lithotripsy have improved. Types of intraureteral lithotripsy include ultrasonic, electrohydraulic, laser, and ballistic methods.
- The recognition and the management of complications have improved. Based on the experience of early investigators, most major complications can be prevented or at least recognized early so the conservative treatment is still possible.

ANATOMY FOR TRANSURETHRAL URETEROSCOPY AND NEPHROSCOPY

A thorough knowledge of the anatomy of the kidney, intrarenal collecting system, and ureter enhances both the safety and the success of ureteroscopic procedures. Although anatomic configuration and location of the ureter and renal pelvis vary among patients, certain endoscopic landmarks remain constant. Similar to the recognition of the bulbus urethrae, verumontanum, bladder neck, and trigone in the lower urinary tract, the endoscopist must recognize the ureteral vesical junction, the pelvic brim, the ureteropelvic junction, and the individual infundibula within the renal pelvis.

This section reviews the gross and microscopic anatomy of the kidney and ureter. A description of the endoscopic anatomy is also presented with an emphasis on the clinical correlation between anatomy of the collecting system and potential hazards encountered during endoscopic procedures performed in the ureter and kidney.

Anatomic Relationships of the Kidney

The right and left kidneys are retroperitoneal organs situated on either side of the vertebral column between the 12th thoracic vertebra and the 3rd lumbar vertebra (Fig. 93–1A) (Markee, 1966; Gray, 1973; Bulger, 1983). The right kidney is slightly more caudal than the left with its renal hilus being directly posterior to the descending portion of the duodenum. The right lobe of the liver covers the bulk of its anterior surface, and hepatic flexure of the colon lies directly anterior

to the lower pole. The upper pole of the right kidney is in direct contact with the adrenal gland.

Immediately anterior to the renal pelvis is the renal vein, which drains into the inferior vena cava medially and the renal artery. Posteriorly the kidney is in contact with psoas quadratus lumborum and transversus abdominis muscles from medial to lateral. The diaphragm and the 12th rib overlie the upper pole of the kidney posteriorly. The left kidney has somewhat different relationships. Posteriorly the same muscles are encountered as for the right kidney, and the diaphragm and the 12th rib overlie the upper pole. Anteriorly the tail of the pancreas extends across the renal hilus, and the inferior tip of the spleen covers its anterior border. The proximal jejunum and the splenic flexure of the colon extend across the lower pole of the left kidney anteriorly, and the greater curvature of the stomach overlies the left upper pole and adrenal gland.

Anatomic Relationships of the Ureter

The ureter is an entirely retroperitoneal structure extending from the renal pelvis to the bladder (Fig. 93–1B). It varies in length from 28 to 34 cm with the right being about 1 cm shorter than the left (Davis et al, 1981). The abdominal portion of the ureter begins superiorly at the ureteropelvic junction where it is covered by the descending duodenum on the right and the beginning portion of the jejunum on the left. As it courses inferiorly from the renal pelvis, it lies lateral to the inferior vena cava and anterior to the psoas major muscle and the genitofemoral nerve. It then courses slightly medially to cross the ventral surface of the transverse processes of the third to fifth lumbar vertebral bodies and then crosses the bifurcation of the common iliac artery at the hypogastric artery. Near this level, it lies directly posterior to the right colic and ileocolic blood vessels and terminal ileum on the right and left colic vessels and the line of attachment of the sigmoid mesocolon on the left. The pelvic portion of the ureter begins as it crosses the bifurcation of the common iliac vessels and enters the true pelvis. As it courses inferiorly, it lies ventral to the hypogastric artery and medial to the obturator nerve and artery. It then runs slightly laterally and posteriorly along the lateral pelvic wall to the region of ischial spine. At this level, it bends medially and anteriorly to reach the bladder at the ureterovesical junction. The ureterovesical junction is the narrowest portion of the ureter and corresponds to the entrance of the ureter through the detrusor hiatus in the bladder wall musculature. At this level, the ureters are approximately 5 cm apart. As the intramural ureter exits this muscular hiatus, it courses submucosally approximately 2 cm within the bladder and ends at the ureteral orifice. It is this anatomic configuration of the submucosal ureter that is thought to allow it to preserve its antireflux mechanism.

Histologic Structure of the Renal Pelvis and Ureter

The renal pelvis and ureter are thin-walled structures (1–2 mm thick when distended) composed of three layers: fibrous, muscular, and mucosal (Figs. 93–2 and 93–3) (Verlando,

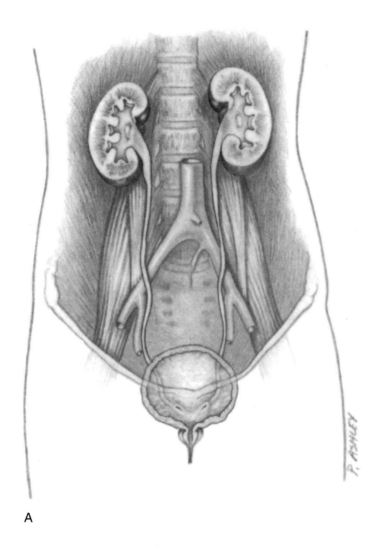

A

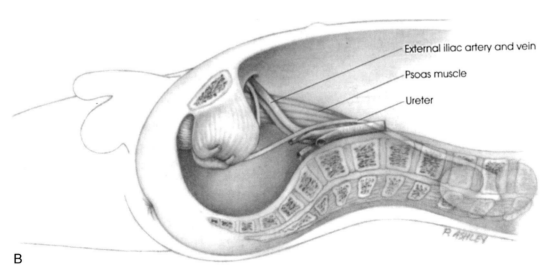

External iliac artery and vein

Psoas muscle

Ureter

B

Figure 93–1. *A,* Anteroposterior view of the bladder, ureters, and kidney. *B,* Lateral view of the bladder, ureter, and kidney. (From Huffman JL, Bagley DH, Lyon ES: Ureteroscopy. Philadelphia, W. B. Saunders, 1988.)

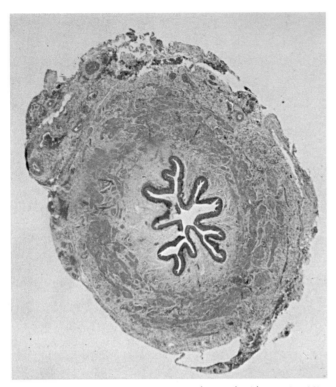

Figure 93–2. Histologic cross section of normal midureter (× 10).

1981). The outermost layer is the fibrous layer or tunica adventitia. This is a continuous fiber structure that runs from the renal sinus along the ureter and inserts into the fibrous coat of the bladder. The most distal aspect of this layer as it inserts into the bladder contains a specialized group of muscle fibers and fibrous tissue known as Waldeyer's sheath. Nerve fibers, lymphatics, and blood vessels are also contained in the tunica adventitia, which is joined externally by adipose tissue surrounding the ureter.

The middle portion is the muscular layer or tunica muscularis. It consists of two poorly defined, thin layers in the renal pelvis and proximal ureter, the inner circular and outer

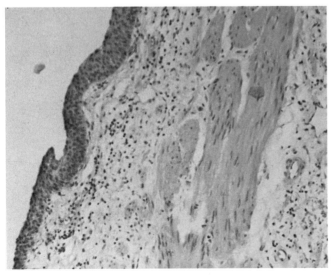

Figure 93–3. Histologic cross section of normal renal pelvis (× 100).

longitudinal. Most often, these layers are indistinct and are found in small bundles and running in oblique directions separated by large amounts of connective tissue. There are three distinct muscle layers in the middle and distal ureter: inner longitudinal, middle circular, and outer longitudinal fibers. The inner longitudinal fibers are more developed near the bladder, and the circular fibers decrease in size at this level. Within the intramural ureter, the longitudinal muscle fibers also decrease in number and size as the ureteral orifice is approached. In the submucosal ureter, there is only a semicircle of longitudinal fibers around the lateral aspect of the ureter with the medial portion having few muscle fibers at this level. This configuration helps to illustrate why great care must be taken when dilating the intramural tunnel in passing any instrument through this area. Perforation or creation of submucosal false passages occurs more easily at this level partly because of the sparse muscular coating.

The innermost lining of the ureter and renal pelvis is the mucosal layer. The anatomic features of this layer give rise to one of the unique properties of the ureter and pelvis: their ability to stretch and distend without rupturing. It consists of epithelium formed by transitional cells and subepithelium (lamina propria) formed by connective tissue. The epithelium becomes thicker in the distal ureter as compared with that found in the minor calyces. It is approximately two cell layers thick in the calyces and becomes about five or six cell layers thick in the distal ureter near the bladder. The lamina propria contains dense collagenous tissue with many elastic fibers and is continuous with the renal interstitial tissue. The mucosal layer also contains many longitudinal folds or rugae. These give the nondistended or contracted ureter its characteristic star-shaped appearance when viewed endoscopically.

Endoscopic Anatomy of the Intrarenal Collecting System

As urine is drained through the collecting ducts within the renal pyramids, it exits into the minor calyces by way of the renal papillae. The papillae form the apex of the renal pyramids and vary in number from 4 to 12 depending on the individual. Endoscopically a papilla appears as a rounded cone with a pink, easily friable epithelium (Huffman et al, 1985a). The cupped minor calyx surrounding each papilla is called the calyceal fornix. Occasionally, more than one papilla may project into a minor calyx. These compound calyces occur more commonly in the upper pole. In a nondistended calyx, the papillae are distinct and polypoid, whereas when the calyx is distended or appears "clubbed" radiographically, the papillae are less distinct and may be totally flattened.

The 4 to 13 minor calyces coalesce at their apices and empty into 2 or 3 major calyces, which drain directly into the renal pelvis. Endoscopically, on entering the renal pelvis from the transureteral route, the bases of the major calyces leading to the upper, middle, and lower pole of the kidney are the first structures visible. They appear as cylindrical openings branching from the pelvis. Often, minor calyces are visible in the background. The tubular portion or infundibulum connects the apex to the base of each major calyx. Separating the major calyces as the branch from the renal pelvis are carinae. Anatomically, these are similar in appearance to the branching of the trachea into the right and left main stem bronchi. There are usually two carinae, however, separating the three major calyceal infundibula.

The endoscopic anatomy of the renal pelvis is extremely variable with many differences in size, shape, and location. The renal pelvis is considered conical, with the apex of the cone representing the ureteropelvic junction. Intrarenal pelves, lying entirely within the renal sinus, are small with short infundibula. Extrarenal pelves are usually capacious, lying entirely outside the renal sinus and often having long, narrow infundibula. The renal pelvis empties urine into the proximal ureter through the ureteropelvic junction. This is one of the naturally narrower portions of the ureter. Endoscopically, it is identified easily as a junction between the relatively narrow ureter and the markedly more capacious renal pelvis. The movement of the pelvis and the proximal ureter with each respiratory excursion of the kidney is also apparent endoscopically. Usually a lip of ureteral mucosa is visible within the lateral ureteral lumen near the ureteropelvic junction. As discussed in the next section, this anatomic landmark signifies the close proximity of the renal pelvis.

Endoscopic Anatomy of the Ureter

A normal ureter is relatively uniform in caliber and easily distensible; however, there are three naturally occurring, relatively narrow sites within the lumen that are recognizable endoscopically: the ureteropelvic junction, the pelvic brim region, and the ureterovesical junction. The degree of narrowing that is encountered endoscopically varies among individuals. Often the narrowing is not noticeable; however, occasionally the amount of narrowing is such to prohibit passage of instruments without mechanical dilation. Besides these anatomic regions, there are other landmarks to be observed. The portion of the ureter as it crosses the termination of the common iliac artery may often be seen pulsating, thus signifying the close approximation of the ureteral and arterial lumen. As discussed previously, the approach to the proximal ureter is signified by movements with respiration. Each inspiration causes the diaphragm to push downward on the kidney leading to simultaneous caudad movement of the renal pelvis and proximal ureter. The junction between the fixed and mobile portions of the ureter has a characteristic appearance and signifies the close proximity of the renal pelvis. A bend or lip of mucosa corresponds to this junction. It is located in the posterolateral lumen and is accentuated during inspiration, becoming barely perceptible during expiration (Huffman et al, 1985a).

Endoscopic Correlation with Anatomy

The clinical availability of small-caliber flexible and rigid ureteroscopes has allowed the indications for ureteroscopy to expand greatly. In addition, the number of unsuccessful procedures has diminished. Previously the tortuous nature of the ureter did not lend itself well to many of the rigid instruments. Smaller-caliber instruments, especially the flexible variety, could be passed more reliably. Thus, anatomic size and configuration have become less restrictive with the

newer smaller, flexible instruments. Young muscular male patients often have a hypertrophied psoas major muscle. This causes the abdominal ureter to be "pushed" more ventrad within the retroperitoneum. This type of ureter was difficult to evaluate with rigid ureteroscopes; however, with the flexible deflectable instrument, it is much easier to traverse this deviation of the ureter and proceed into the kidney.

One must respect the delicate nature of the ureter when performing intraureteral procedures. Initial passage of a guide wire or cone-tipped ureteral catheter may perforate the mucosa and raise a mucosal flap, exposing the underlying submucosal tissue (Fig. 93–4). It is easy to pass a guide wire through the same area and dissect proximally within the ureter in the submucosa. A ureteroscope passed in the submucosal ureter also dissects the ureteral mucosa away from the underlying submucosa and muscle with irrigation fluid. The mucosa derives its blood supply from underlying tissues, and thus when the mucosa is dissected away, it loses its blood supply. The walls of proximal ureter and renal pelvis are thinner than the distal ureter. The mucosal layers contain one to two cell layers versus four to five in the lower ureter. In addition, there are fewer muscle fibers proximally. Any ureteral dilation, biopsy, or even instrument passage in this portion of the ureter is more likely to cause perforation. This is especially noticeable when one attempts to perform balloon dilation in the proximal ureter or ureteropelvic junction. It is much easier to perforate these areas with balloon dilation than in the lower ureter.

INDICATIONS FOR URETEROSCOPY

Table 93–1 lists the indications for ureteroscopy.

Calculi

Transurethral ureteroscopy for treatment of lower ureteral calculi continues to be a common treatment option (Bagley, 1988a). Its use in the lumbar ureter or intrarenal renal collecting system is less common, although, as discussed, there are clear indications for its use. Extracorporeal shock-wave lithotripsy (ESWL) may be used effectively to treat calculi at all locations in the ureter and kidney, and percutaneous techniques may be used to remove large renal or ureteral calculi. Factors such as stone size, composition, location, functional renal anatomy, associated ureteral pathology, and the patient's history need to be considered when deciding on treatment options. A categorical approach to this decision-making process is difficult, and much is left to the judgment of the urologist charged with the patient's care. It is clear that the urologist should be versed in all forms of stone therapy to manage patients effectively.

The success rates for ureteroscopic stone removal depend on stone size, stone location, the availability of ureteroscopic instrumentation, and the experience of the ureteroscopist. Early reported success rates for ureteroscopic stone retrieval in all locations of the ureter ranged from 57% to 97%. Success rates according to stone location vary from 22% to 60% in the upper ureter, 36% to 83% in the midureter, and 84% to 99% in the lower ureter (Ford et al, 1984b; Lyon et al, 1984; Epple and Reuter, 1985; El-Kappany et al, 1986;

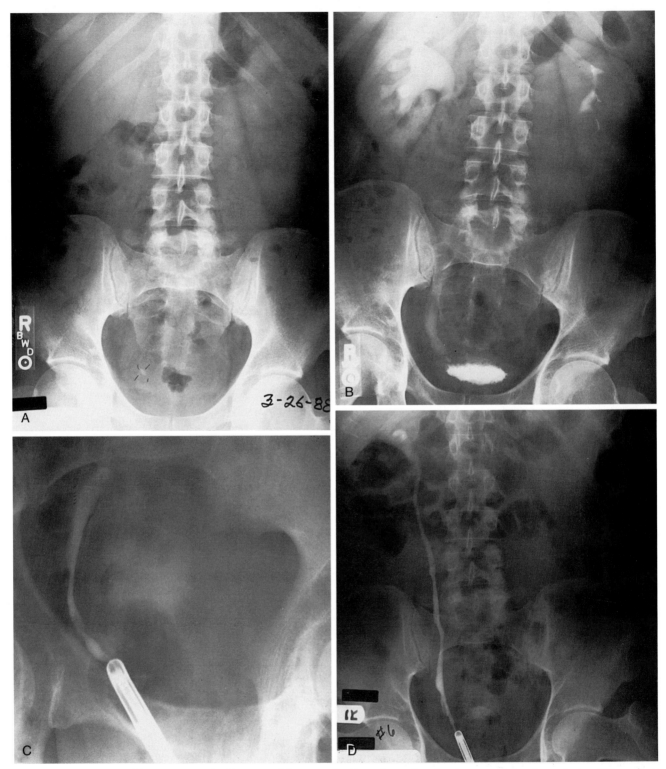

Figure 93–4. *A,* A 36-year-old man presented with severe right ureteral colic and was found to have an obstructing calculus. This preliminary scout x-ray demonstrates a 7 mm × 4 mm calculus in the region of the right lower ureter. *B,* An excretory urogram was performed confirming the diagnosis. The x-ray was taken 2 hours, 10 minutes following the administration of contrast material and shows the stone to be lodged at the right ureteral vesical junction with evidence of partial ureteral obstruction. *C,* The patient was followed with hopes that the stone would pass spontaneously. There was no progression of the stone, however, and the patient continued to have intermittent episodes of severe right ureteral colic. He was considered for ureteroscopic stone removal, and before the procedure an occlusion-tip retrograde pyelogram was performed (shown). The stone can be seen as a negative defect with contrast proximal and distal. There is an area of concentric narrowing just distal to where the stone is lodged. *D,* A sequential radiograph demonstrates the cone-tip catheter advanced proximally a short distance, but now there appears to be a false lumen medial to the stone. Layering of contrast is seen lateral and above the calculus, which most likely represents the true lumen, whereas the contrast medial represents dissection of the mucosa away from the remainder of the ureteral wall.

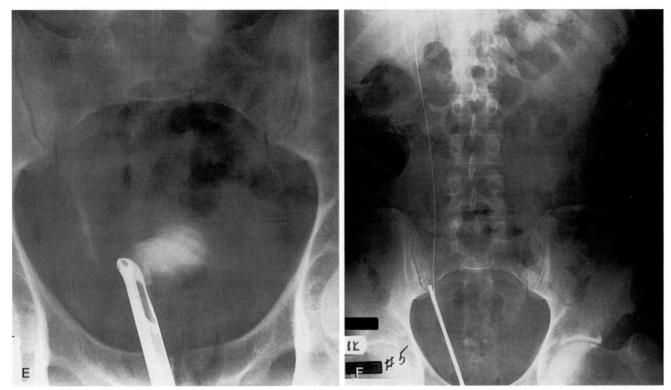

Figure 93–4 *Continued E,* A drainage film from the retrograde study. This again confirms the presence of contrast outside the lumen of the ureter. Residual contrast material is seen within the submucosa of the distal ureter adjacent to the stone. *F,* A guide wire was then inserted over which the ureteroscope was passed. The stone could not be identified with the rigid ureteroscope. Explanation for this phenomenon was that the guide wire was passed submucosally along with the rigid ureteroscope. This explains why the stone could not be seen despite being confirmed to be in the vicinity of the stone by x-ray. (From Huffman JL: Urol Clin North Am 1989; 16:249–254.)

Green and Lytton, 1985; Khuri et al, 1985; Sosa et al, 1985; Kahn, 1986; Aso, 1987; Coptcoat et al, 1987; Keating et al, 1987; El-Faqih et al, 1988; Seeger et al, 1988; Valente et al, 1990; Hernandez et al, 1993; Netto and Claro, 1993; Boline and Belis, 1994; Grasso et al, 1995).

In a large series of 346 ureteroscopic procedures performed at the Mayo Clinic, the success rate was 95% for removing lower ureteral stones and 72% for upper stones, including mid and proximal third ureteral locations (Blute et

Table 93–1. INDICATIONS FOR URETEROSCOPY

Calculi: Removal

   Lower ureteral calculi
   Upper ureteral calculi, after failed ESWL
   Renal calculi, after failed ESWL
   Post ESWL Steinstrasse
   Calculi associated with obstruction
   Calculi plus suspicion of urothelial carcinoma

Diagnosis

   Evaluation of radiographic filling defects or obstruction
   Evaluation of unilateral gross hematuria
   Evaluation of unilateral malignant cytology
   Surveillance after conservative treatment of an upper urinary
     tract tumor

Therapeutic Procedures Other than Calculi

   Passage of a ureteral catheter for obstruction or fistula
   Removal of a foreign body
   Resection/fulguration of selected tumors
   Dilation/incision of strictures

al, 1988). Only eight patients (3%) required ureterolithotomy.

Bagley (1990) reported successful removal of 62 calculi out of 77 attempts (80.5%) using a variety of actively and passively deflectable flexible ureteroscopes. In nine of these patients, stones were repositioned to the lower ureter, where they were removed with a rigid instrument. The successes included extraction of 22 of 23 intrarenal calculi.

Fragments of calculi resulting from ESWL may fill a portion of the ureter causing partial or complete obstruction. Usually, these fragments pass spontaneously with minimal discomfort; however, intervention may become necessary should the patient develop fever, persistent high-grade obstruction, or intractable pain. In these instances, ureteroscopy is a reliable method of removing the debris (Hernandez et al, 1993). The operating instrument with the ultrasonic probe is particularly useful for fragmenting and removing the calculus debris (Fig. 93–5).

Grasso and colleagues compared ESWL with ureteroscopic stone extraction in 112 patients with primary ureteral calculi (Grasso et al, 1995). At 1 month, stone-free rates were 45% versus 95%, and at 3 months they were 62% versus 97%. The mean number of postoperative visits and imaging studies was higher in the ESWL group (2.07 versus 1.13). In addition, overall costs were higher in the ESWL group. Netto and Claro (1993) also compared ESWL to ureteroscopy to remove lower ureteral calculi. Over 3 years, 71 patients underwent ESWL and 161 ureteroscopy to remove lower ureteral calculi. The success rate for ESWL was 82.1% with 19.6% requiring retreatment. The patients

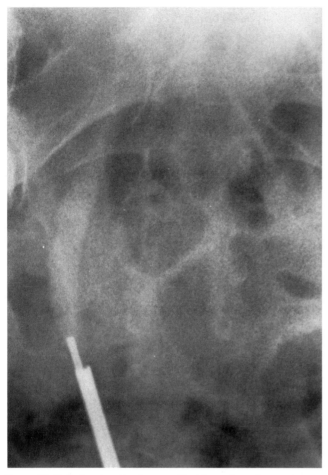

Figure 93–5. Following shock-wave lithotripsy, stone fragments occasionally become lodged in the ureter causing ureteral obstruction. Ultrasonic lithotripsy performed through a rigid ureteroscope is an excellent means of removing these fragments. This radiograph shows a collection of stone particles in the right lower ureter. A rigid ureteroscope and an ultrasonic lithotripsy probe are inserted into the ureter to fragment the particles further and remove them with suction through the probe.

undergoing ureteroscopy were found to have a 95.5% success rate with only 1.2% needing a second procedure.

El-Faqih and co-workers compared ureteroscopy to ESWL for treating stones in the ureter below the level of the sacroiliac joint (El-Faqih et al, 1988). Of 65 patients treated ureteroscopically, 97% had successful stone removal, but 3 required surgery for complications. Of 53 patients treated by ESWL primarily, 90% were stone-free at 6 weeks with no complications. This group suggests that ESWL should be the primary treatment method because of fewer complications, less procedural time, and shorter hospital stay. Anderson and co-workers compared 76 patients undergoing ESWL and 27 patients undergoing ureteroscopy for treatment of stones below the bony pelvis (Anderson et al, 1994). Although the success rate for ureteroscopy was 100% compared with 90% for ESWL, the authors recommended ESWL as first-line therapy because of less treatment time, no need for a stent, and shorter convalescence.

In certain instances, ureteroscopy is clearly indicated: after failed ESWL in the kidney or proximal ureter (Fig. 93–6), if there are stones in calyceal diverticula that are not amena-

ble to percutaneous removal, if there are stones associated with obstruction, and if there are stones asssociated with a suspicion of urothelial malignancy. Again, percutaneous techniques may be preferable for indications with large stone volumes that would be difficult to remove through the ureteroscope. The ureteroscope may be useful, however, to remove stones in upper-pole calyceal diverticula, especially those in anterior locations. Stones in these locations are difficult to approach percutaneously, often requiring supracostal nephrostomy access.

The economics of the two options should also be considered. Kapoor and associates found that ESWL was 60% more expensive than ureterosocopy (P <.005) with no significant differences noted in success or complication rates (Kapoor et al, 1992). For treatment of lower ureteral stones, whether ESWL or ureteroscopy is used, the success rates are high with few complications. There are more ESWL failures that require a second ureteroscopic procedure, and ESWL is more costly. Thus, ureteroscopic stone removal remains an attractive method for removing lower ureteral stones. In the upper ureter or kidney, ureteroscopy is reserved for ESWL failures, stones plus obstruction, or stones plus suspicion of an associated urothelial malignancy.

Suspicion of a Urothelial Tumor

Primary epithelial tumors of the upper urinary tract often pose a formidable diagnostic challenge. In contrast to the cystoscopic approach to the diagnosis of bladder tumors, there previously has not been a satisfactory endoscopic method for the diagnosis of upper tract tumors. The ureteroscope has uses similar to those of the cystoscope including diagnosis of upper tract tumors, surveillance of the urothelium following prior therapy, and occasionally primary treatment of selected tumors. The indications for diagnostic ureteroscopy include radiographic filling defects or obstruction (Fig. 93–7), tumor found cystoscopically near or at the ureteral orifice, unilateral upper tract hematuria (Fig. 93–8), and upper tract urinary cytology suggestive of malignant cells (Fig. 93–9) (Gittes and Varaday, 1981; Huffman et al, 1985c).

The approach to a patient with unilateral essential hematuria may be difficult. Gittes and Varaday (1981) showed the potential for diagnosis and localization of hematuria by operative nephroscopy. Bagley and associates confirmed that this lesion, often a renal hemangioma, may be localized and treated either by coagulation through the flexible ureteroscope or by total or partial nephrectomy (Bagley et al, 1987).

Streem and colleagues analyzed the effects of adding rigid ureteroscopy to standard methods used to diagnose upper tract tumors (Streem et al, 1986). Using intravenous pyelogram, retrograde pyelogram, computed tomography scan, urinary cytology, and cystoscopy, the diagnosis of an upper tract tumor was realized in 7 of 12 patients. Adding rigid ureteroscopy to the diagnostic regimen increased the accuracy to 10 of 12 patients. The prime indication for flexible ureteroscopy has been in the diagnosis within the kidney. The success rate of visualizing the entire intrarenal collecting system was 79% in a prior published report; however, this rate continues to improve with experience. Most lesions in the kidney require biopsy for confirmation of the pathology.

Besides the diagnosis and mapping of urothelial tumors,

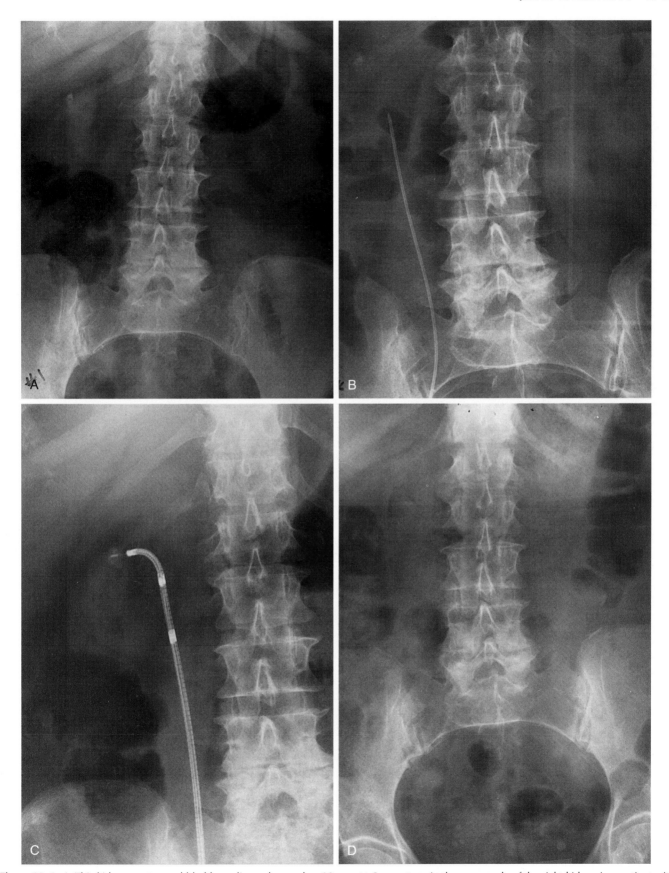

Figure 93–6. *A,* This kidney, ureter, and bladder radiograph reveals a 10 mm × 8 mm stone in the upper pole of the right kidney in a patient with recurrent flank pain and hematuria. *B,* The patient underwent shock-wave lithotripsy, which had little effect in fracturing the calculus. A catheter had been inserted before this procedure to help localize the stone. Because of the failure to fragment the stone, flexible ureteroscopy was performed using an actively deflectable flexible instrument. *C,* A No. 3 Fr electrohydraulic lithotripsy probe was used to fragment the stone, and individual pieces of the stone were removed to render the patient stone-free. *D,* Final abdominal radiograph shows that the patient has been rendered stone-free. (From Huffman JL: Prob Urol 1989; 3:420–434.)

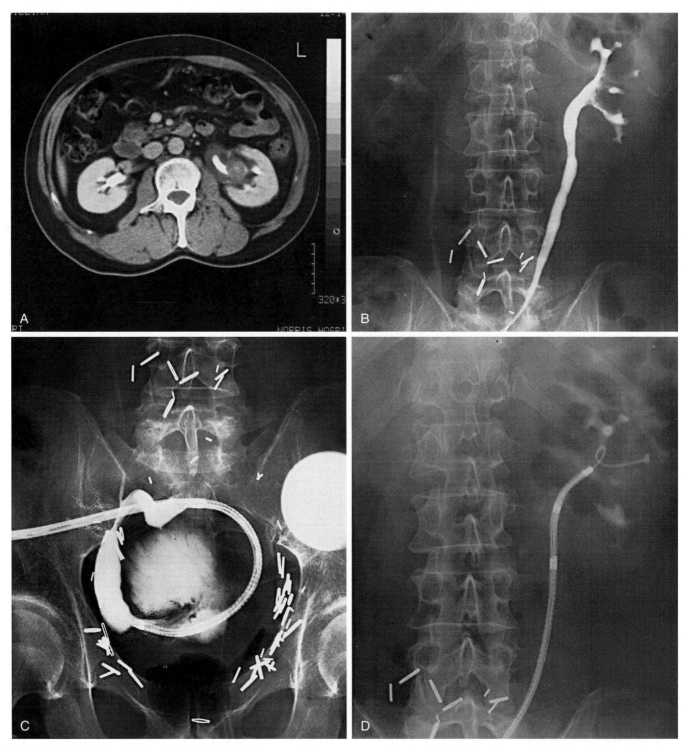

Figure 93–7. A 68-year-old man had previously undergone radical cystectomy, pelvic lymph node dissection, and creation of a continent urinary diversion for P2N0 bladder carcinoma. He presented 4 years later with gross hematuria and was found to have bleeding from the upper urinary tract after endoscopy of the Kock pouch was performed. *A,* Urinary cytology was negative for malignant cells, and a computed tomography (CT) scan was done. This selected view of the CT scan shows a probable mass in the renal pelvis of the left kidney. A retrograde study was then done through the afferent system of the continent diversion. *B,* A selected film from this retrograde study shows the same filling defect in the lateral portion of the renal pelvis. *C,* The flexible cystoscope in the afferent limb of the continent diversion was used to pass a guide wire directly into the left collecting system. *D,* The flexible ureteroscope was passed over a stiff guide wire that had been positioned in the kidney. After the guide wire was removed, the No. 3 Fr biopsy forceps was inserted and tissue obtained. Biopsy confirmed a grade II–III transitional cell carcinoma of the left renal pelvis. The patient underwent a left nephroureterectomy.

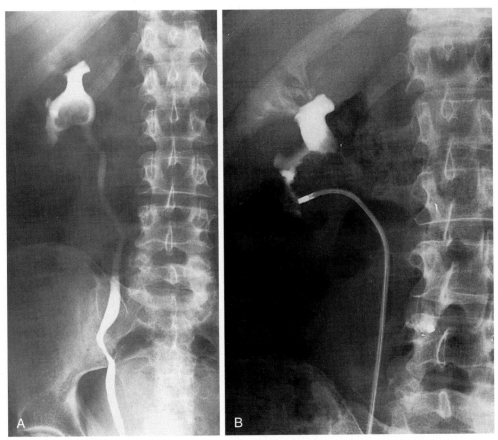

Figure 93–8. A 51-year-old man presented with gross hematuria. An excretory urogram was done initially showing a solitary right kidney with a filling defect in the renal pelvis. A retrograde study was performed documenting the filling defect *(A)*, and at the same setting, flexible ureteropyeloscopy was carried out *(B)*. The tip of the flexible instrument can be identified within the lower pole of the kidney. In fact, multifocal tumor was identified. Biopsy confirmed grade II–III transitional cell carcinoma. Because of the patient's age and the multifocal nature of the tumor within the kidney, it was elected to proceed with nephroureterectomy, removal of a cuff of bladder, and regional lymph node dissection. Final pathology confirmed multifocal carcinoma, including areas of carcinoma in situ in the ureter, which previously had not been identified ureteroscopically. The patient was maintained on long-term hemodialysis for 2.5 years, during which routine surveillance cystoscopy was performed. After remaining free of disease for 2.5 years, living relating renal transplant was performed from one of the patient's brothers. He has now been followed for 2 years, free of tumor recurrence, and he has normal function of his transplanted kidney. (From Huffman JL: Prob Urol 1989; 3:420–434.)

ureteroscopy has been useful in following patients after prior segmental ureterectomies and treating selected patients, especially those with isolated, low-grade lower ureteral tumors and those with solitary kidneys in whom dialysis is not indicated, who are prohibitive anesthesia risks, or who have renal insufficiency to the extent of not allowing nephroureterectomy (Huffman, 1988a). Andersen and Kristensen (1994) reported on results of 31 patients who underwent ureteroscopic diagnosis or treatment or follow-up of upper urinary tract transitional cell carcinoma. Twenty-one of these patients then had open surgery after diagnosis, and ten underwent primary endoscopic management. Of these ten, two eventually required open surgical removal of the kidney, but eight avoided surgery (mean follow-up 25 months).

Nonmalignant lesions of the ureter and renal pelvis may also be diagnosed and treated. For example, benign filling defects such as ureteritis cystica may be identified and biopsied (Suzuki, 1995). In addition, several endoscopists have confirmed the successful use of the ureteroscope to diagnose and remove fibroepithelial polyps (Okamoto et al, 1993; Mikami et al, 1995).

Passage of a Ureteral Catheter

In most instances, ureteral catheters are placed by standard cystoscopic methods. In some patients, however, ureteral tortuosity, obstruction, or an iatrogenic false passage prohibits passage of a catheter. By using the ureteroscopic, direct vision approach, a catheter may pass. Ureteroscopy has also been found to be effective in managing ureterocutaneous fistula, enabling passage of a catheter or stent beyond the fistula site. In these instances, employing either the No. 9.5 Fr instrument with a No. 5 Fr accessory channel or the smaller No. 8.5 Fr instrument with a No. 3.5 Fr channel has been most satisfactory (Huffman, 1989b). These instruments are especially valuable in instances in which dilation of the orifice and tunnel is made impossible by prior trauma. They often may be inserted directly into the orifice without prior dilation.

Another indication for ureteroscopic intervention is for treatment of an iatrogenic ureterovaginal fistula as a complication of hysterectomy. This method may not always be successful depending on the degree of injury, but in some

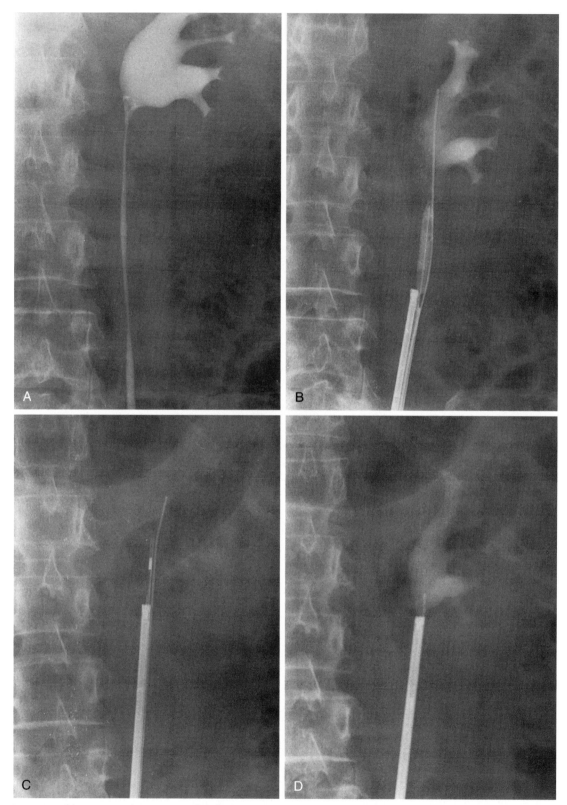

Figure 93–9. A 58-year-old woman with intermittent left flank pain. Excretory urography showed a possible filling defect in the renal pelvis, but urinary cytology was negative for malignant cells. *A,* Retrograde pyelogram revealed a 1.5-cm irregular filling defect at the ureteropelvic junction with an otherwise normal collecting system. *B,* Passage of the diagnostic ureteroscope was prevented by proximal ureteral narrowing, so a 4-mm dilating balloon was used. *C,* Rigid biopsy forceps extending from operating ureteroscope. *D,* After biopsy and fulguration, contrast study obtained via the ureteroscope shows no evidence of extravasation, obstruction, or residual filling defect. (From Huffman JL: Urol Clin North Am 1988; 15:419–424.)

patients subsequent open surgery may be avoided (Koonings et al, 1992)

Retrieval of Foreign Bodies

Another indication for ureteroscopy is the retrieval of ureteral stents that have migrated or of broken instrument parts, such as portions of stone baskets, that are retained in the ureter (Bagley, 1988a; Killeen and Bihrle, 1990). This is not a common indication, and often this method of retrieval is difficult because of associated ureteral edema and inflammation. The three-prong grasping forceps, alligator forceps, or a stone basket should be used for these retrievals (Fig. 93–10).

Incision and Dilation of a Ureteral Stricture

Ureteroscopic methods may be employed to treat postoperative ureteral strictures. The process involves incising the region of narrowing under direct vision using a rigid or flexible ureteroscope (Bagley et al, 1985; Inglis and Tolley, 1986; Clayman et al, 1990). The incision is made with either a cold knife ureterotome or a cutting electrode (Fig. 93–11). The area may then be dilated with a 5- or 6-mm balloon dilating catheter to complete the treatment. Incising the stricture allows controlled splitting of the ureter during the dilation process. An internal ureteral stent, a nephrostomy tube, or both are left in place for 4 to 6 weeks after the procedure. The long-term success of this technique remains to be determined, but preliminary results are encouraging, and it offers definite advantages over repeat open surgery.

Ureteroscopy in Pregnancy

Ureteroscopy has limited applications during pregnancy. The procedure may occasionally be required to help diagnose or treat a ureteral calculus, but in general the risks of medication, radiation exposure, and anesthesia limit any endourology or open surgery. ESWL is contraindicated during pregnancy because of potential harmful effects on the fetus.

Fortunately, most ureteral calculi diagnosed during pregnancy pass spontaneously. In a review by Cass and colleagues, 18 of 24 pregnant patients with stones passed them spontaneously either during pregnancy (14) or postpartum (4) (Cass et al, 1986). Six patients required intervention for persistent pain (two), sepsis (three), and anuria (one). Intervention consisted of stone basket manipulation (two), open surgery (three), or placement of ureteral catheters (one).

The diagnosis of a stone during pregnancy is made difficult because of the desire to limit radiographic exposure (especially in the first trimester) and the inaccuracy of ultrasonography. Diagnostic ultrasound is safe during pregnancy, but the presence of renal pelvic dilation may not be due to an obstructing calculus because upper tract dilation is often associated with pregnancy.

Rittenberg and Bagley (1988) have reported the use of flexible ureteroscopy in two pregnant patients. In one patient at 19 weeks' gestation, the procedure was used to exclude ureteral obstruction, and in another patient at 35 weeks' gestation, a 6-mm obstructing calculus was removed successfully. Both procedures were performed without the use of fluoroscopy, and there were no detrimental effects on the patient or fetus.

Bakke and Ulvik (1988) have reported successful use of

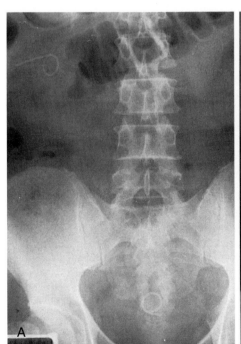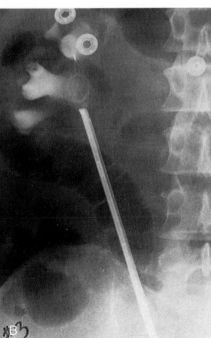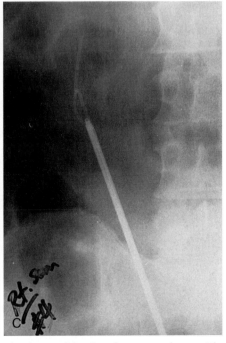

Figure 93–10. A 45-year-old patient presented 3 years after placement of an internal stent before shock-wave lithotripsy for a ureteral stone. The patient admitted to not following up after the procedure as instructed. *A,* Follow-up radiograph revealed that the stent had fractured. Portions of the stent remained in the right urinary system with the proximal coil in the renal pelvis and the distal coil in the bladder. *B* and *C,* The bladder portion was removed cystoscopically, and using a rigid ureteroscope and a stone basket, the renal pelvic fragment was engaged in the basket and then removed.

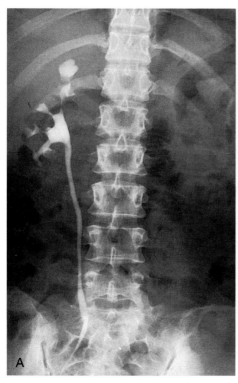
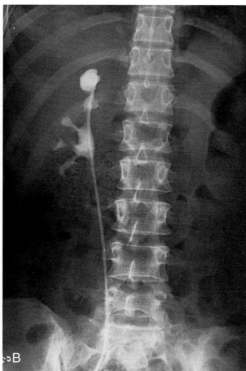

Figure 93–11. A 34-year-old woman presented with recurrent right flank pain and urinary infection localized to the right upper urinary system. An excretory urogram showed a dilated area in the upper pole of the collecting system, which was confirmed by retrograde study *(A)* to be a calyceal diverticulum. A small opening could be detected inferiorly where it drained into an upper pole calyx. Flexible ureteroscopy was performed and the opening identified. Using a cutting electrode, the neck of the diverticulum was incised and opened widely. This allowed placement of a No. 7 Fr internal stent *(B)*. The patient's symptoms and infections resolved immediately, and she has remained asymptomatic for 20 months thus far.

rigid ureteroscopy in eight pregnant patients with the duration of pregnancy ranging from 4 to 35 weeks. All patients were treated with the No. 11 Fr rigid operating ureteroscope. The instrument was passed to the renal pelvis in all patients. Two were found to have excoriations and edema consistent with prior stone passage, one patient had only blood clots in the kidney, and one had no abnormalities detected. Four patients were found to have distal ureteral calculi, and these were removed successfully. Two required ultrasonic lithotripsy before extraction. One pregnancy ended in induced abortion at 8 weeks not associated with the procedure. The remaining seven women had normal babies.

Ureteroscopy in the Pediatric Patient

Ureteroscopy may occasionally be indicated in the pediatric patient for treatment of persistent ureteral calculi. Extreme caution is recommended when performing these procedures because of the smaller size of the upper urinary tract and the narrower safety margin. Certainly, small-caliber instruments should be employed (No. 6–8.5 Fr) and the use of fluoroscopy limited.

Hill and colleagues reported using a No. 8.5 Fr rigid ureteroscope in four children 10 years of age or younger (Hill et al, 1990). In two patients, ureteral calculi were extracted successfully, one requiring fragmentation with laser lithotripsy. The other two patients underwent diagnostic ureteroscopy. In one, an area of stenosis was found and stented, whereas in the other, ureteral polyps were found. The polyps were treated surgically after endoscopic diagnosis. In each patient, follow-up kidney function studies were normal; however, reflux was found by voiding cystogram in two patients. In this report, the authors stressed the importance of adhering to strict ureteroscopic technique, employing an isotonic irrigating solution, and maintaining a stent postoperatively for a minimum of 48 hours.

Thomas and colleagues (1993) and Shroff and Watson (1995) have also reported the success and safety of using small-caliber rigid and flexible ureteroscopes in 16 patients (Thomas and colleagues) and 14 patients (Shroff and Watson) between the ages of 13 months and 15 years. Both authors stress the use of small-caliber instruments and ancillary devices such as baskets and forceps along with a high level of endoscopic skill as key success factors.

PREOPERATIVE PATIENT MANAGEMENT

The preoperative management of a patient before a ureteroscopic procedure includes a thorough history and physical examination, informed consent from the patient, and perioperative antibiotics (Huffman, 1988b). The preoperative patient history is especially important regarding prior pelvic surgery or radiation. Certainly a previous radical prostatectomy or radical hysterectomy may leave the lower ureter fixed in the retroperitoneum and relatively immobile. Similarly a prior history of having a ureteral reimplantation or ureteral lithotomy may make the ureter more difficult to manipulate.

The physical examination may give clues that help predict potential problems in the procedure. A bimanual examination allows assessment of the mobility of the urethra, bladder, and lower ureter. Those that are immobile or frozen may not allow straightening for passage of the rigid instrument and may be angulated, making flexible ureteroscopy more difficult.

The patient consent should inform the patient that ureteroscopy is a relatively new procedure without extremely long patient follow-up. Although the goal of the procedure is to prevent an open operation, surgery may still be necessary if the procedure is unsuccessful or if complications arise. The majority of calculi can be removed in one procedure; however, the patient should be made aware in advance that to become stone-free a second procedure may be necessary. A percutaneous nephrostolithotomy might be done, or an open lithotomy may be required. It is incumbent on the urologist to review all radiographic studies before ureteroscopy. It is also necessary to ensure that the radiographic studies are complete. For example, if the ureter distal to the calculus is not visualized well, it is essential to have a cone-tip retrograde pyelogram done. This allows an appraisal of the ureteral tortuosity and caliber distal to the stone and helps identify the regions within the ureter that may be difficult to negotiate.

Perioperative antibiotics are required. Sterile urine is mandatory before the procedure because intravasation of urine and irrigant is possible, and sepsis has been a complication. Generally, patients are given a broad-spectrum antibiotic (e.g., ampicillin and gentamicin) immediately before the procedure, and this is continued for several dosages after the procedure.

A general or regional anesthetic is normally required because of pain created when passing the rigid instrument or dilating the lower ureter. When performing flexible ureteroscopy or using a small-caliber rigid instrument, it is usually possible to do the procedure under local anesthesia with intravenous sedation. This is especially desirable in a patient undergoing surveillance endoscopy after having prior endoscopic removal of an upper tract tumor or after undergoing segmental removal of the urinary tract. In these instances, flexible ureteroscopy is generally employed and little pain inflicted.

RIGID INSTRUMENTATION

Although first achieved by Young in 1912, rigid ureteroscopy was not performed routinely until Goodman (1977) and Lyon and co-workers (1978) independently demonstrated the feasibility of deliberate excursions into the ureter. A contribution of Hopkins (1960) made this possible. His invention of the rigid rod lens system enabled extremely effective light transmission through rigid endoscopes. Using his principles, it was possible to construct instruments small enough in size to use in the ureter that still provided enough light for effective endoscopy.

The traditional rigid endoscopes before this time were constructed of a field lens system that consisted of a tube of air with thin lenses of glass. There were objective lenses at the distal tip of the endoscope and a succession of thin relay lenses refracting the rays of light through the instrument to the eyepiece, where they were magnified for the observer.

In 1960, Hopkins invented the rod lens system for rigid endoscopes that is used currently. This system relays the image by a succession of rod lenses separated by air. The thin spaces of air serve as lenses, and the glass serves as spaces. The effect of this is twofold: (1) The total light transmitted is increased because of the higher refractive index of glass, and (2) rod lenses are easier to mount than thin lenses, and a greater-diameter lens may be installed for

a given diameter endoscope sheath, thus again increasing light transmission.

Another factor improving light transmission through the rod lens endoscopes was the use of an efficient multilayer antireflection coating on the surfaces of the lens. All these factors added together provide the modern rod lens endoscope with markedly increased light transmission.

Lyon's and Goodman's procedures were performed initially with No. 9.5 Fr pediatric cystoscopes. Although length was a limiting factor, these instruments could be used to examine the distal ureter and intramural tunnel in girls and some boys.

In conjunction with Lyon, Richard Wolf Medical Instruments (Rosemont, IL) designed an instrument modeled after a juvenile cystoscope that was specifically used for ureteroscopy. This instrument had a working length of 23 cm and readily reached the distal ureter in male and female patients (Lyon et al, 1979). There were several different rigid sheaths: No. 13.0, 14.5, and 16.0 Fr with a No. 14.5 Fr resectoscope sheath. The No. 13.0 Fr instrument could be used only for observation. A total of 57 procedures was performed with these instruments between 1978 and 1981 with a success rate of 90%. For the first time, calculi were visualized directly in the ureter, engaged in a basket under vision, and removed (Huffman et al, 1983a).

This instrument was occasionally difficult to pass into the ureteral orifice. Its beak was constructed without much bevel, and to negotiate the orifice, the trigone had to be depressed while advancing the instrument. This often resulted in a blind spot during insertion that prohibited visualization of the ureteral lumen. Insertion was not only difficult and time-consuming, but also often impossible. False passages occasionally resulted because of the blind spot and subsequent improper alignment of the instrument.

Karl Storz Instruments (Culver City, CA) in conjunction with Perez-Castro and Martinez-Pineiro (1980) made the next significant contribution to the field of rigid ureteroscopy. They introduced an instrument with a working length of 39 cm that could reach the renal pelvis in male and female patients after transurethral passage. Often called the ureterorenoscope, or more appropriately the ureteropyeloscope, this instrument could examine the ureter and renal pelvis. The instrument had sheath sizes of No. 9 and 11 Fr, and each had a No. 5 Fr working channel. The No. 9 Fr sheath had an integral 0 degree telescope. In conjunction with the No. 11 Fr sheath, interchangeable 0- and 70-degree telescopes with their bridges were available for visualization within the ureter and renal pelvis. A No. 11 Fr resectoscope sheath that had a partially insulated beak with an inverted bevel allowed ureteroscopic resection.

Wolf developed a similar instrument with a 41-cm working length in sheath sizes of No. 11.5 and 10.0 Fr (Huffman et al, 1983a). The larger operating sheath had a No. 5 Fr channel for accessories, but the smaller sheath was for observation only. A resectoscope sheath was also designed that was No. 11.5 Fr and a completely insulated beak.

Since that time, many new instruments have been introduced by several manufacturers. The trend has been to reduce sheath size and still maintain an accessory channel for forceps, baskets, and intraureteral lithotripsy devices (Huffman, 1989b). The introduction of fiberoptic imaging bundles within a rigid sheath has made this miniaturization possible (Dretler and Cho, 1989). Abdel Razzak and Bagley (1994) have reviewed the features and irrigating capacities of small-caliber rigid ureteroscopes (< No. 10 Fr) with fiberoptic imaging bundles. They found that even the smallest-caliber rigid endoscopes had acceptable flow rates without accessory instruments in their channels. With an accessory device in place, however, the flow rates were reduced significantly (see Appendix A).

FLEXIBLE URETEROSCOPY AND FLEXIBLE INSTRUMENTATION

Flexible ureteroscopy is a valuable addition to the diagnosis and treatment of many lesions in the upper urinary tract including removal of resistant stones. The technique has extended the indications of rigid ureteroscopy and allows virtually any filling defect to be evaluated or any stone to be considered for removal from the ureter or kidney. The rapid advancement of this technology has been made possible by the development of flexible ureteroscopes that are of small enough caliber to extend into the upper urinary tract combined with an instrument channel that accepts wires, baskets, and flexible lithotripsy probes (Fig. 93–12).

Marshall in 1964 reported using a 3-mm fiberscope or ureteroscope that was passed transurethrally through a No. 26 Fr cystoscope and then into the distal ureter, where a ureteral stone was visualized at 9 cm. Although there was excellent transmission of light and images with this instrument, there was no method for changing the direction of the tip of the instrument and no method for irrigation to provide a clear field of view and adequate distention of the ureter. The small size of this instrument, a necessity for passage through the ureter, prevented the incorporation of a deflecting mechanism and a channel for working instruments along with the imaging bundle. This size problem remains somewhat of a limiting factor today.

Takagi and associates began working with a narrow flexible fiberoptic endoscope in 1966 that was 2.7 mm in diameter and 70 cm in length (Takagi et al, 1968). They reported its use in 1968 in a patient undergoing an open operation in which the instrument was passed through the ureterotomy incision to visualize and photograph the renal pelvis and renal papilla. Once again the difficulties of having no irrigation system and no deflecting mechanism were encountered. It became evident, however, that it was possible to visualize portions of the urinary tract that could not be viewed through rigid cystoscopes.

Bush and associates also had been working with flexible instrumentation in the late 1960s (Bush et al, 1970). Their instrument was inserted cystoscopically similar to a ureteral catheter and enabled visualization of the upper urinary tract. Irrigation was provided by means of a forced diuresis, and any manipulation was performed with accessories passed alongside the ureteroscope.

Successful use of a pyeloureteroscope passed transurethrally in 23 patients was reported by Takagi and co-workers in 1971. This instrument, an Olympus model KF (Olympus America Inc, Melville, NY), was 2 mm in diameter and 75 cm long. The addition of a 2.5-cm angulating section at the distal end of the instrument enabled passage of this instrument into the ureteral orifice and through the intramural ureter in the same fashion as a ureteral catheter. It also allowed passage up the ureter and into the intrarenal collecting system with the aid of fluoroscopy. Despite having the advantage of a flexible tip, this instrument still did not have an irrigation system, and as reported by Takagi, there were occasional problems with passage of the instrument through the intramural ureter that resulted in breakage of the glass fibers.

To circumvent this problem of insertion, Takagi (1971) introduced a Teflon guide tube that was passed initially through a special cystoscope with an ocular lens system that protruded at a 45-degree angle from the shaft. The angulation of the lens system helped prevent fracture of the glass fibers as it was pushed through the cystoscope, and a special deflecting bridge limited sharp angulation of the instrument as it passed from the end of the cystoscope. The guide tube was passed into the bladder and engaged by the deflecting bridge. A ureteral catheter was then passed through the guide tube and into the ureteral orifice. Once the catheter was approximately 10 cm within the ureter, the guide tube was pushed over it in a coaxial fashion. The ureteral catheter was then removed and replaced with the flexible pyeloure-

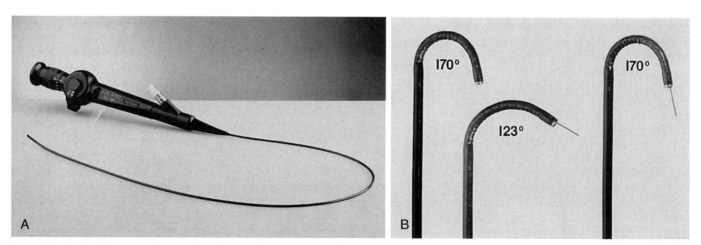

Figure 93–12. A, Karl Storz actively deflectable flexible ureteroscope. The instrument has a No. 7 Fr distal end with deflection 90 degrees and 170 degrees. B, With a No. 1.6 Fr electrohydraulic probe in its channel, deflection is reduced to 123 degrees. (Courtesy of Karl Storz Endoscopy America, Inc., Culver City, CA.)

teroscope. Takayasu and Aso (1974) reported a 100% success rate in 19 patients using this guide tube method compared with an 80% success rate in 50 patients before its use. The only irrigation system, however, was provided by irrigating through the guide tube or by inducing a diuresis. Therefore, observation was often difficult or impossible in the presence of hematuria.

Modern flexible ureteroscopes have been markedly improved by reducing sheath size, increasing channel size, and providing a deflecting mechanism in many designs. The two generic types of instruments are the passively deflectable and the actively deflectable (see Appendix B).

The passively deflectable design does not allow for purposeful movement of its tip, thus depending on a preplaced guide wire for positioning within the urinary tract. The passively deflectable instruments are less expensive. They vary in size from No. 6 to 10 Fr with an irrigation/accessory channel size directly proportional to the overall size. The actively deflectable design has the ability to be purposely deflected within the urinary tract. They also have an irrigation/accessory channel for passage of stone baskets, grasping forceps, biopsy forceps, or guide wires. These actively deflectable instruments have been extremely useful within the kidney, allowing the entire intrarenal collecting system to be visualized in a high percentage of patients.

URETERAL DILATION

Many smaller flexible or rigid instruments may be passed without prior dilation depending on the size of the ureter. Although most orifices are approximately 3 mm in size, some are smaller owing to anatomic variations. Because the size is not predictable, most authorities routinely dilate before a ureteroscopic procedure. Dilation expands the safety margin as the ureteroscopes are passed, and it allows larger fragments of calculi to be removed. Dilation to No. 14 or 15 Fr is sufficient to allow passage of the operating instruments, and thus far, all available experimental and clinical evidence suggest that dilation to this size has no detrimental effect on the structure or function of the orifice (Greene, 1944; Ford et al, 1984a; Huffman and Bagley, 1988).

Methods of Subacute or Passive Dilation of the Ureter

In 1980, Perez-Castro and Martinez-Pineiro described placing a ureteral catheter in the lumen of the ureter 24 hours before the planned ureteroscopic procedure. This was one of the early reports of successful ureteroscopy, and in these patients, the ureter was sufficiently dilated to accept the rigid ureteroscope. If the procedure is being done for stone removal, the catheter is passed to a level above the obstructing calculus to relieve ureteral colic and drain the upper urinary tract. The catheter is secured to a Foley catheter passed into the bladder and left in place for 1 to 3 days depending on the patient's condition and the timing of the ureteroscopic procedure.

An internal ureteral stent may also be employed for passive dilation of the ureter before ureteroscopy. A double-pigtail or double-J stent offers the advantage of being internalized with decreased risk of bacterial contamination when compared with a standard ureteral catheter.

There are several disadvantages of this technique. The major disadvantage is that it makes the ureteroscopic procedure a two-stage procedure with added cost and time for the patient. In addition, the presence of the foreign body in the ureter and bladder does lead to mucosal inflammation and an added risk of urinary tract infection. Passive dilation should not be used when diagnostic ureteroscopy is being performed. The catheter or stent may cause urothelial damage or inflammation and thereby hinder the success of the ureteroscopic procedure.

Methods of Acute Dilation of the Ureter

There are many acceptable methods of acute cystoscopic dilation for ureteroscopy that have been proven by use in large series of patients. These include (1) dilation with successively larger ureteral catheters (Bagley, 1988b), (2) passage of metal bougies, and (3) use of a balloon dilating catheter. Passage of progressively larger ureteral catheters or the cone-shaped metal bougies is done without prior placement of a floppy-tipped guide wire, whereas dilation with fascial dilators, olive-shaped bougies, or balloon dilating catheters is performed after positioning a guide wire in the ureter. Using a dilating method over a prepositioned guide wire has been safest and most satisfactory. Although somewhat more cumbersome than passing a dilator directly, there are fewer false passages and intramural ureteral perforations with this method.

BALLOON DILATION

The successful use of polyethylene balloons for transluminal dilation of arterial narrowings stimulated interest for their use in other areas of medicine. Most recently, these balloons have been used to dilate the ureteral orifice and intramural ureter to facilitate ureteroscopy (Huffman et al, 1983a; Huffman and Bagley, 1988). The advantage of the angioplasty-type balloon is that it provides controlled dilation by radially distributed pressure to a defined length of ureter. The expansion of this balloon is controlled by hand inflation to a predetermined maximum balloon diameter.

Instrumentation

Standard cystoscopes are used for balloon dilation of the ureteral orifice and intramural tunnel. The only requirement is a catheterizing bridge that accepts at least No. 7 Fr accessories. In addition to the balloon catheters discussed subsequently, an inflation syringe and radiographic contrast material (50% solution) are needed for balloon inflation. Along with a pressure gauge and fluoroscopic capabilities, the pressure gauge allows documentation of exact pressure used for dilation and ensures against inflation above the maximum pressure rating of the balloon. Fluoroscopy adds to the safety of the technique by ensuring guide wire posi-

Table 93–2. METHOD OF BALLOON DILATION OF THE URETER

A flexible tip guide wire is positioned cystoscopically and fluoroscopically in renal pelvis
A balloon dilation catheter is placed over the wire and positioned across the orifice and intramural ureteral tunnel
The balloon is inflated at a rate of 2 atm/minute until all "waisting" is eliminated
Once the balloon attains its complete cylindrical shape, it is deflated completely and removed

tioning, balloon placement, and adequate inflation and then deflation.

Selection of a Balloon Catheter

Many manufacturers offer balloon dilating catheters for ureteroscopy. Each is a high-quality product, but it is recommended to use several types and make an individual assessment. A properly sized guide wire accompanies most balloon dilating sets (0.038 or 0.035 inch). The most useful balloons for dilating the ureteral orifice and intramural tunnel have a No. 7 Fr shaft size, 70- to 80-cm shaft length, 5- or 6-mm balloon inflated size, and 4-cm balloon length. These allow satisfactory dilation of the majority of orifices for ureteroscopy. A balloon with maximum inflation pressure of 15 atm is usually sufficient for dilation of normal ureters. Generally, less than 10 atm is needed. Occasional ureters (i.e., reimplanted ureters, scarred ureters, or strictured ureters) require high-pressure balloons for dilation.

Technique

The technique of balloon dilation involves passing a standard cystoscope into the bladder (Table 93–2). The orifice is identified, and the floppy end of the guide wire (sized ac-

cording to the requirements of the balloon catheter) is inserted through the orifice and positioned in the renal pelvis (Fig. 93–13).

The position of the guide wire is monitored fluoroscopically throughout the dilation process. Once the guide wire is positioned, the balloon catheter is passed over the wire and its radiopaque markers positioned across the intramural ureteral tunnel and orifice. The proximal end of the balloon is visualized cystoscopically as it exits the ureteral orifice. The distal end of the balloon cannot be seen, however, and its position is judged fluoroscopically (Fig. 93–14).

Once the dilating balloon is in proper position, the balloon is inflated. Generally a 50% solution radiographic contrast agent is used to inflate the balloon for it to be visible fluoroscopically. A screw-type inflation syringe works well. Inflation is carried out slowly at a rate of 2 atm/minute until all waisting of the balloon is removed. It is deflated completely before being removed over the guide wire. If the entire intramural ureter has not been dilated, the balloon is repositioned, and dilation is repeated. After the balloon is removed, the guide wire is left in place for the ureteroscopic procedure.

Dilation in the Supravesical Ureter

In some patients, dilation is required in a narrow portion of the upper ureter to pass the ureteroscope. Again a guide wire is passed through the ureteroscope, and under vision, a small balloon catheter is then passed over the wire and positioned through the area of narrowing. The distal end of the balloon is judged to be in proper position by fluoroscopic guidance. The balloon is inflated in a similar fashion as described previously while watching endoscopically. Ureteroscope passage is then attempted, and if it is impossible, further dilation is needed. The smaller balloons are fragile, and it is suggested that they not be inflated before passage through the instrument. If redilation is needed after the balloon has been removed, the balloon should be checked

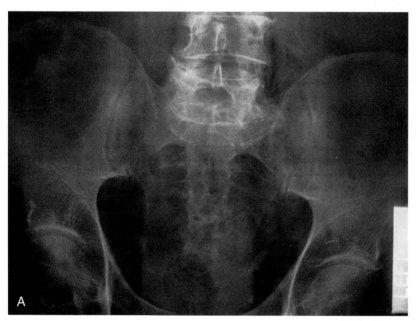

Figure 93–13. The ureteroscopic removal of impacted ureteral calculi is often difficult. The stones become imbedded in the ureteral mucosa, and often only a small portion of the stone is visible endoscopically. *A,* This plain pelvic radiograph shows bilateral large distal ureteral stones. It was impossible to pass a guide wire cystoscopically. Therefore, the orifice was gently dilated with a No. 8 Fr and No. 10 Fr metal cone-shaped dilator, which allowed passage of the No. 8.5 Fr rigid ureteroscope.

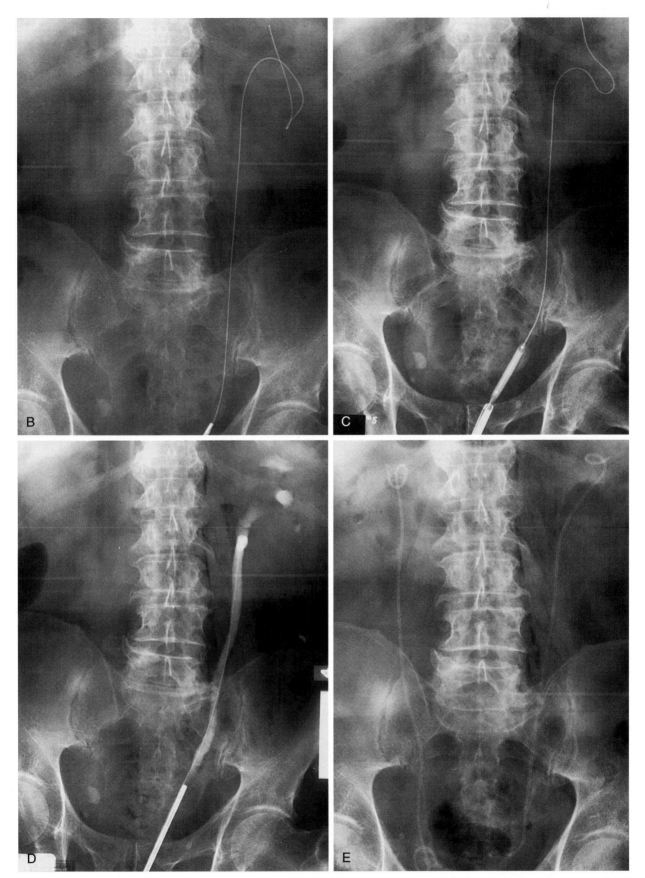

Figure 93–13 *Continued B,* Under direct vision, it was possible to pass a flexible-tipped guide wire above the stone and into the renal pelvis. The ureteroscope was then removed and the cystoscope reinserted. *C,* Balloon dilation was then performed by passing the balloon dilating catheter over the guide wire. The end point of balloon dilation is complete inflation of the balloon without any waisting or hourglass deformity. The operating ureteroscope was then inserted and the stone extracted completely using ultrasonic lithotripsy. Following removal of all stone particles, contrast material was injected through the ureteroscope. *D,* Free flow of contrast material into the left ureter and kidney without evidence of extravasation or obstruction. An internal stent was then placed over the guide wire. This exact procedure was repeated to remove the right-sided stone. *E,* A final radiograph shows internal stents in place bilaterally without any residual stone particles.

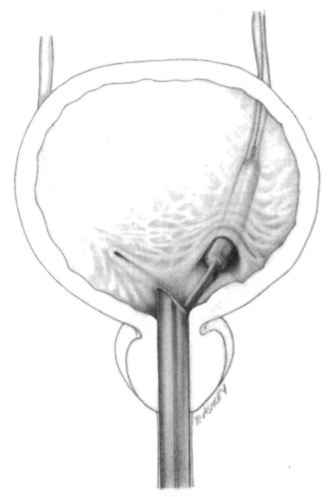

Figure 93–14. Balloon dilating catheter should be placed so that the entire intramural ureter and ureteral orifice are dilated. The proximal cylindrical portion of the balloon should appear in the ureteral orifice. (From Huffman JL, Bagley DH, Lyon ES: Ureteroscopy. Philadelphia, W. B. Saunders, 1988.)

for its integrity and remolded using one of the plastic molds that accompanies the balloon in its package.

Precautions

Caution is advised during several parts of this procedure. The initial placement of the guide wire is crucial to the success of the procedure. This must be done transluminally and not submucosally. The guide wire must pass smoothly into the renal pelvis and should not be forced. Its position in the pelvis is maintained as the balloon catheter is advanced in a coaxial fashion over the guide wire. If buckling occurs or the guide wire slips distally from its correct position, the end of the balloon catheter may perforate the ureter.

The balloon must be deflated completely before trying to advance or withdraw it. Moving a partially inflated balloon may avulse a portion of the ureteral mucosa. It is not unusual, however, to see a small amount of bleeding from the orifice after dilation.

If a balloon is used to dilate an area in the supravesical ureter, it is important to dilate the ureteral orifice first before passing the balloon to more proximal areas of the ureter. Not dilating the orifice may preclude balloon withdrawal after if has been inflated in the upper ureter. The balloon may not resume its preinflation diameter, and it may not be possible to pull it out through a nondilated orifice.

INTRODUCING THE RIGID URETEROSCOPE

The rigid ureteroscope is inserted into the bladder using techniques employed for rigid cystoscopy. Normal saline is used for irrigation. Once the ureteroscope is in the bladder, the orifice is identified and the instrument aligned with the anticipated three-dimensional plane of the distal and intramural ureter if it were extended from the ureteral orifice. In most instances, a guide wire has been positioned in the ureter after dilation. The ureteroscope is passed along the wire into the orifice and advanced through the ureteral lumen. It is often helpful to rotate the rigid ureteroscope 90 to 180 degrees as it enters the ureter. This maneuver enables the beveled tip of the instrument to "lift" the upper lip of the orifice and permit smooth insertion.

The ureteroscope is advanced in the ureter slowly while the operator watches endoscopically. Visualization must be clear; any debris or blood should be removed with irrigation using a syringe attached to the instrument. If there is any question about location of the ureteroscope in the urinary tract, a small amount of dilute contrast material is injected through the instrument while watching fluoroscopically.

INTRODUCING THE FLEXIBLE URETEROSCOPE

Several techniques have been used satisfactorily for introduction of the flexible ureteroscopes into the ureter and kidney (Bagley, 1988c). In most instances, this is done after dilation has been accomplished.

Guide Wire Method

A floppy-tipped guide wire is passed into the lumen of the ureter or left in place after dilation if this was required. Again, this may be a standard 0.035- or 0.038-inch wire or the slippery *glide wire*. The flexible ureteroscope is passed over the guide wire, which is back-loaded through its working channel. The instrument is advanced over the guide wire and into the ureter using fluoroscoping monitoring to ensure proper positioning and to ensure that the guide wire or instrument does not buckle in the bladder (Fig. 93–15). It is also advisable to empty the bladder before attempting passage to help prevent buckling of the flexible instrument in the bladder.

Flexible Introducer Sheath Method

Similar to the technique described by Takayasu and Aso (1974), a flexible guide tube can be passed into the ureter

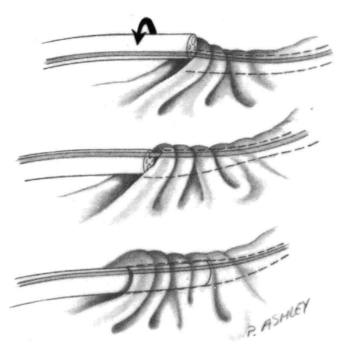

Figure 93–15. Guide wire introduction of flexible ureteroscope. A guide wire can be used to guide flexible endoscopes into the ureteral orifice. Care should be taken as the tip approaches the orifice. Because the channel is located eccentrically at the tip of the instrument, it may impinge on the lip of the orifice. The instrument should be turned to allow it to pass into the lumen. (From Huffman JL, Bagley DH, Lyon ES: Ureteroscopy. Philadelphia, W. B. Saunders, 1988.)

after dilation for the introduction of the flexible instruments. After dilation of the ureter, a No. 12 or 14 Fr flexible dilator with the guide tube as an outer sheath is passed into the ureter. The dilator is removed leaving the outer sheath in place. This acts as a conduit directly from outside the patient into the ureter for passage of the flexible instrument.

Direct Insertion into the Ureter

A flexible ureteroscope may be directed into the ureteral orifice under vision. This method allows manual advancement of the instrument; however, the possibility of buckling of the flexible instrument in the bladder with coiling of its sheath may occur. The most common use of this insertion method is in a patient with a cutaneous ureterostomy.

PASSAGE OF THE FLEXIBLE URETEROSCOPE INTO THE UPPER URINARY TRACT

Once the ureteroscope is in the ureter, the irrigating fluid (0.9% normal saline or sorbitol) is attached to the irrigation channel of the instrument and direct visual advancement performed. For the passively deflectable instruments, it is advisable to pass the instrument directly over the guide wire to the point where the stone or lesion to be biopsied is identified. Buckling and coiling of the flexible instruments may occur, and thus using a stiff guide wire for passage or a guide tube may prove necessary. At this point, the guide

wire is removed. Fluoroscopy is used to ascertain the position of the tip of the instrument, and contrast material is added to the irrigating solution to identify the ureteral lumen and renal anatomy. The tip of the instrument may be adjusted slightly by torquing the sheath of the flexible scope with one hand.

Advancement of the actively deflectable instrument is slightly easier than the passively deflectable design. With one's right hand, the tip of the instrument is deflected with the deflecting lever toward the center of the lumen of the ureter or calyx. The left hand is used to torque the sheath and position the tip after it is deflected. Again, fluoroscopic positioning is mandatory. As one moves to higher levels in the urinary tract, contrast material is again injected to ascertain the position of the ureteral lumen relative to the tip of the instrument. For endoscopic diagnosis in the kidney, each individual calyx must be examined carefully. Thus, fluoroscopy is used to make sure that the tip of the instrument is in the desired calyx.

PERFORMING PROCEDURES THROUGH THE FLEXIBLE URETEROSCOPE

Performing procedures through the flexible ureteroscopes requires a great deal of time and patience. The size of the irrigation/accessory channels is quite limited; thus the size of the accessory instrumentation is also quite small. As one inserts any accessory instrument through the flexible ureteroscope, the position of the tip changes slightly. The accessory instrument acts as a "stiffener" and tends to straighten the tip of the flexible ureteroscope.

Thus, fluoroscopy and constant visual monitoring are essential. It is important to have the appropriate accessory devices available before the procedure. These must fit through the accessory channel, and they must be long enough for the flexible ureteroscope. A tight-fitting rubber nipple is helpful because the amount of irrigating fluid that flows through the ureteroscope with an accessory instrument in place is quite small, and leakage makes visualization difficult. When an accessory instrument is in place, it is also helpful to have a mechanical irrigation device such as a hand syringe system or a blood pump to help ensure adequate fluid flow and visualization within the collecting system. A variety of accessories are available for intrarenal surgery using flexible instruments. These include stone baskets, grasping forceps, biopsy forceps, coagulating electrodes (both Bugbee and bipolar), electrohydraulic lithotripsy probes, and laser lithotripsy probes. Because accessory instruments change tip position when inserted, it is helpful to have them positioned in the field of view and ready for use before locating the stone.

REMOVAL OF LARGE URETERAL CALCULI

Some calculi may be extracted intact without the need of intraureteral lithotripsy. The ureteroscope is advanced toward the stone usually alongside the guide wire placed to dilate

the ureter. On visualizing the stone, a basket is advanced through the ureteroscope and used to engage the stone within its wires. A variety of baskets are available depending on individual preference and instrument channel size. Baskets are made with spiral and double-snare design with either round or flat wires. They are sized from No. 1.9 to 4.5 Fr.

Once the stone is trapped within the wires of the basket, it is withdrawn as a unit with the ureteroscope. It is important to watch this process endoscopically to ensure that there is no binding between the stone and the ureteral wall. If binding does not occur, the stone is removed from the patient. The ureteroscope may then be reinserted to inspect the ureter for evidence of damage and perform a retrograde ureterogram to check for extravasation or injury. An open-end catheter or internal stent is placed over the guide wire and left in place for a minimum of 24 hours. If binding occurs between the ureteral wall and stone, it is important not to pull on the basket any further because of the possibility of ureteral avulsion or injury. A method of intraureteral lithotripsy must then be employed to fragment the stone and allow safe extraction. The types of intraureteral lithotripsy include ultrasonic, electrohydraulic, laser, and ballistic.

METHODS OF INTRAURETERAL LITHOTRIPSY

Ultrasonic Lithotripsy

Stones that are approximately 5 mm in size can often be extracted intact. Stones that are too large to be pulled out intact must be fragmented. Ultrasonic lithotripsy techniques, successfully used in the bladder and with percutaneous approaches, may also be applied ureteroscopically (Huffman et al, 1983b). High-frequency vibrations of a rigid metal transducer provide the energy for stone fragmentation. The energy either fragments a stone completely or carves a path through the calculus, removing the smallest fragments by suction through its hollow central core. The transducer depends on direct contact between its tip and the stone to cause fragmentation. For efficient disintegration, the stone must be secured within a basket and held in a fixed position to provide countertraction. The ultrasonic transducer produces heat while operating. The probe must therefore be cooled throughout the disintegration process to protect against thermal injury to the ureteral mucosa (Howards et al, 1974). Irrigation through the ureteroscope sheath provides an excellent means of cooling and dissipating heat. The irrigant flows in the sheath toward the tip of the probe and then flows out the probe suction port. It is also preferable to negotiate the stone, basket, and instrument into the more proximal ureter, which is usually dilated and more capacious, allowing better heat dissipation.

Technique of Ultrasonic Lithotripsy Using the Rigid Offset Viewing Telescope

The offset viewing telescope offers distinct advantages over the standard method; however, special precautions are necessary. The size of the ultrasonic probe is reduced (1.5 mm) to enable simultaneous passage with the offset telescope. Thus, the size of the suction lumen within the probe is also reduced, and the frequency with which its lumen becomes clogged by debris and stone fragments is increased. When the lumen is clogged, the continuous flow of irrigant stops, and heat is allowed to build up along the probe. In this circumstance, the chance of thermal injury to the ureter becomes much higher. Therefore, patency of these probes must be maintained at all times during the disintegration process. The outflow of irrigant from the probe must be monitored constantly to ensure patency.

It is helpful to have the calculus engaged in a stone basket to provide countertraction with the ultrasonic transducer. This facilitates the disintegration process and then allows the fragments that are still trapped within the basket wires to be removed efficiently. In this instance, a basket No. 3 Fr in size or less must be used to allow simultaneous passage of the smallest ultrasonic probe.

The initial steps of engaging and positioning the calculus are similar to those used for the standard sheath (Fig. 93–16). Instead of replacing the telescope with the probe, however, the probe is applied directly to the stone while watching endoscopically. Again, irrigation is flowing through the sheath, and suction is removing irrigant and fragments through the probe. The stone is either disintegrated completely or fragmented sufficiently to enable it to be pulled down the ureter (Fig. 93–17).

A solid wire probe for transurethral ultrasonic lithotripsy is also available from Karl Storz Medical Instruments (Chaussey et al, 1987). Although this probe is smaller and somewhat more powerful, it does not have a lumen. Thus, fragments are not removed through the probe, and continuous irrigation for cooling is not possible.

Electrohydraulic Lithotripsy

A second method for fragmentation of oversized calculi is electrohydraulic shock-wave lithotripsy (Raney and Handler, 1975; Goodfriend, 1984; Green and Lytton, 1985; Huffman, 1988c; Willscher et al, 1988; Schoborg, 1989; Denstedt and Clayman, 1990). This method, using an electrohydraulic shock-wave generator and a coaxial probe, produces a shock wave that causes cavitation and fragmentation when directed toward a calculus. In conjunction with miniaturization of rigid and flexible ureteroscopes, the sizes of electrohydraulic lithotripsy probes have become smaller and are currently available in sizes No. 1.6 to 5.0 Fr.

A disadvantage is a potential higher incidence of damage to ureteral mucosa. Also, impacted calculi should not be fragmented by this method. The reported rate of perforation when using electrohydraulic lithotripsy on nonimpacted ureteral calculi is 10% to 15%. This rate would be higher if used on impacted calculi, which are often obscured by ureteral mucosa.

The advantages of this method are that standard rigid and flexible ureteroscopes can be used, the procedure is performed under direct visual control, and stone size is effectively reduced to allow subsequent removal or passage of fragments. The cost of electrohydraulic lithotripsy instrumentation is substantially less than laser lithotripsy, thus

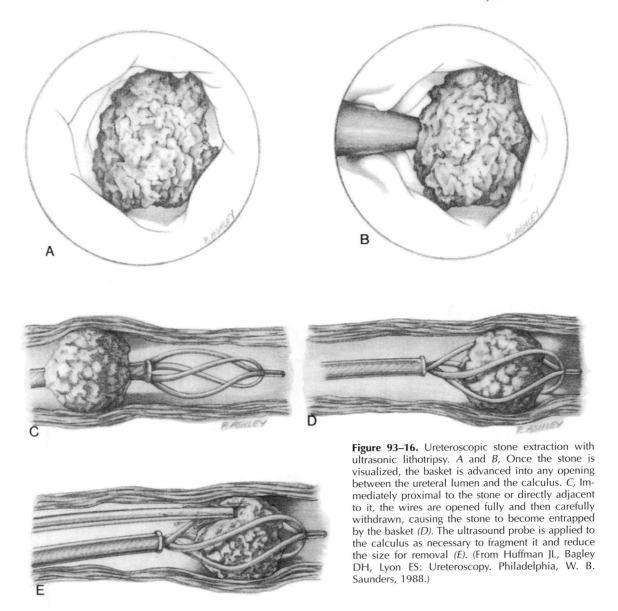

Figure 93–16. Ureteroscopic stone extraction with ultrasonic lithotripsy. *A* and *B,* Once the stone is visualized, the basket is advanced into any opening between the ureteral lumen and the calculus. *C,* Immediately proximal to the stone or directly adjacent to it, the wires are opened fully and then carefully withdrawn, causing the stone to become entrapped by the basket *(D).* The ultrasound probe is applied to the calculus as necessary to fragment it and reduce the size for removal *(E).* (From Huffman JL, Bagley DH, Lyon ES: Ureteroscopy. Philadelphia, W. B. Saunders, 1988.)

making its use preferable at many institutions (Denstedt and Clayman, 1990).

Technique of Ureteroscopic Electrohydraulic Lithotripsy

The rigid or flexible ureteroscope is manipulated into the ureter and the calculus approached using the same technique and precautions described previously. Once the calculus is visualized, the coaxial probe is advanced to a point close to the stone but not quite in contact with it. The generator is set on single impulse (not continuous), and the foot pedal is depressed. After stone fragmentation, the probe is removed and a stone basket inserted. All sizable stone particles are sequentially removed, taking great care not to apply excessive irrigant that might cause migration of the fragments into less accessible intrarenal locations (Fig. 93–18). Alternatively, smaller fragments (1–2 mm) may be left in place and allowed to pass spontaneously. Initially, it was thought that 1/6 normal saline irrigant would allow effective fragmentation with electrohydraulic lithotripsy. Subsequent studies (Miller and Wickham, 1984) have documented that normal saline is a satisfactory irrigant.

Laser Lithotripsy

The most recently introduced method for intraureteral lithotripsy is pulsed-dye laser lithotripsy (Watson and Wickham, 1986; Dretler et al, 1987; Dretler and Cho, 1989; Dretler, 1990). This method employs a small-caliber electrode (250–320 μ) and a pulsed-dye laser (Coumarin green). A laser light at 504 nm is emitted through a quartz fiber 200 to 320 μ in size. The light is absorbed by the stone, and a gaseous plasma forms on the stone surface. The plasma absorbs subsequent laser light, expands between the tip of the fiber and the stone surface, and generates an acoustic shock wave. This shock wave overcomes the tensile strength of the stone, and fragmentation occurs. There is a brief rise

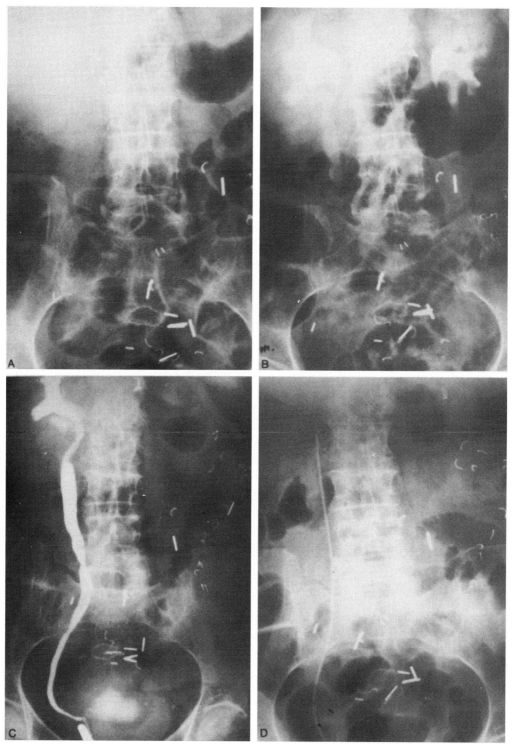

Figure 93–17. A 57-year-old woman who had previously undergone multiple intra-abdominal operations presented with severe right flank pain accompanied by a temperature of 103.5° F and shaking chills. A plain abdominal film *(A)* followed by an excretory urogram *(B)* were done, which showed obstruction at the midportion of the right ureter by a 10 mm × 12 mm radiopaque calculus. *C,* Initially an occlusion-tip retrograde ureteropyelogram was performed. This showed slight medial deviation of the midureter and a narrowed region just distal to the site of stone impaction. *D,* A No. 6 Fr spiral-tip catheter was passed beyond the calculus, and a brisk flow of cloudy urine was obtained.

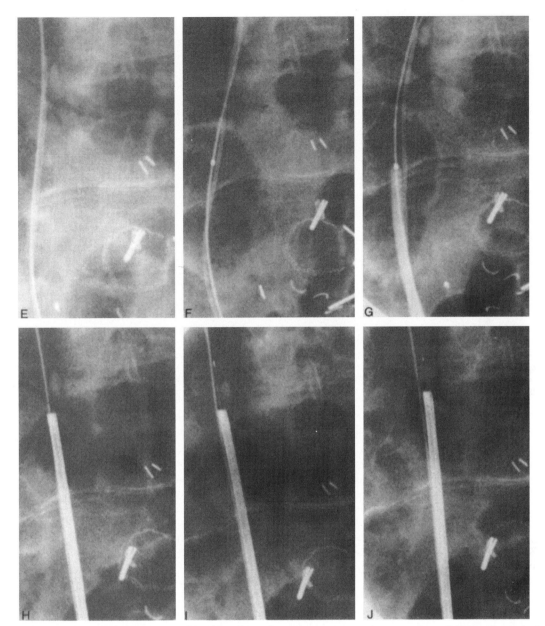

Figure 93–17 *Continued E,* Once the patient was stable clinically, endoscopic stone extraction was planned. This radiograph shows the poorly defined calculus near the vertebral body, with the tip of a spiral catheter alongside. A guide wire has also been passed cystoscopically beyond the calculus and is positioned in the renal pelvis. *F,* A 10 cm × 5 mm ureteral balloon dilation catheter was then positioned across the intramural tunnel and lower ureter. This was passed cystoscopically over the previously passed guide wire. *G,* Inflation of the balloon was carried out, while the maneuver was watched both cystoscopically and fluoroscopically. A 3-ml syringe was used to inflate the balloon to approximately 100 psi. *H,* The spiral-tip catheter was removed and the operating offset ureteroscope inserted. This radiograph shows the tip of the ureteroscope 1 to 2 cm distal to the calculus. *I,* A No. 3.5 Fr stone basket is passed through the catheterizing port of the ureteroscope and positioned above the calculus. *J,* The basket is opened and withdrawn to entrap the stone. This entire process is performed with visual control.

Illustration continued on following page

in temperature on the stone surface but not nearly enough to cause any thermal injury to the surrounding mucosa.

A holmium:yttrium aluminum garnet (Ho:YAG) laser may also be used for fragmenting ureteral and renal calculi. This laser has a wavelength of 2100 nm and has previously shown usefulness in tissue cutting and hemostasis. It is also effective in fragmenting all types of urinary stones but is capable of damaging the ureter if not directly applied to the stone surface. At settings of 0.5 to 1.0 J and 5 to 10 Hz, the Ho:YAG laser is effective at fragmenting stones without proximal stone migration and without damaging the sur-

rounding ureteral tissue (Sayer et al, 1993; Bagley and Erhard, 1995; Denstedt et al, 1995).

Technique of Ureteroscopic Laser Lithotripsy

All operating room personnel, the patient, the anesthesiologist, and the urologist must wear protective eyeglasses when the pulsed-dye laser is in use. An option for the urologist is to attach a protective eyepiece over the endo-

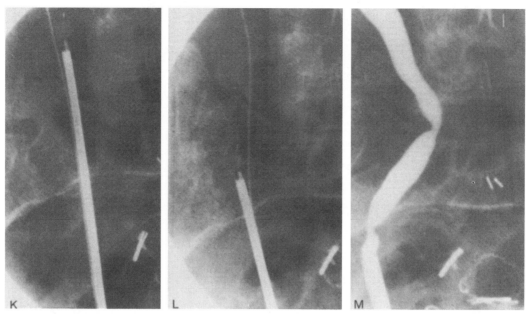

Figure 93–17 *Continued K,* This oversized stone could not be extracted intact; therefore, ultrasonic lithotripsy was necessary. Under direct vision, the ultrasonic probe was applied and used to fragment the calculus partially while it was held in position by the basket. *L,* The calculus could then be pulled partially down the ureter; however, another area of narrowing prohibited passage into the bladder. Therefore, further disintegration was performed at this level. *M,* The stone was removed and the instrument reinserted to check for any damage to the ureter or any residual stone fragments. A retrograde contrast study was performed. This film demonstrates the area of previous stone impaction in the midureter. A ureteral catheter was left in place for 48 hours. (From Huffman JL, Bagley DH, Lyon ES: Ureteroscopy. Philadelphia, W. B. Saunders, 1988.)

scope; however, eyeglasses are preferable in the rare event of breakage of the quartz fiber.

The stone is approached with any rigid or flexible ureteroscope that can accommodate the 200- or 320-μ fiber. Standard normal saline irrigation is employed. Once the stone is visualized, the laser fiber is passed through the endoscope until it makes contact with the stone. It is helpful to pass the fiber through a No. 3 or 4 Fr open-end catheter if the ureteroscope can accommodate this sized accessory. Alternatively the stone may be engaged in a basket and held in position for subsequent laser fragmentation. This method is preferable because it stabilizes the stone and avoids proximal stone migration.

The fiber must be in contact with the stone for effective fragmentation because of rapid dissipation of the laser energy. The pulsed-dye laser is generally set at 60 to 80 mJ of energy initially and increased if necessary for a hard stone (500–1000 mJ for the Ho:YAG laser). A repetition rate of three to five pulses per second is used for the pulsed-dye laser, whereas a higher rate of five to ten appears to be better for the Ho:YAG laser. Laser lithotripsy is initiated by depressing the footswitch while watching endoscopically. A perceptibly louder, high-pitched ticking sound indicates stone fragmentation. The tip of the probe is maneuvered to make contact with different parts of the stone surface as fragmentation proceeds. The fragments may then be removed with a basket or forceps.

Ballistic Lithotripsy

The Swiss Lithoclast is another method used to fragment ureteral stones (Schultze et al, 1993). This method of fragmentation is based on pneumatic shock waves that are trans-mitted through a No. 2.4, 3, or 6 Fr metallic rod. Shock waves are transmitted to the stone by way of the rod at a frequency of 12 to 16 per second. This procedure was used through rigid No. 8.5, 9.5, and 11.5 Fr instruments to treat ureteral stones successfully 95% of the time. Because of proximal migration, the stones are engaged in a basket before fragmentation using a technique similar to that described for ultrasonic lithotripsy.

URETEROSCOPIC BIOPSY, RESECTION, AND FULGURATION

The biopsy of abnormalities within the ureter or pelvis is somewhat awkward for the endoscopist. This is due to the relation of the instrument and forceps to the location of the tumors. In the bladder (a spherical structure), the forceps can be applied perpendicularly to the area being biopsied. The ureter (a tubular structure) requires the forceps to be applied parallel to the ureteral mucosa.

Biopsy is performed during the initial pass of the ureteroscope. If an attempt is made to examine the entire upper tract and then biopsy, the lesion may be traumatized or inadvertently avulsed during instrument passage. When the lesion is identified, the No. 3 or 5 Fr cup forceps is carefully advanced with its jaws parallel to the ureter wall. The intraluminal portion of the lesion is then grasped with the jaws and pulled free from the ureter using gentle traction on the forceps (Fig. 93–19).

The biopsy sample obtained is minute and should be placed into fixative at once. Special notation is transmitted to the pathologist so they are aware of the small size of the biopsy. A potential problem is losing the biopsy specimen as it is pulled through the instrument sheath. To avoid this

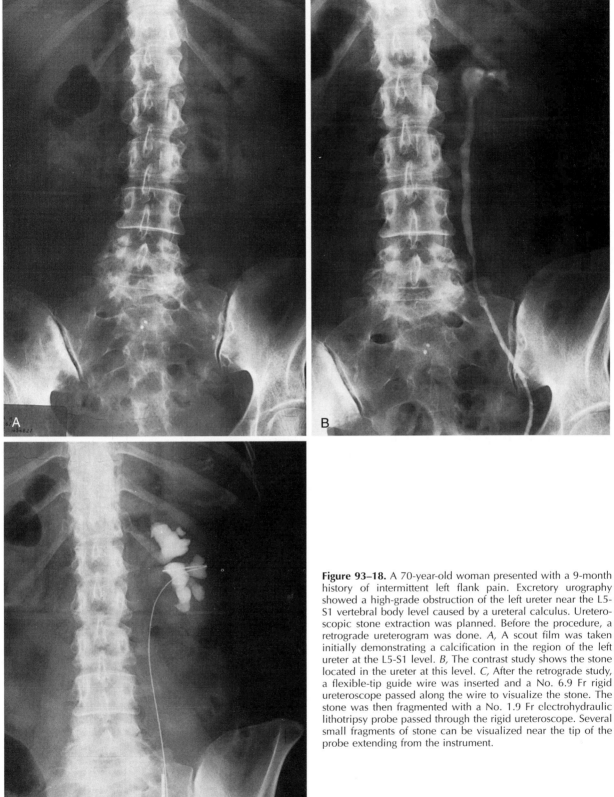

Figure 93–18. A 70-year-old woman presented with a 9-month history of intermittent left flank pain. Excretory urography showed a high-grade obstruction of the left ureter near the L5-S1 vertebral body level caused by a ureteral calculus. Ureteroscopic stone extraction was planned. Before the procedure, a retrograde ureterogram was done. *A,* A scout film was taken initially demonstrating a calcification in the region of the left ureter at the L5-S1 level. *B,* The contrast study shows the stone located in the ureter at this level. *C,* After the retrograde study, a flexible-tip guide wire was inserted and a No. 6.9 Fr rigid ureteroscope passed along the wire to visualize the stone. The stone was then fragmented with a No. 1.9 Fr electrohydraulic lithotripsy probe passed through the rigid ureteroscope. Several small fragments of stone can be visualized near the tip of the probe extending from the instrument.

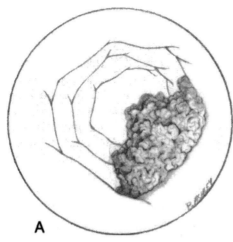
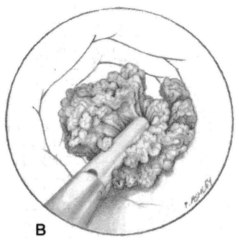

Figure 93–19. When a ureteral lesion is identified ureteroscopically, biopsy is performed during the initial pass of the instrument. *A,* The flexible forceps is extended from the sheath and opened parallel to the ureteral wall. *B,* Once the tissue is within the jaws, the forceps is closed and gently pulled from the ureter. (From Huffman JL, Bagley DH, Lyon ES: Ureteroscopy. Philadelphia, W. B. Saunders, 1988.)

problem, either the telescope is removed first, thus providing more room within the sheath, or the entire scope is removed including the forceps.

The technique of ureteroscopic resection is similar to that of pediatric resection using a pediatric resectoscope. The instrumentation is also similar to pediatric resectoscopes except for added length. The fine construction of the resectoscope loop provides excellent control over depth and location of resection (Fig. 93–20). Basic transurethral electrosurgery principles are maintained: using an irrigant such as glycine or water and using the appropriate setting on the

coagulation and cutting currents to provide the most effective surgery with the least tissue injury.

The actual mechanics of resecting an upper tract tumor are different than those in the bladder or prostate. Only intraluminal tumor is resected, and no attempt is made to take deep arcing bites into the ureteral wall. For this reason, the tip of the resectoscope is positioned directly distal to the tumor. The loop is extended beyond the tumor, and before activating the power, the tissue is drawn back toward the tip insulation or directly outside, the power is started, and the tissue is resected. This method helps to ensure cutting of

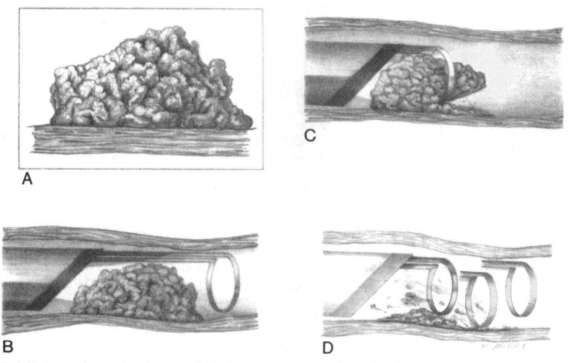

Figure 93–20. *A,* Ureteroscopic resection of a tumor. *B,* The instrument is positioned immediately distal to the lesion, and the resectoscope loop is extended past the tumor. *C,* Before activating the cutting power, the tissue is drawn into the sheath, thus minimizing the chance of ureteral injury. *D,* The base of the tumor and any bleeding sites can be lightly fulgurated. (From Huffman JL, Bagley DH, Lyon ES: Ureteroscopy. Philadelphia, W. B. Saunders, 1988.)

only the desired tissue and prevents injury to the surrounding ureteral wall.

After resection of all intraluminal tumor, the base of the lesion is lightly fulgurated with resectoscope loop. Smooth to-and-fro movements are used to cauterize the region of the resected tumor. Fulguration is also possible with a Bugbee or bipolar electrode. The probe is advanced through the sheath and gently positioned on the area to be fulgurated. With irrigation flowing, the coagulation current is activated. Irrigation is necessary to maintain clear visualization and to dissipate bubbles that are produced.

The operating instruments allow simultaneous passage of two working instruments, such as a stone basket and ultrasonic lithotripsy probe. In addition, a grasping forceps may be passed to secure a polyp or other lesion and a coagulating forceps inserted simultaneously to remove the lesion.

PLACEMENT OF THE URETERAL CATHETER OR STENT AT THE END OF THE PROCEDURE

In most instances, a temporary diversionary catheter or internal stent should be inserted after the ureteroscopic procedure. Many types of catheters may be used, including standard whistle-tip catheters, single-pigtail diversionary stents, open-end ureteral catheters, and double-pigtail internal ureteral stents. The easiest method for insertion of the catheter or stent is directly over the guide wire, which is positioned in the ureter throughout the ureteroscopic procedure. Fluoroscopy is used or a standard radiograph taken to ensure proper position.

The catheter/stent is left in place for a short period of time if no ureteral injury has occurred or for 2 to 3 weeks if there has been evidence of urinary extravasation. If extravasation has been documented during the procedure, a follow-up contrast study should be performed. Either an excretory urogram may be performed with the stent in place or, preferably, a retrograde study may be done at the time of planned stent removal.

COMPLICATIONS

The rapid development of endoscopic instruments for use in the upper urinary tract has expanded the urologist's ability to treat ureteral stones, tumors, and obstructions in these areas. Similar to cystoscopy and transurethral resection of the prostate, ureteroscopy and percutaneous nephroscopy have been associated with iatrogenic injuries. Perforations of the prostatic capsule and formation of a urethral stricture certainly occasionally occur after transurethral resection of the prostate, and after endoscopic surgery within the bladder, there is an incidence of urethral stricture disease and bladder perforation. Thus, it is not surprising that as one advances an endoscope proximally in the urinary tract into the ureter and kidney, similar types of complications and injuries may occur (Kaufman, 1984; Lyon et al, 1984; Biester and Gillenwater, 1986; Carter et al, 1986; Lytton et al, 1987; Schultz et al, 1987; Seeger et al, 1988, Sosa and Huffman, 1988).

There is a smaller margin of safety for endoscopic surgery in the ureter and kidney, mainly because of the smaller anatomic size of the ureter as compared with the urethra. As instrumentation is improved, with the addition of small-caliber rigid endoscopes, dependable flexible ureteroscopes, and newer methods of intraureteral lithotripsy, this safety margin should widen. Operator error, however, whether in judgment or in technique, can still lead to disastrous complications; therefore, it is necessary for the urologist to be familiar with the types of injuries that may occur, the appropriate means for diagnosing these injuries, and their treatment.

This section reviews the incidence of upper tract injuries and the possible etiologic factors in complications during endoscopy of the upper urinary tract. Treatment modalities for iatrogenic injuries are discussed, and various preventive measures are emphasized.

Incidence

It is fortunate that complications of a ureteroscopic procedure do not occur frequently. This is due in part to the caution taken by most endoscopists when performing ureteroscopy, with either rigid or flexible instrumentation. Injuries occurring at the time of the procedure may be recognizable acutely, such as a perforation or avulsion, but occasionally identification is delayed, as in the case of a ureteral stricture (Table 93–3). In a 1984 meeting involving original ureteroscopic investigators, the complication rate in 838 procedures was 4.5% (Sosa and Huffman, 1988). These complications were due to mechanical injury to the ureter in 71%. The injuries included intraoperative perforation because of the guide wire; the beak of an instrument; or an accessory device, such as a biopsy forceps. A false passage may occur in the ureter. This is a partial-thickness injury to the ureteral wall that does not extend through the adventitia of the ureter. An additional injury that is recognized immediately is avulsion of the ureter. This is without doubt the most severe complication.

Reviewing published reports throughout the urologic literature allows one to estimate the incidence of endoscopic injuries (Huffman, 1989a). These data compare the incidence of injury in 15 series totaling 1696 ureteroscopic procedures. Injuries occurred in 9% of all procedures, with 1.6% requiring surgical intervention. These figures are somewhat higher than the original reports and probably represent a more accurate assessment.

Etiology

When one attempts to define the causes of iatrogenic injuries, it is important to consider the anatomy of the upper urinary tract (see Figs. 93–3 and 93–4). The intramural

Table 93–3. TYPES OF IATROGENIC URETERAL INJURIES

Recognized immediately
Perforation
False passage
Avulsion
Delayed recognition
Stricture

ureter and the supravesical ureter have much more muscular support than the proximal ureter or the renal pelvis. Also the number of mucosal cell layers is substantially greater in the lower ureter (3–5) than it is in the renal pelvis (1–2). Thus, there is less likelihood of a complete perforation in the intramural tunnel or distal ureter than there is in the renal pelvis or proximal ureter. It is more common, however, to have a false passage in these areas than in the upper ureter or renal pelvis.

The size and flexibility of the instruments are major determinants of the incidence of ureteral injury. A mucosal flap may become elevated with a cone-tipped catheter, a guide wire, or the beak of the instrument (see Fig. 93–4). This event was more common with original instrumentation, which was larger and more difficult to insert. In addition, flexible instruments are less likely to cause a traumatic injury because they can accommodate to ureteral tortuosity, in contrast to their rigid counterparts.

The blood supply to the ureteral mucosa is also rather tenuous, which underscores the need to be aware of the possibility of dissecting the mucosa away from the muscularis, such as could result with submucosal dissection by the instrument (Chang and Marshall, 1987; Lytton et al, 1987). Coupled with factors such as prior radiation to the ureter, endoscopic manipulation may add to the incidence of devascularization and necrosis, with resulting stricture formation. Other possible causes for stricture formation after ureteroscopy include the initial balloon dilation, mucosal tears, extravasation, and thermal injury secondary to intraureteral lithotripsy. Certainly, stricture formation after ureteral dilation is a potential problem but has not been encountered often. In several large series of patients followed for at least 6 months, there have been no strictures identified because of the initial dilation (Lyon et al, 1984; Stackl and Marberger, 1986). Ureteral wall fibrosis could lead to stricture formation. Fibrosis may occur after a mucosal injury or urinary extravasation.

Electrohydraulic lithotripsy, ultrasonic lithotripsy (Howards et al, 1974), and laser lithotripsy all have the potential of creating a thermal injury to the ureteral wall with secondary stricture formation. Each of these methods causes a local temperature elevation that in the small confines of the ureteral lumen may lead to thermal injury. It appears that electrohydraulic lithotripsy causes the greatest temperature increase, and use of this device has been associated with the greatest incidence of ureteral injury.

Other major determinants of ureteral injuries are poor patient selection and technique. These are more difficult to define but do play a role in many untoward events of ureteroscopy. Proper indications for intervention must be followed and safe methods employed. Inadequate dilation of the orifice and intramural ureter or poor intraoperative judgment, such as forcing an instrument or catheter through a narrow area of the ureter, certainly may lead to injuries. Poor endoscopic visibility, if not corrected, may lead to injuries. If the ureteral lumen is not visible, the chance of a misdirected instrument becomes greater. Improper or inadequate ureteral dilation before the procedure also increases the chance of an injury. With the advent of less traumatic balloon dilating catheters, there have been fewer perforations of the intramural ureteral tunnel than encountered with metal bougie dilators (Huffman and Bagley, 1988).

Treatment

Fortunately, most ureteral injuries can be managed conservatively. The obvious exception to this is avulsion of the ureter, in which the treatment depends on the extent and location of the avulsion. If only the distal ureter is avulsed, a ureteral reimplant may be done with a psoas hitch or Boari flap. With avulsion of the middle or proximal ureter, repair becomes more difficult and may require ureteral substitution with a bowel segment, autotransplantation, or nephrectomy.

Conservative or nonsurgical treatment generally suffices for other injuries (Benjamin et al, 1987). Once a perforation or false passage is recognized, stenting of the ureter with an internal ureteral stent or ureteral catheter most likely allows complete resolution of the injury. If a stent or catheter cannot be inserted, it becomes necessary in most instances to insert a percutaneous nephrostomy tube, thus providing urinary diversion and drainage. Antibiotics are employed to ensure sterilization of the urine. The length of stenting or nephrostomy tube drainage is somewhat debatable; however, one acceptable approach is to divert for 6 weeks after documented perforation. Before removing the catheter, a contrast study is done to document complete healing. Ureteral strictures may be managed conservatively, with balloon dilation. In some instances, open exploration and repair are required.

Prevention of Complications

The reports listed prove that ureteral injuries secondary to upper tract endoscopy do occur. Several factors, however, may lead to fewer injuries (Table 93–4). One important consideration is appropriate patient selection for ureteroscopy after a thorough evaluation. The selection should depend somewhat on the operator's endoscopic experience. For example, one should not approach an oversized upper ureteral calculus and attempt a difficult ureteroscopic extraction without having previously gained experience removing easier, lower ureteral calculi. In addition, a wide selection of instruments allows the urologist to do the procedure more safely. An assortment of small-caliber and large-caliber rigid and flexible instruments, along with a variety of baskets, forceps, and wires, provides more options if problems are encountered. The most common cause of ureteral avulsion is trying to extract a calculus that is too large for the ureter. To avoid this, a method of intraureteral lithotripsy (electrohydraulic lithotripsy, ultrasonic, laser) should be available. Fluoroscopy is mandatory. Either fixed, overhead fluoroscopy or a C-arm unit is acceptable. Not only does fluoroscopy save time during all phases of the procedure, including balloon dilation, instrument passage, stone extraction, or stent passage, but also it adds to the margin of safety. For example, extravasation and guide wire malposition are

Table 93–4. PREVENTION OF URETEROSCOPIC INJURIES

Careful patient selection
Complete urologic work-up
Availability of essential instruments
Availability of fluoroscopy
Sound urologic judgment

JEFFRY L. HUFFMAN **2785**

detected immediately, allowing for quick intraoperative adjustments. Finally, sound endoscopic judgment is imperative. One must be able to judge when to advance the instrument, when to pull on a stone in a basket, and when to terminate the procedure if necessary. Most instances of ureteral avulsion secondary to overzealous basket extractions can be avoided by good judgment based on available information and adequate experience.

SUMMARY

Kaufman reported a severe ureteral injury after ureteroscopy in 1984:

The intent of this report is not to denigrate the splendid advances in nephroscopy and ureteroscopy, but rather to introduce a sobering message that the patient must be informed of the inherent risk of such procedures and that the urologist must be wary of the problems that might occur. Problems have been known ever since endoscopic instrumentation was first introduced, and every experienced urologist has had his share of problems associated with stone extraction and other endoscopic procedures. Traditional teaching in urology has been to eschew manipulation of stones in the upper two thirds of the ureter because the lumbar ureter is mobile and more easily damaged by instrumentation than the pelvic segment. Endoscopic visualization of stones in the upper ureter allowing accurate grasping of calculi would appear at first to provide an element of security heretofore unachievable, but urologists nonetheless should be mindful of the hazards of any type of stone extraction from the upper ureter. Urologists must be ready and equipped to handle emergencies associated with new instruments and techniques, and the patients must be apprised of the exigencies. "Caveat emptor" (buyer beware) could not be a more apt or timely maxim in our specialty.

Nonetheless, ureteroscopy has greatly aided many patients, and a large number of urologists have integrated this procedure into their daily practice. This procedure is no different than any other surgical procedure in that the urologist must be aware of the types of problems that may arise, the ways these problems can be prevented, and the type of treatments required should an injury occur.

REFERENCES

Abdel Razzak OM, Bagley DH: Rigid ureteroscopes with fiberoptic imaging bundles: features and irrigating capacity. J Endourol 1994; 8(6):411–414.
Andersen JR, Kristensen JK: Ureteroscopic management of transitional cell tumors. Scand J Urol Nephrol 1994; 28:153–157.
Anderson KR, Keetch DW, Albala DM, et al: Optimal therapy for the distal ureteral stone: Extracorporeal shock wave lithotripsy versus ureteroscopy. J Urol 1994; 152:62–65.
Aso Y: Use of flexible ureteroscopy to remove upper ureteral and renal calculi. J Urol 1987; 137:629–632.
Bagley DH: Indications for ureteropyeloscopy. In Huffman JL, Bagley DH, Lyon ES, eds: Ureteroscopy. Philadelphia, W. B. Saunders, 1988a, pp 17–30.
Bagley DH: Dilation of the ureterovesical junction and ureter. In Huffman JL, Bagley DH, Lyon ES, eds: Ureteroscopy. Philadelphia, W. B. Saunders, 1988b, pp 51–72.
Bagley DH: Ureteropyeloscopy with flexible fiberoptic instruments. In Huffman JL, Bagley DH, Lyon ES, eds: Ureteroscopy. Philadelphia, W. B. Saunders, 1988c, pp 131–155.
Bagley DH: Removal of upper urinary tract calculi with flexible ureteropyeloscopy. Urology 1990; 35:412–416.
Bagley DH, Erhard M: Use of the holmium laser in the upper urinary tract. Techniques in Urology 1995; 1(1):25–30.
Bagley DH, Huffman JL, Lyon ES: Flexible ureteropyeloscopy: Diagnosis and treatment in the upper urinary tract. J Urol 1987; 138:280–285.
Bagley DH, Huffman JL, Lyon ES, McNamara T: Endoscopic ureteropyelostomy: Opening the obliterated ureteropelvic junction with nephroscopy and flexible ureteropyeloscopy. J Urol 1985; 133:462.
Bakke A, Ulvik NM: Ureterorenoscopy in pregnancy. Scand J Urol Nephrol 1988; 110(suppl):243–244.
Benjamin JC, Donaldson PJ, Hill JT: Ureteric perforation after ureteroscopy—conservative management. Urology 1987; 29:623–624.
Biester R, Gillenwater JY: Complications following ureteroscopy. J Urol 1986; 136:380.
Blute ML, Segura JW, Patterson DE: Ureteroscopy. J Urol 1988; 139:510–512.
Boline GB, Belis JA: Outpatient fragmentation of ureteral calculi with mini-ureteroscopes and laser lithotripsy. J Endourol 1994; 8:341–343.
Bulger RE: The urinary system. In Weiss L, ed: Histology—Cell and Tissue Biology. New York, Elsevier Biomedical, 1983, pp 869–913.
Bush IM, Goldberg E, Javadpour N, et al: Ureteroscopy and renoscopy: A preliminary report. Chicago Med School Q 1970; 30:46.
Carter S St. C, Cox R, Wickham JEA: Complications associated with ureteroscopy. Br J Urol 1986; 58:625–628.
Cass AS, Smith CS, Gleich P: Management of urinary calculi in pregnancy. Urology 1986; 28:370–372.
Chang R, Marshall FF: Management of ureteroscopic injuries. J Urol 1987; 137:1132–1135.
Chaussey C, Fuchs G, Kahn R, et al: Transurethral ultrasonic ureterolithotripsy using a solid wire probe. Urology 1987; 29:531–532.
Clayman RV, Basler JW, Kavoussi L, Picus DD: Ureteronephroscopic endopyelotomy. J Urol 1990; 144:246–252.
Coptcoat MJ, Webb DR, Kellett MJ, et al: The treatment of 100 consecutive patients with ureteral calculi in a British Stone Center. J Urol 1987; 137:1122–1123.
Davis JE, Hagedoorn JP, Bergmann LL: Anatomy of the ureter. In Bergmann H, ed: The Ureter. New York, Springer-Verlag, 1981, pp 55–70.
Denstedt JD, Clayman RV: Electrohydraulic lithotripsy of renal and ureteral calculi. J Urol 1990; 143:13.
Denstedt JD, Razvi HA, Sales JL, Eberwein PM: Preliminary experience with Holmium:YAG laser lithotripsy. J Endourol 1995; 9:255–258.
Dretler SP: An evaluation of ureteral laser lithotripsy: 225 consecutive patients. J Urol 1990; 143:267–273.
Dretler SP, Cho G: Semirigid ureteroscopy: A new genre. J Urol 1989; 141:1314.
Dretler SP, Watson G, Parrish JA, Murray S: Pulsed dye laser fragmentation of ureteral calculi: Initial clinical experience. J Urol 1987; 137:386.
El-Faqih SR, Husain I, Ekman PE, et al: Primary choice of intervention for distal ureteric stone: Ureteroscopy or ESWL? Br J Urol 1988; 62:13–18.
El-Kappany H, Gaballah MA, Ghonheim MA: Rigid ureteroscopy for the treatment of ureteric calculi: Experience in 120 cases. Br J Urol 1986; 58:499–503.
Epple W, Reuter H: Ureterorenoscopy for diagnosis and therapy. Presented at XXth Congress Societe Internationale d'Urologie, Vienna, 1985.
Ford TF, Constance Parkinson M, Wickham JEA: Clinical and experimental evaluation of ureteric dilatation. Br J Urol 1984a; 56:460–463.
Ford TF, Payne SR, Wickham JEA: The impact of transurethral ureteroscopy on the management of ureteric calculi. Br J Urol 1984b; 56:602–603.
Gittes RF, Varaday S: Nephroscopy in chronic unilateral hematuria. J Urol 1981; 126:2297.
Goodfriend R: Ultrasonic and electrohydraulic lithotripsy of ureteral calculi. Urology 1984; 23:5–8.
Goodman TM: Ureteroscopy with pediatric cystoscope in adults. Urology 1977; 9:394.
Grasso M, Loisides P, Beaghler M, Bagley DH: The case for primary endoscopic management of upper urinary tract calculi: I. A critical review of 121 extracorporeal shock-wave lithotripsy failures. Urology 1995; 45(3):363–371.
Gray H: The urogenital system. In Goss CM, ed: Anatomy of the Human Body. Philadelphia, Lea & Febiger, 1973, pp 1265–1339.
Green DF, Lytton B: Early experience with electrohydraulic lithotripsy of ureteral calculi using direct vision ureteroscopy. J Urol 1985; 133:767.
Greene LF: The renal and ureteral changes induced by dilating the ureter: An experimental study. J Urol 1944; 52:505–521.
Hernandez D, Larrea Masvidal E, Castillo M, et al: Ureteroscopy: Our results and complications. Arch Esp Urol 1993; 46:405–409.

Hill DE, Segura JW, Patterson DE, Kramer SA: Ureteroscopy in children. J Urol 1990; 144:481–483.

Hopkins HH: British patent 954,629, and US patent 3,257,902; 1960.

Hosking DH, Ramsey EW: Rigid transurethral ureteroscopy. Br J Urol 1984; 58:621–624.

Howards SS, Merrill E, Harris S, Cohn J: Ultrasonic lithotripsy. Invest Urol 1974; 2:273–277.

Huffman JL: Ureteroscopic management of transitional call carcinoma of the upper urinary tract. Urol Clin North Am 1988a; 15:419–424.

Huffman JL: Preparation for a ureteroscopic procedure. In Huffman JL, Bagley DH, Lyon ES, eds: Ureteroscopy. Philadelphia, W. B. Saunders, 1988b, pp 41–49.

Huffman JL: Approach to upper tract calculi. In Huffman JL, Bagley DH, Lyon ES, eds: Ureteroscopy. Philadelphia, W. B. Saunders, 1988c, p 85.

Huffman JL: Ureteroscopic injuries of the urinary tract. Urol Clin North Am 1989a; 16:45–65.

Huffman JL: Early experience with the 8.5F compact ureteroscope. Surg Endosc 1989b; 3:164–166.

Huffman JL, Bagley DH: Balloon dilation of the ureter for ureteroscopy. J Urol 1988; 140:954–956.

Huffman JL, Bagley DH, Lyon ES: Treatment of distal ureteral stones using a rigid ureteroscope. Urology 1982; 20:574.

Huffman JL, Bagley DH, Lyon ES: Extending cystoscopic techniques into the ureter and renal pelvis: Experience with ureteroscopy and pyeloscopy. JAMA 1983a; 250:2004.

Huffman JL, Bagley DH, Lyon ES: Normal anatomy of the ureter and kidney. In Bagley DH, Huffman JL, Lyon ES, eds: Urologic Endoscopy: A Manual and Atlas. Boston, Little, Brown, 1985a, pp 13–18.

Huffman JL, Bagley DH, Lyon ES: Ureteral catheterization, retrograde ureteropyelography and self-retaining ureteral stents. In Bagley DH, Huffman JL, Lyon ES, eds: Urologic Endoscopy: A Manual and Atlas. Boston, Little, Brown, 1985b, pp 163–176.

Huffman JL, Bagley DH, Schoenberg HW, Lyon ES: Transurethral removal of large ureteral and renal pelvic calculi using ureteroscopic ultrasonic lithotripsy. J Urol 1983b; 130:31–34.

Huffman JL, Morse MJ, Bagley DH, et al: Endoscopic diagnosis and treatment of upper tract urothelial tumors—a preliminary report. Cancer 1985c; 55:1422–1428.

Inglis JA, Tolley DA: Ureteroscopic pyelolysis for pelviureteric junction obstruction. Br J Urol 1986; 58:250.

Kahn RI: Endourological treatment of ureteral calculi. J Urol 1986; 135:239.

Kaufman JJ: Ureteroscopic injury. Urology 1984; 23:267–269.

Kapoor DA, Leech JE, Yap WT, et al: Cost and efficacy of extracorporeal shock wave lithotripsy versus ureteroscopy in the treatment of lower ureteral calculi. J Urol 1992; 148:1095–1096.

Keating MA, Heney NM, Young HH II, et al: Ureteroscopy—the initial experience. J Urol 1987; 135:689–693.

Killeen KP, Bihrle W: Ureteroscopic removal of retained ureteral double-J stents. Urology 1990; 35:354–359.

Koonings PP, Huffman JL, Schlaerth JB: Ureteroscopy: A new asset in the management of post-operative ureterovaginal fistulas. Obstet Gynecol 1992; 80:548–549.

Kramolowsky EV: Ureteral perforation during ureteroscopy. J Urol 1987; 138:36–38.

Khuri FJ, Peartree RJ, Ruotolo RA, Valvo JR: Rigid ureteropyeloscopy. NY State J Med 1985; 85:205.

Lewis B: Discussion. Trans Am Assoc GU Surgeons 1906; 1:124.

Lyon ES, Banno JJ, Schoenberg HW: Transurethral ureteroscopy in men using juvenile cystoscopy equipment. J Urol 1979; 122:152.

Lyon ES, Huffman JL, Bagley DH: Ureteroscopy and pyeloscopy. Urology 1984; 23(suppl):29.

Lyon ES, Kyker JS, Schoenberg HW: Transurethral ureteroscopy in women: A ready addition to urologic armamentarium. J Urol 1978; 119:35.

Lytton B, Weiss RM, Green DF: Complication of ureteral endoscopy. J Urol 1987; 137:649–653.

Markee JE: The urogenital system. In Anson BJ, ed: Morris' Human Anatomy. New York, McGraw-Hill, 1966, pp 1457–1537.

Marshall VF: Fiberoptics in urology. J Urol 1964; 91:110.

Mikami K, Ito H, Kotake T, et al: A case of a ureteral polyp resected transurethrally. Hinyokika Kiyo 1995; 41:219–221.

Miller RA, Wickham JEA: Percutaneous nephrolithotomy: Advances in equipment and endoscopic techniques. Urology 1984; 23(suppl):2.

Netto NR Jr, Claro JF: Extracorporeal lithotripsy or ureteroscopy for the treatment of calculi of the lower ureter. Prog Urol 1993; 3:48–53.

Okamoto M, Inaba Y, Harada M: A case of multiple ureteral polyps treated with ureteroscopy. Hinyokika Kiyo 1993; 39:739–741.

Perez-Castro E, Martinez-Pineiro JA: Transurethral ureteroscopy—a current urological procedure. Arch Esp Urol 1980; 33:445.

Raney AM, Handler J: Electrohydraulic nephrolithotripsy. Urology 1975; 6:439.

Rittenberg MH, Bagley DH: Ureteroscopic diagnosis and treatment of urinary calculi during pregnancy. Urology 1988; 32:427–428.

Sayer J, Johnson DE, Price RE, Cromeens DM: Ureteral lithotripsy with the holmium: YAG laser. J Clin Laser Med Surg 1993; 11:61–65.

Schoborg TW: Efficacy of electrohydraulic and laser lithotripsy in the ureter. J Endourol 1989; 3:361.

Schultz A, Kristenson JK, Bilde T, Eldrup J: Ureteroscopy: Results and complications. J Urol 1987; 137:865–866.

Schultze H, Haupt G, Piergiovanni M, et al: The Swiss Lithoclast: A new device for endoscopic stone disintegration. J Urol 1993; 149:15–18.

Seeger AR, Rittenberg MH, Bagley DH: Ureteropyeloscopic removal of ureteral calculi. J Urol 1988; 139:1180–1183.

Shroff S, Watson GM: Experience with ureteroscopy in children. Br J Urol 1995; 75:395–400.

Sosa RE, Huffman JL: Complications of ureteroscopy. In Huffman JL, Bagley DH, Lyon ES, eds: Ureteroscopy. Philadelphia, W.B. Saunders, 1988, p 157.

Sosa RE, Huffman JL, Riehle RA, Vaughan ED: Ureteropyeloscopy: Pitfalls and early complications of ureteral stone extraction. Presented at XXth Congress Societe Internationale d'Urologie, Vienna, 1985.

Stackl W, Marberger M: Late sequelae of the management of ureteral calculi with the ureterorenoscope. J Urol 1986; 136:386–389.

Streem SB, Pontes JE, Novick AC, Montie J: Ureteropyeloscopy in the evaluation of upper tract filling defects. J Urol 1986; 136:383.

Suzuki K, Kisaki N, Takahashi T: Ureteritis cystica—report of a case diagnosed by biopsy under ureteroscopy. Hinyokika Kiyo 1995; 41(5):379–381.

Takagi T, Go T, Takayasu H, Hioki R: Small caliber fiberscope for visualization of the urinary tract, biliary tract, and spinal canal. Surgery 1968; 64:1933.

Takagi T, Go T, Takayasu H, Aso Y: Fiberoptic pyeloureteroscope. Surgery 1971; 70:661.

Takayasu H, Aso Y: Recent development for pyeloureteroscopy: Guide tube method for its introduction into the ureter. J Urol 1974; 112:176.

Thomas R, Ortenberg J, Lee BR, Harmon EP: Safety and efficacy of pediatric ureteroscopy for management of calculous disease. J Urol 1993; 149:1082–1084.

Valente R, Martino F, Manganini G: Complications and limitations of ureteroscopy. Arch Ital Urol Nephrol Androl 1990; 62:411–417.

Verlando JT: Histology of the ureter. In Bergmann H, ed: The Ureter. New York, Springer-Verlag, 1981, pp 13–54.

Watson GM, Wickham JEA: Initial experience with a pulsed dye laser for ureteric calculi. Lancet 1986; 1:1357.

Willscher MK, Conway JF, Babayan RK, et al: Safety and efficacy of electrohydraulic lithotripsy by ureteroscopy. J Urol 1988; 140:957–958.

Young HH, McKay RW: Congenital valvular obstruction of the prostatic urethra. Surg Gynecol Obstet 1929; 48:509.

Appendix A. RIGID URETEROSCOPY INSTRUMENTS

Ultrasonic Lithotripsy Probes

Karl Storz Endoscopy: 2.5 mm (hollow), 1 mm (hollow)
Richard Wolf Medical Instruments: 1.5 mm, 1.9 mm, 2.4 mm (hollow) (long and short lengths)
Circon ACMI: 1.8 mm (hollow)
Olympus: 1.5 mm (hollow) (long and short lengths)

Long Rigid Ureteroscopes

Circon ACMI

Sheaths (interchangeable): No. 10 Fr (0), No. 12 Fr (5)
Telescopes: 5-degree—straight
Integral sheath with Rigi-Flex 5-degree telescope No. 12.7 Fr (5.4/5 Fr)
Integral sheath with straight 5-degree telescope No. 6.9 Fr (3.4/2.3 Fr)
Integral sheath with straight 5-degree telescope No. 9.4 Fr (5.4/2.1 Fr)
Resectoscope sheath (long and short): No. 12 Fr
Electrodes: cutting and hook
Blades: cold knife

Olympus

Sheaths (interchangeable): No. 10.5 Fr (3) and No. 13.5 Fr (5/4)
Telescopes: 0- and 70-degree—straight
0-degree Vari-flex
Sheaths (Integral): No. 9.8 Fr (5.5 or 4.5/3.5) and No. 7.9 Fr. (3.5)
Telescopes: Angled (No. 9.8 Fr and 7.9 Fr), straight (No. 7.9 Fr), or flexible (No. 9.8 Fr and 7.9 Fr)

Karl Storz Endoscopy

Sheaths (interchangeable): 11.5 (4), 13.5 (5), 14 (6)
Telescopes: 6-, 70-degree—straight
6-degree—angled
Integral sheaths with 6-degree telescope (straight, angled, or adjustable):
No. 11.5 Fr (4)
No. 11.0 Fr (3.7)
No. 12.5 Fr (6)
No. 9.5 Fr (4)
No. 7.0 Fr (3.5)
Resectoscope sheath: No. 12 Fr
Electrodes: cutting and coagulation
Blades: cold knife

Richard Wolf Medical Instruments

Sheaths (interchangeable): No. 10.5 (3.5), 11.5 (5/3), 12.5 (5/3), No. 13.5 Fr (6), 12.5 (5) (continuous flow)
Telescopes: 5-, 25-, 70-degree—straight
5-degree—offset
Resectoscope sheath: No. 12 Fr
Ureterotome sheath: No. 12 Fr

Electrodes: hook, cutting, coagulation
Blades: stricture/scalpel, half-moon blade
Albarron bridge: 13.5 sheath only
Integral sheaths with 0-degree (No. 6 Fr and 7.5 Fr) or 10-degree telescope (No. 9.8 Fr or 11.5 Fr):
No. 6.0 Fr (3.3)—straight
No. 7.5 Fr (3.5)—straight
No. 9.8 Fr (5 or 3/3)—straight
No. 11.5 Fr (5/3)—offset
No. 9.8 Fr (5 or 3.3)—offset

Short Rigid Ureteroscopes

Circon ACMI

Integral sheath with straight 5-degree telescope No. 6.9 Fr (3.4/2.3 Fr)
Integral sheath with straight 5-degree telescope No. 9.4 Fr (5.4/2.1 Fr)

Olympus

Sheaths (interchangeable): No. 10.5 Fr (0), No. 11 Fr (3), and No. 13.5 Fr (5/4)
Telescopes: 0- and 70-degree—straight
0-degree Vari-flex
Sheaths (integral): No. 12.5 Fr (5.5 or 4.5/3.5), No. 9.8 Fr (5.5 or 4.5/3.5), and No. 7.9 Fr (3.5)
Telescopes: Angled (No. 12 Fr, 9.8 Fr, and 7.9 Fr), straight (No. 7.9 Fr), or flexible (No. 9.8 and No. 7.9 Fr)
Ureterotome sheath: No. 13.5 Fr (3)
Blades: stricture/scalpel (long and short lengths)

Karl Storz Endoscopy

Integral sheaths: No. 9.5 Fr (5.0), No. 11.5 Fr (5), and No. 14 Fr (6)
Telescopes: 6-degree—straight
6-degree—angled

Richard Wolf Medical Instruments

Sheaths (interchangeable): No. 10.5 (3.5), 11.5 (5.3), 12.5 (5.3), No. 13.5 (6) Fr, 12.5 (5) continuous flow
Telescopes: 5 degree—straight
5 degree—offset
Integral sheaths with straight 0-degree (No. 6 and 7.5 Fr) or 10-degree telescope (No. 9.8 or 11.5 Fr):
No. 6.0 Fr (3.3)—straight
No. 7.5 Fr (3.5)—straight
No. 9.8 Fr (5 or 3/3)—straight
No. 11.5 Fr (5/3)—offset

Miniscope

Candela

Miniscope: No. 7.2–11.9 Fr (No. 2.1/2.1 Fr)

Appendix B. FLEXIBLE URETEROSCOPES

Actively deflectable			
Circon ACMI	9.8	3.6	160
	8.5	2.5	160
	7.2	3.6	120 & 160
Olympus	9.3	3.6	100 & 180
	10.8	3.6	100 & 160
	12.3	6.0	100 & 160
Karl Storz Endoscopy	10.5	3.6	100 & 180
	7.0	3.0	100 & 180
Surgitek	11.9	4.0	100 & 160
Wolf	9.0	3.0	90 & 180
	7.5	3.6	130 & 160
	12.0	4.2	90 & 180
	10.5	3.6	90 & 180

94

ENDOUROLOGY OF THE UPPER URINARY TRACT: PERCUTANEOUS RENAL AND URETERAL PROCEDURES

Ralph V. Clayman, M.D.
Elspeth M. McDougall, M.D.
Stephen Y. Nakada, M.D.

Today, in urology and in many other surgical specialties, incisional surgery is being replaced by endoscopic surgery (Wickham, 1987). Disease access is being achieved using rigid or flexible endoscopes passed along natural pathways (e.g., ureter, urethra, vein, artery, esophagus) or through keyhole incisions, such as nephrostomy tracts (Fig. 94–1). Surgical therapy is being rendered with diminutive instrumentation capable of incising and excising tissue or concretions, using electrocautery and ultrasonic, electrohydraulic, pneumatic, or laser energy. Indeed, fully 70% to 80% of urologic practice has already become endoscopic in nature.

This chapter reviews the history and current status of percutaneous endosurgery of the upper urinary tract.

INSTRUMENTS OF CHANGE

The development of endosurgery in urology has depended on advances in three areas: **radiologic imaging, endoscopy** (rigid and flexible), and **miniaturization of endoscopic equipment** (e.g., electrocautery probes, lithotriptors, lasers).

Advances in **radiologic imaging** of the urinary tract have been essential to the development of endosurgery. Newer imaging techniques in fluoroscopy, ultrasonography, computed tomography (CT), and magnetic resonance imaging (MRI) have given the urologist the ability to locate and identify accurately various conditions affecting the upper

This chapter is dedicated to Arthur D. Smith, whose energy, enthusiasm, and creativity provided the initial ongoing impetus to the field of endourology, and to Louis R. Kavoussi, who continues to stoke the fires of surgical futures.

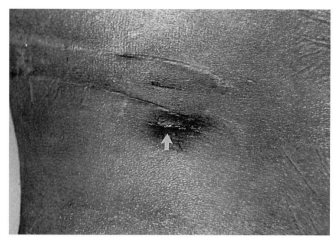

Figure 94–1. Flank incision in patient after two open nephrolithotomies compared with a minute incision *(arrow)* following percutaneous nephrolithotomy.

urinary tract and to access the kidney via either a percutaneous nephrostomy or a ureteroscope.

Of all the radiologic imaging modalities, fluoroscopy is the most important to the endourologist. It is essential to achieving accurate percutaneous access to the kidney. In addition, fluoroscopy is extremely helpful during nephroscopy. The intricacies of the intrarenal collecting system are such that a radiologic map is necessary to plan a route to a particular calyx, to help guide the flexible endoscope into a targeted calyx, and to document the completeness of a nephroscopic examination at the time of second-look nephroscopy (Fig. 94–2). The fluoroscopic view complements the nephroscopic picture because it provides an ongoing dynamic view of the renal collecting system and the location of the endoscope within the kidney, while the endo-

scope provides the visual detail of the immediate surrounding urothelium of each infundibulum and calyx.

In 1955, Goodwin and colleagues reported their initial experience with a percutaneous nephrostomy to drain an obstructed collecting system. Over the ensuing 20 years, marked advances in fluoroscopy and subsequently ultrasonography occurred such that by the early 1970s, percutaneous nephrostomy had largely replaced operative nephrostomy (Goodwin et al, 1955; Stables et al, 1978).

In 1976, Fernstrom and Johansson first used a fluoroscopically developed, percutaneous nephrostomy tract as a means of surgical access to the kidney for removal of a renal calculus. Currently the nephrostomy tract has been adapted as a means of surgical access to a wide range of upper urinary tract diseases: urolithiasis; strictures; renal cysts; calyceal diverticula; and, in some cases, upper tract transitional cell cancer (TCC).

These advances in imaging capabilities were contemporary with developments in antegrade and retrograde endoscopy of the upper urinary tract. For viewing the kidney by way of the nephrostomy tract, specific side-viewing **rigid endoscopes** were developed along with lighter and smaller straight rigid endoscopes. Even with the smallest rigid endoscopes, however, visualization of the collecting system was limited to the renal pelvis, ureteropelvic junction (UPJ), and one or rarely two major calyces (Wickham and Miller, 1983). This problem was subsequently overcome by the introduction into urology of **flexible fiberoptic endoscopes** in 1983 for performing cystoscopy. Shortly afterward, these flexible cystoscopes were used by way of the nephrostomy tract to examine the entire renal collecting system (Clayman, 1984). Within a short period of time, purpose-built flexible nephroscopes became available (Fig. 94–3) (Clayman, 1984).

To apply the percutaneous route and rigid and flexible endoscopes to the treatment of renal and ureteral disease processes, the urologist needed significant advances in in-

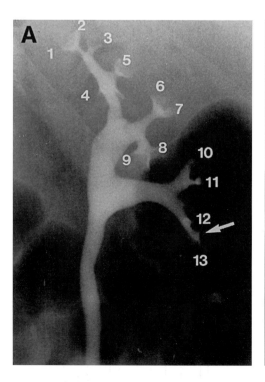

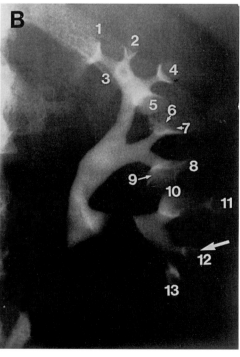

Figure 94–2. *A,* Anteroposterior view of renal collecting system. *B,* Oblique view of the same renal collecting system. This angled view of the collecting system helps delineate more of the calyces; specifically calyces #4 and #12, which are seen "end-on" in the anteroposterior projection, are "laid-out" in the oblique view and thereby more easily viewed.

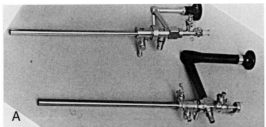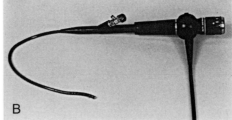

Figure 94–3. *A,* These rigid nephroscopes developed for nephroscopy are lighter than traditional cystoscopes. The tip of the endoscope is rounded to minimize the chance of perforating the intrarenal collecting system. The right-angle viewing system keeps the central portion of the endoscope open for the direct introduction of the rigid ultrasound probe. *B,* Purpose-built flexible nephroscope with an outer diameter of No. 15 Fr and a working port of No. 6 Fr. The tight turning radius allows for inspection of most or all of the calyces and renal pelvis.

strumentation. Specifically, **diminutive equipment** was needed for the fragmentation of renal and ureteral calculi and for the performance of intrarenal surgery. In the former case, ultrasonic, electrohydraulic, pneumatic, and laser probes were developed ranging in diameter from 4 mm (ultrasonic probe) to as small as 320 μ (tunable dye laser probe). In addition, a great number of instruments in the No. 1.6 to 3 Fr range were developed for the flexible endoscope to perform excisional and incisional intrarenal procedures. These instruments include No. 2 Fr stone baskets; No. 2.5 Fr, three-prong grasping forceps; No. 3 Fr biopsy forceps; No. 3 Fr retrieval forceps (rat tooth, alligator tooth); No. 2 Fr, two-prong grasping forceps; less than No. 2 Fr electrohydraulic lithotripsy probes; less than No. 1.5 Fr tunable dye and holmium-yttrium-aluminum-garnet (Ho:YAG) laser lithotripsy probes; No. 2 Fr electrosurgical probes with a 250-μ cutting tip; No. 1.2 Fr neodymium-yttrium-aluminum-garnet (Nd:YAG) probes; and No. 1.2 Fr potassium-titanyl-phosphate (KTP) laser probes (Clayman and Bagley, 1990).

METAMORPHOSIS OF UROLOGIC SURGERY

Bozzini's lichtleiter, developed in 1805, was the initial instrumentation in the realm of endoscopic urologic surgery. It was over 70 years before Nitze in 1877 could create a more practical, less cumbersome, and less dangerous endoscope for exploring the lower urinary tract. The modern age of rigid cystoscopy began in the late 1940s and early 1950s, with the development of the electrosurgical transurethral resectoscope and the discovery of the rod lens system and fiberoptic imaging/light-carrying technology of Hopkins (Desnos, 1972; Wickham and Miller, 1983).

During the past 185 years, there has been a steady transition in the **lower urinary tract** from open to minimally invasive endoscopic procedures. Today, many lower tract, open surgical procedures have been supplanted by their transurethral endoscopic counterparts: prostatectomy, cystolithotomy, suprapubic bladder drainage, urethroplasty, bladder neck contracture repair, and bladder tumor excision.

These "instruments of change" have also affected the treatment of the **upper urinary tract**; however, the transition has been more rapid. Indeed, in the past *decade*, minimally invasive endoscopic and fluoroscopic technology has replaced many formerly open surgical procedures: renal exploration for indeterminate masses, renal and ureteral lithotomy, nephrostomy, renal cyst treatment, drainage of retroper-

itoneal collections (abscess and urinoma), diagnosis and treatment of essential hematuria, and treatment of renal artery stenosis. Currently, other upper tract endoscopic therapies are being evaluated for the following conditions: UPJ obstruction (both primary and secondary); infundibular stenosis; calyceal diverticula; ureteral strictures; ureteroenteric strictures; and low-grade, low-stage TCC of the upper urinary tract.

The current generation of urologists is the beneficiary of the sum total of the aforementioned progress. Because of these advances, urologists have been able to replace the blood and bandage hallmark of the barber surgeon with the endoscope and Band-Aid emblematic of the minimally invasive surgeon. In this manner, urologists have been empowered to heal the disease with minimal harm to the host.

ACCESS: PERCUTANEOUS NEPHROSTOMY

Establishment of the percutaneous nephrostomy is the first step in all upper tract endourologic procedures. In the treatment of upper urinary tract obstruction, the nephrostomy can be placed through any posterior calyx within the kidney. As such, a lower-pole approach is often selected because it is usually infracostal, thereby precluding a transpleural route, and because it traverses the one surface (posterior-inferior) of the kidney that is not usually crossed by a major segmental renal artery. This is especially important in the patient with a pyonephrosis because contamination of the pleural space with infected urine can result in a life-threatening empyema. In contrast, in performing a percutaneous therapeutic procedure (e.g., nephrolithotomy or endopyelotomy), the precise placement of the nephrostomy site is essential to the success of the procedure. A **supracostal** puncture of a posterior calyx in the middle or upper portion of the kidney may be needed (Fig. 94–4) (Castaneda-Zuniga, 1984; Picus et al, 1986).

Patient Preparation

Before placement of a percutaneous nephrostomy, the urine should be sterile. In some cases, **because of the acute nature of the situation,** such as pyocalyx or pyonephrosis, a sterile urine cannot be achieved before emergency nephrostomy tube placement. Regardless, all patients should receive broad-spectrum parenteral antibiotics (most commonly, a

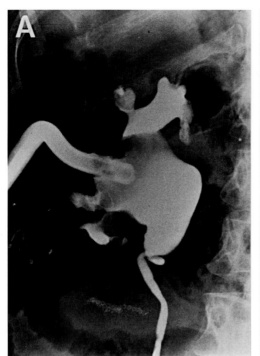
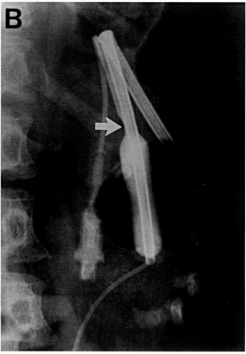

Figure 94–4. *A,* An infracostal nephrostomy tube has been placed into a middle posterior calyx in preparation for a possible endopyelotomy in this patient with a ureteropelvic junction obstruction. *B,* At times, the nephrostomy tube may have to be placed supracostal to provide direct access to the upper pole and the ureteropelvic junction area. In this situation, the nephrostomy tract may traverse the pleural cavity. Note that in this figure, there is marked angulation in this upper-pole, supracostal nephrostomy tube. This is the result of the tube striking the rib *(arrow)* repeatedly during respiration. To help maintain the position of this Kaye tamponade nephrostomy balloon catheter, it has been passed over a No. 7.1 Fr pigtail angiographic catheter, the tip of which is coiled in the bladder. In this patient, there was marked bleeding from the nephrostomy tract when a standard nephrostomy tube was placed; hence the Kaye tube was passed into the tract and the balloon inflated, thereby tamponading the nephrostomy tract and stopping the hemorrhage.

cephalosporin or a combination of penicillin and aminoglycoside) before the nephrostomy procedure.

Also, if time permits, any bleeding diathesis or uncontrolled hypertension should be corrected before the percutaneous procedure. Anticoagulants, especially aspirin, must be stopped. The bleeding time, prothrombin time, platelet count, and partial thromboplastin time should be normal before proceeding. The patient should be normotensive because this may decrease the chance of developing a perirenal hematoma or an extensive renal hemorrhage.

All patients undergoing a percutaneous approach must understand the seriousness of the procedure. Accordingly the patient should be made aware of the following potential complications: acute bleeding requiring transfusion (<5%); emergency embolization (<0.5%); possible nephrectomy (0.19%); delayed hemorrhage (<0.5%); septicemia (<1%); failed access (<5%); periorgan injury (bowel perforation, splenic injury) (<1%); significant loss of functioning renal tissue (<1%); and, in the case of an intercostal approach, possible pleural effusion with the need for chest tube placement (12%) (Picus et al, 1986).

Technique

The technique for performing a percutaneous nephrostomy depends on the **surgeon's preference** and the **circumstances**. With regard to the **surgeon's preference, a one-step procedure** refers to a nephrostomy and therapeutic

procedure done in the operating room under one anesthetic. A **two-step procedure** entails placement of a small, usually No. 10 to 12 Fr, nephrostomy tube in the radiology department followed by nephrostomy tract dilation and a percutaneous therapeutic procedure in the operating room. The **circumstance** of the case refers to one of four situations: drainage, diagnosis, ablative procedure, or reconstructive procedure.

Percutaneous Drainage Procedure

For the patient who requires a tube to drain a hydronephrotic or infected system, associated with distal obstruction, the nephrostomy procedure is quite straightforward. After giving appropriate parenteral antibiotics, the patient is moved to the fluoroscopy suite. The procedure is usually done using intravenous sedation and local anesthesia.

To localize the hydronephrotic system, intravenous contrast material can be given. Alternatively, if the use of contrast material is contraindicated, a 22-gauge Chiba needle can be passed under ultrasonic or fluoroscopic control, approximately one or two fingerbreadths lateral to the first or second lumbar transverse process (Young, 1986a). The needle is initially passed deeply into the flank, attempting to puncture the renal pelvis. Intravenous connecting tubing is placed onto the hub of the needle; an empty 10-ml syringe is placed on the other end of the connecting tubing. As the Chiba needle is withdrawn, gentle suction is applied. When urine appears, another syringe containing radiographic contrast material is connected to the Chiba needle; direct instillation of contrast material then opacifies the collecting system. Once the collecting system is visualized, a nephrostomy needle is passed across **the lower pole** into a posterior lower-pole calyx (see later). The needle is positioned approximately four to six fingerbreadths from the spine. A 0.038-inch Bentson guide wire is coiled in the system. Next the nephrostomy tract is dilated to No. 10 Fr following which a No. 10 or 12 Fr pigtail or self-locking loop (i.e., Cook-Cope) catheter is positioned in the lower-pole calyx. The coiled tip of the locking loop is secured with the retention suture attached to the catheter's shaft; the shaft of the catheter is then separately affixed to the skin of the patient's flank with two 2–0 silk sutures.

Alternatively, to facilitate the procedure, a backloaded single-stick nephrostomy system can be employed. A long, 22-gauge needle is passed through a shorter, 19-gauge needle, onto which a No. 6 Fr catheter has been backloaded (Young, 1986b). Once the collecting system is entered with the 22-gauge needle, the 19-gauge needle and then the No. 6 Fr sheath can be sequentially advanced, thereby establishing immediate access and drainage.

A variety of nephrostomy tubes are available. To drain an acutely obstructed collecting system, a No. 8.2 to 12 Fr pigtail nephrostomy tube can be used (Young, 1986b). The tube comes in two basic forms: nonlocking and locking. The nonlocking tube relies on the strength of the pigtail itself for retention (biliary urinary drainage catheter).

In contrast, the locking Cook-Cope tube (No. 8.2, 10, 12, or 14 Fr) (Fig. 94–5) has a thread running the length of the catheter. The thread exits the tip of the catheter and then re-enters the shaft of the catheter, just distal to the point where the tip is deformed as it coils to create a pigtail (see Fig. 94–5). After passage of the catheter into the collecting system, the tip is allowed to assume a pigtail configuration. The locking thread is pulled taut, thereby fixing the pigtail to the distal shaft of the nephrostomy tube. A knob on the hub of the tube is turned 180 degrees. This action locks the thread and hence the pigtail in place. This type of tube offers

excellent security; however, when removing a locking nephrostomy tube, the thread must be released by either returning the knob to its neutral position or cutting the catheter and thread just below the hub of the catheter. If the thread is cut, it is essential that the entire thread be retrieved along with the nephrostomy tube. If resistance is met in attempting to remove a locking nephrostomy tube, the plastic obturator from a "new" catheter should be obtained and gently introduced into the lumen of the "jammed" catheter to straighten the pigtail and facilitate removal of the catheter. Under no circumstance, however, should the plastic obturator be forcibly introduced.

Percutaneous Nephrostomy for Diagnostic, Ablative, or Reconstructive Intrarenal Procedures

For a patient requiring a diagnostic or therapeutic nephrostomy tract, it is extremely helpful initially to place a **retrograde ureteral catheter.** The retrograde catheter may be placed with a rigid or a flexible cystoscope. With a flexible cystoscope, the retrograde catheter can be placed with the patient already in a prone position on spreader bars. This approach, which is more simply done in females, decreases the procedural time by 15 minutes because the patient does not need to be in a dorsal lithotomy position first and then turned to access the flank (Clayman et al, 1987a). In addition, the prone position provides the urologist with two sterile fields: one for the ureteral catheter and one for the percutaneous nephrostomy (Fig. 94–6) (Clayman et al, 1987a). The retrograde ureteral catheter allows for opacification of the collecting system and provides for drainage of the collecting system should the procedure need to be stopped before securing a nephrostomy tube. In addition, the retrograde ureteral catheter facilitates subsequent endoscopic identification of the UPJ (Castaneda-Zuniga, 1984).

Initially a 0.035-inch, floppy-tipped, 260-cm exchange guide wire is passed. Once the tip of the guide wire is coiled in the renal pelvis, a simple No. 5 Fr angiographic catheter or a No. 7 Fr occlusion balloon catheter (11.5-mm balloon) can be passed over the guide wire until its tip is in the collecting system. If an occlusion balloon catheter is being used, the balloon is slowly inflated in the renal pelvis with 1 ml of dilute contrast material. The catheter is then pulled caudal until the balloon is at the UPJ. A Foley urethral catheter is placed alongside the ureteral catheter, to drain the bladder throughout the procedure.

After placement of the retrograde ureteral catheter and with the patient in a **prone** position, 10 to 15 cc of room air are slowly instilled through the retrograde catheter, thereby outlining the posterior calyces (Fig. 94–7). Alternatively, ionic (Conray 400, i.e., 66.8% iothalamate sodium) or nonionic (Optiray 320, i.e., 68% ioversol) contrast material diluted in half with saline may be used. Because the contrast material is denser than air or urine, however, it usually outlines only the anterior calyces and renal pelvis in the prone patient.

The percutaneous nephrostomy tract before an ablative or reconstructive procedure is most simply and accurately placed using a C-arm fluoroscopy unit (Fig. 94–8). As such, the following description applies to a **C-arm monitored fluoroscopic procedure.** With the C-arm in a straight ante-

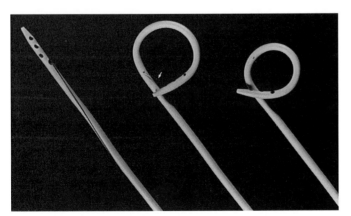

Figure 94–5. Locking pigtail nephrostomy catheter. Note the suture running the length of the locking catheter. When the catheter is in position, the obturator and guide wire, which keep the catheter straight, are removed. The pigtail that subsequently forms is locked in position by pulling on the suture where it exits the shaft, thereby drawing the tip of the pigtail tightly against the distal shaft of the catheter (arrow); by turning the plastic locking knob on the proximal shaft of the catheter, the suture is locked in place, thus securing the pigtail in its coiled state.

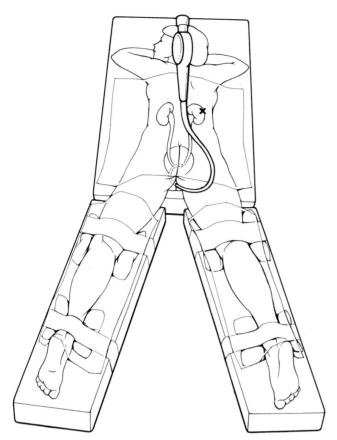

Figure 94–6. Diagram demonstrating prone flexible cystoscopy in preparation for passage of a retrograde 0.035-inch, 260-cm exchange guide wire, followed by removal of the endoscope and passage of a retrograde ureteral catheter (e.g., No. 7 Fr, 11.5-mm occlusion balloon catheter). The patient is lying prone on spreader bars, thereby allowing the urologist more direct access to the perineum because he or she can then stand between the patient's legs. Two sterile fields are simultaneously created: one at the urethral meatus and one at the planned nephrostomy site ("x").

rior-posterior position, a small skin incision is made directly over the desired calyx of entry. An 18-gauge nephrostomy needle is positioned in the incision and vertically aligned, perpendicular to the incision site, until the needle's tip directly overlies the needle's hub; indeed, on the fluoroscopic image, the entire needle should appear only as a radiodense dot overlying the air-filled calyx. The needle is advanced in a straight path, under fluoroscopic control, for approximately 5 cm into the flank, thereby fixing its trajectory. At this point, the C-arm is rotated to a 45-degree oblique or near lateral position. The lateral view of the needle images (i.e., "lays-out") its entire shaft and tip. The tip of the needle can then be clearly seen and monitored fluoroscopically, as it is advanced toward the calyx (Fig. 94–9) (Castaneda-Zuniga, 1984).

Some resistance to passage of the needle occurs, as the renal capsule is encountered and punctured. Once the renal capsule is pierced, the needle should move with respiration because its tip resides within the renal parenchyma. As the calyx is punctured, there is again a sensation of resistance to passage of the needle followed by a "give" or loss of resistance, as the needle tip pops across the urothelium and enters the calyceal space. The needle is advanced another 1

to 2 cm, under fluoroscopic control (C-arm in lateral or oblique orientation), until its tip lies in the center of the calyx (Castaneda-Zuniga, 1984).

Two other types of fluoroscopy units can be used for percutaneous nephrostomy: cephalocaudal movement and fixed (i.e., x-ray tube does not move) (see Fig. 94–8B). Both of these are stationary units and less satisfactory than the C-arm, which provides the physician with multiple views of the collecting system in a variety of planes. A retrograde ureteral catheter and opacification of the collecting system is performed as previously described. With the cephalocaudal or fixed fluoroscopy unit, however, it is necessary to roll the patient into a prone oblique position until the selected posterior calyx lies directly perpendicular to the x-ray tube (see Fig. 94–9A). The calyx is then imaged en face. The nephrostomy needle is positioned, tip over hub (it should appear as a radiodense dot), directly over the calyx. The

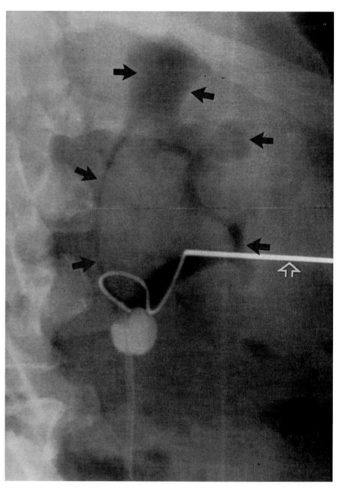

Figure 94–7. Air pyelogram. Air (10–15 cc) has been used to outline the collecting system *(black arrows)* in a patient with a complete staghorn calculus. Note how the air fills out the upper-pole calyces, which lie superiorly and posteriorly when the patient is in the prone position. A No. 7 Fr retrograde occlusion balloon catheter is in the ureter; the 11.5-mm balloon has been inflated with contrast material and pulled caudal to occlude the ureteropelvic junction. An 18-gauge nephrostomy needle *(open arrow)* has been passed into a lower-pole posterior calyx. A 0.035-inch floppy-tipped guide wire has been passed through the nephrostomy needle. The guide wire is just beginning to coil in the renal pelvis. A reasonable, albeit supracostal, alternative path to this stone would be via the uppermost posterior air-filled calyx.

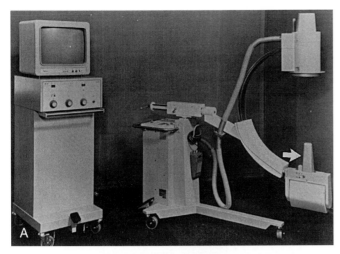

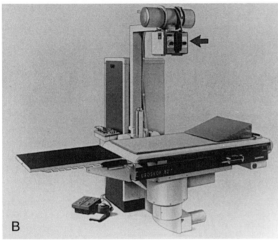

Figure 94–8. *A,* C-arm fluoroscope unit. The x-ray tube *(arrow)* is placed beneath the patient. The equipment has a last image hold and electronic reduction. These features can decrease radiation exposure to the patient by 40-fold and operator by 150-fold compared with an overhead system. *B,* In this stationary overhead fluoroscopy unit, the x-ray tube lies above the patient *(arrow),* thereby exposing the operator to significantly more radiation. The tube can be moved only in a cephalocaudal plane, thereby limiting the operator's ability to visualize the nephrostomy tract. The advantages of a C-arm system are significant from the standpoint of both operator safety and the improved accuracy provided by the unlimited views afforded of the collecting system.

needle is advanced 5 cm into the flank to fix its trajectory. If a cephalocaudal unit is being employed, the x-ray tube can now be moved until the tip of the needle appears to be farthest from the calyx. The needle can be advanced under fluoroscopic control until the tip is seen to enter the calyx.

Alternatively, if a fixed fluoroscopy unit is being used, the physician must rely on the aforementioned "feel" of the needle, as it passes through the resistance of the renal capsule and urothelium to enter the "free space" of the calyx. This approach is significantly more difficult and requires a higher level of skill (Castaneda-Zuniga, 1984).

Ultrasonography can also be helpful in puncturing the collecting system. This technique provides for continuous real-time monitoring of the procedure in multiple planes without involving any radiation. With the ultrasound transducer, the selected calyx can be located, and under continuous ultrasound monitoring, the tip of the needle can be

advanced directly into the calyx (Fig. 94–10) (Thuroff and Alken, 1987). Once the nephrostomy needle is passed into the collecting system, however, the remainder of the procedure is completed under fluoroscopic control.

After entering the collecting system, the next task is to secure a guide wire in the calyx or renal pelvis. The obturator of the needle is withdrawn, and a floppy-tipped guide wire (0.035-inch Bentson) or plastic guide wire (0.035-inch Terumo or glide wire) can be advanced into the collecting system and, if possible, maneuvered down the ureter (Suzuki et al, 1989). Alternatively the guide wire can be coiled in the renal pelvis or secured in the calyx farthest from the site of entry (i.e., for a lower-pole entry, the guide wire is coiled in the upper pole). The needle is removed, and a shovel-shaped No. 13.5 Fr fascial incising needle may be passed into the flank to cut the lumbodorsal fascia. This needle is passed twice. Just before the second passage, it is rotated so that the blades are 90 degrees to the plane of the first pass. This maneuver greatly facilitates subsequent passage of dilators because the lumbodorsal fascia has been widely incised by the No. 13.5 Fr device. Next, semirigid plastic fascial dilators are passed (No. 6, 8, and 10 Fr). A No. 8/10 Fr *safety wire introducer* dilator/sheath assembly is now passed. The dilator is removed, and through the No. 10 Fr sheath, a second guide wire is passed into the collecting system (Fig. 94–11). The No. 10 Fr sheath is removed. The second guide wire is fixed to the skin with a 2–0 silk suture, thereby becoming the *safety guide wire*. The remaining guide wire is now labeled the *working guide wire* because it is used for subsequent dilation of the nephrostomy tract (Castaneda-Zuniga, 1984).

Percutaneous access to the kidney may also be obtained in a **retrograde fashion** with the system developed by Hawkins and associates (1984) or by Lawson and associates (1983). In this approach, a No. 7 or 9 Fr guiding ureteral catheter is passed retrograde and positioned into the calyx of interest. A No. 3 Fr needle-containing catheter is then passed through the retrograde ureteral catheter. The 0.017-inch puncture wire needle is pushed through the kidney and through the retroperitoneal tissue, until it exits the skin of the flank. Once through-and-through access is achieved (i.e., urethral meatus to flank), dilation of the tract is similar to that for antegrade access (see later) (Lawson et al, 1983; Hawkins et al, 1984).

Dilation of the nephrostomy tract can be accomplished with a variety of instruments (Fig. 94–12). The semirigid Amplatz dilators or metal telescoping dilators are quite effective (Marberger et al, 1982; Coleman, 1986). Ireton (1990) has written about a modified Otis urethrotome to enlarge the nephrostomy tract. Balloon dilation of the nephrostomy tract to No. 30 to 36 Fr, however, seems to be the quickest and safest modality (Fig. 94–13) (Clayman et al, 1983a). The balloon dilator, backloaded with a No. 30 Fr Amplatz sheath, is passed over the working guide wire until the tip of the balloon catheter enters the calyx. The radiopaque marker on the balloon is positioned just within the calyx. The balloon is inflated with a syringe capable of developing pressures in the 10 to 12 atm range (LeVeen or power injector).

Once the nephrostomy tract is dilated, the next step is either placement of a sheath through which further therapeutic maneuvers may be accomplished or immediate placement of a nephrostomy tube for drainage. With regard to working

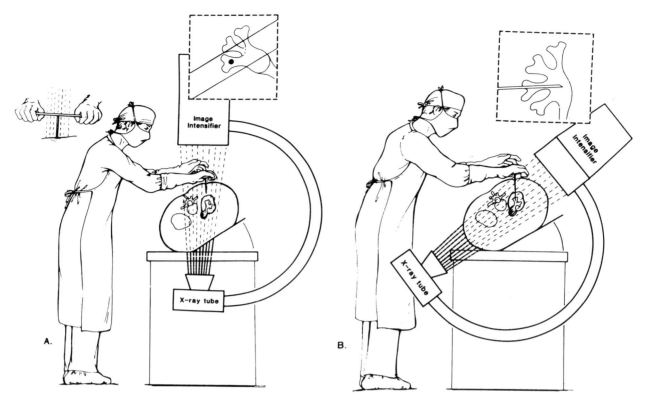

Figure 94–9. *A,* To facilitate a perpendicular entry into a posterior calyx, the prone patient has been placed onto a 45-degree radiolucent wedge, thereby rotating the desired calyx of entry until it is in a direct en face line with the fluoroscope. This is not necessary when using a C-arm fluoroscope; however, this type of positioning is helpful when using a fixed or cephalocaudal imaging unit. The nephrostomy needle is positioned over the desired calyx. With the C-arm fluoroscope in a direct anterior-posterior position, the needle should appear as a dot (i.e., "hub-over-tip" vertical position) on the fluoroscopy screen *(inset). B,* The calyx and needle are now viewed with the fluoroscope rotated to provide a 45-degree oblique view. As the needle is advanced, its tip can be clearly seen, and its entry into the calyx can be fluoroscopically monitored *(inset).* (From Clayman RV, Castaneda-Zuniga WR: Techniques in Endourology: A Guide to Percutaneous Removal of Renal and Ureteral Calculi. Chicago, Year Book Medical Publishers, 1986.)

sheaths, the urologist has many from which to choose. If the nephrostomy tract is being placed solely for diagnostic flexible nephroscopy or for antegrade endopyelotomy using a short rigid ureteroscope, the biliary dilator sheath assembly is sufficient. This allows placement of a No. 18 Fr thin-walled working sheath. Similarly, if antegrade access to the ureter is the goal, a No. 14 Fr ureteral access sheath can be advanced over a previously placed ureteral working guide wire until the sheath rests in the ureter just proximal to the site of pathology.

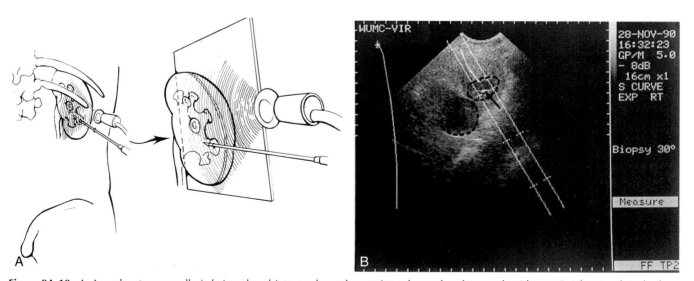

Figure 94–10. *A,* A nephrostomy needle is being placed into a subcostal posterior calyx under ultrasound guidance. *B,* Ultrasound study shows the needle *(arrow)* entering a calyx *(outlined)* of a hydronephrotic kidney. (*A* From Thuroff DW, Alken P: Endourology 1987, 2:1.)

For most cases in which larger instruments are to be used, such as an ultrasonic lithotriptor or the optical urethrotome, a No. 30 Fr Amplatz sheath is passed into the kidney either directly over the inflated No. 30 Fr balloon dilator or using the Amplatz coaxial dilator system (see Fig. 94–12). In the former situation, once the backloaded sheath has been passed over the inflated balloon, the balloon is deflated and removed. Alternatively the sheath can be positioned using a coaxial system. In this case, after balloon dilation, the balloon dilator is removed, and a No. 8 Fr Amplatz catheter is advanced over the working guide wire. A No. 28 Fr Amplatz dilator is passed over the No. 8 Fr catheter. A No. 28 Fr Amplatz sheath is pushed over its No. 28 Fr dilator, until the sheath enters the collecting system. The No. 28 Fr dilator is removed. In passing the large No. 28 Fr sheath, the tip of the sheath should just enter the collecting system. Attempts to put the sheath directly on the calculus may result in an anterior false passage of the collecting system. If desired, the entire dilation and sheath placement can be done with the Amplatz coaxial shear dilators, by serially passing dilators over the No. 8 Fr catheter; each dilator goes up No. 2 Fr in size starting at No. 12 Fr and ending at No. 28 Fr.

After percutaneous intrarenal surgery, a nephrostomy tube that offers excellent drainage, retention, and tamponade is requisite. This can be achieved with a variety of catheters usually of a No. 22 Fr size: Foley urethral, Malecot, Councill, and Cummings tubes. The Foley catheter can be passed through the Amplatz No. 28 Fr sheath; the balloon is inflated with 1 to 2 ml of saline, and the sheath can then be cut and slid off of the catheter. Alternatively a more sure placement of the nephrostomy tube can be obtained with the modified Malecot or Councill catheter. The Malecot catheter has an introducer that collapses the wings of the catheter to facilitate its passage; it also has an end hole so that the catheter can be passed over a pre-existing guide wire.

Likewise, the Councill catheter, with its precut end hole, can be passed directly over a guide wire, and the balloon

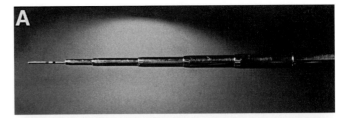

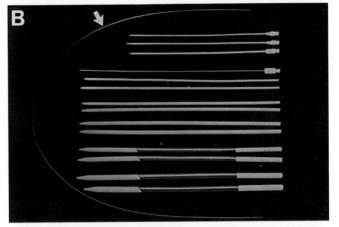

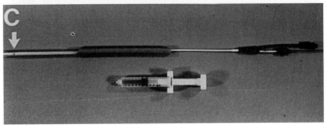

Figure 94–12. *A,* Metal telescoping dilators. *B,* Semirigid fascial dilators: coaxial system. After dilating to No. 10 Fr, each of the remaining dilators is passed over the No. 8 Fr, long Amplatz catheter *(arrow). C,* A 10-mm nephrostomy tract dilating balloon *(arrow)* backloaded with a 10-mm Amplatz sheath. A LeVeen high-pressure inflation syringe is in the foreground.

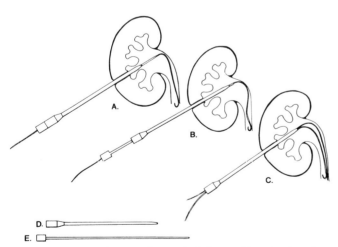

Figure 94–11. Introducer catheter. *A,* Safety guide wire introducer (Amplatz type with No. 8 Fr dilator and a No. 10 Fr sheath) is passed over the initial guide wire. *B,* The No. 8 Fr obturator is removed from the No. 10 Fr sheath. *C,* The second (i.e., "working") wire is introduced through the No. 10 Fr sheath of the introducer catheter. *D,* The No. 10 Fr sheath of the introducer catheter. *E,* No. 8 Fr obturator of the introducer catheter. (From Clayman RV, Castaneda-Zuniga WR: Techniques in Endourology: A Guide to Percutaneous Removal of Renal and Ureteral Calculi. Chicago, Year Book Medical Publishers, 1986.)

can be inflated with 1 to 2 ml of saline once the tip of the catheter has been advanced into the renal pelvis. To secure the Councill catheter further in the collecting system, it can be passed over a No. 5 or 7.1 Fr straight or pigtail catheter that has in turn been passed over a pre-existing through-and-through guide wire or a guide wire that has been passed antegrade and coiled in the bladder. The No. 5 or 7.1 Fr catheter serves as an antegrade ureteral catheter. The Councill catheter is secured to the antegrade ureteral catheter with a side arm adapter, the end of which fits tightly into the end of the Councill catheter. The upper portion of the side arm adapter can be turned until it locks tightly onto the No. 5 or 7.1 Fr catheter. This arrangement provides several means of holding the Councill nephrostomy tube in the system: the balloon of the nephrostomy tube; the side arm adapter, which fixes the nephrostomy tube to the antegrade pigtail ureteral catheter; and the pigtail coil of the tip of the No. 7.1 Fr catheter, which helps to keep the catheter in the bladder (Fig. 94–14). Two ureteral connectors are then used: One is affixed to the side port of the side arm adaptor, thereby draining the renal pelvis, whereas the other is passed over the antegrade ureteral catheter and affixed to the straight end

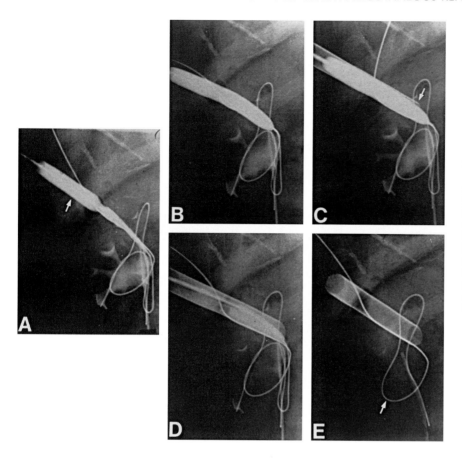

Figure 94–13. *A,* A 10-mm dilating balloon *(arrow)* is being inflated in an upper-pole posterior, supracostal nephrostomy tract. *B,* The balloon has been fully inflated. *C,* Over the balloon, a No. 30 Fr Amplatz nephrostomy sheath *(arrow)* is advanced. *D,* After advancing the No. 30 Fr sheath into the collecting system, the nephrostomy balloon is deflated and removed. *E,* The No. 30 Fr sheath lies in the collecting system and provides a direct conduit to the kidney for passage of the nephroscope. The *safety* guide wire *(arrow)* lies *outside* of the Amplatz sheath. It is sewn to the skin with a 2–0 silk suture.

of the side arm adapter, thereby draining the bladder. A tongue blade is taped at the juncture of the ureteral connectors, side arm adapter (where the No. 7.1 Fr pigtail exits), and proximal end of the Councill catheter. This maneuver precludes any pulling on the connectors, which could dislodge the ureteral catheter. With this arrangement, the Foley catheter can be removed from the bladder because all bladder contents are drained antegrade by way of the pigtail catheter. Patients should be informed that they will likely not void per urethra with this catheter setup; likewise, antispasmotics such as oral oxybutynin or preferably belladonna and opiate suppositories should be ordered to relieve any bladder spasms resulting from the antegrade stent. With this setup, tube dislodgment is distinctly unusual, and loss of access to the collecting system, in the authors' experience, has yet to occur.

Lastly, a one-piece nephrostent can be placed. In this adaptation of a Cummings tube, the antegrade ureteral catheter is an extension of the nephrostomy portion of the catheter. When these tubes are used, the tip usually does not enter the bladder. Although this precludes any bladder spasms, transient obstruction because of tip-induced distal ureteral edema may then occur when the nephrostent is removed.

All nephrostomy tubes are secured to the flank. This step can be done by placing a plastic disc and tape around the nephrostomy tube as it exits the flank or by sewing the tube to the flank with one or preferably two 0 silk sutures. The suture method is recommended. A dressing of gauze sponges covered by laparotomy pads is placed. The dressing can be secured most simply with one large piece of adhesive cut to cover the entire dressing and flank (Cover-Roll), or it can be

secured with Montgomery straps. Dense layers of adhesive tape are discouraged. They can cause marked skin irritation or blisters on removal.

With regard to nephrostomy tubes, in the authors' opinion, **the one type of catheter that must always be immediately available to the urologist performing a percutaneous procedure is a No. 14 Fr Kaye tamponade balloon catheter** (Fig. 94–15) (Kaye and Clayman, 1986). This particular tube is essential when brisk hemorrhage is encountered. Once placed and inflated to its full No. 36 Fr size, it provides immediate, effective tamponade of the tract and satisfactory drainage of the collecting system. As with the previously described nephrostomy tube, it is recommended to pass this catheter over a pre-existing **multiholed** No. 5 or 7 Fr antegrade ureteral catheter and to use a side arm adapter to secure the hub of the Kaye catheter to the ureteral catheter. To preclude kinking, the tube as it exits the skin should be smoothly draped over two rolls of Kerlix on its lateral surface and should be supported by three rolls of Kerlix on its medial surface. Usually, 2 days later, the Kaye tube can be deflated under fluoroscopic control. If there is no nephrostomy tract bleeding, it can be fluoroscopically exchanged for a more comfortable and smaller standard nephrostomy tube (Kaye and Clayman, 1986; Kerbl et al, 1994b).

Results and Complications

Using the aforementioned antegrade or retrograde approaches, percutaneous drainage or access to the kidney can be achieved in more than 90% of patients (Stables et al,

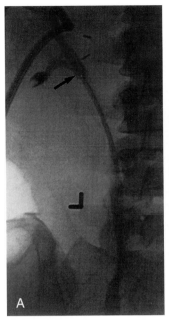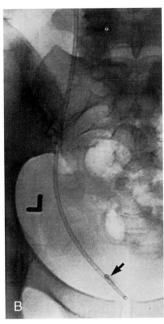

Figure 94–14. *A,* A No. 22 Fr Councill nephrostomy catheter has been passed over a No. 7.1 Fr pigtail antegrade ureteral catheter. The tip of the Councill catheter is positioned in the renal pelvis *(arrow). B,* The distal pigtail end *(arrow)* of the No. 7.1 Fr catheter is positioned in the bladder.

1978). The complications associated with percutaneous nephrostomy, especially if performed only for drainage purposes (i.e., ≤No. 12 Fr nephrostomy tract), are minimal and usually minor in nature. The problems increase when therapeutic endosurgical procedures necessitate a larger (No. 28–30 Fr) nephrostomy tract, extensive intrarenal manipulation, or a supracostal approach. Complications directly attributable to the establishment of a larger nephrostomy tract include the following: hemorrhage, perforation (i.e., false passage) of the renal parenchyma or collecting system, pneumothorax or hydrothorax, infection, injury to neighboring organs, allergic reaction to contrast medium, acute loss of the nephrostomy tract, and dislodgment of the nephrostomy tube (Clayman et al, 1984a; Coleman et al, 1984b; Winfield and Clayman, 1985).

Hemorrhage is best managed by immediate tamponade. Placement of a large nephrostomy tube or of a Kaye catheter is usually effective. Only in rare cases is angiography with arterial embolization or open surgical therapy necessary

(<0.5%) (Fig. 94–16) (Clayman et al, 1984a; Kessaris et al, 1995). Similarly, delayed bleeding occurring after nephrostomy tube removal is rare (<0.5%); however, this problem usually requires angiographic embolization of the postoperative arteriovenous malformation (60% of cases) or pseudoaneurysm (40% of cases) (see Fig. 94–16) (Clayman et al, 1984a; Kessaris et al, 1995).

Perforation of the collecting system occurs commonly (20%–30%); it is managed by the placement of the nephrostomy tube. The tear in the collecting system typically resolves within 48 hours, provided that proper drainage of the collecting system via nephrostomy tube or ureteral catheter is established (Winfield and Clayman, 1985).

In a supracostal approach (i.e., 11th intercostal space), a pleurotomy occurs in approximately 12% of cases (Young et al, 1985; Picus et al, 1986). This complication is more commonly associated with a hydrothorax than a pneumothorax after percutaneous nephrostolithotomy. Chest tube placement (i.e., No. 10 Fr locking Cook-Cope tube) and drainage allow the pleura to seal along the nephrostomy tract such that the chest tube can usually be removed within 48 hours.

Infection or urosepsis is rare, provided that the preoperative urine culture was sterile and perioperative parenteral antibiotic prophylaxis is administered (a penicillin derivative and an aminoglycoside or only a cephalosporin). Oral antibiotics are routinely continued for 1 week after the nephrostomy tube is removed. It is commonplace for the patient to have a fever spike, however, in the evening after surgery.

Injury to an adjacent organ is likewise distinctly unusual during percutaneous procedures. Nephrostomy tract traversal of the spleen, duodenum, and colon, however, has been reported; of these, the organ most commonly injured is the colon (LeRoy et al, 1985; Hopper et al, 1987). Colonic injury is potentially more likely among patients with a megacolon or malpositioned kidney (i.e., jejunoileal bypass, ulcerative colitis, horseshoe kidney). In these patients, preoperative CT is recommended to plan the nephrostomy tract properly. Overall, although only 2% of patients have a retrorenal colon when supine, this increases to 10% when patients are turned prone (LeRoy et al, 1985; Hopper et al, 1987). In most cases, the problem is simply managed by pulling the nephrostomy tube posteriorly until its tip is in the colon (colostomy tube) and by placing an external retrograde ureteral catheter to drain the renal pelvis and divert the urine. Three days later, a gentle retrograde stent study can be done; if there is no fistulous tract remaining, the retrograde stent can be removed. The colostomy tube can be

Figure 94–15. *A,* A No. 14 Fr Kaye tamponade balloon is critical when performing percutaneous work. When bleeding is encountered, it can be inflated to No. 36 Fr to provide immediate hemostasis with satisfactory drainage of the collecting system. This tube should be dressed over a gauze roll to avoid kinking. *B,* Kaye tamponade balloon entering the lower pole of the kidney; the balloon has not yet been fully inflated.

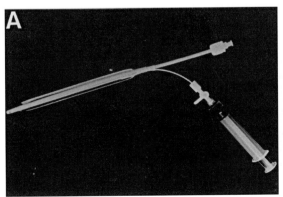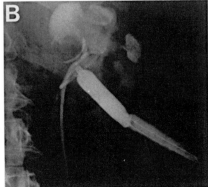

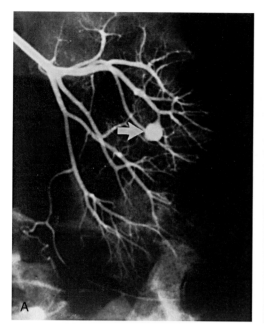
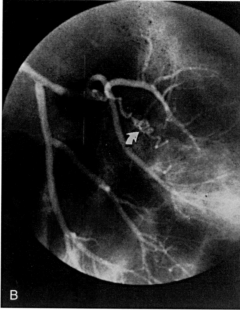

Figure 94–16. *A,* Arteriogram of a patient who developed macroscopic hematuria several weeks after percutaneous stone removal. A pseudoaneurysm of a segmental renal artery is present *(arrow)*. *B,* Embolization with a Gianturco coil *(arrow)* was immediately effective.

removed on the following day. If a leak is still present, it is best to discharge the patient with the tubes in place and to repeat the previously described protocol 1 to 2 weeks later. Only if the patient has signs of peritonitis is it then necessary to proceed with a formal surgical colostomy.

Severe reactions to contrast material are rare (<0.2%), especially because the contrast material is usually instilled directly into the collecting system and not intravenously. If a problem is anticipated based on the patient's history, the preprocedural administration of prednisone and antihistamine is recommended. This regimen consists of giving the patient oral prednisone 50 mg every 6 hours for 24 hours preceding the procedure; a half hour before the procedure the patient is given 50 mg of diphenhydramine hydrochloride orally. Should a minor allergic reaction occur, an antihistamine (diphenhydramine hydrochloride 50 mg intramuscularly) is given; for a severe allergic reaction, epinephrine (0.3–0.5 ml of 1:1000 subcutaneously) is recommended (Siegle and Lieberman, 1978; Winfield and Clayman, 1985).

Acute loss of the nephrostomy tract during the procedure is best prevented by use of a *safety* guide wire. If the tract is lost during the procedure, it can be probed with a Terumo guide wire or directly visualized with the nephroscope while 10 to 15 cc of air is gently instilled through the retrograde ureteral catheter; if the collecting system is regained endoscopically, a guide wire is passed into the system via the endoscope. If a repeat puncture becomes necessary, it will be quite difficult because the collecting system will be decompressed through the initial puncture site. In this circumstance, it is not unreasonable just to leave the preplaced ureteral catheter in position and postpone the procedure for 2 to 3 days, by which time the perforation in the collecting system will have healed, thereby allowing optimal positioning of the nephrostomy tube.

Postoperative displacement of the nephrostomy tube occurs most commonly in obese patients and in patients with supracostal nephrostomy tubes. In these patients, a locking pigtail catheter or, preferably, a nephroureteral stent system that extends to the bladder is recommended. This problem

is approached by gentle probing of the tract with a Terumo guide wire or an endoscope as described for acute tube dislodgment. If this maneuver is unsuccessful, a repeat puncture and creation of a new nephrostomy tract is necessary.

Another concern with regard to percutaneous access to the kidney is the amount of damage to the renal parenchyma. Employing detailed histologic studies and planimetry in pigs, the degree of cortical loss from a percutaneous nephrostomy of No. 36 Fr has been estimated to be less than 0.15% of the total renal cortical surface (Clayman et al, 1987b). Indeed, in a meticulous canine study, Webb and Fitzpatrick (1985) estimated that with a standard No. 24 Fr nephrostomy tract, less than 140 nephrons were injured. This is in agreement with the 1-mm postnephrostomy scar noted at nephrectomy in two patients who had undergone placement of a No. 30 Fr nephrostomy tract 4 and 2 months before kidney removal (Tailly, 1988).

PERCUTANEOUS DRAINAGE PROCEDURES

Pelvocalyceal System

The most common indication for drainage of the collecting system is obstruction. This may be in the form of either intrinsic or extrinsic obstruction affecting the ureter, UPJ, or infundibula. Intrinsic obstruction may be due to a problem in the wall of the ureter (e.g., scarring or dysplastic muscle) or due to an intracollecting system obstructive process, such as a stone, tumor, or inflammatory mass (e.g., fungal bezoar). Extrinsic obstruction has myriad etiologies: a lower-pole anterior crossing vessel, retroperitoneal fibrosis, or retroperitoneal lymphadenopathy, to name a few. The indications for nephrostomy tube placement include preservation of renal function; relief of pain; and, in the most extreme circumstances, the emergency situation of draining a pyocalyx or pyonephrosis in a patient with urosepsis.

Uninfected Obstruction

TECHNIQUE

The goal in these patients is simply to place a small percutaneous drainage tube to decompress the system. These are the easiest percutaneous procedures to perform owing to the dilation of the collecting system. Because of the obstruction, the collecting system often cannot be visualized by administration of intravenous contrast material; in these cases, passage of a 22-gauge Chiba needle opposite the second lumbar process invariably results in puncture of the dilated renal pelvis. The needle is passed deeply so that the collecting system is actually transfixed. A syringe is then placed on the end of the Chiba needle, and the syringe is aspirated as it is slowly withdrawn. The entry of urine into the syringe confirms that the tip is in the collecting system. At this point, contrast material can be injected into the collecting system via the Chiba needle. In addition, a slight amount of air can be injected to outline the posterior calyces.

The safest, most expeditious entry is by way of a posterior lower-pole calyx. A locking No. 10 Fr Cope loop-type catheter is positioned in the renal pelvis and secured to the flank. Alternatively, if one is planning to approach the UPJ therapeutically, the nephrostomy tube should be placed in line with the site of the pathology. For example, if an antegrade endopyelotomy is planned, the nephrostomy tube can be placed in an upper or middle posterior calyx, thereby providing a straight line access to the obstructed UPJ.

RESULTS

Successful antegrade access to the obstructed collecting system is routinely achieved in more than 90% of patients. Failure is most often associated with a collecting system that has become decompressed because of a forniceal rupture. In these rare circumstances, retrograde access is necessary.

Infected Obstruction (Pyonephrosis and Pyocalyx)

A patient with an intracollecting system abscess (i.e., a pyocalyx or pyonephrosis secondary to infection and distal obstruction), usually from a struvite calculus, presents with an **acute septicemia or a chronic condition**, with minimal symptoms. In the **acute case, emergency drainage** of the obstructed collecting system is indicated. Any delay in establishing drainage can be fatal. In the **chronic situation**, however, the patient's symptoms may be so minimal that the diagnosis is not initially entertained. Indeed, the individual may be afebrile and complain of only a slight amount of flank discomfort. These patients may have only a mild leukocytosis. The urine culture is often sterile. In some patients, **nonvisualization** of a stone-bearing calyx (i.e., "missing" or "phantom" calyx) on the intravenous urogram is the first sign of a pyocalyx (Brennan and Pollack, 1979; Meretyk et al, 1992b).

TECHNIQUE

Treatment of pyocalyx or pyonephrosis can be most rapidly done with percutaneous antegrade drainage of the affected calyx or renal pelvis. Initially a 22-gauge Chiba needle is passed into the obstructed system under CT or ultrasound guidance. On return of purulent material, a slight amount of contrast material is introduced to opacify the affected area of obstruction; the amount of contrast material instilled should be less than the amount of purulent material removed to preclude any pyelovenous or pyelosinus backflow and resultant septicemia. The aspirated material is sent for bacterial and fungal cultures.

To avoid an incidental pleurotomy, the recommended approach for the nephrostomy catheter is by way of an **infracostal** puncture, especially if the affected calyx is in the upper pole. As such, when trying to drain an upper-pole calyx, the needle may need to be steeply angled caudad to ensure entry into the calyx below the 12th rib.

Next a No. 10 or 12 Fr locking loop-type catheter is placed using a trocar or guide wire technique as previously described (Meretyk et al, 1992b). No attempt is made at this time to do an antegrade nephrostogram; any injection of contrast material under pressure may result in an iatrogenic septicemia.

After 5 to 7 days of antibiotic coverage, the urine cultured from the bladder and the drainage catheter is usually sterile. At this point, stone therapy can be safely pursued (Meretyk et al, 1992b). In the case of the need for percutaneous removal of a stone in an upper-pole calyx, because of the steep infracostal path of the drainage catheter, it may be necessary to place a new percutaneous tract, one that passes intercostal and enters the stone-bearing upper-pole calyx perpendicularly or slightly angled toward the UPJ.

Attempts at retrograde drainage of a pyonephrotic kidney by way of a ureteral catheter are not recommended. This approach requires significant anesthesia, is more invasive, and provides less effective drainage (i.e., smaller catheter) than a percutaneous antegrade approach. In addition, maneuvering the catheter beyond the obstructing lesion may be difficult and could result in potential ureteral perforation. Also, in the situation of a pyocalyx, placement of a retrograde catheter into the affected obstructed calyx may not be possible, especially if the calyx is in the lower pole.

RESULTS

Among patients with pyocalyx or pyohydronephrosis, adherence to the aforementioned principles can effect an excellent result. The importance of an infracostal approach, however, cannot be overemphasized. Indeed, in one series in which two patients were managed with supracostal (i.e., 11th intercostal space) puncture, pulmonary complications resulted. In one individual, a massive pleural effusion developed, requiring prolonged chest tube drainage. A second individual developed empyema and needed open drainage. Similarly the careful review of intravenous urograms before planned extracorporeal shock wave lithotripsy (ESWL) is the best way for the urologist to identify a phantom calyx. If misdiagnosed, the result of ESWL of a pyocalyx is immediate urosepsis and septicemia necessitating an emergency hospital admission with subsequent percutaneous drainage of the pyocalyx and delayed percutaneous stone removal (Fig. 94–17) (Albala et al, 1991; Meretyk et al, 1992b).

Intrarenal Collections

Renal Cysts

Approximately 25% of adults over the age of 40 years have radiographically detectable renal cysts (≥1 cm); by age 80 years, two thirds of patients have a cyst detectable by CT

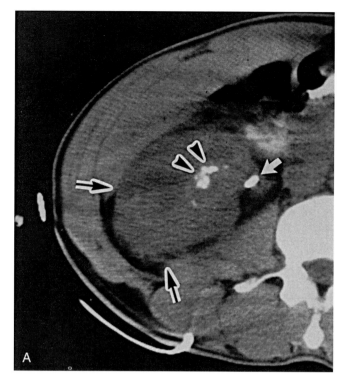
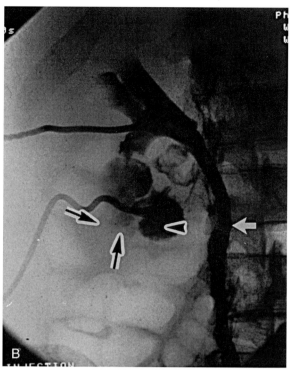

Figure 94–17. *A,* At 24 hours after extracorporeal shock wave lithotripsy, the patient presented with urosepsis. A computed tomography scan reveals stone debris *(arrowheads),* a nephrostent in the ureter *(white arrow),* and a large dilated lower-pole calyx *(black arrows). B,* A percutaneous tube was placed into the lower-pole calyx; purulent material was drained. At a later date, after the urine had been sterilized, the stone material was percutaneously removed via two nephrostomy tracts and continuity between the lower pole infundibulum and the renal pelvis was re-established. *(White arrow,* ureter with a nephrostent; *black arrows,* outline of pyohydrocalyx; *black arrowhead,* location of stone debris.) The black arrows and arrowhead correspond to the level of the computed tomography scan shown in *A.*

(Laucks and McLachlan, 1981). Typically, simple renal cysts increase in number (one third of patients develop more cysts over a 3.5-year period) and only slowly increase in size (6% of patients have progressive increase in size) (Richter et al, 1983; Dalton et al, 1986). Despite this high incidence of renal cysts, fortunately only 8% of patients become symptomatic or develop discernible signs: flank pain, usually secondary to hemorrhage into a cyst; microscopic hematuria; obstruction; or renin-mediated hypertension. Among these few symptomatic patients, percutaneous fluoroscopic cyst puncture with sclerotherapy results in resolution of symptoms in the majority of individuals; it is the rare case that must proceed to percutaneous endoscopic, laparoscopic, or open surgical therapy.

In contrast, among patients with autosomal dominant polycystic kidney disease, cyst-related complications are often encountered. In these patients, cysts are associated with myriad problems: flank pain (30%), pyelonephritis (30%), urolithiasis (34%), hypertension (21%), perinephric abscess (8%), palpable mass (15%), macroscopic hematuria (19%), and renal failure (17%) (Delaney et al, 1985). In these patients, if a single cyst can be targeted as the source of symptoms, it can be approached by percutaneous fluoroscopic needle drainage and sclerotherapy or percutaneous endoscopic electrosurgical scarification. If the painful cyst cannot be localized and a general cyst decortication of the surface cysts is deemed advisable, however, an open or laparoscopic approach is needed.

TECHNIQUE

In the patient with a symptomatic simple peripheral acquired renal cyst, therapy is best achieved by percutaneous drainage during monitoring with ultrasound, fluoroscopy, or CT (Vestby, 1967). Using one of these imaging modalities, the cyst is identified, and a nephrostomy-type needle is placed into the center of the cyst. The cyst contents are drained and sent to the laboratory for cytologic studies, cultures, and chemical evaluation (protein, lactate dehydrogenase, creatinine) (Fig. 94–18). A thin, clear, yellow fluid is indicative of a benign cyst, whereas sanguineous fluid may be associated with a traumatic puncture or a neoplasm. Contrast material is injected into the cyst (i.e., cystogram) to be certain it does not communicate with the collecting system. In addition, a slight amount of air may be injected into the cyst, thereby providing additional contrast for determining if there is any nodularity along the cyst wall; a benign cyst should have a completely smooth wall.

Provided that the cyst appears to be benign and isolated from the collecting system, percutaneous drainage and sclerosis of the cyst can be undertaken. In this regard, it should be noted that simple drainage without sclerosis usually results in only short-lived relief of symptoms because the cyst fluid almost invariably reaccumulates. To proceed with sclerotherapy, the cyst is drained after which 95% ethanol (equal to 25% of cyst volume) is instilled into the cyst and left for 10 to 20 minutes. Apparently the epithelial lining cells are fixed by the ethanol within 3 minutes of exposure. The ethanol is then withdrawn (Bean, 1981; Ozgun et al, 1988). Alternative sclerotherapy can be achieved by injection of 5 to 10 ml of bismuth phosphate (Table 94–1) (Zachrisson, 1982; Holmberg and Hietala, 1989), which remains in the cyst. Other agents that have been used successfully include tetracycline and sodium morrhuate (Zou et al, 1991; Reiner et al, 1992; Ohkawa et al, 1993).

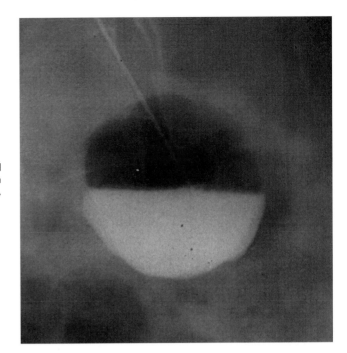

Figure 94–18. A large symptomatic cyst has been filled with air and contrast material. Note the smooth walls of the cyst, indicating its benign nature, and the lack of any contrast or air outside of the cyst boundaries, indicating a lack of communication with the collecting system.

RESULTS

Percutaneous drainage of renal cysts unaccompanied by sclerotherapy is of little therapeutic value (Raskin et al, 1975) (see Table 94–1). Indeed, with drainage alone, only 10% to 20% of the cysts disappear or have a 50% or more reduction in volume over the ensuing follow-up period (Wahlquist and Grumstedt, 1966; Holmberg and Hietala, 1989). Sclerotherapy with ethanol or with bismuth phosphate generally results in a satisfactory outcome in 75% to 100% of patients (Bean, 1981; Zachrisson, 1982; Ozgun et al, 1988; Holmberg and Hietala, 1989). Cysts as large as 600 cc have been effectively sclerosed. Given the simultaneous diagnostic and therapeutic aspects of cyst drainage and sclerotherapy, it is the obvious route of first-line treatment. Long-term data supporting the durability of sclerotherapy out to 5 years or beyond, however, are not available. Also, some physicians have not been able to duplicate the initial sanguine reports previously cited. Indeed, Perugia and associates noted that with a 20% volume of the cyst replaced with 98% ethanol, none of five patients had a satisfactory result (i.e., >50% decrease in the size of the renal cyst) (Perugia et al, 1991) (see Table 94–1).

Renal Abscesses

Intrarenal abscesses are usually due to either lobar nephronia or an infected renal cyst. The responsible organism is most commonly a gram-negative bacterium, such as *Escherichia coli* or less commonly *Proteus mirabilis* or *Klebsiella pneumoniae* (Kaneti and Hertzanu, 1987; Sadi et al, 1988). Although *Staphylococcus aureus* was a common bacterium in renal abscesses in the past, today it accounts for less than 10% of all renal abscesses (Fowler and Perkins, 1994). The major risk of intraparenchymal lesions is life-threatening urosepsis and septicemia. Some patients with infected renal cysts, however, may present with minimal symptoms: mild flank discomfort and low-grade fever.

Other signs of an intrarenal abscess on the intravenous urogram include perirenal gas, calculi, and nonfunction of the affected kidney. The abscess itself can best be outlined by CT or ultrasonography with an accuracy of 96% with CT and 92% with ultrasonography (Fowler and Perkins, 1994). As opposed to the ill-defined wedge-shaped lesions of lobar nephronia, the renal abscess has a well-defined thick-walled margin. The CT density of the abscess contents (i.e., 2–25 HU) is often greater than that of a simple cyst. On ultrasound, these infected collections are hypoechoic with poor development of the posterior wall of the lesion. Intralesional debris may produce ultrasonically detectable intralesional echoes (Weigert et al, 1985).

TECHNIQUE

The most important therapeutic measure with regard to a renal abscess is drainage. Currently, treatment can be most rapidly done with percutaneous drainage. The added benefit of this approach is the minimal morbidity incurred because the entire procedure is performed under local anesthesia supplemented with minimal intravenous sedation.

Initially a 22-gauge Chiba needle is passed into the renal abscess under CT or ultrasound guidance. On confirmation of an abscess (i.e., return of purulent material), a No. 10 or 12 Fr locking loop catheter is placed using a trocar or guide wire technique as described (Meretyk et al, 1992b).

The approach should be **infracostal** even if the affected calyx is in the upper pole. This practice should preclude an incidental pleurotomy and possible empyema. To perform an infracostal puncture, the needle's tip is directed cephalad (i.e., hub of the needle is tilted caudal) at a steep angle. After 5 to 7 days of antibiotic coverage, the urine cultured from the bladder and the abscess drainage catheter is usually sterile. At this point, ESWL or percutaneous stone removal can be safely pursued (Meretyk et al, 1992b). The latter may need to be done via a new nephrostomy tract because the

Table 94–1. RENAL CYSTS: DRAINAGE AND SCLEROTHERAPY

Authors	Agent	Number of Cysts	Cyst with ≥50% Reduction in Size (%)	Cyst Disappearance (%)	Follow-up Data
No Intervention					
Holmberg and Hietala, 1989	No intervention	62	0	0	27 patients ≥24 months
Dalton et al, 1986	No intervention		0	0	
Drainage Alone					
Raskin et al, 1975	Drainage alone	15	13	6	5–48 months
Wahlquist and Grumstedt, 1966	Drainage alone	26	15	19	≥19 months
Holmberg and Hietala, 1989	Drainage alone	57	20	4	25 patients ≥24 months
Sclerosant: Ethanol					
Bean, 1981	Ethanol 95% (4%–44% cyst volume for 10–20 min)	34	—	97	16 patients >1 year
Perugia et al, 1991	Ethanol 98% + fibrin glue	11	0	45	6–24 months
	Ethanol 98% (20% cyst volume for 20 min)	5	0	0	6–24 months
Ozgun et al, 1988	Ethanol 96% (20% cyst volume for 20 min)	16	—	100	3–6 months
Sclerosant: Other					
Vestby, 1967	Pantopaque (3–5 ml)	18	28	56	10 ≥1 year
Raskin et al, 1975	Pantopaque	56	68	—	28 patients ≥2 years
Zachrisson, 1982	Bismuth phosphate (5 ml)	73	100	—	33 patients ≥2 years
Holmberg and Hietala, 1989	Bismuth phosphate (5–10 ml)	59	24	51	37 patients ≥2 years
Zou et al, 1991	Sodium morrhuate	48	77 (reduced ≥33%)	—	4 patients–36 months
Reiner et al, 1992 (children)	Tetracycline	4	—	100	6–36 months
Ohkawa et al, 1993	Minocycline hydrochloride (tetracycline)	154	32	—	≥3 months

steep angle of the drainage tract may not be suitable for stone removal; this is especially true if the stone resides in an upper-pole calyx that projects above the 12th rib. Usually after several days of drainage and after the urine culture is sterile, it is safe to proceed with an intercostal puncture if need be to remove the calculus.

RESULTS

Results of percutaneous drainage of renal abscesses have been satisfactory. The initially reported overall success rate was 82% (22 collected cases), with a complication rate (sepsis, bleeding, secondary nephrectomy, or recurrent abscess) of 18%. Among these 22 cases, there have been two deaths (Cronan et al, 1984; Gerzof et al, 1985; Jaques et al, 1986; Haaga, 1990). More recently, there have been two major series reported on renal abscess. Fowler and Perkins reviewed their experience with renal abscesses from 1972 through 1988. Their overall success rate reached 97% among 57 cases of renal abscesses; only 10% of the patients had a serious complication (Fowler and Perkins, 1994). The majority of these patients were managed by open drainage; only 13% underwent percutaneous drainage. In contrast, Siegel and co-workers reviewed their experience with renal abscess from 1984 through 1993. Among 52 patients, management consisted of intense antibiotic therapy for abscesses less than 3 cm in immunocompetent patients (11%) and percutaneous drainage and antibiotics for all larger abscesses

(63%). Overall cure rates of 100% and 79% were recorded for these two treatment modalities (Siegel et al, 1996). No complications owing to percutaneous drainage were noted; however, one fourth of these patients eventually required a nephrectomy or partial nephrectomy (Siegel et al, 1996).

The key factor affecting the outcome of the percutaneous approach is whether the abscess is simple or loculated. In the simple abscess case, percutaneous drainage yields success rates greater than 80%. In the loculated abscess, a successful percutaneous outcome is noted in only 45%. The presence of air within the mass indicates that the purulent contents may be thick and less amenable to percutaneous drainage (Haaga et al, 1977; Jaques et al, 1986). In addition, fungal infections or infected hematomas respond poorly to percutaneous drainage. In the case of a fungal renal abscess, drainage plus irrigation of the abscess cavity with amphotericin B (50 mg/L/day) may be necessary to achieve a satisfactory result (Haaga, 1990).

Perirenal Collections

Endosurgical Management of a Urinoma (Uriniferous Pseudocyst)

A retroperitoneal urinoma occurs most commonly following renal trauma (Portela et al, 1979; Morano and Burkhalter,

1985). Other causes of urinoma include ureteral obstruction with attendant calyceal forniceal rupture and perforation of the collecting system during an endosurgical procedure. There is one caveat: for a left-sided retroperitoneal fluid collection, the possibility of a pancreatic pseudocyst must be considered.

A retroperitoneal urine collection, by virtue of its size, may cause considerable discomfort. Because of the lipolytic effect of urine, over the next 2 to 5 days, perinephric fat disappears, and an inflammatory reaction follows. The urine collection becomes encapsulated in a fibrous sac within 3 to 6 weeks (Thompson et al, 1976; Healy et al, 1984; Morano and Burkhalter, 1985; Lang and Glorioso, 1986).

Initial studies should include intravenous pyelography (IVP), an antegrade nephrostogram, a retrograde ureterogram, or a CT scan with contrast agent to aid in the identification of the three factors necessary for a urinoma to form: (1) ureteral obstruction, (2) extravasation from the collecting system, and (3) a functioning kidney. Among these studies, the CT scan is the most informative. With a urinoma, in contrast to other retroperitoneal fluid collections, the initial CT attenuation values of approximately 10 to 20 HU may increase after administration of intravenous contrast material (Healy et al, 1984). Also, in contrast to a hematoma or an abscess cavity, the CT attenuation values throughout the urinoma are homogeneous (Lang and Glorioso, 1986). In addition, the CT scan yields important data about the exact location and extent of the urinoma and its relationship to the kidney, ureter, surrounding organs, and retroperitoneal fascial planes.

TECHNIQUE

Percutaneous drainage of a urinoma is performed under ultrasound or CT guidance. The creatinine concentration in the fluid should be identical with the urine creatinine concentration. A No. 10 Fr catheter-bearing needle (biliary urinary drainage catheter with a locking pigtail) is directed into the urinoma. The cavity is drained, and the catheter is left indwelling. The fluid obtained can be cultured; analyzed for creatinine; and, for a left-sided collection, assayed for amylase.

In some instances, no communication between the collecting system and urinoma is identifiable, and no evidence of ureteral obstruction is found. In these cases, drainage from the urinoma usually ceases within 48 to 72 hours, and the cavity rapidly decreases in size. A contrast medium injection via the urinoma catheter is helpful to determine when the cavity has collapsed. Once the cavity is no larger than the drainage catheter itself and is shown radiographically not to communicate with the collecting system, the catheter can be removed.

If ureteral obstruction is present or if over a several-day period the cavity continues to drain without a decrease in the amount of fluid, then it becomes necessary to drain the affected collecting system. In this case, a retrograde ureterogram and placement of an indwelling ureteral stent and Foley catheter or a percutaneous nephrostomy are needed to help divert the urine from the fistulous tract and allow the fistulous communication to heal.

In the rare circumstance in which the fistula persists despite adequate drainage of the urinoma and renal collecting system, ureteroscopy or antegrade nephroscopy is indicated. The fistula tract can be biopsied to rule out a malignancy.

The tract can then be fulgurated in an effort to promote obliterative scarring of the fistulous tract; however, experience with this approach is scant. In these rare cases, surgical exploration and formal closure of the fistulous tract may be necessary.

RESULTS

The largest report on treatment of urinomas is by Thompson and associates (1976); 16 patients were treated surgically. Half of them required nephrectomy. The other half underwent surgical drainage of the urinoma with, at times, resection of the urinoma wall and placement of a nephrostomy tube.

To date, there are only anecdotal reports of percutaneous drainage of urinomas (Morano and Burkhalter, 1985). According to Lang and Glorioso (1986), obstructive urinomas can be successfully treated in more than 90% of patients by percutaneous drainage and relief of the obstruction. Likewise, for nonobstructive (i.e., traumatic) urinomas, drainage of the cavity and establishment of upper tract continuity (retrograde ureteral stent or antegrade nephrostent) are usually successful. In those cases in which an indwelling ureteral stent is placed, a urethral catheter should also be placed, to preclude reflux of urine up the stent and across the fistulous tract. Percutaneous drainage is a reasonable first step, provided that the urinoma can be completely drained (i.e., not multiloculated) and that ureteral or percutaneous drainage of the obstructed collecting system is simultaneously established.

Perinephric Abscess

Perinephric abscess is most commonly associated with disruption of a corticomedullary intranephric renal abscess. This finding is usually seen in conjunction with prior urologic surgery or urolithiasis or most commonly in the presence of diabetes mellitus (60%–90% of cases) (Thorley et al, 1974; Edelstein and McCabe, 1988). The most often noted symptoms of a retroperitoneal abscess are fever (90%) and flank pain (40%–50%) (Saiki et al, 1982). A palpable flank mass occurs in 9% to 47% (Salvatierra et al, 1967; Goldman et al, 1977; Gerzof and Gale, 1982; Sheinfeld et al, 1987; Edelstein and McCabe, 1988). In the 1960s, the predominant organism associated with a perinephric abscess was *S. aureus*; however, today the offending organism is more likely to be a gram-negative bacterium *(E. coli* or *P. mirabilis)* (Thorley et al, 1974). The diagnosis of this entity is best done with CT or ultrasonography (Haaga et al, 1977; Weigert et al, 1985; Jaques et al, 1986). CT is preferred because it is more accurate in diagnosing an intra-abdominal abscess (90%) than ultrasonography, and CT is more effective in defining the extent of the abscess with regard to other retroperitoneal structures. On CT scan, the typical appearance of a perinephric abscess is that of a soft tissue mass (≤20 HU), with a thick wall that may enhance after administration of intravenous contrast material *(rind sign)* (Haaga et al, 1977; Gerzof and Gale, 1982; Sheinfeld et al, 1987). In rare circumstances, a gallium scan or indium-labeled white blood cell scan may be of diagnostic benefit.

TECHNIQUE

Before ultrasound or CT examination, the patient should receive broad-spectrum parenteral antibiotics (e.g., ampicillin and aminoglycoside). Next, a 22-gauge Chiba needle can be passed percutaneously under ultrasound or CT guidance into the abscess cavity. This puncture provides the physician with important information: determination of the presence of infection and consistency of the purulent contents. If the purulent material is too thick, it cannot be drained percutaneously (Gerzof et al, 1985). It is essential that the abscess be punctured below the 12th rib to preclude an inadvertent pleurotomy. If the pleural cavity is traversed, a significant pleural effusion and possible empyema may ensue (Albala et al, 1991). Likewise, the peritoneal cavity should be avoided by planning the access route medial to the posterior axillary line.

Next an 18-gauge needle is passed. Fluid is drained from the abscess and sent to the laboratory for aerobic, anaerobic, and fungal cultures. If the fluid is thick and drains poorly or if the cavity is multiloculated, an open operation is necessary to drain and debride the abscess cavity properly. If the fluid is relatively thin and drains well, however, at the same time as the diagnostic ultrasound or CT study is performed, a catheter (e.g., No. 10 Fr locking loop catheter or a No. 12 or 14 Fr double-lumen sump drain: Van Sonnenberg or Ring-McClean catheter) can be left in the abscess cavity. The double-lumen catheter helps decrease clogging and can be used for infusion and drainage of saline or antibiotic solution.

If need be, a separate tube can be placed to drain the collecting system (i.e., nephrostomy tube) to permit drainage (Fig. 94–19) (Gerzof and Gale, 1982; Elyaderani and Moncman, 1985; Haaga, 1990). The nephrostomy tube is needed only if there is evidence of renal obstruction due to stone or stricture disease. Placement of a nephrostomy tube is preferable to placement of an indwelling stent, and the nephrostomy tube is placed under local anesthesia at the same time as the abscess tube is placed; also, the nephrostomy tube provides for better drainage and control of the collecting system.

Usually within 5 to 7 days, drainage from the abscess ceases (Caldamone and Frank, 1980; Cronan et al, 1980, 1984). If drainage initially decreases, however, then begins to increase and becomes clear, a urinary fistula must be suspected (Caldamone and Frank, 1980; Cronan et al, 1980).

Before removing the drainage tube, a radiographic study of the nondraining cavity can be done by gently injecting contrast material into the drainage catheter. If the cavity has decreased to the size of the catheter, the catheter can be removed. When a large cavity persists, a sclerosant may be instilled, provided that there is no demonstrable communication with the collecting system. Most commonly, tetracycline or 95% ethanol has been chosen for this purpose. The sclerosant effect of tetracycline (50 mg/ml) is attributed to its acid pH of 2 to 3.5. The tetracycline is instilled under gravity drainage into the cavity, and the tube is clamped for 15 minutes and then opened to drainage. The process is repeated on a weekly basis until the only cavity remaining is that which immediately surrounds the pigtail of the drainage tube. At this point, the tube is withdrawn. Alternatively, 95% ethanol may be used as described under sclerosant therapy for renal cysts. The combined sclerosant and antibacterial characteristics of tetracycline, however, make it an ideal choice for treating a persistent retroperitoneal abscess cavity.

Oral antibiotics, appropriate for the responsible bacterium, are given throughout this drainage/sclerosant period and for 1 to 3 weeks after removal of the drainage tube. Repeat urine cultures and repeat CT scans are necessary at 1- and 3-month intervals to rule out recurrent infection or reappearance of a retroperitoneal fluid collection.

Absolute contraindications to a percutaneous approach are few. An uncorrectable or uncorrected bleeding diathesis precludes percutaneous drainage. Likewise, suspicion of a hydatid fluid collection is a direct contraindication to this approach (Gerzof and Gale, 1982).

RESULTS

Perinephric abscess is a life-threatening entity. Left undrained, despite antibiotic administration, the mortality rate approaches 80% (Altemeyer and Alexander, 1961). Even with modern-day surgical therapy (nephrectomy or drainage), the mortality rate is 8% to 22%, and significant morbidity occurs in 35% of patients (Thorley et al, 1974; Haaga, 1990). Major complications, such as sepsis, pleural fistula, bleeding, or need for surgical intervention, are seen in 3% to 22% (Gerzof et al, 1985; Edelstein and McCabe, 1988). Recurrence rates after surgery are as high as 20% (Salvati-

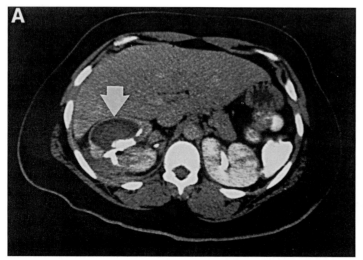
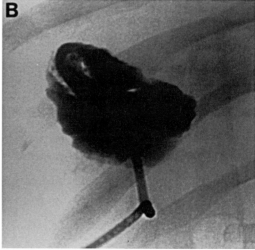

Figure 94–19. *A,* A computed tomography scan of a large retroperitoneal abscess *(arrow)* associated with a staghorn calculus. *B,* Drainage tube in the abscess cavity. Unfortunately, this tube was placed between the 11th and 12th ribs. Ideally the tube should be placed infracostal so that it does not traverse the pleural space.

erra et al, 1967; Haaga et al, 1977; Elyaderani and Monc-man, 1985; Jaques et al, 1986; Edelstein and McCabe, 1988; Haaga, 1990); in contrast, recurrences after percutaneous drainage are relatively rare, 1% to 4% (Gerzof et al, 1985). The need for initial or subsequent nephrectomy after surgical drainage is 25% to 50% and reflects the generally poor renal function of the ipsilateral kidney (Salvatierra et al, 1967; Edelstein and McCabe, 1988).

The results of percutaneous drainage of retroperitoneal abscesses are particularly good. Haaga and associates have reported successful drainage in 39 collected cases of peri-nephric abscess (Haaga et al, 1977; Haaga 1990). This mirrors the 86% success rate for percutaneous drainage of all types of intra-abdominal abscesses (Gerzof et al, 1985; Jaques et al, 1986). Overall the success rate is higher for single than for loculated abscesses, 82% versus 45% (Gerzof et al, 1985).

Unfavorable factors for a percutaneous approach include fungal infection, calcification of the wall of the mass, calcified debris within the mass, thick purulent drainage, multiloculated cavity, markedly diseased nonfunctioning kidney (an indication for nephrectomy), and an infected hematoma. If an enteric fistula is the source of the retroperitoneal abscess, an open surgical repair is necessary (Elyaderani and Moncman, 1985); an air-fluid level within the abscess is identified on CT scan in half of these unusual cases (Jaques et al, 1986).

Lymphocele

Although lymphocele is a complication noted after a variety of procedures, the urologic surgeon most often must manage this problem. Lymphoceles can occur after any extensive retroperitoneal node dissection (testis, kidney, prostate, or bladder cancer) and after renal transplantation (1.2%–14%) (Schweizer et al, 1972; Braun et al, 1974; Morin and Baker, 1977; Brockis et al, 1978; Skinner et al, 1982; Mueller et al, 1984; White et al, 1985). The following symptoms usually are the result of compression of adjacent structures (ureter, colon, and iliac vessels) by the lymphocele: hydronephrosis, ipsilateral lower extremity edema, constipation, decreased bladder volume, and abdominal mass. In transplant patients, a lymphocele may cause a rise in creatinine concentration because of ureteral obstruction (Brockis et al, 1978).

Initial evaluation of these masses includes a CT scan or ultrasonography, either of which is suitable for outlining the lesion (Spring et al, 1981). A definitive diagnosis can be made by needle aspiration of the collection. In the drained, pale yellow or clear fluid, lymphocytes can usually be detected. The values of creatinine and other electrolytes reflect serum values, as opposed to the high creatinine, high potassium, and low sodium values in fluid from a urinoma. In lymphocele fluid from the pelvis, the levels of cholesterol and protein are often lower than those in serum (Braun et al, 1974). However, if the disruption of the lymphatic chain lies in the upper retroperitoneum (celiac axis area), chylous fluid collects. This material is cloudy and has a high content of triglycerides and proteins.

TECHNIQUE

Under CT or ultrasound guidance, a 20- or 22-gauge needle is guided into the cystic collection (Mueller et al,

1984). The fluid obtained is sent to the laboratory for serum electrolytes, creatinine, protein, triglyceride, cholesterol, culture, and cytologic evaluations. Blood and urine samples are obtained for similar chemical evaluations. If more than 150 ml is aspirated, a No. 8 to 14 Fr locking-type, pigtail catheter (Cope loop, Van Sonnenberg sump, or other tube) is guided into the cavity (White et al, 1985). At 1 to 10 days, contrast material is instilled by way of the catheter to assess the size of the cavity. When the cavity has collapsed around the catheter and drainage is less than 10 ml/day, the catheter can be removed. If higher outputs continue, sclerotherapy with tetracycline can be tried (≤50 ml of 50 mg tetracycline per milliliter left in place for 15 minutes) (White et al, 1985); other types of sclerosants include bleomycin, povidone-iodine, or 95% ethanol (Cohan et al, 1987, 1988; McDowell et al, 1991; Khorram and Stern, 1993).

RESULTS

Simple aspiration of a lymphocele appears sufficient for smaller collections (<150 ml). For the larger lymphocele, however, it is usually not effective (<20% success) (Braun et al, 1974). In this case, a drainage tube is necessary. Drainage should cease anytime from days to weeks. Otherwise, sclerotherapy with tetracycline can be attempted. In some cases, it may take up to 4 months before the drainage ceases. Overall the percutaneous approach with or without sclerosant therapy is eventually successful in 70% to 80% of patients (White et al, 1985; Cohan et al, 1987). This approach is much less successful in the patient with a multiloculated lymphocele. Lastly, if the percutaneous approach fails, either open surgical drainage or laparoscopic drainage and marsupialization is the next step. The latter has become the procedure of choice given its excellent results, cost-effectiveness, and low morbidity (Gill et al, 1995).

Hematoma

A retroperitoneal hematoma is most commonly the consequence of blunt renal trauma. Other causes include penetrating renal trauma, anticoagulant therapy, vascular lesions, and tumor or surgical complications (percutaneous surgery, ESWL, renal biopsy). The symptoms include flank mass and discomfort; at times, ureteral obstruction may also occur. The diagnosis is best made by a CT scan, which can both demonstrate the extent of the hematoma and differentiate between a retroperitoneal and subcapsular collection (Fig. 94–20). The latter is of greater concern because it may result in decreased renal function. The attenuation values for clotted blood as found in a hematoma may vary from +18 to +40 HU (±1000 HU scale) (Pollack et al, 1981). Fortunately, these lesions rarely require therapy.

The natural history of a retroperitoneal hematoma is slow, spontaneous resolution of the mass. If the hematoma is overly large (i.e., compromising respiratory function), expanding, impairing renal function, or associated with hypotension, embolization or surgical exploration and drainage are indicated. Percutaneous procedures in these cases are more meddlesome than therapeutic because the blood clot is too thick to drain (Schaner et al, 1977). Likewise, in patients with spontaneous renal hemorrhage in whom there is no history of anticoagulation therapy, vasculitis, or trauma, surgical radical nephrectomy should be considered because 50%

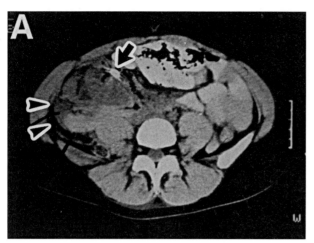 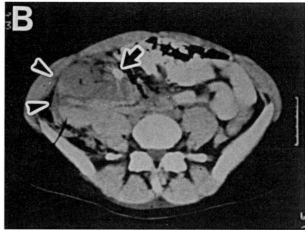

Figure 94–20. *A* and *B*, Massive retroperitoneal hematoma following retrograde endopyelotomy is shown in these two noncontrast computed tomography scans. The kidney was located low in the retroperitoneum. Note the stent in the ureter *(arrow)*. The hematoma is outlined by the *arrowheads.* A total of 4 units of blood was transfused. Ultimately an open pyeloplasty was successful.

to 70% of these kidneys are found to contain a diminutive renal cell cancer (Kendall et al, 1988).

PERCUTANEOUS DIAGNOSTIC PROCEDURES

There are four areas in which endosurgical techniques can be used for diagnostic purposes: indeterminant renal mass, renal biopsy in patients with renal failure or hematuria with suspected medical renal disease, essential hematuria, and intraureteral or upper collecting system lesions. For biopsy of the kidney or of a renal mass, percutaneous radiologic techniques predominate. In patients with essential hematuria or a radiolucent filling defect in the collecting system, noninvasive radiologic evaluation is only the first step. If this evaluation is inconclusive, ureteroscopy becomes the primary means of diagnosis. In these patients, the role of percutaneous techniques, specifically antegrade nephroscopy, is limited to a salvage situation in the rare circumstance that ureteroscopy is inconclusive. Indeed, in the past decade, antegrade nephroscopy has not been employed in any patient in the authors' institution presenting with either essential hematuria or an upper urinary tract ureteral or collecting system lesion. For a complete discussion of these two entities, the reader is referred to Chapter 93.

Renal Mass

An endoscopic approach to a renal mass is rarely necessary. Modern imaging modalities including ultrasound, CT, and MRI have largely supplanted the need to obtain a confirmatory tissue diagnosis.

All renal masses can be separated into three broad categories: cystic, solid, and indeterminant. The vast majority of renal masses are simple cysts. Renal ultrasonography can definitively diagnose a renal cyst, provided that the lesion fulfills the diagnostic criteria of being anechoic at high and low gain and has a strong posterior wall. Similarly, CT criteria for a cyst are likewise reliable: A thin-walled lesion

with a homogeneous interior of low density (i.e., 0 HU) is invariably a simple renal cyst. If these criteria are not met, the lesion is considered indeterminant, and further diagnostic studies are indicated.

For solid, noncystic lesions, the CT or MRI study is essential. One advantage of MRI is in the patient with renal insufficiency or allergy to contrast material; in these patients, the gadolinium-enhanced scan is of particular value (Semelka et al, 1992; Krestin, 1994). For the diagnosis of a solid lesion, the key point is to determine whether or not there is any fat within the lesion. If fat is found within the lesion, an angiomyolipoma is likely present, whereas a solid lesion without any fat is more likely a renal cell cancer. The former, if smaller than 3.5 to 4 cm and asymptomatic, can be followed, whereas the diagnosis of a renal cell cancer leads to surgical ablation (Oesterling et al, 1986; Van Baal et al, 1994).

Technique

Only in the case of an indeterminant or solid renal lesion in a patient with a known nonrenal cancer (i.e., differential diagnosis of primary renal cancer versus a metastatic lesion) does it behoove the urologist to seek a tissue diagnosis. In this regard, an ultrasound-guided or CT-guided puncture or biopsy of the lesion is indicated. If the contents are fluid, cytology, culture, and electrolytes can be obtained on the specimen; if the lesion has a solid component, an aspiration or needle biopsy can be obtained.

Needle biopsy of a renal lesion may be done either percutaneously or via a transrenal approach. The percutaneous approach to biopsy of a renal mass is by far the better-known procedure having been used since 1950. The Vim-Silverman needle and Tru-Cut needle have been the mainstays of percutaneous renal biopsy; however, advances in biopsy guns have provided the physician with much smaller 18-gauge spring-loaded systems, which can be accurately guided to the lesion under ultrasound or CT imaging.

Leal (1992) has described a transurethral, transrenal approach to renal biopsy. Using a torque control guide wire and No. 5 and 8 Fr catheters, the calyx closest to the parenchymal mass is accessed. The guide wire is pushed into the mass, and the No. 8 Fr catheter is then advanced into the mass. The guide wire and No. 5 Fr catheters are removed, and aspiration is applied to the end of the No. 8 Fr catheter during fluoroscopic imaging. The No. 8 Fr catheter is then removed, and the plug of tissue is flushed out of the tip of the catheter and sent for histologic evaluation; an indwelling ureteral stent is placed (Leal, 1992). If all of the aforementioned methods fail to yield a definitive diagnosis, a retroperitoneal laparoscopic or open approach may be necessary, at which time both a diagnostic biopsy and definitive therapy can be accomplished.

Results

Overall the vast majority of incidentally discovered renal masses are cysts. Indeed, a simple renal cyst is identified during abdominal CT in 25% of patients more than 40 years of age. Among incidentally discovered renal masses, a renal cancer is found in approximately 5% or less of patients (Tosaka et al, 1990). When the patient presents with a renal mass in association with macroscopic hematuria, flank pain, or a palpable flank mass, however, the chances of the mass being a renal cell cancer approach 50% (Clayman et al, 1984b). Other renal masses, specifically angiomyolipoma, renal pelvic tumors, and other benign lesions, are all relatively uncommon, accounting for approximately 5% of all renal masses among asymptomatic patients (Tosaka et al, 1990; Van Baal et al, 1994).

Complications from percutaneous renal biopsy with the older, larger 14-gauge needles occurred in 2% to 11% of patients; however, most of these problems were of a minor nature. The nephrectomy rate from renal biopsy is 0.06% with a mortality rate of 0.08%. With the advent of 18-gauge biopsy needles, major complications, mortality, or nephrectomies in some series have been nonexistent; minor complications occur in only 5% (predominantly symptomatic perirenal hematoma or hematuria). Indeed, the improved safety margin of this approach has now made it feasible to pursue a percutaneous biopsy even in the case of a solitary kidney (Dowd et al, 1991; Schow et al, 1992; Doyle et al, 1994).

Concerns about possible postbiopsy malignant seeding of the needle tract are not sufficient to justify a change in course from percutaneous biopsy to laparoscopic or open renal exploration. Indeed, reported cases of seeding of the needle tract are few and are usually associated with unusual circumstances, such as multiple biopsies of a lesion over time, the use of large biopsy needles, or other extenuating circumstances (Levine et al, 1963; Von Schreeb et al, 1970; Gibbons et al, 1977).

Renal Biopsy

Among patients with nephrotic syndrome, nephritic syndrome, or renal allograft dysfunction and in some cases of acute renal failure, a renal biopsy is indicated. Presently, percutaneous renal biopsy has all but replaced the need for an open biopsy. Indeed, even among patients with a solitary kidney, a percutaneous biopsy is now the preferred approach.

A surgical biopsy is used only as a salvage approach should the percutaneous approach fail.

Technique

Before a renal biopsy, routine coagulation studies and a urine culture are performed. For the patient with an eutopic kidney, a prone position is used, whereas for the transplant patient, a supine position is used. The biopsies are most commonly performed under real-time ultrasonography, using a 3.5-MHz ultrasound system equipped with a Tru-Cut needle, Vim-Silverman needle, or spring-loaded biopsy needle (Dowd et al, 1991; Doyle et al, 1994). The biopsy sample is usually taken from the lower pole of the kidney (Bach et al, 1988; Radford et al, 1994). As a rule, two biopsy samples are obtained. The specimens are sent for standard histologic sectioning in 10% buffered formalin, immunofluoresence studies in liquid nitrogen, and electron microscopy in 1% glutaraldehyde at a pH of 7.2 with 4% formaldehyde added. The following stains and preparations highlight various aspects of the kidney: glomerular morphology and inflammatory cells (hematoxylin-eosin), basement membrane (periodic acid–Schiff [PAS] stain, methenamine silver stain, and electron microscopy), extracellular matrix (PAS stain), interstitial fibrosis (trichrome stain), and immune complexes (trichrome stain and immunofluoresence studies) (Radford et al, 1994).

After the biopsy, the patient is placed at bed rest for usually half a day. Discharge is in the morning, provided that the urine is clear.

Results

Percutaneous renal biopsy provides adequate tissue for diagnosis in greater than 90% of patients (Bach et al, 1988). Despite the clinician's overall acumen, renal biopsy provides information that is of the utmost importance. Indeed, in one review, the renal biopsy resulted in a change in clinical diagnosis in 63% of patients and a change in therapy in 34% of patients. The most notable benefit of renal biopsy information was in the areas of nephrotic syndrome and acute renal failure (Cohen et al, 1989).

Clinically significant complications from renal biopsy are unusual now that 15- to 18-gauge needles have replaced the older, larger biopsy needles. Although greater than 90% of patients after renal biopsy have CT-detectable hematomas, bleeding requiring transfusion or other clinical intervention occurs in only 1% to 6% of patients (Ralls et al, 1987; Castoldi et al, 1994; Radford et al, 1994). The need for open surgical treatment of a complication arises in only 0.3%; infection, vascular fistulas, and mortality occur with equal albeit rare frequency: 0.1% (Radford et al, 1994).

PERCUTANEOUS THERAPEUTIC PROCEDURES

Therapeutic endourology can be divided into two broad areas: ablative and reconstructive procedures. Ablative procedures include nephrostolithotomy, renal cyst decortication and fulguration, fulguration and resection of upper urinary tract TCC, and therapy for a fungal bezoar. Reconstructive procedures encompass treatment of the following conditions: calyceal diverticula, hydrocalyx, UPJ obstruction, proximal ureteral strictures, and ureteral fistulas.

Ablative Percutaneous Endourology

Urolithiasis

OVERVIEW

Initially, open surgery was the only treatment available for renal calculi and included anatrophic nephrolithotomy and extended pyelolithotomy (Gil-Vernet, 1965; Boyce and Elkins, 1974). In 1976, Fernstrom and Johansson reported the first percutaneous stone removal through a nephrostomy tract positioned for that specific purpose. Subsequently, Kurth and colleagues used an ultrasonic lithotrite to fragment and retrieve a staghorn calculus successfully, thereby removing a large stone through a small nephrostomy tract (Kurth et al, 1977). Smith and colleagues described the closed manipulation of the urinary tract as *endourology* in 1979 (Smith et al, 1979). Subsequently, Smith and colleagues reported five cases of renal and ureteral calculi treated via a percutaneous nephrostomy tract (Smith et al, 1979). The development and refinement of electrohydraulic and ultrasonic lithotripsy soon made percutaneous nephrostolithotomy (PCNL) of large calculi feasible. The percutaneous approach to all renal calculi became preferred over open surgery because of reduced postoperative discomfort and a quicker convalescence for the patient. The introduction of ESWL to clinical practice in 1984 revolutionized the treatment of urinary calculi. During its early clinical use, ESWL was found to be successful in the treatment of small (i.e., <2 cm) renal pelvis and calyceal calculi of almost all compositions. With regard to calculi greater than 2 cm, other factors come into play: stone diameter, stone location, and stone composition.

With regard to larger renal calculi (i.e., >3 cm), ESWL therapy has been less successful. Indeed, Lam and colleagues demonstrated that ESWL treatment outcome could be accurately determined according to stone surface area and associated hydronephrosis (Lam et al, 1992c). They determined that large renal stones, with surface areas of less than 500 mm^2 in nondilated renal collecting systems, when treated with ESWL monotherapy had a stone-free rate of 92%. The group of patients presenting with this type of stone disease, however, composed only 3% of all patients with large (i.e., staghorn) calculi. When patients with stone surface areas of greater than 500 mm^2 with or without hydronephrosis were considered, the stone-free rate after ESWL monotherapy decreased to 63%. Other investigators have noted similar findings with respect to large stones and treatment outcomes using ESWL monotherapy (Van Deursen and Baert, 1992).

Several investigators have also shown that the position of the stone has a significant effect on the stone-free outcome of ESWL and PCNL (McDougall et al, 1989; Netto et al, 1991a). The success rate of ESWL for lower-pole calculi has been reported at 59% to 79% as compared to the success rate of 85% to 94% for PCNL. Based on these results, PCNL is often considered the treatment of choice for lower-pole renal calculi provided the stone is 2 cm or greater or the lower calyx is dilated.

In addition, stones known to be difficult to fragment may be an indication to treat the patient primarily with PCNL. Cystine and calcium oxalate monohydrate stones are often resistant to fragmentation with many ESWL modalities (Singer and Das, 1991). Therefore, the percutaneous approach to removal of these stones is more successful.

Lastly, it needs to be stressed that advances in the development of flexible ureteroscopes have allowed easier access to the upper ureter and the renal collecting system. As a result, more urologists are reporting successful results treating small intrarenal stones with flexible ureterorenoscopy and intracorporeal electrohydraulic or laser lithotripsy. This approach is preferable to PCNL for calculi 1 cm or less and is becoming competitive with ESWL in certain situations, such as proximal ureteral calculi and even lower-pole calculi.

RENAL CALCULI (LESS THAN 3 CM)

The percutaneous approach to smaller renal calculi is largely a salvage procedure that is used when ESWL and ureteroscopy have either failed or are not feasible. It remains as first-line therapy for smaller renal calculi that are composed of cystine or for 2- to 3-cm stones trapped in a lower-pole calyx. In this regard, work by Lingeman and colleagues suggests that PCNL may be of benefit for lower-pole calyceal calculi even in the 1- to 2-cm range (Lingeman et al, 1994).

TECHNIQUE: PERCUTANEOUS NEPHROSTOLITHOTOMY. Before beginning a PCNL, the patient must have a negative urine culture and normal coagulative indices. Patients presenting with infected urine should have appropriate antibiotic therapy and a confirmatory negative urine culture before proceeding to PCNL. This may necessitate hospital admission for parenteral antibiotics preoperatively. For those patients with a negative urine culture and normal renal function, preventive parenteral antibiotics are administered 1 hour preoperatively and include cephalexin 1 g or ampicillin 1 g plus gentamicin 1 mg/kg. Patients should have a type and screen preoperatively and be offered the opportunity to donate 1 or 2 units of autologous blood or to obtain donor-directed units.

Positioning the patient for simultaneous antegrade and retrograde access of the upper urinary tract reduces the operative time because the time for repositioning from a dorsal lithotomy to a prone position is eliminated (see Fig. 94–6). The patient undergoes general endotracheal intubated anesthesia or spinal regional anesthesia on a standard operative stretcher. After satisfactory control of the airway and establishment of necessary intravenous access, the patient is rolled prone onto the operating table. Two soft rolls are placed under the thorax and upper abdomen on each side of the patient to facilitate ventilation. The operative table is modified with two flat, padded boards (i.e., "spreader" bars) at the end of the table to support and abduct the legs. The patient is positioned such that the genitalia are accessible at the bottom of the table when the leg supporting boards are spread apart at a 45-degree angle. Foam padding is placed under the knees, and a folded pillow is placed under each foot at the ankle to afford slight flexion at the knee and reduce the risk of nerve palsy or pressure injury. Both arms are placed on boards with the shoulders abducted and the

elbows flexed to allow the hands to rest palm down alongside the head. Both the affected flank and the perineum are prepared and draped for access (see Fig. 94–6).

The initial step in performing PCNL is to access the upper collecting system by way of a retrograde approach. Flexible cystoscopy is performed, with the patient in the prone position, and a 0.035-inch polytetrafluoroethylene-coated, floppy-tipped 260-cm exchange guide wire is passed in a retrograde fashion, using C-arm fluoroscopic monitoring. After satisfactory positioning of the guide wire into the upper collecting system, the flexible cystoscope is removed leaving the guide wire in position. A No. 7 Fr, 11.5-mm occlusion balloon catheter is passed over the guide wire and into the upper collecting system, again under fluoroscopic control (Fig. 94–21B). A Touhey-Borst side arm adapter placed over the guide wire and attached to the end of the occlusion balloon catheter allows injection of 10 to 15 cc of

air to outline the renal pelvis and in particular the posterior calyces (see Fig. 94–21B). The air should be delivered slowly so that just enough is given to outline the posterior calyx and not the entire collecting system. Contrast material is avoided because any extravasation might jeopardize subsequent establishment of the nephrotomy tract. The balloon on the occlusion balloon catheter is then inflated with 1 ml dilute contrast material and positioned until it is snug at the UPJ region. The guide wire is removed leaving the occlusion balloon catheter in position in the upper collecting system. The occlusion balloon catheter impedes stone fragments migrating from the kidney to the ureter during the PCNL procedure and facilitates injection of dilute contrast material or air to outline the calyceal system. A Foley catheter is placed alongside the occlusion balloon catheter to provide bladder drainage during the procedure.

Attention is now directed to percutaneous access of the

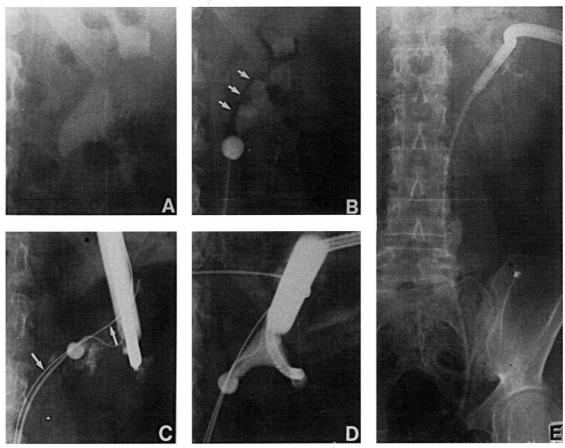

Figure 94–21. *A,* A plain film of the abdomen reveals a near-complete staghorn calculus in the left kidney. *B,* A No. 7 Fr, 11.5-mm occlusion balloon catheter has been passed retrograde up the ureter; the balloon has been inflated with 1 ml of contrast material just beneath the lowermost portion of the stone, at the ureteropelvic junction. Note that 10 to 15 cc of air has been instilled through the occlusion balloon catheter, providing an air pyelogram *(arrows)* and excellent visualization of the upper-pole posterior calyces. *C,* Via an upper-pole approach, a No. 30 Fr Amplatz sheath has been passed across the newly established nephrostomy tract. Note the presence of a safety guide wire *(arrows)* lying outside the No. 30 Fr sheath and passing down the ureter. Using the No. 26 Fr ultrasonic lithotriptor unit, the entire upper pole, renal pelvis, and lower pole have been accessed and largely cleared of stone debris. A rigid No. 24 Fr McCarthy panendoscope equipped with a No. 10 Fr grasping forceps has been passed through the No. 30 Fr sheath and is being used to remove stone debris from a lower-pole calyx. *D,* The flexible nephroscope has been introduced via the No. 30 Fr upper-pole nephrostomy sheath and passed into the lower-pole calyceal system, where additional stone material can be grasped and removed. *E,* At the end of this procedure, the kidney was free of stones by both rigid and flexible nephroscope inspection. A No. 22 Fr Councill balloon catheter has been passed over a No. 7.1 Fr pigtail catheter; the pigtail catheter has been advanced over the safety guide wire, which has been coiled in the bladder. The pigtail catheter was advanced until it was well in the bladder, at which point the guide wire was pulled back slightly, thereby allowing the pigtail in the distal tip of the catheter to form in the bladder. At this point, 1 to 2 ml of water can be placed into the balloon of the Councill catheter to secure its place in the renal pelvis, following which the guide wire can be removed and the Councill tube secured with two 0 silk sutures to the flank.

upper collecting system. If the stone to be managed is in a lower-pole calyx, the percutaneous approach is best performed directly onto the posterior lower-pole calyx. Upper and middle calyceal stones are also best approached directly into the respective calyceal system. Renal pelvis stones may be approached through the middle-pole or upper-pole posterior calyx to provide the most direct line of access to the bulk of the stone (see Fig. 94–21). Upper-pole and middle-pole approaches may require intercostal space nephrostomy placement (Picus et al, 1986) (see Fig. 94–21).

After selecting the calyx of entry, the skin site is selected. For upper-pole access, a skin site in the middle of the 11th to 12th intercostal space may be necessary because the point of entry into the calyx is better if it is done in a 30-degree caudad rather than perpendicular angle. A small skin incision is performed, and puncture is made with an 18-gauge needle with the x-ray beam angled parallel to the needle's path (Fig. 94–22B). Accurate placement of the needle is confirmed by aspiration of air or urine. A 0.035-inch Bentson guide wire is directed through the needle and coiled in the renal pelvis or, if possible, directed down the ureter. After removal of the 18-gauge needle, the No. 8 to 10 Fr coaxial dilator sheath introducer is passed over the guide wire. The No. 8 Fr catheter is removed, and a second guide wire is placed through the No. 10 Fr catheter. An attempt can again be made to direct this guide wire into the ureter; at this point, it is helpful to deflate the balloon on the occlusion balloon catheter. The No. 10 Fr catheter is removed. The guide wire, which is down the ureter or has the greatest amount of itself coiled in the renal pelvis, serves as a safety guide wire and is sutured to the skin. The 10-mm dilating balloon catheter

backloaded with a No. 30 Fr Amplatz nephrostomy sheath is placed over the nonsutured or "working" guide wire to dilate the nephrostomy tract as previously described. The No. 30 Fr Amplatz nephrostomy sheath is then positioned over the inflated balloon and passed into the collecting system (see Fig. 94–12C). The nephrostomy balloon is deflated and removed, leaving the No. 30 Fr Amplatz nephrostomy sheath in position (see Fig. 94–13).

Now the rigid nephroscope can be passed through the No. 30 Fr sheath and into the collecting system. The working guide wire, which still passes through the nephrostomy sheath, assists in directing the nephroscopist into the collecting system and to the region of the stone. If the stone is less than 1 cm in diameter, grasping forceps may be used to secure the stone and extract it through the No. 30 Fr Amplatz sheath. Larger stones require fragmentation before extraction. In this case, the occlusion balloon is reinflated and pulled caudad until it rests snugly against the UPJ. The rigid nephroscope facilitates ultrasonic, electrohydraulic, pneumatic, or laser lithotripsy of the stone. The ultrasonic lithotriptor has the advantage of using simultaneous suction to clear smaller stone fragments, thereby expediting stone clearance. Residual stone fragments less than 10 mm or stone material resistant to lithotripsy may be removed using grasping forceps.

After the removal of the stone material, the entire collecting system should be thoroughly examined with a flexible nephroscope for any residual stone material. The entire collecting system is systematically examined using injection of 50% contrast material through the working channel of the nephroscope to confirm that each calyceal system has been

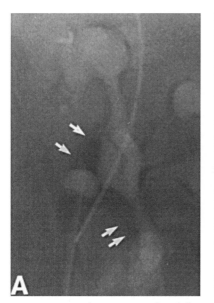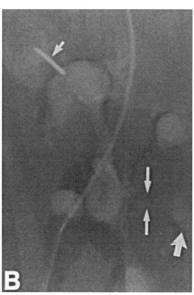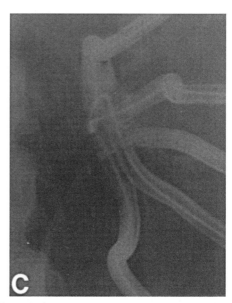

Figure 94–22. *A,* In this patient with a full staghorn calculus in a relatively nonhydronephrotic kidney, a No. 7 Fr 11.5-mm occlusion balloon catheter has been passed up the ureter; the balloon has been inflated with 1 ml of contrast material and pulled downward until it was snug at the ureteropelvic junction. In this image, 10 to 15 cc of air has been instilled through the retrograde catheter, thereby outlining the areas of the collecting system unoccupied by the stone *(arrows). B,* A nephrostomy needle *(uppermost arrow)* is directed at the upper pole in preparation for establishing upper-pole access. Note that the branches of the stone *(large arrow),* "dumbbell" across the infundibulae *(two middle arrows),* thereby precluding any chance of delivering the calyceal portions of the stone into the renal pelvis. *C,* In this patient, the calyceal extensions of the stone could not be delivered into the collecting system; hence at the initial percutaneous session, four additional nephrostomy tracts were established and the calyceal stones removed. Alternatively, after debulking the stone via the upper pole nephrostomy tract, one or two extracorporeal shock wave lithotripsy sessions could have been planned for the calyceal remnants, before a second-look nephroscopy session. By the same token, a stone such as this would also be reasonable to approach with an open anatrophic nephrolithotomy or extended pyelolithotomy and multiple radial nephrotomies.

thoroughly accessed and examined. Small residual fragments may be extracted using a No. 5 Fr, three- or four-pronged grasping forceps through the flexible nephroscope; larger stones can be fragmented with the No. 1.6 to 1.9 Fr electrohydraulic or one of the less than 400 μ laser (tunable dye or Ho:YAG) probes.

At the completion of the PCNL, a No. 7.1 Fr pigtail antegrade ureteral catheter and a coaxial No. 22 Fr Councill catheter are passed to the bladder and renal pelvis, as previously described (see Fig. 94–21E). The bladder catheter can be removed.

Twenty-four to 48 hours postoperatively, renal radiographs with tomograms are performed to check for removal of all stone material from the upper tract. A nephrostogram is performed to ensure patency of the ureter and resolution of any upper tract extravasation. If residual extravasation is present, the catheters are maintained for another 2 to 7 days until the repeat nephrostogram is normal.

Any residual stone fragments in the upper tract should be evaluated with a second-look nephroscopy (see Fig. 94–23). Likewise, if intracorporeal lithotripsy was done, a second-look procedure is always indicated because even with negative tomograms, 14% of patients still have small stone fragments remaining, some of which may have been hidden on the radiographic studies because of the nephrostomy tube.

The second-look nephroscopy can be performed with intravenous sedation on the second postoperative day, provided that the nephrostomy urine is clear to light pink. A bladder catheter is placed. Then the patient is placed prone on the operative table with padded support along either side of the thorax so that the chest is not compressed. The affected flank is prepared and draped with the nephrostomy tube and ureteral catheter in the sterile field. A 0.035-inch Bentson guide wire is passed through the No. 7.1 Fr pigtail catheter and fluoroscopically positioned in the bladder. The ureteral catheter and nephrostomy tube are removed. The flexible nephroscope is passed through the bare nephrostomy tract using the guide wire to direct the instrument into the renal pelvis (see Fig. 94–23).

If there were multiple residual calculi on the tomograms, however, the first step is to backload a No. 26 Fr Amplatz sheath on the No. 24 Fr rigid endoscope; the endoscope and sheath combination are passed down the bare nephrostomy tract. When the collecting system is entered, the No. 26 Fr sheath is slid forward slightly. The endoscope is withdrawn, thereby leaving the No. 26 Fr sheath in optimal position. Multiple stones can now be removed without traumatizing the nephrostomy tract and without losing fragments in the retroperitoneum. Systematic examination of the entire calyceal system is then performed. Injection of 50% contrast material identifies each calyx and helps to assure the urologist that the entire kidney has been thoroughly examined. Small stone fragments may be secured in grasping forceps and removed from the upper collecting system. Minimal manipulation of the upper collecting system during this procedure allows the nephroscope and guide wire to be removed without replacement of the nephrostomy. If manipulation has resulted in bleeding, however, the No. 22 Fr nephrostomy tube is replaced for 24 hours. Alternatively, if there is significant edema at the UPJ, an indwelling ureteral stent is placed. The nephrostomy tube usually can be removed either the next day or on an outpatient basis after an imaging study

confirms ureteral patency. The indwelling stent, if placed, is removed in the office 1 week later. Approximately 2 weeks after the procedure, an IVP can be obtained to assess for any missed stones or postoperative UPJ, ureteral, or infundibular stricture.

RESULTS. ESWL is considered the recommended treatment for calculi less than 1 cm regardless of composition or location. Calculi between 1 and 2 cm are still largely treated with ESWL as the first-line management except for cystine calculi and, possibly, some lower-pole calyceal calculi. Stones 2 to 3 cm are in somewhat of a gray zone, with treatment dependent on the stone composition and location; again, PCNL is preferred for the cystine or calcium oxalate monohydrate stone as well as for the 2- to 3-cm stone trapped in a lower-pole calyx.

Symptomatic, obstructing, and medically resistant **cystine** renal calculi require endourologic intervention, usually PCNL. Kachel and colleagues reviewed 19 patients with renal cystine stones between 1984 and 1988 (Kachel et al, 1991). From evaluation of their results, they recommended ESWL monotherapy for cystine renal calculi less than 15 mm because this was associated with successful fragmentation in 90% of the patients. For stones greater than 15 mm in size, percutaneous ultrasonic lithotripsy was recommended. Other investigators have noted similar failure of ESWL on greater than 1.5 cm cystine calculi (Knoll et al, 1988). Even with PCNL, however, it is difficult to clear the kidney of cystine stones because these patients usually have many small "radiographically unseen" stones in addition to larger calculi. Indeed, in nine patients with renal cystine stones greater than 15 mm who underwent percutaneous ultrasonic lithotripsy monotherapy, a stone-free rate of 58% was noted in a series from the Mayo Clinic (Segura, 1990). The cystine stone is quite hard, and at times the smooth-tip ultrasound probe is not capable of efficiently fragmenting the stone; in these patients, use of electrohydraulic, pneumatic, or Ho:YAG laser lithotripsy is needed. Residual calculi need to be approached with the flexible nephroscope (see Fig. 94–23). Skill with this instrument can increase the stone-free rate by upwards of 20%. Inaccessible cystine stones following percutaneous ultrasonic lithotripsy may be successfully treated with ESWL alone or in combination with medical dissolution (Kachel et al, 1991). At present, PCNL for cystine calculi is performed for all cystine calculi greater than 1.5 cm in diameter. For smaller cystine stones (i.e., <1.5 cm), ESWL is a reasonable option; however, if ESWL fails, ureteroscopy with a flexible ureteroscope and Ho:YAG laser or electrohydraulic lithotripsy is the next step.

Several investigators have shown that the clearance of stone fragments from the dependent **lower pole of the kidney** after ESWL may be significantly less successful than after PCNL (McDougall et al, 1989; Netto et al, 1991a; Lingeman et al, 1994). Review of the literature shows that the stone-free rate after ESWL for smaller lower-pole calculi averages 61% compared with an average stone-free rate of 91% for lower-pole calculi treated with PCNL (Table 94–2) (White and Smith, 1984; Drach et al, 1986; Servadio et al, 1986; Graff et al, 1988, 1989; Clayman et al, 1989; Lingeman et al, 1989; McDougall et al, 1989; Rigatti et al, 1989; El-Damanhoury et al, 1991; Netto et al, 1991a; Maggio et al, 1992; Mays et al, 1992; Lingeman et al, 1994). The

Table 94–2. PERCUTANEOUS NEPHROLITHOTOMY THERAPY FOR LOWER-POLE CALCULI

Authors	Number of Patients	Lithotripsy Modality	Stone Size ≦10 mm	Stone Size 11–20 mm	Stone Size 21–30 mm	Stone-Free Rate (%)	Retreatment Rate* (%)	Auxiliary Procedure (%)	Mean Follow-up
White and Smith, 1984	85	Ultrasound	—	—	—	95	—	—	—
Servadio et al, 1986	17	Ultrasound	—	—	—	70.5	16	—	—
McDougall et al, 1989	29	—	13	9	7	86	10	14	22 months
Netto et al, 1991a	23	Ultrasound	4	15	4	96	0	4	18 months
Mays et al, 1992	38	Electrohydraulic	—	—	—	82	—	—	24 months
Lingeman et al, 1994	32	Ultrasound	16	11	5	100	59	3	12 months
Total	224	—	—	—	—	91	25	7	19 months

*Includes second-look nephroscopy.

ESWL-treated patients, in general, had a similar or lower rate of auxiliary procedures compared to the PCNL group. The retreatment rate was similar for the two treatment groups; however, retreatment in the PCNL patients was usually a planned second-look flexible nephroscopy. Overall, although ESWL is attractive to the physician and patient because of its accessibility, ease of use, and noninvasive nature, there is increasing evidence that the results of ESWL for lower-pole calculi are perhaps even less successful than was heretofore appreciated (Lingeman et al, 1994). Lingeman and colleagues demonstrated that the success of ESWL for lower-pole calculi was directly related to the stone burden, yielding a favorable stone clearance rate when calculi were 10 mm or smaller. As stone size increased, PCNL had significantly better results than ESWL.

With regard to morbidity of PCNL, on review of their own group of patients between 1990 and 1992 who underwent PCNL for lower-pole calculi, Lingeman and colleagues had no blood transfusions or failures to achieve satisfactory access (Lingeman et al, 1994). PCNL in the lower pole is more easily accomplished than in other areas of the kidney; also, experience improves the clinical results and reduces the complication rate. Meta-analysis in the Lingeman and colleagues' review showed that, overall, patients with lower-pole stones are 6.27 times more likely to be rendered stone-free with PCNL compared with ESWL.

Sampaio and Aragao (1994) analyzed the inferior pole collecting system anatomy in 146 three-dimensional polyester resin corrosion endocasts of the pelvicalyceal system. They suggested that anatomic features, including an angle of less than 90 degrees formed between the lower-pole major infundibulum and the renal pelvis, a lower-pole infundibulum smaller than 4 mm in diameter, and multiple calyces (i.e., greater than three), may inhibit the evacuation of lower pole stone fragments after ESWL. They believe that the association of at least two of these anatomic restrictions is sufficient to contraindicate ESWL. Indeed, they tested their hypothesis in a prospective study of 74 patients. Patients with favorable anatomy had a 75% stone-free rate after ESWL versus a 23% stone-free rate among patients with unfavorable anatomy (Sampaio et al, 1995).

The use of PCNL in patients with lower-pole renal calculi or as salvage therapy after failed ESWL must also be viewed in light of ureteroscopic data, especially with regard to use of the flexible ureteroscope. For smaller renal calculi, in the less than 1.5 cm range, flexible ureteroscopy may be a less invasive yet effective approach than PCNL. In this regard, Bagley (1990a) performed ureteroscopy on 23 patients with intrarenal calculi and successfully removed or fragmented, with electrohydraulic or laser lithotripsy, 20 (87%) of the calculi. Fuchs and Fuchs (1990) treated 208 patients with renal calculi using flexible ureterorenoscopy for a variety of indications, including failed ESWL, radiolucent calculi, stones in patients with urinary diversion, and stones associated with infundibular stenosis. They achieved a stone-free rate of 87% in patients with normal renal anatomy and a 47% stone-free rate in patients with urinary diversion. They reported two complications of urosepsis and no deaths.

The experience with ureteroscopic intracorporeal electrohydraulic lithotripsy of lower-pole and renal calculi, between February 1990 and February 1995, was reviewed at Washington University Medical School (Elashry et al, 1996).

Seventeen patients with 31 lower-pole calculi were evaluated. In this group, one third of the patients were ESWL failures. Several patients had failed attempts at laser lithotripsy because the laser probe, albeit less than 400 μ in diameter, was too stiff to allow access of the flexible ureteroscope to the lower pole. In contrast, the No. 1.9 Fr electrohydraulic probe is extremely malleable resulting in minimal loss of deflection of the flexible ureteroscope. The mean stone size of the lower-pole calculi was 7.8 mm (range 3–15 mm). Using the flexible ureteroscope (No. 7.5 or 9.4 Fr) and electrohydraulic probe, a fragmentation rate of 94% was achieved. At follow-up of 8.7 months, the stone-free rate was 88%. Aside from two patients (4.4%) with postoperative fever, there were no other complications. The flexible ureteroscope with the small flexible electrohydraulic probes provides a safe, effective, and economical method for performing intracorporeal lithotripsy. Electrohydraulic lithotripsy is presently the only form of intracorporeal lithotripsy sufficiently malleable to allow routine access and successful fragmentation of lower-pole renal calculi.

At present, for lower-pole renal calculi greater than 2 cm, PCNL is front-line therapy, whereas for calculi 1 cm or less, ESWL is the first step. For lower-pole stones in the 1- to 2-cm range, there is still much controversy; however, PCNL seems the more favored option, especially if there are confounding factors, such as a narrow infundibulum, acute infundibular-pelvis angle, or a stone of hard composition. Lastly, for lower-pole stones 1.5 cm or less that fail ESWL, flexible ureteroscopic intracorporeal lithotripsy may eventually become the most reasonable next step.

A Canadian group of investigators evaluated the cost-effectiveness of ESWL and PCNL for the treatment of renal calculus disease (Jewett et al, 1995). They compared 1000 cases of ESWL and 133 cases of PCNL and assessed cost to include (1) instrumentation capital costs; (2) equipment maintenance service costs; (3) operating costs; (4) hospital costs of admission, floor stay, health records, patient accounts, and intravenous service costs; (5) costs for ancillary procedures; and (6) professional fees, laboratory costs, x-ray costs, and stone analysis costs. This study determined that effectiveness, defined as stone-free rates, was higher with PCNL than with ESWL (96% success versus 70%). The total costs for ESWL treatment varied widely with the annual volume of cases (from $3197 per treatment for 500 cases per year to $2219 per treatment for 2500 cases per year); this variation was less pronounced with PCNL. PCNL was associated with a lower incidence of additional therapy compared to the higher retreatment rate for ESWL. The total costs per case for ESWL, however, were lower than those for PCNL ($2746 per case versus $4087). Therefore, although ESWL is less expensive than PCNL, it is also less effective in rendering patients stone-free. The final advice for selecting one technology over the other is to choose wisely. PCNL for a 1-cm renal pelvis calculus is not likely to be cost-effective because ESWL is highly effective and less expensive. ESWL for a greater than 2 cm lower-pole stone is similarly not going to be cost-effective because the low success rate and need for additional procedures makes PCNL the better first-line treatment.

COMPLICATIONS. Although PCNL is less invasive than open surgical techniques, complications may occur during **access** of the collecting system, **dilation** of the nephrostomy tract, or **removal** of the calculus. An awareness of the potential complications assists the surgeon in prevention or early management to minimize the impact on the patient.

Complications of access and dilation have already been discussed in the percutaneous nephrostomy section. Certain relatively unique problems in this regard, however, may arise during PCNL. Because of the site-specific nature of PCNL, the nephrostomy tube may at times follow a somewhat precarious course. Specifically, patients with organomegaly, malrotated kidneys, marked scoliosis or kyphosis, or extremes of body fat (i.e., morbid obesity and emaciation) may be at increased risk for injury of the bowel, duodenum, liver, or spleen during PCNL. Occasionally the colon may be retroperitoneal. The incidence of colon perforation during percutaneous nephrolithotomy has been reported at 0.2% (Vallencien et al, 1985; Lee et al, 1987). The injury is usually recognized on the postprocedure nephrostogram, which demonstrates contrast material in the colon. If the perforation is extraperitoneal, an indwelling ureteral stent and bladder catheter are placed to decompress the urinary tract, and the nephrostomy tube is drawn back into the colon as a colostomy tube. This allows the renal parenchyma to seal. After several days, if injection of the colostomy tube shows no renal communication, the colostomy tube can be removed. Parenteral antibiotic coverage against coliform organisms should be instituted when the injury is recognized. If intraperitoneal extravasation of contrast material is present, however, a laparotomy and repair of the bowel is recommended to avoid peritonitis (Vallencien et al, 1985). Colon injuries are more likely in morbidly obese patients who have had a jejunoileal bypass resulting in an enlarged colon owing to water dumping, in extremely thin patients in whom the percutaneous access is made too laterally, and in patients with a horseshoe kidney when an upper-pole approach is performed. A preoperative CT scan may be helpful to delineate the position of the bowel with respect to the kidney in these patients. In the morbidly obese patient, performing PCNL in the lateral decubitus position may also allow the abdominal pannus and abdominal contents to fall anteriorly away from the flank and region of the kidney (Kerbl et al, 1994a). This approach is technically challenging, and a longer tract results because the kidney has the tendency to move anteriorly as the nephrostomy tract is dilated.

On the right side, duodenal injuries occur during percutaneous access secondary to guide wire or dilator perforation through the renal pelvis and into the duodenum. These injuries are also recognized during the postprocedure nephrostogram. They are best managed with nasogastric suction and nephrostomy tube drainage of the kidney. Interestingly, to date, there have been no reported hepatic injuries.

On the left side, splenomegaly may be a contraindication to percutaneous left nephrostomy. Preoperative CT scan delineates the feasibility of the left-sided percutaneous access. Percutaneous splenic injury requires emergency laparotomy and splenectomy. Splenic abscess is a rare complication of PCNL (Reinberg et al, 1989).

During the actual process of **stone removal**, several problems may arise. Bleeding equivalent to that encountered with transurethral resection of the prostate can be expected. Venous bleeding is suspected when the visual field is clear while the irrigating fluid is flowing but quickly obscured by dark blood when the irrigation is slowed or stopped. Arterial bleeding or major venous bleeding obscures the field even with gravity irrigation; in this situation, it is advisable to stop and place a large nephrostomy tube. If this is not done, the patient may rapidly become fluid overloaded with resultant bradycardia and hypotension. In this regard, it is essential that the irrigant always be normal saline and not water, glycine, or sorbitol. These alternative irrigants are indicated only in the rare case when intrarenal electrosurgery is needed. If the bleeding is not adequately controlled by placement of the nephrostomy tube, a Kaye tamponade balloon catheter should be placed and fully inflated (Kerbl et al, 1994b). Alternatively the nephrostomy tube may be clamped for 20 minutes and mannitol administered. The renal pelvis should fill with clot, which should tamponade the venous bleeding. If despite these efforts the patient becomes hemodynamically unstable or bleeding continues, emergency angiography with embolization or open exploration is indicated. After a significant hemorrhage, the procedure is postponed for at least 48 hours to allow the clot to lyse and clear and to allow a clear field. In some cases, it is prudent to discharge the patient with the nephrostomy tube in place and delay stone removal for 1 to 2 weeks to allow the nephrostomy tract to mature. The clinician should be aware that the immediate postoperative hematocrit done in the postanesthesia recovery room underestimates the true hematocrit by 4 to 6 points.

A large perforation of the collecting system can occur at any time during stone removal, thereby resulting in retroperitoneal extravasation of fluid. For this reason, normal saline is the preferred irrigant. Water should be avoided because of the hyponatremia and hemolysis associated with absorption of extravasated water. Glycine has been responsible for ammonium intoxication when associated with intravascular extravasation (Schultz et al, 1983). Perforations of the upper collecting system, even those made with the endoscope, usually seal completely within 24 hours of adequate drainage via the nephrostomy tube.

During stone removal, extravasation of irrigating fluid may occur into the peritoneal cavity, retroperitoneum, or intravascular space. Intraperitoneal extravasation is rare and usually is mobilized and excreted over 2 to 3 days with the assistance of diuretics (Dunnick et al, 1985). Rarely, it may be necessary to place an intraperitoneal drain. Intravascular extravasation is manifested by hypertension, dyspnea, bradycardia, cyanosis, confusion, and seizures. Treatment consists of prompt diuresis with mannitol or furosemide, fluid restriction, and monitoring of serum electrolytes.

Other problems relatively unique to PCNL include urosepsis, retained stone fragments, ureteral injury, and delayed bleeding. Despite sterilization of the urine with appropriate antibiotic therapy preoperatively, up to 30% of patients undergoing PCNL have bacteriuria after nephrolithotomy of struvite calculi (Segura et al, 1985). Septic shock has been reported in 0.25% to 1% of patients treated with percutaneous stone removal. Those patients with obstruction of the collecting system at the time of surgery are certainly at higher risk of developing sepsis. If on puncture of the collecting system cloudy or purulent urine is obtained, a small nephrostomy tube should be placed immediately. Tract dilation and stone manipulation are postponed for several days until a sterile urine culture is obtained from the nephrostomy tube and bladder urine samples. With regard to suspected struvite stones, if all urine cultures have been sterile, it is advisable to send some of the retrieved stone material from the nephrolithotomy for culture to determine the responsible organism and to facilitate appropriate antibiotic therapy. Patients who have prolonged nephrostomy drainage and extended antibiotic therapy preoperatively may present with candiduria. This should be treated with intravenous amphotericin or fluconazole (Diflucan) before instrumentation to reduce the risk of candidemia (Segura and Rosen, 1993). Again, in all cases, the urine must be sterile before proceeding with PCNL.

The objective of PCNL is to render the patient entirely stone-free. As the complexity of the stone disease increases, however, so does the risk of residual or retained stone fragments following the primary procedure. Most residual calculi can be removed using flexible nephroscopy through the established nephrostomy tract 48 hours after the initial procedure. Occasionally, it may be necessary to place additional nephrostomy tracts and institute auxiliary procedures such as ESWL to complete the stone removal procedure. There remains some debate as to the importance of residual stone fragments, especially those that are nonobstructive and uninfected. Segura and Rosen (1993) have reported that small residual fragments that would be expected to pass spontaneously after ESWL pass equally well after PCNL and are not associated with any increase in the rate of stone formation. The passage of stone fragments in the immediate postoperative period may result in partial obstruction of the upper tract and persistent urine leakage from the nephrostomy site. A nephrostogram to confirm the absence of edematous or residual stone fragment obstruction of the ureter before removal of the nephrostomy tube reduces the risk of persistent nephrostomy drainage. For patients in whom significant stone fragments remain postoperatively or in whom ureteral patency is questionable, the nephrostomy tube is maintained or an internal ureteral stent is placed until the fragments are resolved (i.e., passage or ESWL) or the ureteral edema subsides.

Ureteral injuries associated with PCNL are relatively uncommon. A ureteral tear may occur from misplacement or overdistention of the occlusion balloon or during extraction of stones from the proximal ureter. The latter may occur in 5% of patients (Roth and Beckman, 1988). These injuries are best managed by placement of an internal ureteral stent for 4 to 6 weeks to allow proper healing. Ureteral avulsion is extremely rare and mandates an open repair.

Delayed bleeding after PCNL is usually secondary to pseudoaneurysm formation or an arteriovenous fistula and occurs in less than 1% of patients (Segura et al, 1985). Factors that predispose to delayed bleeding include medial rather than posterolateral puncture, arteriosclerosis, and hypertension. Arteriography confirms the diagnosis, and embolization is usually curative, although rarely open exploration with partial or total nephrectomy may be necessary (Patterson et al, 1985).

Finally, the complications of PCNL must also be related to the relative health of the patient undergoing the procedure. Patients with concomitant cardiovascular disease and respiratory compromise may be at increased risk for intraoperative and postoperative complications associated with PCNL. Myocardial infarction and dysrhythmias are reported in less than 1% of patients undergoing PCNL (Lee et al, 1987). Morbidly obese patients undergoing PCNL may be more likely to have respiratory complications intraoperatively and postoperatively. Maintaining an airway in these patients when they are in the prone position may be particularly difficult.

STAGHORN CALCULI

Historically, investigators have shown improved survival rates for unilateral staghorn calculus patients treated by primary nephrectomy compared to those treated by conservative observation or delayed nephrectomy (Singh et al, 1973). The advent of percutaneous techniques and ESWL has significantly changed the management of staghorn calculus patients. Teichman and colleagues reviewed 177 consecutive staghorn calculus patients and determined risk factors for ultimate renal deterioration and renal cause–specific death (Teichman et al, 1995). Over a mean follow-up of 7.7 years, they noted that the overall rate of renal deterioration was 28%. Renal deterioration was more frequently associated with solitary versus nonsolitary kidneys (77% versus 21%), previous versus initial stones (39% versus 14%), recurrent versus nonrecurrent calculi (39% versus 22%), hypertension versus normotension (50% versus 22%), complete versus partial staghorn calculi (34% versus 13%), urinary diversion versus no diversion (58% versus 19%), and neurogenic versus non-neurogenic bladder (47% versus 21%). Also, patients who refused treatment were at a significantly higher risk of renal deterioration compared with treated patients (100% versus 28%). No patient with complete clearance of fragments died of renal related causes compared with 3% of those with residual fragments and 67% of those who refused treatment. An untreated struvite staghorn calculus may destroy the kidney over time and has a significant chance of causing the death of the patient from renal failure or sepsis (Rous and Turner, 1977; Koga et al, 1991). The goal of therapy is to render the patient stone-free and eradicate any urinary tract infection. Failure to achieve either of these results is associated with a significantly higher incidence of stone recurrence (Saad et al, 1993; Teichman et al, 1995).

The American Urological Association Nephrolithiasis Clinical Guidelines (AUA-NCG) panel recommends that a newly diagnosed struvite staghorn calculus should be actively treated rather than followed with conservative observation (Segura et al, 1994). After considering all treatment options and completing an exhaustive review of the literature, the AUA-NCG panel recommended that percutaneous stone removal, followed by ESWL or repeat percutaneous procedures as necessary, should be used for most staghorn calculi patients. ESWL monotherapy should be considered only in the rare circumstance of a small-volume staghorn calculus ($\leq$500 mm^2) in a nondilated or minimally dilated collecting system. Open surgery is not considered a first-line therapy option but may be an appropriate treatment alternative when a struvite staghorn calculus is not expected to be removable by a reasonable number of percutaneous or ESWL procedures or when intrarenal reconstruction is deemed necessary. Nephrectomy is considered a reasonable treatment alternative for the patient with a poorly functioning (i.e., <20% function), stone-bearing kidney.

TECHNIQUE: PERCUTANEOUS NEPHROSTOLI-THOTOMY. PCNL for staghorn calculi can be performed through a single access tract in the majority of cases without the addition of ESWL. Lam and colleagues found that successful staghorn calculus removal through a single access required special consideration in selection and placement of the nephrostomy tract, dexterity with a variety of rigid and flexible endoscopes, and access to a variety of intracorporeal lithotripsy devices (Lam et al, 1992a, 1992b).

Selection of the appropriate calyx is crucial to successful PCNL and should be determined preoperatively after careful inspection of the intrarenal anatomy on anteroposterior and oblique intravenous urogram studies. After achieving a sterile urine and while receiving parenteral antibiotic prophylaxis, the percutaneous access is obtained. Access is usually best achieved in the operating room by the urologist or radiologist using biplanar or C-arm fluoroscopy with the patient under general anesthesia. The latter is preferable. As described previously, under general anesthesia, the patient is positioned prone, with the legs supported on spreader bars to allow sterile access to both the bladder and the flank throughout the procedure. As previously described, using a flexible cystoscopy, a No. 7 Fr, 11.5-mm occlusion balloon catheter is passed, inflated, and secured at the UPJ. A Foley catheter is placed to drain the bladder. A percutaneous nephrostomy is performed into the selected calyx, and the tract is dilated to No. 30 Fr as described earlier. A No. 30 Fr Amplatz sheath is placed; this allows for free drainage of the irrigating fluid.

For staghorn calculi, the upper calyceal access is often preferable to optimize the visualization of the entire collecting system and facilitate access to the calculus with rigid instruments because the posterior upper-pole calyx is in the most posterior portion of the kidney and thus provides the most direct access to the renal pelvis, upper ureter, upper-pole calyces, and at times lower-pole calyces (see Fig. 94–21). After placement of the nephrostomy tube, a No. 20 or 24 Fr McCarthy panendoscope is inserted to confirm positioning within the collecting system and identify the calculus. If the sheath is not completely within the calyx, a No. 28 Fr cystoscope can be passed, using the "working" guide wire to direct passage through the dilated tract, into the collecting system. The No. 30 Fr nephrostomy sheath can then be advanced over the No. 28 Fr cystoscope into the calyx.

After establishing satisfactory renal access, intracorporeal lithotripsy is performed under nephroscopic visualization. The ultrasonic lithotriptor is most expedient because it performs fragmentation of the calculus and simultaneous suction removal of the smaller fragments. The stone occupying the initial access calyx and infundibulum is cleared first, allowing advancement of the No. 30 Fr Amplatz sheath deeper into the collecting system for stabilization and to decrease retroperitoneal or intrapleural collection of irrigant. The calculus is progressively fragmented and removed from the renal pelvis and calyces. The stone is best cleared by working progressively from medial to lateral. The ultrasonic probe is used to manipulate and roll the stone material out of the infundibula and calyces as lithotripsy proceeds. Drilling straight into the stone material in the infundibulum or shaving the stone off at the infundibulum leaves chunks of stone within the calyx, which may be difficult to reach with the rigid endoscope. Leaving a small protrusion of stone at the entrance to the infundibulum acts as a handle allowing the stone to be maneuvered out of the calyx and into the renal pelvis, where it can more easily be accessed and fragmented.

Pressurized irrigation (50 mm Hg) is necessary to distend the collecting system and optimize visualization during the procedure. Warmed saline is most commonly used to preclude reduced core temperature and chilling during the procedure. As much as 40 to 60 L of irrigant may be used during a typical 2- to 3-hour staghorn stone procedure.

Multiple percutaneous nephrostomy tracts may be necessary in large staghorn calculi when there is intrarenal anatomy restricting access to the peripheral calyces from a single nephrostomy tract or when the stone "dumbbells" across otherwise normal-sized infundibula (see Fig. 94–22). Excessive torquing or angulation of the nephroscope may result in parenchymal and vascular injury of the kidney and cause significant bleeding, especially in the previously operated kidney. Because of acute angulation, the middle-pole calyces may not be accessible by way of an upper-pole nephrostomy tract and may require a second percutaneous puncture.

After the majority of the calculus has been removed using the rigid nephroscope and ultrasonic lithotripsy, the flexible nephroscope is used to inspect all of the calyces systematically while injecting 50% contrast material to delineate the collecting system fluoroscopically. This can be most easily done by attaching tubing to the inflow channel of the flexible nephroscope, at the end of which is a three-way stopcock. Tubing for irrigant flow is attached into one of the arms of the stopcock, while a 60-ml syringe containing a 50:50 mixture of contrast material and saline is connected to a second arm of the stopcock. As each calyx is entered, the assistant turns the stopcock and proceeds to instill contrast material. This allows the surgeon to map out the entire renal collecting system fluoroscopically and confirm endoscope entry into each calyx. Small residual pieces of calculus can be removed using a three- or four-pronged grasping forceps through the flexible nephroscope. Larger stone fragments accessible by only flexible nephroscopy can be fragmented with electrohydraulic lithotripsy or laser lithotripsy.

Every attempt is made to clear the stone material completely at the initial percutaneous nephroscopy procedure. At the completion of the procedure, a No. 22 Fr Councill nephrostomy tube is positioned over a No. 7.1 Fr pigtail antegrade ureteral catheter as previously described (see Fig. 94–21E). The Foley bladder catheter is removed. If multiple nephrostomy tracts have been used to complete the nephrolithotomy, nephrostomy tube drainage of the kidney with a No. 22 Fr Councill catheter is performed through each tract (see Fig. 94–22). Usually 1 to 2 cc of saline is placed in the balloon of each Councill nephrostomy catheter. The backloaded antegrade pigtail catheter is affixed to the Councill catheter with a side arm adapter. The nephrostomy tube(s) is sewn to the flank with two sutures of 0 silk.

Postoperatively the patient is told that he or she may pass no urine per urethra as the pigtail antegrade catheter usually drains all the bladder urine. Additionally the patient is given belladonna and opiate suppositories every 4 to 6 hours on a per request basis for bladder spasms that may occur because of the ureteral catheter. Twenty-four to 48 hours later, the patient undergoes nephrotomography and nephrostogram evaluation. The nephrotomogram helps to delineate the presence and location of residual stone material, and the nephrostogram evaluates for extravasation. If no extravasation is present, the patient can undergo a second-look procedure performed under intravenous sedation, when indicated (vide infra).

If there is a stone or stones 1 cm or greater remaining in one or more peripheral calyces, ESWL is usually performed. If no definite calculi are seen on tomograms or the remaining stone material is scant and small (i.e., in the 5-mm range), flexible nephroscopy is performed (Fig. 94–23). Likewise, if ESWL is done, 1 to 2 days later, flexible nephroscopy is

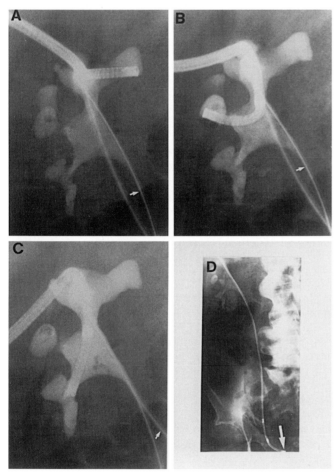

Figure 94–23. Second-look flexible nephroscopy. *A,* The flexible nephroscope has been introduced across the bare upper-pole nephrostomy tract and into the upper-pole calyces. The tip of the endoscope is maneuvered such that all three minor upper-pole calyces are examined. Note that there is a guide wire traversing the ureteropelvic junction *(arrow)* and traveling down the ureter; its distal tip has been coiled in the bladder. A Foley bladder catheter has been passed just before the procedure to drain the bladder. The part of the guide wire lateral to the portion traveling down the ureter is actually lying on the patient's flank. *B,* The flexible nephroscope has been introduced into the infundibulum servicing the middle calyces. One of two minor middle calyces has been entered and is being examined. Contrast material has been injected via the flexible nephroscope to confirm entry into this calyx. *C,* The flexible nephroscope has been maneuvered into the lower-pole major infundibulum in preparation for examining the minor calyces. *D,* A flexible No. 7.5 Fr ureteroscope has been advanced antegrade over the initially placed guide wire into the bladder *(arrow)* in preparation for inspecting the entire ureter immediately before removing all catheters and guide wires from the collecting system.

performed as a final check of the collecting system to make sure all stone debris has been flushed or endoscopically removed from the kidney. Indeed, even if the tomograms are negative for remnant calculi, a final flexible nephroscopy session is indicated because nearly 14% of patients still have significant stone debris either missed on the 1-cm tomogram cuts or obscured by the nephrostomy tube(s).

At the outset of the second-look flexible nephroscopy session, a Foley bladder catheter is placed. At the outset of the flexible nephroscopy session, a guide wire is positioned down the ureter by way of the No. 7.1 Fr ureteral catheter, and the ureteral catheter and nephrostomy tube are removed. If there are no stones on the nephrotomograms or only one or two fragments, the flexible nephroscope is passed alongside the guide wire, through the bare nephrostomy tract, and used to examine the entire collecting system systematically, confirming visualization with fluoroscopic injection of 50% contrast material via the previously described three-way stopcock irrigant/contrast system. The irrigant is pressurized to 150 mm Hg to facilitate "washing" debris from the calyces and visualization. Small stone fragments can be removed with grasping forceps or treated with intracorporeal lithotripsy. If before the flexible nephroscopy the patient had ESWL or there are multiple calculi that need to be removed, second-look nephroscopy is initiated with a rigid No. 24 Fr endoscope (e.g., McCarthy cystoscope) backloaded with a No. 26 Fr Amplatz sheath. The endoscope is visually guided along the guide wire until the collecting system is entered. The No. 26 Fr sheath is then slid forward until it is "seen" to enter the collecting system. The No. 24 Fr endoscope is withdrawn. All subsequent stone manipulation is performed through the sheath with the flexible nephroscope or a No. 20 Fr or smaller rigid endoscope (e.g., No. 20 Fr McCarthy cystoscope or No. 12 Fr short rigid ureteroscope). The sheath protects the nephrostomy tract and allows for the flushing of any smaller stone debris from the collecting system.

At the end of the procedure, a No. 10 Fr or smaller flexible ureteroscope is advanced antegrade over the guide wire until it is shown fluoroscopically to enter the bladder. The guide wire is removed, and the entire ureter is inspected, as the ureteroscope is withdrawn, for any calculi, which if found are immediately removed (see Fig. 94–23D).

At the completion of the second-look nephroscopy, an internal ureteral stent is placed if blood clots or edema at the UPJ are noted. This stent can be removed in the office 1 week later. If the UPJ appears normal and there is no bleeding, ureteral stent placement is not necessary. The nephrostomy tube is not replaced unless there is significant bleeding from the nephrostomy tract.

If a chest tube was placed during the initial operative procedure for management of hydrothorax, it should be left open during the second-look procedure. At the completion of the procedure, the chest tube is placed to water seal. A chest x-ray in the morning demonstrating clear lung fields is an indication for chest tube removal.

RESULTS. There has been no uniform system or method of categorizing staghorn calculi and the collecting system. Lam and colleagues have demonstrated that computer image analysis of standard radiographs can provide an accurate, rapid, and easy method to determine stone surface area (Lam et al, 1992c). Stone surface area closely correlates to stone volume as measured by three-dimensional CT. The technique for calculating surface area uses an electronic pen or mouse to trace the outline of the staghorn calculus onto a digitizing pad linked to a microcomputer. An image analysis software program instantly quantifies the stone area within the contour drawn on the grid. Stolk and Ettershank (1987) have shown the error of stone surface area assessment using a computer program to be less than 1% and the reproducibility of the measurement to be within 5%. Stone surface area provides a more objective means to compare treatment results for staghorn calculi.

Several investigators have shown that experience with PCNL improves successful access and stone-free rates and reduces the complication rates associated with this procedure. Lee and colleagues noted an increase in their success rate for PCNL for all calculi from 89% in the first 100 patients to 95% to 98% when the series was expanded to 500 patients. In this series, failed access occurred in less than 2% of patients overall (Lee et al, 1986). Lam and colleagues reviewed 252 patients with staghorn calculi treated from 1984 to 1987 and 91 patients with the same diagnosis treated from 1988 to 1990 (Lam et al, 1992a). They noted marked decrease in the proportion of cases managed by combination therapy (PCNL plus ESWL) in the latter group (35%) compared to the early group (65%). The use of multiple nephrostomy tracts, however, increased significantly in the latter group (13% versus 9%). There were no blood transfusion requirements in the most contemporary group compared to an 11% transfusion rate in the initial group. The higher incidence of pulmonary complications (9%) in the more recent group, mainly hydrothorax, was attributed to the more liberal use of supracostal punctures in 30.6% of the patients. The mean stone surface area was greater in the more recent group, but despite this finding the stone-free rate tended to increase (87% versus 83%). This was likely due to the more frequent use of upper-pole access and multiple percutaneous nephrostomy tracts, combined with common use of flexible nephroscopy to clear the collecting system.

PCNL is considered the treatment of choice for patients with staghorn calculi. The overall stone-free rates for PCNL monotherapy range between 60% and 92% (Table 94–3). The retreatment rates are high at 21% to 80%; however, this usually consists of flexible nephroscopy through the established nephrostomy tract under intravenous anesthesia, which although counted as a secondary procedure is a preoperatively planned procedure. The average hospital stay varies from 4 to 18 days. Residual stone fragments remain on average in 16% of patients. Snyder and Smith (1986) prospectively studied PCNL versus anatrophic nephrolithotomy for management of staghorn calculi. They reported that although PCNL results in a higher frequency of retained stone fragments compared to anatrophic nephrolithotomy (13% versus 4%), the patients required fewer blood transfusions (2 units in 53% of PCNL patients versus 3.5 units in 70% of anatrophic patients), used less analgesics (16 doses of narcotics versus 33 doses), had a shorter postoperative hospital stay (9.5 days versus 12.8 days), and returned more quickly to regular activities (14 days versus 55 days). This is comparable to the landmark anatrophic nephrolithotomy series of Boyce and Elkins (1974). In 100 cases over 5 years, a stone-free rate of 80% was obtained. The cost to

the patient for this therapy, however, was considerable: 10.7 days in the hospital, 4% transfusion rate of greater than 5 units per patient, 3% pneumothorax rate, and an indwelling ureteral stent in 77% of the patients for an average of 8 days postoperatively.

ESWL was initially applied to a variety of complex renal calculi, with variable results. Monotherapy ESWL for staghorn calculi has a stone-free rate ranging from 44% to 62% and usually requires placement of an internal ureteral stent or percutaneous nephrostomy tube. Residual stone fragments remain in 22% to 70% of cases. Retreatments are commonly necessary in 32% to 88% of cases because of the large stone burden. Auxiliary post-treatment procedures are required in 17% to 40% of cases. As such, it is the exceptional patient who becomes stone-free with only one ESWL session and without the need for auxiliary procedures.

The success of ESWL for staghorn calculi is directly related to the stone burden, the degree of the hydronephrosis, and stone composition. The seminal work in this area can be found in the paper by Lam and colleagues, who have identified a favorable subgroup of patients with staghorn calculi among whom ESWL monotherapy is successful (Lam et al, 1992a). They were able to achieve a 92% stone-free rate in patients with a **500 mm² or smaller stone burden in a nondilated collecting system.** In their experience, this subgroup of patients composed only 3% of their staghorn patient population. These findings further serve to corroborate the importance of measuring stone surface and assessing collecting system anatomy before embarking on a course of ESWL monotherapy.

The development of the *sandwich* technique has been an attempt to combine the success rate of PCNL with the reduced morbidity of ESWL. Sandwich therapy refers to any staged combination of PCNL and ESWL but most commonly involves PCNL debulking of the calculus followed by ESWL, followed by PCNL flexible and rigid nephroscopy. The various stages are each separated by 1 to 2 days. Stone-free rates with this approach are variable, ranging from 52% to 85% (Table 94–4) (Eisenberger et al, 1987; Segura et al, 1987; Lam et al, 1992a). Planned treatments, in addition to a single ESWL and PCNL session, were required to clear stones in 44% to 53% of patients. On analysis, it would appear that the aggressiveness of the PCNL procedures and the skilled use of flexible nephroscopy to remove residual stone fragments had the greatest positive impact on the ultimate stone-free rate.

Saad and colleagues reviewed 57 patients treated by PCNL for staghorn calculi and determined risk factors associated with stone recurrence after treatment (Saad et al, 1993). Factors associated with an increased rate of stone recurrence were positive urine cultures during follow-up, stone remnant greater than 5 mm, and stone complexity. Aggressive follow-up and interventional therapy should be directed at patients with these risk factors at presentation.

COMPLICATIONS. Complication rates associated with PCNL for staghorn calculi are relatively high, although few are major complications. The most common complication after PCNL is fever or infection. Kerlan and colleagues reported complications in 9 of 20 PCNL patients, including 20% pyelonephritis and urosepsis and 20% involving a temperature greater than 38°C (Kerlan et al, 1985). Winfield and associates reported complications in 19 of 23 patients treated

Table 94–3. PERCUTANEOUS NEPHROLITHOTOMY MONOTHERAPY FOR STAGHORN CALCULI

Author	Number of Patients	Average Hospital Stay (days)	Stone-Free Rate (%)	Residual Stones (%)	Retreatment Rate (%)	Auxiliary Procedures (%)	Transfusion Rate (%)	Complications
Snyder and Smith, 1986	75	13.3	86	13.3	22	1	53	Urosepsis 27%
Patterson et al, 1987	68	—	84	16	—	5	—	—
Winfield et al, 1988	23	10.4	86	14	—	5	Average 2 units/patient	Fever 11% Pneumo/hydrothorax 11% Ileus 11% Deep venous thrombosis 5%
Gleeson et al, 1991	30	—	60	13	—	—	0	Fever 42% Pneumo/hydrothorax 6% Respiratory 4% Sepsis 2%
Lam et al, 1992a	103	11.4	91	—	—	—	8	Fever > 100°F 21% Perforation 7% Obstruction 3% Colonic perforation 0.9% Hydrothorax 4%
Chibber, 1993	878	—	93	7	—	—	12	Urinary tract infection 1.4% Angiography 0.7% Prolonged leak 1.3% Hydrothorax 0.5% Bowel fistula 0.1%
Netto et al, 1994	102	3.4	83	16	25	—	13	Urosepsis 16% Cardiac dysrythmia 1% Colonic perforation 1%
Total	1279	9.6	90	9	23	4	14	

Table 94–4. PERCUTANEOUS NEPHROSTOLITHOTOMY/EXTRACORPOREAL SHOCK WAVE LITHOTRIPSY COMBINATION THERAPY FOR STAGHORN CALCULI

Author	Number of Patients	Lithotriptor	Stone-Free Rate (%)	Residual Stones (%)	Average Treatment Sessions PCNL/ESWL	Transfusion Rate (%)	PCNL Complications	ESWL Complications
Eisenberger et al, 1987	78	—	60	34	14% auxiliary procedures	17	Fever 37% Colic 15%	—
Karlsen and Gjolberg, 1989	51	HM3	56	31	1.8/1.1	—	—	—
Schulze et al, 1989	87	HM3	61	23	1.8/1.0	—	—	—
Gleeson et al, 1991	23	—	52	—	overall 2.4	—	Fever 42% Pneumo/hydrothorax 6%	Fever 15% Obstruction 12%
Lam et al, 1992a	195	HM3	85	—	overall 2.8	—	—	—
Streem and Lammert, 1992	28	HM3	57	—	1.6/1.4	—	—	—
Prajsner et al, 1993	110	Lithostar	70	20	1.7/1.8	25	Fever/sepsis 35% Pneumothorax 2% Obstruction 6%	Hematuria 80% Fever 11% Colic 20% Renal hematoma 2%
Total	572		70	25	1.7/1.3	23		

PCNL, percutaneous nephrostolithotomy; ESWL, extracorporeal shock wave lithotomy.

with PCNL monotherapy for staghorn calculi, including 2 with hemothorax or pneumothorax, 2 with displaced nephrostomy tubes, 2 with respiratory distress, and 1 with a deep vein thrombosis (Winfield et al, 1988). Pulmonary complications occur more commonly when upper-pole, supracostal nephrostomy access is used and overall are noted in 25% of upper-pole access PCNL cases (Lam et al, 1992a).

The reported transfusion rates in PCNL staghorn patients have been variable. In early series, the transfusion rate was reported as high as 53%. Lam and colleagues, however, reported no need for transfusion in their 91 contemporary PCNL patients compared with 11% of their PCNL patients before 1988 (Lam et al, 1992a). The need for surgical intervention or nephrectomy for complications of PCNL remains rare: 0% to 2.6% and 0% to 0.1%. The mortality rate for PCNL is 0.1% to 0.7% and is usually related to myocardial infarction and associated dysrhythmias (Lee et al, 1987).

Complications associated with the sandwich technique reflect the emphasis of the selected approach. Aggressive PCNL as the primary treatment modality is associated with transfusion rates of 2.5% to 35%, fever greater than 37.8°C in 13% to 62% of patients, urosepsis in 1% to 4% of patients, and a less than 10% incidence of collecting system perforation. The problems related to passage of stone fragments were less commonly associated with the sandwich technique compared to ESWL monotherapy. No nephrectomies were necessary in any of the sandwich series.

URETERAL CALCULI

The plethora of management options for the ureteric calculus patient may make the appropriate treatment choice somewhat confusing. Certain aspects of the minimally invasive surgical options remain controversial and vehemently debated. Advances in the endourologic and minimally invasive treatment of ureteral calculi have revolutionized management of these patients. Spontaneous passage of the majority of ureteral calculi, however, supports conservative management as a prudent and reasonable option for many patients. Hubner and colleagues reviewed the literature and compared the results with their last 100 patients presenting with ureteral calculi (Hubner et al, 1993). In 2804 patients reviewed, the spontaneous passage rate for all ureteral stones was 38%. The spontaneous stone passage rate was directly correlated to the stone size and the location at the time of presentation. Stones smaller than 4 mm had a spontaneous passage rate of 57%, stones between 4 and 6 mm in size had a spontaneous passage rate of 56%, and stones greater than 6 mm had a spontaneous passage rate of only 8%. Calculus location significantly affected the spontaneous passage rate: The distal third ureteral stone passage rate was 45%, the middle third passage rate was 22%, and the proximal third passage rate was 12%. In Hubner and colleagues' group of 100 patients, the time between onset of symptoms and spontaneous passage of the stone averaged 1.6 weeks (range 1–4 weeks) for stones less than 4 mm and 2.8 weeks (range 1–7 weeks) for stones between 4 and 6 mm in size (Hubner et al, 1993).

Most urologists agree that ESWL is the first line of therapy for proximal ureteral calculi that either are greater than 6 mm or have failed to pass spontaneously. Many urologists also advocate ESWL as first-line therapy for middle and distal ureteral calculi because the noninvasive nature and minimal morbidity of ESWL outweigh the decreased stone-free rate when compared to ureteroscopic procedures. In most American medical centers today, open or laparoscopic ureteral surgery for stone disease has become a phenomenon, accounting for less than 1% of all ureteral stone treatments. As such, there are scant indications for PCNL in patients with ureteral calculi. Indeed, the percutaneous approach is entertained only when ESWL, ureteroscopy, or both have failed. The only indication for an initial percutaneous approach is in the patient with a greater than 1.5 cm, densely impacted proximal ureteral calculus; a ureteral stone proximal to a dense ureteral stricture; or a ureteral stone causing pyonephrosis or complete obstruction. In the last case, the PCNL is a two-step procedure because for pyonephrosis the system must be drained and sterilized before stone manipulation. Even in these few cases, there would be alternative views with regard to the benefit of a rapid open ureterolithotomy or, were the stone located in the middle ureter, laparoscopic ureterolithotomy. Again, it must be stressed that in 1996 for ureteral calculi, PCNL and open or laparoscopic ureterolithotomy are largely salvage procedures that are rarely indicated.

TECHNIQUE: PERCUTANEOUS NEPHROSTOLITHOTOMY. For ureteral calculi, percutaneous access to the kidney is best performed through a posterior upper or middle calyx to provide a direct, straight-line approach to the proximal ureter. The technique is otherwise exactly as described for PCNL in general.

Securing retrograde access to the renal collecting system involves bypassing the ureteral calculus. This can at times be difficult. For this purpose, a 0.035-inch Terumo or plastic guide wire is recommended; an angled instead of straight tip is helpful to pass the stone and enter the renal pelvis. If difficulty is encountered, a Kumpe catheter (angled tip) can be passed over the guide wire until it lies just below the stone on the fluoroscope monitor. With this catheter, the ureteral sidewall around the stone can be probed with the Terumo guide wire. Alternatively, if the ureter is particularly tortuous, a No. 7 Fr, 11.5-mm occlusion balloon can be placed just beneath the stone and inflated with only 0.5 ml of contrast material so that it is fixed in position. The balloon catheter can then be gently pulled retrograde. This should straighten the ureter. While maintaining gentle traction on the occlusion balloon catheter, the Terumo guide wire is advanced into the renal pelvis. Once a guide wire is in the renal pelvis, the No. 7 Fr, 11.5-mm balloon occlusion catheter, in its deflated state, can be advanced to the renal pelvis. If there is resistance to passage of the No. 7 Fr catheter, a No. 5 Fr angiographic catheter should be advanced to the renal pelvis over the Terumo guide wire. Once the No. 5 Fr catheter enters the renal pelvis, the Terumo guide wire is exchanged for a 0.035-inch Amplatz superstiff guide wire. The No. 5 Fr catheter is removed, and the No. 7 Fr occlusion balloon catheter is passed. Once the balloon catheter is in position, the 0.035-inch Amplatz superstiff guide wire is exchanged for a 260-cm-long, 0.035-inch exchange guide wire. If nothing can be passed beyond the stone, the occlusion balloon catheter is inflated with 0.5 ml of contrast material just distal to the stone. Initial injection of saline through the ureteral catheter may displace the calculus into the renal pelvis, which makes the percutaneous extraction easier. A bladder Foley catheter is placed.

A transparenchymal No. 24 to 30 Fr nephrostomy tract is established, as described for PCNL. The smaller tract is sufficient for passage of the flexible or rigid ureteroscope or flexible nephroscope and any intracorporeal electrohydraulic or laser lithotripsy device; a larger tract is needed to access a proximal ureteral stone with the No. 26 Fr ultrasonic lithotriptor.

On examining the collecting system with the rigid nephroscope, the tip of the exchange guide wire should be identified, grasped, and delivered from the nephrostomy tract, thereby providing through-and-through access to the entire ipsilateral urinary tract, bladder, and urethra. Next, if the stone has not moved up the ureter into the renal pelvis, the occlusion balloon catheter should be removed. A No. 8/10 Fr Amplatz dilator/sheath is passed up the ureter; the No. 8 Fr catheter bypasses the stone. The No. 8 Fr catheter is removed, and through the No. 8 Fr lumen of the No. 10 Fr sheath, a 0.035-inch Amplatz superstiff guide wire is passed. The No. 10 Fr sheath is removed. The deflated No. 7 Fr, 11.5-mm occlusion balloon catheter is passed over the superstiff guide wire, until it lies just distal to the calculus. The balloon is filled with 0.5 ml of dilute contrast material and is thus fixed in place. The superstiff guide wire is removed. Now while the surgeon gazes via the nephrostomy tract at the cephalad surface of the stone, the assistant can forcefully flush 10-ml boluses of normal saline through the retrograde occlusion balloon catheter and either dislodge the stone proximal or at least loosen the stone from the ureteral wall. The ureteral stone can then be removed with grasping forceps (e.g., No. 5 Fr, four-prong grasper), or the stone can be fragmented using electrohydraulic, Ho:YAG or tunable dye laser, ultrasonic, or pneumatic lithotripsy. After extraction of the ureteral calculus, the occlusion balloon catheter is removed. A nephrostomy and ureteral catheter drainage system is placed antegrade over a guide wire passed into the bladder, as previously described.

The semirigid or flexible ureteroscope may be necessary to achieve antegrade percutaneous access to the ureter. The small semirigid ureteroscopes are now available with an outside diameter between No. 4.5 and 6.9 Fr. By the use of fiberoptic bundles for both visualization and illumination, these diminutive endoscopes accommodate one or two working channels. The latter situation, found in the No. 6.9 Fr endoscope, provides the surgeon with a No. 2.3 and 3.4 Fr working channel for simultaneous irrigation and passage of instruments. The flexible ureteroscopes are available in diameters as small as No. 7.5 Fr and feature a No. 3.6 Fr working channel. These smaller instruments allow access to the entire undilated ureter.

Impacted ureteral calculi require intracorporeal lithotripsy. Ultrasonic disintegration is used only if the stone is in the proximal ureter and can be accessed with the No. 24 to 26 Fr rigid ultrasonic nephroscope. For all other ureteral calculi, usually a flexible endoscope is needed to access them; as such, either electrohydraulic or laser lithotripsy is used.

Electrohydraulic lithotripsy uses a spark-gap–generated cavitation bubble to cause fragmentation of the surface of the stone. Ureteral injury may occur from direct contact with the probe. Hence, when intraureteral electrohydraulic

lithotripsy is performed, certain guidelines should be followed (Denstedt and Clayman, 1990). The tip of the No. 1.6, 1.7, or 1.9 Fr electrohydraulic probe should be smooth. The tip of the probe should extend 5 mm beyond the ureteroscope during use to eliminate damage to the lens. A rapid flow of normal saline irrigant should be maintained during electrohydraulic lithotripsy (Miller and Wickham, 1984). Before activating the electrohydraulic probe, the stone must be clearly visualized, and the entire tip of the probe must rest on or less than 1 mm from the center of the stone with no intervening urothelium. The stone is reduced to small (<2 mm) fragments. The development of small electrohydraulic probes (No. 1.6 to 1.9 Fr) and a 0.05-second built-in time cutoff in the electrohydraulic machine or single-pulse firing mode has made this method of intracorporeal lithotripsy efficient, safe, and easy to perform. The small electrohydraulic probes provide the power required to fragment hard stones while using the smaller semirigid and flexible ureteroscopes, as the No. 2 Fr working channel easily accommodates the No. 1.9 Fr or smaller electrohydraulic probe and allows the No. 3 Fr channel to be used for irrigation. Likewise with these probes, there is ample room for irrigant flow through the No. 3.6 Fr channel of the flexible ureteroscopes. In addition, if the flow is too sluggish, it is helpful to pressurize the irrigant bag with a blood pressure cuff or other pressure apparatus (e.g., Alton-Dean). Pressures between 50 and 300 mm Hg are sufficient.

Laser lithotripsy is available in two forms: tunable pulsed-dye and Ho:YAG. The tunable pulsed-dye laser consists of a 250-μ, silica-coated quartz fiber through which coumarin green light (wavelength 504 nm) is transmitted. The fiber is applied directly to the stone, and light energy produces activation of electrons, thereby forming a plasma, which results in an acoustic expansion-contraction cycle and creates stone fragmentation. A short pulse-repeat cycle (10 per second) is delivered at 30 to 140 mJ until the stone is reduced to 1- to 2-mm fragments, which pass spontaneously. The specific wavelength of the pulsed-dye laser ensures that the stone and not the urothelium absorbs the laser energy, eliminating the risk of thermal injury.

The Ho:YAG laser has a 200-μ or a 400-μ fiber and operates at a wavelength of 2100 nm. The fiber is applied directly to the stone. A pulse repetition of 5 times per second at 500 mJ is usually used; however, the energy can be raised as high as 2000 mJ. The stone is again reduced to 1- to 2-mm fragments. With this laser, it is essential not to fix it directly on the ureteral wall because the wavelength of 2100 nm allows it to coagulate or even cut the ureteral wall depending on the probe's distance from the ureteral wall.

The latest development in rigid intracorporeal lithotriptors is the rigid pneumatic lithotriptor. This lithotriptor consists of a central pin that is driven by compressed air at a frequency of 12 cycles per second and a pressure between 3 and 5 bars against a restraining outer sheath. The pin projects beyond the outer sheath. When brought into contact with a calculus, it is an efficient lithotriptor. The probe can be used through miniaturized ureteroscopes with working channels of No. 3.4 Fr or larger. It is relatively inexpensive and has no disposable pieces. When used on an impacted calculus, there is negligible bleeding and no ureteral wall injury. The pneumatic lithotriptor, however, does tend to propel an unrestrained calculus proximally, particularly in a dilated ureter (Denstedt, 1993).

A postoperative nephrostogram 48 hours after the surgical procedure usually demonstrates relief of the obstruction. In the absence of any residual extravasation, the nephrostomy tube and ureteral catheter may be removed. The presence of persistent extravasation or marked ureteral edema necessitates placement of an indwelling ureteral stent or maintenance of the nephrostomy tube and antegrade external ureteral stent drainage until resolution of the extravasation is noted on a repeat nephrostogram or IVP. Stone removal with a larger endoscope is usually easier because it provides better visualization; better irrigation; and larger, more versatile extracting instrumentation. The larger endoscope, however, may induce more trauma to the proximal ureter. The size of the most appropriate endoscope can usually be estimated by matching the endoscope to the stone size and position on the preoperative imaging studies. Stones smaller than 1 cm can usually be extracted intact. Stones lying caudal to the first few centimeters of the proximal ureter require use of a flexible endoscope.

RESULTS: UPPER URETERAL CALCULI. The majority of upper ureteral calculi are successfully treated with ESWL. Earlier recommendations to displace the stone to the renal pelvis or to bypass the stone with a ureteral stent have been tested in randomized clinical trials. Neither stone pushback nor stone bypass is indicated. In situ ESWL is as effective as bypass or pushback and entails less expense and less patient discomfort.

Danuser and colleagues prospectively randomized 110 patients with proximal ureteral calculi to in situ treatment versus pretreatment manipulation followed by ESWL on the Dornier HM-3 (Danuser et al, 1993). In the 48 patients who underwent retrograde manipulation, 44 stones were successfully pushed back into the kidney, and 1 was bypassed with a stent; in 3 patients, the ureteral catheter could be positioned only to a level just below the stone. Three-month follow-up was available on 94 patients, and the stone-free rates were 96% for the in situ ESWL group and 94% for the manipulated ESWL group. Only one patient from the in situ ESWL group and none from the manipulated group required more than one ESWL treatment; no ancillary procedures were necessary in either group. Stones treated in situ required significantly more shock waves at a higher voltage than those treated with pre-ESWL manipulation. Also of note, the success rate of in situ ESWL for upper ureteral calculi is equivalent for the first-generation and second-generation lithotriptors.

Hence, contemporary clinical experience strongly supports in situ ESWL as the initial treatment for the majority of upper ureteral calculi, even those that appear to be totally obstructing. The only exceptions include large (greater than 1.5 cm) ureteral calculi or urosepsis necessitating stent bypass or nephrostomy tube placement to preserve renal function or to drain an infected kidney.

Ureteroscopy is presently considered a first-line salvage therapy procedure for upper ureteral calculi that have failed ESWL. The early experience with ureteroscopic management of upper ureteral calculi demonstrated success rates of only 52% to 80% for retrieval or fragmentation of the calculus using rigid ureteroscopes. The development of the flexible ureteroscope and smaller ancillary equipment (e.g.,

laser and electrohydraulic probes) paralleled improvement in the successful ureteroscopic management of proximal ureteral calculi. A review of the literature shows that the stone-free rate for upper ureteral calculi managed ureteroscopically now ranges between 80% and 95% (Abdel-Razzak and Bagley, 1993).

Upper ureteral calculi that fail ESWL and retrograde ureteroscopic manipulation may be candidates for a percutaneous antegrade procedure. PCNL is often easily performed in these dilated renal systems and is highly effective, albeit invasive. The stone-free rate using this approach ranges between 88% and 100% (Reddy et al, 1985; Segura et al, 1985; Liong et al, 1989). A multicenter study comparing various treatment options for upper ureteral calculi reported 100% stone-free rate in 18 patients undergoing single-stage nephrostolithotomy (Liong et al, 1989). A transparenchymal No. 36 Fr nephrostomy tract was established through the upper (84%), middle (11%), or lower (5%) calyx depending on the location of the UPJ. In 22% of the patients, the nephrostomy tract was above the 12th rib. To retrieve the stone in the proximal ureter, 79% of the patients underwent flexible nephroscopy, and all of these stones were removed with grasping forceps; no ultrasonic or electrohydraulic lithotripsy was used. The patients were treated using epidural (47%), general (6%), and intravenous sedation and local (47%) anesthesia. The median procedural time was 90 minutes, and no auxiliary procedures for stone remnant removal were required. The complication rate was 43%. The patients stayed in the hospital an average of 8 days and had a median convalescence time of 14 days.

Although the percutaneous nephrostomy approach for upper ureteral calculi has a high success rate, the associated postoperative morbidity, the significant operative and postoperative complication rates, and the long convalescence time make it only a salvage procedure for patients who have failed ESWL and ureteroscopic manipulation.

RESULTS: MIDDLE URETERAL CALCULI. The middle ureteral calculus is the most accessible for an open surgical extraction. Although ESWL has revolutionized the management of urolithiasis, the middle ureteral calculus presents the most difficult problem for ESWL treatment. The introduction of the Stryker frame modification of the Dornier HM-3 and the bathless lithotriptors has made the middle ureteral stone more easily positioned for more effective treatment with ESWL. Review of the literature shows that the success rate for treating middle ureteral calculi with ESWL ranges between 42% and 97%, with a retreatment rate of 6% to 34%. Mobley and colleagues conclusively showed that stents did not significantly affect the stone-free rate or the need for auxiliary procedures when middle ureteral stones were treated with ESWL (Mobley et al, 1994). Their 3077 patients with middle ureteral calculi had a stone-free rate of 83% following in situ ESWL. As Jenkins points out, the appeal of in situ ESWL for the patient is that no urinary tract instrumentation is required (Jenkins, 1994).

The development of the small, semirigid and flexible ureteroscopes has made the middle ureteral calculus more accessible to ureteroscopic manipulation. A review of the literature shows that the stone-free rate for ureteroscopy combined with intracorporeal lithotripsy for middle ureteral calculi ranges between 57% and 94%.

In most cases, intracorporeal lithotripsy is used through

the ureteroscope. Wills and Burns (1994) used the No. 3 Fr electrohydraulic probe through the No. 7.2 or 9.5 Fr rigid ureteroscope or the No. 10.5 Fr flexible ureteroscope for 62 middle ureteral calculi. They reported a 90% stone-free rate. Dretler and Bhatta (1991), using a 140-mJ pulsed-dye laser fiber, achieved complete fragmentation in 82% of middle ureteral calculi. The remaining three partially fragmented stones migrated into the kidney and were successfully treated with ESWL.

In contrast to electrohydraulic or laser therapy, ultrasonic lithotripsy must be performed through the larger rigid ureteroscope. Netto and colleagues have demonstrated that this treatment modality has a 94% success rate for middle ureteral calculi (Netto et al, 1991b).

Lastly the pneumatic lithotriptor has been described for treatment of renal and ureteral calculi. Hofbauer and colleagues used the No. 2 Fr pneumatic lithotriptor probe through the No. 6.5 Fr rigid ureteroscope to treat four middle ureteral calculi successfully (Hofbauer et al, 1992).

Percutaneous, antegrade ureteroscopy is rarely used for treatment of middle ureteral calculi. Clayman and colleagues reported on 26 patients, with middle and distal ureteral calculi, treated with PCNL with a resultant stone-free rate of only 58% (Clayman et al, 1984c). In this patient group, the complication rate was 65%; five patients required a blood transfusion, nine demonstrated ureteral extravasation at the time of the procedure, one developed a perirenal hematoma, and two developed clot retention. Although PCNL is feasible and effective for middle ureteral calculi, it is technically more difficult with increased procedure-related morbidity compared to ESWL or retrograde ureteroscopy. As such, as with proximal ureteral calculi, the percutaneous approach is a salvage technique activated only in the face of failed ESWL and ureteroscopy.

RESULTS: DISTAL URETERAL CALCULI. Ureteroscopy has been the treatment of choice for most distal ureteral calculi. Reports have suggested, however, that ESWL may be equally effective and have subsequently generated considerable controversy as to the best treatment for this group of stone patients.

A review of the literature shows that the stone-free rate for ESWL treatment of distal ureteral calculi ranges between 59% and 97%. Several investigators, with large numbers of patients treated on the HM-3 for distal ureteral calculi, have shown stone-free rates of greater than 90%, with retreatment rates between 5% and 23% and auxiliary treatment rates between 3% and 11% (Erturke et al, 1993; Tiselius, 1993). Similarly, Thomas and colleagues reported a stone-free rate of 87% in 130 distal ureteral stone patients treated on the Medstone STS 1050 (Thomas et al, 1993b). As with stones at higher levels in the ureter, stinting does not improve the success rate of ESWL for distal ureteral calculi (Tiselius, 1993; Mobley et al, 1994).

Ureteroscopic management of the lower ureteral calculus can be performed with the rigid or rarely, a flexible ureteroscope. Review of the literature indicates that 90% to 100% of patients undergoing ureteroscopy require a general or regional anesthetic. There is great variability in the postprocedure hospital stay (1–4 days). Wills and Burns (1994) were able to treat 82% of distal ureteral stone patients on an outpatient basis, with a 3.5% rehospitalization rate within 72 hours of the ureteroscopy. The overall stone-free rate for ureteroscopic management of distal ureteral calculi approaches 95%, with a retreatment rate ranging between 0 and 6%. Finally, for distal ureteral calculi that fail ESWL and ureteroscopy or that are too large (>2 cm) to be managed with these treatment options, PCNL, open ureterolithotomy, and laparoscopic ureterolithotomy are valid alternatives. The need for this form of therapy should arise in less than 1% of cases. There are no reports of any series of distal ureteral stones, however, treated by antegrade percutaneous ureteroscopy.

COMPLICATIONS. The complications of percutaneous antegrade ureteroscopy and stone extraction for ureteral calculi are the same as those associated with PCNL, including bleeding and possible transfusion, urinary tract infection, septicemia, and injury to adjacent organs. The majority of ureteral calculi necessitate an upper calyx nephrostomy, thereby making pneumothorax and hydrothorax more common owing to the supracostal approach. Ureteral strictures may occur from traumatic manipulation or lithotripsy of the stone. Liong and colleagues reported a 43% immediate complication rate associated with PCNL of proximal ureteral calculi, including ureteral perforations, pleural effusion, and postoperative fever (>38.5°C) (Liong et al, 1989). All of the ureteral injuries were successfully managed with an indwelling ureteral stent; no delayed ureteral strictures were reported.

Urolithiasis: Special Circumstances

RENAL CALCULI IN PATIENTS WITH RENAL COMPROMISE: RENAL INSUFFICIENCY OR SOLITARY KIDNEY

The question has frequently arisen as to the danger of performing PCNL in the patient with compromised renal function because of renal disease or the presence of a solitary kidney. Clayman and colleagues, in a carefully done histologic laboratory evaluation of chronic changes associated with PCNL, noted a 0.15% loss of cortical surface area from a No. 36 Fr nephrostomy tract (Clayman et al, 1987b). To answer this question clinically, Chandhoke and colleagues compared the long-term effects of ESWL and PCNL monotherapy on renal function in 31 patients with a solitary kidney or chronic renal insufficiency (Chandhoke et al, 1992). The patients were studied a mean of 3.5 years after treatment for stone disease. The decrease in glomerular filtration rate in patients with a solitary kidney and creatinine less than 2 mg/dl was 5% for ESWL and 9% for PCNL. All patients with a creatinine between 2 and 3 mg/dl demonstrated long-term improvement of renal function regardless of the treatment modality. The study group had only five patients with a creatinine greater than 3 mg/dl. In four of these patients treated with ESWL, all had initial improvement but eventual deterioration of renal function, and three required dialysis within 2 years of the treatment date. One patient with a creatinine value greater than 3 mg/dl underwent PCNL with stabilization of the renal function after treatment. Therefore, neither ESWL nor PCNL appears to result in long-term deterioration of renal function in patients with chronic renal insufficiency. In patients with a solitary kidney, a slight decrease in function is noted with either modality.

Similarly, in a review of 2000 consecutive urolithiasis patients, the prevalence of mild to moderate chronic renal insufficiency was 1% (Gupta et al, 1994). Complete or partial staghorn calculi were noted in 64% (21 of 33) of these patients. All patients except one managed with alkalinization of the urine required numerous surgical procedures to render them stone-free; 7 patients required 1 procedure, and 25 required an average of 3.5 procedures. The mean serum creatinine level before surgical intervention and after ureteral stent placement or percutaneous nephrostomy in patients with obstruction was 3.2 mg/dl (range 2.0–7.5). There was a significant mean decrease in serum creatinine of 1.2 mg/dl after a mean follow-up of 6 months in the patients. There was no significant difference in the rate of creatinine decrease between patients with pretreatment serum creatinine levels of 2.0 to 2.9 mg/dl and those with initial values of 3.0 mg/dl or higher. Three of 13 patients subsequently developed end-stage renal disease between 4 and 5 years after the stone treatment procedure. All of these patients had severely compromised renal function (serum creatinine ≥3.0 mg/dl) at presentation.

HORSESHOE KIDNEY AND UROLITHIASIS

The most common fusion anomaly is the horseshoe kidney, with an incidence of 0.25% in the general population. The fusion of the lower pole prevents normal ascent and rotation of the kidneys during embryogenesis. The collecting system is displaced anteriorly, and the ureters arise high on the renal pelvis and pass anterior to the isthmus. Drainage of the collecting system may be impaired because of compression of the proximal ureter against the isthmus, and stasis and infection predispose to stone formation. The incidence of stone formation in the horseshoe kidney is 20% (Bauer et al, 1992).

The presenting complaints of patients with calculi in a horseshoe kidney include abdominal pain radiating to the lumbar region, hematuria, and infection. As with stones in normal kidneys, horseshoe kidney calculi may be treated with PCNL, ESWL, combination therapy, and open stone surgery. PCNL, although requiring minor modifications for nephrostomy placement in the anteriorly and inferiorly placed kidneys (i.e., a more medial and more perpendicular access), is highly successful. Jones and colleagues reported successful access in all of their 15 patients with horseshoe kidneys (18 kidneys) undergoing PCNL (Jones DJ et al, 1991). Two patients required an auxiliary ESWL, for an overall stone-free rate of 89%. The overall complication rate was 22%, including blood transfusion (two patients), urosepsis (one patient), and a urethral stricture (one patient). Clinical results support PCNL for calculi in horseshoe kidneys as comparable to the results seen in series of PCNL in normal kidneys (Table 94–5).

Similarly, ESWL of calculi in horseshoe kidneys has demonstrated satisfactory results despite concerns over drainage and stone elimination from the abnormal collecting system. On review of the literature, the overall stone-free rate of 53% (rate 50%–79%) can be achieved with ESWL of calculi in the horseshoe kidney (see Table 94–5). To achieve this stone-free status, however, an auxiliary procedure rate and retreatment rate of 55% and 58% are necessary. Complica-

tions were usually minor and included obstruction or renal colic (25%–43%) and urinary tract infection (14%).

Treatment selection in the horseshoe kidney with high stone burden must consider the ease and low morbidity of ESWL versus the significantly higher stone-free rate of PCNL. For calculi 2 cm or smaller, review of the literature suggests that ESWL and PCNL are both reasonable first-line therapies. For stones greater than 2 cm, PCNL appears to be preferable to ESWL. Open surgery is usually reserved for those cases in which collecting system reconstruction is required in addition to stone removal or in those cases that fail primary ESWL or PCNL.

PEDIATRIC UROLITHIASIS: APPLICATION OF PERCUTANEOUS NEPHROSTOLITHOTOMY

Pediatric urolithiasis is a relatively rare clinical entity in the United States. The Mayo Clinic reported 1 instance of urinary tract calculus in 1400 pediatric admissions (Malek, 1985). In children, percutaneous extraction and ESWL have been described for renal and upper ureteral calculi. Modifications of the gantry chair on the Dornier HM-3 and the second-generation ESWL machines have facilitated application of ESWL to the pediatric patient (Newman et al, 1986; Kramolowsky et al, 1987b; Starr and Middleton, 1992).

On review of the literature, PCNL has a higher stone-free rate than ESWL but is associated with more significant complications. The overall stone-free rate for PCNL in the pediatric patient averages 90% (range 80%–100%) with an average retreatment rate and auxiliary procedure rate of 17% and 24% (Table 94–6). The complications seen in the pediatric stone patient after PCNL are similar to these seen in the adult, including fever and bleeding in 10% to 14% of patients. In comparison, ESWL has an average overall success rate of 81% (range 50%–100%) with an average retreatment rate of 10% and an auxiliary procedure rate of 18% (see Table 94–6). In this patient population, ESWL usually requires general anesthesia, although some investigators have used intravenous sedation techniques successfully. The hospital stay for ESWL is usually shorter than that for the PCNL procedure. Several investigators, however, report pain requiring narcotic medication after ESWL in between 17% and 50% of pediatric patients. The most common complications after ESWL for calculi in the pediatric population are fever and pain. Because of the small size of these patients and difficulties with patient positioning, however, pulmonary and cardiac effects of ESWL may occur in these patients. Pulmonary edema and hemoptysis have been reported by two investigators as a result of the pulmonary effect of the shock waves (Kramolowsky et al, 1987b; Kroovand et al, 1987). Boddy and colleagues reported two patients who developed cardiac arrhythmias during the ESWL treatment for renal calculi (Boddy et al, 1987). Hematuria is also commonly seen after ESWL of the pediatric patient, and one study reported an asymptomatic perirenal hematoma, which resolved without sequelae (Newman et al, 1986).

Several investigators have reported ureteroscopic management of urolithiasis in the pediatric patient. All of these reports have been with the small rigid ureteroscopes and often without balloon dilation of the ureter. The success rate of 100% in all of these reports is encouraging, although most

Table 94-5. PERCUTANEOUS NEPHROSTOLITHOTOMY AND EXTRACORPOREAL SHOCK WAVE LITHOTRIPSY THERAPY FOR CALCULI IN HORSESHOE KIDNEYS

Author	Number of Patients	Lithotriptor	Stone-Free Rate (%)	Retreatment Rate (%)	Auxiliary Procedures (%)	Complications
Percutaneous Nephrostolithotomy						
Tawney, 1989	8		71	—	—	0
Esuvaranathan et al, 1991	2		100	33	67	Urosepsis 33%
Jones DJ et al, 1991	15		89	11	11	Transfusion 13%
						Fever 7%
						Urethral stricture 7%
Total	25		86	14	19	
Extracorporeal Shock Wave Lithotripsy						
Smith et al, 1989	14	HM3	79	29	50	Bowel hematoma (1)
Esuvaranathan et al, 1991	7	HM3	50	86	—	Colic 43%
						Urinary tract infection 14%
Van Deursen and Baert, 1992	10	Lithostar	55	69	—	0
Knopf et al, 1993	20	HM3	55	35	65	Obstruction or colic 25%
		MFL 5000				
Total	51		60	55	58	

Table 94–6. MANAGEMENT OF CALCULI IN THE PEDIATRIC PATIENT

Author	Number of Patients	Stone-Free Rate (%)	Retreatment Rate (%)	Auxiliary Procedure (%)	Complications	Lithotriptor (Average Shocks)	Age (Years)
Percutaneous Nephrolithotomy							
Woodside et al, 1985	7	100	0	43	Fever 14%		
Boddy et al, 1987	10	90	30	10	Bleeding 10%		
Shepherd et al, 1988	5	80	—	—	—		
Zattoni et al, 1989	6	83	17	—	—		
Burns and Joseph, 1993	1	100	—	SWL-Piezolith 2300	Fever 101°F with hemacidrin irrigation		
Total	29	90	17	24			
Extracorporeal Shock Wave Lithotripsy							
Newman et al, 1986	15	72	0	—	Perirenal hematoma 7% Pain 33%	HM3 (960)	3–17
Boddy et al, 1987	6	50	0	—	Arrhythmias 33% Pain and nausea 17%	HM3	6–15
Kramolowsky et al, 1987	14	71	7	7	Pulmonary edema 7% Pain 21%	HM3 (1250)	3–17
Kroovand et al, 1987	18	82	27	39	Hemoptysis 11% Pain 50%	HM3 (1753)	3–20
Shepherd et al, 1988	9	89	—	100	Fever 11% Hemorrhage 11%	HM3 (1675)	<16
Starr and Middleton, 1992	8	100	11	13	None	Piezolith 2300 (2000–4000)	5–17
Total	70	81	10	18			

of the investigators advocated extensive adult ureteroscopic experience before attempting pediatric ureteroscopy (Caione et al, 1990; Hill et al, 1990; Thomas et al, 1993c). Most investigators routinely placed ureteral stents after the ureteroscopy. Hill and colleagues reported a 50% incidence of reflux after ureteroscopic manipulation and recommended prophylactic antibiotic therapy postureteroscopy in the pediatric patient (Hill et al, 1990).

MANAGEMENT OF RENAL CALCULI IN THE MORBIDLY OBESE: USE OF PERCUTANEOUS NEPHROSTOLITHOTOMY

The extremely obese patient is not an uncommon occurrence in urologic practice, and these patients often have complicated stone disease requiring PCNL therapy if the stone is too large to approach ureteroscopically. Often the patient's weight dictates the treatment choice because the HM-3 ESWL machine has a weight limitation of 300 pounds owing to the hydraulic lift system. In addition, the patient's skin-to-stone distance must be equal to or only slightly longer (i.e., "blast path") than the focal length of the specific lithotriptor for effective treatment. With regard to PCNL therapy, general anesthesia may also be a concern in these patients, who may have restricted respiratory capacity, which becomes more pronounced after induction and necessitates higher airway pressures intraoperatively. Also, difficult neck anatomy in these patients makes them a challenge to intubate. Prolonged patient positioning and the extreme weight may rarely result in tissue necrosis and rhabdomyolysis in the obese patient. Likewise, ureteroscopy may be difficult, because these patients often have concomitant osteoarthritis of the hips, which limits abduction. The placement of a ureteral access sheath may facilitate ureteroscopy and retrograde lithotripsy. Also, the use of the flexible ureteroscope

may be necessary to overcome some of the aforementioned anatomic difficulties owing to patient size.

Obese patients undergoing PCNL may be more likely to have respiratory complications intraoperatively and postoperatively. The prone position for PCNL may severely restrict the intraoperative ventilatory capacity. In this regard, Kerbl and colleagues reported the implementation of the flank position for PCNL in two very obese patients. This position resulted in less restriction of the respiratory-dependent movements of the chest wall and facilitated ventilation and anesthesiologic access to the endotracheal tube (Kerbl et al, 1994a). The lateral decubitus position allowed the pannus to fall anteriorly; however, this resulted in greater renal mobility, and thus the nephrostomy tract was longer than anticipated, necessitating in one patient an entirely flexible endoscopic approach. Also, percutaneous access in the flank position is technically more difficult and requires preoperative placement of a ureteral catheter for air or contrast material injection and C-arm fluoroscopy. Overall, it is recommended only if the patient is absolutely unable to lie in the prone position.

In general, the rigid nephroscopes are 17.8 cm long and in very obese patients may not reach the collecting system. Extra-long nephrostomy sheaths (e.g., 20 cm) are available and facilitate percutaneous access. A suture placed in the percutaneous end of the nephrostomy sheath allows retrieval of the sheath if it is pushed too deeply into the patient's back.

Hofmann and Stoller (1992) reported on five morbidly obese patients who underwent a variety of endourologic procedures for calculus disease. All of the patients required at least two procedures, usually because of an initial failed procedure, to complete their treatment. The complication rate was 75%, and complications included rhabdomyolysis and temporary renal failure (one patient) and wound or skin infection (two patients). Three of the patients were rendered stone-free, but one patient was considered such a poor surgical risk that no further intervention could be tolerated. It is interesting that the obese patient does not appear to be at any increased risk of postoperative thrombosis or pulmonary embolism compared to the nonobese patient (Carson et al, 1987).

BILATERAL SIMULTANEOUS PERCUTANEOUS NEPHROSTOLITHOTOMY

Patients with struvite calculi often present with bilateral disease. Rendering these patients stone-free can be a formidable task and involve multiple trips to the operating room. Bilateral PCNL was first reported by Colon-Perez and later expanded on by several groups (Colon-Perez et al, 1987; Regan et al, 1992; Ahlawat, et al, 1995). The authors have also adopted the bilateral, simultaneous approach to PCNL in patients with bilateral staghorn calculi (Nadler et al, 1995a).

Immediately before the procedure, the patient is given a single dose of subarachnoid morphine sulfate (Duramorph), which provides 24 to 36 hours of postoperative pain relief. The procedure is performed in the same manner as the unilateral PCNL. The patient undergoes flexible cystoscopy and guide wire placement of both collecting systems in the prone position. The first side is selected according to worse renal function, larger stone burden, and need for auxiliary procedures. If the initial PCNL is completed without complication and within a reasonable time limit (2–3 hours), the contralateral side is addressed during the same anesthetic after securing nephrostomy drainage of the initial kidney. To date, the authors have performed bilateral simultaneous PCNL in four patients with staghorn calculus disease. The average operative time was 5.3 hours, more than 3.5 hours shorter than the combined operative time for two separate PCNL sessions (9.06 hours). The stone-free rate after the second-look nephroscopy of both kidneys was 100%. The transfusion rate was 1 unit in one of four patients (25%), which was the same transfusion rate noted for similar patients done in two separate sessions. No major or minor complications or deaths occurred. The bilateral, simultaneous PCNL patients required an average of 34 mg morphine postoperatively compared to an average of 1079 mg morphine for the two-session PCNL patients.

Renal Cysts

The incidence, diagnostic studies, and drainage methods as they apply to renal cysts have already been addressed. Percutaneous endoscopic therapy of renal cysts has been ongoing for the past decade albeit in highly select patients. Specifically, this approach is usually reserved for patients in whom there is an absolute contraindication to percutaneous drainage and sclerosis (e.g., peripelvic or communicating cyst) or patients in whom sclerotherapy has failed.

TECHNIQUE

In the **direct** approach, a retrograde ureteral catheter is passed, and the collecting system is opacified via the ureteral catheter by injecting contrast material mixed with indigo carmine and sorbitol (50 ml sorbitol, 25 ml contrast material, and 1–2 ml indigo carmine). Next the radiologist percutane-

ously punctures the cyst with a nephrostomy needle. Clear or thin yellow fluid should drain from the needle; if the drainage fluid is blue, the collecting system has been inadvertently entered, and the needle needs to be passed again. Next, a safety and working guide wire (e.g., 0.035-inch Bentson) are coiled in the cyst; the intracystic nephrostomy tract is dilated, and a No. 30 Fr Amplatz working sheath is placed into the cyst.

Alternatively, after a needle and catheter has been passed into the cyst, an **indirect** approach can be taken. In this case, a separate nephrostomy tract is placed into a calyx, which provides a direct path to the cyst. The nephrostomy tract is dilated to No. 30 Fr, and a No. 30 Fr sheath is placed alongside a safety guide wire. The interior of the cyst is opacified via the previously placed intracystic nephrostomy needle; a mixture of contrast material and indigo carmine mixed with sorbitol is instilled into the cyst. This step facilitates identification of the cyst during nephroscopy and aids any subsequent electrosurgical incision into the cyst.

The next step is to operate on the cyst wall. The thin portion of the cyst wall abutting the renal collecting system can be either **incised** from within the cyst outward and into the distended, blue-stained collecting system (i.e., direct approach) or sharply entered from the collecting system inward into the blue-stained cyst (i.e., indirect approach) with a cutting electrode (Collings knife) or resectoscope loop. Next the opening between the cyst and the collecting system is widened, thereby marsupializing the cyst into the collecting system (Hulbert et al, 1988c). This can be done electrosurgically or by balloon or shear dilation to No. 30 F. A roller electrode is then used through a No. 24 or 26 Fr resectoscope, to fulgurate the walls of the cyst that do not border the collecting system to promote obliteration of the cystic cavity (Fig. 94–24*(1, 3)*.

Following a direct approach to the cyst, a transcystic nephrostomy tube may be placed into the collecting system. With the indirect approach, the nephrostomy tube resides within the renal pelvis and does not enter the cyst. The drainage tube can be removed when a nephrostogram reveals satisfactory obliteration of the cystic cavity; this may require days to weeks.

A third approach has been described by Hubner and coworkers (1990). Instead of entering the collecting system, only the cyst is entered by way of the area of the cyst that abuts the renal parenchyma. Next the transparenchymal intracystic tract is dilated, and an operating nephroscope or resectoscope is introduced. The thin peripheral wall of the cyst is resected, thereby effectively decorticating the cyst and marsupializing it into the retroperitoneum (see Fig. 94–24*(2)* (Hubner et al, 1990). The major advantage of this approach is that in contrast to the direct or indirect nephrostomy-based approaches, it precludes accumulation of stagnant urine in the remaining cyst cavity.

RESULTS

Reports of an endoscopic approach to simple renal cysts have appeared sporadically in the literature (Eickenberg, 1985; Hulbert et al, 1988c; Chehval et al, 1990). Hubner and colleagues (1990) reported one of the largest experiences and noted an early 93% success rate; however, when follow-up was extended in 10 patients out to 46 months, 50% of

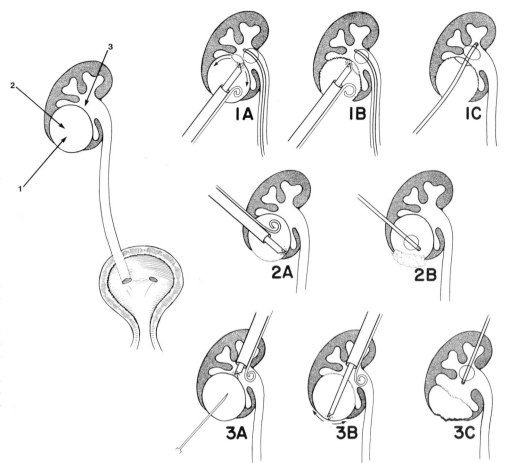

Figure 94–24. Three approaches for endoscopic therapy of a renal cyst. *1. Direct approach: transcystic. A,* Cyst is directly punctured and a No. 30 Fr Amplatz sheath is placed. The cyst wall abutting the renal pelvis is incised. *B,* The remaining cyst wall is fulgurated. *C,* The nephrostomy tube traverses the cyst.

2. Direct approach: transparenchymal. A, Cyst is punctured through the renal parenchyma. A No. 30 Fr Amplatz sheath is placed. The cyst wall abutting the retroperitoneum is resected. *B,* A tube is placed in the cyst; no communication is created between the cyst and the collecting system.

3. Indirect approach. A, The collecting system is entered away from the cyst. A No. 30 Fr Amplatz sheath is placed. An 18-gauge needle is passed into the cyst for instillation of fluid. This distends the cyst and makes the wall of the cyst that abuts the collecting system more apparent to the endoscopist. The cyst is sharply entered and marsupialized into the renal pelvis. *B,* The far wall of the cyst is fulgurated. *C,* A nephrostomy tube is placed.

the treated cysts were again either detectable or close to their preoperative size (Plas and Hubner, 1993). In this instance, if the patient's symptoms reappeared, the next step would be open or laparoscopic cyst decortication.

Transitional Cell Cancer of the Upper Urinary Tract

No area of endosurgery is more controversial than the application of newer endoscopic techniques to TCC affecting the ureter or renal pelvis. The rationale behind this therapy is based on the conservative approach to low-grade, low-stage bladder cancer. Certainly for superficial TCC of the bladder, a transurethral approach is acceptable, whereas cystectomy and urinary diversion are reserved only for those individuals with high-grade or muscle-invasive disease (Catalona, 1987). When superficial or low-stage bladder tumors recur, they are similarly of low grade and stage in nearly 85% to 90% of patients (Kaye and Lange, 1982). The question then arises: Should the same regimen used for treating low-grade, superficial lesions of the bladder be applied to low-grade, superficial TCC affecting the upper urinary tract?

Objections to an endoscopic approach to upper tract cancer center on five issues: (1) the need for renal preservation, (2) accuracy of diagnosis (i.e., grade and stage), (3) tumor implantation, (4) surveillance, and (5) recurrent disease. First, in the patient with two kidneys, why **preserve** the tumor-bearing renal unit? TCC occurs bilateral and metach-

ronously in the renal pelvis in only 1% to 2% of patients (Clayman et al, 1983b). The removal of a kidney in the adult patient population is well tolerated. Although proteinuria may slowly develop, no associated increase occurs in the frequency of renal failure or hypertension among individuals with an iatrogenic solitary kidney. This observation is well documented in patients who survive radical nephrectomy for renal cell cancer and in those who are renal donors (Fotino, 1989; Wishnow et al, 1990). At first glance, renal preservation appears to be a laudable goal; however, its true value to the patient with a healthy contralateral kidney is questionable.

The **accuracy of the diagnosis** of a superficial, noninvasive transitional cell lesion is of paramount importance. In this regard, it is of note that although 85% of bladder cancers present as low-grade superficial disease, only 40% of renal pelvic and 50% to 60% of ureteral tumors initially appear as low-grade, noninvasive disease (Wagle et al, 1974; Batata et al, 1975; Johansson and Wahlquist, 1979).

Unfortunately the reliability of a diagnosis of superficial or noninvasive disease in the upper tract is wanting. Neither urine cytology nor flow cytometry is sufficiently accurate. Although helpful in revealing high-grade tumors, negative urine cytology findings may occur in 60% of patients with low-grade disease and in 10% of patients with high-grade lesions (Sarnacki et al, 1971). Flow cytometry, which measures cellular DNA and RNA content, is also not infallible. A false-negative histogram commonly occurs with predominantly diploid tumors. This problem is noted in 66% of superficial papillomas and in 8% of invasive lesions (Denovic et al, 1982; Melamed, 1984).

Furthermore, TCC affecting the renal pelvis, in contrast to ureteral TCC, is often not a solitary lesion. Overall, 30% of these tumors may be multicentric at the time of presentation (Mazeman, 1976; Wallace et al, 1981; Huffman, 1988). Likewise, in a patient with a low-grade (1, 2), low-stage (O, A) renal *pelvic* tumor, the tumor may be associated with urothelial dysplasia in the renal pelvis in 90% of patients and with actual carcinoma in situ in 3% to 9% of cases (Nocks et al, 1982). Likewise, a low-grade, low-stage *ureteral* tumor may be associated with urothelial dysplasia and carcinoma in situ in other areas of the ureter in 50% and 9% to 13%, respectively (Heney et al, 1981). These pathologic changes may be missed during an endoscopic approach. Indeed, in those series in which an endoscopic diagnosis of TCC of the renal pelvis was followed by surgical extirpation, the error in undergrading and understaging was 60%. In contrast, for TCC of the ureter, tumor grade and stage were correctly diagnosed ureteroscopically (Huffman et al, 1985a, b; Huffman, 1990). Thus, at least for TCC of the renal pelvis, a significant problem with regard to staging and grading the tumor exists.

Another significant concern is the possibility of **tumor implantation** after endosurgical procedures. Implantation may take two forms: (1) confined within the upper tract collecting system and (2) retroperitoneal. Any urothelial abrasion may provide a fertile site for tumor implantation. This finding has been demonstrated in an animal model by Soloway and Masters (1980). In their study, cauterization of part of the mouse bladder increased implantation of transitional cell tumors by fourfold. The same problem may apply during ureteroscopy or nephroscopy of an upper tract tumor. With ureteroscopy, the dilation of the distal ureter and passage of the rigid or flexible ureteroscope may result in multiple abrasions along the ureter. Similar problems may occur with antegrade nephroscopy. Reports of this problem, however, are rare. Superficial studding of the ureter with transitional cell tumors has been noted by the authors in one individual at 9 months after a percutaneous procedure for a low-grade renal pelvic tumor (Clayman RV, unpublished data, 1994). Before the procedure, the patient also underwent diagnostic ureteroscopy. Whether this effect is coincidence (i.e., the natural history of the tumor) or consequence of the ureteroscopy or percutaneous resection is difficult to discern.

Retroperitoneal tumor implantation is a significant concern whenever a percutaneous approach to treat an upper urinary tract transitional cell tumor is undertaken; hypothetically, this could occur either from the nephrostomy tract itself or if the renal pelvis is perforated during tract dilation or tumor resection. Surgical pyelotomy to resect a transitional cell tumor has been shown to result in retroperitoneal seeding and recurrent extrarenal disease in nearly 11% of patients (retroperitoneal recurrence noted at 6 months and 3 years) (Tomera et al, 1982). In contrast, with regard to percutaneous endosurgery, Guz and co-workers, in a series of 14 patients who were undergoing percutaneous nephrostomy to drain a malignant obstruction (13 cases) or resect an upper tract TCC (one case), grossly noted no seeding of the nephrostomy tract at 1 to 121 months' follow-up (average 27.8 months) (Guz et al, 1991). Likewise, other investi-

gators have independently noted no discernible seeding (Blute et al, 1989; Nurse et al, 1989; Huffman, 1990). At present, the only report of nephrostomy tract seeding comes from Huang and co-workers; their patient had a large, grade 3 midureteral tumor that was approached through a No. 36 Fr nephrostomy tract. Seeding of the tract was noted 5 weeks later (Huang et al, 1995). Although this is an isolated case, it is important to realize that most patients in these series have been followed for a relatively brief period of time, usually less than 2 years, and follow-up has not included routine CT scanning of the retroperitoneum to detect asymptomatic retroperitoneal masses. A minimum of a 5-year follow-up period is necessary to evaluate fully whether concerns over tract seeding or retroperitoneal recurrence can be discounted as being extremely rare. In this regard, it is important for these patients to undergo periodic surveillance CT of the retroperitoneum.

The next issue among patients treated with an endoscopic approach is **surveillance**. Logically, if upper tract and lower tract TCC are to be treated similarly, the subsequent follow-up should be similar. Nearly 85% of recurrences after resection of an initial bladder tumor occur within the first year of follow-up (Varkarakis et al, 1974; Loening et al, 1980). Hence, a routine in which cystoscopy is performed every 3 months for at least the first 1 to 2 years, then every 6 months for 1 to 2 years, and then annually thereafter appears to be reasonable (Varkarakis et al, 1974; Droller, 1986). This regimen is reinstituted if a recurrent tumor occurs during the follow-up period. It appears prudent to initiate a similar regimen among patients undergoing endosurgical management of TCC of the ureter or renal pelvis. In support of surveillance ureteroscopy are reports on the inadequacy of upper tract radiographic studies for detecting small TCC recurrences (Huffman et al, 1985a; Gerber and Lyon, 1993; Seaman et al, 1993). In Huffman's experience as well as in the authors' experience, recurrent tumors that were not apparent radiographically have been detected endoscopically. Intravenous urography or retrograde ureterography alone is no more an acceptable replacement for surveillance ureteroscopy than cystography would be an acceptable replacement for follow-up cystoscopy among patients with TCC of the bladder.

The need for postoperative surveillance ureteronephroscopy detracts from the initial benefits of endoscopic therapy. For the 50-year-old patient with an average life expectancy, surveillance ureteroscopy, under the best of circumstances (i.e., assuming no recurrences), might result in more than 30 separate outpatient or short hospital stay ureteroscopic procedures, complete with ureteral dilation and the need to place an indwelling ureteral stent for 2 to 3 days. For example, one of the longest reported follow-ups of a patient undergoing endoscopic resection of upper tract TCC is 6.5 years. During that time period, the patient underwent 14 general anesthetics for 14 surveillance ureteroscopies and fulguration of six low-grade upper tract TCC recurrences (Huffman et al, 1985b). As such, the overall expense and convalescence (i.e., total time off from work and overall discomfort) of the surveillance necessitated by a minimally invasive endourologic approach might well exceed that incurred acutely by a standard surgical nephroureterectomy.

In an effort to simplify the performance of follow-up surveillance ureteroscopy, Kerbl and Clayman (1993) have begun a routine of incising the ipsilateral ureteral orifice and tunnel. The incision and subsequent low-grade reflux ensure a patulous ureteral orifice such that flexible ureteroscopy can be accomplished in the office setting. Indeed, in two patients, over a greater than 2-year period, surveillance ureteroscopy was performed at the same time as surveillance cystoscopy in the office; no fluoroscopy or intravenous or oral sedation was used. Early recurrences in both patients, in advance of radiographic findings, were identified and subsequently treated on an outpatient basis. The downside of this approach is the concern of possibly increasing the chances of upper tract seeding from a subsequent bladder tumor. In this regard, conflicting reports exist in the literature; upper tract disease among patients with TCC of the bladder and reflux have been noted in 0% to 20% of patients over a 2- to 9-year follow-up period (Krogh et al, 1991; Palou et al, 1992).

Also, with regard to follow-up after a percutaneous therapy for TCC of the renal pelvis, it might be reasonable to include an annual CT study of the retroperitoneum to rule out a retroperitoneal recurrence. Only in this manner can retroperitoneal disease secondary to tumor cell extravasation at the time of the procedure be detected early. This would again, however, add to the overall cost of the "less invasive" endourologic approach and increase the time lost from gainful employment.

Lastly, with regard to conservative therapy for TCC of the renal pelvis and ureter, the **tumor recurrence rate** is of great concern. Based on earlier series in which a simple nephrectomy rather than nephroureterectomy was performed for TCC of the renal pelvis, it is reasonable to anticipate rapid and likely multiple recurrences among patients undergoing endoscopic therapy. Indeed, recurrent transitional cell tumors develop in a retained ureteral stump in 30% of patients (48% after simple nephrectomy and 24% after nephrectomy, with subtotal ureterectomy) (Mazeman, 1976; Strong et al, 1976). These recurrent tumors are of a higher grade in approximately 25% of patients (Mazeman, 1976; Strong et al, 1976). Obviously the more urothelium that remains intact, the higher the incidence of recurrence. Indeed, in one series in which endoscopic therapy was used to treat TCC of the renal pelvis and ureter, 46% of 11 patients developed a recurrent tumor in the renal pelvis and ureter within 9 months of the procedure (Orihuela and Smith, 1988). In another series on endourologic TCC of the renal pelvis and the ureter, 38% of patients experienced an upper tract recurrence within a 21-month follow-up period (Huffman et al, 1985a). In general, the incidence of recurrence is higher for TCC of the renal pelvis (30%–75%) than for TCC of the ureter (6%–20%) with follow-up at only 1 to 2 years. Even with adjunctive instillation chemotherapy, recurrences within 2 years can be expected in 30% to 40% of patients.

For all of these reasons, the urologist interested in endoscopic therapy for upper tract TCC is cautioned about broadening the indications for this approach to include otherwise healthy patients with two kidneys who have TCC of the ureter or renal pelvis. Presently, endosurgery for upper tract TCC takes the form of ureteroscopy for ureteral lesions or small, less than 1 cm renal lesions and percutaneous antegrade nephroscopy for larger renal lesions. Overall, either endosurgical approach should be limited to individuals with a **solitary kidney** and a low-grade, apparently low-stage tumor confined to a single focus or to those few individuals with two kidneys who either are too ill or have significant

renal insufficiency such that standard surgical therapy is contraindicated. Given these guidelines, for the majority of patients with TCC of the renal pelvis or ureter, surgical therapy (i.e., distal ureterectomy or nephroureterectomy, dependent on the location of the tumor) remains the treatment of choice.

TECHNIQUE

A percutaneous approach to upper tract TCC necessitates perforation of the collecting system with the attendant concerns over *seeding* of the retroperitoneum with tumor cells. The instrumentation used in the percutaneous approach, however, is the standard resectoscope and biopsy equipment used in the bladder, thereby greatly facilitating biopsy and tumor removal. With these instruments, tumor grade and stage can be accurately determined.

The **antegrade percutaneous** method for resecting a low-grade, presumably low-stage tumor of the renal pelvis or proximal ureter must be carefully planned. Initially a No. 7 Fr retrograde ureteral occlusion balloon (11.5 mm) catheter is passed to the renal pelvis. Air or contrast material can be instilled by way of the retrograde catheter to opacify the collecting system. The balloon is inflated in the renal pelvis and gently pulled caudal to occlude the UPJ. The nephrostomy tract can be made such that either it is in a direct line with the tumor yet enters the collecting system via a remote calyx, or it enters the tumor-bearing calyx itself. Although the authors favor the former approach (Fig. 94–25), Smith and colleagues prefer the latter (Jarrett et al, 1995). Both groups agree, however, that for a renal pelvic or UPJ tumor, an upper or middle posterior calyx provides the best access. The nephrostomy tract is established under C-arm fluoroscopic control in an effort to avoid an anterior false passage and extravasation. The nephrostomy tract is dilated with a 10-mm nephrostomy tract balloon dilator, and an Amplatz working sheath is placed. This maneuver should result in the least amount of trauma to normal urothelium and should protect the tract from subsequent extravasation during the procedure.

The resection of the tumor may be done in several ways. A standard resectoscope can be used and the tumor resected and evacuated piece by piece. The base of the tumor can be separately biopsied and fulgurated. Alternatively a no-touch technique can be employed with the Nd:YAG laser set at 25 to 30 watts. The entire tumor is treated with the laser, and the tumor fronds are removed with cold cup biopsy forceps and sent for histologic analysis. The base of the tumor is biopsied and treated with the Nd:YAG laser. A third approach is to use the resectoscope to resect the bulk of the tumor; the base of the tumor is then biopsied with a cold cup forceps, after which Nd:YAG laser treatment of the base is done at 20 to 30 watts for 3-second exposures, or electrocoagulation can be done at 50 watts coagulating current (Grossman et al, 1992; Jarrett et al, 1995). Throughout the procedure, the irrigation pressure is not allowed to rise above 40 cm H_2O to preclude pyelosinus or pyelovenous backflow of any irrigant laden with tumor cells (Kulp and Bagley, 1994). Indeed, if the irrigant is pressurized or a hand-held syringe is used to push irrigant into the collecting system, pressures as high as 200 mm Hg may occur with resultant backflow of tumor cells (Lim et al, 1993).

After treatment of the tumor, random biopsy samples

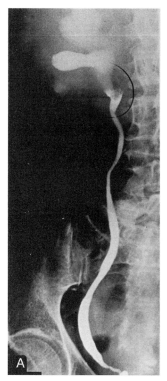
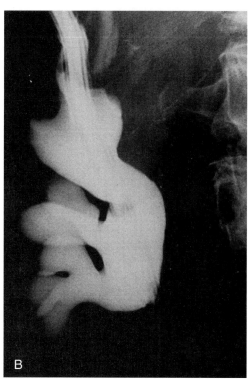
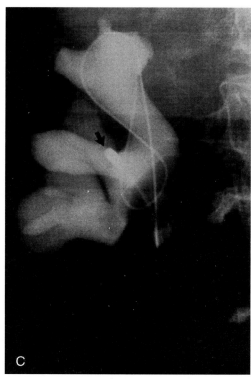

Figure 94–25. *A,* Retrograde ureterogram reveals a filling defect at the ureteropelvic junction *(circle).* A ureteroscopic biopsy sample showed that the tumor was a grade 2 papillary transitional cell carcinoma. *B,* A percutaneous approach was used to resect the tumor. Note that access has been achieved via an upper-pole calyx, distant from the lesion itself. The nephrostogram reveals no anterior extravasation, and the lesion is now absent. The nephrostomy tube was subsequently removed. *C,* Two months later, a retrograde ureterogram showed no recurrent lesions. Surveillance ureteroscopy performed at the same time, however, revealed a radiographically undetected 2- to 3-mm papillary tumor *(arrow);* this was treated with the Nd:YAG laser. In this case, a follow-up intravenous urogram, 1 year later, revealed a recurrent tumor in the renal pelvis. Before any further therapy could be rendered, the patient died from a cardiac event. The autopsy report on the right kidney revealed *recurrent superficial low-grade transitional cell cancer at the ureteropelvic junction.* In addition, new tumors were noted in the calyceal system, midureter, and bladder (dome and left side wall). No evidence of metastatic disease was noted.

of the surrounding urothelium in four separate peritumor quadrants and biopsy samples of any other suspicious areas of urothelium are recommended. The retrograde ureteral occlusion balloon catheter is removed at the end of the procedure. An indwelling nephrostomy tube is placed (see Fig. 94–25).

Postoperatively the nephrostomy tube may be handled in one of two ways. In one scenario, it is removed 2 to 5 days later, provided that a nephrostogram reveals no evidence of extravasation (see Fig. 94–25). Alternatively, several days later, the patient is returned to the operating room for second-look nephroscopy, biopsy of the base of the tumor, and possible retreatment of the tumor bed. The patient is then discharged from the hospital with the nephrostomy tube still in place pending bacille Calmette-Guérin (BCG) or other instillation chemotherapy for 2 to 8 weeks followed by a third-look nephroscopy with biopsy and possible further treatment of the tumor's base (Jarrett et al, 1995).

With regard to endourologic therapy for TCC, a whole host of adjunctive therapies have arisen in an attempt to decrease the incidence of tumor recurrence. Based on work by Gittes, the authors have instilled thiotepa into the retrograde ureteral catheter just before creation of the nephrostomy tract in the patient who is undergoing endourologic therapy for upper tract TCC. At the end of the procedure and for 2 to 3 days during the early postoperative period, thiotepa (30–60 mg in 60–150 ml of normal saline) can be

instilled via the indwelling nephrostomy tube, **provided that a postoperative nephrostogram shows no extravasation** (Gittes, 1980). Alternatively, Orihuela and Smith (1988) have reported using two to eight BCG weekly instillations via the nephrostomy tract beginning 7 days after the percutaneous resection. In contrast, Huffman and associates as well as others have described the use of mitomycin C in the upper urinary tract either as a single 20-hour instillation via the percutaneous nephrostomy tube (40 mg mitomycin C in 1000 ml of normal saline at 50 ml/hour) or as two acute doses via a ureteral catheter, which is then clamped for 30 minutes (5 mg instillation on postoperative day 1 and 2) (Streem and Pontes, 1986; Inglis and Tolley, 1988; Grossman et al, 1992; Eastham and Huffman, 1993). During instillation therapy, the pressure in the collecting system should not be allowed to exceed 40 cm H_2O.

Another adjunctive measure has been reported to be of some benefit after percutaneous resection of TCC of the renal pelvis. Nurse and Patel and their colleagues have described using an iridium wire placed in the nephrostomy tract postoperatively for 3 to 8 days; the radioactive iridium 192 delivers 4000 to 45000 cGy to a 0.5-cm radius (Nurse et al, 1989; Patel et al, 1994).

RESULTS

The results of endosurgical management of upper tract TCC are remarkably similar to open conservative therapy for

upper tract transitional cell disease (Table 94–7) (Huffman et al, 1985a; Orihuela and Smith, 1988; Blute et al, 1989; Nurse et al, 1989; Huffman, 1990; Tasca and Zattoni, 1990; Martinez-Pineiro, et al, 1991). Overall, ureteral tumors appear to respond somewhat better than pelvic tumors to endosurgical management. Ureteral tumors are usually treated ureteroscopically. Both the recurrence rate in TCC of the ureter cases at approximately 2 years (15%) and the progression to open ablative surgery (13%) are low.

In contrast, the renal pelvic tumor is more commonly approached percutaneously, especially if it is larger than 1 cm. In patients with TCC of the renal pelvis, the incidence of multicentricity, the associated urothelial dysplasia, and the more vast and at times poorly accessible urothelium of the renal pelvis "conspire" against definitive endosurgical treatment. Recurrence (30%–70%) and open surgery (30%) rates at 2 years in patients with TCC of the renal pelvis are at least twice those in patients with ureteral tumors. Interestingly, reports of distant metastatic disease or seeding of the nephrostomy tract are exceedingly rare. To date,

there has been only one reported retroperitoneal recurrence (Huang et al, 1995). The follow-up periods in most clinical series of upper tract TCC managed endosurgically, however, remain short: 1.5 to 2.5 years. Only three series have data beyond 4 years' follow-up (Patel et al, 1994; Jarrett et al, 1995; Vasavada et al, 1995). The largest experience is from Long Island Jewish Hospital, in which 36 patients were treated by percutaneous resection and adjunctive BCG instillation therapy and were subsequently followed an average of 4.5 years (9–111 months). Local recurrences occurred in 33% with progression to open nephroureterectomy in 17%. Another 17% of the patients in this series developed metastatic disease (Jarrett et al, 1995).

With regard to topical chemotherapy, it appears that BCG administration in the upper urinary tract is effective in controlling local disease and preventing recurrences. Herr (1985) and Ramsey and Soloway (1990) independently reported giving five or six weekly doses of BCG to the upper urinary tract; both patients were followed beyond 1 year. The lesions in both of these cases responded to BCG despite the fact

Table 94–7. ENDOSURGICAL THERAPY AND OPEN CONSERVATIVE SURGERY FOR UPPER TRACT TRANSITIONAL CELL CARCINOMA

Authors	Patients	Approach	Adjunctive Local Therapy	Local Recurrence (%)	Open Surgical Ablation (%)	Metastases (%)	Follow-up (Months)
Endosurgical Therapy							
Orihuela and Smith, 1988	4 (pelvis)	Percutaneous	No	75	25	0	19
	7 (pelvis)	Percutaneous	Yes (BCG [6]; mitomycin C [1])	29	29	14	22
Nurse et al, 1989	15	Percutaneous	Iridium wire (4000–4500 cGy) (14); mitomycin C (1)	39	33	0	24
Blute et al, 1989	8 (pelvis)	Percutaneous (3)	—	0	0	0	18
	13 (ureter)	Ureteroscopic (5)	—	20	0	0	28
		Ureteroscopic (13)	—	15	0	0	21
Huffman, 1990	5	Percutaneous and ureteroscopic	—	40	40	0	>12
Huffman, 1985a	8	Ureteroscopic	Mitomycin C (1)	38	13	0	21
Tasca and Zattoni, 1990	4	Percutaneous	—	0	0	0	11–24
Papadopoulos et al, 1990	2	Ureteroscopic	—	0	—	0	3
Carson, 1991	8	Ureteroscopic	—	0	—	0	6–40
Eastham and Huffman, 1993	7	Ureteroscopic	Mitomycin C (7)	0	0	0	1–12
Vasavada et al, 1995	6	Percutaneous	BCG	17	0	33	9–59
Patel et al, 1994	26	Percutaneous	Iridium wire (12) or thiotepa (1)	23	4	NA	Up to 5.9 years
Jarrett et al, 1995	36	Percutaneous	BCG	33	17	17	9–111 (56.4)
Surgical Therapy							
Wallace, 1981	7 (pelvis)	Local excision	—	35	NA	29	9.6 years
	7 (ureter)	Segmental ureterectomy	—	14	NA	0	5.9 years
Mazeman, 1976	23 (pelvis)	Local excision	—	35	NA	—	>12
	50 (ureter)	Segmental/distal ureterectomy	—	6	NA	—	>12
Vasavada et al, 1995	2	Partial nephrectomy	—	50	NA	0	17–20
Papadopoulos et al, 1994	1	Local excision segmental ureterectomy	—	0	0	0	3

BCG, Bacillus Calmette-Guérin.

that both were of a high-grade nature (carcinoma in situ and grade 3). Similarly, Sharpe and colleagues gave a 6-week course of upper tract BCG via ureteral catheter to 17 kidneys in patients with positive selective upper tract cytology but negative radiographic studies. At an average follow-up of 3 years, 75% of the patients had a negative urine cytology (Sharpe et al, 1993).

The largest experience with BCG use in the upper urinary tract for documented TCC comes from Orihuela and Smith, who treated seven patients with two to eight weekly instillations. At 22 months' follow-up (range 8–29 months), two of their patients (29%) who received BCG had local recurrences. Both of these individuals underwent successful nephroureterectomy, and there were no deaths in this group. In the non-BCG group (four patients), the results were less favorable: the recurrence rate was 75% within the first 9 months of follow-up. Two of these patients died within 19 months of the initial percutaneous procedure. This favorable BCG experience has held up with extension of follow-up to an average of 56.4 months: 33% recurrence rate (Jarrett et al, 1995). It is of note, however, that a survival advantage for their patients treated with adjunctive BCG could not be identified (Jarrett et al, 1995).

Of note, BCG therapy appears to be well tolerated in the upper urinary tract. There has been only one report of fever and transient BCG bacteremia (Sharpe et al, 1993). Indeed, in Bellman and associates' series, the BCG therapy did not require interruption because of any side effects, although dysuria and transient hematuria were not uncommon (Bellman et al, 1994). Interestingly, one fourth of their patients developed granuloma formation in the renal pelvis. The presence of these granulomas was not a harbinger of improved responsiveness to the BCG therapy; indeed, they can be troublesome in that it is difficult to differentiate between these lesions and recurrent sessile TCC without a biopsy (Bellman et al, 1994).

At present, in the realm of endosurgical therapy for upper tract TCC, there is both consensus and controversy. Endosurgical resection as described appears to be a reasonable option for the patient with a grade 1 or 2, solitary, papillary **renal pelvic** or calyceal solitary lesion (<2 cm), or solitary ureteral lesion (<1 cm) in a solitary kidney; the patient with pre-existing renal compromise in whom cytology findings are negative; or the patient who is a high surgical risk. Likewise, for the patient with grade 3 disease, a standard nephroureterectomy with a cuff of bladder is indicated even if this results in the need for long-term dialysis. Indeed, in Jarrett and colleagues' series on endourologic therapy for upper tract TCC, within 5 years, half of the grade 3 patients developed recurrences, and half of the grade 3 group died of metastatic disease (Jarrett et al, 1995).

Controversy in this field pertains to the patient with grade 1 disease with a normal contralateral kidney and with normal renal function. The current recommendations remain that these patients should undergo a standard nephroureterectomy with a cuff of bladder; however, the findings in the endosurgical series with regard to these low-grade tumors in patients with two kidneys are worth noting. Indeed, for grade 1, solitary upper tract tumors, the endosurgical outcome is excellent. Recurrence rates are relatively low (18% at 54 months), as is the need for subsequent nephrectomy (9%) (Jarrett et al, 1995). Neither metastatic disease nor a cancer-related death has occurred in this group. Accordingly, at some centers, percutaneous therapy for even low-grade tumors in patients with a normal contralateral kidney is now being offered as first-line therapy (Jarrett et al, 1995). Further follow-up and cost-effective outcome data are needed to determine if this "new" approach is indeed a better approach than definitive surgical extirpation.

Fungal Bezoar

Both *Candida* pyelonephritis (associated with cortical abscesses or diffuse involvement of the medullary rays) and asymptomatic *Candida* infestation of the urine can be associated with the development of intrarenal fungal concretions (Beland and Piette, 1973). The pseudomycelia that are characteristic of *Candida albicans* may aggregate to form a significant mass within the renal pelvis. Similarly, *Torulopsis glabrata* can form a fungal conglomeration albeit without pseudohyphae. In these patients, the masses consist of fungus, necrotic tissue, inflammatory cells, and on occasion stone matrix (Abramowitz et al, 1986; Beland and Piette, 1973).

Patients who are especially predisposed to developing fungal bezoars are those who have diabetes mellitus, who use antibiotics chronically, who have urinary tract catheters, and who are immunosuppressed (Schonebeck and Ansehn, 1972). About half the reported cases of fungal concretions are in diabetic patients (Dembner and Pfister, 1977). Upward of 20% of renal transplant patients may develop funguria (Schonebeck and Ansehn, 1972). These individuals present with a variety of symptoms and signs ranging from obstruction to sepsis (Schonebeck and Ansehn, 1972; Beland and Piette, 1973).

The diagnosis of a fungal concretion is suspected when an intravenous urogram or a retrograde ureterogram reveals a noncalcified *filling defect* within the renal pelvis. The pseudomycelia or yeast forms characteristic of a *Candida* infection can be noted on a freshly prepared urinalysis sample. A urine culture likewise reveals the presence of *C. albicans* or *T. glabrata*.

Therapy for the fungal concretion is both medical and surgical. In the preoperative or seriously ill patient, a course of amphotericin B or 5-fluorocytosine is initiated. Once adequate serum levels are obtained, topical irrigation of the affected collecting system with amphotericin B (50 mg/L at 25–50 ml/hour) can be given via either two retrograde ureteral catheters (one for inflow; one for outflow) or an antegrade nephrostomy tube (Blum, 1966; Harrach et al, 1970; Wise, 1990). Next, once antibiotic coverage has resulted in sterile urine cultures, the bezoar can be removed percutaneously or by open surgery (Karlin et al, 1987).

TECHNIQUE

The percutaneous removal of a fungal bezoar requires meticulous attention to detail. Initially a retrograde ureteral catheter is placed. The renal pelvis is gently irrigated with amphotericin B (50 mg/L) to decrease the hypothetical possibility of retroperitoneal seeding of the fungus. The volume instilled should not exceed the drained volume of the renal pelvis.

The percutaneous nephrostomy technique follows the same principles for placement of a nephrostomy tract as previously described. An **infracostal** lower-pole approach to the renal pelvis is secured; a working and a safety guide wire are secured. A supracostal approach is never used because traversal of the pleural cavity could result in a fungal empyema. Because the goal is to minimize both the manipulation of the renal parenchyma and the potential of retroperitoneal extravasation, dilation of the tract is most simply done with a 10-mm nephrostomy tract dilating balloon. In an effort to limit retroperitoneal extravasation of urine and fragments of the fungal concretion, a No. 30 Fr Amplatz sheath is positioned in the collecting system.

The fungal bezoar has a gray-white or yellow-gray appearance. The consistency is similar to a blood clot. If it is smaller than 1.0 cm, it can be extracted intact from the collecting system; however, for the larger concretions, the suction on the ultrasonic lithotriptor probe is useful for bezoar evacuation. The flexible nephroscope is helpful to determine if all fungal concretions have been cleared from the collecting system.

At the end of the procedure, a No. 22 Fr Councill catheter is secured as a nephrostomy tube. The retrograde ureteral catheter is left in place. On postoperative day 1, a nephrostogram is obtained. If there are no extravasation and no remaining concretions, irrigation with amphotericin B (50 mg/ L at 50 ml/hour) is performed via the ureteral catheter for 48 to 72 hours (Wise, 1990; Wise et al, 1982). Provided that the urine culture is free of *Candida*, the ureteral catheter and nephrostomy tube can be removed on postoperative day 3 or 4. If the nephrostogram reveals any remaining filling defects, however, the patient is scheduled for repeat nephroscopy. Again the goal of percutaneous therapy in these patients is to clear the collecting system of all fungal bezoars.

RESULTS

In general, reports of fungal bezoars are rare (Table 94–8). Indeed, in a review of the literature, Schonebeck and Ansehn (1972) noted only 24 cases of upper tract fungal concretions; to this list, they added five more cases from their own

experience. Presence of an upper tract fungal bezoar in association with an unrelieved ureteral obstruction has a mortality rate in the 80% range. Placement of ureteral catheters with and without irrigation with amphotericin B as well as **surgical** removal of the fungal concretion is curative, albeit in a small number of reviewed cases (Gillam and Wadelton, 1958; Blum, 1966; Harrach et al, 1970; Beland and Piette, 1973; Keane et al, 1993).

Given the infrequent occurrence of this problem, it is not surprising that there is a paucity of experience with regard to the percutaneous management and removal of fungal concretions (Dembner and Pfister, 1977; Abramowitz et al, 1986; Karlin et al, 1987; Banner et al, 1988; Doemeny et al, 1988; Keane et al, 1993). Over the last 10 years, fewer than a dozen cases of percutaneous therapy for renal fungal bezoars have been reported. In some cases (i.e., few and small fungal aggregates), this has involved only the establishment of a percutaneous nephrostomy for drainage. In others, with larger fungal masses, the bezoar has been either fragmented (with a guide wire) or extracted directly (Blum, 1966; Harrach et al, 1970; Bartone et al, 1988; Irby et al, 1990). In this limited group of patients, successful endourologic treatment has occurred in approximately 80% with minimal attendant morbidity and mortality (see Table 94–8).

Reconstructive Percutaneous Endourology

Calyceal Diverticulum

The calyceal diverticulum is a relatively rare entity, diagnosed in 4.5 per 1000 intravenous urograms. The diverticulum arises from the fornix of a minor calyx and hence is lined with transitional cell epithelium. Approximately a third to a half of these lesions are associated with pain, infection, hematuria, or calculi (Timmons et al, 1975). In contradistinction to a hydrocalyx, the calyceal diverticulum is believed to be a congenital rather than an acquired lesion. The surgical

Table 94–8. PERCUTANEOUS EXTRACTION OF FUNGAL BEZOAR

Authors	Sex	Age	Fever	Flank Pain	Diabetes Mellitus	Renal Transplant	Immuno-suppression	History of Lithiasis or Renal Surgery	Method	Urine Culture	Long-Term Follow-up
Karlin et al, 1987	F	49	Yes	Yes	Yes	No	No	Yes	Percutaneous extraction/ systemic and percutaneous irrigation with amphotericin B	*Candida albicans Pseudomonas aeruginosa*	—
Abramowitz et al, 1986	F	72	Yes	No	Yes	No	No	No	Percutaneous extraction	*Torulopsis glabrata*	Sterile urine culture at 4 months
Doemeny et al, 1988	F	65	Yes	Yes	Yes	No	No	No	Percutaneous extraction	*T. glabrata*	—
Ireton et al, 1985	F	49	Yes	No	No	Yes	Yes	Yes	Percutaneous extraction	*C. albicans*	6 months
Irby et al, 1990	M	28	—	—	Yes	No	No	No	Percutaneous extraction	*C. albicans*	—
	M	50	—	—	Yes	No	No	No	Percutaneous extraction	*Aspergillus*	Required nephrectomy
Keane et al, 1993	M	67	—	No	No	No	No	No	Percutaneous nephrostomy and fluconazole orally	*C. albicans*	3 months

approach to these lesions involves either excision or marsupialization of the diverticulum with occlusion of the neck of the diverticulum by suture or electrocautery. If the diverticulum is large, a partial nephrectomy may be necessary (Abeshouse and Abeshouse, 1963). Over the past decade, the treatment for calyceal diverticula has shifted to endourologic therapy (Fig. 94–26) (Clayman and Castaneda-Zuniga, 1984; Hulbert et al, 1988a).

TECHNIQUE

The first step in the percutaneous approach to a calyceal diverticulum is the cystoscopic placement of a retrograde ureteral catheter. A 0.035-inch floppy-tipped guide wire is passed retrograde. Over this guide wire, a No. 7 Fr, 11.5-mm occlusion balloon is passed into the renal pelvis; the balloon is inflated with 1 ml of half-strength contrast material, and the entire catheter is then pulled down to the UPJ until the balloon is snug. Next, air or contrast material is gently infused by way of the retrograde catheter until the calyceal diverticulum is well outlined. Then, using an 18-gauge nephrostomy needle, a fluoroscopically guided puncture is made directly into the calyceal diverticulum itself. The guide wire is coiled in the diverticulum because the neck of the diverticulum is usually too small to cannulate. If the diverticulum is particularly large, a second guide wire can be placed (see under "Percutaneous Nephrostomy"), thereby providing the surgeon with both a safety and a

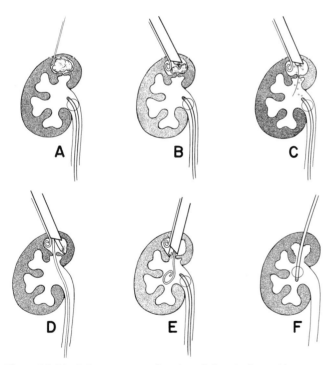

Figure 94–26. *A,* Large upper-pole calyceal diverticulum with a stone. The diverticulum has been punctured directly. *B,* Ultrasonic nephrolithotripsy is used to remove the calculus. *C,* Air injected retrograde is used to identify the diverticular neck. A 0.035-inch Bentson-type guide wire is passed across the diverticular neck. *D,* An electrosurgical probe is used to fulgurate the walls of the diverticulum. *E,* The electrosurgical probe is now used to incise the neck of the diverticulum. Note that a nonconducting catheter has been passed over the guide wire (e.g., a No. 5 Fr angiographic catheter) to preclude current from traveling along the guide wire. *F,* A transdiverticular nephrostomy tube is placed.

working guide wire. The tract into the diverticulum is dilated with a 10-mm balloon dilator. Dilating the tract with shear dilators (i.e., Amplatz coaxial system, separate Teflon dilators, or metal telescoping dilators) is more difficult and may result in an anterior false passage of the diverticulum. A 10-mm Amplatz sheath is placed into the diverticulum, after which the rigid nephroscope is introduced. Any calculus present is treated by either intact removal or ultrasonic nephrolithotripsy (Clayman and Castaneda-Zuniga, 1984).

Next, saline stained with indigo carmine or room air is gently instilled through the retrograde ureteral occlusion balloon catheter while the surgeon examines the interior of the calyceal diverticulum with the rigid or flexible nephroscope. Air bubbles or blue fluid should be seen traversing the neck of the diverticulum. If this is not the case, the Amplatz sheath may be too deep into the diverticulum. The sheath should be carefully withdrawn 1 to 2 cm under endoscopic control, while the assistant continues to instill air (N.B.: 10-cc bolus gently injected) or fluid gently into the retrograde ureteral catheter. Once the neck of the diverticulum is visualized, a 0.035-inch floppy-tipped guide wire or a plastic (i.e., Terumo) guide wire can be passed across the neck of the diverticulum and coiled in the renal pelvis (see Fig. 94–26) (Clayman and Castaneda-Zuniga, 1984). If a metal guide wire is used, following its passage across the diverticular neck, a No. 5 Fr angiographic catheter is passed over the guide wire to insulate it.

At this point, the roller electrode mounted on a standard No. 24 or 26 Fr resectoscope is introduced into the diverticular cavity. The entire surface of the diverticulum is then electrocoagulated except for the immediate area surrounding the diverticular neck (see Fig. 94–26) (Hulbert et al, 1987).

Next the neck of the diverticulum is treated. This can be done most simply by balloon dilation of the neck of the diverticulum with an 8-mm, 4-cm-long ureteral dilating balloon. Some urologists prefer to cut the neck of the diverticulum under direct vision with either a cold knife (i.e., direct vision urethrotome) or an electrosurgical probe (No. 2 or 3 Fr Greenwald electrode). Again, if electrosurgery is to be used, any metal guide wire in the surgical field must be covered with a No. 5 Fr angiographic catheter so that no electrical current is transmitted to the guide wire. Several shallow incisions (2–4 mm) are made in the neck of the diverticulum in a radial fashion (12, 3, 6, and 9 o'clock). A solitary deep cut into the diverticular neck should be avoided because this may result in significant hemorrhage (Clayman and Castaneda-Zuniga, 1984).

After opening the neck of the diverticulum, a large-bore (No. 22 Fr) nephrostomy tube is placed such that its shaft traverses the diverticulum and the tip of the catheter lies in the renal pelvis (see Fig. 94–26). The nephrostomy tube can be removed as early as 3 days after the procedure (Hulbert et al, 1986). Indeed, prolonged drainage of the kidney and stenting of the diverticular neck do not appear to improve results (Hulbert et al, 1988a; Jones et al, 1991).

An alternative and perhaps simpler method is not to spend time trying to identify the diverticular neck. Instead the entire surface of the diverticulum, including the area of the unidentified diverticular neck, is thoroughly cauterized using the roller electrode (Segura J, personal communication, 1988). A No. 22 Fr drainage catheter is placed only to tamponade the percutaneous tract; the tip of the catheter thus resides in the calyceal diverticulum. The "calycostomy" tube is removed on the following morning, provided that there is no drainage.

Three other endosurgical alternatives are possible for treating a calyceal diverticulum: indirect percutaneous approach, ureteroscopic approach, and ESWL. An **indirect percutaneous approach** can be problematic and is mentioned only to be condemned because it results in making the procedure more difficult and less successful. First, a usually nonhydronephrotic collecting system must be punctured. Next the surgeon must locate the diminutive communication between the calyceal diverticulum and the collecting system. After this step, the neck must be opened and the diverticulum entered. Incising the neck of the diverticulum, however, often results in bleeding, which obscures the surgeon's vision and impairs subsequent treatment of the diverticular wall. In addition, the removal of any stones within the diverticulum becomes more difficult because of the angle of entry into the diverticulum and any bleeding incurred by dilating or cutting the neck of the diverticulum. Ureteroscopic and ESWL techniques for dealing with the stone-laden calyceal diverticulum are discussed in Chapters 93 and 94.

RESULTS

In comparing all of the endosurgical methods for treating a calyceal diverticulum, it becomes quite clear that an antegrade (i.e., direct puncture) percutaneous approach is safe and effective. Among 134 patients, in several clinical series, with a calyceal diverticulum and a stone, a percutaneous approach resulted in removal of the stone in 86% of patients and obliteration of the diverticulum in 80% (Table 94–9) (Eshghi et al, 1987; Hulbert et al, 1988a; Janetschek, 1988; Ellis et al, 1991; Jones JA et al, 1991; Lang, 1991; Schneider et al, 1991; Hendrikx et al, 1992; Bellman et al, 1993; Van Cangh et al, 1994a; Grasso et al, 1995; Soble et al, 1995).

The indirect percutaneous method results in poorer results. Hulbert and colleagues noted that in three patients approached with indirect punctures, the diverticula were still present in all three on follow-up radiographic studies, 4 to 14 months later (Hulbert et al, 1986).

The nonpercutaneous alternatives include ureteroscopy, ESWL, or a combination of ureteroscopy and ESWL. Using a ureteroscopic approach, Mikkelsen and co-workers could successfully treat only two of six calyceal diverticula (Mikkelsen et al, 1989). In one of the successful cases, two ureteroscopic procedures were required because of postoperative bleeding from the diverticulum. Similarly, with ESWL as frontline therapy, Psihramis and Dretler (1987) noted that 70% of patients became asymptomatic after treatment. At the time of follow-up, however, 80% still had stone fragments within the diverticula. In all patients studied, the diverticula remained intact. Indeed, even under the most favorable of circumstances, the stone-free rate is only 40% (Streem and Yost, 1992; Van Cangh et al, 1994a) and can be as poor as 6% (Jones JA et al, 1991). In none of the ESWL patients did the calyceal diverticulum disappear.

Fuchs and David (1989) have combined ESWL with ureteroscopy for dilation of the calyceal neck and stone extraction in 15 patients with stone-containing calyceal diverticula. Their overall stone-free rate of 73% is an improvement over ESWL monotherapy; however, although less morbid, it is not as effective as an antegrade percutaneous approach. Likewise, treatment of the diverticulum was limited to balloon dilation of the neck of the diverticulum; in only 47% of the cases was obliteration or a decrease in the size of the diverticulum noted. Of note, with this technique, only diverticula in the upper and middle portion of the kidney can be effectively accessed.

Hydrocalyx

Infundibular stenosis and hydrocalyx are usually an acquired condition associated with inflammation, renal tuber-

Table 94–9. ENDOSURGICAL THERAPY FOR CALYCEAL DIVERTICULA

Authors	Number of Patients	% with Stones	Method of Treatment	Stent Size	Stent Duration	% Stone-Free	% Obliterated Diverticulum	Follow-up (Months)
Percutaneous Approach								
Hulbert et al, 1988a	17	100	Antegrade PCN (14) Retrograde PCN (3) Dilation (17) Fulguration (1)	—	2 weeks	100	80% (all failures had indirect approach)	9 (3–15)
Ellis et al, 1991	10	80	Antegrade PCN Balloon dilation	—	2–4 days	100	75	4–72
Jones JA et al, 1991	14	100	Antegrade PCN Balloon dilation Fulguration	—	3 days	86	100	35 (6–60)
Hendrikx et al, 1992	13	100	Antegrade PCN and dilation	No. 12 Fr	3–6 weeks	77	—	3–36
Bellman et al, 1993	20	95	Antegrade PCN; balloon dilation	No. 24 Fr	2 days	95	80	6 (3–30)
Van Cangh et al, 1994a	36	100	Antegrade PCN	—	—	72	67	56
Soble et al, 1995	21	100	Antegrade PCN; endoincision fulguration	No. 22 Fr	2–7 days	90	86	39 (11–85)
Grasso et al, 1995	3	100	Antegrade PCN; balloon dilation	No. 24 Fr	2 weeks	100	—	5
Overall	134	98		No. 12–24 Fr	2 days–6 weeks	86	80	3–85

PCN, Percutaneous nephrostomy.

culosis, obstructive calculus, or prior renal surgery (Abeshouse and Abeshouse, 1963; Hwang and Park, 1994). Rarely, infundibular stenosis may be caused by an upper pole crossing segmental renal artery (Fraley's syndrome) (Fraley, 1969; Eshghi et al, 1987). If one suspects the presence of an obstructing crossing segmental renal artery, an arteriogram should be obtained before any endourologic therapeutic maneuvers because this condition mandates an open surgical repair (Eshghi et al, 1987). The hydrocalyx should be differentiated from a calyceal diverticulum because the treatments are different. At times, this distinction can be made only by nephroscopy because the presence (hydrocalyx) or absence (calyceal diverticulum) of a renal papilla is diagnostic.

TECHNIQUE

The percutaneous antegrade technique for infundibular stenosis is initially similar to the approach for treating a calyceal diverticulum (Fig. 94–27). First, a retrograde ureteral occlusion balloon (11.5 mm) catheter is placed. The balloon is inflated in the renal pelvis and pulled caudad to place it snugly against the UPJ. Via the flank, the hydrocalyx is punctured directly, and a 0.035-inch floppy-tipped guide wire is coiled in the affected calyx. The nephrostomy tract into the hydrocalyx is dilated with a 10-mm nephrostomy balloon, and an Amplatz 10-mm sheath is placed into the calyx. Alternatively, if one is anticipating placing a large indwelling ureteral stent (a situation that applies only to upper pole or middle affected calyces), the nephrostomy tract can be dilated to only No. 18 Fr, and a No. 18 Fr Amplatz biliary sheath can be placed. Careful inspection with the rigid or flexible nephroscope or, in the case of a No. 18 Fr tract, the No. 12.5 Fr short operating ureteroscope enables the endoscopist to visualize the stenotic infundibulum and cannulate it with a 0.035-inch floppy-tipped or Terumo guide wire. This second (i.e., working) guide wire is coiled in the renal pelvis or, if possible, passed down the ureter. If difficulty is encountered in locating the mouth of the infundibulum, air (10–15 cc bolus gently injected and repeated as needed) or saline mixed with a small amount of indigo carmine can be infused by way of the retrograde occlusion balloon catheter (see Fig. 94–27). Usually, bubbles or blue fluid can be endoscopically traced to the stenotic infundibulum, thereby facilitating cannulation of the infundibulum.

The infundibular narrowing can be resolved in several ways. The least difficult approach is to dilate the infundibulum to 8 mm with an 8-mm ureteral dilating balloon passed over the working guide wire. Alternatively the infundibulum can be cut under endoscopic control with a cold knife through a direct vision urethrotome or with a No. 2 or 3 Fr electrosurgical probe passed via the flexible nephroscope or the short rigid ureteroscope. In the latter case, a No. 5 Fr angiographic catheter is passed over the working guide wire to insulate it, or the working guide wire is exchanged for a nonconducting plastic wire (i.e., Terumo guide wire) (see Fig. 94–27). According to anatomic studies by Sampaio (1992), the incision should be made along the less vascular superior and inferior aspects of the middle calyceal infundibulum or the medial and lateral aspects of the upper calyceal infundibulum. Usually a 2-mm incision is made on the superior and the inferior aspect of the infundibulum. A single deep cut is to be avoided because this may result in marked

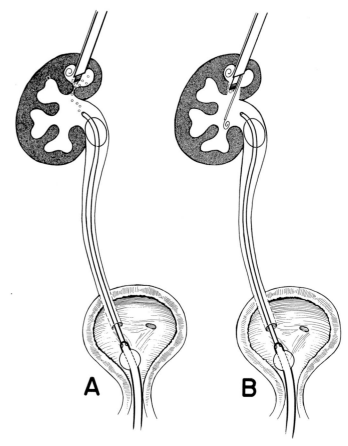

Figure 94–27. *A,* Arrangement for endoscopic treatment of an upper-pole stenotic infundibulum. Note the retrograde occlusion balloon catheter in the ureter, the safety wire coiled in the hydrocalyx, and the air from the ureteral catheter bubbling across the stenotic infundibulum. Via the No. 30 Fr Amplatz sheath, a No. 12.5 Fr therapeutic short ureteroscope with an insulated tip has been introduced. A 0.035-inch metal guide wire has been passed through the ureteroscope and is being directed at the narrowed infundibulum. *B,* A guide wire and No. 5 Fr angiographic catheter have been passed across the stenotic infundibulum. A No. 2 Fr electrosurgical probe with a less than 400-μ tip is passed via the No. 12.5 Fr short therapeutic ureteroscope. The electrosurgical probe has been used to make 2- to 4-mm incisions (3 and 9 o'clock) (pure cut, 50–100 watts) into the stenotic infundibulum, thereby widely opening the infundibulum.

bleeding. Before making an incision, the area to be incised should be carefully inspected for the presence of any arterial pulsations.

After the incision is completed, the patency of the infundibulum can be further gauged by passing an 8-mm dilating balloon catheter across the incised infundibulum. The balloon should inflate to No. 24 Fr at low pressure (<1 atm).

Next the endoscope is passed into the collecting system; a 260-cm exchange guide wire is passed up the occlusion balloon and retrieved with a grasping forceps, thereby providing a through-and-through guide wire. A No. 22 Fr Councill catheter is obtained, and an extra side hole is cut just proximal to the catheter's retention balloon. Now a No. 7.1 Fr pigtail catheter can be advanced through a side arm adapter; a No. 22 Fr Councill nephrostomy tube is advanced over the 260-cm guide wire, and the pigtail catheter is then advanced over the 260-cm guide wire and through the center of the Councill catheter until the tip of the pigtail catheter exits the tip of the Councill catheter. The pigtail catheter is advanced into the bladder under fluoroscopic monitoring, while the Councill catheter is advanced until its tip is in the renal pelvis. The guide wire is now removed, and the side arm adapter is plugged into the butt end of the Councill catheter, and its collar is turned until the side arm adapter is securely affixed to the shaft of the No. 7.1 Fr pigtail catheter. The Councill catheter is sewn to the skin of the flank with 2–0 silk sutures. The urethral catheter is removed. The nephrostomy and antegrade ureteral catheter is left in place for 4 to 6 weeks.

Alternatively, if the procedure was performed on an upper pole or middle calyx, a No. 7/14 Fr variable-sized indwelling stent can be placed, such that one end of the pigtail is in the affected calyx, and the No. 14 Fr portion of the stent traverses the incised infundibulum and coils in the affected calyx. In this case, if only a No. 18 Fr tract was developed, a No. 10 Fr locking loop catheter serves as the nephrostomy tube. The coil of the nephrostomy tube is placed in the calyx or in the renal pelvis. A nephrostogram is obtained 2 to 3 days later. If there is no extravasation, the nephrostomy tube is removed under fluoroscopic control. The indwelling No. 7/14 Fr stent is removed through the bladder 4 to 6 weeks later.

Another therapeutic approach to infundibular stenosis is an **indirect** percutaneous approach. Puncturing the collecting system through an unaffected calyx and trying to approach the stenotic infundibulum in a retrograde fashion with a nephroscope is tedious and may be less efficacious than a direct antegrade approach. As with the calyceal diverticulum, this approach should be avoided.

RESULTS

Reported series of endourologically treated infundibular stenoses are few. Commonly, reports on calyceal diverticula are mixed with cases of hydrocalyx, such that the "true" success rate may appear overly sanguine (Table 94–10) (Eshghi et al, 1987; Janetschek, 1988). Lang (1991) reported a 66% success rate in six patients with an isolated hydrocalyx using simple balloon dilation and a 4-week period of stenting; follow-up ranged from 2 to 7 years. With regard to actual incision of the infundibulum, Schneider and co-workers reported a 67% success rate in nine patients with infundibular stenosis during an average follow-up of 15 months (Schneider et al, 1991). More recently, Hwang and Park (1994) recorded an 80% success rate in 10 patients with

tuberculous infundibular strictures who had undergone a cold knife incision; follow-up in this series was greater than 1 year. It appears that in contrast to the calyceal diverticulum, in which a successful outcome is obtainable in nearly 90%, the infundibular stenosis is a more difficult entity to treat endourologically with only a 60% to 80% success rate.

Strictures of the Upper Urinary Tract

Overview of Endoincision for Upper Urinary Tract Stricture

"In evaluating one's clinical results, I think the relief of symptoms is a very poor guidepost. I think, unless we can demonstrate better renal drainage, we have not accomplished the success which we hope to."

R. B. HENLINE
JULY 1, 1947
AMERICAN UROLOGICAL ASSOCIATION ANNUAL MEETING

In the field of endourology, there is no more difficult area in which to establish a preoperative diagnosis and to judge a postoperative result than that of upper urinary tract strictures. The **diagnosis** of a stricture itself may often be in doubt. **Anatomic** obstruction as noted on an intravenous urogram may not represent **functional** obstruction as delineated by a diuretic washout renogram or a Whitaker bladder and renal pelvis pressure study. Indeed, it is only the documented **functional** obstruction that mandates corrective surgery.

Also, the urologist must be careful to examine the characterization of each stricture in the reported patient population. Coexisting conditions may result in a transient stricture. For example, a renal pelvic calculus or a urinary tract infection may result in inflammation sufficient to obstruct the UPJ. This problem usually resolves spontaneously, however, on removal of the calculus or appropriate antibiotic therapy. In this setting, the "success" of a premature endoincision becomes inflated. Conversely a preponderance of postirradiation ureteral strictures in a series may negatively prejudice the results. Furthermore, both the length and the location of a stricture influence the success of an endoincision. Short (<1 cm) strictures and strictures in the proximal or distal ureter fare better than longer strictures or strictures in the middle ureter.

It is also difficult to ascertain the **success** of an endoincision. Subjective and objective follow-up should be carefully

Table 94–10. ENDOSURGICAL THERAPY FOR INFUNDIBULAR STENOSIS WITH ASSOCIATED HYDROCALYX

Authors	Number of Patients	% with Stones	Method of Treatment	Stent Size	Stent Duration (weeks)	Outcome		Follow-up (Months)
						% Stone-Free	% Patent	
Schneider et al, 1991	9	—	Antegrade PCN; cold knife	—	3–6	—	67	15 (7–45)
Lang, 1991	6	100	Antegrade PCN; balloon dilation	No. 8–10 Fr	4–8	100	60	24–48
Hwang and Park, 1994	10	10	Antegrade PCN; cold knife	No. 14 Fr	6–8	NA	80	>3
Overall	25	—	—	No. 8–14 fr	3–8	—	72	3–48

PCN, Percutaneous nephrostomy.

differentiated. Although a telephone call to the patient or to the primary physician can provide some data as to how the patient has fared, these data are largely anecdotal. To discern the subjective outcome of the procedure, it is helpful for the patient to complete a pain and quality of life analog scale (Nadler et al, 1995b). With this approach, one can numerically assess subjective data, thereby allowing subclassification of patients into three categories: failures (<50% pain relief), improved (50%–90% pain relief), and cured (90%–100%) pain relief. In addition, this type of questionnaire allows the urologist to gauge whether the procedure has allowed the patient to return completely to full activity. Even quantifiable subjective data, however, if unaccompanied by objective studies, are seriously flawed. For example, complaints of minor musculoskeletal back discomfort may negatively prejudice results, whereas some patients with significant recurrent stricture disease or even total obstruction may actually be asymptomatic because of nonfunction of the affected kidney, thereby casting a positive bias on the results.

Hence, objective **functional** tests of patency, such as the diuretic washout renogram or the Whitaker test, although not ideal, are necessary to provide accurate information on the ultimate outcome of the procedure. Alone, the IVP can be misleading because the hydronephrosis associated with chronic UPJ obstruction in the adult usually does not resolve. Certainly, among these patients, when a postoperative IVP is suggestive of recurrent obstruction, a functional test should follow.

Another problem in evaluating the outcome of an endoincision is to discern the **durability** of the "successful" endoincision. In contrast to stone disease, in which the result is immediately evident, with obstructive uropathy it takes at least a year before one can be confident that the problem has resolved in the majority of patients. Shorter follow-up usually provides overly optimistic results. In one series of endoureterotomy patients, late failure (i.e., in this series defined as beyond 6 months) occurred in 15%, thereby lowering the overall success rate from 79% to 64% (Meretyk et al, 1992a). Likewise in some endopyelotomy series, the late failure rate was as high as 13% (Van Cangh et al, 1994b).

Also, incomplete patient follow-up data may likewise result in inaccurate conclusions. To have a series of 100 patients undergoing endoincisions and report follow-up information on only 50 patients, in all of whom the procedure "succeeded," provides one with the uneasy task of attempting to decide whether the success rate is actually 100% or perhaps only 50%. Do the "unreported" failures seek self-exile in the care of another physician? Do the "lost" successes merely declare independence from the "healing" profession? Meticulous follow-up in all patients, albeit tedious, is essential; follow-up rates of less than 75% seriously impair the investigator's ability to make any valid conclusions.

Diagnosis of Obstruction of the Upper Urinary Tract

The classic symptom of obstruction of the upper urinary tract is flank discomfort exacerbated by intake of fluids or diuretics. Interestingly, some patients may be pain-free, the diagnosis being made serendipitously during the evaluation for a nonrenal condition (e.g., cholelithiasis, metastatic evaluation for a nonrenal malignancy). The incidental discovery of UPJ obstruction may lead to repair, if compromise of renal function is documented during conservative follow-up management (Gillenwater, 1996).

The objective diagnosis of obstruction of the upper urinary tract can, at times, be quite difficult. The IVP, with delayed films, usually shows the point of obstruction. This is an anatomic abnormality only, however, and not necessarily a functional obstruction. Indeed, the collecting system may appear to be narrowed at a particular point, yet the patient is asymptomatic. To differentiate between anatomic and functional obstruction, the two longest standing tests available are the diuretic washout renogram and the Whitaker renal pelvic and bladder differential pressure study.

With the diuresis renogram (furosemide [Lasix] washout), [131]I Hippuran (o-iodohippurate), [123]I Hippuran, or technetium-99m diethylenetriamine penta-acetic acid (DTPA) is given, and renal images are taken at 2, 5, 10, 15, 20, 25, and 30 minutes (Talner, 1990). If the curve appears to demonstrate obstruction, furosemide (0.5–1.0 mg/kg) is given intravenously at 30 minutes. After furosemide administration, in a normal nonobstructed situation, with two kid-

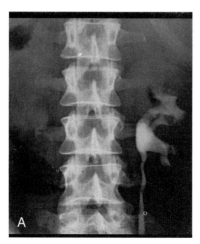
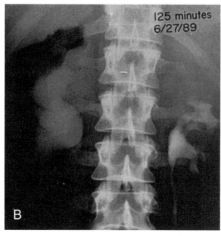
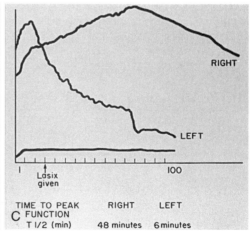

Figure 94–28. *A* and *B,* Intravenous urogram in a 37-year-old woman with intermittent right flank pain. A marked delay occurs in visualization of the right collecting system. *C,* Furosemide (Lasix) washout renogram demonstrating normal clearance from the left kidney but a prolonged clearance of radionuclide from the right kidney with a half-time clearance (T 1/2) of 48 minutes.

neys, 50% of the radionuclide tracer should drain from each kidney within 10 minutes (T 1/2). If it takes longer than 20 minutes, obstruction is likely (Fig. 94–28). Drainage times between 10 and 20 minutes are considered equivocal for obstruction (Talner, 1990). Problems in interpretation of the diuretic washout renogram usually result in a false-positive conclusion; medical renal disease, renal artery disease, decreased renal function owing to chronic obstruction, or massive hydronephrosis may blunt the response to furosemide or adversely affect the dilution of the excreted radionuclide (O'Reilly et al, 1979; Maizels et al, 1986; Talner, 1990).

In cases in which the diuretic washout renogram is equivocal, a renal perfusion pressure flow study (i.e., Whitaker test) can be performed (Fig. 94–29) (Whitaker, 1976; Whitaker, 1979; Newhouse et al, 1981). This invasive study involves placement of a needle (20- or 22-gauge) or a small

nephrostomy tube (No. 8 Fr) into the renal collecting system. A urethral catheter is also placed to drain the bladder. The collecting system is perfused via the percutaneously placed needle or catheter at a rate of 10 ml/minute with dilute contrast material. After the collecting system is fully distended, separate pressure readings of the renal pelvis and the bladder are recorded every 5 minutes until a steady pressure is reached in both areas. If the difference in the pressure between the renal pelvis and bladder is less than 13 to 15 cm H$_2$O, the system is unobstructed. In contrast, a renal pelvis/bladder pressure differential greater than 22 cm H$_2$O indicates obstruction. A pressure difference of 15 to 22 cm H$_2$O is considered equivocal. To test the patency of the system further, the inflow can be increased to 15 ml/minute; in this case, the normal differential pressure should be 18 cm H$_2$O or less (Newhouse et al, 1981).

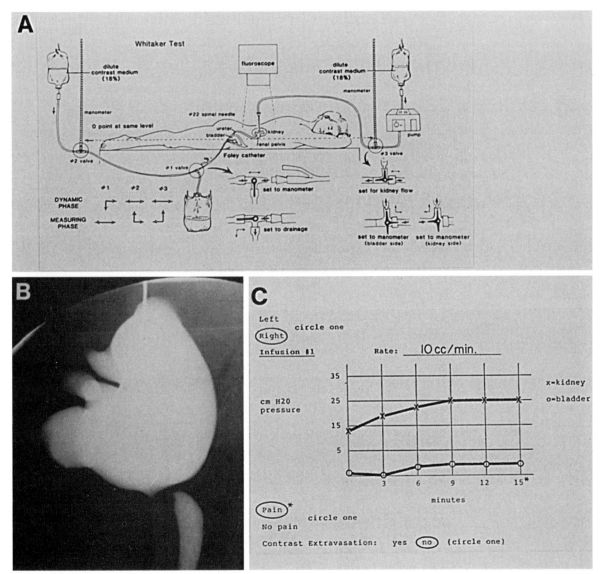

Figure 94–29. *A,* The setup for a Whitaker test. Through the needle in the renal pelvis, fluid is perfused at a constant rate. Once the collecting system is fully distended, the pressure is measured simultaneously in the bladder and renal pelvis. *B,* In this Whitaker test, the collecting system is fully distended. The ureteropelvic junction is markedly narrowed. At 10 ml/minute, the pressure differential is 22 cm H$_2$O, indicating significant obstruction. *C,* Graph of the Whitaker test showing that after a steady state was reached at 9 minutes, the pressure differential remained elevated (22 cm). (*A* From Clayman RV, Castaneda-Zuniga WR: *Techniques in Endourology: A Guide to Percutaneous Removal of Renal and Ureteral Calculi.* Chicago, Year Book Medical Publishers, 1986.)

Problems with the Whitaker test usually result in a false-negative study. Two sources of false-negative test results are extravasation during the test and failure to fill the renal pelvis system completely before obtaining pressure readings. Also, if the obstruction is positional in nature, it may not be evident during the Whitaker test because the patient is studied in the prone position (O'Reilly, 1986).

Overall the diuretic washout renal scan and the Whitaker test are complementary. Although a normal diuretic washout renal scan is a reliable indicator of a nonobstructed system, an abnormal result must be viewed with caution. In this case, a Whitaker test is indicated because it helps differentiate between the true-positive and false-positive renal scan (O'Reilly, 1986). In 9% to 30% of patients, a positive diuretic washout renal scan is discredited by a concomitantly normal perfusion pressure flow study. Conversely, the Whitaker test may be clinically unreliable in 15% of patients, primarily owing to a false-negative result (Krueger et al, 1980).

A third test has been brought to bear on the problem of diagnosis of chronic upper tract obstruction: duplex Doppler renal ultrasonography (Vaughan, 1995). By measuring the peak systolic and end diastolic velocity in the interlobar and arcuate arteries, a *resistive index* can be determined (peak systolic velocity − end diastolic velocity ÷ the peak systolic velocity). In the unobstructed kidney, the resistive index should be less than 0.70, and the difference in resistive indices between the two kidneys should be less than 0.05; resistive indices greater than 0.75 and differential indices greater than 0.10 are indicative of obstruction (Rodgers et al, 1992; Ordorica et al, 1993). Gilbert and colleagues noted that the results with duplex Doppler renal ultrasonography and diuresis renography were similar in a group of patients studied with both modalities (Gilbert et al, 1993). However, false-positive problems are prevalent with this study, as medical renal disease also elevates the resistive indices.

Ureteropelvic Junction Obstruction: Endopyelotomy

The surgical correction of UPJ obstruction spans a century of operations both creative and effective. In 1886, Trendelenburg performed the first reconstructive procedure for UPJ obstruction; however, the patient died in the early postoperative period (Murphy, 1972). The first successful pyeloplasty was reported by Kuster in 1891. He repaired the pelvis using a dismembered procedure (Murphy, 1972). Subsequently, myriad operations were devised to repair the obstruction: renal pelvic plication, Foley Y-V advancement, the Anderson-Hynes dismembered pyeloplasty, the Culp flap, and the Scardino flap. With almost all of the aforementioned approaches, success rates in the 80% to 90% range were reported, albeit rarely with attendant long-term functional follow-up studies (Scardino and Scardino, 1984; Schaefffer and Grayhack, 1986).

Endopyelotomy, albeit seemingly "new," is a contemporary of pyeloplasty. The basis for the technique was developed well before the classic operations of Foley, Anderson, Hynes, and others. In 1909, Albarran in France described a procedure he entitled *ureterotome externe*, in which a scarred or narrowed ureter was incised through its entire thickness, after which a catheter was placed in the ureter, and a large

drain was placed in the retroperitoneum (Murphy, 1972). The incised ureter was left to heal in situ, or sutures could be used to close the periureteric tissues over the stent.

Keyes brought this technique to the United States in 1915 (Murphy, 1972). It was not until the 1940s, however, that Davis (1943) popularized this approach and renamed it the *intubated ureterotomy*. In his technique, after opening the ureter, a stent was placed, and a few "loose" sutures were employed to guide the growth of the incised ureter around the indwelling tube. The cut ureteral edges were not coapted. The stent was removed in 4 to 5 weeks. Success with this approach was achieved in 89% and 60% of 47 patients based on subjective and objective follow-up, respectively, with a mean follow-up of 1 to 2 years (Davis, 1943; Davis et al, 1948).

It appears that although contracture plays a role in the healing process, urothelium and hyperplastic ureteral smooth muscle regeneration are the major ongoing processes. This appears to occur, in animal studies, with or without a ureteral stent. Without a stent, a retroperitoneal drain is placed. Drainage usually ceases within 5 days, indicating a watertight urothelial covering (Hamm and Weinberg, 1955; Webb et al, 1957). Peristalsis returns to the incised area in approximately 6 weeks (Oppenheimer and Hinman, 1955; Hamm and Weinberg, 1955, 1956; Webb et al, 1957; Mahoney et al, 1962). The establishment of a complete muscle layer requires 6 to 12 weeks (Oppenheimer and Hinman, 1955). Despite the initial enthusiastic interest in this method, use of the intubated ureterotomy began to wane when more effective methods of surgical pyeloplasty were perfected.

In 1983, Wickham and Miller, at the Institute of Urology in London, brought Albarran's procedure into the modern era (Wickham, 1983). The nephrostomy tract and a cold knife urethrotome were used to incise an obstructed UPJ percutaneously from the inside outward, thereby accomplishing the same effect as the classic intubated ureterotomy, only via a 1-cm flank incision. Wickham named the procedure *pyelolysis*. An indwelling stent was left in place for 4 weeks. Success with this approach was achieved in 65% (Ramsey et al, 1984). Interestingly, at about this same time (1982), Kadir and associates reported successful balloon dilation of a secondary UPJ.

Subsequently, Smith popularized the endourologic incisional approach in the United States. He renamed the procedure an *endopyelotomy* (Greek endo—within; Greek tome—to cut) because the renal pelvis and ureteral junction were being incised under endoscopic control (Badlani et al, 1986; Karlin et al, 1988; Motola et al, 1993a). Smith's success rate of 87% is remarkably similar to that of Davis.

TECHNIQUE

For an **antegrade endoscopic** endopyelotomy, the initial step is the retrograde passage of a 0.035-inch floppy-tipped or Terumo guide wire. Next a percutaneous nephrostomy is performed into an upper or middle **posterior** calyx to provide a straight-line, direct access to the UPJ. With the cold knife endopyelotomy technique, the nephrostomy tract is dilated and a No. 30 Fr Amplatz sheath is placed. A second (i.e., working) guide wire is now advanced, albeit antegrade, through the UPJ. The knife of the direct vision urethrotome or a pyelotome (hooked blade) may be used to cut in be-

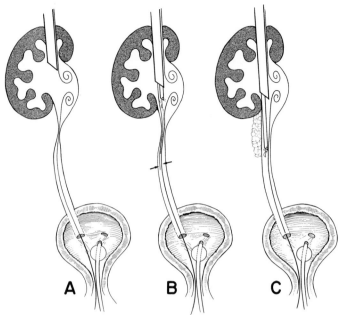

Figure 94–30. *A,* For an endopyelotomy, the nephrostomy tract is placed through an upper-pole or middle posterior calyx. A retrograde guide wire has been passed across the stenotic primary ureteropelvic junction (UPJ). *B,* A second guide wire has been passed, albeit antegrade, across the stenotic UPJ, thereby providing a clear guide for incising the UPJ (*arrows* point to the two guide wires). Endoscope with cold knife is in place. *Hatch marks* outline the planned site of incision, which would be lateral. *C,* A straight cold knife has been used to incise the UPJ until normal ureter can be seen distally. The incision is made through the full thickness of the ureter until retroperitoneal fat is clearly visible.

tween the ''rails'' of the guide wires (Fig. 94–30) (Karlin and Smith, 1988; Van Cangh et al, 1989).

If electrosurgery is selected to make the endopyelotomy, a smaller nephrostomy tract can be created, and a No. 18 Fr biliary dilator sheath can be placed. The electrosurgery probe can be used through a No. 12 Fr short, rigid ureteroscope with an insulated sheath. In this case, a second guide wire may be passed antegrade into the ureter, and a lateral incision in the UPJ can be made by cutting in between the guide wires; the beak of the scope serves nicely to separate the wires while the incision is being made. A No. 2 or 3 Fr Greenwald-type electrode or the cutting element that comes with one of the operating ureteroscopes can be used (50–75 watts pure cut). If electrosurgical current is to be used, both guide wires must be constructed with a nonconducting material (i.e., plastic or Terumo guide wires rather than Teflon-coated metal guide wires) or covered with a No. 5 Fr angiographic catheter.

There are two variations on performing an endopyelotomy by using a 6-mm, 4-cm-long ureteral dilating balloon to facilitate the procedure. In one method, the 6-mm ureteral dilating balloon is passed over the initial retrograde guide wire until the balloon straddles the UPJ area. The balloon is inflated (with a mixture of contrast material and a few drops of indigo carmine) to less than 1 atm. Using one of the aforementioned electrosurgical units, an incision in the UPJ is made laterally alongside the ''blue'' balloon. The inflated balloon facilitates incising the UPJ area because it places the UPJ tissue under tension and to some extent immobilizes the UPJ area, thereby providing for a more controlled incision (Fig. 94–31). The other method, called the **invagination** technique, is best used in patients with a dependent UPJ obstruction. In this procedure, the 6-mm dilating balloon is again passed retrograde; however, it is now gently inflated just beneath the UPJ obstruction. By pushing the inflated catheter cephalad, the balloon invaginates the strictured UPJ area into the renal pelvis. Now, when the tissue overlying the balloon is incised laterally, two layers of tissue are cut

because the UPJ has been folded over on the tissue of the renal pelvis. This method may well displace the UPJ up and away from any crossing vessels, thereby hypothetically decreasing any chance of hemorrhage (Gelet et al, 1991).

In all cases, the incision in the UPJ is made through the full thickness of the ureter, until retroperitoneal fat is clearly seen (Karlin and Smith, 1988). Based on the anatomic stud-

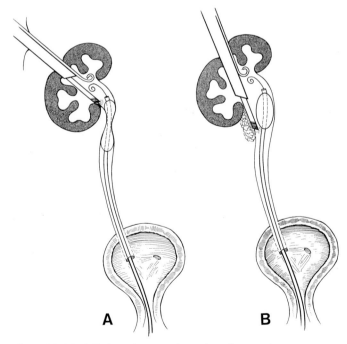

Figure 94–31. *A,* Endopyelotomy using a short therapeutic ureteroscope and a No. 3 Fr electrosurgical probe. Note how the balloon, inflated to ≤1 atm, clearly outlines the area of obstruction. *B,* The incision is made laterally and carried down along the balloon to 1 cm distal to the ureteropelvic junction obstruction. The depth of the incision is through the full thickness of the ureter, such that retroperitoneal fat is clearly seen.

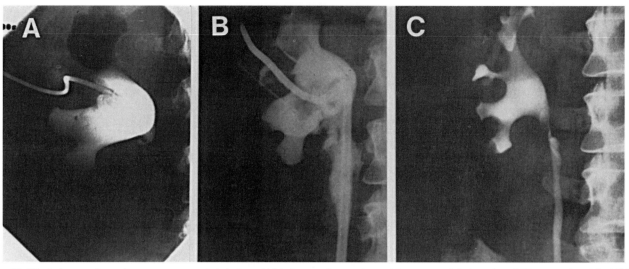

Figure 94–32. *A,* Antegrade nephrostogram recorded during a Whitaker test in a patient with ureteropelvic junction (UPJ) narrowing. The Whitaker test was positive. Note the hooking of the UPJ and lack of filling of the ureter. *B,* At the completion of an antegrade endopyelotomy using an electrosurgical probe, there is marked extravasation of contrast material from the area of the incision. A nephrostomy tube and a No. 14 Fr/7 Fr indwelling stent are in place. *C,* An intravenous urogram 6 months later shows that the UPJ area, albeit irregular, is patent. No remaining hydronephrosis is noted. The patient is asymptomatic.

ies of Sampaio and the spiral CT scan findings reported by Quillin and colleagues, the safest place to make the incision in a patient with a **primary** UPJ obstruction is along the lateral border of the UPJ (Quillin et al, 1995). In patients with a **secondary** UPJ obstruction, the incision site is determined after reviewing the operative note and the spiral CT scan or endoluminal ultrasound study to see where any vessels may be lying in proximity to the UPJ and to judge the proximity of the lateral border of the UPJ to the medial surface of the kidney; based on this assessment, a lateral, posteromedial, posterolateral, or straight posterior incision is made. The incision is carried caudad for approximately 1 cm beyond the point of UPJ obstruction. To confirm the adequacy of the incision, dilute contrast material is instilled by way of the endoscope—there should be rapid extravasation of contrast material through the incised UPJ (Fig. 94–32). To confirm the adequacy of the incision further, an 8-mm ureteral dilating balloon can be passed over one of the

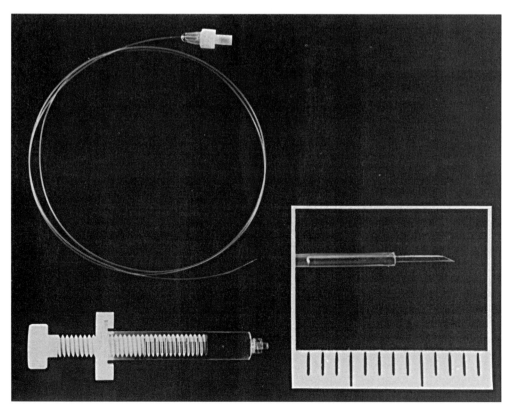

Figure 94–33. A No. 3 Fr Greenwald injection needle (*inset,* closeup of the <1 mm needle) used for triamcinolone injection. A LeVeen pressure syringe is helpful to inject the medication forcefully into the scarred area.

guide wires until the balloon straddles the UPJ area. If the UPJ has been properly incised, the 8-mm balloon should inflate to full size at low pressure (<1 atm).

Two other methods of performing an antegrade percutaneous endopyelotomy have been described independently by Ono and Schneider. Ono and co-workers have developed a **transpelvic** approach to endopyelotomy. In their technique, the renal pelvis is incised laterally, and the urethrotome is deliberately passed outside of the renal pelvis and into the retroperitoneum. The incision in the UPJ is now made from the outside inward (Ono et al, 1992). Another and seemingly simple method for making the incision in the UPJ has been described by Schneider and colleagues. Instead of using a cutting modality controlled by the free hand of the surgeon and passed through the endoscope, Schneider and colleagues have reported on a wire-guided knife that can be passed antegrade over the antegrade ureteral guide wire, thereby incising the narrowed UPJ as it is pushed along the guide wire (Schneider et al, 1991; Gutierrez et al, 1994).

When the UPJ obstruction is of a secondary rather than a primary nature, dense scar tissue may be encountered. A deeper incision than normal may be necessary to access retroperitoneal fat. If, despite a generous incision, no fat is seen, it may be worthwhile to inject 3 to 5 ml of triamcinolone (40 mg/ml) into the scar tissue bordering the incision in the UPJ area (Fig. 94–33) (Clayman RV, unpublished data, 1996). A No. 3 Fr Greenwald needle or standard cystoscopic needle can be chosen for this purpose; a pressure syringe (e.g., LeVeen syringe) is used to inject the triamcinolone forcefully into the scar tissue. The triamcinolone is slowly absorbed over 3 months; its peak effect is at 3 weeks (Damico et al, 1973; Farah et al, 1979). In theory, the triamcinolone serves as a catalyst for endogenous collagenase, thereby limiting collagen formation. Although triamcinolone administration has received favorable comments in association with treating contractures at the bladder neck, there are scant data on its effectiveness in dealing with ureteral strictures (Farah et al, 1979). It is as yet undetermined, however, whether the injection of triamcinolone is truly beneficial in reducing recurrent scarring of the UPJ area.

After the procedure, the incised UPJ may be stented in one of two manners: nephrostent or indwelling ureteral stent (Fig. 94–34). The nephrostent is a No. 14 Fr catheter that tapers to a No. 8.2 Fr pigtail tip. The No. 14 Fr proximal portion of the nephrostent traverses the nephrostomy tract and the incised UPJ area; the No. 8.2 Fr distal portion traverses the middle and distal ureter and enters the bladder (Badlani and Smith, 1988). Alternatively an indwelling ureteral stent may be placed along with a separate nephrostomy tube. The nephrostomy tube may vary from No. 12 to 24 Fr depending on the degree of nephrostomy tract dilation. The indwelling stent may vary among No. 7, 8, 10, or 7/14 Fr graduated stent (Van Cangh et al, 1989). The last stent has a No. 7 Fr pigtail on either end; however, half of the stent's shaft is No. 14 Fr, and the rest of the shaft is No. 7 Fr. After an endopyelotomy, the stent is placed such that the No. 14 Fr portion traverses the incised UPJ (Meretyk et al, 1992).

On the second postoperative day, a nephrostogram is obtained. If this study shows no evidence of extravasation, the nephrostent can be capped, or if an indwelling stent was placed, the nephrostomy tube can be removed. The latter

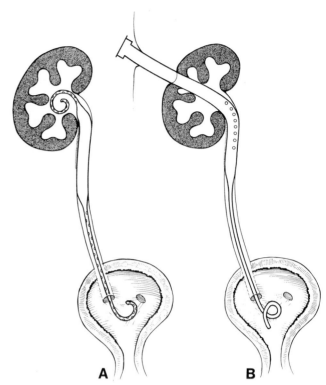

Figure 94–34. *A,* Indwelling variable-sized endopyelotomy stent. The pigtail and distal shaft of the stent are No. 7 Fr, but the part of the stent that traverses the ureteropelvic junction (UPJ) area is No. 14 Fr. The stent is removed via the bladder at the end of 6 weeks. The *hatch marks* indicate the site of the lateral incision made in the UPJ. *B,* Smith nephrostent for use after endopyelotomy. The UPJ area is stinted by the No. 14 Fr portion of the stent, whereas the No. 8.2 Fr portion of the stent traverses the normal ureter. The No. 14 Fr nephrostomy portion of the stent is left capped for the ensuing 6 weeks. *Hatch marks* indicate the site of the endopyelotomy.

should be done under fluoroscopic monitoring to avoid dislodgment of the indwelling ureteral stent. The nephrostent or indwelling ureteral stent is removed 4 to 6 weeks later. Follow-up studies usually consist of a furosemide washout renogram or an intravenous urogram 1 to 2 weeks after the stent has been removed.

In **complete** obstruction of the UPJ, the area of stenosis can still be overcome with endourologic techniques (Hulbert, 1990). A combined antegrade percutaneous nephroscopic and retrograde ureteroscopic approach is necessary. To make a new opening, the first step is to pass a flexible nephroscope or a short rigid No. 12 Fr ureteroscope by way of the nephrostomy tract and a flexible ureteroscope by way of the ureter. The light from the antegrade endoscope is disconnected, and the light from the retrograde ureteroscope is sought (i.e., a "cut-to-the-light" procedure). When the glow through the obstructing tissue is light pink to white and the C-arm fluoroscope shows the tips of the two endoscopes to be aligned in two planes, a direct incision (rigid endoscope, cold knife or flexible endoscope, electrosurgical probe) of the ureter can be made via the nephroscope at the brightest point of light. The light on the nephroscope is then reconnected to look for a guide wire passed through the retrograde ureteroscope. This procedure can also be done in reverse, with the light disconnected from the ureteroscope and the light from the nephroscope sought. In this case, the incision is made via the ureteroscope. It appears to be simpler, however, to make an incision with the larger, rigid endoscope passed antegrade through the nephrostomy tract whenever possible.

After contact is established, a 260-cm, 0.035-inch exchange guide wire is passed by way of the ureteroscope and retrieved by the nephroscope, thereby providing a through-and-through guide wire. A No. 5 Fr angiographic catheter is passed over the guide wire in preparation for extending the electrosurgical incision. The incision is deepened alongside the No. 5 Fr catheter until retroperitoneal fat is seen. An 8-mm balloon catheter is passed and inflated (<1 atm) to gauge the adequacy of the incision.

Alternatively, a No. 5 or 8 Fr straight-tip angiographic catheter is passed retrograde. A stiff guide wire (Lunderquist) or stylet (rocket wire with a sharp tip from the Lawson retrograde nephrostomy kit) can be passed through the retrograde catheter and its indentation on the ureteral tissue noted with the antegrade nephroscope. The wire can then be forced across the occluded ureter, grasped with the antegrade nephroscope, and pulled out through the nephrostomy tract, thereby establishing a through-and-through guide wire. At this point, the stricture can be balloon dilated or incised, as previously described. A nephrostent or a nephrostomy tube plus an indwelling standard No. 7 or 8 Fr pigtail stent or a No. 7/14 Fr stent is placed. In the latter case, 2 days after the procedure, a nephrostogram is obtained. If there is no extravasation, the nephrostomy tube can be removed under fluoroscopic monitoring. If there is extravasation, the nephrostomy tube is left in place for 1 week, and the nephrostogram is repeated on an outpatient basis. Because the obstruction was complete, the indwelling ureteral stent is left in place for 6 to 12 weeks (Bagley, 1990b). In some patients, a permanent indwelling ureteral stent is placed to preclude recurrent occlusion; the stent is changed every 3 to 6 months.

Some controversy has arisen as to the best type of cutting modality for incising the UPJ. Concern has been expressed with regard to possible tissue damage from employing electrosurgical current to make incisions in the UPJ area. Of interest is that data from Korth, Smith, and Van Cangh, in which only a cold knife was used to make the endopyelotomy, are similar to independent reports from Meretyk and Hulbert, in which monopolar electrosurgery was used (No. 2 and 3 Fr electrocautery probes) (Hulbert et al, 1988b; Karlin et al, 1988; Van Cangh et al, 1989; Kuenkel and Korth, 1990; Meretyk I et al, 1992c; Motola et al, 1993a). Current clinical data regarding a bipolar electrocautery system, Nd:YAG laser, KTP laser, or Ho:YAG laser to make an incision in the UPJ are lacking. Laboratory data in pigs reveal that larger electrosurgical probes (i.e., >400-μ tip) cause considerably more peri-incisional injury than a cold knife, Nd:YAG laser, or KTP laser. The monopolar No. 2 Fr electrosurgical probe with a 250-μ cutting surface, however, produces an incision similar to a cold knife or laser incision with regard to peri-incisional tissue damage (Dierks et al, 1990).

Lastly, for all patients undergoing an endopyelotomy, maintenance of a sterile urine throughout the postoperative period is important. As such, an oral antibiotic is continued for a few days after the procedure, and a urine culture is obtained 3 weeks and 6 weeks after the procedure. The urine must be sterile before removal of the ureteral stent. After stent removal, an oral antibiotic is usually given for several days.

RESULTS

The results of endourologic therapy for UPJ obstruction have been excellent. By far the largest endourologic experience (more than 700 cases reported) has been with **antegrade endoscopic** endopyelotomy (Table 94–11). Many different investigators have reported success rates in the 61% to 88% range (Van Cangh et al, 1989; Kuenkel and Korth, 1990; Cassis et al, 1991; Meretyk I et al, 1992; Motola et al, 1993a; Kletscher et al, 1995). There does not appear to be a significant difference in success rates for primary versus secondary UPJ obstruction (Meretyk I et al, 1992; Gerber and Lyon, 1994).

The average operative time in Smith's large series was 90 minutes with a hospital stay of 6.2 days. In other series, the hospital stay has been only 3 to 4 days; however, average operating room times in these other series have been as long as 200 minutes (Cassis et al, 1991; Meretyk I et al, 1992; Motola et al, 1993a; Kletscher et al, 1995). Complications have been few; the transfusion rate varies from 1% to 4%, and reports of arteriovenous fistula or pseudoaneurysm formation are rare (Badlani et al, 1988; Malden et al, 1992; Motola et al, 1993a; Kletscher et al, 1995). The need for open operation because of a complication from the procedure (e.g., avulsion, bleeding) has been less than 1% (Sutherland et al, 1992; Motola et al, 1993a). Finally, when endopyelotomy fails, subsequent salvage by open pyeloplasty is uniformly successful, albeit slightly more difficult than operating on a primary UPJ obstruction; Motola and co-workers noted no difference between pyeloplasty for secondary UPJ after failed endopyelotomy in 15 patients and open pyeloplasty for primary UPJ obstruction with regard to operative time, blood loss, hospitalization, or outcome (Motola et al, 1993b). Likewise, Kavoussi and co-workers noted that all six failed endopyelotomies in their series could successfully be salvaged with an open pyeloplasty (Kavoussi et al, 1993).

The success rate for **antegrade endoscopic** endopyelotomy appears to be durable. The average duration of follow-up in the reported series is from 1 to 5 years (see Table 94–11). The majority of failures occur within 3 months of the procedure (Brannen et al, 1988; Kuenkel and Korth, 1990; Cassis et al, 1991; Meretyk I et al, 1992; Motola et al, 1993a); however, both Cuzin and Van Cangh and their colleagues have independently noted late failures, some as long as 5 years later (Cuzin et al, 1992; Van Cangh et al, 1994b). As such, there exists a significant disparity between Smith's data of a 1% failure rate at 1 to 8 years and Van Cangh's data showing a 13% late failure rate at 1 to 10 years.

Experience with a retrograde approach to endopyelotomy has trailed the antegrade approach. Also, given the three approaches to retrograde therapy of UPJ obstruction—balloon dilation, endoscopic incision, and cutting balloon—it is not surprising that series on each of these approaches have been few, and follow-up in general has been brief (Table 94–12). Early results with each type of approach, however, have been quite favorable.

Success with **balloon dilation** up to No. 30 Fr for treating primary and secondary UPJ obstruction is in the 64% to

Table 94–11. ANTEGRADE ENDOPYELOTOMY: URETEROPELVIC JUNCTION OBSTRUCTION

Authors	Number of Patients	Method of Incision	Stent Size (Fr)	Stent Duration (Weeks)	Success Rate			Hospital Stay (Days)	Secondary Pyeloplasty (%)	Secondary Nephrectomy (%)	Average Follow-up (Months)
					Overall (%)	Primary UPJ (%)	Secondary UPJ (%)				
Cassis et al, 1991	27	Cold knife (pyelotome)	8–10	6–8	78	80	—	4.1	4	0	6–48
Kuenkel and Korth, 1990	175	Cold knife (urethrotome)	10–14	3–6	78	83	75	—	—	0	12
Meretyk I et al, 1992	23	Electrocautery	14	6	78	—	—	4	9	0	22 (2–39)
Ramsay, Miller et al, 1984	28	Cold knife (urethrotome)	8–10	4–10	65	61	80	—	32	—	18 (9–48)
Schneider et al, 1991	26	Cold knife (urethrotome)	14	3–6	81	—	—	—	19	0	15 (7–45)
Motola et al, 1993a	189	Cold knife (pyelotome)	12–14	6	86	85	86	6.2	12	0	6 months–8 years
Cuzin et al, 1993	25	Electrocautery	—	8	84	—	—	—	16	0	20 (7–27)
Gutierrez et al, 1994	41	Cold knife (over the guide wire)	—	—	88	84	94	2–8	7	0	—
Streitz et al, 1992	52	Electrocautery (hooked)	—	—	61	—	—	—	15 (including ureterocalicostomy)	15	6 months–7 years
Van Cangh et al, 1994b	102	Cold knife (urethrotome)	10–12	6	73	—	—	6.7	12	0	5 years (1–10)
Kletscher et al, 1995	50	Cold knife	7–14; 8–8.5	6	88	90	82	3.8	10 (including ureterocalicostomy)	0	12
Overall	738		7–14	6	79	—	—	5.4	12	0–15	>6

UPJ, Ureteropelvic junction.

Table 94–12. RETROGRADE ENDOPYELOTOMY: URETEROPELVIC JUNCTION OBSTRUCTION

Authors	Number of Patients	Method of Treatment	Stent Size (Fr)	Stent Duration (Weeks)	Success Rate Overall (%)	Primary UPJ (%)	Secondary UPJ (%)	Hospital Stay (Days)	Secondary Pyeloplasty (%)	Secondary Nephrectomy (%)	Average Follow-up (Months)
Cutting Balloon Catheter											
Gelet et al, 1994	22	Cutting balloon catheter (electrocautery)	7–12	5.2	81	—	—	—	5	9	5.4 (3–12)
Nadler et al, 1995b	28	Cutting balloon catheter (electrocautery)	7/14	4–6	81	78	100	1.6	0	0	33 (24–43)
Preminger et al, 1996	58	Cutting balloon catheter (electrocautery)	6–14	5	76	74	82	—	0	0	8 (1–18)
Overall	108		6–14	5	79	—	—	1–2	0–5	0–9	>6
Ureteroscopic Incision											
Gallucci et al, 1991	11	Cold knife (three-ring blade)	—	—	82	—	—	—	0	0	12 (4–18)
Chowdhury and Kenogbon, 1992	12	Cold knife ureterotome	6–7	6	83	—	—	3	0	0	
Meretyk I et al, 1992	20	Electrocautery	7/14	6	80	—	—	3.4	5	5	17 (4–36)
Thomas et al, 1995	51	Electrocautery	14	6.5	85	—	—	1.2	0	5	17 (6–51)
Overall	94		6–14	6	83	—	—	2	0–5	0–5	>6
Balloon Dilation											
Beckman, 1989	11	Balloon dilation	8–10	4–8	73	86	50	—	—	—	10 (2–22)
Lanigan et al, 1992	10	Balloon dilation No. 36 Fr	6	—	70	—	—	—	20	0	7 (1–16)
McClinton et al, 1993	43	Balloon dilation No. 30 Fr	8–10	6	80	85	56	1	2	12	18 (5–49)
Snow et al, 1994	26	Balloon dilation No. 36 Fr	7	6	64	—	—	—	15	0	21 (3–44)
Deane et al, 1992	30	Balloon dilation	—	—	73	—	—	—	17	0	20 (4–26)
Overall	120		6–10	6	73	—	—	0–1	2–20	0–12	>6

UPJ, Ureteropelvic junction.

80% range (Beckman et al, 1987, 1989; Deane et al, 1992; McClinton et al, 1993; Snow et al, 1994). Although initially performed in an antegrade manner in earlier series (Beckman et al, 1987; O'Flynn et al, 1989), in later series, the retrograde approach has been used uniformly (Deane et al, 1992; McClinton et al, 1993; Snow et al, 1994). The largest series with the longest follow-up is by McClinton and colleagues; however, there was a marked difference between the success rate for primary (85%) versus the success rate for secondary (56%) UPJ obstruction at a mean follow-up of 18 months. Of note is Snow's observation that during inflation the presence of a well-demarcated area of narrowing in the balloon just before full inflation of the balloon is a favorable prognostic sign; among patients with this so-called waisting sign, a successful outcome was noted in 75% versus only a 43% success rate among patients without waisting during balloon dilation (Snow et al, 1994). With balloon dilation, operative time (estimated at 20–30 minutes) and morbidity (0% transfusion or embolization) are the least of any method (O'Flynn et al, 1989). Complications have all been minor, occurring in 14%, and largely due to stent migration, lower urinary tract infection, or stent-related hematuria. Hospital stay is ≤1 day (see Table 94–12) (Kadir et al, 1982; O'Flynn et al, 1989; Snow et al, 1994). As yet, there have been no comparative studies of balloon dilation versus an endopyelotomy.

Although the success with a **retrograde endoscopic** approach is similar to that with the antegrade approach, initial technical difficulties and delayed complications were discouraging (Inglis and Tolley, 1986). In the first reported series on retrograde endoscopic endopyelotomy, the average procedural time was 188 minutes, and the hospital stay was 3.4 days. Immediate complications consisting of bleeding requiring blood transfusion occurred in 16% of patients (Meretyk I et al, 1992). Most worrisome was the late postoperative development of distal ureteral strictures in 20% of patients (Meretyk I et al, 1992).

With the advent of smaller ureteroscopes and with the use of presstenting to allow the ureter to dilate slowly before the procedure, however, far more sanguine results have been reported. Thomas (1993a, 1995), using a regimen of presstenting for 1 week before endopyelotomy, reported an 85% success rate among 51 patients with a follow-up beyond 6 months. Of note, the average hospital stay was 1.2 days; 55% of the cases were completed on an outpatient basis. Similarly, Chowdhury and Kenogbon (1992) and Gallucci and colleagues (1991) have independently reported success rates of 82% to 83% with a retrograde endoscopic approach; of note, in neither series was a period of presstenting employed. As yet, there have been no studies in which a retrograde endoscopic approach using either a presstenting period or the newer smaller ureteroscopes has been directly compared with an antegrade approach.

Similar to the other types of retrograde treatment for UPJ obstruction, experience with the **retrograde fluoroscopic** approach for performing endopyelotomy is relatively small. Following the initial report of this method in 1993, a multicenter trial with this device was initiated (Chandhoke et al, 1993; Preminger et al, 1996). Among 58 patients with UPJ obstruction, the success rate was 76% overall (74% for primary UPJ obstruction and 82% for secondary UPJ obstruction) at a mean follow-up of only 8 months (Chandhoke et al, 1993; Preminger et al, 1996). Subsequently, Gelet

and associates have reported an 81% success rate with the cutting balloon in 21 patients with UPJ obstruction (Gelet et al, 1994). Most patients were prestented before the procedure. Average hospital stay ranges from outpatient to 2 days (Brooks et al, 1995). Operative time is routinely under 1 hour (Brooks et al, 1995; Preminger et al, 1996). Serious complications requiring transfusion or embolization have occurred rarely: 3.4% in Preminger's multi-institutional review. Likewise an isolated case report of embolization and wire fracture has been published (Floth and Anzbock, 1995; Streem and Geisinger, 1995). The most common problem has been stent-related complications, which occurred in 8.6% of patients in the multicenter study; actual stent replacement was needed in only two cases (Preminger et al, 1996). No patient required an open operation owing to a complication of the procedure. Of note is the report by Nadler and colleagues in which 29 patients undergoing Acucise endopyelotomy were restudied at a **minimum of 2 years after the procedure** (mean follow-up of 32 months) (Nadler et al, 1995b). In this study, subjective data were obtained by using analog scale questionnaires, and objective data were obtained solely through furosemide washout renal scans. Subjectively, 40% of patients were cured, and 48% were markedly improved. The latter designation was applied to patients who reported a 50% to 90% reduction in preoperative discomfort. Objectively a normal renal scan was noted in 81% of the patients. Of interest, 78% of patients with primary UPJ obstruction had a normal renal scan; all three patients in the study with a secondary UPJ obstruction had a normal renal scan.

With regard to the Acucise cutting balloon endopyelotomy, there has been one comparative, albeit nonrandomized retrospective study. In their limited study, Brooks and colleagues noted that the Acucise endopyelotomy provided results identical to an antegrade endopyelotomy with a 77% to 78% success rate (Brooks et al, 1995). However, the hospital stay (0.2 days) and recovery time (1 week) were markedly shorter than for patients undergoing an antegrade endopyelotomy (3 days and 4.7 weeks). They concluded that among patients who were candidates for endopyelotomy, the Acucise endopyelotomy was the preferred method (Brooks et al, 1995).

ENDOPYELOTOMY: CONCERNS AND CONTROVERSIES

Patient selection for endopyelotomy has raised several areas of concern with regard to selecting which patients with UPJ obstruction would best benefit from an endourologic approach. These areas of concern include the etiology of the UPJ obstruction, the site of UPJ insertion, the presence of impaired renal function, and the degree of hydronephrosis.

Among these defining characteristics, the greatest amount of interest has centered around the cause of the UPJ obstruction, specifically intrinsic versus extrinsic obstruction. The **intrinsically** "diseased" UPJ area has been evaluated by Hanna and other investigators. In UPJ obstruction of childhood, the pathology of the obstructed UPJ is, at least in part, due to the presence of dysfunctional muscle cells, secondary to excessive intercellular deposits of collagen, incapable of properly propelling urine (Murnaghan, 1958; Hanna et al, 1976a, 1976b; Whitaker, 1976). An **extrinsic** cause for UPJ obstruction is noted in more than one third of pediatric and adult cases. Given the advent of intraureteral retrograde endoluminal ultrasound and spiral CT, an extrinsic cause is found in 40% of adult patients with UPJ obstruction (Bagley et al, 1994; Quillin et al, 1995). Usually, this is due to a branching lower-pole renal artery and/or vein crossing the UPJ **anteriorly**. In addition to the physical obstruction induced by the crossing vessel, the problem is compounded by the development of fibrous tissue between the area of the vessel crossing and the adjacent UPJ.

The impact of a crossing vessel on the subsequent outcome of an endopyelotomy has been only recently studied. In Van Cangh and colleagues' landmark study, a crossing vessel identified by arteriography was found in 39% of patients undergoing an antegrade endopyelotomy (Van Cangh et al, 1994b). Among this group, the presence of a crossing vessel was associated with a favorable outcome in only 42%, whereas in the group with no crossing vessel the success rate was 86%. Subsequently, Bagley and co-workers as well as the Washington University group have sought to use endoluminal ultrasound and spiral CT scanning to identify crossing vessels preoperatively in patients with UPJ obstruction scheduled to undergo an endopyelotomy (Bagley et al, 1994; Quillin et al, 1995). A crossing vessel of greater than 2 mm diameter was identified in approximately 40% of patients; almost all of the vessels crossed anterior to the UPJ (Quillin et al, 1995). In Bagley and co-workers' series, only the simultaneous presence of an anterior and posterior crossing vessel, a rare event, resulted in uniformly poor results: 0% success among two patients. In their series, however, a solitary anterior or solitary posterior crossing vessel did not appear to affect the immediate outcome adversely (Bagley et al, 1994).

The Washington University group has subsequently looked at **two questions**. Firstly, among failed endopyelotomy patients coming to open pyeloplasty, what percentage have an associated crossing vessel? Among five failed patients, all five had an anterior crossing vessel; thus in their series, 100% of failed endopyelotomy patients had a crossing vessel. The second question was the converse of the initial question: Specifically, among patients with a durable successful endopyelotomy, what percentage had a crossing vessel? Long-term (i.e., >2 years) successful cutting balloon patients underwent spiral CT more than 2 years after their initial Acucise procedure. Among 16 patients in whom a successful Acucise procedure had been performed more than 2 years earlier, 38% had a crossing vessel: 84% an anterior, 16% a posterior, and none had both an anterior and a posterior crossing vessel. There was no correlation with vessel size or vessel type (i.e., artery versus vein) and subsequent outcome (Nakada et al, 1995). Further analysis of these data revealed that 64% of patients with a crossing vessel would have a favorable result from endopyelotomy. As such, these data corroborate Van Cangh's initial findings that among patients with a crossing vessel the incidence of a successful outcome is markedly reduced; however, there is no apparent way to preselect which patients with a crossing vessel will have a favorable outcome versus those patients with a crossing vessel in whom the procedure will fail. Hence, one must ask whether it is better on a routine basis to expend the time and money preoperatively to seek out the crossing vessel and inform the patient of the reduced chances of success, or to proceed with endopyelotomy in all adult patients knowing

that the overall success rate is in the 80% range. Although the former approach allows for more patient information, the expense necessary to obtain these data can be justified only if, based on this knowledge, the patient and physician will uniformly select a different treatment approach. Indeed, even with only a 42% to 64% success rate, many patients when faced with the choice of an outpatient, retrograde procedure with minimal convalescence versus an inpatient, open or laparoscopic procedure (although >90% successful) often choose the former.

Concern over the effectiveness of this procedure in a patient with a "high insertion" of the ureter into the renal pelvis has been addressed by Van Cangh and associates (1989). The procedure appears to be effective in these individuals. To date, however, no investigator has subdivided an endopyelotomy series into patients with a high versus a low insertion and then looked at the success rate using the site of UPJ insertion as the primary independent variable.

Another question with regard to patient selection is: Does poor renal function negatively affect the subsequent outcome of an endopyelotomy? To date, as with concerns over the high insertion, no formal studies have been completed in this area. It is the stated opinion of some investigators, however, that renal function less than 20% augurs poorly. Indeed, in the adult with this situation, a nephrectomy may be preferable to an endopyelotomy (Meretyk I et al, 1992).

Lastly, in selecting an adult patient for an endopyelotomy, the presence of chronic massive hydronephrosis appears to be an undesirable situation (Badlani et al, 1988; Glinz et al, 1994a; Van Cangh et al, 1994b). This problem accounted for 30% of the failures in the series reported by Badlani and associates (1988). Also, Glinz and colleagues noted that among patients with a successful antegrade endopyelotomy, the renal pelvis volume was on average less than 60 ml, whereas among patients with a failed endopyelotomy the renal pelvis volume was on average greater than 90 ml. Likewise, in van Cangh's series, patients with grade 3–4 hydronephrosis had a success rate of only 77%, versus a 95% successful endopyelotomy outcome in patients with grade 1–2 hydronephrosis.

Areas of controversy with regard to endopyelotomy are based on three questions: the application of endopyelotomy techniques to children, the size of the stent to leave, and the duration of postoperative ureteral stinting. With regard to the pediatric population, experience in this age group is scant. Towbin and colleagues reported on antegrade endopyelotomy in three patients with primary UPJ obstructions, two of whom had a subjectively successful result at 10 and 27 months (Towbin et al, 1987). Lingeman and co-workers reported excellent results (100% success) for an antegrade endopyelotomy in seven children with a primary UPJ obstruction followed for an average of 13 months (Lingeman et al, 1993). Neither Figenshau and colleagues nor Tan and colleagues could independently corroborate this outcome; in their combined experience of 21 patients with primary UPJ obstruction, the success rate was only 52% when the follow-up was extended to 1.3 to 3.2 years (Tan et al, 1993; Figenshau et al, 1995). The failure rate could not be equated to patient age because patients as young as 2 years and as old as 17 years were counted among the failures.

The situation is totally different, however, for pediatric patients with a secondary UPJ obstruction. In these patients, the results have been excellent. Among nine patients in Figenshau's report and two patients in Tan's report, the success rate in treating secondary UPJ obstruction with an endopyelotomy was 100%; the follow-up in Tan's series was 15 months, whereas in Figenshau's report, the patients had been followed for an average of 4.5 years. Accordingly, although endopyelotomy for secondary UPJ obstruction in the child appears to be effective and durable, its role in children with a primary UPJ obstruction remains unsettled.

The role of the stent continues to stimulate debate. At first, the stent was thought to serve as a mold for ureteral healing, and hence a large stent, in the No. 14 Fr range, was preferred (Davis, 1951). Other investigators, however, have stated their belief that the stent serves only as a scaffold along which the ureter heals; as such, a small stent would provide results similar to a large stent, albeit with greater ease of insertion and perhaps less patient discomfort (Oppenheimer and Hinman, 1955; McDonald and Calams, 1960). In an attempt to settle this controversy, Moon and associates studied ureteral healing in a porcine secondary ureteral stricture model; no difference in outcome occurred when either a No. 14 or a 7 Fr stent was used (Moon et al, 1994). Clinically, Chowdury, McClinton, and Kletscher and their colleagues all have independently noted favorable outcomes using No. 8 F to 10 Fr stents after endourologic therapy for UPJ obstruction (Chowdhury and Kenogbon, 1992; McClinton et al, 1993; Kletscher et al, 1995). As yet, a prospective, randomized study has not been done to answer this question of stent size.

Likewise, it is uncertain how long a stent should remain within the ureter to promote ureteral healing. On the one hand, the stent serves to help guide ureteral healing, yet on the other hand, all stents result in ureteral inflammation, which may impair ureteral healing. Although the literature of the 1940s and 1950s suggested stent dwell times of 6 to 12 weeks (canine studies), other studies from the same era suggested that no stent was needed (Davis, 1951; Oppenheimer and Hinman, 1955; Mahoney et al, 1962). Kerbl and associates completed several studies in the porcine secondary ureteral stricture model; in their report, stinting for 1 week provided results identical to or better than stinting for 6 weeks after an endoureterotomy (Kerbl et al, 1993). Gardner and colleagues completed a study on ureteral healing in the porcine secondary ureteral stricture model; they found that the ureters that were left unstinted healed better than those ureters in which an indwelling stent was left for 6 weeks (Gardner et al, 1995). Clinically, successful endopyelotomy has occurred in patients stinted for 4 days or for 3 weeks in two separate reports (Abdel-Hakim, 1987; Kuenkel and Korth, 1990).

Ureteral Strictures: Endoureterotomy

In dealing with ureteral strictures, it is helpful to divide the ureter into three unequal areas: the proximal ureter (≤ 3 cm below the UPJ), the distal ureter (≤ 5 cm above the ureteral orifice), and the middle ureter. By this classification, the majority of the ureter falls under the designation of middle ureter. Most strictures occur in the distal ureter owing to injury sustained during ureteroscopy, gynecologic surgery, or other types of pelvic surgery.

TECHNIQUE

Percutaneous procedures among patients with ureteral strictures usually take one of two forms: palliative (i.e., placement of a nephrostomy tube to relieve symptoms and preserve renal function) and therapeutic (i.e., use of the nephrostomy tract to approach the stricture in an antegrade fashion). The latter approach is usually used in conjunction with a retrograde approach. Three general endosurgical techniques exist for treating ureteral strictures: catheter dilation, balloon dilation, and endoincision (Glanz et al, 1983; Banner and Pollack, 1984; Lang, 1984; Gothlin et al, 1988; Smith, 1988; Beckman et al, 1989; Eshghi, 1989; Eshghi et al, 1989; Netto et al, 1990; Farah et al, 1991; Meretyk et al, 1992a; Benoit et al, 1993; Kim et al, 1993; Kwak et al, 1995; Preminger et al, 1996). In each situation, the first step is to pass a guide wire beyond the stricture until its tip is coiled in the renal pelvis. The simplest guide wire to pass under these circumstances is often a 0.035-inch Terumo. Its plastic hydrophilic coating greatly facilitates its passage through even a tight ureteral stricture. The surface of this guide wire must always be kept wet. Once this guide wire has been passed, a No. 5 Fr angiographic catheter can be passed over it. The Terumo guide wire is then exchanged for a stiffer guide wire, such as a 0.035-inch Bentson guide wire or the most rigid guide wire available, a 0.035-inch Amplatz superstiff guide wire.

Once a guide wire has been passed, a variety of retrograde approaches to treating the stricture may be used: catheter dilation, balloon dilation, or retrograde incision via a ureteroscopic or fluoroscopic approach (Witherington and Shelor, 1980; Banner and Pollack, 1984; Johnson et al, 1987; Beckman et al, 1989; Meretyk et al, 1992a; Kwak et al, 1995; Preminger et al, 1996). These approaches are similar to the retrograde techniques already described for treating UPJ obstruction. Likewise the percutaneous approach to the proximal ureteral stricture is identical to an antegrade endopyelotomy (Fig. 94–35). In this case, however, the incision, based on the peristricture anatomy, defined by spiral computed tomography or endoluminal ultrasound, is continued cephalad into the area of the UPJ and renal pelvis. As such, the proximal ureteral stricture is marsupialized into the renal pelvis (Fig. 94–36). The antegrade approach may also be used in combination with a flexible nephroscope to approach middle ureteral strictures. In these cases, the incision is usually done with a No. 2 Fr electrosurgical probe. Side-firing KTP laser probe, end-firing KTP probe, and Ho:YAG laser probes have become available for this same purpose, although experience with these newer modalities is scant. In the middle ureter, the incision is again made laterally except in the region of the iliac vessels, in which case the incision is made anteromedially (see Fig. 94–35). In rare circumstances, the antegrade approach is used for distal ureteral strictures, the incision being made medially just proximal to the ureterovesical junction and directly anteriorly in the area of the ureteral tunnel (see Fig. 94–35). Again in the distal ureter, access is usually easier with the ureteroscope (Cubelli and Smith, 1987). In these cases, the strictured ureter is incised caudad until it is marsupialized into the bladder.

For performing an endoincision, the same cutting modalities can be used that were discussed for performing an endopyelotomy: cold knife, electrosurgical probe, or laser

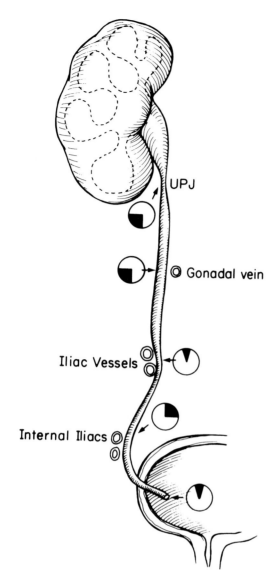

Figure 94–35. Endoureterotomy. The site of the incision *(black quadrant)* is dependent on the location of the stricture. In cases of secondary ureteral strictures, a preoperative spiral computed tomography scan can demonstrate the peristricture anatomy, allowing the urologist to make an incision in the "safest" plane. UPJ, ureteropelvic junction. (From Eshghi M: AUA Update Series Vol 8, Lesson 38, 1989.)

energy (Nd:YAG, KTP, or Ho:YAG). The majority of cases have been done with a cold knife; electrosurgical endoureterotomy has been reported by Meretyk and colleagues (1992a). To date, there are no series on laser incision of ureteral strictures (see Table 94–13). Korth and Kuenkel (1988) have developed a cold knife, flexible ureterotome for incising strictures in the middle portion of the ureter. Similarly, Selikowitz (1990) developed a diminutive No. 4.5 Fr coaxial cold knife. Netto and colleagues reported on a ureteroscopic back-cutting endoscopic scissors, in which the outer edges of the blades of the scissors were sharpened (Netto et al, 1990). On passing the scissors beyond the stricture, the blades were opened, and the open scissors were drawn through the stricture, thereby incising the stricture in two places. Electrosurgical probes (No. 2 or 3 Fr) have had either a straight-tip or right-angle configuration; the tip size should not be larger than 400 μ (Figenshau et al, 1991).

The depth of the incision should be through the full thickness of the stricture and ureteral wall. In the upper distal and the remaining middle and proximal ureter, retroperitoneal fat should be seen. If, after incising deeply enough to see fat along the peristricture area of the ureter, there is still no fat noted in the depth of the incised stricture, the surgeon may consider injecting triamcinolone as previously described in the endopyelotomy technique section. Cutting deeper may result in significant hemorrhage; in these cases, it is more than likely that the entire area of the stricture is encased in fibrotic tissue, and no normal retroperitoneal fat is present.

After the incision, a No. 14 Fr nephrostent or an indwelling ureteral stent (No. 7 or 8 Fr double pigtail or a No. 7/14 Fr variable size stent) and a small No. 10 Fr nephrostomy tube are placed. A urethral catheter drains the bladder for 24 to 36 hours. Two days later, a nephrostogram is performed. If the nephrostogram reveals an intact collecting system, the nephrostent can be capped; if an indwelling ureteral stent is present, the nephrostomy tube can be removed. The nephrostent or ureteral stent is maintained for a total of 4 to 6 weeks.

The most difficult situation occurs when the ureteral obstruction is **complete** (Bagley et al, 1985). In this case, neither contrast agent nor a guide wire can be made to traverse the stricture. A nephrostomy tract must therefore be established. The exact limits of the total occlusion are defined by a combined nephrostogram and retrograde ureterogram. If the occlusion is short (<1 cm), an endosurgical approach can be tried; however, if the occlusion is long (>1 cm), an open surgical procedure is recommended (Bagley, 1990). Bagley (1990) has reported successful recannulation of complete ureteral obstructions as long as 5 cm.

When **complete obstruction occurs in the proximal or**

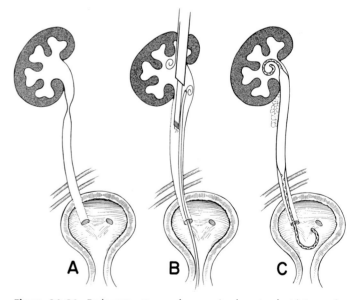

Figure 94–36. Endoureterotomy of a proximal ureteral stricture. *A,* Proximal ureteral stricture: the stricture and the ureteropelvic junction are in close proximity. *B,* A hot knife incision is being made on the lateral surface of the ureteral stricture using a No. 2 Fr electrode passed through a No. 12.5 Fr insulated therapeutic ureteroscope. *C,* Two days after the endoincision, a nephrostogram is performed. If there is no extravasation, the nephrostomy tube is removed. The ureteral stent (No. 7 Fr/14 Fr) is left in place for 6 weeks.

middle ureter, the technique is identical to that described for approaching the completely obstructed UPJ. The only difference is that in these patients the indwelling ureteral stent is left in place for a longer period of time, usually up to 12 weeks (Bagley, 1990).

If the site of **total occlusion** is **in the distal ureter,** a nephrostomy tube is placed. The approach to this problem can be solely fluoroscopic or a combination of fluoroscopy and endoscopic incision. In the fluoroscopic approach, via a percutaneous nephrostomy, a stiff guide wire or a sharpened wire, such as the rocket wire from a retrograde percutaneous access kit, is passed antegrade to the site of obstruction (Lang, 1984; Chao et al, 1987). The bladder is filled with contrast material. Using the C-arm, the tip of the antegrade guide wire is maneuvered until it is pointed directly at the bladder in both the anterior-posterior and lateral planes. The guide wire is then forcefully advanced into the bladder. Using the flexible or rigid cystoscope to monitor the procedure greatly increases the safety of this maneuver; likewise, as soon as the wire enters the bladder, it is grasped and pulled caudad until it exits the urethral meatus, thereby providing a through-and-through guide wire from flank to urethral meatus. Next a 4- to 8-mm, 4-cm-long polyethylene balloon can be passed antegrade and used to dilate the obstructed site. It is left inflated for 10 minutes and exchanged for a No. 10 Fr or larger antegrade biliary urinary drainage or multiholed locking loop nephrostent or for an indwelling ureteral stent and a small nephrostomy tube. The latter situation permits removal of the nephrostomy tube on the second or third postoperative day, provided that a nephrostogram reveals no extravasation. The nephrostent or indwelling stent is removed 6 to 12 weeks later.

Alternatively the distal ureteral stricture may be approached by the antegrade passage of a guide wire; a flexible ureteroscope or a 6- or 8-mm ureteral dilating catheter with no protruding tip is passed over the guide wire to the level of obstruction. The balloon can be inflated with contrast material mixed with indigo carmine. Next an Iglesias resectoscope equipped with a Collings knife or an Orandi knife or a direct vision urethrotome is passed through the urethra. Using the fluoroscope, the endoscope in the bladder is positioned until it directly overlies the antegrade endoscope or the contrast medium–containing balloon. If the first method is chosen, the light in the retrograde endoscope (i.e., cystoscope) is turned off, and the incision is made to the bright light coming from the antegrade flexible ureteroscope. Alternatively, if the contrast agent–filled balloon is selected as a target, the fluoroscope is used to align the cystoscope over the No. 5 Fr catheter or balloon. An incision is directed toward the contrast-filled balloon (Fig. 94–37). Once the nephroscope or antegrade balloon catheter is uncovered in the proximal ureter, a 260-cm, 0.035-inch exchange guide wire is passed and retrieved through the urethra, thereby providing a longer through-and-through guide wire. As previously described, an indwelling stent and nephrostomy tube or a nephrostent can be placed. In the former circumstance, the nephrostomy tube is removed on postoperative day 2 (provided that a nephrostogram reveals no extravasation). If there was no extravasation at the time of the ureteral incision, the urethral catheter is removed on the first or second postoperative day; however, if during the incision perivesical fat is seen, the urethral catheter is left indwelling for a full

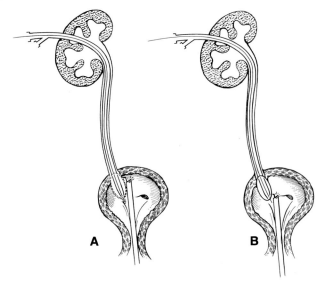

Figure 94–37. Distal ureteral obstruction complete. *A,* A 0.035-inch guide wire has been advanced via a percutaneous nephrostomy until its tip lies at the cephalad border of a distal ureteral occlusion. A 6-mm ureteral dilating balloon (no tip) has been advanced over the guide wire and inflated. An Orandi electrosurgical knife has been aligned under fluoroscopic guidance, such that the tip of the knife directly overlies the inflated balloon. *B,* The overlying tissue has been incised, thereby uncovering the balloon. At this point, a 260-cm exchange guide wire is passed antegrade through the balloon catheter and pulled via the cystoscope through the urethra, thereby establishing a "through-and-through" guide wire extending from the flank to the urethral meatus. An indwelling stent and nephrostomy tube or a nephrostent is positioned across the incised stricture. The stent is removed after 6 weeks.

week to prevent any extravasation of urine during voiding. At 1 week, on an outpatient basis, a cystogram is obtained. If there is no extravasation, the urethral catheter is removed. The indwelling ureteral stent or nephrostent remains in place for 4 to 6 weeks (Cubelli and Smith, 1987).

Despite the seemingly straightforward nature of the previously described methods for treating ureteral strictures, the urologist is actually beset by a bewildering array of technical details with regard to either endodilation or endoincision. Indeed, with regard to endodilation with a balloon, the size of the balloon (4–8 mm), duration of inflation (15 seconds to 60 minutes), and number of inflation cycles (one to three) are different in each reported series (Banner and Pollack, 1984; Coleman et al, 1984a; Finnerty et al, 1984; Chang et al, 1987; Johnson et al, 1987; Lang and Glorioso, 1988; O'Brien et al, 1988; Kramolowsky et al, 1989; Netto et al, 1990). With regard to the endoincision, the method may vary among cold knife, electrosurgical, and laser energy.

For the relief of the totally obstructed ureter when chances of recannulation appear small or prior endourologic procedures have been unsuccessful, a nephrovesical stent is of value (Desgrandchamps et al, 1993, 1995; Lingam et al, 1994; Nakada et al, 1995). One end of the stent is inserted into the renal pelvis via a percutaneous nephrostomy puncture, and the body of the stent is tunneled subcutaneously toward the bladder. The distal end of the stent is then passed via a percutaneous puncture into the bladder (Fig. 94–38). The stent is changed every 4 months using a combined cystoscopic and percutaneous cutdown technique, over the flank portion of the stent.

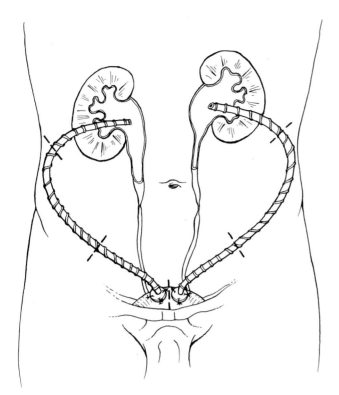

Figure 94–38. Nephrovesical stent. The stents shown are each made of two coaxial tubes: The inner tube is No. 18 Fr and made of silicone, whereas the outer tube is No. 28.5 Fr and made of polytetrafluoroethylene. The two pairs of dashed lines are skin incision sites used to create the subcutaneous tunnel for the nephrovesical stent. The bladder end of the stent is passed through a silicone nipple, which, in turn, is sewn to the outer wall of the bladder; a small midline incision *(vertical dashed line)* is made to access the bladder. (Drawn after Desgrandchamps F, Cussenot O, Meria P, et al: J Urol 1995; 154:367.)

RESULTS

In reviewing the results of endourologic management of ureteral strictures, the most striking aspect is the tremendous variability in reported results (Table 94–13). From a strict therapeutic standpoint, success rates with balloon dilation vary from 45% to 88%, with an average success rate of 55% among 340 patients reviewed. In contrast, endoureterotomy has a success range of 55% to 88%, with an average patency rate of 70% albeit in a total of only 132 patients (Banner and Pollack, 1984; Chang et al, 1987; Johnson et al, 1987; Gothlin et al, 1988; Lang and Glorioso, 1988; O'Brien et al, 1988; Beckman et al, 1989; Kramolowsky et al, 1989; Netto et al, 1990; Meretyk S et al, 1992a; Glinz et al, 1994). There are three reasons for the tremendous variability in outcome data among the reported series: differences in technique, differences in method of data collection and reporting, and differences in the nature of the strictures treated.

With regard to differences in technique, this is obvious from the previously described variations for balloon dilation and endoureterotomy. In the former group, balloon size, length, duration of inflation, and number of inflation cycles are different in each study, whereas in the endoureterotomy group, the type of energy source and method of energy delivery (e.g., endoscopic versus fluoroscopic cutting balloon) to make the incision are significant variables. Also, the controversy of stent duration and stent size plays a significant role among these patients, as it does among the endopyelotomy patients. The duration of stent placement (2 days to 2 months) is different in each reported series (Banner and Pollack, 1984; Coleman et al, 1984a; Finnerty et al, 1984; Chang et al, 1987; Johnson et al, 1987; Lang and Glorioso, 1988; O'Brien et al, 1988; Kramolowsky et al, 1989; Netto et al, 1990). Likewise the stent size varies from No. 7 to 14 Fr (Glanz et al, 1983; Banner and Pollack, 1984; Finnerty et al, 1984; Chang et al, 1987; Johnson et al, 1987). In one study, no indwelling stent was used after endoureterotomy (Reimer and Oswalt, 1981). Optimal stent size and duration remain an enigma.

Another major variable with regard to outcome data is the method of analysis and length of follow-up period for determining treatment success. Subjective follow-up, although not difficult to secure, is hardly reliable. Analog questionnaires, which enable the investigator to characterize accurately the impact of an intervention on a patient's quality of life, have yet to be introduced into studies on the outcome of ureteral stricture therapy. In addition, it must be noted that an asymptomatic state, in the absence of confirmatory objective studies, is not indicative of a successful outcome; indeed, in one series of ureteral strictures, 25% of patients were asymptomatic **at the time of presentation** (Meretyk S et al, 1992a). Similarly, there are problems with the objective data collected on these patients. Unfortunately, these data are often incomplete, the follow-up is brief (i.e., <1 year), or both. In Meretyk and colleagues' series, an additional 15% of patients undergoing an endoincision failed between the 6th and 12th month of follow-up, thereby lowering the successful outcome to 64% (Meretyk S et al, 1992a).

The third and perhaps most telling variable among ureteral stricture series is the variability in the type of stricture treated. Each stricture has its own unique set of characteristics determined by its length, etiology, and location. These factors significantly influence the final result. Currently the most important determinant of the outcome of an endoureterotomy appears to be the length of the stricture. Strictures longer than 1 cm rarely respond well to an endosurgical approach (11%–18%), whereas the success rate for strictures 1 cm or smaller is 90% to 100% in three series comprising 43 patients (Chang et al, 1987; Netto et al, 1990; Meretyk S et al, 1992a).

Another, albeit lesser, factor that affects the outcome of endoureterotomy is the etiology of the strictured area. Intrinsic ureteral strictures are currently most commonly (upward of 75%) caused by postoperative fibrosis following open pelvic surgery or a ureteroscopic procedure (Netto et al, 1990). Other causes of intrinsic ureteral strictures include inflammatory processes associated with schistosomiasis, retroperitoneal fibrosis, tuberculosis, malignancy, submucosal calculus, and radiation (ischemic injury) (Johnson et al, 1987; Kramolowsky et al, 1989; Netto et al, 1990; Dretler and Young, 1993). A stricture caused by an ischemic problem appears to respond less well than a benign nonischemic stricture—40% versus 58% (Lang, 1984; O'Brien et al, 1988; Meretyk S et al, 1992a).

With regard to stricture location and subsequent outcome of an endoureterotomy, those strictures that are of a proximal or distal nature and can be marsupialized at either their upper or their lower border into the renal pelvis or bladder, respectively, have a better success rate than strictures that are

Table 94–13. ENDOSURGERY FOR URETERAL STRICTURES

Authors	Patients	Approach	Stent Size (Fr)	Stent Duration	Patent (%)	Follow-up (months)
Balloon Dilation						
Banner and Pollack, 1984	44	4 mm balloon	7–10	4 days–3 months	48	—
Beckman et al, 1989	17	4–8 mm balloon	7–10	4–8 weeks	82	1–40
Johnson et al, 1987	30	4–10 mm balloon	6–10	2 days–months	58	≥6
Lang and Glorioso, 1988	127	4–6 mm balloon	7–10	3–6 weeks	50	≥15
Netto et al, 1990	19	4–6 mm balloon	8.5	2–8 weeks	53	≥18
Chang et al, 1987	11	5–8 mm balloon	8–16	4–8 weeks	88	10 (average)
O'Brien et al, 1988	24	4–6 mm balloon	—	—	45	2–36
Kramolowsky et al, 1989	20	5–10 mm balloon	6–12	6 weeks	64	22
Farah et al, 1991 (transplant)	17	8–12 mm balloon	6–7	4–15 weeks	53	3–44 (mean 16)
Benoit et al, 1993 (transplant)	16	10 mm balloon	10	8 weeks	75	≥12
Kim et al, 1993 (transplant)	10	4–10 mm balloon	7–12	4 days–5 months	40	15–40 (mean 29)
Kwak et al, 1995	5	8 mm balloon	10	—	0	9
Overall	340	4–12 mm	6–16	2 days–5 months	55	>6
Endoureterotomy						
Schneider et al, 1991	12	Cold knife	14	3–6 weeks	67	7–45 (mean 15)
Eshghi et al, 1989	40	Cold knife	6–10	4–6 weeks	88	—
Glinz et al, 1994	18	Cutting balloon catheter (electrocautery)	—	6 weeks	83	≥6
Meretyk et al, 1992a	13	Electrocautery (endoscopic); 2 patients free graft of urothelium	14	3–7 weeks	62	≥12 (mean 20)
Preminger et al, 1996	49	Electrocautery (cutting balloon catheter)	6–14	5 weeks	55	1–17 (mean 8.7)
Overall	132	—	6–14	3–7 weeks	70	>12

midureteral and bounded by normal-caliber ureter on either end—80% versus 25% (Meretyk S et al, 1992a). In Smith's (1988) series, all four patients with a midureteral stricture failed balloon dilation.

Although concern has been raised that strictures of a chronic nature fare less well than strictures that have been present for only a short while, there are no data to substantiate this hypothesis. Indeed, when the aforementioned factors of stricture length, vascularity, and location are taken into consideration, the duration of the stricture appears to have little or no effect on the subsequent outcome of an endoureterotomy (Finnerty et al, 1984; Netto et al, 1990). Success has been recorded with strictures as old as 18 months, and failure has been recorded with strictures diagnosed within 8 weeks of the initiating event (Netto et al, 1990).

More detailed studies with meticulous long-term follow-up data and proper separation of strictures according to length, etiology, and location are necessary to define better the indications for an endourologic approach. At present, endourologic management is most applicable for those "favorable" ureteral strictures in which the obstruction is short in length (<1 cm), not associated with radiation or other ischemic injury, and preferably located in the proximal or distal ureter.

The question of what to do with the "unfavorable" stricture is a vexing one. Short of open surgery, there are few endourologic options. These options are all in the investigational stages and include injection of triamcinolone, placement of a "free" urothelial graft, use of metal stents, and nephrovesical diversion.

The injection of triamcinolone into the incised bed of a ureteral stricture has been reported by the group at Washington University. Meretyk S and co-workers noted that among 13 patients with ureteral strictures, a remarkable 80% patency rate was obtained among 5 patients injected with triamcinolone and followed for 19 months, whereas the patency rate in the more favorable, noninjected group of 8 patients was 50% at 22 months. This was an anecdotal, nonrandomized series, however, encompassing strictures of diverse length, etiology, and location (Meretyk S et al, 1992a). To date, there have been no additional studies to test this treatment alternative.

Clayman and Denstedt (1989) initially reported on the endourologic "free" urothelial graft. In four patients with long distal strictures (5–7 cm), a patch of urothelium was cystoscopically harvested from the bladder (up to 2 cm × 4 cm in size). This patch of urothelium was defatted and sewn onto a No. 7 Fr ureteral stent with the urothelium facing the stent. The graft-bearing stent was positioned in the bed of the incised stricture, such that the free graft of urothelium covered the incised area. The stent was removed 6 weeks later (Clayman and Denstedt, 1989). Urban and associates have updated the Washington University series to six patients followed for a mean of 30 months. Overall, 83% have had a successful result (Urban et al, 1994). These investigators to date have been unable to provide any data showing that the graft has actually "taken." Future developments in the area of biologically compatible prosthetics in combination with cell and tissue culture may eventually render an acceptable ureteral substitute.

Metal stents have also been used to overcome unfavorable dense ureteral strictures. Cussenot and associates noted that three of four patients failed use of one metal stent because of ingrowth of hyperplastic mucosa (Cussenot et al, 1993). In contrast, Pauer and Lugmayr (1992) had a more favorable outcome using a Wallstent (i.e., a self-expanding stainless steel alloy 7-mm stent) in 12 patients. Despite some mild initial hyperplasia, overall, at 27 weeks, 87% of the stents remained patent (Pauer and Lugmayr, 1992).

Lastly, for the patient with total ureteral obstruction or failed endourologic therapy who is not considered a surgical candidate, a final effort before a lifetime commitment to a nephrostomy tube is the placement of a nephrovesical or pyelovesical stent (Desgrandchamps et al, 1993). Lingam and Nakada and their colleagues have independently reported successful use of this stent in a total of seven patients, all with metastatic disease; these stents have remained in situ for as long as 12 months (Lingam et al, 1994; Nakada et al, 1995). Desgrandchamps and colleagues have updated their series to 19 pyelovesical bypasses in 13 patients with a malignancy and a life expectancy of less than 1 year; in each case, attempted indwelling ureteral stent bypass had failed. In all 13 patients, the pyelovesical bypass functioned well at an average follow-up of 7 months; only one patient in this group had follow-up beyond 1 year (Desgrandchamps et al, 1995).

Other Applications

URETEROENTERIC STRICTURES: ENDOURETEROTOMY

A ureteroenteric stricture occurs in 4% to 8% of patients who are undergoing urinary conduit procedures (Engel, 1969; Schmidt et al, 1973; Vandenbroucke et al, 1993). These strictures are usually noted within the first year of follow-up; however, as many as 20% may occur beyond a year and as late as 5 years postoperatively (Vandenbroucke et al, 1993). Fortunately, it appears that the large majority of these strictures are of a benign nature and associated with distal ureteral vascular compromise and necrosis; an underlying recurrent malignancy is distinctly unusual and was present in none of 27 ureteroileal stenoses noted by Vandenbroucke and colleagues over a 10-year period. The standard surgical repair of these strictures can be tedious and in some cases may lead to the need to create an entirely new conduit; as such, in properly selected patients, the endosurgical therapy of these strictures can offer a welcome alternative to open surgical therapy (Meretyk et al, 1991).

In dealing with a ureteroenteric stricture, the initial evaluation includes an intravenous urogram and a radiographic contrast study of the conduit (i.e., loopogram). For further evaluation of the degree of obstruction and the remaining renal function in the affected kidney, a furosemide washout renogram is indicated; if inconclusive, a Whitaker renal pelvis and loop pressure study can be performed. The latter is also of value to help outline the length of the stricture. In patients with a history of bladder cancer, a full metastatic evaluation is completed: CT of the abdomen and pelvis, along with a chest radiograph, serum liver function studies, and a serum alkaline phosphatase and calcium. Any abnormality in the last two blood chemistries necessitates obtaining a bone scan to rule out metastases. In addition, endoscopy of the ileal conduit with a flexible endoscope is helpful to rule out the unlikely presence of malignant disease in the conduit, at the site of the ureteroenteric anastomosis.

If the stricture is **complete or of malignant origin,** the goal of endourologic therapy is to place a retrograde **external ureteral catheter.** The ureteral drainage catheter is changed on an outpatient basis every 3 to 4 months (Horgan et al, 1988). If the **stricture is benign and partial,** however, the goal of endosurgical therapy is to re-establish continuity in such a manner that a permanent indwelling stent is not necessary.

TECHNIQUE. Before endosurgical therapy for a ureteroenteric stricture, the patient is advised of the following: a 60% success rate; the 5% risk of either hemorrhage or bowel injury, either one of which may necessitate an emergency open procedure; and the possibility of nephrectomy should excessive bleeding from the nephrostomy tract occur (Meretyk et al, 1991).

The position of the patient must allow access both to the flank on the affected side and to the stoma of the conduit. The patient is thus placed in a flank position, with the affected side superior (Fig. 94–39). Both the planned nephrostomy site on the flank and the abdominal stoma are prepared and draped with a nephrostomy drape.

As with other upper urinary tract strictures, there are two methods and two approaches for management of an ureteroenteric stricture: balloon dilation or endoincision, via an antegrade or a retrograde approach (Figs. 94–40 and 94–41). **Balloon dilation** is by far the older and simpler of the two techniques (Banner and Pollack, 1984; Lang, 1984). For this technique, no preoperative bowel preparation is needed. A guide wire is passed either antegrade via a small nephrostomy tract or retrograde at the time of looposcopy. The preferred guide wire for this purpose is a 0.035-inch Terumo guide wire, usually with an angled tip. A torque control device attached to the back end of the guide wire enables the urologist to rotate it without difficulty. This extremely lubricious guide wire has a tendency to bypass even the tightest strictures. When passed retrograde, the guide wire is coiled in the renal pelvis; however, if an

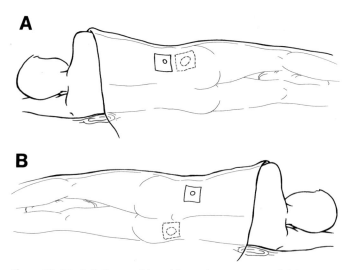

Figure 94–39. A, Patient positioned for endoureterotomy of right ureteroenteric stricture (*dotted circle,* ileal stoma on anterior abdominal wall; *solid circle,* nephrostomy site). B, Patient positioned for endoureterotomy of left ureteroenteric stricture (*dotted circle,* ileal stoma on anterior abdominal wall; *solid circle,* nephrostomy site). In both cases, the nephrostomy tube site is superior. Two separate nephrostomy drapes are used to prepare the stoma site and nephrostomy site, respectively.

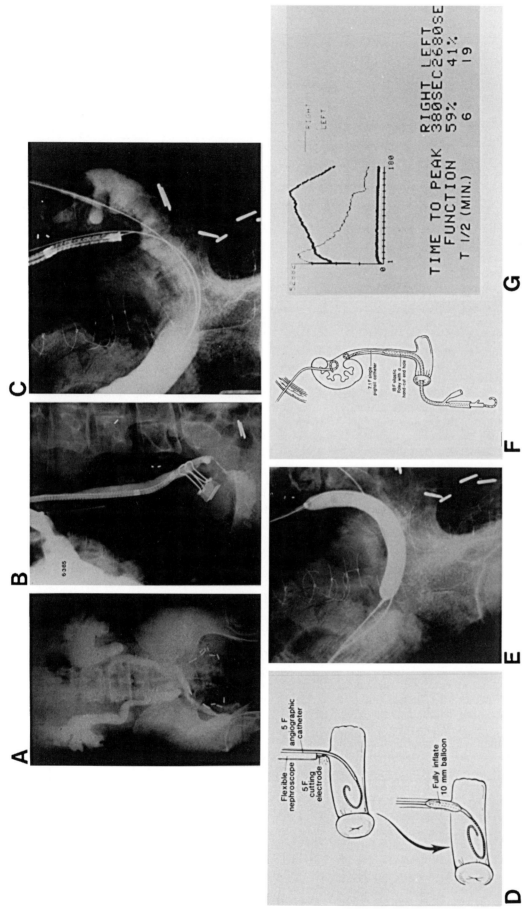

Figure 94–40. Steps in performing an endoincision of ureteroenteric strictures via an *antegrade* approach. *A,* Bilateral ureteroenteric anastomotic strictures occurring 10 years after a total exenteration for rectal cancer (June 1985). *B,* Antegrade approach is performed with a flexible nephroscope. *C,* A No. 3 Fr electrosurgery probe has been passed through the flexible nephroscope and is protruding from the working channel. *D,* Before activating the electrosurgical probe, a No. 5 Fr angiographic catheter is passed over the guide wire to insulate it from any current. The incision is continued until the ileal conduit is entered. The incised ureter is then balloon dilated to No. 30 Fr. *E,* Radiograph showing balloon dilation of the incised stricture to No. 30 Fr. *F,* The endoincision is stinted with an No. 18 Fr Councill-type Silastic Foley catheter backloaded over a No. 7.1 Fr pigtail catheter. A nephrostomy tube is also placed. The stent is left in place for at least 6 weeks; the nephrostomy tube can be removed on the second postoperative day, provided that a nephrostogram shows no extravasation. Alternatively a No. 10 Fr or No. 16 Fr biliary urinary drainage catheter with a pigtail coil may be passed retrograde and positioned in the renal pelvis. *G,* A renal scan, 14 months later, reveals acceptable clearance on the right and slightly prolonged clearance on the left. The patient is asymptomatic, and the serum creatinine is normal. (From Kramolowsky EV, Clayman RV, Weyman PJ: J Urol 1987; 137:390. Copyright by Williams & Wilkins, 1992.)

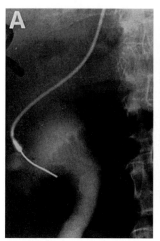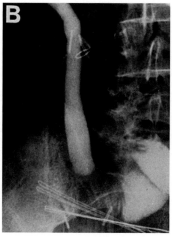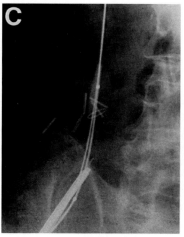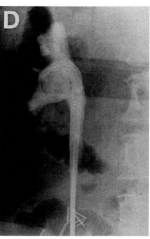

Figure 94–41. A retrograde approach to a ureteroenteric stricture. *A* and *B,* Antegrade nephrostogram demonstrates ureteroenteric stricture. *A,* Nephrostomy needle in kidney. *B,* Distal ureter at ureteroenteric juncture. *C,* The stricture was incised via a retrograde approach. A No. 3 Fr Greenwald needle is being used via a No. 12 Fr short rigid ureteroscope to inject the area of the incision with 3 to 5 ml of triamcinolone (40 mg/ ml). *D,* Two retrograde pigtail catheters (each No. 8 Fr) have been positioned with their distal coils in the renal pelvis. The shaft of each pigtail exits the stoma to preclude obstruction from mucus. Holes are only in the coiled renal pelvic portions of the pigtail biliary urinary drainage catheters. In this case, the nephrostomy tube was not replaced.

antegrade approach is taken, the tip of the guide wire is passed into the loop, where it can be retrieved with an endoscope, thereby creating a through-and-through Terumo guide wire. The latter situation provides the surgeon with the benefit of complete control over the collecting system.

Next a No. 5 Fr angiographic catheter is passed over the Terumo guide wire, and the Terumo guide wire is exchanged for a 0.035-inch Amplatz superstiff guide wire (retrograde approach) or a 0.035-inch, 260-cm exchange guide wire (antegrade approach). The No. 5 Fr angiographic catheter is removed. An 8-mm or a 10-mm, 4-cm-long balloon dilating catheter is passed over the guide wire, until it straddles the stricture. The dilating balloon, rated to at least 15 atm, is slowly inflated with a pressure syringe (LeVeen type). Once the waist (i.e., stricture) disappears, the balloon is left inflated for 1 minute; the balloon is deflated, and the inflation/ deflation cycle may be repeated once or twice.

After this, when a **retrograde** approach is used, two No. 8 Fr or a single No. 10 to 16 Fr single pigtail catheter (usually a biliary urinary drainage catheter) is passed retrograde over the Amplatz superstiff guide wire and positioned in the renal pelvis. The flush end of the pigtail catheter, as it exits the stoma, can be sewn with 2–0 Prolene to the lateral edge of the peristomal skin to prevent its premature dislodgment. When an **antegrade** approach is used, the biliary urinary drainage catheter(s) is placed retrograde, as described, and a separate percutaneous nephrostomy tube (No. 10 Fr) is also positioned. Alternatively a No. 16 Fr Silastic Foley catheter, converted to a Councill-type catheter by punching a hole in the tip of the catheter, can be used to stint the ureter. In this case, a No. 7.1 Fr pigtail catheter is first passed retrograde to the renal pelvis; next the No. 16 Fr Silastic catheter is backloaded over the No. 7.1 Fr pigtail catheter and passed until its tip is in the midureter. The pigtail catheter is affixed to the Silastic catheter by backloading a side arm adapter over the pigtail catheter and firmly pushing the adapter into the butt end of the Silastic catheter. The adjustable rubber diaphragm portion of the side arm adapter is then tightened onto the shaft of the No. 7.1 Fr pigtail catheter. The No. 16

Fr Silastic catheter can then be sewn to the peristomal skin as described; the balloon of the Silastic catheter is not inflated. If a nephrostomy tube was placed, 2 days postoperatively a nephrostogram is obtained. If the collecting system is intact and there is no extravasation from the former ureteral stricture site, the nephrostomy tube is removed. The retrograde ureteral stent is either removed after 6 weeks or exchanged under fluoroscopic control after 3 to 4 months, depending on whether the stricture was benign and partial versus malignant or complete (Meretyk et al, 1991).

For performing an endoincision of a ureteroenteric stricture, a **retrograde** approach is simpler (see Fig. 94–41) (Meretyk et al, 1991). Paradoxically the initial step in a retrograde approach is to secure control of the kidney by way of a No. 10 Fr nephrostomy catheter. A guide wire (usually a 0.035-inch Terumo guide wire) can then be passed antegrade, across the area of stricture and into the conduit, thereby allowing establishment of a through-and-through guide wire. If this is not possible, a nephrostomy tube should still be placed to allow for repeated injection of indigo carmine–stained saline to enable the endoscopist to localize the narrowed ureteroenteric anastomosis.

Endoscopy of the conduit is performed with a rigid endoscope (i.e., direct vision urethrotome or a No. 12.5 Fr short, rigid therapeutic ureteroscope with an insulated tip). If a guide wire has not been passed antegrade, attempts are made to pass a guide wire retrograde until its tip is coiled in the renal pelvis. The endoscope is removed and then reinserted alongside the guide wire. A 10-mm, 4-cm-long ureteral dilating balloon catheter is passed either antegrade or retrograde, until the balloon straddles the stricture. The balloon is inflated to 1 atm, with 50:50 contrast agent and saline stained with indigo carmine; fluoroscopically the full length of the narrow waist of the stricture is thereby well outlined. Next the balloon is deflated, and the area of the stricture is deeply incised with a cold knife via the rigid endoscope. Alternatively the balloon can be left inflated and an electrosurgical incision (75 watts pure cut) made along the balloon, using a No. 2 or 3 Fr Greenwald electrosurgical probe. In either case, the incision should extend through the entire thickness of the ureter. Occasionally, retroperitoneal fat can be seen. At the completion of the incision, the 10-mm balloon is reinflated to be certain that at low pressure (i.e., 1 atm), the previously strictured area completely expands. A No. 10 or 16 Fr single pigtail catheter (biliary urinary drainage) is passed over the guide wire and its pigtail end is positioned in the renal pelvis. The pigtail catheter, as it exits the stoma, is secured to the lateral edge of the peristomal skin with a 2–0 Prolene suture.

Under no circumstances should any of the currently available **internal** ureteral stents be placed. These catheters have drainage holes all along the shaft; as such, they may become occluded with mucus. The resulting obstruction may lead to fatal urosepsis (Walther et al, 1985). In contrast, the described types of external ureteral catheters have drainage holes only in the portion that resides within the renal pelvis and the drainage bag.

Retrograde endoincision has also been accomplished using a cutting balloon catheter (i.e., Acucise device) (Preminger et al, 1996). The placement of the cutting balloon catheter proceeds exactly as described for balloon dilation; the direction of the cutting wire is usually lateral or medial. This method, although seemingly simple, has the potential for major complications because of the proximity of bowel and major vascular structures, especially on the left side. In general, this modality is better reserved for endopyelotomy or the typical ureteral stricture; for ureteroenteric strictures, an endoscopic incision is recommended.

At the end of the procedure, the urinary drainage appliance is replaced onto the stoma. A No. 10 Fr percutaneous nephrostomy catheter is also placed. Two days postoperatively, with the patient still receiving parenteral antibiotics, a nephrostogram is performed. If there is no extravasation, the nephrostomy tube can be removed, **under fluoroscopic guidance.** The retrograde pigtail catheter can be removed or exchanged 6 weeks postoperatively, depending on the goal of therapy. During the 6-week period and for 2 weeks after stent removal, the patient takes a nightly antibiotic tablet, usually nitrofurantoin or a trimethoprim-sulfamethoxazole combination.

When a retrograde approach cannot be performed because of the tortuosity of the conduit or failure to identify and cannulate the stenotic ureteroenteric anastomosis, an **antegrade** approach is necessary (see Fig. 94–40) (Meretyk et al, 1991). The nephrostomy tract is placed in an upper or a middle posterior calyx to provide a direct line of access to the UPJ. The nephrostomy tract is dilated to No. 18 Fr, and a No. 18 Fr Amplatz sheath is placed. A No. 15 Fr flexible nephroscope or, if this is too short, a flexible ureteroscope is passed, down the nephrostomy tract and into the dilated proximal ureter. It is advanced under direct endoscopic control until the lumen of the strictured ureter is identified. Next a 0.035-inch Terumo guide wire is passed through the working channel of the endoscope, beyond the stricture and coiled in the conduit. A rigid endoscope is passed by way of the abdominal stoma into the conduit, and the guide wire is grasped and pulled until its tip exits the stoma, thereby creating a through-and-through guide wire. The flexible endoscope is withdrawn and passed again via the sheath, albeit alongside the through-and-through guide wire. Over the through-and-through Terumo guide wire, a No. 5 Fr angio-

graphic catheter is passed, and the Terumo guide wire is exchanged for a 0.035-inch, 260-cm exchange guide wire. The No. 5 Fr catheter is removed, and a 10-mm, 4-cm-long balloon dilating catheter is positioned so that the balloon straddles the stricture. The balloon is inflated with dilute radiographic contrast material stained with indigo carmine to 1 atm or less using a LeVeen syringe connected to an in-line pressure gauge. Next, with the balloon inflated, a No. 2 or 3 Fr electrosurgical probe is passed via the flexible antegrade endoscope, and an incision (75 watts, pure cut) is made along the ureter until the conduit is entered.

The incision is made through the full thickness of the ureter; however, only occasionally is retroperitoneal fat seen. The 10-mm, 4-cm-long ureteral dilating balloon should now fully inflate to No. 30 Fr at only 1 to 2 atm. This indicates that the depth of the incision into the stricture was sufficient. As previously described, a nephrostomy tube, in this case a No. 10 Fr pigtail or No. 16 Fr Council catheter, is placed, along with a separate retrograde No. 10 or 16 Fr biliary urinary drainage catheter. The postoperative regimen is identical to that described for the retrograde approach.

If the scar tissue is particularly dense, 3 to 5 ml of triamcinolone (40 mg/ml) may be injected into the bed of the incised stricture. This step is done with a No. 3 Fr Greenwald needle catheter (see Fig. 94–33). It is helpful to inject the scar tissue using a LeVeen pressure syringe because otherwise the scar tissue may be too dense to allow the triamcinolone to penetrate. Although conceptually appealing, the benefit of this maneuver remains anecdotal (Meretyk S et al, 1991).

A third and latest alternative to balloon dilation and endoincision is to place a metallic stent across the strictured area. There have now been two reports of using metallic stents to treat ureteroileal strictures (Gort et al, 1990; Reinberg et al, 1994). These stents can be placed in either a retrograde or an antegrade manner. Reinberg and colleagues described placement of an 8-mm self-expanding metallic stent in two patients with ureteroileal strictures: one right-sided and one left-sided (Reinberg et al, 1994). In both cases, the stent was placed in a retrograde manner. Both patients had failed multiple balloon dilations; however, neither had previously undergone an endoincision. In both patients, stent deployment was uneventful, and both patients were asymptomatic at 12 to 13 months' follow-up; objective follow-up at 3 to 12 months revealed evidence of a patent ureter. More patients and longer follow-up are needed to test this intriguingly simple treatment further.

When the ureteroenteric obstruction is **complete,** a combined antegrade and retrograde approach is required. In this case, a rigid endoscope is passed by way of the bowel conduit, and a flexible endoscope is passed by way of the nephrostomy tract. The light from the antegrade endoscope is turned off. The examiner then seeks the light coming from the rigid retrograde endoscope within the conduit. When the tips of the two endoscopes are fluoroscopically close (<5 mm), the initial pink hue transilluminating the intervening tissue should change to an intense white light. In this regard, a C-arm fluoroscope is essential because the position of the tips of the endoscopes must appear aligned in **two** separate projections (e.g., anterior-posterior and an oblique plane) to **ensure** that their tips are in close proximity to one another.

At this point, several methods can be selected to re-establish a communication between the ureter and the conduit. The stiff end of a 0.035-inch, 260-cm exchange guide wire can be passed via the antegrade flexible endoscope, guided fluoroscopically and endoscopically to perforate the brightest (i.e., "white") area of light and thereby enter the conduit (Muench et al, 1987). Alternatively a No. 2 or 3 Fr electrosurgical probe can be employed via the flexible antegrade endoscope to "cut to the light" and uncover the rigid retrograde endoscope. A third approach is to turn off the light of the rigid retrograde endoscope while maintaining the light of the flexible endoscope. If the conduit is not tortuous, a cold knife urethrotome can be used via the retrograde endoscope to cut to the white light cast by the antegrade flexible endoscope.

As soon as a recommunication is established between the ureter and enteric conduit, a 0.035-inch, 260-cm exchange guide wire is passed by way of the flexible antegrade endoscope, grasped via the retrograde rigid endoscope, and pulled through the stoma of the conduit, thereby providing a through-and-through guide wire. Subsequent incision of the stricture is accomplished, as previously described.

The ureteroenteric stricture is the most difficult type of stricture to approach endourologically. No landmarks, as with a UPJ obstruction or standard ureteral stricture, are present to guide the urologist as to where to make the incision. Accordingly, it is important for the surgeon to review the original operative notes to determine if the conduit is intraperitoneal or retroperitoneal; likewise the CT scan should be carefully reviewed to see if there is any bowel or vascular structure in close proximity to the area of the stricture. The incision in the ureter should be deepened slowly **under constant endoscopic monitoring** to avoid inadvertent injury to an underlying artery or the bowel. If during the incision a new smooth-walled tissue surface is seen, this is more than likely the serosal surface of the adjacent bowel.

If the bowel is entered, placement of the ureteral pigtail drainage catheter across the incised stricture and into the renal pelvis should be done immediately. For bowel decompression, a nasogastric tube is placed, and the patient is kept without food or drink for several days, after which an oral hyperalimentation diet is begun. A follow-up CT scan with oral contrast material is helpful in determining when the fistulous tract has healed; however, given that there is no obstruction distal to the bowel fistula, healing is usually complete within 1 to 3 weeks (Meretyk S et al, 1991).

If excessive bleeding is encountered, a 10-mm ureteral dilating balloon can be placed over the through-and-through guide wire until it straddles the incised stricture; the balloon is inflated. Tamponade usually stops the bleeding. With excessive bleeding, it is helpful to leave the through-and-through guide wire in place. A separate nephrostomy tube is positioned alongside the through-and-through guide wire. With a suture, the through-and-through guide wire can be sewn to the skin of the flank, and with a side-arm adapter, the guide wire can be secured to the hub of the balloon tamponade catheter, thereby maintaining the position of the inflated balloon catheter on the incised portion of ureter. The balloon can usually be deflated 2 days later and removed and a No. 10 to 16 Fr pigtail catheter placed retrograde. The through-and-through guide wire can also be removed. If despite the aforementioned measures bleeding continues or

recurs at the time of placing the pigtail catheter, angiography and embolization or open exploration is the next step.

A final word of caution is indicated. If the ureteral stricture is on the left side and lies above the ureteroenteric anastomosis, the area of narrowing is likely occurring where the left ureter tunnels under the sigmoid mesocolon. Endoincision in this area is contraindicated because it is fraught with potential complications: enterotomy into the sigmoid colon lying anteriorly or arteriotomy or venotomy into the common iliac vessels lying posteriorly. Hence, although balloon dilation may be tried, the majority of these patients require an open repair.

RESULTS. Reports on the **open surgical** results of treating ureteroenteric strictures are scant. In one report of a total of nine patients (with 33 months of objective follow-up), the patency rate was 89%. The complication rate in this series, however, was high. Indeed, in these seven patients, two (29%) required reoperation in the immediate postoperative period for urine leakage from the conduit or from the ureteroenteric anastomosis (Kramolowsky et al, 1988).

In 1982, Martin and co-workers as well as Dixon and colleagues published reports of successful **balloon dilation** of ureteroenteric strictures in four patients (Dixon et al, 1982; Martin et al, 1982). Since then, only a few series of balloon dilation of ureteroenteric strictures have been reported (Table 94–14) (Banner and Pollack, 1984; Kwak et al, 1994; Lang, 1984; Chang et al, 1987). In these studies, the size of the balloon for dilation varied from 4 to 10 mm, the number of cycles of dilation varied from one to four (during one session or over several days or months) (Martin et al, 1982; Kwak et al, 1995), and the balloon was left inflated from 30 seconds to 15 minutes (Banner and Pollack, 1984; Chang et al, 1987; Kramolowsky et al, 1987a; O'Brien et al, 1988; Beckman et al, 1989; Kwak, et al, 1994). The stent size varied from No. 7 to 16 Fr, and the duration of stent placement was from 1 week to 3 months (average, 6 weeks). Follow-up at approximately 6 months showed a patency rate of 58%; however, longer follow-up revealed an ongoing deterioration of patency: 33% patent at 11 months and less than 20% patent, in two series, at 1 year or more (Lang, 1984; Chang et al, 1987; Kramolowsky et al, 1987a; Shapiro et al, 1988). Of note, in none of the reports was any significant morbidity incurred with balloon dilation.

With regard to **endoincision** of ureteroenteric strictures, Kramolowsky and co-workers and subsequently Meretyk S and co-workers at Washington University have reported the largest series (Kramolowsky et al, 1988; Meretyk S et al, 1991). Among 19 ureteroenteric strictures in 15 patients, 25% of the strictures were managed only by placement of a permanent external ureteral stent because of the presence of metastatic disease or because of complete obliteration of the ureteroenteric anastomosis. Of the remaining 14 strictures, all were treated by endoincision usually by way of an antegrade approach employing a No. 2 or 3 Fr monopolar electrosurgical probe. The average procedural time was 175 minutes. Blood loss was minimal in all patients, estimated at 50 to 200 ml. Among these patients, long-term objective follow-up (average, 2.5 years; all patients, >9 months postoperatively) revealed a patency rate of 57%.

Of those six patients who experienced a failed procedure, two developed metastatic disease within a year, two were

Table 94–14. URETEROENTERIC STRICTURES: ENDOSURGICAL THERAPY

Authors	Number of Patients	Size Balloon (Fr)	Stent Size (Fr)	Stent Duration (Weeks)	Patency (%)	Follow-up (Months)
Balloon Dilation						
Shapiro et al, 1988	37	12–30	8–10	1–6	16	≥12
Chang et al, 1987	6	15–24	8–16	5–12	33	≥11 (average 14)
O'Brien et al, 1988	6	12–18	—	—	17	≥12
Beckman et al, 1989	5	12–24	7–10	4–8	60	≥20 (mean 22)
Kwak et al, 1995	10	24	10	—	50	9
Overall	64	12–30	7–16	6	27	>6
Endoincision		**Method**				
Meretyk et al, 1991	15	Electrocautery (Greenwald electrode)	12–22	4–28	57	≥9 (average 29)
Cornud et al, 1992	9	Electrocautery (papillotome)	18	8	67	2–3
Ahmadzadeh, 1992	5	Electrocautery (needle electrode)	7	4	60	14
Germinale et al, 1992	4	Electrocautery/cold knife (Greenwald electrode)	10	8	75	10
Murray and Wilkinson, 1993	2	Electrocautery	7 (1)	2 (1)	100	6–18
Preminger et al, 1996	6	Electrocautery (cutting balloon catheter)	6–14	5	50	1–7
Overall	41	—	6–22	6	63	1–29

too debilitated to undergo an open repair and were managed with a long-term external retrograde ureteral stent, and two would have been candidates for an open surgical correction. Of these last two patients, one patient experienced restricture of the anastomosis soon after endosurgery and was advised to have an open procedure; however, he refused. He continues with a long-term external ureteral catheter. The other patient developed restricturing of the left ureteroileal anastomosis 4.5 years after endoincision. The recurrent left ureteroenteric stricture was managed by balloon dilation; the ureteroenteric anastomosis has remained patent during the subsequent 6 years of follow-up. Complications with an endoincision occurred in 7% of the patients (ureteroenteric fistula managed conservatively and closing without intervention). No blood transfusions were necessary in any of the patients. With the aforementioned techniques and guidelines, only 7% to 13% of all patients presenting with ureteroenteric strictures would have required open surgical procedures.

Similarly satisfactory results with endoincision of ureteroenteric anastomotic strictures have been reported independently by Ahmadzadeh, Germinale, Cornud, and Murray (see Table 94–14) (Ahmadzadeh, 1992; Cornud et al, 1992; Germinale et al, 1992; Murray and Wilkinson, 1993). Using a cold knife technique or electrosurgery, a successful result was achieved in 63% of patients with follow-up of 1 to 29 months.

With regard to the use of a metallic endoprosthesis, experience is scant. Among four patients with follow-up of 7 to 13 months, the stents have remained patent. Further follow-up and more patients are needed to assess this approach; however, these early data are most encouraging (Gort et al, 1990; Sanders et al, 1993; Reinberg et al, 1994).

VESICOCUTANEOUS FISTULAS

Few problems are as vexing to surgeon and patient alike as inoperable vesicovaginal or vesicocutaneous fistulas re-

sulting from pelvic malignancy. This situation most often occurs in women with recurrent or inoperable cervical or uterine cancer (34% of cases) or in men with bladder cancer (18% of cases) or prostate cancer (8% of cases) in whom the tumor has eroded into the floor of the bladder (Papanicolaou et al, 1985; Kinn et al, 1986; Darcy et al, 1987; Reddy et al, 1987; Smith et al, 1987; Schild et al, 1994). The constant leakage of urine results in the maceration and eventual destruction of the perineal skin with ensuing infection, discomfort, and malodor.

TECHNIQUE. Although bilateral nephrostomy tubes can divert the urine, enough urine traverses the ureter to result in continued leakage. Nephrostomy tube drainage can become a solution only when it is coupled with concomitant occlusion or diversion of the ureters. A variety of endosurgical solutions are available to accomplish this goal by either a percutaneous **transrenal intraluminal** or a percutaneous **retroperitoneal extraluminal** approach to the ureter (Moldwin and Smith, 1988).

Intraluminal ureteral occlusion via a nephrostomy tract is most commonly accomplished today by one of two methods: (1) the fluoroscopic placement of an obstructing foreign body or (2) the application of electrocautery to the ureteral wall. Fluoroscopically guided occlusion has in the past been achieved using a detachable or nondetachable balloon to block the distal ureter; of the two types of balloons, it would appear that the detachable balloon is the favored and more reliable method for producing an effective and durable occlusion (Papanicolaou et al, 1985; Brandl, 1987; Schild et al, 1994). Alternatively, multiple 8 mm × 5 cm and 5 mm × 3 cm Gianturco coils plus gelatin sponge (3/8-inch thick × 3/4-inch long × 1/4-inch wide) material can be introduced under fluoroscopic control via a nephrostomy tract to occlude the ureter. This described method is simple, effective, and nontoxic (Gaylord and Johnsrude, 1989; Schild et al, 1994).

Another method for achieving intraluminal occlusion is by endoscopically monitored (i.e., antegrade nephroscopy) application of electrocoagulation current to the inner wall of the ureter. In this technique, developed by Reddy and associates (1987), a No. 24 Fr nephrostomy tract is created in an upper-pole or middle posterior calyx, thereby providing direct access to the UPJ and proximal ureter. Next a No. 20 Fr rigid cystoscope; a No. 12.5 Fr short, rigid ureteroscope; or a No. 15 Fr flexible nephroscope is passed by way of this tract into the UPJ and proximal ureter. Through the endoscope, a No. 5 Fr electrode is passed, and the ureteral lumen is circumferentially electrocoagulated (50 watts, pure coagulation current), for a distance of 2 cm along the most proximal portion of the ureter. As the mucosa is electrocoagulated, it turns white. The operative time for the coagulation process is in the range of 15 minutes (Fig. 94–42) (Reddy et al, 1987).

Two **direct extraluminal** approaches have been described to occlude the ureter in patients with incurable vesicovaginal fistulas: creation of a cutaneous ureterostomy and direct extraluminal occlusion of the ureter via a metallic clip. Experience with both techniques is limited. The former is best performed in thin patients with a tortuous ureter, whereas the latter requires procedure-specific special equipment. Neither is more effective nor simpler to perform than the two previously described intraluminal techniques (Darcy et al, 1987; Smith et al, 1987).

RESULTS. The occurrence of a vesicovaginal or vesicocutaneous fistula in the patient with a pelvic malignancy is often the final degrading event in a life that has already become nearly intolerable. The resulting malodor and perineal ulceration force these individuals into a state of self-exile precisely at the time when they are in greatest need of both professional care and family support. The aforementioned minimally invasive techniques can substantially add to the quality of the brief life that remains.

As can be seen from Table 94–15, many of these individuals die from their underlying malignancy within a short period of the development of urinary tract fistula. Accordingly, any therapy rendered must be simple, be preferably on an outpatient basis, involve minimal anesthesia, and yet be highly and immediately effective. In this regard, only the intraluminal techniques for ureteral occlusion are recommended: fluoroscopic occlusion (with a detachable balloon or Gianturco coils and gelatin sponge) or endoscopic application of electrocoagulation current to the ureter (Hubner et al, 1992). Both therapies are less expensive, are less time-consuming, and require a lesser degree of anesthesia than the extraluminal alternatives. The endoscopic technique appears to be quite reliable given its 100% success rate albeit in only four patients. More data on endoscopic electrocoagulation are needed to determine its status compared to the aforementioned fluoroscopic techniques. Given the advent of the No. 7.5 Fr flexible ureteroscope, however, this procedure can now be accomplished with a No. 2 Fr electrode through only a No. 10 Fr nephrostomy tract. Similarly, ureteral occlusion under fluoroscopic guidance using a detachable balloon or Gianturco coils in combination with a gelatin sponge, in some series, provided equally excellent results to endoscopic occlusion (Gaylord and Johnsrude, 1989; Hubner et al, 1992).

ENDOUROLOGIC MANAGEMENT OF COMPLICATIONS OF RENAL TRANSPLANTATION

Patients undergoing renal transplantation are at risk for developing a variety of urinary tract problems: urolithiasis,

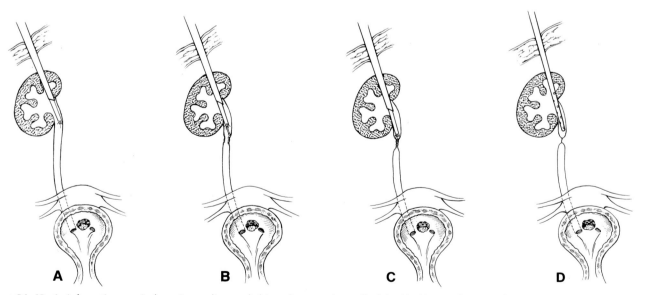

Figure 94–42. *A,* A fungating cervical carcinoma has eroded into the posterior wall of the bladder resulting in a large vesicovaginal fistula. Via an upper posterior calyx, a percutaneous nephrostomy has been placed and dilated to No. 24 Fr. A No. 24 Fr Amplatz sheath has been placed, through which a rigid No. 20 Fr endoscope has been passed into the proximal ureter. *B,* A No. 5 Fr electrosurgical probe (50 watts, coagulating current) is used to fulgurate *circumferentially* the right ureteral wall for a distance of 2 cm. *C,* Immediately after fulguration, the proximal right ureter is just barely patent. *D,* One week later, the right proximal ureter has completely closed; the kidney is drained via a No. 20 Fr nephrostomy tube. A similar procedure is simultaneously performed on the left ureter, thereby resolving any urine leakage from the fistula.

Table 94–15. ENDOUROLOGY: URETERIC OCCLUSION

Authors	Approach	Method	Nephrostomy Tube (Fr)	Patients	Ureter Successfully Occluded (%)	Procedures Per Patient	Complications	Follow-up
Fluoroscopically Guided Occlusion								
Kinn et al, 1986	Intraluminal	Polidocanol intramural injection nylon plugs	Yes (24–26)	15	67	1–2	Nausea, pain at injection site; 46% with plug migration	8 months (mean) (58% died at 7 months of primary disease)
Papanicolaou et al, 1985	Intraluminal	Nondetachable balloon	Yes (7–8)	3	33	1	Bleeding necessitating nephrectomy	≤4 weeks
Gaylord et al, 1989	Intraluminal	Gianturco coils with gelatin sponges	Yes (8–12)	5	100	1	2 urinary tract infections (responded to oral antibiotics)	9 months (1–22 months)
Hubner et al, 1992	Intramural	Detachable balloon	—	9	100	1–2	—	6–14 weeks
Schild et al, 1994	Intraluminal	Tissue adhesive and Gianturco coils	Yes	76	55	1–2	Perforation of ureteropelvic junction (2), septicemia (1), bleeding requiring embolization (1)	3.6 months (1 week–38 months)
		Detachable silicone-filled balloons			69			7.9 months (1 week–61 months)
Endoscopically Guided Occlusion								
Reddy and Sidi, 1990	Intraluminal	No. 5 Fr probe via No. 15 Fr flexible nephroscope to electrocoagulate proximal ureter	Yes (20)	4	100	1	None	2–21 months (3 died at 2, 3, and 21 months)

ureteral strictures (3%), ureteral fistulas, and funguria with associated fungal concretions (Oosterhof et al, 1989). Each of these problems can be approached endourologically. Urolithiasis in the transplant patient can be managed by standard percutaneous techniques. The technique for percutaneous stone removal in the transplant patient is almost identical to that in the nontransplant patient. Indeed, because of the proximity of the kidney to the skin surface and its anterior location, placement of the nephrostomy tract is simpler. It may be difficult to preplace a retrograde ureteral occlusion balloon catheter, however, because of the poorly accessible ureteral reimplantation site.

For **ureteral strictures,** antegrade catheter or balloon dilation from 4 to 10 mm using the **aforementioned techniques** and placement of a No. 6 to 12 Fr internal stent for 6 to 8 weeks can be therapeutic, especially if the stricture is in the distal ureter. Success rates for this approach range from 50% to 79% (Streem et al, 1986; Voegeli et al, 1988; Oosterhof et al, 1989). If this fails, the next step is endosurgical incision as previously described for other types of distal ureteral strictures.

The placement of a percutaneous nephroureterostomy tube can be beneficial in resolving a postoperative ureteral fistula. Streem and colleagues noted a satisfactory response in two of three patients managed in this way (Streem et al, 1986).

Lastly the percutaneous approach has been helpful in managing fungal complications of renal transplantation. Fungal growths within the collecting system can be percutaneously extracted, and topical antifungal agents (e.g., amphotericin B) can be administered via the nephrostomy tube (see "Fungal Bezoar") (Wise et al, 1982; Ireton et al, 1985).

ROLE OF PERCUTANEOUS RENAL SURGERY IN THE YEAR 2000

The simple percutaneous approach to the kidney will continue to have broad application through the next decade. For simple drainage procedures necessitated by obstruction or infection, the percutaneous nephrostomy will continue to offer the simplest yet most effective solution. For ablative procedures, such as percutaneous stone removal of large renal stones, there will likewise continue to be a significant and perhaps expanding role as more urologists become disenchanted with the results of ESWL for large or lower-pole renal calculi. Percutaneous ablative procedures for noncalculus entities, such as renal cysts and transitional cell cancer, will likely give way to laparoscopy and ureteroscopic approaches. In the realm of reconstructive renal and ureteral surgery, the percutaneous approach will likely again fall from favor as advances in ureteroscopic and retrograde fluoroscopic manipulation of the ureter become perfected.

The goal of the practical surgical sciences is to afford patients a surgical cure with minimal surgical morbidity. To this end, open surgery is being replaced by minimally invasive surgery; minimally invasive surgery eventually needs to be replaced in turn by noninvasive surgical techniques. This paradigm shift is what has largely happened to surgical urolithiasis; during the next decade, a similar change for ablative surgery will occur. For reconstructive surgery, a noninvasive solution is difficult to imagine; yet the hope of urology and surgery rests in the imagination of future urolo-

gists who will carry forward to realization ideas inconceivable to those of us in a position to write "definitive" book chapters. Urologists of today are both travelers and guides on an exciting journey leading us from blood and blades to terminals and telepresence.

REFERENCES

Abdel-Hakim AM: Endopyelotomy for UPJ obstruction: Is long-term stenting mandatory? J Endourol 1987; 1:265.
Abdel-Razzak O, Bagley DH: The 6.9F semirigid ureteroscope in clinical use. Urology 1993; 41:45.
Abeshouse BS, Abeshouse GA: Calyceal diverticulum: A report of sixteen cases and review of the literature. Urol Int 1963; 15:329.
Abramowitz J, Fowler JE Jr, Falhuni K, et al: Percutaneous identification and removal of fungus ball from renal pelvis. J Urol 1986; 135:1232.
Ahlawat R, Banerjee GK, Dalela D: Bilateral simultaneous percutaneous nephrolithotomy. Eur Urol 1995; 28:166.
Ahmadzadeh M: Use of a prototype 3-Fr needle electrode with flexible ureteroscopy for antegrade management of stenosed ureteroileal anastomosis. Urol Int 1992; 49:215.
Albala D, Meretyk S, Clayman RV, et al: Percutaneous procedures for purulent perirenal/renal processes: Pleural precautions. J Urol 1991; 145:235a.
Altemeyer WA, Alexander J: Retroperitoneal abscess. Arch Surg 1961; 83:512.
Bach D, Hanraths M, Maar K, Grabensee B: Ultrasound guided percutaneous biopsy or operative biopsy in patients with renal impairment? Int Urol Nephrol 1988; 20:519.
Badlani G, Eshghi M, Smith AD: Percutaneous surgery for UPJ obstruction (endopyelotomy): Technique and early results. J Urol 1986; 135:26.
Badlani G, Karlin G, Smith AD: Complications of endopyelotomy: Analysis in series of 64. J Urol 1988; 140:473.
Badlani GH, Smith A: Stent for endopyelotomy. Urol Clin North Am 1988; 15:445.
Bagley DH: Removal of upper urinary calculi with flexible ureteropyeloscopy. Urology 1990a; 35:412.
Bagley DH: Endoscopic ureteroureterostomy. J Urol 1990b; 143:235a.
Bagley DH, Huffman J, Lyon E, et al: Endoscopic ureteropyelotomy: Opening the obliterated ureteropelvic junction with nephroscopy and flexible ureteropyeloscopy. J Urol 1985; 133:462.
Bagley DH, Liu J, Grasso M, Goldberg BB: Endoluminal sonography in evaluation of the obstructed ureteropelvic junction. J Endourol 1994; 8:287.
Banner MP, Pollack HM: Dilation of ureteral stenoses: Techniques and experience in 44 patients. AJR 1984; 143:789.
Banner MP, Pollack HM, Amendola MA, et al: Percutaneous extraction of renal fungus ball (Letter to the editor). Am J Radiol 1988; 152:1342.
Bartone FF, Hurwitz RS, Rojas EL, et al: The role of percutaneous nephrostomy in the management of obstructing candidiasis of the urinary tract in infants. J Urol 1988; 140:338.
Batata MA, Whitmore WF Jr, Hilaris BS, et al: Primary carcinoma of the ureter: A prognostic study. Cancer 1975; 35:1626.
Bauer SB, Perlmutter AD, Retik AB: Anomalies of the upper urinary tract. In Walsh PC, Retik AB, Stamey TA, Vaughn ED Jr, eds: Cambell's Urology, 6th ed. Philadelphia, W.B. Saunders, 1992, pp 1376–1388.
Bean WJ: Renal cysts: Treatment with alcohol. Radiology 1981; 138:329.
Beckman CF, Roth RA: Secondary ureteropelvic junction stricture: Percutaneous dilation. Radiology 1987; 164:365.
Beckman CF, Roth RA, Bihrle W III: Dilation of benign ureteral strictures. Radiology 1989; 172:437.
Beland G, Piette Y: Urinary tract candidiasis: Report of a case with bilateral ureteral obstruction. Can Med Assoc J 1973; 108:472.
Bellman GC, Silverstein JI, Blickensderfer S, et al: Technique and follow-up of percutaneous management of caliceal diverticula. Urology 1993; 42:21.
Bellman GC, Sweetser P, Smith AD: Complications of intracavitary bacillus Calmette-Guerin after percutaneous resection of upper tract transitional cell carcinoma. J Urol 1994; 151:13.
Benoit G, Alexandre L, Moukarzel M, et al: Percutaneous antegrade dilation of ureteral strictures in kidney transplants. J Urol 1993; 150:37.
Blum JA: Acute monilial pyelohydronephrosis: Report of a case success-

fully treated with amphotericin B continuous renal pelvis irrigation. J Urol 1966; 96:614.

Blute ML, Segura JW, Patterson DE, et al: Impact of endourology on diagnosis and management of upper urinary tract urothelial cancer. J Urol 1989; 141:1298.

Boddy SAM, Kellett MS, Ransley PG, et al: Extracorporeal shock wave lithotripsy and percutaneous nephrolithotomy in children. J Pediatr Surg 1987; 22:223.

Boyce WH, Elkins IB: Reconstructive renal surgery following anatrophic nephrolithotomy: Follow up of 100 consecutive cases. J Urol 1974; 111:307.

Brandl H: Percutaneous ureteral occlusion with silicone olive. Fifth World Congress on Endourology and ESWL, Cairo, Egypt, 1987, p 90.

Brannen GE, Bush WH, Lewis GP: Endopyelotomy for primary repair of UPJ obstruction. J Urol 1988; 139:29.

Braun WE, Banowsky LH, Straffon RA, et al: Lymphoceles associated with renal transplantation: Report of 15 cases and review of the literature. Am J Med 1974; 57:714.

Brennan RE, Pollack HM: Nonvisualized ("phantom") renal calyx: Causes and radiological approach to diagnosis. Urol Radiol 1979; 1:17.

Brockis JG, Hulbert JC, Patel AS, et al: The diagnosis and treatment of lymphoceles associated with renal transplantation. Br J Urol 1978; 50:307.

Brooks JD, Kavoussi LR, Preminger GM, et al: Comparison of open and endourologic approaches to the obstructed ureteropelvic junction. Urology 1995; 46:791.

Burns JR, Joseph DB: Combination therapy for a partial staghorn calculus in an infant. J Endourol 1993; 7:469.

Caione P, Degennaro M, Capozza N, et al: Endoscopic manipulation of ureteral calculi in children by rigid operative ureteroscopy. J Urol 1990; 144:484.

Caldamone AA, Frank IN: Percutaneous aspiration in the treatment of renal abscess. J Urol 1980; 123:92.

Carson CC III: Endoscopic treatment of upper and lower urinary tract lesions using lasers. Semin Urol 1991; 9:185.

Carson CC III, Danneberger JE, Weinerth JL: Percutaneous lithotripsy in morbid obesity. J Urol 1987; 139:243.

Cassis AN, Brannen GE, Bush WH, et al: Endopyelotomy: Review of results and complications. J Urol 1991; 146:1492.

Castaneda-Zuniga WR: Establishing access: The percutaneous nephrostomy. *In* Clayman RV, Castaneda-Zuniga WR, eds: Techniques in Endourology: A Guide to the Percutaneous Removal of Renal and Ureteral Calculi. Chicago, Year Book Medical Publishers, 1984, p 73.

Castoldi MC, Del Moro RM, D'Urbano ML, et al: Sonography after renal biopsy: Assessment of its role in 230 consecutive cases. Abdom Imaging 1994; 19:72.

Catalona WM: Bladder cancer. *In* Gillenwater JY, Grayhack JT, Howards SS, Duckett JW, eds: Adult and Pediatric Urology. Chicago, Year Book Medical Publishers, 1987, p 1000.

Chandhoke PS, Albala DM, Clayman RV: Long-term comparison of renal function in patients with solitary kidneys and/or moderate renal insufficiency undergoing extracorporeal shock wave lithotripsy or percutaneous nephrolithotomy. J Urol 1992; 147:1226.

Chandhoke PS, Clayman RV, Stone AM, et al: Endopyelotomy and endoureterotomy with the Acucise ureteral cutting balloon device: Preliminary experience. J Endourol 1993; 7:45.

Chang R, Marshall FF, Mitchell S: Percutaneous management of benign ureteral strictures and fistulas. J Urol 1987; 137:1126.

Chao PW, Glanz S, Gordon DH, et al: Percutaneous ureteroneocystotomy for treatment of postoperative distal-ureteral stricture. J Endourol 1987; 1:55.

Chehval MJ, Nepute JQ, Purcell MH: Nephroscopic obliteration of an obstructing peripelvic renal cyst in conjunction with stone removal. J Endourol 1990; 4:259.

Chibber PJ: Percutaneous nephrolithotomy for large and staghorn calculi. J Endourol 1993; 7:293.

Chowdhury SD, Kenogbon J: Rigid ureteroscopic endopyelotomy without external drainage. J Endourol 1992; 6:357.

Clayman RV: Rigid and flexible nephroscopy. *In* Clayman RV, Castaneda-Zuniga Wr, eds: Techniques in Endourology: A Guide to the Percutaneous Removal of Renal and Ureteral Calculi. Chicago, Year Book Medical Publishers, 1984, p 153.

Clayman RV, Bagley DH: Ureteronephroscopy. *In* Gillenwater JY, Grayhack JT, Howards SS, Duckett JW, eds: Adult and Pediatric Urology. Chicago, Year Book Medical Publishers, 1990.

Clayman RV, Bub P, Haaff E, et al: Prone flexible cystoscopy: An adjunct to percutaneous stone removal. J Urol 1987a; 137:65.

Clayman RV, Castaneda-Zuniga WR: Calyceal diverticulum. *In* Techniques in Endourology: A Guide to the Percutaneous Removal of Renal and Ureteral Calculi. Dallas, Heritage Press, 1984, p 45.

Clayman RV, Castaneda-Zuniga WR, Hunter DW, et al: Rapid balloon dilatation of the nephrostomy tract for nephrostolithotomy. Radiology 1983a; 147:884.

Clayman RV, Denstedt JD: New technique: Ureteronephroscopic urothelial endoureteroplasty: Case report. J Endourol 1989; 3:425.

Clayman RV, Elbers J, Miller RP, et al: Percutaneous nephrostomy: Assessment of renal damage associated with semi-rigid (24F) and balloon (36F) dilation. Invest Urol 1987b; 138:203.

Clayman RV, Lange PH, Fraley EE: Cancer of the upper urinary tract. *In* Javadpour N, ed: Principles and Management of Urologic Cancer, 2nd ed. Baltimore, Williams & Wilkins, 1983b, p 544.

Clayman RV, McClennan BL, Garvin TJ, et al: Lithostar: An electromagnetic acoustic shock wave unit for extracorporeal lithotripsy. J Endourol 1989; 3:307.

Clayman RV, Surya V, Hunter D, et al: Renal vascular complications associated with percutaneous removal of renal calculi. J Urol 1984a; 132:228.

Clayman RV, Surya V, Miller RP, et al: Percutaneous nephrostolithotomy: Extraction of renal and ureteral calculi from 100 patients. J Urol 1984c; 131:868.

Clayman RV, Surya V, Miller RP, et al: Pursuit of the renal mass: Is ultrasound enough? Am J Med 1984; 77:218.

Cohan RH, Saeed M, Schwab SJ, et al: Povidone-iodine sclerosis of pelvic lymphoceles: A prospective study. Urol Radiol 1988; 10:203.

Cohan RH, Saeed M, Sussman SK, et al: Percutaneous drainage of pelvic lymphatic fluid collections in the renal transplant patient. Invest Radiol 1987; 11:864.

Cohen AH, Nast CC, Adler SG, et al: Clinical utility of kidney biopsies in the diagnosis and management of renal disease. Am J Nephrol 1989; 9:309.

Coleman CC: Percutaneous nephrolithotomy: Dilation techniques. *In* Amplatz K, Lange PH, eds: Atlas of Endourology. Chicago, Year Book Medical Publishers, 1986, p 131.

Coleman CC, Kimura Y, Castaneda-Zuniga WR, et al: Interventional techniques in the ureter. Semin Intervent Radiol 1984a; 1:24.

Coleman CC, Kimura Y, Reddy P, et al: Complications of nephrostolithotomy. Semin Intervent Radiol 1984b; 1:70.

Colon-Perez B, Canto RJ, Ramos ME: Simultaneous bilateral nephrostolithotomies: Immediate results in three cases. J Endourol 1987; 1:209.

Cornud Fr, Mendelsberg M, Chretien Y, et al: Fluoroscopically guided percutaneous transrenal electroincision of ureterointestinal anastomotic strictures. J Urol 1992; 147:578.

Cronan JJ, Amic ES, Dorfman GS: Percutaneous drainage of renal abscess. J Urol 1980; 123:92.

Cronan JJ, Armiag ES Jr, Dorfman GS: Percutaneous drainage of renal abscesses. Am J Radiol 1984; 142:351.

Cubelli V, Smith AD: Transurethral ureteral surgery guided by fluoroscopy. Endourology 1987; 2:8.

Cussenot O, Bassi S, Desgrandchamps F, et al: Outcomes of non-self-expandable metal prosthesis in strictured human ureter: Suggestions for future developments. J Endourol 1993; 7:205.

Cuzin B, Abbar M, Dawahra M, et al: 100 percutaneous endopyelotomies: Technique, indications, results. Prog Urol 1992; 2:559.

Dalton D, Neiman H, Grayhack JT: The natural history of simple renal cysts: A preliminary study. J Urol 1986; 135:905.

Damico CF, Mebust WK, Valk WL, et al: Triamcinolone: Adjuvant therapy for vesical neck contracture. J Urol 1973; 110:203.

Danuser H, Ackerman DK, Marth DC, et al: Extracorporeal shock wave lithotripsy in situ or after push-up for upper ureteral calculi: A prospective randomized trial. J Urol 1993; 150:824.

Darcy MD, Jung GB, Smith TP, et al: Percutaneously applied ureteral clips: Treatment of vesicovaginal fistula. Radiology 1987; 163:819.

Davis DM: Intubated ureterotomy: A new operation for ureteral and ureteropelvic stricture. Surg Gynecol Obstet 1943; 76:513.

Davis DM: Intubated ureterotomy. J Urol 1951; 66:77.

Davis DM, Strong GH, Drake WM: Intubated ureterotomy: Experimental work and clinical results. J Urol 1948; 59:851.

Deane RF, Buckley JF, Scott R, et al: Retrograde balloon rupture for pelviureteric junction obstruction. J Urol 1992; 147:434a.

Delaney VB, Adler S, Bruns FJ, et al: Autosomal dominant polycystic kidney disease: Presentation, complications, and prognosis. Am J Kidney Dis 1985; 5:104.

Dembner AG, Pfister RC: Fungal infection of the urinary tract: Demonstration by antegrade pyelography and drainage by percutaneous nephrostomy. AJR 1977; 129:415.

Denovic M, Darzynkiewicz A, Kostryrka-Claps ML, et al: Flow cytometry of low stage bladder tumors. Cancer 1982; 48:109.

Denstedt JD: Use of Swiss lithoclast for percutaneous nephrolithotomy. J Endourol 1993; 7:477.

Denstedt JD, Clayman RV: Electrohydraulic lithotripsy of renal and ureteral calculi. J Urol 1990; 143:13.

Desgrandchamps F, Cussenot O, Bassi S, et al: Percutaneous extra-anatomic nephrovesical diversion: Preliminary report. J Endourol 1993; 7:323.

Desgrandchamps F, Cussenot O, Meria P, et al: Subcutaneous urinary diversions for palliative treatment of pelvic malignancies. J Urol 1995; 154:367.

Desnos E: The nineteenth century. In Murphy LJT, ed: The History of Urology. Springfield, IL, Charles C Thomas, 1972, p 180.

Dierks SM, Clayman RV, Kavoussi LR, et al: Intraureteral surgery: Appropriate cutting modality. J Endourol 1990; 4:s114.

Dixon GD, Moore JD, Stockton R: Successful dilatation of ureteroileal anastomotic stenosis using Gruntzig catheter. Urology 1982; 19:555.

Doemeny JM, Banner MP, Shapiro MJ, et al: Percutaneous extraction of renal fungus ball. Am J Radiol 1988; 150:1331.

Dowd PE, Mata JA, Arden C, et al: Ultrasound guided percutaneous renal biopsy using an automatic core biopsy system. J Urol 1991; 135:912.

Doyle AJ, Gregory MC, Terreros DA: Percutaneous native renal biopsy: Comparison of a 1.2 mm spring-driven system with a traditional 2 mm hand-driven system. Am J Kidney Dis 1994; 23:498.

Drach GW, Dretler S, Fair W, et al: Report of the United States cooperative study of extracorporeal shock wave lithotripsy. J Urol 1986; 135:1127.

Dretler SP, Bhatta KM: Clinical experience with high power (140mj) large fiber (320 micron) pulsed dye laser lithotripsy. J Urol 1991; 146:1228–1231.

Dretler SP, Young RH: Stone granuloma: A cause of ureteral stricture. J Urol 1993; 150:1800.

Droller MJ: TCC: Upper tracts and bladder. In Walsh PC, Gittes RF, Perlmutter AD, Stamey TA, eds: Campbell's Urology, 5th ed. Philadelphia, W.B. Saunders, 1986, p 1382.

Dunnick NR, Carson CC III, Braun SD, et al: Complications of percutaneous nephrostolithotomy. Radiology 1985; 157:51.

Eastham JA, Huffman JL: Technique of mitomycin C instillation in the treatment of upper urinary tract urothelial tumors. J Urol 1993; 150(2 part 1):324.

Edelstein H, McCabe RE: Perinephric abscess: Modern diagnosis and treatment in 47 cases. Medicine 1988; 67:118.

Eickenberg HU: Percutaneous surgery of renal cysts. J Urol 1985; 133:200a.

Eisenberger Fr, Rassweiler J, Bub P, et al: Differentiated approach to staghorn calculi using extra-corporeal shock wave lithotripsy and percutaneous nephrolithotomy: An analysis of 151 consecutive cases. World J Urol 1987; 5:248.

Elashry OM, Nakada SY, Dimeglio R, et al: Intracorporeal electrohydraulic lithotripsy (electrohydraulic) of ureteral and renal calculi using small caliber (< 1.9F) electrohydraulic probes. J Urol 1996; (in press).

El-Damanhoury H, Scharfe T, Ruth J, et al: Extracorporeal shock wave lithotripsy of urinary calculi: Experience in treatment of 3,278 patients using the Siemens lithostar and lithostar plus. J Urol 1991; 145:484.

Ellis JH, Patterson SK, Sonda LP, et al: Stones and infection in renal caliceal diverticula: Treatment with percutaneous procedures. AJR 1991; 156:995.

Elyaderani MK, Moncman J: Value of ultrasonography, fine needle aspiration and percutaneous drainage of perinephric abscesses. South Med J 1985; 78:685.

Engel RM: Complications of bilateral uretero-ileo cutaneous urinary diversion: A review of 208 cases. J Urol 1969; 101:508.

Erturke E, Herrman E, Cockett ATK: Extracorporeal shock wave lithotripsy for distal ureteral stones. J Urol 1993; 149:1425.

Eshghi M: Endoscopic incisions of the urinary tract. AUA Update Series 1989; Vol 8, Lesson 37–39.

Eshghi M, Franco I, Schwalb D, et al: Cold knife endoureterotomy of 40 strictures (Abstract P6-4). Seventh World Congress on Endourology and ESWL, Kyoto, Japan, 1989.

Eshghi M, Tuong W, Fernandez R, et al: Percutaneous (endo) infundibulotomy. J Endourol 1987; 1:107.

Esuvaranathan K, Tan EC, Tung KH, et al: Stones in horseshoe kidneys: Results of treatment by extracorporeal shock wave lithotripsy and endourology. J Urol 1991; 146:1213.

Farah NB, Roddie M, Lord RHH, et al: Ureteric obstruction in renal transplants: The role of percutaneous balloon dilatation. Nephrol Dial Transplant 1991; 6:977.

Farah RN, Diloreto RR, Cerny JC: Transurethral resection combined with steroid injection in treatment of recurrent vesical neck contracture. Urology 1979; 13:395.

Fernstrom I, Johansson B: Percutaneous pyelolithotomy. Scand J Urol Nephrol 1976; 10:257.

Figenshau RS, Clayman RV, Colberg JW, et al: Pediatric endopyelotomy: The Washington University experience. J Urol 1996; (in press).

Figenshau RS, Clayman RV, Wick MR, et al: Acute histologic changes associated with endoureterotomy in the normal pig ureter. J Endourol 1991; 5:357.

Finnerty DP, Trulock TS, Berkman W, et al: Transluminal balloon dilation of ureteral stricture. J Urol 1984; 131:1056.

Floth A, Anzbock W: Melting and fracture of the cutting wire: A possible complication of Acucise endopyelotomy. J Endourol 1995; 9:s97.

Fotino S: The solitary kidney: A model of chronic hyperfiltration in humans. Am J Kidney Dis 1989; 13:88.

Fowler JE Jr, Perkins T: Presentation, diagnosis and treatment of renal abscesses: 1972–1988. J Urol 1994; 151:847.

Fraley EE: Dismembered infundibulopyelostomy: Improved technique for correcting vascular obstruction of the superior infundibulum. J Urol 1969; 101:144.

Fuchs AM, Fuchs GJ: Retrograde intrarenal surgery for calculus disease: New minimally invasive treatment approach. J Endourol 1990; 4:337.

Fuchs GJ, David RD: Flexible ureterorenoscopy, dilation of narrow caliceal neck, and ESWL: A new, minimally invasive approach to stones in caliceal diverticula. J Endourol 1989; 3:255.

Gallucci M, Alpi G, Ricciuti GP, et al: Retrograde cold-knife endopyelotomy in secondary stenosis of the UPJ. J Endourol 1991; 5:49.

Gardner SM, Wolf JS Jr, Nakada SY, et al: The unintubated endoureterotomy endourologically revisited. J Endourol 1995; 9:s51.

Gaylord GM, Johnsrude IS: Transrenal ureteral occlusion with Gianturco coils and gelatin sponge. Radiology 1989; 172:1047.

Gelet A, Lo'pez JG, Cuzin B, et al: Endopyelotomy with the Acucise balloon device: Preliminary results (Abstract 59). XI Congress of the European Association of Urology, Berlin, 1994, p 31.

Gelet A, Martin X, Dessouki T: Ureteropelvic invagination: Reliable technique of endopyelotomy. J Endourol 1991; 5:223.

Gerber GS, Lyon ES: Endopyelotomy: Patient selection, results, and complications. Urology 1994; 43:2.

Gerber GS, Lyon ES: Endourological management of upper tract urothelial tumors. J Urol 1993; 150:2.

Germinale Fr, Bottino P, Caviglia C, et al: Endourologic treatment of ureterointestinal strictures. J Endourol 1992; 6:439.

Gerzof SC, Johnson WC, Robbins AH, et al: Expanded criteria for percutaneous abscess drainage. Arch Surg 1985; 120:227.

Gerzof SG, Gale ME: Computed tomography and ultrasonography for the diagnosis and treatment of renal and retroperitoneal abscesses. Urol Clin North Am 1982; 9:185.

Gibbons RP, Bush WH Jr, Burnett LL: Needle tract seeding following aspiration of renal cell carcinoma. J Urol 1977; 118:865.

Gilbert R, Garra B, Gibbons MD: Renal duplex Doppler ultrasound: An adjunct in the evaluation of hydronephrosis in the child. J Urol 1993; 150:1192.

Gill IS, Clayman RV, McDougall EM: Advances in urological laparoscopy. J Urol 1995; 154:1275.

Gillam JFE, Wadelton DH: A case of renal moniliasis. Br Med J 1958; 1:985.

Gillenwater JY: Hydronephrosis. In Gillenwater JY, Grayhack JT, Howards SS, Duckett JW, eds: Hydronephrosis in Adult and Pediatric Urology, 3rd ed. Chicago, Year Book Medical Publishers, 1996, p 973.

Gil-Vernet J: New surgical concepts in removing renal calculi. Urol Int 1965; 20:255.

Gittes RF: Management of transitional cell carcinoma of the upper tract: Case for conservative local excision. Urol Clin North Am 1980; 7:559.

Glanz S, Gordon PH, Butt K, et al: Percutaneous transrenal balloon dilation of the ureter. Radiology 1983; 149:101.

Gleeson M, Lerner SP, Griffith DP: Treatment of staghorn calculi with extracorporeal shock-wave lithotripsy and percutaneous nephrolithotomy. Urology 1991; 38:145.

Glinz M, Ackermann D, Zingg EJ: The balloon-catheter Acucise: An important instrument for endoureterotomy (Abstract 62). XI Congress of the European Association of Urology, Berlin, 1994, p 32.

Glinz M, Merz V, Ackermann D, et al: Impact of the pelvicaliceal size on the success rate of endopyelotomy (Abstract 63). XI Congress of the European Association of Urology, Berlin, 1994, p 33.

Goldman SM, Minkin SD, Naraval DC, et al: Renal carbuncle: The use of ultrasound in its diagnosis and management. J Urol 1977; 118:525.

Goodwin WE, Casey WC, Woolfe W: Percutaneous trocar (needle) nephrostomy in hydronephrosis. JAMA 1955; 157:891.

Gort HB, Mali WP, van Wases PF, et al: Metallic self-expandable stenting of a ureteroileal stricture. AJR 1990; 152:422.

Gothlin JH, Gadeholt G, Farsund T, et al: Percutaneous antegrade dilatation of distal ureteral strictures and obstruction. Eur J Radiol 1988; 8:217.

Graff J, Benkert S, Pastor J, et al: Experience with a new multi functional lithotriptor, the Dorneir MFL 5000: Results of 415 treatments. J Endourol 1989; 3:315.

Graff J, Diederichs W, Schulze H: Long term follow up in 1,003 extracorporeal shock wave lithotripsy patients. J Urol 1988; 140:479.

Grasso M, Lang G, Loisides P, et al: Endoscopic management of the symptomatic caliceal diverticular calculus. J Urol 1995; 153:1878.

Grossman HB, Schwartz SL, Konnak JW: Ureteroscopic treatment of urothelial carcinoma of the ureter and renal pelvis. J Urol 1992; 148:275.

Gupta M, Bolton DM, Gupta PN, et al: Improved renal function following aggressive treatment of urolithiasis and concurrent mild to moderate renal insufficiency. J Urol 1994; 152:1086.

Gutierrez J, Munoz A, Sedano I: Percutaneous endopyelotomy: Results with the over the wire guide cold knife technique. J Endourol 1994; 8:s100.

Guz B, Streem SB, Novick AC, et al: Role of percutaneous nephrostomy in patients with upper tract transitional cell carcinoma. Urology 1991; 37:331.

Haaga JR: Imaging intra-abdominal abscesses and nonoperative drainage procedures. World J Surg 1990; 14:204.

Haaga JR, Alfidi RJ, Harvilla TR: CT detection and aspiration of abdominal abscess. AJR 1977; 128:465.

Hamm FC, Weinberg SR: Renal and ureteral surgery without intubation. J Urol 1955; 73:475.

Hamm FC, Weinberg SR: Experimental studies of regeneration of the ureter without intubation. J Urol 1956; 75:43.

Hanna MK, Jeffs RD, Sturgess JM, et al: Ureteral structure and ultrastructure: I. The normal human ureter. J Urol 1976a; 116:718.

Hanna MJ, Jeffs RD, Sturgess JM, et al: Ureteral structure and ultrastructure: II. Congenital ureteropelvic junction obstruction and primary obstructive megaureter. J Urol 1976b; 116:725.

Harrach LB, Burkholder GV, Goodwin WE: Renal candidiasis—a cause of anuria. Br J Urol 1970; 42:258.

Hawkins IF Jr, Hunter P, Leal J, et al: Retrograde nephrostomy for stone removal: Combined cystoscopic/percutaneous technique. Am J Radiol 1984; 143:299.

Healy ME, Teng SS, Moss AA: Uriniferous pseudocyst? Computed tomographic findings. Radiology 1984; 153:757.

Hendrikx AJM, Bierkens AF, Bos R, et al: Treatment of stones in caliceal diverticula: Extracorporeal shock wave lithotripsy versus percutaneous nephrolitholapaxy. Br J Urol 1992; 70:478.

Heney NM, Nocks BN, Daly JJ, et al: Prognostic factors in carcinoma of the ureter. J Urol 1981; 125:632.

Herr HW: Durable response of a carcinoma in situ of the renal pelvis to topical bacillus Calmette-Guerin. J Urol 1985; 134:531.

Hill DE, Segura JW, Patterson DE, et al: Ureteroscopy in children. J Urol 1990; 144:481.

Hofbauer J, Hobarth K, Marberger M: Lithoclast: New and inexpensive mode of intracorporeal lithotripsy. J Endourol 1992; 6:429.

Hofmann R, Stoller ML: Endoscopic and open stone surgery in morbidly obese patients. J Urol 1992; 148:1108.

Holmberg G, Hietala SO: Treatment of simple renal cysts by percutaneous puncture and instillation of bismuth phosphate. Scand J Urol Nephrol 1989; 23:207.

Hopper KD, Sherman JL, Luethke JM, et al: The retrorenal colon in the supine and prone patient. Radiology 1987; 162:443.

Horgan J, Cubelli V, Lee WJ, et al: Endourologic stenting of ureteroileal anastomotic stricture: Cope modification. J Endourol 1988; 1:275.

Huang A, Low RK, White RD: Nephrostomy tract tumor seeding following percutaneous manipulation of a ureteral carcinoma. J Urol 1995; 153:1041.

Hubner WA, Irby P, Stoller ML: Natural history and current concepts for the treatment of small ureteral calculi. Eur Urol 1993; 24:172.

Hubner W, Knoll M, Porpaczy P: Percutaneous transrenal ureteral occlusion: Indication and technique. Urol Radiol 1992; 13:177.

Hubner W, Pfab R, Porpaczy P, et al: Renal cysts: Percutaneous resection with standard urologic instruments. J Endourol 1990; 4:61.

Huffman JL: Ureteroscopic management of transitional cell carcinoma of the upper urinary tract. Urol Clin North Am 1988; 15:419.

Huffman JL: Endoscopic management of upper urinary tract urothelial cancer. J Endourol 1990; 4:s-141.

Huffman JL, Bagley DH, Lyon ES, et al: Endoscopic diagnosis and treatment of upper tract urothelial tumors: A preliminary report. Cancer 1985a; 55:1422.

Huffman JL, Morse MJ, Herr HW, et al: Ureteropyeloscopy: The diagnostic and therapeutic approach to upper tract urothelial tumors. World J Urol 1985b; 3:58.

Hulbert JC: Percutaneous endoscopic management of the completely obliterated ureteropelvic junction. J Endourol 1990; 4:s142.

Hulbert JC, Hernandez J, Hunter DW, et al: Current concepts in the management of pyelocaliceal diverticula. J Endourol 1988a; 2:11.

Hulbert JC, Hunter D, Castaneda-Zuniga WR: Classification of and techniques for the reconstitution of acquired strictures in the region of the ureteropelvic junction. J Urol 1988b; 140:468.

Hulbert JC, Hunter D, Young AT, et al: Percutaneous intrarenal marsupialization of a perirenal cystic collection—endocystolysis. J Urol 1988c; 139:1039.

Hulbert JC, Lapointe S, Reddy PK, et al: Percutaneous endoscopic fulguration of a large volume caliceal diverticulum. J Urol 1987; 138:116.

Hulbert JC, Reddy PK, Hunter DW, et al: Percutaneous techniques for the management of caliceal diverticula containing calculi. J Urol 1986; 135:225.

Hwang T, Park Y: Endoscopic infundibulotomy in tuberculous renal infundibular stricture. J Urol 1994; 151:852.

Inglis JA, Tolley DA: Ureteroscopic pyelolysis for pelviureteric junction obstruction. Br J Urol 1986; 58:250.

Inglis JA, Tolley DA: Conservative management of transitional cell carcinoma of the renal pelvis. J Endourol 1988; 2:27.

Irby PB, Stoller ML, McAninch JW: Fungal bezoars of the upper urinary tract. J Urol 1990; 143:447.

Ireton RC: Percutaneous nephrostomy tract incision using modified Otis urethrotome. Urol Clin North Am 1990; 17:95.

Ireton RC, Krieger JN, Rudd TG, et al: Percutaneous endoscopic treatment of fungus ball obstruction in a renal allograft. Transplantation 1985; 39:453.

Janetschek G: Percutaneous intrarenal surgery for calyceal stones, infundibular stenosis, calyceal diverticula, and obstruction of the ureteropelvic junction. J Urol 1988; 139:187a.

Jaques P, Mauro M, Safrit H, et al: CT features of intraabdominal abscesses. AJR 1986; 146:1041.

Jarrett TW, Sweetser PM, Weiss GH, et al: Percutaneous management of transitional cell carcinoma of the renal collecting system: 9-year experience. J Urol 1995; 154:1629.

Jenkins JM: Editorial comment. Urology 1994; 43:186.

Jewitt MAS, Bombardier C, Menchoins CWB: Comparative costs of the various strategies of urinary stone disease management. Urology 1995; 46(suppl 3a):15.

Johansson S, Wahlquist L: A prognostic study of urothelial renal pelvic tumors. Cancer 1979; 43:2525.

Johnson DC, Oke EJ, Dunnick RN, et al: Percutaneous balloon dilation of ureteral strictures. AJR 1987; 148:181.

Jones DJ, Wickham JA, Kellett MJ: Percutaneous nephrolithotomy for calculi in horseshoe kidneys. J Urol 1991; 145:481.

Jones JA, Lingeman JE, Steidle CP: The roles of extracorporeal shock wave lithotripsy and percutaneous nephrolithotomy in the management of pyelocaliceal diverticula. J Urol 1991; 146:724.

Kachel TA, Vijan SR, Dretler SP: Endourological experience with cystine calculi and a treatment algorithm. J Urol 1991; 145:25.

Kadir S, White RI Jr, Engel R: Balloon dilatation of a UPJ obstruction. Radiology 1982; 143:263.

Kaneti J, Hertzanu Y: Renal abscess owing to *Salmonella* septicemia: Percutaneous drainage. J Urol 1987; 138:395.

Karlin GS, Rich M, Lee W, et al: Endourological management of upper-tract fungal infection. J Endourol 1987; 1:49.

Karlin GS, Smith AD: Endopyelotomy. Urol Clin North Am 1988; 15:433.

Karlsen S, Gjolberg T: Branched renal calculi treated by percutaneous nephrolithotomy and extracorporeal shock waves. Scand J Urol Nephrol 1989; 23:201.

Kavoussi LR, Albala DM, Clayman RV: Outcome of a secondary open surgical procedure in patients who failed primary endopyelotomy. Br J Urol 1993; 72:157.

Kaye KW, Clayman RV: Tamponade nephrostomy catheter for percutaneous nephrostolithotomy. Urology 1986; 27:441.

Kaye KW, Lange PH: Mode of presentation of invasive bladder cancer: Reassessment of the problem. J Urol 1982; 128:31.

Keane PF, McKenna M, Johnston SR: Fungal bezoar causing ureteric obstruction. Br J Urol 1993; 72:247.

Kendall AR, Senay BA, Coll ME: Spontaneous subcapsular renal hematoma: Diagnosis and management. J Urol 1988; 139:246.

Kerbl K, Chandhoke PS, Figenshau RS, et al: Effect of stent duration on ureteral healing following endoureterotomy in an animal model. J Urol 1993; 150:1302.

Kerbl K, Clayman RV, Chandhoke PS, et al: Percutaneous stone removal with the patient in a flank position. J Urol 1994a; 151:686.

Kerbl K, Clayman RV: Incision of the ureterovesical junction for endoscopic surveillance of transitional cell carcinoma of the upper urinary tract. J Urol 1993; 150:1440.

Kerbl K, Picus DD, Clayman RV: Clinical experience with the Kaye nephrostomy tamponade catheter. Eur Urol 1994b; 25:94.

Kerlan RK Jr, Kahn RK, Laberge JM, et al: Percutaneous removal of renal staghorn calculi. AJR 1985; 145:797.

Kessaris DN, Bellman GC, Pardalidis NP, et al: Management of hemorrhage after percutaneous renal surgery. J Urol 1995; 153:604.

Khorram O, Stern JL: Bleomycin sclerotherapy of an intractable inguinal lymphocyst. Gynecol Oncol 1993; 50:244.

Kim J, Banner MP, Ramchandani P, et al: Balloon dilation of ureteral strictures after renal transplantation. Radiology 1993; 186:717.

Kinn A, Ohlsen H, Brehmer-Andersson E, et al: Therapeutic ureteral occlusion in advanced pelvic malignant tumors. J Urol 1986; 135:29.

Kletscher BA, Segura JW, Leroy AJ, et al: Percutaneous antegrade endoscopic pyelotomy: Review of 50 consecutive cases. J Urol 1995; 153:701.

Knoll LD, Segura JW, Patterson DE, et al: Long-term follow-up in patients with cystine urinary calculi treated by percutaneous ultrasonic lithotripsy. J Urol 1988; 140:246.

Knopf HJ, Diederich R, Sommerfeld HJ: Extracorporeal shock wave lithotripsy (ESWL) in horseshoe kidneys. J Endourol 1993; 7(suppl 1):s15.

Koga S, Arakaki V, Matsuoka M, et al: Staghorn calculi—long-term results of management. Br J Urol 1991; 68:122.

Korth K, Kuenkel J: Unusual applications of ureteroscopy. Urol Clin North Am 1988; 15:459.

Kramolowsky EV, Clayman RV, Weyman PJ: Endourologic management of ureteroileal anastomotic strictures: Is it effective? J Urol 1987a; 137:390.

Kramolowsky EV, Clayman RV, Weyman PJ: Management of ureterointestinal anastomotic strictures: Comparison of open surgical and endourological repair. J Urol 1988; 139:1195.

Kramolowsky EV, Tucker RD, Nelson CMK: Management of benign ureteral strictures: Open surgical repair on endoscopic dilation? J Urol 1989; 141:285.

Kramolowsky EV, Willoughby BL, Loening SA: Extracorporeal shock wave lithotripsy in children. J Urol 1987b; 137:939.

Krestin GP: Magnetic resonance imaging of the kidneys: Current status. Magn Reson Q 1994; 10:2.

Krogh J, Kvist E, Rye B: Transitional cell carcinoma of the upper urinary tract: Prognostic variables and post-operative recurrences. Br J Urol 1991; 67:32.

Kroovand RL, Harrison LH, McCullough DL: Extracorporeal shock wave lithotripsy in childhood. J Urol 1987; 138:1106.

Krueger RP, Ash JM, Silver MM, et al: Primary hydronephrosis: Assessment of diuretic renography, pelvis perfusion pressure, operative findings, and renal and ureteral histology. Urol Clin North Am 1980; 7:231.

Kuenkel M, Korth K: Endopyelotomy: Results after long-term follow-up of 135 patients. J Endourol 1990; 4:109.

Kulp DA, Bagley DH: Does flexible ureteropyeloscopy promote local recurrence of transitional cell carcinoma? J Endourol 1994; 8:111.

Kurth K, Hohenfellner R, Altwein JE: Ultrasound litholapaxy of a staghorn calculus. J Urol 1977; 117:242.

Kwak S, Leef JA, Rosenblum JD: Percutaneous balloon catheter dilatation of benign ureteral strictures: Effect of multiple dilatation procedures on long-term patency. AJR 1995; 165:97.

Lam HS, Lingeman JE, Barron M, et al: Staghorn calculi: Analysis of treatment results between initial percutaneous nephrostolithotomy and extracorporeal shock wave lithotripsy monotherapy with reference to surface area. J Urol 1992a; 147:1219.

Lam HS, Lingeman JE, Mosbaugh PG, et al: Evolution of the technique of combination therapy for staghorn calculi: A decreasing role for extracorporeal shock wave lithotripsy. J Urol 1992b; 148:1058.

Lam H, Lingeman JE, Russo R, et al: Stone surface area determination techniques: A unifying concept of staghorn stone burden assessment. J Urol 1992c; 148:1026–1029.

Lang EK: Antegrade ureteral stenting for dehiscence, strictures, and fistulae. AJR 1984; 143:795.

Lang EK: Percutaneous infundibuloplasty: Management of calyceal diverticula and infundibular stenosis. Radiology 1991; 181:871.

Lang EK, Glorioso LW III: Management of urinomas by percutaneous drainage procedures. Radiol Clin North Am 1986; 24:551.

Lang EK, Glorioso LW III: Antegrade transluminal dilation of benign ureteral strictures: Long term results. AJR 1988; 150:131.

Lanigan D, Wells IP, Choa RG, et al: Endoscopic balloon lysis of pelviureteric junction obstruction. Society of Minimally Invasive Therapy, Fourth International Meeting, Dublin, E-94, 1992.

Laucks SP Jr, McLachlan MSF: Aging and simple cysts of the kidney. Br J Radiol 1981; 54:12.

Lawson RK, Murphy JB, Taylor AJ, et al: Retrograde method for percutaneous access to kidney. Urology 1983; 22:580.

Leal JJ: A new procedure for biopsy of a solid renal mass: Transurethral approach under fluoroscopic control. J Urol 1992; 148:98.

Lee WJ, Smith AD, Cubelli V, et al: Percutaneous nephrolithotomy: Analysis of 500 consecutive patients. Urol Radiol 1986; 8:61.

Lee WJ, Smith AD, Cubelli V, et al: Complications of percutaneous nephrolithotomy. AJR 1987; 148:177.

Leroy AJ, Williams HJ Jr, Bender CE, et al: Colon perforation following percutaneous nephrostomy and renal calculus removal. Radiology 1985; 155:83.

Levine SR, Emmett JL, Woolner LB: Cyst and tumor occurring in the same kidney (discussion). Trans Am Assoc Genitourin Surg 1963; 55:126.

Lim DJ, Shattuck MC, Cook WA: Pyelovenous lymphatic migration of transitional cell carcinoma following flexible ureterorenoscopy. J Urol 1993; 149:109.

Lingam K, Paterson PJ, Lingam MK, et al: Subcutaneous urinary diversion: An alternative to percutaneous nephrostomy. J Urol 1994; 152:70.

Lingeman JE, Siegel YI, Newman DM: Endopyelotomy for primary UPJ obstruction in the pediatric population. J Urol 1993; 149:423a.

Lingeman JE, Siegel YI, Steele B, et al: Management of lower pole nephrolithiasis: A critical analysis. J Urol 1994; 151:663.

Lingeman JE, Smith LH, Woods JR, et al: Bioeffects and long-term results of ESWL. In Lingeman JE, Smith LH, Woods JR, Newman DM, eds: Urinary Calculi: ESWL, Endourology, and Medical Therapy. Philadelphia, Lea & Febiger, 1989, pp 273–292.

Liong ML, Clayman RV, Gittes RF, et al: Treatment options for proximal ureteral urolithiasis: Review and recommendations. J Urol 1989; 141:504.

Loening S, Narayana A, Yoder L, et al: Factors influencing the recurrence rate of bladder cancer. J Urol 1980; 123:29.

Maggio MI, Nicely ER, Peppas DS, et al: An evaluation of 646 stone patients treated on the HM4 extracorporeal shock wave lithotriptor. J Urol 1992; 148:1114.

Mahoney SA, Koletsky S, Persky L: Approximation and dilatation: The mode of healing of an intubated ureterostomy. J Urol 1962; 88:197.

Maizels M, Firlit CF, Conway JJ, et al: Troubleshooting the diuretic renogram. Urology 1986; 28:355.

Malden ES, Picus D, Clayman RV: Arteriovenous fistula complicating endopyelotomy. J Urol 1992; 148:1520.

Malek RS: Urolithiasis. In Kelalis PP, King LR, Belman AB, eds: Clinical Pediatric Urology, 2nd ed. Philadelphia, W.B. Saunders, 1985, p 1093.

Marberger M, Stackl W, Hruby W: Percutaneous litholapaxy of renal calculi with ultrasound. Eur Urol 1982; 8:236.

Martin EC, Fankuchen EI, Casarella WJ: Percutaneous dilatation of ureteroenteric strictures or occlusions in ileal conduits. Urol Radiol 1982; 4:19.

Martinez-Pineiro JA, Togores LH, Martinez-Piniero L, et al: Endourologic surgery of urothelial tumors of the upper urinary tract. Arch Esp de Urol 1991; 44:529.

Mays N, Petruckevitch A, Burney PG: Results of one and two year follow-up in a clinical comparison of extracorporeal shock wave lithotripsy and percutaneous nephrolithotomy in the treatment of renal calculi. Scand J Urol Nephrol 1992; 26:43.

Mazeman E: Tumors of the upper urinary tract calyces, renal pelvis and ureter. Eur Urol 1976; 2:120.

McClinton S, Steyn JH, Hussey JK: Retrograde balloon dilatation for pelviureteric junction obstruction. Br J Urol 1993; 71:152.

McDonald JH, Calams JA: Experimental ureteral stricture: Ureteral regrowth following ureterotomy with and without intubation. J Urol 1960; 84:52.

McDougall EM, Denstedt JD, Brown RD, et al: Comparison of extracorporeal shock wave lithotripsy and percutaneous nephrolithotomy for the treatment of renal calculi in lower pole calices. J Endourol 1989; 3:265.

McDowell GC, Babaian RJ, Johnson DE: Management of symptomatic lymphocele via percutaneous drainage and sclerotherapy with tetracycline. Urology 1991; 37:237.

Melamed MR: Flow cytometry of the urinary bladder. Urol Clin North Am 1984; 11:599.

Meretyk I, Meretyk S, Clayman R: Endopyelotomy: Comparison of ureteroscopic retrograde and antegrade percutaneous techniques. J Urol 1992; 148:775.

Meretyk S, Albala DM, Clayman RV, et al: Endoureterotomy for treatment of ureteral strictures. J Urol 1992a; 147:1502.

Meretyk S, Clayman RV, Kavoussi LR, et al: Endourological treatment of ureteroenteric anastomotic strictures: Long-term follow-up. J Urol 1991; 145:723.

Meretyk S, Clayman RV, Kavoussi LR, et al: Caveat emptor: Caliceal stones and the missing calix. J Urol 1992b; 147:1091.

Mikkelsen DJ, Kavoussi LR, Clayman RV, et al: Advances in flexible deflectable ureteronephroscopy (FDU): Intrarenal surgery. J Urol 1989; 141:192a.

Miller RA, Wickham JEA: Percutaneous nephrolithotomy: Advances in equipment and endoscopic techniques. Urology 1984; 23(suppl 5):2.

Mobley TB, Myers DA, Jenkins JM, et al: Effects of stents on lithotripsy of ureteral calculi: Treatment results in 18,825 calculi using the Lithostar lithotriptor. J Urol 1994; 152:53.

Moldwin RM, Smith AD: Percutaneous management of ureteral fistulas. Urol Clin North Am 1988; 15:453.

Moon YT, Kerbl K, Gardner SM, et al: Evaluation of optimal stent size after endourologic incision of ureteral strictures. J Urol 1994; 151:338a.

Morano JU, Burkhalter JL: Percutaneous catheter drainage of post-traumatic urinoma. J Urol 1985; 134:319.

Morin ME, Baker DA: Lymphocele: A complication of surgical staging of carcinoma of the prostate. Am J Radiol 1977; 129:333.

Motola JA, Badlani GH, Smith AD: Results of 212 consecutive endopyelotomies: An 8-year follow-up. J Urol 1993a; 149:453.

Motola JA, Fried R, Badlani GH, et al: Failed endopyelotomy: Implications for future surgery on the UPJ. J Urol 1993b; 150:821.

Mueller PR, van Sonnenberg E, Ferrucci JT Jr: Percutaneous drainage of 250 abdominal abscesses and fluid collections: II. Current procedural concepts. Radiology 1984; 151:343.

Muench PJ, Haynes CB, Raney AM, et al: Endoscopic management of the obliterated ureteroileal anastomosis. J Urol 1987; 137:277.

Murnaghan GF: The mechanism of congenital hydronephrosis with reference to the factors influencing surgical treatment. Ann R Coll Surg Eng 1958; 23:25.

Murphy LJT: The kidney. In Murphy LJT, ed: The History of Urology. Springfield, IL, Charles C Thomas, 1972, p 201.

Murray KHA, Wilkinson ML: Endoscopic transurostomy diathermy anastomotomy: A combined approach to uretero-ileal stenoses. Br J Urol 1993; 72:23.

Nadler RB, Nakada SY, Monk TG, et al: Bilateral percutaneous nephrolithotomy with subarachnoid spinal anesthesia. J Endourol 1995a; 9:S119.

Nadler RB, Pearle MS, Nakada SY, et al: Acucise endopyelotomy: Two-year follow-up report. J Urol 1995b; 153:366a.

Nakada SY, Gerber AJ, Wolf JS Jr, et al: Subcutaneous urinary diversion utilizing a nephrovesical stent: A superior alternative to long-term external drainage? Urology 1995; 45:538.

Nakada SY, Wolf JS Jr, Brink JA, et al: Retrospective analysis of the effect of crossing vessels on retrograde endopyelotomy outcomes using spiral CT angiography. J Endourol 1995; 9(Suppl 1):S88.

Netto NR, Dealmeida-Claro JF, Ferreira U: Is percutaneous monotherapy for staghorn calculus still indicated in the era of extracorporeal shock wave lithotripsy? J Endourol 1994; 8:195.

Netto NR Jr, Claro JFA, Lemos GC, et al: Renal calculi in lower pole calices: What is the best method of treatment. J Urol 1991a; 146:721.

Netto NR Jr, Claro JFA, Lemos GC, et al: Treatment options for ureteral calculi: Endourology or extracorporeal shock wave lithotripsy. J Urol 1991b; 146:5.

Netto NR Jr, Ferreira U, Lemos GC, et al: Endourological management of ureteral strictures. J Urol 1990; 144:631.

Newhouse JH, Pfister RC, Hendren WH, et al: Whitaker test after pyeloplasty: Establishment of normal ureteral perfusion pressures. Am J Radiol 1981; 137:223.

Newman DM, Coury T, Lingeman JE, et al: Extracorporeal shock wave lithotripsy experience in children. J Urol 1986; 136:238.

Nocks BN, Heney NM, Daly JJ, et al: Transitional cell carcinoma of the renal pelvis. Urology 1982; 19:472.

Nurse DE, Woodhouse CRJ, Kellett MJ, et al: Percutaneous removal of upper tract tumors. World J Urol 1989; 7:131.

O'Brien WM, Maxted WC, Pahira JJ: Ureteral stricture: Experience with 31 cases. J Urol 1988; 140:737.

Oesterling JE, Fishman EK, Goldman SM, et al: The management of renal angiomyolipoma. J Urol 1986; 135:1121.

O'Flynn K, Hehin M, McKelvie G, et al: Endoballoon rupture and stenting for pelviureteric junction obstruction: Technique and early results. Br J Urol 1989; 64:572.

Ohkawa M, Tokunaga S, Orito M, et al: Percutaneous injection sclerotherapy with minocycline hydrochloride for simple renal cysts. Int Urol Nephrol 1993; 25:37.

Ono Y, Ohshima S, Kinukawa T, et al: Endopyeloureterotomy via a transpelvic extraureteral approach. J Urol 1992; 147:352.

Oosterhof GON, Hoitsma AJ, Debruyne FRJ: Antegrade percutaneous dilation of ureteral strictures after kidney transplantation. Transplant Int 1989; 2:36.

Oppenheimer R, Hinman F Jr: Ureteral regeneration: Contracture vs. hyperplasia of smooth muscle. J Urol 1955; 74:476.

Ordorica RC, Lindfors KK, Palmer JM: Diuretic Doppler sonography following successful repair of renal obstruction in children. J Urol 1993; 150:774.

O'Reilly PH: Diuresis renography 8 years later: An update. J Urol 1986; 136:993.

O'Reilly PH, Lawson RS, Testa HJ: Idiopathic hydronephrosis: The diuresis renogram: A new non-invasive method of assessing equivocal pelvioureteral junction obstruction. J Urol 1979; 121:1531.

Orihuela E, Smith AD: Percutaneous treatment of transitional cell carcinoma of the upper urinary tract. Urol Clin North Am 1988; 15:425.

Ozgun S, Cetin S, Ilken Y: Percutaneous renal cyst aspiration and treatment with alcohol. Int Urol Nephrol 1988; 20:481.

Palou J, Farina LA, Villavicencio JH, et al: Upper tract urothelial tumor after transurethral resection for bladder tumor. Eur Urol 1992; 21:110.

Papadopoulos I, Wirth B, Bertermann H, Wand H: Diagnosis and treatment of urothelial tumors by ureteropyeloscopy. J Endourol 1990; 4:55.

Papanicolaou N, Pfister RC, Yoder IC: Percutaneous occlusion of ureteral leaks and fistulae using nondetachable balloons. Urol Radiol 1985; 7:28.

Patel A, Soonawalla P, Shepherd S, et al: Long term outcome after percutaneous treatment of TCC of the renal pelvis. J Endourol 1994; 8(suppl 1):S125.

Patterson DE, Segura JW, Leroy AJ: Long term follow up of patients treated with percutaneous ultrasonic lithotripsy for struvite staghorn calculi. J Endourol 1987; 1:177.

Patterson DE, Segura JW, Leroy AJ, et al: The etiology and treatment of delayed bleeding following percutaneous lithotripsy. J Urol 1985; 133:447.

Pauer W, Lugmayr H: Metallic wall stents: A new therapy for extrinsic ureteral obstruction. J Urol 1992; 148:281.

Perugia G, Drudi FM, Carbone A, et al: Role of fibrin glue in percutaneous treatment of renal cysts. J Endourol 1991; 5:225.

Picus DD, Weyman PJ, Clayman RV, et al: Intercostal-space nephrostomy for percutaneous stone removal. Am J Radiol 1986; 147:393.

Plas EG, Hubner WA: Percutaneous resection of renal cysts: A long-term followup. J Urol 1993; 149:703.

Pollack HM, Arger PH, Banner MP, et al: Computed tomography of renal pelvic filling defects. Radiology 1981; 138:645.

Portela LA, Patel SK, Callahan DH: Pararenal pseudocyst (urinoma) as complication of percutaneous nephrostomy. Urology 1979; 13:570.

Prajsner A, Szkodny A, Szewczyk W, et al: Long-term results of kidney staghorn stone treatment with percutaneous nephrolithotripsy and extracorporeal shock wave lithotripsy. Int Urol Nephrol 1993; 25:533.

Preminger GM, Nakada SY, Babayan RK, et al: A multicenter clinical trial investigating the use of a fluoroscopically controlled cutting balloon catheter for the management of ureteral and ureteropelvic junction obstruction. In preparation, 1996.

Psihramis KE, Dretler SP: Extracorporeal shock wave lithotripsy of caliceal diverticula calculi. J Urol 1987; 138:707.

Quillin SP, Brink JA, Nakada SY, et al: Detection of crossing vessels at the ureteropelvic junction with spiral CT angiography. J Urol 1995; 153:367a.

Radford MG Jr, Donadio JV Jr, Holley KE, et al: Renal biopsy in clinical practice. Mayo Clin Proc 1994; 69:983.

Ralls PW, Barakos JA, Kaptein EM, et al: Renal biopsy-related hemorrhage: Frequency and comparison of CT and sonography. J Comput Assist Tomogr 1987; 11:1031.

Ramsey JC, Soloway MS: Instillation of bacillus Calmette-Guerin into the renal pelvis of a solitary kidney for the treatment of transitional cell carcinoma. J Urol 1990; 143:1220.

Ramsey JWA, Miller RA, Kellet MJ, et al: Percutaneous pyelolysis: Indications, complications, and results. Br J Urol 1984; 56:586.

Raskin MM, Poole DO, Roen SA, et al: Percutaneous management of renal cysts: Results of a four year study. Radiology 1975; 1150:551.

Reddy PK, Hulbert JC, Lange PH, et al: Percutaneous removal of renal and ureteral calculi: Experience with 400 cases. J Urol 1985; 134:662.

Reddy PK, Moore L, Hunter D, et al: Percutaneous ureteral fulguration: A nonsurgical technique for ureteral occlusion. J Urol 1987; 138:724.

Reddy PK, Sidi AA: Endoscopic ureteral occlusion for urinary diversion in patients with lower urinary tract fistulas. Urol Clin North Am 1990; 17:103.

Regan JS, Lam HS, Lingeman JE: Simultaneous bilateral percutaneous nephrolithotomy. J Endourol 1992; 6:245.

Reimer DE, Oswalt GC Jr: Iatrogenic ureteral obstruction treated with balloon dilation. J Urol 1981; 126:689.

Reinberg Y, Ferral H, Gonzalez R, et al: Intraureteral metallic self-expanding endoprosthesis (Wallstent) in the treatment of difficult ureteral strictures. J Urol 1994; 151:1619.

Reinberg Y, Moore SL, Lange PH: Splenic abscess as a complication of percutaneous nephrostomy. Urology 1989; 34:274.

Reiner I, Donnell S, Jones M, et al: Percutaneous sclerotherapy for simple renal cysts in children. Br J Radiol 1992; 65:281.

Richter S, Karbel G, Bechar R, et al: Should a benign renal cyst be treated? Br J Urol 1983; 55:457.

Rigatti P, Francesca F, Montorsi F, et al: Extracorporeal lithotripsy and combined surgical procedures in the treatment of renoureteral stone disease: Our experience with 2,955 patients. World J Surg 1989; 13:765.

Rodgers PM, Bates JA, Irving HC: Intrarenal Doppler ultrasound studies in normal and acutely obstructed kidneys. Br J Radiol 1992; 65:207.

Roth RA, Beckmann CF: Complications of extracorporeal shockwave lithotripsy and percutaneous nephrolithotomy. Urol Clin North Am 1988; 15:155.

Rous SN, Turner WR: Retrospective study of 95 patients with staghorn calculus disease. J Urol 1977; 118:902.

Saad F, Faucher R, Mauffette F, et al: Staghorn calculi treated by percutaneous nephrolithotomy: Risk factors for recurrence. Urology 1993; 41:141.

Sadi MV, Nardozza A Jr, Gianotti I: Percutaneous drainage of retroperitoneal abscesses. J Endourol 1988; 2:293.

Saiki J, Vaziri ND, Barton C: Perinephric and intranephric abscesses: A review of the literature. West J Med 1982; 136:96.

Salvatierra O Jr, Bucklew WB, Morrow JW: Perinephric abscess: A report of 71 cases. J Urol 1967; 98:296.

Sampaio FJB: Review: Anatomic background for intrarenal endourologic surgery. J Endourol 1992; 6:301.

Sampaio FJB, Aragao AHM: Limitations of extracorporeal shockwave lithotripsy for lower caliceal stones: Anatomic insight. J Endourol 1994; 8:241.

Sampaio FJB, D'Anunciacoa AL, Bianco M: Comparative follow up of patients with acute and obtuse infundibulum-pelvic angle submitted for SWL for treatment of lower pole nephrolithiasis. J Endourol 1995; 9:s63.

Sanders R, Bissada NK, Bielsky S: Ureteroenteric anastomotic strictures: Treatment with Palmaz permanent indwelling stents. J Urol 1993; 150:469.

Sarnacki CT, McCormack LJ, Kiser WS, et al: Urinary cytology and the clinical diagnosis of urinary tract malignancy: A clinicopathological study of 1400 patients. J Urol 1971; 106:761.

Scardino PT, Scardino PL: Obstruction of the ureteropelvic junction. In Bergman H, ed: The Ureter. New York, Springer-Verlag, 1984, p 697.

Schaeffer AJ, Grayhack JT: Surgical management of ureteropelvic junction obstruction. In Walsh PC, Gittes RF, Perlmutter AD, Stamey TA, eds: Campbell's Urology, 5th ed. Philadelphia, W.B. Saunders, 1986, p 2505.

Schaner EG, Balow JE, Doppman JL: Computed tomography in the diagnosis of subcapsular and perirenal hematoma. Am J Radiol 1977; 128:83.

Schild HH, Gunther R, Thelen M: Transrenal ureteral occlusion: Results and problems. J Vasc Interv Radiol 1994; 5:321.

Schmidt JD, Hawtrey CE, Flocks RH, et al: Complications, results, and problems of ileal conduit diversions. J Urol 1973; 109:210.

Schneider AW, Conrad S, Busch R, et al: The cold-knife technique for endourological management of stenoses in the upper urinary tract. J Urol 1991; 146:961.

Schonebeck J, Ansehn S: The occurrence of yeast-like fungi in the urine under normal conditions and in various types of urinary tract pathology. Scand J Urol Nephrol 1972; 6:123.

Schow DA, Vinson RK, Morrisseau PM: Percutaneous renal biopsy of the solitary kidney: A contraindication? J Urol 1992; 147:1235.

Schultz RE, Hanno PM, Wein AJ, et al: Percutaneous ultrasonic lithotripsy: Choice of irrigant. J Urol 1983; 130:858.

Schulze H, Hertle L, Kutta A, et al: Critical evaluation of treatment of staghorn calculi by percutaneous nephrolithotomy and extracorporeal shock wave lithotripsy. J Urol 1989; 141:822.

Schweizer RT, Cho S, Korentz SL, et al: Lymphoceles following renal transplantation. Arch Surg 1972; 104:42.

Seaman EK, Slawin KM, Benson MC: Treatment options for upper tract transitional-cell carcinoma. Urol Clin North Am 1993; 20:349.

Segura JW, Patterson DE, Leroy AJ: Combined percutaneous ultrasonic lithotripsy and extracorporeal shock wave lithotripsy for struvite staghorn calculi. World J Urol 1987; 5:245.

Segura JW, Patterson DE, Leroy AJ, et al: Percutaneous removal of kidney stones: Review of 1,000 cases. J Urol 1985; 134:1077.

Segura JW, Preminger GM, Assimos DG, et al: Nephrolithiasis clinical guideline panel summary report on the management of staghorn calculi. J Urol 1994; 151:1648.

Segura JW, Rosen C: Percutaneous nephrolithotomy: Technique, indications and complications. AUA Update Series 1993; 20:154.

Selikowitz SM: New coaxial ureteral stricture knife. Urol Clin North Am 1990; 17:83.

Semelka RC, Shoenut JP, Kroeker MA, et al: Renal lesions: Controlled comparison between CT and 1.5-t MR imaging with nonenhanced and gadolinium-enhanced fat-suppressed spin-echo and breath-hold FLASH techniques. Radiology 1992; 182:425.

Servadio C, Winkler H, Neuman M, et al: Percutaneous nephrolithotomy. Israel J Med Soc 1986; 22:541.

Shapiro MJ, Banner MP, Amendola MA, et al: Balloon catheter dilation of ureteroenteric strictures: Long-term results. Radiology 1988; 168:385.

Sharpe JR, Duffy G, Chin JL: Intrarenal bacillus Calmette-Guerin therapy for upper urinary tract carcinoma in situ. J Urol 1993; 149:457.

Sheinfeld J, Erturk ERF, Cockett ATK: Perinephric abscess: Current concepts. J Urol 1987; 137:191.

Shepherd P, Thomas R, Harmon EP: Urolithiasis in children: Innovations in management. J Urol 1988; 140:790.

Siegel JF, Smith A, Moldwin R: Minimally invasive treatment of renal abscess. J Urol 1996; 155:52.

Siegle RL, Lieberman P: A review of untoward reactions to iodinated contrast material. J Urol 1978; 119:581.

Singer A, Das S: Therapeutic dilemmas in management of cystine calculi. Urology 1991; 37:322.

Singh M, Chapman R, Tresidder GC, et al: The fate of the unoperated staghorn calculus. Br J Urol 1973; 45:581.

Skinner DG, Melamud A, Lieskovsky G: Complications of thoracoabdominal retroperitoneal lymph node dissection. J Urol 1982; 127:1107.

Smith AD: Management of iatrogenic ureteral strictures after urological procedures. J Urol 1988; 140:1372.

Smith AD, Lange PH, Fraley EE: Application of percutaneous nephrostomy: New challenges and opportunities in endo-urology. J Urol 1979; 121:382.

Smith AD, Moldwin RM, Karlin GS: Percutaneous ureterostomy. J Urol 1987; 138:286.

Smith JE, Vanarsdalen KN, Hanno PM, et al: Extracorporeal shock wave lithotripsy treatment of calculi in horseshoe kidneys. J Urol 1989; 142:683.

Snow M, Wells IP, Hammond JC: Balloon rupture and stenting for pelviureteric junction obstruction: Abolition of waisting is a prognostic marker. Clin Radiol 1994; 49:708.

Snyder JA, Smith AD: Staghorn calculi: Percutaneous extraction versus anatrophic nephrolithotomy. J Urol 1986; 136:351.

Soble J, Nakada SY, Wolf JS Jr, et al: Long-term outcome of pyelocaliceal diverticula after endosurgical management. J Urol 1995; 153:286a.

Soloway MS, Masters S: Urothelial susceptibility to tumor cell implantation: Influence of cauterization. Cancer 1980; 46:1158.

Spring DB, Schroeder D, Babu S, et al: Ultrasonic evaluation of lymphocele formation after staging lymphadenectomy for prostatic carcinoma. Radiology 1981; 141:479.

Stables DP, Ginsberg NJ, Johnson ML: Percutaneous nephrostomy: A series and review of the literature. AJR 1978; 130:75.

Starr NT, Middleton RG: Extracorporeal piezoelectric lithotripsy in unanesthesized children. Pediatrics 1992; 89:1226.

Stolk R, Ettershank G: Calculating the area of an irregular shape. Byte 1987; 12:135.

Streem SB, Geisinger MA: Prevention and management of hemorrhage associated with cautery wire balloon incision of ureteropelvic junction obstruction. J Urol 1995; 153:1904.

Streem SB, Lammert G: Long-term efficacy of combination therapy for struvite staghorn calculi. J Urol 1992; 147:563.

Streem SB, Novick AC, Steinmuller DR, et al: Percutaneous techniques for the management of urological renal transplant complications. J Urol 1986; 135:456.

Streem SB, Pontes EJ: Percutaneous management of upper tract TCC. J Urol 1986; 135:773.

Streem SB, Yost A: Treatment of caliceal diverticular calculi with extracorporeal shock wave lithotripsy: Patient selection and extended followup. J Urol 1992; 148:1043.

Streitz D, Hulbert JC, Hunter D: Long-term follow-up of the results of percutaneous treatment of strictures in the region of the ureteropelvic junction. J Urol 1992; 147:434a.

Strong DW, Pearse HD, Tank ES Jr, et al: The ureteral stump after nephroureterectomy. J Urol 1976; 115:654.

Sutherland RS, Pfister RR, Koyle MA: Endopyelotomy associated ureteral necrosis: Complete ureteral replacement using the Boari flap. J Urol 1992; 148:1490.

Suzuki K, Tanaka T, Ikeda R, et al: Terumo guide wire in endourologic treatment. J Endourol 1989; 3:69.

Tailly G: Tract healing after percutaneous nephrolithotomy. J Endourol 1988; 2:71.

Talner LB: Obstructive uropathy. In Pollack HM, ed: Nuclear Medicine Techniques in Clinical Urography. Philadelphia, W.B. Saunders, 1990, p 1570.

Tan HL, Najmaldin A, Webb DR: Endopyelotomy for pelvi-ureteric junction obstruction in children. Eur Urol 1993; 24:84.

Tasca A, Zattoni Fr: The case for a percutaneous approach to transitional cell carcinoma of the renal pelvis. J Urol 1990; 143:902.

Tawney RH: Special challenges. In Lingeman JE, Smith LH, Woods JR, Newman DM, eds: Urinary Calculi: ESWL, Endourology and Medical Therapy. Philadelphia, Lea & Febiger, 1989, pp 207–220.

Teichman JMH, Long RD, Hulbert JC: Long-term renal fate and prognosis after staghorn calculus management. J Urol 1995; 153:1403.

Thomas R: Ureteroscopic retrograde endopyelotomy for uretero-pelvic junction (UPJ) obstruction: Long term statistical functional analysis. J Endourol 1995; 9:S98.

Thomas R, Cherry R, Vandenberg T: Long term efficacy of retrograde ureteroscopic endopyelotomy. J Urol 1993a; 149:276a.

Thomas R, Macaluso JN, Vandenberg T, et al: An innovative approach to management of lower third ureteral calculi. J Urol 1993b; 149:1427.

Thomas R, Ortenberg J, Lee BR, et al: Safety and efficacy of pediatric ureteroscopy for management of calculous disease. J Urol 1993c; 149:1082.

Thompson IM, Ross G Jr, Habib EH, et al: Experiences with 16 cases of pararenal pseudocyst. J Urol 1976; 116:289.

Thorley JD, Jones SR, Sanford JP: Perinephric abscess. Medicine 1974; 53:441.

Thuroff JW, Alken P: Ultrasound for renal puncture and fluoroscopy for tract dilation and catheter placement: A combined approach. Endourology 1987; 2:1.

Timmons JW Jr, Malek RS, Hattery RR, et al: Caliceal diverticulum. J Urol 1975; 114:6.

Tiselius H: Anesthesia-free in situ extracorporeal shock wave lithotripsy of distal ureteral stones without a ureteral catheter. J Endourol 1993; 7:185.

Tomera KM, Leary FJ, Zincke H: Pyeloscopy in urothelial tumors. J Urol 1982; 127:1088.

Tosaka A, Ohya K, Yamada K, et al: Incidence and properties of renal masses and asymptomatic renal cell carcinoma detected by abdominal ultrasonography. J Urol 1990; 144:1097.

Towbin RB, Wacksman J, Ball WS: Percutaneous pyeloplasty in children: Experience in three patients. Radiology 1987; 163:381.

Urban DA, Kerbl K, Clayman RV, et al: Endo-ureteroplasty with a free urothelial graft. J Urol 1994; 152:910.

Vallencien G, Capdeville R, Viellon B, et al: Colonic perforation during percutaneous nephrostomy. J Urol 1985; 134:1185.

Van Baal JG, Smits NJ, Keeman JN, et al: The evolution of renal angiomyolipomas in patients with tuberous sclerosis. J Urol 1994; 152:35.

Van Cangh PJ, Jorion JL, Wese FX, et al: Endoureteropyelotomy: Percutaneous treatment of ureteropelvic junction obstruction. J Urol 1989; 141:1317.

Van Cangh PJ, Lorge PFF, Abi Aad A, et al: Symptomatic caliceal diverticula: Long term follow-up. J Endourol 1994a; 8:S121.

Van Cangh PJ, Wilmart JF, Opsomer RJ, et al: Long-term results and late recurrence after endoureteropyelotomy: A critical analysis of prognostic factors. J Urol 1994b; 151:934.

Vandenbroucke F, van Poppel H, Van Deursen H, et al: Surgical versus endoscopic treatment of nonmalignant uretero-ileal anastomotic strictures. Br J Urol 1993; 71:408.

Van Deursen J, Baert L: Electromagnetic extracorporeal shock wave lithotripsy for calculi in horseshoe kidneys. J Urol 1992; 148:1120.

Varkarakis MJ, Gaeta J, Moore RH, et al: Superficial bladder tumor: Aspects of clinical progression. Urology 1974; 4:414.

Vasavada SP, Streem SB, Novick AC: Definitive tumor resection and percutaneous bacille Calmette-Guerin for management of renal pelvic transitional cell carcinoma in solitary kidneys. Urology 1995; 45:381.

Vaughan ED: Commentary on the renal resistive index. J Urol 1995; 154:922.

Vestby GW: Percutaneous needle-puncture of renal cysts: New method in therapeutic management. Invest Radiol 1967; 2:449.

Voegeli DR, Crummy AB, McDermott JC, et al: Percutaneous dilation of ureteral strictures in renal transplant patients. Radiology 1988; 169:185.

Von Schreeb T, Arner O, Skovsted G, et al: Renal adenocarcinoma: Is there a risk of spreading tumor cells in diagnostic puncture? Scand J Urol Nephrol 1970; 1:270.

Wagle DG, Moore RH, Murphy GP: Primary carcinoma of the renal pelvis. Cancer 1974; 33:1642.

Wahlquist L, Grumstedt B: Therapeutic effect of percutaneous puncture of simple renal cyst. Acta Chir Scand 1966; 132:340.

Wallace DMA, Wallace DM, Whitfield HN, et al: The late results of conservative surgery for upper tract urothelial carcinomas. Br J Urol 1981; 53:537.

Walther PJ, Robertson CN, Paulson DF: Lethal complications of standard self-retaining ureteral stents in patients with ileal conduit urinary diversion. J Urol 1985; 133:851.

Webb DR, Fitzpatrick JM: Percutaneous nephrolithotripsy: A functional and morphological study. J Urol 1985; 134:587.

Webb EA, Smith BA Jr, Price WE: Plastic operations on the ureter without intubation. J Urol 1957; 77:821.

Weigert F, Schulz V, Kromer HD: Renal abscess: Report of a case with sonographic, urographic, and CT evaluation. Eur J Radiol 1985; 5:224.

Whitaker RH: Pathophysiology of ureteric obstruction. In Williams DI, ed: Scientific Foundations of Urology. London, Blackwell Scientific, 1976, p 18.

Whitaker RH: An evaluation of 170 diagnostic pressure flow studies of the upper urinary tract. J Urol 1979; 121:602.

White EC, Smith AD: Percutaneous stone extraction from 200 patients. J Urol 1984; 132:437.

White M, Mueller PR, Ferucci JT, et al: Percutaneous drainage of postoperative abdominal and pelvic lymphoceles. Am J Radiol 1985; 145:1065.

Wickham JEA: Percutaneous pyelolysis. In Wickham JEA, Miller RA, eds: Percutaneous Renal Surgery. New York, Churchill Livingstone, 1983, p 148.

Wickham JEA: Minimally invasive surgery. J Endourol 1987; 1:71.

Wickham JEA, Miller RA: Nephroscopy: Endoscopic instruments and their accessories. In Wickham JEA, Miller RA, eds: Percutaneous Renal Surgery. New York, Churchill Livingstone, 1983, p 45.

Wills TE, Burns JR: Ureteroscopy: An outpatient procedure? J Urol 1994; 151:1185.

Winfield HN, Clayman RV: Complications of percutaneous removal of renal and ureteral calculi: Part I. World Urology Update Series 1985; Vol 2, Lesson 37.

Winfield HN, Clayman RV, Chaussy CG, et al: Monotherapy of staghorn renal calculi: A comparative study between percutaneous nephrolithotomy and extracorporeal shock wave lithotripsy. J Urol 1988; 139:895.

Wise GJ: Amphotericin B in urological practice. J Urol 1990; 144:215.

Wise GJ, Kozinn PJ, Goldberg P: Amphotericin B as a urologic irrigant in the management of noninvasive candiduria. J Urol 1982; 128:82.

Wishnow KI, Johnson DE, Preston D, et al: Long-term serum creatinine values after radical nephrectomy. Urology 1990; 35:114.

Witherington R, Shelor WC: Treatment of postoperative ureteral stricture by catheter dilation: A forgotten procedure. Urology 1980; 16:592.

Woodside JP, Sevens GF, Stark GL, et al: Percutaneous stone removal in children. J Urol 1985; 134:1166.

Young AT: Percutaneous nephrostomy: Opacification of collecting system.

In Amplatz K, Lange PH, eds: Atlas of Endourology. Chicago, Year Book Medical Publishers, 1986a, p 39.

Young AT: Percutaneous nephrostomy: Puncture techniques. *In* Amplatz K, Lange PH, eds: Atlas of Endourology. Chicago, Year Book Medical Publishers, 1986b, p 55.

Young AT, Hunter DW, Castaneda-Zuniga WR, et al: Percutaneous extraction of urinary calculi: Use of the intercostal approach. Radiology 1985; 154:633.

Zachrisson L: Simple renal cysts treated with bismuth phosphate at the diagnostic puncture. Acta Radiol Diagn 1982; 23:209.

Zattoni F, Passerini-Glanzel G, Tascas A, et al: Pediatric nephroscope for percutaneous stone removal. Urology 1989; 33:404.

Zou SZ, Fan WN, He XH: Percutaneous ultrasound-guided injection of sodium morrhuate in the treatment of cystic renal masses. Br J Urol 1991; 68:441.

95
LAPAROSCOPY IN CHILDREN AND ADULTS

Craig A. Peters, M.D.
Louis R. Kavoussi, M.D.

Laparoscopy has been an important part of gynecologic practice for more than 50 years; however, only recently has it been regularly applied as a minimally invasive alternative to treat urologic pathology. Initial urologic applications explored the diagnostic capabilities of a laparoscopic approach in select patients (e.g., nonpalpable testicle, intersex conditions) (Gans and Berci, 1973; Cortesi et al, 1976). The phenomenal success of laparoscopic cholecystectomy sparked investigators to examine the potential for therapeutic applications in other surgical specialties, including urology. Several laparoscopic urologic applications have demonstrated similar therapeutic results with less postoperative discomfort and disfigurement compared with traditional open techniques (Gill et al, 1995a).

Laparoscopic methods are distinct from conventional incisional surgery and require physicians to use novel operative skills. Unfortunately, most urologists have not had access to extensive resources and training in laparoscopic techniques. This chapter serves as an in-depth introduction to basic laparoscopic techniques. Current applications are reviewed and contrasted with traditional open surgery.

BASIC PRINCIPLES OF LAPAROSCOPY

Indications and Contraindications

Although most transabdominal or retroperitoneal urologic procedures have been successfully completed laparoscopically, this does not currently imply that all surgical urologic pathology should be approached laparoscopically. Some procedures (e.g., laparoscopic renal biopsy, diagnostic evaluation of nonpalpable testicle) have clear benefits, whereas others (e.g., radical prostatectomy) currently have no defined role in standard practice (Gaur et al, 1992; Schuessler et al, 1992; Peters, 1993; Docimo et al, 1995c). Moreover, before proceeding, every surgeon must recognize his or her own level of expertise. A surgeon with limited experience should not undertake a complex laparoscopic procedure without additional support.

The paramount factor in ensuring safe, effective laparoscopic intervention is appropriate patient selection. Each case must be individualized, and patient expectations need to be considered. Although pain is less, there is still postoperative discomfort and required convalescence.

A thorough medical history is mandatory to reveal any contraindications to a laparoscopic approach. Because of the nature and length of current urologic procedures, a general endotracheal anesthetic is usually required (Monk and Weldon, 1992). Thus, **patients who are not candidates for a general anesthetic, such as those with severe cardiopulmonary disease, should not undergo laparoscopy.** Physicians must be cognizant of conditions that may alter a patient's physiology, such as the pneumoperitoneum, which may further compromise ventilation, and compression of the vena cava, which may limit venous return (Arthure, 1970; Hodgson et al, 1970; Nunn, 1987; Lew et al, 1992). Patients with mild to moderate chronic obstructive pulmonary disease may have difficulty compensating for the hypercarbia, and the pneumoperitoneum may need to be kept at lower pressures than usual (Monk and Weldon, 1992; Adams et al, 1995a). **Laparoscopy should also be avoided in patients with severely dilated bowels from either functional or obstructive ileus.** In these cases, the dilated intestines take up working space and may be injured during access and dissection (Borten, 1986). **Other absolute contraindications include uncorrected coagulopathy, untreated infection, and hypovolemic shock** (Capelouto and Kavoussi, 1993).

Several conditions require caution when considering a laparoscopic approach. Prior intra-abdominal or retroperitoneal surgery is not a contraindication to laparoscopy; however, each case must be carefully assessed. Prior transperitoneal surgery can cause bowel adhesions to the abdominal wall or scar tissue formation about the operative site, increasing the possibility of injury during insertion of the Veress needle, trocar placement, or dissection (Borten, 1986). In approaching these patients, the Veress needle should be placed away from any scars and any prior surgical fields. Alternatively, open trocar placement can be undertaken to minimize access injuries (Hassan, 1971).

Obese patients should also be approached with discretion because abdominal wall fat may make trocar placement difficult and mask anatomic landmarks (Mendoza et al, 1996). Moreover, the weight of the pannus may raise the intra-abdominal pressure and limit the working space.

Early literature cautioned against performing laparoscopy in patients with an acute abdomen because of the risk of the pneumoperitoneum's causing sepsis. Studies have demonstrated, however, that laparoscopy can be performed in select acute settings (Chardavoyne and Wise, 1994; Tanaka et al, 1994).

Patient Preparation

In general, patient preparation is similar to that for comparable open surgery. **Informed consent must be obtained with discussion of possible complications, including conversion to an open surgical approach.** All patients should be typed and screened for blood, and when performing an advanced procedure, cross-matched blood should be made available. Bowel preparation varies with operative procedure as well as physician preference. For pelvic procedures, an enema the night before surgery may help decompress the sigmoid colon and rectum to facilitate visualization.

Patient and equipment positioning varies with each procedure. In general, the patient is supine with the monitor at the foot of the table when approaching pelvic organs or the lower ureter (Fig. 95–1). For upper ureteral, renal, and adrenal access, the patient should be in a modified lateral position and monitors placed on each side at the level of the chest (see Fig. 95–1*B*). When positioning patients, care must be taken to pad pressure points adequately. During laparoscopic procedures, the operating table is actively tilted, and gravity acts as a retractor to move bowel and fluid out of the operative field. Hence, patients must be adequately secured to the operating table.

The patient should undergo a full abdominal preparation in the event that an emergent laparotomy is required. For pelvic procedures in men, gas may dissect into the scrotum, resulting in pneumoscrotum or pneumopenis. This is not harmful but may be obtrusive in the operative field and disconcerting to the patient. Wrapping the genitalia with a gauze roll can avert this problem. A Foley catheter and nasogastric tube are placed to decompress the bladder and stomach, minimizing inadvertent injury during access. Lower extremity sequential compression stockings should be used to decrease the risk of venous thrombosis.

Intra-abdominal Access

During conventional surgery, the working space is obtained by opening the patient and bringing the operative field into the surgeon's environment. In contrast, laparoscopic pathology is approached in situ by creating a working space in the patient. This space is obtained by establishing a pneumoperitoneum: instilling gas into an existing body cavity (e.g., the peritoneal cavity) or into a cavity created by separating tissue planes (e.g., space of Retzius). This can be accomplished through open or closed techniques.

Closed Access

The first step in closed abdominal access involves placing a Veress needle into the peritoneal cavity. The Veress needle is a sharp beveled needle with a retractable inner blunt tip (Fig. 95–2). When pressure is placed against the inner core, it retracts, exposing the sharp outer core, which can pierce through the abdominal wall fascia. Once in the abdominal cavity, the blunt core snaps forward to protect underlying organs from injury by the sharp outer tip.

In patients who have had prior surgery, **attempts should be made to avoid placing the Veress needle or initial trocar over the scar or area of prior surgery.** At these sites, there is a high likelihood that omentum or viscus is adherent to the anterior abdominal wall, increasing the possibility of unsuccessful insufflation and bowel injury. Alternative sites for initial access include any quadrant just lateral to the rectus muscle, the 11th intracostal space, and the anterior vaginal wall.

The surgeon's hand dominance and patient position dictate where the surgeon should stand relative to the patient when accessing the abdomen. When the patient is supine, a right-handed physician should stand on the patient's left side and

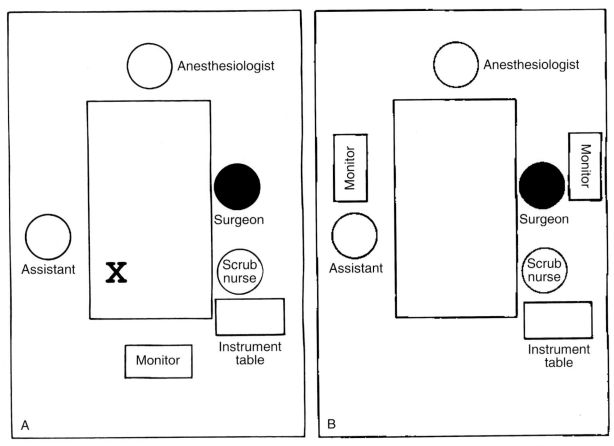

Figure 95–1. Room setup for laparoscopic pelvic procedures. Note the video monitor is positioned at the patient's foot (*A*). Note the surgeon on the contralateral side of the pathology (x). With upper urinary tract surgery, the camera monitor is placed near the head of the table (*B*).

a left-handed surgeon on the patient's right side (see Fig. 95–1). The needle should be held like a pencil near midshaft during placement. The needle is passed perpendicular to the skin in the base of the umbilicus with patients in the supine position. Three areas of resistance are felt in this location: skin, fascia, and peritoneum.

Surgeon location is somewhat different with the patient in the lateral position. The surgeon should stand opposite the side of the patient that is elevated (i.e., when the left side of the patient is elevated, the surgeon should be on the patient's right side and vice versa) (see Fig. 95–1*B*). The needle is again placed in the dominant hand and passed perpendicular to the abdominal wall in the midclavicular line at the level of the iliac crest.

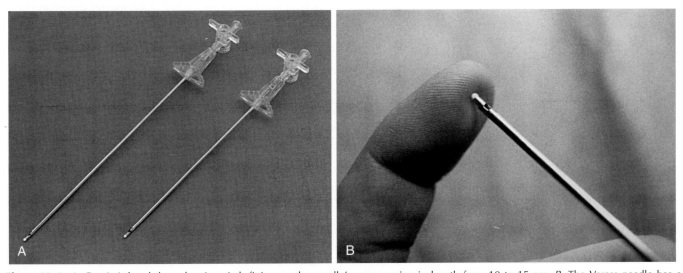

Figure 95–2. *A,* Gas is infused through a Luer-Lok fitting on the needle's core varying in length from 10 to 15 cm. *B,* The Veress needle has a blunt retractable inner core to minimize the risk of injury to intra-abdominal organs.

Once the needle is passed, proper tip location needs to be ensured before insufflation. A 10-ml syringe should first be connected to the needle and aspiration performed to be sure the needle is not within a vessel or hollow viscus. Next, injected saline (2–5 ml) should pass easily through the needle. A drop of water placed at the tip of the needle should flow into the peritoneal cavity owing to the negative pressure generated during expiration. **The most sensitive indicator of correct needle position is how the needle feels as it is gently pivoted.** This maneuver should reveal free motion and the characteristic tactile sensation of the needle balloting the bowel.

Once correct needle placement is verified, gas is insufflated into the peritoneal cavity. Carbon dioxide and nitrous oxide are the two gases most commonly used for laparoscopy. Carbon dioxide is preferred because it is highly soluble in blood, decreasing the risk of a gas pulmonary embolus (Graff et al, 1959). Unfortunately, carbon dioxide is converted to carbonic acid on the peritoneal surface and if not completely evacuated can lead to significant postoperative abdominal, chest, back, and shoulder discomfort. Moreover, hypercarbia can lead to significant metabolic abnormalities (see later).

Because of the shortcomings of carbon dioxide, some laparoscopists prefer nitrous oxide as the insufflant because it is not a peritoneal irritant and does not result in metabolic abnormalities (Sogge et al, 1980; Minoli et al, 1982). Nitrous oxide, however, is less soluble in blood and theoretically represents a higher risk for gas embolization. Also, in contrast to carbon dioxide, nitrous oxide supports combustion. Hence, there is a small risk of explosion when it is used in the presence of electrocautery (Steptoe, 1976). Nitrous oxide is well suited for short procedures performed under a local anesthetic.

Gas is transferred from the source (a pressurized tank) to the patient by way of an insufflator. The insufflator is an electronically controlled mechanical valve that regulates the rate at which the pressurized gas flows from the gas tank into the patient's abdomen. While instilling gas, the insufflator also measures intra-abdominal pressure. As a safety feature, insufflators are designed such that when a preset intra-abdominal pressure is reached, gas stops flowing. Initial settings should allow gas to flow in at 1 L/minute and stop if measured intra-abdominal pressure is greater than 15 to 20 mm Hg. Gas flows from the insufflator to the patient by way of a sterile plastic tube.

Opening pressures can vary with patient body habitus and level of muscle relaxation but should be less than 10 mm Hg (preferably less than 5 mm Hg). Rapid rise in pressure may indicate incorrect needle placement or obstruction by omentum. If this occurs, insufflation should stop, and the needle position should be reassessed. Once 500 ml has been insufflated, symmetric distention and tympany in all four quadrants usually can be noted. **Asymmetric distention can occur when the needle is incorrectly placed (in an extraperitoneal location or a loop of bowel) or in patients who have abdominal wall weakness from prior surgery.** Symmetric tympany implies correct position, and the flow rate may be increased to 10 L/minute to expedite reaching the set intra-abdominal pressure. Of note, the maximal flow rate through a Veress needle is 2.5 L/minute (Clayman RV, unpublished data).

Trocar Placement

Proper trocar placement is pivotal in facilitating a successful laparoscopic intervention. Trocars act as the conduit into the peritoneal cavity allowing passage of instruments for dissection and tissue removal. They also allow for maintenance of the pneumoperitoneum once the Veress needle is removed.

A trocar is a hollow tube with a removable sharpened inner obturator that is used to pierce through the abdominal wall (Fig. 95–3). A gasket and built-in valve mechanism prevent escape of gas once the trocar is placed into the insufflated peritoneal cavity. To maintain the pneumoperitoneum, most trocars have an external valve with a Luer-Lok fitting. This allows for continuous monitoring of the intra-abdominal pressure and insufflation.

Both disposable and nondisposable trocars are available from several manufacturers. The reusable units are more cost-effective but have certain limitations compared with their disposable counterparts. The nondisposable trocars are made of metal and thus are heavier than the plastic disposable units. They are also radiopaque, which may be problematic when intraoperative radiography is required. Moreover, the tip of the nondisposable obturator dulls with time and needs routine sharpening. Finally, Corson and colleagues have demonstrated that significantly more force is needed to introduce these trocars compared with disposable units (Corson et al, 1989). The potential thus exists for inadvertently transmitting this force to underlying organs. The disposable units have a safety shield that snaps into place once the obturator has pierced the peritoneal cavity to protect underlying structures from injury (Fig. 95–4).

Once the pneumoperitoneum has been achieved with the Veress needle, trocar placement can commence. A skin incision is made parallel to Langer's lines or along natural skin folds to provide an optimal cosmetic result. The incision should be made just sufficient to allow for placement of the trocar; too large an incision can result in continuous loss of the pneumoperitoneum, whereas too small an incision can necessitate excessive force to move the trocar through the skin. Once the skin incision is made, a curved clamp can be used to spread away vessels in the subcutaneous tissue.

The surgeon takes the trocar in his or her dominant hand with the index finger extended to act as a break to prevent

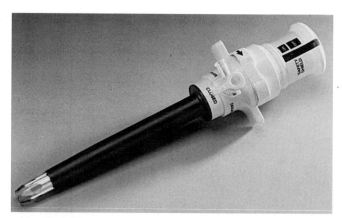

Figure 95–3. The trocar consists of a hollow tube with seals and an active valve to maintain the pneumoperitoneum. The Luer-Lok fitting allows for maintenance of the pneumoperitoneum.

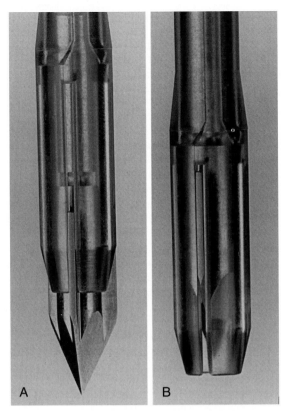

Figure 95–4. Trocars come with a sharp obturator to perforate the abdominal wall fascia. Disposable trocars have a safety shield to prevent bowel injury during placement. During placement, the inner sharp core is exposed to pierce the fascia (*A*). Once the fascia is traversed, the outer shield slides over the blade to protect underlying organs (*B*).

where 2–0 silk stay sutures are placed. The fascia and peritoneum are incised just wide enough to allow a finger into the peritoneal cavity to be sure no bowel or omentum is adherent to the abdominal wall. A specially designed blunt-tipped trocar (Hassan trocar) is then passed into the incision (Hassan, 1971). The stay sutures are wrapped about holders built onto the trocar sleeve, which is snugged down to the incision (Fig. 95–5). This prevents the trocar from dislodging and creates a seal that preserves the pneumoperitoneum.

Gasless Laparoscopy

Because of potential risks of the pneumoperitoneum, some investigators prefer alternative methods to create the working space. Gasless laparoscopy uses mechanical means to tent up the abdominal wall (Akimaru et al, 1993; Araki et al, 1993; Etwaru et al, 1994). One such gasless technique involves passing a blunt blade through an incision into the peritoneal cavity and placing upward traction on the blade by connecting it to an arm clamped to the operating table (Etwaru et al, 1994). Another method involves placing sutures through the abdominal wall fascia and suspending the suture from the ceiling (Araki et al, 1993). These gasless techniques eliminate the need for using trocars and allow for standard surgical instruments to be placed through small incisions. The primary disadvantage of these approaches is an asymmetric limited working space compared with traditional laparoscopy; however, further modification of these devices may lead to more widespread application.

the trocar from advancing too deeply. The nondominant hand is also used to guide the trocar in a controlled manner. Constant steady pressure is placed while using a twisting motion until the trocar is felt to pop into the peritoneal cavity. Once the trocar enters the peritoneal cavity, a rush of gas is heard escaping from the external valve. The insufflator is then connected to the external valve of the trocar, and the laparoscope is inserted. The peritoneal cavity is inspected for possible injury because of Veress needle or trocar placement.

Disposable trocars have become available with visual obturators such that the laparoscope can be placed down the center of the trocar. This allows for direct visualization of all abdominal wall layers during passage and potentially provides safer placement under direct vision.

Trocar placement without first creating a pneumoperitoneum has been described in large series with minimal morbidity (Jarrett, 1990). The trocar is directly placed while lifting the abdominal wall with the nondominant hand. The peritoneal cavity is then inflated through the trocar.

Open Access

Some surgeons prefer to obtain initial access using open trocar placement. This technique is favored for patients who have undergone multiple prior surgeries and in patients in whom difficulty is encountered with Veress needle placement. A 2- to 3-cm incision is made down to the fascia,

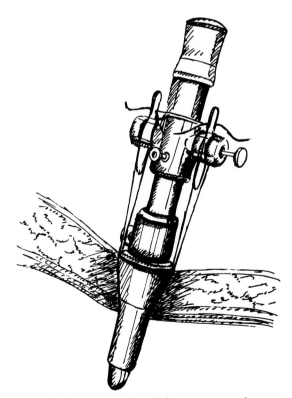

Figure 95–5. A Hassan trocar is used for open trocar placement. Stay sutures are placed in the fascia and wrapped about the outer sleeve of the trocar to prevent trocar migration or gas leakage.

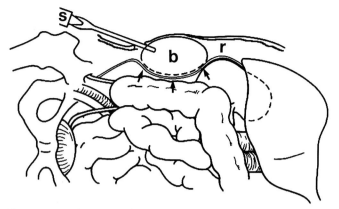

Figure 95–6. Placement of an extraperitoneal balloon (b) to create a working space. A syringe (s) is used to fill the balloon placed in the retroperitoneum (r). Inflation results in separation of the peritoneum (*arrows*) from the posterior abdominal musculature. When performing renal surgery, this balloon can be placed within Gerota's fascia.

Extraperitoneal Laparoscopy

Several investigators have advocated using a direct approach to the retroperitoneum to minimize potential risks associated with transperitoneal surgery (Gaur, 1992, 1993; Gaur et al, 1993; Capelouto et al, 1994; McDougall et al, 1994b). The first direct percutaneous approach to the retroperitoneum was by Wickham in 1979 (Wickham and Miller, 1983). Using a nephroscope, he reported a case of retroperitoneoscopy for the purpose of removing a ureteral calculus. Kerbl and associates used blunt dissection in their initial report on retroperitoneoscopic nephrectomy (Kerbl et al, 1993d). This technique was refined by Gaur, who described the use of a dilating balloon after bluntly entering the retroperitoneal space at the superior lumbar triangle (Fig. 95–6) (Gaur, 1992). Balloon dilation facilitates the creation of the operative space by separating and compressing the loose connective tissue. A variety of commercially built balloons are currently available. Alternatively, "homemade" balloons fashioned from catheters and parts of surgical gloves, rectal sheaths, or condoms have been reported (McDougall et al, 1994b).

Balloon dilation is not without risk, and **incorrect placement or rupture can result in tissue damage** (Adams et al, 1996). Filling with fluid under low pressure with a large-diameter syringe minimizes damage in the event of rupture (Moore et al, 1995a).

Secondary Trocar Placement

After the initial trocar is secured in place, secondary trocars should be passed under direct vision. The abdominal wall is inspected under the selected trocar site to identify underlying vessels. The abdominal wall is then transilluminated to avoid injuring superficial abdominal wall vessels. During placement, the tip of the secondary trocar must be continuously monitored. Once all secondary trocars are placed, the camera is repositioned to inspect the initial trocar site for injury to an abdominal wall vessel.

All trocars should be fixed to the abdominal wall to avoid dislodgment during surgery. Special sleeves that screw into the abdominal wall can be used. Alternatively, trocars are available with balloon or Malecot tips to prevent accidental removal. The authors prefer to secure the trocar with a 2–0 polyglactin 910 (Vicryl) suture to the abdominal wall (Kavoussi and Clayman, 1992). If gas leaks about a trocar site, petroleum jelly gauze can be wrapped around the base and a purse-string suture placed to help obtain a tight seal.

Trocar Configuration

One of the most crucial factors in facilitating laparoscopic dissection is choosing the most advantageous trocar arrangement in aligning the surgeon, laparoscope, and video monitor to the operative field. The camera is the surgeon's eyes in viewing the operative field, so proper orientation is mandatory. **The laparoscope must always be held such that the image is upright relative to the floor, not the operating table. With the tip of the laparoscope aimed at the opera-**

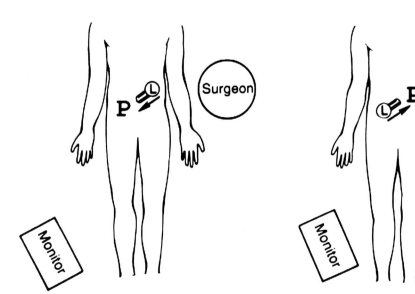

Figure 95–7. When performing laparoscopy, the surgeon should be positioned across the patient from the video monitor. The laparoscope (L) acts as the surgeon's eyes and thus should be placed between the surgeon and the operative field (P). Placement behind the pathology results in viewing the operative field in a mirror image.

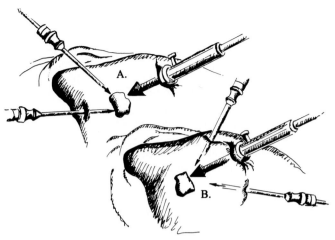

Figure 95–8. Trocars should be placed between the surgeon and the operative field *(B)*. If they are positioned behind the operative field *(A)*, instrument motion is as if one were operating on a mirror image.

tive field, the surgeon should be standing facing the eyepiece (Fig. 95–7). **The video monitor is placed directly across the table in line with the surgeon, laparoscope, and operative field. Primary working trocars should not be placed behind the vertical plane of the operative field** (Fig. 95–8). This creates an awkward situation with instruments behaving as if one were operating on a mirror image (i.e., hand motions to the left cause instruments to move to the left).

Patient positioning and trocar configuration depend on the pathology being approached, patient body habitus, and prior surgical history. In general, when approaching pelvic pathology, the patient should be positioned supine on the operative table and the Veress needle placed in the base of the umbilicus. Once trocars are placed, the patient should be put in a steep Trendelenburg position to allow bowel to shift from the operative field. Lateral tilting of the table also helps expose the pathology. The upper ureter, kidney, and adrenal gland are best approached with the patient in a modified or full flank position. In these instances, the Veress needle is placed just lateral to the rectus muscle at the level of the iliac crest. Again, tilting the table may be helpful in exposing the operative field.

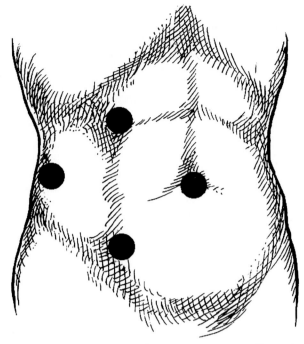

Figure 95–10. Trocar placement for upper tract surgery: diamond configuration.

Care should be taken not to place trocar sites too close together or between the laparoscope and pathology. In general, **a fan or diamond configuration allows for optimal access when working in the pelvis** (Fig. 95–9). When working on the upper urinary tract, a diamond or pentagon configuration is advisable (Fig. 95–10).

Concluding Laparoscopic Procedures

All laparoscopic procedures should be concluded in a sequential fashion. The pneumoperitoneum can tamponade bleeding at higher pressures. Hence, the intra-abdominal pressure should be lowered to 7 mm Hg and the operative field inspected for adequate hemostasis at the conclusion of the case.

Trocars may also tamponade abdominal wall bleeding and

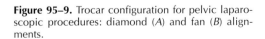

Figure 95–9. Trocar configuration for pelvic laparoscopic procedures: diamond *(A)* and fan *(B)* alignments.

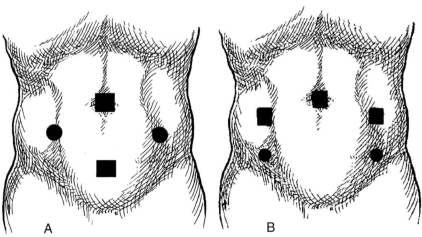

A   B

thus should be removed under direct vision. **The anterior fascia of 10 mm or greater trocar sites in adults and all trocar sites in children should be closed under visual control to avoid postoperative hernia formation** (Bloom and Ehrlich, 1993). This may be readily accomplished in thin individuals by standard extracorporeal suture placement; however, in heavier patients, suture placement can be challenging. A variety of suturing devices have been developed to facilitate fascial closure.

Before removing the final trocar, all carbon dioxide should be evacuated from the peritoneal cavity. Residual gas can irritate the peritoneum and cause postoperative abdominal, back, shoulder, and chest pain. The final trocar should be backed out over the laparoscope and the laparoscope removed slowly to inspect for tract bleeding and prevent bowel from being pulled into the incision.

Postoperative Care

The orogastric tube is removed at the conclusion of the procedure. The Foley catheter, stents, and any drains are left indwelling according to each operation. Oral intake and usual activity are advanced as tolerated.

LAPAROSCOPIC APPLICATIONS IN THE ADULT

The potential advantages of a laparoscopic approach have led to reports of treating essentially all surgical abdominal and pelvic urologic pathology in a laparoscopic manner; however, several shortcomings have limited widespread advocation. First, technical boundaries have restricted global endorsement: Limited outcomes data exist, and current techniques do not allow all procedures to be completed in a cost-effective time frame. When applied to treat malignancy, predominantly small series with short follow-up are available for comparison. Moreover, laparoscopic procedures require a general anesthetic, whereas open approaches to pelvic pathology can be done with a regional anesthetic. Many laparoscopic approaches currently require longer operative time when compared to open procedures, raising the overall cost of the procedure (Troxel and Winfield, 1994; Winfield et al, 1994b; Bishoff et al, 1996). Finally, laparoscopy requires technical expertise that has not been taught during residency training of the majority of practicing urologists. The relative degree of difficulty and limited number of appropriate cases compared to those available in general surgery or gynecology markedly restrict the ability of most urologists to feel comfortable with a laparoscopic approach.

Despite these shortcomings, the advantages of a laparoscopic approach make it an attractive alternative for many patients. In many applications, the decrease in postoperative morbidity can be obtained while achieving equivalent operative results to those of open surgery. Time will help determine which disease processes in which patient population would be best served by a laparoscopic approach. This section reviews the more common diseases to which laparoscopy has been applied and found to be useful.

Varicocelectomy

Laparoscopy has been used as an approach to treat a symptomatic varicocele (Donovan and Winfield, 1992a; Donovan and Winfield, 1992b; Hagood et al, 1992; Jarow et al, 1993; Reissigl et al, 1993; Mischinger et al, 1994). It is the least technically demanding interventional laparoscopic procedure performed by urologists and perhaps the most controversial. The indications for a laparoscopic repair are similar to those for an open repair and include varicoceles associated with pain, infertility, and impaired testicular growth.

With the patient in a supine position, three trocars are placed: a 10-mm umbilical trocar, a 10-mm trocar on the contralateral side at the level of the umbilicus just lateral to the rectus muscle, and a 5-mm trocar on the contralateral side in the left lower quadrant. The camera is placed in the lateral 10-mm trocar, whereas the other trocars are used for dissection and clip application.

Once all trocars are in place, the spermatic vessels and vas are identified entering the slit-like internal ring. A peritoneal incision is made lateral to the spermatic vessels, 2 cm away from the internal ring (Fig. 95–11). The incision is taken 4 cm proximally, and midway across the incision the peritoneum is transected over the cord to create a T. The spermatic cord is then freed from the underlying psoas muscle and is gently split to dissect out the veins and artery.

Careful observation allows for visualization of the artery;

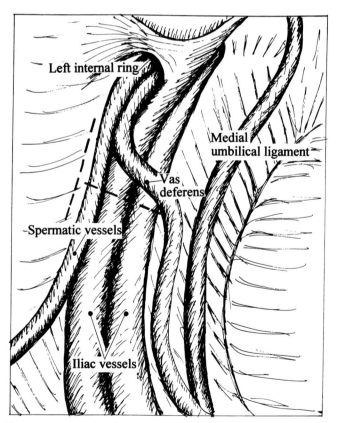

Figure 95–11. Landmarks for varix ligation: the intimal inguinal ring, vas deferens, and spermatic cord. A T-incision is made beginning lateral to the cord to expose the spermatic veins, which are clipped and transected.

however, if there is uncertainty, a laparoscopic Doppler probe may be used. Alternatively, dripping papaverine on the vessel may be helpful to allow identification of vessels put into spasm by manipulation. Once the artery is identified, all nonarterial tissue is clipped and transected.

Data indicate that a laparoscopic approach offers equivalent results as that obtained with open ligation. Donovan and Winfield (1992a, 1992b) reported on 50 patients with 71 varicoceles: 29 unilateral (58%) and 21 bilateral (42%). The spermatic artery was preserved in 67 (94.3%) patients. They found no major complications, and in only one patient was a persistent varix noted. In 29 cases of infertility, they had 6-month follow-up and found improvement in sperm density in 82%, found improvement in motility in 50%, and achieved pregnancy in 34%. The procedure was accomplished on an outpatient basis in 88% of cases, with patients returning to usual activity on average 4.3 days postoperatively.

Ogura and associates performed a comparative study of 97 patients undergoing either laparoscopic or open high varicocele ligation (Ogura et al, 1994). They found no difference in improvement in semen parameters and pregnancy but did note a statistical decrease in postoperative recovery time for the laparoscopic group.

These results are similar to what has been reported for open varix ligation. Pryor and Howards (1987) reviewed 15 series of open varix ligation and found improvement in semen parameters in 66% of patients and pregnancy rates ranging from 24% to 53%.

Laparoscopic varix ligation does have several disadvantages compared with open dissection. The average operative times tend to be longer for a laparoscopic approach (Ross and Ruppman, 1993; Ogura et al, 1994). In the University of Iowa series, operative times were 107 minutes for unilateral and 164 minutes for bilateral varix ligation (Donovan and Winfield, 1992b). Moreover, the laparoscopic approach requires a general anesthetic compared with many open ligations, which can be performed under a regional or local anesthetic. Several centers have reported the postoperative morbidity and recovery of a laparoscopic approach to be greater than vascular embolization or subinguinal varicocelectomy (Ross and Ruppman, 1993; Enquist et al, 1994). Thus, the decision to choose a laparoscopic approach to varix ligation must be individualized.

Lymphadenectomy

Limitations with noninvasive radiographic methods (computed tomography, magnetic resonance imaging) to assess accurately the status of pelvic lymph nodes in patients with prostate cancer led to the development of the laparoscopic pelvic lymphadenectomy (LPLND) (Loughlin and Kavoussi, 1992; Moore et al, 1996). The use of this technique depends on one's philosophy in treating the primary lesion. If one believes that only patients with organ-confined disease are candidates for curative therapy, lymphadenectomy is useful. Conversely, lymphadenectomy is unwarranted if treatment recommendation is not based on pathologic assessment.

When initially introduced, LPLND was applied to all patients who were candidates for local curative therapy. Contemporary series, however, that used screening criteria (i.e., prostate-specific antigen [PSA], Gleason grade, clinical

stage) demonstrated that the incidence of pathologically positive pelvic lymph nodes was much lower than described in earlier reports (Petros and Catalona, 1992; Danella et al, 1993; Partin et al, 1993). It has been recommended that LPLND be used only in individuals who are at an increased risk of having lymph node metastasis based on probability nomograms (Moore et al, 1996).

Technique

Patient preparation consists of a Fleet enema the evening before surgery to decompress the sigmoid colon. The patient is positioned supine with a Foley catheter in place. A compression dressing is wrapped around the scrotum and penis to prevent pneumoscrotum from developing.

Once a pneumoperitoneum is achieved, trocars can be placed in either a diamond or a fan configuration (see Fig. 95–9). **In relatively obese patients, the fan configuration is preferable because fatty tissue may be more prominent overlying the urachus.** The patient should be placed in the Trendelenburg position with the operative field tilted upward to shift bowel out of the way.

After trocar placement, pelvic landmarks should be identified, including the medial umbilical ligament, inguinal ring, spermatic vessels, and urachus (Fig. 95–12). In thin patients, the vas deferens and pulsating iliac vessels may also be identified. Often the sigmoid colon and cecum encroach on the operative field. Adhesions and peritoneal reflections may need to be incised to have clear access to the obturator fossa.

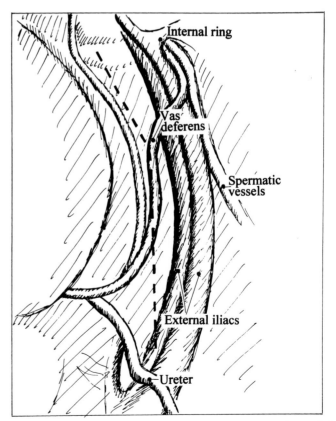

Figure 95–12. Landmarks for the pelvic lymphadenectomy: the medial umbilical ligament, vas deferens, and spermatic vessels. The initial incision is made just lateral to the medial umbilical ligament.

A longitudinal incision is made just lateral to the medial umbilical ligament extending from the pubic bone proximally to the bifurcation of the iliac vessels (see Fig. 95–12). Using blunt dissection, the vas deferens is identified, clipped, and divided. The medial border of the iliac vein is next identified and cleared distally to the pubis and proximally to the iliac bifurcation. This maneuver establishes the lateral border of the nodal tissue. The packet is then grasped distally, and while placing medial traction on the medial umbilical ligament, the tissues are spread to identify the underlying pubic bone and create the medial border of the dissection. The distal extent of the packet is then ligated with clips and transected (Fig. 95–13).

The packet is grasped and pulled proximally, revealing the obturator nerve (see Fig. 95–13). Blunt dissection is usually sufficient to free the packet to the iliac bifurcation, where the remaining attachments are ligated and transected. A 10-mm spoon grasper is used to remove the packet under direct vision. Large specimens may be placed in a laparoscopic sac to facilitate extraction and minimize the risk of tissue loss. The sac is grasped by the neck and brought into the trocar, where the trocar and sac can be removed en bloc through the incision.

In some patients, an extended pelvic lymphadenectomy may be warranted. These include patients with carcinoma of the bladder, penis, and urethra (Bowsher et al, 1992; Winfield et al, 1992; Holevas et al, 1993; Assimos and Jarow, 1994). Moreover, in select patients with prostate cancer (i.e., high-risk patients in whom obturator nodes are negative), a more extensive dissection may be preferred by the surgeon (Schuessler et al, 1993). In an extended dissection, tissue is removed from the iliac vessels laterally to the genitofemoral nerve and proximally to the aortic bifurcation. In these cases, further bowel mobilization is necessary, and care must be taken to identify and preserve the ureters.

Results

Comparative investigations with open pelvic lymph node dissection (OPLND) have verified the applicability of LPLND as an accurate staging tool (Schuessler et al, 1991; Winfield et al, 1992; Kerbl et al, 1993c; Rukstalis et al, 1994). Studies examining tissue yield confirm it to be equivalent to OPLND; however, false-negative studies can occur during the learning phase (Winfield et al, 1992; Guazzoni et al, 1994a; Rukstalis et al, 1994). Guazzoni and associates have estimated this learning curve to be less than 30 cases and recommend open surgical verification for physicians with less experience (Guazzoni et al, 1994a).

These studies have demonstrated significantly less postoperative morbidity with LPLND compared to OPLND. Kerbl and co-workers showed lower narcotic requirements (1.55 versus 47 mg morphine), shorter hospital stay (1.7 versus 5.37 days), and quicker return to normal activity (10.8 versus 65.5 days) for laparoscopic versus open procedures (Kerbl et al, 1993c).

Several series have demonstrated an initial overall complication rate of 15% with LPLND; however, with experience, it appears to be less than 4% (Parra et al, 1992a; Kavoussi et al, 1993c; Lang et al, 1994). This compares to complication rates of 0% to 33% reported in series of OPLND (Freiha and Salzman, 1977; Babaian et al, 1981; Donohue et al, 1990; McDowell et al, 1990).

Extraperitoneal endoscopic pelvic lymphadenectomy (EELND) has been championed as an alternative to transperitoneal dissection to avoid potential injury to intraperitoneal structures (Villers et al, 1993; Das and Tashima, 1994; Etwaru et al, 1994). Anecdotal experience indicates that in rare instances a transperitoneal approach can result in bowel adhesions to the pelvic sidewall, making secondary radical surgery more complicated (Williams R, personal communication, 1996). This procedure has been found to be comparable to LPLND in completeness, operative time, postoperative pain, and complications (Etwaru et al, 1994). It may be a useful alternative in patients who have had prior intra-abdominal surgery; however, lack of anatomic landmarks and decreased working space make this approach more difficult. Moreover, studies have demonstrated that risk of postoperative intra-abdominal adhesion formation is not as great as postulated with a transabdominal approach (Moore et al, 1995b, 1995c). Thus far, no studies have shown a distinct advantage of EELND over LPLND.

As with most laparoscopic procedures, operative time for LPLND is longer than traditional open dissection (Troxel and Winfield, 1994). This factor has continued to make hospital charges for LPLND higher than OPLND even though postoperative charges were less for LPLND. Although postoperative charges were 280% greater for OPLND, Troxel and Winfield found the more expensive operative costs to be 52% higher for LPLND, resulting in greater overall costs of LPLND (Troxel and Winfield, 1996).

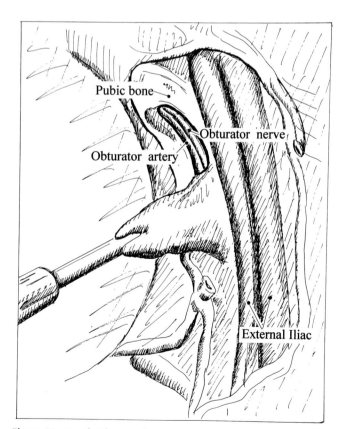

Figure 95–13. After ligating the vas deferens, the nodal packet is freed off the iliac vein laterally and perivesical fat medially. The nodal tissue is reflected proximally to expose the obturator nerve and vessels.

Nephrectomy

The first upper urinary tract application of laparoscopy was by Clayman and associates, who performed a laparoscopic nephrectomy in 1990 for benign disease (Clayman et al, 1991). Since this report, several centers have verified the advantages of this technique in treating select patients with both benign and malignant processes affecting the upper urinary tract (Coptcoat et al, 1992; Kavoussi et al, 1993a; Kerbl et al, 1993a; Kerbl et al, 1993b; Rassweiler et al, 1993; Eraky et al, 1994).

Technique

The procedure is performed with the patient in the flank position as if to undergo an open nephrectomy. Five trocars are positioned in the flank with the camera starting in the lower midclavicular line (see Fig. 95–10). The peritoneum is incised to reflect the colon medially to expose Gerota's fascia (Fig. 95–14). Lateral attachments are freed so that the kidney can be retracted anteriorly, and the camera is moved to the posterior port to view the renal hilum. The artery is clipped with 9-mm clips and transected (Fig. 95–15). The vein is ligated with a vascular GIA (gastrointestinal anastomosis) stapler, and the ureter is clipped and cut. When treating malignancy, the adrenal vessels can also be ligated with clips. The kidney is then freed from surrounding tissue using a combination of blunt and sharp dissection.

When performing nephroureterectomy, the ureter is freed to the level of the bladder (McDougall et al, 1995a). A GIA stapler is used to transect the ureter with a cuff of bladder. Cystoscopy is performed at the conclusion of the procedure to be sure a watertight closure has been obtained.

Once free, the kidney is manipulated into an organ entrapment sack (Fig. 95–16). The neck of the sack is brought out through the lower midclavicular trocar site. The kidney is then morcellated under direct vision using ring forceps or an electric tissue morcellator.

Results

Laparoscopic nephrectomy has been successfully completed at several centers (Coptcoat et al, 1992; Kavoussi et

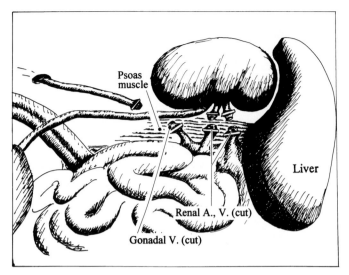

Figure 95–15. Endoscopic clips are used to control the renal artery and vein.

al, 1993a; Kerbl et al, 1993a; Rassweiler et al, 1993; Eraky et al, 1994). Postoperative results are similar to that of open nephrectomy with markedly less pain and convalescence (Perez et al, 1994). In the Washington University experience of 47 patients undergoing laparoscopic nephrectomy, the mean operative time was 355 minutes (Kerbl et al, 1994). Postoperative pain medicine requirements were four times less than traditional open procedures. Mean hospital stay was less than 4 days, and all patients achieved **full convalescence at 1.8 months.** Of note, **full convalescence in patients undergoing open nephrectomy averaged 9.9 months.**

Gill and co-workers summarized the results of laparoscopic nephrectomy in a multi-institutional review of 185 patients (Gill et al, 1995b). Ten patients (5.4%) required conversion to open surgery: two emergent and eight elective. The emergent cases were opened because of hemorrhage, whereas elective conversion was performed because of difficulty of dissection from fibrosis (five) or size (two). In one case, conversion was performed because of injury to the superior mesenteric artery.

In Gill's series, there was no mortality; however, 16% of patients had complications. The complication rate for benign disease (12%) was less than that for malignancy (34%). The incidence of complications decreased markedly with experience: 71% of complications occurred during the initial 20 cases at each institution.

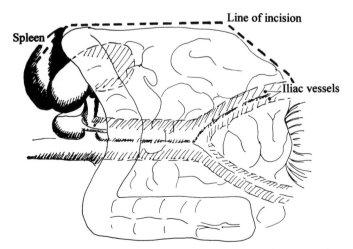

Figure 95–14. For a transperitoneal approach to the kidney, the colon must be reflected medially. The splenic flexure must be incised on the left and hepatic flexure on the right.

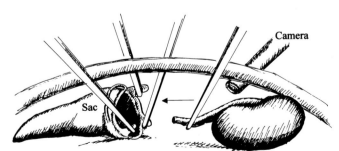

Figure 95–16. Graspers are used to triangulate the endoscopic sack to facilitate organ entrapment.

The use of laparoscopic nephrectomy has been extended to treat patients with malignant disease of the upper urinary tract (Kavoussi et al, 1993a; Ono et al, 1993; Gill et al, 1995a). Similar convalesence results have been achieved as when approaching benign disease. Capelouto and associates reported on nine patients with upper tract malignancies with at least 1 year follow-up (Capelouto et al, 1995). Overall, survival was no different than if patients were treated with incisional nephrectomy. One patient with nodal positive disease died of metastatic disease in 1 year, and two patients had bladder recurrences treated by transurethral resection.

Limited data are available regarding laparoscopic nephroureterectomy for upper tract transitional cell carcinoma (Rassweiler et al, 1992; Das et al, 1993; McDougall et al, 1995a). McDougall and associates performed laparoscopic nephroureterectomy in ten patients (average age 68 years), all of whom were followed for at least 1 year (McDougall et al, 1995a). They were successful in removing the entire ureter in all but the first patient. The specimen was placed in an entrapment sac and removed intact by extending a dorsal or lower trocar site 5 cm to obtain a specimen for assessing pathologic margins. Pathology revealed organ-confined disease in all but one patient, who subsequently died of disease. Three patients developed subsequent bladder recurrences away from the cuff that were managed transurethrally. They compared their results with 13 similar patients undergoing open nephroureterectomy during the same time period and found that the laparoscopic group had significantly less blood loss, needed less pain medication, and had a shorter hospital stay. Moreover, the period to full recovery was 6 weeks in the laparoscopic group compared with 7.4 months in the open group.

A novel approach to live donor transplantation has been reported by Schulam and co-workers (1996). They performed laparoscopic live donor nephrectomy in seven patients in whom they delivered the kidney through an 8-cm lower midline incision. The warm ischemic time was less than 5 minutes, and the lengths of renal vessels and ureter were adequate for routine transplantation. All harvested kidneys were successfully transplanted without complication, and donors required minimal postoperative analgesia and convalescence.

Upper Urinary Tract Applications

Laparoscopy has been successfully used to treat a variety of pathologies affecting the upper urinary tract (Kavoussi et al, 1992a; Atala et al, 1993; Baba et al, 1993; Puppo et al, 1994; Brooks et al, 1995). Both ablative and reconstructive procedures have been demonstrated to be feasible and efficacious by several investigators worldwide.

Partial Nephrectomy

Successful studies in porcine models have led to limited clinical attempts to perform partial nephrectomy (Gill et al, 1993; Jordan and Winslow, 1993a; McDougall et al, 1993b; Winfield et al, 1994a). For these procedures, purpose-designed equipment (i.e., plastic tourniquets, pedicle clamps) has been suggested as means to control intraoperative bleeding and facilitate renal manipulation (Gill et al, 1993;

Kletscher et al, 1995). After parenchymal excision, absorbable gelatin sponge (Gelfoam), oxidized cellulose (Surgicel), and argon beam coagulation have been found to be helpful to achieve adequate hemostasis.

Winfield and colleagues have reported successful partial nephrectomy in four of five patients with mean postoperative convalescence of less than 3 weeks (Winfield et al, 1994a). McDougall and co-workers described two patients who underwent a retroperitoneal approach to excise benign lesions (McDougall et al, 1994b).

Successful reports of partial nephrectomy with ureterectomy have been described in children with duplicated collecting systems (Ehrlich et al, 1993a; Jordan and Winslow, 1993a). In these cases, dissection in the avascular plain between normal kidney and the obstructed segment decreased the potential for bleeding.

Cyst Ablation

Symptomatic simple renal cysts (i.e., pain, hypertension, decreased function owing to compression) have been ablated by both the transperitoneal and the retroperitoneal laparoscopic routes (Rubenstein et al, 1993; Guazzoni et al, 1993; Munch et al, 1994). Laparoscopy is reserved for patients who have failed prior aspiration with sclerosis or those who are at risk for complications of fibrosis with sclerosis (i.e., peripelvic cyst). This approach may also be helpful in evaluating patients with indeterminant cystic renal masses (Yamaguchi et al, 1995).

The surface of the cyst should be completely exposed and cyst fluid aspirated for cytology. **The cyst wall is sharply excised completely, and the cyst and any suspicious areas in the base are sent for pathologic analysis.** To prevent recurrence, the base can be lightly fulgurated with the argon beam coagulator, packed with Surgicel, or filled with surrounding fat.

Limited series have demonstrated success in greater than 95% of cases and complication rates of less than 4% (Guazzoni et al, 1993; Rubenstein et al, 1993; Munch et al, 1994). Reports exist on patients who were found intraoperatively or postoperatively to have an unsuspected neoplasm (Rubenstein et al, 1993; Stanley et al, 1993). These patients were subsequently treated by open nephrectomy with wide excision. Short-term follow-up did not reveal evidence of tumor recurrence.

Limited data appear promising in using laparoscopy to treat patients with symptomatic polycystic kidney disease (Elashry et al, 1996). In reported cases, all visible cysts were excised. Intraoperative ultrasonography has been useful in locating cysts. Long-term follow-up is lacking to demonstrate the durability of this operative approach.

Adrenalectomy

The fragility and anatomic location of the adrenal gland deep within the retroperitoneum initially intimidated surgeons from using laparoscopy to treat surgical pathology. Once attempted, however, it became quickly apparent that laparoscopy offers a straightforward and delicate means to remove the adrenal gland (Albala and Prinz, 1994; Guazzoni et al, 1994b; Suzuki et al, 1994; Takeda et al, 1994). Functional adenomas, adrenocortical carcinomas, Cushing's syndrome, and pheochromocytomas have all been laparoscopically.

Nakagawa and associates reported on 25 patients undergoing laparoscopic adrenalectomy and compared them to 15 patients undergoing open removal (Nakagawa et al, 1995). Blood loss was minimal, and they found the mean operative time to be 254 minutes for the laparoscopic group compared to 190 minutes for the open cases. Postoperative pain medication requirement and convalescence were statistically significantly less in the laparoscopic group. These data are similar to what have been reported in cumulative series (Gill et al, 1995a).

Reconstructive Lower Tract Applications

The gold standard for the treatment of stress urinary incontinence has been retropubic bladder suspension. The evolution of surgical approaches for the correction of stress urinary incontinence has focused on minimally invasive techniques to place the urethra in a high, well-supported retropubic position. Laparoscopy has evolved as an alternative technique that allows for placement of suture under visual control without the morbidity associated with an open retropubic repair (Albala et al, 1992; Breda et al, 1993; Liu, 1993; Das and Palmer, 1995; McDougall et al, 1995c; Polascik et al, 1995).

Early reports using laparoscopy have demonstrated hospital stay and pain medication requirements similar to transvaginal approaches; however, success rates at 2 years are roughly 75% (McDougall et al, 1995c; Polascik et al, 1995). This is **no better** than what is obtained with the minimally invasive transvaginal approaches (Rodriguez et al, 1995; Trockman et al, 1995). Greater understanding of the pathophysiology of female stress incontinence is needed to help guide new surgical therapies.

Laparoscopic cystectomy and ileal conduit urinary diversion have been performed for pyocystis and invasive bladder cancer (Kozminski and Partamian, 1992; Parra et al, 1992b; Sanchez-de-Badajoz et al, 1993). Cases of laparoscopic partial cystectomy for diverticula or tumor and autoaugmentation have also been reported (Das, 1992; Ehrlich and Gershman, 1993; Docimo et al, 1995b; McDougall et al, 1995b). The technical complexity of these procedures, potential risks, and unknown long-term results markedly limit the utility of these procedures.

Schuessler and associates have demonstrated the feasibility of laparoscopic radical prostatectomy in five patients (Schuessler et al, 1994). Unfortunately, difficulties with the creation of the vesicourethral anastomosis lead to lengthy operative times, and thus far the advantages of minimizing postoperative morbidity have not been demonstrated.

Reconstructive Upper Tract Applications

The development of laparoscopic suturing techniques and evolution of purpose-built instrumentation have allowed for the application of laparoscopic reconstructive techniques

(Adams et al, 1995b). The efficacy and safety of pyeloplasty, ureterolithotomy, pyelolithotomy, and ureterolysis have been confirmed, and data have demonstrated success rates similar to comparable open series with much less morbidity (Gaur, 1993; Brooks et al, 1995). The greatest limiting factors to widespread application have been increased operative time and technical expertise needed to perform these complex procedures. Limited reports on ureteral reimplantation, ureterosigmoidostomy, and ileal conduit urinary diversion in highly select patients and in experimental models have also been published (Kozminski and Partamian, 1992; Anderson et al, 1993; Atala et al, 1993; Ehrlich et al, 1993b; Sanchez-de-Badajoz et al, 1993; Janetschek et al, 1995b).

Laparoscopy has also revived interest in renal ptosis. The historical overdiagnosis of this condition and lack of defined pathophysiology for symptoms (i.e., pain) caused most urologists to question this entity as a true medical condition. Careful evaluation implies that in select patients renal ptosis can result in pain (Hubner et al, 1994; Urban et al, 1993). Laparoscopic fixation allows for a minimally morbid approach to secure the renal capsule to the retroperitoneum.

Laparoscopy as Applied to the Male Genital Tract

The genital system offers a wide variety of pathologic conditions for which laparoscopic techniques have proven efficacious. Laparoscopic techniques have been developed to approach the seminal vesicles. These have been shown to be helpful in isolating the seminal vesicles in preparation for a perineal prostatectomy or in treating congenital pathology (symptomatic seminal vesicle cyst) (Kavoussi et al, 1993b; McDougall et al, 1994a).

Retroperitoneal lymph node sampling has also been advocated for select patients with primary testicular carcinoma (Janetschek et al, 1993; Gerber et al, 1994; Rassweiler et al, 1994). Studies have demonstrated the ability to perform both lymph node sampling and complete dissection. Thus far, most cases have been in patients with low-stage disease; however, Janetschek and colleagues have demonstrated the feasibility of removing bulky disease after chemotherapy (Janetschek et al, 1995a).

LAPAROSCOPIC APPLICATIONS IN THE CHILD

Diagnostic Laparoscopy for Cryptorchidism

Indications

Laparoscopic evaluation permits precise and accurate localization of the nonpalpable testis (NPT). Representing approximately 25% of all boys with cryptorchidism, those with NPT pose a clinical challenge. The initial goal of the surgeon should be the specific definition of the presence or absence of a testis and its precise location to permit subsequent surgical planning. It is important to document that a testis is nonpalpable by way of careful preoperative examination and subsequent examination under anesthesia. Occasionally, what may be cord structures are felt over the pubic tubercle, or a nubbin of tissue is noted in the scrotum. Although these may represent a testicular remnant, they may also be a looping vas or simply a nodule of fatty tissue. Unless a testis is distinctly palpable, laparoscopic evaluation has emerged as an important factor in preparation for definitive management at the same operative setting (Boddy et al, 1985; Manson et al, 1985; Garibyan, 1987; Weiss and Seashore, 1987; Bloom et al, 1988; Doig, 1989; Guiney et al, 1989; Peloquin et al, 1991; Atlas and Stone, 1992; Holcomb et al, 1994; Moore et al, 1994; Tennenbaum et al, 1994; Cortes et al, 1995).

In the boy with **bilateral** NPT, laparoscopy is a useful diagnostic modality. The endocrinologic diagnosis of anorchia is reviewed elsewhere, and controversy remains as to the accuracy of human chorionic gonadotropin–stimulation tests in boys. At present, the availability of müllerian inhibiting substance assays appears to permit more accurate determination of anorchia (Yamanaka et al, 1991; Gustafson et al, 1993). It is useful to note the level of gonadotropins in the prepubertal boy with bilateral NPT. If luteinizing hormone or follicle-stimulating hormone is elevated and the testosterone level is low, it is unlikely that any testicular tissue is present. If the gonadotropins are low, it is more likely, although not absolute, that testicular tissue is present. Given this uncertainty as to the definitive diagnosis of anorchia, **the authors have recommended diagnostic laparoscopy in almost all patients with bilateral NPT.**

Unusual situations of NPTs can arise for which laparoscopy may afford clinically useful information. In a boy with a prior inguinal exploration without a testis being found and without definitive pathologic identification of remnant testicular structures, laparoscopy may be able to provide the reassurance that a testis is not being left in the abdomen (Tennenbaum et al, 1994). Older boys with a possible intra-abdominal testis are well served by laparoscopic diagnosis because surgical planning is more complex in these boys, in whom testicular mobilization is much more difficult than it is in younger boys.

Technique

A mild bowel cleansing (clear liquids for 24 hours and 1 suppository) is given preoperatively to boys in whom laparoscopic dissection of an intra-abdominal testis may be undertaken. At the time of laparoscopy, the abdomen is prepared so as to permit any form of orchiopexy. A rectal tube is placed to decompress the left colon during pneumoperitoneum, and a bladder catheter is placed. Access is achieved using open technique, although Veress technique is safe in experienced hands. A 5-mm laparoscope is used to visualize the lower abdomen and pelvis.

It is of critical importance for the operator to be familiar with the normal anatomic laparoscopic appearance of the pelvis and internal inguinal ring (Fig. 95–17). The most prominent landmark is the obliterated umbilical artery (medial umbilical ligament), running from the pelvic sidewall up to the dome of the bladder and urachus. It is a prominent white structure, covered by peritoneum. Coursing over the obliterated umbilical should be the vas deferens, the first of two critical landmarks. It is white and paralleled by multiple small vessels. It crosses the obliterated umbilical artery at

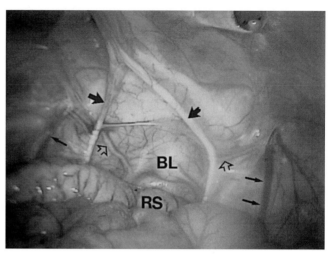

Figure 95–17. Laparoscopic view of a boy's pelvis from a right upper quadrant port. The obliterated umbilical arteries are indicated by *closed arrows,* the vasa deferentia by *open arrows.* The bladder (BL) is seen decompressed at the base of the pelvis, and just behind is the rectosigmoid (RS). The spermatic vessels are indicated by the *small arrows.*

right angles as it runs to the internal ring. Joining it at the internal inguinal ring should be the spermatic vascular pedicle, the second critical landmark (Fig. 95–18). It is usually prominent and parallels the iliac vessels at the level of the pelvic brim. Often the ureter may be seen running over the iliac vessels. The colon may mask the view of the spermatic vessels and may be moved with the telescope or by placing the patient in Trendelenburg position and tilting the table to the appropriate side up position.

The normal side should be examined first to gain a visual impression of the anatomy and the affected side then examined. Similar landmarks are used to locate the internal inguinal ring, lateral to the obliterated umbilical artery and superior to the inferior epigastric vessels. The vas and vessels

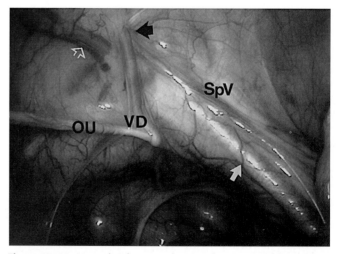

Figure 95–18. Normal right internal inguinal ring viewed laparoscopically. The vas deferens (VD) is readily seen crossing the obliterated umbilical artery (OU) and exiting the abdomen at the internal inguinal ring (*black arrow*) at the same point it joins the spermatic vessels (SpV), which run parallel to the iliac vessels (*white arrow*). The inferior epigastric vessels are seen medial to the vas deferens on the anterior abdominal wall (*open white arrow*).

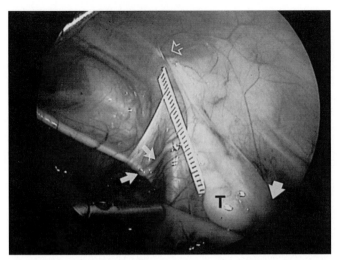

Figure 95–19. Intra-abdominal testis whose position is being measured with a laparoscopic ruler. The testis is approximately 3 cm from the internal inguinal ring (*open arrow*). The vas deferens (*small arrows*) runs over the obliterated umbilical artery and iliac vessels to join the testis (T). The *large arrow* marks the epididymis.

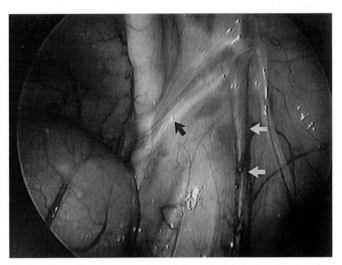

Figure 95–21. Laparoscopic view of the right inguinal region in a boy with a nonpalpable right testis. The vas (*black arrow*) appears normal as it approaches the internal ring, where it is joined by an unusual-appearing structure where the spermatic vessels should be (*white arrows*). This structure was traced cephalad and joined a testis near the inferior liver edge.

should be searched for. An intra-abdominal testis is usually readily apparent (Fig. 95–19) yet may be hidden behind the colon (Fig. 95–20), which may need to be mobilized. **To find the testis, it is critical to identify the vas deferens and the spermatic vessels.** An intra-abdominal testis may not be immediately seen, but it is usually found lateral to the iliac vessels, then cephalad along the line of the normal spermatic vessels. In such cases, the vas deferens crosses the iliac vessels more cephalad than usual, often adjacent to the ureter. The vas may also be hidden by a loop of bowel. In the setting of an intra-abdominal vanishing testis, the end of the vas and vessels are not much above the inguinal ring. Indeed, an intra-abdominal testis may appear to be a

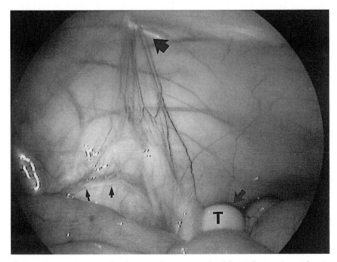

Figure 95–20. View of a boy with a nonpalpable right testis and prior negative inguinal exploration. Small vessels approach the internal ring (*large arrow*) and might be mistaken for a vanishing testis, yet the vas is not seen in association with the vessels but is more proximal and marked by the *small arrows*. The testis (T) was found behind the small bowel and cecum (*arrow*). Unless both vas deferens and vessels are seen, the diagnosis of vanishing testis cannot be made.

vanishing testis at first look (Fig. 95–21). In 104 diagnostic laparoscopies for nonpalpable testes, only one case was noted of the vas and vessels being absent on both laparoscopy and open exploration (Moore et al, 1994). In the unusual case of no identifiable vas deferens or spermatic vessels on diagnostic laparoscopy, laparoscopic retroperitoneal exploration is necessary, using two laparoscopic instrument ports in addition to the camera port. This extra effort is needed to exclude the possibility of a high intra-abdominal or perirenal testis. Other areas to inspect include the deep pelvis and paravesical area or a crossed ectopic testis (Gornall and Pender, 1987; Fairfax and Skoog, 1995). An anecdotal case of a testis passing through the obturator foramen highlights the need to examine the entire pelvis and retroperitoneum carefully (Thomas M, personal communication, 1991).

In the situation in which the vas deferens and spermatic vessels definitely fade away, indicating an intra-abdominal vanishing testis, no further exploration is necessary (Fig. 95–22) (Moore et al, 1994). One must be certain of this diagnosis. When the vas and vessels are seen to exit the internal inguinal ring, inguinal exploration is recommended. Even though it may be possible to identify the small vessels of a canalicular vanishing testis (Figs. 95–23 and 95–24), the remnant should be removed because viable germ cells have been seen in the resected testicular nubbin in 5% of cases (Plotzker et al, 1992).

Results

The initial report of the use of laparoscopy for NPT was published in 1976 by Cortesi and associates (1976), and the technique has gained steady acceptance since that time. Series have reported excellent accuracy rates and few, if any, complications (Manson et al, 1985; Garibyan, 1987; Weiss and Seashore, 1987; Bloom et al, 1988; Guiney et al, 1989; Castilho, 1990; Peloquin et al, 1991; Diamond and Caldamone, 1992; Froeling et al, 1994; Moore et al, 1994; Tennen-

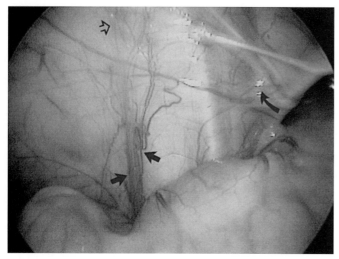

Figure 95–22. Vanishing testis in a boy with a nonpalpable left testis. The spermatic vessels (*arrows*) are clearly seen and thin out rapidly near the inguinal ring (*open arrow,*) as does the vas deferens (*curved arrow*).

baum et al, 1994; Cortes et al, 1995). A meta-analytic review of reported cases from 1976 to 1992 demonstrated an accuracy rate of 93%, representing more than 750 cases (Peters et al, 1992). To confirm the claims of accuracy, open surgical exploration was performed in all of 104 patients (122 testes) undergoing diagnostic laparoscopy and could demonstrate an accuracy of 97% (Moore et al, 1994). In two cases, an intra-abdominal testis might not have been identified laparoscopically. In each case, however, the vas deferens and spermatic vessels had not been specifically identified. **It is clear that these two structures must be specifically seen without question to permit an accurate diagnosis.** The incidences of the various diagnostic groups are shown in Figure 95–25, drawn from many reports. The high incidence

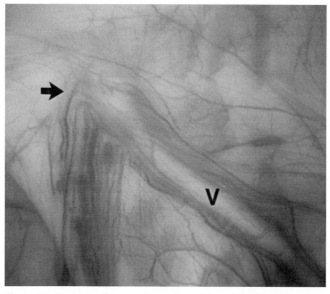

Figure 95–23. Normal inguinal ring viewed laparoscopically in the left side of a boy with a right nonpalpable testis. The spermatic vessels are a distinct structure with valvular dilations seen in the veins, running to the internal inguinal ring (*arrow*), joining the vas deferens (V). This is in contrast to Figure 95–24 of the opposite side.

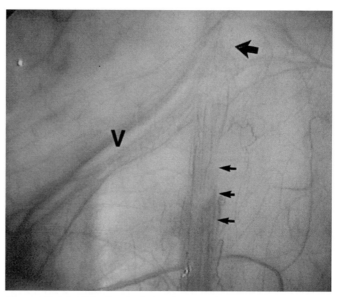

Figure 95–24. Right inguinal ring in same boy as Figure 95–23, in which the vas deferens (V) is seen to pass through the internal ring (*large arrow*) associated with attenuated spermatic vessels (*small arrows*). A nubbin of testicular tissue was removed from the inguinal canal. This image indicates that a salvageable testis is unlikely to be found, and a limited exploration may be performed to remove the nubbin of tissue.

of salvageable testes being found in the inguinal canal has been criticized by some as indicative of suboptimal clinical examinations preoperatively. Even with a cooperative patient, a careful examination, and a skilled examiner, not all salvageable extra-abdominal testes are palpable.

The high incidence of inguinal testes has prompted some to suggest preoperative inguinal ultrasound to look for those testes in the canal to obviate laparoscopy (Cain et al, 1995). A testis would be found at most in 30% to 40% of cases, all of which would need surgery, and all the other patients would undergo laparoscopy after an unrevealing ultrasound study. It is difficult to assess the relative cost-benefit balance of this possibility. Others have suggested primary surgical exploration for all boys and laparoscopy only if no structures are found in the canal. This would limit the surgical exposure for those patients with an intra-abdominal testis and cause an unnecessary incision in those with an intra-abdominal vanishing testis. It might be possible to perform further diagnostic laparoscopy through the inguinal canal (Horgan and Brock, 1994), although this would induce an extra incision in those patients with intra-abdominal testes.

Operative Laparoscopy for Cryptorchidism

Indications

There are many options for the management of the intra-abdominal testis (Waldschmidt and Schier, 1991b; Wright, 1986; Zerella and McGill, 1993). Open surgical techniques are well described and have acceptable results, yet they remain imperfect (Docimo, 1995). More certain testicular salvage should be possible. Early results suggest that laparo-scopic surgical techniques may be able to provide some of

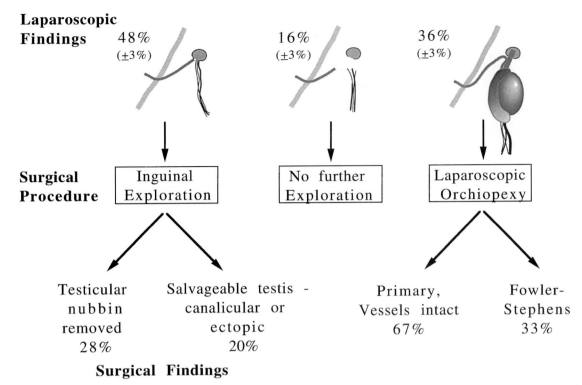

Figure 95–25. Chart illustrating distribution of laparoscopic and surgical findings in boys with nonpalpable testes, based on meta-analysis of 1044 reported cases.

that improvement. Operative laparoscopic orchiopexy was first described by Jordan and colleagues (1992), and a similar technique has been used by several authors (Bogaert et al, 1993; Diamond, 1994; Jordan and Winslow, 1994; Peters et al, 1994).

Operative laparoscopic orchiopexy has been generally reserved for the intra-abdominal testis, although some have reported its use for canalicular testes (Docimo et al, 1995c). The decision regarding salvage or removal is a difficult one; the authors' approach is to offer salvage in virtually all cases. A dysplastic-appearing testis, high in the abdomen, or with aberrant vascular or epididymal attachments is a poor candidate for repair. The patient should be able to tolerate a pneumoperitoneum without cardiorespiratory compromise. The authors have performed laparoscopic orchiopexy on several young children who were sensitive to the pneumoperitoneum yet did well with lower pressures. In a child with bilateral intra-abdominal testes, the authors believe it is useful to obtain a preoperative laboratory assessment of potential testicular function. This is to prognosticate about testicular function to some degree as well as to provide an indication of the response to surgery.

Once testicular location is known and operative laparoscopic orchiopexy is deemed appropriate, two secondary cannulae are placed depending on the location of the testis. For right-sided testes, a 5-mm cannula is inserted in the right upper quadrant at the midclavicular line, just below the costal margin. On the left, the cannula is placed in the midclavicular line below the umbilicus, at the level of the anterior superior iliac spine. Three 5-mm cannulae are acceptable if there is to be no vessel clipping, which requires a 10-mm cannula to permit insertion of the more common multiple-fire endoscopic clip applicator, although a 5-mm

multifire, disposable clip applier is now available (Ethicon, Cincinnati, OH). In some situations, the spermatic vessels may be clipped using a single working port in which scissors are used to create a passage under the vessels and the clips applied through the passage. In single-stage procedures, a fourth cannula may be placed in the ipsilateral side of the patient to provide traction.

The decision whether to perform a primary orchiopexy with intact spermatic vessels or a Fowler-Stephens orchiopexy is usually based on the position of the testis and the age of the patient. By empirical evidence, the authors have found in children less than 3 years of age that testes located more than 2.5 cm cephalad to the internal inguinal ring require a Fowler-Stephens technique (see Fig. 95–19), whereas testes within that distance all have been able to be mobilized to the scrotum with the spermatic vessels intact. Older children appear to have less "stretch" to their spermatic vessels, and even if the testes are at the internal inguinal ring, the authors have found them difficult to move into the scrotum without dividing the vessels. Establishing this distinction before mobilization has begun is important because the Fowler-Stephens orchiopexy is based on an intact vasal peritoneal flap to permit development of collateral circulation.

If a primary orchiopexy is to be performed, the operation begins at the internal inguinal ring with careful dissection of the gubernacular attachments (Fig. 95–26) that usually pass through the ring into the canal. It is essential to identify the path of the vas deferens in these cases because it may loop down into the canal and is therefore at risk for injury during this mobilization. Once the gubernacular attachments are free, they may be used as a handle for further testicular mobilization. Incision of the peritoneum lateral to the

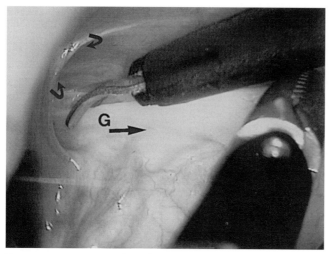

Figure 95–26. Dissecting the gubernaculum (G) from the inguinal canal during a laparoscopic orchiopexy. The dissection is seen just at the patent processus vaginalis (*curved arrows*) and must be done cautiously to avoid injury to a potentially looping vas deferens. Countertraction on the gubernaculum (*arrow*) facilitates teasing away the peritoneal attachments.

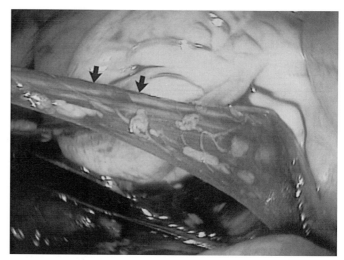

Figure 95–28. High dissection of the retroperitoneal attachments of the spermatic vessels during laparoscopic orchiopexy. The vessels are clearly seen and indicated by the *arrows,* whereas the web of retroperitoneal connective tissue is seen in preparation to being taken down.

spermatic vessels in a cephalad direction is next, while gently pulling the testis medially (Fig. 95–27). This dissection continues as far cephalad as possible, usually until the bowel obscures the view (Fig. 95–28). Following this, the peritoneum on the lateral aspect of the vas is incised, permitting the testis and a triangular flap, defined by the vas inferiorly and the vessels superiorly, to be mobilized medially by bluntly sweeping it off the lateral pelvic sidewall, away from the iliac vessels, ureter, and obturator fossa. This triangular flap of peritoneum is incised at the junction of the vas and vessels medial to the testis (Fig. 95–29) and cut superiorly along the vessels to the maximal level of dissection. The peritoneum is cut over the vessels proximally and swept superiorly. It may be necessary to grasp the peritoneal

tissues adjacent to the vessels to facilitate dissection at this time. Periodically the testis is moved toward the contralateral internal inguinal ring as a rough estimate of whether sufficient length has been attained to move it to the scrotum. Once this is achieved, the passage into the scrotum is created.

A passage for the testis into the scrotum is created over the pubic tubercle by gently guiding a dissecting instrument under direct laparoscopic vision and palpation externally, medial to the obliterated umbilical vein but lateral to the bladder edge, over the tubercle, and into the scrotum (Fig. 95–30). The passage is best established using the ipsilateral supraumbilical port, which permits a straight-line passage from the abdomen. Steady pressure with some spreading of the instrument facilitates this maneuver and develops a passageway sufficiently wide to permit the testis to move through. Once the instrument is in the scrotum, a dartos pouch is developed from the outside in the usual fashion,

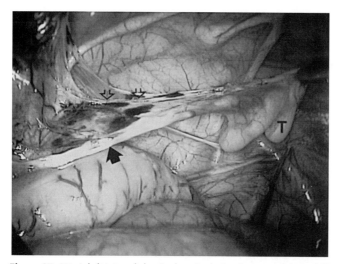

Figure 95–27. A left intra-abdominal testis during laparoscopic mobilization. The testis (T) can be moved easily to the contralateral inguinal ring, which has served as a rule of thumb to indicate adequate mobilization for scrotal positioning. The spermatic vessels are indicated by the *closed arrow* and the vas deferens by the *open arrows.* The web of peritoneum between the two remains intact at this point.

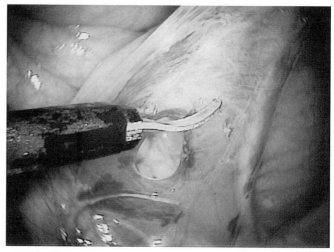

Figure 95–29. Laparoscopic view of incision of the peritoneal web between the vas deferens and spermatic vessels. This permits better spermatic vessel mobilization.

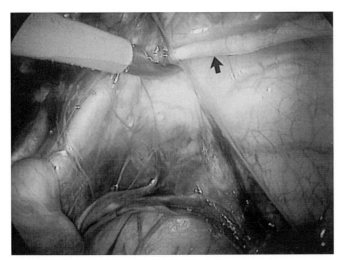

Figure 95–30. A laparoscopic dissecting instrument is being used to create a new left inguinal ring, just over the pubic tubercle and lateral to the bladder. The obliterated umbilical artery (*arrow*) is being pushed laterally to avoid bladder injury. Medial passage of the testis facilitates placement into the scrotum, which might otherwise be under tension from the vas deferens crossing the obliterated umbilical artery.

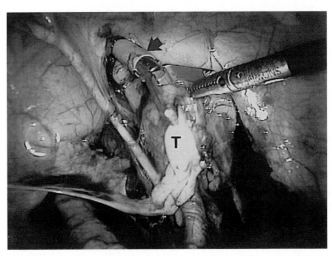

Figure 95–32. Intra-abdominal view showing the right testis (T) being grasped from the scrotal port (*arrow*) after establishing the passage between the scrotum and pelvis. This passageway is lateral to the obliterated umbilical artery in this patient.

and two sutures are preplaced in the floor of the pouch. The instrument is passed through the pouch (Fig. 95–31), and a 5-mm cannula is backloaded over it and passed into the abdomen under direct vision. This cannula serves as the access port for a grasping instrument to draw the testis from the abdomen into the scrotum. The testis should be grasped

at the gubernacular attachments and gently pulled through the new canal (Fig. 95–32). Occasionally, further spreading or even sharp dissection is needed to widen the passage. If there is insufficient length to move the testis into the scrotum, the scrotal access port may be used to facilitate further proximal dissection of the spermatic vessels, with two free instrument ports to expose and mobilize the vessels. Care should be taken not to skeletonize the vessels too aggressively because they are thin and may be torn. It is useful to inspect the mobilization of the vas deferens because it may actually be restricting movement of the testis. For this reason, the authors recommend passing the testis medial to the obliterated umbilical artery. When testes were passed lateral to the obliterated umbilical artery, tethering was noted by the vas deferens. The obliterated umbilical artery can be transected between ties or clips in such cases. Once the testis is in the scrotum (Fig. 95–33), it may be fixed in place in the usual fashion, although in cases with any tension, an external fixation button with Prolene suture is placed for 1 to 2 weeks.

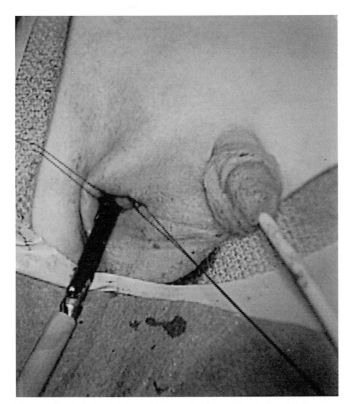

Figure 95–31. Exterior view of boy undergoing right laparoscopic orchiopexy with a dissecting instrument having passed out of the scrotum from the abdomen after creation of a dartos scrotal pouch and placement of fixation sutures.

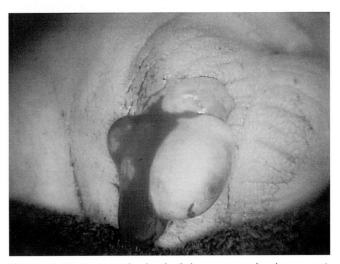

Figure 95–33. Testis at the level of the scrotum after laparoscopic orchiopexy.

If the testis is thought to be too far away from the internal inguinal ring, a Fowler-Stephens orchiopexy may be performed, using laparoscopic techniques. This was the initial operative aspect of laparoscopy with intra-abdominal testis. When a testis was found in the abdomen, its vessels were clipped in the first stage of a Fowler-Stephens orchiopexy performed in a two-stage fashion as suggested by Ransley and colleagues (1984). It remains to be definitively established whether the staged Fowler-Stephens is superior to the single-stage Fowler-Stephens procedure, as originally described (Fowler and Stephens, 1959). A review of orchiopexy techniques (Docimo, 1995) and outcomes suggests a success rate of only 75% for single-stage Fowler-Stephens, in contrast to 85% for staged Fowler-Stephens. Ransley's original report indicated 100% success for staged Fowler-Stephens, based on 13 testes in 10 patients, which may explain the enthusiasm for this approach. Eight of the patients had the prune-belly syndrome as the basis for their cryptorchidism. These numbers are difficult to assess because the criteria for success are variable and dependent on an observer who is usually the surgeon. Staged Fowler-Stephens was soon embraced for laparoscopy because the first stage could be done laparoscopically (Bloom et al, 1988), and the second stage was usually done open. Both may be done laparoscopically, and the success rate to date for the staged technique has been good. A direct comparison between single-stage and two-stage techniques has not been performed. It is more cost-effective to perform these procedures in one stage, but this may reduce operative successes.

The laparoscopic Fowler-Stephens is begun by gentle dissection of the spermatic vessels 1 to 2 cm above the testis and occlusion with clips or sutures (Fig. 95–34). If performed in the context of a staged Fowler-Stephens, there is no testicular mobilization, and the vessels are left in continuity. At the second stage, the vessels are transected, and the testis is mobilized on a broad peritoneal pedicle surrounding the vas deferens (Fig. 95–35). There is seldom any trouble moving the testis into the scrotum in this configuration. The basic technique is identical to that used for primary orchiopexy. It is important to preserve the vas deferens

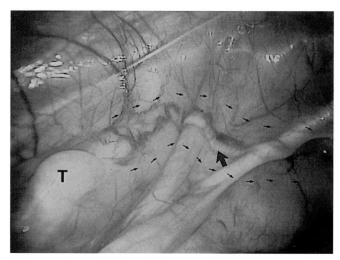

Figure 95–35. Intra-abdominal left testis (T) seen 6 months after spermatic vessel ligation in preparation for staged laparoscopic Fowler-Stephens orchiopexy. The vas (*large arrow*) may be seen with a prominent vasal artery The *small arrows* indicate the lines of incision to create the peritoneal pedicle for the testis. Medial to the obliterated umbilical artery, the pedicle should spread out and become more triangular.

pedicle, yet to mobilize it well into the deep pelvis to avoid any tension on the pedicle. Often the spermatic vessels are cut so as to leave them open, permitting backbleeding as an indication of collateral circulation.

There are few objective guidelines about the appropriate interval between stages. **The authors recommend that the interval between stages be 6 months.** It is presumed that this interval permits enhanced development of collateral circulation around the vas deferens to the epididymis, without the testis being stressed. The advantage of performing the Fowler-Stephens in a two-stage procedure, as opposed to the initially described single-stage operation, remains to be strictly defined. As yet, there have not been any reports of single-stage laparoscopic Fowler-Stephens orchiopexies, although a report of open Fowler-Stephens single-stage procedures claimed a 90% success rate (Koff and Sethi, 1995). This is better than the average report of Fowler-Stephens orchiopexies and was accomplished using a low vascular ligation, in contrast to the high ligation classically described.

Technique Selection

Determination of the optimal method of laparoscopic orchiopexy may be hindered by relatively poor objective outcomes parameters. Doppler ultrasound of the testes has been applied to permit accurate measurement of size as well as an assessment of vascular perfusion (Paltiel et al, 1994). With skilled ultrasonographers, a vascular signal may usually be obtained in normal testes and has been found in almost all of the operated testes in the authors' group experience. It has not been proven that short-term perfusion predicts ultimate functional potential, but this is as good as any other series relating to orchiopexy has reported. It is difficult to justify the use of radionuclide testicular imaging in such cases because there is little benefit to the patient to justify an invasive diagnostic test. Use of an objective observer

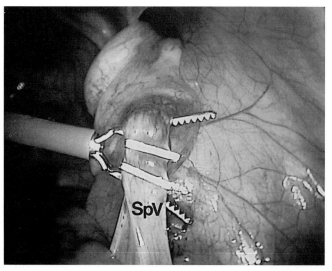

Figure 95–34. First stage of laparoscopic staged Fowler-Stephens orchiopexy. The spermatic vessel (SpV) is being clipped laparoscopically.

other than the operating surgeon to assess testicular size or growth may also be helpful in this regard.

It is important to recognize that the choice of primary orchiopexy with vessels intact in contrast to a staged Fowler-Stephens has usually been made without objective criteria. The criteria that the authors' group has reported are also somewhat subjective and rely on an assessment of the difficulty in surgically mobilizing the testis into the scrotum, and they are not based on outcomes. When bilateral intra-abdominal testes are found, the lowest testis should be mobilized to the scrotum with vessels intact, if at all possible. The other testis should then have its vessels ligated, unless it is well within the distance for a primary orchiopexy or if the first orchiopexy was complicated in some way. Both testes may be mobilized at one time if within an appropriate distance from the internal ring.

The use of microvascular testicular autotransplant has been advocated by some for intra-abdominal testes (Silber and Kelly, 1976; Upton et al, 1983; Frey and Bianchi, 1987, 1989; Harrison et al, 1990; Oesterwitz and Fahlenkamp, 1993), and this may be performed adjunctively with laparoscopic techniques (Sanchez et al, 1992; Wacksman et al, 1995). The testis may be mobilized initially as well as the spermatic vessels and the inferior epigastric vessels if they are to be the source vessels to which the testicular vessels are anastomosed. This requires close coordination between the laparoscopist and microvascular surgeon if they are not the same person. This may be facilitated by making the initial diagnosis at a separate setting and preparing for the procedure in advance. Results of microvascular surgery are reported to be as high as 84% (Docimo, 1995) for intra-abdominal testes. This is better than the reported success rates for any other technique. Whether this is indeed the best means of bringing an intra-abdominal testis into the scrotum is unclear. In several cases, the authors have had teenage boys with a solitary intra-abdominal testis, in whom microvascular techniques are clearly the best option and probably the only way the testis could be moved into the scrotum with vessels intact.

Results

Results of laparoscopic orchiopexy have been good in the few reported series to date (Table 95–1). No serious complications have been reported. The length of the procedure is longer than with most open cases, but most practitioners report it to be decreasing with experience. Hospitalization is brief but not significantly less than most with open surgery. When a two-stage Fowler-Stephens orchiopexy is chosen, the expense owing to operative time and use of hospital resources increases because of there being two procedures. In many ways, this is an issue separate from laparoscopy because both stages may be performed using open or laparoscopic methods. The utility of two-stage Fowler-Stephens orchiopexy rests on whether it provides a better result than single-stage Fowler-Stephens; as noted previously, that issue remains to be proved. In general, the subjective opinion of practitioners has been positive in terms of the ability to mobilize the intra-abdominal testis and potentially to enhance the surgical outcome of the procedure. The testicular outcomes have been assessed to a limited degree and with short-term follow-up (see Table 95–1). In one case, the authors noted a healthy scrotal testis 3 months after laparoscopic primary orchiopexy, only to find it to be atrophic 6 months later, emphasizing the importance of longer follow-up. Although testicular atrophy is usually apparent soon after surgery, the absence of growth may be evident only at puberty. **The ultimate utility of laparoscopic orchiopexy will depend on long-range studies assessing testicular growth after the various procedures and will need to be controlled for initial position of the testis.**

Laparoscopic techniques for the undescended testis will likely continue to expand with improved selection of cases and, it is hoped, better means of assessing outcomes. Although the techniques may not change markedly, it is likely that as understanding of the physiology of the undescended testis improves, adjunctive hormonal or pharmacologic methods will enhance the ultimate results of this surgical approach.

Intersex

The diagnosis and management of various intersexuality conditions is well suited to laparoscopic methods, which offer the capability of minimally invasive diagnosis, biopsy, and definitive intervention in specific cases (Waldschmidt and Schier, 1991a; Ferreira et al, 1993; Yu et al, 1995). Laparoscopic diagnosis is seldom necessary as an urgent

Table 95–1. REPORTED EXPERIENCE WITH LAPAROSCOPIC ORCHIOPEXY

Authors	Technique	Patients	Testes	Age	(%) Success*	Follow-up
Jordan and Winslow, 1994	Primary	13	13	<15 years	100	6 months
	Staged FS	3	3	<15 years	100	6 months
Bogaert et al, 1993	Primary	2	2	<16 years	100	<9 months
	Staged FS	8/3†	3	<16 years	100	<9 months
Caldamone and Amaral, 1994	Second-stage FS	5	5	<15 years	100	6–18 months
Peters et al, 1994	Primary	8	10	<5 years	100	6 months
	Staged FS	7	7	<7 years	100	6 months
Poppas et al, 1995	Primary	9	10		100	3.5 months
	Staged FS	2	2		100	3.5 months

*Success usually defined as scrotal location of testis and absence of atrophy.
†Number of first-stage procedures/number of second-stage procedures.
FS, Fowler-Stephens orchiopexy.

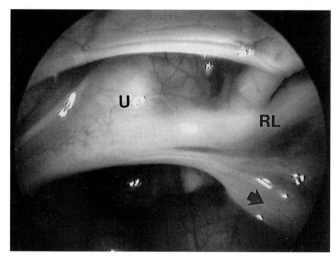

Figure 95–36. Laparoscopic view of the uterus (U) of an infant with a complex intersex condition. The round ligament (RL) passes over the obliterated umbilical artery and is adjacent to the rudimentary fallopian tube and gonad (*arrow*).

modality to permit sex assignment, although in unusual cases of true hermaphroditism and gonadal dysgenesis, the need for anatomic definition of the pelvic organs as well as gonadal biopsy may be critical to sex assignment. **In general, laparoscopy provides for definitive diagnosis of the gonadal anatomy and location and permits biopsy or removal of gonads.** This is particularly important in the various gonadal dysgenesis syndromes in which the risk of gonadoblastoma in retained gonads is high (Droesch et al, 1990; Wilson et al, 1992). In testicular feminization syndromes in which female sex of rearing is chosen, gonadectomy is generally recommended in the young child, and laparoscopic orchiectomy is readily accomplished (Mahadevan and Shaxted, 1992; Gililland et al, 1993; Long and Wingfield, 1993; McDougall et al, 1993a). When gonadal biopsies are necessary, as in hermaphroditic states, deep longitudinal biopsies are possible, even in the small child. These procedures are transperitoneal and may be accomplished with an umbilical cannula and two lower quadrant cannulae just below the umbilicus in the midclavicular lines. Assessment and documentation of any müllerian structures can be carried out (Fig. 95–36). Table 95–2 indicates specific applications for laparoscopic diagnosis and treatment in various intersexuality conditions.

Laparoscopy has been reported in the creation of an intestinal vagina in a case of testicular feminization (Jordan G, personal communication, 1993); laparoscopic access to the posterior vesical space is excellent and may be better than

Table 95–2. LAPAROSCOPIC EVALUATION AND MANAGEMENT OF INTERSEX CONDITIONS

Diagnosis	Laparoscopic Procedures
Congenital adrenal hyperplasia	None
Female pseudohermaphrodite	Assessment of müllerian structures
Male pseudohermaphrodite	Assessment of müllerian structures
Mixed gonadal dysgenesis	Gonadal biopsy, removal
True hermaphrodite	Gonadal biopsy
Testicular feminization	Gonadectomy

that achieved with open surgery, even using the posterior sagittal approach.

Hernia and Hydrocele

Laparoscopic techniques have shown utility in the evaluation of contralateral pediatric hernia and hydrocele, an area of enduring controversy. The incidence of contralateral hernia, found at exploration, is inversely dependent on age, ranging from about 60% in the young infant to 20% in schoolchildren (Kiesewetter and Parenzan, 1959; Rowe et al, 1969; Bock and Sobye, 1970). The incidence of clinically apparent new contralateral hernia after surgical repair of a unilateral hernia is about 16% to 20%, without breakdown for age (Sparkman, 1962; Bock and Sobye, 1970; McGregor et al, 1980). The practice of contralateral inguinal exploration has been a part of surgical technique for 40 years, but the practice remains variable, with some practitioners exploring all patients and others not exploring the uninvolved side in any patients. Various diagnostic techniques have been explored to assess the patency of the contralateral processus vaginalis, including pneumoperitoneum and peritoneal instillation of contrast material (herniogram). None are in common practice.

Diagnostic laparoscopy affords a superb view of the internal inguinal ring, and a patent processus vaginalis is readily apparent. Umbilical laparoscopy has been reported to diagnose the presence of a patent processus, yet it entails the risks of umbilical access (Holcomb et al, 1993). Inguinal laparoscopy, using the access afforded by the surgically mobilized hernia sac, offers an efficient means of creating a pneumoperitoneum and examining the contralateral internal inguinal ring without risk. This has been reported by several groups with satisfactory results (Hatch and Trockman, 1994; Peters and Bauer, 1995). The procedure should require only 5 to 10 minutes and may be performed with reusable equipment. An oblique lens enhances the view of the internal inguinal ring from the opposite groin (Fig. 95–37). The authors have used an integrated pediatric cys-

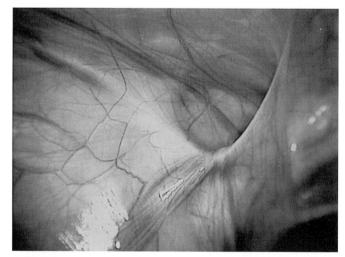

Figure 95–37. Laparoscopic view of internal inguinal ring in a boy with a left inguinal hernia. The ring is wide open, the processus vaginalis (hernia sac) is gaping, and one can see the spermatic vessels and vas deferens passing out of the ring, closely associated with the hernia sac.

toureteroscope with insufflation through a working port and a smooth leading edge with good results and efficient operation. As indicated in Figure 95–38, a substantial fraction of young children would be spared an inguinal exploration. Widely patent hernia sacs may be found in otherwise asymptomatic older children in whom contralateral exploration might not otherwise be performed. The precise accuracy of a negative examination is important to assess with long-term follow-up to ensure that no clinically evident hernias develop in those without exploration. It is difficult to assess the converse, without a controlled study of nonoperation in those with a patent processus.

Approaches to the Kidney

Laparoscopic techniques offer enormous potential advantages in the area of renal surgery. The advantages include rapid access to the kidney in a less invasive manner than open surgery in almost all ages and superb exposure and visualization of all anatomic structures of the kidney. **Laparoscopy provides a surgical approach to the entire upper urinary tract through one access arrangement, in contrast to the need for two incisions to deal with the kidney and distal ureter.** These elements should permit safe, accurate surgery with a significant reduction in surgical morbidity from muscle-cutting incisions as are commonly practiced in many centers.

Several limitations remain to be efficiently dealt with to permit the realization of the potential advantages of a laparoscopic approach noted earlier. Most laparoscopic renal surgery in children remains transperitoneal with the concerns of intraperitoneal adhesions and intestinal obstruction. Retroperitoneal laparoscopic renal surgery has been reported in children but remains to be developed (Chandhoke et al, 1993; Diamond et al, 1995). This surgery is likely to be dependent on experience, improved dissecting techniques to minimize peritoneal injury, and better tools to permit working within the smaller operative spaces of the retroperitoneum. A second limitation to pediatric laparoscopic renal

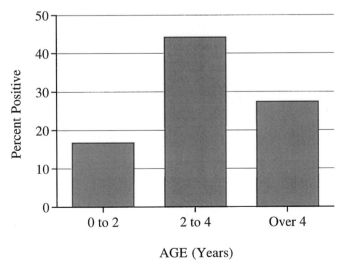

Figure 95–38. Incidence of contralateral patent processus observed at the time of inguinal hernia repair with laparoscopic examination of the opposite internal inguinal ring.

surgery is in tissue approximation techniques that need to be extremely precise and delicate. An infant pyeloplasty is usually performed with 12 to 16 7–0 sutures being placed at the anastomosis. This is a formidable task through the laparoscope. Suturing devices are available to facilitate this, but they have not yet been down-sized below a 4–0 absorbable suture, which is completely unsuitable for a child's pyeloplasty. Improved suturing techniques (both suture placement and knot tying) are needed as well as laparoscopic suturing instruments that permit precise needle placement and yet are delicate enough to use with fine suture. Alternative tissue-joining techniques also hold promise and are being developed (Poppas et al, 1993). These include laser tissue welding and tissue adhesives. Each of these, separately or in combination, is ideally suited to laparoscopic techniques and holds promise to make delicate reconstructive laparoscopic renal surgery efficient and cost-effective. If these elements are not developed, it is difficult to justify the duration and expense of many laparoscopic techniques for renal surgery in children.

The initial experience in laparoscopic renal surgery in children strongly suggests the enormous potential for improving the surgical outcomes in renal surgery for children using laparoscopic techniques (Ehrlich et al, 1994). Reported procedures include laparoscopic nephrectomy (Ehrlich et al, 1992; Chandhoke et al, 1993; Peters et al, 1993; Koyle et al, 1994; Diamond et al, 1995), partial nephrectomy (Ehrlich et al, 1992; Jordan and Winslow, 1993a), nephroureterectomy (Ehrlich et al, 1992; Peters et al, 1993), and pyeloplasty (Peters et al, 1995b). Although the initial cases have been prolonged, probably owing to the new territory as well as a healthy dose of caution, the rapid application of progressively more complex techniques is a good indicator of the potential for further development.

Techniques

INDICATIONS

Laparoscopic nephrectomy has been performed mostly for multicystic dysplastic kidney disease and nonfunctioning kidneys associated with hydronephrosis. Although the controversy regarding the management of multicystic dysplastic kidneys will continue, some parents have strong conviction that the kidney should be removed, and in such cases laparoscopic nephrectomy has developed as a possible alternative to open surgery. In situations of a large multicystic dysplastic kidney, with a palpable mass, laparoscopic removal is not contraindicated. The nonfunctioning hydronephrotic kidney is well suited to laparoscopic removal. Indications for laparoscopic renal surgery should be the same as those for open renal surgery. Contraindications to laparoscopic nephrectomy include malignant disease in children, suppurative lesions of the kidney (unless retroperitoneal techniques are used), or the previously operated kidney likely to be encased in a significant amount of scar tissue. The last-mentioned is a relative contraindication and is likely to diminish in importance, as have the contraindications to laparoscopy in patients with prior abdominal surgery.

PATIENT PREPARATION

Little specific preparation is needed for laparoscopic renal surgery, although the authors recommend a liquid diet the day before and a suppository the night before surgery. Consent must include the possibility of conversion to an open procedure, although this has been unusual. A sample of blood should be with the blood bank, although the authors do not routinely have blood set up for these procedures. A bladder catheter and a rectal tube are placed. Nitrous anesthesia is avoided. Epidural anesthetics are not usually used because they do not seem to have any extra benefit as they have with open renal surgery. Parenteral antibiotics are given.

Several options exist in terms of patient positioning. The authors prefer to perform a total lower body surgical preparation in small children. Pneumoperitoneum is achieved in the supine position, and the patient is then turned into the flank position. This affords the opportunity to create the pneumoperitoneum in the supine position, which is a bit easier, but also allows quick return to the supine position if rapid conversion to an open procedure is needed. Alternatively the patient may be lifted partially into the flank position by a wedge under the operative side and the table counter-rotated to have the patient flat for creation of the pneumoperitoneum. The table is then steeply angled in the opposite direction so that the patient is in an almost full flank position (Fig. 95–39). This is useful for older patients. Finally, patients may be prepared in the flank position and pneumoperitoneum created through flank cannulae using open technique. This latter approach is useful for retroperitoneal access.

CANNULA POSITION

Placement of the operative cannulas is critical in laparoscopic renal surgery in children. The smaller operative area limits movement and cannulas placed too close hinder each other, as does the camera. The angle of approach to critical portions of the renal anatomy must be optimal, particularly if suturing is required. The most useful configuration has been with an umbilical port and two ipsilateral ports in the midclavicular line above and below the umbilicus (Fig. 95–40). A fourth port may be placed in the midaxillary line if needed for exposure. This is particularly useful to retract

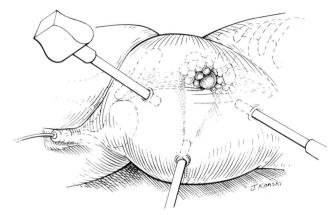

Figure 95–40. Diagram indicating the positioning of laparoscopic ports for simple nephrectomy in an infant.

the liver or spleen to permit access to the upper pole of the kidney.

BASIC TECHNIQUES

Most renal procedures begin with exposure of the kidney by medial mobilization of the colon (Fig. 95–41). Incision of the lateral peritoneal reflection of the colon (right or left) with blunt dissection to sweep the colon off the kidney is readily accomplished when a transperitoneal exposure is used. Identification of the ureter as it crosses the iliac vessels is the next step to gain access to the kidney. In a simple nephrectomy, the ureter may be grasped and lifted as a handle to bring the lower pole downward (Fig. 95–42). Otherwise, it may serve as a guide up to the lower pole of the kidney, at which most of the procedures diverge to address their particular components.

Nephrectomy

TECHNIQUE

Once the lower pole of the kidney is identified, it is often most efficient to mobilize the renal hilum and gain vascular

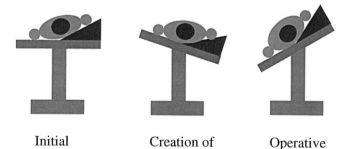

Initial   Creation of   Operative
Positioning   pneumoperitoneum   Position

Figure 95–39. Diagram showing a positioning technique for laparoscopic renal surgery in a teenager or adult. A 30-degree or 45-degree soft wedge is placed under one side of the patient. With the table rotated to put the wedge down, the pneumoperitoneum is created, and the table is counter-rotated to put the patient into a flank-up position to perform the surgery. The advantages include the ability to create the pneumoperitoneum in the supine position, to operate in the flank-up position without having to reposition the patient relative to the table, and to move rapidly back to a supine position if emergency access to the peritoneum is needed.

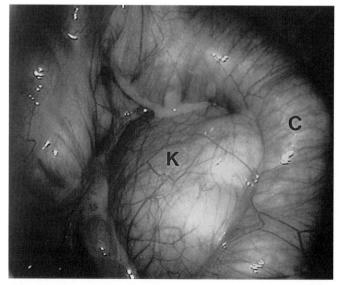

Figure 95–41. Large renal cyst associated with multicystic dysplastic kidney (K) seen laparoscopically behind the mesentery of the large bowel (C).

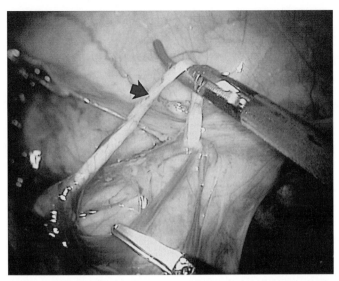

Figure 95–42. Mobilization of the ureter of a nonfunctioning dysplastic kidney just over the iliac vessels in preparation for a laparoscopic nephrectomy. The ureter (*arrow*) serves well as a handle to dissect up to the kidney and retract it inferiorly during dissection.

control. Vessels are ligated individually using metal clips. Some have advocated absorbable clips for children, although the rationale is unclear, and the reliability of metal clips is reassuring. Multiple small aberrant vessels are frequently associated with dysplastic kidneys, and they should be sought out carefully. The posterior of the kidney may then be mobilized with both sharp and blunt dissection. The upper pole may require control of some small vessels, and care must be take to avoid injury to the adrenal vessels. After the upper pole is free, the kidney should be ready for removal. The ureter is cut with or without clipping, and the specimen is removed through the largest available port. Large cysts should be needle punctured and aspirated before removal (Fig. 95–43). The renal fossa should be inspected at low pneumoperitoneum pressure to look for venous bleeding. **No specific attempt is made to reclose the peritoneum be-**

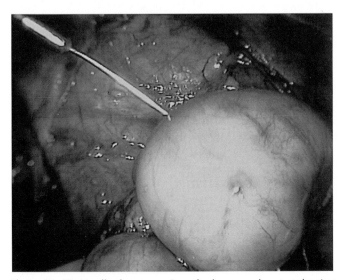

Figure 95–43. Needle decompression of a large renal cyst at the time of laparoscopic nephrectomy to permit easy removal of the kidney.

cause the colon falls back in place after the patient is returned to the supine position. No drains are left. Patients usually return home the next morning.

RESULTS

A limited number of reports of pediatric laparoscopic nephrectomy are available in the literature (Ehrlich et al, 1992; Chandhoke et al, 1993; Koyle et al, 1993, 1994; Peters et al, 1993; Diamond et al, 1995). These reports indicate the technical feasibility of the procedure as well as its relative safety. Patients as young as 3 months have undergone laparoscopic nephrectomy, and no significant complications have been reported. A comparative study of laparoscopic and open nephrectomy for multicystic kidneys indicated shorter hospital stays for laparoscopic nephrectomy but longer operative times. Both of these are relative values and unlikely to be inherent to the procedures specifically. Operative time is likely to decrease with experience, and improved instruments and hospital stay can always be limited if this is the aim. There is no difference in the efficacy of the procedures for simple nephrectomy, and the comparison becomes one of the risks of laparoscopy as compared to the morbidity of open nephrectomy. These are difficult parameters to quantitate and may be influenced by parental interests and impressions of the morbidity of such things as scars. **Laparoscopic nephrectomy has served an important role in facilitating the development of more complex laparoscopic renal surgery, for which distinct advantages may be ultimately realized.**

Partial Nephrectomy

The indications for partial nephrectomy or nephroureterectomy are well described and include nonfunctioning upper-pole segments associated with obstruction, ectopic ureters, or ureteroceles. **Removal of the ureter associated with the upper pole is usually necessary, and in this context laparoscopy offers a significant advantage in place of two incisions to remove the entire system. Lower-pole partial nephrectomy is usually performed for vesicoureteral reflux into the lower pole, and this necessitates removal of the distal ureter.** In small children, it is possible to remove a fair amount of the distal ureter from a flank incision; however, laparoscopy can provide for complete removal using the basic cannula sites.

Partial nephrectomy is a more complex procedure than simple nephrectomy and requires great care to protect the vascularity and drainage of the remaining segment (Jordan and Winslow, 1993a). The basic strategy involves identification of the affected ureter, separation from the unaffected ureter, and dissection to expose the hilum of the pole to be removed. The vasculature to the upper pole is usually evident and can be ligated and divided in the usual fashion. Separation of the two renal poles is often best accomplished by creation of a plane of dissection between the renal pelves. This is readily accomplished in hydronephrotic segments. The crescent of parenchyma surrounding the affected pole is then cut using electrocautery and specific control of any larger vessels encountered. Alternatively, use of the argon beam coagulator has been described for hemostasis of the parenchyma. It is important to provide for venting of gases when using the argon beam coagulator through the laparoscope because it emits high volumes of gas during operation. Ehrlich and associates reported using the GIA stapling device to remove the upper pole laparoscopically, providing hemostasis and division of the poles (Ehrlich et al, 1994). Until absorbable staples are available for endoscopic use, the authors are hesitant to use this technique out of concern for development of stones in the remaining pole owing to the metal staples. The resected segment is then removed in the usual fashion. The cut segment may be closed with mattress sutures, including either a patch of fat or absorbable hemostatic material. The surgical area should be drained briefly, and a suction drain may be placed laparoscopically.

The distal ureter can be dissected out to the level of the bladder, at which point it develops a commonly vascularized wall with the unaffected ureter. This segment of wall can be left on the other ureter to avoid injury to the vascularity and the stump of ureter closed with a single stitch. Markedly ectopic ureters are more separated from the unaffected ureter and can be removed as far down as readily accomplished; in most cases, they do not reflux. Much of the dissection of the distal ureter can be carried out within a peritoneal sheath unless exposure is hindered.

Pyeloplasty

INDICATIONS AND TECHNIQUE

Radiographic evaluation of ureteropelvic junction obstruction should be no different for a case to be performed laparoscopically. An adequate assessment of function (radionuclide studies or intravenous pyelogram) combined with anatomic definition (intravenous pyelogram, retrograde pyelogram) is necessary. The possibility of an extrinsic obstruction because of a crossing vessel should be considered but would not contraindicate laparoscopic repair.

The indications for pyeloplasty in children remain in evolution and cannot be reviewed here (Peters et al, 1995b), **although they would not be different between open or laparoscopic techniques.** Present application of laparoscopic pyeloplasty has been in older children, in whom the indications of pain, hematuria, or decreased function are less controversial.

A ureteral stent may be placed before the start of the laparoscopic aspect of the procedure, but the authors have not found this to be essential. Laparoscopic pyeloplasty is performed in the flank position with access being gained as for any renal operation. Three to four cannulas are used for manipulation, in a fan distribution with a lateral holding port. The ureteropelvic junction is exposed through the retroperitoneum. The point of obstruction is excised, the proximal ureter is spatulated, and the anastomosis is performed using interrupted or running suture. Knot tying remains the major time-consuming element of the procedure. The kidney may be drained using a nephroureteral stent or with a simple nephrostomy. The operative site is drained. The basic principles of pediatric pyeloplasty should be followed.

RESULTS

The outcomes of pediatric laparoscopic pyeloplasty can be assessed only on the basis of anecdotal reports (Peters et

al, 1995b; Jordan G, personal communication, 1995). All have been successfully accomplished with adequate clinical outcomes in short-term follow-up. Although there is probably no reason to suspect that these procedures should be any more likely to have late stenosis if initial findings are satisfactory, an adequate assessment of the technical success has to await age-matched comparative studies with objective outcome criteria.

Laparoscopic pyeloplasty is less morbid in the older patient, who is spared a flank or dorsal lumbotomy incision and may be home and back to normal activities more quickly. In the infant, in whom recovery from open pyeloplasty is rapid, the advantages of laparoscopic techniques depend on elimination of the scar and the theoretical potential for an enhanced procedure owing to the better exposure and visibility and reduced renal manipulation. These are currently offset, however, by the inefficiency of the anastomosis. It is clear that better methods of tissue approximation are needed if laparoscopic pyeloplasty is ever to have an advantage over open surgery.

Approaches to the Bladder

Laparoscopic bladder surgery in children has developed slowly and has included antireflux surgery, creation of a continent catheterizable stoma, autoaugmentation, and gastrocystoplasty. It is likely that applications will continue to develop in the three basic areas of pediatric bladder surgery. These are antireflux surgery, bladder reconstruction (such as augmentation cystoplasty), and continence procedures at the bladder neck.

The bladder may be approached transperitoneally or through the preperitoneal space. Antireflux and bladder neck surgery is conventionally preperitoneal, and this is the preferred laparoscopic approach, yet this limits working space and hinders efficiency. Both methods have been reported for these procedures. In smaller children, bladder access is enhanced because of the relatively intra-abdominal position of the bladder yet is limited by the smaller relative size of the pelvis. Cannula position needs to be adjusted to the laterality of the operation but in general is best arranged using a fan configuration. The anatomic complexity of the posterior perivesical region must be fully understood from the new perspective of the laparoscope. Once these new perspectives are mastered, however, the access to the deep pelvis, particularly the posterior aspect of the bladder, is excellent, considering the difficulty of access to this area using conventional surgical approaches. Bowel decompression is essential for bladder access as well as the ability to control bladder filling with an indwelling catheter in the surgical field.

Laparoscopic Procedures for Vesicoureteral Reflux

The high frequency of antireflux surgical procedures indicates the potential for significant contribution from an efficient laparoscopic antireflux procedure. For such a procedure to be beneficial, however, it needs to have a high success rate to match open surgical cure rates of greater than 95%; it must have low morbidity because conventional open surgical techniques have low complication rates, and many patients are discharged after 2 to 3 days with a rapidly healing lower abdominal Pfannenstiel incision. It would be difficult to devise an operation that could claim to be a technical improvement on one with such a high therapeutic index (success rate versus morbidity).

Several reports of experimental laparoscopic antireflux procedures have been published, and all applied the Lich-Grégoir, extravesical method of creating an antireflux mechanism for the ureter (Atala et al, 1993; Schimberg et al, 1994; McDougall et al, 1995d). This was a logical application because the bladder did not need to be opened (Fig. 95–44). Studies in the pig model of induced reflux were the most convincing because they were able to demonstrate actual resolution of reflux as well as absence of obstruction.

Ehrlich and co-workers (1993b) reported the first application of the Lich-Grégoir antireflux operation in children and was soon followed by Janetschek and associates (1995b). Ureteral stenting was used by Ehrlich, which is an extra addition to conventional surgery, but was brief. It was clear that the procedure in humans is more complex than in the animal model. The human bladder, even in children, is settled in the pelvis, in contrast to animals, in which it is suspended in the abdominal wall in an envelope of peritoneum. Janetschek and associates have reported uniform success in six children, including bilateral procedures, and have performed the procedure extraperitoneally (Janetschek et al, 1994, 1995b). Janetschek, however, abandoned the procedure because of the time required (3–4 hours for unilateral repair and 6–7 hours for bilateral), the lack of a substantial surgical advantage, and minimal decrease in morbidity.

The reported technique (Ehrlich et al, 1993b; Janetschek et al, 1995b) involves mobilization of the distal ureter up to the insertion of the ureter into the bladder musculature. The line of incision into the bladder wall is marked with cautery, and the muscle is divided with cautery to the level of the mucosa, which usually bulges outward and has a bluish color. The trough is developed for the length needed to create an antireflux tunnel and is extended beyond the actual insertion of the ureter into the mucosa for a short distance. With completion of the trough, the ureter may be fixed into the tunnel with an advancing stitch or simply laid into the trough. Use of the advancing stitch as a modification of the Lich-Grégoir technique was described by Zaontz and colleagues to prevent prolapse of the ureter out the tunnel and is termed *detrusorrhaphy* (Zaontz et al, 1987). The tunnel is created by closing the muscular wall over the ureter using sutures or absorbable clips. Although the bladder has not been entered, it seems advisable to avoid use of permanent sutures or staples in this repair. Once the tunnel is created, the procedure is complete, and the bladder is left to temporary drainage by catheter. Stents have been left in place for 2 to 5 days (Ehrlich et al, 1993b).

Several aspects of the procedure present a sufficient challenge so as to hinder efficient application of this technique. Ureteral dissection from the peritoneal approach is tedious and must be done cautiously. Preperitoneal access may reduce some of this difficulty but must be performed within a smaller operative field. Most approaches have been described as being from above the bladder, along the line of the ureter. It may be preferable to approach the ureter and its new tunnel from the lateral aspect, at right angles to the ureter itself. It is clear that laparoscopic antireflux surgery can be effective, yet it is limited by its reduced efficiency and does not demonstrate a clear-cut benefit. It is necessary to show significant advantages in terms of patient comfort postoperatively as well as shortened recovery times. At present, laparoscopic antireflux surgery remains in development, limited by the inefficiency of creating the muscular trough and securing the muscle edges over the ureter. An interesting possible developmental area is an integration of laparoscopic and endoscopic techniques to approach the ureter. This might

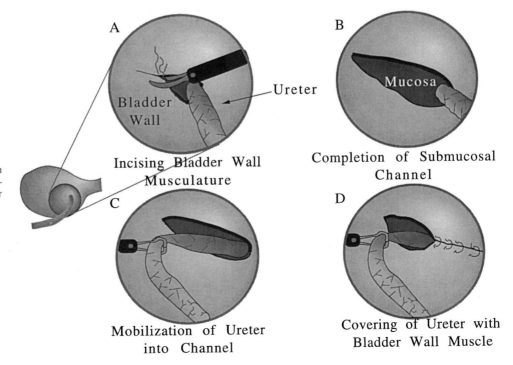

Figure 95–44. *A* through *D,* Steps in laparoscopic correction of vesicoureteral reflux using the Lich-Grégoir technique.

A
Bladder Wall

Ureter

Incising Bladder Wall Musculature

B
Mucosa

Completion of Submucosal Channel

C
Mobilization of Ureter into Channel

D
Covering of Ureter with Bladder Wall Muscle

entail simultaneous laparoscopic and cystoscopic access as well as percutaneous intravesical instrumentation to assist in the procedure.

One approach along these lines has been the performance of an unusual type of antireflux procedure, the Gil-Vernet ureteroplasty. This method, originally described using open surgical methods, involves a vertical incision in the trigone and placement of a horizontal mattress suture to draw the ureters toward the midline (De Gennaro et al, 1991). This elongates their intramural tunnels, increases ureteral stability, and should eliminate reflux. In the laparoendoscopic method, this has been reported using cystoscopic control and two percutaneous bladder cannulas for suture positioning (Oka-mura et al, 1995). The technique has not achieved wide acceptance and does not have the reported high success rates needed for an efficient substitute for more commonly performed methods but hints at the possibilities of combining technologies. More extensive laboratory investigation is needed to develop this potential fully.

Augmentation Cystoplasty

ENTEROCYSTOPLASTY

Bladder augmentation using gastrointestinal segments is well described and developed in pediatric urology. Development of these techniques to laparoscopic means requires much ingenuity. Bowel harvesting techniques have been established in laparoscopy using endoscopic GIA stapling devices. These have a good reported record, with safety that should equal that of conventional intestinal stapling devices. The manipulation necessary for fashioning the harvested bowel segment into a detubularized augmentation patch is a challenge to any laparoscopist but is technically feasible. Performing the bowel-to-bladder anastomosis requires a significant amount of suturing or the use of an endoscopic stapling device that delivers absorbable staples. These are available for open surgery and have been developed for endoscopic applications. Pediatric laparoscopic gastrocystoplasty has been described (Docimo et al, 1995b) and indicates the technical potential for major reconstructive surgery using laparoscopic techniques. The efficiency of the procedure requires development, yet the reduction in morbidity may be substantial. It is important to consider the possibility of decreased intraperitoneal adhesions after laparoscopic augmentation cystoplasty as compared with an open surgical approach. It has been seen that laparoscopic intraperitoneal surgery produces relatively few adhesions in children, although the reason remains unknown (Moore et al, 1995b). It may simply be due to reduced handling of the bowel during the surgical procedure, particularly the application of sponges and retractors onto the serosal surface. Whether this would be of any clinical significance when performing major reconstructive surgery is unclear, but the possibility of reducing the incidence of adhesion formation and postoperative intestinal obstruction is attractive.

AUTOAUGMENTATION

Bladder autoaugmentation is a procedure in which the bladder wall musculature is stripped away from the underlying uroepithelium and partially removed to reduce intravesi-

cal pressures (Cartwright and Snow, 1989). It has achieved marginal success with open surgical techniques and is limited by an inability to predict the response of any particular patient. It is an attractive alternative to enterocystoplasty because there is no intestinal epithelium in the urinary tract. It is much less morbid a procedure than conventional augmentation. Laparoscopic autoaugmentation is even more attractive, but the success rates are not consistent. Several preliminary reports and animal studies have been published (Ehrlich and Gershman, 1993; Britanisky et al, 1995; McDougall et al, 1995b). The animal studies are fraught with the problem of being performed in animals with essentially normal bladders, in contrast to the human situation of a diseased bladder, which is likely to respond differently to the procedure. Laser technology has been applied to the technically difficult aspect of the procedure laparoscopically, the dissection of the muscularis away from the epithelium in an animal model (Britanisky et al, 1995) as well as in two children (Poppas et al, 1996). The procedure was technically successful, but the long-term benefit was limited. Improved patient selection criteria are necessary for laparoscopic autoaugmentation to become an effective part of the management of bladder dysfunction in children, yet it is suited to laparoscopic methods.

Horizons of Reconstructive Surgery

Other reconstructive techniques have been reported anecdotally. These include creation of a continent catheterizable stoma (Mitrofanoff) in a teenage girl with a surgically unreconstructable bladder neck (Jordan and Winslow, 1993b). This was performed using both laparoscopic and open techniques. Intestinal vaginoplasty has been reported using laparoscopic harvesting of the bowel segment and preparation of the pelvic bed for the bowel segment (Jordan G, video presentation, Pediatric Endourology and Laparoscopy Course, Harvard Medical School, 1993). The perineal anastomosis was performed using open technique. These cases indicate the potential and technical feasibility of complex reconstructive surgery in children using laparoscopic methods. Efficient development of this potential depends on technical and conceptual improvements in the way laparoscopic surgery is performed (Peters, 1996). This includes methods of tissue handling, tissue joining, and improved exposure and visualization techniques. Combined laparoscopic and endoscopic methods may facilitate these procedures.

PHYSIOLOGIC CONSIDERATIONS IN CHILDREN AND ADULTS

The creation of a pneumoperitoneum produces significant alterations in respiratory and circulatory function, including alterations in renal blood flow. In adults, this can potentially result in challenging anesthesia management; in contrast, pediatric laparoscopy has not been associated with clinically significant complications. In part, this is due to the ability of the child to compensate for these changes as well as the relatively moderate degree of severity of changes. A knowledge of the limits of tolerance in healthy and compromised patients is therefore essential. As laparoscopic applications are expanding, more children and adults with various degrees of cardiopulmonary or renal functional limitations have become candidates for laparoscopic surgery. Determining the risks of pneumoperitoneum in those individuals is necessary for further application of laparoscopic methods (Peters et al, 1995a).

The principal physiologic effects of pneumoperitoneum are similar in children and adults, whereas the ramifications are distinct (Holzman, 1996). The increased metabolic rate of children produces a greater oxygen demand, which is combined with a reduced oxygen reserve within the lungs. This is due to the underdeveloped pulmonary tree of the child with less compliance than the adult. **The child's baseline functional reserve capacity (FRC) of the lung is less than in the adult.** As intra-abdominal pressure increases, FRC further declines. Loss of FRC reduces the safety net of oxygenation should loss of airway control occur. Oxygen desaturation may occur more rapidly, with early effects. Some of these effects have been observed in patients with chest wall deformities who have reduced pulmonary capacity at the start. Desaturation was observed as intraperitoneal pressures exceeded 10 mm Hg but were adequate at 8 mm Hg. Increases in airway pressure are not of significance within certain limits but were of concern in a patient with a previously repaired tracheoesophageal fistula and the potential for barotrauma at the tracheal closure site.

When carbon dioxide is used for insufflation, it is absorbed into the blood stream and released into the expired breath (Wolf et al, 1995). **This is seen with increases in end-tidal carbon dioxide ($ETCO_2$) during laparoscopy** (Fig. 95–45). Increased $ETCO_2$ is associated with acidosis in extremes but has not been seen to be a clinical issue in children. Elevated carbon dioxide increases catecholamine release, vasoconstriction, and central venous pressure. There are inotropic and chronotropic effects on the heart, and there may be a lower threshold to arrhythmias. No specific attempt has been made in the authors' unit to correct the increased $ETCO_2$ using increased minute ventilation, although some anesthesiologists do so. In contrast to the adult, the slight metabolic alteration of increased $ETCO_2$ is not generally a risk in children. In those sensitive to acidosis or

catecholamine release because of cardiac dysrhythmias, an increased minute ventilation may be appropriate.

The authors performed transesophageal echocardiography in a child with mild left ventricular hypertrophy during creation of pneumoperitoneum. Right-sided heart filling and function could be assessed by examining changes in right ventricle cross-sectional diameter. Surprisingly, there were no changes evident as insufflation pressures rose from 5 to 20 mm Hg in 5-mm steps. This indicates that normal cardiac function is not markedly affected despite significant increases in intra-abdominal pressure.

No significant alteration in lower extremity circulation was detected in a group of children undergoing pneumoperitoneum for laparoscopy using simultaneous upper and lower extremity pulse oximetry. Some changes in venous circulation may be induced in the lower limbs, but these did not appear to have any effect on tissue oxygenation.

Renal function is affected by pneumoperitoneum in patients with decreased urinary output during laparoscopic procedures, despite vigorous fluid resuscitation. This effect has been reported in adults and anecdotally in children. **Laboratory studies have suggested this to be due to compression of the renal parenchyma causing a reduction in renal blood flow** (Chiu et al, 1994; Kirsch et al, 1994; McDougall et al, 1996; Razvi et al, 1996). It does not appear to be due to compression of the ureters or the renal vein. The possibility of hormonal or neural mechanisms has not been fully investigated, yet these are important in that they may be manipulated pharmacologically if needed. Although there have been no reports of negative consequences with pneumoperitoneum on renal function, in two independent pilot studies, one in adults and one in children, evidence of subtle renal injury because of laparoscopy has been demonstrated. The renal tubular enzyme N-β-acetyl glucosaminidase (NAG) is a nonspecific indicator of tubular injury and may be seen to be elevated after extracorporeal shock-wave lithotripsy, drug nephrotoxicity, or infection. Elevated levels of urinary NAG (indexed to creatinine) were found in patients following laparoscopy relative to normal postoperative patients. The degree of increase was not extreme, and no clinical consequences were detected, but this observation

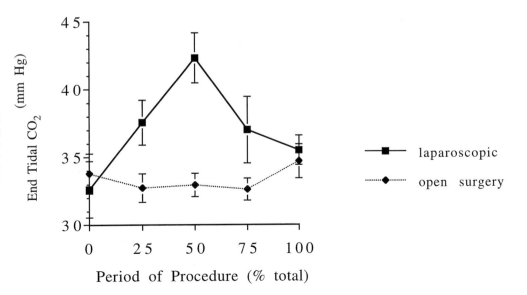

Figure 95–45. Increases in end-tidal CO_2 during laparoscopic procedures in infants less than 1 year old, as compared to comparable procedures (nephrectomy and orchiopexy) performed using open surgical techniques.

suggests that pneumoperitoneum may pose some risk to the kidney. In children with compromised renal function, this might actually have clinical consequences. The limits of tolerance remain to be determined as well as any age dependency on these effects. Just as the infant kidney is more susceptible to infectious injury, so may it be at risk for injury from increased intra-abdominal pressure. Of note, no increase in injury has been noted in the authors' experience with laparoscopic live donor nephrectomy.

A surprising observation about pediatric physiologic response to laparoscopy has been an increase in body temperature. Concern had often been expressed that children would be at greater risk for hypothermia during laparoscopy because of instillation of cold insufflating gas, yet the contrary has been observed in the absence of specific heat conservation measures (Fig. 95–46). The effect is not sufficient to pose a risk but indicates that aggressive heat conservation measures do not necessarily need to be instituted without regard for the patient's status, and it raises interesting physiologic questions about the mechanisms. Activation of retroperitoneal brown fat, mediated through catecholamine release, has been a postulated mechanism. This might be important in children with cardiac disease who are sensitive to catecholamines.

It is apparent that most adults and children tolerate laparoscopy well, yet the limits of that tolerance, and the generality of that observation, remain to be determined. Definition of these limits is important to the expansion of laparoscopic techniques to more patients with compromised renal and cardiopulmonary function.

COMPLICATIONS

Complications in the Adult

As outlined previously, **proper patient selection is critical in minimizing complications.** One must be certain that for a given patient's pathology, laparoscopy is the most appropriate form of surgical treatment.

Equally important is each surgeon's abilities and laparoscopic experience. Laparoscopy is an operative approach that requires different technical skills than traditional open surgery. During laparoscopy, the normal hand-eye axis used in surgery is dissociated: The eyes are not directly watching hand motions. Developing the ability to operate off of a video image as well as obtaining a feel for how the various instruments interact with tissue takes a great deal of practice. Moreover, anatomy is viewed from novel perspectives, and experience is needed to identify tissue planes and structures accurately.

Several studies have demonstrated that **complications are directly related to surgical experience** (Kavoussi et al, 1993c; See et al, 1993; Gill et al, 1995b; Peters, 1995a). The exact number of cases varies from surgeon to surgeon; however, the learning curve is less for experienced laparoscopic surgeons learning a new procedure.

Many complications from laparoscopic procedures are similar to those seen with open surgery. Anesthetic risks should be discussed in detail. Improper patient positioning and padding can lead to neuromuscular injury during prolonged procedures. Specific to laparoscopy, complications are related to initial abdominal access, the pneumoperitoneum, tissue dissection, or concluding the procedure.

Abdominal Access Injuries

Major abdominal vessels, viscous structures, and solid organs can be injured during initial Veress needle or trocar placement. At the initiation of any laparoscopic procedure, the abdomen should be palpated and inspected for scars. One should **refrain from placing a needle or trocar in the area of a palpable mass.** Moreover, scars from prior intra-abdominal surgery should be avoided because underlying bowel may be adherent. In these instances, one should entertain the use of open trocar placement. A Foley catheter and oral gastric tube are placed to minimize perforation of the bladder and stomach. When placing the initial trocar, a blunt visual obturator can be helpful to identify entry into the peritoneal cavity while minimizing risk to underlying viscera. All secondary trocars should be placed under direct vision.

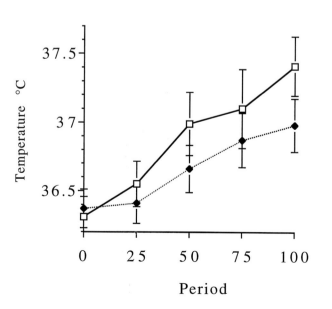

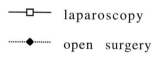

Figure 95–46. Increases in body temperature during laparoscopic procedures were greater than with comparable open procedures (nephrectomy and orchiopexy), without specific warming measures. Aggressive warming of children during laparoscopy is not necessary, and such increases in temperature should be anticipated.

Even in the most controlled circumstances, Veress needle and trocar injuries to the bowel can occur (Borten, 1986). A **straightforward Veress needle injury can heal with conservative management; however, trocar injuries require formal repair.** If one is facile with endoscopic suturing techniques, a laparoscopic repair may be chosen. In cases of gross spillage of large bowel content, an open repair may be preferable.

Bladder injuries can occur with placement of lower midline trocars. These usually present intraoperatively as hematuria or with gas distending the Foley drainage bag (Kavoussi et al, 1993c). If suspected, methylene blue injected through the catheter can be used to identify the injury site. Veress needle injuries can be observed, and small leaks may be managed using clips to approximate the edges of the bladder. Larger injuries require endoscopic or open repair. In patients with persistent gross hematuria, a bladder injury must be suspected.

Unfortunately, many visceral injuries may not be noted at the time of occurrence. In patients with persistent postoperative pain, drainage from a trocar site, fever, or peritoneal signs, one must suspect an occult bowel injury. Prompt radiographic evaluation and surgical exploration is mandatory.

Vascular injuries represent a significant cause of operative morbidity and in severe cases can develop into a life-threatening surgical emergency (Hulka, 1985). **Anterior abdominal wall vessels are the most frequently injured vascular structures** during laparoscopic surgery (Kavoussi et al, 1992b). For minor bleeding, laparoscopic guided fulguration can be attempted. In severe cases, a transcutaneous stitch can be passed using a Keith or Stamey needle (Green et al, 1992). In rare instances, a cut-down over the bleeding trocar site may be needed. Abdominal wall vessels can be avoided by placing trocars lateral to the rectus muscle and identifying superficial vessels with transillumination from the laparoscope light.

Major vascular structures may be perforated during intra-abdominal access. The safest course of action to take when blood is aspirated from a Veress needle is immediate laparotomy. The needle should be left in place because it acts as a guide to the area of injury and may serve to tamponade bleeding. Injuries may be through-and-through; thus, sites of perforation must be inspected circumferentially. Trocar injuries can present with significant intra-abdominal or retroperitoneal hemorrhage and clinical signs of acute blood loss. Again, **immediate** laparotomy and vascular repair is crucial.

Injuries Related to the Pneumoperitoneum

Problems with the pneumoperitoneum can cause significant technical and physiologic challenges. Incorrect Veress needle position can result in subcutaneous emphysema, preperitoneal insufflation, or inflation of a viscus. **Subcutaneous and preperitoneal insufflation is more common in obese individuals** and results in an increase in the distance between the skin and the true peritoneal cavity (Mendoza et al, 1996). This can make trocar placement difficult and distort intraperitoneal anatomy. Open trocar placement may be necessary to achieve intra-abdominal access.

Visceral insufflation usually presents as asymmetric abdominal wall distention with insufflation pressures rising quickly relative to the amount of gas infused. In these instances, the distended bowel markedly inhibits visualization, and the laparoscopic procedure should be aborted. One may consider proceeding with open laparotomy or rescheduling the laparoscopic procedure at a later date.

The pneumoperitoneum can cause physiologic problems as a result of both **mechanical and biochemical effects. The increased intra-abdominal pressure may impede ventilation because of pressure on the diaphragm** (Nunn, 1987; Monk and Weldon, 1992). **Moreover, hypotension can develop secondary to decreased venous return secondary to pneumoperitoneum compression of the vena cava** (Arthure, 1970; Lew et al, 1992). In patients with a hiatal hernia, abdominal contents can be pushed into the chest leading to decreased cardiac output and impaired ventilation.

Severe subcutaneous emphysema may result in hypercarbia, especially in patients with minimal cardiac reserve (Kent, 1991). Gas tracking through the subcutaneous tissue can dissect along abdominal wall fascial planes. Gas dissecting to the neck can potentially track into the mediastinum, resulting in cardiac tamponade (Brantley and Riley, 1988; Ostman et al, 1990).

Although relatively uncommon, one of the most frightening complications of the pneumoperitoneum is a gas pulmonary embolism (Diakun, 1974; Yacoub et al, 1982; Shulman and Aronson, 1984). **It is crucial to recognize a gas embolism promptly and institute immediate therapy to avoid a fatal outcome.** Accumulated gas in the right atrium can migrate into the pulmonary artery and cause interruption of pulmonary blood flow. **Patients present with sudden cardiovascular collapse. The anesthesiologist notices a mill-wheel murmur and a rapid decrease in the $ETCO_2$.** This latter occurrence is due to decreased pulmonary blood flow caused by the embolism (Shulman and Aronson, 1984). If a gas embolism is suspected, the procedure should be terminated, and **cardiopulmonary resuscitation** should commence. A **left lateral decubitus position** may be helpful to prevent further gas from entering the pulmonary artery. A central line or percutaneous puncture may be used in an attempt to aspirate the gas. Open surgical evacuation and bypass have been reported to be successful in reviving patients (Diakun, 1974).

Dissection Injuries

As with all surgical procedures, inadvertent injuries may occur with dissection. Early recognition and prompt repair are pivotal components to minimize patient morbidity. Depending on each surgeon's experience and type of injury, an open or laparoscopic repair should be undertaken.

In the event of a vascular injury, pressure should be placed under direct vision, and rapid assessment should be made to determine the type of injury and best route of repair. If it is well controlled, a laparoscopic clip or suture repair may be undertaken; however, if this is not readily possible, emergent laparotomy is necessary (Theil et al, 1996). Rapid entry to the abdominal cavity can be achieved by torquing the laparoscope up against the abdominal wall and cutting down on it with a knife.

Bowel injuries should be approached as outlined in the

section on access injuries; however, special considerations should be given to **electrocautery injuries.** In these cases, **the zone of thermal injury may be much greater than what is visually apparent, and wide débridement is necessary** (Schwimmer, 1974).

Ureteral injuries usually occur during gynecologic procedures or dissection deep in the pelvis (laparoscopic pelvic lymphadenectomy) (Gomel and Christopher, 1991; Kavoussi et al, 1993c). Minor injuries can be managed with stenting; however, complete transection or cautery injuries may require formal repair (Grainger et al, 1990; Nezhat et al, 1992).

Closure Injuries

Concentration must be maintained at the conclusion of any laparoscopic procedure because the potential for significant injury remains. After dissection, the intra-abdominal pressure should be lowered to 7 mm Hg to **inspect for any venous bleeding that may have been tamponaded by the pneumoperitoneum.** Moreover, careful examination must be made to rule out unsuspected injury.

The anterior abdominal wall fascia of larger (>10 mm) trocar sites in adults and all trocar sites in children must be closed to prevent incisional hernia formation (Thomas et al, 1990; Bloom and Ehrlich, 1993). Similar occurrences have been reported in adults, both acutely and postoperatively (Vaughan ED Jr, personal communication, 1996). These sites should be closed using endoscopic monitoring to avoid inadvertent injury to underlying bowel.

Each trocar should also be removed under direct vision to exclude the possibility of occult bleeding. Before removing the last trocar, all carbon dioxide should be evacuated from the abdominal cavity to prevent postoperative abdominal, chest, and shoulder pain caused by diaphragmatic irritation.

Trocar sites should be irrigated and inspected for hemostasis to minimize the risk of wound infection. Larger sites can be sutured closed, whereas smaller sites can be reapproximated with tape strips.

Complications in the Child

Many of the technical issues related to prevention and management of complications in children are similar to those in adults. Although several studies report the incidence of laparoscopic complications in adult urologic patients, there have been few reports of pediatric complications, despite the use of diagnostic laparoscopy in pediatric urology since 1974 (Cortesi et al, 1976). As operative laparoscopy has developed, several reports have been published (Bloom and Ehrlich, 1993; Sadeghi-Nejad et al, 1994). A survey of the AAP Section on Pediatric Urology was conducted to assess the incidence of complications in pediatric urology (Peters, 1995a). In addition to indicating wide usage—75% of respondents (61% response to a mailed anonymous survey) stated they were using laparoscopy in their practice—the survey showed that complications do occur in pediatric urologic laparoscopy. These ranged from trivial complications such as preperitoneal insufflation and subcutaneous insufflation, to major vascular injuries, bowel injury, and bladder injury. These were reported to occur with diagnostic and operative laparoscopy (Table 95–3).

Table 95–3. INCIDENCE OF REPORTED COMPLICATIONS IN PEDIATRIC LAPAROSCOPY

Complication	All Cases (%)	Diagnostic Only (%)
Preperitoneal insufflation	3.2	3.1
Subcutaneous emphysema	0.94	0.63
Bowel injury	0.17	0.09
Great vessel injury	0.06	0.09
Abdominal wall vessel	0.37	0.18
Bladder injury	0.17	0.09
Cannula site hernia	0.15	0.09
Death	0	0
Major complication	1.18	0.54
Surgical complication	0.39	0.09

From Peters CA: Complications in pediatric urologic laparoscopy: Results of a survey. J Urol 1995a; 155:1070–1073.

Predictors of the incidence of complications were identified, with the most important being experience of the operator (Fig. 95–47). The learning curve appears to be such that the incidence of complications does not significantly decline until after 50 cases. This is expressed as an aggregate rate of complications, however, and not the current or ongoing rate. The method of training was not found to be a significant predictor of complications. Laparoscopic access technique was found to be a predictor of complications, with practitioners using exclusively the Veress technique having a higher rate than those using only the open technique or a combination of techniques. This effect was seen when the experience of the practitioner was accounted for also. It was important to note that even with open technique (Hassan),

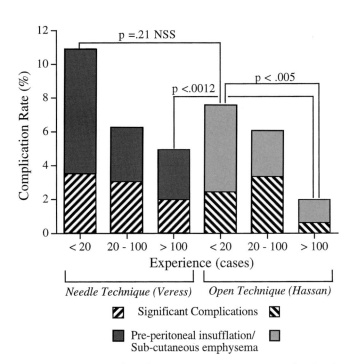

(comparisons based upon rates of significant complications)

Figure 95–47. Incidence of reported complications in pediatric urologic laparoscopic procedures. The experience of the operator was an important predictor of complications, as was the technique used for creation of the pneumoperitoneum. (From Peters CA: J Urol 1995; 155:1070–1073.)

complications did occur (Sadeghi-Nejad et al, 1994), although at a low rate. It is essential that care be taken in all steps of the laparoscopic procedure, particularly in children, in whom the operating spaces are small and the abdominal wall is much more pliable than in the adult.

CONCLUSIONS

Laparoscopy is a powerful tool to treat urologic pathology in that it can markedly reduce postoperative morbidity compared with many traditional surgical approaches and may hold the potential for improving surgical outcomes. Laparoscopy has not been applied to its fullest potential because of the associated learning curve and difficulty of most urologic applications. The technical challenges have limited extensive use, and only a small portion of urologists who have taken a training course use laparoscopy in clinical practice (See et al, 1993). Moreover, operative time is longer, increasing overall patient costs and decreasing the financial incentive for urologists to consider this approach (Winfield et al, 1994b; Bishoff et al, 1996; Troxel and Winfield, 1996).

For laparoscopy to become an integral part of mainstream urology, several advances in teaching and technology are needed. Current teaching practices (i.e., a weekend laboratory course) are not sufficient to impart the necessary skills to allow most urologic surgeons to become comfortable with laparoscopic techniques. Methods need to be developed to support surgeons when they return to their home institutions. Advances in telemedical systems may provide a means of support for beginning laparoscopists. Moreover, technical progress needs to be made to create a transparent interface when moving from open surgery to a minimally invasive approach. Automated and robotic devices may help standardize skill among urologists to help provide all patients with the same excellent surgical outcome. Improving skills also decreases operative times and associated costs.

Perhaps the greatest contribution of laparoscopic surgery has been that it has emphasized to surgeons the need to consider the patient as a whole. Urologists must begin looking at factors in addition to outcomes when recommending a surgical approach. Postoperative pain, convalescence, and disfigurement are all important to patients and should be weighed when recommending a surgical approach. Laparoscopy begins to address these issues; however, it is only a stepping stone in the evolution of surgery.

REFERENCES

Adams JB, Marco AD, Averch TD et al: Physiologic changes during laparoscopy utilizing 20 mmHg intra-abdominal pressure. J Endourol 1995a; 9:S152.

Adams JB, Micali S, Moore RG et al: Complications of extraperitoneal balloon dilation. J Endourol 1996; 10:375–378.

Adams JB, Schulam PG, Moore RG et al: New laparoscopic suturing device: Initial clinical experience. Urology 1995b; 46:242–245.

Akimaru K, Ide M, Saitoh M, et al: Subcutaneous wire traction technique without CO_2 insufflation for laparoscopic cholecystectomy. J Laparoendosc Surg 1993; 3:59.

Albala DA, Prinz RA: Laparoscopic adrenalectomy: Results of eight patients. J Urol 1994; 2:661.

Albala DM, Schuessler WW, Vancaille TG: Laparoscopic bladder neck suspension. J Endourol 1992; 2:137.

Anderson KR, Fadden PA, Kerbl K, et al: Laparoscopic continent urinary diversion in a porcine model. J Endourol 1993; 7:S197.

Araki K, Namikawa K, Yamamoto H, et al: Abdominal wall retraction during laparoscopic cholecystectomy. World J Surg 1993; 17:105.

Arthure H: Laparoscopy hazard. Br Med J 1970; 4:492.

Assimos DG, Jarow JP: Role of laparoscopic pelvic lymph node dissection in the management of patients with penile cancer and inguinal adenopathy. J Endourol 1994; 8:365.

Atala A, Kavoussi LR, Goldstein DS, et al: Laparoscopic correction of vesicoureteral reflux. J Urol 1993; 150:748–751.

Atlas I, Stone N: Laparoscopy for evaluation of cryptorchid testis. Urology 1992; 40:256–258.

Baba S, Ohya M, Deguchi N, Tazaki H: Laparoscopic management of retrocaval ureter. J Endourol 1993; 7:S238.

Babaian RJ, Bracken RB, Johnson DE: Complications of transabdominal retroperitoneal lymphadenectomy. Urology 1981; 17:126.

Bishoff J, O'Sullivan D, Schulam P, et al: Comparative cost analysis of laparoscopic and open nephrectomy. 1997. Submitted.

Bloom DA, Ayers JW, McGuire EJ: The role of laparoscopy in management of nonpalpable testes. J Urol (Paris) 1988; 94:465–470.

Bloom DA, Ehrlich RM: Omental evisceration through small laparoscopy port sites. J Endourol 1993; 7:31–33.

Bock JE, Sobye JV: Frequency of contralateral inguinal hernia in children. Acta Chir Scand 1970; 136:707.

Boddy SA, Corkery JJ, Gornall P: The place of laparoscopy in the management of the impalpable testis. Br J Surg 1985; 72:918–919.

Bogaert GA, Kogan BA, Mevorach RA: Therapeutic laparoscopy for intraabdominal testes. Urology 1993; 42:182–188.

Borten M: Laparoscopic Complications: Prevention and Management. Toronto, B.C. Decker, 1986, pp 317–329.

Bowsher WG, Clarke A, Clarke DG, Costello AJ: Laparoscopic pelvic lymph node dissection for carcinoma of the prostate and bladder. Aust N Z J Surg 1992; 62:634.

Brantley JC, Riley PM: Cardiovascular collapse during laparoscopy: A report of two cases. Am J Obstet Gynecol 1988; 159:735.

Breda G, Tamai A, Xausa D, et al: Pelvioscopic colposuspension. J Endourol 1993; 7:S247.

Britanisky RG, Poppas DP, Shichman SN, et al: Laparoscopic laser-assisted bladder autoaugmentation. Urology 1995; 46:31–35.

Brooks JD, Preminger GM, Kavoussi LR, et al: Comparison of open and endourologic approaches to the obstructed ureteropelvic junction. Urology 1995; 46:791.

Cain MP, Garra B, Gibbons MD: Scrotal/inguinal ultrasonography: A technique for identifying nonpalpable inguinal testes without laparoscopy. J Urol 1996; 156(part 2):791–794.

Caldamone AA, Amaral JF: Laparoscopic stage 2 Fowler-Stephens orchiopexy. J Urol 1994; 152:1253–1256.

Capelouto CC, Adams JB, Moore RG, Kavoussi LR: Intermediate follow-up in patients undergoing laparoscopic removal of renal malignancy. J Urol 1995; 153:255A.

Capelouto CC, Kavoussi LR: Complications of laparoscopic surgery. Urology 1993; 42:2–12.

Capelouto CC, Moore RG, Silverman SG, Kavoussi LR: Retroperitoneoscopy: Anatomic rationale for direct retroperitoneal access. J Urol 1994; 152:2008.

Cartwright P, Snow B: Bladder autoaugmentation: Early clinical experience. J Urol 1989; 142(Part 2):505–508.

Castilho LN: Laparoscopy for the nonpalpable testis: How to interpret the endoscopic findings. J Urol 1990; 144:1215–1218.

Chandhoke PS, Galansky S, Koyle M, Kaula NF: Pediatric retroperitoneal laparoscopic nephrectomy. J Endourol 1993; 7(Suppl 1):S138.

Chardavoyne R, Wise L: Exploratory laparoscopy for perforation following colonoscopy. Surg Laparosc Endosc 1994; 4:241.

Chiu AW, Azadzoi KM, Hatzichristou DG, et al: Effects of intra-abdominal pressure on renal tissue perfusion during laparoscopy. J Endourol 1994; 8:99–103.

Clayman RV, Kavoussi LR, Soper NJ, et al: Laparoscopic nephrectomy. N Engl J Med 1991; 324:1370.

Coptcoat MJ, Joyce AJ, Popert R, et al: Laparoscopic nephrectomy—the King's experience. Min Inv Ther 1992; (Suppl)1:67.

Corson SL, Batzer FR, Gocial G, Maislin G: Measurement of the force necessary for laparoscopic trocar entry. J Reprod Med 1989; 34:282.

Cortes D, Thorup JM, Lenz K, et al: Laparoscopy in 100 consecutive patients with 128 impalpable testes. Br J Urol 1995; 75:281–287.

Cortesi N, Ferrari P, Zambarda E, et al: Diagnosis of bilateral abdominal cryptorchidism by laparoscopy. Endoscopy 1976; 8:33.

Danella JF, deKernion JB, Smith RB, Steckel J: The contemporary incidence of lymph node metastases in prostate cancer: Implications for laparoscopic lymph node dissection. J Urol 1993; 149:1488.

Das S: Laparoscopic removal of bladder diverticulum. J Urol 1992; 148:1837.

Das S, Keizur JJ, Tashima M: Laparoscopic nephroureterectomy for end-stage reflux nephropathy in a child. Surg Laparosc Endosc 1993; 3:462–465.

Das S, Palmer JK: Laparoscopic colpo-suspension. J Urol 1995; 154:1119–1121.

Das S, Tashima M: Extraperitoneal laparoscopic staging pelvic lymph node dissection. J Urol 1994; 151:1321.

De Gennaro M, Appetito C, Lais A, et al: Effectiveness of trigonoplasty to treat primary vesicoureteral reflux. J Urol 1991; 146(Part 2):636–638.

Diakun TA: Carbon dioxide embolism: Successful resuscitation with cardiopulmonary bypass. Anesthesiology 1974; 74:1151.

Diamond DA: Laparoscopic orchiopexy for the intra-abdominal testis. J Urol 1994; 152:1257–1258.

Diamond DA, Caldamone AA: The value of laparoscopy for 106 impalpable testes relative to clinical presentation. J Urol 1992; 148(Part 2):632–634.

Diamond DA, Price HM, McDougall EM, Bloom DA: Retroperitoneal laparoscopic nephrectomy in children. J Urol 1995; 153:1966–1968.

Docimo SG: The results of surgical therapy for cryptorchidism: A literature review and analysis. J Urol 1995; 154:1148–1152.

Docimo SG, Moore RG, Adams J, Kavoussi LR: Laparoscopic bladder augmentation using stomach. Urology 1995a; 46:565–569.

Docimo SG, Moore RG, Adams J, Kavoussi LR: Laparoscopic orchiopexy for the high palpable undescended testis: Preliminary experience. J Urol 1995b; 154:1513–1515.

Docimo S, Moore RG, Kavoussi LR: Laparoscopic orchiopexy. Urology 1995c; 46:715.

Doig CM: Use of laparoscopy in children with impalpable testes. Int J Androl 1989; 12:420–422.

Donohue RE, Mani JH, Whitesel JA: Intraoperative and early complications of staging pelvic lymph node dissection in prostatic adenocarcinoma. Urology 1990; 35:223.

Donovan JF, Winfield HN: Laparoscopic varix ligation. J Urol 1992a; 147:77–81.

Donovan JF Jr, Winfield HN: Laparoscopic varix ligation with the Nd:YAG laser. J Endourol 1992b; 6:165–171.

Droesch K, Droesch J, Chumas J, Bronson R: Laparoscopic gonadectomy for gonadal dysgenesis. Fertil Steril 1990; 53:360–361.

Ehrlich RM, Gershman A: Laparoscopic seromyotomy (auto-augmentation) for non-neurogenic neurogenic bladder in a child: Initial case report. Urology 1993; 42:175–178.

Ehrlich RM, Gershman A, Fuchs G: Expanding indications for laparoscopy in pediatric urology: An update. J Endourol 1993a; 7:S140.

Ehrlich RM, Gershman A, Fuchs G: Laparoscopic ureteral reimplantation for vesicoureteral reflux: Initial case reports. J Endourol 1993b; 7:S171.

Ehrlich RM, Gershman A, Fuchs G: Laparoscopic renal surgery in children. J Urol 1994; 151:735–739.

Ehrlich RM, Gershman A, Mee S, Fuchs G: Laparoscopic nephrectomy in a child: Expanding horizons for laparoscopy in pediatric urology. J Endourol 1992; 6:463–465.

Elashry OM, Nakada SY, Wolf JS, et al: Laparoscopy for adult polycystic kidney disease: A promising alternative. Am J Kidney Dis 1996. In press.

Enquist E, Stein BS, Sigman M: Laparoscopic versus subinguinal varicocelectomy: A comparative study. Fertil Steril 1994; 61:1092.

Eraky I, el-Kappany H, Shamaa MA, Ghoneim MA: Laparoscopic nephrectomy: An established routine procedure. J Endourol 1994; 8:275.

Etwaru D, Raboy A, Ferzli G, Albert P: Extraperitoneal endoscopic gasless pelvic lymph node dissection. J Laparoendosc Surg 1994; 4:113.

Fairfax CA, Skoog SJ: The laparoscopic diagnosis of transverse testicular ectopia. J Urol 1995; 153:477–478.

Ferreira U, Cassiano ES, Nogueira CL, Rodrigues NNJ: Laparoscopy in the management of nonpalpable testes and intersex states. Arch Esp Urol 1993; 46:638–641.

Fowler R, Stephens FD: The role of testicular vascular anatomy in the salvage of high undescended testes. Aust N Z J Surg 1959; 29:92.

Freiha FS, Salzman J: Surgical staging of prostatic cancer: Transperitoneal versus extraperitoneal lymphadenectomy. J Urol 1977; 118:616.

Frey P, Bianchi A: Microvascular orchiopexy. Eur J Pediatr 1987; 2:S51–52.

Frey P, Bianchi A: Microvascular autotransplantation of intra-abdominal testes. Prog Pediatr Surg 1989; 23:115–125.

Froeling FM, Sorber MJ, de la Rosette JJ, de Vries JD: The nonpalpable testis and the changing role of laparoscopy. Urology 1994; 43:222–227.

Gans SL, Berci G: Peritoneoscopy in infants and children. J Pediatr Surg 1973; 8:399–405.

Garibyan H: Use of laparoscopy for the localization of impalpable testes. Neth J Surg 1987; 39:68–71.

Gaur DD: Laparoscopic operative retroperitoneoscopy: Use of a new device. J Urol 1992; 148:1137.

Gaur DD: Retroperitoneal endoscopic ureterolithotomy: Our experience in 12 patients. J Endourol 1993; 7:501.

Gaur DD, Agarwal DK, Purohit KC: Retroperitoneal laparoscopic ureterolithotomy and renal biopsy. J Urol 1992; 2:149.

Gaur DD, Agarwal DK, Purohit KC: Retroperitoneal laparoscopic nephrectomy: Initial case report. J Urol 1993; 149:103–105.

Gerber G, Bissada NK, Hulbert JC, et al: Laparoscopic retroperitoneal lymphadenectomy: Multi-institutional analysis. J Urol 1994; 152:1188.

Gililland J, Cummings D, Hibbert ML, et al: Laparoscopic orchiectomy in a patient with complete androgen insensitivity. J Laparoendosc Surg 1993; 3:51–54.

Gill IS, Clayman RV, McDougall EM: Advances in urological laparoscopy. J Urol 1995a; 154:1275.

Gill IS, Kavoussi LR, Clayman RV, et al: Complications of laparoscopic nephrectomy in 185 patients: A multi-institutional review. J Urol 1995b; 154:479.

Gill IS, Munch LC, McRoberts JW, Clayman RV: A new laparoscopic kidney entrapment and tourniquet device. J Endourol 1993; 7:S197.

Gomel V, Christopher J: Intraoperative management of ureteral injury by operative laparoscopy. Fertil Steril 1991; 55:416.

Gornall PG, Pender DJ: Crossed testicular ectopia detected by laparoscopy. Br J Urol 1987; 59:283.

Graff TD, Arbegast NR, Phillips OC: Gas embolism: A comparative study of air and carbon dioxide as embolic agents in the systemic venous system. Am J Obstet Gynecol 1959; 78:259.

Grainger DA, Soderstrom RM, Schiff SF, et al: Ureteral injuries at laparoscopy: Insights into diagnosis, management and prevention. Obstet Gynecol 1990; 75:839.

Green LS, Loughlin KR, Kavoussi LR: Management of epigastric vessel injury during laparoscopy. J Endourol 1992; 6:99.

Guazzoni G, Montorsi F, Bergamaschi F, et al: Open surgical revision of laparoscopic pelvic lymphadenectomy for staging of prostate cancer: The impact of laparoscopic learning curve. J Urol 1994a; 151:930.

Guazzoni G, Montorsi F, Bergamaschi F, et al: Long-term assessment of laparoscopic decortication of simple renal cysts. J Endourol 1993; 7:S174.

Guazzoni G, Montorsi F, Lanzi R, et al: Operative morbidity and clinical efficacy of laparoscopic vs open adrenalectomy. J Urol 1994b; 2:151.

Guiney EJ, Corbally M, Malone PS: Laparoscopy and the management of the impalpable testis. Br J Urol 1989; 63:313–316.

Gustafson ML, Lee MM, Asmundson L, et al: Mullerian inhibiting substance in the diagnosis and management of intersex and gonadal abnormalities. J Pediatr Surg 1993; 28:439–444.

Hagood PG, Mehan DJ, Worischeck JH, et al: Laparoscopic varicocelectomy: Preliminary report of a new technique. J Urol 1992; 147:73.

Harrison CB, Kaplan GW, Scherz HC, et al: Microvascular autotransplantation of the intra-abdominal testis. J Urol 1990; 144:506–507.

Hassan HM: A modified instrument and method for laparoscopy. Am J Obstet Gynecol 1971; 110:886–887.

Hatch DA, Trockman B: Laparoscopy via patent processus vaginalis to prevent unnecessary contralateral exploration in boys with unilateral inguinal hernia or hydrocele. J Urol 1994; 151:237A.

Hodgson C, McClelland RMA, Newton JR: Some effects of the peritoneal insufflation of carbon dioxide at laparoscopy. Anaesthesia 1970; 25:382.

Holcomb GW 3d: Laparoscopic evaluation for a contralateral inguinal hernia or a nonpalpable testis. Pediatr Ann 1993; 22:678–684.

Holcomb GW, Brock JW, Neblett WW, et al: Laparoscopy for the nonpalpable testis. Am Surg 1994; 60:143–147.

Holevas R, Lui P, Hadley R, et al: Laparoscopic management of metastatic penile carcinoma. J Urol 1993; 2:149.

Holzman RS: Special considerations of anesthesia for endourologic procedures and laparoscopy in children. In Smith AD, ed: Smith's Textbook of Endourology. St. Louis, Quality Medical Publishing, 1996, pp 1293–1306.

Horgan JD, Brock WA: Transinguinal laparoscopy for nonpalpable testis. J Urol 1994; 151:473–474.

Hubner WA, Schramek P, Pflger H: Laparoscopic nephropexy. J Urol 1994; 152:1184.

Hulka JF: Textbook of Laparoscopy. New York, Grune & Stratton, 1985, p 119.

Janetschek G, Hobisch A, Bartsch G: Diagnostic laparoscopic retroperitoneal lymphadenectomy for clinical stage II B nonseminomatous testicular cancer treated by primary chemotherapy. J Endourol 1995a; 9:S153.

Janetschek G, Radmayr C, Bartsch G: Laparoscopic ureteral reimplantation: First clinical experience. J Endourol 1994; 8(Suppl 1):S94.

Janetschek G, Radmayr C, Bartsch G: Laparoscopic ureteral anti-reflux plasty reimplantation—first clinical experience. Ann Urol 1995b; 29:101–105.

Janetschek G, Reissigl A, Peschel R, Bartsch G: Laparoscopic retroperitoneal lymphadenectomy for clinical stage I testicular tumor. J Endourol 1993; 7:S175.

Jarow JP, Assimos DG, Pittaway DE: Effectiveness of laparoscopic varicocelectomy. Urology 1993; 42:544.

Jarrett JC II: Laparoscopy: Direct trocar insertion without pneumoperitoneum. Obstet Gynecol 1990; 75:725–727.

Jordan GH, Robey EL, Winslow BH: Laparoendoscopic surgical management of the abdominal/transinguinal undescended testicle. J Endourol 1992; 6:157–161.

Jordan GH, Winslow BH: Laparoendoscopic upper pole partial nephrectomy. J Urol 1993a; 150:940–943.

Jordan GH, Winslow BH: Laparoscopically assisted continent catheterizable cutaneous appendicovesicostomy. J Endourol 1993b; 7:517–520.

Jordan GH, Winslow BH: Laparoscopic single stage and staged orchiopexy. J Urol 1994; 152:1249–1252.

Kavoussi LR, Clayman RV: Trocar fixation during laparoscopy. J Endourol 1992; 6:71.

Kavoussi LR, Clayman RV, Brunt LM, Soper NJ: Laparoscopic ureterolysis. J Urol 1992a; 147:425.

Kavoussi LR, Kerbl K, Capelouto CC, et al: Laparoscopic nephrectomy for renal neoplasms. Urology 1993a; 42:603–609.

Kavoussi LR, Schuessler WW, Clayman RV, Vancaillie T: Laparoscopic approach to the seminal vesicles. J Urol 1993b; 150:417.

Kavoussi LR, Sosa RE, Capelouto C: Complications of laparoscopic surgery. J Endourol 1992b; 2:95.

Kavoussi LR, Sosa E, Chandhoke G, et al: Complications of laparoscopic pelvic lymph node dissection. J Urol 1993c; 149:322–325.

Kent RB III: Subcutaneous emphysema and hypercarbia following laparoscopic cholecystectomy. Arch Surg 1991; 126:1154–1156.

Kerbl K, Clayman RV, McDougall DE, Kavoussi LR: Laparoscopic nephrectomy: Current status. Arch Esp Urol 1993a; 46:581–584.

Kerbl K, Clayman RV, McDougall EM, Kavoussi LR: Laparoscopic nephrectomy. Br Med J 1993b; 307:1488–1489.

Kerbl K, Clayman RV, McDougall EM, Kavoussi LR: Laparoscopic nephrectomy: The Washington University experience. Br J Urol 1994; 73:231–236.

Kerbl K, Clayman RV, Petros JA, et al: Staging pelvic lymphadenectomy for prostate cancer: A comparison of laparoscopic and open techniques. J Urol 1993c; 150:396.

Kerbl K, Figenshau RS, Clayman RV: Retroperitoneal laparoscopic nephrectomy: Laboratory and clinical experience. J Endourol 1993d; 7:23.

Kiesewetter WB, Parenzan L: When should hernia in the infant be treated bilaterally? JAMA 1959; 171:287.

Kirsch AJ, Hensle TW, Chang DT, et al: Renal effects of CO_2 insufflation: Oliguria and acute renal dysfunction in a rat pneumoperitoneum model. Urology 1994; 43:453–459.

Kletscher BA, Lauvetz RW, Segura JW: Nephron-sparing laparoscopic surgery: Techniques to control the renal pedicle and manage parenchymal bleeding. J Endourol 1995; 9:23.

Koff SA, Sethi PS: Treatment of high undescended testes by low spermatic vessel ligation: Alternative to Fowler-Stephens technique. J Urol 1996; 156(part 2):799–803.

Koyle M, Chandhoke P, Galensky S: Pediatric retroperitoneal laparoscopic nephrectomy. J Endourol 1994; 8(Suppl 1):S94.

Koyle MA, Woo HH, Kavoussi LR: Laparoscopic nephrectomy in the first year of life. J Pediatr Surg 1993; 28:693–695.

Kozminski M, Partamian KO: Case report of laparoscopic ileal loop conduit. J Endourol 1992; 6:147–150.

Lang GS, Ruckle HC, Hadley HR, et al: One hundred consecutive laparoscopic pelvic lymph node dissections: Comparing complications of the first 50 cases to the second 50 cases. Urology 1994; 44:221.

Lew JKL, Gin T, Oh TE: Anaesthetic problems during laparoscopic cholecystectomy. Anaesth Intens Care 1992; 20:91.

Liu CY: Laparoscopic retropubic colposuspension (Burch procedure): A review of 58 cases. J Reprod Med 1993; 38:526.

Long MG, Wingfield JG: Laparoscopic gonadectomy in testicular feminization syndrome: A technique for the removal of testes firmly situated within the inguinal canal. Gynecol Endosc 1993; 2:43.

Loughlin KR, Kavoussi LR: Laparoscopic lymphadenectomy in the staging of prostate cancer. Contemp Urol 1992; 4:69.

Mahadevan N, Shaxted EJ: Laparoscopic gonadectomy in complete androgen insensitivity: A novel approach to management. Gynecol Endosc 1992; 1:51–52.

Manson AL, Terhune D, Jordan G, et al: Preoperative laparoscopic localization of the nonpalpable testis. J Urol 1985; 134:919–920.

McDougall EM, Clayman RV, Anderson K, et al: Laparoscopic gonadectomy in a case of testicular feminization. Urology 1993a; 42:201–204.

McDougall EM, Clayman RV, Bowles WT: Laparoscopic excision of mullerian duct remnant. J Urol 1994a; 152:482.

McDougall EM, Clayman RV, Chandhoke PS, et al: Laparoscopic partial nephrectomy in the pig model. J Urol 1993b; 149:1633.

McDougall EM, Clayman RV, Elashry O: Laparoscopic nephro-ureterectomy for upper tract transitional cell cancer: The Washington University experience. J Urol 1995a; 154:975–980.

McDougall EM, Clayman RV, Fadden PT: Retroperitoneoscopy: The Washington University Medical School experience. Urology 1994b; 43:446.

McDougall EM, Clayman RV, Figenshau RS, Pearle MS: Laparoscopic retropubic auto-augmentation of the bladder. J Urol 1995b; 153:123–126.

McDougall EM, Klute CG, Cornell T: Comparison of transvaginal versus laparoscopic bladder neck suspension for stress urinary incontinence. Urology 1995c; 45:641–646.

McDougall EM, Monk TG, Wolf JS, et al: The effect of prolonged pneumoperitoneum on renal function in an animal model. J Am Coll Surg 1996; 182:317–328.

McDougall EM, Urban DA, Kerbl K, et al: Laparoscopic repair of vesicoureteral reflux utilizing the Lich-Grégoir technique in the pig model. J Urol 1995d; 153:497–500.

McDowell GC II, Johnson JW, Tenney DM, Johnson DE: Pelvic lymphadenectomy for staging clinically localized prostate cancer: Indications, complications, and results in 217 cases. Urology 1990; 35:476.

McGregor DB, Halverson K, McVay CB: The unilateral pediatric inguinal hernia: Should the contralateral side be explored? J Pediatr Surg 1980; 15:313.

Mendoza D, Newman R, Cohen M, et al: Laparoscopic complications in markedly obese urologic patients: A multi-institutional review. J Urol 1996; 48:562–567.

Minoli G, Terruzzi V, Spinzi GC: The influence of carbon dioxide and nitrous oxide on pain during laparoscopy: A double-blind, controlled trial. Gastrointest Endosc 1982; 28:173.

Mischinger HJ, Colombo T, Rauchenwald M, et al: Laparoscopic procedure for varicocelectomy. Br J Urol 1994; 74:112.

Monk TG, Weldon BC: Anesthetic considerations for laparoscopic surgery. J Endourol 1992; 6:89.

Moore RG, Demaree RD, Sanda MG, Kavoussi LR: Retroperitoneoscopy: Effects of insufflation media on surrounding tissue during balloon rupture. J Endourol 1995a; 9:67.

Moore RG, Kavoussi LR, Bloom DA, et al: Postoperative adhesion formation after urologic laparoscopy in the pediatric population. J Urol 1995b; 153:792–795.

Moore RG, Partin AW, Adams JB, Kavoussi LR: Adhesion formation following transperitoneal nephrectomy: Laparoscopic vs open approach. J Endourol 1995c; 9:277.

Moore RG, Partin AW, Kavoussi LR: The role of laparoscopy in the diagnosis and treatment of prostate cancer. Semin Surg Oncol 1996; 12:139–144.

Moore RG, Peters CA, Bauer SB, et al: Laparoscopic evaluation of the nonpalpable testis: A prospective assessment of accuracy. J Urol 1994; 151:728–731.

Munch LC, Gill IS, McRoberts JW: Laparoscopic retroperitoneal renal cystectomy. J Urol 1994; 151:135–138.

Nakagawa K, Murai M, Deguchi N, et al: Laparoscopic adrenalectomy: Results in 25 patients. J Endourol 1995; 9:265.

Nezhat C, Nezhat F, Green B, Gonzalez G: Laparoscopic ureteroureterostomy. J Endourol 1992; 6:143.

Nunn J: Respiratory aspects of anesthesia. In Applied Respiratory Pysiology. London, Butterworths, 1987, p 350.

Oesterwitz H, Fahlenkamp D: Microsurgical technique and results of testicular autotransplantation in children—essential venous anastomosis. Int Urol Nephrol 1993; 25:587.

Ogura K, Matsuda T, Terachi T, et al: Laparoscopic varicocelectomy: Invasiveness and effectiveness compared with conventional open retroperitoneal high ligation. Int J Urol 1994; 1:1.

Okamura K, Ono Y, Yamada Y, et al: Endoscopic trigonoplasty for primary vesico-ureteric reflux. Br J Urol 1995; 75:390–394.

Ono Y, Sahashi M, Yamada S, Ohshima S: Laparoscopic nephrectomy without morcellation for renal cell carcinoma: Report of initial 2 cases. J Urol 1993; 150:1222.

Ostman PL, Pantie-Fisher FH, Faure EA, Glosten B: Circulatory collapse during laparoscopy. J Clin Anesthesiol 1990; 2:129.

Paltiel HJ, Rupich RC, Babcock DS: Maturational changes in arterial impedance of the normal testis in boys: Doppler sonographic study. AJR 1994; 163:1189–1193.

Parra RO, Andrus C, Boullier J: Staging laparoscopic pelvic lymph node dissection: Comparison of results with open pelvic lymphadenectomy. J Urol 1992a; 147:875.

Parra RO, Andrus CH, Jones JP, Boullier JA: Laparoscopic cystectomy: Initial report on a new treatment for the retained bladder. J Urol 1992b; 148:1140.

Partin AW, Yoo J, Carter HB, et al: The use of prostate specific antigen. J Urol 1993; 150:110.

Peloquin F, Kiruluta G, Quiros E: Management of an impalpable testis: The role of laparoscopy. Can J Surg 1991; 34:587–590.

Perez MG, Parra RO, Boullier JA, et al: Comparison between standard flank versus laparoscopic nephrectomy for benign renal disease. J Urol 1994; 2:151.

Peters CA: Laparoscopy in pediatric urology. Urology 1993; 41:33–37.

Peters CA: Complications in pediatric urologic laparoscopy: Results of a survey. J Urol 1995a; 155:1070–1073.

Peters CA: Urinary tract obstruction in children. J Urol 1995b; 154:1874–1884.

Peters CA: Innovations in pediatric urologic laparoscopy. In Smith AD, ed: Smith's Textbook of Endourology. St. Louis, Quality Medical Publishing, 1996, pp 1507–1517.

Peters CA, Bauer SB: Laparoscopic evaluation of contralateral hernia using inguinal access (Abstract 150). AAP, Section on Urology, San Francisco, 1995.

Peters CA, Joseph RG, Holzman RS: Physiologic effects of laparoscopy in children (Abstract 145). AAP, Section on Urology, San Francisco, 1995a.

Peters CA, Kavoussi LR, Atala A, et al: Laparoscopic management of intra-abdominal testes. J Urol 1994; 151:236A.

Peters CA, Kavoussi LR, Retik AB: Laparoscopic nephrectomy and nephroureterectomy in children. J Endourol 1993; 7(Suppl 1):S174.

Peters CA, Moore RG, Retik AB: Meta-analysis of laparoscopic diagnosis of 720 non-palpable testes. J Endourol 1992; 6:S145.

Peters CA, Shlussel RN, Retik AB: Pediatric laparoscopic dismembered pyeloplasty. J Urol 1995b; 153:1962–1965.

Petros JA, Catalona WJ: Lower incidence of unsuspected lymph node metastases in 521 consecutive patients with clinically localized prostate cancer. J Urol 1992; 147:1574.

Plotzker ED, Rushton HG, Belman AB, Skoog SJ: Laparoscopy for nonpalpable testes in childhood: Is inguinal exploration also necessary when vas and vessels exit the inguinal ring? J Urol 1992; 148:635–637.

Polascik TJ, Moore RG, Rosenberg MT, Kavoussi LR: Comparison of laparoscopic and open retropubic urethropexy for treatment of stress urinary incontinence. Urology 1995; 45:647.

Poppas D, Sutaria P, Sosa RE, et al: Chromophore enhanced laser welding of canine ureters in vitro using a human protein solder: A preliminary step for laparoscopic tissue welding. J Urol 1993; 150:1052.

Poppas DP, Lemack GE, Mininberg DT: Laparoscopic orchiopexy: Clinical experience and description of technique. J Urol 1995; 155:708–711.

Poppas DP, Uzzo RG, Britanisky RG, Mininberg DT: Laparoscopic laser assisted auto-augmentation of the pediatric neurogenic bladder: Early experience with urodynamic follow-up. J Urol 1996; 155:1057–1060.

Pryor JL, Howards SS: Varicocele. Urol Clin North Am 1987; 14:499.

Puppo P, Carmignani G, Gallucci M, et al: Bilateral laparoscopic ureterolysis. Eur Urol 1994; 25:82–84.

Ransley PG, Vordermark JS, Caldamone AA: Preliminary ligation of the gonadal vessels prior to orchidopexy for the intra-abdominal testicle: A staged Fowler-Stephens procedure. World J Urol 1984; 2:226–268.

Rassweiler J, Henkel T, Tschda R, et al: Modified laparoscopic retroperitoneal lymphadenectomy for testicular cancer—the lessons learned. J Urol 1994; 2:151.

Rassweiler J, Potempa DM, Henkel TO, et al: The technical aspects of transperitoneal laparoscopic nephrectomy (TLN) adrenalectomy (TLA) and nephroureterectomy. J Endourol 1992; 6:S58.

Rassweiler JJ, Henkel TO, Stock C, et al: Transperitoneal and retroperitoneal laparoscopic nephrectomy: Indications and results. J Endourol 1993; 7:S175.

Razvi HA, Fields D, Vargas JC, et al: Oliguria during laparoscopic surgery: Evidence for direct renal parenchymal compression as an etiologic factor. J Endourol 1996; 10:1–4.

Reissigl A, Janetschek G, Pointner S, et al: Results of varicocele treatment: A comparison of embolotherapy and laparoscopic varix ligation. J Endourol 1993; S168.

Rodriguez R, Partin AW, Mostwin JL, Kavoussi LR: Long term follow-up of surgically treated stress urinary incontinence. J Urol 1995; 153.

Ross LS, Ruppman N: Varicocele vein ligation in 565 patients under local anesthesia: A long-term review of technique results and complications in light of proposed management by laparoscopy. J Urol 1993; 149:1361.

Rowe MI, Copelson LW, Clatworthy HW: The patent processus vaginalis and the inguinal hernia. J Pediatr Surg 1969; 4:102.

Rubenstein SC, Hulbert JC, Pharand D, et al: Laparoscopic ablation of symptomatic renal cysts. J Urol 1993; 150:1103.

Rukstalis DB, Gerber GS, Vogelzang NJ, et al: Laparoscopic pelvic lymph node dissection: A review of 103 consecutive cases. J Urol 1994; 151:670.

Sadeghi-Nejad H, Kavoussi LR, Peters CA: Bowel injury in open technique laparoscopic cannula placement. Urology 1994; 43:559–560.

Sanchez-de-Badajoz E, Miauelez E, Lago C, et al: Laparoscopic testicular autotransplantation. Arch Esp Urol 1992; 45:1011–1014.

Sanchez-de-Badajoz E, Gallego JL, Reche A, et al: Laparoscopic cystectomy. J Endourol 1993; 7:S227.

Schimberg W, Wacksman J, Rudd R, et al: Laparoscopic correction of vesicoureteral reflux in the pig. J Urol 1994; 151:1664–1667.

Schuessler WW, Kavoussi LR, Clayman RV, Vancaillie TH: Laparoscopic radical prostatectomy: Initial case report. J Urol 1992; 147.

Schuessler WW, Pharand D, Vancaillie TG: Laparoscopic standard pelvic node dissection for carcinoma of the prostate: Is it accurate? J Urol 1993; 150:898.

Schuessler WW, Tecuanhuey L, Vancaillie TG, et al: Laparoscopic prostatic surgery: An evolving surgical technique. J Urol 1994; 151:343A.

Schuessler WW, Vancaillie TG, Reich H, Griffith DP: Transperitoneal endosurgical lymphadenectomy in patients with localized prostate cancer. J Urol 1991; 145:988.

Schulam PG, Kavoussi LR, Cheriff AD, et al: Laparoscopic live donor nephrectomy: The initial 3 cases. J Urol 1996; 155:1857–1859.

Schwimmer WB: Electrosurgical burn injuries during laparoscopy sterilization. Treatment and prevention. Obstet Gynecol 1974; 44:526.

See WA, Cooper CS, Fisher RJ: Predictors of laparoscopic complications after formal training in laparoscopic surgery. JAMA 1993; 270:2689–2692.

Shulman B, Aronson HB: Capnography in the early diagnosis of carbon dioxide embolism during laparoscopy. Can Anaesth Soc J 1984; 31:455.

Silber SJ, Kelly J: Successful autotransplantation of an intra-abdominal testis to the scrotum by microvascular technique. J Urol 1976; 115:452.

Sogge MR, Goldner FH, Butler ML: Pain response comparison between carbon dioxide and nitrous oxide in peritoneoscopy. Gastrointest Endosc 1980; 26:78.

Sparkman RS: Bilateral exploration in inguinal hernia in juvenile patients. Surgery 1962; 51:393.

Stanley KE, Winfield HN, Donovan JF: Laparoscopic marsupialization of renal cysts. J Urol 1993; 149:452A.

Steptoe P: Laparoscopy explosion hazards with nitrous oxide. Br Med J 1976; 1:833.

Suzuki K, Ihara H, Ishikawa A, et al: Laparoscopic adrenalectomy—clinical analysis of 25 cases. J Urol 1994; 2:151.

Takeda M, Go H, Imai T, Komeyama T: Experience with 17 cases of laparoscopic adrenalectomy: Use of ultrasonic aspirator and argon beam coagulator. J Urol 1994; 152:902.

Tanaka J, Kato Y, Umezawa A, Koyama K: Laparoscopic management of percutaneous transhepatic biliary drainage catheter dislodgement accompanied by bile peritonitis. J Am Coll Surg 1994; 197:480.

Tennenbaum SY, Lerner SE, McAleer IM, et al: Preoperative laparoscopic localization of the nonpalpable testis: A critical analysis of a 10-year experience. J Urol 1994; 151:732–734.

Theil R, Adams JB, Schulam PG, et al: Venous dissection injuries during laparoscopic urologic surgery. J Urol 1996; 155:1874–1876.

Thomas AG, McLymont F, Moshipur J: Incarcerated hernia after laparoscopic sterilization: A case report. J Reprod Med 1990; 35:639.

Trockman BA, Leach GE, Hamilton J, et al: Modified Pereyra bladder neck suspension: 10-year mean follow-up using outcomes analysis in 125 patients. J Urol 1995; 154:1841.

Troxel S, Winfield HN: Comparative financial analysis of laparoscopic versus open pelvic lymph node dissection for men with cancer of the prostate. J Urol 1994; 151:675.

Troxel SA, Winfield HN: Comparative financial analysis of laparoscopic pelvic lymph node dissection performed in 1990-'92 versus 1993-'94. J Urol 1995; 153:357A.

Upton J, Schuster SR, Colodny AH, Murray JE: Testicular autotransplantation in children. Am J Surg 1983; 145:514–519.

Urban DA, Clayman RV, Kerbl K, et al: Laparoscopic nephropexy for symptomatic nephroptosis: Initial case report. J Endourol 1993; 7:27.

Villers A, Vannier JL, Abecassis R, et al: Extraperitoneal endosurgical lymphadenectomy with insufflation in the staging of bladder and prostate cancer. J Endourol 1993; 7:229.

Wacksman J, Billmore DA, Sheldon CA, Lewis AG: Laparoscopically assisted testicular autotransplantation for management of intra-abdominal undescended testis. J Urol 1996; 156(part 2):772–774.

Waldschmidt J, Schier F: Laparoscopic surgery in neonates and infants. Eur J Pediatr Surg 1991a; 1:145–150.

Waldschmidt J, Schier F: Surgical correction of abdominal testes after Fowler-Stephens using the neodymium: YAG laser for preliminary vessel dissection. Eur J Pediatr Surg 1991b; 1:54–57.

Weiss RM, Seashore JH: Laparoscopy in the management of the nonpalpable testis. J Urol 1987; 138:382–384.

Wickham JEA, Miller RA: Percutaneous renal access. In Percutaneous Renal Surgery. New York, Churchill Livingstone, 1983, p 33.

Wilson EE, Vuitch F, Carr BR: Laparoscopic removal of dysgenetic gonads containing gonadoblastoma in a patient with Swyer syndrome. Obstet Gynecol 1992; 79:842–844.

Winfield HN, Donovan JF, Loening SA, et al: Laparoscopic partial nephrectomy—lessons learned. J Urol 1994a; 151:496A.

Winfield HN, Donovan JF, See WA, et al: Laparoscopic pelvic lymph node dissection for genitourinary malignancies: Indications, techniques, and results. J Endourol 1992; 6:103.

Winfield HN, Rashid TM, Lund GI, et al: Comparative financial analysis of laparoscopic versus open nephrectomy. J Urol 1994b; 151.

Wolf JS, Clayman RV, Monk TG, et al: Carbon dioxide absorption during laparoscopic pelvic operation. J Am Coll Surg 1995; 180:555–560.

Wright JE: Impalpable testes: A review of 100 boys. J Pediatr Surg 1986; 21:151–153.

Yacoub OF, Cardona I, Coverler LA, Dodson MG: Carbon dioxide embolism during laparoscopy. Anesthesiology 1982; 57:533.

Yamaguchi Y, Kaswick J, Bellman GC: Laparoscopic evaluation of indeterminate renal cysts. J Urol 1995; 153:481A.

Yamanaka J, Baker M, Metcalfe S, Hutson JM: Serum levels of Mullerian inhibiting substance in boys with cryptorchidism. J Pediatr Surg 1991; 26:621–623.

Yu TJ, Shu K, Kung FT, et al: Use of laparoscopy in intersex patients. J Urol 1995; 154:1193–1196.

Zaontz MR, Maizels M, Sugar EC, Firlit CF: Detrusorrhaphy: Extravesical ureteral advancement to correct vesicoureteral reflux in children. J Urol 1987; 138:947.

Zerella JT, McGill LC: Survival of nonpalpable undescended testicles after orchiopexy. J Pediatr Surg 1993; 28:251–253.

XIV
UROLOGIC
SURGERY

96
THE ADRENALS

E. Darracott Vaughan, Jr., M.D.
Jon D. Blumenfeld, M.D.

HISTORICAL BACKGROUND

The understanding of the essential physiologic role of the adrenal glands has evolved from the initial description in *Opuscula Anatomica* in 1563 (Eustachius, 1563) to the elegant biochemical analysis of adrenal secretory products and precise radiologic imaging studies currently available (Vaughan and Carey, 1989a; Janus and Mendelson, 1991).

Despite earlier recognition of the presence of the adrenals and the division into cortex and medulla (Cuvier, 1800–1805), it was not until the precise observations of Addison in 1855 that the essential role of these glands was recognized in patients who died with adrenal destruction secondary to tuberculosis. Soon thereafter, Brown-Sequard (1856) performed bilateral adrenalectomies in animals and predicted that the adrenals were essential for life.

Hyperfunction of the adrenal cortex was not documented until 1912, with the definitive report on 11 patients describ-

ing the now-classic characteristics of Cushing's syndrome being reported in 1932 in patients with basophilic adenomas of the pituitary (Cushing, 1912, 1932). It was not until the purification of adrenocortical extracts, however, that adrenalectomized animals could be maintained; the adrenal cortex was then documented as the site of critical and essential steroid production (Hartman et al, 1927). Progressive and sequential advances in the understanding of adrenal steroid production have led to the development of precise diagnostic tests to identify patients with Cushing's syndrome (Orth, 1995), adrenocortical forms of hypertension (Biglieri et al, 1990), congenital adrenal hyperplasia (New and Speiser, 1989), adrenal carcinoma (Vaughan and Carey, 1989b), and other adrenal disorders.

Fränkel first described a medullary adrenal tumor in 1886. London physiologists demonstrated a pressor substance from the adrenal medulla, which they named *adrenalin* (Oliver and Sharpey-Schafer, 1895). Subsequently, Abel coined the term *epinephrine* (Abel, 1897), and Kohn described the *chromaffin system* (Kohn, 1902). In 1912, the pathologist Pick formulated the descriptive term *pheochromocytoma* from the Greek *phaios* (dark or dusty) and *chroma* (color) to describe adrenal medullary tumors with their chromaffin reaction (Pick, 1912).

The development of precise urinary and plasma tests led to the accurate identification of patients with adrenal medullary disorders (Stein and Black, 1990). Moreover, it is particularly in the identification and localization of pheochromocytomas that imaging techniques have become highly accurate and essential (Markisz and Kazam, 1989; Rosano et al, 1991; Vaughan, 1991).

The diagnosis of the major adrenal disorders is now actually simpler than in the past because of precise diagnostic assays and radiologic tests. The evaluation of a patient for a potential adrenal disorder can be performed efficiently, usually without hospitalization by a practicing urologist knowledgeable in adrenal disease. Moreover, the surgical approaches are well within the expertise of the urologist and are now precisely described (Libertino and Novick, 1989; Vaughan and Carey, 1989a; Scott, 1990b; Vaughan, 1991).

This chapter reviews the relevant adrenal anatomy, pathology, and physiology that serve as the bases for the clinical, biologic, and radiologic diagnoses of the major adrenal disorders. In addition, current medical and surgical strategies are reviewed. The adrenal disorders of neuroblastoma and congenital adrenal hyperplasia are reviewed in detail elsewhere and are mentioned only briefly in this chapter.

ANATOMY, HISTOLOGY, AND EMBRYOLOGY

The adrenal glands are paired retroperitoneal organs that lie within perinephric fat at the anterosuperior and medial aspects of the kidneys. They measure up to 5 cm in length by 3 cm in width and are 1 cm thick. In the healthy nonstressed adult, the glands weigh about 5 g each. **In contrast, the adrenal weight at birth is quite large (5–10 g) because of the fetal adrenal cortex, which may play a major role in fetal embryogenesis and homeostasis** (Fig. 96–1) (Pepe and Albrecht, 1990). The fetal adrenal regresses rapidly during the first 6 weeks of life (Scott et al, 1990) but is susceptible to **adrenal hemorrhage at the time of birth, a condition now readily diagnosed by magnetic resonance imaging (MRI)** (Fig. 96–2). The presence of a neuroblastoma has been diagnosed by intrauterine ultrasonography, differentiated from the fetal adrenal or adrenal hemorrhage, and confirmed at birth, resulting in a successful early removal (Kogan, personal communication).

Sectional imaging has provided a better understanding of the precise appearance of the adrenals. Both glands are flattened anteriorly with a thick central ridge and thinner medial and lateral rami (Kazam et al, 1989). Cortical infoldings, especially seen on sagittal sections, may be confused for small adenomas, especially in primary aldosteronism in which the lesions are small.

The right adrenal lies above the kidney posterolateral to the inferior vena cava. The anterior surface is in immediate

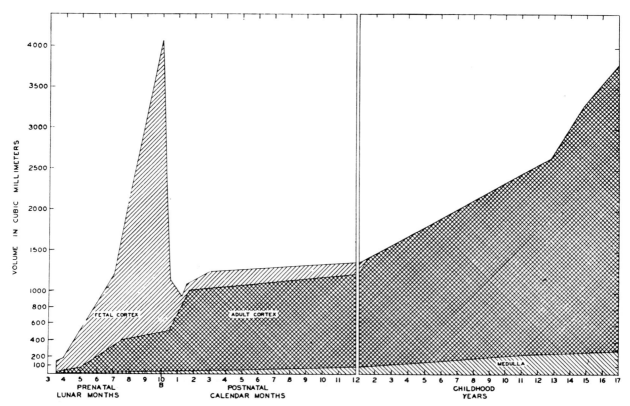

Figure 96–1. Growth of the adrenal cortex including the fetal cortex in utero and after birth. A striking decrease occurs in the size of the fetal cortex after birth, and a gradual increase occurs in the adult cortex with aging. (From Bethune JE: The Adrenal Cortex. A Scope Monograph. Kalamazoo, MI, The Upjohn Co.)

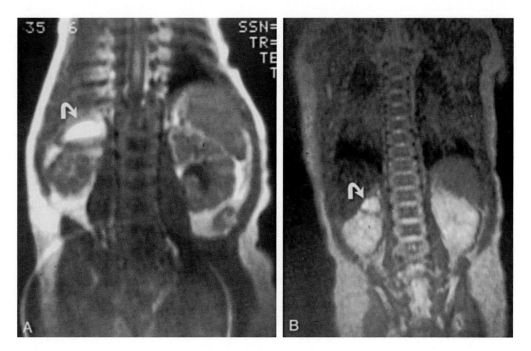

Figure 96–2. Adrenal hemorrhage *(A)* bright on magnetic resonance imaging *(arrow)* showing later resolution *(B).*

contact with the inferior-posterior surface of the liver. Thus, from an anterior approach, the anterior surface of the adrenal can be exposed by remaining extraperitoneal and by gently lifting the liver cephalad, the inferior vena cava being medial. The posterior surface of both adrenals is in contact with the posterior diaphragm (Fig. 96–3). Both adrenals lie more posteriorly as they follow the lumbar curve of the spine, thus falling away from the surgeon for the superior dissection.

The left adrenal is in more intimate contact with the kidney, and the main left renal artery often lies deep to the left adrenal vein as it enters the left renal vein. The gland overlies the upper pole of the kidney with its anterior surface and medial aspect behind the pancreas and splenic artery (see Fig. 96–3). The anterior surface of the left adrenal can be exposed by remaining retroperitoneal and by gently retracting the spleen cephalad within the peritoneum. Division of the splenorenal ligament facilitates this dissection.

The adrenals have a delicate and rich blood supply estimated to be 6 to 7 ml/g per minute, without a dominant single artery. The inferior phrenic artery is the main blood supply with additional branches from the aorta and the renal artery (Fig. 96–4) (Pick and Anson, 1940; Anson et al, 1947). In addition, there can be an adrenal arterial supply arising from the gonadal arteries in 60% of fetal adrenal vascular dissections (Bianchi and Ferrari, 1991). The small arteries penetrate the gland in a circumferential stellate fashion, leaving both anterior and posterior surfaces avascular. The venous drainage is usually a common vein on the right exiting the apex of the gland and **entering the posterior surface of the inferior vena cava; this vein is short, fragile, and the most common source of troublesome bleeding during right adrenalectomy (Fig. 96–5).** The left vein empties directly into the left renal vein about 3 cm from the inferior vena cava and often opposite to the gonadal

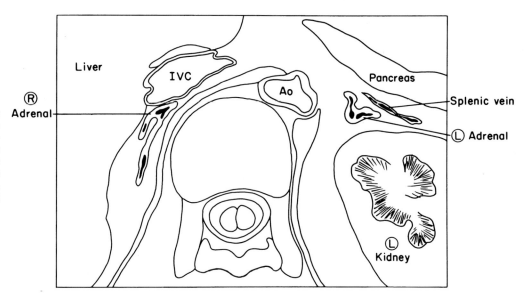

Figure 96–3. Line schematic of an anatomic specimen showing position of the adrenal glands in relation to the diaphragm, inferior vena cava, and kidneys. (From Vaughan ED Jr, Carey RM, eds: Adrenal Disorders. New York, Thieme Medical Publishers, 1989.)

vein (Johnstone, 1957). **Not well recognized is the left inferior phrenic vein, which typically communicates with the adrenal vein but then courses medially and can be injured during dissection of the medial edge of the gland.**

The adrenal cortex develops from mesoderm and the medulla from neuroectoderm. During the fifth week of development, mesothelial cells located between the root of the mesentery and the developing gonad proliferate and invade the mesenchyme. These cells form the fetal cortex, whereas a second migration of cells forms the definitive cortex; an additional cell type comes from mesonephric origin (Crowder, 1957). The intimate relationship with developing gonad, kidney, and adrenal generally explains the finding of ectopic or aberrant adrenal tissue. Heterotopic adrenal tissue is usually associated with the kidney but is also reported to be associated with the broad ligament, gonadal vessels, spermatic cord, canal of Zuck, uterus, testis, and sites of peritoneal attachment (Culp, 1959; Schechter, 1968).

Microscopically the mature adrenal cortex constitutes 90% of the gland and is divided into three zones: zona glomerulosa, zona fasciculata, and zona reticularis (Fig. 96–6). Zonation is complete by 18 months, although adult configuration is not reached until 10 to 12 years (Moore et al, 1989). The zona glomerulosa is less prominent in humans than in other species and is the site of aldosterone production. The zonae fasciculata and reticularis form a single functional zone that produces glucocorticoids, androgens, and estrogens.

The adrenal medulla is derived from cells of the neural crest that migrate at the seventh week to form collections, which enter the fetal cortex leaving nodules of neuroblasts scattered throughout the cortex. Neuroblastic cortical nodules regress as the medulla forms, but they can persist and should not be confused with an in situ neuroblastoma. By

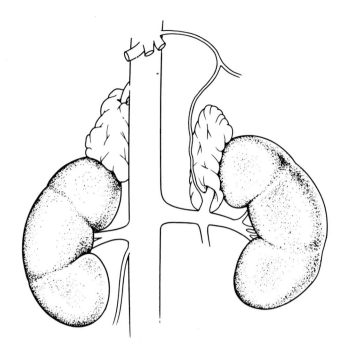

Figure 96–5. Venous drainage of the left and right adrenal glands with particular attention to the intercommunicating vein on the left, which is medial and drains into the phrenic system. (From Vaughan ED Jr, Carey RM: Adrenal Disorders. New York, Thieme Medical Publishers, 1989.)

the 20th week, there is a primitive medulla, but the distinct medulla is not present until atrophy of the fetal cortex.

The medulla is soft currant jelly–like and can be bluntly dissected free from cortex for adrenal medullary transplantation (Madrazo et al, 1987). The medulla produces both norepinephrine and epinephrine, with the reaction facilitated in the presence of glucocorticoids. Moreover, there is morphologic evidence for a close interaction of chromaffin cells with cortical cells of the adrenal gland, suggesting a possible paracrine role for neuroregulation of the adrenal cortex (Bornstein et al, 1991). The chromaffin cells are polyhedral, arranged in cords, and richly ennervated. Epinephrine-secreting and norepinephrine-secreting cells are distinct (Tannebaum, 1970).

ADRENAL PHYSIOLOGY

The adrenal can be thought of functionally as two distinct organs: cortex and medulla. Each has its own unique physiology and hormonally active secretory products.

Adrenal Cortex

From a common precursor, the zones of the adrenal cortex produce a series of steroid hormones that have an array of actions, including salt retention, metabolic homeostasis, and adrenarche development. The basic steroid structure of pregnenolone as derived from cholesterol is shown in Figure 96–7. The zona glomerulosa is the only source of the major mineralocorticoid aldosterone, which regulates sodium resorption in the kidney, gut, and salivary and sweat glands

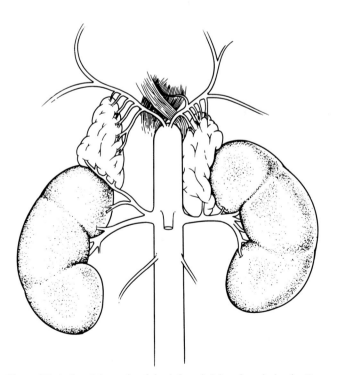

Figure 96–4. Arterial supply of the left and right adrenal glands. (From Vaughan ED Jr, Carey RM: Adrenal Disorders. New York, Thieme Medical Publishers, 1989.)

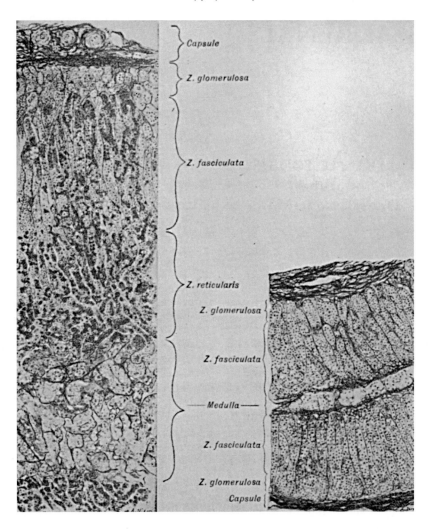

Figure 96–6. Section of an adrenal *(left)* of a man and *(right)* of a 6-month-old infant (Mallory azan stain, about × 105). (From Fawcett DW: Bloom and Fawcett A Textbook of Histology, 11th ed. Philadelphia, W.B. Saunders, 1986. By permission from Don W. Fawcett, MD.)

(Carey and Sen, 1986). The other zones produce and secrete cortisol, the major glucocorticoid in humans and the **principal androgens dehydroepiandrosterone (DHEA), dehydroepiandrosterone sulfate (DHEAS), and androstenedione.** The pathways for production of these steroids are

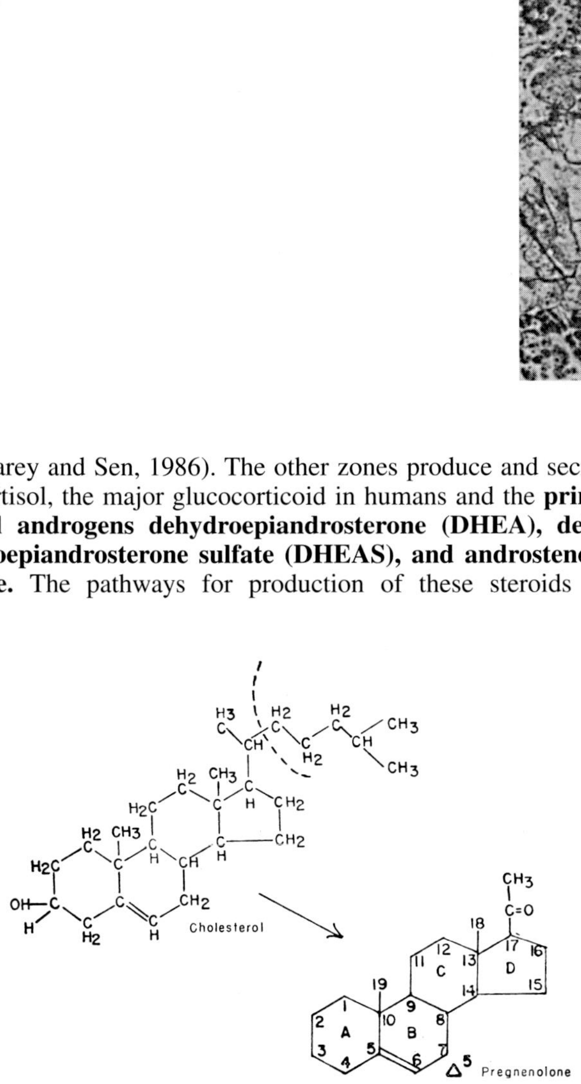

shown in Figures 96–8 and 96–9. The rate-limiting step for the formation of all these hormones is the production of pregnenolone (see Fig. 96–7) (Nelson, 1980).

As is discussed in detail elsewhere in this text, it is the deficiency of one of the five enzymes necessary to convert cholesterol to cortisol that leads to the family of diseases termed *congenital adrenal hyperplasia* (New and Speiser, 1989; Speiser et al, 1991). The presenting symptom complexes depend on the specific enzyme deficiency, the lack of necessary pituitary feedback, and the resultant adrenal hyperplasia and proximal precursor excess.

The excess of one or numerous steroid products gives the characteristic signs and symptoms of Cushing's syndrome, primary hyperaldosteronism (Conn's syndrome), or adrenal carcinoma.

Now that these pathways have been established clearly, it is possible to perturb the system purposely for diagnostic purposes. Thus, the system can be stimulated with adrenocorticotropic hormone (ACTH), also known as corticotropin, to search for adrenal insufficiency; suppressed with dexamethasone, a synthetic glucocorticoid, to identify different types of Cushing's syndrome; or interrupted with a drug such as metyrapone, which inhibits the enzyme 11β-hydroxylase, thus decreasing circulating cortisol and thereby stimulating the hypothalamic-pituitary axis to increase ACTH (Dolan and Carey, 1989).

Figure 96–7. Conversion of cholesterol to pregnenolone. The cholesterol formula shows the complete steroid structure; the pregnenolone formula shows the conventional representation of the steroid molecule with the rings designated by letter and the carbon atoms numbered.

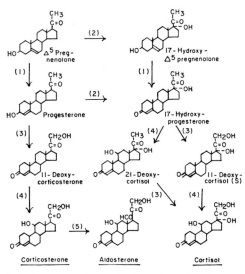

Figure 96–8. Corticosteroid synthesis in the adrenal cortex. Enzyme systems are numbered: (1) β-hydroxysteroid dehydrogenase: Δ5-oxosteroid isomerase complex, (2) C-17-hydroxylase, (3) C-21-hydroxylase, (4) C-11-hydroxylase, (5) C-18-hydroxylase. The Δ signifies a double bond, and the attached number shows its position in the nucleus.

Regulation of Hormone Release

The regulation of corticosteroid release involves a complex interaction of the hypothalamus, pituitary gland, and adrenal gland. ACTH is a 39–amino acid polypeptide that exerts a major influence on the adrenal cortex (Hoffman, 1974). ACTH is produced from a large protein (290 amino acids) termed *proopiomelanocortin* (POMC). Other POMC-derived peptides include beta-lipotropin (β-LPH), alpha-melanocyte stimulating hormone (α-MSH), beta-melanocyte stimulating hormone (β-MSH), beta-endorphin, and methionine enkephalin (Fig. 96–10) (Mains and Eipper, 1980; Tep-

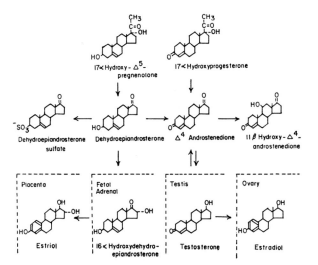

Figure 96–9. Sex hormone synthesis. The upper two panels of the scheme show the synthesis of adrenal androgens. The lower panel shows conversion of androstenedione to testosterone (testis, adrenal cortex, and, to a small degree, the liver); 16 α-hydroxylation of dehydroepiandrosterone by the fetal adrenal and conversion to estrogen in the placenta; and conversion of androgen to estrogen in the ovary. Note that the initial steps in sex hormone synthesis are the same in all these organs.

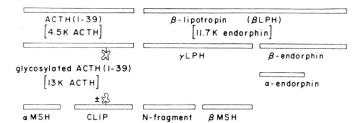

Figure 96–10. Structural relationships of peptides with a parental compound of proopiomelanocortin. (Adapted from Eipper BA, Mains RE: Endocr Rev 1980; 1:2. Copyright The Endocrine Society.)

perman and Tepperman, 1987). ACTH secretion is characterized by an inherent diurnal rhythm leading to parallel changes in cortisol and ACTH (Fig. 96–11) (Orth et al, 1967; Kreiger, 1975). The absence of the normal diurnal variation of plasma cortisol is a critical finding in a patient with Cushing's syndrome. **Corticotropin-releasing hormone (CRH) is synthesized in the hypothalamus and carried to the anterior pituitary in the portal blood** (Taylor & Fishman, 1988). **CRH is a 41–amino acid linear peptide** (Speiss et al, 1981; Vale et al, 1981), **which stimulates ACTH release** as well as other POMC products, proba-

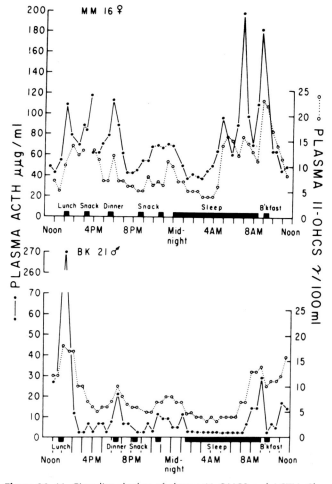

Figure 96–11. Circadian rhythm of plasma 11-OHCS and ACTH. Characterization of the normal temporal pattern of plasma corticosteroid levels. (Adapted from Kreiger DT, et al: J Clin Endocrinol Metab 1971; 32:269. Copyright The Endocrine Society.)

bly working through a cAMP-dependent process requiring calcium (Vale et al, 1981). Other stimulators of ACTH include vasopressin, oxytocin, epinephrine, angiotensin II (AII), vasoactive intestinal peptide (VIP), serotonin, gastrin-releasing peptide, atrial natriuretic factor (ANF), and gamma-aminobutyric acid (GABA) (Antoni, 1986). **Finally, ACTH secretion is reciprocally related to the circulating cortisol level.**

Adrenal androgen production in the zonae reticularis and fasciculata is also under the influence of ACTH, but other mechanisms are involved. DHEA level rises after administration of ACTH; a later elevation of DHEAS level occurs, presumably because of the slow peripheral conversion (Vaitukaitis et al, 1969). There clearly are situations, however, whereby adrenal androgen stimulation is disassociated from ACTH. These include adrenarche, puberty, aging, fasting, and stress (Parker and Odell, 1980).

In contrast to glucocorticoids and adrenal androgens, the **primary physiologic control of aldosterone secretion is AII** (Laragh et al, 1960; Laragh and Sealey, 1992). **ACTH control is secondary.** The physiology of the renin-angiotensin-aldosterone system (RAAS) is thoroughly reviewed in Chapters 7 and 11. A clear knowledge of the system is mandatory to understand the pathophysiology and to evaluate patients with primary hyperaldosteronism.

The critical sensor of the RAAS resides in the

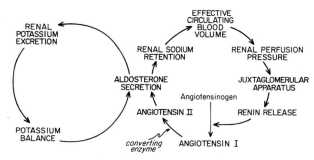

Figure 96–13. Control of aldosterone secretion by means of interrelationships between the potassium and renin-angiotensin feedback loops.

juxtaglomerular apparatus within the kidney. Thus, in response to a variety of stimuli but primarily decreased renal perfusion (Fig. 96–12), there is renin release, angiotensin II formation, and subsequent aldosterone secretion resulting in sodium retention in an attempt to restore renal perfusion (Fig. 96–13). Conversely, if there is sodium retention, renin secretion is suppressed, aldosterone secretion falls, and urinary sodium rises. The inverse relationship found between plasma renin activity (PRA) or aldosterone and urinary sodium excretion in normal volunteers is shown in Figure 96–14.

A second, less potent stimulus for aldosterone release is potassium; thus there is a second cybernetic system for the control of serum potassium involving the RAAS (Laragh and Sealey, 1992). Hypokalemia blunts the adrenal's ability to synthesize aldosterone and can result in the lowering of the plasma aldosterone to a normal range in a patient with hypokalemia and hyperaldosteronism (Herf et al, 1979).

Hormonal Actions

All steroid hormones diffuse passively into cells and then bind to the amino terminal end of a high-affinity protein receptor in the cystosol to form a steroid-receptor complex. The complex slowly converts to an active form and then migrates to the nucleus (Rousseau et al, 1972). In the nucleus, a second activation results in a stimulation of transcription, which is regulated by interaction with a specific group of steroid-regulated genes, resulting in new RNA and specific protein synthesis (Johnson and Baxter, 1987).

In addition, glucocorticoids have a non-nuclear pathway that is important in the control of ACTH. The numerous activities of this pathway include inhibition of prostaglandin synthesis, inhibition of calcium flux, inhibition of cAMP protein kinase, and others (Hubbard et al, 1990).

Glucocorticoids are essential for life, even following mineralocorticoid replacement. Glucocorticoids exert their effects on a wide spectrum of cellular metabolism, including accumulation of glycogen in the liver and muscle, enhanced gluconeogenesis, impaired peripheral glucose utilization, muscle wasting and myopathy, osteopenia, immune-mediated inflammation, and numerous interactions with other hormones (Table 96–1) (Howards and Carey, 1991; Chrousos, 1995).

Aldosterone accounts for 95% of adrenal mineralocorticoid activity and serves to maintain sodium and potassium balance as previously stated. The active sites include the kidney, gut, salivary glands, and sweat glands. In all sites,

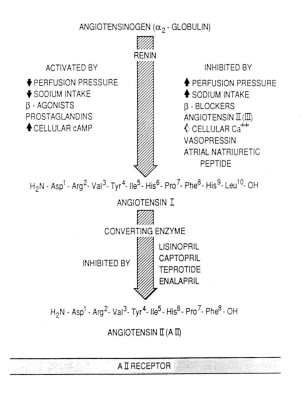

Figure 96–12. Factors activating and inhibiting the renin-angiotensin-aldosterone system.

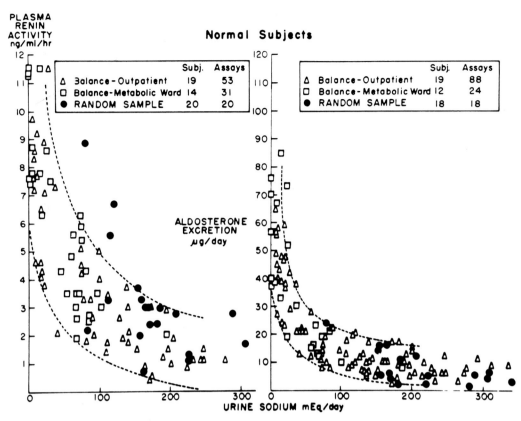

Figure 96–14. Relation of renin activity in plasma samples obtained at noon, and the corresponding 24-hour urinary excretion of aldosterone, to the concurrent daily rate of sodium excretion. For these normal subjects, the data describe a dynamic hyperbolic relationship between each hormone and sodium excretion.

The dynamic fluctuations in renin in response to changes in sodium intake help to maintain constant blood pressure in the presence of wide changes in sodium balance. The renin and aldosterone responses work together in the kidney to conserve or eliminate sodium in response to changes in dietary sodium intake.

Subjects who were studied while on random diets outside the hospital or on carefully controlled diets in the hospital exhibited similar relationships—a finding that validates the use of this nomogram in the study of outpatients or subjects who were not on controlled diets. (From Laragh JH, et al: *In* Hypertension Manual. Stoneham, Butterworth, Yorke Medical Publishers, 1974, p 313.)

there is the effect of stimulating sodium reabsorption and the increased secretion of potassium and hydrogen via activation of Na-K-ATPase activity, or activation of permease in the luminal membrane (Biglieri et al, 1990).

Adrenal androgens are only weakly active in contrast to testosterone and appear to be relevant only in pathologic states, such as congenital adrenal hyperplasia, in which there may be excess production.

Table 96–1. EFFECTS AND IMPLICATIONS OF GLUCOCORTICOIDS

Effects	Clinical Implications
Enhance skeletal and cardiac muscle contraction	Absence results in weakness
Cause protein catabolism	Excess results in wastage and weakness
Inhibit bone formation	Excess decreases bone mass
Inhibit collagen synthesis	Excess causes thin skin and fragile capillaries
Increase vascular contractility and decrease permeability	Absence makes it difficult to maintain blood pressure
Have anti-inflammatory activity	Exogenous steroid useful in treating inflammatory diseases
Have anti-immune system activity	Exogenous steroids useful in treating transplantation and various immune diseases
Maintain normal glomerular filtration	Absence reduces glomerular filtration

From Howards SS, Carey RM: The adrenals. *In* Gillenwater JY, Grayhack JT, Howards SS, Duckett JW, eds; Adult and Pediatric Urology, 2nd ed. Chicago, Year Book Medical Publishers, 1991.

Metabolism

The release of these steroids and their metabolism and route of excretion play a critical role in understanding of the tests used to diagnose adrenal disorders. In the circulation, 80% of cortisol is bound to corticosterone-binding globulin (CBG, transcortin); 10% to 15% is bound to albumin; and 7% to 10% is free.

Thus, variations in binding proteins influence the total plasma cortisol value but not the free cortisol, which is metabolically active (Baxter and Tyrrell, 1981). Accurate plasma cortisol assays are now available, using the fluorometric assay (Nielson and Asfeldt, 1967) or the radioimmunoassay (Kreiger, 1979). Thus, the diurnal variation of plasma cortisol (see Fig. 96–11) and its response to dexamethasone suppression have evolved as critical tests in the evaluation of patients for possible Cushing's syndrome (Orth, 1995). Urinary-free cortisol is also used as a screening test, although about 3.3% of lean, obese, or chronically ill individuals have elevated values, and values are not well established in children (Crapo, 1979). Difficulties have also been found in establishing upper limits of 17-hydroxysteroid secretion. They are most valuable in evaluating normal adrenal function, particularly in looking for adrenal insufficiency or congenital adrenal hyperplasia, in which 17-hydroxysteroid levels are low and 11-hydroxylase levels are high.

The precise control of adrenal androgens is not totally understood, although there is some ACTH control. Peripheral conversion of DHEA to DHEAS contributes to the DHEAS level (Nelson, 1980). DHEA does show some diurnal variation. DHEA is not produced in significant quantities by other tissues except occasionally in polycystic ovarian disease and gonadal androgen-producing tumors (Osborn and Yannone, 1971; Nelson, 1980). Patients with high DHEA levels also have high 17-ketosteroids, whereas those with virilization caused by elevated testosterone do not. Elevated levels of DHEA, androstenedione, or 17-ketosteroids out of proportion to glucocorticoid production call to mind the diagnosis of adrenal carcinoma (Cohn et al, 1986). Of these tests of adrenal androgen function, the plasma DHEAS value is more commonly used today and is more accurate than the androstenedione value. **Elevated serum concentrations of testosterone and DHEA are the hallmark of the presence of adrenal tumors in women who present with hirsutism** and are used as screening tests to identify the 5% of women with hirsutism who have a significant adrenal pathology (Derksen et al, 1994).

Aldosterone, the major sodium-retaining hormone secreted by the zona glomerulosa, is poorly bound to albumin and plasma protein (Laragh and Sealey, 1992) and has a short half-life of 20 to 30 minutes. Plasma aldosterone can be measured by radioimmunoassay. The plasma value has to be related to the sodium status of the patient and should be measured in conjunction with the PRA. Equally accurate is urinary aldosterone excretion analyzed in a similar fashion (see Fig. 96–14).

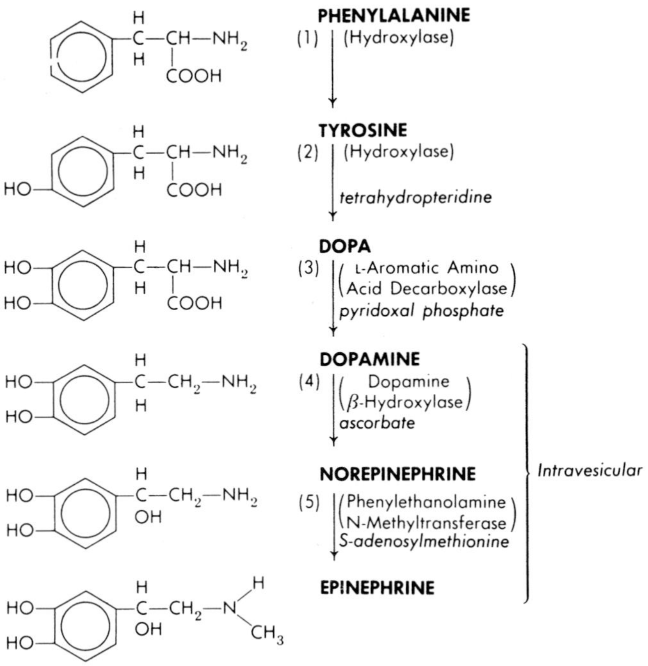

Adrenal Medulla

The adrenal medulla is composed of large chromaffin cells, which primarily secrete epinephrine but also secrete norepinephrine and dopamine. The fact that the cells stain brown when exposed to chromium salts as the result of oxidation of epinephrine and norepinephrine is the derivation of the term *chromaffin cell* (Fig. 96–15). The enzyme phenylethanolamine-*N*-methyltransferase (PNMT), which catalyzes the methylation of norepinephrine to form epinephrine, is almost solely localized to the adrenal medulla (Axelrod, 1962). Thus, if there is excessive production of both norepinephrine and epinephrine, the offending lesion is almost always within the adrenal and not other sites of chromaffin tissue. Data suggest that high levels of glucocorticoids are necessary to maintain high levels of PNMT and thus epinephrine secretion (Wurtman and Axelrod, 1965). These

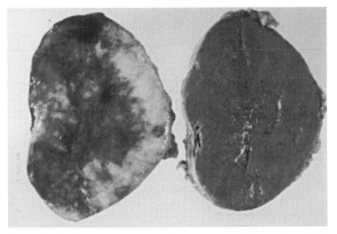

Figure 96–15. Pheochromocytoma showing chromaffin reaction *(right).*

Figure 96–16. Enzymatic pathway for dopamine, norepinephrine, and epinephrine synthesis. Enzymes are in parentheses; cofactors are in italics. (Adapted from Goodman AG, Goodman LS, Gillman A, eds: The Pharmacologic Basis of Therapeutics, 6th ed. New York, Macmillan, 1980, p 72.)

observations explain the unique location of the adrenal medulla and the central venous drainage system within the adrenal bathing the medullary cells with high levels of glucocorticoids.

Catecholamine synthesis begins with dietary tyrosine and phenylalanine, which are the substrates (Fig. 96–16). Catecholamine synthesis occurs in the adrenal, the central nervous system, and the adrenergic nerve terminals. Activation and suppression of tyrosine hydroxylase activity are the major regulators of catecholamine biosynthesis (Levitt et al, 1965) and may be influenced by the adrenal cortex (Mueller et al, 1970). Norepinephrine is the major catecholamine secreted by sympathetic neurons. Studies of healthy humans indicate that plasma dopamine accounts for 13% of the free catechols; epinephrine, 14%; and norepinephrine, 73% (Manger and Gifford, 1990).

Catecholamines are stored in separate vesicles along with ATP, chromogranins, and the enzyme dopamine β-hydroxylase. Stimulation of the preganglionic sympathetic nerves during stress, pain, cold, heat, asphyxia, hypotension, hypoglycemia, and sodium depletion increases catecholamine release (Lewis, 1975). Following stimulation, the contents of the vesicles are released by exocytosis (Winkler and Smith, 1975). In addition, catechols may be released without sympathetic stimulation and possibly without exocytosis—a phenomenon postulated in patients with pheochromocytomas.

Catecholamine Metabolism

Catecholamines are rapidly removed from the circulation with a plasma half-life less than 20 seconds (Ferrerira and Vane, 1967). The metabolic pathways for catecholamines are shown in Figure 96–17. Neuronal re-uptake is of major

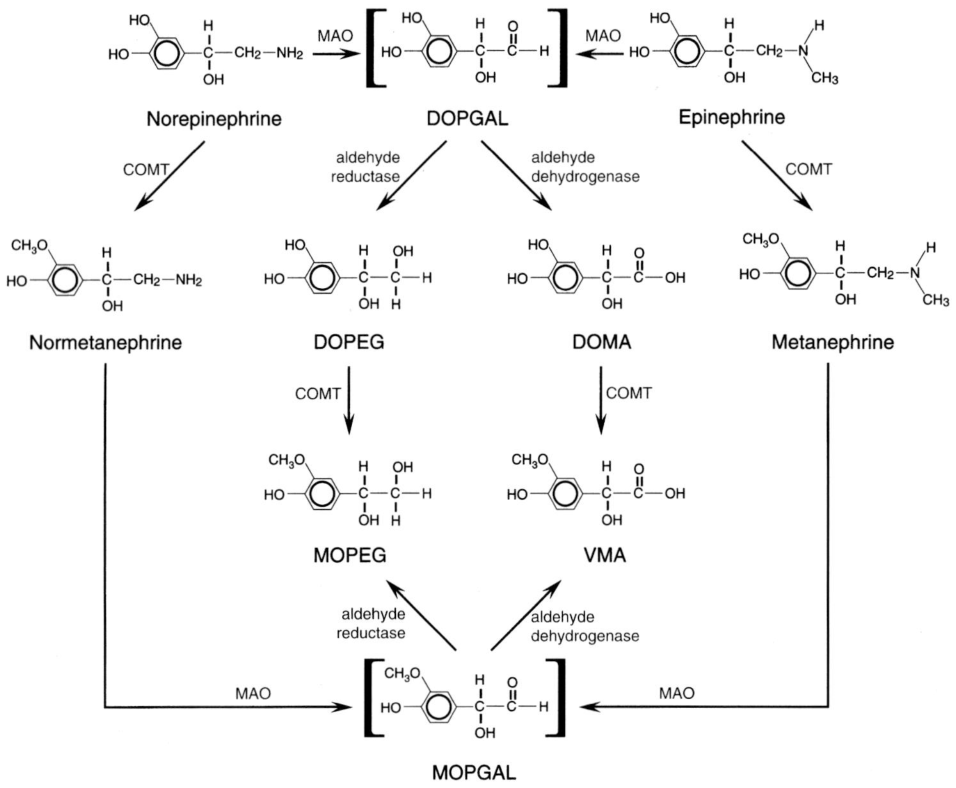

Figure 96–17. Steps in the metabolic disposition of catecholamines. Both norepinephrine and epinephrine are first oxidatively deanimated by mono-amine oxidase (MAO) to 3,4-dihydroxy-phenylglycoaldehyde (DOPGAL) and then either reduced to 3,4-dihydroxy-phenylethylene glycol (DOPEG) or oxidized to 3,4-dihydroxymandelic acid (DOMA). Alternatively, they can be initially methylated by catechol-O-methyl-transferase (COMT) to normetanephrine and metanephrine, respectively. Most of the products of either type of reaction are then metabolized by the other enzyme to form the major excretory products, 3-methoxy-4-hydroxyphenylethy-lene glycol (MOPEG or MHPG) and 3-methoxy-4-hydroxymandelic acid (VMA). Free MOPEG is largely converted to VMA. The glycol and, to some extent, the O-methylated amines and the catecholamines may be conjugated to the corresponding sulfates or glucu-ronides. (Modified from Axelrod, and others. From Hardman JG et al: Goodman and Gilman's the Pharmacological Basis of Therapeutics, 9th ed. New York, McGraw-Hill, 1996, p 124.)

importance in the removal of norepinephrine from the synaptic gap for re-release and has been termed *uptake* (Iverson, 1975). Catecholamines are degraded by the action of catechol-*O*-methyltransferase (COMT) and monoamine oxidase (MAO) (see Fig. 96–17), with either enzyme beginning the degradative process. **The primary metabolite in the urine is vanillylmandelic acid (VMA), with metanephrine, normetanephrine, and their derivatives contributing to total metabolic products,** which are often measured while evaluating patients with pheochromocytomas (Reckler et al, 1989).

Catecholamine Actions

Catecholamines exert varied effects by stimulating specific cellular receptors (adrenoreceptors), which are protein-binding sites (Table 96–2). The diversity of effects of circulating catecholamines on various organs acting at specific receptors accounts for the diversity of symptoms exhibited by patients with pheochromocytomas. Moreover, different tumors can produce different proportions of norepinephrine, epinephrine, or dopamine.

The actions of epinephrine and norepinephrine are not totally independent and are dose dependent. Hence, the classification of naturally occurring adrenergic hormones as alpha or beta or as a blocking agent, such as an *alpha₁ antagonist,* is useful but does not fully characterize the activity of the hormone or antagonist in all clinical settings.

CUSHING'S SYNDROME

Cushing's syndrome is the term used to describe the symptom complex caused by excess circulating glucocorticoids (Cushing, 1912, 1932). The term is all-encompassing and includes patients with pituitary hypersecretion of ACTH,

Cushing's disease, which accounts for 75% to 85% of patients with endogenous Cushing's; patients with adrenal adenomas or carcinomas; and patients with ectopic secretion of ACTH or CRH (Carey et al, 1984), or about 20% of those with ACTH-dependent disease (Meador et al, 1962; Hardy, 1982; Howlet et al, 1985; Carpenter, 1986; Scott, 1990b) (Tables 96–3 and 96–4).

The entity is rare, occurs most often in young adults, and is more common in females. **An exogenous source of Cushing's syndrome should always first be excluded**

Table 96–2. CATECHOLAMINE RECEPTORS

Adrenoreceptors	
Alpha-Adrenergic	
Alpha₁	Postsynaptic agonists
	Vascular smooth muscle—vasoconstriction
	Prostate—contraction
	Liver glycogenesis
Alpha₂	Presynaptic—inhibit norepinephrine release
	Postsynaptic—agonist
	Large veins—venoconstrictor
	Brain—decrease sympathetic outflow
	Pancreas—inhibit insulin secretion
	Gut—relaxation
	Adipocyte—inhibit lipolysis
Beta-Adrenergic	
Beta₁	Heart—inotrophic and chromotrophic effect
	Adipocyte—lipolysis
	Kidney—stimulate renin release
Beta₂	Lung—bronchodilatation
	Vascular smooth muscle—vasodilatation
	Liver—gluconeogenesis
	Uterus—relaxation
	Gut—relaxation
Dopaminergic	
DA₁	Vascular—vasodilatation
DA₂	Presynaptic—inhibit norepinephrine release

Table 96–3. RELATIVE PREVALENCE OF VARIOUS TYPES OF CUSHING'S SYNDROME AMONG 630 PATIENTS STUDIED AT DIFFERENT TIMES*

Diagnosis	Percent of Patients
Corticotropin-dependent Cushing's syndrome	
Cushing's disease	68
Ectopic corticotropin syndrome	12
Ectopic CRH syndrome	<1
Corticotropin-dependent Cushing's syndrome	
Adrenal adenoma	10
Adrenal carcinoma	8
Micronodular hyperplasia	1
Macronodular hyperplasia	<1
Pseudo–Cushing's syndrome	
Major depressive disorder	1
Alcoholism	<1

Data are based on a study of 146 consecutive patients seen at Vanderbilt University Medical Center before 1993 and on published reports describing a total of 484 patients. Because these and most other published series were reported by major referral centers, the proportion of patients with unusual diagnoses may be exaggerated as compared with that of patients with more common diagnoses. The prevalence of pseudo–Cushing's syndrome depends largely on the individual physician's threshold of clinical suspicion. The proportions of children and adolescents with the different causes of Cushing's syndrome may differ slightly from the proportions of adults; for example, the ectopic corticotropin syndrome is less common in children.
CRH, corticotropin-releasing hormone.
From Orth DN: N Eng J Med 1995; 32:791.

Table 96–4. SOURCES OF ECTOPIC ACTH IN 100 CASES

Tumor	Number
Carcinoma of lung	52
Carcinoma of pancreas (including carcinoid)	11
Thymoma	11
Benign bronchial adenoma (including carcinoid)	5
Pheochromocytoma	3
Carcinoma of thyroid	2
Carcinoma of liver	2
Carcinoma of prostate	2
Carcinoma of ovary	2
Undifferentiated carcinoma of mediastinum	2
Carcinoma of breast	1
Carcinoma of parotid gland	1
Carcinoma of esophagus	1
Paraganglioma	1
Ganglioma	1
Primary site uncertain	3

ACTH, adrenocorticotropic hormone.
From Scott HW Jr, Orth DN: Hypercortisolism (Cushing's syndrome). *In* Scott HW, ed: Surgery of the Adrenal Glands. Philadelphia, J. B. Lippincott, 1990, p 145.

because therapeutic steroids are the most common cause. Often the patient does not even realize he or she is using a steroid-containing preparation, especially creams or lotions (Champion, 1974; Flavin et al, 1983). The manifestations of the disease are legion and are the result of the manifold actions of glucocorticoids (see Table 96–1). There are few diseases in which the clinical appearance of the patient can be as useful in suspecting the diagnosis (Figs. 96–18 and 96–19). Old photographs are helpful in documenting the changes in appearance that have occurred. The more common clinical manifestations of Cushing's syndrome found in several series of patients are shown in Table 96–5. The clinical findings do not distinguish patients with Cushing's disease from those with adrenal adenomas or carcinomas. Most patients with ectopic ACTH do not present with the typical features (Bagshaw, 1960) but exhibit cachexia owing to underlying tumor as well as hypertension, hypokalemic alkalosis, and skin pigmentation (Bagshaw, 1960; Schambelan et al, 1971). The most common characteristics in children are weight gain and growth retardation (Magiakou et al, 1994). Virilization in the female or feminization in the male should raise the question of adrenal carcinoma, although more patients present with traditional manifestations of glucocorticoid excess (Luton et al, 1990).

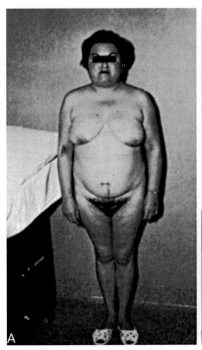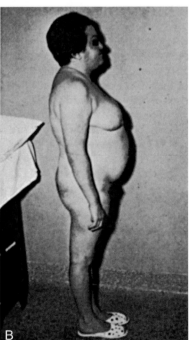

Figure 96–18. *A,* A 34-year-old woman with Cushing's syndrome. The patient shows truncal obesity and mild hirsutism. *B,* Note that cutaneous striae and ecchymoses are absent, in contrast to most cases shown in textbooks.

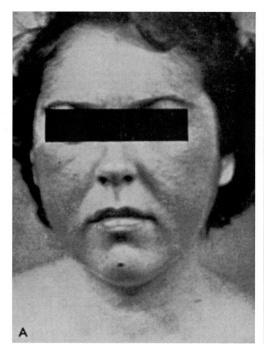
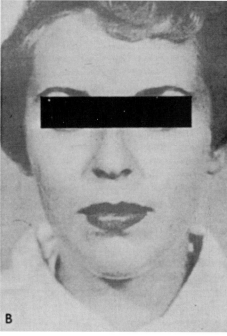

Figure 96–19. *A,* A 23-year-old woman 6 months after the development of moon face and other early signs of Cushing's syndrome owing to an adrenocortical adenoma on the left side. *B,* Same patient 6 months after surgical removal of adenoma of the adrenal cortex. (From Harrison JH: Surgery of the adrenals. *In* Davis L, ed. Christopher's Textbook of Surgery, 8th ed. Philadelphia, W. B. Saunders, 1964.)

The goals of managing patients with Cushing's syndrome have been articulated by investigators who have a long-standing interest in this disease: (1) lowering daily cortisol secretion to normal, (2) eradicating any tumor threatening health, (3) producing no permanent endocrine deficiency, and (4) avoiding permanent dependence on medications (Orth and Liddle, 1971). Obviously, all of these goals cannot be met in all patients; however, they serve as a thoughtful frame of reference. To initiate evaluation, the cause of Cushing's syndrome in a given patient must be established.

Table 96–5. CLINICAL MANIFESTATIONS OF CUSHING'S SYNDROME

	All[1] %	Disease[2] %	Adenoma/Carcinoma[3] %
Obesity	90	91	93
Hypertension	80	63	93
Diabetes	80	32	79
Centripetal obesity	80	—	—
Weakness	80	25	82
Muscle atrophy	70	34	—
Hirsutism	70	59	79
Menstrual abnormalities/sexual dysfunction	70	46	75
Purple striae	70	46	36
Moon facies	60	—	—
Osteoporosis	50	29	54
Early bruising	50	54	57
Acne/pigmentation	50	32	—
Mental changes	50	47	57
Edema	50	15	—
Headache	40	21	46
Poor healing	40	—	—

[1]Hunt and Tyrrell, 1978.
[2]Wilson, 1984.
[3]Scott, 1973.
From Scott HW Jr: *In* Scott HW, ed: Surgery of the Adrenal Glands. Philadelphia, J. B. Lippincott, 1990.

Importantly, patients with nonendocrine disorders who mimic the clinical and sometimes biochemical manifestations of Cushing's syndrome must be separated from those patients with true Cushing's syndrome; these patients have been termed to have pseudo–Cushing's syndrome. Abnormally regulated cortical secretion, albeit mild, may exist in as many as 80% of patients with major depression and can occur commonly in patients with chronic alcoholism (Gold et al, 1986; Stewart et al, 1993).

Laboratory Diagnosis

A panoply of tests of glucocorticoid function have evolved that are used to establish the presence of Cushing's syndrome and to distinguish between pituitary and adrenal causes as well as ectopic ACTH secretion (Orth et al, 1995) (Fig. 96–20). Moreover, medical institutions have developed their own set of tests, which time has proved most helpful, particularly in the sometimes difficult task of distinguishing bilateral adrenal hyperplasia from adenoma. The clinical diagnosis of Cushing's syndrome is confirmed by the demonstration of cortisol hypersecretion. **At the present time, the determination of 24-hour excretion of cortisol in the urine is the most direct and reliable index of cortisol secretion.** Orth (1995) recommends that urinary cortisol should be measured in two and preferably three consecutive 24-hour urine specimens collected on an outpatient basis. He believes that multiple collections are necessary because of the possibility of errors in collection and because of variations in hour-to-hour or day-to-day cortisol excretion. As for other 24-hour urine collections, the cortisol excretion should be calculated as a function of creatinine excretion.

In the patient with an elevated 24-hour urinary cortisol, the authors advocate determining the presence or absence of the normal circadian rhythm in plasma cortisol by obtaining ambulatory AM and PM plasma cortisol levels to continue the

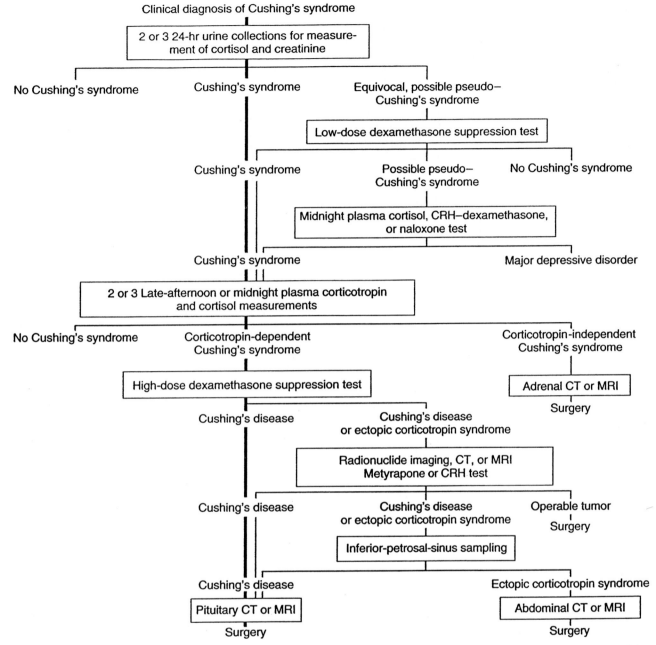

Figure 96–20. Identifying Cushing's syndrome and its causes. (From Orth DN: N Engl J Med 1995; 332:791. Reprinted by permission of the New England Journal of Medicine. Copyright 1995, Massachusetts Medical Society.)

diagnosis. Following ACTH release (see Fig. 96–10), healthy subjects show the characteristic rise in plasma cortisol in the morning with a fall to less than 5 ng/dl in the evening (Fig. 96–21). Patients with Cushing's syndrome lose the diurnal variation (Besser and Edwards, 1972) or show some variations but at higher basal levels (Glass et al, 1984).

Commonly the next test used is the dexamethasone suppression test as developed by Liddle (1960). Pituitary ACTH secretion is regulated with a negative feedback inhibition by cortisol. Liddle used the synthetic steroid dexamethasone, 30 times as potent as cortisol, to study the pituitary feedback mechanism in patients with suspected Cushing's syndrome. In normal subjects, 0.5 mg orally every 6 hours for 2 days causes a dramatic fall in 17-hydroxycorticosteroid, urinary free cortisol, or plasma cortisol (<5 ng/dl). A simplification

of the test is to administer a single 1-mg oral dose between 11:00 PM and midnight and to measure the plasma cortisol level between 8:00 AM and 9:00 AM (Fig. 96–22) (Paulotos et al, 1965; Sarvin et al, 1968). The test is less reliable, however, than the formal "low-dose" 2-day test as described previously, especially in obese patients. Patients with Cushing's syndrome show resistance to suppression to low-dose dexamethasone. This failure of suppression has been found to be characteristic of all patients with Cushing's syndrome studied by Scott and Orth (1990). These low-dose suppression tests are now reserved primarily for patients with equivocal 24-hour urinary cortisol excretion (Orth, 1995) and are especially useful for identifying patients with pseudo–Cushing's syndrome.

Alternatively, **if available, the ideal way to determine**

whether a patient has **ACTH-dependent or ACTH-independent hypercortisolism is the concurrent measurement of both plasma ACTH (corticotropin) and cortisol by two-site immunoradiometric assay** (Raff and Findling, 1989). Despite the fact that the ideal time to measure these hormones is between midnight and 2:00 AM, when the concentrations are at the lowest, a more practical approach is to measure the test late in the afternoon. Again, Orth (1995) recommends the measurement of the two hormones at least on two and preferably three separate days. If the plasma cortisol concentration is greater than 50 μg/dl and the corticotropin concentration is less than 5 pg/ml, cortical secretion is ACTH-independent (the patient has primary adrenal Cushing's syndrome). If the plasma ACTH level is greater than 50 pg/ml, the cortical secretion is ACTH-dependent (the patient has Cushing's disease or ectopic ACTH or CRH syndrome) (Orth, 1995). In situations in which the two-site immunoradiometric assay test is not available, the high-dose dexamethasone suppression test has always been the standard test to differentiate between pituitary and adrenal Cushing's syndrome. Patients are given high-dose dexamethasone (2 mg every 6 hours for 2 days) and plasma cortisol, and urinary free cortisol levels are measured. In patients with pituitary disease, there should be a 50% or greater suppression in cortisol. Patients with adrenal adenomas or carcinomas fail to suppress cortisol secretion. In addition, the tests usually distinguished Cushing's disease, in which there is only relative resistance to glucocorticoid negative feedback, from ectopic ACTH syndrome, in which there is usually complete resistance. A number of different criteria have been established to try to obtain greater sensitivity in correctly identifying patients with Cushing's disease, but in almost all of the different studies, patients with ectopic ACTH as well as those with primary adrenal disease have uniformly failed to suppress cortisol (Avgerinos et al, 1994; Miller and Crapo, 1994).

Additional tests currently in use to differentiate between pituitary Cushing's and ectopic ACTH secretion are the metapyrone stimulation tests and petrosal venous sinus catheterization. The metapyrone stimulation test was originally

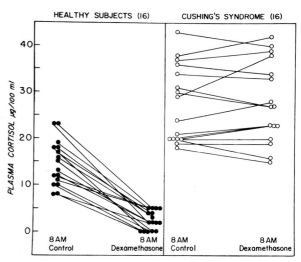

Figure 96–22. The rapid dexamethasone suppression test distinguishes patients with Cushing's syndrome from healthy subjects or other obese subjects. Note the overlap in cortisol levels between the two groups before suppression. The patients with high basal cortisol levels were those with ectopic ACTH production by a nonendocrine tumor as the underlying cause. (From Melby J: N Engl J Med 1971;285:735. Reprinted with material from the New England Journal of Medicine.)

used to determine pituitary insufficiency. Metapyrone blocks conversion of 11-desoxycortisol to cortisol, and as the plasma cortisol concentration falls, the pituitary secretes more ACTH and there is an increase in urinary 17-hydroxycorticosteroid concentration. Patients with Cushing's disease have a normal or supernormal increase in urinary excretion of 17-hydroxycorticosteroids, in contrast to patients with ectopic ACTH-secreting tumors, who have little or no increase in either value because of the suppression of pituitary ACTH (Avgerinos et al, 1994). **Obviously the most direct way to demonstrate pituitary hypersecretion of ACTH is to measure its level in the petrosal venous sinus and compare the level to the peripheral level.** Sampling can also be done before and after stimulation with CRH. This is an invasive procedure, however, and significant complications have been reported (Oldfield et al, 1991; Miller et al, 1992). Before petrosal sinus catheterization is indicated, thorough studies should be performed to identify occult ACTH-secreting tumors. Many of these tumors can be identified with standard computed tomography (CT) or MRI scanning and, more recently, unique radionuclide imaging for somatostatin receptors, which are present in small cell lung carcinomas and thymic carcinoid tumors (Phlipponneau et al, 1994).

At this point, despite the availability of numerous other stimulatory or inhibitory tests (Dolan and Carey, 1989), the dramatic advances in radiologic localizing tests usually make further biochemical studies unnecessary (Mezrich et al, 1986; Reinig et al, 1986; Kazam et al, 1989; Korobkin, 1989; Dunnick, 1990; Newhouse, 1990).

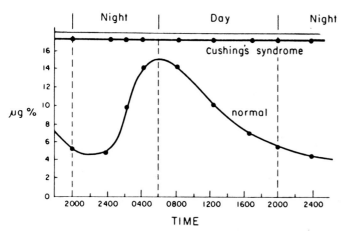

Figure 96–21. Circadian rhythm in cortisol secretion of plasma in a normal subject contrasted with absence of rhythm in patient with Cushing's syndrome. (From Bergland RM, Harrison TS: Pituitary and adrenal. *In* Schwartz SI, ed: Principles of Surgery, 3rd ed. New York, McGraw-Hill, 1979, p 1493. Reproduced by permission of the McGraw-Hill Companies.)

Radiographic Localization

The development of computer-aided sectional imaging and MRI has revolutionized adrenal imaging. Accordingly, older tests such as intravenous urography with tomography,

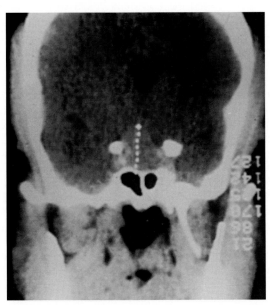

Figure 96–23. Computed tomography scan of a chromophobe adenoma in the sella turcica of a patient with Cushing's syndrome presenting with hyperpigmentation, headaches, and a visual field defect.

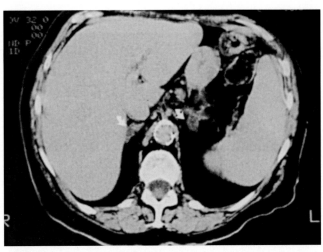

Figure 96–25. Computed tomography scan showing a patient with macronodular adrenal hyperplasia.

ultrasound, and adrenal arteriography and venography are only rarely used today. In general, CT has become the initial imaging procedure.

In patients with Cushing's disease, additional information can be obtained with CT or MRI of the sella turcica in search of a pituitary adenoma (Fig. 96–23) (Mitty and Yeh, 1982). More recently, both unenhanced and gadolinium-enhanced MRI are used; however, only 50% of microadenomas are detected (Klibanski and Zervas, 1991; Hall et al, 1994).

Patients with hyperplasia can show diffuse thickening and elongation of the adrenal rami (Fig. 96–24) or, unfortunately, prominent glands bilaterally that fall within normal range (Kazam et al, 1989). A second variant, found in 10% to 20% of cases, is nodular cortical hyperplasia characterized by multinodularity of both adrenals (Fig. 96–25). The CT appearance does not distinguish between patients with glucocorticoid excess or idiopathic hyperaldosteronism (pseudo–primary hyperaldosteronism), owing to bilateral adrenal hyperplasia. The small size (<2 cm) and multiplicity of the nodules as well as the bilateral distribution are the distinguishing features from Cushing's adenomas. Rarely, patients with macronodular hyperplasia develop autonomous glucocorticoid secretion and may require adrenalectomy.

Adrenal adenomas are usually larger than 2 cm, solitary, and associated with atrophy of the opposite gland. The density is low because of the high concentration of lipid. Sonography and study after contrast showing enhancement avoid misdiagnosis of an adrenal cyst (Fig. 96–26) (Huebener and Treugut, 1984).

Adrenal carcinomas are often indistinguishable from adenomas except for the larger size (>6 cm) (Fig. 96–27) (Belldegrun and deKernion, 1989). Necrosis and calcification are also more common in association with adrenal carcinoma but are not diagnostic. Clearly, large irregular adrenal lesions with invasion represent carcinoma; however, metastatic carcinoma to the adrenal has the same appearance.

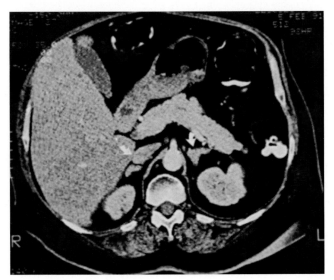

Figure 96–24. Computed tomography scan showing bilateral adrenal hyperplasia in a patient with Cushing's disease.

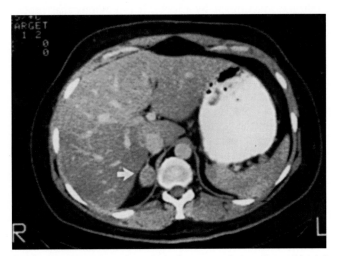

Figure 96–26. Computed tomography scan of a patient with right adrenal adenoma.

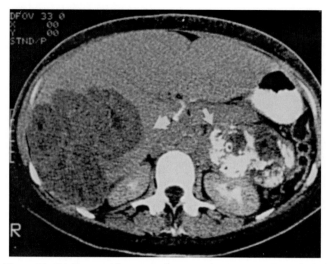

Figure 96–27. Computed tomography scan of a patient with a calcified left adrenal carcinoma and hepatic metastasis.

MRI is not usually necessary in patients with Cushing's syndrome unless adrenal carcinoma is suspected. In that clinical setting, the signal intensity may be much higher with carcinoma than that in the spleen, accurately differentiating adenomas from carcinomas (Bilbey et al, 1995). MRI also may provide useful information about adjacent organ or vascular invasion.

Adrenal cortical scanning with iodinated cholesterol agents is no longer routinely used but can be helpful in differentiating functional adrenal tissue from other retroperitoneal lesions (Kazerooni et al., 1990; Nakajo et al, 1993) and in identifying residual cortical tissues. It is not useful for the identification of adrenal carcinoma (Pasieka et al, 1992).

Treatment

Cushing's Disease and Ectopic Adrenocorticotropic Hormone

When recalling the goals of management of Cushing's syndrome as outlined by Liddle, it is obvious that precise diagnosis is critical. Accordingly, in the patient with ectopic ACTH syndrome, treatment is directed to the primary tumor. Reduction of secretion of functional steroids by use of blocking agents can further ameliorate symptoms. Agents used include aminoglutethimide, which blocks the conversion of cholesterol to pregnenolone, and metyrapone, which blocks the conversion of 11-desoxycortisol to cortisone and ketoconazole, the antifungal agent that blocks cytochrome P-450–mediated side chain cleavage and hydroxylation at both the early and late steps in steroid biosynthesis (Loose et al, 1983; Farwell et al, 1988; Mortimer et al, 1991). Patients given aminoglutethimide must be observed for adrenocortical insufficiency because aldosterone production is also impaired. Metyrapone does not usually result in salt wasting at the usual dose of 250 to 500 mg three times daily because of increased production of desoxycorticosterone—a potent mineralocorticoid (see Figs. 96–8 and 96–9) (Scott and Orth, 1990). Other agents used with some success are

ketoconazole (Sonino et al, 1991) and the cortisol receptor blocker mifepristone (Bertagna et al, 1986).

The synthesis of cortisol in 1950 (Wendler et al, 1950) led to the availability of replacement steroids not only for patients with Addison's disease but also for those following bilateral adrenalectomy for Cushing's disease. Thus, bilateral adrenalectomy through a bilateral posterior approach was used in patients with severe Cushing's disease. Generally, patients did well with resolution of the disease (Scott et al, 1977, 1990). **Ten percent to 20% of patients, however, subsequently developed pituitary tumors, usually chromophobe adenomas perhaps caused by the lack of hypothalamic/pituitary feedback and high ACTH and related compounds** (Nelson et al, 1958; Cohen et al, 1978). **This entity, termed Nelson's syndrome, may arise many years after bilateral adrenalectomy.** Thus, patients must be followed with the determination of ACTH levels and the evaluation of the sella turcica (Fig. 96–28). The development of Nelson's syndrome may be prevented by prophylactic pituitary radiotherapy (Jenkins et al, 1995).

The development of pituitary irradiation subsequently limited the utilization of bilateral adrenalectomy for Cushing's disease beginning in the 1950s (Orth and Liddle, 1971).

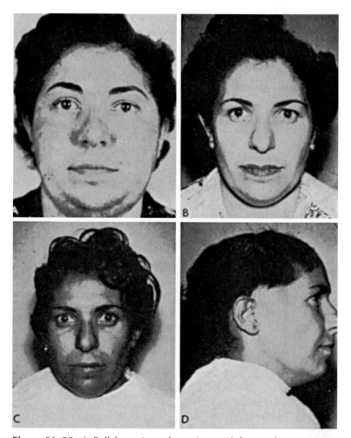

Figure 96–28. *A,* Full-face view of a patient with hyperadrenocorticism in 1954, treated by total adrenalectomy at that time. *B,* The same patient 6 months after total adrenalectomy, showing striking improvement. All symptoms and signs of Cushing's syndrome had disappeared. *C,* Deep pigmentation, headache, and failing vision supervened in 1957; emergency craniotomy was necessary after radiation therapy. *D,* Disappearance of pigmentation is shown in the facial view after removal of chromophobe adenoma of pituitary by Dr. Donald Matson. (From Rothenberg RE, ed: Reoperative Surgery New York, McGraw-Hill, 1969. Reproduced by permission of the McGraw-Hill Companies.)

Long-term follow-up, however, revealed about a third of patients were cured, a third improved, and a third failed to respond. The results appear to be better in children (Jennings et al, 1977). Irradiation is useful to treat Nelson's syndrome. Heavy particle proton beam therapy may be more effective but also is more likely to induce panhypopituitarism (Burch, 1985).

In 1971, Hardy reported his experience with transphenoidal hypophysial microsurgery for removal of pituitary adenomas with preservation of pituitary function. Subsequently, this technique evolved as the single most effective and safest treatment of Cushing's disease. The cure rates are 85% to 95%, the results immediate, the complications low, and the recurrences rare (Bigos et al, 1980; Styne et al, 1984; Ludecke, 1991). Patients often have transient decreases in cortisol levels and may need replacement therapy and monitoring for some months (Fitzgerald et al, 1982). Transient diabetes mellitus may also occur. In adults, irradiation now is reserved for patients not cured by transphenoidal surgery. Finally, although unusual, there may be spontaneous regression of Cushing's disease (Dickstein et al, 1991).

Cushing's Syndrome During Pregnancy

Cushing's syndrome during pregnancy is rare (Mulder et al, 1990; Guilhaum et al, 1992) because of the menstrual irregularities characteristic of the disease. Of cases reported, 59% have been ACTH-independent and 33% ACTH-dependent. The others were not classified. During normal pregnancy, plasma cortisol binding protein and plasma protein bound and unbound cortisone levels rise; however, the normal diurnal variation persists (Siragy et al, 1989). Urinary free cortisol level also rises slightly. Moreover, there is some resistance to dexamethasone suppression that progresses with each trimester; however, some suppression remains so that the total absence of suppression to low-dose dexamethasone is compatible with Cushing's syndrome.

Obviously, imaging studies are contraindicated during pregnancy, especially in the first trimester. **The authors have used MRI to identify an adenoma in a pregnant patient with Cushing's syndrome (Fig. 96–29).**

Both fetal and maternal morbidity are reduced with treatment. Surgical removal of an adenoma can be successfully achieved during pregnancy, as was done in the authors' patient, especially during the second trimester. Alternatively, some patients have been treated with metyrapone or transphenoidal adenomectomy when indicated (Casson et al, 1987).

Fortunately, because of the low transplacental transfer of adrenal corticosteroids, the fetus is not affected in most cases and does not require steroid replacement following birth; however, the prematurity rate is high.

Adrenal Adenoma

Adrenal adenomas causing Cushing's syndrome are treated by surgical removal, which is discussed in the section on adrenal surgery (van Heerden et al, 1995).

ADRENAL CARCINOMA

Adrenal carcinoma is a rare disease and has a poor prognosis (Vaughan and Carey, 1989b; Luton et al, 1990). The incidence is estimated as 1 case per 1.7 million, accounting for 0.02% of cancers and 0.2% of all cancer deaths (Nader et al, 1983; Plager, 1984; Brennan, 1987).

A practical subclassification for adrenal carcinomas is according to their ability to produce adrenal hormones. The varieties of functioning tumors are shown in Table 96–6. Most tumors secrete multiple compounds. In a series by Luton and co-workers, 79% of adrenal tumors were functional—a higher percentage than previously reported

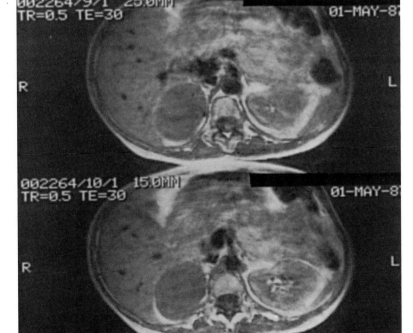

Figure 96–29. *A* and *B,* Magnetic resonance T1 and T2 weighted images of patient who developed Cushing's syndrome during pregnancy showing the large right adrenal adenoma. (From Vaughan ED Jr, Carey RM, eds: Adrenal Disorders. New York, Thieme Medical Publishers Inc., 1989.)

Table 96–6. CLASSIFICATION OF ADRENAL CARCINOMA

Functional
    Cushing's syndrome
    Virilization in females
        Increased DHEA 17-ketosteroids
        Increased testosterone
    Feminizing syndrome in males
    Hyperaldosteronism
    Mixed combination of above
Nonfunctional

DHEA, Dehydroepiandrosterone.

probably because of more sensitive assays (Luton et al, 1990). In addition, nonfunctional tumors may become functional, or a tumor may subsequently produce multiple hormones (Grunberg, 1982; Arteaga et al, 1984). Moreover, tumors may produce metabolites that are nonfunctional or in such low amounts so as not to cause physiologic changes. Thus, although convenient, a classification of tumors by product is somewhat contrived, and debate exists as to whether "nonfunctioning" tumors carry a worse prognosis for the patient than functioning tumors (Heinbecker et al, 1957; Lewinsky et al, 1974).

Incidentally Discovered Adrenal Masses

The increased utilization of abdominal ultrasound and CT scanning is leading to the frequent finding of an unexpected adrenal mass, or an "incidentaloma" (Fig. 96–30) (Belldegrun et al, 1986; Belldegrun and deKernion, 1989).

Adrenal malignancies are usually larger than 6 cm in size. Belldegrun and co-workers (1986), reviewing six series, found that 105 of 114 adrenocortical carcinomas were more than 6 cm in size (Heinbecker et al, 1957; Knight et al, 1960; Lewinsky et al, 1974; Sullivan et al, 1978; Bertagna and Orth, 1981). Accordingly, solid adrenal lesions of more than 6 cm should be considered malignant until proven otherwise by exploration and adrenalectomy.

The problem arises in the management of incidentally found adrenal lesions smaller than 6 cm. Unsuspected adre-

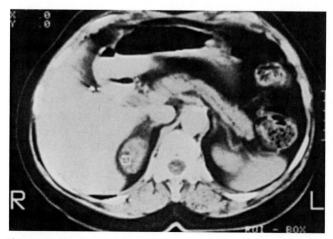

Figure 96–30. Computed tomography scan of patient with a 5-cm nonfunctioning adrenal mass found incidentally.

nal masses have been detected on 0.6% to 1.3% of upper abdominal CT studies (Copeland, 1983; Abecassis et al, 1985; Ross and Aron, 1990). Moreover, the prevalence of benign, clinically silent, adrenal adenomas found on autopsy series ranges from 1.4% to 8.7% (Russi et al, 1945; Hedeland et al, 1968). In contrast, occult nonfunctioning adrenocortical carcinoma is rarely found on autopsy. Accordingly, attention has turned to the appropriate management of the "incidentaloma" (Prinz et al, 1982; Copeland, 1983; Belldegrun et al, 1986; Ross and Aron, 1990; Osella et al, 1994).

One approach is shown in Table 96–7. Several points do not engender controversy. First, there is agreement that all patients with solid adrenal masses should undergo biochemical assessment. If biochemical abnormalities are identified, the lesions should be treated appropriately as described elsewhere in this chapter—usually by removal of the offending lesion. The extent of the biochemical evaluation has been reviewed (Ross and Aron, 1990). A selective approach has been outlined, which markedly limits cost without sacrificing diagnostic accuracy. A limited evaluation is recommended, including only the tests to rule out pheochromocytoma, potassium levels in hypertensive cases, and glucocorticoid evaluation only in the presence of clinical stigmata of Cushing's syndrome or virilization. Because of the likelihood that nonfunctioning solid lesions larger than 6 cm are malignant, these lesions should be removed. **CT scanning may underestimate the size of an adrenal lesion, and the authors suggest that exploration be performed when the lesion is more than 5 cm on CT or MRI** (Cerfolio et al, 1993). Furthermore, lesions clearly proved to be cystic by CT, MRI, or cyst puncture, which is often not necessary, can also be followed.

The controversy arises in the management strategy for the solid adrenal lesion smaller than 5 cm in size. Glazer and co-workers have suggested that adrenalectomy be considered for solid lesions more than 3 to 4 cm in size (Glazer et al, 1982). Prinz and associates have also suggested a surgical approach, especially in younger patients (Prinz et al, 1982). Copeland (1983) challenges the "3- to 4-cm" criterion and suggests observation for all patients with nonfunctioning lesions less than 6 cm in size. These workers estimate that more than 4000 adrenalectomies would have to be done on patients with masses 1.5 cm in diameter or larger to remove one carcinoma. It is undeniable, however, that most of the major reviews of adrenal malignancies reveal the occasional lesion smaller than 6 cm.

The 3- to 6-cm solid, nonfunctioning adrenal mass incidentally found remains the major area of controversy. Certainly on statistical ground, the majority are benign. The occasional one, however, is malignant and potentially curable, a situation not frequently encountered in patients with adrenal carcinomas. Fine needle adrenal biopsy guided by ultrasound and CT is now available and is well tolerated by the patient and associated with minimal complications. In a large series of 56 patients in Finland, significant cytologic material was obtained in 96.4%, and the accuracy to differentiate benign from malignant disease was 85.7% (Tikkakoski et al, 1991). These authors had no complications; however, pancreatitis has been reported, which can result in death (Kane et al, 1991). The risk of tumor spread following percutaneous biopsy is unknown.

An additional test that may prove useful is MRI, whereby

Table 96–7. EVALUATION OF INCIDENTALLY FOUND ADRENAL MASS

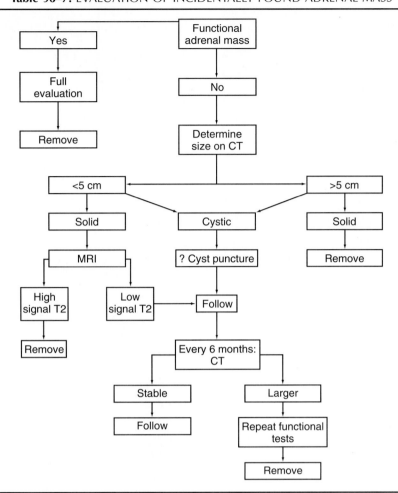

a high signal intensity ratio on T2 images suggests that the lesion is not a benign adenoma (Fig. 96–31) (Reinig et al, 1986). Currently, there is controversy over the ability of signal characteristics to reliably differentiate benign from malignant masses (Lubat and Weinreb, 1990; Bilbey et al, 1995). The most accurate reference standard at the moment seems to be the spleen, and if the mean signal intensity ratio is over 0.8, it is unlikely that the lesion is a benign adenoma. There are **a number of entities other than adrenal carcinoma, however, that can cause high intensity, including neural tumors, metastatic tumors to the adrenal, and hemorrhage into a variety of adrenal lesions** (Lubat and Weinreb, 1990).

Myelolipoma

In the past, these nonfunctioning benign lesions were incidentally found at autopsy. They are generally small (<5 cm), unilateral, asymptomatic, and benign, containing hematopoietic and fatty elements (DelGaudio and Solidoro, 1986, 1991; Sanders et al, 1995).

The lesion has been recognized with increasing frequency because it has a characteristic appearance on CT scanning and MRI (Casey et al, 1994) that establishes the diagnosis

and excludes the need for surgical exploration. The exception may be the case of the large lesion (Fig. 96–32), in which confusion with a necrotic adrenal carcinoma could exist (Wilhelmus et al, 1981).

The cause of the lesion is unknown but may be a part of a group of entities characterized by deposition of myeloid and adipose tissue (Papavasiliou et al, 1990). Patients have been predominantly obese with a 1.75:1.0 male-to-female ratio. Pain is the most common presenting symptom. The lesions are rarely calcified or hormonally active. Hormonal levels should be obtained, however, because coexisting cortical adenoma and myelolipoma have been reported (Vyberg and Sestof, 1986).

Adrenal Metastasis

Actually, primary adrenocortical carcinoma is less common than metastatic tumors to the adrenal. In a series of 500 autopsy cases, Willis (1952) found adrenal metastasis in 9%. Specifically the adrenal has been found to be a site of metastasis in more than 50% of patients with melanomas and carcinomas of the breast and lung; 40% with renal cell carcinomas; and, in order of frequency, carcinomas of the contralateral adrenal, bladder, colon, esophagus, gallbladder,

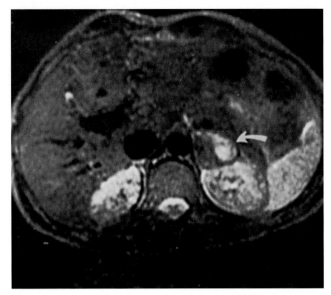

Figure 96–31. Ganglioneuroma. Nonfunctioning left adrenal tumor *(arrow)*, bright on T2, found incidentally.

liver, pancreas, prostate, stomach, and uterus (Bullock and Hirst, 1953).

Now that adrenal imaging with CT and MRI is commonplace, more adrenal lesions are identified earlier in the course of patients with cancer (Thomas et al, 1982). Management is obviously predicated on the underlying malignancy. The major clinical point is not to confuse a metastatic adrenal lesion for a primary adrenal process. Generally the adrenal lesion is part of the clinical picture of diffuse metastatic disease. Long-term survival following adrenalectomy and aggressive treatment of the primary process, however, has been reported in patients with pulmonary carcinoma and adrenal metastasis (Twomey et al, 1982; Reyes et al, 1990). Moreover, the finding of an unsuspected adrenal mass should heighten the clinical suspicion of a neoplasm elsewhere. The MRI pattern not characteristic of a benign adenoma raises the index of suspicion for metastatic disease (Fig. 96–33) (Reinig et al, 1986; Bilbey et al, 1995). Adrenal insufficiency has been reported secondary to both benign adenomas and bilateral adrenal metastases (Sheeler et al, 1983).

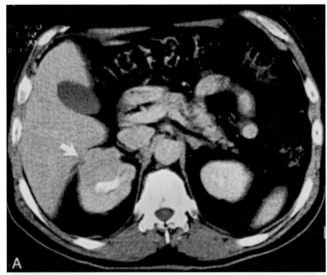

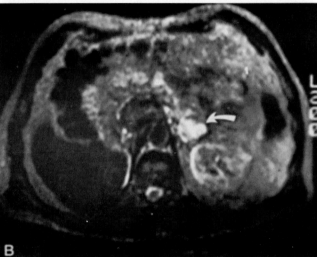

Figure 96–33. *A,* Computed tomography scan showing a left renal cell carcinoma. *B,* Subsequent right adrenal metastasis with high intensity. Pathology was proved by excision.

Benign Adenoma

The difficulty in discriminating by pathologic examination adenoma from carcinoma is a major problem for pathologists (Amberson and Gray, 1989; Medeiros and Weiss, 1992). All large adrenal lesions do not behave biologically as carcinomas. Some lesions that appear benign on histologic evaluation eventually metastasize. Hence, as discussed previously, surgical removal is recommended for all lesions larger than 5 cm in size.

Weiss (1984) has compared the histology of 43 clinically benign and malignant adrenal tumors. Using a multifactorial analysis of nine criteria, he was able to differentiate metastasizing from nonmetastasizing tumors.

Klein and co-workers have reported that flow cytometry accurately demonstrated aneuploid stem lines in four cases classified histologically as carcinoma (Klein et al, 1985). The authors have also found that all but one patient exhibiting subsequent metastatic disease have had aneuploid primary tumors (Fig. 96–34).

Others also have shown that adrenal carcinomas can show

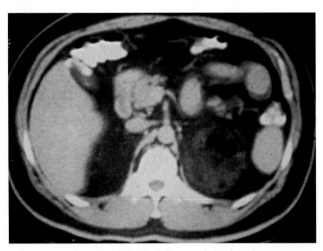

Figure 96–32. Myelolipoma, left adrenal.

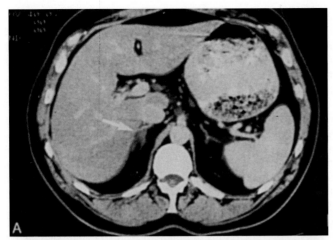

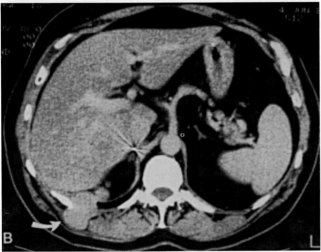

Figure 96–34. Patient with a small right aldosterone-producing adenoma *(A)*, which was malignant and recurred in the adrenal bed and at the site of the flank incision *(B)*. The disease caused the death of the patient.

either aneuploid or diploid characteristics; however, there is some evidence that there may be a longer disease-free survival in patients with hypodiploid or hyperdiploid carcinomas in contrast to those with aneuploid patterns (Haak et al, 1993a). Abnormalities in DNA content may not be as useful in children with adrenal cortical tumors (Moore et al, 1993). Other pathologic markers that are being investigated to help in understanding the cause of adrenal adenomas and carcinomas as well as to delineate between the two include studies of clonal composition of human adrenal cortical neoplasms (Beuschlein et al, 1994; Gicquel et al, 1994), neuroendocrine differentiation (Haak and Fleuren, 1995), mutations of P53 (Sameshima et al, 1992; Reincke et al, 1994), and immuno-histochemical monoclonal antibody studies (Tartour et al, 1993).

Functional Tumors

Cushing's Syndrome

Cushing's syndrome has been discussed in detail—adrenal carcinoma being one of the causes of corticosteroid excess.

This form of functional tumor is the most common in its pure form or with associated virilization. In a study comparing the clinical and laboratory studies of patients with Cushing's syndrome caused by adenoma and carcinoma, Bertagna and Orth (1981) found that virilization without evidence of cortisol excess was indicative of carcinoma except in children. Other clinical parameters were not helpful except for hirsutism, being more common in patients with carcinoma. Thin skin, purple striae, thin hair, and temporal hair loss were more common in patients with adenomas. From a metabolic standpoint, 17-ketosteroid (Forbes and Albright, 1951) and DHEAS levels (Yamaji et al, 1984) are often high in patients with carcinomas, usually in conjunction with elevated glucocorticoid production (Luton et al, 1990). Patient prognosis is poor.

Testosterone-Secreting Adrenal Cortical Tumors

Virilization is the hallmark of Cushing's syndrome secondary to adrenal carcinoma. Virilization in the absence of elevated urinary 17-ketosteroids, however, is uncommon and should raise the possibility of testosterone-secreting ovarian or adrenal lesions (Imperato-McGinley et al, 1981; Del Gaudio and Del Gaudio, 1993). Of the two sites of origin, adrenal cortical tumors that secrete testosterone are exceedingly rare. Most adrenal tumors have been adenomas, but several have been ganglioneuromas with Leydig cell nodules (Aguirre and Sculley, 1983) or a Leydig cell adenoma (Trost et al, 1981). The majority of tumors have been found in women, although cases in men and in children have been reported. The testosterone secretion can be autonomous, under gonadotropin control (Werk et al, 1973), or under ACTH control (Trost et al, 1981).

In contrast to the other tumors described in this chapter, these tumors are usually small, less than 6 cm, and they behave in a benign fashion. In a review of 47 documented cases of testosterone-producing neoplasms, however, 8 were virilizing carcinomas (Gabrilove et al, 1981; Mattox and Phelan, 1987).

Estrogen-Secreting Adrenal Cortical Tumors

Most feminizing tumors occur in men 25 to 50 years old, and, in contradistinction to testosterone-secreting tumors, they are usually larger, often palpable, and highly malignant (Gabrilove et al, 1965). Characteristically the patients present with gynecomastia. In addition, they may exhibit testicular atrophy, impotence, or decreased libido. In one of the authors' patients, the clinical presentation was infertility and oligospermia.

These tumors secrete androstenedione, which is converted peripherally to estrogens. Other steroids may also be secreted, and the clinical picture may be mixed with associated cushingoid features.

Of these tumors, 80% have been malignant. Half the patients with this disease expire within 18 months of diagnosis. The 3-year survival is less than 20%.

The prime therapy is surgical, usually employing a thoracoabdominal approach with wide excision of the tumor, adjacent organs, if necessary, and regional lymph nodes.

Despite wide resection, the patient's prognosis remains poor, and no effective adjunctive therapy has been developed to date.

Aldosterone-Secreting Adrenal Cortical Carcinoma

Primary hyperaldosteronism is almost always due to a small benign solitary adenoma, Conn's syndrome, or bilateral adrenal hyperplasia. The syndrome in its pure form, however, may rarely be caused by adrenal carcinoma (Vaughan and Carey, 1989b). In fact, in most cases with evidence of mineralocorticoid excess and hypokalemia owing to adrenal carcinoma, there are also signs of abnormalities in glucocorticoid or androgen secretion.

On review of the cases, the striking difference between the tumors found in these patients and in those with Conn's syndrome caused by benign adenomas is the size of the tumor. Benign adenomas are rarely larger than 3 cm in size. In contrast, all but two reported aldosterone-secreting carcinomas were larger than 3 cm (Vaughan et al, 1989). Accordingly the clinical and biochemical syndrome of hyperaldosteronism and the CT evidence of a large adrenal mass should strongly suggest carcinoma. Similar to most of the other patients with tumors as described, these patients do poorly despite initial resection of the tumor. Adjunctive therapy is ineffective.

Adrenocortical Carcinoma in Children

Adrenocortical carcinoma constitutes only 0.002% of all childhood malignancies (Young and Miller, 1975) and only 6% of childhood malignant adrenal tumors—the majority being neuroblastomas (Stewart et al, 1974) (see Chapter 74). Despite the somewhat tenuous feeling that survival is better in children, double that in adults, the entity is still highly lethal and refractory to adjunctive therapy, although adequate trials have not been carried out (Kay et al, 1983).

In contrast to adults, in children most of these tumors are hormonally active, and perhaps earlier detection is the reason for their better survival. The clinical syndromes include Cushing's syndrome, commonly as a result of carcinoma— not adenoma—in children, virilization in females, and isosexual precocious puberty in males. Evaluation follows the same lines as that described in adults with careful examination for steroid precursors and by-products. These may be of later use as tumor markers after initial tumor removal. In addition to recurrence, the late occurrence of other tumors has also been reported (Andler et al, 1978). Adrenocortical carcinoma is also found in excess in children with Beckwith-Wiedemann syndrome, among children with isolated hemihypertrophy, and in association with the Li-Fraumeni syndrome. Tumors have been found to show a high frequency of germ line P53 mutations, as are found in the Li-Fraumeni syndrome, suggesting a potential relationship (Wagner et al, 1994).

Management of Adrenocortical Carcinoma

Except for testosterone-secreting tumors, adrenocortical carcinomas are highly malignant with both local and hematogenous spread and a 5-year survival rate of about 35% (Icard et al, 1992; Pommier and Brennan, 1992). In the series by Richie and Gittes, the most common sites of metastasis were lung, liver, and lymph nodes (Richie and Gittes, 1980). A large autopsy study of 132 cases showed metastases to lungs (60%), liver (50%), lymph nodes (48%), bone (24%), and pleura and heart (10%) (Didolkar et al, 1981). In addition, these tumors often extend directly into adjacent structures, especially the kidney, and may involve the inferior vena cava (Long et al, 1993). The treatment is surgical removal of the primary tumor with attempt to remove the entire lesion even if resection of adjacent organs (e.g., kidney and spleen) is necessary as well as resection of local lymph nodes en bloc. In one series, patients with complete resection had a higher (47%) 5-year survival rate (35% overall) (Pommier and Brennan, 1992). After surgical removal of functioning adrenal tumors, the patient can be followed with appropriate hormonal levels as markers for tumor recurrence.

Medical Therapy

Despite the current accuracy in anatomic and biochemical definition of adrenal carcinoma, many patients present with metastatic disease. Most patients with locally resectable disease eventually die from recurrent local or distant disease. The search for effective adjunctive therapy has been frustrating; radiation therapy has not been useful except for palliation (Percarpio and Knowlton, 1976). In addition, conventional chemotherapy, although not widely studied in a systematic fashion, has not been effective, probably because of p glycoprotein expression (Flynn et al, 1992; Haak et al, 1993b).

The most success reported has been with the adrenolytic drug (1,1-dichloro-2-[o-chlorophenyl]-2-[p-chlorophenyl]-ethane) (o,p'-DDD) or mitotane (Bergenstal et al, 1960). This DDT derivative has been shown to induce tumor response in 34% (Hutter and Kayhoe, 1966) and 35% in a review of 551 cases reported in the literature (Wooten and King, 1993). The major use has been for patients with metastatic disease, and despite the response rates given, survival time has not been prolonged (Hoffman and Mattox, 1972; Luton et al, 1990), unless high serum levels are obtained (Haak et al, 1994) or it is given postoperatively in an adjuvant fashion (Vassilopoulou-Sellin et al, 1993). Moreover, the usual treatment regimen is to increase the dosage to 8 to 10 g per day until toxicity occurs. Toxicity that is significant includes gastrointestinal, neurologic, and dermatologic disorders, most of which regress on cessation of therapy.

During management, adrenal insufficiency can occur, and cortisol and aldosterone levels should be monitored. Because of the high fat solubility of the drug, traces of it can be found several months after the drug has been discontinued, warranting continued steroid monitoring during this period.

The overall response to o,p'-DDD has been disappointing, even in combination regimens (Bukowski et al, 1993). Suramin, the antiparasitic agent, also has limited efficacy (Arit et al, 1994). The antifungal drug ketoconazole, which has an adrenolytic effect, has also induced regression in metastatic adrenal carcinoma (Contreras et al, 1985), as have cis-platin and etoposide (Johnson and Greco, 1986).

Thus, drugs such as mitotane, ketoconazole, metyrapone,

and aminoglutethimide may help relieve the devastating symptoms of glucocorticoid or mineralocorticoid excess. Little evidence exists, however, that survival is extended in most cases.

Transarterial embolization has been reported to achieve partial remission of symptoms in a patient with metastatic disease (Koh et al, 1991).

ADRENAL CYSTS

These are usually unilateral lesions discovered incidentally during imaging procedures or surgery and at autopsy. Calci-

fications may be found in approximately 15% of cases and need not imply malignancy. Endothelial or lymphangiomatous cysts account for nearly 45% of these lesions and are usually small, measuring 0.1 to 1.5 cm in diameter. Adrenal pseudocysts that lack an epithelial lining are the next most common variety (39%) and most likely represent encapsulated residua of previous adrenal hemorrhages. Pseudocysts may become massive and may cause symptoms because of the compression of adjacent structures (Fig. 96–35). The acute hemorrhage in the case shown was readily distinguished by MRI (see Fig. 96–35). Parasitic cysts owing to

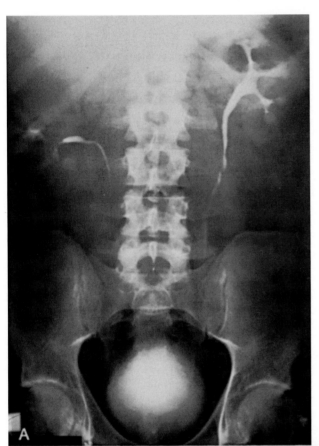

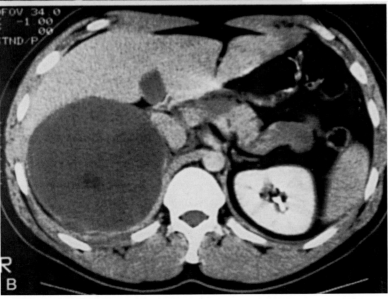

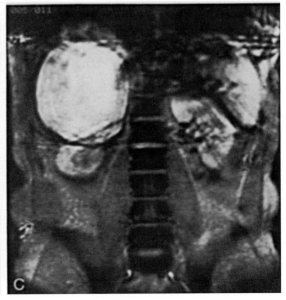

Figure 96–35. *A,* Massive right adrenal cyst. The patient presented with fever, pain, and anemia. *B,* Computed tomography scan of cyst. *C,* Bright hemorrhage into the lumen, cyst proved at exploration, shown on magnetic resonance image.

echinococcal disease (7%) and true epithelial cysts (9%) account for the remainder of adrenal cysts (Kazam et al, 1989; Sroujieh et al, 1990).

ADRENAL INSUFFICIENCY

Adrenal insufficiency is rarely encountered in the practice of urology. Because it is potentially fatal if not recognized, the salient features of the entity are worthy of review.

Addison's disease is rare, the death rate being approximately 0.3 per 100,000 with the most common cause being either tuberculosis or adrenal atrophy (Dunlop, 1963; Irvine and Barnes, 1972; Eason et al, 1982). Other causes include malignant infiltration (Cedermark et al, 1977), sarcoidosis (Rickards and Barrett, 1954; Irvine and Barnes, 1972), histoplasmosis (Crispel et al, 1956), North American blastomycosis (Fish et al, 1960), South American blastomycosis (Osa et al, 1981), and coccidioidomycosis (Moloney, 1952). The general term *adrenal atrophy* actually refers to a pathologic process of lymphocytic adenitis with fibrosis (Maisey and Stevens, 1969). From a clinical point of view, however, symptoms of adrenal insufficiency usually appear in hospitalized patients in whom a history of the long-term use of exogenous steroids has not been obtained and acute withdrawal from steroids has occurred. Adrenal insufficiency may be an important aspect of the care of a patient with cancer and may be due to replacement of the adrenals with metastases, infiltration with lymphoma, hemorrhagic necrosis in association with anticoagulation, or sepsis as well as impaired adrenal steroidogenesis in patients receiving aminoglutethimide, ketoconazole, mitotane, or suramin (Ihde et al, 1990).

The symptoms and signs of chronic adrenal insufficiency are nonspecific and may be associated with numerous other diseases (Table 96–8). Similarly, abnormalities determined with routine laboratory tests are also nonspecific. The most common abnormalities are hyponatremia and hyperkalemia, with at least one electrolyte abnormality being found in 99 of 108 patients in one series (Nerup, 1974). The classic triad of hyponatremia, hyperkalemia, and azotemia was present in only 50% to 60% of cases. Hypercalcemia may also be an initial abnormality. Other endocrine disorders, including hyperthyroidism or hypothyroidism (17%), diabetes mellitus (12%), gonadal dysfunction (12%), and hypothyroidism (5%), occur in about 10% to 30% of patients with Addison's disease (May et al, 1989).

The symptoms of acute adrenal insufficiency "crisis," usually due to withdrawal of exogenous steroids, sepsis, bilateral adrenal hemorrhage, or postadrenalectomy, differ somewhat from those of Addison's disease, particularly fever, which occurs in 70% of patients (see Table 96–8) (Liu et al, 1982). Abdominal pain is also often present and may be due to unilateral or bilateral adrenal hemorrhage, which can be diagnosed by CT (Liu et al, 1982) or MRI (Falke et al, 1987).

The critical test to confirm the presence of Addison's disease is the demonstration of a failure to increase plasma (Perkoff et al, 1954) or urinary corticosteroid level into the normal range with ACTH infusions (Renold et al, 1952; Schlaghecke et al, 1992). A provocative test is particularly important because there are numerous reports of patients

Table 96–8. SIGNS AND SYMPTOMS OF CHRONIC ADDISON'S DISEASE AND ACUTE ADRENAL INSUFFICIENCY

Prevalence		Symptom
Number	Percent	
Addison's Disease		
435/462	94	Weakness, tiredness, fatigue
393/438	90	Weight loss
303/351	86	Anorexia
178/268	66	Nausea, vomiting
100/164	61	Unspecified gastrointestinal complaints
35/127	28	Abdominal pain
44/246	18	Diarrhea
15/94	16	Muscle pain
24/168	14	Salt craving
24/166	14	Orthostatic hypotension, dizziness, or syncope
4/33	12	Lethargy, disorientation
Acute Adrenal Insufficiency		
165/165	100	Severe clinical deterioration
98/140	70	Fever
20/31	64	Nausea, vomiting
21/46	46	Abdominal or flank pain
59/165	36	Hypotension
9/28	32	Abdominal distention
25/96	26	Lethargy, obtundation
55/122	45	Hyponatremia
21/83	25	Hyperkalemia

From May ME, Vaughan ED Jr, Carey RM: Adrenocortical insufficiency—clinical aspects. *In* Vaughan ED Jr, Carey RM, eds: Adrenal Disorders. New York, Thieme Medical Publishers, 1989.

with primary adrenal insufficiency having normal-based plasma cortisol or urinary 17-hydroxycorticoid levels (May et al, 1989). Plasma ACTH levels may be markedly elevated, but such an assay is not always available. The simplest screening test is the rapid ACTH test, whereby plasma cortisol levels are measured before and 60 minutes after 0.25 mg of cosyntropin is given intravenously; cortisol levels should be greater than 18 μg/dl at 60 minutes (Fig. 96–36) (Speckard et al, 1971). Alternatively, 100 μg of human CRH can be used (Schlaghecke et al, 1992). A patient with a relative or an absolute lack of ACTH may respond normally to cosyntropin but not respond properly to surgical stress (Jasani et al, 1968; Kehlet and Binder, 1973). Most of these patients, however, tolerate surgical stress without steroid coverage. If treatment is mandated in a patient with suspected adrenal insufficiency, the ACTH stimulation test can be performed when treatment is with the synthetic steroid dexamethasone (Sheridan and Mattingly, 1975). Other more definitive but more complex and longer infusion tests also can be used (Dolan and Carey, 1989).

The treatment of acute or chronic adrenal insufficiency is obviously the acute administration of glucocorticoids. In acute adrenal crisis, stress level dexamethasone (8–12 mg/day) is given along with replacement saline (Smith and Byrne, 1981) and a simultaneous ACTH stimulation test to confirm the diagnosis (Sheridan and Mattingly, 1975) (Table 96–9).

The treatment of chronic Addison's disease is maintenance therapy—approximately 30 mg of hydrocortisone plus 0.05 to 0.1 μg fluorohydrocortisone per day orally or a synthetic steroid (Table 96–10).

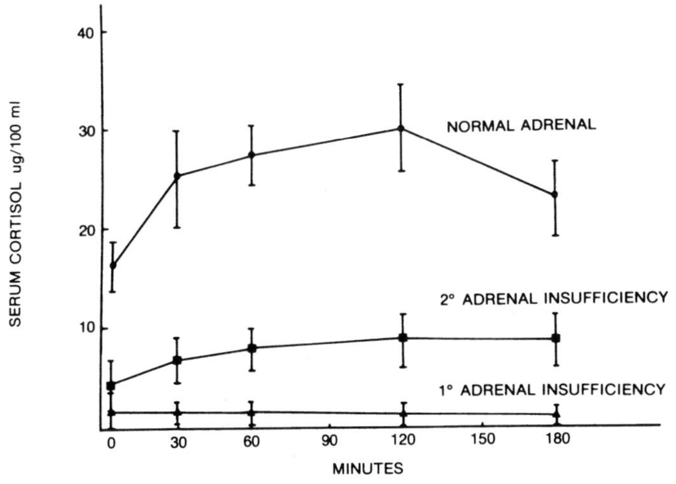

Figure 96–36. Serum cortisol response and response to ACTH infusion in normal persons and in patients with primary and secondary adrenal insufficiency and adrenal insufficiency. (From Vaughan ED Jr, Carey RM, eds: Adrenal Disorders. New York, Thieme Medical Publishers, 1989.)

Replacement therapy following unilateral adrenalectomy is discussed elsewhere. The same guidelines pertain, however, and it is helpful to maintain patients on dexamethasone so that the ACTH test can be used to follow the recovery of the contralateral gland.

Selective Adrenal Insufficiency

Selective hypoaldosteronism is rare and usually is due to hyporeninemia or functional "hypoaldosteronism" caused by tubular insensitivity to normal aldosterone levels (Schambelan et al, 1972; Williams et al, 1983). The urologist occasionally observes this phenomenon in an adult or a child who exhibits unexplained hyperkalemia following relief of

Table 96–9. TREATMENT OF ADRENAL CRISIS

Emergency Treatment

Establish 19-gauge IV line. Obtain stat serum electrolytes, glucose, cortisol, and plasma ACTH. Do not wait for results

Infuse 2–3 L 0.9% saline solution (154 mmol/L) or 5% dextrose (50 g/L) in 0.9% saline solution as quickly as possible. Monitor for fluid overload by observing central or peripheral venous pressure or listening for pulmonary rales. Reduce infusion rate if indicated

Inject 4 mg dexamethasone sodium phosphate (Decadron) IV at beginning of IV infusion or give 100 mg hydrocortisone sodium succinate (Solu-Cortef) or hydrocortisone sodium phosphate (Hydrocortone) IV and 100 mg every 8 hours thereafter

Provide supportive measures as needed

Mineralocorticoids are unnecessary; ACTH is useless

Subacute Treatment After Stabilization of Patient

Continue IV infusion of 0.9% saline solution at a lower rate for 24–48 hours as needed

Search for and treat, if possible, precipitating cause of adrenal crisis

In patient not known to have Addison's disease, and if not already done, perform short ACTH stimulation test to confirm diagnosis of adrenal insufficiency

Taper glucocorticoid to maintenance dosage over 1–3 days if precipitating or complicating disease permits

Begin or resume mineralocorticoid replacement with fludrocortisone (Florinef) 0.1 mg orally daily when saline infusion is stopped

IV, Intravenous; ACTH, adrenocorticotropic hormone.
From Magiakou MA, Chrousos GP: Corticosteroid therapy, nonendocrine disease, and corticosteroid withdrawal. In Bardin CW, ed: Current Therapy in Endocrinology and Metabolism, 5th ed. St. Louis, C.V. Mosby, 1994, p 120.

chronic obstructive uropathy, especially in association with azotemia (Schambelan et al, 1980; Pelleya et al, 1983; Kozeny et al, 1986).

Other selective hypoaldosteronism may occur from primary disturbances of the zona glomerulosa, endogenous impairment of AII production (Findling et al, 1987), or aldosterone receptor deficiency (Armanini et al, 1985). Congenital primary hypoaldosteronism may be sporadic or familial (May et al, 1989).

Selective familial glucocorticoid deficiency has been well described, almost totally in the pediatric literature (May et al, 1989). The clinical presentation is dominated by recurrent hypoglycemia, both fasting and reactive with subsequent seizures. The children usually have normal findings of electrolytes, which often delays the proper diagnosis.

PRIMARY HYPERALDOSTERONISM

The term *primary hyperaldosteronism* was originally coined by Conn (1955a, 1955b) to describe the clinical syndrome characterized by hypertension, hypokalemia, hypernatremia, alkalosis, and periodic paralysis caused by an aldosterone-secreting adenoma. As precise methodology for quantifying the components of the RAAS has become available, the syndrome of primary hyperaldosteronism is now identified by the combined findings of hypokalemia, suppressed PRA, and high urinary and plasma aldosterone levels in hypertensive patients. Moreover, the term *primary aldosteronism* should be extended to contain a family of adrenal forms of hyperaldosteronism, including but not exclusive to adrenal adenomas (Biglieri et al, 1990; Brownie, 1990).

Addison (1855) first associated the syndrome of weakness, prostration, dehydration, and coma to adrenal insufficiency. Subsequently, Loeb (1933) demonstrated renal sodium wastage in patients with Addison's disease and in dogs with adrenal insufficiency as well as the therapeutic effect of sodium replacement.

The first demonstration by Hench and associates, in 1949, that cortisol administration restored sodium balance and initiated kaliuresis as well as reversing characteristics of glucocorticoid deficiency led to the hypothesis that cortisol was the sole and omnipotent adrenal cortical hormone. The vari-

Table 96–10. COMPARISON OF HALF-LIFE AND BILOGIC ACTIVITY OF VARIOUS NATURAL AND SYNTHETIC STEROIDS

Compound	Biologic Half-Life (h)	Plasma Half-Life (h)	Equivalent Dose (mg)	Relative Sodium-Retaining Activity
Cortisone*	8–12	0.5	25	0.8
Cortisol (hydrocortisone)	8–12	1.5	20	1.0
Prednisone*	12–36	1	5	0.8
Prednisolone	12–36	2–4	5	0.8
6-Alpha-methylprednisolone	12–36	1–3	4	0.5
Dexamethasone	36–72	2–3	0.75	0–2
Betamethasone	36–72		0.60	0
Deoxycorticosterone†			0	20
9-Alpha-fluorohydrocortisone			2	125–400
Aldosterone		0.2	0.1	400

*Require hepatic metabolism for bioactivity.
†Inactivated on oral administration.
From May ME, Vaughan ED Jr, Carey RM: Adrenocortical insufficiency—clinical aspects. In Vaughan ED Jr, Carey RM, eds: Adrenal Disorders. New York, Thieme Medical Publishers, 1989.

ances among glucocorticoid excess, Cushing's syndrome, and toxicity from excess administration of the mineralocorticoid 11-deoxycorticosterone, however, led Luetscher and associates to search for the presence of another steroid. Such activity was demonstrated in large amounts in patients exhibiting renal sodium retention (Deming and Luetscher, 1950; Luetscher and Johnson, 1954). This substance also exhibited sodium-retaining activity in adrenalectomized rats. At about the same time, Simpson and associates began a series of studies that were to culminate in the isolation and identification of 18-oxycorticosterone, electrocortin, or aldosterone (Simpson et al, 1954). The clinical impact of this information is best described in Conn's own words (Conn, 1977):

In April, 1954, a 34-year-old female patient with a bizarre constellation of clinical and laboratory manifestations was presented to me on ward rounds. They included periodic paralysis, intermittent muscular weakness, episodic tetanic manifestations, polydipsia and nocturnal polyuria, headache, hypertension, positive Chvostek and Trousseau signs, hypokalemia, hypernatremia, alkalosis, alkaline urine with mild proteinuria, and a ward note suggesting a diagnosis of hyperventilation tetany.

Although that morning at the bedside I made the correct diagnosis, namely, excessive activity of the, then, newly described adrenal steroid, electrocortin, I was not unaware of the raised eyebrows and of the slow to-and-fro motion of the heads of my staff. It required 8 months of continuous metabolic study of that patient to put all the multiple manifestations satisfactorily into the syndrome that I then called "primary aldosteronism." It was only then that I mounted sufficient courage to request adrenal exploration for indications that had never before been employed. My head rang with the objections of my associates: "What if it turns out to be simple potassium-losing nephritis?" But it did not turn out that way and, with time, the so-called potassium-losing nephritis has turned out, in most cases, to be primary aldosteronism.

Pathophysiology

The normal physiology of the RAAS including the stimuli for aldosterone release has been reviewed in Chapters 7 and 11. When aldosterone is secreted in amounts inappropriately high for the state of sodium balance, there is additional sodium reabsorption by the distal nephron (O'Neil, 1990; Verrey, 1990). Extracellular sodium is increased and is ac-

companied by water so that isotonicity is maintained. **Mild increases in serum sodium may occur, and accompanying hypokalemia and mild alkalosis are characteristic.** The sodium accumulation is usually gradual and is dependent on the availability of sodium and the degree of hyperaldosteronism. After a gain of about 1.5 kg of extracellular fluid, however, there is diminished proximal tubular reabsorption of sodium, and the phenomenon of *renal escape* occurs (Espiner et al, 1967). The mechanism of renal escape remains unclear, but there appears to be decreased sodium reabsorption at sites not responsible for the initial sodium reabsorption. Escape is associated with increased renal arterial pressure and increased ANF, which may play critical roles (Haas and Knox, 1990; Rocco et al, 1990; Atlas and Maack, 1991). This limitation of sodium retention explains the characteristic clinical findings in patients with primary aldosteronism of mild hypertension, the rarity of malignant hypertension, and the absence of edema.

In contrast to the escape from further aldosterone-induced sodium retention, there is no escape from potassium loss. In addition, aldosterone increases potassium secretion from all sites in which it enhances sodium absorption: renal tubule, sweat and salivary glands, and intestine. Hence, overactivity of aldosterone can be determined by analyzing salivary electrolyte content (Wotman et al, 1970) or transluminal potential differences across the intestine (Carey et al, 1974). Aldosterone also increases renal tubular secretion of hydrogen ion, which escapes mainly as ammonium ion. The alkalosis that ensues appears to correlate with the degree of potassium depletion. Taken together, these physiologic derangements explain the clinical and biochemical findings of patients with hyperaldosteronism. At the present time, however, the clinical syndrome as first described by Conn is rarely observed because physicians are more suspicious of this entity in hypertensive patients and now usually establish the diagnosis and treatment earlier in the evolution of the disease.

As the understanding of adrenal physiology, biochemistry, histopathology, and molecular biology and genetics has advanced, it has become evident that there are distinct subsets of the primary hyperaldosteronism syndrome. Reports from several centers indicate that the majority of patients with primary aldosteronism can have hypertension and related metabolic abnormalities ameliorated by unilateral adrenalectomy (Bravo et al, 1988; Irony et al, 1990; Blumenfeld et al, 1994). **Patients who are most likely to respond favorably to surgery are those in whom aldosterone production is autonomous** (see under Diagnostic Studies). **Among the features that identify autonomy are (1) limited stimulation of aldosterone production by maneuvers that increase angiotensin II levels (e.g., angiotensin infusion or postural stimulation) or decrease angiotensin II levels (e.g., saline infusion or angiotensin converting enzyme inhibition), (2) increased levels of aldosterone biosynthetic precursors (e.g., 18-hydroxycorticosterone-to-cortisol ratio), and (3) elevated levels of unusual steroids (e.g., urinary C-18 cortisol methyloxygenated metabolites [18-hydroxycortisol and 18-oxocortisol])** (Biglieri et al, 1995). Identifying patients with these diagnostic features has important implications for determining clinical management and for predicting response to treatment (see Treatment, following).

The response of PRA to the aldosterone-induced sodium retention and blood pressure elevation is the cornerstone of early diagnosis of the entity (Fig. 96–37). Accordingly the normal renal juxtaglomerular responses to increased blood pressure (the baroreceptor mechanism) and the increased distal delivery of sodium chloride (the macula densa mechanism) result in suppression of PRA (Conn et al, 1964; Laragh and Sealey, 1992; Briggs et al, 1995). Moreover, the PRA remains low even in the presence of sodium depletion or acute furosemide administration (Spark and Melby, 1968; Carey et al, 1972; Weinberger et al, 1979). This observation is in marked contrast to the elevated PRA seen in patients with secondary aldosteronism, usually caused by renal arterial or parenchymal disease. In this last clinical setting, the oversecretion of aldosterone is secondary to the excess production of angiotensin II, stimulating the adrenal zona glomerulosa (see Chapter 11).

The ability to measure urinary and plasma aldosterone has given further insight to abnormalities of aldosterone secretion (Dolan and Carey, 1989). Hence, the oversecretion of aldosterone is not suppressed by sodium loading (Espiner et al, 1967; Weinberger et al, 1979) as in healthy subjects. Conversely, with ambulation, patients with an aldosterone-producing adenoma (APA) do not exhibit the characteristic rise in aldosterone secretion found in healthy subjects, and there may be a paradoxical fall in plasma aldosterone levels (Herf et al, 1979; Ganguly et al, 1981). These observations highlight the autonomous secretion that is present in patients with APA and begin to highlight the differences in the pathophysiology of APA and idiopathic adrenal hyperplasia (Fontes et al, 1991; Biglieri et al, 1995).

In a subset of APAs, aldosterone production is stimulated by the RAAS, as determined by AII infusion and postural stimulation (Gordon et al, 1987). Gordon and colleagues found that shortly after adrenalectomy AII infusion no longer stimulated aldosterone release, suggesting that the adenoma was the sole source of aldosterone. This variant, referred to as AII-responsive (AII-R) APA, has other unique biochemical and histologic features (Tunny et al, 1991). In contrast to the typical APA, which is unresponsive to angiotensin (AII-U APA) and in which there is overproduction of cortisol C-18-oxygenated metabolites (i.e., 18-oxocortisol, 18-hydroxycortisol), AII-R APA is not associated with increased levels of these hybrid steroids. In addition, plasma cortisol levels were suppressible in AII-U APA but not in AII-R APA. These findings, together with earlier reports, indicate that autonomous overproduction of cortisol occurs from some aldosterone-producing adenomas (Imai et al, 1991). These heterogeneous biochemical responses are consistent with the histologic characteristics: AII-U APA consisted predominantly of fasciculata-like cells, whereas AII-R APA were primarily composed of glomerulosa-like cells. Tunny and co-workers found a reciprocal relationship between the increment in plasma aldosterone during AII infusion and the percentage of fasciculata-type cells in the adenoma and concluded that the aldosterone responsiveness to AII was related to the predominant tumor cell type (Tunny et al, 1991).

Biglieri and associates (1995) have characterized a subset of patients with autonomous aldosterone production in whom an adrenal adenoma could be not identified (Banks et al, 1984; Irony et al, 1990). This variant has been referred to as *primary adrenal hyperplasia* (PAH). The adrenal glands in PAH are hyperplastic, frequently with a dominant nodule. As in patients with AII-R APAs, aldosterone production in PAH is autonomous. Furthermore, correction of the metabolic abnormalities and hypertension in this subset occurs after unilateral adrenalectomy.

Adrenal carcinoma is an extremely rare cause of primary aldosteronism (Arteaga et al, 1984; Isles et al, 1987). Aldosterone production is autonomous, with high levels causing severe hypokalemia. In contrast to benign APA, malignant tumors are larger (>3 cm), have internal calcification that is

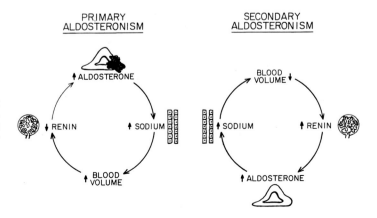

Figure 96–37. Hyperaldosteronism may be seen in association with elevated (secondary) or depressed (primary) levels of plasma renin activity. In primary aldosteronism, an adrenal neoplasm or bilateral hyperplasia is the initiating event. Secondary aldosteronism is most commonly seen in edematous disorders (e.g., cirrhosis, renal failure), in which the elevated renin levels are a physiologic adjustment to a contracted blood volume; it is also present in renal artery stenosis, secondary to the stimulus of elevated levels of renin and angiotensin II.

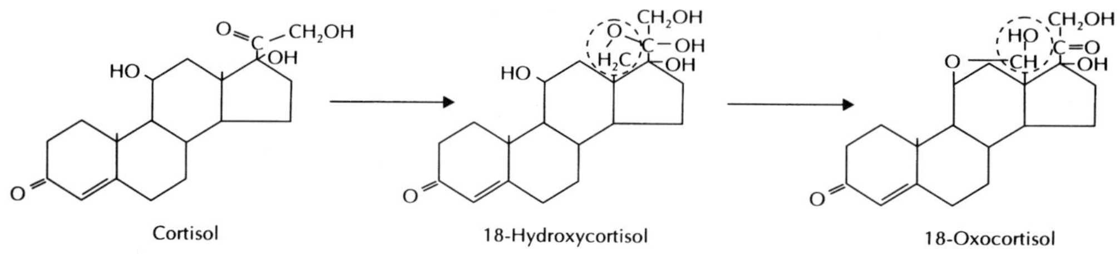

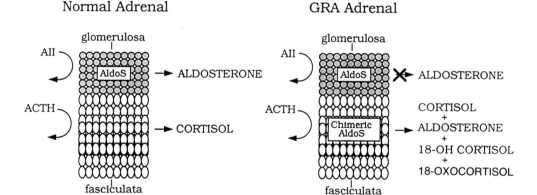

Figure 96–38. Biosynthesis of the C-18 methyloxygenation metabolites of cortisol. (From Blumenfeld JD: Curr Opin Nephrol Hypertens 1993;2:274. Copyright Rapid Science Publishers.)

Cortisol   18-Hydroxycortisol   18-Oxocortisol

evident on CT scan, and may produce excess amounts of androgens and cortisol. The pathogenesis of adrenal nodular hyperplasia remains uncertain, but the fact that the lesions are bilateral suggests the presence of some stimulus other than AII or ACTH inducing adrenal hyperplasia and hyperaldosteronism.

Less common disorders associated with bilateral adrenal hyperplasia and hyperaldosteronism have been identified and characterized (Blumenfeld, 1993; Biglieri et al, 1995). One example is glucocorticoid remediable aldosteronism (GRA), an autosomal dominant form of mineralocorticoid hypertension in which aldosterone biosynthesis is regulated by ACTH, rather than the RAAS (Sutherland et al, 1966; Lifton et al, 1992). Clinical features include early-onset hypertension, which may be complicated by cerebral hemorrhage or aortic dissection, and a strong family history of hypertension. The most common, routine laboratory finding is a low plasma renin activity level, although other evidence of aldosterone excess may be absent (e.g., 24-hour urine aldosterone levels, hypokalemia, metabolic alkalosis [Rich et al, 1992]). A key diagnostic feature is the overproduction of the C-18 cortisol-aldosterone structural hybrids, 18-hydroxycortisol and 18-oxocortisol, which are formed when cortisol is accepted by aldosterone synthase (P-450$_{C18}$) as a substrate for methyloxidation (Ulick and Chan, 1989) (Fig. 96–38). Normally, this enzyme is expressed predominantly in the glomerular zone (White, 1994). Based on these biochemical features and hyperplasia of the fascicular zone characteristic of GRA, Ulick and associates proposed that the fascicular zone acquires P-450$_{C18}$ activity, thereby abrogating the normal zonation of adrenal function (Ulick and Chan, 1989; Ulick et al, 1992). This hypothesis was supported by the finding of a chimeric P-450$_{11β}$/P-450$_{C18}$ gene that arose from unequal crossing over between the 5' regulatory region of P-450$_{11β}$ and the coding sequences of P-450$_{C18}$ (Lifton et al, 1992) (Fig. 96–39). This hybrid gene can catalyze the termi-

nal methyloxidation reactions required for aldosterone synthesis but is regulated as the P-450$_{11β}$ by ACTH instead of the RAAS. Furthermore, because of its aberrant expression in the fascicular zone, the enzymatic product of this chimeric gene uses cortisol as a substrate for C-18 oxidation to the cortisol-aldosterone hybrid steroids. Treatment of this syndrome with low doses of exogenous glucocorticoid inhibits ACTH secretion, suppresses aldosterone production, normalizes PRA, and consequently corrects the hypertension and other metabolic abnormalities.

GRA is a rare disorder. When elevated urinary levels of 18-hydroxycortisol and 18-oxocortisol were used to screen the relatives of a proband, however, 11 previously undiagnosed patients spanning three generations were discovered (Rich et al, 1992). All affected adults were hypertensive before age 20 years and had lower PRA than their unaffected family members. Surprisingly, none of those affected were hypokalemic, and their urinary aldosterone excretion overlapped with the unaffected group. Thus, a diagnostic test for this disorder is a 24-hour urine collection demonstrating overproduction of cortisol C-18 oxidation metabolites. One implication from that study is that GRA is more common than previously considered, with some affected patients diagnosed incorrectly as having essential hypertension (Rich et al, 1992).

Gordon and colleagues have described a familial form of primary aldosteronism (termed FHII), distinct from GRA (FHI), in which aldosterone production was not suppressed by exogenous glucocorticoid (Gordon et al, 1992). The FHII group was not defined by a common histologic presentation and included family members with AII-R APA, AII-U APA, and bilateral hypersecretion of aldosterone. These investigators have proposed that a genetic basis exists for all forms of primary aldosteronism (Stowasser et al, 1991). According to this hypothesis, cortisol-aldosterone hybrid steroids are overproduced in AII-U APA, in which a gene mutation is

Normal Adrenal   GRA Adrenal

glomerulosa

AII

AldoS → ALDOSTERONE

ACTH

→ CORTISOL

fasciculata

glomerulosa

AII

AldoS ✗ ALDOSTERONE

ACTH

Chimeric AldoS

→ CORTISOL
+
ALDOSTERONE
+
18-OH CORTISOL
+
18-OXOCORTISOL

fasciculata

Figure 96–39. Adrenal cortex responsiveness to ACTH and angiotensin II in normal subjects and in glucocorticoid remediable aldosteronism (GRA). (From Lifton RP, Dluhy RG, Powers M, et al: Nature Genet 1992;2:66–74.)

Table 96–11. AGE DISTRIBUTION OF 266 TUMORS OF THE ADRENAL CORTEX IN HYPERALDOSTERONISM WITH LOW PLASMA RENIN

Adrenal Changes (No. of Cases)	Sex	Age (Years)							Total
		15–20	*21–30*	*31–40*	*41–50*	*51–60*	*61–70*	*>70*	
Adenoma (241)	Female	6	16	59	67	17	5	1	171
	Male	2	7	20	28	9	3	1	70
Carcinomas (25)	Female	—	2	5	3	5	1	—	16
	Male	—	1	4	1	2	1	—	9

From Neville AM, O'Hare MJ: The Human Adrenal Cortex: Pathology and Biology—An Integrated Approach. New York, Springer-Verlag, 1982.

present with features similar to that of GRA. This hypothesis is not supported by the report that the chimeric CYP11B1/CYP11B2 gene was not present in a series of APAs (Fallo et al, 1995). The specific C-18 methyloxygenated cortisol metabolites, however, were not measured in that study.

Clinical Characteristics

Primary aldosteronism is relatively uncommon, occurring in only about 1% of the hypertensive population, with APAs being more prevalent than nonadenomatous adrenal hyperplasia. The clinical findings in patients with this syndrome are primarily due to the increased total body sodium content and deficit in total body potassium (Ferriss et al, 1978) (see Chapter 7). Symptoms include, in approximate order of frequency, nocturia, urinary frequency, muscular weakness, frontal headaches, polydipsia, paresthesias, visual disturbances, temporary paralysis, cramps, and tetany. If the patient is normokalemic, these characteristic symptoms are usually mild or absent. Renal potassium wasting is attenuated during sodium restriction, and the observant patient may recognize that he or she feels better when eating a low-salt diet (Pedrinelli et al, 1988) (see Chapter 7).

An adenoma is more likely to occur in younger patients and in women. The age and gender distribution of 266 tumors in patients with hyperaldosteronism is shown in Table 96–11 (Neville and O'Hare, 1982). The weights and sites of adrenal adenomas and adrenal carcinomas is shown in Table 96–12. The genetic basis for one hereditary form of primary aldosteronism, GRA, has been established and is now being reported with increasing frequency because efficient screening methods are available (see earlier) (Lifton et al, 1992). Whether there is a hereditary pattern for APAs is less well established (Gordon et al, 1992).

Patients with primary aldosterone excess are not edematous because sodium retention in this syndrome is limited by the *mineralocorticoid escape* phenomenon (Nakada et al, 1989) (see Chapter 7). Patients with an adenoma, however, usually have more extensive manifestations of mineralocorticoid excess than those with hyperplasia, including more severe hypertension (Ferriss et al, 1978; Blumenfeld et al, 1994). The physical examination is not usually distinguishable from essential hypertension, unless hypokalemia is severe. Malignant hypertension occurs rarely (Tarazi et al, 1973).

APA is the most common cause of primary aldosteronism (Weinberger, 1979; Bravo et al, 1983; Melby, 1984; Quinn et al, 1990; Gleason et al, 1993). In a review of 82 patients with primary aldosteronism followed at the New York Hospital–Cornell Medical Center, Blumenfeld and colleagues found that 63% had APAs (Blumenfeld et al, 1994). Additional diagnostic studies were performed in 56 patients (34 adenoma, 22 hyperplasia) after antihypertensive medications were withdrawn. In that study, patients with an adenoma had significantly higher systolic (184 versus 161 mm Hg) and diastolic (112 versus 105 mm Hg) pressures than those with hyperplasia. Systolic blood pressure was 175 mm Hg or greater in 66% with adenoma, compared with only 15% with hyperplasia. Diastolic pressure was 114 mm Hg or greater in 50% of patients with adenoma, compared with only 19% of those in the hyperplasia group. There was a direct relationship (r = 0.58) between the urinary aldosterone excretion rate and the mean arterial pressure among the adenoma patients.

In contrast to the escape from sodium retention that occurs

Table 96–12. HYPERALDOSTERONISM

Weights of 151 Adrenal Adenomas			Weights of 25 Adrenal Carcinomas	
Weight (g)	*No.*	*Percent*	*Weight (g)*	*No.*
<2	51	(34)	<30	1
2–4	36	(24)	30–100	5
4–5	16	(11)	100–200	3
5–10	26	(17)	200–500	4
10–20	11	(7)	500–1000	6
20–30	3	(3.5)	1000–2000	5
>30	8	(3.5)	>2000	1
Total	151	(100)		

Site Distribution of Adrenal Adenomas in 218 Patients

	No. of Patients		
Site	*Male*	*Female*	*Total*
Single			
Right adrenal	22	37	59
Left adrenal	25	70	95
Bilateral	2	1	3
Unknown	14	40	54
Subtotal	63 (91%)	148 (93%)	201 (92%)
Multiple			
Right adrenal	4	2	6
Left adrenal	1	8	9
Bilateral	1	1	2
Unknown	—	—	—
Subtotal	6 (9%)	11 (7%)	17 (8%)
Total	69 (30%)	159 (70%)	218 (100%)

From Neville AM, O'Hare MJ: The Human Adrenal Cortex: Pathology and Biology—An Integrated Approach. New York, Springer-Verlag, 1982.

in this syndrome, aldosterone-mediated renal secretion of potassium is persistent and causes total body potassium deficit, hypokalemia, and related symptoms (Ferriss et al, 1978). In the Cornell study, serum potassium levels were significantly lower in the adenoma patients (3.0 versus 3.5 mEq/L). Levels below 2.8 mEq/L occurred in 44% of the adenoma group compared with only 6% of the group with hyperplasia (Fig. 96–40). The profound hypokalemia that occurs in patients with an adenoma contributes to the more marked metabolic alkalosis, indicated by the higher plasma carbon dioxide level, observed in this and other studies. Conversely, 18% of the hyperplasia group had a serum potassium concentration above 3.5 mEq/L compared with only 6% of those with an adenoma. Several previous studies have also reported normal serum potassium levels in approximately 20% of patients with primary aldosteronism (Conn, 1967; Bravo, 1983; Melby, 1984), most commonly in patients with adrenal hyperplasia. **Because severe hypokalemia occurs less frequently in patients with restricted dietary sodium intake, the authors do not recommend screening patients for this syndrome unless they are adequately salt loaded** (see under Diagnostic Studies). Normokalemic hyperaldosteronism was recognized by Conn and co-workers, however, and has been reported by others during sodium loading (Conn, 1967; Bravo et al, 1983).

Diagnostic Studies

The diagnostic studies described are designed to accomplish two goals: to screen the large hypertensive population for primary hyperaldosteronism and to distinguish the patients with adrenal adenoma from those with bilateral hyperplasia. The absence of a reliable clinical picture of hyperaldosteronism has led to a battery of tests suggested to

accomplish these goals. The authors' approach is shown in Figure 96–41.

Screening Tests

Certainly unprovoked hypokalemia is the hallmark of hyperaldosteronism, but as already discussed, serum K^+ levels between 3.5 and 4.0 mEq/L are commonly found in patients subsequently proven to have primary aldosteronism. Patients with essential hypertension may exhibit hypokalemia. Monitoring serum K^+ following salt loading lowers the false-negative normokalemic finding, but the entity of normokalemic primary aldosteronism is well recognized (Weinberger et al, 1979; Bravo et al, 1983). In addition, following sodium loading, patients with primary aldosteronism excrete more sodium and potassium in the urine. Adjunctive measurements such as salivary sodium-to-potassium ratios and oral-rectal electrical potential differences are too cumbersome and inaccurate to be used as screening tests (Espiner et al, 1967; Wotman et al, 1970; Christlieb et al, 1971).

A combination of studies is necessary to identify the entity accurately. The first breakthrough followed the ability to determine PRA accurately. In 1964, Conn and associates demonstrated the suppression of PRA in patients with primary aldosteronism. At that time, a major diagnostic dilemma was distinction of patients with primary aldosteronism from patients with excessive secretion of aldosterone secondary to primary renal disease and oversecretion of renin (secondary hyperaldosteronism). This single measurement has survived the test of time as critical to the differentiation of patients with these two disorders (Streeten et al, 1979; Weinberger et al, 1979; Vaughan et al, 1989; McDougal et al, 1990). The test has subsequently been refined by demonstrating that the PRA remains low in patients with primary hyperaldosteronism despite sodium depletion (Baer

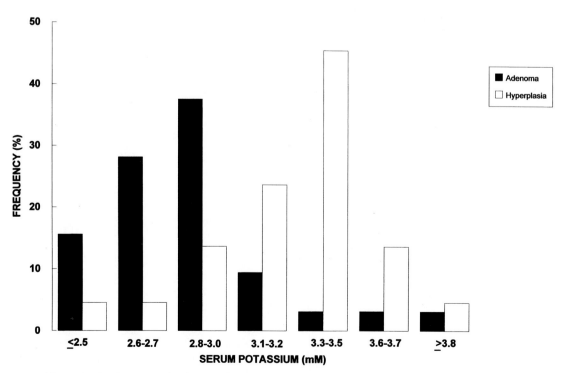

Figure 96–40. Frequency distribution of serum potassium in patients with primary hyperaldosteronism.

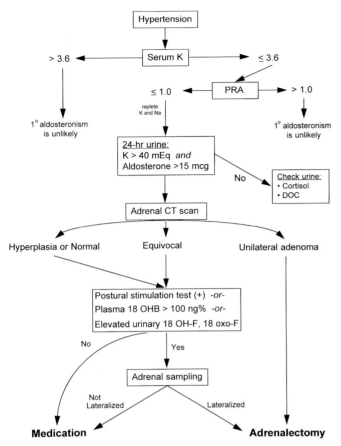

Figure 96–41. Algorithm for the diagnosis and treatment of primary aldosteronism. (From Blumenfeld JD, Schlussel Y, Sealey JE, et al: Ann Intern Med 1994;121:877–885.)

et al, 1970), ambulation (Ganguly et al, 1973), and administration of furosemide (Carey et al, 1972). Twenty-five percent of patients with essential hypertension, however, exhibit low PRA (Brunner et al, 1972). Although most of these patients are normokalemic, additional screening tests are necessary.

The development of an accurate methodology to measure plasma aldosterone has led to accurate screening. **Elevated plasma or urinary aldosterone level indexed against urinary sodium excretion, measured following sodium loading in combination with previously demonstrated low PRA during sodium depletion, is the biochemical hallmark of the entity** (see Fig. 98–14). This measurement does not distinguish patients with APA from those with idiopathic hyperaldosteronism.

ALDOSTERONE-TO-RENIN RATIO. An elevated ratio of plasma aldosterone to PRA is another indicator of autonomous aldosterone secretion that has been proposed as a screening test for primary aldosteronism (Hamlet et al, 1985; Hiramatsu et al, 1991; McKenna et al, 1991), and it may be particularly useful to identify patients with the syndrome who are not hypokalemic (Gordon et al 1992). In the Cornell study, a plasma aldosterone-to-renin ratio greater than 50 (aldosterone ng/dl-to-PRA ng/ml/hour) was more commonly observed in primary aldosteronism than in either essential hypertension or renovascular disease (Blumenfeld et al, 1994). There was considerable overlap, however, be-

tween the hyperplasia and adenoma subsets; therefore, this is not a useful index for differentiating these diagnostic groups. Furthermore, this ratio was not predictive of surgical cure (Blumenfeld et al, 1994).

POSTURE TEST. Stimulation of renin secretion and, in turn, increases in plasma aldosterone levels occur in normal individuals during upright posture (Herf et al, 1979; Laragh and Sealey, 1992). In subsets of primary aldosteronism associated with autonomous aldosterone production, however, including AII-U adenoma and PAH, postural stimulation of aldosterone does not occur (Ganguly et al, 1973; Fontes et al, 1991). The postural stimulation test is conducted by drawing plasma cortisol and aldosterone levels at 8:00 AM with the patient supine after an overnight recumbency and again while upright after 2 to 4 hours of ambulation. In patients with primary aldosteronism with highly autonomous aldosterone production, plasma aldosterone levels *decrease* during this test, reflecting the influence of the diurnal fall in ACTH, which is normally a relatively minor stimulus for aldosterone production (Schambelan et al, 1976). A false-negative response, which might occur during a stress-related increase in ACTH, can be detected if plasma cortisol levels increase during upright posture. By contrast, in patients with idiopathic hyperaldosteronism or AII-R adenoma, aldosterone production increases during upright posture because of the increase in AII formation and increased sensitivity of the zona glomerulosa to AII. In GRA, aldosterone production falls during the test because of the ACTH dependency of aldosterone biosynthesis and may, therefore, lead to an inaccurate diagnosis.

SODIUM LOADING. Sodium-loading maneuvers are useful for identifying patients with primary aldosteronism (Weinberger, 1979; Arteaga et al, 1985). Accordingly, during volume expansion in normal individuals or in patients with essential hypertension, PRA levels decrease, and, consequently, aldosterone secretion falls. In patients with primary aldosteronism, renin secretion is suppressed before salt loading, and, therefore, additional volume expansion does not decrease aldosterone levels to the same extent as in normal subjects or patients with essential hypertension. Several salt-loading protocols have been validated for diagnostic screening, including dietary sodium loading for 3 days ($\geq$200 mEq/day) and oral fludrocortisone (0.4 mg/day) for 5 days. On a high-sodium diet, 24-hour urinary aldosterone excretion is below 10 μg/day in normal individuals but exceeds 14 μg/day in patients with primary hyperaldosteronism (Bravo et al, 1983).

Although these maneuvers are useful for identifying patients with primary aldosteronism, they do not adequately discriminate patients with APAs from those with nonadenomatous adrenal hyperplasia. By contrast, measurement of morning levels of plasma cortisol, aldosterone, and 18-hydroxycorticosterone after intravenous saline loading (1.25–2.0 l over 90–120 minutes) can distinguish these diagnostic subsets: In APA, the ratio of aldosterone to cortisol is greater than 2.2, or 18-hydroxycorticosterone to cortisol is greater than 3, whereas for patients with idiopathic hyperaldosteronism, the ratios are lower (Arteaga et al, 1985). Alternatively, acute sodium depletion after furosemide stimulates renin in normal subjects but not in patients with primary aldosteronism (Weinberger, 1979). On a normal sodium intake, supine morning 18-hydroxycorticosterone level plasma greater than

50 ng/dl is characteristic of primary aldosteronism, and a level 100 ng/dl or greater is diagnostic of aldosteronoma (Biglieri and Schambelan, 1979; Bravo et al, 1983).

CORTISOL METABOLITES. C-18-methyloxygenated metabolites of cortisol, 18-hydroxycortisol and 18-oxocortisol, are increased in primary aldosteronism when it is caused by adenoma but not by nonadenomatous adrenal hyperplasia (Ulick and Chan, 1989; Ulick et al, 1992). This steroid pattern appears to reflect the loss of normal functional zonation of the adrenal gland (see previously). In the Cornell study, two of the adenoma patients with hybrid steroid levels in hyperplasia range also had a negative postural stimulation test, and their blood pressures were improved but not cured by surgery (Blumenfeld et al, 1994). These findings are in accord with a previous report that patients with adenomas who increase aldosterone production during upright posture or infusion of exogenous AII have low levels of these hybrid cortisol metabolites (Gordon et al, 1987).

Lateralizing Tests

APAs are usually small, and they often defied identification by studies such as intravenous pyelography, retroperitoneal air insufflation, and arteriography. The first major advance in this regard followed the demonstration that it was relatively simple to catheterize the adrenal veins for radiocontrast retrograde injection, outlining the venous circulation of the adrenal (Bucht et al, 1964). Obviously, larger tumors are most easily visualized, but clearly many APAs can be visualized by this method. Inaccuracies of venography and reports of inadvertent adrenal infarction, however, led to a search for more accurate tests (Fisher et al, 1971).

The ability to measure plasma aldosterone concentration added a new and highly useful dimension to adrenal vein catheterization (Horton and Finck, 1972; Dunnick et al, 1982; Geisinger et al, 1983). The major problems encountered involve the difficulty in catheterizing the short right adrenal vein, the risk of trauma, the dilution of blood by blood from nonadrenal sources, and the episodic changes in aldosterone secretion coincident with changes in cortisol (Weinberger et al, 1979). Most of these problems can be controlled by careful catheter localization, simultaneous plasma cortisol measurements to document appropriate catheter placement, collecting blood by gravity flow, or collecting during ACTH administration. Weinberger and co-workers have found this last maneuver to increase sensitivity of aldosterone production to such an extent that their technique consistently identified patients with APA (Weinberger et al, 1979).

Adrenal vein sampling of aldosterone remains the cornerstone for localization of aldosterone production. In patients with APA, there is a high aldosterone concentration from the involved gland with contralateral suppression of aldosterone from the normal gland. In contrast, in idiopathic hyperaldosteronism, there is bilateral secretion, albeit asymmetric in some cases. The results of the various lateralizing studies are shown in Table 96–13.

The problems with adrenal vein sampling and the search for a noninvasive test led to the development of a radioiodinated analogue of cholesterol, which concentrated in the adrenal. In 1971, Beirwaltes and colleagues reported visualization of human adrenal glands using ^{131}I-6-iodomethyl-19-

Table 96–13. RESULTS OF LOCALIZATION STUDIES

	Unilateral Adenoma
Blood pressure response to adrenalectomy	
Normotensive	26/38
No change	0/38
Adrenal venography*	16/27
Adrenal scan*	13/28
Adrenal hormones*	35/35
Postural decline in plasma aldosterone*	23/32

*Positive/total.
From Weinberger MH, Grim CE, Hollifield JW, et al: Ann Intern Med 1979; 93:86.

nor-cholesterol. Despite refinements, however, the accuracy of adrenal scanning has been limited by both subjective interpretation and asymmetric uptake in healthy subjects as well as in patients with primary aldosteronism. The unreliability of the test in relation to other modalities as found by Weinberger and co-workers is shown in Table 96–13. Scanning now holds an adjunctive role when other tests are inconclusive and clearly has been superseded by CT (White et al, 1980; Dunnick et al, 1982; Geisinger et al, 1983; Kazam et al, 1989).

The CT scan has evolved as the most accurate anatomic test for adrenal disease. Earlier the small lesions of APA could not be defined by CT, **but further refinements in technology allow a highly accurate identification of APA as small as 1 cm. CT coupled with adrenal venous sampling for plasma aldosterone has become the authors' preferred technique for localization.** In contrast, small adrenal lesions are often not well visualized with adrenal MRI (Newhouse, 1990).

The sensitivity and specificity of these imaging techniques may differ substantially among medical centers, depending on the local resources and expertise. It is important to recognize that incidental, nonfunctioning adrenal masses are relatively common: They are found in 0.6% of all CT scans of the abdomen, and 2% to 9% of adults have grossly visible adenomas at autopsy. Conversely, a subset of patients with surgically curable primary hyperaldosteronism have radiographically normal adrenal glands (Robbins and Cotran, 1979; Glazer et al, 1982; Radin et al, 1992). Therefore, to minimize confusion during diagnostic evaluation, radiographic imaging procedures should be withheld until after biochemical confirmation of primary aldosteronism has been accomplished.

Diagnostic Strategy

The results of diagnostic screening of patients with this syndrome are often ambiguous, especially when the serum potassium level is in the normal range. Relatively simple tests that can improve the diagnostic accuracy include (1) 24-hour urinary aldosterone excretion rate 14 µg or greater, after sodium loading for at least 3 days (urinary sodium content >250 mEq/day [Bravo et al, 1983]); (2) ratio of plasma aldosterone to renin activity greater than 50 (Hiramatsu et al, 1981; Hamlet et al, 1985; Blumenfeld et al, 1994); (3) failure to increase PRA after sodium restriction, furosemide-induced diuresis (Weinberger, 1979); and (4) supine plasma 18-hydroxycorticosterone levels above 50 ng/dl or ratio of plasma 18-hydroxycorticosterone to cortisol greater than 3 after saline infusion (Biglieri et al, 1979; Bravo et al, 1983; Arteaga et al, 1985). Measurements of aldosterone should be performed only after potassium supplementation because aldosterone secretion is attenuated by the potassium deficit and, thus, may obfuscate the diagnosis.

The sensitivity and specificity of each of these diagnostic maneuvers can be adversely influenced by concurrent use of antihypertensive medications. For example, β-adrenoceptor antagonists markedly decrease PRA in essential hypertension and may alter the interpretation of these tests (Buhler et al, 1972; Blumenfeld et al, 1995). Hypokalemia when caused by thiazide diuretics may be difficult to distinguish from primary aldosteronism, although the PRA level is often elevated during diuretic use in patients with essential hypertension (Laragh and Sealey, 1992). Angiotensin converting enzyme inhibitors and calcium channel antagonists reportedly reduce aldosterone biosynthesis and improve hypokalemia in some patients with primary aldosteronism (Melby, 1984; Nadler et al, 1985) (see later). Therefore, antihypertensive medications should be discontinued for at least 2 weeks before diagnostic evaluation and potassium supplements provided to hypokalemic patients. Spironolactone should be discontinued for at least 1 month before these biochemical assessments because it has a long duration of action.

Figure 96–41 is a diagnostic algorithm that can be useful for directing treatment when biochemical screening tests are indicative of primary aldosteronism (Blumenfeld et al, 1994). If a solitary unilateral adrenal mass is identified unequivocally on adrenal CT scan in a patient with biochemical criteria for primary aldosteronism, surgery is indicated. Adrenal vein sampling is not essential, although lateralization of aldosterone secretion confirms the diagnosis and is therefore warranted. **Adrenalectomy should be preceded by several weeks of adequate control of hypertension and correction of hypokalemia and other metabolic abnormalities** (see later).

In the patient with biochemical criteria for primary aldosteronism but with an adrenal CT scan that is normal or indicates hyperplasia, additional evaluation is required because a **subgroup can be cured by unilateral adrenalectomy** (McCleod et al, 1989; Fontes et al, 1991). **Additional diagnostic tests that suggest the potential for surgical cure include a positive postural stimulation test, elevated levels of plasma 18-hydroxycorticosterone and urinary 18-methyloxygenated cortisol metabolites, and lateralization of aldosterone secretion.** If the patient has bilateral aldosterone secretion, a negative postural stimulation test, and low levels of cortisol metabolites, adrenalectomy is not indicated. If secretion is bilateral or sampling is unsuccessful and the ancillary diagnostic tests described previously indicate autonomous aldosterone production, the patient should be treated medically and re-evaluated in 6 to 12 months, including adrenal vein sampling.

Treatment

The cornerstone of medical therapy in primary aldosteronism caused by bilateral hyperplasia is spironolactone (Aldactone), a competitive antagonist of the aldosterone receptor. The efficacy of this drug relates to the reduction in plasma volume in disorders associated with aldosterone excess. Although a favorable blood pressure response to spironolactone has been associated with improved chances of surgical cure, it does not reliably predict outcome (Bravo et al, 1988). Amiloride can also effectively lower blood pressure and correct hypokalemia in patients with gynecomastia or other side effects associated with spironolactone. The dihydropyridine calcium channel antagonists can acutely decrease blood pressure and aldosterone secretion in patients with this syndrome (Melby, 1984; Nadler et al, 1985). Other studies of longer duration, however, have failed to demonstrate these beneficial effects when nifedipine was used as monotherapy (Bravo et al, 1986; Bursztyn et al, 1988). Angiotensin converting enzyme inhibitors have been reported to treat successfully some patients with hyperplasia in whom aldosterone production is not completely autonomous from A-II stimulation (Melby, 1984). Phentolamine did not acutely reduce blood pressure; therefore, a role for alpha-adrenergic receptor blockade has not been established (Bravo et al, 1985). Nevertheless, long-term treatment with prazosin is effective in low-renin essential hypertension, suggesting that alpha-adrenergic receptor antagonists may have an ancillary role in the treatment of primary aldosteronism (Bolli et al, 1980).

Subsets of patients with primary aldosteronism who demonstrate autonomous aldosterone production should be managed with excision of the adrenal gland containing the adenoma or, in the case of nonadenomatous adrenal hyperplasia, the gland from which aldosterone secretion is predominant. This rationale is based on the observation that both the metabolic abnormalities and the hypertension are alleviated by unilateral adrenalectomy in a vast majority of these patients. By contrast, patients with idiopathic hyperaldosteronism usually do not have significant improvement in hypertension after unilateral or bilateral adrenalectomy.

In the Cornell study, blood pressure decreased below 140/90 mm Hg postoperatively, *without concurrent antihypertensive medication* in 35% of patients with an adenoma (Blumenfeld et al, 1994). These patients were designated as cured. Postoperatively, hypertension improved in another 55.8% in the adenoma group, with blood pressure decreasing to 140/90 mm Hg or lower in 60% after medication was added following adrenalectomy. **Thus, hypertension was either cured or improved to an acceptable target in more than 90% of the patients with an adenoma.** By contrast, hypertension was more difficult to control in patients with an adenoma who were unable or unwilling to have an adrenalectomy.

Of the eight patients with nonadenomatous hyperplasia who underwent adrenalectomy, three were cured and one was improved. When data were pooled from those adenoma and hyperplasia patients who were cured by adrenalectomy, they were found to be significantly younger than those who required antihypertensive medication postoperatively (43 versus 54 years). Streeten and colleagues also reported that hypertension persisted after adrenalectomy in patients older than 50 years at the time of surgery (Streeten et al, 1990).

In the Cornell study, preoperative renin system activity was an important predictor of blood pressure outcome. Cured patients had lower pretreatment PRA levels (0.17 versus 0.50 ng/ml/hour) than those who were not cured. Furthermore, in cured patients, there was also a correlation between the preoperative urinary aldosterone excretion and the relative decrease in diastolic blood pressure following adrenalectomy (r = 0.59). All patients in whom lateralization of aldosterone secretion occurred had hypertension cured or improved by adrenalectomy (Blumenfeld et al, 1994).

Summary

Establishing the diagnosis of primary aldosteronism is important because hypertension and metabolic disturbances are potentially curable by unilateral adrenalectomy in subsets of patients with adenoma and nonadenomatous hyperplasia. Furthermore, the hypertension is often severe and can be difficult to control solely with antihypertensive medication. The diagnosis may be obscured, however, because the complete clinical and biochemical expression of mineralocorticoid hypertension may not be present, particularly in those with nonadenomatous hyperplasia who present with serum potassium in the normal range. Support for the diagnosis is provided by a low PRA, elevated 24-hour urinary aldosterone level and ratio of plasma aldosterone to renin activity, positive postural stimulation test, and elevated urinary excretion of 18-oxocortisol and 18-hydroxycortisol. Adrenal vein sampling has an important role in the diagnostic evaluation of primary aldosteronism because lateralization of aldosterone secretion can indicate the presence of a curable lesion regardless of the radiographic findings (Radin et al, 1992).

PHEOCHROMOCYTOMA

Pheochromocytoma is an uncommon entity but one that has fascinated both clinicians and investigators who have worked together to derive effective means for detection, localization, and management (Bravo and Gifford, 1984; Manger and Gifford, 1990). **Although the causative factor of hypertension in less than 1% of the hypertensive population, detection is mandatory not only for the potential of cure of the hypertension, but also to avoid the potentially lethal effects of the unrecognized tumor.**

Clinical manifestations of pheochromocytoma are all due to the physiologic effects of the amines produced by the lesion. Epinephrine and norepinephrine are similar in their metabolic action, although epinephrine is more potent. The symptom complex manifested by the patient depends somewhat on the secretory products, both type and amount, including the more unusual products dopa and dopamine as well as a variety of peptides produced from amine precursor uptake and decarboxylation (APUD)–type cells (Pearse and Polak, 1971; Bolande, 1974). The peptides are ACTH, somatostatin, serotonin, enkephalins, calcitonin, VIP, neuropeptide, lipotropin, beta endorphin, and dynorphin (Robertson et al, 1990). Small tumors generally bind catecholamine poorly. Thus, the severity of symptoms, despite the small size of these tumors, results from direct release of most of catecholamines directly into the circulation. Large lesions have high catecholamine content but bind them well and metabolize substantial quantities directly within the tumors. Thus, only relatively small amounts of the vasoactive amines

mixed with large amounts of inactive metabolites are secreted (see Fig. 96–17).

Signs and Symptoms

Signs and symptoms of patients with pheochromocytoma, all secondary to secretion of the neurohumoral agents, epinephrine and norepinephrine, may be extraordinarily variable. In all reported series, hypertension is by far the most consistent sign (Tables 96–14 and 96–15). Of 106 patients

Table 96–14. SYMPTOMS REPORTED BY 76 PATIENTS (ALMOST ALL ADULTS) WITH PHEOCHROMOCYTOMA ASSOCIATED WITH PAROXYSMAL OR PERSISTENT HYPERTENSION

Symptoms	Percent Paroxysmal (37 Patients)	Percent Persistent (39 Patients)
Symptoms presumably due to excessive catecholamines or hypertension		
Headache (severe)	92	72
Excessive sweating (generalized)	65	69
Palpitations ± tachycardia	73	51
Anxiety or nervousness (± fear of impending death, panic)	60	28
Tremulousness	51	26
Pain in chest, abdomen (usually epigastric), lumbar regions, lower abdomen, or groin	48	28
Nausea ± vomiting	43	26
Weakness, fatigue, prostration	38	15
Weight loss (severe)	14	15
Dyspnea	11	18
Warmth ± heat intolerance	13	15
Visual disturbances	3	21
Dizziness or faintness	11	3
Constipation	0	13
Paresthesia or pain in arms	11	0
Bradycardia (noted by patient)	8	3
Grand mal	5	3
Manifestations due to complications		
Congestive heart failure ± cardiomyopathy		
Myocardial infarction		
Cerebrovascular accident		
Ischemic enterocolitis ± megacolon		
Azotemia		
Dissecting aneurysm		
Encephalopathy		
Shock		
Hemorrhagic necrosis in a pheochromocytoma		
Manifestations due to coexisting diseases or syndromes		
Cholelithiasis		
Medullary thyroid carcinoma ± effects of secretions of serotonin, calcitonin, prostaglandin, or ACTH-like substance		
Hyperparathyroidism		
Mucocutaneous neuromas with characteristic facies		
Thickened corneal nerves (seen only with slit lamp)		
Marfanoid habitus		
Alimentary tract ganglioneuromatosis		
Neurofibromatosis and its complications		
Cushing's syndrome (rare)		
Von Hippel–Lindau disease (rare)		
Virilism, Addison's disease, acromegaly (extremely rare)		
Symptoms caused by encroachment on adjacent structures or by invasion and pressure effects of metastases		

From Manger WM, Gifford RW Jr: Pheochromocytoma. *In* Laragh JH, Brenner BM, eds: Hypertension: Pathophysiology, Diagnosis, and Management. New York, Raven Press, 1990.

Table 96–15. SIGNS OBSERVED IN PATIENTS WITH PHEOCHROMOCYTOMA

Blood pressure changes
  ± Hypertension ± wide fluctuations (rarely, paroxysmal hypotension or hypertension alternating with hypotension)
  Hypertension induced by physical maneuver such as exercise, postural change, or palpation and massage of flank or mass elsewhere
  Orthostatic hypotension ± postural tachycardia
  Paradoxical blood pressure response to certain antihypertensive drugs; marked pressor response with induction of anesthesia
Other signs of catecholamine excess
  Hyperhidrosis
  Tachycardia or reflex bradycardia, forceful heartbeat, arrhythmia
  Pallor of face and upper part of body (rarely flushing; mottled cyanosis)
  Anxious, frightened, troubled appearance
  Hypertensive retinopathy
  Dilated pupils (rarely exophthalmos, lacrimation, scleral pallor, or injection; pupils may not react to light)
  Leanness or underweight
  Tremor (± shaking)
  Raynaud's phenomenon or livedo reticularis (occasionally puffy, red, cyanotic hands in children); skin of extremities wet, cold, clammy, or pale; gooseflesh; occasionally cyanotic nail beds
  Fever
Mass lesion (rarely palpable)
  Tumor in abdomen or neck (pheochromocytoma, chemodectoma, thyroid carcinoma, or thyroid swelling that is rare and only during hypertensive paroxysm)
  Signs caused by encroachment on adjacent structures or by invasion and pressure effects of metastases
  Manifestations related to complications or to coexisting diseases or syndromes

From Manger WM, Gifford RW Jr: Pheochromocytoma. *In* Laragh JH, Brenner BM, eds: Hypertension: Pathophysiology, Diagnosis, and Management. New York, Raven Press, 1990.

reported by Van Heerden and colleagues, 84% were hypertensive (Van Heerden et al, 1982). As a sign itself, hypertension may have a variety of manifestations. The three common patterns are as follows:

1. **Sustained hypertension**—37% of Van Heerden's patients manifest sustained hypertension with little fluctuation, much as in patients with essential hypertension. This form is most common in children and patients with multiple endocrine adenoma type 2 (MEA 2).

2. **Paroxysmal hypertension**—"dramatic attacks" of hypertension, usually associated with other signs and symptoms, punctuating the patient's usual asymptomatic, normotensive status. This pattern more readily provokes the suspicion of and work-up for the possibility of an underlying pheochromocytoma and was reported to affect 47% of the patients. Females are more likely than males to manifest paroxysmal hypertension.

3. **Sustained hypertension with superimposed paroxysms**—the phenomenon is self-explanatory. Manger and Gifford (1990) have reported a 50% incidence of this manifestation. Scott and co-workers reported 66% (Scott et al, 1976, 1990).

The frequency of attacks among patients is quite variable, ranging from a few times per year to multiple daily episodes. Their duration may be minutes to hours, usually with rapid onset and slower subsidence. One or more episodes a week occur in 75% of patients. Daily attacks, or more than one

attack each day, occur in nearly all other patients. Among patients with pheochromocytoma, half experience symptoms for a duration of less than 15 minutes. In 80% of patients, attacks last less than an hour. With passage of time after the initial appearance of symptoms, frequency of attacks tends to increase, although severity may or may not change.

Attacks may occur in the absence of recognizable stimuli. A multitude of associated factors, however, have been reported: compression of the tumor elicited by massage; physical exercise, particularly a certain posture or lying in a certain position; and direct trauma. Similar precursors of attacks are the wearing of tight clothing, straining to defecate or to void, micturition itself, bladder distention, sexual intercourse, laughing, sneezing, coughing, retching, Valsalva maneuver, and hyperventilation, which cause increased intraabdominal pressure. Foods that are rich in tyramine may elicit attacks: beer, wine, and aged cheese. Potentially provocative drugs are tyramine, histamine, epinephrine and norepinephrine, nicotine, glucagon, tetraethylammonium, methacholine, succinylcholine, phenothiazine, ACTH, and beta-blockers such as propranolol.

Additional signs and symptoms are numerous but not specific. Among these are headaches, sweating, pallor or flushing, palpitations, tachycardia, abdominal or chest pain, and postural hypotension. Also common are weakness, nausea, emesis, and anorexia. Profound psychologic changes are frequently observed. The occasional patient in whom the diagnosis has not been recognized has sometimes been referred for psychiatric evaluation of what was thought to have been functional symptoms.

Some patients are symptomatic for years before diagnosis. Others may present with convulsions, cerebrovascular accidents, and coma. Others have died of massive intracranial bleeding. The appearance of sudden, severe hypertension during the induction of anesthesia or during the course of a surgical procedure may herald underlying pheochromocytoma.

Patients may have pheochromocytomas without manifesting hypertension. **About 10% of pheochromocytomas are found in normotensive patients** (Scott et al, 1976). On occasion, during a severe paroxysmal attack, blood pressure may be unobtainable. Herein, the patient is not hypotensive. Marked peripheral vasoconstriction occurs; therefore, one cannot measure the blood pressure with a sphygmomanometer. Hypertension may also be modest in nature, less serious than other signs and symptoms. Flushing, pallor, and signs of hypermetabolism closely mimic the classic appearance of thyrotoxicosis, leading to surgery of the thyroid gland before recognition of the underlying cause of the disease process.

Many reports exist of pheochromocytoma diagnosed during pregnancy (Schenker and Chowers, 1971; Fudge et al, 1980). Symptoms commonly mimic those of eclampsia, preeclampsia, and toxemia. Headache, visual disturbances, palpitations, diaphoresis, and hypertension (paroxysmal or sustained) are common. According to Fudge and associates, the diagnosis of pheochromocytoma in association with pregnancy has been made before delivery in only one third of patients (Fudge et al, 1980). All too often, it is only with stress of labor and delivery, although more commonly during the postpartum period, that resultant fulminant hypertension or shock leads to the diagnosis of an underlying pheochromocytoma (Hume, 1960). Maternal and infant mortality rates exceed 40%. Despite a history of prior successful pregnancy, in the presence of hypertension, the diagnosis of pheochromocytoma should be considered in the pregnant patient with labile or postural hypertension, congestive heart failure, or arrhythmias. Appropriate diagnostic studies must be carried out.

Pheochromocytoma may be the underlying causative agent in patients afflicted by other various disease states with conditions that may result from excess catecholamine secretion. Common manifestations are cerebrovascular accident, encephalopathy, retinopathy, congestive heart failure, cardiomyopathy, dissecting aneurysm, acute respiratory distress syndrome, shock, renal failure, azotemia, ischemic enterocolitis, and megacolon. Conversely, numerous entities mimic some of the symptoms and signs of pheochromocytoma (Table 96–16).

One specific entity that has gained more recognition is catecholamine-induced cardiomyopathy (Imperato-McGinley et al, 1987, Quigg and Om, 1994; Vaughan, 1996). Experimentally injected catecholamines can cause foci of myocardial necrosis, with inflammation and fibrosis (Van Vliet et al, 1966; Rosenbaum et al, 1988). These patients may have a reduction in blood pressure because of a global reduction in myocardial pump functions, considered to be due to both a down-regulation of beta-receptors and a decrease of viable myofibrils (Sardesai et al, 1990). Fortunately the lesion is usually reversible with the combination of alpha-blockade and alpha-methylparatyrosine (Imperato-McGinley et al, 1987). All patients with pheochromocytoma should have a complete cardiac evaluation with echocardiograms and radionuclide scans before corrective surgery.

An appreciable number of pheochromocytomas have been found in association with several disease entities and hereditary syndromes (see Table 96–16). Among these unusual conditions are the association of tumors of the glomus jugulare region and either pheochromocytoma or ectopic paragangliomas (Hamberger et al, 1967; Sato et al, 1974; Blumenfeld et al, 1993; Mena et al, 1993). It is now recognized that both the tumor in the glomus jugulare region and the other adrenal or nonadrenal chromaffin tumors can secrete catecholamines. It is also apparent that these patients can have multiple lesions (Fig. 96–42). Accordingly, the patients have to have sequential procedures with appropriate blockade and determination of catecholamine secretion after each procedure to determine residual activity. Tank and Gelbard (1982) estimate that 95% of pheochromocytomas are sporadic in occurrence but that the remaining 5% have a familial pattern. Ten percent is often reported. Calkins and Howard (1947) published the first report of familial pheochromocytoma. Familial transmission is believed to be through autosomal dominance, with a locus on chromosome 10 (Simpson et al, 1987) found in the subset designated multiple endocrine neoplasia (MEN) type 2.

Familial pheochromocytomas may be divided into different types of genetic abnormalities. In 1961, Sipple described the combination of pheochromocytoma and medullary carcinoma of the thyroid (MCT) that came to be known as Sipple's syndrome. In subsequent years, as more cases came to light, new terminology—MEA or MEN—has been popularized as has a subclassification system: MEA 1, MEA 2, and MEA 3 or MEA 2b (Raue et al, 1985; Larsson and Nordenskjold, 1990). Pheochromocytomas occur in MEA 2,

Table 96–16. DIFFERENTIAL DIAGNOSIS*

All hypertensives (sustained and paroxysmal)
Anxiety, tension states, psychoneurosis, psychosis
Hyperthyroidism
Paroxysmal tachycardia
Hyperdynamic beta-adrenergic circulatory state
Menopause
Vasodilating headache (migraine and cluster headaches)
Coronary insufficiency syndrome
Acute hypertensive encephalopathy
Diabetes mellitus
Renal parenchymal or renal arterial disease with hypertension
Focal arterial insufficiency of the brain
Intracranial lesions (with or without increased intracranial pressure)
Autonomic hyperreflexia
Diencephalic seizures and syndrome
Toxemia of pregnancy (or *eclampsia with convulsions*)
Hypertensive crises associated with monoamine oxidase inhibitors
Carcinoid
Hypoglycemia
Mastocytosis
Familial dysautonomia
Acrodynia
Neuroblastoma; ganglioneuroblastoma; ganglioneuroma
Neurofibromatosis (with or without renal arterial disease)
Adrenocortical carcinoma
Acute infectious disease

Rare causes of paroxysmal hypertension (*adrenal medullary hyperplasia, acute porphyria, lead poisoning,* tabetic crisis, encephalitis, *clonidine withdrawal,* hypovolemia with inappropriate vasoconstriction, pulmonary artery fibrosarcoma, portal hypersensitivity, dysregulation of hypothalamus, *tetanus, Guillain-Barré syndrome, factitious*)

Fortuitous circumstances simulating pheochromocytoma
Conditions sometimes associated with pheochromocytoma
    Coexisting disease or syndromes
    Cholelithiasis
    Medullary thyroid carcinoma
    Hyperparathyroidism
    Mucosal neuromas
    Thickened corneal nerves
    Marfanoid habitus
    Alimentary tract ganglioneuromatosis
    Neurofibromatosis
    Cushing's syndrome
    Von Hippel–Lindau disease
    Polycythemia
    Virilism, Addison's disease, acromegaly
    Complications
    Cardiovascular disease†
    Cerebrovascular disease
    Renovascular disease
    Circulatory shock
    Renal insufficiency
    Hemorrhagic necrosis of pheochromocytoma†
    Dissecting aneurysm†
    Ischemic enterocolitis with or without intestinal obstruction†

*Conditions in italics may have increased excretion of catecholamines or metabolites (or both).
†Patient may present as having abdominal or cardiovascular catastrophe.
From Manger WM, Gifford RW Jr: Pheochromocytoma. *In* Laragh JH, Brenner BM, eds: Hypertension: Pathophysiology, Diagnosis, and Management. New York, Raven Press, 1990.

a triad including pheochromocytoma, MCT, and parathyroid adenomas. The last may be a secondary phenomenon. The parafollicular cells of MCT elaborate thyrocalcitonin. The resulting decrease in serum calcium concentration leads to parathyroid stimulation with subsequent hyperplasia or development of adenomas. Pheochromocytoma may also be a part of MEN 3, which also includes MCT, mucosal neuromas, thickened corneal nerves, alimentary tract, ganglioneuromatosis, and frequently a marfanoid habitus (Manger and Gifford, 1990).

Recognition of MEA 2 and aggressive evaluation of MEA 2 kindreds are mandatory. Carney and associates report 22% mortality from complications of pheochromocytoma in a

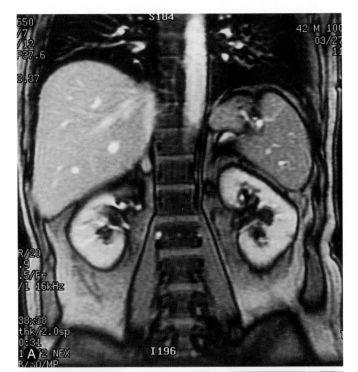
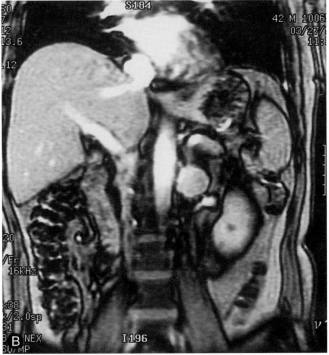

Figure 96–42. Magnetic resonance imaging scan showing bilateral adrenal pheochromocytomas in a patient with bilateral glomus jugulare tumors. The patient was treated with left adrenalectomy and enucleation of the smaller right pheochromocytoma. *A,* Small right pheochromocytoma; *B,* larger left pheochromocytoma.

review of 149 patients with MEA 2 (Carney et al, 1976). MCT has an expected incidence of 50% in MEA 2 kindred. The development of DNA technology to identify carriers of the MEN 2A gene (Lips et al, 1994) and the awareness of patients with pheochromocytomas as a component of MEN 2A or von Hippel–Lindau disease has resulted in the recommendation that all patients with pheochromocytoma be screened for these syndromes as well as family members of patients with these diseases (Neumann et al, 1993; Lips et al, 1994).

The neuroectodermal dysplasias are a group of related diseases: von Recklinghausen's disease (neurofibromatosis), tuberous sclerosis, Sturge-Weber syndrome, and von Hippel–Lindau disease. All are strongly familial and associated with each other and with pheochromocytoma.

The prevalence of pheochromocytoma in patients with neurofibromatosis is reported as 1% to 2%. Of those patients with pheochromocytoma, 5% have von Recklinghausen's disease. Kalff and associates, having seen ten patients with pheochromocytoma and neurofibromatosis, reviewed the sample population, selecting patients with both von Recklinghausen's disease and hypertension (Kalff et al, 1982). They found 17 such patients, 53% of whom had pheochromocytomas.

Pheochromocytoma is distinctly less common than the other neuroectodermal dysplasias (Kalff et al, 1982). The rare association of a somatostatin-rich duodenal carcinoid tumor and pheochromocytoma has also been reported (Wheeler et al, 1986).

The increased incidence of pheochromocytomas in association with the neuroectodermal dysplasias and MCT may be explained by the APUD cell system of Pearse. The APUD cells derive from the neural crest of the embryo, sharing common ultrastructural and cytochemical features and elaborating amines by precursor uptake and decarboxylation (Pearse and Polak; 1971; Bolande, 1974). The products of these cells have been previously listed. Immunochemical techniques showing both neuron-specific enolase and chromogranin A in a variety of polypeptide hormone-producing tissues support the concept of the APUD system (Fig. 96–43) (Lloyd et al, 1984; O'Connor and Deftos, 1986; Hsiao et al, 1991).

Children

Manifestations of pheochromocytoma in children vary somewhat from those in adults. Headache, nausea or vomiting, weight loss, and visual complaints occur more commonly in children than in adults. Manger and Gifford (1977) report polydypsia, polyuria, and convulsions—rarely observed in adults—occurring in 25% of children. Puffy, red, and cyanotic appearance of the hands is reported in 11% of children. Of children with pheochromocytomas, 90% have sustained hypertension. Paroxysmal hypertension occurs in less than 10% of children.

In contrast to adults, children manifest a higher incidence of familial pheochromocytomas (10%) and bilaterality (24%). Multiple pheochromocytomas have been reported in children with an incidence of 15% to 32%, and extra-adrenal location of pheochromocytomas has been reported in 15% to 31% of the children (Glenn et al, 1968).

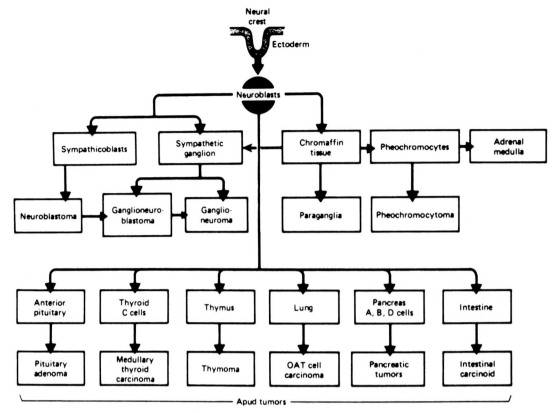

Figure 96–43. Ectodermal origin of APUD (amine precursor uptake and decarboxylation) tumors. (From Manger WM, Gifford RW Jr: *In* Laragh JH, Brenner BM, eds: Hypertensions: Pathophysiology, Diagnosis, and Management. New York, Raven Press, 1990.)

Glenn and co-workers believed that on a histologic basis, there was a higher incidence of malignant pheochromocytomas in children (Glenn et al, 1968). Stackpole's review found a random distribution of age at diagnosis among boys. In girls, the diagnosis was made in 62% during menarche (Stackpole et al, 1963). Because of the tendency toward multiplicity and thus asynchronous recurrence, close follow-up for recurrent symptoms and hypertension is mandatory in children (Ein et al, 1990).

Laboratory Diagnosis

The clinical diagnosis of pheochromocytoma is based on the subjective evaluation of signs and symptoms. Laboratory confirmation of the clinical diagnosis is mandatory and may be divided into two general categories: biochemical diagnosis and radiologic diagnosis (Fig. 96–44).

Confirmation of the diagnosis is by demonstrating elevated levels of catecholamines in the blood or urine,

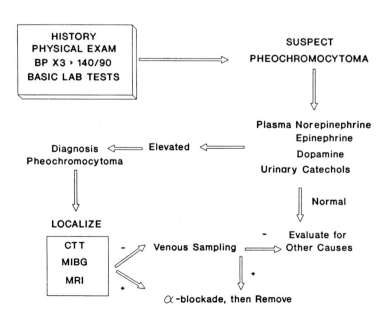

Figure 96–44. Identifying pheochromocytoma. (From Vaughan ED Jr: Diagnosis of adrenal disorders in hypertension. World J Urol, 1989;7:111–116.)

which occur in 95% to 99% of patients with pheochromocytoma. Extremely accurate assays exist (Dolan and Carey, 1989; Bravo, 1991). There are a considerable number of foods and drugs that can affect urinary levels of catecholamines or breakdown products (Table 96–17). Plasma catecholamines are highly responsive to stress, activity, blood loss, and other stimuli.

Because of the severe consequences of the undiagnosed pheochromocytoma, it is recommended that all hypertensive patients be screened. Measurement of urinary catecholamines and metanephrines are adequate in most patients (Bravo, 1991).

Rarely the concentrations of plasma and urinary catecholamines and their metabolites are not elevated, especially if the patient is normotensive at the time of study. In this clinical setting, if there is a high index of suspicion, imaging studies with ^{131}I-metaiodobenzylguanidine (Shapiro et al, 1985), MRI (Newhouse, 1990), or repeating sampling when the patient is hypertensive is indicated. Provocative tests with histamine, glucagon, or phentolamine are rarely used (Dolan and Carey, 1989).

In contrast, some patients with essential hypertension and signs or symptoms of pheochromocytoma have slightly elevated plasma catecholamine levels, probably representing a neurogenic component to the hypertension. The clonidine suppression test distinguishes these patients (Bravo et al, 1981; Karlberg and Hedman, 1986). Two to 3 hours after a single 0.3-mg oral dose of clonidine, patients with neurogenic hypertension at rest show a fall in plasma norepinephrine plus epinephrine to a level below 500 pg/ml (Bravo, 1991), whereas patients with pheochromocytoma do not.

Radiologic Tests

Similar to other adrenal tumors, the development of sectional imaging was a major advancement in the diagnosis and localization of pheochromocytoma (Kazam et al, 1989). For adrenal pheochromocytomas, the CT accuracy for detection is more than 90% (Thomas et al, 1980; Abrams et al, 1982), and CT has rapidly replaced angiography, venography, and ultrasonography for extra-adrenal pheochromocytoma, in which the detection is less (about 75%). CT, however, does not aid in differentiating pheochromocytomas from other adrenal lesions or in predicting malignancy.

The authors have been impressed with the multiple uses of MRI in patients with pheochromocytoma. The test appears to be as accurate as CT in identifying lesions, while having a characteristically bright, "light bulb" image on T2-weighted study (Fig. 96–45) (Reinig et al, 1986). In addition, sagittal and coronal imaging can give excellent anatomic information about the relationship between the tumor and the surrounding vasculature as well as the draining venous channels (Figs. 96–46 and 96–47). The authors believe that MRI should be the initial scanning procedure in patients with biochemical findings of a pheochromocytoma.

An alternative approach that is also useful at times, particularly in the search for residual or multiple pheochromocytoma, is the metaiodobenzylguanidine (MIBG) scan that images medullary tissue (Shapiro et al, 1985; Campeau, et al, 1991). In the experience in 400 cases, the developers of the technique found a 78.4% sensitivity in primary sporadic tumors, 92.4% in malignant lesions, and 94.3% in familial cases, giving an overall sensitivity of 87.4% with 99% specificity. Thus, the test may be more sensitive than CT in patients with extra-adrenal lesions. The isotope may be picked up by other APUD cell–type tumors. In a smaller series involving children, the MIBG scan findings were positive in all cases (Deal et al, 1990). The MIBG scan is highly sensitive and is a useful tool, especially if CT and MRI findings are negative or confusing (Fig. 96–48). Sequential venous sampling has been used successfully to identify small extra-adrenal lesions (Newbould et al, 1991).

Preoperative Management

There is unanimity of opinion that surgical extirpation is the only effective treatment for pheochromocytoma. The one

Table 96–17. EFFECTS OF DRUGS AND INTERFERING SUBSTANCES ON CONCENTRATIONS OF URINARY CATECHOLAMINES AND METABOLITES*

Upper Limit of Normal Adult (mg/24 h)		Effects	
		Increases Apparent Value	Decreases Apparent Value
Catecholamines		Catecholamines	Fenfluramine (large doses)
Epinephrine	0.02	Drugs containing catecholamines	
Norepinephrine	0.08	Isoprenolol (isoproterenol)†	
Total	0.10	Levodopa	
Dopamine	0.20	Labetalol†	
Methyldopa		Tetracyclines†	
		Erythromycin†	
		Chlorpromazine†	
		Other fluorescent substances† (e.g., quinine, quinidine, bile in urine)	
		Rapid clonidine withdrawal	
		Ethanol	
Metanephrine		Catecholamines	Methylglucamine (in Renovist, Renografin)
Metanephrine	0.4	Drugs containing catecholamines	
Normetanephrine	0.9	Monoamine oxidase inhibitors	Fenfluramine (large doses)
Total	1.3	Benzodiazepines	
		Rapid clonidine withdrawal	
		Ethanol	
Vanillylmandelic acid	6.5	Catecholamines (minimal increase)	Clofibrate
			Disulfiram
			Ethanol
		Drugs containing catecholamines (minimal increase)	Monoamine oxidase inhibitors
		Levodopa	Fenfluramine (large doses)
		Nalidixic acid†	
		Rapid clonidine withdrawal	

*As determined by most reliable assays.
†Probably spurious interference with fluorescence assays.
From Manger WM, Gifford RW Jr: Pheochromocytoma. In Laragh JH, Brenner BM, eds: Hypertension: Pathophysiology, Diagnosis, and Management. New York, Raven Press, 1990.

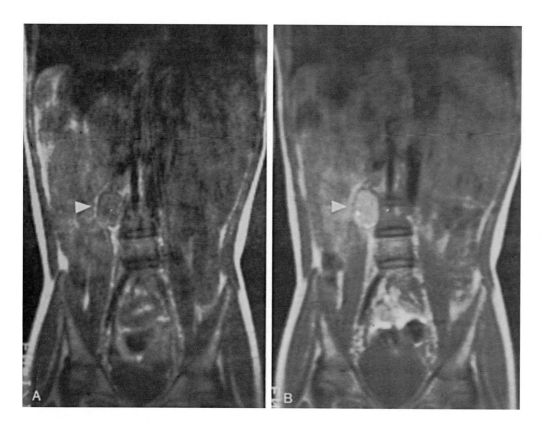

Figure 96–45. Extra-adrenal pheochromocytoma showing a T1 image *(A)* and a bright T2 image *(B)*.

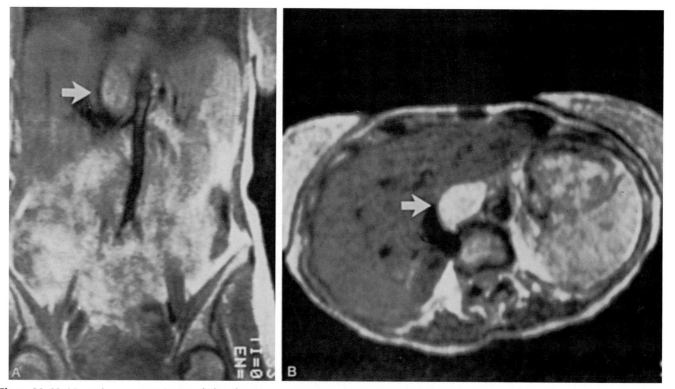

Figure 96–46. Magnetic resonance image of pheochromocytoma *(arrows)*. Right adrenal arising from the medial limb, which grew medial to the inferior vena cava above the celiac axis under the caudate lobe of the liver and was missed at first abdominal exploration. Intra-aorticocaval location is clearly seen on these films. *A,* Coronal image; *B,* transverse image.

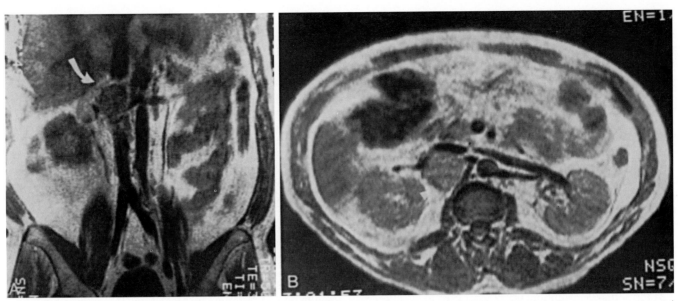

Figure 96–47. Magnetic resonance image of recurrent pheochromocytoma *(arrow)* with an excellent demonstration of an anterior-crossing right renal vein, a feeding lumbar vein, and involvement of right renal artery. *A,* Coronal image; *B,* transverse image.

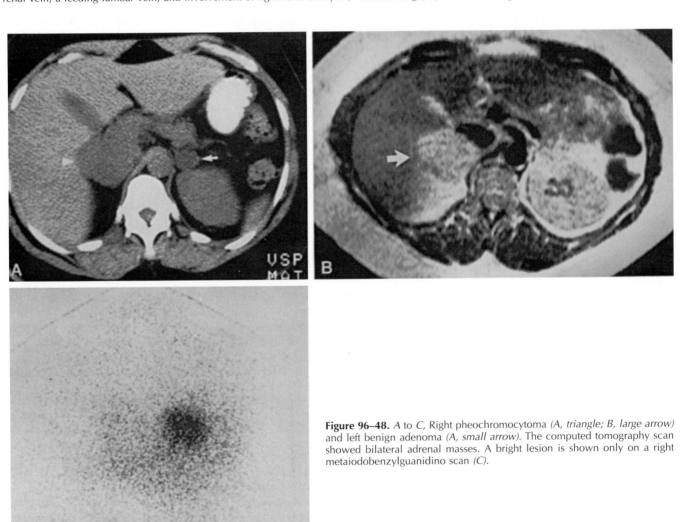

Figure 96–48. *A* to *C,* Right pheochromocytoma *(A, triangle; B, large arrow)* and left benign adenoma *(A, small arrow).* The computed tomography scan showed bilateral adrenal masses. A bright lesion is shown only on a right metaiodobenzylguanidino scan *(C).*

accepted exception to this principle is treatment late in pregnancy. The patient should be treated with alpha-adrenergic blockade via oral administration of phenoxybenzamine until the fetus has reached maturity. At this point, cesarean section with tumor excision in one operation should be carried out, without allowing the patient to undergo the stress of vaginal delivery.

In the past, one of the most controversial issues in the management of patients with pheochromocytoma was whether to employ pharmacologic blockade preoperatively (Boutros et al, 1990). **The authors do not believe that there is an issue at the present time. The evolution of an accurate localization test weakens the argument that alpha blockade limits the ability to identify the lesion at the time of exploration.**

Moreover, the greater stability of the patient with adequate preoperative preparation greatly facilitates the procedure for both surgeon and anesthesiologist as well as increasing the safety to the patient.

At the authors' institution, the preoperative medical preparation is of utmost importance to provide an ideal anesthetic and operative environment (Malhotra, 1995). The perioperative course is smoother with adequate preoperative preparation. **Phenoxybenzamine hydrochloride (Dibenzyline), a long-acting alpha-adrenergic blocker, controls blood pressure in patients with pheochromocytoma.** The initial divided dose of 20 to 30 mg is given orally and is increased by 10 to 20 mg per day, until the blood pressure has been stabilized and there is mild postural hypotension. Usually a dose of 40 to 100 mg per day is required.

Beta-adrenergic blockers, such as propranolol, have been added to alpha-blockers to prepare patients for anesthesia and surgery. Beta-blockers protect against arrhythmias and permit reduction in the amount of alpha-adrenergic blockers necessary to control blood pressure (Ross et al, 1967). Beta-blockers have also been given when tachyphylaxis to alpha-blockers occurs. However, they must be used carefully (Salem and Ivankovic, 1969). A beta-adrenergic blocker should be administered only when alpha blockade is established. Beta blockade alone may cause a marked rise in the total peripheral vascular resistance secondary to unopposed alpha-adrenergic activity. Accordingly, the authors do not routinely prepare patients with propranolol. A beta-adrenergic blocker is provided only when cardiac arrhythmias are prominent. Propranolol is given orally in doses of 20 to 40 mg three or four times daily. Labetalol, an alpha-adrenergic and beta-adrenergic blocking agent, has been used but may not control hypertension (Rosen et al, 1976; Briggs et al, 1978).

Alpha-methylparatyrosine (metyrosine, a tyrosine hydroxylase inhibitor) has been recommended in addition to phenoxybenzamine or propranolol during preparation of the patient for anesthesia and surgery (Sjoerdsma et al, 1965; Engleman et al, 1968). Metyrosine decreases the rate of catecholamine synthesis—the conversion of tyrosine to dihydroxyphenylalanine (DOPA). Adverse effects include crystalluria, sedation, diarrhea, anxiety, psychic disturbance, and extrapyramidal signs. Experience with alpha-methylparatyrosine is limited, although its combination with alpha-adrenergic blockade has been recommended (Perry et al, 1990). The authors therefore do not use it routinely. The authors reserve the drug for patients who have myocardiopathy, multiple catecholamine-secreting paragangliomas, or re-

sistance to alpha-adrenergic blockers. Alpha-methylparatyrosine is given in doses of 0.5 to 1.0 g orally three or four times daily and is usually started before surgery (Reckler et al, 1989). The dose is determined by repeat catecholamine evaluations.

Prazosin, a specific postsynaptic alpha$_1$-adrenergic blocker, has gained rapid acceptance as an effective antihypertensive agent. The drug has been evaluated in the medical management of patients with pheochromocytoma either alone (Wallace and Gill, 1978) or in combination with a beta-blocker. The authors, however, have experience with four patients who were prepared with prazosin alone for surgical removal of adrenal pheochromocytoma. The control of blood pressure was effective preoperatively but was not adequate during surgical removal of the tumor. Marked blood pressure elevations were present in all four patients. In contrast to phenoxybenzamine, which binds irreversibly to alpha-adrenergic receptors, prazosin blockade is reversible and may be overwhelmed by the surge in catecholamine secretion during intubation and surgical manipulation. The authors have since abandoned prazosin in preparing patients for anesthesia and surgery (Nicholson et al, 1983).

In addition to the alpha-blocking and beta-blocking agents, it is important that the state of hydration and blood volume be evaluated because many patients have decreased intravascular volume. Crystalloids may be needed to raise the intravascular volume to accommodate the expanded vascular bed produced by alpha-blocking agents. To avoid this potential problem, patients receive at least a liter of 5% glucose in Ringer's lactate preoperatively. The alpha-blocking agent and beta-blocking agent (if used) should be continued up to and including the day of surgery.

Anesthetic Management

Anesthetic management of the patient undergoing surgical removal of a pheochromocytoma is directed toward control of the cardiovascular system (Robertson et al, 1990; Artusio, 1995). Close monitoring is of utmost importance and includes attention to the electrocardiogram, blood pressure (arterial line for continuous arterial pressure reading), urinary output, and central venous pressure. A Swan-Ganz catheter may be employed to measure pulmonary capillary wedge pressure if the patient has left ventricular dysfunction.

Patients should arrive in the operating room in a relaxed state, and therefore some form of preanesthesia medication such as a barbiturate (pentobarbital at a dose of 100–300 mg) should be given an hour before the patient's arrival to the operating room. **The authors recommend general anesthesia with a combined approach, induction with an intravenous agent such as thiopental, followed by isoflurane as the agent of choice as an inhalation agent.** At the time of induction of anesthesia, there may be a marked vasopressor response and appropriate alpha-adrenergic and beta-adrenergic blocking agents should be available for intravenous use. Acutely, it is recommended that phentolamine (Regitine), a short-acting alpha-blocker, be used to control blood pressure during the induction of anesthesia. Phentolamine can be given in boluses of 1 to 5 mg or by continuous infusion (50 mg of phentolamine per 500 ml of Ringer's lactate). Alternatively, sodium nitroprusside may be needed to control severe hypertension, and it should be present in a solution of 50 mg in 250 ml of 5% dextrose and water.

Throughout the procedure, particularly during any manipulations of the tumor, hypertensive episodes may occur as well as arrhythmias. The use of general anesthesia allows the anesthesiologist to follow the progress of the surgery, and as the blood supply of the tumor is diminished, fluids can be increased, and the depth of anesthesia can be decreased. Beta-adrenergic blockers, such as esmolol or propranolol, should be reserved for persistent tachycardias or arrhythmias that persist despite alpha-blockade.

A variety of anesthetic agents and drugs should be avoided in patients with pheochromocytoma (Table 96–18). Using this approach and adequate preoperative blockade, at times with both alpha-adrenergic blocking agents and alpha-methylparatyrosine, hypotension following removal of the tumor now rarely occurs. If the systolic blood pressure falls below 100 mm Hg, however, norepinephrine (4–8 mg/500 ml normal saline) should be started and blood pressure stabilized above the 100 mm Hg level. Usually the norepinephrine can be withdrawn after further fluid resuscitation.

ADRENAL SURGERY

Surgical Options

There are numerous approaches to the adrenal gland (Table 96–19). The proper approach depends on the underlying cause of the adrenal pathology, the size of the adrenal, the size of the lesion, the habitus of the patient, and the experience and preference of the operating surgeon (Vaughan, 1991). In some cases, options and a careful review of all these variables are required before a choice is made. Thus, each case should be considered individually, although there are preferred approaches for given diseases. For example, the posterior or modified posterior approach is preferred for small well-localized lesions. An abdominal approach is used for a patient with multiple pheochromocytomas. In contrast, a large adrenal carcinoma may require a thoracoabdominal approach, and a well-localized large pheochromocytoma may best be excised through a similar incision if there is no evidence for multiple lesions.

Table 96–18. ANESTHETICS AND DRUGS TO BE AVOIDED IN PHEOCHROMOCYTOMA

Inhalation agents	Halothane
Intravenous agents	Propofol
	Ketamine
Tranquilizers	Droperidol
Narcotics	Morphine
Local anesthetics	Cocaine
Muscle relaxants	Tubocurarine
	Atracurium
	Pancuronium
Vasopressors	Ephedrine
Adjuvants	Chlorpromazine
	Metoclopramide

From Artusio JF Jr: Anesthesia for pheochromocytoma. In Malhotra V, ed: Anesthesia for Renal and Genitourinary Surgery. New York, McGraw-Hill, 1995. Reproduced by permission of the McGraw-Hill Companies.

Table 96–19. SURGICAL OPTIONS

Disease	Approach
Primary hyperaldosteronism	Posterior (left or right)
	Modified posterior (right)
	11th rib (left > right)
	Posterior transthoracic
Cushing's adenoma	11th rib (left or right)
	Thoracoabdominal (large)
	Posterior (small)
Cushing's disease	Bilateral posterior
Bilateral hyperplasia	Bilateral 11th rib (alternating)
Adrenal carcinoma	Thoracoabdominal
	11th rib
	Transabdominal
Bilateral adrenal ablation	Bilateral posterior
Pheochromocytoma	Transabdominal chevron
	Thoracoabdominal
	(large—usually right)
	11th rib
Neuroblastoma	Transabdominal
	11th rib

From Vaughan ED Jr: Adrenal surgery. In Marshall F, ed: Operative Urology. Philadelphia, W.B. Saunders, 1991.

Operative Techniques

Before describing specific techniques, some unifying concepts warrant attention. Adequate visualization with the use of head lamps is critical. Hemostasis should be rigorously maintained. The operator should bring the adrenal down by initially exposing the cranial attachments and by dividing the rich blood supply between right-angle clips, using the forceps cautery for additional control. The blood supply bounds the gland in a stellate fashion. It is often simplest to begin dissection laterally, identifying the vascular supply and then working around the cranial edge of the gland. Interestingly the posterior surface of the adrenal is usually devoid of vasculature. The gland then can be drawn caudally with gentle traction on the kidney. The gland is extremely friable and fractures easily, which causes troublesome bleeding. In essence, the patient should be dissected from the tumor, a concept particularly true during removal of a pheochromocytoma when the gland should not be manipulated and early venous control is preferred.

Posterior Approach

The posterior position can be used for either bilateral adrenal exploration or unilateral removal of small tumors (Fig. 96–49). In the past, all patients with primary aldosteronism were explored in this fashion because of the inability to localize the lesion. Today, localization is mandatory before exploration is recommended. The bilateral approach is primarily used for ablative total adrenalectomy. The options for incisions are shown, and generally rib resection is preferable to obtain high exposure. Following standard subperiosteal rib resection, care must be taken with the diaphragmatic release. The pleura should be avoided and the diaphragm swept cranially.

The fibrofatty contents within Gerota's fascia are swept away from the paraspinal musculature exposing a subdiaphragmatic "open space," which is the apex of the resection. The liver, within the peritoneum, is dissected off the

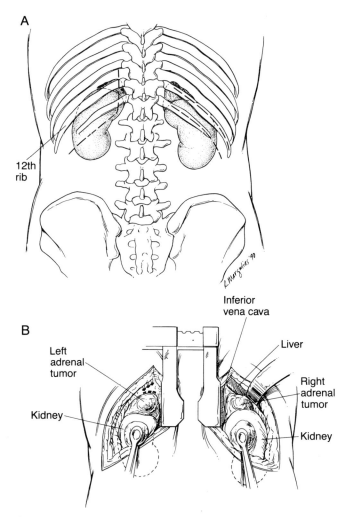

Figure 96–49. Posterior approach to the adrenals. (From Vaughan ED Jr: Adrenal surgery. *In* Marshall FF, ed: Operative Urology. Philadelphia, W. B. Saunders, 1991.)

anterior surface of the adrenal, and the cranial blood supply is divided. Medially, on the right, the inferior vena cava is visualized. The short, high adrenal vein, entering the cava in dorsolateral fashion, is identified and can be clipped or ligated. The adrenal can be drawn caudally by traction on the kidney. Care must be taken to avoid apical branches of the renal artery. On the left, the approach is similar with division of the splenorenal ligament giving initial lateral exposure.

The posterior approach can also be modified for a transthoracic adrenal exposure through the diaphragm (Novick et al, 1989). The authors rarely find this more extensive approach necessary for small adrenal tumors.

Modified Posterior Approach

Although the posterior position has the advantages of rapid adrenal exposure and low morbidity, there are definite disadvantages. The jackknife position may impair respiration, the abdominal contents are compressed posteriorly, and the visual field is limited. The advantage of the posterior approach is primarily for control of the short, right adrenal vein (Fig. 96–50A); therefore, the authors have developed a

modified approach for right adrenalectomy (Vaughan and Phillips, 1987).

The approach is based on the anatomic relationship of the right adrenal, which lies deeply posterior and high in the retroperitoneum behind the liver (see Fig. 96–50A). In addition, the short, stubby right adrenal vein enters the inferior vena cava posteriorly at the apex of the adrenal. Hence, the authors use an approach that is posterior but with the patient in a modified position, similar to that for a Gil-Vernet dorsal lombotomy incision (Fig. 96–50B) (Gil-Vernet, 1965). The patient is placed in this position, and the 11th or 12th rib is resected with care to avoid the pleura. The diaphragm is resected off the underlying peritoneum and liver and should be sharply dissected free to gain mobility. Similarly the inferior surface of the peritoneum, closely associated with the liver, is sharply dissected from Gerota's fascia, which is gently retracted inferiorly.

The adrenal becomes visible in the depth of the incision, as the final hepatic attachments are divided. A lateral space can be found exposing the posterior abdominal musculature. The adrenal lies against the paraspinal muscles and multiple small adrenal arteries that actually course behind the inferior vena cava, emerge over these muscles, and are clipped and divided (Fig. 96–50C). At this point, the adrenal can usually be moved against the paraspinal musculature, exposing the inferior vena cava below the adrenal gland.

The major advantage of this approach is that the adrenal vein is identified without difficulty because it emerges from the segment of the inferior vena cava exposed and courses up to the adrenal, which now rises toward the operating surgeon. In other flank or anterior approaches, the adrenal vein resides in its posterior relationship, requiring caval rotation with the chance of adrenal vein avulsion. After adrenal vein exposure, it is doubly tied and divided or clipped with right-angle clips and divided (Fig. 96–50D).

The adrenal can now be retracted inferiorly for division of the remaining arteries and total removal. The wound is not drained and is closed with interrupted 0 polydioxanone sutures.

The authors select this technique for all patients with right adrenal aldosterone-secreting tumors and for other patients with benign adenomas less than 6 cm. The authors do not recommend the approach in the patient with pheochromocytoma or malignant adrenal neoplasm.

Flank Approach

The standard extrapleural, extraperitoneal 11th rib resection is excellent for either left or right adrenalectomy (Fig. 96–51) (Riehle and Lavengood, 1985). This approach is described in detail in Chapter 97, and only the adrenal dissection is described here.

Following the completion of the incision, the lumbocostal arch is used as a landmark showing the point of attachment of the posterior diaphragm to the posterior abdominal musculature. Gerota's fascia containing the adrenal and kidney can be swept medially.

On the right side, the liver within the peritoneum is lifted off the anterior surface of the adrenal (see Fig. 96–51). Quite often, the adrenal gland cannot be identified precisely until these maneuvers are performed. **One should not attempt to** dissect into the body of the adrenal or to dissect the **inferior surface of the adrenal off the kidney. The kidney is quite useful for retraction. The dissection should continue from lateral to medial along the posterior abdominal and diaphragmatic musculature with precise ligation or clipping of the small but multiple adrenal arteries (Fig. 96–52A).** While the operator clips these arteries with one hand, the opposite hand is used to retract both adrenal and kidney inferiorly. With release of the superior vasculature, the adrenal becomes visualized.

Following the release of the adrenal from the superior vasculature, it is helpful to expose the inferior vena cava and to divide the medial arterial supply, allowing mobilization of the cava for better exposure of the high posterior adrenal vein. This vein then is again doubly tied or clipped and divided (Fig. 96–52B). Patients with large adrenal carcinomas or pheochromocytomas may require en bloc resections of the adrenal and kidney, following the principles of radical nephrectomy (Fig. 96–52C).

A major deviation from this technique is used in patients with pheochromocytoma, in whom the initial dissection should be aimed toward early control and division of the main adrenal vein on either side. Obviously, in this clinical setting, the anesthesiologist should be notified when the adrenal vein is divided because there often is a marked drop in blood pressure even if the patient is adequately hydrated and treated with alpha-adrenergic blockade.

On the left side, the lumbocostal arch also is used as a landmark. Gerota's fascia can be swept medially and inferiorly, giving exposure to the splenorenal ligament, which

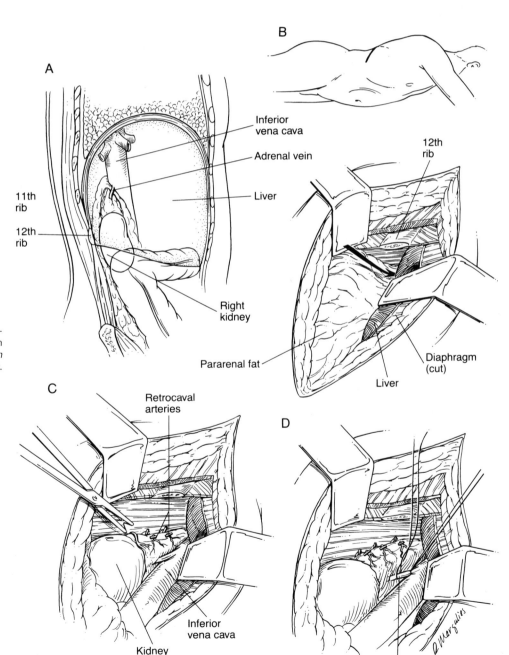

Figure 96–50. Modified posterior approach to the right adrenal. (From Vaughan ED Jr: Adrenal surgery. *In* Marshall FF, ed: Operative Urology. Philadelphia, W. B. Saunders, 1991.)

A

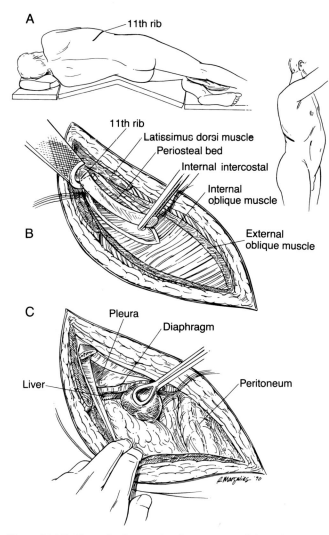

Figure 96–51. Eleventh rib resection for exposure of the right adrenal. (From Vaughan ED Jr: Adrenal surgery. *In* Marshall FF, ed: Operative Urology. Philadelphia, W. B. Saunders, 1991.)

should be divided to avoid splenic injury (Fig. 96–53). While the surgeon works anteriorly, the spleen and pancreas within the peritoneum can be lifted cranially, exposing the anterior surface of the adrenal gland. The superior dissection is performed first, drawing the adrenal and kidney down inferiorly. On the left medially, the phrenic branch of the venous drainage must be carefully clipped or ligated (Fig. 96–54). This vessel is not noted in most surgical atlases and can cause troublesome bleeding if divided. The medial dissection along the crus of the diaphragm and aorta leads to the renal vein, and finally the adrenal vein is controlled, doubly tied, and divided. The adrenal is then removed from the kidney with care to avoid the apical branches of the renal artery.

After removal of the adrenal, inspection should be made for any bleeding. Also, inspection of the diaphragm for pleural tear and inspection of the kidney should be done. The incision is closed without drains with interrupted 0 polydioxanone sutures.

Thoracoabdominal Approach

The thoracoabdominal 9th- or 10th-rib approach is used for **large adenomas, some large adrenal carcinomas, and**

well-localized pheochromocytomas especially on the right side. The incision and exposure is standard, with a radial incision through the diaphragm and a generous intraperitoneal extension. The techniques described for adrenalectomy with the 11th-rib approach are used.

Transabdominal Approach

The transabdominal approach is commonly chosen for patients with pheochromocytomas, for pediatric patients, and for some patients with adrenal carcinomas. The obvious concept is to have the ability for complete abdominal exploration to identify either multiple pheochromocytomas or adrenal metastases.

The authors use the transverse or chevron incision, which they believe gives better exposure of both adrenal glands than does a midline incision. The rectus muscles and lateral abdominal musculature are divided, exposing the peritoneum. On entering the peritoneal cavity, the surgeon should gently palpate the para-aortic areas and the adrenal areas. Close attention is paid to blood pressure changes, in an attempt to identify any unsuspected lesions if the patient has a pheochromocytoma. This maneuver is less important today because excellent localization techniques are available, as previously discussed. In fact, with precise preoperative localization of the offending tumor, the chevron incision does not need to be completely symmetric and can be limited on the contralateral side.

If the patient has a lesion on the right adrenal, the hepatic flexure of the colon is reflected inferiorly. The incision is made in the posterior peritoneum lateral to the kidney and carried superiorly, allowing the liver to be reflected cranially (Fig. 96–55). Incision in the peritoneum is carried downward, exposing the anterior surface of the inferior vena cava to the entrance of the right renal vein. Once the vena cava is cleared, there are often one or two accessory hepatic veins that should be secured (Fig. 96–56B). These veins are easily avulsed from the vena cava and can cause troublesome bleeding. Ligation of these veins gives 1 to 2 cm of additional vena caval exposure, which often is quite useful during the exposure of the short posterior right adrenal vein. Small accessory adrenal veins may also be encountered. The cava is rolled medially, exposing the adrenal vein, which should be doubly tied or clipped and divided (Fig. 96–56C).

As mentioned, the surgeon should inform the anesthesiologist when the vein is ligated in a patient with a pheochromocytoma because a precipitous fall in blood pressure can occur at this point, requiring volume expansion or even vasopressors. Following control of the adrenal vein, it is then simplest to proceed with the superior dissection, lifting the liver off the adrenal and securing the multiple small adrenal arteries arising from the inferior phrenic artery, which is rarely seen. The adrenal can then be drawn inferiorly with retraction on the kidney. The adrenal arteries traversing to the adrenal from under the cava can be secured with right-angle clips. The final step is removing the adrenal from the kidney.

The left adrenal vein is simpler to approach because it lies lower, partially anterior to the upper pole of the kidney. The adrenal vein empties into the left renal vein. Accordingly, on the left side, the colon is reflected medially, exposing the anterior surface of Gerota's capsule. The initial

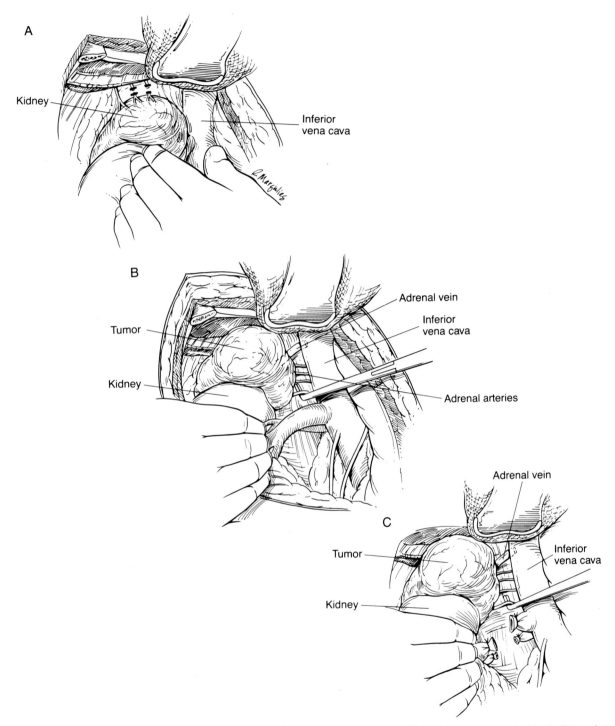

Figure 96–52. Exposure of the right adrenal with and without nephrectomy. (From Vaughan ED Jr: Adrenal surgery. *In* Marshall FF, ed: Operative Urology. Philadelphia, W. B. Saunders, 1991.)

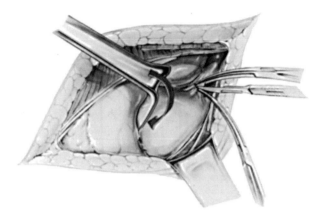

Figure 96–53. Release of the splenorenal ligament early in exposure of the left adrenal. (From Vaughan ED Jr: Adrenal surgery. *In* Marshall FF, ed: Operative Urology. Philadelphia, W. B. Saunders, 1991.)

dissection should be directed toward identification of the renal vein (see Fig. 96–55*B*). In essence, the dissection is the same as that used for a radical nephrectomy for renal carcinoma. Once the renal vein is exposed, the adrenal vein is identified and doubly ligated and divided. Following this maneuver, the pancreas and splenic vasculature are lifted off the anterior surface of the adrenal gland. Because of additional drainage from the adrenal into the phrenic system, the authors generally carry on with the medial dissection and control of the phrenic vein. The authors then work cephalad and lateral to release the splenorenal ligament and the supe-

rior attachments of the adrenal. The remaining dissection is carried out as previously described (Fig. 96–57).

Following removal of the tumor, regardless of size, careful inspection is made to ensure hemostasis and the absence of injury to adjacent organs. Careful abdominal exploration is carried out, after which the wound is closed with the suture material of choice. No drains are used.

Patients with MEA, those with a familial history of pheochromocytoma, or pediatric patients should be considered at high risk for multiple lesions. It is hoped that the preoperative evaluation would identify these lesions. Regardless, a careful abdominal exploration should be carried out.

In patients with suspected malignant pheochromocytomas, en bloc dissections may be necessary to obtain adequate

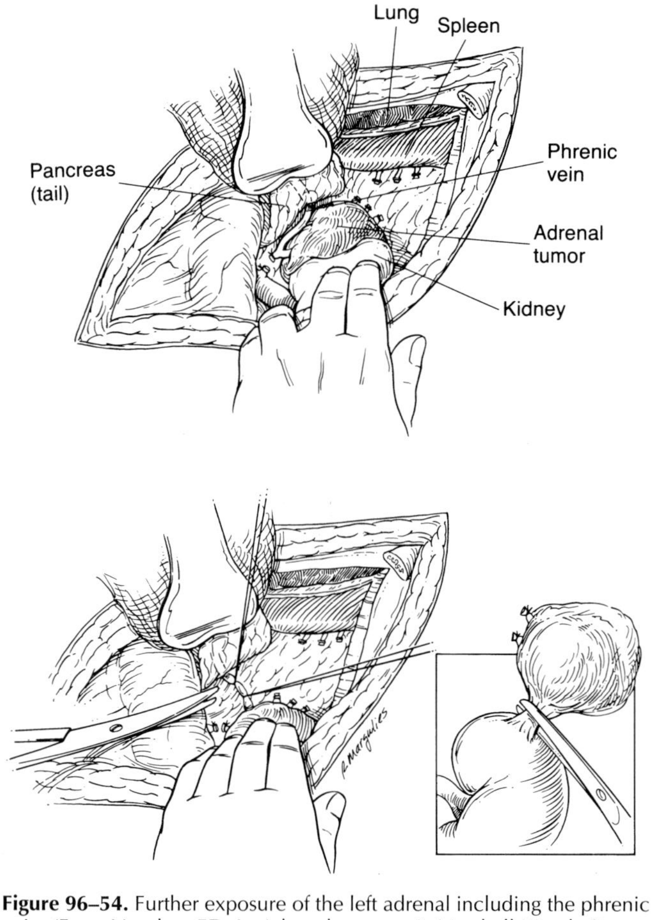

Figure 96–54. Further exposure of the left adrenal including the phrenic vein. (From Vaughan ED, Jr: Adrenal surgery. *In* Marshall FF, ed: Operative Urology. Philadelphia, W. B. Saunders, 1991.)

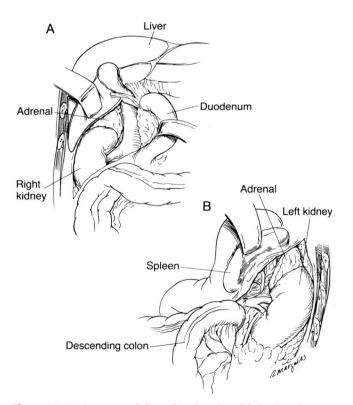

Figure 96–55. Exposure of the right adrenal and left adrenal using a transabdominal approach. (From Vaughan ED Jr: Adrenal surgery. *In* Marshall FF, ed: Operative Urology. Philadelphia, W. B. Saunders, 1991.)

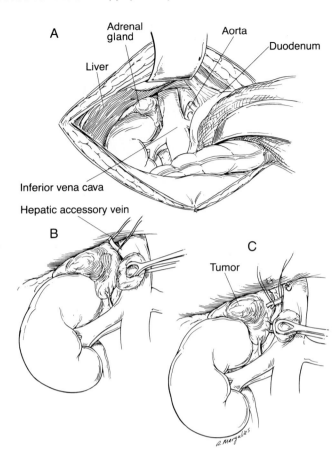

Figure 96–56. Further transabdominal exposure of the right adrenal with ligation of an accessory right hepatic vein. (From Vaughan ED Jr: Adrenal surgery. *In* Marshall FF, ed: Operative Urology. Philadelphia, W. B. Saunders, 1991.)

margins, a concept that is also true of patients with adrenal carcinomas (Fig. 96–58).

The results of adrenal surgery are extremely satisfying to both the treating physicians and the patients. Rarely in medicine do clinicians have a better understanding of the underlying pathophysiology than with adrenal disorders. Moreover, highly sophisticated analytic and radiographic diagnostic techniques are available that confirm clinical impressions. Elegant surgical approaches have been developed to the adrenal, which can be individualized for the specific clinical setting and can be successfully performed at minimum risk to the patient.

Partial Adrenalectomy

Nakada and co-workers have compared the therapeutic outcome of partial adrenalectomy versus total adrenalectomy in a series of patients with primary hyperaldosteronism. In their hands, there was no recurrent hyperaldosteronism in either group in a total of 48 patients who were followed for 5 years. Accordingly, it appears that partial adrenalectomy is an option that can be used in patients with primary hyperaldosteronism (Nakada et al, 1995). The need for adrenal preservation with *adrenal sparing surgery* is unclear in the patient with the normally functioning contralateral adrenal (Vaughan, 1995). There is no evidence that there is difficulty with adrenal function in a patient with a solitary functioning adrenal gland, and indeed there is evidence for compensatory adrenal hypertrophy following adrenalectomy (Gross et al, 1991).

The authors have used partial adrenalectomy in patients with bilateral disease, for example, in one patient in whom there was a pheochromocytoma and a contralateral nonfunctioning adenoma in which the adenoma was enucleated (see Fig. 96–48) and in a patient with bilateral pheochromocytomas (see Fig. 96–42) in whom the smaller lesion was enucleated, leaving functional cortical tissue. Certainly this technique is useful in the rare patient with a solitary adrenal.

Laparoscopic Adrenalectomy

In view of the maturation of laparoscopic surgery and the development of an exciting array of instruments, it is apparent that all of the surgical principles described herein, which are mandatory for successful open adrenalectomy, can be applied to the technique of laparoscopic adrenalectomy. The specific techniques for laparoscopic adrenalectomy are described elsewhere (see Chapter 95). This technique, however, now can be offered to patients as an alternative to open adrenalectomy. Patients with small adrenal tumors, incidentally found tumors, and even small pheochromocytomas have been treated successfully with this technique. The approach can be either retroperitoneal or transperitoneal, and with the evolution of the different techniques, operating times are being reduced, as is the need for transformation to an open procedure (Gagner et al, 1992; Suzuki et al, 1993; Go et al, 1993; Higashihara et al, 1993; Takeda et al, 1994; Brunt et al, 1996).

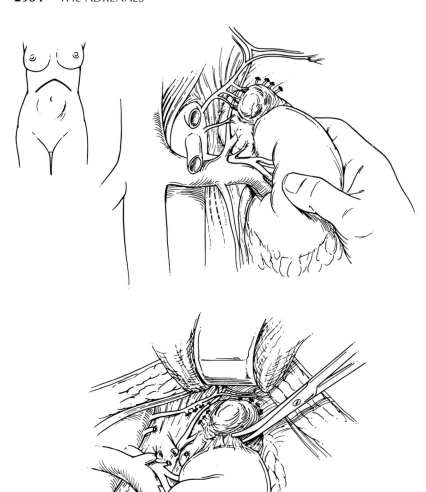

Figure 96–57. Further exposure of the left adrenal. (From Vaughan ED Jr: Adrenal surgery. *In* Marshall FF, ed: Operative Urology. Philadelphia, W. B. Saunders, 1991.)

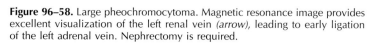

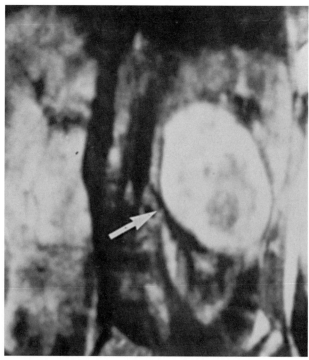

Figure 96–58. Large pheochromocytoma. Magnetic resonance image provides excellent visualization of the left renal vein *(arrow)*, leading to early ligation of the left adrenal vein. Nephrectomy is required.

ACKNOWLEDGMENT

Acknowledgment is made to all the contributors to the text *Adrenal Disorders,* edited by E. D. Vaughan, Jr., and R. M. Carey, which served as the basis for much of this chapter.

REFERENCES

Abecassis M, McLoughlin MJ, Langer B, Kudlow JE: Serendipitous adrenal masses: Prevalence, significance, and management. Am J Surg, 1985;149:783.

Abel JJ, Crawford AC: On the blood-pressure raising constituent of the suprarenal capsule. Johns Hopkins Hosp Bull 1897;8:151.

Abrams HL, Siegelman S, Adams DF, et al: Computed tomography versus ultrasound of the adrenal gland: A prospective study. Radiology 1982;143:121.

Addison T: On the Constitutional and Local Effects of Disease of the Suprarenal Capsules. London, Samuel Highley, 1855.

Aguirre P, Scully RE: Testosterone-secreting adrenal ganglioneuroma containing Leydig cells. Am J Surg Pathol 1983;7:699.

Amberson JB, Gray GF: Adrenal pathology in adrenal disorders. In Vaughan ED Jr, Carey RM, eds: Adrenal Disorders. New York, Thieme Medical Publishers, 1989.

Amberson JB, Vaughan ED Jr, Gray GF, Naus GJ: Flow cytometric analysis of nuclear DNA from adrenocorticoid tumors: A retrospective study using paraffin-imbedded tissue. Cancer 1987;59:2091.

Andler W, Havers W, Stambolis C, et al: Renal cell carcinoma following irradiation therapy for adrenal cortical carcinoma. J Pediatr 1978;93:634.

Angermeier KW, Montie JE: Perioperative complications of adrenal surgery. Urol Clin North Am 1989;16:597–606.

Anson BJ, Caldwell EW, Pick JW, Beaton LE: The blood supply of the kidney suprarenal gland and associated structures. Surg Gynecol Obstet 1947;84:313.

Antoni F: Hypothalamic control of adrenocorticotropin secretion: Advances since the discovery of 41-residue corticotropin-releasing factor. Endocr Rev 1986;7:351.

Arit W, Reincke M, Siekmann L, et al: Suramin in adrenocortical cancer: Limited efficacy and serious toxicity. Clin Endocrinol 1994;41:299–307.

Armanini D, Kuhnle U, Strasser T, et al: Aldosterone-receptor deficiency in pseudohypoaldosteronism. N Engl J Med 1985;313:1178–1181.

Arteaga E, Biglieri EG, Kater CE, et al: Aldosterone-producing adrenocortical carcinoma; Preoperative recognition and course in 3 cases. Ann Intern Med 1984;101:316.

Arteaga E, Klein R, Biglieri EG: Use of the saline infusion test to diagnose the cause of primary aldosteronism. Am J Med 1985;78:722–727.

Artusio JF Jr: Anesthesia for pheochromocytoma. In Malhotra V, ed: Anesthesia for Renal and Genitourinary Surgery. New York, McGraw-Hill; 1995, pp 79–92.

Atlas SA, Maack T: Atrial natriuretic factor. In Windhager EE, ed: Handbook of Physiology. New York, Oxford University Press, 1991.

Avgerinos PC, Yanovski JA, Oldfield EH, et al: The metrapone and dexamethasone suppression tests for the differential diagnosis of the adrenocorticotropin-dependent Cushing syndrome: A comparison. Ann Intern Med 1994;121:318–327.

Axelrod J: Purification and properties of phenylethanolamine-N-methyl transferase. J Biol Chem 1962;237:1657.

Baer L, Sommers SC, Krakoff LR, et al: Pseudoprimary aldosteronism: An entity distinct from true primary aldosteronism. Circ Res 1970;27(suppl):203.

Bagshaw EKD: Hypokalemia carcinoma and Cushing's syndrome. Lancet 1960;2:284.

Banks WA, Kastin HA, Biglieri EG, Ruiz EA: Primary adrenal hyperplasia: A new subset of primary hyperaldosteronism. J Clin Endocrinol Metab 1984;58:783.

Baxter JD, Tyrrell JB: The adrenal cortex. In Felig P, Baxter JD, Broadus AE, Frohman LA, eds: Endocrinology and Metabolism. New York, McGraw-Hill, 1981, p 408.

Beierwaltes WH, Lieberman LM, Ansari AN, Nishiyama H: Visualization of human adrenal glands in vivo by scintillation scanning. JAMA 1971;216:275–277.

Belldegrun A, deKernion JB: What to do about the incidentally found adrenal mass. World J Urol 1989;7:117–120.

Belldegrun A, Hussain S, Seltzer SE, et al: The incidentally discovered adrenal mass: A therapeutic dilemma—BWH experience 1976–1983. Surg Gynecol Obstet 1986;163:203.

Bergenstal DM, Hurtz R, Lipsett MB, Moy RH: Chemotherapy of adrenal cortical cancer with o,p'DDD. Ann Intern Med 1960;53:672.

Bergland RM, Harrison PS: Pituitary and adrenal. In Schwartz SI, ed: Principles of Surgery. New York, McGraw-Hill, 1983.

Berkoff GT, Sandberg AA, Nelson DH, Tyler FH: Clinical usefulness of determination of circulating 17-hydroxycorticosteroid levels. Arch Intern Med 1954;93:1.

Bertagna C, Orth DN: Clinical and laboratory findings and results of therapy in 58 patients with adrenocortical tumors admitted to a single medical center (1951 to 1978). Am J Med 1981;71:855–875.

Bertagna X, Bertagna C, Laudat MH, et al: Pituitary-adrenal response to the antiglucocorticoid action of RU 486 in Cushing's syndrome. J Clin Endocrinol Metab 1986;63:639–643.

Besser GM, Edwards CRW: Cushing's syndrome. J Clin Endocrinol Metab 1972;1:451.

Beuschlein F, Reincke M, Karl M, et al: Clonal composition of human adrenocortical neoplasms. Cancer Res 1994;54:4927–4932.

Bianchi H, Ferrari A: The arterial circulation of the left suprarenal gland. Surg Radiol Anat 1991;13:113–116.

Biglieri EG, Irony I, Kater CE: Adrenocortical forms of human hypertension. In Laragh JH, Brenner BM, eds: Hypertension: Pathophysiology, Diagnosis, and Management. New York, Raven Press, 1990.

Biglieri EG, Kater CE, Mantero F: Adrenocortical forms of human hypertension. In Laragh JH, Brenner BM, eds: Hypertension: Pathophysiology, Diagnosis, and Management, 2nd ed. New York, Raven Press, 1995, pp 2145–2162.

Biglieri EG, Schambelan M: The significance of elevated levels of plasma 18-hydroxycorticosterone in patients with primary aldosteronism. J Clin Endocrinol Metab 1979;49:87–91.

Bigos ST, Somma M, Rasio E, et al: Cushing's disease: Management by transphenoidal pituitary microsurgery. J Clin Endocrinol Metab 1980;50:348.

Bilbey JH, McLoughlin RF, Kurkjian PS, et al: MR imaging of adrenal masses: Value of chemical-shift imaging for distinguishing adenomas from other tumors. AJR 1995;164:637–642.

Blumenfeld J, Cohen N, Laragh JH, Ruggiero DA: Hypertension and catecholamine biosynthesis associated with a glomus jugulare tumor. N Engl J Med 1992;327:894–895.

Blumenfeld J, Cohen N, Anwar M, et al: Hypertension and a tumor of the glomus jugulare region: Evidence for epinephrine biosynthesis. Am J Hypertens 1993;6:382–387.

Blumenfeld JD: Hypertension and adrenal disorders. Curr Opin Nephrol Hypertens 1993;2:274–282.

Blumenfeld JD, Schlussel Y, Sealey JE, et al: Diagnosis and treatment of primary hyperaldosteronism. Ann Intern Med 1994;121:877–885.

Blumenfeld JD, Sealey JE, Bragat AC, et al: Effects of β-blockade on blood pressure, prorenin, renin and angiotensin II and its interaction with captopril in normotensives and essential hypertensives. Presented at Annual Meeting of the American Society of Nephrology, 1995.

Bolande RP: The neurocrestopathias: A unifying concept of disease arising in neurocrest maldevelopment. Hum Pathol 1974;5:409.

Bolli P, Amann FW, Buhler FR: Antihypertensive response to postsynaptic alpha-blockade with prazosin in low and normal renin hypertension. J Cardiovasc Pharmacol 1980;2(suppl 3):S399–S405.

Bornstein SR, Ehrhart-Bornstein M, Usadel H, et al: Morphological evidence for a close interaction of chromaffin cells with cortical cells within the adrenal gland. Cell Tissue Res 1991;265:1–9.

Boutros AR, Bravo EL, Zanettin G, Straffon RA: Perioperative management of 63 patients with pheochromocytoma. Cleve Clin J Med 1990;57:613–617.

Bravo EL, Gifford RW Jr: Pheochromocytoma: Diagnosis, localization and management. N Engl J Med 1984;311:1298.

Bravo EL: Pheochromocytoma: New concepts and future trends. Kidney Int 1991;40:544–556.

Bravo EL, Fouad FM, Tarazi RC: Calcium channel blockade with nifedipine in primary aldosteronism. Hypertension 1986;8(suppl I):I-91–I-94.

Bravo EL, Fouad-Tarazi FM, Tarazi RC, et al: Clinical implications of primary aldosteronism with resistant hypertension. Hypertension 1988;11(suppl I):I-207–I-211.

Bravo EL, Tarazi RC, Dustan HP, et al: The changing clinical spectrum of primary aldosteronism. Am J Med 1983;74:641.

Bravo EL, Tarazi RC, Dustan HP, Fouad FM: The sympathetic nervous system and hypertension in primary aldosteronism. Hypertension 1985;7:90–96.

Bravo EL, Tarazi RC, Fouad FM, et al: Clonidine-suppression test: A useful aid in the diagnosis of pheochromocytoma. N Engl J Med 1981;305:623.

Brennan MF: Adrenocorticoid carcinoma. Cancer 1987;37:348.

Briggs RSJ, Birtwell, AJ, Pohl JEF: Hypertensive response to labetalol in pheochromocytoma. Lancet 1978;1:1045.

Briggs JP, Schnermann J: Control of renin release and glomerular vascular tone by the juxtaglomerular apparatus. In Laragh JH, Brenner BM, eds: Hypertension: Pathophysiology, Diagnosis, and Management, 2nd ed. New York, Raven Press, 1995, pp 1359–1383.

Brownie AC: The adrenal cortex and hypertension DOCA/salt hypertension and beyond. In Laragh JH, Brenner BM, eds: Hypertension: Pathophysiology, Diagnosis, and Management. New York, Raven Press, 1990.

Brown-Sequard CE: Recherches experimentales sur la physiologie et la pathologie des capsules surrenales. Arch Gen Med 1856;2:385.

Brunner HR, Laragh JH, Baer L, et al: Essential hypertension: Renin and aldosterone, heart attack and stroke. N Engl J Med 1972;286:441.

Brunt LM, Doherty GM, Norton JA, et al: Laparoscopic adrenalectomy compared to open adrenalectomy for benign adrenal neoplasms. J Am Coll Surg 1996;183:1–10.

Bucht H, Bergstrom J, Lindholmar G, et al: Catheterization of left adrenal vein for contrast injection and steroid analysis in a case of Conn's syndrome. Acta Med Scand 1964;176:233.

Buhler FR, Laragh JH, Baer L, et al: Propranolol inhibition of renin secretion: A specific approach to diagnosis and treatment of renin-dependent hypertensive diseases. N Engl J Med 1972;287:1209–1214.

Bukowski RM, Wolfe M, Levine HS, et al: Phase II trial of mitotane and cisplatin in patients with adrenal carcinoma: A Southwest Oncology Group study. J Clin Oncol 1993;11:161–165.

Bullock WK, Hirst AE: Metastatic carcinoma of the adrenal. Am J Med Sci 1953;226:521.

Burch WM: Cushing's disease: A review. Intern Med 1985;145:1106.

Bursztyn M, Grossman E, Rosental T: The absence of long-term therapeutic effect of calcium channel blockade in the primary aldosteronism of adrenal adenomas. Am J Hypertens 1988;1:88S–90S.

Calkins E, Howard JE: Bilateral familiar pheochromocytoma with paroxysmal hypertension: Successful surgical removal of tumors in two cases, with discussion of certain diagnostic procedures and physiological considerations. J Clin Endocrinol Metab 1947;7:475.

Campeau RJ, Garcia OM, Correa OA, Rege AB: Pheochromocytoma: Diagnosis by scintigraphy using iodine I131 metaiodobenzyl-guanidine. Southern Med J 1991;84:1221–1230.

Carey RM, Douglas JG, Schweikert JR: The syndrome of essential hypertension with suppressed plasma renin activity: Normalization of blood pressure with spironolactone. Arch Intern Med 1972;130:849.

Carey RM, Estratopoluos AD, Peart WS, Wilson GA: Effect of aldosterone on colonic potential difference in renal electrolyte excretion in normal man. Clin Sci 1974;46:488.

Carey RM, Sen S: Recent progress in the control of aldosterone secretion. Rec Prog Hormone Res 1986;42:251.

Carey RM, Varma SK, Drake CR Jr, et al: Ectopic secretion of corticotropin-releasing factor as a cause of Cushing's syndrome: A clinical, morphologic and biochemical study. N Engl J Med 1984;311:13–20.

Carney JA, Sizemore GW, Sheps GS: Adrenal medullary disease in multiple endocrine neoplasia type 2. Am J Clin Pathol 1976;66:279.

Carpenter PC: Cushing syndrome: Update of diagnosis and management. Mayo Clin Proc 1986;61:49.

Casey LR, Cohen AJ, Wile AG, Dietrich RB: Giant adrenal myelolipomas: CT and MRI findings. Abdom Imaging 1994;19:165–167.

Casson IF, Davis JC, Jeffreys RV, et al: Successful management of Cushing's disease during pregnancy by transsphenoidal adenectomy. Clin Endocrinol 1987;27:423–428.

Cedermark BJ, Blumenson LE, Pickering JW, et al: The significance of metastasis to the adrenal glands in adenocarcinoma of the colon and rectum. Surg Gynecol Obstet 1977;144:537.

Cerfolio RJ, Vaughan ED Jr, Brennan TG, Hirvela ER: Accuracy of computed tomography in predicting adrenal tumor size. Surg Gynecol Obstet 1993;176:307.

Champion PK: Cushing's syndrome secondary to abuse of dexamethasone nasal spray. Arch Intern Med 1974;134:750.

Christlieb AR, Espiner EA, Amsterdam EA, et al: The pattern of electrolyte excretion in normal and hypertensive subjects before and after saline infusions: A simple electrolyte formula for the diagnosis of primary aldosteronism. Am J Cardiol 1971;27:595.

Chrousos GP: The hypothalamic-pituitary-adrenal axis and immune-mediated inflammation. N Engl J Med 1995;332:1351–1362.

Cohen KL, Noth RH, Pechinski T: Incidence of pituitary tumors following adrenalectomy: A long-term follow-up study of patients treated for Cushing's disease. Arch Intern Med 1978;138:575.

Cohn K, Gottesman L, Brennan M: Adrenocortical carcinoma. Surgery 1986;100:1170.

Conn JW: Primary hyperaldosteronism: A new clinical syndrome. J Lab Clin Med 1955a;45:3.

Conn JW: Primary aldosteronism. J Lab Clin Med, 1955b;45:661.

Conn JW: The evolution of primary aldosteronism: 1954–1967. Harvey Lect 1967;62:257.

Conn JW: Primary aldosteronism. In Genest J, Koiw E, Kuchel O, eds: Hypertension: Physiopathology and Treatment. New York, McGraw-Hill, 1977, pp 768–780.

Conn JW, Cohen EL, Rovner DR: Suppression of plasma renin activity in primary aldosteronism: Distinguishing primary from secondary aldosteronism in hypertensive disease. JAMA 1964;190:125.

Conn JW, Rovner DR, Cohen EL, Nesbit RM: Normokalemic primary aldosteronism: Its masquerade as "essential" hypertension. JAMA 1966;195:111.

Contreras P, Rojas HA, Biagini L, et al: Regression of metastatic adrenal carcinoma during palliative ketoconazole. Lancet 1985;2:151.

Copeland PM: The incidentally discovered adrenal mass. Ann Intern Med 1983;98:940.

Crapo L: Cushing's syndrome: A review of diagnostic tests. Metabolism 1979;28:955.

Crispel KR, Parson W, Hamlin J, Hollifield G: Addison's disease associated with histoplasmosis. Am J Med 1956;20:23.

Crowder RE: The development of the adrenal gland in man. Carnegie Contrib Embryol 1957;36:193.

Culp OS: Adrenal hetertopia: A survey of the literature and a report of a case. J Urol 1959;41:303.

Cushing H: The Pituitary Body and Its Disorders: Clinical States Produced by Disorders of the Hypophysis Cerebri. Philadelphia, J. B. Lippincott, 1912.

Cushing H: The basophil adenomas of the pituitary body and their clinical manifestations (pituitary basophilism). Johns Hopkins Hosp Bull 1932;50:137.

Cuvier GLCFD, Baron: Lecons d'Anatomie Comparee. Five volumes. Paris, Baudonin, 1800–1805.

Deal JE, Sever PS, Barratt TM, Dillon MJ: Pheochromocytoma—investigation and management of 10 cases. Arch Dis Child 1990;65:269–274.

DelGaudio A, DelGaudio G-A: Virilizing adrenocortical tumors in adult women: Report of 10 patients, 2 of whom each had a tumor secreting only testosterone. Cancer 1993;72:1997–2003.

DelGaudio A, Solidoro G: Myelolipoma of the adrenal gland: Report of 2 cases with the review of the literature. Surgery 1986;99:293.

DelGaudio A, Solidoro G: Myelolipoma of the adrenal gland: Two further observations and update of literature. J Urol. In press.

Deming QB, Luetscher JA Jr: Bioassay of desoxycorticosterone-like material in urine. Proc Soc Exp Biol Med 1950;73:171.

Derksen J, Nagesser SK, Meinders AE, et al: Identification of virilizing adrenal tumors in hirsute women. N Engl J Med 1994;331:968–973.

Dickstein G, Spindel A, Shechner C, et al: Spontaneous remission in Cushing's disease. Arch Intern Med 1991;151:185–189.

Didolkar MS, Bescher AR, Elias EG, Moore RH: Natural history of adrenal cortical carcinoma: A clinical pathologic study of 42 patients. Cancer 1981;47:2153.

Dolan LM, Carey RM: Adrenal cortical and medullary function: Diagnostic tests. In Vaughan ED Jr, Carey RM, eds: Adrenal Disorders. New York, Thieme Medical Publishers, Inc. 1989, p 81.

Dunlop D: 86 cases of Addison's disease. BMJ 1963;2:887.

Dunnick NR: Adrenal imaging: Current status. Am J Radiol 1990;154:927.

Dunnick NR, Doppman JL, Gill JR Jr, et al: Localization of functional adrenal tumors by computed tomography and venous sampling. Radiology 1982;142:429.

Eason RJ, Croxson MS, Perry MC, Somerfield SD: Addison's disease, adrenal autoantibodies and computerized adrenal tomography. NZ Med J 1982;95:569.

Eddy RL, Jones AL, Gilliland PF, et al: Cushing's syndrome: A perspective study of diagnostic methods. Am J Med 1973;55:621.

Ein SH, Shandling B, Wesson D, Filler RM: Recurrent pheochromocytomas in children. J Pediatr Surg 1990;25:1063–1065.

Engelman K, Horowitz D, Jequier E, Sjoerdsma A: Biochemical and pharmacologic effects of alpha-methyl-tyrosine in man. J Clin Invest 1968;47:577.

Espiner EA, Tucci JR, Yagger PI, Lauler DP: Effect of saline infusions on aldosterone secretion and electrolyte excretion in normal subjects and patients with primary aldosteronism. N Engl J Med 1967;277:1.

Eustachius B: Opuscula anatomica Venice vicentius luchinus. 1563.

Falke THM, Strakel TE, Sandler MP: Magnetic resonance imaging of the adrenal glands. Radio Graphics 1987;7:343.

Fallo F, Dluhy R, Carroll J, et al: Aldosterone-producing adenomas do not contain glucocorticoid remediable aldosteronism chimeric gene duplication. Twenty-first International Aldosterone Conference, 1995.

Farwell AP, Devlin JT, Stewart JA: Total suppression of cortisol excretion by ketoconazole in the therapy of the ectopic adrenocorticotropic hormone syndrome. Am J Med 1988;84:1063.

Ferrerira SH, Vane JR: Half lives of peptides and amines in the circulation. Nature 1967;215:1237.

Ferriss JB, Beevers DG, Brown JJ, et al: Clinical, biochemcial, and pathological features of low-renin ("primary") hyperaldosteronism. Am Heart J 1978;95:375–388.

Findling JW, Adams AH, Raff H: Selective hypoaldosteronism due to an endogenous impairment in angiotensin II production. N Engl J Med 1987;316:1632–1635.

Fish RG, Takaro T, Lovell M: Coexistent Addison's disease and American blastomycosis. Am J Med 1960;28:152.

Fisher CE, Turner FA, Horton R: Remission of primary hyperaldosteronism after adrenal venography. N Engl J Med 1971;285:334.

Fitzgerald PA, Aron DC, Findling JW, et al: Cushing's disease transient adrenal insufficiency after selective removal of the pituitary microadenomas: Evidence for pituitary origin. J Clin Endocrinol Metab 1982;54:413.

Flavin DK, Fredrickson PA, Richardson JW: An unusual manifestation of drug dependence. Mayo Clin Proc 1983;58:764.

Flynn SD, Murren JR, Kirby WM, et al: P-glycoprotein expression and multidrug resistance in adrenocortical carcinoma. Surgery 1992;112:981–986.

Fontes R, Kater C, Biglieri EG, Irony II: Reassessment of the predictive value of the postural stimulation test in primary aldosteronism. Am J Hypertens 1991;4:786–791.

Forbes AP, Albright F: A comparison of the 17-keto steroid excretion in Cushing's syndrome associated with adrenal tumor and with adrenal hyperplasia. J Clin Endocrinol Metab 1951;11:926.

Fränkel F: Ein fall von doppelseitigen vollig latent verlaufenen Nebennierentumor und gleichseitigen Nephritis mit Veranderungen am circulations—Apparat und Retinitis. Arch Pathol Anat 1886;103.

Fries JG, Chamberlin JA: Extra-adrenal pheochromocytoma: Literature review and report of a cervical pheochromocytoma. Surgery 1968;63:268–279.

Fudge TL, McKinnon WMP, Geary WL: Current surgical management of pheochromocytoma during pregnancy. Arch Surg 1980;15:1224.

Gabrilove JL, Seeman AT, Saba T: Virilizing adrenal adenoma with studies on the steroid content of the adrenal venous effluent and review of the literature. Endocrinol Rev 1981;2:462.

Gabrilove JL, Sharma DC, Waitz HH, Dorfman R: Feminizing adrenal cortical tumors in the male: A review of 52 cases including a case report. Medicine 1965;44:37.

Gagner M, Lacroix A, Bolte E: Laparoscopic adrenalectomy in Cushing's syndrome and pheochromocytoma (Letter to the Editor). N Engl J Med 1992;327:1033.

Ganguly A, Dowdy AJ, Luetscher JA, Melada GA: Anomalous postural response of plasma aldosterone concentration in patients with aldosterone-producing adrenal adenomas. J Clin Endocrinol Metab 1973;36:401.

Ganguly A, Grim CE, Weinberger MH: Anomalous postural aldosterone response in glucocorticoid-suppressible hyperaldosteronism. N Engl J Med 1981;305:991.

Geisinger MA, Zelch MG, Bravo EL, et al: Primary hyperaldosteronism: Comparison of CT, adrenal venography and venous sampling. AJR 1983;141:299.

Gicquel C, Leblond-Francillard M, Bertagna X, et al: Clonal analysis of human adrenocortical carcinomas and secreting adenomas. Clin Endocrinol 1994;40:465–477.

Gil-Vernet J: New surgical concepts in removing renal calculi. Urol Int 1965;20:255–262.

Glass AR, Zavadil AP, Halberg F, et al: Circadian rhythm of serum cortisol in Cushing's disease. J Clin Endocrinol Metab 1984;59:161.

Glazer HS, Weyman PJ, Sagal SS, et al: Nonfunctioning adrenal masses: Incidental discovery on computed tomography. AJR 1982;139:81.

Gleason PE, Weinberger MH, Pratt JH, et al: Evaluation of diagnostic test in the differential diagnosis of primary aldosteronism: Unilateral adenoma versus bilateral micronodular hyperplasia. J Urol 1993;150:1365–1368.

Glenn F, Peterson RE, Mannix H Jr, eds: Surgery of the Adrenal Glands. New York, Macmillan, 1968.

Go H, Takeda M, Takahashi H, et al: Laparoscopic adrenalectomy for primary aldosteronism: A new operative method. J Laparoendosc Surg 1993;3:455.

Gold PW, Loriaux DL, Roy A: Responses to corticotropin-releasing hormone in the hypercortisolism of depression and Cushing's disease: Pathophysiologic and diagnostic implications. N Engl J Med 1986;314:1329–1335.

Gordon RD, Gomez-Sanchez CE, Hamlet SM, et al: Angiotensin-responsive aldosterone producing adenoma masquerades as idiopathic aldosteronism or low renin essential hypertension. J Hypertens 1987;5(suppl 5):S103–S106.

Gordon RD, Klemm SA, Tunny T, Stowasser M: Primary aldosteronism: Hypertension with a genetic basis. Lancet 1992;340:159–161.

Gross MD, Shapiro B, Freitas JE, et al: Clinical significance of the solitary functioning adrenal gland. J Nucl Med 1991;32:1882–1887.

Grunberg SM: Development of Cushing's syndrome and virilization after presentation of a nonfunctioning adrenocortical carcinoma. Cancer 1982;50:815.

Guilhaume B, Sanson ML, Billaud L, et al: Cushing's syndrome and pregnancy: Aetiologies and prognosis in twenty-two patients. Eur J Med 1992;1:83–89.

Haak HR, Cornelisse CJ, Hermans J, et al: Nuclear DNA content and morphological characteristics in the prognosis of adrenocortical carcinoma. Br J Cancer 1993a;68:151–155.

Haak HR, Fleuren G-J: Neuroendocrine differentiation of adrenocortical tumors. Cancer 1995;75:860–864.

Haak HR, Hermans J, van de Velde CJH, et al: Optimal treatment of adrenocortical carcinoma with mitotane: Results in a consecutive series of 96 patients. Br J Cancer 1994;69:947–951.

Haak HR, van Seters AP, Moolenaar AJ, Fleuren GJ: Expression of P-glycoprotein in relation to clinical manifestation, treatment and prognosis of adrenocortical cancer. Eur J Cancer 1993b;29A:1036–1038.

Haas JA, Knox FG: Mechanism for escape from salt-retaining effects of mineralocorticoids: Role of the nephrons. Semin Nephrol 1990;10:380.

Hall WA, Luciano MG, Doppman JL, et al: Pituitary magnetic resonance imaging in normal human volunteers: Occult adenomas in the general population. Ann Intern Med 1994;120:817–820.

Hamberger C-A, Hamberger CB, Wersall J, Wagermark J: Malignant catecholamine-producing tumour of the carotid body. Acta Pathol Microbiol Scand 1967;69:489–492.

Hamlet SM, Tunny TJ, Woodland E, Gordon RD: Is aldosterone/renin ratio useful to screen a hypertensive population for primary aldosteronism? Clin Exp Pharmacol Physiol 1985;12:249–252.

Hardy J: Transphenoidal hypophysectomy. J Neurosurg 1971;34:582

Hardy J: Cushing's disease—50 years later. Can J Neurol Sci 1982;9:375.

Hartman FA, MacArthur CG, Hartman WE: A substance which prolongs the life of adrenalectomized cats. Proc Soc Exp Biol Med 1927;25:69.

Hedeland H, Ostberg G, Hokfeld B: On the prevalence of adrenal cortical adenomas in an autopsy and autopsy material in relation to hypertension and diabetes. Acta Med Scand 1968;184:211.

Heinbecker P, O'Neal LW, Ackerman LV: Functioning and nonfunctioning adrenocortical tumors. Surg Gynecol Obstet 1957;105:21.

Hench PS, Kendall EC, Slocumb CH, Polley HF: The effect of a hormone of the adrenal cortex (17-hydroxy-11-dehydrocorticosterone: compound E) and of pituitary adrenocorticotropic hormone on rheumatoid arthritis. Proc Staff Meetings Mayo Clin 1949;24:181–197.

Herf SM, Teates DC, Tegtmeyer CJ, et al: Identification and differentiation of surgically correctable hypertension due to primary aldosteronism. Am J Med 1979;67:397.

Higashihara E, Tanaka Y, Horie S, et al: Laparoscopic adrenalectomy: The initial 3 cases. J Urol 1993;149:973.

Hiramatsu K, Yamada T, Yukimura Y, et al: A screening test to identify aldosterone-producing adenoma by measuring plasma renin activity: Results in hypertensive patients. Arch Intern Med 1981;141:1589–1593.

Hoffman DL, Mattox VL: Treatment of adrenal cortical carcinoma with o,p' DDD. Med Clin North Am 1972;50:999.

Hoffman K: Relations between chemical structure and function of adrenocorticotropin and melanocyte stimulating hormones. In Knobil E, Sawyer WH, eds: Handbook of Physiology, Endocrinology, Vol. 4. The Pituitary and Its Neuroendocrine Control, section 7, part 2. Washington, D.C., American Physiological Society, 1974.

Horton R, Finck E: Diagnosis and localization in primary aldosteronism. Ann Intern Med 1972;76:885.

Howards SS, Carey RM: The adrenals. *In* Gillenwater JY, Grayhack JT, Howards SS, Duckett JW, eds: Adult and Pediatric Urology, 2nd ed. Chicago, Year Book Medical Publishers, 1991.

Howlet TA, Rees LH, Besser GM: Cushing's syndrome. J Clin Endocrinol Metab 1985;14:911.

Hsiao RJ, Parmer RJ, Takiyyuddin MA, O'Connor DT: Chromogranin A storage and secretion: Sensitivity and specificity for the diagnosis of pheochromocytoma. Medicine 1991;70:33–45.

Hubbard MM, Kulaylat MM, Amabumrad NN: Adrenocorticoids—physiology regulation function and metabolism. *In* Scott HW Jr, ed: Surgery of the Adrenal Glands. Philadelphia, J. B. Lippincott, 1990.

Huebener KH, Treugut H: Adrenal cortex dysfunction: CT findings. Radiology 1984;150:195.

Hume TM: Pheochromocytoma in the adult and in the child. Am J Surg 1960;99:458.

Hunt TK, Tyrrell JB: Cushing's syndrome: Hypercortisolism. *In* Friesen SR, ed: Surgical Endocrinology: Clinical Syndromes. Philadelphia, J. B. Lippincott, 1978.

Hutter AM, Kayhoe DE: Adrenal cortical carcinoma: Results of treatment with o,p'DDD in 138 patients. Am J Med 1966;41:581.

Icard P, Chapuis Y, Andreassian B, et al: Adrenocortical carcinoma in surgically treated patients: A retrospective study on 156 cases by the French Association of Endocrine Surgery. Surgery 1992;112:972–980.

Ihde JA, Turnbull ADM, Bajorunas DR: Adrenal insufficiency in the cancer patient: Implications for the surgeon. Br J Surg 1990;77:1335–1337.

Imai T, Seo H, Murata Y, et al: Dexamethasone-nonsuppressible cortisol in two cases with aldosterone-producing adenoma. J Clin Endocrinol Metab 1991;72:575–581.

Imperato-McGinley J, Gautier T, Ehlers K, et al: Reversibility of catecholamine-induced dilated cardiomyopathy in a child with a pheochromocytoma. N Engl J Med 1987;316:793–797.

Imperato-McGinley J, Young IS, Huang T, et al: Testosterone secreting adrenal cortical adenomas. Int J Gynaecol Obstet 1981;19:421.

Irony I, Kater CE, Arteaga E, Biglieri EG: Characteristics of correctable subtypes of primary aldosteronism. Am J Hypertens 1988;1:50A.

Irony I, Kater C, Biglieri EG, Shackelton CHL: Correctable subsets of primary aldosteronism: Primary adrenal hyperplasia and renin responsive adenoma. Am J Hypertens 1990;3:576–582.

Irvine WJ, Barnes EW: Adrenocortical insufficiency. J Clin Endocrinol Metab 1972;1:549.

Isles CG, MacDougall IC, Lever AF, et al: Hypermineralocorticoidism due to adrenal carcinoma: Plasma corticosteroids and their response to ACTH and angiotensin II. Clin Endocrinol 1987;26:239–251.

Iverson LL: Uptake of circulating catecholamines. *In* Blaschko H, Sayers G, Smith AD, eds: Handbook of Physiology. Washington, D.C., American Physiological Society, 1975, p 713.

Janus CL, Mendelson DS: Comparison of MRI and CT for study of renal and perirenal masses. Crit Rev Diag Imaging 1991;32:69–118.

Jasani MK, Freeman PA, Boyle JA, et al: Studies of the rise in plasma 11-hydroxycorticosteroids in corticosteroid-treated patients with rheumatoid arthritis during surgery: Correlations with the functional integrity of the hypothalamic-pituitary-adrenal axis. Q J Med 1968;37:407.

Jenkins PJ, Trainer PJ, Plowman PN, et al: The long-term outcome after adrenalectomy and prophylactic pituitary radiotherapy in adrenocorticotropin-dependent Cushing's syndrome. J Clin Endocrinol Metab 1995;80:165–171.

Jennings AS, Liddle GW, Orth DN: Results of treating childhood Cushing's disease with pituitary radiation. N Engl J Med 1977;29:957.

Johnson DH, Greco FA: Treatment of metastatic adrenal cortical carcinoma with cisplatin and etoposide (vp16). Cancer 1986;58:2198.

Johnson LK, Baxter JD: Regulation of gene expression by glucocorticoid hormones: Early effects preserved in insulin chromatin. J Biol Chem 1987;254:1991.

Johnstone FR: The suprarenal veins. Am J Surg 1957;94:615.

Junqueira LC, Ncearneir OJ: Adrenal islets of Langerhans, parathyroids and pineal body. *In* Junqueira LC, Carneiro J; eds: Basic Histology, 4th ed. Los Altos, CA, Lange Medical Publications, 1983.

Kalff V, Shapiro B, Lloyd R, et al: The spectrum of pheochromocytoma in hypertensive patients with neurofibromatosis. Arch Intern Med 1982;142:209.

Kane NM, Korobkin M, Francis IR, et al: Percutaneous biopsy of left adrenal masses: Prevalence of pancreatitis after anterior approach. AJR 1991;157:777–780.

Kaplan NM, Kramer NJ, Holland OB, et al: Single-voided urine metanephrine assays in screening for pheochromocytoma. Arch Intern Med 1977;137:190.

Karlberg BE, Hedman L: Value of clonidine suppression test in the diagnosis of pheochromocytoma. Acta Med Scand 1986;714(suppl):15.

Kay R, Schumacker OP, Pank ES: Adrenal cortical carcinoma in children. J Urol 1983;130:1130.

Kazam E, Engel IA, Zirinsky K, et al: Sectional imaging of the adrenal glands, computed tomography and ultrasound. *In* Vaughan ED Jr, Carey RM, eds: Adrenal Disorders. New York, Thieme Medical Publishers, 1989.

Kazerooni EA, Sisson JC, Shapiro B, et al: Diagnostic accuracy and pitfalls of (iodine-131) 6-beta-iodomethyl-119-norcholesterol (np59) imaging. J Nucl Med 1990;31:526.

Kehlet H, Binder C: Value of an ACTH test in assessing hypothalamic-pituitary-adrenal cortical function in glucocorticoid-treated patients. BMJ 1973;2:147.

Klein FA, Kay S, Ratliff JE, et al: Flow cytometric determinations of ploidy and proliferation patterns of adrenal neoplasms: An adjunct to histological classification. J Urol 1985;9:33.

Klibanski A, Zervas NT: Diagnosis and management of hormone-secreting pituitary adenomas. N Engl J Med 1991;324:822–830.

Knight CD, Trichel BE, Mathews WR: Nonfunctioning carcinoma of the adrenal cortex. Ann Surg 1960;151:349–358.

Koh MS, Lee M-S, Hong SW, Lim D: Partial remission with transarterial embolization in a case of metastatic adrenal cortical carcinoma. J Korean Med Sci 1991;6:173–176.

Kohn A: Das chromaffin Gewebe. Anat entwicklungsgeschicte 1902;12:253.

Korobkin M: Overview of adrenal imaging/adrenal CT. Urol Radiol 1989;11:221.

Kozeny GA, Hurley RM, Vertuno LL, et al: Hypertension, mineralocorticoid-resistant hyperkalemia, and hyperchloremic acidosis in an infant with obstructive uropathy. Am J Nephrol 1986;6:476–481.

Kreiger DT: Rhythms of ACTH and corticosteroid secretion in health and disease and their experimental modification. J Steroid Biochem 1975;6:785.

Kreiger DT: Plasma ACTH and corticosteroids. *In* deGroot L, ed: Endocrinology. New York, Grune & Stratton, 1979.

Kreiger DT, Allen W, Rizzo F, Kreiger HP: Characterization of the normal temporal pattern of plasma corticosteroid levels. J Clin Endocrinol Metab 1971;32:266.

Laragh JH, Angers M, Kelly WG, et al: The effect of epinephrine, norepinephrine, angiotensin II, and others on the secretory rate of aldosterone in man. JAMA 1960;174:234.

Laragh JH, Sealey JE: Renin-angiotensin-aldosterone system and the renal regulation of sodium, potassium, and blood pressure homeostasis. *In* Windhager EE, ed: Handbook of Physiology. Section 8: Renal Physiology, Vol II. New York, Oxford University Press; 1992: pp 1409–1541.

Larsson C, Nordenskjold M: Multiple endocrine neoplasia. Cancer Surveys 1990;9:703–723.

Levitt M, Spector S, Sjoredsma A, Udenfriend S: Elucidation of the rate-limiting step in norepinephrine biosynthesis in the profuse guinea pig heart. J Pharmacol Exp Ther 1965;148:1.

Lewinsky BS, Grigor KM, Symington T, Nelville AM: The clinical and pathologic features of "non-hormonal" adrenocortical tumors: Report of 20 new cases and review of the literature. Cancer 1974;33:778.

Lewis GP: Physiological mechanisms controlling secretory activity of adrenal medulla. *In* Blaschko H, Sayer G, Smith AD, eds: Handbook of Physiology. Washington, D.C., American Phyisological Society, 1975, p 309.

Libertino JA, Novick JE: Adrenal surgery. Urol Clin North Am 1989;16:

Liddle GW: Test of pituitary-adrenal suppressibility in the diagnosis of Cushing's syndrome. J Clin Endocrinol Metab 1960;20:1539.

Lifton RP, Dluhy RG, Powers M, et al: A chimeric 11 β-hydroxylase/aldosterone synthase gene causes glucocorticoid remediable aldosteronism and human hypertension. Nature Genetics 1992;16:262–265.

Lifton RP, Dluhy RG: Inherited forms of mineralocorticoid hypertension: Glucocorticoid remediable aldosteronism and the syndrome of apparent mineralocorticoid excess. *In* Laragh JH, Brenner, BM, eds: Hypertension: Pathophysiology, Diagnosis, and Management, 2nd ed. New York, Raven Press, 1995, pp 2163–2166.

Lim RC, Nakayama DT, Biglieri EG, et al: Primary aldosteronism: Changing concepts and diagnosis and management. Am J Surg 1986;152:116.

Lips CJM, Landsvater RM, Hoppener JWM, et al: Clinical screening as compared with DNA analysis in families with multiple endocrine neoplasia type 2A. N Engl J Med 1994;331:828–835.

Liu L, Haskin ME, Rose LA, Beemus CE: Diagnosis of bilateral adrenal cortical hemorrhage by computerized tomography. Ann Intern Med 1982;97:720.

Lloyd RV, Shapiro B, Sisson JC: An immunohistochemical survey of pheochromocytomas. Arch Pathol Lab Med 1984;108:541.

Loeb RF: Effect of sodium chloride in treatment of patients with Addison's disease. Proc Soc Exp Biol Med 1933;380:8.

Long JP, Choyke PL, Shawker TA, et al: Intraoperative ultrasound in the evaluation of tumor involvement of the inferior vena cava. J Urol 1993;150:13–17.

Loose DS, Kan PB, Hirst MA, et al: Ketoconazole blocks adrenal steroidogenesis by inhibiting cytochrome P450-dependent enzymes. J Clin Invest 1983;71:1495.

Lubat E, Weinreb JC: Magnetic resonance imaging of the kidneys and adrenals. Top Magn Reson Imag 1990;2:17–36.

Lubitz JA, Freeman L, Okun R: Mitotane use in inoperable adrenal cortical carcinoma. JAMA 1973;223:1109.

Ludecke DK: Transnasal microsurgery of Cushing's disease 1990. Overview including personal experiences with 256 patients. Pathol Res Pract 1991;187:608–612.

Luetscher JA Jr, Johnson BB: Observations on the sodium-retaining corticoid (aldosterone) in the urine of children and adults in relation to sodium balance and edema. J Clin Invest 1954;23:1441.

Luton J-P, Cerdas S, Billaud L, et al: Clinical features of adrenocortical carcinoma, prognostic factors, and the effect of mitotane therapy. N Engl J Med 1990;322:1195.

Mador CK, Liddle GW, Island DP, et al: Cause of Cushing's syndrome in patients with tumors arising from "non-endocrine" tissue. J Clin Endocrinol Metab 1962;22:693.

Madrazo I, Drucker-Colin RH, Diaz V, et al: Open microsurgical autograph of adrenal medulla to the right caudate nucleus into patients with intractable Parkinson's disease. N Engl J Med 1987;316:3831.

Magiakou MA, Chrousos GP: Corticosteroid therapy, nonendocrine disease, and corticosteroid withdrawal. In Bardin CW, ed: Current Therapy in Endocrinology and Metabolism, 5th ed. St. Louis, C.V. Mosby, 1994, p 120.

Magiakou MA, Mastorakos G, Oldfield EH, et al: Cushing's syndrome in children and adolescents. Presentation, diagnosis and therapy. N Engl J Med 1994;331:629–636.

Mains RE, Eipper BA: Structure and biosynthesis of proadrenocorticotropin/ endorphin and related peptides. Endocr Rev 1980;1:1.

Maisey I, Stevens A: Addison's disease at Guys Hospital: A pathologic study. Guys Hosp Rep 1969;118:373.

Malhotra V, ed: Anesthesia for Renal and Genitourinary Surgery. New York, McGraw-Hill, 1995.

Manger WM, Gifford RW Jr: Pheochromocytoma. New York, Springer-Verlag, 1977.

Manger WM, Gifford RW Jr: Pheochromocytoma. In Laragh JH, Brenner BM, eds: Hypertension: Pathophysiology, Diagnosis, and Management. New York, Raven Press, 1990.

Markisz JA, Kazam E: Magnetic resonance imaging of the adrenal glands. In Vaughan ED Jr, Carey RM, eds: Adrenal Disorders. New York, Thieme Medical Publishers, 1989.

Mattox JH, Phelan S: The evaluation of adult females with testosterone-producing neoplasms of the adrenal cortex. Surg Gynecol Obstet 1987;164:98.

May ME, Vaughan ED Jr, Carey RM: Adrenocortical insufficiency—clinical aspects. In Vaughan ED Jr, Carey RM, eds: Adrenal Disorders. New York, Thieme Medical Publishers, 1989.

Mazze RI, Calverley RK, Smith NT: Inorganic fluoride and nephrotoxicity: Prolonged enflurane and halothane anesthesia in volunteers. Anesthesiology 1977;46:265–271.

McCleod MK, Thompson NW, Gross MD, Grekin RJ: Idiopathic aldosteronism masquerading as discrete aldosterone-secreting adrenal cortical neoplasms among patients with primary aldosteronism. Surgery 1989;106:1161–1168.

McDougal WS, Kirchner FK Jr, Scott HW Jr, Nadeau JH: Primary aldosteronism (Conn's syndrome). In Scott HW Jr, ed: Surgery of the Adrenal Glands. Philadelphia, J. B. Lippincott, 1990.

McKenna TJ, Sequeira SJ, Heffernan A, et al: Diagnosis under random conditions of all disorders of the renin-angiotensin aldosterone axis, including primary aldosteronism. J Clin Endocrinol 1991;73:952–957.

Meador CK, Liddle GW, Island DP, et al: Cause of Cushing's syndrome in patients with tumors arising from "nonendocrine tumors." J Clin Endocrinol Metab 1962;22:693.

Medeiros LJ, Weiss LM: New developments in the pathologic diagnosis of adrenal cortical neoplasms: A review. Am J Clin Pathol 1992;97:73–83.

Melby J: Assessment of adrenocortical function. N Engl J Med 1971;285:735–739.

Melby JC: Primary aldosteronism. Kidney Int 1984;26:769–778.

Mena J, Bowen JC, Hollier LH: Metachronous bilateral nonfunctional intercarotid paraganglioma (carotid body tumor) and functional retroperitoneal paraganglioma: Report of a case and review of the literature. Surgery 1993;114:107–111.

Mezrich R, Banner MP, Pollack HM: Magnetic resonance imaging of the adrenal glands. Urol Radiol 1986;8:127.

Miller J, Crapo L: The biochemical analysis of hypercortisolism. Endocrinologist 1994;4:7–16.

Miller DL, Doppman JL, Peterman SB, et al: Neurologic complications of petrosal sinus sampling. Radiology 1992;185:143–147.

Mitty HA, Yeh HC: Radiology of the Adrenals for Sonography and CT. Philadelphia, W. B. Saunders, 1982.

Moloney BJ: Addison's disease due to chronic disseminating coccidioidomycosis. Arch Intern Med 1952;90:869.

Moore L, Bramwell NH, Byard RW: DNA analysis and clinical outcome in pediatric adrenal cortical tumors. Pathology 1993;25:144–147.

Moore M, Amberson JB, Kazam E, Vaughan ED Jr: Anatomy, histology, embryology. In Vaughan ED Jr, Carey RM, eds: Adrenal Disorders. New York, Thieme Medical Publishers, 1989.

Morimoto S, Hakeda R, Murakami M: Does prolonged pretreatment with large dosage of spironolactone hasten a recovery from juxtaglomerular-adrenal suppression in primary aldosteronism? J Clin Endocrinol Metab, 1970;31:659.

Mortimer RH, Cannell GR, Thew CM, Galligan JP: Ketoconazole and plasma and urine steroid levels in Cushing's disease. Clin Exp Pharmacol Physiol 1991;18:563–569.

Mueller RA, Thoenen H, Axelrod J: Effect of the pituitary and ACTH on the maintenance of basal tyrosine hydroxylase activity in the rat adrenal gland. Endocrinology 1970;86:751.

Mulder WJ, Berghout A, Wiersinga WM: Cushing's syndrome during pregnancy. Neth J Med 1990;36:234–241.

Nader S, Hickey RC, Sellin RV, Samaan NA: Adrenal cortical carcinoma: The study of 77 cases. Cancer 1983;52:707.

Nadler JL, Hseueh W, Horton R: Therapeutic effect of calcium channel blockade in primary aldosteronism. J Clin Endocrinol Metab 1985;60:896–899.

Nakada T, Furuta H, Katayama T, et al: The effect of adrenal surgery on plasma atria natriuretic factor and sodium escape phenomenon in patients with primary aldosteronism. J Urol 1989;142:13–18.

Nakada T, Kubota Y, Sasagawa I, et al: Therapeutic outcome of primary aldosteronism: Adrenalectomy versus enucleation of aldosterone-producing adenoma. J Urol 1995;153:1775–1780.

Nakajo M, Nakabeppu Y, Yonekura R, et al: The role of adrenocortical scintigraphy in the evaluation of unilateral incidentally discovered adrenal and juxtaadrenal masses. Ann Nucl Med 1993;7:157–166.

Nelson DH: The adrenal cortex: physiological function and disease. Major Probl Intern Med 1980;18:15.

Nelson DH, Meakin JW, Dealy JB Jr, et al: ACTH-producing tumor of the pituitary gland. N Engl J Med 1958;259:161.

Nerup J: Addison's disease—clinical studies: A report of 108 cases. Acta Endocrinol 1974;76:127.

Neumann HPH, Berger DP, Sigmund G, et al: Pheochromocytomas, multiple endocrine neoplasia type 2, and von Hippel–Lindau disease. N Engl J Med 1993;329:1531–1538.

Neville AM, O'Hare MJ: The Human Adrenal Cortex: Pathology and Biology—An Integrated Approach. New York, Springer-Verlag, 1982.

New MI, Speiser PW: Disorders of adrenal steroidogenesis. In Vaughan ED Jr, Carey RM, eds: Adrenal Disorders. New York, Thieme Medical Publishers, 1989.

Newbould EC, Ross GA, Dacie JE, et al: The use of venous catheterisation in the diagnosis and localization of bilateral phaeochromocytomas. Clin Endocrinol 1991;35:55–59.

Newhouse JH: MRI of the adrenal gland. Urol Radiol 1990;12:1.

Nicholson JP, Vaughan ED Jr, Pickering TG, et al: Pheochromocytoma and prazosin. Ann Intern Med 1983;99:477–479.

Nielson E, Asfeldt VH: Studies on the specificity of fluorimetric determination of plasma corticosteroids. Scand J Clin Lab Invest 1967;20:185.

Novick AC, Straffon RA, Kaylor W: Posterior transthoracic approach for adrenal surgery. J Urol 1989;141:254.

O'Connor DT, Deftos LJ: Secretion of chromogranin A by peptide-producing endocrine neoplasms. N Engl J Med 1986;314:1145–1151.

Oldfield EH, Doppman JL, Nieman LK, et al: Petrosal sinus sampling with and without corticotropin-releasing hormone for the differential diagnosis of Cushing's syndrome. N Engl J Med 1991;325:897–905.

Oliver G, Sharpey-Schafer EA: The physiological effects of extracts on the suprarenal capsules. J Physiol (London) 1895;18:230.

O'Neil RG: Aldosterone regulation of sodium and potassium transport in the cortical collecting duct. Semin Nephrol 1990;10:365.

Orth DN: Cushing's syndrome. N Engl J Med 1995;332:791.

Orth DN, Island DP, Liddle GW: Experimental alteration of the circadian rhythm in plasma cortisol concentration in man. J Clin Endocrinol Metab 1967;27:549.

Orth DN, Kovacs WJ, DeBold CR: The adrenal cortex. In Wilson JD, Foster DW, eds: Williams Textbook of Endocrinology, 8th ed. Philadelphia, W. B. Saunders, 1992, pp 489–619.

Orth DN, Liddle GW: Results of treatment in 108 patients with Cushing's syndrome. N Engl J Med 1971;285:243.

Osa SR, Peterson RE, Roberts SBRB: Recovery of adrenal reserve following treatment of disseminated South American blastomytosis. Am J Med 1981;71:298.

Osborn RH, Yannone ME: Plasma androgens in the normal and androgenic female. Obstet Gynecol Surg 1971;26:195.

Osella G, Terzolo M, Borretta G, et al: Endocrine evaluation of incidentally discovered adrenal masses (incidentalomas). J Clin Endocrinol Metab 1994;79:1532–1539.

Papavasiliou C, Gouliamos A, Deligiorgi E: Masses of myeloadipose tissue: Radiological and clinical considerations. Int J Radiat Oncol Biol Phys 1990;19:985–993.

Parker L, Odell W: Control of adrenal androgen secretion. Endocr Rev 1980;1:392.

Pasieka JL, McLeod MK, Thompson NW, et al: Adrenal scintigraphy of well-differentiated (functioning) adrenocortical carcinomas: Potential surgical pitfalls. Surgery 1992;112:884–890.

Paulotos FC, Smilo RP, Forchamp H: A rapid screening test of Cushing's syndrome. JAMA 1965;193:720.

Pearse AG, Polak JM: Cytochemical evidence for the neural crest origin of mammalian ultimobranchial C cells. Histochemie 1971;27:96.

Pedrinelli R, Bruschi G, Grazidei L, et al: Dietary sodium change in primary aldosteronism: Atrial natriuretic factor, hormonal, and vascular responses. Hypertension 1988;12:192–198.

Pelleya R, Oster JR, Perez GO: Hyporeninemic hypoaldosteronism, sodium wasting and mineralocorticoid-resistant hyperkalemia in two patients with obstructive uropathy. Am J Nephrol 1983;3:223–227.

Pepe GJ, Albrecht ED: Regulation of the primate fetal adrenal cortex. Endocr Rev 1990;11:151.

Percarpio B, and Knowlton AH: Radiation therapy of adrenal cortical carcinoma. Acta Radiol [Ther] (Stockh) 1976;15:288.

Perkoff GT, Sandberg AA, Nelson DH, Tyler FH: Clinical usefulness of determination of circulation 17-hydroxycorticosteroid levels. Arch Intern Med 1954;93:1–8.

Perry RR, Keiser HR, Norton JA, et al: Surgical management of pheochromocytoma with the use of metyrosine. Ann Surg 1990;212:621–628.

Phlipponneau M, Nocaudie M, Epelbaum J, et al: Somatostatin analogs for the localization and preoperative treatment of an adrenocorticotropin-secreting bronchial carcinoid tumor. J Clin Endocrinol Metab 1994;78:20–24.

Pick JW, Anson BJ: The inferior phrenic artery: Origin and suprarenal branches. Anat Rec 1940;78:413.

Pick L: Das Ganglioma embryonale sympathicum. Klin Wochenschr 1912;19:16.

Plager JE: Carcinoma of the adrenal cortex: Clinical description, diagnosis and treatment. Int Adv Surg Oncol 1984;7:329.

Pommier RF, Brennan MF: An eleven-year experience with adrenocortical carcinoma. Surgery 1992;112:963–971.

Prinz RA, Brooks MH, Churchill R, et al: Incidental asymptomatic adrenal masses detected by computed tomographic scanning—is operation required? JAMA 1982;248:701.

Quigg RJ, Om A: Reversal of severe cardiac systolic dysfunction caused by pheochromocytoma in a heart transplant candidate. J Heart Lung Transplant 1994;13:525–532.

Quinn WF, Hogan MJ, Klee GG, et al: Primary aldosteronism: Diagnosis and treatment. Mayo Clin Proc 1990;65:96–110.

Radin DRR, Manoogian C, Nadler J: Diagnosis of primary aldosteronism: Importance of correlating CT findings with endocrinologic studies. AJR 1992;158:553–557.

Raff H, Findling JW: A new immunoradiometric assay for corticotropin evaluated in normal subjects in patients with Cushing's syndrome. Clin Chem 1989;35:596–600.

Raue F, Frank K, Meybeir H, Ziegler R: Pheochromocytoma in multiple endocrine neoplasia. Cardiology 1985;72(suppl):147.

Reckler JM, Vaughan ED Jr, Tjeuw M, Carey RM: Pheochromocytoma. In Vaughan ED Jr, Carey RM, eds: Adrenal Disorders. New York, Thieme Medical Publishers, 1989.

Reincke M, Karl M, Travis WH, et al: p53 mutations in human adrenocortical neoplasms: Immunohistochemical and molecular studies. J Clin Endocrinol Metab 1994;78:790–794.

Reinig JW, Doppelman JL, Dwyer AJ, et al: Adrenal masses differentiated by MR. Radiology 1986;158:81.

Renold AE, Jenkins D, Forsham PH, Thorn GW: The use of intravenous ACTH: A study in quantitative adrenocortical stimulation. J Clin Endocrinol Metab 1952;12:763.

Reyes L, Parvez Z, Nemoto P, et al: Adrenalectomy for adrenal metastases from lung carcinoma. J Surg Oncol 1990;44:32.

Rich GM, Ulick S, Cook S, et al: Glucocorticoid-remediable aldosteronism in a large kindred: Clinical spectrum and diagnosis using a characteristic biochemical phenotype. Ann Intern Med 1992;116:813–820.

Richie JP, Gittes RF: Carcinoma of the adrenal cortex. Cancer 1980;45:1957.

Rickards AG, Parrett GM: Non-tuberculous Addison's disease and its relationship to giant cell granuloma and multiple glandular disease. Q J Med 1954;43:403.

Riehle RA Jr, Lavengood RW: An extrapleural approach with rib removal for the 11th rib flank incision. Surg Gynecol Obstet 1985;161:276–279.

Robbins SL, Cotran RS: Pathologic Basis of Disease, 2nd ed. Philadelphia, W. B. Saunders, 1979.

Robertson D: The adrenal medulla and adrenomedullary hormones. In Scott HW ed: Surgery of the Adrenal Glands. Philadelphia, J. B. Lippincott, 1990.

Robertson D, Oates JA, Jr, Berman ML: Preoperative and anesthetic management of pheochromocytoma. In Scott HW, ed: Surgery of the Adrenal Glands. Philadelphia, J. B. Lippincott, 1990.

Rocco S, Opocher G, Carpene G, Mantero F: Atrial natriuretic peptide infusion in primary hyperaldosteronism renal hemodynamic and hormonal effects. Am J Hypertens 1990;3:688.

Rosano G, Swift TA, Hayes LW: Advances in catecholamine and metabolite measurement as diagnosis of pheochromcytoma. Clin Chem 1991;37/10(B):1854.

Rosen AE, Brown JJ, Lever AF: Treatment of pheochromocytoma and of clonidine withdrawal hypertension with labetalol. Br J Clin Pharmacol 1976;3(suppl 3):809.

Rosenbaum JS, Billingham ME, Ginsberg R: Cardiomyopathy in a rat model of pheochromocytoma morphological and functional alterations. Am J Cardiovasc Pathol 1988;1:389.

Ross EJ, Prichard BNC, Kaufman L, et al: Preoperative and operative management of patients with pheochromocytoma. BMJ 1967;1:191.

Ross NS, Aron DC: Hormonal evaluation of the patient with an incidentally discovered adrenal mass. N Engl J Med 1990;323:1401.

Rousseau GG, Baxter JD, Tomkins GM: Glucocorticoid receptors: Relationship between steroid binding and biological effects. J Mol Biol 1972;67:99.

Russi S, Blumenthal HT, Gray SH: Small adenomas of the adrenal cortex in hypertension and diabetes. Arch Intern Med 1945;76:284.

Salem MR, Ivankovic AD: Management of phentolamine-resistant pheochromocytoma with beta adrenergic blockade. Br J Anaesth 1969;41:1087–1090.

Sameshima Y, Tsunematsu Y, Watanabe S, et al: Detection of novel germline p53 mutations in diverse-cancer-prone families identified by selecting patients with childhood adrenocortical carcinoma. J Natl Cancer Inst 1992;84:703–707.

Sanders R, Bissada N, Curry N, Gordon B: Clinical spectrum of adrenal myelolipoma: Analysis of 8 tumors in 7 patients. J Urol 1995;6:1791–1793.

Sardesai SH, Mourant AJ, Sivathandon Y, et al: Pheochromocytoma and catecholamine-induced myocardiopathy presenting as heart failure. Br Heart J 1990;63:234.

Sarvin CT, Bray GA, Idelson BA: Overnight suppression test with dexamethasone in Cushing's syndrome. J Clin Endocrinol Metab 1968;28:422.

Sato T, Saito H, Yoshinaga K, et al: Concurrence of carotid body tumor and pheochromocytoma. Cancer 1974;34:1787–1795.

Scasheeler LR, Myers JH, Eversman JJ, Taylor HC: Adrenal insufficiency secondary to carcinoma metastatic in the adrenal gland. Cancer 1983;52:1312.

Schambelan M, Brust NL, Chang BCF, et al: Circadian rhythm and effect of posture on plasma aldosterone concentration in primary aldosteronism. J Clin Endocrinol Metab 1976;43:115–131.

Schambelan M, Sebastin A, Biglieri EG, et al: Prevalence, pathogenesis and functional significance of aldosterone deficiency in hyperkalemic patients with chronic renal insufficiency. Kidney Int 1980;17:89.

Schambelan M, Slaton PE Jr, Biglieri EG: Mineralocorticoid production in hyperadrenocorticism. A role in pathogenesis of hypokalemic alkalosis. Am J Med 1971;51:299.

Schambelan M, Stockigt JR, Biglieri EG: Isolated hypoaldosteronism in adults, a renin deficiency syndrome. N Engl J Med 1972;287:573.

Schechter DC: Aberrant adrenal tissue. Ann Surg 1968;167:421.

Schenker JG, Chowers I: Pheochromocytoma and pregnancy. Obstet Gynecol Surg 1971;26:739.

Schlaghecke R, Kornely E, Santen RT, Ridderskamp P: The effect of long-term glucocorticoid therapy on pituitary-adrenal responses to exogenous corticotropin-releasing hormone. N Engl J Med 1992;326:226–230.

Schteingert DE, Motazedi A, Noonan RA, Thompson NW: Treatment of adrenal carcinomas. Arch Surg 1982;117:1142.

Scott EM, Thomas A, McGarrigle HHG, Lachelin GCL: Serial adrenal ultrasonography in normal neonates. J Ultrasound Med 1990;9:279.

Scott HW Jr: In Scott HW, ed: Surgery of the Adrenal Glands. Philadelphia, J. B. Lippincott, 1990b.

Scott HW Jr: Tumors of the adrenal cortex and Cushing's syndrome. In Seventh National Cancer Conference Proceedings. Philadelphia, J. B. Lippincott, 1973.

Scott HW Jr: Historical background of the adrenal glands. In Scott HW ed.: Surgery of the Adrenal Glands. Philadelphia, J. B. Lippincott, 1990a.

Scott HW Jr, Liddle GW, Mulherin JL Jr, et al: Surgical experience with Cushing's disease. Ann Surg 1977;185:524.

Scott HW Jr, Oates JA, Nies AS, et al: Pheochromocytoma: Present diagnosis and management. Ann Surg 1976;183:587.

Scott HW Jr, Orth DN: Hypercortisolism (Cushing's syndrome). In Scott HW ed: Surgery of the Adrenal Glands. Philadelphia J. B. Lippincott, 1990.

Scott HW Jr, Van Way CW III, Gray GF, Sussman CR: Pheochromocytoma. In Scott HW ed: Surgery of the Adrenal Glands. Philadelphia, J. B. Lippincott, 1990.

Sealey JE, Laragh JH: Measurement of urinary aldosterone excretion in man. In Laragh JH, ed: Hypertension Manual. New York, Yorke Medical Books, 1974.

Selem MR, Ivankovic AD: Management of phentolamine-resistant pheochromocytoma with beta-adrenergic blockade. Br J Anaesth 1969; 41:1087.

Shapiro B, Copp JE, Sisson JC, et al: Iodine-131 metaiodobenzylguanidine for the locating of suspected pheochromocytoma: Experience in 400 cases. J Nucl Med 1985;26:576.

Sheeler LR, Myers JH, Eversman JJ, Taylor HC: Adrenal insufficiency secondary to carcinoma metastatic to the adrenal gland. Cancer 1983;52:1312–1316.

Sheridan P, Mattingly P: Simultaneous investigative treatment of suspected acute adrenal insufficiency. Lancet 1975;2:676.

Simpson NE, Kidd KK, Goodfellow PJ: Assignment of multiple endocrine neoplasia type 2a to chromosome 10 by linkage. Nature 1987;328:528.

Simpson SA, Tait JR, Wettstein A, et al: Konstitution des aldosterons des neuen. Mineralocorticoids Experientia 1954;10:132.

Sipple JH: The association of pheochromocytoma with carcinoma of the thyroid gland. Am J Med 1961;31:163.

Siragy HM, Vaughan ED Jr, Carey RM: Cushing syndrome. In Vaughan ED Jr, Carey RM eds: Adrenal Disorders. New York, Thieme Medical Publishers, 1989.

Sjoerdsma A, Engelman K, Spector S, Undenfriend S: Inhibition of catecholamine synthesis in man with alpha-methyl tyrosine, an inhibitor to tyrosine hydroxylase. Lancet 1965;1:1092.

Smith MG, Byrne AJ: An Addisonian crisis complicating anesthesia. Anesthesia 1981;36:681.

Sonino N, Boscaro M, Paoletta A, et al: Ketoconazole treatment in Cushing's syndrome: Experience in 34 patients. Clin Endocrinol 1991;35:347–352.

Spark RF, Melby JC: Aldosteronism and hypertension: The spironolactone response test. Ann Intern Med 1968;69:685.

Speckard PF, Nicoloff JT, Bethune JE: Screening for adrenocortical insufficiency with corticosyntrophin. Arch Intern Med 1971;128:761.

Speiser PW, Agdere L, Ueshiba H, et al: Aldosterone synthesis in salt-wasting congenital adrenal hyperplasia with complete absence of adrenal 21-hydroxylase. N Engl J Med 1991;324:145–149.

Speiss J, Rivier J, Rivier C, Vale W: Primary structure of corticotropin-releasing factor from ovine hypothalamus. Proc Natl Acad Sci (USA) 1981;78:6517.

Sroujieh AS, Farah GR, Haddad MJ, Abu-Khalaf MM: Adrenal cysts: Diagnosis and management. Br J Urol 1990;65:570–575.

Stackpole RH, Melicow MM, Uson AC: Pheochromocytomas in children. J Pediatr 1963;63:315.

Stein PP, Black HR: A simplified diagnostic approach to pheochromocytoma. A review of the literature and report of one institution's experience. Medicine 1990;70:46.

Stewart DR, Jones PH, Jolley SA: Carcinoma of the adrenal gland in children. J Pediatr Surg 1974;9:59.

Stewart PM, Burra P, Shackleton CHL, et al: 11β-hydroxysteroid dehydrogenase deficiency and glucocorticoid status in patients with alcoholic and non-alcoholic chronic liver diease. J Clin Endocrinol Metab 1993;76:748–751.

Stowasser M, Gordon RD, Tunny T, et al: Primary aldosteronism: Implications of a new familial variety. J Hypertens 1991;9(suppl 6):S264–265.

Streeten DHP, Andersen GH, Wagner S: Effect of age on response of secondary hypertension to specific treatment. Am J Hypertens 1990;3:360–365.

Streeten DHP, Tomycz N, Anderson GH Jr: Reliability of screening test for the diagnosis of primary aldosteronism. Am J Med 1979;67:403.

Styne DM, Grumbach MM, Kaplan SL, et al: Treatment of Cushing's disease in childhood and adolescence by transsphenoidal microadenomectomy. N Engl J Med 1984;310:889.

Sullivan M, Boileau M, Hodges CV: Adrenal cortical carcinoma. J Urol 1978;120:600–665.

Sutherland DJ, Ruse JL, Laidlaw JC: Hypertension, increased aldosterone secretion and low plasma renin activity relieved by dexamethasone. Can Med Assoc J 1966;95:1109–1119.

Sutton MG, Sheps SG, Lie JT: Prevalence of clinically unsuspected pheochromocytoma: A review of a 50-year autopsy series. Mayo Clin Proc 1981;56:354.

Suzuki K, Kageyama S, Ueda D, et al: Laparoscopic adrenalectomy: Clinical experience with 12 cases. J Urol 1993;150:1099–1102.

Takeda M, Go H, Imai T, et al: Laparoscopic adrenalectomy for primary aldosteronism: Report of initial 10 cases. Surgery 1994;115:621–625.

Tank ES, Gelbard MK, Blank B: Familial pheochromocytomas. J Urol 1982;128:1013.

Tannenbaum M: Ultrastructural pathology of the adrenal medullary tumor. In Sommers, SC ed.: Pathology Annual, Vol 5. New York, Appleton-Century-Crofts, 1970, pp 145–171.

Tarazi RC, Ibrahim MM, Bravo EL, Dustan HP: Hemodynamic characteristics of primary aldosteronism. N Engl J Med 1973;289:1330.

Tartour E, Caillou B, Tenenbaum F, et al: Immunohistochemical study of adrenocortical carcinoma. Predictive value of the D11 monoclonal antibody. Cancer 1993;72:3296–3303.

Taylor AL, Fishman LM: Corticotropin-releasing hormone. N Engl J Med 1988;319:213–222.

Tepperman J, Tepperman H: Metabolic and Endocrine Physiology, 5th ed. Chicago, Year Book Medical Publishers, 1987.

Thomas JL, Barnes PA, Bernardino ME, Lewis E: Diagnostic approaches to adrenal and renal metastases. Radiol Clin North Am 1982;20:531.

Thomas JL, Bernardino ME, Samaan NA, Hickey RC: CT of pheochromocytoma. AJR 1980;135:477.

Tikkakoski T, Taavitsainen M, Paivansalo M, et al: Accuracy of adrenal biopsy guided by ultrasound and CT. Acta Radiol 1991;32:371–374.

Trost BN, Koenig MP, Zimmerman A, et al: Virilization of a post-menopausal woman by a testosterone-secreting Leydig cell type adrenal adenoma. Acta Endocrinol 1981;98:274–282.

Tunny T, Gordon RD, Klemm S, Cohn D: Histological and biochemical distinctiveness of atypical aldosterone producing adenoma responsive to upright posture and angiotensin. Clin Endocrinol (Oxford) 1991;34:363–369.

Twomey P, Montgomery C, Clark O: Successful treatment of adrenal metastasis from large-cell carcinoma of the lung. JAMA 1982;248:581.

Ulick S, Blumenfeld JD, Atlas SA, et al: The unique steroidogenesis of the aldosteronoma in the differential diagnosis of primary aldosteronism. J Clin Endocrinol Metab 1992;76:873–878.

Ulick S, Chan C: Physiologic insights derived from the search for unknown steroids in low renin essential hypertension. In Mantero F, Takeda R, Scoggins BA, et al, eds: The Adrenal and Hypertension: From Cloning to Clinic, Serono Symposia, No. 57. New York, Raven Press, 1989, pp 313–322.

Vaitukaitis JL, Dale SL, Malby JC: Role of ACTH in the secretion of free dehydroepiandrosterone and its sulfate ester in man. J Clin Endocrinol Metab 1969;29:1443.

Vale W, Speiss J, Rivier C, Rivier J: Characterization of a 41 residue ovine hypothalmic peptide that stimulates secretion of corticotropin and beta endorphin. Science 1981;213:1394.

van der Mey AGL, Maaswinkel-Mooy PD, Cornelisse CJ, et al: Genomic imprinting in hereditary glomus tumours: Evidence for new genetic theory. Lancet 1989;2:1291–1294.

Van Heerden JA, Sheps SG, Hamberger B, et al: Pheochromocytoma: Current status and changing trends. Surgery 1982;91:367.

van Heerden JA, Young WF Jr, Grant CS, Carpenter PC: Adrenal surgery for hypercortisolism—surgical aspects. Surgery 1995;117:466–472.

Van Vliet PD, Burchell HB, Titus JL: Focal myocarditis associated with pheochromocytoma. N Engl J Med 1966;274:1102.

Vassilopoulou-Sellin R, Guinee VF, Klein MJ, et al: Impact of adjuvant mitotane on the clinical course of patients with adrenocortical cancer. Cancer 1993;71:3119–3123.

Vaughan ED Jr: Diagnosis of adrenal disorders in hypertension. World J Urol 1989;7:111–116.

Vaughan ED Jr: Adrenal surgery. In Marshall FF ed.: Atlas of Urologic Surgery. Philadelphia, W. B. Saunders, 1991.

Vaughan ED Jr: Imaging of the adrenal gland. World J Urol 1992;10:190.

Vaughan ED Jr: Editorial overview: New techniques in the diagnosis and management of prostate cancer. Semin Urol 1995;13:95.

Vaughan ED Jr: Catecholamine cardiomyopathy. In Manger WM, Gifford RW Jr, eds: Clinical and Experimental Pheochromocytoma, 2nd ed. Cambridge, Blackwell Science, 1996, pp 421–422.

Vaughan ED Jr, Atlas S, Carey RM: Hyderaldosteronism. In Vaughan ED Jr, Carey RM, eds: Adrenal Disorders. New York, Thieme Medical Publishers, 1989.

Vaughan ED Jr, Carey RM: Adrenal Disorders. New York, Thieme Medical Publishers, 1989a.

Vaughan ED Jr, Carey RM: Adrenal carcinoma. In Vaughan ED Jr, Carey RM, eds: Adrenal Disorders. New York, Thieme Medical Publishers, 1989b.

Vaughan ED Jr, Phillips H: Modified posterior approach for right adrenalectomy. Surg Gynecol Obstet 1987;165:453–455.

Vaughan ED Jr, Laragh JH, Gavras I, et al: Volume factor in low and normal renin essential hypertension. Am J Cardiol 1973;32:523.

Verrey F: Regulation of gene expression by aldosterone in tight epithelia. Semin Nephrol 1990;10:410.

Vyberg M, Sestof TL: Combined adrenal myelolipoma and adenoma associated with Cushing's syndrome. Am J Clin Pathol 1986;86:541.

Wagner J, Portwine C, Rabin K, et al: High frequency of germline p53 mutations in childhood adrenocortical cancer. J Natl Cancer Inst 1994;86:1707–1710.

Wallace JM, Gill DP: Prazosin in the diagnosis and treatment of pheochromocytoma. JAMA 1978;240:2752.

Weinberger MH, Grim CE, Hollifield JW, et al: Primary aldosteronism: Diagnosis, localization and treatment. Ann Intern Med 1979;93:86.

Weiss JM: Comparative histologic study of 43 metastasizing and non-metastasizing adrenal cortical tumors. Am J Surg Pathol 1984;8:163.

Wendler NL, Graber RP, Jones RE, Tischler M: Synthesis of 11 hydroxylated steroids: 17 hydroxycorticosterone. J Am Chem Soc 1950;72:5793.

Werk EE Jr, Sholiton LJ, Kalejs L: Testosterone-secreting adrenal adenoma under gonadotropin control. N Engl J Med, 1973;289:767–770.

Wheeler MH, Curley IR, Williams ED: The association of neurofibromatosis, pheochromocytoma, and somatostatin-rich aduodenal carcinoid tumor. Surgery 1986;100:1163.

White EA, Schambelan M, Rost LR, et al: Use of computed tomography in diagnosing the cause of primary aldosteronism. N Engl J Med 1980;303:1503–1507.

White PC: Disorders of aldosterone biosynthesis and action. N Engl J Med 1994;331:250–258.

Wilhelmus JL, Schrodt GR, Alberhasky MT, Alcorn MO: Giant adrenal myelolipoma: Case report and review of the literature. Arch Pathol Lab Med 1981;105:532.

Williams FA Jr, Schambelan M, Biglieri EG, Carey RM: Acquired primary hypoaldosteronism due to an isolated zona glomerulosa defect. N Engl J Med 1983;309:1623–1627.

Willis RA: The Spread of Tumors in the Human Body, 2nd ed. St. Louis, C. V. Mosby, 1952.

Winkler H, Smith AD: The chromaffin granule and the storage of catecholamines. In Blaschko H, Sayers G, Smith AD, eds: Handbook of Physiology. Washington, D.C., American Physiological Society, 1975, p 321.

Wooten MD, King DK: Adrenal cortical carcinoma: Epidemiology and treatment with mitotane and a review of the literature. Cancer 1993;72:3145–3155.

Wotman S, Baer L, Mendel ID, Laragh JH: Submaxillary potassium concentration in true and pseudoprimary hyperaldosteronism. Arch Intern Med 1970;129:248.

Wurtman RJ, Axelrod J: Adrenalin synthesis: Control by the pituitary gland and adrenoglucosteroids. Science 1965;150:1464.

Yamaji T, Ishibashi M, Sekihara H, et al: Serum dehydroepiandrosterone sulfate in Cushing's syndrome. J Clin Endocrinol Metab 1984;59:1164.

Young JL Jr, Miller RW: Incidence of malignant tumors in U.S. children. J Pediatr 1975;86:254.

97
SURGERY OF THE KIDNEY

Andrew C. Novick, M.D.
Stevan B. Streem, M.D.

HISTORICAL ASPECTS

The first nephrectomies were probably performed seren-dipitously. Early reports of removal of large ovarian tumors indicate that the surgeon was occasionally surprised to find the kidney included in the surgical specimen. Definitive renal surgery was first performed in 1869 by Gustav Simon, who carried out a planned nephrectomy for treatment of a ureterovaginal fistula. The operation was preceded by extensive experimental investigation of uninephrectomy in dogs to demonstrate that they could survive normally with only one kidney. This application of an experimental model to a clinical problem was the forerunner of the method by which many current surgical procedures were developed.

In 1881, Morris was the first to perform nephrolithotomy in an otherwise healthy kidney, and he later defined the terms *nephrolithiasis, nephrolithotomy, nephrectomy,* and *nephrotomy.* The first partial nephrectomy was performed in 1884 by Wells for removal of a perirenal fibrolipoma. In 1890, Czerny was the first to use partial nephrectomy for excision of a renal neoplasm. Kuster performed the first successful pyeloplasty (a dismembered procedure) in 1891 on the solitary kidney of a 13-year-old boy (Kuster, 1892). In 1892, Fenger applied the Heinecke-Mikulicz principle for pyloric stenosis to ureteropelvic junction obstruction (Fenger, 1894). In 1903, Zondek emphasized the importance of a thorough knowledge of the renal arterial circulation when performing partial nephrectomy.

There was great controversy among early surgeons regarding the relative merits of retroperitoneal versus transperitoneal exposure of the kidney. Kocher performed an anterior transperitoneal nephrectomy through a midline incision as early as 1878 (Kocher and Langham, 1878). A transverse abdominal incision was employed in 1913 by Berg, who also mobilized the colon laterally to expose the great vessels and thus secure the renal pedicle with greater safety. Berg was able to remove vena caval tumor thrombi through a cavotomy after control of the veins by vascular clamps. Rehn actually reimplanted the contralateral renal vein after resecting the inferior vena cava in 1922. The high incidence of peritonitis and other abdominal complications, however, led most urologists to adopt a retroperitoneal flank approach to the kidney during the first half of this century. During the late 1950s, the development of safe abdominal and vascular surgical techniques led to a revival of the anterior approach in patients undergoing renal surgery (Culp and DeWeerd, 1951; Poutasse, 1961).

SURGICAL ANATOMY

The kidneys are paired vital organs located on each side of the vertebral column in the lumbar fossa of the retroperitoneal space. Each kidney is surrounded by a layer of perinephric fat, which is, in turn, covered by a distinct fascial layer termed *Gerota's fascia.* Posteriorly, both kidneys lie on the psoas major and quadratus lumborum muscles. They are also in relationship with the medial and lateral lumbocostal arches and the tendon of the transversus abdominis. Posteriorly and superiorly the upper pole of each kidney is in contact with the diaphragm (Fig. 97–1).

A small segment of the anterior medial surface of the right kidney is in contact with the right adrenal gland. The major anterior relationships of the right kidney, however, are the liver, which overlies the upper two thirds of the anterior surface, and the hepatic flexure of the colon, which overlies the lower one third. The second portion of the duodenum covers the right renal hilum.

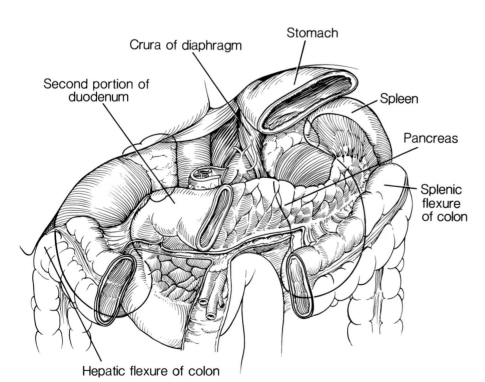

Figure 97–1. The anatomic relationship of the kidneys to surrounding structures. The liver is retracted superiorly in this illustration.

A small segment of the anterior medial surface of the left kidney is also covered by the left adrenal gland. The major anterior relationships of the left kidney are the spleen, body of the pancreas, stomach, and splenic flexure of the colon.

The kidney has four constant vascular segments, which are termed *apical, anterior, posterior,* **and** *basilar* (Boyce and Smith, 1967). The anterior segment is the largest and extends beyond the midplane of the kidney onto the posterior surface. A true avascular line exists at the junction of the anterior and posterior segments on the posterior surface of the kidney.

Each vascular segment of the kidney is supplied by one or more major arterial branches (Fig. 97–2). Although the origin of the branches supplying these segments may vary, the anatomic position of the segments is constant (Graves, 1954). All segmental arteries are end-arteries with no collateral circulation; therefore, when performing renal surgery, failure to preserve one of these branches leads to devitalization of functioning renal tissue. Most individuals have a single main artery to each kidney originating from the lateral aspect of the aorta just below the superior mesenteric artery.

Multiple renal arteries occur unilaterally in 23% and bilaterally in 10% of the population.

The normal renal venous anatomy is depicted in Figure 97–3. Both the left and right renal veins terminate in the lateral aspect of the inferior vena cava. The left renal vein is longer and has a thicker muscular layer than the right renal vein. Several important nonrenal branches empty into the left renal vein. These are the gonadal vein inferiorly, the left adrenal vein superiorly, and one or two large lumbar veins posteriorly. There are no significant branches draining into the right renal vein. Multiple renal veins are less common than multiple renal arteries.

The renal venous drainage system differs significantly from the arterial blood supply in that the intrarenal venous branches intercommunicate freely between the various renal segments. Ligation of a branch of the renal vein, therefore, does not result in segmental infarction of the kidney because collateral venous blood supply provides adequate drainage. This is important clinically because it enables one to obtain surgical access to structures in the renal hilus by ligating and dividing small adjacent or overlying venous branches.

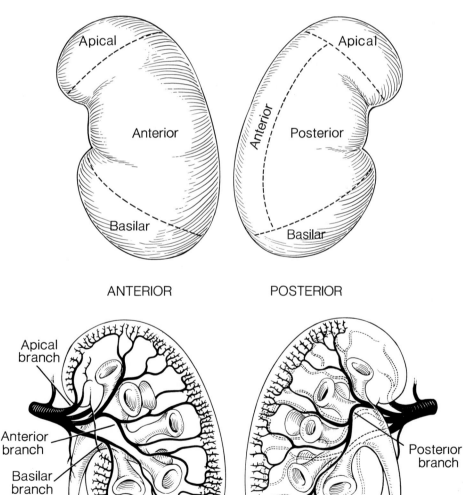

Figure 97–2. The vascular segments of the left kidney, as shown in the anterior and posterior projections, and the corresponding segmental arterial supply to each segment.

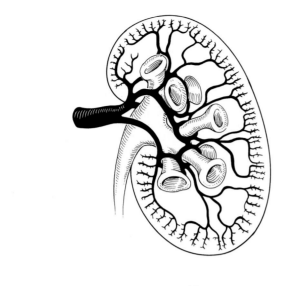

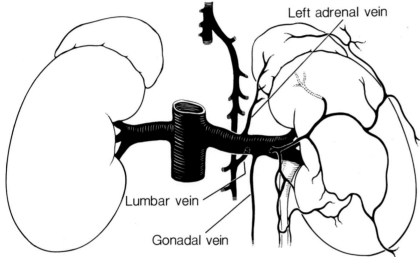

Left adrenal vein

Lumbar vein

Gonadal vein

Figure 97–3. The normal renal venous anatomy including branches of the left renal vein *(bottom)*. The intrarenal venous drainage parallels the segmental arterial supply and is depicted for the left kidney *(top)*.

This allows major venous branches to be completely mobilized and freely retracted in either direction to expose the renal hilus safely with no vascular compromise of renal parenchyma.

With regard to the intrarenal collecting system, there are eight to ten major calyces that open into the renal pelvis (Fig. 97–4). The apical segment has one major calyx that lies in the midfrontal plane and receives two minor calyces, which are lateral and medial. The basilar segment has a single major calyx in the median plane and receives two minor calyces, which are anterior and posterior. There are three major calyces in the anterior segment that enter the renal pelvis at a 20-degree angle to the midfrontal plane and three major calyces in the posterior segment that enter the renal pelvis at a 75-degree angle to the midfrontal plane.

PREOPERATIVE PREPARATION

A thorough preoperative evaluation is important in patients undergoing renal surgery because of the special positions in which the patient may have to be placed intraoperatively and the systemic disturbances that may occur

secondary to renal infections and impairment of renal function. Cardiorespiratory function is evaluated by eliciting any history of heart disease, chest pain, smoking, or respiratory distress on exertion. An electrocardiogram, chest film, and complete blood count should be obtained on all patients. The flank position with lateral flexion of the spine is known to cause embarrassment of ventilatory capacity, and the venous return may be significantly diminished in this position, resulting in hypotension. Therefore, alternatives to the flank approach should be used whenever possible in patients with a decreased pulmonary reserve. Preoperative pulmonary function studies and blood gas analysis are mandatory in patients suspected of having impaired respiratory function. In the event of the latter, use of an anterior surgical approach with the patient in the supine position is preferred.

Regardless of the surgical incision used, respiration may be seriously impaired postoperatively because of transection of upper abdominal or flank muscles and, occasionally, because of removal of a rib. Also the upper poles of the kidneys encroach on the undersurface of the diaphragm, and the removal of a large upper pole renal mass may interfere temporarily with its function. Preoperative breathing exercises, alleviation of bronchospasm, cessation of smoking,

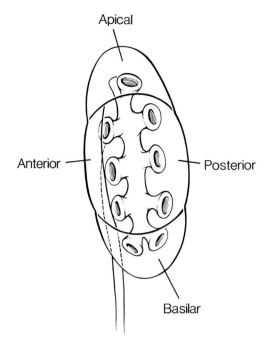

Figure 97–4. The intrarenal collecting system in relation to major vascular segments of the kidney.

and evaluation of cardiopulmonary function are helpful in improving respiratory function and in preventing postoperative cardiorespiratory problems.

Bleeding tendencies are assessed by examination of platelet function and coagulation factors. Patients should be questioned about excess alcohol intake and ingestion of drugs, such as aspirin, that can influence blood clotting.

A thorough anatomic examination of the urinary tract should be made in all patients undergoing renal surgery. Available studies include intravenous pyelography, cystoscopy, retrograde pyelography, ureteroscopy, cystourethrography, computed tomography, ultrasonography, magnetic resonance imaging, renal arteriography, and renal venography. These studies are reviewed in detail in Chapter 6 and their usefulness in evaluating patients for specific renal operations is described in subsequent sections of this chapter.

Overall renal function is evaluated by estimation of the serum creatinine level and either endogenous creatinine clearance or iothalamate glomerular filtration rate. Differential renal function can be assessed noninvasively with computerized isotope renography using radioactive iodine (^{131}I) or technetium Tc-99m. Hippuran I 131 is cleared by both glomeruli and tubules and is most useful for measuring unilateral renal dysfunction when overall renal function is normal. Technetium chelated with diethylenetriaminepentaacetic acid (DTPA) is filtered only by the glomeruli and is thus more helpful in assessing differential renal perfusion. Both of these isotopes are excreted in the urine, and, in the presence of obstruction, parenchymal concentration is obscured by the high concentration of isotope in the accumulated urine. Selective ureteral catheterization to determine differential renal function is an invasive study that is used rarely.

Patients with either upper or lower urinary tract infection should receive organism-specific antibiotic therapy preoperatively. With suspected or proven upper tract infection, at least 48 hours of antibiotic therapy is indicated before renal surgery. Severe bacteremia can occur during operation on an infected kidney with significant resulting morbidity and potential mortality.

Percutaneous embolization of the kidney is occasionally helpful before performing radical nephrectomy for large renal malignancies. The major value of this adjunct is in patients with an arterialized vena caval tumor thrombus or medial extension of tumor that interferes with early ligation of the renal artery. Currently, absolute ethanol injected directly into the renal artery appears to be the most satisfactory material for angioinfarction. Subsequent transient flank pain is common and often requires analgesic medication.

Patients are often concerned about how the removal of a kidney will affect their renal function. After nephrectomy for unilateral renal disease, the opposite kidney undergoes compensatory hypertrophy, and the glomerular filtration rate is ultimately maintained at 75% of the normal value (Aperia et al, 1977; Robitaille et al, 1985). Several long-term studies have shown no increase in hypertension or proteinuria, stable overall renal function, and normal life expectancy after unilateral nephrectomy with a normal contralateral kidney (Kretschmer, 1943; Goldstein, 1956; Anderson and Hansen, 1968). This information should be shared with patients to alleviate their anxiety before surgery.

INTRAOPERATIVE RENAL ISCHEMIA

Temporary occlusion of the renal artery is necessary for a variety of operations, such as partial nephrectomy, renal vascular reconstruction, anatrophic nephrolithotomy, and repair of traumatic renal injury. In such cases, temporary arterial occlusion not only diminishes intraoperative renal bleeding but also improves access to intrarenal structures by causing the kidney to contract and reducing renal tissue turgor. Performance of these operations requires an understanding of renal responses to warm ischemia and available methods of protecting the kidney when the period of arterial occlusion exceeds that which may be safely tolerated.

Renal Tolerance to Warm Ischemia

Because renal metabolic activities are predominantly aerobic, the kidney is susceptible to damage from warm ischemia. Almost immediately after renal arterial occlusion, energy-rich adenosine triphosphates (ATP) within the kidney cells begin to break down into monophosphate nucleotides to provide the energy required for maintenance of structural and functional cellular integrity (Collste et al, 1971; Collins et al, 1977). When energy sources have been depleted, cellular membrane transport mechanisms fail, causing an influx of salt and water, which ultimately results in severe cellular edema and cell death.

The extent of renal damage after normothermic arterial occlusion depends on the duration of the ischemic insult. Canine studies have shown that warm ischemic intervals of up to 30 minutes can be sustained with eventual full recovery of renal function (Ward, 1975). **For periods of warm ischemia beyond 30 minutes, there is significant immediate functional loss, and late recovery of renal function is**

either incomplete or absent. Histologically, renal ischemia is most damaging to the proximal tubular cells, which may show varying degrees of necrosis and regeneration, whereas the glomeruli and blood vessels generally are spared.

Human tolerance to warm renal ischemia closely parallels experimental canine observations, and in general 30 minutes is the maximum tolerable period of arterial occlusion before permanent damage is sustained. In some clinical situations, the latter admonition may not apply, and a longer period of ischemia may be safely tolerated. It is acknowledged that the solitary kidney is more resistant to ischemic damage than the paired kidney, although precise limits have not been defined (Askari et al, 1982). Another situation that may enhance renal tolerance to temporary arterial occlusion is the presence of an extensive collateral vascular supply. This is generally observed only in patients with renal arterial occlusive disease (Schefft et al, 1980).

Another determinant of renal ischemic damage is the method employed to achieve vascular control of the kidney. Animal studies have shown that functional impairment is least when the renal artery alone is continuously occluded. Continuous occlusion of both the renal artery and the renal vein for an equivalent time interval is more damaging because this prevents retrograde perfusion of the kidney through the renal vein and may produce venous congestion of the kidney (Neely and Turner, 1959; Leary et al, 1963; Schirmer et al, 1966). Intermittent clamping of the renal artery with short periods of recirculation is also more damaging than continuous arterial occlusion, possibly because of the release and trapping of damaging vasoconstrictor agents within the kidney (Neely and Turner, 1959; Schirmer et al, 1966; Wilson et al, 1971; McLaughlin et al, 1978). Animal studies have further demonstrated that the use of manual renal compression to control intraoperative hemorrhage is more deleterious than simple arterial occlusion (Neely and Turner, 1959).

Prevention of Ischemic Renal Damage

Several general adjunctive measures should be employed in all patients undergoing operations that involve a period of temporary renal arterial occlusion. These include generous preoperative and intraoperative hydration, prevention of hypotension during the period of anesthesia, avoidance of unnecessary manipulation or traction on the renal artery, and intraoperative administration of mannitol. These measures help to limit postischemic renal injury by ensuring optimal perfusion with absence of cortical vasospasm at the time of arterial occlusion, which allows uniform restoration of blood flow throughout the kidney when the renal artery is unclamped. Mannitol is most effective when given 5 to 15 minutes before arterial occlusion (Collins et al, 1980) and is beneficial by increasing renal plasma flow, decreasing intrarenal vascular resistance, minimizing intracellular edema, and promoting an osmotic diuresis when the renal circulation is restored (Nosowsky and Kaufmann, 1963). Systemic or regional heparinization before renal arterial occlusion is not necessary, unless there is existing small vessel or parenchymal renal disease.

When the anticipated period of intraoperative renal ischemia is longer than 30 minutes, additional specific protective measures are indicated to prevent permanent damage to the kidney. Local hypothermia is the most efficacious and commonly employed method for protecting the kidney from ischemic damage. Lowering renal temperature reduces energy-dependent metabolic activity of the cortical cells, with a resultant decrease in both the consumption of oxygen and the breakdown of ATP (Harvey, 1959; Levy, 1959). The optimum temperature for hypothermic in situ renal preservation is 15°C based on canine experiments conducted by Ward (1975). In clinical renal surgery, it is difficult to achieve uniform cooling to this level because of the temperature of adjacent tissues and the need to have a portion of the kidney exposed to perform the operation. For practical reasons, a temperature of 20 to 25°C is easier to maintain and represents a compromise that renders renal surgery technically feasible while still allowing a renal preservative effect. Both animal and human studies have shown that this level of hypothermia provides complete renal protection from up to 3 hours of arterial occlusion (Wickham et al, 1967; Luttrop et al, 1976; Petersen et al, 1977; Wagenknecht et al, 1977; Marberger et al, 1978; Stubbs et al, 1978; Kyriakidis et al, 1979).

In situ renal hypothermia can be achieved with external surface cooling or perfusion of the kidney with a cold solution instilled into the renal artery. These two methods are equally effective; however, the latter is an invasive technique that requires direct entry into the renal artery (Leary et al, 1963; Farcon et al, 1974; Kyriakidis et al, 1979; Abele et al, 1981). Surface cooling of the kidney is a simpler and more widely used method that has been accomplished by a variety of techniques, such as surrounding the kidney with ice slush (Metzner and Boyce, 1972; Gibbons et al, 1976; Stubbs et al, 1978), immersing the kidney in a cold solution (Mitchell, 1959), or applying an external cooling device to the kidney (Cockett, 1961). These methods all require complete renal mobilization to achieve effective surface cooling.

Most urologists currently prefer ice slush cooling for surface renal hypothermia because of its relative ease and simplicity. The mobilized kidney is surrounded with a rubber sheet on which sterile ice slush is placed to immerse the kidney completely. **An important caveat with this method is to keep the entire kidney covered with ice for 10 to 15 minutes immediately after occluding the renal artery and before commencing the renal operation.** This amount of time is needed to obtain core renal cooling to a temperature (approximately 20°C) that optimizes in situ renal preservation. During performance of the renal operation, invariably large portions of the kidney are no longer covered with ice slush, and, in the absence of adequate prior core renal cooling, rapid rewarming and ischemic renal injury can occur. This technique is effective for in situ renal preservation. Stubbs and associates reported 30 patients with a solitary kidney in whom anatrophic nephrolithotomy was performed with ice slush surface hypothermia; despite a mean renal artery clamp time of longer than 2 hours, and as long as 4 hours in some cases, renal function was completely preserved in all patients (Stubbs et al, 1978).

Another approach to in situ renal preservation that does not involve hypothermia has been pretreatment with one or more pharmacologic agents to prevent postischemic renal failure (Novick, 1983). Agents that have been tested include vasoactive drugs, membrane-stabilizing drugs, calcium channel blockers, and agents that act to preserve or replenish intracellular levels of ATP. A review of this field is beyond the scope of this chapter. Experimental studies have shown that several of these agents can help to prevent postischemic renal failure. Thus far, however, no pharmacologic regimen has proven to be as effective as local hypothermia for ischemic intervals of 2 hours or more.

SURGICAL APPROACHES TO THE KIDNEY

Exposure of the kidney during surgery must be adequate to perform the operation and to deal with any possible complications. This is particularly important in renal surgery because the kidney is deeply placed in the upper retroperitoneum with access limited by the lower ribs, liver, and spleen. Injuries to large renal vessels may be difficult to control or repair through small incisions, particularly in the presence of a large tumor or inflamed perinephric tissues. Poor exposure renders the operation unnecessarily difficult and leads to excessive retraction, with bruising of the muscles and possible injury to the intercostal nerves, which can increase postoperative pain.

Factors to consider in selecting an appropriate incision for renal surgery include the operation to be performed, underlying renal pathology, previous operations, concurrent extrarenal pathology that requires another operation to be done simultaneously, the need for bilateral renal operations, and body habitus. Physical abnormalities in the patient, such as kyphoscoliosis or severe pulmonary disease, may also dictate that certain approaches, such as the standard flank incision, not be used.

The kidney may be approached by four principal routes: an extraperitoneal flank approach, a dorsal lumbotomy, an abdominal incision, or a thoracoabdominal incision. The indications, relative advantages, and technical performance of each approach are reviewed separately.

Flank Approach

This approach provides good access to the renal parenchyma and collecting system (Woodruff, 1955). It is an extraperitoneal approach and involves minimal disturbance to other viscera. Contamination of the peritoneal cavity is avoided, and drainage of the perirenal space is readily established. This approach is particularly useful in the obese patient because most of the panniculus falls forward, making this incision relatively straightforward even in a large person. **The principal disadvantage of the flank incision is that exposure in the area of the renal pedicle is not as good as with anterior transperitoneal approaches.** In addition, the flank incision may prove unsuitable for the patient with scoliosis or cardiorespiratory problems.

The most commonly used flank approach to the kidney is through the bed of the 11th or 12th rib (Hess, 1939; Hughes, 1949; Bodner and Briskin, 1950). The choice of rib depends on the position of the kidney and on whether the upper or lower pole is the site of disease. With a flank incision, the midportion of the wound and the site of maximum exposure

are in the midaxillary line. Access in the posterior part, at the neck of the rib, is limited by the sacrospinalis muscle. The appropriate level of the incision is therefore best determined by drawing a horizontal line on the urogram from the hilum of the kidney to the most lateral rib that it intersects (Fig. 97–5). When access to the upper renal pole is required, the rib above is selected.

The patient is placed in the lateral position after being anesthetized and having an endotracheal tube inserted. The back should be placed fairly close to the edge of the operating table to ensure unimpeded access by the surgeon, and the patient should be positioned so that the tip of the 12th rib is over the kidney rest. The bottom leg is flexed to 90 degrees, with the top leg straight to maintain stability. A pillow is placed between the knees, and a sponge pad is placed under the axilla to prevent compression of the axillary vessels and nerves. The patient is secured in this position with a wide adhesive tape passed over the greater trochanter and attached to the movable portion of the table (Fig. 97–6). The extended upper arm can be supported on a padded Mayo stand, which is adjusted to the appropriate height to maintain the arm in a horizontal position with the shoulder rotated slightly forward.

Flexion of the table and elevation of the kidney rest should be performed slowly and may be delayed until the surgeon is ready to make the skin incision to minimize the time spent in this position. The flexion increases the space between the costal margin and iliac crest and puts the flank muscles and skin on tension. Care must be taken with patients who have stiff spines to ensure that their extremities remain in contact with the table because their range of lateral flexion is limited. This position may not be well tolerated in elderly patients or in those with impaired cardiopulmonary function because it results in decreased venous return owing to compression of the inferior vena cava and the dependent position of the legs. It also limits aeration of the lung on the dependent side. It is important to determine the patient's blood pressure after the patient has been turned on his or her side and again after the table has been flexed and the kidney rest elevated. The rest may have to be lowered and the table unflexed if hypotension is observed.

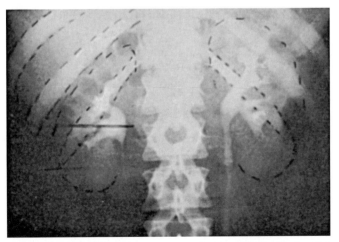

Figure 97–5. The right kidney is traversed at its midpoint by the 12th rib. The ideal incision is chosen by drawing a horizontal line from the hilum to the lateral rib cage.

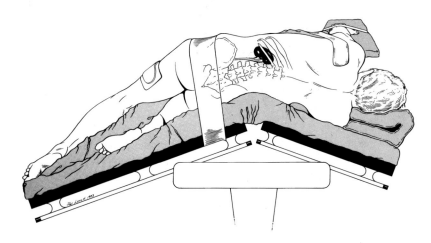

Figure 97–6. Position of the patient for the flank approach. Note the axillary pad. The kidney rest may be elevated if further lateral extension is needed.

The flank incision is made directly over the appropriate rib, beginning at the lateral border of the sacrospinalis muscle (Fig. 97–7). A left-sided 12th rib incision is demonstrated in Figures 97–7 to 97–12. After dividing the external oblique, latissimus dorsi, and slips of the underlying serratus posterior inferior muscles (Fig. 97–8), the periosteum over the rib is incised with a scalpel or by diathermy. The flat periosteal elevator is used to reflect the periosteum off the rib (Fig. 97–9). Mobilization of the periosteum is completed

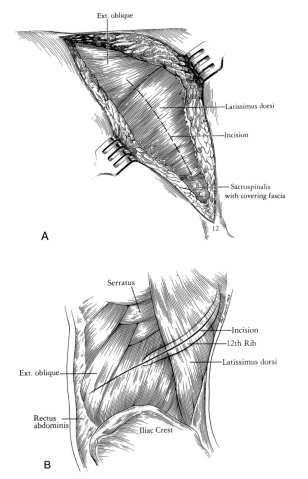

Figure 97–7. *A,* Left flank incision. Anterior edge of the latissimus dorsi muscle overlies the posterior edge of the external oblique muscle. *B,* The relationship of the 12th rib to the overlying muscles is depicted.

by separating it from the inner aspect of the rib, using a Doyen periosteal elevator (Fig. 97–10). The proximal end of the rib is then transected as far back as possible with the guillotine rib resector. The retracted muscle mass is allowed to fall back over the sharp cut edge, protecting the operator from injury. The rib is grasped with a Kocher clamp and is separated from the muscles attached anteriorly by sharp dissection to complete its removal.

When the 11th rib is resected, attention must be directed at the pleural reflection, which crosses its lower border at the junction of the anterior and middle thirds and which occupies the posterior part of the wound as it lies on the lower fibers of the diaphragm. The pleura may be reflected upward by sharply dividing the fascial attachments to the diaphragm. Alternatively the lower fibers of the diaphragm can be detached from their insertion into the posterior inner aspect of the 12th rib. This allows the lower diaphragm and pleura to be retracted upward, out of the wound.

An incision is now made through the periosteal bed of the rib to expose Gerota's fascia (Fig. 97–11). The incision is completed anteriorly by incising the lumbar fascia and inserting two fingers into the perinephric space to push the underlying peritoneum forward. The lateral peritoneal reflection is peeled off the undersurface of the anterior abdominal wall and transverse fascia by sweeping it forward with the fingers. The external and internal oblique muscles are divided by incising them sharply or with electrocautery while they are tented up over the two fingers inserted below the transversus muscle (Fig. 97–12). A little upward pressure controls bleeding from the severed vessels, allowing them to be clamped or cauterized by the assistant. This should expose the intercostal neurovascular bundle as it courses forward and downward between the internal oblique and transversus muscles. The transverse fibers of the transversus muscle may be split by blunt dissection below the nerve, allowing it to fall away with the upper margin of the incision.

A Finochietto retractor is used to maintain the exposure. The blades of the retractor are placed over moistened gauze sponges to avoid breaking a rib. The perinephric space is entered by incising Gerota's fascia posteriorly to avoid injury to the peritoneum. Care should be taken to avoid injury to the iliohypogastric and ilioinguinal nerves as they emerge from behind the lateral border of the psoas muscle and pass down over the anterior surface of the quadratus lumborum in the renal fossa.

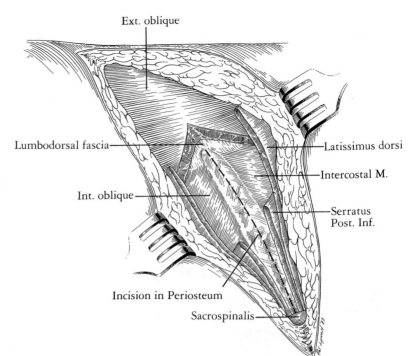

Figure 97–8. The muscles in the posterior part of the wound have been divided to expose the rib for incision of the periosteum.

The incision is closed by careful approximation of the corresponding muscle and fascial layers. To facilitate this, the kidney rest is lowered, and the table is returned to the horizontal position. Care must be taken to avoid inclusion of any intercostal nerves or branches during closure of the transversus muscle. Injection of 0.5% bupivacaine (Marcaine) into the fascial sheath around the intercostal nerves as they emerge from the intervertebral foramina is helpful in diminishing postoperative pain and involuntary splinting of the lower chest. Drains are usually brought out posteriorly through a separate stab incision below the wound.

Occasionally a subcostal flank incision is indicated for surgery on the lower renal pole or upper ureter, insertion of a nephrostomy tube, or drainage of a perinephric abscess. It has the disadvantage of being rather low in relation to the usual position of the kidney, which makes access to the pedicle and renal pelvis more difficult. Exposure may be hampered by the iliac crest and subcostal nerve. The subcostal incision does not have these disadvantages in children, in whom it provides good access to the kidney because the lower ribs are soft and easily displaced upward.

The subcostal incision is begun at the lateral border of the sacrospinalis muscle, where it crosses the inferior edge of the 12th rib, and is carried forward about a fingerbreadth below the lower border of the last rib onto the anterior abdominal wall. The medial end of the incision is curved slightly downward as it passes the midaxillary line to avoid the subcostal nerve and may be extended as far as the lateral border of the rectus abdominis muscle. The extent of the incision is modified, depending on the location of the kidney and the nature of the disease.

With a subcostal incision, the latissimus dorsi muscle is

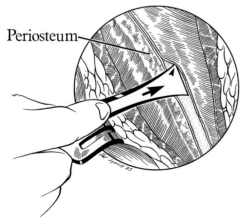

Figure 97–9. The periosteum is reflected off the upper surface of the rib. Note that the periosteal elevator is moved distally or downward on the upper edge of the rib against the direction of the intercostal muscle fibers.

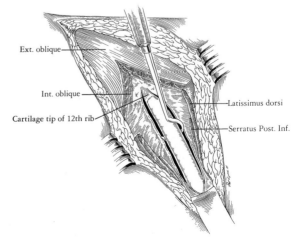

Figure 97–10. The periosteum is dissected off the rib, using a Doyen periosteal elevator, before resection of the rib.

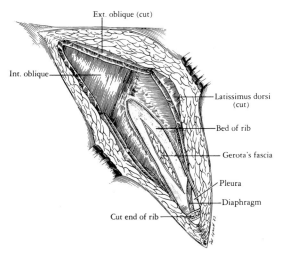

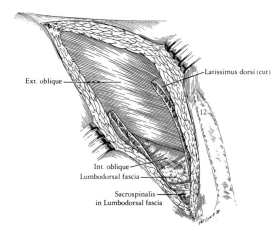

Figure 97–11. The rib has been resected, exposing the diaphragm and pleura in the posterior part of the wound. The slips of the diaphragm inserting into the rib have been divided, allowing the pleura to be displaced upward. An incision is made through the periosteal bed of the wound to expose Gerota's fascia.

Figure 97–13. Left subcostal incision. The latissimus dorsi muscle has been divided to expose the lumbodorsal fascia and posterior aspects of the abdominal muscles.

divided in the posterior part of the wound to expose the posterior edge of the external oblique muscle (Fig. 97–13). The serratus posterior-inferior muscles, arising from the lumbar fascia and inserting into the lower four ribs, are divided in the posterior portion of the wound. The external oblique muscle is divided anteriorly. The fused layers of the lumbodorsal fascia are now exposed because they give origin to the internal oblique and transversus muscles. After the internal oblique muscle is divided, the transversus is separated bluntly either above or below the subcostal nerve depending on the course of the nerve in relation to the incision (Fig. 97–14). Every effort should be made to avoid injury to the intercostal nerves because this may cause persistent postoperative pain or bulging in the flank as a result of paresis of

the denervated muscle. The lumbar fascia and the lateral border of the sacrospinalis may need to be incised to improve exposure in the posterior part of the wound. Division of the costotransverse ligament, as it passes up to the neck of the 12th rib, allows the rib to be retracted upward to improve the exposure further. The closure is as described for a flank incision.

Dorsal Lumbotomy

The dorsal lumbotomy incision is a useful approach for removal of a small kidney, for bilateral nephrectomy in patients with end-stage renal disease, for open renal biopsy, for pyeloplasty, for pyelolithotomy, and for an upper ureterolithotomy when the stone is firmly impacted (Gil-Vernet, 1965; Novick, 1980). This approach offers several advantages when performing these operations (Gardiner et al,

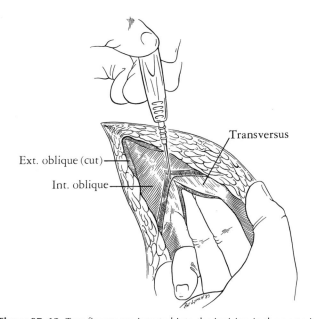

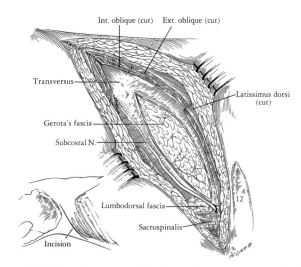

Figure 97–12. Two fingers are inserted into the incision in the posterior part of the transversus muscle to sweep the peritoneal reflection forward and divide the anterior abdominal muscles.

Figure 97–14. The lumbodorsal fascia and transversus muscles have been divided to expose Gerota's fascia. The subcostal nerve and vessels pierce the lumbodorsal fascia posteriorly and course forward on the transversus muscle.

1979). In contrast to the standard flank incision, no muscles are transected, and access to the kidney is obtained by simply incising the posterior fascial layers. This approach is more rapid, provides a strong wound closure with less postoperative pain, and obviates anterolateral bulging of the abdomen that commonly results from flank incisions. With detachment of the costovertebral ligament, the 12th rib can be retracted widely laterally, rendering resection of the rib unnecessary. The dorsal lumbotomy approach is also advantageous in patients with prior abdominal or flank operations on the kidney because it permits dissection of fresh tissue planes. **The major disadvantage of the dorsal lumbotomy is the limited access to the kidney and renal vessels,** which can pose a problem if there are intraoperative complications, such as migration of a calculus or injury to major renal vessels with bleeding.

When bilateral nephrectomy is done, the patient is placed in the prone position with the table flexed to increase the distance between the 12th rib and the iliac crest. In this position, the patient is supported over the sternum and pubis so that there is free excursion of the anterior abdominal wall to prevent embarrassment of respiration and venous return. For unilateral renal operations, the patient may be placed in the lateral position with the table flexed to extend the lumbar region. In this position, a sandbag is placed between the abdomen and the table for support and to help push the kidney posteriorly.

A vertical lumbar incision is made along the lateral margin of the sacrospinalis muscle. The incision begins at the upper margin of the 12th rib superiorly and follows a gentle lateral curve to the iliac crest inferiorly (Fig. 97–15A). The incision is carried through the lumbodorsal fascia just lateral to the sacrospinalis and quadratus lumborum muscles, which are then retracted medially to approach the renal fossa (Fig. 97–15B). The transverse fascia is incised to expose the kidney contained within Gerota's fascia (Fig. 97–15C). Exposure of the kidney is thus obtained without transection of any muscle fibers. If additional superior exposure is needed, the costovertebral ligamentous attachment of the 12th rib is divided to allow lateral and superior retraction of the rib (Fig. 97–15D and E). The kidney can be mobilized and delivered down into the incision, provided that the lower third of the kidney is located below the 12th rib on preoperative x-ray films. For high-lying or enlarged kidneys, however, the dorsal lumbotomy approach is cumbersome, and either a flank or an anterior incision provides better exposure. To close the incision, the retracted muscles are allowed to return to their original position, and the lumbodorsal fascia is reapproximated.

Abdominal Incisions

The principal advantage of the abdominal approach is that exposure in the area of the renal pedicle is excellent. The principal disadvantage is the somewhat longer period of postoperative ileus and the possible long-term complication of intra-abdominal adhesions leading to bowel obstruction. The choice between a vertical or a transverse type of abdominal incision is determined by the patient's anatomy and disease entity. A vertical incision is

easier and quicker to perform and repair because it involves only division of the linea alba or the anterior and posterior layers of the rectus sheath rather than several muscle layers. The vertical incision may be used in patients with a narrow subcostal angle and is preferred in patients with renal injury because it allows better access for inspection of the remainder of the abdominal contents for associated injuries. A transverse incision is preferable for patients with a wide subcostal angle and for the exploration or removal of renal mass lesions (Chute et al, 1967). This incision provides better access to the lateral and superior portion of the kidney. A unilateral subcostal incision can be extended across the midline as a chevron incision to provide excellent exposure of both kidneys along with the aorta and inferior vena cava.

When employing an anterior subcostal incision, the patient is in the supine position with a rolled sheet beneath the upper lumbar spine. The incision begins approximately 1 to 2 fingerbreadths below the costal margin in the anterior axillary line and then extends with a gentle curve across the midline, ending at the midportion of the opposite rectus muscle. The incision is carried through the subcutaneous tissues to the anterior fascia, which is divided in the direction of the incision. In the lateral aspect of the incision, a portion of the latissimus dorsi muscle is divided. The external oblique muscle is divided, exposing the fibers of the internal oblique muscle (Fig. 97–16A). The rectus, internal oblique, and transversus abdominis muscles are divided along with the posterior rectus sheath (Fig. 97–16B and C). The peritoneal cavity is entered in the midline, and the ligamentum teres is divided (Fig. 97–16D).

The bilateral subcostal incision is performed as described for the unilateral incision except that both sides are involved (Fig. 97–17). It extends from one anterior axillary line to the opposite anterior axillary line, with a gentle upward curve as it crosses the midline. This incision provides better exposure of both kidneys than a midline incision, particularly in obese patients with a wide subcostal angle. The disadvantage is that it involves extensive transection of the abdominal wall musculature.

An extraperitoneal anterior subcostal approach may be useful to perform open renal biopsy or nephrectomy, particularly when there has been a previous intra-abdominal procedure or when there is a possibility that the patient may require peritoneal dialysis postoperatively (Lyon, 1958). The peritoneal cavity is not entered, thereby minimizing postoperative ileus and the chance of an intra-abdominal complication. Reflection of the peritoneum off the anterior abdominal wall may at times be difficult, and access to the renal pedicle may be less satisfactory than with a transperitoneal incision. The patient is placed in a semioblique position with a rolled sheet beneath the side in which the incision is to be made. The muscle layers are divided as they are for a unilateral subcostal incision except that the peritoneal cavity is not entered. The peritoneum is mobilized intact from the undersurface of the lateral musculature and rectus sheath and is then retracted medially to expose the retroperitoneal space (Fig. 97–18).

When employing a midline upper abdominal incision, the patient is placed supine on the operating table with a rolled sheet beneath the upper lumbar spine. The incision extends from the xiphoid to the umbilicus and can be extended around the umbilicus on one side if necessary. The incision

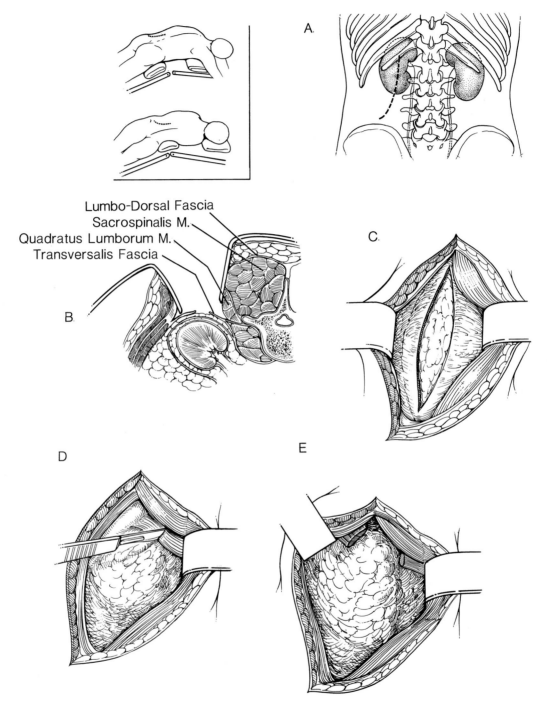

Lumbo-Dorsal Fascia
Sacrospinalis M.
Quadratus Lumborum M.
Transversalis Fascia

Figure 97–15. *A* to *E*, The dorsal lumbotomy incision.

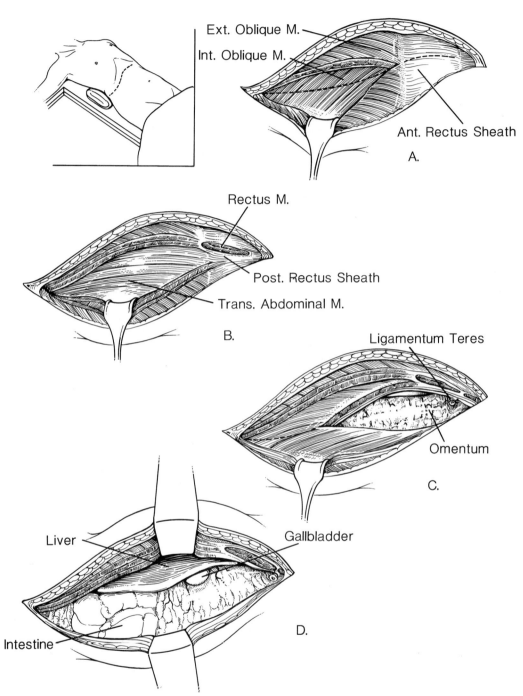

Figure 97–16. *A* to *D*, Unilateral anterior subcostal transperitoneal incision.

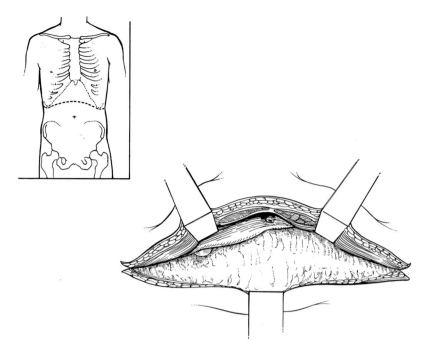

Figure 97–17. Bilateral anterior subcostal transperitoneal incision.

is carried down through the subcutaneous tissues to the linea alba, which is the midline fusion of the tendinous fibers of the anterior rectus sheath. The linea alba is divided to expose the extraperitoneal fat and peritoneum, which is then entered (Fig. 97–19).

A paramedian incision is another type of vertical abdominal incision that may be preferred because the separate closure of the two layers of the rectus sheath makes the wound more secure. The incision is made about 3 cm lateral to the midline to provide an adequate margin of rectus sheath medially (Fig. 97–20). The anterior sheath is divided and reflected medially off the underlying muscle by sharp division of the tendinous intersections. The free medial edge of the muscle is retracted laterally to allow the posterior rectus sheath and peritoneum to be incised (Fig. 97–21). An extraperitoneal approach to the kidney can also be made through a paramedian incision by carefully reflecting the peritoneum off the posterior rectus sheath after it has been divided (Tessler et al, 1975).

Thoracoabdominal Incision

The thoracoabdominal approach is desirable for performing radical nephrectomy in patients with large tumors involving the upper portion of the kidney (Clarke et al, 1958; Khoury, 1966; Chute et al, 1967; Middleton and Presto, 1973). It is particularly advantageous on the right side where the liver and its venous drainage into the upper vena cava can limit exposure and impair vascular control as the tumor mass is being removed. There is less need for a thoracoabdominal incision on the left side because the spleen and pancreas can usually be readily elevated away from the tumor mass. The thoracoabdominal incision optimizes exposure of the suprarenal area. Nevertheless, because it involves additional operative time and greater potential pulmonary morbidity, the authors reserve this approach for patients in whom the additional exposure over that provided by an anterior subcostal incision is considered important to achieve complete, safe tumor removal.

The patient is placed in a semioblique position with a rolled sheet placed longitudinally beneath the flank. The lower leg is flexed, and the upper one is extended with a pillow beneath the legs. The pelvis assumes a more horizontal position, being tilted only about 10 to 15 degrees, which allows free access to the anterior abdominal wall. The incision is begun in the eighth or ninth intercostal space near the angle of the rib and is carried across the costal margin to the midpoint of the opposite rectus muscle just above the umbilicus. The incision is carried down to the fascia, which is divided in the direction of the incision (Fig. 97–22A). The latissimus dorsi, external oblique, rectus, and intercostal muscles are also divided in the direction of the incision. The costal cartilage between the tips of the adjacent ribs is divided (Fig. 97–22B). The pleura in the posterior portion of the incision is opened to obtain complete exposure of the diaphragm (Fig. 97–22C).

The diaphragmatic incision is begun at the periphery about 2 cm inside its attachment to the chest wall, with the incision then being carried around circumferentially to the posterior aspect of the diaphragm (Fig. 97–22D). In doing this, there must be at least 2 or 3 cm of diaphragm left attached to the rib cage to allow later reconstruction. By dividing the diaphragm in a circumferential manner from anterior to posterior, damage to the phrenic nerve is avoided. This also creates a diaphragmatic flap that can be pushed into the chest to provide complete exposure of the liver, which is then simply retracted upward (Fig. 97–22E). If further mobilization of the liver is needed, the right triangular ligament and coronary ligament can be incised to mobilize the entire right lobe of the liver upward. This provides excellent additional exposure of the suprarenal vena cava. Medial to the ribs, the internal oblique and transversus abdominis muscles

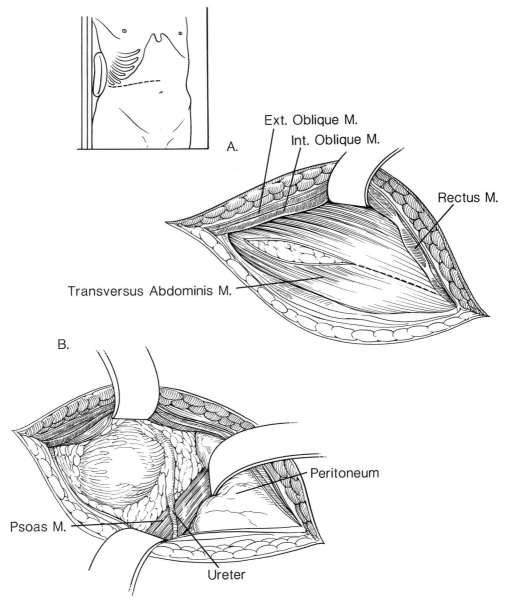

Figure 97–18. *A* and *B*, Extraperitoneal anterior subcostal incision.

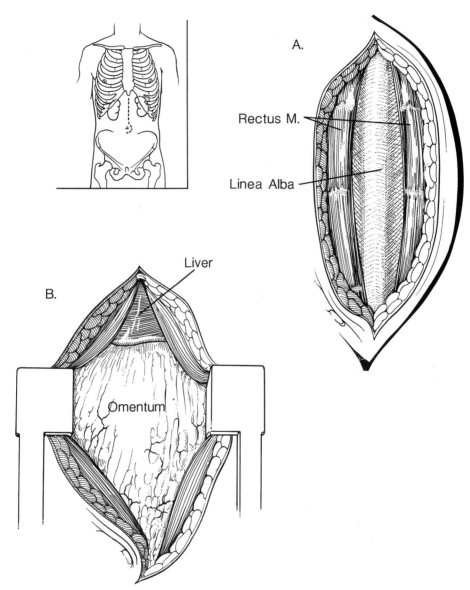

Rectus M.

Linea Alba

Liver

Omentum

A.

B.

Figure 97–19. *A* and *B*, Midline upper abdominal incision.

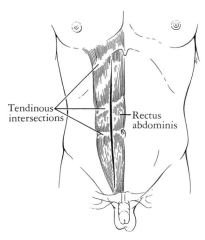

Figure 97–20. Right paramedian incision with division of the anterior rectus sheath.

are divided, and the peritoneal cavity is entered. The colon and duodenum are mobilized medially and the liver is retracted upward to expose the kidney and great vessels (Fig. 97–22*F*).

At the completion of the procedure, the abdominal viscera are replaced in their anatomic position. The diaphragm is repaired with interrupted 2–0 silk or PDS mattress sutures with the knots tied on the undersurface. The chest wall is reapproximated by passing 0 polyglycolic sutures around the ribs above and below. These sutures should be passed on a tapered needle to avoid cutting any vessels, with care taken to avoid the neurovascular bundle. Before closing the pleura, a No. 20 Fr chest tube is placed in the pleural cavity and brought out through a stab wound below the incision in the posterior axillary line. The transected muscle and fascial layers are reapproximated separately. The chest tube is con-

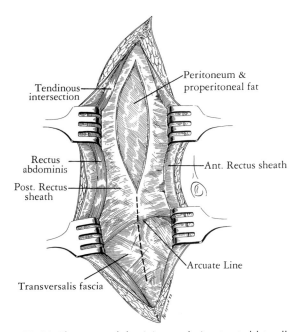

Figure 97–21. The rectus abdominis muscle is retracted laterally, and the posterior rectus sheath and transversalis fascia are then incised to expose the properitoneal space.

nected to an underwater drain and is usually removed 24 to 48 hours postoperatively, provided that there is no persistent leakage of air and a chest film shows satisfactory lung expansion.

SIMPLE NEPHRECTOMY

Indications

Simple nephrectomy is indicated in patients with an irreversibly damaged kidney because of symptomatic chronic infection, obstruction, calculus disease, or severe traumatic injury. It is occasionally appropriate to remove a functioning kidney involved with one of these conditions when the patient's age or general condition is too poor to permit a reconstructive operation and provided that the opposite kidney is normal. Nephrectomy may also be indicated to treat renovascular hypertension owing to noncorrectable renal artery disease or severe unilateral parenchymal damage owing to nephrosclerosis, pyelonephritis, reflux dysplasia, or congenital dysplasia.

Simple nephrectomy can be performed through a variety of incisions. **An extraperitoneal flank approach is usually preferable when the kidney is chronically infected, when the patient is obese, or when multiple prior abdominal operations have been performed.** A subcapsular approach is indicated when severe perirenal inflammation or adhesions obscure anatomic relationships between the kidney and surrounding structures. A transperitoneal approach is preferable in patients who cannot tolerate the flank position, in patients with end-stage renal disease undergoing bilateral nephrectomy for polycystic kidney disease, and in patients with traumatic renal injury in whom early access to the pedicle is necessary. The transperitoneal approach is also useful when multiple operations have been performed previously through the flank with resulting dense adhesions around the kidney. Bilateral nephrectomy in patients with small end-stage kidneys can be done through a bilateral simultaneous posterior approach (Novick, 1980).

Flank Approach

Once the perinephric space is entered, access to the kidney is obtained by incising Gerota's fascia on the lateral aspect of the kidney to avoid injury to the overlying peritoneum (Fig. 97–23*A*). The plane of cleavage between the perinephric fat and the renal capsule is usually developed easily. The kidney is mobilized by blunt dissection, and, on the left side, the pancreas and duodenum are carefully reflected medially along with the peritoneum. The ureter is identified during mobilization of the lower renal pole. It is preferable to divide the ureter after ligation of the pedicle to avoid congestion of the kidney. The kidney is now pulled downward, and the upper pole is dissected free. There is normally a separate compartment in Gerota's fascia for the adrenal gland, which enables it to be readily separated from the upper pole.

The kidney is now pulled laterally to identify the renal

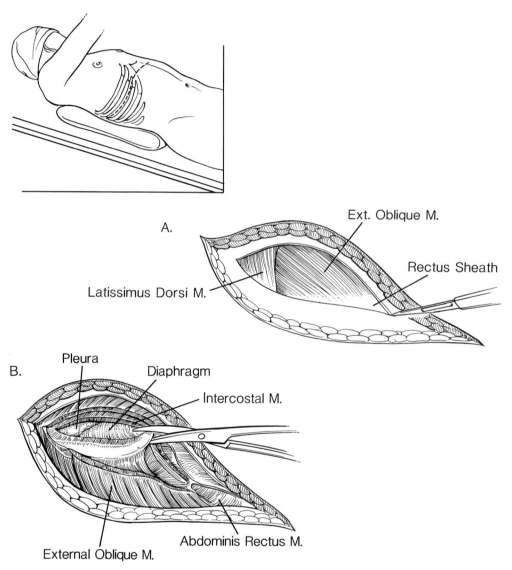

A.

Ext. Oblique M.

Rectus Sheath

Latissimus Dorsi M.

B.

Pleura

Diaphragm

Intercostal M.

External Oblique M.

Abdominis Rectus M.

Figure 97–22. *A to F,* Right thoracoabdominal incision.

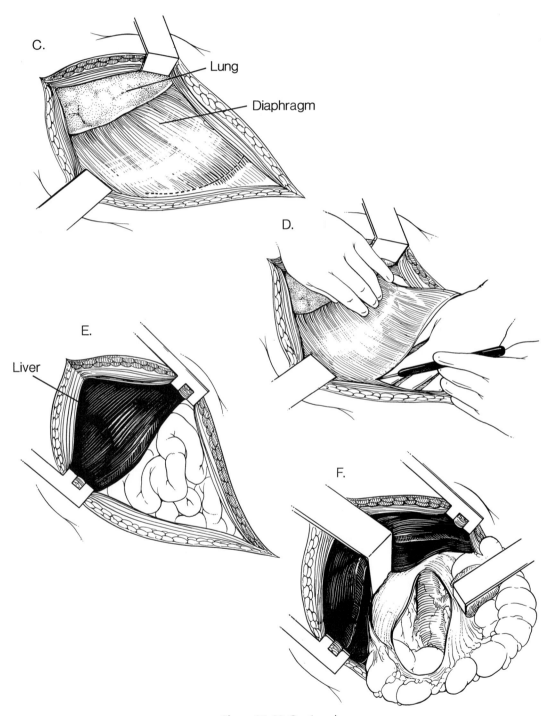

Figure 97–22 *Continued*

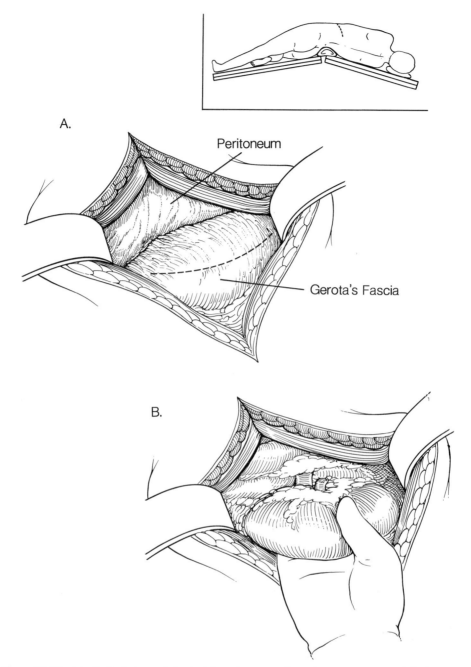

Figure 97–23. *A* to *D,* Technique of simple left nephrectomy through an extraperitoneal flank incision.

artery and vein, which are separated from surrounding fatty and lymphatic tissues by blunt dissection (Fig. 97–23*B*). Whenever possible, it is preferable to secure the vessels individually away from the hilus, and the artery should always be ligated first. The renal vein is usually visualized easily and is mobilized by ligating and dividing the gonadal, adrenal, and lumbar branches. The vein can then be retracted to expose the artery, which lies posteriorly. Alternatively the renal vein can be approached posteriorly by mobilizing the kidney and retracting it up into the wound. The renal artery and vein are individually secured with 2–0 silk ligatures and are then divided (Fig. 97–23*C*). The ureter is now clamped and divided, and the distal end is ligated with 2–0 chromic catgut to complete the nephrectomy (Fig. 97–23*D*).

Subcapsular Technique

Subcapsular nephrectomy is indicated when severe perirenal inflammation precludes satisfactory dissection between the kidney and surrounding structures (Kimbrough and Morse, 1953; Kittredge and Fridge, 1958). After the retroperitoneal space has been entered, the renal capsule is identified, and a longitudinal incision is made over the lateral surface of the kidney (Fig. 97–24*A*). Once the capsule has been entered, a plane is developed between the renal parenchyma and capsule over the entire surface of the kidney down to the level of the hilus (Fig. 97–24*B* and *C*). The renal parenchyma is retracted laterally to expose the major renal vessels as they enter the hilus. Vascular branches are ligated and

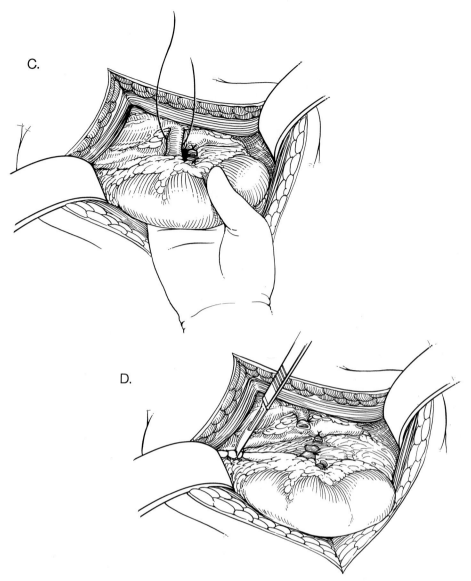

Figure 97–23 *Continued*

transected as far laterally as possible to allow satisfactory proximal control of each branch (Fig. 97–24D). The upper ureter is then ligated and divided to complete the nephrectomy.

Transperitoneal Approach

When performing transperitoneal simple nephrectomy, a subcostal incision is made, and the peritoneal cavity is entered. On the left side, the colon, pancreas, and spleen are reflected upward and medially to expose the left renal vein. A self-retaining ring retractor is useful to maintain exposure of the surgical field (Fig. 97–25A).

The renal vein and artery are mobilized, ligated, and transected (Fig. 97–25B). The artery is occluded first to avoid excessive blood loss into the kidney. The kidney is then mobilized laterally, superiorly, and inferiorly by sharp and blunt dissection. It is best to initiate the dissection laterally to obtain maximum mobilization before ap-

proaching the posterior renal hilus where friable lumbar veins may be present (Fig. 97–25C). In cases of severe perirenal fibrosis, it may be necessary to remove some of the posterior psoas fascia together with the kidney. After complete renal mobilization, the ureter is ligated and divided to complete the nephrectomy.

RADICAL NEPHRECTOMY

Indications and Evaluation

Radical nephrectomy is the treatment of choice for patients with localized renal cell carcinoma (Robson et al, 1969; Skinner et al, 1971). The preoperative evaluation of patients with renal cell carcinoma has changed considerably as a result of the advent of new imaging modalities such as ultrasonography, computed tomography scanning, and magnetic resonance imaging. In many patients, a complete preliminary evaluation can be performed using these noninva-

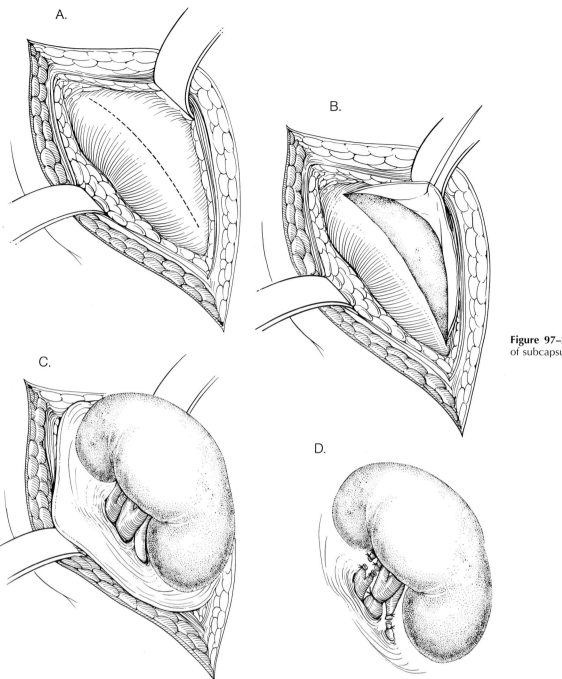

A.

B.

C.

D.

Figure 97–24. *A* to *D*, Technique of subcapsular nephrectomy.

sive modalities. Renal arteriography is no longer routinely necessary before performing radical nephrectomy. All patients should undergo a metastatic evaluation including a chest film, abdominal computed tomography scan, and occasionally a bone scan; the last-mentioned is necessary only in patients with bone pain or an elevated serum alkaline phosphatase. Radical nephrectomy is occasionally done in patients with metastatic disease to palliate severe associated local symptoms or to allow entry into a biologic response modifier protocol or concomitant to resection of a solitary metastatic lesion.

Involvement of the inferior vena cava with renal cell carcinoma occurs in 3% to 7% of cases and renders the task

of complete surgical excision more complicated (Schefft et al, 1978). Yet operative removal offers the only hope for cure, and when there are no metastases, an aggressive approach is justified. Five-year survival rates of 40% to 68% have been reported after complete surgical excision (Libertino et al, 1987; Neves and Zincke, 1987; Skinner et al, 1989, Novick et al, 1990). The best results have been achieved when the tumor does not involve the perinephric fat and regional lymph nodes (Cherrie et al, 1982). The cephalad extent of vena caval involvement is not prognostically important, and even with intra-atrial tumor thrombi, extended cancer-free survival is possible after surgical treatment when there is no nodal or distant metastasis (Glazer

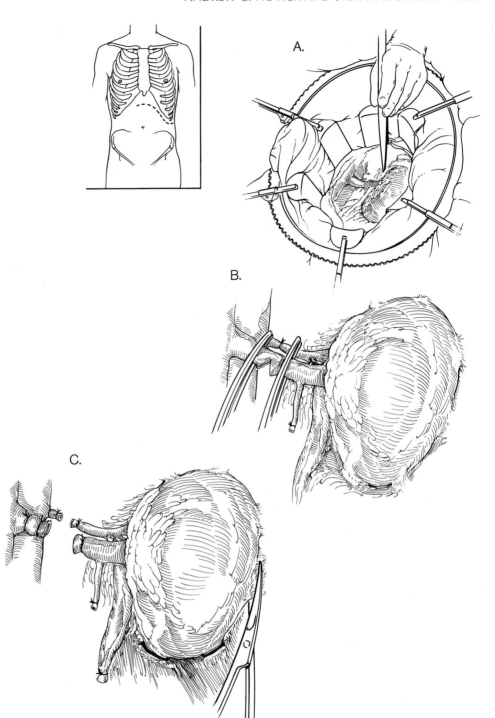

Figure 97–25. *A to C,* Technique of transperitoneal simple nephrectomy through an anterior subcostal incision.

and Novick, 1996). In planning the appropriate operative approach for tumor removal, it is essential for preoperative radiographic studies to define accurately the distal limits of a vena caval tumor thrombus.

Renal cell carcinoma involving the inferior vena cava should be suspected in patients who have lower extremity edema, a varicocele, dilated superficial abdominal veins, proteinuria, pulmonary embolism, a right atrial mass, or nonfunction of the involved kidney. Currently, magnetic resonance imaging is the preferred diagnostic study for demonstrating both the presence and the distal extent of inferior

vena caval involvement (Pritchett et al, 1987; Goldfarb et al, 1990). Transesophageal echocardiography (Fig. 97–26) (Treiger et al, 1991) and transabdominal color flow Doppler ultrasonography (McGahan et al, 1993) have also proven to be useful diagnostic studies in this regard. Inferior vena cavography is reserved for patients in whom a magnetic resonance imaging or ultrasound study is either nondiagnostic or contraindicated. Renal arteriography is particularly helpful in patients with renal cell carcinoma involving the inferior vena cava because in 35% to 40% of cases, distinct arterialization of a tumor thrombus is observed. When this

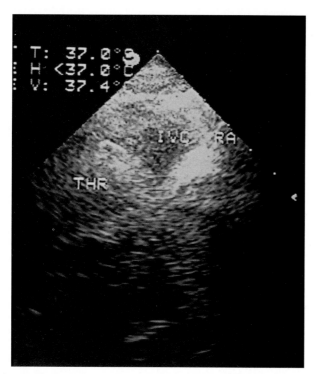

Figure 97–26. Transesophageal ultrasound demonstrating thrombus (THR) in intrahepatic inferior vena cava (IVC) proximal to the right atrium (RA).

finding is present, preoperative embolization of the kidney often causes shrinkage of the thrombus, which facilitates its intraoperative removal. When adjunctive cardiopulmonary bypass with deep hypothermic circulatory arrest is considered, coronary angiography is also performed preoperatively (Belis et al, 1989; Novick et al, 1990). If significant obstructing coronary lesions are found, these can be repaired simultaneously during cardiopulmonary bypass.

Standard Technique

Radical nephrectomy encompasses the basic principles of early ligation of the renal artery and vein, removal of the kidney outside Gerota's fascia, removal of the ipsilateral adrenal gland, and performance of a complete regional lymphadenectomy from the crus of the diaphragm to the aortic bifurcation (Robson et al, 1969). **Perhaps the most important aspect of radical nephrectomy is removal of the kidney outside Gerota's fascia because capsular invasion with perinephric fat involvement occurs in 25% of patients.** It has been shown that removal of the ipsilateral adrenal gland is not routinely necessary unless the malignancy either extensively involves the kidney or is located in the upper portion of the kidney (Sagalowsky et al, 1994). Although lymphadenectomy allows for more accurate pathologic staging, the therapeutic value remains controversial. Nevertheless, there may be a subset of patients with micrometastatic lymph node involvement that can benefit from performance of a lymphadenectomy (Giuliani et al, 1990). At the present time, the need for routine performance of a complete lymphadenectomy in all cases is unresolved, and

there remains a divergence of clinical practice among urologists with respect to this aspect of radical nephrectomy.

The surgical approach for radical nephrectomy is determined by the size and location of the tumor as well as the habitus of the patient. The operation is usually performed through a transperitoneal incision to allow abdominal exploration for metastatic disease and early access to the renal vessels with minimal manipulation of the tumor. **The authors prefer an extended subcostal or bilateral subcostal incision for most patients. A thoracoabdominal incision is used for patients with large upper pole tumors (Fig. 97–27). The authors occasionally employ an extraperitoneal flank incision to perform radical nephrectomy in elderly or poor risk patients with a small tumor.**

When performing radical nephrectomy through a subcostal transperitoneal incision, a thorough exploration for metastatic disease is performed after opening the abdominal cavity. On the left side, the colon is reflected medially to expose the great vessels. This is facilitated by division of the splenocolic ligaments, which also helps to avoid excessive traction and injury to the spleen. On the right side, the colon and duodenum are reflected medially to expose the vena cava and aorta (Fig. 97–28).

The operation is initiated with dissection of the renal pedicle. On the right side, the renal vein is short, and care must be taken not to injure the vena cava. The right renal artery may be mobilized either lateral to the vena cava or, with a large medial tumor, between the vena cava and the aorta (Fig. 97–29).

On the left side, the renal vein is quite long as it passes over the aorta. The vein is mobilized completely by ligating and dividing gonadal, adrenal, and lumbar tributaries. The vein can then be retracted to expose the artery posteriorly, which is then mobilized toward the aorta (Fig. 97–30). The renal artery is ligated with 2–0 silk ligatures and divided, and the renal vein is then similarly managed (Fig. 97–31).

The kidney is then mobilized outside Gerota's fascia with blunt and sharp dissection as needed. Remaining vascular attachments are secured with nonabsorbable sutures or metal

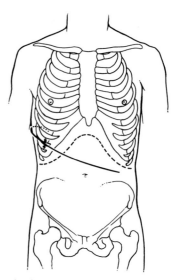

Figure 97–27. Radical nephrectomy is performed through either a bilateral subcostal or a thoracoabdominal incision.

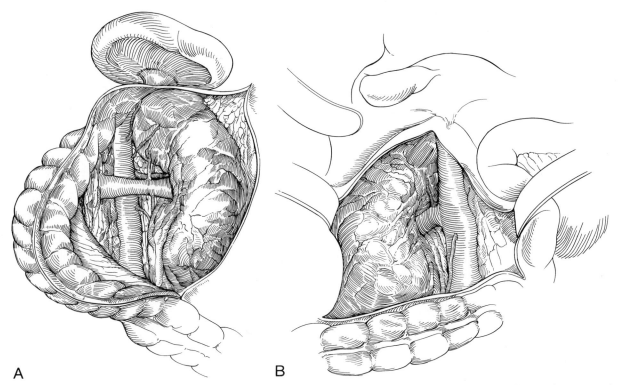

Figure 97–28. After entering the peritoneal cavity, the colon is reflected medially to expose the left *(A)* or right *(B)* kidney and great vessels. (From Novick AC, Streem SB, Pontes E, eds: Stewart's Operative Urology, 2nd ed. Baltimore, Williams & Wilkins, 1989.)

clips. The ureter is then ligated and divided to complete the removal of the kidney and adrenal gland (Fig. 97–32).

The classic description of radical nephrectomy includes the performance of a complete regional lymphadenectomy. The lymph nodes can be removed either en bloc with the kidney and adrenal gland or separately after the nephrec-

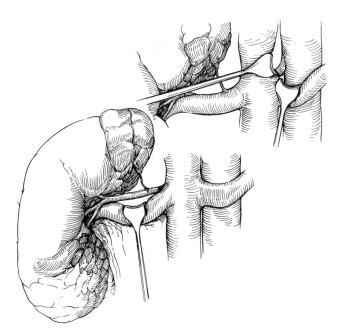

Figure 97–29. The right renal artery may be mobilized either lateral to the vena cava or between the vena cava and the aorta. (From Novick AC, Streem SB, Pontes E, eds: Stewart's Operative Urology, 2nd ed. Baltimore, Williams & Wilkins, 1989.)

tomy. The lymph node dissection is begun at the crura of the diaphragm just below the origin of the superior mesenteric artery. There is a readily definable periadventitial plane close to the aorta that can be entered so that the dissection may be carried along the aorta and onto the origin of the major vessels to remove all the periaortic lymphatic tissue. Care must be taken to avoid injury to the origins of the celiac and superior mesenteric arteries superiorly as they arise from the anterior surface of the aorta. The dissection of the periaortic and pericaval lymph nodes is then carried downward en bloc to the origin of the inferior mesenteric artery. The sympathetic ganglia and nerves are removed together with the lymphatic tissue. The cisterna chyli is identified medial to the right crus, and entering lymphatic vessels are secured to prevent the development of chylous ascites.

A thoracoabdominal incision is preferable when performing radical nephrectomy for a large upper pole tumor. This approach is demonstrated in Figures 97–32 through 97–34 for a right-sided tumor. Once the liver has been retracted upward into the chest, the hepatic flexure of the colon and the duodenum are reflected medially to expose the anterior surface of the kidney and great vessels (Fig. 97–33). The renal artery is secured with 2–0 silk ligatures and divided, and the renal vein is then similarly managed (Fig. 97–34). The ureter and right gonadal vein are ligated and divided, and the kidney is mobilized outside Gerota's fascia. Downward and lateral traction of the kidney exposes the superior vascular attachments of the tumor and adrenal gland. Exposure of these vessels is also facilitated by medial retraction of the inferior vena cava (Fig. 97–35). Care is taken to preserve small hepatic venous branches entering the vena cava at the superior margin of the tumor mass. The

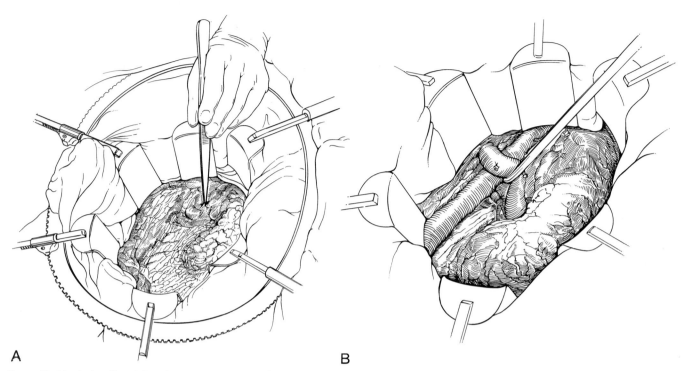

A   B

Figure 97–30. *A,* A self-retaining ring retractor is inserted to maintain exposure. *B,* The left renal vein is mobilized by ligating its major branches to expose the artery posteriorly. (From Novick AC, Streem SB, Pontes E, eds: Stewart's Operative Urology, 2nd ed. Baltimore, Williams & Wilkins, 1989.)

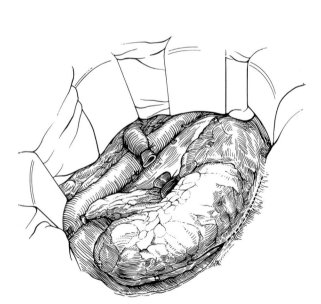

Figure 97–31. After the pedicle is secured and the ureter divided, the kidney is mobilized outside Gerota's fascia. (From Novick AC, Streem SB, Pontes E, eds: Stewart's Operative Urology, 2nd ed. Baltimore, Williams & Wilkins, 1989.)

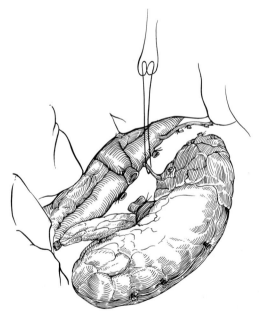

Figure 97–32. Remaining medial vascular attachments are secured and divided to complete the nephrectomy. (From Novick AC, Streem SB, Pontes E, eds: Stewart's Operative Urology, 2nd ed. Baltimore, Williams & Wilkins, 1989.)

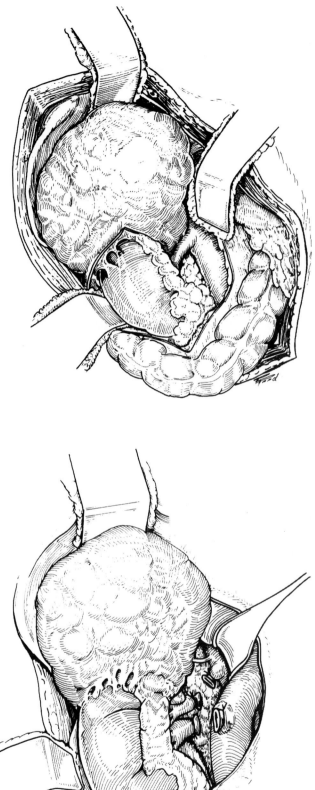

Figure 97–33. Exposure of a large right upper pole tumor through a thoracoabdominal incision. (From Novick AC, Streem SB, Pontes E, eds: Stewart's Operative Urology, 2nd ed. Baltimore, Williams & Wilkins, 1989.)

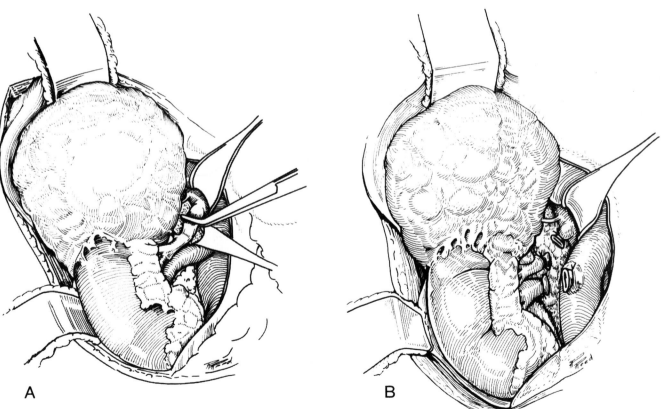

A

B

Figure 97–34. *A* and *B,* The renal artery and vein are secured and divided. (From Novick AC, Streem SB, Pontes E, eds: Stewart's Operative Urology, 2nd ed. Baltimore, Williams & Wilkins, 1989.)

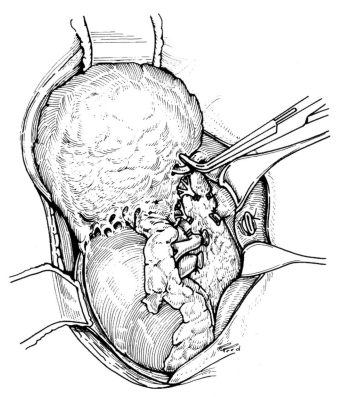

Figure 97–35. The vena cava is retracted medially to expose remaining superior vascular attachments, which are secured and divided. (From Novick AC, Streem SB, Pontes E, eds: Stewart's Operative Urology, 2nd ed. Baltimore, Williams & Wilkins, 1989.)

tumor mass is then gently separated from the undersurface of the liver to complete the resection.

Management of Retroperitoneal Hemorrhage

During performance of radical nephrectomy, intraoperative hemorrhage can occur from the inferior vena cava or its tributaries. The urologist should be familiar with methods of preventing or controlling this problem. In most cases, vena caval hemorrhage is caused by the laceration or avulsion of large yet fragile veins entering the vena cava at predictable locations.

Lumbar veins enter the posterolateral aspect of the vena cava at each vertebral level, and undue traction on the cava can result in their avulsion with troublesome bleeding. To prevent this, care should be taken to retract the vena cava gently with curved vein retractors during its dissection; if additional mobilization is necessary, these veins should be dissected free from surrounding structures, ligated, and divided. In ligating venous tributaries entering the vena cava, 3–0 to 4–0 suture material should be used, and the ligatures should not be tied too tightly because this can cause shearing through the fragile venous wall with further hemorrhage. After the ligature has been applied, it should not be pulled too tightly before the ends of the ligature are cut, again for fear of avulsing the entrance of the vein into the vena cava.

A second predictable bleeding site is the entry of the right gonadal vein into the anterolateral surface of the vena cava. This is an extremely thin-walled vein, and excessive traction or mobilization of the cava at this level can lead to its avulsion, with resulting hemorrhage.

A third predictable site of bleeding lies at the level of the renal veins, where large lumbar veins often course posteriorly from the left renal vein just lateral to the aorta or from the posterior aspect of the vena cava close to the entry of the right renal vein. Injudicious mobilization of the renal veins, without consideration of these fragile and often large-caliber veins, can result in severe hemorrhage that may be difficult to control.

A fourth predictable site of bleeding is at the level of the right adrenal vein, which enters the inferior vena cava. This vein is large and friable, frequently lies higher than the surgeon expects, and must be carefully dissected free from surrounding structures to avoid avulsion from the vena cava.

Finally, excessive vena caval hemorrhage can be prevented by careful dissection in proper tissue planes along the vena cava. This may be difficult when tumor involves the vena cava, but usually a plane can be established along the vena caval wall that, if followed, allows safe, relatively bloodless exposure. One should follow the general principle of isolating a relatively normal area of vena cava and working upward or downward from that level to expose the diseased portion.

If inadvertent vena caval lacerations or avulsion of entering veins occurs, control of hemorrhage can be accomplished by a variety of techniques. Direct pressure on the site of bleeding gives immediate control until additional exposure can be gained, the field properly illuminated, and additional suckers or retractors brought in if necessary. If the laceration involves the anterior or lateral caval wall and is of considerable length, it can be readily controlled by applying a series of Allis clamps over the edges of the laceration in serial fashion. The edges of the laceration are then oversewn with running 5–0 vascular suture material (Fig. 97–36).

If avulsion of an entering lumbar vein is the cause of bleeding, the vena cava should be rolled medially, with digital compression above and below the site of bleeding, until the posterolateral entry of the avulsed vein is exposed. This is then grasped with one or two Allis clamps, which can be used as tractors to bring the avulsion into better view for oversewing with vascular suture material. Persistent bleeding can occur from the proximal end of an avulsed lumbar vein, which may retract into the psoas muscle and be difficult to secure. This can be controlled in some cases by grasping the end of the vein with a hemostat, then twisting the hemostat to bring the end of the vein into better view for suture ligation (Fig. 97–37). If this is not possible, bleeding can be controlled by inserting a figure-of-eight 2–0 silk suture through the muscle overlying the vein.

Bleeding from large lumbar veins entering the posterior aspect of the left renal vein or the posterior wall of the vena cava near the entry of the right renal vein can be particularly troublesome (Fig. 97–38). Further mobilization of the vena cava and renal veins is often needed while compression is maintained on the bleeding site. It may be necessary to apply a Satinsky side clamp across the entry of the renal vein as well as a distal bulldog clamp beyond the bleeding point in the renal vein to control the hemorrhage and allow closure

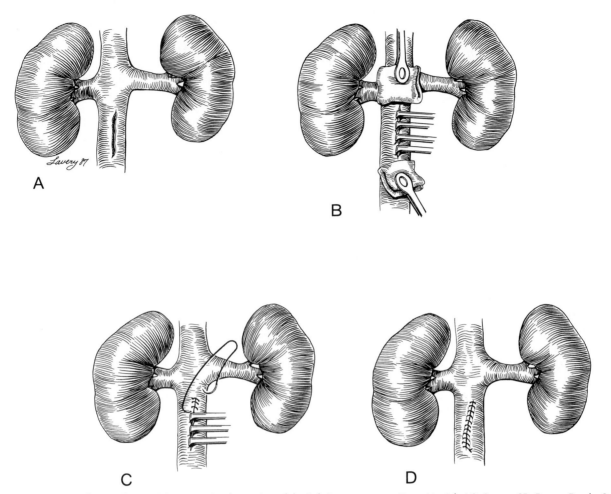

Figure 97–36. *A* to *D*, Technique for repairing extensive laceration of the inferior vena cava. (From Novick AC, Streem SB, Pontes E, eds: Stewart's Operative Urology, 2nd ed. Baltimore, Williams & Wilkins, 1989.)

of the venous defect. Mobilization and gentle rotation of the vena cava or renal veins may also be necessary to gain optimal exposure. In this situation as well, the distal entry of the lumbar vein into the posterior musculature can cause

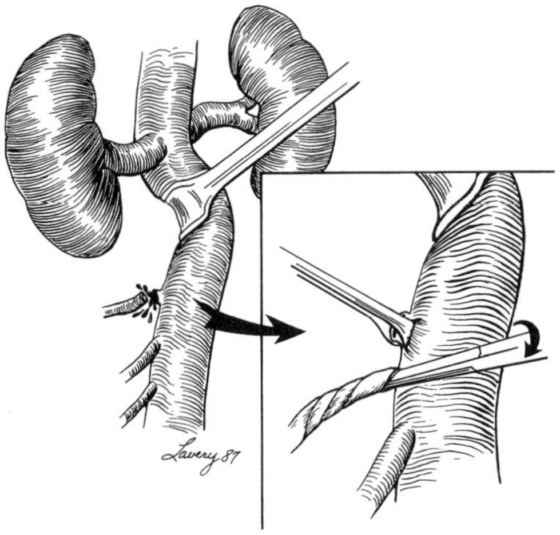

Figure 97–37. Technique for securing ends of the lumbar vein avulsed from the inferior vena cava. (From Novick AC, Streem SB, Pontes E, eds: Stewart's Operative Urology, 2nd ed. Baltimore, Williams & Wilkins, 1989.)

troublesome bleeding and must be controlled as described previously.

Radical Nephrectomy with Infrahepatic Vena Caval Involvement

There are four levels of vena caval involvement in renal cell carcinoma that are characterized according to the distal extent of the tumor thrombus (Fig. 97–39). **A bilateral subcostal transperitoneal incision usually provides excellent exposure for performing radical nephrectomy and removal of a perirenal or infrahepatic inferior vena caval thrombus. For extremely large tumors involving the upper pole of the kidney, a thoracoabdominal incision may alternatively be used.** After the abdomen is entered, the colon is reflected medially, and a self-retaining ring retractor is inserted to maintain exposure of the retroperitoneum (Fig. 97–40A). The renal artery and the ureter are ligated and divided, and the entire kidney is mobilized outside Gerota's fascia leaving the kidney attached only by the renal vein (Fig. 97–40B and C). During the initial dissection, care is taken to avoid unnecessary manipulation of the renal vein and vena cava.

The vena cava is then completely dissected from sur-

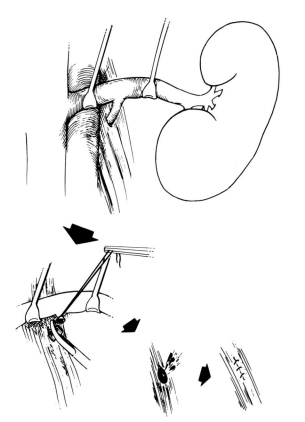

Figure 97–38. Technique for securing ends of the lumbar vein avulsed from the left renal vein. (From Novick AC, Streem SB, Pontes E, eds: Stewart's Operative Urology, 2nd ed. Baltimore, Williams & Wilkins, 1989.)

rounding structures above and below the renal vein, and the opposite renal vein is also mobilized. It is essential to obtain exposure and control of the suprarenal vena cava above the level of the tumor thrombus. If necessary, perforating veins to the caudate lobe of the liver are secured and divided to allow separation of the caudate lobe from the vena cava. This maneuver can allow an additional 2- to 3-cm length of vena cava to be exposed superiorly. The infrarenal vena cava is then occluded below the thrombus with a Satinsky venous clamp, and the opposite renal vein is gently secured with a small bulldog vascular clamp. Finally, in preparation for tumor thrombectomy, a curved Satinsky clamp is placed around the suprarenal vena cava above the level of the thrombus (Fig. 90–40D).

The anterior surface of the renal vein is then incised over the tumor thrombus, and the incision is continued posteriorly with scissors, passing just beneath the thrombus (Fig. 97–40E). In most cases, there is no attachment of the thrombus to the wall of the vena cava. After the renal vein has been circumscribed, gentle downward traction is exerted on the kidney to extract the tumor thrombus from the vena cava (Fig. 97–40F). After removal of the gross specimen, the suprarenal vena caval clamp may be released temporarily as the anesthetist applies positive pulmonary pressure; this maneuver can ensure that any small remaining fragments of thrombus are flushed free from the vena cava. When the tumor thrombectomy is completed, the cavotomy incision is repaired with a continuous 5–0 vascular suture (Fig. 97–40G).

In occasional cases, there is direct caval invasion of the tumor at the level of the entrance of the renal vein and for varying distances. This requires resection of a portion of the vena caval wall. Narrowing of the caval lumen by up to 50% does not adversely affect maintenance of caval patency. If further narrowing appears likely, caval reconstruction can be performed with a free graft of pericardium.

In some patients, more extensive direct growth of tumor into the wall of the vena cava is found at surgery. The prognosis for these patients is generally poor, particularly when hepatic venous tributaries are also involved, and the decision to proceed with radical surgical excision must be carefully considered. Several important principles must be kept in mind when undertaking en bloc vena caval resection. Resection of the infrarenal portion of the vena cava usually can be done safely because an extensive collateral venous supply has developed in most cases. With right-sided kidney tumors, resection of the suprarenal vena cava is also possible, provided that the left renal vein is ligated distal to the gonadal and adrenal tributaries, which then provide collateral venous drainage from the left kidney. With left-sided kidney tumors, the suprarenal vena cava cannot be resected safely owing to the paucity of collateral venous drainage from the right kidney. In such cases, right renal venous drainage can be maintained by preserving a tumor-free strip of vena cava (Fig. 97–41) augmented, if necessary, with a pericardial patch; alternatively the right kidney can be autotransplanted to the pelvis, or an interposition graft of saphenous vein may be placed from the right renal vein to the splenic, inferior mesenteric, or portal vein.

Radical Nephrectomy with Intrahepatic or Suprahepatic Vena Caval Involvement

In patients with renal cell carcinoma and an intrahepatic or suprahepatic inferior vena caval thrombus, the difficulty of surgical excision is significantly increased. In such cases, the operative technique must be modified because it is not possible to obtain subdiaphragmatic control of the vena cava above the tumor thrombus. Several different surgical maneuvers have been used to provide adequate exposure, prevent severe bleeding, and achieve complete tumor removal in this setting (Cummings et al, 1979; Novick, 1980; Foster et al, 1988; Skinner et al, 1989; Burt, 1991).

One described technique for obtaining vascular control involves temporary occlusion of the suprahepatic intraperi-cardial portion of the inferior vena cava. To reduce hepatic venous congestion and troublesome backbleeding, the porta hepatis and superior mesenteric artery are also temporarily occluded (Skinner et al, 1989). A disadvantage of this approach is that occlusion of the latter vessels can be safely tolerated for only 20 minutes. This approach is also not applicable in cases of tumor extension into the right atrium. **At the Cleveland Clinic, the authors have preferred to employ cardiopulmonary bypass with deep hypothermic circulatory arrest for most patients with supradiaphragmatic tumor thrombi and for all patients with right atrial tumor thrombi** (Marshall and Reitz, 1986). The authors initially reported a favorable experience with this approach in 43 patients (Novick et al, 1990), and a subsequent study

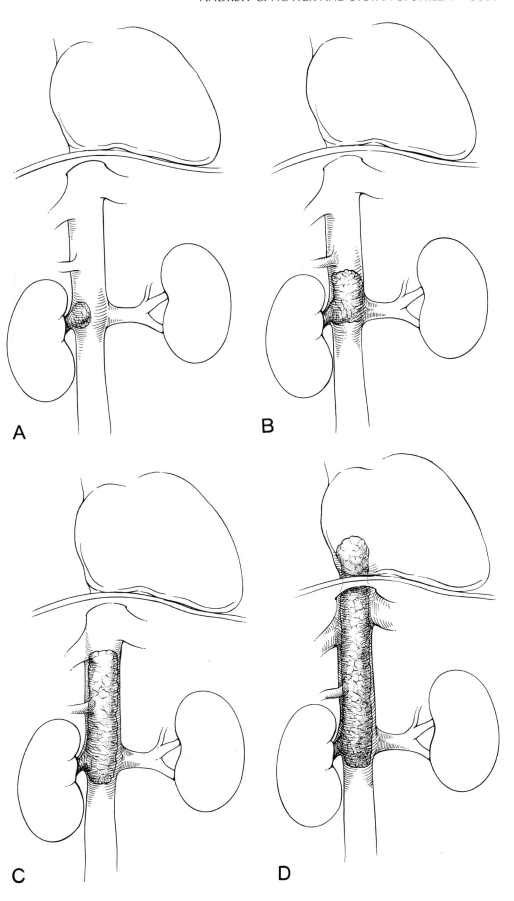

Figure 97–39. Classification of inferior vena caval tumor thrombus from renal cell carcinoma, according to the distal extent of the thrombus, as *(A)* perirenal, *(B)* infrahepatic, *(C)* intrahepatic, and *(D)* suprahepatic. (From Novick AC, Streem SB, Pontes E, eds: Stewart's Operative Urology, 2nd ed. Baltimore, Williams & Wilkins, 1989.)

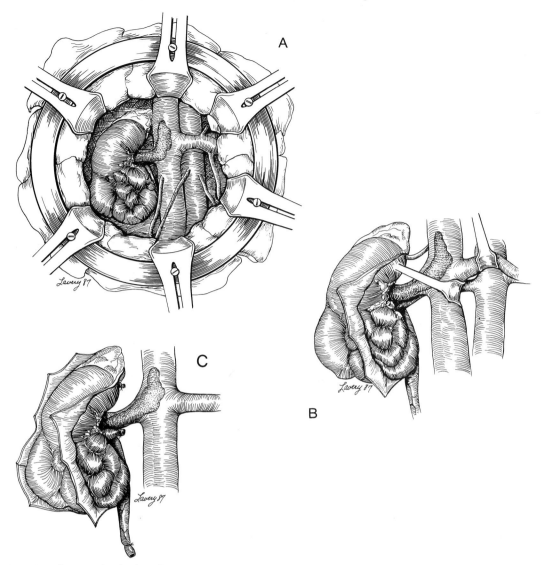

Figure 97–40. *A* to *G*, Technique of radical nephrectomy and vena caval tumor thrombectomy with infrahepatic tumor thrombus. (From Novick AC, Streem SB, Pontes E, eds: Stewart's Operative Urology, 2nd ed. Baltimore, Williams & Wilkins, 1989.)

has shown excellent long-term cancer-free survival after its use in patients with right atrial thrombi (Glazer and Novick, 1996). The relevant technical aspects are subsequently described.

A bilateral subcostal incision is used for the abdominal portion of the operation. After confirming resectability, a median sternotomy is made (Fig. 97–42). Intraoperative monitoring is accomplished with an arterial line, a multiple-lumen central venous pressure catheter, transesophageal ultrasound, and a pulmonary artery catheter. Nasopharyngeal and bladder temperatures are monitored. Anesthesia is induced with fentanyl, sufentanil, or thiopental and maintained with a narcotic inhalation agent (Welch et al, 1989).

The kidney is completely mobilized outside Gerota's fascia with division of the renal artery and ureter, such that the kidney is left attached only by the renal vein. The infrarenal vena cava and contralateral renal vein are also exposed. Extensive dissection and mobilization of the suprarenal vena cava are not necessary with this approach. Adequate exposure is somewhat more difficult to achieve for a left renal tumor. Simultaneous exposure of the vena cava on the right and the tumor on the left is not readily accomplished simply by reflecting the left colon medially. The authors have dealt with this by transposing the mobilized left kidney anteriorly through a window in the mesentery of the left colon, while leaving the renal vein attached. This maneuver yields excellent exposure of the abdominal vena cava with the attached left renal vein and kidney. Precise retroperitoneal hemostasis is essential before proceeding with cardiopulmonary bypass because of the risk of bleeding associated with systemic heparinization.

The heart and great vessels are now exposed through the median sternotomy. The patient is heparinized, ascending aortic and right atrial venous cannulas are placed, and cardiopulmonary bypass is initiated (Fig. 97–43). When the heart fibrillates, the aorta is clamped, and crystalloid cardioplegic solution is infused. Under circulatory arrest, deep hypothermia is initiated by reducing arterial inflow blood temperature as low as 10°C. The head and abdomen are packed in ice during the cooling process. After approximately 15 to 30

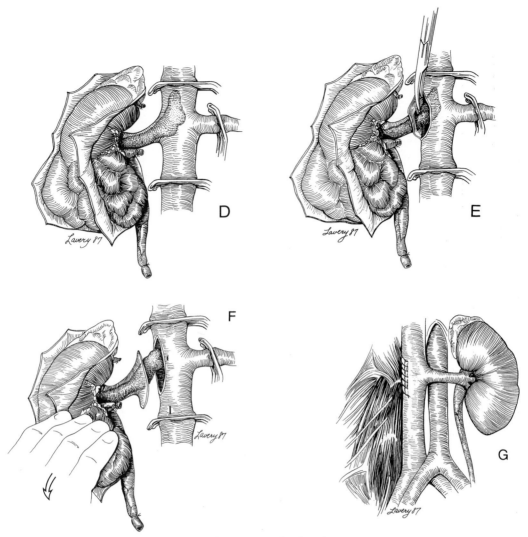

Figure 97–40 *Continued*

minutes, a core temperature of 18 to 20°C is achieved. At this point, flow through the perfusion machine is stopped, and 95% of the blood volume is drained into the pump with no flow to any organ.

The tumor thrombus can now be removed in an essentially bloodless operative field. An incision is made in the inferior vena cava at the entrance of the involved renal vein, and the ostium is circumscribed. When the tumor extends into the

right atrium, the atrium is opened at the same time (Fig. 97–44A). If possible, the tumor thrombus is removed intact with the kidney. Frequently, this step is not possible because of the friability of the thrombus and its adherence to the vena caval wall. In such cases, piecemeal removal of the thrombus from above and below is necessary. Occasionally a venous Fogarty catheter can be inserted into the vena cava to assist in extraction of the thrombus. Under deep

Figure 97–41. With vena caval resection, right renal venous drainage can be maintained by preserving a tumor-free strip of vena cava. (From Novick AC, Streem SB, Pontes E, eds: Stewart's Operative Urology, 2nd ed. Baltimore, Williams & Wilkins, 1989.)

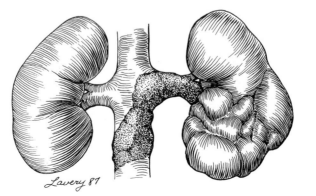
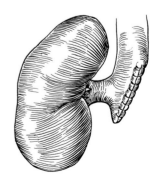

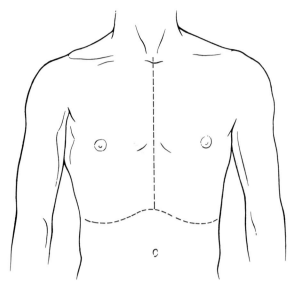

Figure 97–42. Surgical incision for performing radical nephrectomy with removal of a suprahepatic vena caval tumor thrombus. (From Novick AC, Streem SB, Pontes E, eds: Stewart's Operative Urology, 2nd ed. Baltimore, Williams & Wilkins, 1989.)

hypothermic circulatory arrest, the entire interior lumen of the vena cava can be directly inspected to ensure that all fragments of thrombus are completely removed. **Hypothermic circulatory arrest can be safely maintained for at least 40 minutes without incurring a cerebral ischemic event** (Svensson et al, 1993). In difficult cases, this interval can be extended either by maintaining "trickle" blood flow at a rate of 5 to 10 ml/kg/minute (Mault et al, 1993) or by adjunctive retrograde cerebral perfusion (Pagano et al, 1995).

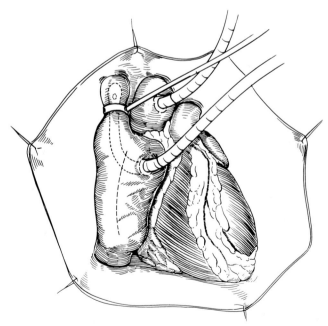

Figure 97–43. Cannulas are placed in the ascending aorta and right atrium in preparation for cardiopulmonary bypass. The planned incision into the right atrium is shown. (From Novick AC, Streem SB, Pontes E, eds: Stewart's Operative Urology, 2nd ed. Baltimore, Williams & Wilkins, 1989.)

After complete removal of all tumor thrombus, the vena cava is closed with a continuous 5–0 vascular suture, and the right atrium is closed (Fig. 97–44*B*). As soon as the vena cava and right atrium have been repaired, rewarming of the patient is initiated. If coronary artery bypass grafting is necessary, this procedure is done during the rewarming period. Rewarming takes 20 to 45 minutes and is continued until a core temperature of approximately 37°C is obtained. Cardiopulmonary bypass is then terminated. Decannulation takes place, and protamine sulfate is administered to reverse the effects of the heparin. Platelets, fresh frozen plasma, desmopressin acetate, or their combination may be provided when coagulopathy is suspected (Harker, 1986). Aprotinin has also proven effective in reversing the coagulopathy associated with cardiopulmonary bypass (Bidstrup et al, 1989) but may induce thrombotic complications. Mediastinal chest tubes are placed, but the abdomen is not routinely drained.

In patients with supradiaphragmatic vena caval tumor thrombi that do not extend into the right atrium, venovenous bypass in the form of a caval-atrial shunt may be employed (Foster et al, 1988; Burt, 1991). In this approach, the intrapericardiac vena cava, infrarenal vena cava, and opposite renal vein are temporarily occluded. Cannulas are then inserted into the right atrium and infrarenal vena cava. These cannulas are connected to a primed pump to maintain adequate flow from the vena cava to the right side of the heart (Fig. 97–45). This avoids the obligatory hypotension associated with temporary occlusion alone of the intrapericardiac and infrarenal vena cava. Following the initiation of venovenous bypass, the abdominal vena cava is opened, and the thrombus is removed. If bleeding from the hepatic veins is troublesome during extraction of the thrombus, the porta hepatis may also be occluded (Pringle's maneuver). After removal of the thrombus, repair of the vena cava is performed as previously described. This technique is simpler than cardiopulmonary bypass with hypothermic circulatory arrest but may entail more operative bleeding.

Complications

After radical nephrectomy, postoperative complications occur in approximately 20% of patients, and the operative mortality rate is approximately 2% (Swanson and Borges, 1983). Systemic complications may occur as after any surgical procedure. These include myocardial infarction, cerebrovascular accident, congestive heart failure, pulmonary embolism, atelectasis, pneumonia, and thrombophlebitis. The incidence of these problems can be reduced by adequate preoperative preparation, avoidance of intraoperative hypotension, appropriate blood and fluid replacement, postoperative breathing exercises, early mobilization, and elastic support of the legs both during and after surgery.

An intraoperative gastrointestinal injury should always be checked for during the procedure, and lacerations should be repaired and drained. Tears of the livers may be repaired with mattress sutures. Splenic injuries usually require splenectomy, although small lacerations may be managed by application of Avitene or Oxycel. Injuries to the tail of the pancreas, which may occur with left radical nephrectomy, are best managed by partial amputation.

A particularly distressing postoperative complication is

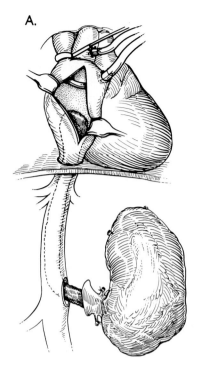

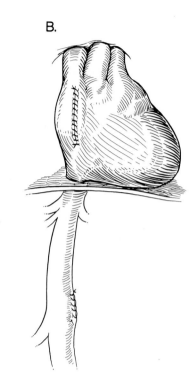

Figure 97–44. *A,* The ostium of the renal vein is circumferentially incised, and the right atrium is opened. *B,* Following removal of the tumor thrombus, the atriotomy and vena cavotomy incisions are closed.

the development of a pancreatic fistula because of unrecognized intraoperative injury to the pancreas. This is usually manifested in the immediate postoperative period with signs and symptoms of acute pancreatitis and drainage of alkaline fluid from the incision. A computed tomography scan of the abdomen demonstrates a fluid collection in the retroperitoneum. Fluid draining from the incision should be analyzed for pH and the presence of amylase. Treatment involves percutaneous or surgical drainage of the fluid collection to avoid the development of a pancreatic pseudocyst or abscess (Zinner et al, 1974; Spirnak et al, 1984). The majority of fistulas close spontaneously with the establishment of adequate drainage. Because the healing of a pancreatic fistula is usually a slow process, the patient is also supported with hyperalimentation. Surgical closure by excising the fistulous tract and creating an anastomosis between the pancreas and a Roux-en-Y limb of the jejunum is only occasionally necessary in patients with prolonged drainage.

Other gastrointestinal problems that may occur include a generalized ileus or a functional obstruction caused by a localized ileus of the colon overlying the operated renal fossa. Oral feedings should not be given until adequate bowel sounds are present and the patient has passed flatus. Nasogastric suction is used in more severe cases. When a prolonged period of ileus is anticipated or if the patient is in a poor nutritional state, parenteral hyperalimentation should be instituted.

Secondary hemorrhage may occur after radical nephrectomy and is manifested by pain, signs of shock, abdominal or flank swelling, and drainage of blood through the incision or a drain site. Bleeding may be from the kidney or renal pedicle but is occasionally from an unrecognized injury to a neighboring structure, such as the spleen, liver, or a mesenteric vessel. Patients should be given blood and fluid replacement as needed. In most cases, it is best to reopen the wound, evacuate the hematoma, and secure the bleeding point. In the event of diffuse bleeding from a clotting disorder, it may be necessary to pack the wound temporarily with gauze, which can then be gradually removed after 24 to 48 hours.

Pneumothorax may occur during thoracoabdominal or flank incisions. Pleural injuries are usually recognized immediately and repaired with a running 3–0 or 4–0 chromic suture. Before complete closure of the incision, a red rubber catheter is inserted into the pleural cavity and a purse-string suture is tied around the catheter. The anesthesiologist is then asked to hyperinflate the lungs. With hyperinflation and suction on the catheter, air and fluid in the hemithorax are forced out through the red rubber catheter, which is then removed, and the purse-string suture is secured. An alternative method is to place the distal end of the catheter in a basin of water. As the anesthesiologist hyperinflates the lung, air and fluid are forced out of the pleural cavity through the red rubber catheter and into the basin of water. When the pleura is entered, a chest film should be obtained in the recovery room to ensure adequate re-expansion of the lung. A pneumothorax greater than 10%, tension pneumothorax, or one that is causing respiratory distress requires insertion of a chest tube.

Postoperative atelectasis is common in patients undergo-

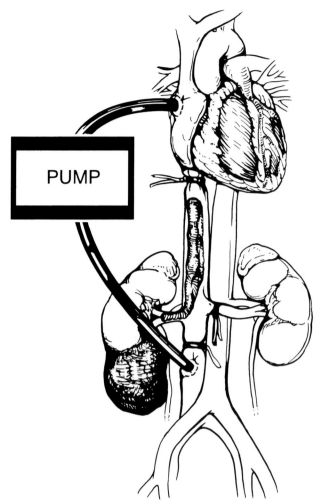

Figure 97–45. Technique of veno-venous bypass for removal of supradiaphragmatic vena caval tumor thrombus.

ing radical nephrectomy and is probably secondary to the positioning of the patient during the procedure. This is a common cause of fever postoperatively and may be effectively treated with pulmonary physiotherapy, including deep breathing, coughing, and incentive spirometry.

Infection is a common complication encountered in the postoperative period. Superficial wound infections are best managed by removal of skin sutures or staples to allow for drainage. Deeper infections must be treated by the establishment of adequate drainage and the administration of appropriate antibiotics when there are systemic manifestations of the infection. If the drainage is persistent and profuse, the possibility of a retained foreign body or a fistulous communication with the intestine should be considered. Accumulations of lymph or serous fluid in the renal fossa or pleura are best managed expectantly unless they are causing respiratory embarrassment. Such accumulations may become infected or may be complicated by bleeding if treated by needle aspiration.

Temporary renal insufficiency may develop postoperatively after ligation of the left renal vein in conjunction with right radical nephrectomy and extraction of a vena caval tumor thrombus (Clark, 1961; Pathak, 1971). Renal failure in this setting is probably secondary to venous obstruction and usually resolves as drainage improves with the development of venous collaterals, although temporary hemodialysis may occasionally be needed. It is always preferable, if possible, to preserve left renal venous drainage into the vena cava to diminish the risk of this complication. As previously mentioned, ligation of the right renal vein leads to permanent, complete renal failure.

When a flank incision is used to perform nephrectomy, an incisional hernia or bulge may occur postoperatively. The intracostal nerve lies immediately below the corresponding rib between the internal oblique and the transverse abdominal muscle. At surgery, an effort should be made to spare this nerve by dissecting both proximally and distally, enabling careful padding and retraction of the nerve out of the operative field, because transection may lead to muscle denervation. Postoperatively, muscle denervation with flank bulging must be differentiated from a flank incisional hernia, which is rare. In the latter, a fascial defect is usually palpable.

PARTIAL NEPHRECTOMY FOR MALIGNANCY

Interest in partial nephrectomy or nephron-sparing surgery for renal cell carcinoma has been stimulated by advances in renal imaging, improved surgical techniques, the increasing number of incidentally discovered low-stage renal cell carcinomas, and good long-term survival in patients undergoing this form of treatment. Partial nephrectomy entails complete local resection of a renal tumor while leaving the largest possible amount of normal functioning parenchyma in the involved kidney.

Accepted indications for partial nephrectomy include situations in which radical nephrectomy would render the patient anephric with subsequent immediate need for dialysis. This encompasses patients with bilateral renal cell carcinoma or renal cell carcinoma involving a solitary functioning kidney. The latter circumstance may be present because of unilateral renal agenesis, prior removal of the contralateral kidney, or irreversible impairment of contralateral renal function from a benign disorder. Another indication for partial nephrectomy is represented by patients with unilateral renal cell carcinoma and a functioning opposite kidney, when the opposite kidney is affected by a condition that might threaten its future function, such as calculus disease, chronic pyelonephritis, renal artery stenosis, ureteral reflux, or systemic diseases such as diabetes and nephrosclerosis (Licht and Novick, 1993).

Studies have clarified the role of partial nephrectomy in patients with localized unilateral renal cell carcinoma and a normal contralateral kidney. **These data indicate that radical nephrectomy and partial nephrectomy provide equally effective curative treatment for such patients who present with a single, small (<4 cm), and clearly localized renal cell carcinoma** (Butler et al, 1995). The results of partial nephrectomy are less satisfactory in patients with larger (>4 cm) or multiple localized renal cell carcinomas, and radical nephrectomy remains the treatment of choice in such cases when the opposite kidney is normal. The long-term renal functional advantage of partial nephrectomy with a normal opposite kidney requires further study. Partial nephrectomy is also occasionally indicated in the management of patients with renal pelvic transitional cell carcinoma or Wilms' tumor when preservation of functioning renal parenchyma is a clinically relevant consideration (Zincke and Neves, 1984; Ziegelbaum et al, 1987).

The technical success rate with partial nephrectomy for renal cell carcinoma is excellent, and several large studies have reported 5-year cancer-specific survival rates of 87% to 90% in such patients (Morgan and Zincke, 1990; Steinbach et al, 1992; Licht et al, 1994). These survival rates are comparable to those obtained after radical nephrectomy, particularly for low-stage renal cell carcinoma. The major disadvantage of partial nephrectomy for renal cell carcinoma is the risk of postoperative local tumor recurrence in the operated kidney, which has been observed in 4% to 6% of patients (Morgan and Zincke, 1990; Steinbach et al, 1992; Licht et al, 1994). These local recurrences are most likely a manifestation of undetected microscopic multifocal renal cell carcinoma in the renal remnant. The risk of local tumor recurrence after radical nephrectomy has not been studied, but it is presumably low.

Evaluation of patients with renal cell carcinoma for partial nephrectomy should include preoperative testing to rule out locally extensive or metastatic disease. For most patients, preoperative renal arteriography to delineate the intrarenal vasculature aids in excising the tumor with minimal blood loss and damage to adjacent normal parenchyma. This test can be deferred in patients with small peripheral tumors. **Selective renal venography is performed in patients with large or centrally located tumors to evaluate for intrarenal venous thrombosis secondary to malignancy** (Angermeier et al, 1990). The latter, if present, implies a more advanced local tumor stage and increases the technical complexity of tumor excision. Preoperative hydration and mannitol administration are important adjuncts to ensure optimal renal perfusion at operation.

In patients with bilateral synchronous renal cell carcinoma, the kidney most amenable to a partial nephrectomy is usually approached first by the authors. Then, approximately 1 month after a technically successful result has been documented, radical nephrectomy or a second partial nephrectomy is performed on the opposite kidney. Staging surgery in this fashion obviates the need for temporary dialysis if ischemic renal failure occurs after nephron-sparing excision of renal cell carcinoma.

It is usually possible to perform partial nephrectomy for malignancy in situ by using an operative approach that optimizes exposure of the kidney and by combining meticulous surgical technique with an understanding of the renal vascular anatomy in relation to the tumor. The authors employ an extraperitoneal flank incision through the bed of the 11th or 12th rib for almost all of these operations; the authors occasionally use a thoracoabdominal incision for large tumors involving the upper portion of the kidney. These incisions allow the surgeon to operate on the mobilized kidney almost at skin level and provide excellent exposure of the peripheral renal vessels. With an anterior subcostal transperitoneal incision, the kidney is invariably located in the depth of the wound, and the surgical exposure is simply not as good.

With in situ partial nephrectomy for malignancy, the kidney is mobilized within Gerota's fascia while leaving intact the perirenal fat around the tumor. For small peripheral renal tumors, it may not be necessary to control the renal artery. In most cases, however, partial nephrectomy is most effectively performed after temporary renal arterial occlusion. This measure not only limits intraoperative bleeding but, by reducing renal tissue turgor, also improves access to intrarenal structures. In most cases, the authors believe that it is important to leave the renal vein patent throughout the operation. This measure decreases intraoperative renal ischemia and, by allowing venous backbleeding, facilitates hemostasis by enabling identification of small transected renal veins. In patients with centrally located tumors, it is helpful to occlude the renal vein temporarily to minimize intraoperative bleeding from transected major venous branches.

When the renal circulation is temporarily interrupted, in situ renal hypothermia is used to protect against postischemic renal injury. Surface cooling of the kidney with ice slush allows up to 3 hours of safe ischemia without permanent renal injury. An important caveat with this method is to keep the entire kidney covered with ice slush for 10 to 15 minutes immediately after occluding the renal artery and before commencing the partial nephrectomy. This amount of time is needed to obtain core renal cooling to a temperature (approximately 20°C) that optimizes in situ renal preservation. During excision of the tumor, invariably large portions of the kidney are no longer covered with ice slush, and, in the absence of adequate prior renal cooling, rapid rewarming and ischemic renal injury can occur. Cooling by perfusion of the kidney with a cold solution instilled via the renal artery is not recommended because of the theoretical risk of tumor dissemination. Mannitol is given intravenously 5 to 10 minutes before temporary renal arterial occlusion. Systemic or regional anticoagulation to prevent intrarenal vascular thrombosis is not necessary.

A variety of surgical techniques are available for performing partial nephrectomy in patients with malignancy (Novick, 1987). These include simple enucleation, polar segmental nephrectomy with preliminary ligation of the appropriate renal arterial branch, wedge resection, major transverse resection, and extracorporeal partial nephrectomy with renal autotransplantation. All of these techniques require adherence to basic principles of early vascular control; avoidance of ischemic renal damage; complete tumor excision with free margins; precise closure of the collecting system; careful hemostasis; and closure or coverage of the renal defect with adjacent fat, fascia, peritoneum, or Oxycel. Whichever technique is employed, the tumor is removed with at least a 1-cm surrounding margin of grossly normal renal parenchyma. Intraoperative ultrasound is helpful in achieving accurate tumor localization, particularly for intrarenal lesions that are not visible or palpable from the external surface of the kidney (Fig. 97–46) (Assimos et al, 1991a; Campbell et al, 1995). The argon beam coagulator is a useful adjunct for achieving hemostasis on the transected renal surface (Hernandez et al, 1990). **If possible, the renal defect created by the excision is closed as an additional hemostatic measure.** A retroperitoneal drain is always left in place for at least 7 days. An intraoperative ureteral stent is placed only when major reconstruction of the intrarenal collecting system has been performed.

In patients with renal cell carcinoma or transitional cell

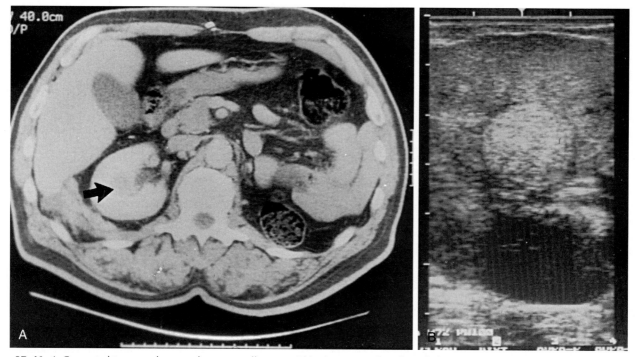

Figure 97–46. *A*, Computed tomography scan shows a small tumor within the center of a solitary kidney. *B*, Intraoperative ultrasound demonstrating localization of this intrarenal tumor.

carcinoma, partial nephrectomy is contraindicated in the presence of lymph node metastasis because the prognosis for these patients is poor. Biopsy specimens of enlarged or suspicious-looking lymph nodes should be obtained before initiating the renal resection. When partial nephrectomy is performed, after excision of all gross tumor, absence of malignancy in the remaining portion of the kidney should be verified intraoperatively by frozen-section examinations of biopsy specimens obtained at random from the renal margin of excision. It is usual for such specimens to demonstrate residual tumor, but, if so, additional renal tissue must be excised.

Segmental Polar Nephrectomy

In a patient with malignancy confined to the upper or lower pole of the kidney, partial nephrectomy can be performed by isolating and ligating the segmental apical or basilar arterial branch while allowing unimpaired perfusion to the remainder of the kidney from the main renal artery. This procedure is illustrated in Figure 97–47 for a tumor confined to the apical vascular segment. The apical artery is dissected away from the adjacent structures, ligated, and divided. Often a corresponding venous branch is present, which is similarly ligated and divided. An ischemic line of demarcation then generally appears on the surface of the kidney and outlines the segment to be excised. If this area is not obvious, a few milliliters of methylene blue can be directly injected distally into the ligated apical artery to outline better the limits of the involved renal segment. An incision is then made in the renal cortex at the line of demarcation, which should be at least 1 cm away from the

visible edge of the cancer. The parenchyma is divided by sharp and blunt dissection, and the polar segment is removed. In cases of malignancy, it is not possible to preserve a strip of capsule beyond the parenchymal line of resection for use in closing the renal defect.

Often a portion of the collecting system has been removed with the cancer during a segmental polar nephrectomy. The collecting system is carefully closed with interrupted or continuous 4–0 chromic sutures to ensure a watertight repair. Small transected blood vessels on the renal surface are identified and ligated with shallow figure-of-eight 4–0 chromic sutures. The edges of the kidney are reapproximated as an additional hemostatic measure, using simple interrupted 3–0 chromic sutures inserted through the capsule and a small amount of parenchyma. Before these sutures are tied, perirenal fat or Oxycel can be inserted into the defect for inclusion in the renal closure. If the collecting system has been entered, a Penrose drain is left in the perinephric space.

Wedge Resection

Wedge resection is an appropriate technique for removing peripheral tumors on the surface of the kidney, particularly tumors that are larger or not confined to either renal pole. Because these lesions often encompass more than one renal segment and because this technique is generally associated with heavier bleeding, it is best to perform wedge resection with temporary renal arterial occlusion and surface hypothermia.

In performing a wedge resection, the tumor is removed with a 1-cm surrounding margin of grossly normal renal parenchyma (Fig. 97–48). The parenchyma is divided by a combination of sharp and blunt dissection. Invariably the

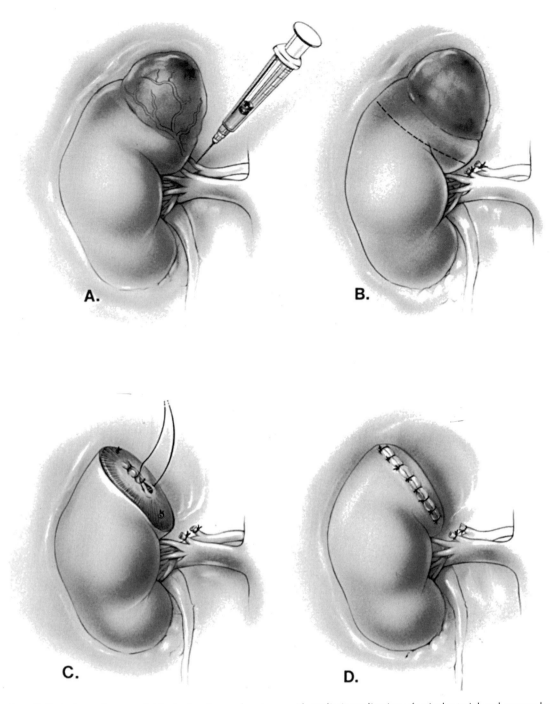

Figure 97–47. *A* to *D,* Technique of segmental (apical) polar nephrectomy with preliminary ligation of apical arterial and venous branches. (From Novick AC: Urol Clin North Am 1987; 14:419.)

tumor extends deeply into the kidney, and the collecting system is entered. Often, prominent intrarenal vessels are identified as the parenchyma is being incised. These may be directly suture-ligated at that time, while they are most visible. After excision of the tumor, the collecting system is closed with interrupted or continuous 4–0 chromic sutures. Remaining transected blood vessels on the renal surface are secured with figure-of-eight 4–0 chromic sutures. Bleeding at this point is usually minimal, and the operative field can be kept satisfactorily clear by gentle suction during placement of hemostatic sutures.

The renal defect can be closed in one of two ways (see Fig. 97–48). The kidney may be closed on itself by approximating the transected cortical margins with simple interrupted 3–0 chromic sutures, after placing a small piece of Oxycel at the base of the defect. If this is done, there must be no tension on the suture line and no significant angulation or kinking of blood vessels supplying the kidney. Alternatively a portion of perirenal fat may simply be inserted into the base of the renal defect as a hemostatic measure and sutured to the parenchymal margins with interrupted 4–0 chromic sutures. After closure or coverage of the renal

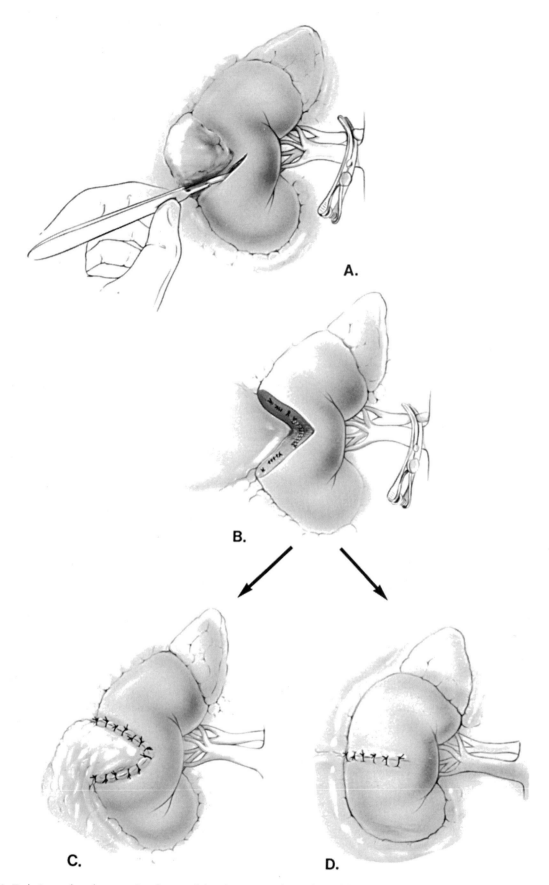

Figure 97–48. Technique of wedge resection for a peripheral tumor on the surface of the kidney (*A* and *B*). The renal defect may be closed on itself *(D)* or covered with perirenal fat *(C)*. (From Novick AC: Urol Clin North Am 1987; 14:419.)

defect, the renal artery is unclamped, and circulation to the kidney is restored. A Penrose drain is left in the perinephric space.

Major Transverse Resection

A transverse resection is done to remove large tumors that extensively involve the upper or lower portion of the kidney. This technique is performed using surface hypothermia after temporary occlusion of the renal artery. Major branches of the renal artery and vein supplying the tumor-bearing portion of the kidney are identified in the renal hilus, ligated, and divided (Fig. 97–49A). If possible, this should be done before temporarily occluding the renal artery to minimize the overall period of renal ischemia.

After occluding the renal artery, the parenchyma is divided by blunt and sharp dissection, leaving a 1-cm margin of grossly normal tissue around the tumor (Fig. 97–49B). Transected blood vessels on the renal surface are secured as previously described, and the hilus is inspected carefully for remaining unligated segmental vessels. An internal ureteral stent may be inserted if extensive reconstruction of the collecting system is necessary. If possible, the renal defect is sutured together with one of the techniques previously described (Fig. 97–49C). If this suture cannot be placed without tension or without distorting the renal vessels, a

piece of peritoneum or perirenal fat is sutured in place to cover the defect. Circulation to the kidney is restored, and a Penrose drain is left in the perirenal space.

Simple Enucleation

Some renal cell carcinomas are surrounded by a distinct pseudocapsule of fibrous tissue (Vermooten, 1950). The technique of simple enucleation implies circumferential incision of the renal parenchyma around the tumors simply and rapidly at any location, often with no vascular occlusion and with maximal preservation of normal parenchyma.

Initial reports indicated satisfactory short-term clinical results after enucleation with good patient survival and low rate of local tumor recurrence (Graham and Glenn, 1979; Jaeger et al, 1985). Most studies, however, have suggested a higher risk of leaving residual malignancy in the kidney when enucleation is performed (Rosenthal et al, 1984; Marshall et al, 1986; Blackley et al, 1988).

These latter reports include several carefully done histopathologic studies that have demonstrated frequent microscopic tumor penetration of the pseudocapsule that surrounds the neoplasm. These data indicate that it is not always possible to be assured of complete tumor encapsulation before surgery. Local recurrence of tumor in the treated kidney is a grave complication of partial nephrectomy for renal cell

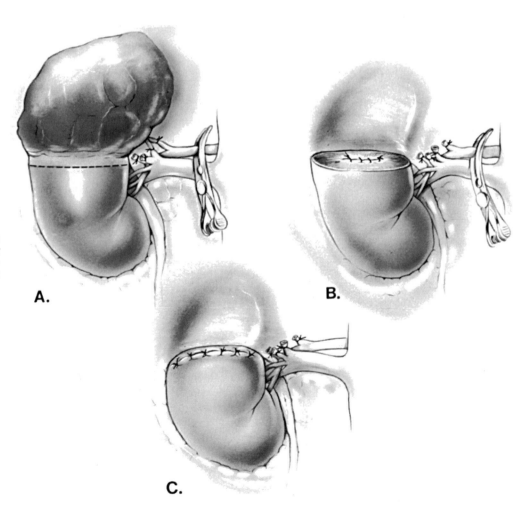

Figure 97–49. *A* to *C,* Technique of transverse resection for a tumor involving the upper half of the kidney. (From Novick AC: Urol Clin North Am 1987; 14:419.)

A.

B.

C.

carcinoma, and every attempt should be made to prevent it. Therefore, it is the authors' view that a surrounding margin of normal parenchyma should be removed with the tumor whenever possible. This provides an added margin of safety against the development of local tumor recurrence and, in most cases, does not appreciably increase the technical difficulty of the operation. The technique of enucleation is currently employed only in occasional patients with von Hippel–Lindau disease and multiple low-stage encapsulated tumors involving both kidneys (Spencer et al, 1988).

Extracorporeal Partial Nephrectomy and Autotransplantation

Extracorporeal partial nephrectomy for renal cell carcinoma with autotransplantation of the renal remnant was initially described by several surgeons (Calne, 1973; Gittes and McCullough, 1975). **This surgical technique allows for the successful excision of large complex tumors involving the renal hilus. Reconstruction of kidneys with renal cell carcinoma as well as renal artery disease may be facilitated with this approach** (Campbell et al, 1993). The advantages of an extracorporeal approach include optimum exposure, a bloodless surgical field, the ability to perform a more precise operation with maximum conservation of renal parenchyma, and a greater protection of the kidney from prolonged ischemia. Disadvantages of extracorporeal surgery include longer operative time with the need for vascular and ureteral anastomoses and an increased risk of temporary and permanent renal failure (Campbell et al, 1994); the latter presumably reflects a more severe intraoperative ischemic insult to the kidney. Although some urologic surgeons have found that almost all patients undergoing partial nephrectomy for renal cell carcinoma can be managed satisfactorily in situ (Novick et al, 1989), others have continued to recommend an extracorporeal approach for selected patients (Morgan and Zincke, 1990).

Extracorporeal partial nephrectomy and renal autotransplantation are generally performed through a single midline incision. The kidney is mobilized and removed outside Gerota's fascia with ligation and division of the renal artery and vein as the last steps in the operation (Fig. 97–50A). Immediately after dividing the renal vessels, the removed kidney is flushed with 500 ml of a chilled intracellular electrolyte solution and is submerged in a basin of ice slush saline solution to maintain hypothermia. Under these conditions, if warm renal ischemia has been minimal, the kidney can safely be preserved outside the body for as much time as needed to perform extracorporeal partial nephrectomy.

If possible, it is best to leave the ureter attached in such cases to preserve its distal collateral vascular supply, particularly with large hilar or lower renal tumors in which complex excision may unavoidably compromise the blood supply to the pelvis, ureter, or both. When this procedure is done, the extracorporeal operation is performed on the abdominal wall. If the ureter is left attached, it must be occluded temporarily to prevent retrograde blood flow to the kidney when it is outside the body. Often, unless the patient is thin, working on the abdominal wall with the ureter attached is cumbersome because of the tethering and restricted movement of the kidney. If these are observed, the ureter should be divided and the kidney placed on a separate workbench. This practice provides better exposure for the extracorporeal operation, and while this is being done, a second surgical team can be preparing the iliac fossa for autotransplantation. If concern exists about the adequacy of ureteral blood supply, the risk of postoperative urinary extravasation can be diminished by restoring urinary continuity through direct anastomosis of the renal pelvis to the retained distal ureter.

Extracorporeal partial nephrectomy is done with the flushed kidney preserved under surface hypothermia. The kidney is first divested of all perinephric fat to appreciate the full extent of the neoplasm. Because such tumors are usually centrally located, dissection is generally begun in the renal hilus with identification of major segmental arterial and venous branches. Vessels clearly directed toward the neoplasm are secured and divided, and those supplying uninvolved renal parenchyma are preserved. The tumor is then removed by incising the capsule and parenchyma to preserve a 1-cm surrounding margin of normal renal tissue (Fig. 97–50B). Transected blood vessels visible on the renal surface are secured, and the collecting system is closed as described for in situ partial nephrectomy.

At this point, the renal remnant may be reflushed or placed on the pulsatile perfusion unit to facilitate identification and suture ligation of remaining potential bleeding points (Fig. 97–50C). The kidney can be perfused alternately through the renal artery and vein to ensure both arterial and venous hemostasis. Because the flushing solution and perfusate lack clotting ability, there may continue to be some parenchymal oozing, which can safely be ignored. If possible, the defect created by the partial nephrectomy is closed by suturing the kidney on itself to ensure further a watertight repair (Fig. 97–50D).

Autotransplantation into the iliac fossa is done, employing the same vascular technique as that in renal allotransplantation. Urinary continuity may be restored with ureteroneocystostomy or pyeloureterostomy, leaving an internal ureteral stent in place. When removal of the neoplasm has necessitated extensive hilar dissection of vessels supplying the renal pelvis, an indwelling nephrostomy tube is also left for postoperative drainage. After autotransplantation, a Penrose drain is positioned extraperitoneally in the iliac fossa away from the vascular anastomotic sites.

Complications

Complications of partial nephrectomy include hemorrhage, urinary fistula formation, ureteral obstruction, renal insufficiency, and infection. Significant intraoperative bleeding can occur in patients who are undergoing partial nephrectomy. The need for early control and ready access to the renal artery is emphasized. Postoperative hemorrhage may be self-limiting if confined to the retroperitoneum, or it may be associated with gross hematuria. The initial management of postoperative hemorrhage is expectant with bed rest, serial hemoglobin and hematocrit determinations, frequent monitoring of vital signs, and blood transfusions as needed. Angiography may be helpful in some patients to localize actively bleeding segmental renal arteries, which may be

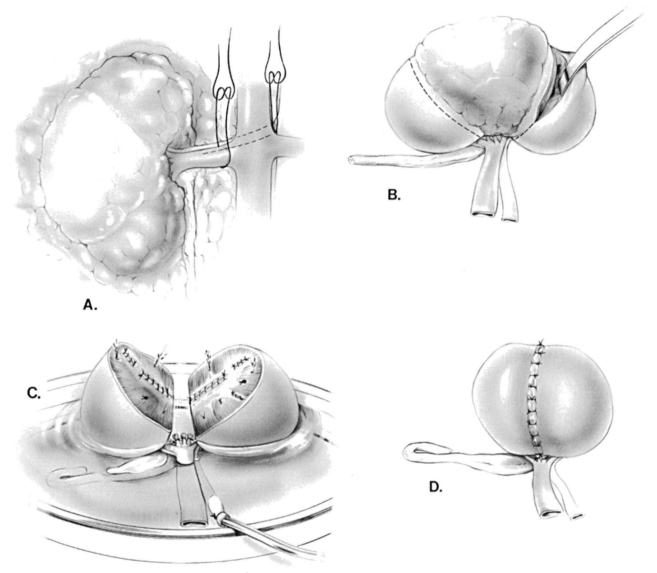

Figure 97–50. Technique of extracorporeal partial nephrectomy for a large central tumor. *A,* The kidney is removed outside Gerota's fascia. *B,* The tumor is excised extracorporeally while preserving the vascular branches to uninvolved parenchyma. *C,* Pulsatile perfusion or reflushing is used to identify transected blood vessels. *D,* The kidney is closed on itself. (From Novick AC: Urol Clin North Am 1987; 14:419.)

controlled via angioinfarction. Severe intractable hemorrhage may necessitate re-exploration with early control of the renal vessels and ligation of the active bleeding points.

Postoperative urinary flank drainage after a partial nephrectomy is common and usually resolves as the collecting system closes with healing. Persistent drainage suggests the development of a urinary cutaneous fistula. This diagnosis can be confirmed by determination of the creatinine level of the drainage fluid and intravenous injection of indigo carmine with subsequent appearance of the dye in the drainage fluid. The majority of urinary fistulas resolve spontaneously if there is no obstruction of urinary drainage from the involved renal unit. If the perirenal space is not adequately drained, a urinoma or abscess may develop. An intravenous pyelogram or a retrograde pyelogram should be obtained to rule out obstruction of the involved urinary collecting system. In the event of hydronephrosis or persistent urinary leakage, an internal ureteral stent is placed. If this is not

possible, a percutaneous nephrostomy may be inserted. The majority of urinary fistulas resolve spontaneously with proper conservative management, although this may take several weeks in some cases. A second operation to close the urinary fistula is rarely necessary.

Ureteral obstruction can occur after partial nephrectomy because of postoperative bleeding into the collecting system with resulting clot obstruction of the ureter and pelvis. This obstruction can lead to temporary extravasation of urine from the renal suture line. In most cases, expectant management is appropriate, and the obstruction resolves spontaneously with lysis of the clots. When urinary leakage is excessive or in the presence of intercurrent urinary infection, placement of an internal ureteral stent can help to maintain antegrade ureteral drainage.

Varying degrees of renal insufficiency often occur postoperatively when partial nephrectomy is performed in a patient with a solitary kidney. This insufficiency is a consequence of both intraoperative renal ischemia and removal of some normal parenchyma along with the diseased portion of the kidney. Such renal insufficiency is usually mild and resolves spontaneously with proper fluid and electrolyte management. Also, in most cases, the remaining parenchyma undergoes compensatory hypertrophy that serves to improve renal function further. Severe renal insufficiency may require temporary or permanent hemodialysis, and the patients should be aware of this possibility preoperatively.

Postoperative infections are usually self-limiting if the operative site is well drained and in the absence of existing untreated urinary infection at the time of surgery. Unusual complications of partial nephrectomy include transient postoperative hypertension and aneurysm or arteriovenous fistula in the remaining portion of the parenchyma (Snodgrass and Robinson, 1964; Rezvani et al, 1973).

A study detailed the incidence and clinical outcome of technical or renal-related complications occurring after 259 partial nephrectomies for renal tumors at the Cleveland Clinic (Campbell et al, 1994). In the overall series, local or renal-related complications occurred after 78 operations (30.1%). The incidence of complications was significantly less for operations performed after 1988 and significantly less for incidentally detected versus suspected tumors. The most common complications were urinary fistula formation and acute renal failure. A urinary fistula occurred after 45 of 259 operations (17%). Significant predisposing factors for a urinary fistula included central tumor location, tumor size greater than 4 cm, the need for major reconstruction of the collecting system, and ex vivo surgery. Only one urinary fistula required open operative repair, whereas the remainder resolved either spontaneously (n = 30) or with endoscopic management (n = 14).

Acute renal failure occurred after 30 of 115 operations (26%) performed on a solitary kidney. Significant predisposing factors for acute renal failure were tumor size greater than 7 cm, greater than 50% parenchymal excision, greater than 60 minutes ischemia time, and ex vivo surgery. Acute renal failure resolved completely in 25 patients, of whom 9 (8%) required temporary dialysis; 5 patients (4%) required permanent dialysis.

Overall, only eight complications (3.1%) required repeat open surgery for treatment, whereas all other complications resolved with noninterventive or endourologic management. Surgical complications contributed to an adverse clinical outcome in only seven patients (2.9%). These data indicate that partial nephrectomy can be performed safely with preservation of renal function in most patients with renal tumors.

Postoperative Follow-up

Patients who undergo a partial nephrectomy for renal malignancy are advised to return for initial follow-up 4 to 6 weeks postoperatively. At this time, a serum creatinine measurement and intravenous pyelogram are obtained to document renal function and anatomy; in patients with impaired overall renal function, a renal ultrasound study is obtained instead of an intravenous pyelogram. **Subsequent surveillance for recurrent malignancy is performed at 6-month intervals for 4 years and at yearly intervals thereafter.** Such surveillance entails biochemical liver and renal function studies, a chest film, and an abdominal imaging study to rule out local tumor recurrence; concerning the last-mentioned, computed tomography remains the most accurate study for detecting recurrent malignancy in a renal remnant after partial nephrectomy. If such local recurrence is found without metastatic disease, either a second partial nephrectomy or a total nephrectomy may be performed (Novick and Straffon, 1987).

Emerging data suggest that patients with less than one kidney are at higher risk for developing proteinuria, glomerular damage, and impaired renal function as a result of glomerular hyperfiltration (Solomon et al, 1985; Foster et al, 1991). In one study, long-term renal function was evaluated in 14 patients with a solitary kidney who underwent partial nephrectomy for localized malignancy (Novick et al, 1991). Preoperatively, there was no clinical or histopathologic evidence of primary renal disease. Postoperative renal function remained stable in 12 patients, and 2 patients developed end-stage renal failure. A total of nine patients had proteinuria, low grade (<750 mg/day) in four and moderate to severe (930–6740 mg/day) in five patients. A statistically significant association was found between more proteinuria and a lesser amount of remaining renal tissue as well as a longer follow-up interval. A renal biopsy was done in four patients with moderate-to-severe proteinuria, which, in each case, showed focal segmental or global glomerulosclerosis.

These data suggest that patients with greater than 50% reduction in overall renal mass are at increased risk for proteinuria, glomerulopathy, and progressive renal failure. Structural or functional renal damage in such cases is usually antedated by the appearance of proteinuria. Therefore, the follow-up of patients after partial nephrectomy in a solitary kidney should include a 24-hour urinary protein determination in addition to the usual renal function and tumor surveillance studies. Patients who have proteinuria (>150 mg/day) may be treated with a low-protein diet and a converting enzyme inhibitor agent, which appear to be beneficial in preventing glomerulopathy caused by reduced renal mass (Meyer et al, 1985; Novick and Schreiber, 1995).

PARTIAL NEPHRECTOMY FOR BENIGN DISEASE

Partial nephrectomy is also indicated in selected patients with localized benign pathology of the kidney (Leach and Kieber, 1980). The indications include (1) hydronephrosis with parenchymal atrophy or atrophic pyelonephritis in a duplicated renal segment; (2) calyceal diverticulum complicated by infection or stones, or both; (3) calculus disease with obstruction of the lower pole calyx or segmental parenchymal disease with impaired drainage (Papathanassiadis and Swinney, 1966; Bates et al, 1981); (4) renovascular hypertension caused by segmental parenchymal damage or noncorrectable branch renal artery disease (Aoi et al, 1981; Parrott et al, 1984); (5) traumatic renal injury with irreversible damage to a portion of the kidney (Gibson et al, 1982); and (6) removal of a benign renal tumor, such as an angiomyolipoma or oncocytoma (Maatman et al, 1984).

The preoperative considerations are similar to those in patients undergoing partial nephrectomy for malignancy. In most cases, renal arteriography should be performed to delineate the main and segmental renal arterial supply. The same measures should be taken to minimize intraoperative renal damage from ischemia. The preferred surgical approach is usually through an extraperitoneal flank incision except for cases of renal trauma, which are best approached anteriorly. The surgical techniques are also similar to those described for malignant renal disease.

When performing an apical or basilar partial nephrectomy for benign disease, the segmental apical or basilar arterial branch is secured, and the parenchyma is divided at the ischemic line of demarcation, without the need for temporary renal arterial occlusion. More complex transverse or wedge renal resections are best performed with temporary renal arterial occlusion and ice slush surface hypothermia. When employing the technique of transverse renal resection for a benign disorder, the renal capsule is excised and reflected off the diseased parenchyma for subsequent use in covering the renal defect (Fig. 97–51). The technical aspects of partial nephrectomy for benign disease are otherwise the same as those described for malignancy with adherence to the same basic principles of appropriate vascular control, avoidance of ischemic renal damage, precise closure of the collecting system, careful hemostasis, and closure or coverage of the renal defect.

Heminephrectomy in Duplicated Collecting Systems

Because the indications for partial nephrectomy in this setting are usually hydronephrosis and parenchymal atrophy of one of the two segments, the demarcation of the tissue to be removed is usually evident. The atrophic parenchyma lining the dilated system can be further delineated by blue pyelotubular backflow if the ureter is ligated and the affected collecting system is distended by blue dye under pressure. In such cases, there is also often a dual arterial supply with distinct segmental branches to the upper and lower halves of the kidney. Segmental arterial and venous branches to the diseased portion of the kidney are ligated and divided. After preserving a strip of renal capsule, the parenchyma is divided at the observed line of demarcation. There is usually minimal bleeding from the renal surface, and temporary occlusion of the arterial supply to the nondiseased segment is often unnecessary. There should be no entry into the collecting system over the transected renal surface, which is then closed or covered as described previously.

RENAL STONE DISEASE

The surgical management of renal calculus disease has changed dramatically since the introduction of percutaneous and extracorporeal shock wave technology. Clearly, well over 95% of patients previously requiring open operative intervention may now be managed with either of these less invasive modalities, either alone or in combination (Assimos et al, 1989; Kane et al, 1995).

Although technologic advances have changed the manner in which urologic surgeons approach renal calculi, **the basic indications for intervention remain the same. These in-**clude obstruction, pain, infection, or significant hematuria associated with the stone or stone growth despite appropriate medical therapy. Within these settings, the indications for open operative intervention are much more confined and include

- **An associated anatomic abnormality requiring open operative intervention.**
- **A stone so large and extensive that in the judgment of an experienced urologic surgeon a single open operative procedure would, with less risk, more likely render the patient stone-free than would the option of multiple percutaneous and extracorporeal shock wave procedures.**
- **Failure of or contraindication to both extracorporeal shock wave lithotripsy (ESWL) and percutaneous nephrostolithotomy.**

Radiographic and Renal Function Evaluation

In most cases, intravenous urography is the initial radiographic study obtained. Ideally, this provides adequate anatomic and functional information. Specifically the number, size, and location of the stones are evident from this study alone. Oblique views and nephrotomograms should be included both before and after contrast material injection.

At times, renal function may be compromised either from intrinsic renal disease or from obstruction so that intravenous urography does not allow adequate visualization of the upper tracts. In those cases, retrograde or antegrade pyelography can delineate the renal anatomy. When obstruction is found, an internal stent or percutaneous nephrostomy tube should be left indwelling to relieve symptoms, enhance treatment of any associated infection, and allow recovery of renal function. For select patients, further assessment of renal function may be attained with a differential renal function scan (computerized renogram) using technetium Tc-99m DTPA or MAG 3 technetium.

Planning or surgical intervention for complex stone disease may also include a computed tomography scan obtained both before and after intravenous contrast material injection because this provides valuable information about three-dimensional location of the stone. Computed tomography scanning also allows evaluation of renal cortical thickness, which is especially useful when consideration is being given to an ablative procedure such as partial or total nephrectomy. Currently, standard catheter angiography has only a limited role in the preoperative evaluation of stone patients. When information about the number and location of the main renal arteries is desired, intra-arterial or intravenous digital subtraction angiography is generally adequate (Zabbo et al, 1988).

Anatrophic Nephrolithotomy

Although the approach to managing staghorn calculi has changed dramatically, the rationale for intervention remains the same. Most staghorn calculi are composed of magnesium-ammonium-calcium phosphate and are associated with

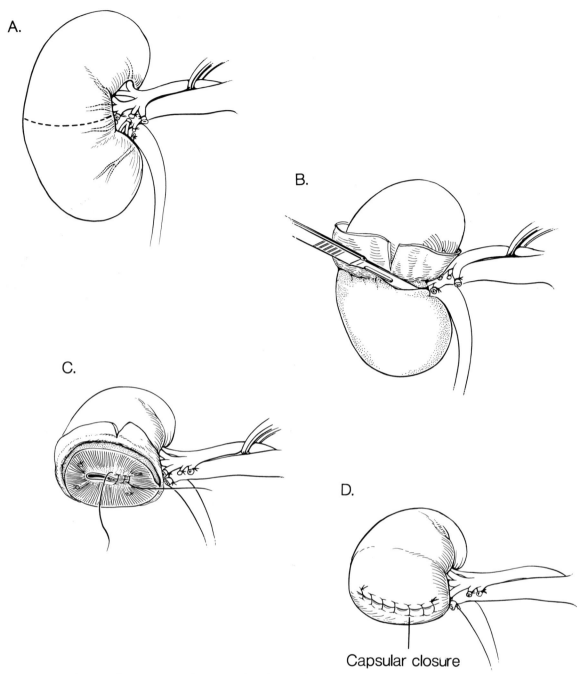

Figure 97–51. *A* to *D*, Technique of transverse renal resection for a benign disorder. The renal capsule from the diseased parenchyma is preserved and used to cover the transected renal surface.

chronic urinary tract infection that is virtually impossible to eradicate as long as the stone is present. Although a controlled, prospective study of conservative medical management versus operative intervention has yet to be done, there is strong clinical evidence that in all but the poorest-risk surgical patients, renal function and overall clinical status are improved by removing the stone (Blandy and Singh, 1976; Rous and Turner, 1977; Vargas et al, 1982; Teichman et al, 1995).

The American Urological Association Nephrolithiasis Clinical Guidelines Panel made recommendations about the management of struvite staghorn calculi and stressed that an untreated struvite staghorn stone is almost invari- **ably associated with recurrent infection, loss of renal function, and high rates of renal-related morbidity or even mortality** (Segura et al, 1994). Furthermore, the panel suggested that adequate treatment of a struvite stone requires its complete removal because intact residual stones are associated with high rates of recurrent infection and stone growth.

In performing a meta-analysis of available studies, several conclusions and recommendations about appropriate management were offered by the panel. The most important considerations in the analysis were the probability of a stone-free renal unit after treatment and the probabilities of requiring a secondary unplanned treatment or developing complications. The four treatment alternatives studied were open surgery, percutaneous nephrolithotomy, ESWL, and combined percutaneous nephrolithotomy/ESWL.

In reviewing the outcome probabilities of these four modalities, the panel made nine conclusive statements, summarized here:

1. The risk of residual stone fragments after initial treatment is highest after ESWL monotherapy.

2. Post-ESWL residual struvite fragments may be associated with recurrent infection and stone growth, although literature support for that is scarce.

3. The need for unplanned secondary intervention is high with ESWL monotherapy.

4. Percutaneous nephrolithotomy, combined percutaneous nephrolithotomy/ESWL, and open surgery are most likely to require general or regional anesthesia.

5. ESWL monotherapy is the least likely modality to result in bleeding requiring transfusion.

6. The patient should be involved in a discussion of potential complications or the need for secondary treatments.

7. Although ESWL monotherapy has the highest rate of complications and need for unplanned secondary intervention, the complications associated with it tend to be less severe than those associated with the other treatment options.

8. In determining the optimal treatment option, factors such as stone size, composition, and anatomy of the collecting system should be considered.

9. In choosing a treatment option, patient factors such as overall health, body habitus, and associated medical problems should be considered.

From this analysis, the panel made recommendations for treatment of a struvite staghorn calculus in a *standard* patient, which they defined as an adult with two equally functioning kidneys or with a normally functioning solitary kidney, in whom overall medical condition and body habitus permit performance of any of the four studied treatment modalities and the use of anesthesia. For the *nonstandard* patient, the choice of treatment options may be more limited. The recommendations for treatment were made at three levels based on the strength of available scientific evidence for estimating the outcome. These recommendations were classified as *standard*, a *guideline*, or an *option*. **As a standard, the panel recommended that a newly diagnosed struvite staghorn calculus was of and by itself an indication for intervention and that any affected patient must be informed of the four active treatment modalities and the relative benefits and risks associated with each.** As a guideline, the panel recommended percutaneous stone removal followed by ESWL or repeat percutaneous procedures as needed to achieve a stone-free renal unit and emphasized that a percutaneous procedure should be the first part of any combination therapy. As a general guideline, percutaneous nephrolithotomy or combined percutaneous nephrolithotomy/ESWL is preferable to ESWL monotherapy or to open surgery. As an option, the panel recommended ESWL monotherapy or percutaneous monotherapy as equally effective treatment choices for small-volume struvite staghorn calculi in anatomically normal or near-normal collecting systems. **The panel recommended open surgery as an appropriate treatment option only in unusual situations, such as a staghorn calculus so extensive that an unreasonable number of percutaneous or ESWL procedures would be required to achieve a stone-free renal unit.**

Clearly the majority of staghorn calculi, even extensive ones, can and should be managed by combinations of percutaneous debulking and ESWL (Kahnoski et al, 1986; Schulze et al, 1986; Streem et al, 1987; Streem and Lammert, 1992). Occasionally, however, specific circumstances may dictate open operative intervention, although such an approach to staghorn calculi is recommended only rarely. **The most frequent relative indication for an open procedure to manage these patients is the finding of a massively sized, complete staghorn calculus with multiple dumbbell-shaped infundibulocalyceal extensions associated with relatively narrow infundibula** (Fig. 97–52). In such patients, the option of a single, open operative procedure, especially in a previously unoperated kidney, may be a reasonable one when weighed against the alternative of multiple percutaneous tracts just to attain significant debulking and the need for multiple additional sessions of ESWL and possible percutaneous chemolysis (Assimos et al, 1991b). **In these cases, the open operative approach of choice is the anatrophic nephrolithotomy initially described by Boyce and Smith in 1967.**

Complete radiographic and renal function evaluation of these patients is accomplished as outlined earlier in this section. Because most of these stones are associated with chronic infection, it is important to search for underlying anatomic or functional urinary tract abnormalities predisposing to infection. Metabolic evaluation should also be performed because a significant proportion of struvite stones form secondarily (Resnick, 1981; Lingeman et al, 1995). Vigorous treatment of associated urinary tract infection is an important part of preoperative care, and intravenous antibiotics are generally begun 36 to 48 hours before surgery. Adequate intravenous hydration is also a standard part of the immediate preoperative regimen.

The technique of anatrophic nephrolithotomy follows the basic principles set forth by Boyce and Smith. Essentially, all stone is to be removed through an incision that is least traumatic to overall renal function. Because temporary occlusion of the renal artery is required for a bloodless field, the kidney must be protected from an ischemic insult. Finally, areas of true, functionally significant infundibular stenosis must be addressed to provide adequate drainage from all parts of the collecting system.

A flank approach is used with resection of the 12th or 11th rib. Medially the incision should extend to the lateral border of the rectus muscle. The peritoneum is reflected medially to gain access to the retroperitoneum. The proximal ureter is identified and surrounded with a vessel loop to prevent distal migration of any stone fragments during the subsequent nephrolithotomy. The kidney is then completely mobilized, leaving only the renal pedicle and ureter intact. A surgical tape placed around the upper and lower poles at this time provides a useful sling to facilitate handling of the kidney. Medial retraction of the kidney then affords exposure to the hilar vessels posteriorly, where the renal artery is dissected free and surrounded with a vessel loop (Fig. 97–53). Mannitol 12.5 g is now given intravenously to help protect the kidney from the subsequent period of ischemia. The renal artery is further dissected until the anterior and

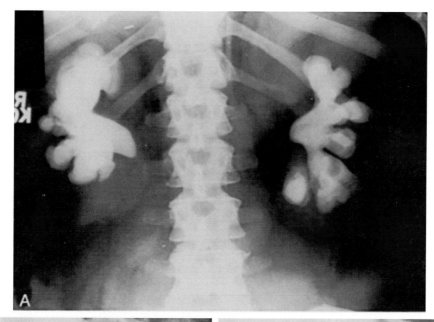

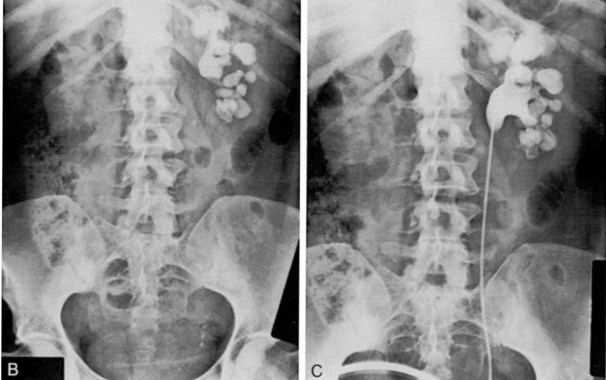

Figure 97–52. *A,* Scout film reveals bilateral staghorn calculi. There is no infundibular stenosis, however. Therefore, a combination of percutaneous nephrostolithotomy and extracorporeal shock wave lithotripsy is an excellent contemporary treatment option. *B* and *C,* Scout film reveals staghorn calculus on the left side. In contrast to the patient in *A,* the retrograde study reveals multiple areas of relative infundibular narrowing. Therefore, significant debulking would be difficult without multiple percutaneous tracts. In addition, multiple sessions of extracorporeal shock wave lithotripsy may also be required. In such cases, anatrophic nephrolithotomy still provides a reasonable therapeutic option.

posterior divisional branches are identified. Generally the first major branch of the main renal artery represents the posterior division. This dissection is required to identify precisely the junction of the blood supply to the anterior and posterior segments of the kidney. As first described by Brodell in 1901 and then delineated further by Graves in 1954, this junction, at the surface of the kidney, generally lies on the posterior aspect approximately two thirds of the distance

from the hilum to the true lateral border of the kidney (Fig. 97–54).

A vascular clamp may now be placed temporarily on the anterior division of the renal artery and 10 ml methylene blue injected intravenously in the systemic circulation. This stains the posterior renal segment, thus helping to identify the appropriate line of incision and subsequent dissection into the renal parenchyma. A plastic dam is placed beneath

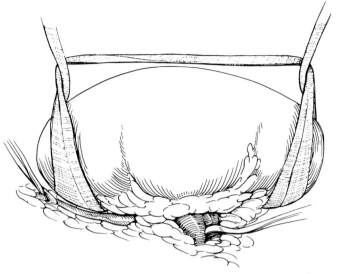

Figure 97–53. The kidney is retracted medially after it is completely mobilized. Vessel loops surround the renal artery and ureter, and a sling facilitates handling of the kidney.

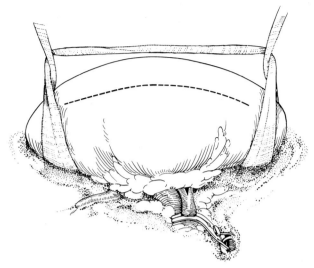

Figure 97–55. After the renal artery has been clamped and the kidney cooled in ice slush, the nephrotomy incision is made through the capsule between the anterior and the posterior segments. This nephrotomy incision extends only to the apical and basilar renal segments.

the kidney and wrapped around the pedicle as a reservoir for ice slush. The main renal artery is clamped, and the kidney packed in slush with a goal of obtaining a core temperature of 10°C, again as protection from subsequent ischemia. Once the kidney is cooled, a longitudinal incision is made through the capsule between the anterior and posterior segments, extending only to the apical and basilar renal segments (Fig. 97–55). Blunt dissection is then used to continue the dissection through the parenchyma. The correct plane is along the line of demarcation between the anterior and posterior arterial segments down toward the renal pelvis in a plane just anterior to the posterior row of infundibula and calyces (Fig. 97–56). At this time and throughout the subsequent dissection, any venous bleeding is managed by suture ligation with fine chromic sutures. If small arterioles have been cut, they are managed in the same manner. The stone is now usually identified by palpation in one of the involved posterior infundibula or calyces. A longitudinal infundibulotomy is then performed and extended down to

the renal pelvis (Fig. 97–57). In a similar manner, each posterior infundibulocalyx is opened longitudinally on its anterior aspect with the infundibulotomy extending out from the renal pelvis toward the calyx.

On completion of the longitudinal nephrotomy and exposure of the pelvic and posterior aspect of the stone, the anterior and polar portions are exposed by sequential longitudinal infundibulotomies made on the posterior aspect of the anterior segmental infundibula and medial aspects of the polar infundibula (Fig. 97–58A) (Boyce et al, 1979). These infundibulotomies should begin at each infundibulopelvic junction and extend outward toward the calyx as far as necessary to provide adequate exposure for subsequent removal of the calculus. Gradually then, the entire staghorn calculus is exposed and is now ready for removal (Fig.

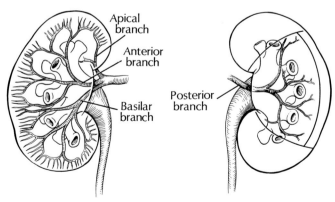

Figure 97–54. The avascular line of incision is defined by the junction of the anterior and posterior segments of the renal artery. On the surface of the kidney, this avascular plane generally lies on the posterior aspect approximately two thirds of the distance from the renal hilum to the true lateral border of the kidney.

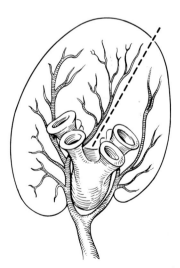

Figure 97–56. The nephrotomy incision is continued in a plane along the line of demarcation between the anterior and the posterior arterial segments and extended down toward the renal pelvis. The correct line dissection generally lies just anterior to the posterior row of infundibula and calyces.

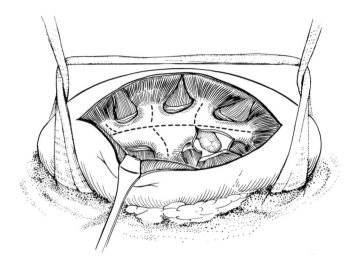

Figure 97–57. A longitudinal infundibulotomy is performed on the anterior aspect of one of the posterior infundibula through which the stone is palpable. The infundibulotomy is extended down to the renal pelvis, and the pelvis itself is then opened. A longitudinal infundibulotomy is subsequently performed on each posterior infundibulum.

97–58*B*). During this portion of the procedure, invaluable exposure may be obtained using malleable brain retractors and nerve hooks. At times, the stone may be delivered intact (Fig. 97–58*C*). Although this is a laudable achievement, piecemeal extraction is, in practice, more often the rule because infundibulocalyceal extensions may break off and require separate removal. This may result from the relatively soft and friable nature of the stone, or, alternatively, the entire stone may not have been in continuity to begin with. When infundibulocalyceal extensions of the stone remain, the involved infundibulum should be further incised out toward the calyx. Blunt dissection between the stone and urothelium with a tonsil clamp or similar instrument helps free the stone, which, because of a local inflammatory reaction, may be densely adherent.

After removal of the bulk of the stone, each infundibulocalyceal system should be individually explored for residual fragments. This requires both visual inspection and palpation. Occasionally, residual fragments can be palpated through thin parenchyma, but the infundibulum leading to the stone cannot be localized. In such cases, the fragment is removed by making a small nephrotomy directly over the stone. The nephrotomy is then closed with absorbable sutures in one or two layers, depending on the thickness of the parenchyma. The entire collecting system is now thoroughly lavaged with cold saline, using an appropriate-sized red rubber catheter placed sequentially in each infundibulocalyceal system. During this portion of the procedure, a No. 8 Fr catheter should be placed antegrade from within the renal pelvis down the ureter again to help prevent distal migration of stone fragments.

Because removal of all stone fragments is an important goal of this operation, intraoperative x-ray with organ films remains an integral part of the procedure. X-O-mat KS film is ideal, and sterile cassettes should be a routine part of the available instrumentation (Fig. 97–59). When residual stone fragments are noted, intraoperative ultrasonography may allow their localization (Cook and Lytton, 1977). In the authors' experience, however, intraoperative nephroscopy with a flexible nephroscope provides a more direct route for rapid localization (Miki et al, 1978).

When all stone has been removed, closure of the collecting system is begun. At this point, the red rubber catheter is

withdrawn from the ureter. In selected patients, especially those who may have residual fragments, an internal stent is placed antegrade with the proximal portion positioned in the lower infundibulocalyceal system or renal pelvis. Nephrostomy tubes are used rarely and generally only for those patients with severely compromised renal function and thin parenchyma or when residual stones may be present that could then be treated with either percutaneous extraction or chemolysis.

Separate closure of the collecting system with a running, fine chromic suture is generally recommended. In most cases, this involves simple closure of each infundibulotomy and the renal pelvis (Fig. 97–60). Close attention, however, must be paid to areas of significant infundibular stenosis that require infundibuloplasty. In previous years, infundibular stenosis was believed to be a common sequela of staghorn calculi. The success of percutaneous and extracorporeal techniques alone or in combination for most of these patients, however, has proven to the authors that infundibular stenosis is more often apparent than real and is usually not of any functional significance once the stone is removed. As an analogy, this is perhaps best compared to the patient with a stone impacted at the ureteropelvic junction. Intravenous or retrograde pyelograms in these cases often reveal apparent narrowing just distal to the stone, which can suggest intrinsic ureteropelvic junction obstruction. In the vast majority of cases, however, such patients can be managed successfully by ESWL or percutaneous techniques alone, without a concomitant procedure on the ureteropelvic junction, and follow-up studies show complete resolution of the apparent intrinsic obstruction. Occasionally, however, infundibular stenosis may require reconstruction in the form of infundibuloplasty. In fact, multiple areas of true infundibular stenosis (Fig. 97–61) associated with an extensive staghorn calculus is one of the few primary indications for an anatrophic nephrolithotomy rather than a combined endourologic approach. In such cases, internal reconstruction of the collecting system is an integral part of the operative procedure.

When there is stenosis of adjacent infundibula, infundibuloplasty is performed by joining the sides of each to one another, using running fine chromic sutures. These sutures begin at the level of the renal pelvis and are carried out distally to the involved calyx (Fig. 97–62*A*). In this proce-

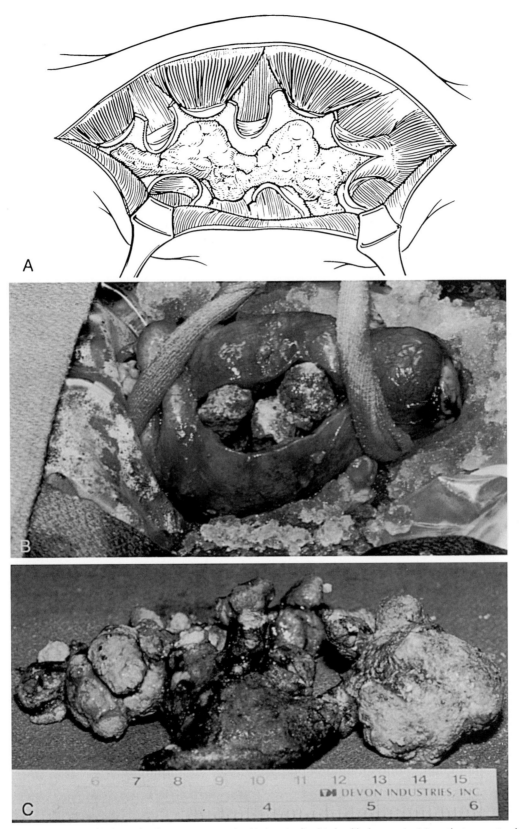

Figure 97–58. *A,* The anterior infundibula and calyces are opened with longitudinal infundibulotomy incisions that are extended from the renal pelvis out toward the calyces. The anterior infundibula are opened on their posterior aspects, whereas the polar infundibula are opened on their medial aspects. Eventually the entire stone is exposed. *B,* Intraoperative view of a mobilized kidney packed in ice slush. The nephrotomy incision has been made and the stone exposed. *C,* Complete staghorn calculus removed with an anatrophic nephrolithotomy.

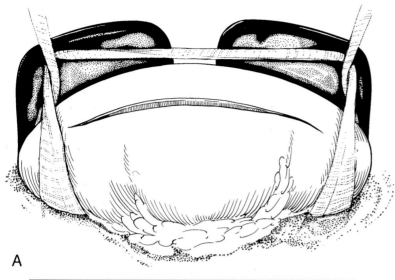

A

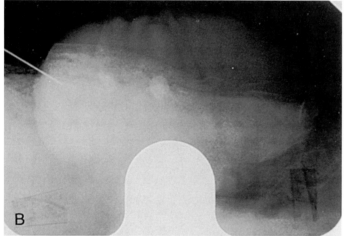

B

Figure 97–59. Before closure of the collecting system, an intraoperative organ film is obtained to exclude the presence of residual stones. X-O-mat KS film is ideal for this purpose. *B*, Residual calculi noted on X-O-mat organ film. Needle localization is a useful adjunct at this time.

dure, the mirroring anterior or posterior infundibula must also be joined. This in effect converts two or more stenotic infundibulocalyceal systems to one large portion of the renal pelvis (Fig. 97–62*B*).

Alternatively, stenosis of isolated infundibula may be managed with infundibulorrhaphy. This involves horizontal

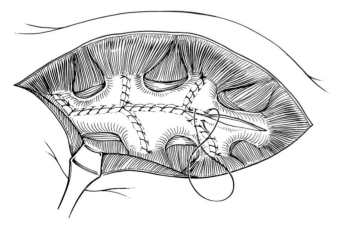

Figure 97–60. Simple closure of the collecting system with running absorbable suture.

closure of the primary vertical infundibulotomy in a Heineke-Mikulicz fashion (Fig. 97–63). This effectively shortens and widens the stenotic infundibulum and brings the renal pelvis closer to the calyx.

After reconstruction of the collecting system, the renal capsule is approximated with running or interrupted 3–0 chromic suture (Fig. 97–64). At this time, an additional 12 to 15 g of mannitol is given intravenously, and the vascular clamp is removed. Whenever possible, Gerota's fascia and the perirenal fat are reapproximated over the nephrotomy incision. External drainage is accomplished with a Penrose or closed-suction drain placed near, but not directly on, the nephrotomy itself. The wound is thoroughly irrigated and then closed in layers in a standard fashion.

Standard Pyelolithotomy

This first use of an incision through the renal pelvis for removal of a stone is credited to Czerny, who performed the procedure in 1880. That approach remained controversial for many years, however, because most surgeons favored nephrolithotomy. In 1913, Lower, at the Cleveland Clinic, popularized the vertical pyelotomy, which became the preferred method for removal of uncomplicated renal pelvic

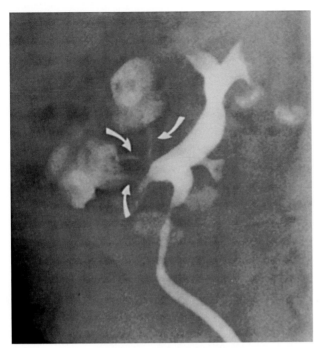

Figure 97–61. Retrograde study in this patient with chronic infection and stones reveals multiple areas of true infundibular stenosis *(arrows).*

calculi. In 1965, Gil-Vernet published his studies on the functional anatomy of the renal pelvic musculature. With this work, he advocated a transverse rather than a vertical pyelotomy. This variation of a pyelolithotomy was rapidly accepted as the approach of choice for the vast majority of patients with renal pelvic calculi. Currently, however, almost any patient whose stone could be removed via a pyelotomy incision can and should be managed with either percutaneous or extracorporeal shock wave technology. Thus, the role for a pyelolithotomy, once performed routinely as part of every urologic surgeon's armamentarium, is now exceedingly limited.

Although a standard pyelolithotomy had been the procedure of choice for most patients with uncomplicated renal pelvic calculi, there are currently only two indications for this procedure. The first is failure of or contraindication to both ESWL and percutaneous nephrostolithotomy. The other indication is the presence of an associated anatomic abnormality requiring open operative intervention, such as ureteropelvic junction obstruction.

A pyelolithotomy is generally performed through a standard flank incision with 12th rib resection or through a dorsal lumbotomy. Either approach allows rapid access to the renal pelvis posteriorly. With either approach, the retroperitoneum is entered and Gerota's fascia opened posteriorly at the lower pole of the kidney. The proximal ureter is identified and surrounded with a vessel loop to prevent distal migration of the stone during the subsequent dissection. The dissection is carried proximally toward the renal pelvis, along the posterior aspect of the ureter (Fig. 97–65*A*). In uncomplicated cases, the kidney need not (and should not) be mobilized any more than is necessary to provide adequate exposure of the renal pelvis. Excessive mobilization may

result in significant perirenal scarring, which could complicate subsequent interventional procedures.

Once the renal pelvis is adequately exposed posteriorly, stay sutures are placed in preparation for a transverse pyelotomy, which should be made well away from the ureteropelvic junction. This pyelotomy is initiated with a curved "banana blade" and extended with a Potts scissors as far as necessary to extract the calculus under direct vision (Fig. 97–65*B*). The stone is then removed with a standard Randall's forceps (Fig. 97–65*C*), and a No. 8 Fr catheter is passed antegrade to the bladder to ensure ureteral patency. With the catheter left in place to prevent distal migration of any stone fragments, the renal pelvis is thoroughly irrigated with saline. The pyelotomy is then closed in a single layer using interrupted or running 4–0 chromic sutures through the full thickness of the renal pelvic wall (Fig. 97–65*D*). If the dissection has been difficult, as may occur in previously operated kidneys, or if the procedure has been performed in the presence of infection, consideration should be given to placement of an internal stent before closure of the pyelotomy. Nephrostomy tubes are indicated only in the rarest of cases but can be considered when there is a question of distal ureteral patency or residual calculi. This then allows

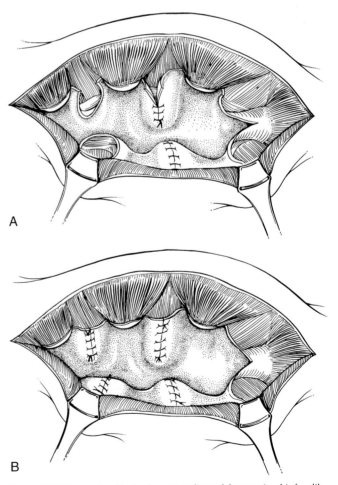

Figure 97–62. *A,* Infundibuloplasty is indicated for repair of infundibular stenosis involving two or more adjacent infundibula. Rather than simple closure of the initial longitudinal infundibulotomies, the sides of the adjacent involved infundibula are sutured to each other. The mirroring anterior or posterior infundibula must also be joined. *B,* This in effect creates a large, well-drained infundibulopelvis.

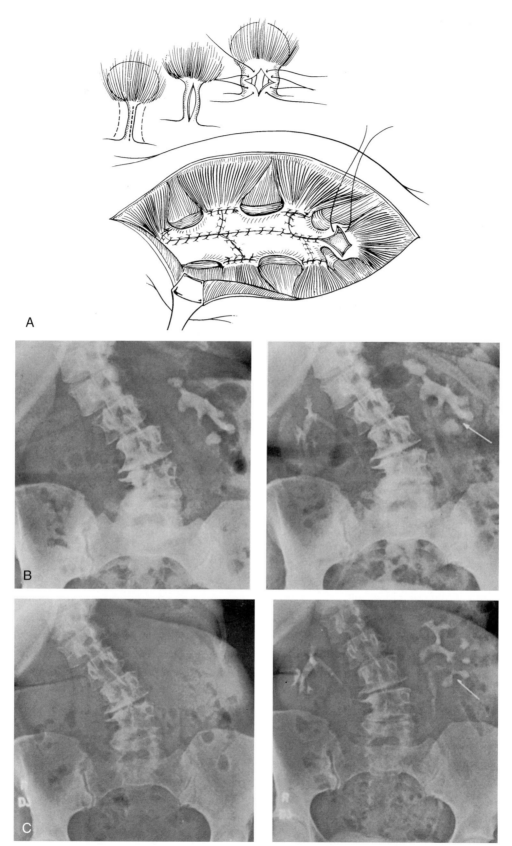

Figure 97–63. *A,* Alternatively, stenosis of isolated infundibula are managed with infundibulorrhaphy. The stenotic infundibulum, which has been opened longitudinally, is closed horizontally in a Heineke-Mikulicz fashion. *B,* Intravenous pyelography (scout and 20-minute film) reveals extensive left staghorn calculus. There is isolated infundibular stenosis of the lower medial infundibulum *(arrow). C,* Following anatrophic nephrolithotomy and infundibulorrhaphy, the lower medial infundibulum is widely patent and the calyx well drained *(arrow).*

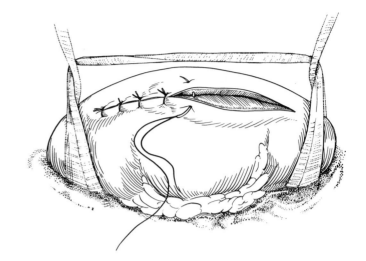

Figure 97–64. Following closure of the collecting system, the renal capsule is approximated with running or interrupted absorbable suture.

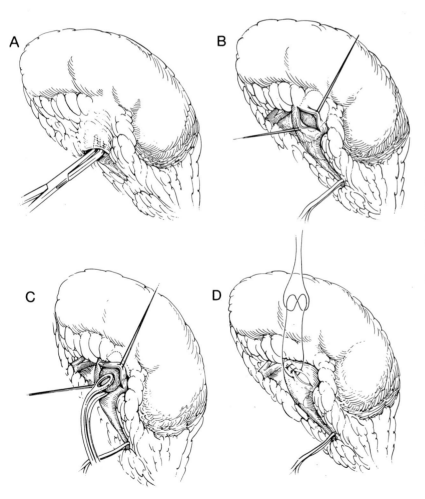

A

B

C

D

Figure 97–65. *A,* For a standard pyelolithotomy, the proximal ureter and renal pelvis are exposed posteriorly. *B,* Stay sutures are placed on the renal pelvis and a horizontal pyelotomy incision is made, well away from the ureteropelvic junction. *C,* The stone is extracted with standard Randall's or other stone forceps. *D,* Following irrigation of the collecting system, the pyelotomy incision is closed with running or interrupted absorbable suture placed through the full thickness of the renal pelvic wall.

easy access in the postoperative period for subsequent antegrade radiographic studies or percutaneous stone extraction. External drainage is routinely provided with a Penrose or closed-suction drain placed near but not on the pyelotomy, and the wound is closed in a standard fashion.

Extended Pyelolithotomy

Gil-Vernet, in 1965, advocated the use of an extended transverse pyelotomy for management of many patients with complicated stone disease, including those with extensive staghorn calculi. His approach was based on studies that defined the renal sinus as a rectangular space containing the intrarenal collecting system, vessels, nerves, and lymphatics. Disse, in 1891, described fibrous extensions from the renal capsule to the posterior renal pelvis that normally act to separate the renal sinus from the retroperitoneal space. An extended pyelolithotomy uses dissection into the renal sinus to gain access to the intrarenal collecting system.

The extended pyelolithotomy was used much more frequently for management of extensive staghorn calculi in Europe than in the United States, where the anatrophic nephrolithotomy was favored. There had been general agreement, however, that **an extended pyelolithotomy was indicated for relatively large renal pelvic stones, especially those in an intrarenal pelvis, and for partial staghorn calculi that extend into one or more infundibula without multiple dumbbell-shaped calyceal extensions or associated infundibular stenosis. Again, however, the vast majority of patients who had been good candidates for an extended pyelolithotomy are now managed with ESWL or percutaneous techniques. Thus, specific indications to use an extended pyelolithotomy as a primary approach again include only failure of or contraindication to both of the less invasive modalities or an associated anatomic abnormality requiring operative intervention.**

The posterior aspect of the renal pelvis is exposed as described for a standard pyelolithotomy. Dissection is then carried into the renal sinus by first incising the fibrous tissue between the posterior hilar lip of the renal parenchyma and the pelvis itself and entering the plane between the renal pelvis and peripelvic fat (Fig. 97–66A). Further exposure of the intrarenal collecting system is accomplished using vein retractors or Gil-Vernet renal sinus retractors to elevate the posterior parenchymal lip while dissecting into the sinus with a moist gauze (Fig. 97–66B). In select cases, temporary occlusion of the renal artery, which should be done in conjunction with local hypothermia, softens the renal parenchyma and allows further exposure of the intrarenal collecting system. This also facilitates palpation of any infundibulocalyceal extensions of the stone (Wulfsohn, 1981).

A transverse pyelotomy is made in a curvilinear fashion between stay sutures, well away from the ureteropelvic junction. The pyelotomy is then extended along both the upper and the lower infundibula. Thus, a renal pelvic flap is created that affords access for removal of the stone (Fig. 97–66C).

If infundibular extensions of the calculus remain after extraction of the pelvic portion, these can generally be removed with Randall's forceps after gentle dilation of the infundibulopelvic junction. Removal of dumbbell-shaped calyceal extensions near the midportion or superior pole of the kidney, however, may require a local nephrotomy made directly over the stone (Fig. 97–66D). Lower pole infundibulolicalyceal extensions, however, may be managed by extending the inferior aspect of the pyeloinfundibulotomy into the posterior parenchyma itself, directly over the lower infundibulum. This infundibulonephrotomy is thus performed in an avascular plane between the junction of the posterior and basilar segments of the kidney (Fig. 97–66E).

When all stone material has been removed, a small catheter is passed antegrade down the ureter, and the intrarenal collecting system is thoroughly irrigated. If multiple stones had been present, an intraoperative x-ray film should be taken to exclude residual fragments. Again, flexible nephroscopy may be a valuable adjunctive maneuver at this time.

Nephrostomy tube drainage is rarely indicated, although if the dissection was extensive, an internal stent may be left in place. The pyelotomy incision is closed as described for a standard pyelotomy, with external drainage routinely provided by a Penrose or closed-suction drain.

Coagulum Pyelolithotomy

The coagulum pyelolithotomy was first reported by Dees in 1943, who used human fibrinogen and clotting globulin to form an extractable cast of the upper collecting system. Since that time, several authors have reported modifications of the coagulum "recipe" in attempts both to simplify the procedure and to reduce the risk of complications (Kalash et al, 1983; Watson et al, 1984). The technique favored at the authors' institution is that described by Fischer and associates in 1980 (Table 97–1). This protocol uses cryoprecipitate as the source of fibrinogen, which is converted to fibrin, with thrombin acting as the catalyst. Calcium chloride increases the tensile strength of the coagulum by neutralizing the citrate (an anticoagulant) present in the cryoprecipitate and acting as a cofactor in the conversion of prothrombin to thrombin. In elective cases, autogenous cryoprecipitate can be used to eliminate entirely the risk of any viral disease transmission (McVary and O'Conor, 1989).

Classically the indication for coagulum pyelolithotomy is the presence of multiple stones scattered throughout the collecting system. Stones located in calyces drained

Table 97–1. PREPARATION OF CONSTITUENTS FOR A COAGULUM PYELOLITHOTOMY

Calcium chloride: 1 g/10 ml (Upjohn ampule = 100 mg/ml)
  Aspirate contents into a sterile 10-ml syringe and warm to room temperature
  Draw required volume directly into a sterile tuberculin syringe: 0.25 ml = 25 mg of calcium chloride
Topical bovine thrombin: 5000 U/vial (Parke-Davis) plus 5 ml of standard diluent = 1000 U/ml
  Using a sterile 10-ml syringe, draw up 1 ml of thrombin and 9 ml of saline (= 100 U/ml)
Cryoprecipitate: Arrives from the blood bank and is thawed to room temperature
  Draw required volume into a sterile syringe

Reprinted by permission of the publisher from Fischer CP, Sonda LP III, Diokno AC: Urology 1980; 15:6. Copyright 1980 by Elsevier Science Inc.

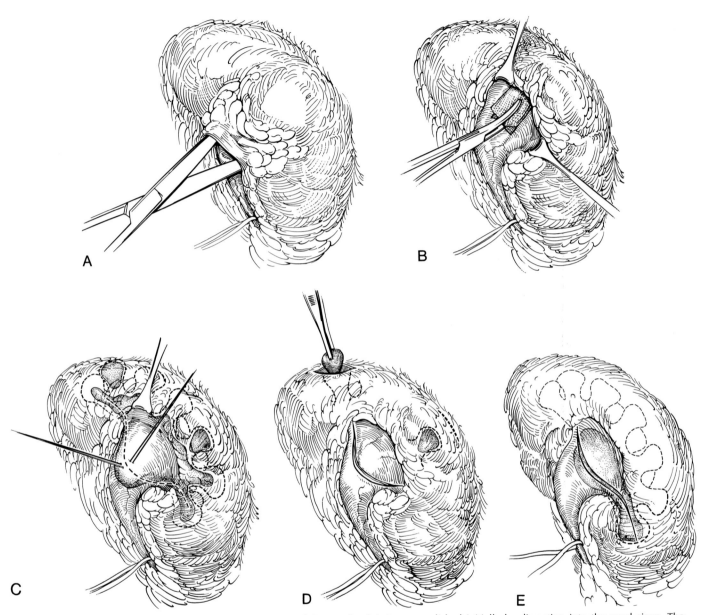

Figure 97–66. *A,* For an extended pyelolithotomy, exposure of the renal pelvis is accomplished initially by dissection into the renal sinus. The correct plane is between the renal pelvis and peripelvic fat. *B,* Gil-Vernet or renal vein retractors are used to elevate the posterior parenchymal lip, while dissection into the sinus is continued with a moist gauze. *C,* Stay sutures are again placed. A curvilinear pyelotomy is then performed and extended through the upper and lower infundibula, creating a renal pelvic flap. The stone is then delivered. *D,* Dumbbell-shaped calyceal extensions of the stone in the superior pole or midportion of the kidney may be removed with a local nephrotomy made directly over the stone. *E,* For lower pole infundibulocalyceal extensions, however, the lower pole infundibulotomy may be extended through the parenchyma itself as an infundibulonephrotomy. This area of the parenchyma is in an avascular plane between the junction of the posterior and basilar arterial segments of the kidney.

by relatively stenotic infundibula are not extracted with this method because the dumbbell-shaped calyceal extensions of the coagulum simply break off as the pelvic portion is removed. Any residual coagulum left this way, however, is of no consequence because it dissolves within 24 to 48 hours in response to the normally present urokinase.

As is true for all stone procedures described in this section, almost any patient who would have been a candidate for a coagulum pyelolithotomy may now be managed with percutaneous or extracorporeal shock wave technology, either alone or in combination. Currently, then, coagulum pyelolithotomy is reserved for patients who fail those techniques or in whom they are contraindicated. Again, however, coagulum pyelolithotomy may be indicated as a primary procedure if there is a coexistent anatomic abnormality requiring open operative reconstruction.

The renal pelvis is exposed in the manner described for a standard or extended pyelolithotomy. An occluding vessel loop is then placed around the proximal ureter to prevent subsequent distal migration of stone fragments or the coagulum itself. The capacity of the pelvicalyceal system is now estimated by puncturing and draining the renal pelvis with a 14-gauge angiocatheter. The pelvis is then refilled to capacity with a measured amount of saline. The volume of coagulum to be prepared is based on the amount of saline required to distend the renal pelvis gently.

The appropriate amount of cryoprecipitate is then drawn up in one large syringe with requisite volumes of thrombin and calcium chloride combined together in a second syringe (Table 97–2). This formulation is based on a ratio 1 ml cryoprecipitate to 2 units thrombin to 1 mg calcium chloride.

The angiocatheter, which has been left in place in the renal pelvis, is used again to drain completely the pelvicalyceal system. Additionally the vessel loop around the proximal ureter can be temporarily loosened to allow complete drainage. This is then resecured before injection of the coagulum.

The thrombin and calcium chloride are then injected into the syringe with the cryoprecipitate, and the mixture, which

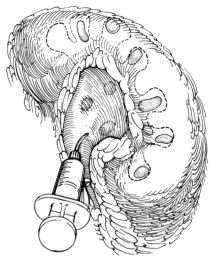

Figure 97–67. The mixture of thrombin, calcium chloride, and cryoprecipitate are injected via a large angiocatheter or red rubber catheter into the renal pelvis. The proximal ureter has been occluded with a vessel loop. The amount of coagulum to be injected has been predetermined, as described in the text.

clots within 45 seconds, is immediately introduced via the angiocatheter into the pelvicalyceal system (Fig. 97–67).

If the measured capacity was correct, there should be complete filling and gentle distention of the renal pelvis. Care must be taken not to overdistend the collecting system because this could result in pyelovenous backflow or, rarely, pulmonary embolus (Pence et al, 1981).

After 5 to 10 minutes, the coagulum is well established. A standard or extended pyelotomy incision is made, and the coagulum is extracted (Fig. 97–68). When performed correctly, the coagulum has formed a cast of the collecting system, with multiple stones trapped within its substance (Fig. 97–69).

Intraoperative radiographs and nephroscopy are then performed as necessary to exclude residual calculi. If internal stents are used, they are placed antegrade at this time, and the renal pelvis is then closed as described earlier. External drainage is routinely provided with a Penrose or closed-suction drain.

Calyceal Diverticulolithotomy

Calyceal diverticula are cavities in the renal parenchyma lined by transitional epithelium. Although communication with a calyx is implied by definition, the communication may not be demonstrable at the time of patient presentation. Failure to demonstrate the area of communication may be the result of localized obstruction from edema or true stricture formation secondary to chronic inflammation or infection. Because calyceal diverticula are associated with localized urinary stasis, they may be a source of stone formation.

As for any upper tract stone, indications to intervene for calculi in calyceal diverticula include pain, obstruction, or infection associated with it. In properly selected patients, stones in calyceal diverticula can be treated successfully with ESWL (Psihramis and Dretler, 1987). The best candidates for that are those in whom the stone is relatively

Table 97–2. CONSTITUENTS USED IN COAGULUM PYELOLITHOTOMY RELATED TO MEASURED VOLUME OF RENAL COLLECTING SYSTEM

Measured Capacity of Renal Pelvis (ml)	Volume of Cryoprecipitate (ml)*	Calcium Chloride (100 mg/ml)	Thrombin (100 U/ml)
10	9	9 (0.10 ml)	18 (0.20 ml)
15	14	14 (0.15 ml)	28 (0.30 ml)
20	19	19 (0.20 ml)	38 (0.40 ml)
25	24	24 (0.25 ml)	48 (0.50 ml)
30	28	28 (0.30 ml)	56 (0.55 ml)
35	33	33 (0.35 ml)	66 (0.65 ml)
40	38	38 (0.40 ml)	76 (0.75 ml)
45	43	43 (0.45 ml)	86 (0.85 ml)
50	48	48 (0.50 ml)	96 (1.00 ml)

(qs with saline to make 1, 2, or 3 ml)

*Ratio of 1 ml cryoprecipitate to 2 U thrombin to 1 mg calcium chloride is maintained regardless of the volume required to fill the collecting system.
qs, Sufficient quantity.
Reprinted by permission of the publisher from Fischer CP, Sonda LP III, Diokno AC: Urology 1980; 15:6. Copyright 1980 by Elsevier Science Inc.

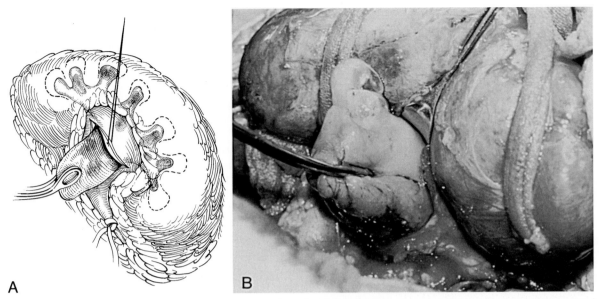

Figure 97–68. *A,* A standard or extended pyelotomy incision is performed and the coagulum extracted. *B,* Intraoperative view of coagulum being extracted through a pyelotomy incision.

small and in whom a patent calyceal communication can be demonstrated by filling of the diverticulum with contrast material by either intravenous or retrograde pyelography (Streem and Yost, 1992). **ESWL remains a controversial treatment for stones in calyceal diverticula, however, because the source of the stone persists, even when the stone itself has been resolved.**

Alternatively a percutaneous approach may be used. Although this is more invasive than ESWL, it does allow the primary problem to be addressed directly with either dilatation or fulguration and obliteration of the diverticular neck (Hulbert et al, 1986). A transureteropyeloscopic approach has also been reported, although experience has been limited. **More recently, laparoscopic techniques have been adapted to management of calyceal diverticular calculi.** This approach is most suitable for those located anteriorly and in which the overlying parenchyma is relatively thin (Ruckle and Segura, 1994).

Currently, indications for open diverticulolithotomy are still changing. **Clearly, failures of or contraindications to both ESWL and percutaneous techniques dictate an open approach. In addition, open surgery may still be recommended as a primary procedure when local anatomy dictates.** To determine the feasibility of a percutaneous or open surgical approach, three-dimensional radiographic localization of the diverticulum is required. Oblique and lateral films obtained during intravenous or retrograde pyelography are helpful and should be a routine part of the evaluation. More precise localization, however, is available through the use of computed tomography scanning (Fig. 97–70).

Exposure of the kidney is accomplished through a standard flank incision, generally with resection of a lower rib. On entering Gerota's fascia, the diverticulum is usually evident by palpation of a soft or fluctuant area in the parenchyma or by inspection alone (Fig. 90–70D). If not, intraoperative radiographs with organ films and needle localization or intraoperative ultrasonography is valuable. In all cases, confirmation that a suspicious area represents the diverticu-

lum can be accomplished with a small-gauge needle, either by aspiration of urine or "sounding" of the calculus.

In most cases, the diverticulum may be managed with marsupialization, similar to that performed for a simple renal cyst. To accomplish this, the thinned parenchyma overlying the diverticulum is excised, and the calculi are removed (Fig. 90–70E). The diverticular neck should then be identified. If this is difficult, injection of methylene blue either intravenously or retrograde via a ureteral catheter placed at the outset of the procedure may prove to be a useful adjunctive maneuver. The neck is then oversewn with absorbable suture, as is the rim of remaining parenchyma (Fig. 97–70F). Alternatively the urothelial lining of the diverticulum may be excised, although this can be associated with bleeding that is difficult to control. Another alternative is simple fulguration of the entire lining and diverticular neck.

A Penrose or closed-suction drain is placed, and the wound is irrigated and closed in a standard fashion.

Partial Nephrectomy

Percutaneous and extracorporeal shock wave technology have virtually eliminated the role of partial nephrectomy for removal of otherwise uncomplicated infundibular or calyceal calculi. Furthermore, as reviewed by Roth and Findlayson in 1983, partial nephrectomy is no longer accepted as a reliable method of preventing stone recurrences. Currently, **partial nephrectomy is considered only when less invasive techniques fail or are contraindicated. In such cases, if the stone is associated with a localized area of irrecoverable renal function, as may occur with chronic obstruction or infection, removal of the diseased portion of the kidney along with the stone may be the best option** (Fig. 97–71). In these cases, partial nephrectomy is performed as described earlier.

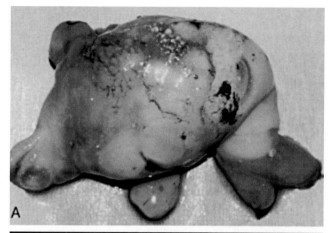

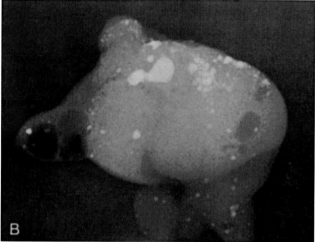

Figure 97–69. *A,* The extracted coagulum forms a cast of the collecting system. Multiple small calculi can be seen near the surface of the coagulum. *B,* An x-ray of the coagulum reveals multiple larger stones trapped within its substance.

Nephrectomy

Nephrectomy is indicated only rarely for management of renal calculi. It does have a role, however, in well-defined patients. **Specifically, if the stone is associated with a nonfunctioning or poorly functioning kidney that is unlikely to recover adequate function with removal of the stone alone, nephrectomy may be the best option.** This is especially true for older patients with significant concomitant medical problems in whom the contralateral kidney is normal. **Obviously, however, if overall renal function would be significantly compromised by nephrectomy, every attempt should be made to salvage the kidney instead.**

Salvageability of the kidney is determined preoperatively with a complete radiographic evaluation. The possibility that irrecoverable loss of renal function has occurred is generally suggested first when an intravenous pyelogram reveals nonvisualization of the involved kidney, even on delayed films (Fig. 97–72A). In such cases, neither a pyelogram nor a nephrogram phase is perceived. A computed tomography scan should then be performed to determine the degree of parenchymal atrophy because significant cortical

thinning is also consistent with irrecoverable loss of function from obstruction (Fig. 97–72B). Finally, a technetium Tc-99m DTPA scan may also be helpful because it can estimate differential renal function (Fig. 97–72C). With a normally functioning contralateral kidney, nephrectomy is considered a primary option when the scan reveals that less than 10% of overall function is being contributed by the involved kidney (Fig. 97–72D).

When there remains any question as to recoverability of function, especially in the presence of obstruction, placement of a percutaneous nephrostomy may provide valuable information. After relief of obstruction and treatment of any associated infection, differential creatinine clearances may be attained and nuclear scans repeated.

Once the decision for nephrectomy is made, it is performed as described earlier. Generally a flank incision is used, although an anterior approach may be preferential in the face of previous flank surgery.

Complications

Bleeding into the collecting system or the perinephric space generally resolves spontaneously. Accordingly, conservative, supportive measures should be the primary treatment. When intervention is required, selective or supraselective transcatheter embolization is the treatment of choice. Surgical exploration is reserved only for refractory cases because it generally results in partial or complete nephrectomy (Assimos et al, 1986).

Persistent fistulas are uncommon and generally imply a devascularized renal segment or distal obstruction. Again, conservatism is the rule because most fistulas resolve as long as they are properly drained. If urinary leakage persists after 10 to 14 days, further investigation is indicated. Intravenous or retrograde pyelography is then used to define the area of extravasation and to rule out distal obstruction. If obstruction is found distal to the level of the fistula, passage of an internal stent generally allows rapid resolution of the problem.

Retained calculi is a discouraging complication that occurs in up to 20% of patients. Those stones, associated with obstruction, pain, chronic infection, or active stone growth, require further intervention. Currently, essentially all residual calculi may be managed with percutaneous techniques or ESWL. Whenever possible, such treatment should be delayed for at least 4 to 6 weeks after the initial operative intervention.

URETEROPELVIC JUNCTION OBSTRUCTION

The diagnosis of ureteropelvic junction obstruction implies functionally significant impairment of urinary transport from the renal pelvis to the ureter. Although most cases are probably congenital in origin, the problem may not become clinically apparent until much later in life (Jacobs et al, 1979). Acquired conditions such as stone disease, postoperative or inflammatory stricture, or urothelial neoplasms may also present clinically with symptoms and

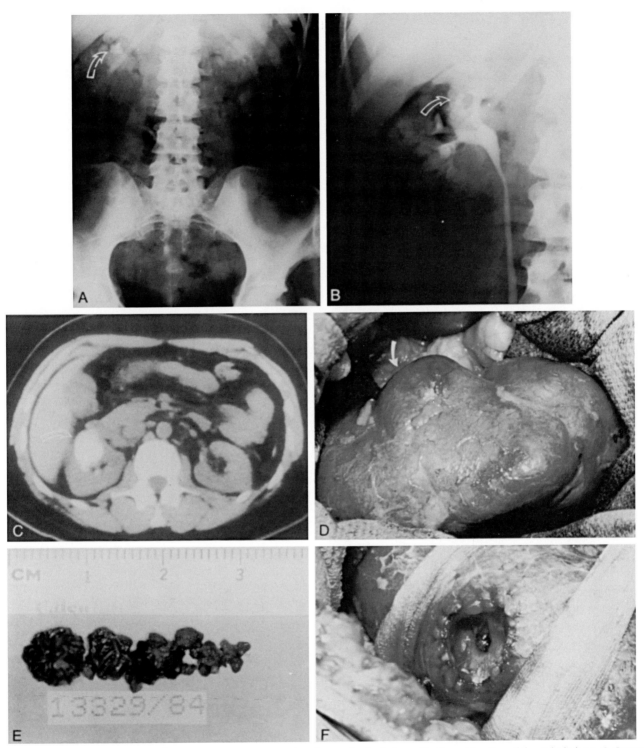

Figure 97–70. *A* and *B,* Scout film and intravenous urogram reveal a cluster of calculi *(arrow)* in the midportion of the right kidney. *C,* Computed tomography (CT) scan in the same patient 1 day following the urogram clearly reveals contrast material remaining in the area surrounding the stones, consistent with a partially obstructed calyceal diverticulum *(arrow).* The anatomic location of this diverticulum in the anterior midportion of the kidney is well visualized on the CT scan. *D,* Intraoperative view of the same patient reveals the calyceal diverticulum bulging from the anterior midportion of the kidney *(arrow).* *E,* Following diverticulotomy, multiple "jackstone" calculi were removed. The configuration of these stones is consistent with urinary stasis as the etiology. *F,* The diverticular cavity is marsupialized. In this intraoperative view, the diverticular neck is evident at the base of the diverticulum. The neck is then oversewn or fulgurated.

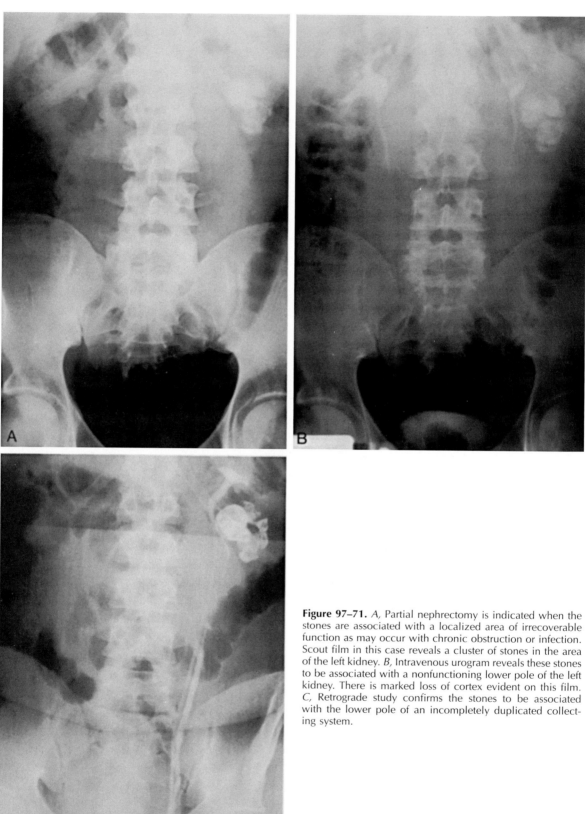

Figure 97–71. *A,* Partial nephrectomy is indicated when the stones are associated with a localized area of irrecoverable function as may occur with chronic obstruction or infection. Scout film in this case reveals a cluster of stones in the area of the left kidney. *B,* Intravenous urogram reveals these stones to be associated with a nonfunctioning lower pole of the left kidney. There is marked loss of cortex evident on this film. *C,* Retrograde study confirms the stones to be associated with the lower pole of an incompletely duplicated collecting system.

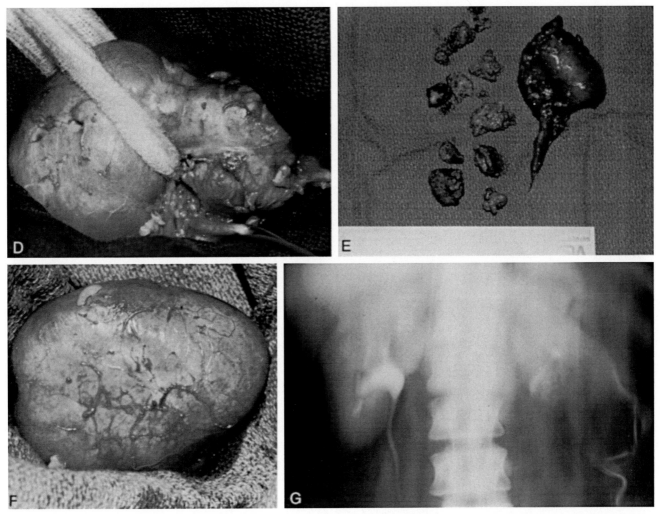

Figure 97–71 *Continued D,* Left renal exploration through the flank confirms marked loss of cortex in the lower pole associated with the stones. *E,* Excised lower pole and stones. *F,* Intraoperative view of the remaining, well-functioning upper pole. *G,* Early postoperative study reveals excellent function in the remaining upper pole on the left side.

signs of obstruction at the level of the ureteropelvic junction. This section is limited primarily to a discussion of the diagnosis and treatment of congenital ureteropelvic junction obstruction, although at times these techniques may be applied appropriately to the management of some of the acquired conditions.

Pathogenesis

Congenital ureteropelvic junction obstruction most often results from intrinsic disease. A frequently found defect is the presence of an aperistaltic segment of the ureter, perhaps similar to that found in primary obstructive megaloureter. **In these cases, histopathologic studies reveal that the normally present spiral musculature has been replaced by abnormal longitudinal muscle bundles or fibrous tissue** (Allen, 1970; Foote et al, 1970; Hanna et al, 1976; Gosling and Dixon, 1978). This results in failure to develop a normal peristaltic wave for propagation of urine from the renal pelvis to the ureter. Recognition that this type of segmental defect is often responsible for ureteropelvic junction obstruction is of utmost importance clinically be-

cause such ureters may appear grossly normal at the time of surgery and in fact may often be calibrated to No. 14 Fr or greater. A less frequent intrinsic cause of congenital ureteropelvic junction obstruction is true ureteral stricture. Such congenital ureteral strictures are most frequently found at the ureteropelvic junction, although they may be located at multiple sites anywhere along the lumbar ureter. Abnormalities of ureteral musculature are again implicated because electron microscopy has demonstrated excessive collagen deposition at the site of the stricture (Hanna et al, 1976).

Intrinsic obstruction at the ureteropelvic junction may also result from kinks or valves produced by infoldings of the ureteral mucosa and musculature (Maizels and Stephens, 1980). In these cases, the obstruction may actually be at the level of the most proximal ureter. This phenomenon appears to result from retention or exaggeration of congenital folds normally found in the ureter of developing fetuses. In some of these cases, the defects are bridged by ureteral adventitia. Grossly, this can appear as external bands or adhesions that appear to be causing the obstruction. In fact, Johnston and associates (1977) reported that lysis of external adhesions can at times re-establish nonobstructed flow without formal pyeloplasty. In the majority of cases, however, these bands

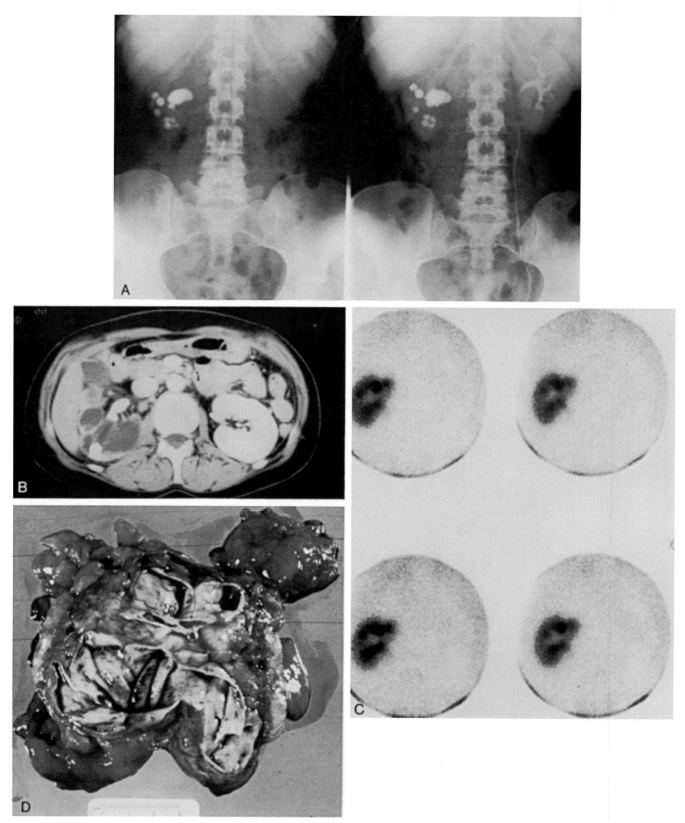

Figure 97–72. *A,* Nephrectomy is indicated for stone disease when the stones are associated with a nonfunctioning or poorly functioning kidney that is unlikely to recover with removal of the stone alone. The contralateral kidney should be normal; otherwise every attempt should be made to salvage the kidney. The scout film in this case reveals multiple right renal calculi. With contrast injection, there is no discernible uptake in the right kidney. The left kidney appears normal. *B,* A computed tomography scan performed with contrast material again reveals the left kidney to be normal. On the right, however, there is only a thin shell of parenchyma. Stones are evident in the renal pelvis and in one of the markedly dilated calyces in this view. *C,* A technetium Tc-99m DTPA scan reveals nonfunction of the right kidney. All of these studies together suggest clearly that this is a nonsalvageable right kidney. *D,* Gross appearance of right kidney following nephrectomy reveals marked cortical loss and parenchymal thinning, confirming that this was a nonsalvageable kidney.

or adhesions are likely to be a secondary phenomenon associated with intrinsic obstruction so that formal pyeloplasty is generally warranted. The presence of these kinks, valves, bands, or adhesions may also produce angulation of the ureter at the lower margin of the renal pelvis in such a manner that as the pelvis dilates anteriorly and inferiorly, the ureteral insertion is carried farther proximally. In these cases, the most dependent portion of the pelvis is inadequately drained, and the apparent "high insertion" of the ureteral ostium is actually a secondary phenomenon (Kelalis, 1976). In at least some cases, however, the high insertion itself is likely the primary obstructing lesion because this phenomenon is found more frequently in the presence of renal ectopia or fusion anomalies (Zincke et al, 1974; Das and Amar, 1984).

Controversy persists regarding the potential role of aberrant vessels in the cause of ureteropelvic junction obstruction. Arteries entering directly into the lower pole of the kidney have been noted in up to one third of cases of ureteropelvic junction obstruction, which represents an incidence higher than that of the normal population. In this setting, these lower pole vessels have often been referred to as *aberrant*. These segmental vessels, however, which may be branches from the main renal artery or arise directly from the aorta, are, in fact, usually normal variants (Stephens, 1982). In a minority of patients, these lower pole vessels cross the ureter posteriorly and as such truly have an aberrant course. In any case, as reviewed by Hanna in 1978, it is unlikely that the associated vessel alone is causing the primary obstruction. Rather, there is probably an intrinsic lesion at the ureteropelvic junction or proximal ureter that causes dilatation and ballooning of the renal pelvis over the polar vessel. **The presence of crossing vessels, however, may have functional significance, especially in the era of less invasive endourologic management** (Van Cangh et al, 1994).

As mentioned earlier, ureteropelvic junction obstruction may also result from acquired lesions. In children, vesicoureteral reflux can lead to upper tract dilatation with subsequent elongation, tortuosity, and kinking of the ureter. In some cases, these changes may only mimic the radiographic findings of true ureteropelvic junction obstruction. True ureteropelvic junction obstruction, however, may definitely coexist with vesicoureteral reflux, although it may be difficult to determine whether the anomalies are merely coincident or whether the upper tract ureteral obstruction has resulted from the reflux (Lebowitz and Johan, 1982). Other acquired causes of obstruction at the ureteropelvic junction include benign tumors such as fibroepithelial polyps (Berger et al, 1982; Macksood et al, 1985), urothelial malignancy, stone disease, and postinflammatory or postoperative scarring or ischemia. For these acquired diseases, the surgical techniques discussed in this section may be useful adjuncts for management of the obstruction as long as the primary problem is also addressed where appropriate.

Patient Presentation and Diagnostic Studies

Ureteropelvic junction obstruction, although generally the result of a congenital problem, can present at any time from prenatally to geriatrically. Classically the most common presentation in neonates and infants was the finding of a palpable flank mass. The current widespread use of maternal ultrasonography, however, has led to a dramatic increase in the number of asymptomatic newborns being diagnosed with hydronephrosis, many of whom are subsequently found to have ureteropelvic junction obstruction (Bernstein et al, 1988; Wolpert et al, 1989). A relatively small number of cases may also be found during evaluation of azotemia, which may result from bilateral obstruction in a functionally or anatomically solitary kidney. Ureteropelvic junction obstruction may also be incidentally found during contrast studies performed to evaluate unrelated anomalies, such as congenital heart disease (Roth and Gonzales, 1983). In older children or adults, intermittent abdominal or flank pain, at times associated with nausea or vomiting, is a frequent presenting symptom. Hematuria, either spontaneous or associated with otherwise relatively minor trauma, may also be an initial symptom. Laboratory findings of microhematuria, pyuria, or frank urinary tract infection might also bring an otherwise asymptomatic patient to the attention of a urologist. Rarely, hypertension may be a presenting finding (Riehle and Vaughan, 1981).

Radiographic studies should be performed with a goal of determining both the anatomic site and the functional significance of an apparent obstruction. Excretory urography remains a cornerstone of radiographic diagnosis. Classically, findings on the affected side include delay in function associated with a dilated pelvicalyceal symptom (Fig. 97–73). If the ureter is visualized, it should be of normal caliber. **In some patients, symptoms may be intermittent, and intravenous pyelography between painful episodes may be normal. In such cases, the study should be repeated during an acute episode when the patient is symptomatic (Nesbit, 1956). Alternatively, provocative testing with a diuretic urogram may allow accurate diagnosis. The patient should be well hydrated and the study then performed by injecting furosemide 0.3 to 0.5 mg/kg intravenously at the time of intravenous urography** (Malek, 1983) (Fig. 97–74).

Ultrasonography has also maintained an important role in diagnosis. Obviously, it is a valuable initial diagnostic study under any circumstance in which overall renal function is inadequate to perform intravenous urography. It should also be performed in any patient in whom the initial intravenous urogram revealed nonvisualization of the affected collecting system to differentiate obstruction from other causes of nonfunction. In some patients, computed tomography scanning may be performed in addition to or in place of ultrasonography, although, in general, the information obtained is similar. Both ultrasonography and computed tomography scanning also have a role in differentiating potential acquired causes of obstruction such as radiolucent calculi or urothelial tumors.

In neonates and infants, the diagnosis of ureteropelvic junction obstruction has generally been suggested either by routine performance of maternal ultrasonography or by the finding of a flank mass. In either setting, renal ultrasonography is usually the first radiographic study performed. Ideally, ultrasonography should be able to visualize dilatation of the collecting system, help differentiate ureteropelvic junction obstruction from multicystic

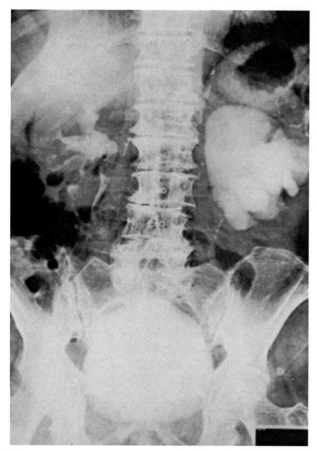

Figure 97–73. Intravenous urogram in this older patient with left flank pain reveals marked hydronephrosis on the left to the level of the ureteropelvic junction consistent with ureteropelvic junction obstruction.

kidney, and help determine the level of obstruction. Ureteropelvic junction obstruction and multicystic kidneys should, in fact, be distinguishable in the majority of cases by ultrasound alone. With ureteropelvic junction obstruction, the pelvis is visualized as a large, medial sonolucent area surrounded by smaller, rounded sonolucent structures representing dilated calyces. At times, dilated calyces are seen connecting to the pelvis via dilated infundibula. Occasionally a solid-appearing renal cortex can be seen surrounding the sonolucent areas or separating the dilated calyces. In contrast, the cysts of multicystic kidneys are visualized as variably sized sonolucent areas in random distribution. Although the cysts may be connected, this is rarely visualized sonographically. Furthermore, little solid tissue is seen, and that which is present has a random distribution among the cysts. **Rarely a large centrally located cyst may cause confusion in the diagnosis** (King et al, 1984). In this setting, nuclear renography should be performed.

Specifically a technetium Tc-99m scan allows differentiation of these two entities. Multicystic kidneys rarely reveal concentration of this isotope. When uptake is seen, the areas of functioning tissue are discrete initially and are usually medial to the bulk of the mass, which itself remains a "cold" area. In contrast, neonatal kidneys with ureteropelvic junction obstruction generally exhibit good concentration of

the isotope. Furthermore, even with severe obstruction in which only a cortical rim remains, uptake of the isotope is seen peripherally in the cortex, again helping to differentiate this from multicystic kidney (King et al, 1984). **A nuclear scan is also of value in predicting recoverability of function in these cases when intravenous urography has revealed nonvisualization. In this setting, a technetium Tc-99m DTPA scan can help predict recoverability of function because essentially all kidneys that function on such scans improve after relief of obstruction** (King et al, 1983). A technetium Tc-99m DTPA scan is also of value in differentiating dilated, nonobstructed systems from those with functional obstruction by combining the renogram with injection of furosemide 0.5 mg/kg to obtain a diuretic renogram. This study allows quantification of the degree of obstruction and, when standard studies are equivocal, helps differentiate the level of obstruction (O'Reilly et al, 1978; Koff et al, 1979, 1980; O'Reilly, 1986) (Fig. 97–75).

The diagnosis of ureteropelvic junction obstruction can generally be made with a high degree of certainty based on the clinical presentation and the results of any one or more of the relatively noninvasive studies just discussed. Retrograde pyelography, however, remains the procedure of choice for confirmation of the diagnosis and demonstration of the exact site and nature of obstruction before surgical repair. In most cases, this study is performed at the time of planned operative intervention to avoid the risk of introducing infection in the face of obstruction. Retrograde pyelography is indicated emergently, however, in any setting in which the ureteropelvic junction obstruction requires acute decompression, such as in the presence of infection or when renal function is compromised. In such cases, an attempt can be made to pass a floppy-tipped guide wire followed by an open-ended ureteral catheter or internal stent to allow decompression of the system and thus better prepare the patient for reconstruction at a later date.

In cases in which cystoscopic retrograde manipulation has been unsuccessful or may be hazardous, such as in male neonates or infants, placement of a percutaneous nephrostomy is an excellent alternative. This allows the performance of antegrade studies, which help define the nature and exact anatomic site of obstruction. It also allows decompression of the system in cases of associated infection or compromised renal function and allows assessment of recoverability of renal function after decompression. Finally, when there remains some doubt as to the clinical significance of a dilated collecting system, placement of percutaneous nephrostomy allows access for pressure perfusion studies. As described and later modified by Whitaker (1973, 1978), the renal pelvis is perfused at 10 ml/minute with normal saline. Alternatively a dilute radiographic contrast solution may be used and the procedure performed under fluoroscopic control. Renal pelvic pressure is monitored during the infusion, and the pressure gradient across the presumed area of obstruction is then determined. During the infusion, the bladder is continuously drained with an indwelling catheter to prevent transmission of intravesical pressures. Renal pelvic pressure ranging up to 12 to 15 cm H_2O during this infusion suggests a nonobstructed system. In contrast, pressures in excess of 15 to 22 cm H_2O are highly suggestive of a functional obstruction. Pressures between these extremes may be nondiagnostic (O'Reilly, 1986).

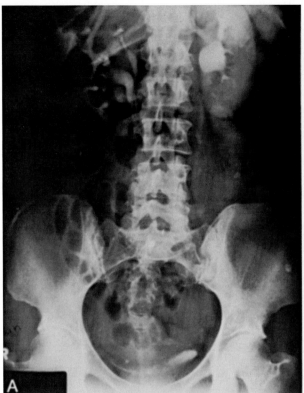

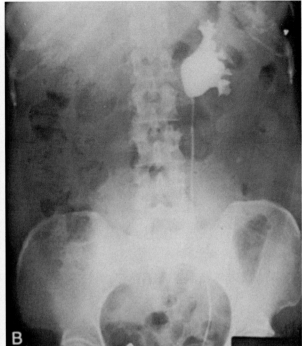

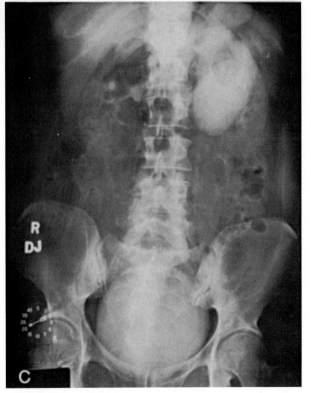

Figure 97–74. *A,* This patient with intermittent left flank pain underwent intravenous urography. The calyces are sharp bilaterally without evidence of obstruction. There is a box-shaped pelvis on the left side, however, which may be associated with intermittent obstruction. *B,* Retrograde study again confirms sharp calyces, although the presence of an extrarenal, box-shaped pelvis is still evident. *C,* This intravenous urogram in the same patient was performed along with injection of intravenous furosemide, which brought out the obvious left-sided ureteropelvic junction obstruction. The patient's symptoms were subsequently relieved with a left pyeloplasty.

Although pressure perfusion studies can often provide valuable information on the functional significance of an apparent obstruction, these studies, similar to any other test currently available for assessing obstruction, can at times be inaccurate owing to variation in renal pelvic anatomy and compliance (Koff et al, 1986). Accordingly, there remains an important role for the urologist as a diagnostician to collate the results of the clinical presentation and multitude of diagnostic studies available to prescribe appropriately the timing and nature of subsequent intervention.

Indications and Options for Intervention

Indications for intervention include the presence of symptoms from the obstruction, impairment of renal function, or development of stones or infection. In such cases, the primary goal of intervention is relief of symptoms and preservation or improvement of renal function. In general, such intervention should be a reconstructive

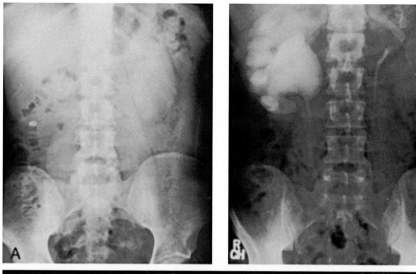

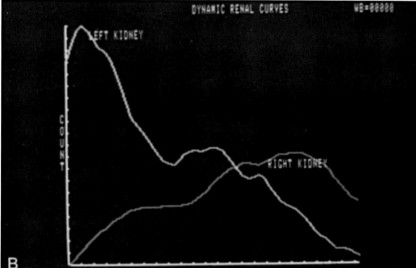

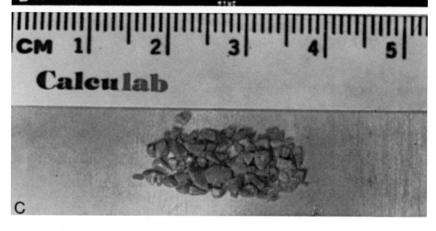

Figure 97–75. *A,* A diuretic renogram can help differentiate dilatation of the collecting system from functional obstruction. This patient had undergone a pyeloplasty as a child several years earlier. Scout film now reveals a 1-cm ovoid calcification in the area of the right lower pole. Following contrast material injection, there is obvious dilatation of the collecting system with a normal-caliber ureter. Differentiation of residual dilatation from ongoing obstruction is of utmost importance in this case before recommending definitive treatment. *B,* A diuretic renogram reveals a shift to the right in uptake by the right kidney, followed by a rapid fall-off of the radionuclide after injection of furosemide. This is consistent with dilatation without obstruction. *C,* The patient was subsequently treated wiht extracorporeal shock wave lithotripsy. Multiple fragments (pictured here) passed without difficulty, and at 1 month follow-up he was symptom-free and stone-free. The ease with which this patient passed these fragments supports the diagnosis of residual dilatation without obstruction.

procedure aimed at restoring nonobstructed urinary flow. This is especially true for neonates, infants, or children, in whom early repair is desirable because these patients have the best chance for improvement in renal function after relief of obstruction (Bejjani and Belman, 1982; Roth and Gonzales, 1983; Wolpert et al, 1989). **Timing of the repair in neonates remains controversial, however, mostly because of difficulty in defining those kidneys truly at risk**

for functional obstruction. In a prospective study of 104 neonates with primary unilateral hydronephrosis suspected of being caused by ureteropelvic junction obstruction, after a mean follow-up of 21 months, only 7 (7%) required pyeloplasty for functional obstruction, defined as a progression of hydronephrosis or a 10% reduction in differential glomerular filtration rate on serial ultrasonography and diuretic renography (Koff and Campbell, 1994). All operated patients had a return of renal function to predetermination levels. Thus, **because of the inaccuracy associated with contemporary diagnostic studies used to assess obstruction in this age group and the low risk of developing obstructive injury, at least some investigators believe it is safe to follow closely neonatal hydronephrosis nonoperatively. Obviously, for a patient of any age, a reconstructive procedure is always indicated whenever overall renal function is compromised because of involvement in a solitary kidney or bilateral disease (Kumar et al, 1988).**

Ureteropelvic junction obstruction may not become apparent until middle age or later (Jacobs et al, 1979). Occasionally, if the patient is asymptomatic and the physiologic significance of the obstruction seems indeterminate, careful observation with serial follow-up studies may be appropriate. The majority of affected patients can, in fact, benefit from reconstructive intervention (Jacobs et al, 1979; Clark and Malek, 1987; O'Reilly, 1989).

When intervention is indicated, the procedure of choice has generally been an open repair of the ureteropelvic junction, that is, a pyeloplasty. Percutaneous procedures (endopyelotomies) clearly have a proven role now that longer-term follow-up has become available in a larger number of patients (Brannen et al, 1988; Motola et al, 1993; Kletscher et al, 1995). Although long-term success rates with percutaneous procedures have not been comparable to standard open pyeloplasty, the results can be improved with careful patient selection. In a prospective study, Van Cangh and associates achieved an overall success rate for endopyelotomy of 73% (Van Cangh et al, 1994). These investigators, however, found the presence of crossing vessels to be a major determinant of outcome (42% success rate versus 86% success rate without a crossing vessel). Furthermore, when endopyelotomy was applied to patients with "a high degree of obstruction," the success rate was only 60% compared with an 81% success rate for those patients with low-grade obstruction. When patients with both a crossing vessel and a high degree of obstruction were excluded from analysis, the success rate improved to 95%, which is comparable to open pyeloplasty.

Other less invasive approaches to management of ureteropelvic junction obstruction have also been introduced into clinical practice, including laparoscopic management (Schuessler et al, 1993), **retrograde ureteroscopic management** (Meretyk et al, 1992), **and cautery wire balloon incision** (Chandhoke et al, 1993). **Again, the potential risks and benefits of these approaches are still being defined** (Streem and Geisinger, 1995), **while the long-term results in a large number of patients are pending.**

Currently the indications for open versus endourologic management of ureteropelvic junction obstruction are still under development. It would seem appropriate, however, to discuss the risks and benefits of all available options with each patient and to advise patients individually based on all the anatomic and functional information available preoperatively. For secondary ureteropelvic junction obstruction, it is the authors' preference to recommend an open approach for any patient who has failed primary endourologic management and an endourologic approach to those who have failed open repair.

Rarely, nephrectomy may be the procedure of choice. Indications for this ablative approach as primary therapy include nonfunction of the involved renal unit on both radiographic and radionuclide studies. In such cases, ultrasonography or computed tomography scanning should also be performed and should reveal only a thin shell of parenchyma remaining. If the potential for salvageability of function is still unclear, an internal stent or percutaneous nephrostomy may be placed for temporary relief of obstruction and renal function studies subsequently repeated. Nephrectomy may also be considered for patients in whom the obstruction has led to extensive stone disease with chronic infection and significant loss of function in the presence of a normal contralateral kidney (Fig. 97–76). Removal of the kidney may also be chosen over reconstruction for patients in whom repeated attempts at repair have already failed and in whom further intervention would therefore be extremely complicated. Again, however, this option should be considered only when the contralateral kidney is normal. Finally, if the patient's life expectancy is limited either because of advanced age or because of significant associated medical problems, nephrectomy may be the best option, again provided that the contralateral kidney is normal.

General Surgical Principles of Pyeloplasty

A variety of incisions have been described for performance of a pyeloplasty. An anterior extraperitoneal approach is preferred by some because it allows an in situ repair with minimal mobilization of the pelvis and proximal ureter. An anterior transperitoneal approach may also be of value, especially in the presence of previous flank incisions or for repair of bilateral disease. Alternatively, a posterior lumbotomy offers direct exposure to the ureteropelvic junction and again allows repair with minimal mobilization of surrounding tissue. Similar to the anterior extraperitoneal approach, however, this is best suited to relatively thin patients in whom there has been no previous ipsilateral surgery. Although a posterior lumbotomy is an attractive approach for an uncomplicated pyeloplasty, its use has been limited, at least in the United States. The authors' preference for most patients undergoing primary surgical repair is an extraperitoneal flank approach. This may be subcostal, although in adults it usually is performed through the bed of the 12th rib or carried anteriorly to its tip. This incision is advantageous in that it is familiar to all urologists and provides excellent exposure without regard to body habitus. In the presence of other renal anomalies associated with the ureteropelvic junction, such as horseshoe or pelvic kidney, alternative incisions may be required because the ureter and pelvis are generally oriented anteriorly. In such cases, anterior extraperitoneal approaches are preferable (Fig. 97–77).

Preoperative drainage of a kidney with ureteropelvic junction obstruction is recommended only in specific instances. These include infection associated with the obstruction or azotemia resulting from obstruction in a solitary kidney or bilateral disease. In either case, preliminary drainage results in better healing with less risk of complications. **Rarely the patient presents with severe, unrelenting pain requiring emergent relief of obstruction, and, again, preliminary drainage is of value.** For any of these problems, such drainage can be provided by passage

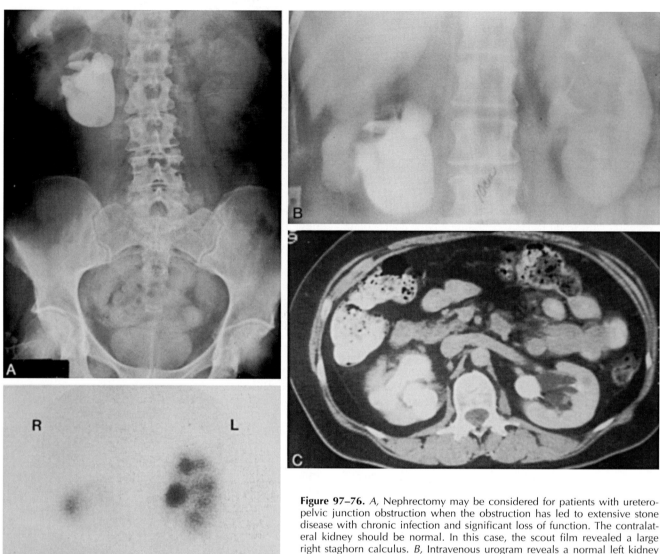

Figure 97–76. *A,* Nephrectomy may be considered for patients with ureteropelvic junction obstruction when the obstruction has led to extensive stone disease with chronic infection and significant loss of function. The contralateral kidney should be normal. In this case, the scout film revealed a large right staghorn calculus. *B,* Intravenous urogram reveals a normal left kidney with some evidence of compensatory hypertrophy. On the right, there is little discernible function and marked parenchymal loss, especially in the midportion and upper pole. *C,* Computed tomography scan in this patient confirms the marked parenchymal loss associated with the stones and obstruction on the right side. *D,* Technetium renogram was performed and revealed that less than 10% of overall function was being contributed by the right kidney. The patient subsequently underwent simple right nephrectomy.

of an internal stent or placement of a percutaneous nephrostomy.

The indications for placement of stents or nephrostomy tubes intraoperatively remain controversial and may be different in pediatric and adult practices. In the past, ureteral stents and nephrostomy tubes were used almost routinely in neonates and infants (Perlmutter et al, 1980). Most pediatric urologists now believe, however, that routine use of stents and nephrostomy tubes is no longer indicated. Rather, such diversion is reserved for complicated cases, such as those involving secondary repairs or active inflammation (Bejjani and Belman, 1982; Roth and Gonzales, 1983; King et al, 1984; Nguyen et al, 1989). For adults, however, the authors' preference is for routine placement of a soft, inert, self-retaining internal stent, which is removed

4 to 6 weeks postoperatively. In contrast to their use in infants or children, such stents in adults are easily removed in an outpatient setting without the need for general anesthesia and without the risk of urethral injury. Also, the adult-size ureter easily accepts these stents without risk of local ischemia. Routine use of internal stents offers several advantages, especially in the early postoperative period. Most importantly, they appear to decrease the amount and length of time of urinary extravasation, thereby decreasing the risk of secondary fibrosis. Decreased extravasation also allows earlier removal of external drains and generally decreases the length of hospital stay. Routine use of internal stents may also help prevent kinking of the ureter in the early postoperative period, which again could lead to secondary obstruction.

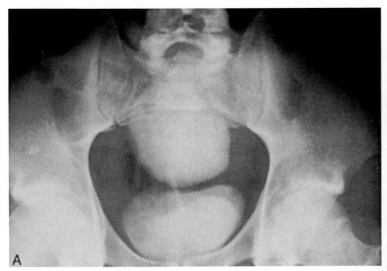

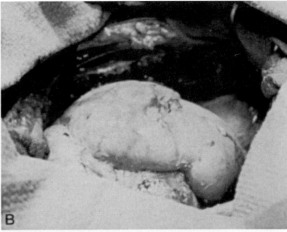

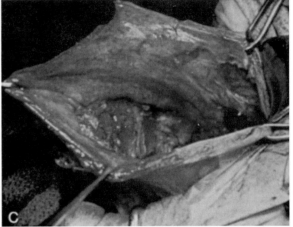

Figure 97–77. *A,* Intravenous urogram in this patient with lower abdominal pain revealed a hydronephrotic left pelvic kidney. *B,* Exposure was obtained through an anterior extraperitoneal Gibson incision in the left lower quadrant. *C,* This incision provided excellent exposure to the anteriorly located renal pelvis and proximal ureter. This intraoperative photograph shows the dilated renal pelvis after it has been opened in preparation for reduction pyeloplasty.

For the uncomplicated pyeloplasty in adults, there appears to be no advantage to using both a nephrostomy and a stent because this may result in a prolonged hospital stay and increased incidence of infection (Wollin et al, 1989). Rather, nephrostomy tubes are reserved for complicated procedures, such as those required for secondary repairs or associated with active inflammation. If a percutaneous nephrostomy had been placed preoperatively, however, it should generally be left indwelling to allow proximal diversion and access for antegrade radiographic studies during the postoperative period.

Although the use of internal stents and nephrostomy tubes remains somewhat controversial, **provision of external drainage from the line of repair is mandatory.** This prevents urinoma formation and its possible subsequent disruption of the suture line, scarring, or sepsis. Such external drainage is accomplished with a Penrose or closed-suction drain placed near but not on the suture line and brought out through a separate stab incision.

In the past, proximal diversion was often accomplished with a slash pyelotomy made transversely in the renal pelvis above the suture line (Schaeffer and Grayhack, 1986). Theoretically, this vented the suture line and allowed adequate drainage during the period of edema associated with the repair. This practice is now rarely used, however, because most reconstructive surgeons believe the increased extravasation, although perhaps "controlled," leads to excessive fibrosis and scar formation.

Historical Notes

Historical aspects of ureteropelvic junction repair have been reviewed by Kay (1989) and Schaeffer and Grayhack (1986). The first reconstructive procedure was performed by Trendelenberg in 1886, although the patient died of postoperative complications. Kuster is credited with the first successful pyeloplasty. In 1891, he divided the ureter and reanastomosed it to the renal pelvis, thus apparently performing the first dismembered pyeloplasty. His technique, however, was prone to recurrent stricture. In 1894, Fenger applied the Heineke-Mickulicz principle to reconstruction of the ureteropelvic junction. This technique involves transverse closure of a longitudinal incision. Unfortunately, for repair of ureteropelvic junction obstruction, this technique can cause shortening of the suture line on one side of the ureteropelvic junction, thus resulting in buckling or kinking with recurrent obstruction. Flap techniques were introduced by Schwyzer in 1923. His Y-V pyeloplasty was then modified successfully by Foley in 1937. This procedure was best applied to high insertions and was essentially unsuitable when the ureteropelvic junction itself was already in a dependent position. Subsequently, flap techniques were developed that were more universally applicable. These included the spiral flap of Culp and DeWeerd in 1951 and the vertical flap of Scardino and Prince reported in 1953. Later, Thompson and associates reported the use of a renal capsular flap for complex cases in which an adequate amount of renal pelvis is not available for repair (Thompson et al, 1969).

Nesbit (1949) modified Kuster's dismembered procedure by using an elliptic anastomosis to decrease the likelihood of stricture formation at the site of repair. Also in 1949, Anderson and Hynes, two English surgeons, described their modification of this technique, which involved anastomosis of the spatulated ureter to a projection of the lower aspect of the pelvis after a redundant portion was excised.

A separate issue has been the development of techniques for repair of extensive or multiple strictures of the proximal ureter. These techniques of intubated ureterotomy were popularized by Davis in 1943 but had been previously described by Fiori in 1905, Albarran in 1909, and Keyes in 1915.

Although a variety of procedures have been described for management of the obstructed ureteropelvic junction, there are several basic principles that must always be applied to ensure successful repair. For any technique, the resultant anastomosis should be widely patent and performed in a watertight fashion without tension. Finally, the reconstructed ureteropelvic junction should allow a funnel-shaped transition between the pelvis and ureter that is in a position of dependent drainage.

Dismembered Pyeloplasty

Currently, **most urologists rely on a variation of a dismembered pyeloplasty for the majority of patients because this procedure is almost universally applicable for repair of the ureteropelvic junction. Specifically, it can be used regardless of whether the ureteral insertion is high on the pelvis or already dependent. It also allows** reduction of a redundant pelvis when necessary or straightening of a lengthy or tortuous proximal ureter. In addition, anterior or posterior transposition of the ureteropelvic junction can be accomplished when the obstruction is associated with accessory or aberrant lower pole vessels. Finally, in contrast to all flap techniques, only a dismembered pyeloplasty allows complete excision of the anatomically or functionally abnormal ureteropelvic junction. **A dismembered pyeloplasty is, however, poorly suited to ureteropelvic junction obstruction associated with lengthy or multiple proximal ureteral strictures or to patients in whom the ureteropelvic junction is associated with a small, relatively inaccessible intrarenal pelvis.**

Exposure to the ureteropelvic junction is obtained by first identifying the proximal ureter in the retroperitoneum. The ureter is dissected cephalad to the renal pelvis, leaving a large amount of periureteral tissue to preserve ureteral blood supply. A marking stitch of fine suture is then placed on the lateral aspect of the proximal ureter, below the level of the obstruction, to maintain proper orientation subsequently for the repair. In a similar fashion, the medial and lateral aspects of the dependent portion of the renal pelvis are delineated with traction sutures (Fig. 97–78A). The ureteropelvic junction is excised, and the proximal ureter is then spatulated on its lateral aspect. The apex of this lateral, spatulated aspect of the ureter is brought to the inferior border of the pelvis, while the medial side of the ureter is brought to the superior edge of the pelvis (Fig. 97–78B). The anastomosis is then performed with fine interrupted or running absorbable sutures, placed full thickness through the ureteral and renal pelvic walls, in a watertight fashion (Fig. 97–78C). As mentioned earlier, the authors' preference for adult patients is to perform the anastomosis routinely over an internal

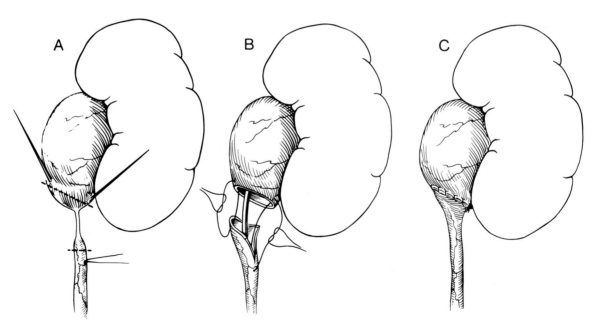

Figure 97–78. *A,* Traction sutures are placed on the medial and lateral aspects of the dependent portion of the renal pelvis in preparation for dismembered pyeloplasty. A traction suture is also placed on the lateral aspect of the proximal ureter, below the level of obstruction. This helps maintain proper orientation for the subsequent repair. *B,* The ureteropelvic junction is excised. The proximal ureter is spatulated on its lateral aspect. The apex of this lateral, spatulated aspect of the ureter is then brought to the inferior border of the pelvis, whereas the medial side of the ureter is brought to the superior edge of the pelvis. *C,* The anastomosis is then performed with fine interrupted or running absorbable sutures placed full thickness through the ureteral and renal pelvic walls in a watertight fashion. In general, the authors prefer to leave an indwelling internal stent for adult patients. The stent is removed 4 to 6 weeks later.

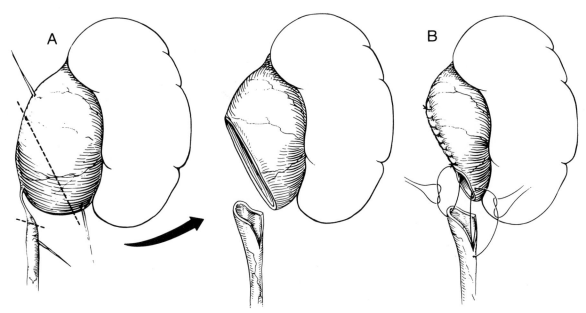

Figure 97–79. *A,* For large or redundant renal pelves, a reduction pyeloplasty is performed by excising the redundant portion between traction sutures. *B,* The cephalic aspect of the pelvis is then closed with running absorbable suture down to the dependent portion. The dependent aspect of the pelvis is then anastomosed to the proximal ureter as described in Figure 97–78.

stent, which is left indwelling. Alternatively the anastomosis can be performed over a ureteral catheter, which is simply removed before the last few sutures are placed.

If the renal pelvis is particularly large or redundant, a reduction pyeloplasty is performed by excising the redundant portion of the pelvis (Fig. 97–79*A*). The cephalic aspect of the pelvis is then closed with running absorbable sutures down to the dependent portion, which is subsequently joined to the ureter (Fig. 97–79*B*).

When aberrant or accessory lower pole vessels are found in association with the ureteropelvic junction obstruction, a dismembered pyeloplasty allows proper repositioning of the ureteropelvic junction in relation to these vessels (Fig. 97–80).

Foley Y-V Plasty

The Foley Y-V plasty was originally designed for reconstruction of a ureteropelvic junction obstruction associated with a high ureteral insertion. As for other flap techniques, however, its use has generally been supplanted by the more versatile dismembered pyeloplasty. Similar to other nondismembered flap techniques, the Foley Y-V plasty is specifically contraindicated when transposition of lower pole vessels is required. The Foley Y-V plasty is also of little value when significant reduction of renal pelvic size is required.

The pelvis and proximal ureter are exposed as previously described. A widely based triangular or V-shaped flap is

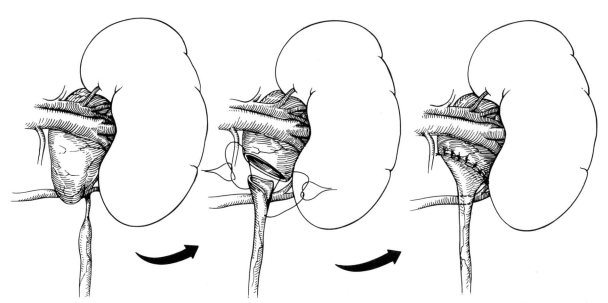

Figure 97–80. When aberrant or accessory lower pole vessels are found in association with the ureteropelvic junction obstruction, a dismembered pyeloplasty allows transposition of the ureteropelvic junction in relation to the vessels.

outlined with methylene blue or other tissue marker or fine stay sutures. The base of the V is positioned on the dependent, medial aspect of the renal pelvis and the apex at the ureteropelvic junction. The incision from the apex of the flap (the stem of the Y) is then carried out along the lateral aspect of the proximal ureter. The incision in the ureter should be long enough to traverse completely the area of stenosis and extend for several millimeters into the normal-caliber ureter (Fig. 97–81A).

The pelvic flap and ureterotomy are then developed. A fine scalpel blade is used for the initial pelvic incision. A Potts or fine Metzenbaum scissors completes the flap and ureterotomy (Fig. 97–81B). An internal stent is placed and the repair performed over it. First, the apex of the pelvic flap is brought to the apex (inferior aspect) of the ureterotomy incision using fine absorbable suture. The posterior walls are then approximated using interrupted or running suture (Fig. 97–81C). As for all pyeloplasty repairs, however, the authors' preference is generally for interrupted suture technique because they believe this decreases the likelihood of pursing or buckling of the suture line. Inter-

rupted technique is also less likely to cause local ischemia. Anastomosis of the anterior walls is then accomplished, thus completing the repair (Fig. 97–81D).

Culp-DeWeerd Spiral Flap Technique

The Culp-DeWeerd spiral flap is best suited to large, readily accessible extrarenal pelves in which the ureteral insertion is already in a dependent, oblique position. Although most such patients are generally also good candidates for a standard or reduction dismembered pyeloplasty, **the spiral flap may be of particular value when the ureteropelvic junction obstruction is associated with a relatively long segment of proximal ureteral narrowing or stricture.**

The spiral flap is outlined with a broad base situated obliquely on the dependent aspect of the renal pelvis. To preserve blood supply to the flap, the base is situated in a position anatomically lateral to the ureteropelvic junction, that is, between the ureteral insertion and the renal parenchyma. The flap itself may be spiraled posteriorly to anteriorly or vice versa. In either case, the anatomically medial line of incision (furthest from the parenchyma) is carried down the ureter, completely through the obstructed segment (Fig. 97–82A). Proper placement of the apex of the flap is determined by the length of flap needed. This is, in turn, a function of the length of proximal ureter to be bridged. The longer the flap required, the further away is the apex from the base. To preserve vascular integrity of the flap, however, the ratio of flap length to width should not exceed 3:1. In general, the outline of the flap should be made longer than what may initially be perceived as necessary because the flap shrinks once the pelvis is incised. If the flap is then too long, excess length can safely be reduced by trimming back the apex, thus keeping blood supply intact. Once the flap is developed, the apex is rotated down to the inferiormost aspect of the ureterotomy (Fig. 97–82B). The anastomosis is then performed over an internal stent, again using fine absorbable sutures (Fig. 97–82C).

Scardino-Prince Vertical Flap

The Scardino-Prince vertical flap technique has limited application today. It may appropriately be used only when a dependent ureteropelvic junction is situated at the medial margin of a large, square (box-shaped) extrarenal pelvis (Fig. 97–83A). **Its use in most instances has been supplanted by a standard dismembered pyeloplasty, although the verticle flap may be preferable for relatively long areas of proximal ureteral narrowing.** Although the verticle flap can bridge stenotic areas of average length, the procedure cannot produce as long a flap, and thus bridge as long a stricture, as the spiral flap.

The vertical flap technique itself is similar to the spiral flap procedure except that the base of the flap is situated more horizontally on the dependent aspect of the renal pelvis, between the ureteropelvic junction and the renal parenchyma. The flap itself is formed by straight incisions converging from the base vertically to the apex on either the anterior or posterior aspects of the renal pelvis. Again, the site of the apex, and thus the length of the flap, is determined

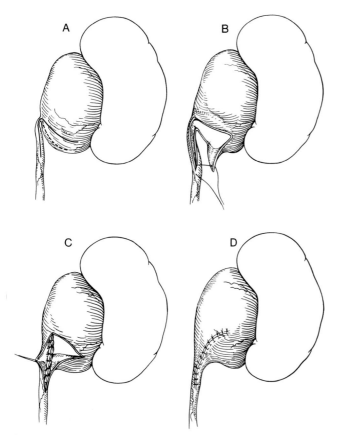

Figure 97–81. *A,* A Foley Y-V plasty is best applied to a ureteropelvic junction obstruction associated with a high insertion of the ureter. The flap is outlined with tissue marker or stay sutures. The base of the V is positioned on the dependent, medial aspect of the renal pelvis and the apex at the ureteropelvic junction. The incision from the apex of the flap, which represents the stem of the Y, is then carried along the lateral aspect of the proximal ureter well into an area of normal caliber. *B,* The flap is developed with a fine scissors. The apex of the pelvic flap is then brought to the inferiormost aspect of the ureterotomy incision. *C,* The posterior walls are then approximated using interrupted or running fine absorbable suture. *D,* The anastomosis is completed with approximation of the anterior walls of the pelvic flap and ureterotomy.

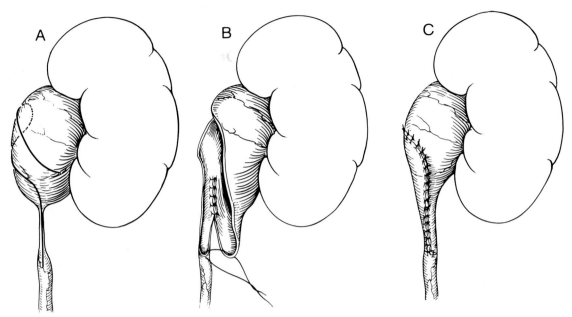

Figure 97–82. *A,* A spiral flap may be indicated for relatively long areas of proximal ureteral obstruction when the ureteropelvic junction is already in a dependent position. The spiral flap is outlined with the base situated obliquely on the dependent aspect of the renal pelvis. The base of the flap is positioned anatomically lateral to the ureteropelvic junction, between the ureteral insertion and the renal parenchyma. The flap is spiraled posteriorly to anteriorly or vice versa. The anatomically medial line of incision is carried down completely through the obstructed proximal ureteral segment into normal-caliber ureter. The site of the apex for the flap is determined by the length of flap required to bridge the obstruction. The longer the segment of proximal ureteral obstruction, the farther away is the apex because this makes the flap longer. To preserve vascular integrity to the flap, however, the ratio of flap length to width should not exceed 3:1. *B,* Once the flap is developed, the apex is rotated down to the inferiormost aspect of the ureterotomy. *C,* The anastomosis is then completed, usually over an internal stent, again using fine absorbable sutures.

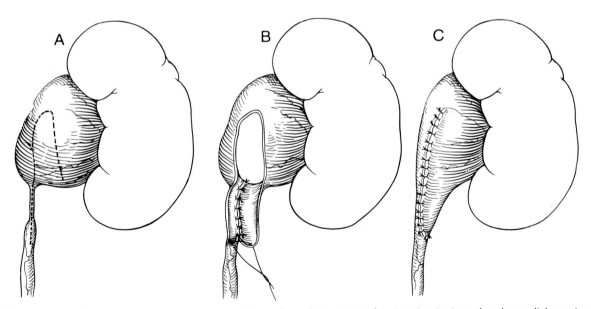

Figure 97–83. *A,* The vertical flap technique may be used when a dependent ureteropelvic junction is situated at the medial margin of a large, box-shaped extrarenal pelvis. In contrast to the spiral flap, the base of the vertical flap is situated more horizontally on the dependent aspect of the renal pelvis, between the ureteropelvic junction and the renal parenchyma. The flap itself is formed by two straight incisions converging from the base vertically up to apex on either the anterior or the posterior aspect of the renal pelvis. As for the spiral flap, the position of the apex determines the length of the flap, which should be a function of the length of the proximal ureter to be bridged. The medial incision of the flap is carried down the proximal ureter completely through the strictured area into normal-caliber ureter. *B,* The apex of the flap is rotated down to the inferiormost aspect of the ureterotomy. *C,* The flap is then closed by approximating the edges with interrupted or running fine absorbable sutures.

by the length of proximal ureter to be bridged. The medial incision is carried down the proximal ureter, completely through the strictured area and into normal-caliber ureter (Fig. 97–83*B*). The flap is developed with fine scissors. The apex of the flap is then rotated down and sutured to the inferiormost aspect of the ureterotomy. Closure of the flap is then completed with interrupted or running fine absorbable sutures (Fig. 97–83*C*).

Intubated Ureterotomy

The intubated ureterotomy, popularized by Davis in 1943, is rarely used today. Its primary role was for repair of lengthy or multiple ureteral strictures. If these strictures are found in association with ureteropelvic junction obstruction, the intubated ureterotomy may be combined with any of the standard pyeloplasty techniques. At least in principle, however, the Davis intubated ureterotomy is best combined with a spiral flap procedure. Compared with the vertical flap, the spiral flap can be made longer, thus allowing more of the strictured area to be bridged by a pelvic flap. Thus, a shorter area is left to rely on healing by secondary intention. Any flap technique, however, is preferable to a dismembered repair, at least in regard to preservation of blood supply and subsequent healing.

A flap is outlined as described earlier, with the ureterotomy to be carried completely through the long, strictured area (Fig. 97–84*A*). The flap is then developed, taking care to use minimal dissection of the ureter to preserve its blood supply. In contrast to uncomplicated pyeloplasties, nephrostomy tube drainage is routinely accomplished in these cases to divert the urine and prevent subsequent urinoma formation. Nephrostomy drainage in these cases also allows access for antegrade radiographic studies as necessary during the postoperative period. Originally the ureteral intubation was accomplished with a stenting catheter that was placed across the strictured area to the distal ureter or bladder. Proximally, it was brought out through the cortex alongside a nephrostomy tube. Currently, most urologists use a self-retaining, soft, inert internal ureteral stent instead. The apex of the flap is brought as far down as possible over the stent on the ureterotomy, and the flap is closed with interrupted or running absorbable suture (Fig. 97–84*B*). The distal aspect of the ureterotomy is left open to heal secondarily by ureteral regeneration, although a few fine absorbable sutures may be placed loosely to keep the sides of the ureter in accurate relation to the stent (Fig. 97–84*C*).

A nephrostogram should be obtained after 6 to 8 weeks. If there is no extravasation, the internal stent is removed cystoscopically, and antegrade radiographic studies are then repeated. When adequate ureteral patency has been ensured, without evidence of extravasation, the nephrostomy tube is clamped and subsequently removed.

Salvage Procedures

Management of the failed pyeloplasty is a challenging problem. At times, successful reconstruction can be achieved

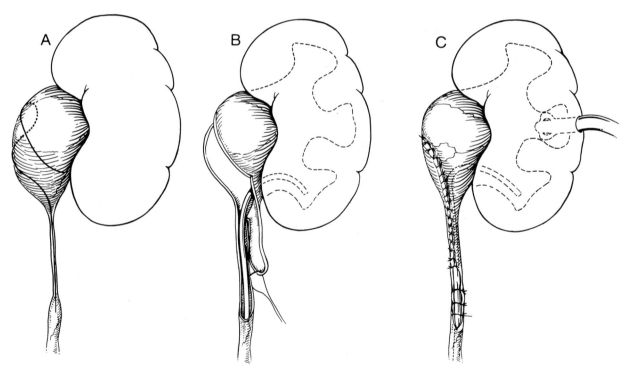

Figure 97–84. *A,* The intubated ureterotomy may be of value when a ureteropelvic junction obstruction is associated with extremely long or multiple ureteral strictures. A spiral flap is outlined and developed as described in Figure 97–82. The ureterotomy incision is carried completely through the long strictured area or through each of the multiple areas of stricture. *B,* The flap is developed, taking care to use minimal dissection of the ureter to preserve its blood supply. In contrast to uncomplicated repairs, nephrostomy tube drainage is used routinely. A self-retaining, soft, inert internal ureteral stent is then placed and positioned proximally in the renal pelvis or lower infundibulum and distally in the bladder. The apex of the flap is then brought as far down as possible over the stent on the ureterotomy, and the flap is closed with interrupted or running absorbable suture. *C,* The distal aspect of the ureterotomy is left open to heal secondarily by ureteral regeneration. A few fine absorbable sutures may be placed loosely to keep the sides of the ureter in apposition with the stent.

using one of the flap or dismembered techniques already described. In this setting, the secondary reconstruction is aided by preliminary cystoscopic or antegrade placement of a ureteral catheter to help intraoperative identification and subsequent dissection of the ureter and renal pelvis. In these cases, there is often a relatively long length of proximal ureteral stenosis to repair. Accordingly, in contrast to primary repairs in which dissection of the kidney and ureter is to be minimized, wide mobilization of both is generally a necessity. This allows the kidney to be displaced downward and the ureter upward, thus helping to bridge the area of stenosis and perform the secondary pyeloplasty without tension.

Several other options are available for these secondary, often complex repairs. Many of these surgical alternatives are those generally available for any extensive ureteral problem. The standard options for preserving renal function include an ileoureteral replacement and autotransplantation with a Boari flap pyelovesicostomy. For cases in which function of the involved kidney is already significantly compromised and the contralateral kidney is normal, consideration can also be given to nephrectomy, especially when previous attempts at salvage have already failed or the repair would be particularly complex for any reason. Other options, more specific for the failed pyeloplasty, include the renal capsule flap and ureterocalycostomy.

Renal Capsular Flap Technique

The use of a renal capsule flap for repair of complicated or secondary ureteropelvic junction obstruction was described by Thompson and associates in 1969. The kidney itself can be approached anteriorly or posteriorly, depending on local anatomy and type of previous surgery, although a posterior approach through the flank is generally preferable. In either case, the corresponding surfaces of the kidney, renal pelvis, and ureter are exposed. An inverted V- or U-shaped flap is then outlined on the renal capsule, with a wide base oriented medially at the renal sinus. A vertical incision is then made through the ureteropelvic junction into normal proximal ureter (Fig. 97–85A). The apex of the flap is brought down to the inferior aspect of the ureterotomy.

The edges of the pyeloureterotomy incision are then sutured to the corresponding sides of the flap with running or interrupted fine absorbable sutures (Fig. 97–85B). These complex repairs should generally include routine use of both nephrostomy tubes and internal stents.

Ureterocalycostomy

Anastomosis of the proximal ureter directly to the lower calyceal system has become a well-accepted salvage technique for the failed pyeloplasty (Ross et al, 1990). **Ureterocalycostomy may also be used as a primary reconstructive procedure whenever a ureteropelvic junction obstruction or proximal ureteral stricture is associated with a relatively small intrarenal pelvis or when the ureteropelvic junction is associated with rotational anomalies such as horseshoe kidney** (Levitt et al, 1981). In those cases, it may be of particular value because it provides completely dependent drainage. Many of the indications for a ureterocalycostomy are illustrated in Figure 97–86.

The ureter is isolated in the retroperitoneum and dissected proximally as far as possible with a large amount of periureteral tissue. For secondary procedures, extensive scarring may preclude identification and dissection of the renal pelvis itself (Fig. 97–87A). The kidney is then mobilized as much as necessary to gain access to the lower pole. An important technical point to be emphasized is that the parenchyma overlying the lower pole calyx must be resected rather than simply incised (Couvelair et al, 1964). The amount of parenchyma to be removed depends on the extent of cortical thinning already present. Again, however, a simple nephrotomy over a calyx is not adequate because a secondary stricture may result.

The proximal ureter is spatulated laterally and the ureterocalyceal anastomosis then performed over an internal stent. Consideration should also be given to leaving a nephrostomy tube in these cases. The first suture is placed at the apex of the ureteral spatulation and lateral wall of the calyx, and the second one is placed 180 degrees away. The remainder of the anastomosis is then completed using an interrupted, open suture technique. That is, each suture is placed but is left

Figure 97–85. *A,* A renal capsule flap may be valuable as a salvage procedure in the presence of failed previous attempts at repair or whenever there is inadequate renal pelvis associated with the ureteropelvic junction obstruction. An inverted V-shaped or U-shaped flap is outlined on the renal capsule. The base of this flap is oriented medially at the renal sinus to preserve its blood supply. A vertical ureteropyelotomy is then made completely through the ureteropelvic junction into normal-caliber proximal ureter. *B,* The renal capsule flap is developed by sharp dissection and the apex brought down to the inferior aspect of the ureterotomy, over an internal stent. Nephrostomy tube drainage is also of value in these complicated repairs. The edges of the pyeloureterotomy incision are then sutured to the corresponding sides of the flap with running or interrupted fine absorbable suture.

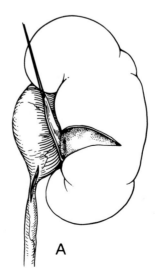
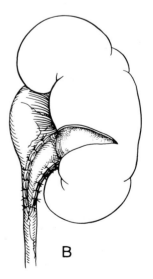

A   B

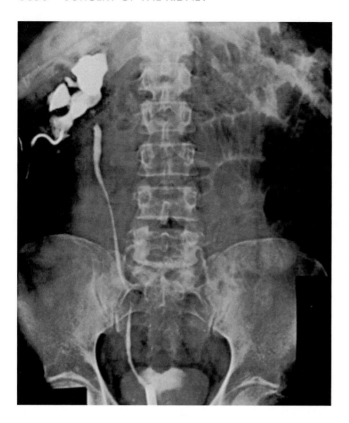

Figure 97–86. This man was referred with persistent urinary drainage following an open pyelolithotomy and pyeloplasty. A percutaneous nephrostomy was placed. Several indications for ureterocalycostomy are demonstrated by this simultaneous antegrade and retrograde pyelogram. These include the fact that the patient has undergone previous surgery, suggesting that there will be a significant amount of peripelvic fibrosis. The obstruction is also associated with an intrarenal pelvis. Finally, there is a relatively long gap between the renal pelvis and nonobstructed proximal ureter. Note, however, that the normal proximal ureter reaches the lower calyx without tension, especially if the kidney is mobilized downward and the ureter dissected distally for additional length.

untied until the final one is in place (Fig. 97–87B). This allows a more accurate anastomosis to be performed under direct vision. When the full set of circumferential sutures has been placed, they are secured down together (Fig. 97–87C and D).

Whenever possible, the renal capsule is closed over the cut surface of the parenchyma but not close enough to the anastomosis itself to compromise its lumen by extrinsic compression. Rather the anastomosis should be protected by surrounding it with perinephric fat or a peritoneal or omental flap (Fig. 97–87E).

Postoperative Care and Management of Complications

In general, external drains are advanced and removed 24 to 48 hours after urinary drainage has ceased. When internal stents have been placed, the authors' preference is to remove them on an outpatient basis in 4 to 6 weeks. If a nephrostomy tube is present, a nephrostogram is obtained no sooner than 7 to 10 days postoperatively or even later for particularly complicated repairs. When that study demonstrates a patent anastomosis without obstruction or extravasation, the tube is clamped for 12 to 24 hours and removed if there is no flank pain, fever, or leakage around the tube.

If an internal stent had not been left indwelling and urinary drainage persists after 7 to 10 days or recurs after the external drain has been removed, retrograde studies should be obtained and an attempt made to pass an internal stent. The problem then generally resolves immediately, and, again, the internal stent is removed 1 month later. If an attempt at passing an internal stent is unsuccessful, a percuta-

neous nephrostomy is placed and then managed as if it had been left intraoperatively. If drainage then persists despite nephrostomy tube placement, an internal or internal/external stent should be placed in an antegrade fashion. At times, despite appropriate use of stents, drains, and nephrostomy tubes, urinary extravasation results in urinoma formation. This is best managed with direct percutaneous drainage of the fluid collection using ultrasound or computed tomography guidance.

Standard follow-up of the functional result is accomplished with a urogram or renogram obtained approximately 4 weeks postoperatively or after any stents or nephrostomy tubes have been removed. Earlier studies are indicated if the patient becomes symptomatic. Compared to preoperative studies, radiographic evaluation at this time should show a definite improvement in any hydronephrosis (Fig. 97–88). If a question remains as to the functional significance of any residual calicectasis, further evaluation can be performed with any of the studies outlined earlier for evaluation of ureteropelvic junction obstruction.

MISCELLANEOUS RENAL OPERATIONS

Open Renal Biopsy

Open renal biopsy may be necessary to establish a tissue diagnosis in patients with renal disease, to assess the severity of such disease, or to evaluate the potential for salvageable renal function in patients with a known correctable disorder who are candidates for a reconstructive operation. Open biopsy is usually preferred over the percutaneous technique

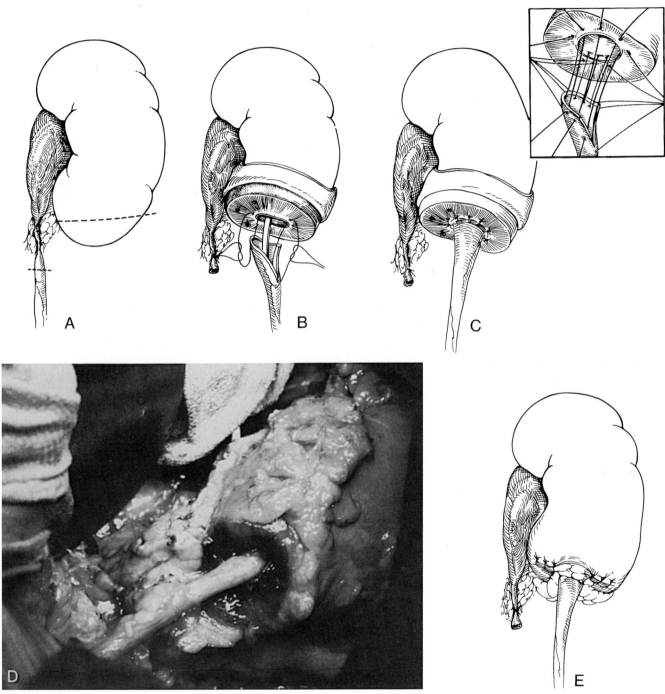

Figure 97–87. *A,* The ureter is identified in the retroperitoneum and dissected proximally as far as possible. The kidney is mobilized as much as necessary to gain access to the lower pole and to perform subsequently the anastomosis without tension. A lower pole nephrectomy is performed, removing as much parenchyma as necessary to expose widely a dilated lower pole calyx. *B,* The proximal ureter is spatulated laterally. The anastomosis should subsequently be performed over an internal stent and consideration also given to leaving a nephrostomy tube. The initial sutures are placed at the apex of the ureteral spatulation and the lateral wall of the calyx with a second suture placed 180 degrees from that. *C,* The anastomosis is then completed in a open fashion, placing each suture circumferentially but not securing them until the anastomosis has been completed. *D,* Intraoperative view of completed ureterocalycostomy. *E,* The renal capsule is closed over the cut surface of the parenchyma whenever possible. The capsule should not be closed close to the anastomosis itself, however, because that may compromise the lumen by extrinsic compression. Instead the anastomosis should be protected with a graft of perinephric fat or a peritoneal or omental flap.

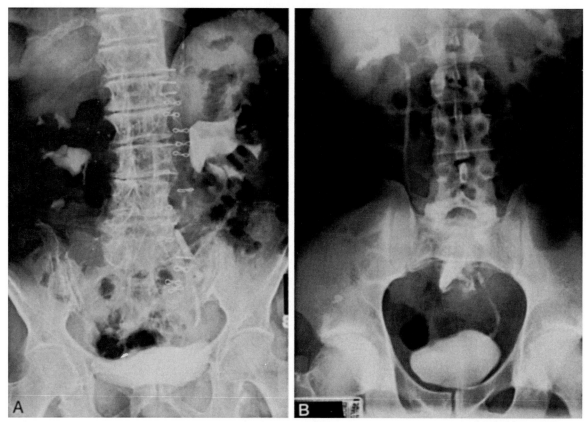

Figure 97–88. *A,* Intravenous urogram 2 months following left dismembered pyeloplasty reveals sharp calyces without any residual obstruction. Compare to this patient's preoperative urogram (see Fig. 97–73). *B,* Intravenous urogram following dismembered pyeloplasty of a left pelvic kidney. Compare to this patient's preoperative urogram (see Fig. 97–77*A*).

in patients with a solitary kidney, coagulopathy, atypical anatomy, or other factors that may increase the risk of a closed biopsy. An open biopsy also provides more tissue for study and minimizes the potential for complications, such as arteriovenous fistula, perirenal hematoma, and gross hematuria.

An open renal biopsy may be performed through an extraperitoneal flank or posterior incision. A general anesthetic is preferable; however, in a thin cooperative patient, local anesthesia may be employed. The right kidney is usually preferentially used for biopsy because of its more caudad location.

After the surgical incision is made, Gerota's fascia is opened, and the lower pole of the kidney is exposed. An elliptic incision is made in the renal capsule, which is usually 1 to 2 cm long and 0.5 to 1.0 cm wide (Fig. 97–89*A*). The incision is deepened on each side with a scalpel and beveled so that the final wedge depth includes an adequate segment of cortical tissue, usually 5 to 8 mm deep. A fine Metzenbaum scissor is used to complete the transection of cortex at the bottom of the wedge, and the tissue is then gently lifted out using the slightly spread scissor blades rather than a forceps, which might crush the specimen (Fig. 97–89*B*). Suction is avoided during this final maneuver to prevent loss of tissue into the suction tip. This technique of elliptic wedge biopsy is preferred over an open needle biopsy because bleeding is more readily controlled and more renal tissue is obtained. The renal incision is closed with absorbable 2–0

or 3–0 sutures placed across the defect and gently tied over Oxycel (Fig. 97–89*C*).

Surgery for Simple Renal Cysts

Simple renal cysts usually present as mass lesions and are often detected during renal imaging studies performed for unrelated reasons. A small number of patients require exploration to distinguish between a cyst and an atypical tumor mass. Large renal cysts causing obstruction may also occasionally require open surgical drainage with unroofing (Stanisic et al, 1977).

The preferred surgical approach for drainage of a renal cyst is through an extraperitoneal posterior, flank, or anterior incision, according to the number and location of lesions that are present. Gerota's fascia is opened, and the cystic lesion is exposed by dissection of perirenal fat from the cyst and adjacent parenchyma (Fig. 97–90*A*). The surrounding area is packed off, and cyst fluid is aspirated for diagnostic study. The cyst wall is then entered sharply and is resected near its junction with normal parenchyma (Fig. 97–90*B*). The base of the cyst cavity is inspected, and biopsy specimens of any suspicious areas are obtained with immediate frozen section examination. After unroofing, the perimeter of the cyst wall is oversewn with an absorbable 3–0 or 4–0 continuous suture to achieve hemostasis (Fig. 97–90*C*). Alternatively the edge of the cyst wall may be cauterized

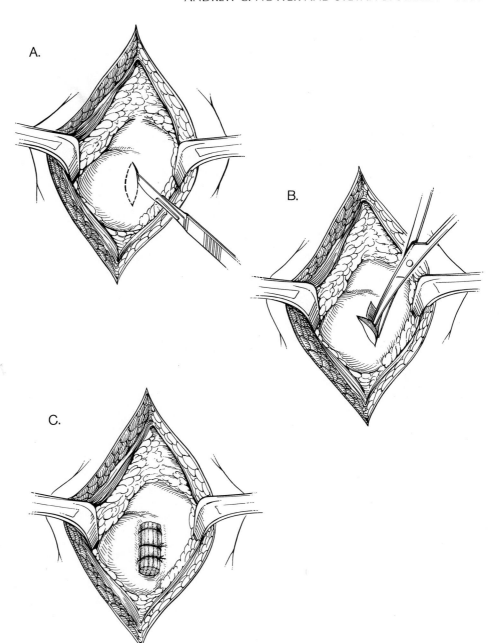

Figure 97–89. *A* to *C,* Technique of open renal biopsy.

and persistent bleeders controlled with interrupted figure-of-eight absorbable sutures. Drainage is not required unless the cyst is infected.

Open Nephrostomy Insertion

Nephrostomy tube drainage is usually achieved by the percutaneous approach, but there are occasional instances when an open operation is necessary because of difficult anatomy or a minimally dilated upper urinary tract. Open nephrostomy insertion may also be performed intraoperatively at the time of a reconstructive procedure, such as a pyeloplasty or ureterocalicostomy.

Primary nephrostomy insertion is usually performed through an extraperitoneal flank incision. After mobilizing the kidney, the renal pelvis is exposed and opened. A

Willscher nephrostomy tube, as illustrated in Figure 97–91, is particularly simple to place because of a built-in malleable stylet within a smoothly tapered sheath (Noble, 1989). The stylet of the catheter is passed through the pyelotomy and is then used to puncture the cortex from within a calyx (see Fig. 97–91A). It is important to ensure that the nephrostomy is made near the convex border of the kidney and not in the anterior or posterior surface because this allows for a better lie of the tube and minimizes the risk of injury to large intrarenal vessels. Usually a No. 22 Fr or 24 Fr catheter is used. The Willscher tube has a flared portion with wide openings followed by a long tip, which may be used as a splint through the ureteropelvic junction if necessary. The catheter is pulled through the cortex until the flared portion lies in good position within the collecting system, usually in the pelvis or a dependent calyx (see Fig. 97–91B). The nephrostomy tube is secured to the renal capsule with a 3–0

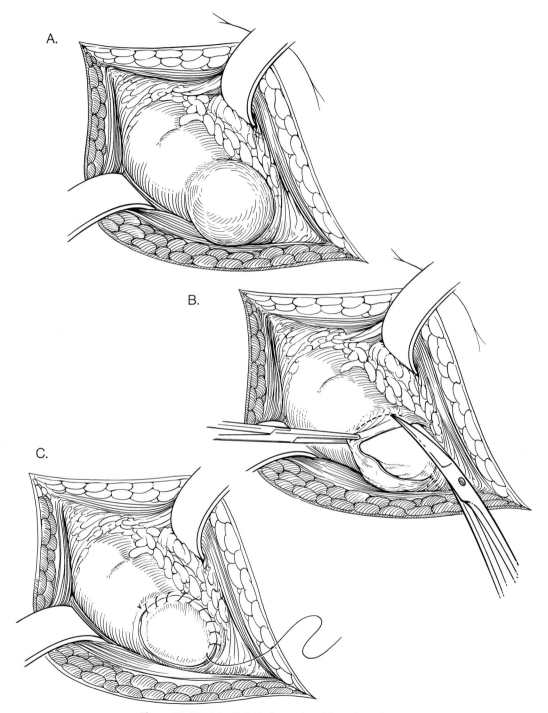

Figure 97–90. *A* to *C,* Technique of excision of renal cyst.

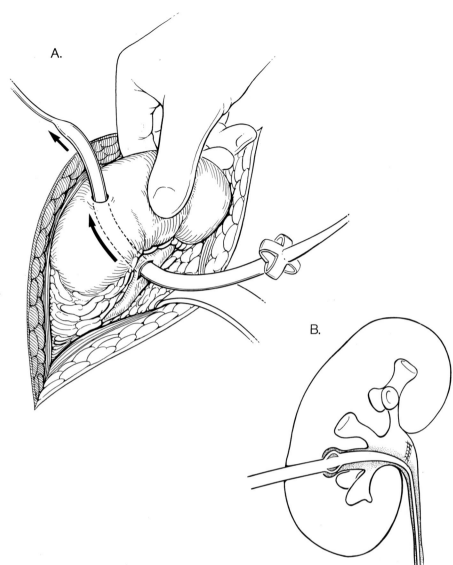

Figure 97–91. *A* and *B,* Technique of open nephrostomy tube insertion.

absorbable purse-string suture. The pyelotomy is closed with 3–0 or 4–0 absorbable suture. The stylet of the nephrostomy tube is passed through the flank muscles, subcutaneous tissue, and skin with care taken to ensure proper alignment of the tube as it passes from the kidney to the exterior. Heavy 2–0 skin sutures are inserted to secure the tube near the flank wall exit point to prevent inadvertent dislodgment. A Penrose drain is placed near the pyelotomy site and brought out through a separate stab wound in the flank.

Ongoing care of a nephrostomy tube is important to prevent infection and ensure unobstructed drainage. Periodic urine cultures are obtained, and significant intercurrent urinary infection is appropriately treated. If the tube is dislodged within 7 to 10 days of its insertion, it may not be possible to replace it through the tract, and a secondary procedure may be necessary. Even with the best of care, encrustations form around the tube and require tube replacement at 6- to 8-week intervals. This is usually readily performed under fluoroscopic guidance once a chronic tract has been established.

Surgery for Polycystic Kidney Disease

Bilateral nephrectomy may be necessary in selected patients with end-stage renal failure from polycystic kidney disease who are candidates for renal transplantation. The indications for bilateral nephrectomy in this setting are a history of significant bleeding or renal infection or massively enlarged kidneys that may interfere with placement of an allograft in the pelvis. This operation is best performed through an anterior bilateral subcostal or midline transperitoneal incision.

Occasionally, unilateral nephrectomy is required before the patient develops end-stage renal failure when the polycystic kidney is a site of complications such as infection, severe pain because of bleeding or obstruction, or development of a tumor. Cyst puncture and unroofing of cysts may be helpful when they obstruct the collecting system or cause flank pain (Lue et al, 1966). **Multiple cyst punctures and unroofing of cysts (Rovsing's operation) do not appear to improve renal function or prevent further deterioration**

(Milam et al, 1963). This approach, however, can provide long-term pain relief in symptomatic patients (Elzinga et al, 1993).

Isthmectomy for Horseshoe Kidney

Horseshoe kidney occurs in about 1 in 700 individuals and is frequently associated with other urologic anomalies. The isthmus that joins the kidneys usually lies anterior to the great vessels. Ureteral obstruction with hydronephrosis, some formation, or infection is the most common associated problem in this condition and may require surgical treatment (Culp and Winterringen, 1955). In patients with ureteral or ureteropelvic junction obstruction, division of the isthmus alone is insufficient, and appropriate correction of the obstruction is required; in such cases, isthmectomy may be a useful adjunctive measure to allow repositioning of the kidney and maintenance of an unobstructed upper urinary tract. Abdominal pain in the absence of any demonstrable renal symptoms is rarely due to the presence of polar fusion alone and is not an indication of isthmectomy.

When performing surgery on a horseshoe kidney, an anterior subcostal extraperitoneal approach is preferred. This provides good access to the isthmus as well as to the pelvis and ureter, which are rotated anteriorly. Horseshoe kidneys are generally supplied by multiple renal vessels, which, in some cases, can enter the isthmus directly. The isthmus may be fibrous but often consists of parenchymal tissue.

Isthmectomy is performed by mobilizing the isthmus from the great vessels, being careful to avoid injury to any anomalous vessels and placing mattress sutures of 0 chromic catgut through the parenchyma about 1 cm on each side of the line of section to control bleeding. The divided ends can subsequently be further oversewn with sutures passed through the capsule of the cut edges. Two or three sutures through the divided isthmus and into the fascia overlying the muscles of the posterior abdominal wall are used to fix the lower pole, which is rotated outward to allow room for the ureter to lie on the posterior abdominal wall.

Local Excision of Renal Pelvic Tumor

In patients with localized transitional cell carcinoma of the renal pelvis, nephroureterectomy with a bladder cuff is the treatment of choice. A nephron-sparing operation may be indicated in selected patients with low-grade, noninvasive malignancy present bilaterally or in a solitary kidney to avoid the need for dialytic renal replacement therapy. A variety of conservative surgical approaches are available in such cases, including open pyelotomy with tumor excision and fulguration, partial nephrectomy (Fig. 97–92), and endourologic techniques with or without adjunctive topical chemotherapy (Zincke and Neves, 1984; Huffman et al, 1985; Streem and Pontes, 1986; Smith et al, 1987; Ziegelbaum et al, 1987; Vasavada et al, 1995). The latter two approaches are reviewed elsewhere in this text.

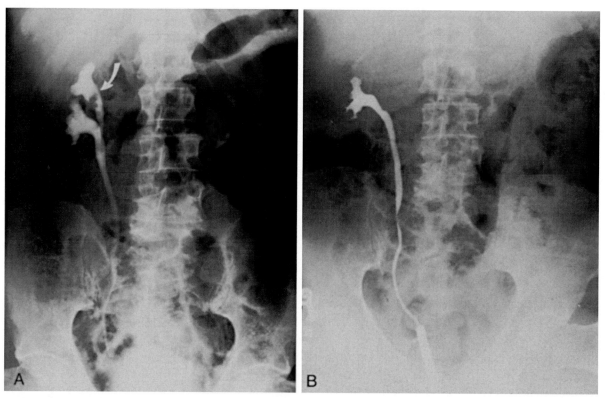

Figure 97–92. *A,* This patient had undergone left nephroureterectomy for transitional cell carcinoma of the left renal pelvis. Intravenous pyelography now suggested a lesion in the upper infundibulum of the remaining right kidney *(arrow).* This was confirmed at the time of retrograde pyelography. *B,* Upper pole partial nephrectomy was performed, leaving the pelvis and lower infundibulocalyceal system intact, as demonstrated on this postoperative retrograde pyelogram. (From Novick AC, Streem SB, Pontes E, eds: Stewart's Operative Urology, 2nd ed. Baltimore, Williams & Wilkins, 1989.)

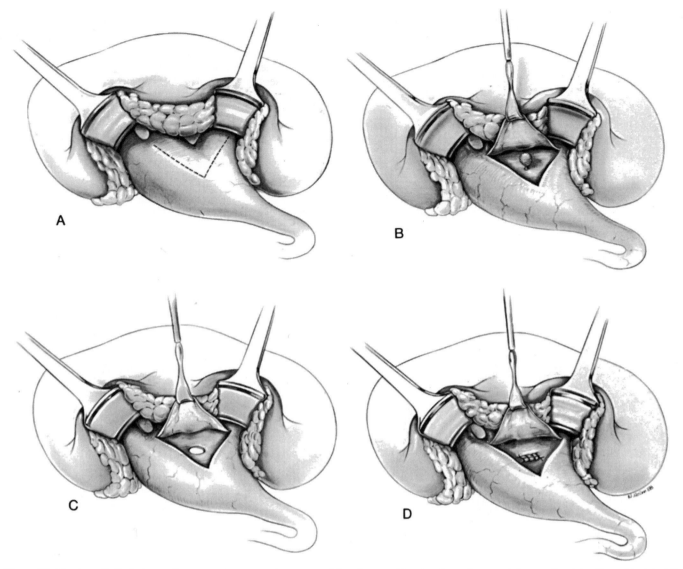

Figure 97–93. *A* to *D,* Technique of open pyelotomy and tumor excision for transitional cell carcinoma of the renal pelvis. (From Novick AC, Streem SB, Pontes E, eds: Stewart's Operative Urology, 2nd ed. Baltimore, Williams & Wilkins, 1989.)

Open pyelotomy and tumor excision may be employed in patients with noninvasive transitional cell carcinoma confined to a portion of the renal pelvis. Occasionally, small lesions involving an infundibulum may be accessible for this approach. This operation is performed through an extraperitoneal flank incision after mobilization of the entire kidney within Gerota's fascia.

The upper ureter and renal pelvis are mobilized along the posterior renal aspect. The renal pelvic dissection is carried into the renal sinus, which often also exposes one or more infundibula. Small vein or Gil-Vernet retractors are used to maintain this operative exposure (Fig. 97–93*A*). The renal pelvic incision is made to expose the tumor-bearing portion of the renal pelvis (Fig. 97–93*B*). This incision may be extended into an infundibulum if necessary. It is preferable to excise a full-thickness segment of the renal pelvis encompassing the tumor (Fig. 97–93*C*). Frozen sections are prepared to ensure that the resected margins are free of disease. An alternative approach is to excise the tumor sharply at its base while preserving the integrity of the renal pelvic wall

and then to fulgurate the base and surrounding area extensively. Following excision of all gross tumor, operative pyeloscopy is used to examine the intrarenal collecting system for any remaining lesions. The site of renal pelvic tumor excision is repaired with 4–0 chromic suture (Fig. 97–93*D*), and the pyelotomy incision is then similarly closed. A Penrose drain is placed near the pyelotomy and brought out through a separate stab wound in the flank.

REFERENCES

Abele RP, Novick AC, Ishigami N, et al: Comparison of flushing solutions for in situ renal preservation. Urology 1981; 18:485.

Allen TD: Congenital ureteral strictures. J Urol 1970; 104:196.

Anderson B, Hansen JB, Jorgensen SJ: Survival after nephrectomy. Scand J Urol Nephrol 1968; 2:91.

Anderson JC, Hynes W: Retrocaval ureter: A case diagnosed preoperatively and treated successfully by a plastic operation. Br J Urol 1949; 21:209.

Angerweier KW, Novick AC, Streem SB: Nephron-sparing surgery for renal cell carcinoma with venous involvement. J Urol 1990; 144:1352.

Aoi W, Akahoshi M, Seto S, et al: Correction of hypertension by partial nephrectomy in segmental renal artery stenosis and electron microscopic studies of renin. Jpn Heart J 1981; 22:686.

Aperia A, Broberger O, Wikstad I, Witon P: Renal growth and function in patients nephrectomized in childhood. Acta Paediatr Scand 1977; 66:185.

Askari A, Novick AC, Stewart BH, et al: Surgical treatment of renovascular disease in the solitary kidney: Results in 43 cases. J Urol 1982; 127:20.

Assimos DG, Boyce WH, Harrison LH, et al: Postoperative anatrophic nephrolithotomy bleeding. J Urol 1986; 135:1153.

Assimos DG, Boyce WH, Harrison LH, et al: The role of open stone surgery since extracorporeal shockwave lithotripsy. J Urol 1989; 142:263.

Assimos DG, Boyce WH, Woodruff RD, et al: Intraoperative renal ultrasonography: A useful adjunct to partial nephrectomy. J Urol 1991a; 146:1218.

Assimos DG, Wrenn JJ, Harrison LH, et al: A comparison of anatrophic nephrolithotomy and percutaneous nephrolithotomy with and without extracorporeal shockwave lithotripsy for management of patients with staghorn calculi. J Urol 1991b; 145:710.

Bates RJ, Heaney JA, Kerr WS Jr: Segmental calculus disease: Potential of partial nephrectomy. Urology 1981; 17:409.

Bejjani B, Belman AB: Ureteropelvic junction obstruction in newborns and infants. J Urol 1982; 128:770.

Belis JA, Pae WE, Rohner TJ, et al: Cardiovascular evaluation before circulatory arrest for removal of vena cava extension of renal carcinoma. J Urol 1989; 141:1302.

Berg AA: Malignant hypernephroma of the kidney, its clinical course and diagnosis, with a description of the author's method of radical operative cure. Surg Gynecol Obstet 1913; 17:463.

Berger RM, Lebowitz JM, Carroll PA: Ureteral polyps presenting as ureteropelvic junction obstruction in children. J Urol 1982; 128:805.

Bernstein GT, Mandell J, Lebowitz RL, et al: Ureteropelvic junction obstruction in the neonate. J Urol 1988; 140:1216.

Bidstrup BP, Royston D, Sapsford RN, et al: Reduction in blood loss and blood use after cardiopulmonary bypass with high dose aprotinin (Trasylol). J Thorac Cardiovasc Surg 1989; 97:364.

Blackley SK, Ladaga L, Woolfit RA, Schellhammer PF: Ex situ study of the effectiveness of enucleation in patients with renal cell carcinoma. J Urol 1988; 140:6.

Blandy JP, Singh M: The case for a more aggressive approach to staghorn stones. J Urol 1976; 115:505.

Bodner H, Briskin HJ: Subdiaphragmatic renal exposure by resection of the eleventh rib. Urol Cutan Rev 1950; 54:272.

Boyce WH, Russell JM, Webb R: Management of the papillae during intrarenal surgery. Trans Am Assoc Genitourin Surg 1979; 71:76.

Boyce WH, Smith MGV: Anatrophic nephrotomy and plastic calyrrhaphy. Trans Am Assoc Genitourin Surg 1967; 59:18.

Brannen GE, Bush WH, Lewis GP: Endopyelotomy for primary repair of ureteropelvic junction obstruction. J Urol 1988; 139:29.

Brodell M: The intrinsic blood vessels of the kidney and their significance in nephrotomy. Bull Johns Hopkins Hosp 1901; 12:10.

Burt M: Inferior vena caval involvement by renal cell carcinoma: Use of venovenous bypass as adjunct during resection. Urol Clin North Am 1991; 18:437.

Butler BP, Novick AC, Miller DP, et al: Management of small unilateral renal cell carcinomas: Radical versus nephron-sparing surgery. Urology 1995; 45:34.

Calne RY: Treatment of bilateral hypernephromas by nephrectomy, excision of tumor, and autotransplantation. Lancet 1973; 2:1164.

Campbell S, Novick AC, Steinbach F, et al: Intraoperative evaluation of renal cell carcinoma: A prospective study of the role of ultrasonography and histopathological frozen sections. J Urol 1996; 155:1191.

Campbell SC, Novick AC, Streem SB, et al: Complications of nephron-sparing surgery for renal tumors. J Urol 1994; 151:1177.

Campbell SC, Novick AC, Streem SB, Klein EA: Management of renal cell carcinoma with coexistent renal artery disease. J Urol 1993; 150:808.

Chandhoke PS, Clayman RV, Stone AM, et al: Endopyelotomy and endoureterotomy with the acucise ureteral cutting balloon device: Preliminary experience. J Endourol 1993; 7:45.

Cherrie RJ, Goldman DG, Linder A, deKernion JG: Prognostic implications of vena caval extension of renal cell carcinoma. J Urol 1982; 128:910.

Chute R, Baron JA Jr, Olsson CA: The transverse upper abdominal "chevron" incision in urological surgery. Trans Am Assoc Genitourin Surg 1967; 59:15.

Chute R, Soutter T, Kerr W: The value of thoracoabdominal incision in the removal of kidney tumors. N Engl J Med 1956; 241:951.

Clark CD: Survival after excision of a kidney, segmental resection of vena cava, and division of the opposite renal vein. Lancet 1961; 2:105.

Clark WR, Malek RS: Ureteropelvic junction obstruction: Observations on the classic type in adults. J Urol 1987; 138:276.

Clarke BG, Rudy HA, Leadbetter WF: Thoracoabdominal incision for surgery of renal, adrenal and testicular neoplasms. Surg Gynecol Obstet 1958; 106:363.

Cockett ATK: The kidney and regional hypothermia. Surgery 1961; 50:905.

Collins GM, Green RD, Boyer D, et al: Protection of kidneys from warm ischemic injury: Dosage and timing of mannitol administration. Transplantation 1980; 29:83.

Collins GM, Taft P, Green RD, et al: Adenine nucleotide levels in preserved and ischemically injured canine kidneys. World J Surg 1977; 1:237.

Collste H, et al: ATP in cortex of canine kidneys undergoing hypothermic storage. Life Sci 1971; 10:1201.

Cook JH, Lytton B: Intraoperative localization of calculi during nephrolithotomy by ultrasound scanning. J Urol 1977; 117:543.

Couvelair R, Auvert J, Moulonguet A: Implantations et anastomoses ureter-ocalicielles: Techniques et indications. J Urol Nephrol 1964; 70:437.

Culp OS, DeWeerd JH: A pelvic flap operation for certain types of ureteropelvic obstruction: Preliminary report. Mayo Clinic Proc 1951; 26:483.

Culp OS, Winterringen JR: Surgical treatment of horseshoe kidney: Comparison of results after various types of operations. J Urol 1955; 73:747.

Cummings KB, Li WI, Ryan JA, et al: Intraoperative management of renal cell carcinoma with supradiaphragmatic caval excision. J Urol 1979; 122:829.

Czerny HE: Cited by Herczel E: Ueber nierenextirpation beitr 2. Klin Chir 1890; 6:485.

Czerny V: Veber Nierenextripation. Zentralbl Chir 1897; 6:737.

Das S, Amar AD: Ureteropelvic junction obstruction with associated renal anomalies. J Urol 1984; 131:872.

Davis DM: Intubated ureterotomy: A new operation for ureteral and ureteropelvic stricture. Surg Gynecol Obstet 1943; 76:513.

Dees JE: The use of intrapelvic coagulum in pyelolithotomy: Preliminary report. South Med J 1943; 36:167.

Elzinga LW, Barry JM, Bennett WM: Surgical management of painful polycystic kidneys. Am J Kidney Dis 1993; 22:532.

Farcon EM, Morales P, Al-Askari S: In vivo hypothermic perfusion during renal surgery. Urology 1974; 3:414.

Fenger C: Operation for the relief of valve formation and stricture of the ureter in hydro or pyonephrosis. JAMA 1894; 22:335.

Fischer GP, Sonda LP, Diokno AC: Use of cryoprecipitate coagulum in extracting renal calculi. Urology 1980; 15:6.

Foley FEB: New plastic operation for stricture at the ureteropelvic junction. J Urol 1937; 38:643.

Foote JW, Blennerhassett JB, Wigglesworth FW, MacKinnon KJ: Observations on the ureteropelvic junction. J Urol 1970; 104:252.

Foster MH, Sant GR, Donohoe JF, Harrington JT: Prolonged survival with a remnant kidney. Am J Kidney Dis 1991; 17:261.

Foster RS, Mahomed Y, Bihrle R, Strup S: Use of a caval-atrial shunt for resection of a caval tumor thrombus in real cell carcinoma. J Urol 1988; 140:1370.

Gardiner RA, Naunton-Morgan TC, Whitefield HN, et al: The modified lumbotomy versus the oblique loin incision for renal surgery. Br J Urol 1979; 51:256.

Gibbons RP, Correa RJ, Cummings KB, et al: Surgical management of renal lesions using in situ hypothermia and ischemia. J Urol 1976; 115:12.

Gibson S, Kuzmarov IW, McClure DR, Morehouse DD: Blunt renal trauma: The valve of a conservative approach to major injuries in clinically stable patients. Can J Surg 1982; 25:25.

Gil-Vernet J: New surgical concepts in removing renal calculi. Urol Int 1965; 20:255.

Gittes RF, McCullough DL: Bench surgery for tumor in a solitary kidney. J Urol 1975; 113:12.

Giuliani L, Giberti C, Martorama G, Rovida S: Radical extensive surgery for renal cell carcinoma. J Urol 1990; 143:468.

Glazer AA, Novick AC: Long-term follow-up after surgical treatment for renal cell carcinoma extending into the right atrium. J Urol 1996; 155:448.

Goldfarb DA, Novick AC, Lorig R, et al: Magnetic resonance imaging for assessment of vena caval tumor thrombi: A comparative study with vena cavography and CT scanning. J Urol 1990; 144:1110.

Goldstein AE: Longevity following nephrectomy. J Urol 1956; 76:31.

Gosling JA, Dixon JS: Functional obstruction of the ureter and renal pelvis: A histological and electron microscopic study. Br J Urol 1978; 50:145.

Graham SD Jr, Glenn JF: Enucleation surgery for renal malignancy. J Urol 1979; 122:546.

Graves FT: The anatomy of the intrarenal arteries and its application to segmental resection of the kidney. Br J Surg 1954; 42:132.

Hanna MK: Some observations on congenital ureteropelvic junction obstruction. Urology 1978; 12:151.

Hanna MK, Jeffs RD, Sturgess JM, Baskin M: Ureteral structure and ultrastructure: Part II. Congenital ureteropelvic junction obstruction and primary obstructive megaureter. J Urol 1976; 116:725.

Harker LA: Bleeding after cardiopulmonary bypass. N Engl J Med 1986; 314:1446.

Harvey RB: Effect of temperature on function of isolated dog kidney. Am J Physiol 1959; 197:181.

Hernandez AD, Smith JA Jr, Jeppson KG, Terreros DA: A controlled study of the argon beam coagulator for partial nephrectomy. J Urol 1990; 143:1062.

Hess E: Resection of the rib in renal operations. J Urol 1939; 42:943.

Huffman JL, Bagley DH, Lyon ES, et al: Endoscopic diagnosis and treatment of upper tract urothelial tumors. Cancer 1985; 55:1422.

Hughes FA: Resection of the twelfth rib in surgical approach to the renal fossa. J Urol 1949; 61:159.

Hulbert JC, Reddy PK, Hunter DW, et al: Percutaneous techniques for the management of calyceal diverticula containing calculi. J Urol 1986; 135:225.

Jacobs JA, Berger BW, Goldman SM, et al: Ureteropelvic obstruction in adults with previously normal pyelograms: A report of five cases. J Urol 1979; 121:242.

Jaeger N, Weissbach L, Vahelensieck W: Valve of enucleation of tumor in solitary kidneys. Eur Urol 1985; 11:369.

Johnston JH, Evans JP, Glassberg KI, Shapiro SR: Pelvic hydronephrosis in children: A review of 219 personal cases. J Urol 1977; 117:97.

Kahnoski RJ, Lingeman JE, Coury TA, et al: Combined percutaneous and extracorporeal shockwave lithotripsy for staghorn calculi: An alternative to anatrophic nephrolithotomy. J Urol 1986; 135:679.

Kalash SS, Campbell EW Jr, Young JD Jr: Further simplification of cryoprecipitate coagulum pyelolithotomy without thrombin. Urology 1983; 22:483.

Kane CJ, Bolton DM, Stoller ML: Current indications for open stone surgery in an endourology center. Urology 1995; 45:218.

Kay R: Procedures for ureteropelvic junction obstruction. In Novick AC, Streem SB, Pontes JE, eds: Stewart's Operative Urology, ed 2. Baltimore, Williams & Wilkins, 1989, pp 220–233.

Kelalis PP: Ureteropelvic junction. In Kelalis PP, King LR, eds: Clinical Pediatric Urology. Philadelphia, W. B. Saunders, 1976.

Khoury EN: Thoraco-abdominal approach in lesions of kidney, adrenal and testis: Morbidity studies. J Urol 1966; 96:631.

Kimbrough JC, Morse WH: Subcapsular nephrectomy. Surg Gynecol Obstet 1953; 96:235.

King LR, Coughlin PWF, Bloch EC, et al: The case for immediate pyeloplasty in the neonate with ureteropelvic junction obstruction. J Urol 1984; 132:725.

King LR, Kozlowski JM, Schacht MJ: Ureteroceles in children: A simplified and successful approach to management. JAMA 1983; 249:1461.

Kittredge WE, Fridge JC: Subcapsular nephrectomy. JAMA 1958; 168:758.

Kletscher BA, Segura JW, LeRoy AJ, Patterson DE: Percutaneous antegrade endoscopic pyelotomy: Review of 50 consecutive cases. J Urol 1995; 153:701.

Kocher T, Langham T: Ein Nephrotome wegen neirnsarkom: Zugleich ein beitrag zur histologie des nierenkrebses. Deutsch Z Chirc (Leipzig) 1878; 9:312.

Koff SA, Campbell KD: The nonoperative management of unilateral neonatal hydronephrosis: Natural history of poorly functioning kidneys. J Urol 1994; 152:593.

Koff SA, Hayden LJ, Cirulli C, Short R: Pathophysiology of ureteropelvic junction obstruction: Experimental and clinical observations. J Urol 1986; 136:336.

Koff SA, Thrall JH, Keyes JW Jr: Diuretic radionuclide urography: A non-invasive method for evaluating nephroureteral dilatation. J Urol 1979; 122:451.

Koff SA, Thrall JH, Keyes JW Jr: Assessment of hydroureteronephrosis in children using diuretic radionuclide urography. J Urol 1980; 123:531.

Kretschmer HL: Life after nephrectomy. JAMA 1943; 121:473.

Kumar A, Sharma SK, Vaigyanathan S: Results of surgical reconstruction in patients with renal failure owing to ureteropelvic junction obstruction. J Urol 1988; 140:484.

Kuster: Ein fall von resection des ureter. Arch Klin Chir 1892; 44:850.

Kyriakidis A, Karidis G, Papachaialambous A, et al: Surgical management of renal staghorn calculi by selective hypothermic perfusion. Eur Urol 1979; 5:173.

Leach GE, Kieber MM: Partial nephrectomy: Mayo Clinic experience 1957–1977. Urology 1980; 15:219.

Leary FJ, Utz DC, Wakim KGP: Effects of continuous and intermittent ischemia on renal function. Surg Gynecol Obstet 1963; 116:311.

Lebowitz RL, Johan BG: The coexistence of ureteropelvic junction obstruction and reflux. Am J Radiol 1982; 140:231.

Levitt SB, Nabizadeh I, Javaid M, et al: Primary calicoureterostomy for pelvioureteral junction obstruction: Indications and results. J Urol 1981; 126:382.

Levy M: Oxygen consumption and blood flow in the hypothermic perfused kidney. Am J Physiol 1959; 197:111.

Libertino JA, Zinman L, Watkins E: Long-term results of resection of renal cell cancer with extension into inferior vena cava. J Urol 1987; 137:21.

Licht MR, Novick AC: Nephron-sparing surgery for renal cell carcinoma. J Urol 1993; 145:1.

Licht MR, Novick AC, Goormastic M: Nephron-sparing surgery in incidental versus suspected renal cell carcinoma. J Urol 1994; 152:39.

Lingeman JE, Siegel YI, Steele B: Metabolic evaluation of infected renal lithiasis: Clinical relevance. J Endourol 1995; 9:51.

Lower WE: Conservative surgical methods in operating for stone in the kidney. Cleve Med J 1913; 12:260.

Lue YB, Anderson EE, Harrison JH: The surgical management of polycystic renal disease. Gynecol Obstet 1966; 122:45.

Luttrop W, Nelson CE, Nilsson T, et al: Study of glomerular and tubular function after in situ cooling of the kidney. J Urol 1976; 115:133.

Lyon RP: An anterior extraperitoneal incision for kidney surgery. J Urol 1958; 79:383.

Maatman TJ, Novick AC, Tanzinco BF, et al: Renal oncocytoma: A diagnostic dilemma. J Urol 1984; 132:878.

Macksood MJ, Roth DR, Chang CH, Perlmutter AD: Benign fibroepithelial polyps as a cause of intermittent ureteropelvic junction obstruction in a child: A case report and review of the literature. J Urol 1985; 134:951.

Maizels M, Stephens FD: Valves of the ureter as a cause of primary obstruction of the ureter: Anatomic, embryologic and clinical aspects. J Urol 1980; 123:742.

Malek RS: Intermittent hydronephrosis: The occult ureteropelvic obstruction. J Urol 1983; 130:863.

Marberger M, Georgi M, Guenther R, et al: Simultaneous balloon occlusion of the renal artery and hypothermic perfusion in in situ surgery of the kidney. J Urol 1978; 119:463.

Marshall FF, Powell KC: Lymphadenectomy for renal cell carcinoma: Anatomical and therapeutic considerations. J Urol 1982; 128:677.

Marshall FF, Reitz BA: Technique for removal of renal cell carcinoma with suprahepatic vena caval tumor thrombus. Urol Clin North Am 1986; 13:551.

Marshall FF, Taxy JB, Fishman EK, Chang R: The feasibility of surgical enucleation for renal cell carcinoma. J Urol 1986; 135:231.

Mault JR, Ohtake S, Klingensmith M, et al: Cerebral metabolism and circulatory arrest: Effects of duration and strategies for protection. Ann Thorac Surg 1993; 55:57.

McGahan JP, Blake LC, DeVere White R, et al: Color flow sonographic mapping of intravascular extension of malignant renal tumors. J Ultrasound Med 1993; 12:403.

McLaughlin GA, Heal MR, Tyrell IM: An evaluation of techniques used for production of temporary renal ischemia. Br J Urol 1978; 50:371.

McVary KT, O'Conor VJ: Transmission of non-A non-B hepatitis during coagulum pyelolithotomy. J Urol 1989; 141:923.

Meretyk I, Meretyk S, Clayman RV: Endopyelotomy: Comparison of ureteroscopic retrograde and antegrade percutaneous techniques. J Urol 1992; 148:775.

Metzner PJ, Boyce WH: Simplified renal hypothermia: An adjunct to conservative renal surgery. Br J Urol 1972; 44:76.

Meyer TW, Anderson S, Rennke HG, Brenner BM: Converting enzyme inhibitor therapy limits progressive glomerular injury in rats with renal insufficiency. Am J Med 1985; 79(suppl 3C):31.

Middleton RG, Presto AJ III: Radical thoracoabdominal nephrectomy for renal cell carcinoma. J Urol 1973; 110:36.

Miki M, Inaba Y, Machia T: Operative nephroscopy with fiberoptic scope: Preliminary report. J Urol 1978; 119:166.

Milam JH, Magee JH, Bunts RC: Evaluation of surgical decompression of polycystic kidneys by differential renal clearance. J Urol 1963; 90:144.

Mitchell RM: Renal cooling and ischemia. Br J Surg 1959; 46:593.

Morgan WR, Zincke H: Progression and survival after renal conserving surgery of renal cell carcinoma: Experience in 104 patients and extended follow-up. J Urol 1990; 144:857.

Morris H: A case of nephrolithotomy or the extraction of a calculus from an undilated kidney. Trans Clin Soc (London) 1881; 14:31.

Motola JA, Badlani GH, Smith AD: Results of 212 consecutive endopyelotomies: An 8-year follow-up. J Urol 1993; 149:453.

Neely WA, Turner MD: The effect of arterial venous and arteriovenous occlusion on renal blood flow. Surg Gynecol Obstet 1959; 108:669.

Nesbit RM: Elliptical anastomosis in urologic surgery. Ann Surg 1949; 130:796.

Nesbit RM: Diagnosis of intermittent hydronephrosis: Importance of pyelography during episodes of pain. J Urol 1956; 75:767.

Neves RJ, Zincke H: Surgical treatment of renal cancer with vena cava extension. Br J Urol 1987; 59:390.

Nguyen DH, Aliabadi H, Ercole CJ, Gonzales R: Non-intubated Anderson-Hynes repair of ureteropelvic junction obstruction in 60 patients. J Urol 1989; 142:704.

Noble M: Miscellaneous renal operations. *In* Novick AC, Streem SB, Pontes JE, eds: Stewart's Operative Urology, ed 2. Baltimore, Williams & Wilkins, 1989, pp 240–249.

Nosowsky EE, Kaufmann JJ: The protection action of mannitol in renal artery occlusion. J Urol 1963; 89:295.

Novick AC: Posterior surgical approach to the kidney and ureter. J Urol 1980; 124:192.

Novick AC: Renal hypothermia: In vivo and ex vivo. Urol Clin North Am 1983; 10:637.

Novick AC: Partial nephrectomy for renal cell carcinoma. Urol Clin North Am 1987; 14:419.

Novick AC, Cosgrove DM: Surgical approach for removal of renal cell carcinoma extending into the vena cava and the right atrium. J Urol 1980; 123:947.

Novick AC, Gephardt G, Guz B, et al: Long-term follow-up after partial removal of a solitary kidney. N Engl J Med 1991; 325:1058.

Novick AC, Kaye M, Cosgrove D, et al: Experience with cardiopulmonary bypass and deep hypothermic circulatory arrest in the management of retroperitoneal tumors with large vena caval thrombi. Ann Surg 1990; 212:472.

Novick AC, Schreiber MJ: The effect of angiotensin-converting-enzyme inhibition on nephropathy in patients with a remnant kidney. Urology 1995; 46:785.

Novick AC, Straffon RA: Management of locally recurrent renal cell carcinoma after partial nephrectomy. J Urol 1987; 138:607.

Novick AC, Streem SB, Montie JE, et al: Conservative surgery for renal cell carcinoma: A single-center experience with 100 cases. J Urol 1989; 141:835.

O'Reilly PH: Diuresis renography eight years later: An update. J Urol 1986; 136:993.

O'Reilly PH: Functional outcome of pyeloplasty for ureteropelvic junction obstruction: Prospective study in 30 consecutive cases. J Urol 1989; 142:273.

O'Reilly PH, Testa JH, Lawson RS, et al: Diuresis renography in equivocal urinary tract obstruction. Br J Urol 1978; 50:76.

Pagano D, Carey JA, Patel RL, et al: Retrograde cerebral perfusion: Clinical experience in emergency and elective aortic operations. Ann Thorac Surg 1995; 59:393.

Papathanassiadis S, Swinney J: Results of partial nephrectomy compared with pyelolithotomy and nephrolithotomy. Br J Urol 1966; 38:403.

Parrott TS, Woodard JR, Trulock TS, Glenn JF: Segmental renal vein renins and partial nephrectomy for hypertension in children. J Urol 1984; 131:736.

Pathak IC: Survival after right nephrectomy, excision of infrahepatic vena cava and ligation of left renal vein: A case report. J Urol 1971; 106:599.

Pence JR, Airhart RA, Novicki DE: Coagulum pyelolithotomy (Letter). J Urol 1981; 125:134.

Perlmutter AD, Kroovand RL, Lai YW: Management of ureteropelvic obstruction in the first year of life. J Urol 1980; 123:535.

Petersen HK, Moller BB, Iverson HJ: Regional hypothermia in renal surgery for severe lithiasis. Scand J Urol Nephrol 1977; 11:27.

Poutasse EF: Anterior approach to the upper urinary tracts. J Urol 1961; 85:199.

Pritchett TR, Raval JK, Benson RC, et al: Preoperative magnetic resonance imaging of vena caval tumor thrombi: Experience with 5 cases. J Urol 1987; 138:1220.

Psihramis KE, Dretler SP: Extracorporeal shockwave lithotripsy of calyceal diverticula calculi. J Urol 1987; 138:707.

Rehn E: Gefasskimplikationem und ihre beherrschung bei dem hypernephrom. Z Urol Chir 1922; 10:326.

Resnick MI: Evaluation and management of infection stones. Urol Clin North Am 1981; 8:265.

Rezvani A, Ward JN, Lavengood RW Jr: Intrarenal aneurysm following partial nephrectomy. Urology 1973; 2:286.

Riehle RA Jr, Vaughan ED Jr: Renin participation in hypertension associated with unilateral hydronephrosis. J Urol 1981; 126:243.

Robitaille P, Mongeau JG, Lortie L, Sinnassamy P: Long-term follow-up of patients who underwent unilateral nephrectomy in childhood. Lancet 1985; 1:1297.

Robson CJ, Churchill BM, Anderson W: The results of radical nephrectomy for renal cell carcinoma. J Urol 1969; 101:297.

Rosenthal CL, Kraft R, Zingg EJ: Organ-preserving surgery in renal cell carcinoma: Tumor enucleation versus partial kidney resection. Eur Urol 1984; 10:222.

Ross JH, Streem SB, Novick AC, et al: Ureterocalicostomy for reconstruction of complicated pelviureteric junction obstruction. Br J Urol 1990; 65:322.

Roth DR, Gonzales ET Jr: Management of ureteropelvic junction obstruction in infants. J Urol 1983; 129:108.

Roth RA, Findlayson B: Partial nephrectomy and nephrectomy for stones. *In* Roth RA, Findlayson B, eds: Stones: Clinical Management of Urolithiasis. Baltimore, Williams & Wilkins, 1983.

Rous SN, Turner WR: Retrospective study of 95 patients with staghorn calculus disease. J Urol 1977; 118:902.

Ruckle HC, Segura JW: Laparoscopic treatment of a stone-filled, caliceal diverticulum: A definitive, minimally invasive therapeutic option. J Urol 1994; 151:122.

Sagalowsky AI, Kadesky KT, Ewalt DM, Kennedy TJ: Factors influencing adrenal metastasis in renal cell carcinoma. J Urol 1994; 151:1181.

Scardino PL, Prince CL: Vertical flap ureteropelvioplasty: Preliminary report. South Med J 1953; 46:325.

Schaeffer AJ, Grayhack JT: Surgical management of ureteropelvic junction obstruction. *In* Walsh PC, Gittes RF, Perlmutter AD, Stamey TA, eds: Campbell's Urology, 5th ed. Philadelphia, W. B. Saunders, 1986, pp 2505–2533.

Schefft P, Novick AC, Stewart BH, et al: Renal revascularization in patients with total occlusion of the renal artery. J Urol 1980; 124:184.

Schefft P, Novick AC, Straffon RA, Stewart BH: Surgery for renal cell carcinoma extending into the vena cava. J Urol 1978; 120:28.

Schirmer H, Taft JL, Scott WW: Renal metabolism after occlusion of the renal artery and after occlusion of the renal artery and vein. J Urol 1966; 96:136.

Schuessler WW, Grune MT, Tecuanhuey LV, Preminger GM: Laparoscopic dismembered pyeloplasty. J Urol 1993; 150:1795.

Schulze H, Hertle L, Graff J, et al: Combined treatment of branched calculi by percutaneous nephrolithotomy and extracorporeal shockwave lithotripsy. J Urol 1986; 135:1138.

Schwyzer A: New pyeloureteral plastic operation for hydronephrosis. Surg Clin North Am 1923; 3:1441.

Segura JW, Preminger GM, Assimos DG, et al: Nephrolithiasis clinical guidelines panel summary report on the management of staghorn calculi. J Urol 1994; 151:1648.

Simon G: Extirpation einer allere am menschen. Deutsch Klin 1870; 22:137.

Skinner DG, Colvin RB, Vermillion CD, et al: Diagnosis and management of renal cell carcinoma: A clinical and pathological study of 309 cases. Cancer 1971; 28:1165.

Skinner DG, Pritchett TR, Lieskovsky G, et al: Vena caval involvement by renal cell carcinoma: Surgical resection provides meaningful long-term survival. Ann Surg 1989; 210:387.

Smith AD, Orihada E, Crowly AR: Percutaneous management of renal pelvic tumors: A treatment option in selected cases. J Urol 1987; 137:852.

Snodgrass WT, Robinson MJ: Intrarenal arteriovenous fistula: A complication of partial nephrectomy. J Urol 1964; 91:135.

Solomon LR, Mallick NP, Lawler W: Progressive renal failure in a remnant kidney. Med J 1985; 291:1610.

Spencer WF, Novick A, Montie JE, et al: Surgical treatment of localized renal carcinoma in von Hippel-Lindau disease. J Urol 1988; 139:507.

Spirnak JP, Resnick MI, Persky L: Cutaneous pancreatic fistula as a complication of left nephrectomy. J Urol 1984; 132:329.

Stanisic THE, Babcock JR, Grayhack JT: Morbidity and mortality of renal exploration for cyst. Surg Gynecol Obstet 1977; 145:733.

Steinbach F, Stockle M, Muller SC, et al: Conservative surgery of renal tumors in 140 patients: 21 years of experience. J Urol 1992; 148:24.

Stephens FD: Ureterovascular hydronephrosis and the "aberrant" renal vessels. J Urol 1982; 128:984.

Streem SB, Geisinger MA: Prevention and management of hemorrhage associated with cautery-wire balloon incision of ureteropelvic junction obstruction. J Urol 1995.

Streem SB, Geisinger MA, Risius B, et al: Endourologic "sandwich" therapy for extensive staghorn calculi. J Endourol 1987; 1:253.

Streem SB, Lammert G: Long-term efficacy of combination therapy for struvite staghorn calculi. J Urol 1992; 147:563.

Streem SB, Pontes JE: Percutaneous management of upper tract transitional cell carcinoma. J Urol 1986; 135:773.

Streem SB, Yost A: Treatment of caliceal diverticular calculi with ESWL: Patient selection and extended follow-up. J Urol 1992; 148:1043.

Stubbs AJ, Resnick MI, Boyce WH: Antrophic nephrolithotomy in the solitary kidney. J Urol 1978; 119:457.

Svensson LG, Crawford E, Hess K, et al: Deep hypothermia with circulatory arrest. Determinants of stroke and early mortality in 656 patients. J Thorac Cardiovasc Surg 1993; 106:19.

Swanson DA, Borges PM: Complications of transabdominal radical nephrectomy for renal cell carcinoma. J Urol 1983; 129:704.

Teichman JMH, Long RD, Hulbert JC: Long-term renal fate and prognosis after staghorn calculus management. J Urol 1995; 153:1403.

Tessler AN, Yuvienco F, Farcon E: Paramedian extraperitoneal incision for total nephroureterectomy. Urology 1975; 5:397.

Thompson IM, Baker J, Robards VL Jr, et al: Clinical experience with renal capsule flap pyeloplasty. J Urol 1969; 101:487.

Treiger BFG, Humphrey LS, Peterson CV, et al: Transesophageal echocardiography in renal cell carcinoma: An accurate diagnostic technique for intracaval neoplastic extension. J Urol 1991; 145:1138.

Van Cangh PJ, Wilmart JF, Opsomer RJ, et al: Long-term results and late recurrence after endoureteropyelotomy: A critical analysis of prognostic factors. J Urol 1994; 151:934.

Vargas AD, Bragin SD, Mendez R: Staghorn calculus: Its clinical presentation, complications and management. J Urol 1982; 127:860.

Vasavada SP, Streem SB, Novick AC: Definitive tumor resection and percutaneous BCG for management of renal pelvic transitional cell carcinoma in solitary kidneys. Urology 1995; 45:381.

Vermooten V: Indications for conservative surgery in certain renal tumors: A study based on the growth pattern of clear cell carcinoma. J Urol 1950; 64:200.

Wagenknecht LV, Lupe W, Bucheler E, et al: Selective hypothermic perfusion of the kidney for intrarenal surgery. Eur Urol 1977; 3:62.

Ward JP: Determination of optimum temperature for regional renal hypothermia during temporary renal ischemia. Br J Urol 1975; 47:17.

Watson GM, Wickham JEA, Colvin B: Does calcium contribute to the effectiveness of a coagulum pyelolithotomy? Br J Urol 1984; 56:131.

Welch M, Bazaral MG, Schmidt R, et al: Anesthetic management for surgical removal of renal cell carcinoma with caval or atrial tumor thrombus using deep hypothermic circulatory arrest. J Cardiothorac Anesth 1989; 3:580.

Wells S: Successful removal of two solid circum-renal tumors. BMJ 1884; 1:758.

Whitaker RH: Methods of assessing obstruction in dilated ureters. Br J Urol 1973; 45:15.

Whitaker RH: Clinical assessment of pelvic and ureteral function. Urol 1978; 12:146.

Wickham JEA, Hanley HG, Joekes AM: Regional renal hypothermia. Br J Urol 1967; 39:727.

Wilson DH, Barton BB, Parry WL, et al: Effects of intermittent versus continuous renal arterial occlusion on hemodynamics and function of the kidney. Invest Urol 1971; 8:507.

Wollin M, Duffy PG, Diamond DA, et al: Priorities in urinary diversion following pyeloplasty. J Urol 1989; 142:576.

Wolpert JJ, Woodard JR, Parrott TS: Pyeloplasty in the young infant. J Urol 1989; 142:573.

Woodruff LM: Eleventh rib, extrapleural approach to the kidney. J Urol 1955; 73:183.

Wulfsohn MA: Extended pyelolithotomy: The use of renal artery clamping and regional hypothermia. J Urol 1981; 125:467.

Zabbo A, Streem SB, Novick AC, Risius B: Intravenous digital subtraction angiography for preoperative evaluation of patients with extensive calculus disease. Cleve Clin J Med 1988; 55:263.

Ziegelbaum M, Novick AC, Streem SB, et al: Conservative surgery for transitional cell carcinoma of the renal pelvis. J Urol 1987; 138:1146.

Zincke H, Kelalis PP, Culp OS: Ureteropelvic obstruction in children. Surg Gynecol Obstet 1974; 139:873.

Zincke H, Neves RJ: Feasibility of conservative surgery for transitional cell cancer of the upper urinary tract. Urol Clin North Am 1984; 11:717.

Zinner MJ, Baker RR, Cameron JL: Pancreatic cutaneous fistulas. Surg Gynecol Obstet 1974; 138:710.

98
SURGERY OF THE URETER

Jenny J. Franke, M.D.
Joseph A. Smith, Jr., M.D.

Surgical Anatomy

Ureteral Physiology
Healing and Regeneration of the Ureter
Ureteral Stenting and Drainage

Endoscopic Ureteral Surgery
Ureteroscopic Application of Laser Energy
Endopyelotomy

Surgical Approaches to the Ureter
Approach to the Upper Ureter
Approach to the Middle Ureter
Approach to the Distal Ureter

Surgical Repair of Ureteral Injuries
Ureteroureterostomy

Ureteroneocystostomy
Psoas Hitch
Boari Flap
Transureteroureterostomy
Renal Descensus
Ileal Ureteral Substitution
Autotransplantation

Surgical Techniques
Ureterolysis
Intubated Ureterotomy
Ureterolithotomy
Cutaneous Ureterostomy
Ureterectomy

Technologic Advances

Surgery of the ureter requires an understanding by the surgeon of ureteral anatomy and physiology as well as surgical principles regarding tissue handling and repair. Minimizing ureteral trauma and preservation of adequate blood supply are key concepts that can contribute to a successful outcome. Although appropriate preoperative assessment and planning are mandatory, operative versatility is equally important because the surgeon may be required to perform any of a number of procedures for repair or reconstruction of the ureter.

This chapter discusses the pertinent aspects of anatomy and physiology related to ureteral surgery. Attention is directed to the use of indwelling stents or a nephrostomy tube, which can facilitate healing and sometimes are the keys to a successful outcome. Relevant aspects of surgical technique are presented along with a discussion of the indications for and results of various surgical maneuvers.

SURGICAL ANATOMY

The ureter is a muscular tube 20 to 30 cm in length that propels and transports urine from the ureteropelvic junction to the bladder. **Its caliber varies from 2 to 10 mm with**

three anatomic points of narrowing—the ureteropelvic junction, the crossing of the iliac vessels, and the ureterovesical junction. Consequently, these are also the most common sites of stone impaction. The ureter has been arbitrarily divided into the upper portion, which extends from the ureteropelvic junction to the superior sacrum; the middle portion, which overlies the sacrum; and the lower portion, which traverses the pelvis. Alternatively the ureter can be categorized as abdominal and pelvic segments, with the division being the iliac vessels.

In the retroperitoneum, the ureter lies anterior to the psoas muscle and lateral to the tip of the transverse processes of the lumbar vertebrae (Fig. 98–1). The gonadal vessels cross anteriorly as they run obliquely toward the pelvis. At the pelvic brim, the ureter crosses anterior to the common iliac vessels, just at their point of bifurcation. Intra-abdominal structures that lie anterior to the right ureter include the duodenum, terminal ileum, cecum, appendix, and the ascending colon and its mesentery. The descending and sigmoid colons and their mesenteries are anterior to the left ureter.

In the female pelvis, the ureter lies anterior to the hypogastric artery and directly posterior to the ovary. It then courses under the broad ligament just posterior to the uterine vessels. **The greatest risk of ureteral injury during gyne-**

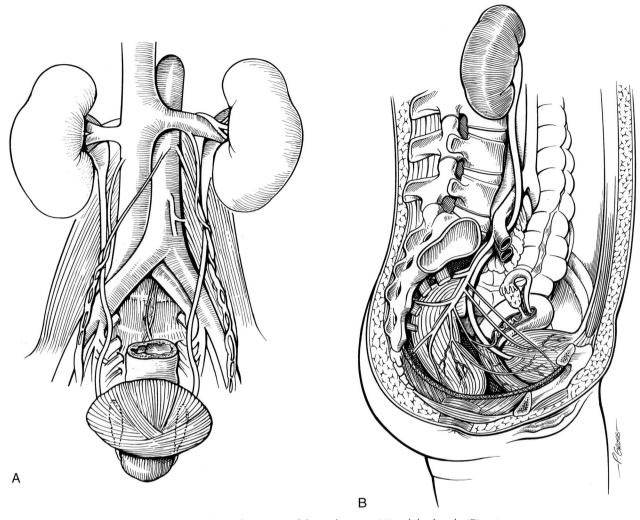

A

B

Figure 98–1. Surgical anatomy of the male ureter *(A)* and the female *(B)* ureter.

cologic procedures is at the point where the ureter lies only 1 to 2 cm from the uterine cervix. In the male, the vas deferens loops anterior-superior to the ureter just before the ureter enters the bladder. The intramural ureter in both sexes has an oblique course within a submucosal tunnel, preventing vesicoureteral reflux by compression during bladder filling (Noordzij and Dabhoiwala, 1993; Thompson et al, 1994).

Histologically the ureter's mucosal lining consists of transitional cell epithelium and a connective tissue lamina propria. The smooth muscle layer is a complex network of interweaving bundles that become more longitudinally oriented as they approach the ureterovesical junction. The outer adventitia contains loose connective tissue, blood vessels, lymphatics, and nerves.

Multiple sources contribute to the blood supply of the ureter. From superior to inferior, they include the renal and gonadal arteries; the aorta; and the iliac, vesical, uterine, vaginal, and hemorrhoidal arteries. The venous and lymphatic drainage parallel the arterial supply. Autonomic nerves are present within the ureteral wall, primarily from the sympathetic plexus. The role of autonomic nerve modulation of ureteral peristalsis, however, is poorly understood.

URETERAL PHYSIOLOGY

The ureter functions as a conduit, propelling urine in boluses from the renal pelvis to the bladder. The smooth muscle of the ureter is a functional syncytium (Weiss, 1987). **Spontaneous depolarization of pacing cells at the pelvicalyceal junction creates a wave of depolarization that continues down the muscular syncytium, leading to increased intracellular calcium and a coordinated peristaltic contraction.** Smooth muscle cells throughout the ureter have pacing potential, becoming dominant when the ureter has been injured or transected (Woolfson et al, 1994). The average human ureter generates three contractions per minute, with both the volume of each bolus and the frequency of contractions increasing during diuresis (Wemyss-Holden et al, 1993).

Histochemistry studies have identified the distribution of acetylcholinesterase and numerous neuropeptides throughout the ureter (Prieto et al, 1994). This rich innervation, however, is not necessary for ureteral peristalsis and only modulates the frequency and volume of contractions. The concentration of these neurotransmitters is greatest at the ureterovesical junction. This observation, in addition to the anatomic description of a relatively short intramural tunnel, suggests that the ureteral smooth muscle at the ureterovesical junction may play an active role in preventing reflux.

Prostaglandins and calcium also appear to alter ureteral peristalsis. Horgan and colleagues demonstrated that extracorporeal shock wave lithotripsy to renal and upper calculi results in the release of prostaglandins into the urine with an increase in ureteric peristalsis (Horgan et al, 1993). Nonsteroidal anti-inflammatory drugs decrease renal blood flow and ureteral pressure in the acutely obstructed canine model (Perlmutter et al, 1993). In addition to the effects of nonsteroidal anti-inflammatory drugs, Sahin and co-workers found that calcium channel blockers decrease peristaltic contractions (Sahin et al, 1993). Overall, the normal pacemaker activity of the ureter appears to be modulated by innervation from fibers containing acetylcholine and neuropeptides, the presence of endogenous prostaglandins, and the influx of calcium.

Healing and Regeneration of the Ureter

Studies of ureteral healing were prompted by the reported success of the intubated ureterotomy in 1943 (Boyarsky and Duque, 1955; Schlossberg, 1987; Lennon and Fitzpatrick, 1994). Davis (1943) described treating ureteral strictures by creating a longitudinal incision through the full thickness of the ureter and allowing healing to occur around a ureteral stent. Lapides and Caffrey (1955) subsequently studied the regeneration of ureteral components after intubated ureterotomy in dogs. **Mucosal integrity was established at 3 weeks with smooth muscle bridging completed at 6 weeks.** Begin and co-workers evaluated healing after balloon rupture of the ureter (Begin et al, 1993). At 4 weeks, a fibrous central zone was found to be contiguous with the adjacent muscularis propria. Myofibroblasts in this zone were thought to play a contractile and perhaps inductive role, leading to near-total muscular continuity at 7 weeks.

The return of normal peristaltic activity parallels muscular regeneration. Immediately after end-to-end ureteroureterostomy, the action potential proceeds to the anastomosis and stops, creating completely independent peristaltic activity of the proximal and distal segments (Butcher and Sleator, 1956). **Conduction of action potentials across the anastomosis is present by 28 days, at which time coordinated peristalsis is seen fluoroscopically, and hydronephrosis improves** (Caine and Hermann, 1970).

Fibrotic tissue neither conducts an action potential nor allows peristalsis. Optimal surgical conditions and technique, therefore, are crucial in allowing normal ureteral regeneration and subsequent restoration of function. Eradicating a urinary tract infection before surgery reduces the inflammation within tissues being used for repair and consequently improves the longevity and tensile strength of absorbable suture. **The ureter should be mobilized carefully, preserving the adventitia and the ureteral vessels within it, and handled with fine vascular forceps to avoid ischemia. A watertight, tension-free, mucosa-to-mucosa anastomosis using fine absorbable suture is generally performed in a spatulated fashion to minimize postoperative fibrosis and stricture formation.** The tissue surrounding the ureter is important because retroperitoneal adipose tissue allows the ureter to slide within it during peristalsis, whereas adjacent

bone or fascia lacks pliability. In surgical practice, wrapping the ureter with omentum not only allows mobility but also surrounds it with well-vascularized tissue with rich lymphatics, which can absorb periureteral fluid. Extravasated urine may lead to inflammation, fibrosis of periureteral tissue, stricture formation, and obstruction.

Ureteral Stenting and Drainage

The need for stenting during and after ureteral surgery remains controversial (Persky and Carlton, 1972; Shore et al, 1987; Lee and Smith, 1993; Selmy et al, 1993). Progressive miniaturization of endoscopic equipment not only provides better upper urinary tract visualization but also permits manipulation with minimal trauma. Additionally, many congenital ureteral anomalies in children are successfully performed without the need for stenting. In contrast, however, infection, scarring, and diminished blood supply represent circumstances in which placement of a ureteral stent may be essential for proper healing. **A stent used during open ureteral surgery serves to align the area of anastomosis, provide a mold around which ureteral healing can occur, prevent extravasation by diverting the urine past the anastomosis, and alleviate obstruction from postoperative edema.**

Potential complications of ureteral stents include irritative voiding symptoms, hematuria, infection, migration, fragmentation, reflux with flank pain, and encrustation with stone formation and obstruction. Animal studies have demonstrated deleterious effects of long-term stenting on renal function, emphasizing the importance of the judicious use of a ureteral stent. El-Deen and associates, examining the effects of stenting on normal rabbit ureters, demonstrated that the hydronephrosis and stasis present at 1 week were reversible after stent removal (el-Deen et al, 1993). At 3 weeks, hydronephrosis had progressed, and renal function was lost in 2 of 18 renal units. Significant histopathologic changes included dilated renal tubules, inflammatory infiltration of the kidney and ureter, mucosal ulceration, and ureteral muscular hypertrophy. Stents in normal dog ureters caused decreased peristalsis and low pressure reflux. Similarly, stenting after ureteral balloon dilation in the pig model was associated with an increased incidence of urinary tract infection and a resultant decrease in renal function as compared with those animals that underwent balloon dilation without placement of a stent. **It appears that, in the animal model, irreversible deleterious renal and ureteral changes can take place with prolonged ureteral stenting, particularly when infection is present.**

The biocompatibility of a stent is determined by its composition (Saltzman, 1988). Silicone stents, which are softer and cause fewer irritative voiding symptoms, are also fairly resistant to encrustation. Because of their pliability, these stents are more difficult to place past a stricture or through a tortuous ureter and are more prone to obstruction from external compression. Polyurethane is stiffer and able to withstand external compression, allowing a thinner sheath of material and a resultant larger inner lumen. Polyurethane is less prone to fragmentation than the polyethylene stents that had been used earlier. Pressure-flow studies performed in patients with different types of stents showed no difference in flow characteristics at physiologic flow rates (Hubner et al, 1992).

Ureteral stents are available in diameters of No. 4.0 to 8.0 Fr and lengths of 8 to 30 cm. **Stents so large as to fit snugly in the ureter and cause ureteral blanching can significantly compromise ureteral blood supply and lead to stricture formation.** Smaller stents with vertical grooves have been suggested to aid in the passage of ureteral stones. Generally, in open ureteral surgery, the largest-diameter stent that fits comfortably within the ureter provides the largest scaffold for healing and adequate diversion without producing ischemia. When using indwelling stents, the length should be tailored to the patient. Ureteral length can be estimated on a plain radiograph or by observing the patient's height and body habitus. A 26- or 28-cm stent is adequate in most adults. Additional length within the bladder may exacerbate irritative voiding symptoms; therefore, precise estimation is preferable.

Most indwelling stents have side holes through the length of the stent. This improves flow characteristics and may blunt the transmission of intravesical pressure from reflux during voiding. Side holes present in single-J stents used during urinary diversion employing bowel can become obstructed with mucus and lead to an increased incidence of pyelonephritis. In addition, a stent without side holes provides more complete diversion of urine, which is optimal for healing after creation of a continent reservoir.

Before the development of indwelling stents, proximal diversion with nephrostomy tubes or internal-external ureteral catheters was commonplace. **Proximal diversion still may be useful when delayed healing is expected from infection, scarring, or tension on the anastomosis or in the presence of a solitary kidney.** An internal-external stent that extends just distal to the anastomosis can avoid instrumentation of a small, distal ureter in pediatric pyeloplasties. **Prolonged, complete proximal diversion should be avoided.** Although extravasation of urine delays organized healing, the flow of urine through the anastomosis stimulates the ingrowth of smooth muscle and provides a volume stenting effect. Before a difficult ureteral reconstruction, most patients already have a nephrostomy tube in place. Many surgeons then place an indwelling stent at the time of surgery and allow the nephrostomy tube to drain for several days. When there is minimal output from the periureteral drains, the nephrostomy tube can be clamped and removed shortly thereafter.

Drainage of the area surrounding ureteral reconstruction may be provided by use of a Penrose or closed-suction drain with equal efficacy. Although more convenient for the patient, a closed-suction drain may promote extravasation by a vacuum effect. If placed too close to the anastomosis, either a Penrose or suction drain can create a wick, which prevents the anastomosis from sealing. Gradually withdrawing the drain allows proper healing while providing adequate periureteral drainage.

Stents or external catheters may be placed preoperatively to aid in ureteral identification. This is most helpful before ureterolysis for retroperitoneal fibrosis or excision of a large pelvic or retroperitoneal mass. The catheters can be removed sequentially soon after the procedure if ureteral blood supply and integrity are not compromised during surgery.

ENDOSCOPIC URETERAL SURGERY

Ureteroscopic Application of Laser Energy

There are two primary issues surrounding endoscopic treatment of ureteral lesions. First, adequate access to and visualization of the appropriate segment of ureter are mandatory. Improvements in both rigid and flexible instruments have facilitated ureteroscopy and increased the potential for endoscopic management.

Second, just as important as access and visualization is a means for effective energy delivery to the ureter. Problems are created by the thin wall of the ureter, which can lead easily to perforation. In addition, even a small amount of bleeding can obscure visualization with small-caliber instruments such as ureteroscopes.

Lasers offer several advantages for use within the ureter. The small, flexible laser fibers can be inserted through virtually any ureteroscope. Often a coagulating form of energy is delivered that decreases the risk of ureteral perforation. The lack of bleeding associated with laser use can be particularly advantageous during ureteroscopy.

A laser can be used to incise a ureteral stricture or ureteropelvic junction obstruction. For tissue incision, a wavelength that produces vaporization is preferable. Of the available surgical lasers, the 10,600-nm wavelength of a carbon dioxide (CO_2) laser provides the best tissue vaporization. Nontoxic, flexible fibers for transmission of CO_2 laser energy, however, are not available. Contact tips on a neodymium:yttrium aluminum garnet (Nd:YAG) laser create a high-energy density and improve the vaporizing characteristics of this wavelength. A KTP laser has a wavelength of 532 nm, which allows more tissue vaporization and separation than a Nd:YAG laser. **Whether a laser actually offers any advantage over cold knife or cautery incision of ureteral strictures is uncertain.** Although bleeding is well controlled, tissue incision is more difficult. From the limited reports available, the contribution of the laser itself to the results obtained cannot be determined.

Although nephroureterectomy has been the standard and accepted treatment for transitional cell carcinoma of the ureter, more conservative approaches with the intent of renal sparing are appropriate in some patients. Endoscopic treatment of transitional cell cancers of the ureter can be accomplished with various forms of energy. Lasers, however, are a particularly effective means for coagulating papillary transitional cell cancer.

Appropriate patient selection is one of the key factors that influences the outcome of laser treatment of ureteral tumors. **High-grade and invasive lesions should not be treated endoscopically in general.** If possible, biopsy specimens should be taken from the lesion to help establish the diagnosis and provide some staging and grading information. Biopsy, however, is often difficult. The visible appearance is important. Low-grade tumors have a characteristic papillary appearance, and a stalk may be present. A more sessile-appearing lesion is typical of a high-grade cancer.

Either a flexible or rigid ureteroscope may be used. The tip of the ureteroscope is positioned just distal to the lesion and at a point where optimal visualization is obtained. Any laser energy that is transmissible by a fiber can be used, but the greatest experience is with the Nd:YAG laser. The laser fiber is visualized at the tip of the ureteroscope and, ideally, should be positioned 2 to 3 mm from the tumor surface. Sometimes, this is not feasible and direct contact is used. The tumor undergoes a characteristic white discoloration indicative of thermal necrosis. If the tumor is bulky, coagulated portions can be dislodged with the tip of the fiber or ureteroscope to expose deeper areas. **Tissue necrosis and coagulation extend beyond the visible changes, so care should be taken to avoid excessive energy application in any given area.**

Ideally a double-J stent should be left indwelling after laser treatment of the ureter. Edema at the site of treatment may otherwise lead to obstruction or perforation of the ureter and result in urinary extravasation. Complete healing and re-epithelialization may take several months. Depending on the circumstances, follow-up ureteroscopic examination of the ureter may be indicated to ensure complete eradication of the tumor.

Endoscopic diagnosis and treatment of upper tract urothelial tumors have developed a role in the management of selected patients with low-grade tumors (Huffman, 1988; Tasca and Zattoni, 1990; Sweetser et al, 1994). In 1989, Schmeller and Pensel reported on the use of a Nd:YAG laser to treat ureteral tumors in 20 patients. Postoperative strictures were noted in four patients, and tumor recurrence was seen in three. Caution was expressed against the use of a laser for treatment of invasive cancers, although the strictures were believed to be related to the ureteroscopy itself rather than the laser treatment (Schmeller and Pensel, 1989).

Endopyelotomy

Successful treatment of renal stones using percutaneous, antegrade techniques has provided a foundation for endoscopic incision of stenoses involving the ureter and ureteropelvic junction. With encouraging early experience with secondary ureteropelvic junction obstruction, endopyelotomy has evolved into a standard method of treatment for adults and older children with primary or secondary ureteropelvic junction obstruction (Szewczyk et al, 1992; Motola et al, 1993a). Adults often present with obstruction associated with pain, infection, stones, or compromised renal function. Preoperative evaluation generally includes an intravenous pyelogram to guide percutaneous access and identify any associated abnormalities, diuretic renogram to assess obstruction and function, and urinalysis and urine culture as indicated. **Patients with strictures greater than 2 cm in length have a significant risk of restenosis and are more appropriate candidates for open pyeloplasty.** Coagulopathy is an absolute contraindication to percutaneous renal surgery. Relative contraindications include a large, redundant renal pelvis and a crossing vessel (Sampaio and Favorito, 1993), although patients with both of these conditions have been successfully treated with endopyelotomy. As with any ureteral surgery, results are optimized by eliminating infection preoperatively.

Patients with proximal ureteral strictures and ureteropelvic junction obstruction are approached similarly. Cystoscopy with placement of a No. 6 Fr ureteral catheter is performed

initially to allow opacification and distention of the renal pelvis and to assist in passage of a guide wire. The patient is then placed in the prone position, and the shoulders and hips are padded to assist in ventilation and prevent pressure complications. **Under two-plane, fluoroscopic control, a posterior, middle calyx is accessed, thus providing adequate visualization of the ureteropelvic junction while minimizing the incidence of pneumothorax.** Treatment of proximal ureteral strictures may require access through a superior calyx. A transparenchymal route avoids injury to major vessels and provides a seal on removal of the nephrostomy tube. A guide wire is then passed into the renal pelvis. After dilation of the tract to accommodate a No. 10 Fr sheath, a safety wire is passed down the ureter into the bladder. If this is unsuccessful, a guide wire may be passed up the ureteral catheter, grasped endoscopically after dilation of the tract, and delivered through the flank.

The nephrostomy tract is dilated to a large size (up to No. 34 Fr) with equal efficacy using either fascial dilators or a balloon system. The balloon dilator is, however, associated with less intraoperative blood loss. A nephroscope is introduced through the polytef (Teflon) sheath and the pelvicaliceal system inspected. A cold knife, laser, or electrocautery may be used to incise the tissue. **The incision is oriented posterolaterally, and the corresponding mucosal lip is elevated and inspected for pulsations. This incision should extend in depth until periureteral fat is visualized and the ureteropelvic junction has a funnel shape.** An endopyelotomy stent with a larger proximal than distal diameter is often used to bridge the incised ureter (Babayan, 1993). The smaller, tapered segment reduces the incidence of distal ureteral stricture from ischemia. A pigtail is present in the bladder and renal pelvis, and the stent exits the flank as a nephrostomy tube. If an antegrade nephrostogram postoperatively shows the stent to be in good position and no extravasation is present, the nephrostomy may be clamped. The stent is generally removed at 6 weeks (Kerbl et al, 1993).

The reported success of endopyelotomy in older children and adults is 60% to 85% (Meretyk I et al, 1992; Perez et al, 1992; Motola et al, 1993a; Kletscher et al, 1995) **compared with 90% to 95% after open pyeloplasty.** The outcome appears to be related to the experience of the surgeon and is similar in primary and secondary repairs. **Endopyelotomy offers substantial advantages over open pyeloplasty with respect to operative time, postoperative hospitalization, and recovery.** Although endopyelotomy has been used successfully for primary treatment of ureteropelvic junction obstruction in children, the reported numbers are small. In addition, infants tolerate an open pyeloplasty with minimal morbidity, thus limiting the pediatric application of endopyelotomy. Endoscopic incision is, however, considered an option in treating pyeloplasty failures in small children.

The most common complication of endoscopic incision is failure to relieve obstruction. Decreased success is seen in stenoses greater than 1.5 cm in length and cases associated with angulation of the ureteropelvic junction. Motola and associates have reported that 85% of restenoses occur in the first 6 months (Motola et al, 1993a). Failed endopyelotomy has not made subsequent open surgery particularly more difficult (Motola et al, 1993b). Intraoperatively, hemorrhage requiring transfusion has been reported in 2% to 3% of patients undergoing endopyelotomy. Significant renal pelvic or ureteral injury is uncommon. Early postoperative problems are generally stent related. Patients presenting with fever, flank pain, and irritative voiding symptoms should undergo antegrade nephrostogram to ensure stent patency and position.

Ureteropelvic junction and ureteral strictures may also be managed using a retrograde endoscopic approach. **Placing a ureteral stent 1 to 2 weeks before the planned procedure allows passive dilation of the ureter, thereby decreasing the incidence of postoperative ureteral stricture from pressure ischemia and facilitating passage of a ureteroscope.** Balloon dilation is generally effective only with strictured segments less than 1 cm in length and of short duration. Endoureterotomy using a cold knife or small-caliber electrode may be employed under direct vision through a rigid ureteroscope. An incision to periureteral fat in this fashion is reported to be successful in 60% to 80% of cases (Meretyk S et al, 1992). A device consisting of a cutting wire that loops over a dilating balloon may be used (Acucise, Applied Medical Resources, Laguna, CA). Under fluoroscopic control, the catheter is passed over a wire and across the stricture. Radiopaque markers allow precise positioning of the balloon. The cutting wire should be directed laterally to avoid vascular injury. As the balloon is inflated to 2 ml, cutting current is applied to the wire at 75 watts for 3 to 5 seconds. The balloon is left inflated for several minutes to tamponade bleeding. An optimal result is achieved when extravasation is noted and wasting of the balloon eliminated. This may require repeat incision. A stent usually is left in place postoperatively (Chandhoke et al, 1993b).

Meretyk and colleagues reported their early experience with the Acucise cutting balloon device (Meretyk I et al, 1992). Eighty-five percent of patients had improvement or resolution in their symptoms and radiographic obstruction.

SURGICAL APPROACHES TO THE URETER

Adequate exposure to the area of pathology is crucial in obtaining an optimal result during ureteral surgery. The most

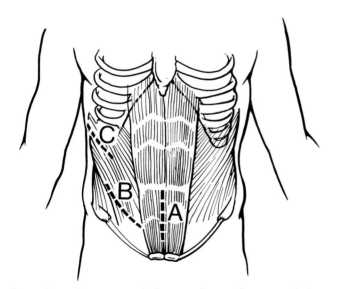

Figure 98–2. Common surgical approaches to the ureter. *A,* Lower midline; *B,* Gibson; *C,* flank.

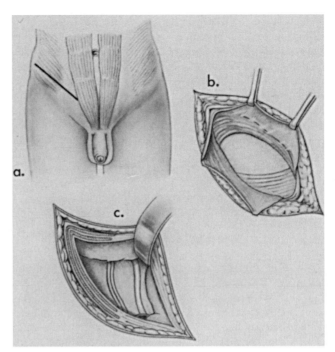

Figure 98–3. Gibson incision.

common surgical approaches to the ureter include a subcostal flank and dorsal lumbotomy for upper ureteral surgery, a Gibson incision for midureteral cases, and a Pfannenstiel or lower midline approach for the lower ureter (Fig. 98–2). Each of these incisions may provide extraperitoneal exposure of the ureter. Confining the surgery and any potential urine extravasation to the extraperitoneal space decreases postoperative ileus. In difficult cases, however, especially those secondary to surgical trauma, a transperitoneal approach offers better exposure and more versatility. If access to the omentum or bowel may be required, a transperitoneal approach is preferable.

Approach to the Upper Ureter

The ureteropelvic junction and upper ureter can be accessed through a flank or dorsal lumbotomy approach. Both incisions are described in detail in Chapter 97. **Because the dorsal lumbotomy is a muscle-splitting incision, postoperative convalescence is shorter. Access to the kidney and renal vessels is poor, however, limiting exposure for managing intraoperative complications or a migrated stone.**

Approach to the Middle Ureter

A midline or paramedian approach allows transperitoneal exposure of the ureter throughout its length. A Gibson incision provides extraperitoneal access to the midureter, allowing extension for more exposure if necessary (Fig. 98–3). With the patient in the supine position, a curvilinear incision is made, beginning 2 to 3 cm medial to the anterior superior iliac spine, running parallel to the inguinal ligament, and ending 2 to 3 cm superior to the pubic tubercle at the lateral edge of the rectus abdominis. The external oblique aponeurosis is incised parallel to its fibers. In sequential fashion, the external oblique, internal oblique, and transversalis muscle and fascia are bluntly divided parallel to their fibers for 4 to 5 cm in length. It is important to understand that the transversalis fascia must be opened to enter the proper plane to identify the ureter. The peritoneum is swept medially to expose the retroperitoneum. The ureter is identified adherent to the posterior peritoneum as it crosses anterior to the iliac vessels. Exposure to the distal ureter is facilitated by sharply dividing the round ligament or processus vaginalis at the internal inguinal ring. The Gibson incision may be extended cephalad for more proximal exposure or medially across the midline for exposure to the bladder.

Approach to the Distal Ureter

The distal ureter is adequately exposed for ureterolithotomy using a Gibson incision. A lower anterior midline or Pfannenstiel approach, however, is more versatile for ureteral reconstruction, providing the ability to mobilize the bladder, create a bladder flap, or gain access to intraperitoneal structures. A Pfannenstiel incision begins with a semilunar, transverse incision 2 to 3 cm cephalad to the pubic tubercle. The anterior rectus sheath is incised horizontally, curving upward on either side to avoid the inguinal canal. Laterally the internal and external oblique and transversalis muscles and fascia are incised for 3 to 4 cm. The edge of the rectus sheath is grasped with clamps, and the rectus muscle is bluntly separated from the sheath. The midline is taken down sharply or with electrocautery. A curved clamp is used bluntly to enter the prevesical space just above the pubis. The attenuated transversalis fascia is incised in the midline. Intraperitoneal or extraperitoneal exposure is provided using a Pfannenstiel approach. A suprapubic V incision, as described by Turner-Warwick (Hinman, 1989), is a modification of the Pfannenstiel incision.

SURGICAL REPAIR OF URETERAL INJURIES

Although the causes of ureteral injury are numerous and varied, an iatrogenic etiology is most common. **Within this group, the incidence of injury secondary to pelvic surgery is 0.5% to 1.0%, with the greatest risk occurring during gynecologic procedures.** The ureter is most susceptible to injury as it passes lateral to the cervix, where it is prone to incorporation into the uterine vessel ligature or closure in the vaginal cuff. In each instance, the ureter is often crushed or kinked. A difficult oophorectomy represents another threat because the ovary may be fibrosed to the posterior peritoneum, which overlies the ureter as it crosses the hypogastric vessels.

Urologic, abdominal, and vascular procedures are associated with ureteral injury in decreasing order (Flam et al, 1988; Adams et al, 1992; Dalsing et al, 1993; Assimos et al, 1994) (Table 98–1). If ureteral injury is suspected at the time of surgery, intravenous indigo carmine may be administered to identify the site and allow immediate repair (Pearse et al, 1985). **Often the injury is not recognized, however, until the patient presents with postoperative**

Table 98–1. COMMON CAUSES OF IATROGENIC URETERAL INJURY

Gynecologic surgery
   Abdominal hysterectomy
   Vaginal hysterectomy
   Salpingo-oophorectomy
   Laparoscopy
   Cystocele repair
Urologic surgery
   Ureteroscopy
   Ureterolithotomy
   Bladder neck suspension
   Retrograde pyelography
   Transurethral resection
   Radical prostatectomy
Abdominal/retroperitoneal surgery
   Colectomy
   Abdominoperineal resection
   Exploratory laparotomy
   Appendectomy
   Retroperitoneal lymphadenectomy
   Excision of retroperitoneal mass
Vascular surgery
   Abdominal aortic aneurysm repair
   Abdominal femoral bypass

fever, flank pain, ileus, or a fistula (Ockerblad and Carlson, 1939; Popescu, 1964; Falandry, 1992). Ureteral injury most often is confirmed by an intravenous pyelogram. The presence of extravasation, decreased function, or hydroureteronephrosis usually requires decompression. Retrograde pyelography provides an assessment of the level and length of the injury. If the injury is incomplete, an attempt can be made to pass a guide wire proximal to the renal pelvis and place a double-J stent (Carlton et al, 1971; Cormio et al, 1993). If passage is not possible, placement of a percutaneous nephrostomy with antegrade stenting may allow adequate healing without open repair. Dowling and associates reported on 27 patients with iatrogenic ureteral injury (Dowling et al, 1986). Percutaneous nephrostomy with or without ureteral stenting was successful as primary treatment in 73% of patients in whom it was used. When a stent cannot be passed, open repair in the early convalescent period is definitive in the majority of patients despite the presence of postoperative inflammation (Badenoch et al, 1987). Repair should be delayed, however, in patients with significant infection or in whom complicated reconstruction is anticipated.

Ureteral injury secondary to penetrating trauma is most commonly a consequence of a gunshot wound (Carlton et al, 1969; Rober et al, 1990). **The surgical approach should begin with débridement of devitalized tissue, although suspicion of significant blast effect should also prompt the excision of a segment of adjacent normal-appearing ureter to minimize late stricture from ischemia.** Stab wounds generally create clean ureteral transection that can be repaired primarily with minimal débridement.

A ureteral stricture as a consequence of external beam irradiation is relatively uncommon but may present many years after therapy. Evaluation to rule out malignancy is indicated in this setting and in patients with strictures of unclear etiology. Preoperatively the extent of the ureteral defect should be evaluated by intravenous pyelogram or antegrade nephrostogram and retrograde ureterogram. Re-

Table 98–2. CATEGORIZATION OF THE USUAL LENGTH OF URETERAL DEFECT THAT CAN BE BRIDGED WITH VARIOUS SURGICAL TECHNIQUES FOR URETERAL RECONSTRUCTION

Procedure	Ureteral Defect
Ureteroureterostomy	2–3 cm
Ureteroneocystostomy alone	4–5 cm
Ureteroneocystostomy with psoas hitch	6–10 cm
Ureteroneocystostomy with Boari flap	12–15 cm
Renal descensus	5–8 cm

nal function determined by nuclear medicine renogram is indicated when nephrectomy is considered as an alternative to reconstruction. The length of the ureteral defect that can be reconstructed using various techniques is presented in Table 98–2 (Hinman, 1989; Koch and McDougal, 1989; Galal et al, 1993). The surgical approach should be planned to allow intraoperative flexibility in choosing an appropriate repair.

Ureteroureterostomy

Although ureteroureterostomy is conceptually the simplest form of ureteral reconstruction, its success depends on strict patient selection criteria and precise surgical technique. Most appropriate is a short defect involving the upper ureter or midureter—presenting as a benign stricture or as a consequence of an intraoperative injury or penetrating trauma. Congenital anomalies such as retrocaval ureter or a duplex system with an ectopic ureter to the upper pole moiety can also be managed with a ureteroureterostomy (Smith et al, 1989; Galmes et al, 1994) (Fig. 98–4). Other indications include a donor ureteral stricture in a renal transplant patient in whom reconstruction by a ureteroureterostomy to a healthy, native ureter is possible and a midureteral tumor in the setting of renal insufficiency or a solitary kidney.

Because tension on the anastomosis nearly always leads to stricture formation, only short defects should be managed by ureteroureterostomy. Determination of whether enough mobility can be achieved to allow adequate ureteroureterostomy can often be made only intraoperatively.

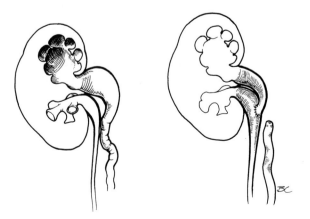

Figure 98–4. Ureteroureterostomy in the duplex kidney. The obstructed upper pole ureter is anastomosed to the lower pole ureter.

Lower ureteral abnormalities are best managed by ureteroneocystostomy with or without a psoas hitch or Boari flap. Preoperative assessment includes an intravenous pyelogram and a retrograde pyelogram if indicated. Further evaluation such as a nuclear medicine renogram to assess renal function and ureteroscopy or ureteral barbotage or brushing to rule out carcinoma should be individualized.

The optimal operative approach depends on the level of the ureteral pathology. A flank approach accesses the upper ureter, and a Gibson incision is suitable for the midureter. The lower ureter can be approached through a lower, midline incision. If, however, the patient has sustained an iatrogenic ureteral injury from previous surgery performed through a Pfannenstiel incision, this prior incision may be used. Proximal ureteral dissection may be difficult through a Pfannenstiel, necessitating cephalad extension of the lateral portion of the incisions in a "hockey stick" fashion. Extraperitoneal dissection is generally employed except in cases of surgical ureteral injury.

After an appropriate incision has been made, the retroperitoneal space is developed, and the peritoneum is mobilized and retracted medially. **The ureter is adherent to the posterior peritoneum and is most easily identified as it crosses the iliac vessels.** A Penrose drain, vessel loop, or Babcock clamp is placed around the ureter. Care must be taken to preserve the adventitia, which loosely attaches the blood supply to the ureter.

The amount of ureteral mobilization required depends on the clinical setting. Generally, enough mobility must be present to avoid tension once the diseased ureter is excised. With a gunshot wound, devitalized tissue and a segment of normal-appearing ureter should be excised to eliminate late ischemia from blast effect. Children undergoing a ureteroureterostomy within a duplex system should have minimal mobilization of the recipient ureter performed to preserve its blood supply. Handling the ureter with forceps should be minimized. Once the ureter has been adequately trimmed to healthy tissue, mobilized, and correctly oriented, it is spatulated for 5 to 6 mm. Spatulation is performed in both ureteral segments 180 degrees apart. A grossly dilated ureter may be transected obliquely and not spatulated to match the circumference of the nondilated segment. A fine, absorbable suture is placed in the corner of one ureteral segment and the apex of the other and tied outside the lumen. The opposite corner and apex are similarly sutured. The anastomosis may then proceed by running these two sutures in 2-mm bites and tying them to each other or in an interrupted fashion (Fig. 98–5). A double-J stent should be placed before completion of the closure.

Observation of reflux of methylene blue irrigant from the bladder to the ureterotomy can be used to verify the placement of the stent in the bladder. Retroperitoneal fat or omentum may be mobilized to surround the anastomosis. The retroperitoneum should be drained, and a Foley catheter is generally left indwelling for 1 to 2 days. The drain may be removed when there has been minimal drainage for 24 to 48 hours. If the drain is not completely retroperitonealized, peritoneal fluid drainage must be differentiated from extravasated urine. The creatinine level of the fluid determines the nature of the drainage and allows safe removal of the drain if there is no urine extravasation. The double-J stent is

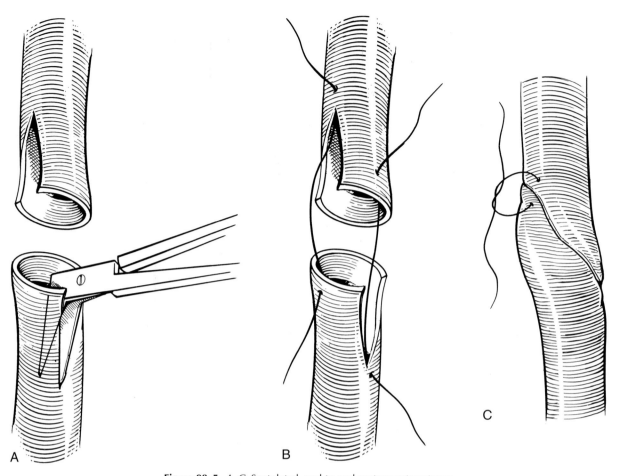

Figure 98–5. *A–C,* Spatulated, end-to-end ureteroureterostomy.

removed endoscopically and usually 4 to 6 weeks postoperatively.

The success rate for a watertight ureteroureterostomy is greater than 90% (Carlton et al, 1969). Guiter and colleagues performed ureteroureterostomy routinely when re-establishing urinary continuity in renal transplant patients (Guiter et al, 1985). No stenoses resulted, and only 4% of patients required surgery for a urinary fistula. If a fistula is suspected, a plain abdominal radiograph should be obtained to verify correct placement of the double-J stent. The proximity of a drain to the anastomosis may exacerbate a leak. A suction device can be taken off suction and a Penrose gradually advanced to allow proper healing. Reflux from voiding or bladder spasms may also contribute to extravasation and can be managed by Foley catheter drainage and anticholinergics. Prolonged drainage may require the placement of a nephrostomy tube for proximal diversion.

Ureteroneocystostomy

Ureteroneocystostomy for vesicoureteral reflux is covered in detail in Chapter 61. Ureteroneocystostomy without a psoas hitch or Boari flap in an adult is indicated for injury or obstruction affecting the distal 3 to 4 cm of the ureter, such as stricture, penetrating trauma, or intraoperative injury. An extravesical, Lich-Gregoire reimplantation may be performed through a lower midline or Pfannenstiel incision.

A Foley catheter should be placed. Using extraperitoneal exploration if possible, the ureter usually is identified as it crosses the iliac vessels and surrounded with a Penrose drain or vessel loop. It is dissected distally and transected at the level of the lesion. The ureter is mobilized proximally with care taken to preserve the ureteral adventitia and blood supply. Direct ureteroneocystotomy is performed if a tension-free anastomosis is possible. Otherwise, a psoas hitch or Boari flap is used. A direct, nontunneled anastomosis may be performed if postoperative reflux is not an issue. Otherwise, a submucosal tunnel is created. A double-J stent may be used postoperatively, and drains generally should be placed.

Stefanovic and co-workers addressed the need to prevent reflux in the adult undergoing ureteral reconstruction (Stefanovic et al, 1991). **In a retrospective review of adults having undergone a ureteroneocystostomy, they concluded there was no difference in the preservation of renal function or risk of stenosis with antireflux versus reflux procedures.** Whether a nonrefluxing anastomosis decreases the risk of pyelonephritis in an adult is uncertain.

Psoas Hitch

The psoas hitch, as popularized by Turner-Warwick and Worth in 1969, is an effective means to bridge a defect of the lower third of the ureter. Indications include distal ureteral injury, ureteral fistulas secondary to pelvic surgery, segmental resection of a distal ureteral tumor, and failed ureteroneocystostomy (Prout and Koontz, 1970; Ehrlich et al, 1978; Rodo Salas et al, 1991). A psoas hitch can also be used in conjunction with a transureteroureterostomy in more complicated urinary tract reconstruction. **A small, contracted bladder generally is a contraindication because sufficient bladder size and mobility may not be present.** Preoperatively the ureteral defect should be characterized with either intravenous pyelogram or antegrade nephrostogram and with retrograde pyelogram. **Ureteral defects proximal to the pelvic brim usually require more than a simple psoas hitch alone.** Urodynamic studies may provide information about detrusor capacity and compliance. Bladder outlet obstruction or neurogenic dysfunction should be treated preoperatively.

A Pfannenstiel or lower midline incision is usually employed. A urethral catheter is placed, and 200 ml of sterile water is instilled into the bladder. The space of Retzius is developed, and the bladder is mobilized by freeing its peritoneal attachments and dividing the vas deferens or round ligament. With traction on the ipsilateral dome, the bladder should be able to reach superior to the iliac vessels. **Additional mobility is gained by dividing the contralateral superior vesical artery.** The affected ureter is identified as it crosses the iliac vessels and divided just proximal to the diseased segment. A fine stay suture is placed on the normal proximal ureter, and the ureter is carefully mobilized. Manual displacement of the bladder toward the ipsilateral ureter may be facilitated by an anterior cystotomy. Although a vertical or oblique cystotomy is generally used, a horizontal incision that is then closed vertically in a Heineke-Mikulicz fashion is advocated by some.

The ureter is delivered into the bladder at the superolateral aspect of the dome and the anastomosis performed, with or without a submucosal tunnel. **The ipsilateral bladder dome is affixed to the psoas minor tendon, if present, or the psoas major muscle using several absorbable sutures. Care should be taken to avoid injury to the genitofemoral nerve when placing these sutures.** Alternatively, psoas fixation may be performed before ureteral reimplantation. A double-J stent generally is placed, and bladder closure is performed with absorbable sutures (Fig. 98–6).

A psoas hitch can provide an additional 5 cm of length as compared with ureteroneocystostomy alone. Its advantages over a Boari flap include simplicity, improved vascularity, ease of endoscopic surveillance, and minimal voiding difficulties. The success rate of ureteral reimplantation with a psoas hitch is greater than 95% in both adults and children (Middleton, 1980). The most common complications are urinary fistula and ureteral obstruction (Fig. 98–7).

Boari Flap

Midureteral defects present a particular surgical challenge because of a tenuous blood supply and potential problems achieving a tension-free repair. When the diseased segment is too long or ureteral mobility too limited to perform a primary ureteroureterostomy, a Boari flap may be a useful alternative. Boari first described the use of this technique in 1894 in the canine model. Boari flaps can be constructed to

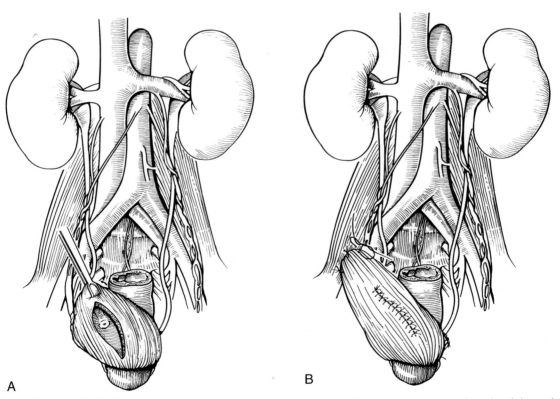

A   B

Figure 98–6. Psoas hitch. *A,* The bladder is mobilized and anterior cystotomy performed. *B,* The ureter is reimplanted and the ipsilateral bladder dome is fixed to the psoas tendon.

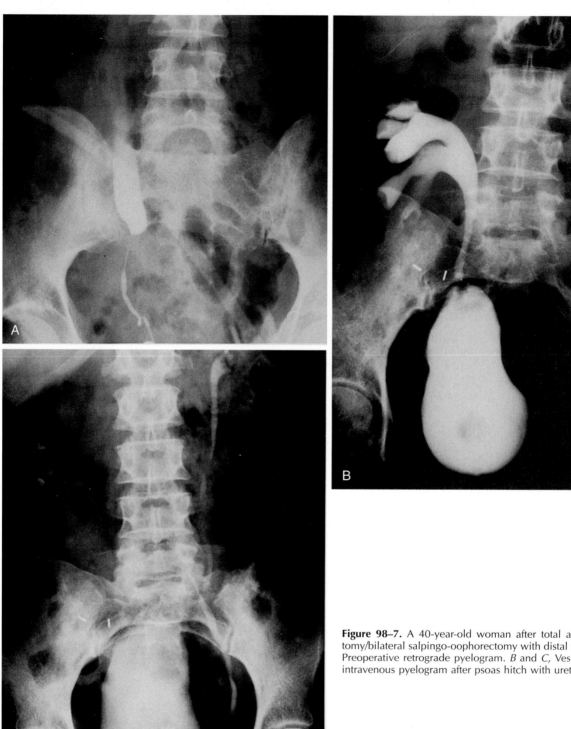

Figure 98–7. A 40-year-old woman after total abdominal hysterectomy/bilateral salpingo-oophorectomy with distal ureteral stricture. *A,* Preoperative retrograde pyelogram. *B* and *C,* Vesicoureterogram and intravenous pyelogram after psoas hitch with ureteroneocystostomy.

bridge a 10- to 15-cm defect comfortably, and spiraled bladder flaps can reach to the renal pelvis in some circumstances. As with a psoas hitch, complete visualization of the ureter and evaluation of bladder function should be performed preoperatively. Bladder outlet obstruction and neurogenic dysfunction should be addressed preoperatively, and a small bladder capacity can be predicted to cause difficulty.

A Pfannenstiel incision may be employed, but a midline incision allows easier access to the upper ureter. The bladder is mobilized from its peritoneal attachments, and the umbilical ligaments are divided. The contralateral bladder pedicle is divided and ligated. The ureter is mobilized with care being taken to preserve its adventitia. **The ipsilateral superior vesicle artery or one of its branches is identified, and a posterolateral bladder flap is outlined based on this vessel.** The base of the flap should be at least 4 cm in width, depending on the size of the flap needed. The flap continues obliquely across the anterior bladder wall with the tip of the flap being at least 3 cm in width. The flap length should equal the estimated ureteral defect plus 3 to 4 cm if a nonrefluxing anastomosis is desired.

The distal end of the flap is secured to the psoas minor tendon or psoas major muscle with several absorbable sutures. The ureter is delivered through the posterior flap, and a standard mucosa-to-mucosa anastomosis is carried out after spatulation. A direct, refluxing anastomosis has been used with no apparent detrimental effect on renal function. Regardless of the anastomosis chosen, there should be no tension. The tube is rolled anteriorly and closed using absorbable suture. The ureteral adventitia may be secured to the distal aspect of the flap and the base of the flap secured to the psoas (Fig. 98–8).

Although the number of reported patients treated with a Boari flap is small, the results are good when well-vascularized tissue is used (Ockerblad, 1947; Benson et al, 1990; Motiwala et al, 1990) (Fig. 98–9). In 1974, Thompson and Ross reported on 25 adults in whom Boari flap reconstruction was performed. Three failures included one patient with recurrent retroperitoneal fibrosis and two with recurrent strictures believed to be ischemic in origin. Scott and Greenberg (1972) performed nonrefluxing Boari flaps in six patients, all of whom had successful short-term outcomes. The most common complication is clearly recurrent stricture formation, resulting from either ischemia or excessive tension on the anastomosis.

Transureteroureterostomy

Since Higgins (1934) described the first successful clinical application of a transureteroureterostomy in 1934, the procedure has undergone intense scrutiny (Schmidt et al, 1972; Ehrlich and Skinner, 1975; Sandoz et al, 1977). Surgeons were initially reluctant to put an otherwise normal contralateral ureter at risk of surgical complications, particularly when successful alternatives for treatment may be available. Transureteroureterostomy remains an important option for complex urinary tract reconstruction of congenital anomalies in children. In adults, a transureteroureterostomy may be used for reconstruction when ureteral length is insufficient for anastomosis to the bladder (Brannan, 1975). **Although the only absolute contraindications are a donor ureter that is too short to reach the contralateral ureter without kinking or tension or a diseased recipient ureter, the relative contraindications include any disease process that may affect both ureters** (Table 98–3). Previous ureteral

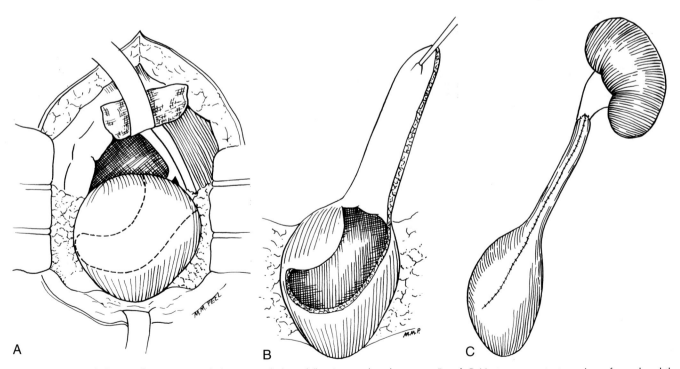

Figure 98–8. Extended Boari flap. *A,* A spiraled, posteriorly based flap is pexed to the psoas. *B* and *C,* Ureteroneocystostomy is performed and the bladder tube is closed longitudinally.

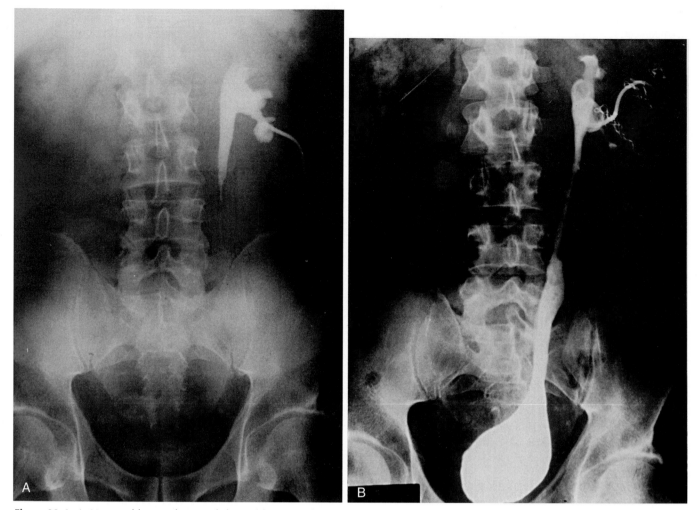

Figure 98–9. A 60-year-old man after aortobifemoral bypass with proximal ureteral injury. *A,* Preoperative nephrostogram. *B,* Vesicoureterogram after Boari flap.

surgery or mobilization may compromise ureteral blood supply, further limiting the application of a transureteroureterostomy. Reflux to the recipient ureter should be identified preoperatively and corrected simultaneously. Therefore, a voiding cystogram should be performed and both ureters thoroughly evaluated with intravenous pyelogram or retrograde pyelography before reconstruction.

A midline, transperitoneal approach allows access to both ureters. The peritoneum is incised and the colon reflected on the side of the diseased ureter. The ureter is mobilized, preserving the adventitia with the ureteral blood supply, and divided at the level of obstruction. The contralateral colon is reflected, exposing only the portion of ureter needed for the anastomosis. This is generally 5 cm cephalad to the level of division of the opposite ureter. **A tunnel under the mesentery of the sigmoid colon is created superior to the inferior mesenteric artery to avoid ureteral tethering by this vessel.** The donor ureter is then brought through the tunnel to the recipient side. A short segment of recipient ureter is dissected free from surrounding tissue at a level where a tension-free anastomosis can be accomplished. **Mobilization of the recipient ureter should be minimized.** An anteromedial ureterotomy is made in the recipient ureter, and a spatulated, watertight anastomosis is performed using either interrupted or running absorbable sutures. A double-J stent is generally passed from the donor renal pelvis, through the anastomosis, and into the bladder. If the recipient ureter is large enough in diameter, another double-J stent may also be placed throughout its length (Fig. 98–10).

Hendren and Hensle (1980) performed 75 pediatric transureteroureterostomies without compromising a single recipient kidney. Hodges and associates had similar success in a large group of children and adults (Hodges et al, 1980). Two patients required revision because of ureteral kinking by the inferior mesenteric artery.

Table 98–3. ABSOLUTE AND RELATIVE CONTRAINDICATIONS TO TRANSURETEROURETEROSTOMY

Absolute
Short donor ureter
Diseased recipient ureter
Relative
Urothelial tumor
Nephrolithiasis
Pelvic or abdominal irradiation
Chronic pyelonephritis
Retroperitoneal fibrosis

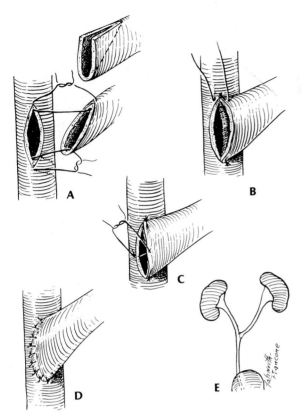

Figure 98–10. Transureteroureterostomy. A 1.5-cm anteromedial ureterotomy is performed. The donor ureter is spatulated, and end-to-side anastomosis is completed. (From Young JD Jr: *In* Glenn JF, ed: Urologic Surgery, 3rd ed. Philadelphia, J.B. Lippincott, 1983.)

Renal Descensus

Mobilization of the kidney as described by Popescu in 1964 is helpful in repairing upper ureteral defects or when additional length is needed to bridge a gap or decrease tension on a ureteral repair (Harada et al, 1964; Passerini-Glazel et al, 1994). A transperitoneal, subcostal, midline, or paramedian incision may be used to approach the kidney and the appropriate level of the ureter. The colon is reflected medially and Gerota's fascia entered. The kidney is completely mobilized and rotated inferiorly and medially on its vascular pedicle. The lower pole of the kidney is secured to the retroperitoneal muscle using several 2–0 absorbable sutures. As much as 8 cm of length can be bridged using this technique (Fig. 98–11).

The renal vessels, especially the renal vein, limit the extent to which the kidney can be mobilized. A technique for division of the renal vein with reanastomosis more inferiorly to the inferior vena cava has been described. Although rarely indicated, this technique may provide additional ureteral length on the right side (Gil-Vernet and Caralps, 1968).

Ileal Ureteral Substitution

Replacement or repair of long-diseased or absent segments of the ureter, especially the proximal ureter, poses a particularly difficult surgical challenge (Benson et al, 1990). Iatro-

genic injury, often as a complication of ureteroscopy, is the major contributing cause. **Reconstruction of the urinary tract with tissue lined with urothelium is preferable because urothelium is not absorptive and is resistant to the inflammatory and potentially carcinogenic effects of urine** (Harzmann et al, 1986). Replacement of the ureter with other tissue is, therefore, reserved for situations in which a defect cannot be bridged by other methods or the bladder is unsuitable for reconstruction. Appendix and fallopian tube have been found to be unreliable ureteral substitutes, whereas ileal interposition has become a satisfactory option for complicated ureteral reconstruction.

In 1909, Shoemaker performed the first ileal ureteral substitution in a woman with tuberculous involvement of the urinary tract. The metabolic and physiologic effects of the ileal ureter have been investigated in dogs (Hinman and Oppenheimer, 1958; Martinez et al, 1965). When an isoperistaltic segment of ileum is directly anastomosed to the bladder, reflux is generally seen only when voiding. Similarly, renal pelvic pressure increases only during voiding. The retrograde transmission of intravesical pressure depends on the length of ileum interposed and the voiding pressure. Waters and co-workers compared dogs with tapered ileal replacement to those with nontapered segments and found no difference in renal perfusion pressure or metabolic derangements (Waters et al, 1981).

Clinical experience in 89 patients was reported in 1979 by Boxer and associates. Preoperative renal function was found to be an important prognostic factor. Only 12% of patients with normal preoperative renal function had significant metabolic problems postoperatively. Nearly half of those with a serum creatinine of greater than 2 mg/dl developed hyperchloremic acidosis, necessitating conversion to a conduit (Koch and McDougal, 1985). Patients with bladder dysfunction also experience more complications. The authors emphasized the value of creating an isoperistaltic anastomosis, leaving a nephrostomy tube and retroperitonealizing the reconstruction. No good data clinically establish the superiority of a tapered segment, a nonrefluxing anastomosis, or a shorter, segmental replacement over a standard ileal substitu-

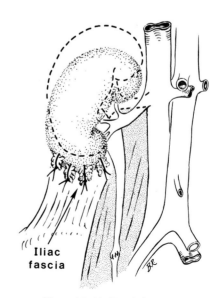

Figure 98–11. Renal descensus.

tion (Waters et al, 1981). **Based on these observations, general contraindications to an ileal ureteral substitution are a serum creatinine of greater than 2 ml/dl, bladder dysfunction or outlet obstruction, inflammatory bowel disease, or radiation enteritis.**

A full mechanical and antibiotic bowel preparation is usually used, and exposure is obtained via a long midline, transperitoneal approach. The ipsilateral colon is reflected, and the ureter is mobilized and dissected proximally to healthy tissue. Often, when the entire ureter is diseased, the proximal anastomosis is performed at the level of the renal pelvis.

The length of the defect is estimated and an appropriate segment of distal ileum chosen. The segment should be at least 15 cm away from the ileocecal valve and have adequate blood supply. The mesentery is divided more extensively than with a standard ileal conduit to allow greater mobility. On occasion, a segment of colon may be more accessible than ileum and is prepared using the same principles. **In the presence of a scarred or intrarenal pelvis, ileocalycostomy may be preferable** (Mesrobian and Kelalis, 1989). In this circumstance, excision of lower pole parenchymal tissue is helpful in preventing stenosis at the anastomosis.

The bowel is divided, the distal end of the loop tagged for orientation, and bowel continuity re-established. A small window is made in the peritoneum of the colonic mesentery and the loop of ileum delivered through it. Alternatively, when performing right ureteral reconstruction, the cecum and ascending colon can be reflected superiorly. The loop is rotated to ensure isoperistaltic orientation, and the anastomoses are performed at the level of the renal pelvis or calyx and at the bladder (Figs. 98–12 and 98–13). Bilateral ileal ureteral substitution may be performed by using a longer segment that loops intraperitoneally from one kidney to the other and then to the bladder. Alternatively, two separate loops may be used.

Complications include early extravasation with fistula or urinoma formation and obstruction from edema, a mucous plug, or a kink in the loop. Ischemic necrosis of the loop may occur and should be considered if signs of an acute abdomen are present. Clinical problems with electrolyte abnormalities and renal insufficiency are unusual if preoperative renal function is normal. **Patients with worsening metabolic abnormalities associated with a progressively dilating loop should be evaluated for vesicourethral dysfunction.**

Autotransplantation

Autotransplantation can be used in situations in which a long ureteral defect is present (Hardy 1963; Novick and Stewart, 1981; Benson et al, 1990). Most often, autotransplantation is considered when the contralateral kidney is absent or poorly functioning and other methods for ureteral substitution or repair are not feasible. The kidney is "harvested" with maximal vessel length, and the iliac vessels are used to re-establish vascular integrity. A healthy segment of ureter is anastomosed to the bladder (Bodie et al, 1986). The renal pelvis may be anastomosed directly to the bladder without apparent long-term adverse effects (Kennelly et al, 1993).

SURGICAL TECHNIQUES

Ureterolysis

External ureteral compression may occur from a number of intraperitoneal and extraperitoneal processes (Table 98–4). Patients may present with symptoms of the primary disease process or with flank pain as a consequence of obstruction.

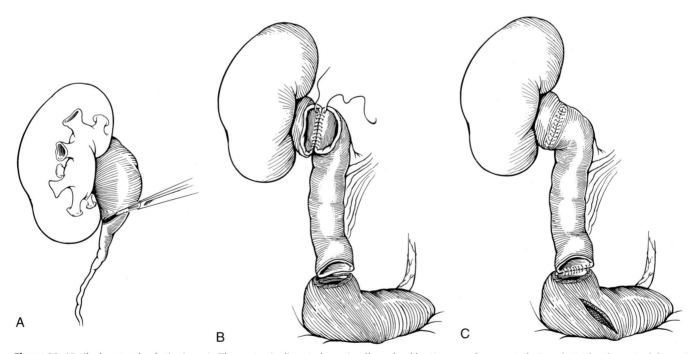

Figure 98–12. Ileal ureteral substitution. *A,* The ureter is dissected proximally to healthy tissue and transected. *B* and *C,* The ileum is delivered through the colonic mesentery; proximal and distal anastomoses are performed in running, full-thickness fashion.

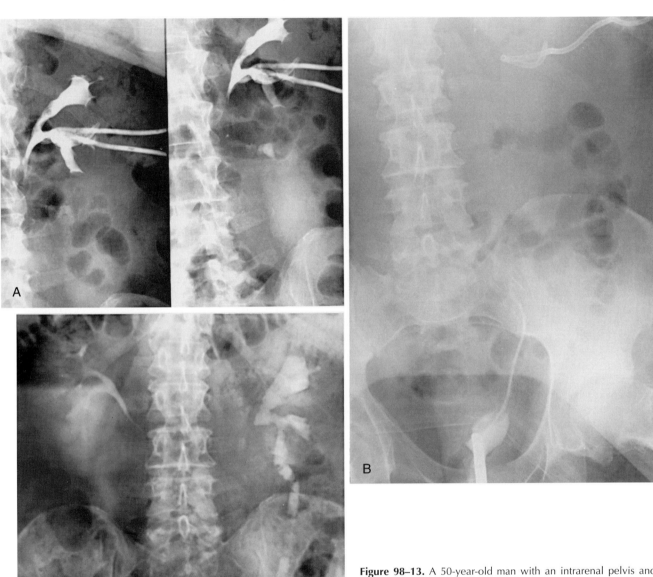

Figure 98–13. A 50-year-old man with an intrarenal pelvis and extensive ureteral loss after complicated ureteroscopy. *A*, Preoperative nephrostogram; *B*, retrograde pyelogram; *C*, IVP after ileal ureteral substitution.

Table 98–4. ETIOLOGY OF EXTRINSIC URETERAL COMPRESSION

Vascular—Abdominal aortic or iliac aneurysm, retrocaval ureter
Gynecologic—Ovarian cyst, tubo-ovarian abscess, endometriosis
Gastrointestinal—Inflammatory bowel disease, diverticulitis, tumor, appendiceal abscess
Retroperitoneal—Tumor, idiopathic retroperitoneal fibrosis, hematoma
Irradiation

Renal compromise and symptoms of uremia may occur if the process is bilateral (Ormond, 1948; Baker et al, 1987). **With benign retroperitoneal fibrosis, intravenous pyelography typically demonstrates unilateral or bilateral hydronephrosis with medial deviation of the ureters. On computed tomography scan, a retroperitoneal mass usually obscures the borders of the great vessels and may extend from the renal hilum to the iliac vessels.** The ureters are surrounded by the mass, with resultant external compression. Lymphoma and sarcoma may have a similar radiographic appearance. Most patients initially undergo a retrograde pyelogram and placement of double-J stents for relief of symptoms and obstructive uropathy. Despite the marked narrowing of the midureter, retrograde placement of a stent can usually be performed without difficulty. The presence of a ureteral stent also aids in ureterolysis.

Preoperative evaluation includes an intravenous pyelogram, abdominal and pelvic computed tomography scan, and careful physical examination to identify any associated peripheral adenopathy. Ureterolysis is indicated in a suitable operative candidate with symptoms of renal insufficiency secondary to ureteral obstruction from extrinsic compression (Lindell and Lehtonen, 1988). Appropriate treatment of the primary disease process, such as antibiotics and drainage for those with an abscess, should be completed preoperatively. Although the technique described is that employed in a patient with idiopathic retroperitoneal fibrosis, the principles are the same regardless of the etiology.

A midline transperitoneal abdominal incision is performed to access both ureters easily. Even if hydronephrosis is demonstrable only unilaterally, the process is generally bilateral. The parietal peritoneum should be incised and both the right and left colon reflected medially. Deep biopsy specimens from the mass should be sent for frozen and permanent section to rule out malignancy. If possible, dissection should begin at the distal, nondilated ureter to avoid injury to the thin, dilated proximal segment. The presence of a ureteral catheter or stent greatly aids in the identification and dissection of the ureter. A right-angle clamp is placed between the ureter and mass parallel to the ureter, and the fibrotic tissue is incised. This is repeated throughout the length of the enveloped ureter, using both blunt and sharp dissection to free the ureter from its fibrous bed. The ureteral wall may become quite thin at times. An inadvertent ureterotomy should be closed with absorbable suture.

Once both ureters are completely lysed, they must be repositioned and protected from further entrapment. A simple option is to retract the ureters laterally and secure the overlying peritoneum medially to the psoas muscle to maintain the ureters in this location. Alternatively the ureters may be displaced anteriorly into the peritoneal cavity with closure of the peritoneum behind them. Closure of the peritoneum

at the ureteral hiatus should not constrict the ureter. When used in the setting of extensive idiopathic retroperitoneal fibrosis, recurrent ureteral obstruction may occur. A more definitive approach is to surround the ureters with omentum once they are repositioned within the peritoneal cavity (Tresidder et al, 1972). The omentum is mobilized from its attachment to the transverse colon. It is then divided down the midline, ligating the small omental vessels up to the gastric attachment. The short gastric vessels are divided and ligated at the level of the stomach wall, so that the omentum can be retracted laterally based on the right and left gastroepiploic arteries. The entire length of the ureter can be wrapped in omentum, which is tacked in place with several absorbable sutures. **The omentum protects the ureter against recurrent extrinsic compression and provides vascularity to a potentially ischemic ureter** (Fig. 98–14). Postoperative steroids may be used in an attempt to decrease the size of the mass and help prevent recurrent upper tract and venous compression (Kearney et al, 1976; Rhee et al, 1994). If no ureterotomies occurred during dissection, the stents may be removed shortly after surgery.

Intubated Ureterotomy

In 1943, Davis described the intubated ureterotomy for treatment of ureteral stricture (Davis, 1943, 1951, 1958; Smart, 1961). Because of the development of more effective alternatives for treatment, the procedure is described primarily for historical interest and as a corollary to endoscopic ureteral incision. An intubated ureterotomy is generally employed for ureteral strictures too long for conventional ureteroureterostomy or ureteroneocystostomy and has been used to treat defects 10 to 12 cm long. The area of strictured ureter is exposed, and a longitudinal ureterotomy is performed in the posterolateral ureter through the entire length of the stricture. Care should be taken not to spiral the incision. As long as a longitudinal bridge of ureteral wall is maintained, the ureteral components can regenerate around a stent. A double-J stent of appropriate length is inserted and a nephrostomy tube placed. To maintain proximity of the stent and the ureter, retroperitoneal fat or omentum may be wrapped around the involved portion of ureter. The retroperitoneum is drained with Penrose or closed-suction drains. The stent is left in place for 6 to 8 weeks or until a nephrostogram demonstrates no extravasation.

Ureterolithotomy

Although advancing technology has provided effective alternatives for the treatment of ureteral stones, an open ureterolithotomy remains the procedure of choice under certain circumstances. Extracorporeal shock wave lithotripsy and ureteroscopy with lithotripsy or stone extraction are effective, less invasive methods of treating most ureteral stones that have not passed spontaneously. **The indications for ureterolithotomy are generally failure of extracorporeal shock wave lithotripsy or ureteroscopic therapy (or both) (i.e., stones too hard to fragment, inability to localize the stone or focus shock waves, inability to access the stone ureteroscopically, or a densely impacted stone)**

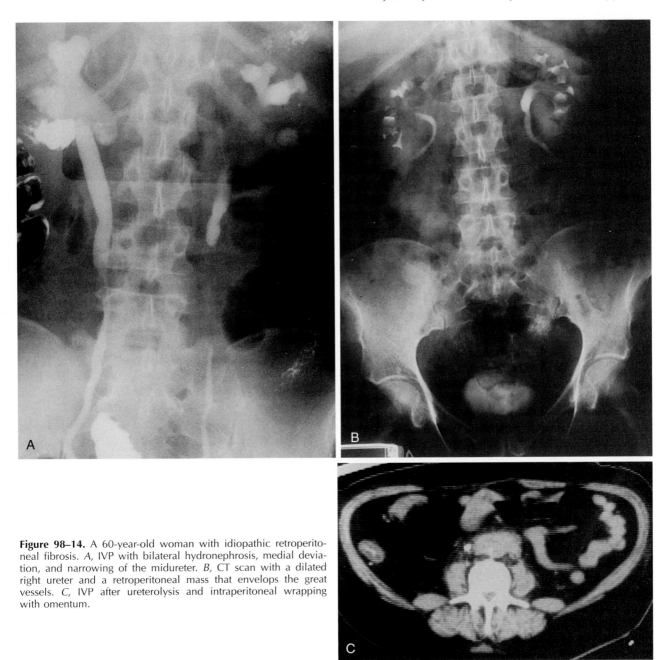

Figure 98–14. A 60-year-old woman with idiopathic retroperitoneal fibrosis. *A,* IVP with bilateral hydronephrosis, medial deviation, and narrowing of the midureter. *B,* CT scan with a dilated right ureter and a retroperitoneal mass that envelops the great vessels. *C,* IVP after ureterolysis and intraperitoneal wrapping with omentum.

(Cohen and Persky, 1983). The presence of a ureteral stricture, urinary diversion, or congenital anomaly may require open ureterolithotomy, especially if concomitant repair of a ureteral disorder is indicated.

Preoperatively a patient should undergo intravenous pyelogram to assess the number of stones, the presence or absence of contralateral stones, or any associated urinary tract anomalies. Because ureteral stones may move up or down unexpectedly, a kidney, ureter, and bladder radiograph should be obtained immediately before surgery to aid in planning the operative approach.

The appropriate incision is determined by the location of the stone. An upper ureteral stone may be accessed through a flank or dorsal lumbotomy incision. A modified Gibson incision provides exposure of the midureter and may be extended proximally or distally if needed. A distal ureteral

stone may be extracted using a Gibson, midline, or Pfannenstiel incision. In addition, a large distal ureteral stone that can be easily palpated on bimanual examination may be removed transvaginally. Although most stones can be removed through a retroperitoneal approach, a ureterolithotomy in a patient who has undergone previous ureteral surgery may require transperitoneal exposure.

After the stone has been radiographically localized and an appropriate incision made, the peritoneum is reflected medially. The proximal ureter and midureter are adherent to the parietal peritoneum. The stone should be palpated carefully so as not to dislodge it. **A Penrose drain, vessel loop, or Babcock clamp is placed around the ureter just proximal and distal to the stone to prevent migration.** Stripping of the adventitia and ureteral blood vessels should be avoided. Traction sutures placed on either side of the planned ureterotomy may be helpful. A vertical ureterotomy is made beginning just at the superior extent of the stone and continuing inferiorly. The ureterotomy should be a few millimeters longer than the stone. Using forceps or a fine clamp, the stone should be gently teased from the mucosa. After complete removal of the stone, a No. 8 Fr feeding tube or rubber catheter is passed through the ureterotomy, both proximally to the renal pelvis and distally to the bladder. The tube is irrigated while withdrawing to ensure ureteral patency and to flush out any residual stone fragments. The ureterotomy is closed by loosely approximating the adventitia with a few interrupted, absorbable sutures. The ureter is surrounded by retroperitoneal fat, and a drain is placed.

In complicated cases, especially those requiring concomitant ureteral repair, a double-J stent should be left in place for 4 to 6 weeks. When drainage has ceased, the drain is advanced and removed. **If significant urinary drainage persists, the patient should be evaluated for distal obstruction. A kidney, ureter, and bladder radiograph may demonstrate residual stone fragments. In addition, the drain may be too close to the ureterotomy.** Percutaneous nephrostomy or placement of a double-J stent generally provides adequate diversion, allowing the ureterotomy to seal. The risk of development of a ureteral stricture at the site of the stone can be minimized by judicious ureteral dissection, adequate periureteral drainage, and proximal diversion in complicated cases.

Distal stones may require more dissection for exposure. Dividing the obliterated umbilical and superior vesical vessels improves access in some instances. Stones in the intramural ureter often require transvesical exposure. An anterior cystotomy is performed. If the stone is visualized or palpated just at the ureteral orifice, a meatotomy alone may allow extraction. Access to the ureter 1 to 2 cm proximal to the orifice can be gained by bimanual palpation of the stone through an open bladder. An incision is made through the bladder and ureteral wall directly onto the stone, and the stone is extracted. The ureteral adventitia is loosely approximated and the bladder closed with absorbable suture. A double-J stent is often left in place.

A transvaginal ureterolithotomy is associated with a shorter, less morbid postoperative course than an abdominal procedure. **It should be used, however, only in a patient with a large, fixed, distal ureteral stone that can be easily palpated bimanually.** In addition, the patient should have an adequate introitus for performing transvaginal surgery. The patient is placed in the dorsal lithotomy position, a Foley catheter and weighted vaginal speculum are placed, and the labia are retracted laterally. The cervix is grasped with a tenaculum and retracted to the side opposite the stone. The stone is palpated, and two stay sutures are placed through the vaginal wall on either side of the stone. The vaginal mucosa is infiltrated with 1% lidocaine with epinephrine. A full-thickness incision is made through the vaginal wall overlying the stone and parallel to the course of the ureter. Using blunt dissection and being careful not to dislodge the stone, the ureter is exposed. The ureter just proximal to the stone is surrounded with a vessel loop to avoid proximal migration. A ureterotomy is made, the stone extracted, and the ureter closed as previously described. The vaginal wall is approximated with running absorbable suture.

A postoperative complication unique to this mode of stone extraction is urinary extravasation manifested by vaginal drainage (i.e., a ureterovaginal fistula). A double-J stent generally allows adequate healing if distal obstruction is not present (Figs. 98–15 and 98–16).

Cutaneous Ureterostomy

The use of cutaneous ureterostomy as either a permanent or a temporary mode of urinary diversion has diminished markedly since the development of intestinal diversion, percutaneous nephrostomy and double-J stents, and early definitive treatment of congenital anomalies. Cutaneous ureterostomy was initially described by Johnston in 1963 as a means of diversion in children with congenital urinary obstruction. It was later used in adults with ureteral obstruction, generally from malignancy; however, a stomal stenosis rate of greater than 50% in an end cutaneous ureterostomy has limited its application (Straffon et al, 1970; MacGregor et al, 1987).

Currently, cutaneous ureterostomy is most commonly performed in children with posterior urethral valves or prune-belly syndrome who have persistent renal insufficiency despite adequate bladder drainage. Even in this population, a cutaneous pyelostomy is often preferred in patients with a large, extrarenal pelvis so as not to compromise ureteral blood supply and complicate further reconstruction. When a ureterostomy is performed as a temporizing measure, a loop stoma is generally created because of its lower stomal stenosis rate and better preservation of ureteral length. Although the indications for cutaneous ureterostomy in adults are limited, the procedure may be useful for the unusual case in which rapid diversion is needed in a patient who is suffering serious intraoperative problems.

An end cutaneous ureterostomy may be performed through a variety of incisions depending on the stoma site, whether one or both ureters are to be diverted, and whether an intraperitoneal or extraperitoneal approach is chosen. Care should be taken to mark the stoma site preoperatively, avoiding skin creases, the belt line, and proximity to a rib.

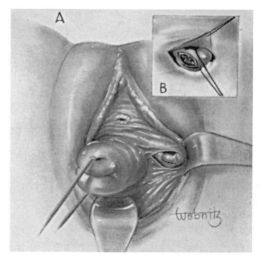

Figure 98–15. Transvaginal ureterolithotomy. *A,* The cervix is retracted to the opposite side of the stone. *B,* After incision of the vaginal wall, the ureter is isolated and the stone extracted.

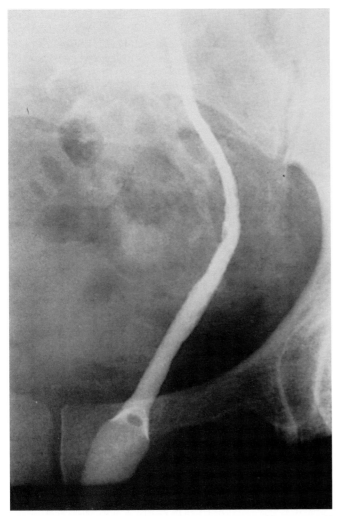

Figure 98–16. Antegrade nephrostogram in a 50-year-old woman with pyelonephritis, a duplex kidney, and a large stone in an ectopic upper-pole ureter. Transvaginal ureterolithotomy was performed on this fixed, easily palpable stone.

The patient's body habitus should be evaluated in the sitting, standing, and lying positions to ensure that the patient can easily access the stoma and that there is adequate muscular backing for application of an appliance. A small child can often wear an extra-large diaper with no stomal appliance. The optimum location for a stoma in an adult is along the lateral aspect of the rectus muscle, one third of the way from the umbilicus to the anterior superior iliac spine. The ureter can generally be mobilized without entering the peritoneal cavity in children. An intraperitoneal approach, however, is advantageous in adults with malignant obstruction, bilateral obstruction, or obesity. The ureter is identified as it crosses the iliac vessels, surrounded with a Penrose drain, and dissected down to the bladder, carefully preserving the adventitia. It is divided as distally as possible and mobilized as far cephalad as necessary to create a gentle curve to the abdominal wall. **Because distal ureteral ischemia with stricture formation and stomal stenosis is the most common complication of a ureterostomy, care must be taken to handle the ureter gently and to avoid abdominal wall compression.** The ureter is delivered through the stomal site, avoiding

rotation or kinking and allowing 2 to 3 cm for a tension-free anastomosis. The lateral ureter is spatulated for 1 to 2 cm. Using absorbable suture, the apex of a V-shaped skin flap is turned in and sutured to the apex of the spatulated ureter. It is preferable to create a slight eversion of the stoma to assist in application of an appliance. Bilateral ureteral diversion may be accomplished using a cutaneous ureterostomy in combination with a transureteroureterostomy or by bringing both ureters out through the same stoma. The ureters may be spatulated, sutured together, and anastomosed to a V-shaped skin flap. Alternatively a Z-plasty of the skin provides two flaps for inversion into the spatulated apex of each ureter.

With a loop cutaneous ureterostomy, a loop of dilated proximal ureter is brought out through a flank incision. The fascia is closed either around or underneath the loop with care taken to avoid constriction of it. The lateral aspect of the ureter is opened for 2 to 3 cm, and the ureter is sutured to the skin edge using interrupted, absorbable suture. A study by Rosen and colleagues of 20 children who underwent loop cutaneous ureterostomy reported no stomal-related complications in patients whose mean duration of diversion with ureterostomy was 12 months (Rosen et al, 1994). The prognosis with respect to renal function was related to the primary disease.

The most common complications of an end cutaneous ureterostomy are all related to distal ureteral ischemia: stomal necrosis, distal ureteral stricture, and stomal stenosis. Two thirds of patients have been reported to develop strictures. Observations made by Feminella and Lattimer (1971) show that dilated ureters (diameter >8 mm) have a lower stricture rate than nondilated ones, everted stomas stenose less often than flush stomas, and stricture rates are greater in patients who have undergone previous pelvic irradiation. A loop cutaneous ureterostomy is an effective means of temporary, proximal urinary diversion in children awaiting definitive reconstruction. **The high complication rate of end cutaneous ureterostomy in adults, obese patients, and those with nondilated ureters or previous irradiation makes its applicability for urinary diversion quite narrow.**

Ureterectomy

A ureterectomy may be performed for tumor, infection, stricture, or congenital anomaly. A radical nephroureterectomy remains the preferred treatment for an upper tract urothelial tumor in a patient with a normal contralateral kidney and is described in Chapter 97. The risk of tumor recurrence after a segmental ureteral resection increases with increasing tumor grade and stage. In addition, the location of multifocal recurrence tends to be distal to the primary tumor. **Therefore, the ideal candidate for segmental resection of an upper tract transitional cell carcinoma is a patient with a low-grade, low-stage, distal ureteral tumor.** The indication for such conservative treatment broadens significantly in the patient with renal insufficiency or a solitary kidney. In this population, local resection with adequate margins and close follow-up is generally preferable to dialysis. Ureterectomy is also indicated for complications related to a retained ureteral stump, at the time of ureteroureterostomy (or pyelopyelostomy) in a duplex system, and in conjunction with ureteral substitution for benign ureteral stricture.

Preoperatively an intravenous pyelogram (or retrograde pyelogram) is performed to rule out multifocal disease. Cystoscopy with ureteral barbotage or brushing or ureteroscopy and biopsy are performed in a patient with a suspected ureteral tumor. Ultrasonography or noncontrasted computed tomography scan can rule out the presence of a stone if this is in question. In patients with congenital anomalies, cystoscopy may assist in surgical planning and the need for additional reconstruction.

Primary Segmental Ureterectomy

A flank, Gibson, Pfannenstiel, or lower midline incision is chosen, depending on the level of ureteral pathology. The peritoneum is reflected medially and the ureter identified. A ureteral stent may have been placed preoperatively to relieve obstruction. The area of stricture or tumor is then visualized or palpated. A vessel loop or Penrose drain is placed around the ureter at the level of the diseased segment. Stay sutures are placed proximal and distal to the planned area of excision for traction and orientation. The ureter is divided obliquely proximal to the tumor or stricture. The ureteral wall opposite the base of the tumor is incised distal to the tumor, and the diseased segment is amputated in an oblique fashion. The excised segment is inspected to ensure adequate tumor resection with at least a 1-cm margin. In the case of a benign stricture, only the area of fibrosis is removed. The ureter is mobilized enough to bring the edges together without tension. Both ends are spatulated, and a watertight anastomosis is performed over a double-J stent with adequate periureteral drainage as described for ureteroureterostomy.

For a distal ureterectomy, the ureter is divided proximal to the lesion and a ligature placed on the distal segment. The ureter is dissected down to its insertion into the bladder. An anterior cystotomy is made, and a 1-cm full-thickness cuff of bladder is excised around the ureteral orifice using the knife or electrocautery. This allows a more precise margin for distal tumors and prevention of injury to the contralateral ureter. After ureteral reimplantation, the ureteral hiatus and cystotomy are closed with absorbable suture, and the area is drained.

Excision of a Retained Ureteral Stump

Most often, the entire ureter is excised for transitional cell carcinoma or a pathologic condition affecting the entire ureter. Occasionally, complications may develop in a retained distal ureteral segment after nephrectomy. Secondary excision of the distal ureter may be indicated for tumor, recurrent infection from reflux or obstruction of the stump, or stones in the stump. Preoperative placement of a ureteral catheter may be of benefit because of previous surgical fibrosis. Chandhoke and associates reported ureteral excision using a combination of laparoscopic dissection of the ureter and endoscopic incision of the ureterovesical junction (Chandhoke et al, 1993a).

TECHNOLOGIC ADVANCES

Progress continues to be made in developing minimally invasive techniques in ureteral surgery. Laser tissue welding

(Kirsch et al, 1994), laparoscopic ureteral repair (Nezhat and Nezhat, 1992), and endoscopic metallic ureteral stents (Pauer and Lugmayr, 1992) have been employed in ureteral surgery. Their practical use as compared with current alternatives is undefined.

REFERENCES

Adams JR Jr, Mata JA, Culkin DJ, Venable DD: Ureteral injury in abdominal vascular reconstructive surgery. Urology 1992; 39:77–81.
Assimos DG, Patterson LC, Taylor CL: Changing incidence and etiology of iatrogenic ureteral injuries. J Urol 1994; 152:2240–2246.
Babayan RK: Stents and catheters in percutaneous renal surgery. J Endourol 1993; 7:163–168.
Badenoch DF, Tiptaft RC, Thakar DR, et al: Early repair of accidental injury to the ureter or bladder following gynaecological surgery. Br J Urol 1987; 59:516–518.
Baker LR, Mallinson WJ, Gregory MC, et al: Idiopathic retroperitoneal fibrosis: A retrospective analysis of 60 cases. Br J Urol 1987; 60:497–503.
Begin LR, Selmy GI, Hassouna MM, et al: Healing and muscular restoration of the ureteral wall following balloon-induced rupture: An experimental animal model with light microscopic and ultrastructural observations. Exp Mol Pathol 1993; 59:58–70.
Benson MC, Ring KS, Olsson CA: Ureteral reconstruction and bypass: Experience with ileal interposition, the Boari flap-psoas hitch and renal autotransplantation. J Urol 1990; 143:20.
Bodie B, Novick AC, Rose M, et al: Long-term results with renal autotransplantation for ureteral replacement. J Urol 1986; 136:1187.
Boxer RJ, Fritzsche P, Skinner DG, et al: Replacement of the ureter by small intestine: Clinical application and results of the ileal ureter in 89 patients. J Urol 1979; 121:728.
Boyarsky S, Duque O: Ureteral regeneration in dogs: An experimental study bearing on the Davis intubated ureterotomy. J Urol 1955; 73:53.
Brannan W: Useful applications of transureteroureterostomy in adults and children. J Urol 1975; 113:460.
Butcher HR Jr, Sleator W Jr: The effect of ureteral anastomosis upon conduction of peristaltic waves: An electroureterographic study. J Urol 1956; 75:650.
Caine M, Hermann G: The return of peristalsis in the anastomosed ureter: A cine-radiographic study. Br J Urol 1970; 42:164.
Carlton CE Jr, Guthrie AG, Scott R Jr: Surgical correction of ureteral injury. J Trauma 1969; 9:457.
Carlton CE Jr, Scott R Jr, Guthrie AG: The initial management of ureteral injuries: A report of 78 cases. J Urol 1971; 105:335.
Chandhoke PS, Clayman RV, Kerbl K, et al: Laparoscopic ureterectomy: Initial clinical experience. J Urol 1993a; 149:992–997.
Chandhoke PS, Clayman RV, Stone AM, McDougall EM: Endopyelotomy and endoureterotomy with the Acucise ureteral cutting balloon device: Preliminary experience. J Endourol 1993b; 7:45–51.
Cohen JD, Persky L: Ureteral stones. Urol Clin North Am 1983; 10:699.
Cormio L, Battaglia M, Traficante A, Selvaggi FP: Endourological treatment of ureteric injuries. Br J Urol 1993; 72:165–168.
Dalsing MC, Bihrle R, Lalka SG, et al: Vascular surgery-associated ureteral injury: Zebras do exist (Review). Ann Vasc Surg 1993; 7:180–186.
Davis DM: Intubated ureterotomy: A new operation for ureteral and ureteropelvic stricture. Surg Gynecol Obstet 1943; 76:513.
Davis DM: Intubated ureterotomy. J Urol 1951; 66:77.
Davis DM: The process of ureteral repair: A recapitulation of the splinting question. J Urol 1958; 79:215.
Dowling RA, Corriere JN Jr, Sandler CM: Iatrogenic ureteral injury. J Urol 1986; 135:912–915.
Ehrlich RM, Melman A, Skinner DG: The use of vesicopsoas hitch in urologic surgery. J Urol 1978; 119:322.
Ehrlich RM, Skinner DG: Complications of transureteroureterostomy. J Urol 1975; 113:467.
el-Deen ME, Khalaf I, Rahim FA: Effect of internal ureteral stenting of normal ureter on the upper urinary tract: An experimental study. J Endourol 1993; 7:399–405.
Falandry L. Ureterovaginal fistulas: diagnosis and surgical tactic. Apropos of 19 personal cases [French]. J Urol 1992; 98:213–220.
Feminella JG Jr, Lattimer JK: A retrospective analysis of 70 cases of cutaneous ureterostomy. J Urol 1971; 106:538.

Flam TA, Malone MJ, Roth RA: Complications of ureteroscopy. Urol Clin North Am 1988; 15:167.

Galal H, Lazica A, Lampel A, et al: Management of ureteral strictures by different modalities and effect of stents on upper tract drainage. J Endourol 1993; 7:411–417.

Galmes Belmonte I, Serrano Pascual A, Garcia Cuerpo E, et al: Abnormalities of the inferior vena cava: the retrocaval ureter [Spanish]. Arch Espan Urol 1994; 47:647–655.

Gil-Vernet JM, Caralps A: Human renal homotransplantation: New surgical technique. Urol Int 1968; 23:201–223.

Guiter J, Cuenant E, Mourad G, et al: Re-establishment of urinary continuity by uretero-ureterostomy in renal transplantation. Apropos of 135 cases [French]. J Urol 1985; 91:27–32.

Harada N, Tanimura M, Fukuyama K, et al: Surgical management of a long ureteral defect: Advancement of the ureter by descent of the kidney. J Urol 1964; 92:192.

Hardy JD: High ureteral injuries: Management by autotransplantation of the kidney. JAMA 1963; 184:111.

Harzmann R, Kopper B, Carl P: Cancer induction by urinary drainage or diversion through intestinal segments? [German]. Urol Ausgabe A 1986; 25:198–203.

Hendren WH, Hensle TW: Transureteroureterostomy: Experience with 75 cases. J Urol 1980; 123:826.

Higgins CC: Transuretero-ureteral anastomosis: Report of clinical case. Trans Am Assoc Genitourin Surg 1934; 27:279.

Hinman F: Ureter. In Hinman F, ed: Reconstruction Atlas Of Urologic Surgery. Philadelphia, W. B. Saunders Company, 1989, pp 636–693.

Hinman F, Oppenheimer R: Functional characteristics of the ileal segment as a valve. J Urol 1958; 80:448.

Hodges CV, Barry JM, Fuchs EF, et al: Transureteroureterostomy: 25-year experience with 100 patients. J Urol 1980; 123:834.

Horgan PG, Hanley D, Burke J, et al: Extracorporeal shock wave lithotripsy induces the release of prostaglandins which increase ureteric peristalsis. Br J Urol 1993; 71:648–652.

Hubner WA, Plas EF, Stoller ML: The double-J ureteral stent: In vivo and in vitro flow studies. J Urol 1992; 148:278–280.

Huffman JL: Ureteroscopic management of transitional cell carcinoma of the urinary tract. Urol Clin North Am 1988; 15:419.

Kearney GP, Mahoney EM, Sciammas FD, et al: Venacavography, corticosteroids and surgery in the management of idiopathic retroperitoneal fibrosis. J Urol 1976; 115:32.

Kennelly MJ, Konnak JW, Herwig KR: Vesicopyeloplasty in renal transplant: A 20 year follow-up. J Urol 1993; 150:1118–1120.

Kerbl K, Chandhoke PS, Figenshau RS, et al: Effect of stent duration on ureteral healing following endoureterotomy in an animal model. J Urol 1993; 150:1302–1305.

Kirsch AJ, Dean GE, Oz MC, et al: Preliminary results of laser tissue welding in extravesical reimplantation of the ureters. J Urol 1994; 151:514–517.

Kletscher BA, Segura JW, LeRoy AJ, Patterson DE: Percutaneous antegrade endoscopic pyelotomy: Review of 50 consecutive cases. J Urol 1995; 153:712–713.

Koch MO, McDougal WS: The pathophysiology of hyperchloremic metabolic acidosis after urinary diversion through intestinal segments. Surgery 1985; 98:561.

Koch MO, McDougal WS: Ureteral substitution. In McDougal WS, ed: Difficult Problems in Urologic Surgery. Chicago, Year Book Medical Publishers, 1989, pp 76–100.

Lapides J, Caffrey EL: Observation on healing of ureteral muscle: Relationship to intubated ureterotomy. J Urol 1955; 73:47.

Lee CK, Smith AD: Role of stents in open ureteral surgery. J Endourol 1993; 7:141–144.

Lennon GM, Fitzpatrick JM: Effects of balloon dilatation on canine ureteric physiology. Eur Urol 1994; 25:248–253.

Lindell OI, Lehtonen TA: Surgical treatment of ureteric obstruction in idiopathic retroperitoneal fibrosis. Scand J Urol Nephrol 1988; 110(suppl):299–302.

MacGregor PS, Montie JE, Straffon RA: Cutaneous ureterostomy as palliative diversion in adults with malignancy. Urology 1987; 30:31.

Martinez J, Kaplan N, Boyarsky S: Laboratory and clinical studies of ureteral replacement by ileum. J Urol 1965; 93:185.

Meretyk I, Meretyk S, Clayman RV: Endopyelotomy: Comparison of ureteroscopic retrograde and antegrade percutaneous techniques. J Urol 1992; 148:775–783.

Meretyk S, Albala DM, Clayman RV, et al: Endoureterotomy for treatment of ureteral strictures. J Urol 1992; 147:1502–1506.

Mesrobian H-GJ, Kelalis PP: Ureterocalicostomy: Indications and results in 21 patients. J Urol 1989; 142:1285.

Middleton RG: Routine use of the psoas hitch in ureteral reimplantation. J Urol 1980; 123:352.

Motiwala HG, Shah SA, Patel SM: Ureteric substitution with Boari bladder flap. Br J Urol 1990; 66:369–371.

Motola JA, Badlani GH, Smith AD: Results of 212 consecutive endopyelotomies: An 8-year follow-up. J Urol 1993a; 149:453–456.

Motola JA, Fried R, Badlani GH, Smith AD: Failed endopyelotomy: Implications for future surgery on the upj. J Urol 1993b; 150:821–823.

Nezhat C, Nezhat F: Laparoscopic repair of ureter resected during operative laparoscopy. Obstet Gynecol 1992; 80:543–544.

Noordzij JW, Dabhoiwala NF: A view on the anatomy of the ureterovesical junction. Scand J Urol Nephrol 1993; 27:371–380.

Novick AC, Stewart BH: Experience with extracorporeal renal operations and autotransplantation in the management of complicated urologic disorders. Surg Gynecol Obstet 1981; 153:10.

Ockerblad NF: Reimplantation of the ureter into the bladder by a flap method. J Urol 1947; 57:845.

Ockerblad NF, Carlson HE: Surgical treatment of ureterovaginal fistula. J Urol 1939; 42:263.

Ormond JK: Bilateral ureteral obstruction due to envelopment and compression by an inflammatory retroperitoneal process. J Urol 1948; 59:1072.

Passerini-Glazel G, Meneghini A, Aragona F, et al: Technical options in complex ureteral lesions: "Ureter-sparing" surgery. Eur Urol 1994; 25:273–280.

Pauer W, Lugmayr H: Metallic Wallstents: A new therapy for extrinsic ureteral obstruction. J Urol 1992; 148:281–284.

Pearse HD, Barry JM, Fuchs EF: Intraoperative consultation of the ureter. Urol Clin North Am 1985; 12:423.

Perez LM, Friedman RM, Carson CC 3d: Endoureteropyelotomy in adults: Review of procedure and results. Urology 1992; 39:71–76.

Perlmutter A, Miller L, Trimble LA, et al: Toradol, an NSAID used for renal colic, decreases renal perfusion and ureteral pressure in a canine model of unilateral ureteral obstruction. J Urol 1993; 149:926–930.

Persky L, Carlton CE Jr: Urinary diversion in ureteral repair. In Scott R Jr, ed: Current Controversies in Urologic Management. Philadelphia, W. B. Saunders Company, 1972, pp 169–175.

Popescu C: The surgical management of postoperative ureteral fistulas. Surg Gynecol Obstet 1964; 119:1079.

Prieto D, Simonsen U, Martin J, et al: Histochemical and functional evidence for a cholinergic innervation of the equine ureter. J Auton Nerv Syst 1994; 47:159–170.

Prout GR Jr, Koontz WW Jr: Partial vesical immobilization: An important adjunct to ureteroneocystostomy. J Urol 1970; 103:147.

Rhee RY, Gloviczki P, Luthra HS, et al: Iliocaval complications of retroperitoneal fibrosis. Am J Surg 1994; 168:179–183.

Rober PE, Smith JB, Pierce JM Jr: Gunshot injuries of the ureter. J Trauma 1990; 30:83.

Rodo Salas J, Martin Hortiguela E, Salarich de Arbell J: Psoas fixation of the bladder: An efficient aid in cases of repeat surgery of the ureterovesical junction [Spanish]. Arch Espan Urol 1991; 44:125–129.

Rosen MA, Roth DR, Gonzales ET: Current indications for cutaneous ureterostomy. Urology 1994; 43:92–96.

Sahin A, Erdemli I, Bakkaloglu M, et al: The effect of nifedipine and verapamil on rhythmic contractions of human isolated ureter. Arch Int Physiol Biochim Biophys 1993; 101:245–247.

Saltzman B: Ureteral stents. Urol Clin North Am 1988; 15:481.

Sampaio FJ, Favorito LA: Upj stenosis: Vascular anatomical background for endopyelotomy. J Urol 1993; 150:1787–1791.

Sandoz IL, Paull DP, MacFarlane CA: Complications with transureteroureterostomy. J Urol 1977; 117:39.

Schlossberg SM: Ureteral healing. Semin Urol 1987; 5:197–199.

Schmeller N, Pensel J: Laser treatment of the ureter. In Smith JA Jr, ed: Lasers in Urologic Surgery, 2nd ed. Chicago, Year Book Medical Publishers, 1989, pp 81–91.

Schmidt JD, Flocks RH, Arduino L: Transureteroureterostomy in the management of distal ureteral disease. J Urol 1972; 108:240.

Scott FB, Greenberg M: Submucosal bladder flap ureteroplasty: Clinical experience. South Med J 1972; 65:1308.

Selmy GI, Hassouna MM, Begin LR, et al: Long-term effects of ureteric stent after ureteric dilation. J Urol 1993; 150:1984–1989.

Shore ND, Bregg KJ, Sosa RB: Indwelling ureteral stents. Semin Urol 1987; 5:200–207.

Smart WR: An evaluation of intubation ureterotomy with a description of surgical technique. J Urol 1961; 85:512.

Smith FL, Ritchie EL, Maizels M, et al: Surgery for duplex kidneys with ectopic ureters: Ipsilateral ureteroureterostomy versus polar nephrectomy. J Urol 1989; 142:532–534.

Stefanovic KB, Bukurov NS, Marinkovic JM: Non-antireflux versus antireflux ureteroneocystostomy in adults. Br J Urol 1991; 67:263–266.

Straffon RA, Kyle K, Corvalan J: Techniques of cutaneous ureterostomy and results in 51 patients. J Urol 1970; 103:138.

Streem SB: Percutaneous management of upper-tract transitional cell carcinoma. Urol Clin North Am 1995; 22:221–229.

Sweetser P, Weiss GH, Smith AD: Percutaneous laser treatment of the kidney and ureter. In Smith JA Jr, ed: Lasers in Urologic Surgery, 3rd ed. St. Louis, Mosby-Year Book, 1994, pp 157–170.

Szewczyk W, Szkodny A, Noga A, et al: Endopyelotomy for upj stenosis. Int Urol Nephrol 1992; 24:105–108.

Tasca A, Zattoni F: The case for a percutaneous approach to transitional cell carcinoma of the renal pelvis. J Urol 1990; 143:902.

Thompson AS, Dabhoiwala NF, Verbeek FJ, Lamers WH: The functional anatomy of the ureterovesical junction. Br J Urol 1994; 73:284–291.

Thompson IM, Ross G Jr: Long-term results of bladder flap repair of ureteral injuries. J Urol 1974; 111:483.

Tresidder GC, Blandy JP, Singh M: Omental sleeve to prevent retroperitoneal fibrosis around the ureter. Urol Int 1972; 27:144.

Turner-Warwick RT, Worth PHL: The psoas bladder-hitch procedure for the replacement of the lower third of the ureter. Br J Urol 1969; 41:701.

Waters WB, Whitmore WF, Lage AL, et al: Segmental replacement of the ureter using tapered and non-tapered ileum. Invest Urol 1981; 18:258.

Weiss RM: Physiology of the upper urinary tract. Semin Urol 1987; 5:148.

Wemyss-Holden GD, Rose MR, Payne SR, Testa HJ: Non-invasive investigation of normal individual ureteric activity in man. Br J Urol 1993; 71:156–160.

Woolfson RG, Hilson AJ, Lewis CA, et al: Scintigraphic evidence of abnormal ureteric peristalsis following urological surgery. Br J Urol 1994; 73:142–146.

Zungri E, Chechile G, Algaba F, et al: Treatment of transitional cell carcinoma of the ureter: Is the controversy justified? Eur Urol 1990; 17:276–280.

99
GENITOURINARY TRAUMA

Arthur I. Sagalowsky, M.D.
Paul C. Peters, M.D.

Optimal management of the trauma patient requires a coordinated team approach. The genitourinary tract frequently is involved in various types of trauma to the chest, abdomen, and pelvis. With the exception of the external genitalia in the male, the genitourinary tract is protected fairly well from external violence and even penetrating trauma because of the surrounding musculoskeletal structures and surrounding viscera. The inherent mobility of most urinary tract structures offers an additional measure of protection.

An accurate history is as important in assessing the trauma victim as in any other type of patient. History should be obtained directly from the patient whenever possible. Additional indirect history from witnesses must be sought in unconscious or severely injured patients. The history may alert the physician to a high likelihood of injury to the genitourinary tract regardless of the findings or lack of findings on the physical examination and urinalysis (see later). The pertinent history suggesting possible injury to the upper (kidneys, ureters) or lower (bladder, urethra, external genitalia) genitourinary tract is presented in each related section.

The urologist as well as the physicians initially called to assess the trauma patient should be certain that priorities in

system care are observed before focusing on the genitourinary tract. First, an adequate airway must be established. Second, any external bleeding is controlled. Third, sufficient lines for patient stabilization and resuscitation are placed. These include large-bore intravenous access for administration of crystalloid fluid and blood or other colloid and a nasogastric tube for decompression of the stomach to prevent vomiting and aspiration. A urinary catheter is inserted routinely unless history of pelvic trauma or the finding of blood at the urethral meatus suggests urethral injury.

The **physical examination** is carried out simultaneously with the preceding steps in the generalized stabilization and resuscitation of the trauma patient. Penetrating wounds and bruises or tenderness over the flank, pelvis, suprapubic region, or external genitalia all suggest possible injury to the underlying genitourinary structures and require a systematic approach for further evaluation, as described subsequently.

KIDNEY

Presentation

History

The kidneys are located high in the retroperitoneum and are protected posteriorly by the psoas and quadratus lum-

3085

borum muscles and anteriorly by the peritoneum and abdominal viscera. In addition, the kidneys are cushioned by perinephric fat inside Gerota's fascia and have a vertical mobility of one to three vertebral bodies. The lower rib cage (ribs 10 to 12) covers and protects the kidneys. In terms of surface anatomy and risk for trauma, the kidneys should be considered intrathoracic as well as retroperitoneal organs. Trauma to the back, flank, lower thorax, or upper abdomen may result in renal injury. Historical details are important in assessing blunt or penetrating trauma. In assessing victims of motor vehicle accidents, knowledge of the vehicle's speed and the patient's role as driver, passenger, or pedestrian is crucial. The size of weapon in stabbings or bullet caliber in gunshots is an important determinant of the severity of penetrating injuries. Flank pain or history of hematuria following trauma requires consideration of possible renal injury. Pre-existing renal abnormality makes renal injury more likely following trauma. History of sudden deceleration in motor vehicle accidents or a fall from a height suggests a high risk for renal injury.

Physical Examination

Physical examination may reveal obvious penetrating trauma from stabs to the lower thorax, back, or flank (Figs. 99–1 and 99–2) or bullet entry or exit wounds in this area. Bruises over the flank suggest possible renal trauma following blunt trauma (Fig. 99–3).

Urinalysis

Urinalysis is the most important laboratory test in the evaluation of renal trauma and should be obtained in every patient unless urethral injury also is suspected. The **degree of hematuria may not predict the severity of renal injury.** Hematuria may be absent in 10% to 25% of renal injuries. In one series of 102 patients with renal trauma, hematuria was absent in 5.8% and 2.8% of cases of minor and major parenchymal injuries and in 64.3% of renovascular injuries (Hai et al, 1977). **In general, however, hematuria is present in greater than 95% of renal trauma, and gross hematuria is associated with more severe renal trauma than is microscopic hematuria.** Hematuria out of proportion to the history of trauma suggests pre-existing renal abnormality, such as hydronephrosis, tumor, cystic disease, or vascular malformation (Fig. 99–4). Urine dipstick is a rapid and economical screen for hematuria and largely replaces the need for microscopic urinalysis. In one study comparing urine dipstick and microscopic urinalysis in 339 patients who underwent renal imaging following blunt trauma, the dipstick result had a specificity and sensitivity of 97.5% each with false-negative and false-positive rates of 2.5% in detection of hematuria (Chandhoke and McAninch, 1988). A urine dipstick reading of trace to 2+ for blood did not correlate with the magnitude of hematuria on microscopic urinalysis, but a 3+ dipstick reading was associated with more than 50 red blood cells per high-power field in greater than 80% of cases. Variability in dipstick results depends on the specific product and accuracy of the interpretation.

Mechanism of Injury

Renal trauma results from shearing forces that exceed the tensile strength of the renal parenchyma. **Blunt renal**

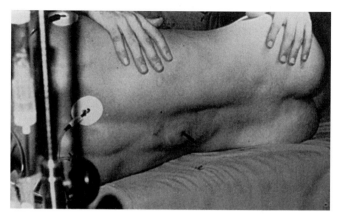

Figure 99–2. Penetrating trauma to the flank raises obvious concern over possible renal injury.

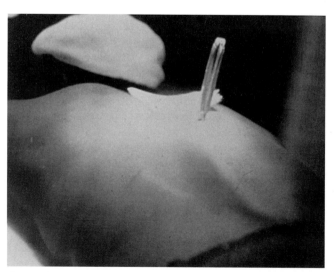

Figure 99–1. Penetrating trauma to the lower thorax may produce renal injury.

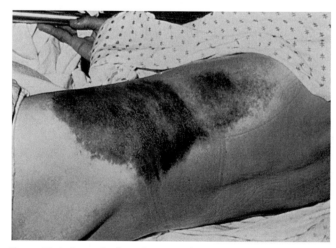

Figure 99–3. Large flank ecchymosis after blunt trauma suggests renal injury.

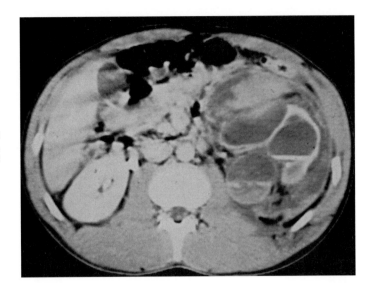

Figure 99–4. This patient had hematuria out of proportion to the magnitude of a flank injury incurred during spring football practice. Computed tomography suggests pre-existing hydronephrosis. Note the cortical rim sign.

trauma usually is associated with sudden deceleration of the human body. Motor vehicle accidents, falls, and blunt physical contact with external objects are the causes of this type of injury (Fig. 99–5). Deceleration or crush injuries may thrust the kidney against the rib cage or vertebrae or against the steering wheel or dashboard of a vehicle or other objects, resulting in contusion, laceration, or avulsion of renal parenchyma. A direct blow to the abdomen or flank during athletics or fisticuffs is a common cause of blunt renal injury. Sudden deceleration may stretch the renal artery and produce a tear in the intima leading to subintimal dissection of blood and renal artery thrombosis unless the defect is repaired promptly (Fig. 99–6). Children are prone to suffer disruption of the ureteropelvic junction following deceleration and hyperextension injuries.

The mechanism of injury for **penetrating trauma** is the obvious tissue disruption to the parenchyma, collecting system, and vasculature. Gunshot wounds produce a radiating current of energy and cavitation known as blast effect, which damages tissue beyond the tract of the projectile. Energy is proportional to the square of missile velocity. High-velocity missiles (>1100 feet per second) generally penetrate and exit from the body. Blast effect may cause delayed tissue necrosis leading to bleeding, urine leak, or abscess from areas that appeared viable at the time of injury.

Classification of Injury

Renal injuries may be classified as minor or major (Fig. 99–7). **Minor injuries** consist of superficial lacerations, small subcapsular hematomas, and contusions (see Fig. 99–7A, B, and C). **Major renal trauma** includes deep parenchymal lacerations through the corticomedullary junction and collecting system (see Fig. 99–7C and D), renovascular pedicle injuries (see Fig. 99–7B), and shattered kidneys

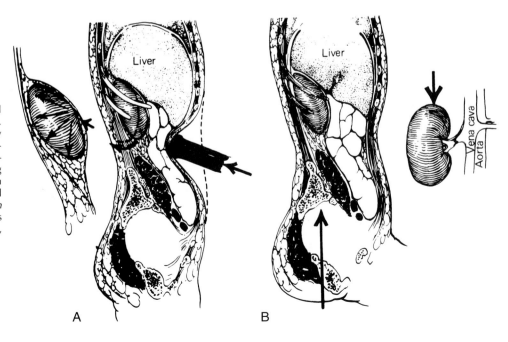

Figure 99–5. Mechanisms of renal injury. *A,* Direct blow to abdomen. Smaller drawing shows force of blow radiating from the renal hilum. *B,* Falling on buttocks from a height (contrecoup of kidney). Smaller drawing shows direction of force exerted on the kidney from above. Tear of renal pedicle. (From McAninch JW: *In* Smith DR, ed: General Urology. Los Altos, Lange Medical Publications, 1981, p 245.)

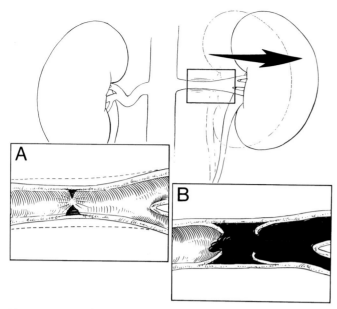

Figure 99–6. Mechanism of renal artery thrombosis in blunt traumatic injury. The kidney remains in motion in reference to the more stationary aorta. *A*, The media and adventitia, because of their elasticity, stretch readily. The intima, being less elastic, tears. *B*, The intimal flap initiates the clotting mechanism, and the thrombus is quickly propagated distally. (From Peters PC, Bright TC III: Urol Clin North Am 1977; 4:17–28.)

ages of cases by mechanism were 89%, 4%, and 7% for blunt, gunshot, and stab injuries, respectively (Nash et al, 1995). Surgery was required for renal trauma in 2.1% of blunt, 72.8% of gunshot, and 41.6% of stab injuries.

The frequency and type of associated nonrenal injuries are related to the mechanism of trauma (Table 99–2). Penetrating renal injuries are associated with other intraabdominal or intrathoracic injuries in 80% to 95% of cases (Carlton et al, 1968; Carlton, 1978; Peters and Bright, 1977; Sagalowsky et al, 1983). In one series, every renal injury caused by gunshots had other associated injuries (Sagalowsky et al, 1983). The reported incidence of associated injuries with renal stabbings varies from a low of 12% for entry wounds posterior to the anterior axillary line (Bernath et al, 1983) up to 30% to 77% for renal stabs overall (Carlton, 1978; Heyns et al, 1983; Sagalowsky et al, 1983). Blunt renal trauma requiring surgery is associated with nonrenal injuries in 44% to 100% of cases (Peters and Bright, 1977; Sagalowsky et al, 1983). Predictably the most common associated injuries are to the organs adjacent to the kidneys— liver, small bowel, spleen, stomach, and pancreas.

Renal pedicle injury warrants special discussion. In some series, blunt trauma with sudden deceleration is the leading cause of injury to the intima of the renal artery leading to thrombosis (Maggio and Brosman, 1978; Cass et al, 1979). In the Parkland experience with renovascular trauma, pene-

(see Fig. 99–7*A*). This schema corresponds closely with the official classification of the Organ Injury Scaling Committee of the American Association for the Surgery of Trauma (Table 99–1) (Moore et al, 1989). Approximately 70% of renal injuries are minor and do not require intervention. Ten percent to 15% of renal injuries are shattered kidneys or injuries to the renal pedicle. These injuries almost always require immediate surgery to control life-threatening bleeding and often result in nephrectomy. The remaining group of major parenchymal injuries generate much controversy in terms of optimal management. These injuries are commonly associated with large intrarenal and perirenal hematomas and extravasation of urine. The decision for initial exploration and repair versus observation alone or with delayed repair taxes the clinician's judgment and is discussed in detail in the section on treatment.

Relationship of Mechanism and Class of Renal and Nonrenal Injuries

The mechanism of injury is an important predictor of the likelihood and severity of renal trauma, the need for surgery, and the risk of associated nonrenal injuries. Renal injury is present in approximately 10% of abdominal trauma. Blunt trauma predominates in civilian populations and accounts for nearly 90% of renal injuries. Penetrating trauma produces the majority of major renal injuries requiring surgery. In a Parkland Hospital series of 185 consecutive cases of renal trauma requiring surgery, 66% were due to gunshots, 18% to stabs, and 16% to blunt injury (Sagalowsky et al, 1983). In a series of more than 2500 patients with renal trauma at the University of California at San Francisco, the percent-

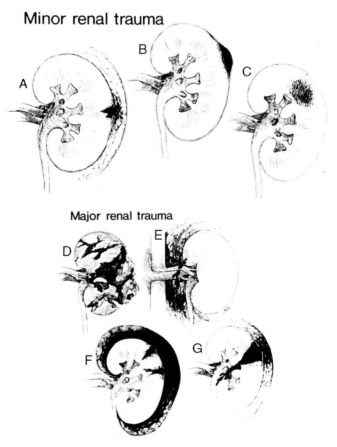

Figure 99–7. Minor and major renal injuries. *Minor injuries: A,* Simple laceration. *B,* Subcapsular hematoma. *C,* Renal contusion. *Major injuries: D,* Renal rupture. *E,* Laceration of renal artery and vein. *F,* Perirenal hematoma. *G,* Laceration through collecting system. (From Peters PC, Bright TC III: Urol Clin North Am 1977; 4:17–28.)

Table 99–1. RENAL INJURY SCALE OF THE AMERICAN ASSOCIATION FOR THE SURGERY OF TRAUMA

Grade*		Description†
I	Contusion	Microscopic or gross hematuria: urologic studies normal
II	Hematoma	Subcapsular, nonexpanding without parenchymal laceration
	Hematoma	Nonexpanding perirenal hematoma confined to renal retroperitoneum
III	Laceration	<1.0 cm parenchymal depth of renal cortex without urinary extravasation
IV	Laceration	>1.0 cm parenchymal depth of renal cortex without collecting system rupture or urinary extravasation
	Laceration	Parenchymal laceration extending through the renal cortex, medulla, and collecting system
V	Vascular	Main renal artery or vein injury with contained hemorrhage
	Laceration	Completely shattered kidney
	Vascular	Avulsion of renal hilum, which devascularizes kidney

*Increase one grade for multiple injuries to the same kidney.
†Based on most accurate degree of assessment: autopsy>surgery>imaging.
Adapted from Moore EE, Shackford SR, Pachtes HL, et al: J Trauma 1989; 29:1664–1666.

trating injuries predominate because of the referral pattern to the urban trauma center. A total of 26 renal pedicle injuries were identified among 185 trauma cases requiring surgery from 1976 to 1980 for a 14% incidence of renovascular injuries (Sagalowsky et al, 1983). The cause was penetrating trauma in 77% of cases from gunshots (58%) or stabs (19%). The specific renovascular injuries were to the renal artery, renal vein, or both in 6, 11, and 9 cases each for an incidence of 3%, 6%, and 5% for the entire series. Nephrectomy was required in 81% of renovascular injuries overall: renal artery, 83%; renal vein, 73%; and combined injury, 89%. The high rate of nephrectomy for all types of renovascular injuries was due to the severity of coexisting renal parenchymal and other nonrenal injuries.

A total of 96 renovascular injuries were identified in a larger Parkland series of all trauma encountered over a 20-year period (Turner et al, 1983). Penetrating trauma produced 67% of these injuries. The distribution of injuries was

Table 99–2. ASSOCIATED NONRENAL INJURIES IN RENAL TRAUMA

Organ	Gunshots, n = 122		Stabs, n = 33		Blunt, n = 30	
	No.	%	No.	%	No.	%
Liver	58	48	6	18	12	40
Small intestine	47	38	4	12	1	3
Stomach	45	37				
Colon	43	35	5	13	2	7
Spleen	28	23	5	13	17	57
Pancreas	25	20			4	13
Chest	12	10			4	13
Vena cava	9	7	1	3		
Aorta	5	4				
Ureter	3	2	1	3		

Adapted from Sagalowsky AI, McConnell JD, Peters PC: J Trauma 1983; 23:128–131.

to the renal artery in 19%, renal vein in 34%, or both in 47% of cases. Repair of the renal artery succeeded in 4 of 12 attempts. The trauma group at the University of California at San Francisco reported a similar predominance of penetrating trauma in renovascular injuries (75%) and a low renal salvage rate primarily as a result of patient hemodynamic instability or shattered kidneys, which precluded prolonged attempts at renovascular repairs (Nash et al, 1995).

The greatest determinant of mortality in patients with renal trauma is the nature and extent of associated nonrenal injuries. During the past two decades, improvements in anesthesia, trauma surgery, and renal repair in particular have resulted in increases in surgical renal salvage rates from 64% to 90% for blunt and 70% to 86% for gunshot injuries (Sagalowsky et al, 1983; Nash et al, 1995). Renal salvage rates after stab injuries remain approximately 85%. Continued improvement in triage and patient resuscitation, however, allows more seriously injured patients to survive to reach trauma centers and undergo exploration than in the past. Consequently, trauma patients who still require nephrectomy continue to have high mortality rates in most series (50%–70%) because of the severity of other injuries.

Evaluation and Diagnosis

From the preceding discussion of presentation, mechanism, and classification of renal injuries, a simplified algorithm for evaluation and diagnosis of renal trauma emerges (Fig. 99–8). The possibility of renal trauma should be considered in all patients with a history of any trauma and hematuria or any of the following historical or physical findings regardless of the presence or absence of hematuria: a direct blow to the flank; sudden deceleration as in a fall or motor vehicle accident; penetrating injury to the flank, back, lower chest, or upper abdomen; or flank bruise, crepitance, or lower rib fracture.

Findings on a plain abdominal film that suggest possible renal injury include lower rib or vertebral fractures (Fig. 99–9A), ground-glass density over the renal area, obliteration of the psoas muscle shadow, and scoliosis to the side opposite the injury because of spasm of the ipsilateral psoas muscle.

The **high-dose intravenous pyelogram (IVP)** remains an excellent initial imaging study for assessing renal trauma. A rapid bolus infusion of 1 ml per pound body weight of 30% iodinated contrast material is given, and films are obtained at 1, 5, 15, and 30 minutes. The goal of the study is to determine if both kidneys are present and functioning and to delineate the renal parenchymal outline and the collecting system. Causes of nonvisualization of the kidney on IVP are shown in Table 99–3. The majority of renal injuries may be staged accurately by high-dose IVP. Nephrotomograms, if available, increase sensitivity for detection of parenchymal lacerations, devitalized segments, and intrarenal hematomas and yield overall staging accuracy in 87% of blunt and 68% of penetrating renal injuries (Nicolaisen et al, 1985). Poor visualization on IVP suggests a major parenchymal injury and the need for further studies (Fig. 99–9B and C).

Computed tomography (CT) provides greater sensitivity and specificity than the IVP in the detection and characterization of the renal injury (Sandler and Toombs, 1981; McAn-

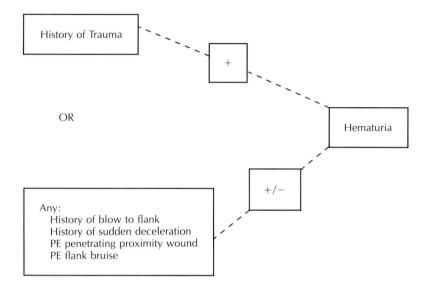

History of Trauma

OR

Any:
    History of blow to flank
    History of sudden deceleration
    PE penetrating proximity wound
    PE flank bruise

\+

\+/−

Hematuria

Figure 99–8. Diagnostic algorithm for renal trauma. (See text for further explanation. PE, physical examination.

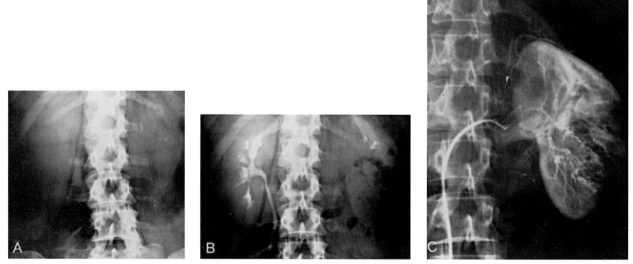

Figure 99–9. *A,* Fractures of transverse processes of left L2–4 vertebrae following blunt trauma. *B,* Intravenous pyelogram demonstrates poor excretion, loss of lower pole outline, and nonvisualization of lower calyces in left kidney. *C,* Arteriogram reveals major laceration through corticomedullary junction. (From Sagalowsky AI, Peters PC, Berman H: A unified approach to renal trauma. *In* Ehrlich RM, ed: Modern Technics in Surgery. Mount Kisco, NY, Futura Publishing, 1984, Chap. 31, pp 1–11.)

Table 99–3. CAUSES OF NONVISUALIZATION ON INTRAVENOUS PYELOGRAM

Renal absence—congenital or surgical
Renal ectopia
Shock
Renovascular spasm because of severe contusion
Renal artery thrombosis
Avulsion of renal pedicle
High-grade obstruction

inch and Federle, 1982; Herschorn et al, 1991). The three-dimensional nature of CT provides valuable information about the major abdominal and retroperitoneal organs in the trauma patient. At major trauma centers, the abdominal CT scan often is the initial imaging study in the multiple injury patient and replaces the IVP. Renal ectopia, minor degrees of urinary extravasation, major parenchymal lacerations, intrarenal and perirenal hematomas, and segmental devascularization are more easily identified on CT than IVP (Table 99–4; Figs. 99–10 to 99–14). Intrarenal hematoma appears as a round, poorly marginated lesion, with decreased contrast enhancement compared with the normal parenchyma (see Figs. 99–10 and 99–11). Perinephric hematoma has a streaked or bubbly appearance from infiltration of blood in the perinephric fat (see Figs. 99–12, 99–13, and 99–14A). Renal lacerations and urine extravasation are well shown after the injection of contrast material (see Fig. 99–14B). Segmental devascularization or arterial spasm reveals a sharp margin on CT, in contrast to a contusion or intrarenal hematoma, and lacks subcapsular hematoma or enhancement with contrast material.

The use of arteriography in the evaluation of patients with renal trauma has diminished greatly because of CT. Nonvisualization on IVP or CT and poor visualization on CT are the main indications for renal arteriography in the trauma patient. Although severe contusion with spasm may produce nonvisualization, renal artery thrombosis is the most common cause (Fig. 99–15). Disruption of the arterial intima is highly disposed to thrombosis unless repaired promptly (Fig. 99–16). In the past, appearance of any nephrogram on IVP had a 95% to 97% positive predictive value that no surgically correctable renal arterial injury was present. This is not true for CT scan because of its greater sensitivity for visualization owing to parasitized collateral vessels, which may produce a cortical rim enhancement in the presence of an occlusion to the main renal artery (Fig. 99–17).

Arteriography may reveal preservation of arterial supply to all renal segments despite complete parenchymal fracture (Fig. 99–18). Such patients heal without surgery. Identification of devascularized renal segments is important because necrosis, urine leak, abscess formation, or hypertension may occur unless the devitalized tissue is débrided and drained

Table 99–4. INDICATIONS FOR SURGERY IN RENAL TRAUMA

Uncontrolled bleeding
Renovascular injury
Nonviable parenchyma
Major urinary extravasation

(Fig. 99–19). Husmann and colleagues have reported on the outcome with expectant versus surgical management of major blunt renal injuries with or without devitalized segments (Husmann and Morris, 1990; Husmann et al, 1993). Delayed urologic complications occurred in 13% of nonoperated patients if all renal segments were vascularized. In the follow-up series, among patients with a devitalized renal segment, delayed urologic complications occurred in 38% who did not undergo a laparotomy. Perinephric abscess occurred in every patient with an unrepaired, devitalized renal segment and a concomitant pancreatic or bowel injury.

Figure 99–20 represents a comprehensive imaging and treatment decision tree for patients with possible renal trauma. During the past decade, numerous investigators have reported on both prospective and retrospective outcome analyses on the need for imaging and intervention in patients with renal trauma. In 1985, the San Francisco trauma group reported a prospective analysis of the need for renal imaging in 359 trauma patients (Nicolaisen et al, 1985). Major renal injuries were common among the 85 patients with blunt trauma and gross hematuria or microscopic hematuria plus shock (defined as systolic blood pressure <90 mm Hg at any time since the injury). The history and clinical findings did not reliably correlate with the presence of major renal injuries in 53 patients with penetrating trauma. The authors concluded that both of these groups need to undergo renal imaging to identify and assess the degree of renal trauma. In 221 patients with blunt trauma and only microscopic hematuria without shock, however, renal imaging revealed only renal contusions, which required no intervention. The authors raised the possibility that renal imaging may be unnecessary in these patients. Selective avoidance of renal imaging would allow enormous cost reduction and minimize toxicity owing to intravenous contrast material without any decrease in renal salvage rates or overall patient safety. These observations apply to adult trauma patients. Children with blunt trauma and hematuria should undergo renal imaging regardless of the blood pressure or the degree of hematuria. The caveats regarding all patients who lack hematuria but are at high risk for renal trauma based on history still apply. Most patients with renovascular injuries have shock, which compels evaluation, and successful renovascular repair is infrequent in the remaining few patients with subtle injuries.

The same group of investigators reported a 10-year prospective analysis on the need for renal imaging in 1146 consecutive patients with blunt (1007 cases) or penetrating (139 cases) trauma (Mee et al, 1989). Major renal injuries were present in 63% of patients (88 of 139) with penetrating trauma and in 4.4% of patients (44 of 1007) with blunt trauma and either gross hematuria or microscopic hematuria plus shock. In the largest group of 812 patients with blunt trauma and only microscopic hematuria without shock, 404 patients underwent renal imaging and 408 patients did not. Among these 812 patients, no major renal injuries were identified, and no delayed operations for renal injury occurred. No late sequelae from untreated renal injuries were identified. Again, **the conclusion is that renal imaging is indicated in all patients with penetrating trauma to the flank, back, or abdomen but only in adult blunt trauma patients with gross hematuria or microscopic hematuria plus shock.**

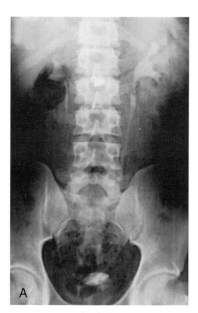
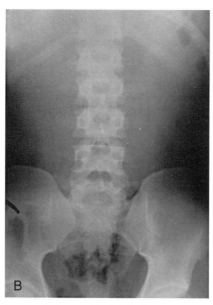
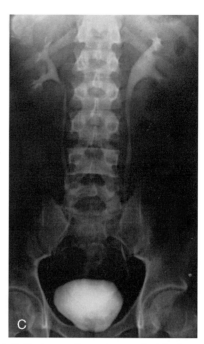

Figure 99–10. *A,* Initial infusion pyelogram following gunshot wound to left flank appears normal. Bullet is noted over L2 vertebral body. No renal injury was identified at the time of exploration. *B,* Abdominal plain film taken 5 days later, when the patient developed fever and pain, shows generalized ground-glass appearance and paucity of bowel gas, suggesting urinary extravasation. *C,* Pyelogram taken the same day as *B* is still normal.

Hardeman and associates reported virtually identical results in a retrospective review of renal imaging in 506 patients with blunt trauma and hematuria seen at Parkland Memorial Hospital (Hardeman et al, 1987). Detectable renal injuries were present in 4.9% (25 of 506) of patients overall, and 21 of 25 patients had gross hematuria. Three patients had microscopic hematuria without shock and had renal contusions or minor laceration. Only one patient had microscopic hematuria plus shock and required surgery. Herschorn and co-workers from Toronto also found no patients (0 of 126) with major renal injury following blunt trauma and microscopic hematuria without shock in a retrospective series of trauma in 3993 patients (Herschorn et al, 1991).

Ultrasonography is of limited use compared with CT in the evaluation of renal trauma. Radionuclide scans may be helpful to document renal blood flow in the trauma patient with severe allergy to iodinated contrast material or in follow-up after repair of renovascular trauma. Retrograde pye-

lography has little role in the diagnosis of renal trauma but is helpful in the evaluation of ureteral trauma (see later).

Treatment

A clear understanding of the importance of the history and physical examination, the influence of differing mechanisms of renal injury for penetrating versus blunt trauma, and how they relate to the frequency and severity of renal injury is essential for treatment planning. **The critical feature of the safe, efficient use of the diagnostic, imaging, and treatment schema depicted in Figures 99–8 and 99–20 is aggressive pursuit of diagnosis and complete classification of injury in patients at risk for major renal trauma.** Better understanding of the natural history of renal trauma allows for more selective use of renal imaging. Better precision in the classification of renal injuries by CT allows for

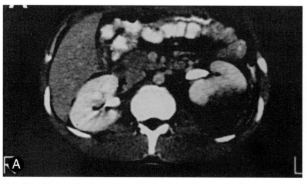
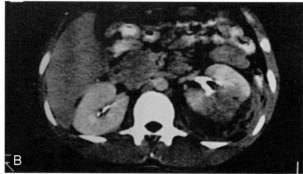

Figure 99–11. Abdominal computed tomography scan of same patient as in Figure 99–10 reveals perirenal hematoma and urinoma *(A)* and intrarenal hematoma *(B).*

Figure 99–12. *A,* Pyelogram reveals poor visualization of left kidney in a patient after an automobile accident. *B,* Flush aortogram reveals left main renal artery and major segmental blood supply to be intact. A small amount of vascular extravasation *(arrows)* is demonstrated.

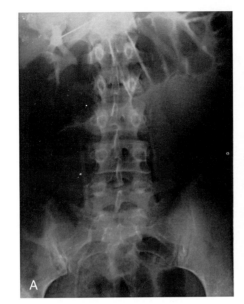

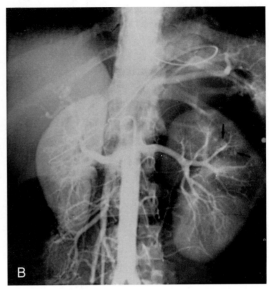

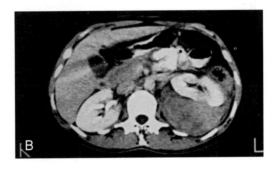

Figure 99–13. *A,* Abdominal computed tomography scan of the same patient as in Figure 99–12 reveals a large perirenal fluid collection. *B,* This view shows a parenchymal laceration and the characteristic bubbly appearance created by dissection of blood and urine in the perinephric fat.

Figure 99–14. *A,* Computed tomography scan following trauma to the right flank shows perinephric collection. *B,* After the injection of intravenous iodinated contrast material, deep parenchymal laceration extending into the collecting system is shown.

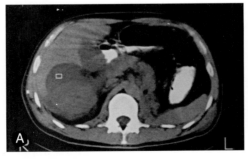

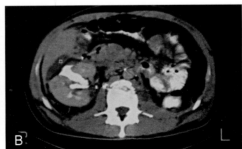

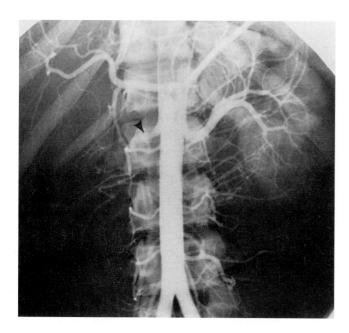

Figure 99–15. Total occlusion of right renal artery *(arrow)* following blunt renal trauma. (From Sagalowsky AI: In Ehrlich RM, ed: Modern Technics in Surgery. Mount Kisco, NY, Futura Publishing, 1984.)

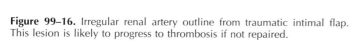

Figure 99–16. Irregular renal artery outline from traumatic intimal flap. This lesion is likely to progress to thrombosis if not repaired.

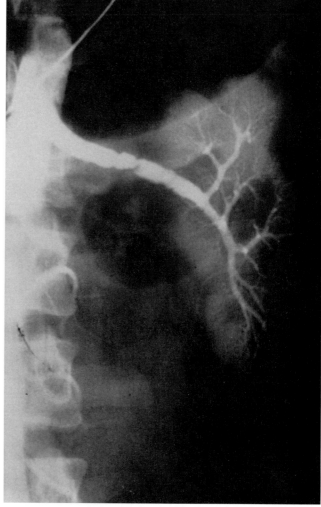

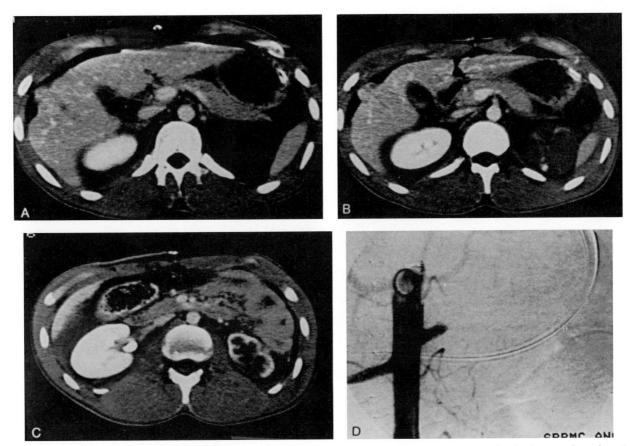

Figure 99–17. A through D, Computed tomography (CT) showing nonenhancement of the left kidney except for the lower pole and cortical rim sign. Digital subtraction arteriogram shows total occlusion of the left renal artery in a kidney in which the cortex is visualized by CT. Such a kidney would have been nonfunctioning by intravenous pyelography. This case shows the need for occasional arteriography to complement CT findings. (Adapted from Cass AS, Luxenberg M: J Urol 1987; 138:266–268. Copyright Williams & Wilkins.)

more selective surgical exploration. The condition of the patient, however, remains the final determinant in the decision for initial observation versus surgical intervention.

The **indications for renal exploration** in trauma patients are shown in Table 99–4 and Figure 99–20. Uncontrolled bleeding manifest as hemodynamic instability requires renal exploration. Some multiple-injury trauma patients need to undergo immediate laparotomy without imaging studies for control of life-threatening hemorrhage. Intraoperative consultation on these cases taxes the judgment of even the most experienced urologist. Following control of nonrenal bleeding, one should consider intraoperative one-shot IVP to document the presence and function of both kidneys. Expanding, pulsatile, or uncontained hematoma in Gerota's fascia indicates major renal bleeding requiring renal exploration. The need for prompt repair of renovascular injuries for salvage of renal function and control of bleeding and débridement of devitalized parenchyma to prevent delayed complications was described earlier. Although small lacerations of the collecting system usually seal without intervention, large urinary extravasation is best treated by draining the urinoma and repairing the injury primarily.

McAninch (1993) reports that surgical exploration of renal injuries caused by gunshots is required in only 77% of cases, provided that appropriate imaging studies completely stage the extent of renal injury and that none of the indications listed previously are present. The authors agree with this in

concept. As a practical matter in a teaching hospital setting with house officers at varying levels of experience, however, the authors continue to recommend exploration of nearly all penetrating renal injuries caused by gunshots because of the high association of intra-abdominal injuries and the unpredictable and serious nature of the renal injuries.

Selective observation of some stab wounds confined to the flank and without apparent major renal injury on complete imaging studies is possible. Investigators at the University of California at San Francisco reported that following complete imaging studies, surgical exploration is required in only 45% of renal injuries caused by stabs (McAninch, 1993). Eastham and colleagues reported a retrospective experience with 244 patients with stabs to the flank over a 5-year period (Eastham et al, 1992, 1993). Excretory urography had an accuracy of 96% in identifying renal stab injuries in 17.6% (43 of 244) of cases. Arteriography, rather than CT, was the second-line study for further classification of the injury. All 20 patients with major parenchymal or renovascular stab injuries underwent surgery or angiographic embolization for control of bleeding. Eleven of 23 patients with minor renal stab injuries were initially observed, and 12 patients underwent exploratory laparotomy either with (5 patients) or without (7 patients) renal exploration and drainage. Subsequent angiographic embolization was required in 16 patients with injuries to segmental renal arteries and provided prompt hemostasis in 14 patients. Partial nephrectomy was required

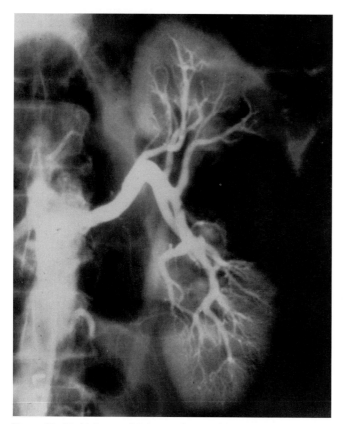

Figure 99–18. Major renal injury with complete parenchymal fracture and preservation of segmental blood supply.

in two patients, and nontarget embolization of portions of the kidney occurred in two patients. Other investigators have reported on initial observation with small numbers of patients with stab wounds confined to the flank, with delayed bleeding occurring in approximately 15% and secondary control of bleeding by angiographic embolization in approximately 85% of cases (Bernath et al, 1983; Heyns and van Vollenhoven, 1992; Teiger et al, 1992).

There is consensus that the 80% to 85% of blunt renal injuries that are minor contusions or lacerations require only observation and bed rest until the urine clears and vital signs stabilize. There also is agreement that the 10% of blunt injuries with renal pedicle trauma almost always require surgery to control hemorrhage. In the past, there was much controversy regarding optimal management of the remaining 10% to 15% of patients with major renal injuries caused by blunt trauma. The proponents of expectant management argued that most of these injuries heal, and initial exploration of the fresh wound risks uncontrolled hemorrhage requiring nephrectomy (Peters and Bright, 1977; Thompson, 1977). Reports continue to favor expectant management for nearly all pediatric patients with major blunt renal parenchymal injuries in the absence of any of the features listed in Table 99–4 (Baumann et al, 1992; Smith et al, 1993). The proponents of routine surgical exploration for this group of blunt renal injuries point out that nearly all of the delayed complications, secondary repairs, and prolonged hospital stays occur in this group of patients (Carlton, 1978).

In 1966, Scott and Selzman noted that the need for nephrectomy to control bleeding during renal exploration for

trauma can be reduced if the renal vessels are isolated before opening Gerota's fascia. Opponents of exposing the renal vessels before opening Gerota's fascia argue that this step is time-consuming and occasionally difficult and that actual temporary occlusion of the renal vessels is rarely necessary in a kidney that is salvageable (Atala et al, 1991; Corriere et al, 1991). A series of publications from the San Francisco trauma group, which routinely obtains preliminary renovascular control, provide valuable insight on this issue. Exposure of the renal vessels did not prolong the operative time significantly. The nephrectomy rate during exploration for trauma declined from 56% to 18% once routine initial isolation of the renal pedicle was obtained (McAninch and Carroll, 1982). Temporary occlusion of the renal pedicle was required in 12% and 17% of 92 and 185 patients, respectively (Carroll et al, 1989, 1994). The preoperative classification of renal injury apart from renovascular injury did not predict which patients required temporary renovascular occlusion. Mortality rate and postoperative renal function were not adversely affected by the need for temporary renovascular occlusion. Repair of the renal injury was possible in 83% of patients (25 of 30) that required temporary renovascular occlusion. **Thus, routine exposure of the renal vessels before opening Gerota's fascia allows a higher renal salvage rate and adds to the safety of the procedure.**

Surgical Technique

A vertical midline incision from xiphoid to pubis is made for speed in opening and closing the wound and to afford maximum exposure. A complete inspection of the intra-abdominal contents is performed, and active bleeding is controlled. The renal vessels are exposed and controlled with vessel loops before Gerota's fascia is opened. An incision is made in the posterior parietal peritoneum medial and parallel to the inferior mesenteric vein (Fig. 99–21A). Additional exposure may be obtained by dividing the inferior mesen-

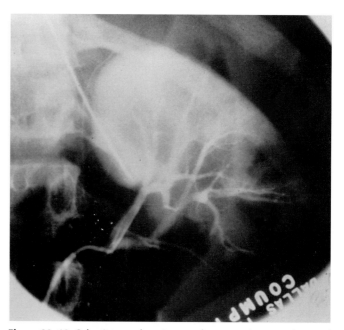

Figure 99–19. Selective renal angiogram demonstrating complete avulsion of the lower pole artery and associated parenchyma.

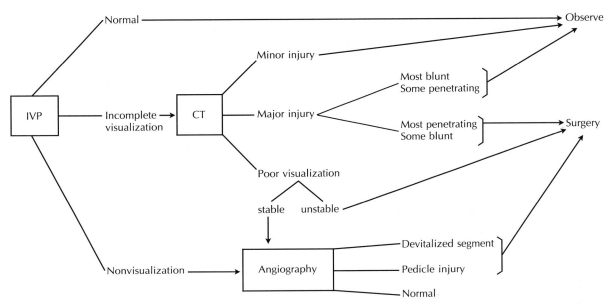

Figure 99–20. Imaging and treatment algorithm for renal trauma. (See text for further explanation.) IVP, intravenous pyelogram; CT, computed tomography.

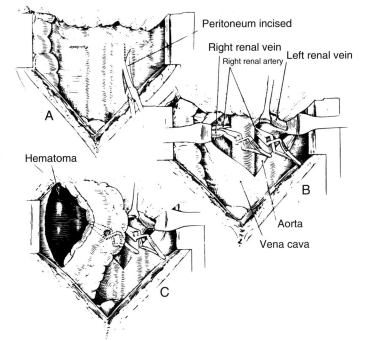

Figure 99–21. *A,* The posterior peritoneum is incised parallel to the inferior mesenteric vein. *B,* The left renal vein is mobilized and retracted cephalad to expose the origin of right and left renal arteries. *C,* The perirenal hematoma is entered only after the renal pedicle is controlled.

teric vein and continuing the peritoneal incision around the cecum (Fig. 99–22). Cephalad retraction on the pancreas exposes the left renal vein as it crosses over the aorta (Figs. 99–21*B* and 99–23). The left renal vein is mobilized and elevated to reveal the renal arteries (see Fig. 99–23).

The origin of both the right and the left main renal arteries is found almost invariably posterior to the junction of the left renal vein and inferior vena cava. This constant relationship allows for rapid exposure of the renal arteries. Farther from the aorta, the course of the renal arteries may encompass a vertical span of several inches (Fig. 99–24). Multiple renal arteries occur in 25% of patients, on right or left sides equally. Multiple renal veins occur in 15% of patients and are on the right side 80% of the time. Vessel loops are placed around the renal arteries so that a temporary vascular clamp can be applied rapidly. Then the colon on the affected side is mobilized off the anterior surface of Gerota's fascia (Fig. 99–21*C*), which is opened, and the kidney is explored. The renal capsule is reflected from traumatized renal tissue and preserved for closure of defects in the parenchyma (Fig. 99–25*A*, *B*, and *C*).

Traumatized parenchyma is débrided sharply. Severe polar injuries are best treated by guillotine amputation to minimize delayed necrosis and fistula formation (see Fig. 99–25*B*). Openings into the collecting system are closed with absorbable suture (4–0 chromic catgut or polyglycolic acid). Injured intraparenchymal vessels are oversewn with the same suture material or with polydioxanone suture. Further hemostasis may be obtained with the argon beam coagulator.

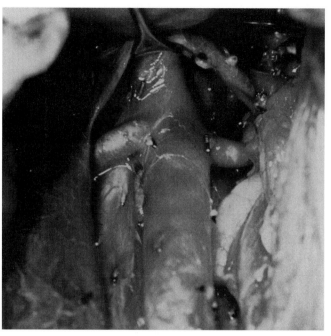

Figure 99–23. Retroperitoneal node dissection demonstrates the nearly constant origin of right and left renal arteries dorsal to the left renal vein (retracted cephalad) as it crosses the aorta.

Approximation of the renal capsule over the injured area is desirable (see Fig. 99–25*C*). Perinephric or omental fat or a free peritoneal graft may be sutured to the capsular edges (Fig. 99–26). Further hemostasis over large parenchymal defects may be obtained by filling the defect with a topical clotting agent such as oxidized cellulose (Oxycel) and placing mattress sutures with 2–0 chromic through the parenchyma.

Most shattered kidneys require nephrectomy to control

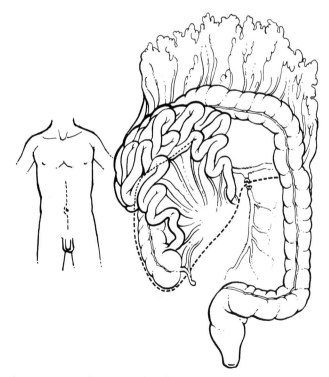

Figure 99–22. A long vertical midline incision allows rapid exposure in renal trauma cases. The entire small bowel and ascending colon may be rapidly mobilized by incising the posterior peritoneum, as shown. The inferior mesenteric vein may be ligated and divided to increase exposure of the renal vessels. (From Sagalowsky AI: *In* Ehrlich RM, ed: Modern Technics in Surgery. Mount Kisco, NY, Futura Publishing, 1984.)

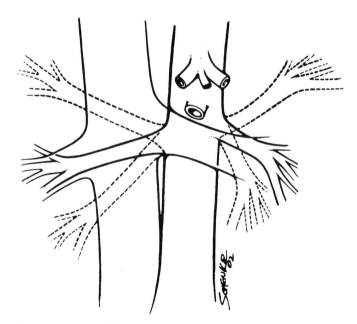

Figure 99–24. Variable course of renal arteries (particularly on the right side) is demonstrated. For rapid control, the renal artery is best located near the aorta.

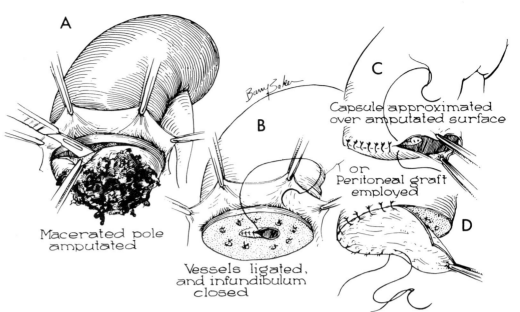

Figure 99–25. Surgical treatment of renal polar injury. *A,* Guillotine amputation of the injured parenchyma. *B,* Watertight closure of the collecting system and suture hemostasis. *C,* Reapproximation of renal capsule. *D,* Denuded surface covered with peritoneal patch graft.

hemorrhage, and the degree of parenchymal injury prevents repair. Occasionally a patient with a solitary kidney or bilateral renal trauma is encountered with multiple stellate fractures and preserved parenchyma, and hemostasis cannot be obtained by the techniques described previously. An absorbable polyglycolic acid mesh may be wrapped around the parenchyma to provide a tamponade effect.

Segmental renal vein injuries may be simply ligated, whereas renal arterial injuries are repaired whenever possible. Major lacerations to the renal vein are repaired directly by venorrhaphy. Repair of renal arterial injuries may require a variety of techniques, including resection and end-to-end anastomosis, bypass graft with autogenous vein or a synthetic graft, and arteriorrhaphy. Renovascular repairs are performed with 5–0, 6–0, or 7–0 polypropylene (Prolene)

sutures. A closed-suction drain is placed in the renal fossa following surgical exploration for renal trauma.

Postoperative Care and Management of Complications

Patients are kept at bed rest until the urine is grossly clear of blood and vital signs have stabilized. The serum hematocrit and creatinine level are measured serially. Flank drains are removed after several days when there is no further evidence of urine leak or bleeding.

Adherence to the diagnostic and surgical principles in the preceding sections prevents most delayed complications of secondary bleed, contained hematoma, abscess, or urinoma following renal trauma. New-onset flank pain, fever, mass,

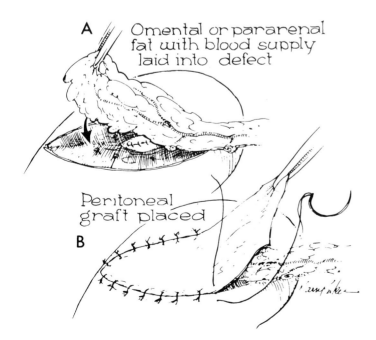

Figure 99–26. *A* and *B,* Placement of viable omentum or perirenal fat in large renal defect.

sudden drop in hematocrit, or rise in creatinine may signal one or more of these complications. Ultrasound and CT are especially helpful in diagnosis. Percutaneous drainage is an effective treatment of perinephric abscess, hematoma, or urinoma. Selective angiographic embolization is the preferred treatment of delayed hemorrhage owing to segmental renal artery injury and false aneurysm (Fig. 99–27). Demonstration of retained renal function before the patient is discharged is desirable because compliance with follow-up often is poor in trauma patients. Hypertension after renal injury resolves within 6 weeks in most cases.

URETER

The ureter is the least commonly injured portion of the genitourinary tract because of its small caliber and mobility and because it is well protected by the back muscles and the retroperitoneal fat.

Causes

The causes of ureteral injury may be categorized as due to external trauma or to iatrogenic events. Isolated ureteral injuries from external trauma are exceedingly rare, with only 24 reported in the United States armed forces for all of World War II. Injury from small-caliber missiles or stab wounds are the usual causes of penetrating ureteral trauma. Blunt trauma to the ureter is even less common with one exception. Children are prone to avulsion of the ureteropelvic junction following severe flexion-hyperextension injuries in high-speed motor vehicle accidents.

Iatrogenic ureteral injuries predominate in most civilian and rural populations. The surgical subspecialties and the associated open pelvic procedures most likely to produce iatrogenic ureteral injury are as follows: gynecology—hysterectomy, oophorectomy, bladder neck suspension; general surgery—colectomy, appendectomy; vascular surgery—aortoiliac bypass; urology—ureterolithotomy, ureteral reimplan-

tation. Lumbar laminectomy is an infrequent cause of ureteral injury. The increasing array of pelvic endoscopic and laparoscopic procedures is associated with a new group of ureteral injuries, as follows: gynecology—laser treatment of endometriosis, tubal ligation; urology—pelvic lymphadenectomy, ureteroscopy, stone removal; general surgery—appendectomy, bowel resection.

Diagnosis

History and physical evidence of trauma to the flank or pelvis raise the possibility of ureteral injury. Hematuria is present in 90% of ureteral trauma owing to external violence but is present in only 11% of iatrogenic cases (Carlton, 1978). Persistent pain, fever, ileus, and rising creatinine in a trauma or postoperative patient suggest urine leak and possible missed ureteral injury.

The diagnosis of ureteral injury is established by demonstration and localization of urinary extravasation or high-grade obstruction on imaging studies. The IVP detects ureteral injury in 94% of cases and localizes the level of injury in 50% of cases (Fig. 99–28A) (Carlton, 1978). Retrograde pyelography establishes the level and extent of the ureteral injury (Fig. 99–28B). **The IVP and retrograde pyelogram are the most useful studies when ureteral injury is suspected during the initial trauma evaluation.** Ultrasound, radionuclide scan, or abdominal CT may provide the first clues for delayed diagnosis of ureteral injury.

Classification

Ureteral injuries are classified based on four criteria that affect the management:

1. **Mechanism**—blunt versus penetrating, with the latter having possible blast effect and a high incidence of associated organ injury.

2. **Level of injury**—upper, middle, or lower ureter. The

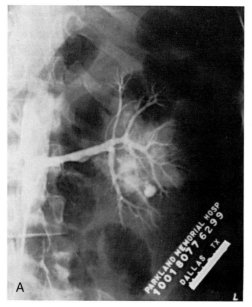 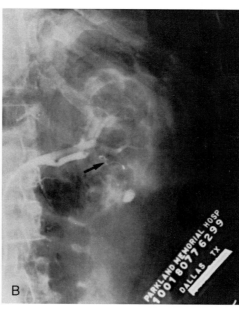

Figure 99–27. *A,* Angiogram obtained after delayed renal bleed following trauma reveals false aneurysm. *B,* Bleeding is controlled by embolization with a steel coil *(arrow).*

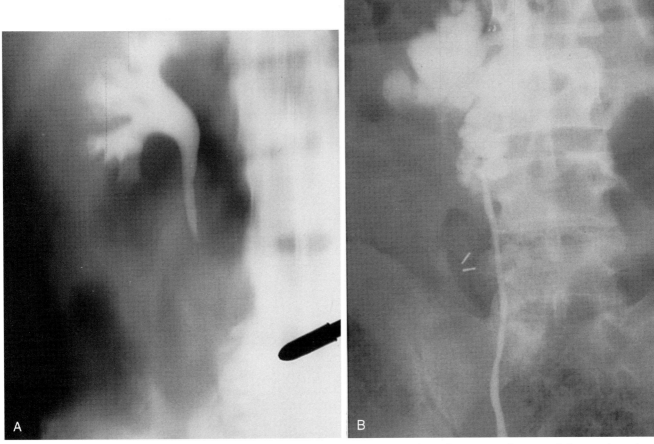

Figure 99–28. *A,* Intravenous pyelogram reveals obstruction of upper ureter in a patient with gunshot injury to the ureter. *B,* Retrograde pyelography reveals the lower ureter is intact, and there is marked extravasation at the level of ureteral injury.

upper and lower thirds receive vascular supply from the renal hilum and iliac vessels. The middle third has the most vulnerable blood supply. Iatrogenic ureteral injury occurs most commonly at the pelvic brim where the ureter crosses the iliac artery and where it courses posterior to the broad ligament and ovarian vessels in women (Daly and Higgins, 1988; Spirnak et al, 1989). Watery vaginal leakage in a patient after pelvic surgery suggests possible ureterovaginal or vesicovaginal fistula secondary to iatrogenic injury.

3. **Time of recognition**—immediate versus delayed. Prompt diagnosis before there is intense tissue inflammation and abscess formation from urinary extravasation may allow primary definitive ureteral repair. Delayed diagnosis may require drainage and proximal urinary diversion before definitive repair. Abdominal pain, fever, and ileus are the most common symptoms of unsuspected ureteral injury. Five percent of such patients are asymptomatic and may be diagnosed years later with a nonfunctioning or hydronephrotic kidney (Peters and Bright, 1977).

4. **Presence of associated injuries.** The patient's overall condition and the specific nonurologic injuries affect management of the ureteral injury. Simple ureteral intubation rather than definitive repair may be lifesaving in a patient with profound shock, massive transfusion, multiple injuries, and prolonged surgical time before the ureteral injury can be addressed (Fig. 99–29). In a patient with a normal contra-

lateral kidney, nephrectomy may be preferable to a complex ureteral repair if there are associated injuries to the colon, pancreas, and aorta.

Treatment

Ureteral injury diagnosed during the initial evaluation of a trauma patient is treated by open surgical repair in most cases. Delayed diagnosis of missed or iatrogenic injuries may be treated by percutaneous drainage of urinoma and retrograde or antegrade placement of a ureteral stent, provided that the ureter is at least partially intact. Following tangential injury to a portion of the ureteral wall by penetrating trauma or following a clamp or suture injury during surgery, passage of an indwelling double-J ureteral catheter may allow complete healing of the ureter. If a large amount of extravasation is present or a large ureteral defect is suspected, however, exploration and repair is preferable. When inadvertent ureteral ligation is suspected in the immediate postoperative period, laparoscopy may allow confirmation and removal of the suture followed by endoscopic placement of a ureteral stent.

The type of open surgical repair depends on the level and extent of ureteral injury (Table 99–5; Fig. 99–30). A tension-free repair must be obtained for optimal results. Partial

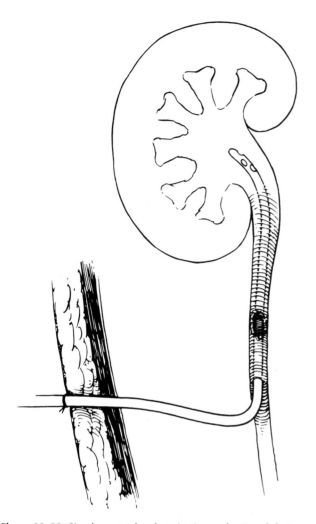

Figure 99–29. Simple ureteral catheterization and external drainage.

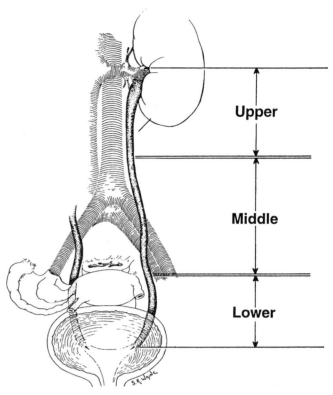

Figure 99–30. Management of ureteral injury, depending on location. (Modified from Orkin LA: Trauma to the Ureter: Pathogenesis and Management. Philadelphia, FA Davis Co, 1964.)

avulsion of the ureteral wall or complete transection with only a short defect is repaired by direct approximation of the ureteral wall or end-to-end direct reanastomosis after dèbridement and spatulation of the ureteral ends (Figs. 99–31 and 99–32) whenever possible for injuries at any level of the ureter. The principles of successful repair are accurate reapproximation of the ureteral wall with small interrupted sutures (4–0 or 5–0 chromic catgut), placement of a ureteral stent (internal double-J is usually preferable), and placement of a closed-suction drain (Jackson-Pratt type) near but not

Table 99–5. SURGICAL REPAIRS BASED ON LEVEL OF URETERAL INJURY

Repair	Level of Injury		
	Upper	*Middle*	*Lower*
Direct reanastomosis	+++	+++	++
Ureteroneocystostomy			+++
Psoas hitch ± Boari flap	+++	+++	+++
Transureteroureterostomy	++	++	+
Ileal ureter	++	++	+
Autotransplant	+	+	

*Number of + signs indicates order of preference.

touching the repair. Placement of a nephrostomy and an external ureteral stent allows greater postoperative control of urinary drainage in complex injuries in which tissue viability and wound contamination are in doubt (Fig. 99–33). Internal ureteral stents and closed-suction wound drains, however, suffice in most cases.

Lower third ureteral injuries are best managed by ureteroneocystostomy of healthy ureter anastomosed into the bladder. When the length of the ureteral defect prevents end-to-end ureteroureterostomy or ureteroneocystostomy, mobilization of the bladder with a psoas-hitch technique allows a tension-free anastomosis of healthy ureter to the bladder in nearly all injuries to the distal or middle ureter. The ureteral reimplant is protected by a ureteral stent in all cases. The addition of a Boari-Ockerblad flap onto a bladder psoas hitch permits repair of large ureteral defects even to the proximal ureter (Figs. 99–34 and 99–35). These techniques are especially helpful in repair of ureteral injuries after obstetric and gynecologic surgeries. The pelvic tissue inflammation, hematoma, and distended postpartum veins may be avoided, and healthy proximal ureter and bladder are repaired above the pelvic field.

Ileal ureteral substitution, transureteroureterostomy, and autotransplantation are alternatives when none of the preceding techniques for ureteral repair are possible. The authors do not recommend these procedures in the acute setting, however, with the possible exception of transureteroureterostomy. Ileal ureteral substitution or renal autotransplantation in a contaminated field and without a bowel preparation (in the case of ileal ureter) is contraindicated. Proximal ureteral ligation and nephrostomy drainage followed by elective de-

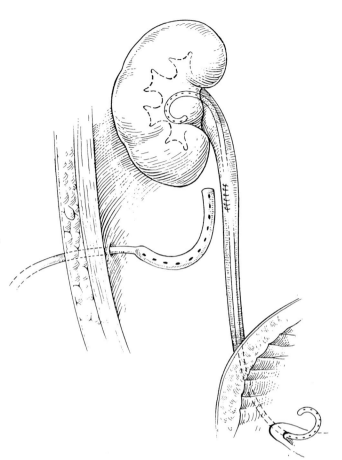

Figure 99–31. Approximation of ureteral edges with interrupted suture and placement of internal ureteral stent and closed-suction drain.

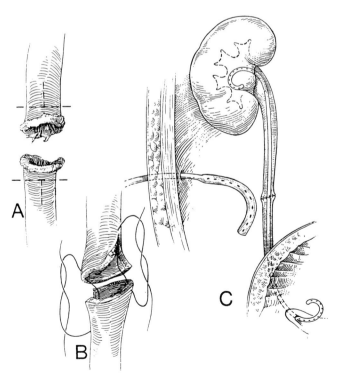

Figure 99–32. *A* through *C,* Direct end-to-end ureteral reanastomosis with interrupted suture and placement of internal ureteral stent and closed-suction drain.

finitive repair are preferred in such cases. Nephrectomy may be preferable if a normal contralateral kidney is present.

Postoperative Care

Drains are maintained until evidence of ongoing urinary leak ceases. Ureteral stents usually are removed 3 to 4 weeks after complex repairs (gunshots, ureteroureterostomy, psoas hitch) or 7 to 10 days after simple repairs (reimplant, closure of ureteral wall). Fever, pain, or prolonged urine leakage suggests a nonhealing repair that may require surgical re-exploration and reconsideration of all of the aforementioned options, including nephrectomy. Ureteral stricture after repair of ureteral injury may be corrected by ureteroscopic balloon dilation or incision or open surgical revision.

BLADDER

Presentation

Anatomic Considerations

In the adult, the bladder is an extraperitoneal organ situated deep in the pelvis protected by the bony pelvis laterally,

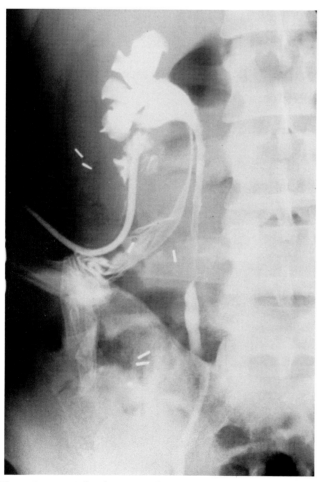

Figure 99–33. High-velocity missile transection of the midureter with much blast effect repaired by end-to-end ureteroureterostomy protected by nephrostomy, external ureteral stent, and closed-suction drain.

the symphysis pubis anteriorly, the pelvic floor fascia and musculature inferiorly, and the rectum posteriorly. The bladder base (and prostate in male patients) is relatively firmly anchored in the pelvis, whereas the body is more mobile. In children, the bulk of the bladder is intraperitoneal.

History and Physical Examination

Patients with blunt or penetrating trauma to the lower abdomen and pelvis are at risk for bladder injury. Sudden bladder deceleration in patients involved in high-speed motor vehicle accidents or application of excessive external force by seat belts, a direct blow, or crush injuries may cause blunt trauma to the bladder. The cause of bladder injury in penetrating trauma from gunshots or stabs is self-evident. Penetrating bladder injury also may occur from bone fragments associated with pelvic fracture (Corriere, 1991). **The type of bladder rupture is somewhat related to the state of bladder filling at the time of injury. The empty bladder is more susceptible to extraperitoneal rupture, whereas the full bladder is prone to intraperitoneal rupture.**

Bladder injury should be suspected when physical examination reveals suprapubic and vague, diffuse lower abdominal tenderness or bruises over the suprapubic and pelvic region. Careful vaginal and rectal examination is indicated in all trauma patients with suspected bladder injury. Intraperitoneal bladder rupture may produce abdominal distention and referred pain to the shoulder as a result of accumulation of urine within the abdomen and under the diaphragm.

Urinalysis

Urine is collected for microscopic or dipstick detection of hematuria in all patients at risk for bladder injury unless there is blood present at the urethral meatus. This latter finding suggests urethral injury (see later) and makes spontaneous voiding or passage of a catheter for urine collection contraindicated. **The importance of hematuria as a finding in patients with bladder injury cannot be overstated because it is present in greater than 95% of cases** (McConnell et al, 1982; Carroll and McAninch, 1984; Corriere, 1986). In one Parkland review of 46 patients seen with bladder rupture over a 6-year period, gross hematuria was present in 98% of cases, and the remaining 2% had microhematuria and a pelvic fracture (McConnell et al, 1982).

Radiologic Evaluation

Cystography is the definitive study for diagnosis of bladder rupture. The bladder must be completely filled for optimal detection of extravasation. At least 300 ml of water-soluble iodinated contrast solution (15%–30%) is instilled by gravity through a Foley catheter placed in the bladder. Films should include filled anteroposterior, oblique or lateral, and postdrain views. Cystography may fail to disclose extravasation if clot occludes the perforation.

Cystography may be obtained by percutaneous suprapubic bladder filling if urethral injury precludes passage of a urethral catheter. Direct surgical inspection of the bladder, however, usually replaces cystography if open placement of a suprapubic catheter is required for management of the urethral injury. Studies comparing the accuracy of CT cystogra-

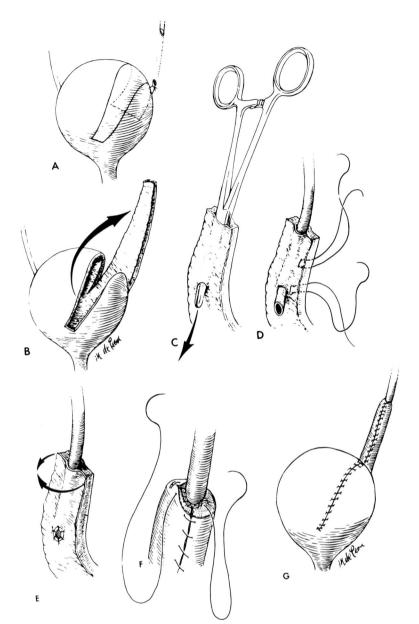

Figure 99–34. Technique of bladder flap ureteroplasty. *A* and *B,* Creation of broad-based bladder flap. *C,* Submucosal tunnel created for antireflux reimplantation of the ureter. *D,* Submucosal reimplantation of the ureter. Sutures in the posterior aspect of the flap rigidly fix the flap to the psoas muscle. *E,* Bladder flap rolled into tube. *F,* Ureter fixed to proximal flap. *G,* Completed bladder flap ureteroplasty.

phy with standard cystography for detection of bladder rupture in trauma patients who also require abdominal CT are not available at this time.

Classification and Mechanism of Injury

In civilian populations, blunt trauma accounts for 67% to 86% and penetrating trauma for 14% to 33% of bladder ruptures (McConnell et al, 1982; Carroll and McAninch, 1984; Corriere, 1986). Approximately 90% of bladder ruptures from blunt trauma are due to motor vehicle accidents. Bladder rupture caused by gunshots is associated with other visceral injuries in greater than 80% of cases. Both blunt and penetrating trauma may cause bladder wall contusion without actual perforation, which may or may not be suspected on cystography.

Extraperitoneal Rupture

Extraperitoneal rupture of the bladder is more common than intraperitoneal rupture in most series (Corriere, 1991). The lower abdominal pain associated with this injury is more diffuse and less severe than that seen with acute intra-abdominal processes, such as appendicitis or superior mesenteric vascular occlusion. Cystography reveals extravasation of contrast material into the pelvis around the base of the bladder (Fig. 99–36). Often the bladder assumes a "teardrop" deformity because of compression by a large pelvic hematoma (see Fig. 99–36*A*).

The strong association of extraperitoneal bladder rupture and pelvic fracture deserves special comment. Pelvic fracture is reported in 89% to 100% of these injuries (McConnell et al, 1982; Carroll and McAninch, 1984; Corriere, 1991). In one series, nonpelvic orthopedic injuries such as femur fracture were seen in 80% of patients with

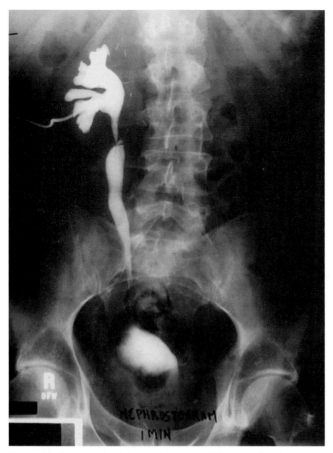

Figure 99-35. Repair of loss of entire middle and distal ureter by bladder psoas hitch plus Boari-Ockerblad flap. One-minute nephrostogram film shows prompt drainage across anastomosis just below the ureteropelvic junction.

extraperitoneal rupture of the bladder (McConnell et al, 1982). Conversely, bladder rupture is present in only 5% to 10% of all patients with pelvic fractures (McConnell et al, 1982; Corriere and Sandler, 1986).

Intraperitoneal Rupture

The weakest point of the bladder is the peritoneal surface across the dome. Sudden blunt force applied to the full bladder produces intraperitoneal rupture at this point. Cystography reveals intraperitoneal extravasation of contrast material outlining loops of bowel, filling the lumbar gutters, or pooling under the diaphragm (Fig. 99–37). Intraperitoneal bladder rupture usually is associated with multiple-injured and more seriously injured patients. In one series, patients with intraperitoneal rupture had a mortality rate of 20.3% owing to associated nonurologic injuries (Peters, 1989). In the Parkland experience, intra-abdominal injuries were only slightly more common with intraperitoneal versus extraperitoneal rupture of the bladder (43% versus 40%) but were more severe.

Combined Injury

Approximately 10% of patients with bladder rupture have combined extraperitoneal and intraperitoneal bladder perfo-

ration. The magnitude of force creating these combined bladder injuries and the high rate of nonurologic injuries are associated with a mortality rate of approximately 60%.

Treatment

Treatment is based both on the mechanism (blunt versus penetrating) and on the extent of injury (extraperitoneal versus intraperitoneal). Bladder wall contusion requires only catheter drainage for a few days. No doubt some contusions are not diagnosed and go untreated without untoward results. Associated pelvic hematoma may distort the bladder neck and interfere with voiding such that temporary catheter drainage is required.

Penetrating Injuries

All penetrating bladder injuries caused by gunshots, stabs, or bone fragments should undergo surgical exploration because of the nature of the bladder and associated injuries. The peritoneum routinely is opened and explored owing to the high rate of associated intra-abdominal injuries. Devitalized or foreign tissue is débrided. The bladder should be opened and formally explored so that all sites of penetrating injury are identified and repaired. Each bladder laceration is repaired from within the bladder with a two-layer closure of 3–0 chromic catgut or polyglycolic acid suture. The intraperitoneal serosal surface of perforations at the bladder dome also is closed from within the abdomen. The trigone, ureteral orifices, and bladder neck are inspected for injury. A ureteral catheter is passed or 5 ml of intravenous indigo carmine is given when injury to the juxtavesical portion of the ureter is suspected. Careful repair of injuries to the bladder neck is required to minimize postoperative extravasation of urine, incontinence, and stricture formation.

After repairing all bladder injuries, a large-bore suprapubic cystostomy (No. 22–24 Fr) is placed through a separate stab wound in the bladder dome. A Malecot catheter functions better than a Foley for this purpose. The catheter is secured to the outside of the bladder wall with 2–0 absorbable suture. Placement of the suprapubic tube through a separate opening allows a more secure closure of the anterior cystotomy, which also is repaired in two layers with running 3–0 absorbable suture. Two principles are important in suprapubic cystostomy: (1) The tube should be placed high in the bladder, well away from the trigone to diminish postoperative urinary frequency and bladder spasms; (2) the tube should be brought obliquely through the abdominal wall to discourage formation of a fistulous tract when the suprapubic tube is removed. The suprapubic catheter should be securely sutured at the skin exit site to prevent dislodgment from the bladder. A closed-suction drain is placed in the prevesical space and brought through a separate wound in the abdominal wall. The suprapubic tube can be safely removed in 10 to 14 days when a voiding cystogram shows that bladder lacerations have healed.

Intraperitoneal Rupture

All intraperitoneal bladder ruptures caused by penetrating trauma and nearly all caused by blunt trauma

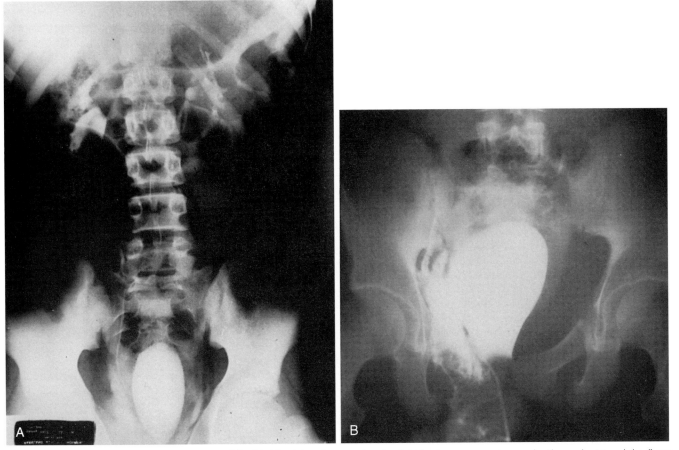

Figure 99–36. *A* and *B,* Extraperitoneal rupture of the bladder. Note the associated pelvic fracture commonly seen by the urologist and the flume-like distribution of the contrast material confined to the pelvis.

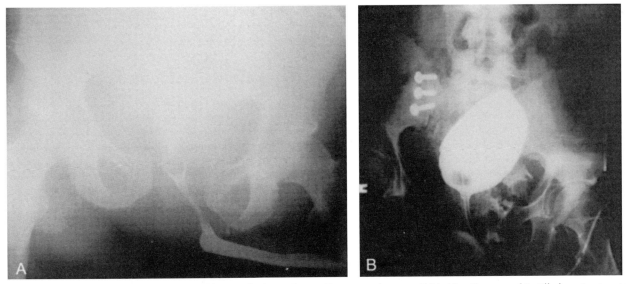

Figure 99–37. Intraperitoneal rupture of the bladder. *A,* Shadow of a small, apparently normal, bladder. Pressure of instilled contrast material is not great enough to disclose previous rent. As volume approaches 250 ml, rent becomes obvious (see *B*). *B,* Note contrast material escaping into peritoneal cavity around loops of bowel. The rupture may be subphrenic and along lumbar gutters and associated with other severe visceral injuries. Isolated intraperitoneal ruptures have been repaired via laparoscope, but, most commonly, exploratory laparotomy is the procedure of choice. At least 250 ml of contrast material needs to be instilled into the bladder. Otherwise, the rent may not be disclosed.

are best managed by surgical exploration and repair as described earlier. Cystoscopy may identify a rare case with blunt intraperitoneal rupture caused by a small bladder perforation in a patient with no other indication for surgery that may be managed by a urethral catheter alone for 7 to 10 days. Most patients, however, have a large perforation that should be repaired. The majority of publications describing successful nonoperative management of intraperitoneal bladder rupture deal with iatrogenic injuries rather than external trauma (Richardson and Leadbetter, 1975; Robards et al, 1976). Laparoscopic repair of an iatrogenic intraperitoneal bladder rupture has been described (Parra, 1994).

Extraperitoneal Rupture

Penetrating extraperitoneal bladder rupture requires exploration for all the reasons listed previously. In these cases, the perivesical hematoma should be opened to exclude other injuries and drained to prevent abscess formation.

Extraperitoneal bladder rupture caused by blunt trauma requires a greater degree of judgment in determining the management. Many injuries heal with urethral catheter drainage for 7 to 10 days. **The degree of extravasation seen on cystography may not correlate with the size of the perforation in the bladder wall.** Flexible cystoscopy may help in this regard. Nevertheless, a policy of repairing cases with a large amount of extravasation is safest. If the patient requires surgery for other nonurologic injuries and is stable, the bladder should be opened and repaired as already described. In blunt trauma, the perivesical hematoma should not be opened or drained to avoid the risk of introducing infection.

Complications

The most serious complications of bladder rupture relate to failure to diagnose or to control urinary extravasation initially. Extensive pelvic and abdominal wall abscess formation and necrosis may occur from unrecognized extraperitoneal urine leak. Peritonitis and intra-abdominal abscess formation results from ongoing intraperitoneal urine leakage. Lesser complications of bladder rupture and treatment include dislodgment of the suprapubic tube, continued leakage around the suprapubic tube or from the areas of injury, and bladder spasms. The position of the suprapubic tube may be checked by cystography or flexible cystoscopy. Percutaneous suprapubic puncture may be used to reposition the catheter over a guide wire if the suprapubic tube is out of position and continued suprapubic drainage is necessary. Pelvic fluid collections and abscess may be treated by ultrasonic controlled puncture and aspiration, and broad-spectrum antibiotics may be instilled into the cavity if necessary. Bladder spasms may be controlled with oral anticholinergic agents such as oxybutynin chloride 5 mg orally three times a day.

URETHRA

The urethra in the male is divided into four areas: (1) prostatic, (2) membranous, (3) bulbous, and (4) penile or pendulous. The anatomic relationships are important because injuries in different areas require different treatment and have distinct outcomes. **For treatment purposes, male urethral injuries are classified into two groups: (1) posterior**—prostatic and membranous injuries above or including the urogenital diaphragm; **(2) anterior**—injuries of the bulbous and penile urethra.

Urethral trauma in the female is much less common than in the male. Severe pelvic fracture and bony displacement along with lacerations through the bladder neck and vagina often are present in cases of urethral trauma in the female.

Posterior Urethra

Presentation and Physical Examination

This is the most severe injury of the lower urinary tract and usually results from violent external force. Strong shearing forces in high-speed blunt and crush injuries or high-velocity penetrating trauma tear the attachments of the prostate and puboprostatic ligaments from the pelvic floor. As a result, the prostatic urethra is torn. Pelvic fracture is present in greater than 90% of patients.

Patients with posterior urethral injury may have attempted to void unsuccessfully before arrival at the hospital. Often the bladder neck remains competent after the injury, and the degree of urinary extravasation may be minimal. Thus, the amount of swelling of the perineum, scrotum, or penis may be small. If the patient voids, gross hematuria is present in nearly all cases. On examination, blood is present at the urethral meatus in the majority of patients with urethral trauma. Patients with suspected urethral injury should be instructed not to void pending further evaluation.

Digital rectal examination is performed in all patients with pelvic trauma. After laceration of the posterior urethra, the bladder and prostate ascend above the normal anatomic position, and the defect fills with blood and urine. On rectal examination, a boggy fluid collection is present in the normal location of the prostate.

Imaging and Classification of Injury

Retrograde urethrography is indicated in all patients with suspected urethral trauma. The initial anteroposterior film of the pelvis serves to identify pelvic fractures, bony displacement of the symphysis, or the presence of foreign objects. Next the patient is placed in a 25-degree to 30-degree oblique position, and 25 ml of water-soluble contrast material is injected into the urethral meatus. The film is taken during the injection so that the urethra is distended. The oblique positioning offers the best demonstration of the entire urethra and any areas of extravasation. The best injection technique is with a small catheter inserted just past the fossa navicularis and the balloon inflated with 1 or 2 ml of water. Simply holding the tip of a syringe in the penile meatus results in the examiner's hands being exposed to radiation. Penile clamps such as the Brodney are awkward to use. If a urethral catheter already was inserted into the bladder, it should not be removed. A retrograde urethrogram may be obtained by inserting a feeding tube, angiocatheter, or Fogarty balloon catheter into the urethral meatus and injecting contrast material alongside the urethral catheter.

The mildest form of posterior urethral injury is stretching and elongation, owing to pelvic hematoma without rupture (type I) (Fig. 99–38). **The type II urethral injury results from partial or complete rupture of the prostatomembranous urethra. Extravasation on the retrograde urethrogram is confined below the urogenital diaphragm. The type III urethral injury is the most severe and is twice as common as each of the other injuries** (Fig. 99–39). **There is partial or complete rupture of the prostatomembranous urethra as well as rupture of the urogenital diaphragm and bulbous urethra.** Extravasation of contrast material is seen in the pelvis and the perineum. The degree (partial versus total rupture) and extent (type II versus type III) of urethral injury may be overestimated or underestimated on urethrography if spasm of the external urethral sphincter occurs and limits the extravasation or proper passage of contrast material into the bladder (Herschorn et al, 1992).

Treatment

Urethral catheterization for 3 to 5 days is recommended for patients with a type I injury because the hematoma distorting the urethra may produce incomplete voiding or actual retention. These mild injuries usually heal without sequelae.

Management of patients with partial or complete rupture of the posterior urethra (types II and III) is one of the most difficult and controversial areas in genitourinary trauma. **The goal of initial therapy is urinary diversion with the least negative impact on long-term rates of stricture formation, incontinence, and impotence.** There should be documentation in the medical records that the patient was advised

that the injury itself may result in these complications regardless of the initial method of treatment.

A urethral catheter may be passed into the bladder in many patients with a small, partial tear of the posterior urethra. The catheter is maintained for 7 to 14 days, and a voiding cystourethrogram is obtained when the catheter is removed. One gentle attempt at passing a catheter is unlikely to convert a partial urethral tear into a complete rupture. If any difficulty passing the catheter occurs, however, the attempt should cease, and a suprapubic catheter should be inserted. After successful initial passage of a urethral catheter, many of these injuries heal without any stricture or with a mild stricture amenable to periodic dilation.

Historical approaches to the patient with posterior urethral rupture emphasized primary exploration and direct urethral realignment, almost at any cost, with interlocking sounds passed antegrade through the bladder neck and retrograde per urethra to avoid complex urethral stricture formation and the need for difficult delayed repairs. The problems with this approach were multiple. Often the patients were hemodynamically unstable, and pelvic bleeding was active and hindered exposure. Infection could be introduced into the pelvic space. The rates of stricture, incontinence, and impotence were high. Beginning around 1960, Morehouse and colleagues followed up on Johansen's idea that posterior urethral rupture could be better handled by initial suprapubic cystostomy alone, acceptance of an inevitable stricture, and delayed repair of the stricture at least 3 months after the injury (Fig. 99–40) (Morehouse et al, 1972). Morehouse reported that delayed rather than primary repair resulted in a decrease of each of the three major complications: permanent stricture—from 14% to 6%; incontinence—from 21% to 6%; impotence—from 33% to 10%. **Avoidance of urethral instrumentation at the time of injury and suprapubic cystostomy alone have been the preferred initial management of nearly all cases of posterior urethral rupture for approximately the last 25 years.** Primary repair, however, is still recommended with severe prostatomembranous dislocation, major bladder neck laceration, and concomitant pelvic vascular or rectal injury (Corriere, 1991; Devine et al, 1992; Herschorn et al, 1992). The length of the stricture is assessed with combined simultaneous antegrade voiding and retrograde urethrograms when the patient is ready for the delayed repair (Fig. 99–41). Details of the surgical techniques for delayed urethral reconstruction are discussed in Chapter 107.

Advances in endoscopic techniques with flexible cystoscopy and the use of guide wires and the Seldinger technique for catheter placement are producing a reappraisal of both the initial management of posterior urethral rupture and the delayed repair of urethral stricture (Webster et al, 1983; Marshall et al, 1987; Herschorn et al, 1992; Spirnak et al, 1993; Quint and Stanisic, 1993). Initial urethral realignment at the time of injury may be accomplished by exploring the bladder and passing cystoscopes from above and below, advancing a flexible guide wire under direct vision across the injury, and advancing a Councill catheter over the guide wire into the bladder (Fig. 99–42). Herschorn and associates reported a single-center experience and presented a literature review of series in which posterior urethral rupture was managed initially either by endoscopic urethral realignment or by suprapubic cystostomy alone (Herschorn

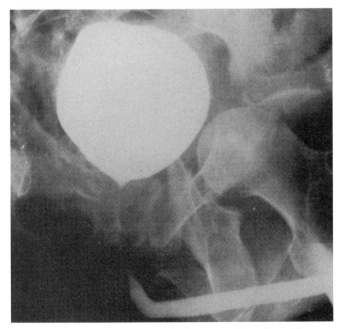

Figure 99–38. Type I posterior urethral injury—elongation without actual rupture.

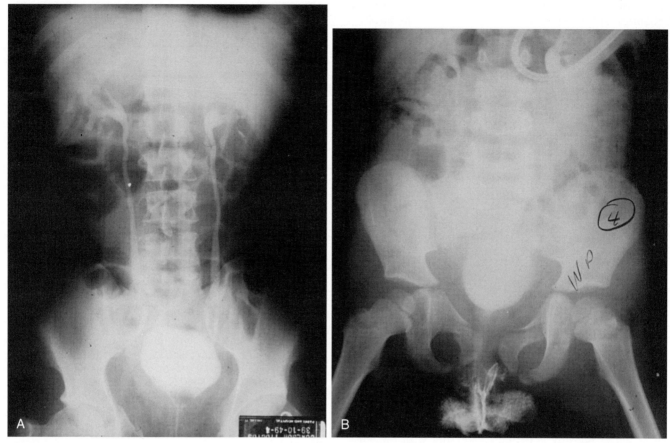

Figure 99–39. *A,* Type III complete posterior urethral rupture in a man. Note floating bladder and prostate giving "pie-in-the-sky" effect of Turner-Warwick. *B,* Rare posterior urethral rupture in a woman. Note that bladder shadow floats in the pelvis and does not come down to the symphysis as in extraperitoneal bladder rupture (see Fig. 99–36). Vesicovaginal fistula may complicate the repair in a woman.

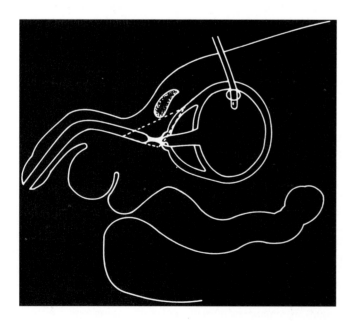

Figure 99–40. A suprapubic tube is in place, and no initial attempt is made to prevent stricture at the site of the posterior urethral rupture. The tube should be placed high in the bladder away from the trigone. It should come through the abdominal wall obliquely and through a separate stab wound in the bladder to avoid or minimize the chance of bladder spasms and the chance of a postoperative fistula.

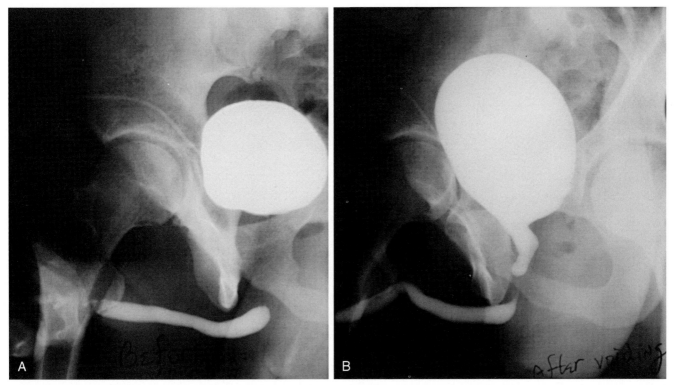

Figure 99–41. *A,* Typical picture of healed type III posterior urethral rupture shown at time of reconstruction 3 months after injury. Note that competent bladder neck prevents one from seeing the true length of the stricture. *B,* When the patient voids through the suprapubic tube and a retrograde urethrogram is done at the same time, the bladder neck is opened, and the true length of the stricture may be more accurately visualized.

et al, 1992). A total of 199 cases of suprapubic cystostomy alone from 7 series and 304 cases of endoscopic realignment from 12 series were identified. Suprapubic cystostomy alone was followed by stricture formation in 95.5% of cases and required urethroplasty in 89.4% of cases. In contrast, successful endoscopic urethral realignment was associated with stricture formation and the need for urethroplasty in 53.9% and 23.2% of cases (Herschorn et al, 1992). In the same literature review, the reported range of impotence was 0% to 60% versus 13% to 50% for suprapubic cystostomy or delayed repair versus primary realignment. The reported range of incontinence was 0% to 14% and 0% to 22% for these same two approaches.

A number of investigators have reported on endoscopic management as the definitive delayed repair of traumatic posterior urethral strictures (Marshall et al, 1987; Spirnak et al, 1993; Quint and Stanisic, 1993). Combined antegrade cystoscopy across the bladder neck via the suprapubic tract and retrograde urethroscopy are performed while a guide wire or needle is inserted across the stricture. Urethral continuity is re-established by dilation or endoscopic incision or resection of the scar. Endoscopic repair is most successful for strictures of less than 3 cm in length. Careful three-dimensional orientation before traversing or cutting the stricture is essential to prevent injury to the rectum or the bladder neck. Most investigators describe placing the surgeon's finger in the rectum and using C-arm fluoroscopy to ensure correct orientation.

Pelvic magnetic resonance imaging in the sagittal, coronal, and transaxial planes reveals the length of the urethral defect as well as adjacent injuries (Dixon et al, 1992). The urethral scar is seen particularly well on transaxial T2-weighted im-ages. Avulsion of the corpora cavernosa from the pubic rami is associated with a high rate of impotence. Pelvic magnetic resonance imaging assessment of the stricture helps one determine whether endoscopic or open perineal versus transpubic repair is required.

The overall results of delayed endoscopic repair of traumatic posterior urethral stricture in 73 patients from seven series were presented by Quint and Stanisic (1993). Complete continence was obtained in 83.6% of patients. Stress incontinence or mild nocturnal leakage occurred in 11% and 1.4% of cases, respectively. Major incontinence was present in 4.1% of patients. Sixty-eight percent of patients required periodic repeat visual internal urethrotomy (VIU) to maintain good urethral patency and urine flow. Patency was maintained in 97.3% of patients who were patent before endoscopic repair of the stricture.

Posterior urethral rupture in children deserves special comment. Vesicostomy may be the best initial management in an infant as the bladder resides in a high intraperitoneal position away from the pelvic injury. Spontaneous urethral healing without a stricture occurs in approximately 5% of injuries (Fig. 99–43).

Boone and co-workers reported on 24 boys with rupture of the posterior urethra who were followed through puberty (Boone et al, 1992). The site of rupture was prostatomembranous in 67%, supraprostatic in 17%, and transprostatic in 17% of cases. In contrast, nearly all urethral ruptures above the urogenital diaphragm in men occur at the prostatomembranous level. In children, the site of injury (i.e., prostatomembranous versus higher) correlated with specific complications as follows: impotence—31% versus 75%; intractable stricture—12% versus 75%; and incontinence—0% versus 25%.

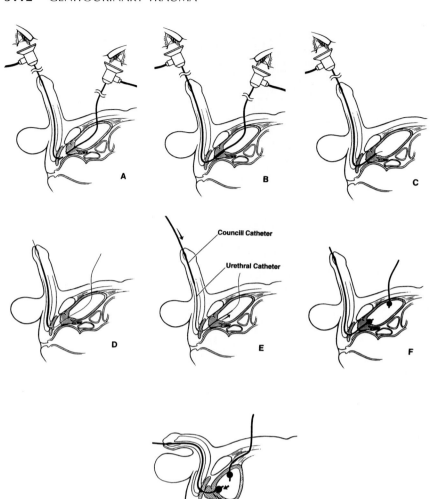

Councill Catheter

Urethral Catheter

Figure 99–42. *A* through *G*, Use of proximal and distal flexible cystoscope to pass wire into bladder and pass Councill catheter to establish urethral continuity.

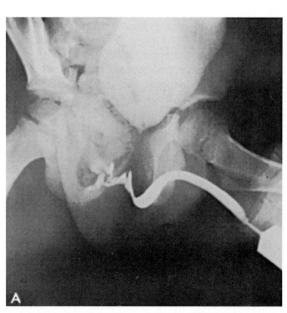
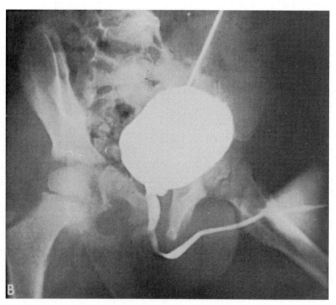

Figure 99–43. *A* and *B*, Posterior urethral rupture in an infant treated by vesicostomy with complete healing in 3 months. Closure of the vesicostomy is the only additional surgery needed.

Anterior Urethra

Presentation and Anatomic Considerations

Injuries of the anterior urethra are more common than of the posterior urethra and result most often from blunt trauma owing to straddle injuries such as falling astride a bicycle or post (Corriere, 1991). Blunt trauma with a direct blow to the perineum is the next most common cause of injury and may produce urethral contusion or actual partial or complete laceration. Pelvic fracture is uncommon in rupture of the anterior urethra. Accidental blunt urethral trauma may occur during sexual activity with associated fracture of the corpora cavernosa (see section on penile trauma later), masturbation, or self-mutilation in mentally deranged patients. Anterior urethral injury may occur as a result of penetrating wounds from gunshots, stabs, or iatrogenic instrumentation. Inflation of a Foley catheter balloon in the urethra and accidental removal of a catheter with the balloon inflated are common causes of partial or complete urethral laceration.

Each of the causes of anterior urethral injury may produce partial or complete disruption of the integrity of the urethra and its fascial coverings. Buck's fascia tightly surrounds the erectile bodies and the corpus spongiosum of the urethra from the suspensory ligament proximally to the coronal

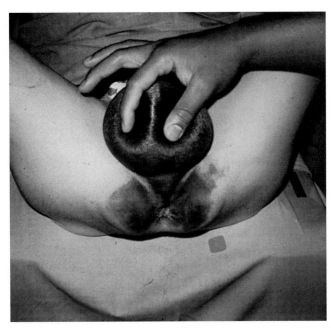

Figure 99–45. Anterior urethral rupture through Buck's fascia confined by Colles' fascia. Posterior extent limited by fusion of Colles' fascia with fascia of transverse perineal muscle.

sulcus distally. **Urethral rupture contained by Buck's fascia leads to dissection of urine and blood along the penile shaft appearing as a sleeve of the penis** (Fig. 99–44). Rupture of the urethra or corpora cavernosa through Buck's fascia results in extravasation of blood and urine corresponding to the attachments of Colles' fascia. Colles' fascia fuses posteromedially with the fascia of the superficial and deep transverse perineal muscles and laterally with the fascia lata of the thigh. Superiorly, Colles' fascia continues on the abdominal wall as Scarpa's fascia, which inserts on the coracoclavicular fascia. **Urethral rupture with extravasation of urine, blood, or pus into the scrotum and contained by Colles' fascia produces a characteristic butterfly configuration in the perineum** (Figs. 99–45 and 99–46).

Imaging

Retrograde urethrography should be performed on all patients in whom the history or physical examination suggests possible injury to the anterior urethra. These findings include blood at the urethral meatus and evidence of penile, scrotal, or perineal contusion, hematoma, or fluid collection (see Figs. 99–44 through 99–46).

Treatment

Blunt contusion of the anterior urethra without laceration may be treated by a few days of catheter drainage. **Surgical exploration, débridement, and direct repair are indicated for most blunt or penetrating ruptures of the anterior urethra.** The incision is placed in the perineum for injuries of the distal bulbous or proximal pendulous urethra. A circumcising incision with degloving of the penile shaft may be suitable for injuries confined to the more distal portion of the pendulous urethra.

Partial urethral lacerations are débrided and closed over a

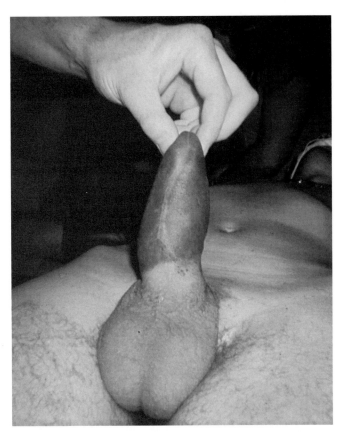

Figure 99–44. Penile injury confined by Buck's fascia. Corporal rupture during intercourse. Note "sleeve of penis" injury. Lesion is palpated in corpus cavernosum and closed with three interrupted nonabsorbable sutures. This minimized the Peyronie-like effect of corporal scarring. Note the scrotum appears normal.

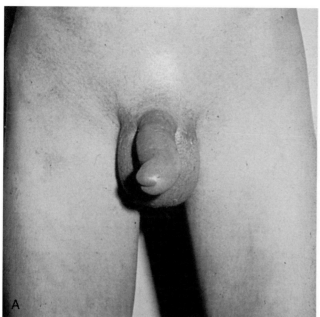 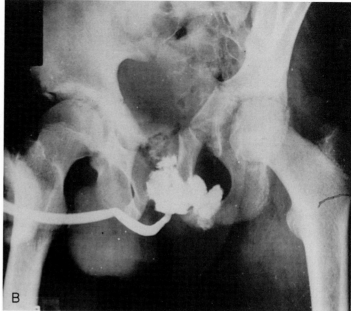

Figure 99–46. *A,* Anterior urethral rupture. Note urine filling penis and scrotum and extending into the abdomen beneath Scarpa's fascia. Note the lack of extension into thigh because of fusion of Scarpa's fascia with the fascia lata of the thigh. *B,* Urethrogram of the anterior urethral rupture. Immediate repair and end-to-end spatulated oblique anastomosis with fixation of proximal urethra to perineal fascia are done to prevent postoperative stricture by stabilizing anastomosis.

urethral catheter with 4–0 or 5–0 chromic catgut or polyglycolic acid suture. The catheter is maintained for 7 to 10 days, and a pullout voiding cystourethrogram is performed to exclude further extravasation.

Complete disruptions of the distal bulbous or pendulous urethra are repaired by direct end-to-end reanastomosis whenever possible (Fig. 99–47). The ends of the urethra are spatulated to provide a large-caliber oblique anastomosis. The proximal end of the urethra is sutured to the underlying perineal fascia to immobilize the repair. A urethral catheter is left in the bladder for 10 to 14 days. A urethrogram is performed around the catheter or as a pullout study to exclude continued extravasation. The bladder catheter is maintained for 7 to 10 days more if extravasation is present on the first postoperative study.

Devastating blowout injuries of the urethra and perineum may occur from shotgun blasts, power machine avulsions, or high-speed blunt contusion. The degree of injury to the urethra and soft tissues may prevent primary repair. Initial management consists of meticulous hemostasis, careful débridement to preserve any viable genital and rectal tissue, and proximal urinary diversion by suprapubic cystostomy. Proctoscopy is mandatory in bullet wounds of the suprapubic area and perineum whether or not the missile can be seen on plain radiography (Franko et al, 1993). The goal of the initial débridement of massive wounds of the perineum is to establish proximal urinary and fecal diversion and to approximate viable tissue in such a manner as to end up with a posterior urethral opening, which may be repaired in a few months by staged urethroplasty (Baskin and McAninch, 1993; Husmann et al, 1993). At the time of delayed repair, vascularized musculocutaneous flaps may be transferred to the perineum to compensate for large tissue defects (Bandt and Khouri, 1993). The omentum also may be used to

provide a well-vascularized pedicle to fill tissue defects in the perineum underneath the perineal skin.

EXTERNAL GENITALIA

Penis

Superficial Injuries to the Penis

Sudden downward flexion of the erect penis may tear the suspensory ligament. The patient often describes hearing a snap accompanied by a painful tearing sensation at the base of the penis. Physical examination reveals minimal or no hematoma in contrast to laceration or fracture of the corpora cavernosa (see later). The suspensory ligament should be surgically repaired to provide future penile stability during intercourse. Injuries to the erectile bodies may result in extravasation of blood corresponding to the extent of Buck's fascia. Such lesions may occur from penetrating wounds, such as a bullet wound or stab wound. The corpora may rupture from blunt trauma caused by sudden flexion of the erect penis against the partner's pubic bone during intercourse (see Fig. 99–44). Ruptures through Buck's fascia result in a distribution of extravasation of blood or urine corresponding to the attachments of Colles' fascia (see Fig. 99–45). The anatomic attachments of Buck's and Colles' fasciae are described in the section on trauma of the anterior urethra. Ongoing extravasation of blood or urine through Buck's fascia may spread onto the abdominal wall laterally to the fascia lata of the thigh and superiorly and anteriorly to the attachments of the coracoclavicular fascia. The defect in the corpus cavernosum may be palpable. The injury should be explored and repaired with 2–0 or 3–0 polypropylene or polydioxanone suture with the knots inverted. Prompt

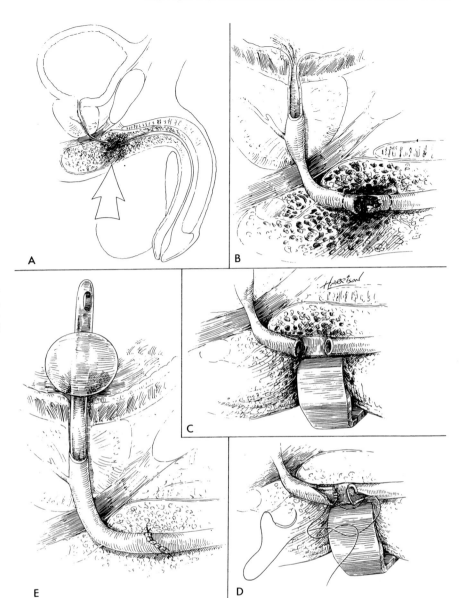

Figure 99–47. *A* through *E,* Repair of anterior urethral rupture. A spatulated oblique anastomosis. The authors prefer interrupted suture technique with slowly absorbed suture such as 4–0 chromic or polyglycolic acid.

repair tends to minimize scar and penile deviation, which may produce curvature during erection similar to Peyronie's disease.

Strangulating lesions of the penis may occur when self-mutilation or masturbation is carried out by the patient and objects are placed around the circumference of the penis. Accidental penile strangulation may occur in children or elderly nursing home patients from hair or condom catheters wrapped too tightly. Solid objects around the penis usually are removed by applying soap and water to the penis or applying a string beginning at the meatus and wrapping around the glans circumferentially until the offending object is released by constriction of the distal edema by the string (Fig. 99–48) (Vähäsarja et al, 1993). At times, it is necessary to anesthetize the patient and use metal cutting tools to remove some materials used for masturbation (Fig. 99–49). Priapism may result after superficial or deep trauma to the penis. DeStafani and colleagues have successfully treated post-traumatic priapism by autologous clot embolization of the dorsal artery on the affected side(s) with subsequent recovery of potency (DeStafani et al, 1993).

Degloving Injuries of the Penis

Degloving injuries of the penis occur when the genitalia are caught in machinery such as industrial, garden, or farming tools. There may be considerable loss of skin, subcutaneous tissue, and even portions of the urethra and corporal bodies. Gross contamination from soil and pieces of clothing complicate repair of these injuries. One should débride the distal penile skin and excise it to the level of the coronal sulcus if incomplete destruction of the skin has occurred and simple end-to-end anastomosis is not possible. If split-thickness grafting is deemed necessary, one should graft proximally from the coronal sulcus to the intact body skin and should not leave spare pieces of skin distally on the penis to diminish the amount of graft material needed (Fig. 99–50). Split-thickness skin grafts of approximately 0.15-cm thickness allow for normal expansion of the healed penis during erection. Split-thickness grafts greater than 0.15-cm thickness to the shaft of the penis sometimes do not permit proper corporal expansion during erection and become a source of discomfort to the patient.

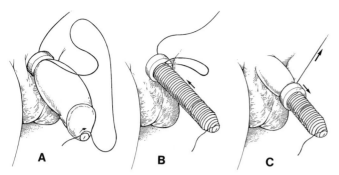

Figure 99–48. *A,* Edematous penis with metal ring trapped at base of penis. Note heavy string has been passed beneath the metal ring using a small curved clamp. *B,* String has been wrapped from meatus to the level of the ring thereby compressing the edema out of the distal penis. The authors prefer this method to pharmacologic agents to relieve edema. *C,* Ring is now being pushed distally over the shaft of the penis, which has been constricted by ring.

Partial or complete penile amputation may occur by accident or as the result of an attack by an assailant or by a self-inflicted wound. In 1968, McRoberts and co-workers reported the first successful reanastomosis of a traumatically amputated penis. The largest series on management of penile amputation described 100 cases that occurred in Thailand during the 7-year period 1973–1980 (Bhangarada et al, 1983). From this concentrated experience in the management of a relatively rare event, the authors were able to identify several general principles important in penile salvage. The amputated part should be cleansed vigorously and then placed in a sterile bag containing a sterile balanced salt solution and the closed bag placed on ice for transportation to a medical facility. Patients routinely have ongoing active bleeding when first seen and should have a tourniquet placed

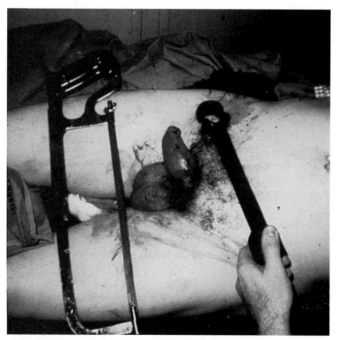

Figure 99–49. Self-mutilation with wrench on penis. Lesion may be treated by use of metal saw under anesthesia or string technique (see Fig. 99–48) from distal meatus to the point of narrowing.

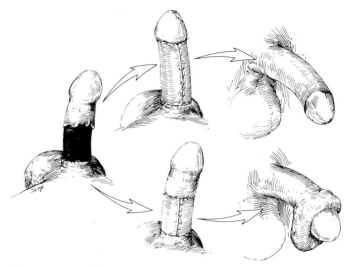

Figure 99–50. Problem in using distal penile skin. In reconstruction of penile skin, distal penile skin should be excised and a split-thickness graft applied from coronal sulcus to intact body skin to avoid poor cosmetic result.

about the base of the penile shaft. Microsurgical repair of the dorsal penile arteries and vein should be performed with 8–0 to 11–0 nonabsorbable suture. The corpora cavernosa are reapproximated with 2–0 or 3–0 polypropylene or polydioxanone suture with the knots buried (Fig. 99–51). The penile shaft skin usually is grossly contaminated and is best managed by excision and subsequent split-thickness skin grafting to cover the penile shaft if the distal reimplantation survives. If the distal penis sloughs, delayed penile reconstruction may be carried out according to techniques described by Jordan and colleagues (Chapter 107) to obtain a sensate penis. Successful temporary ectopic implantation of an amputated penis has been described when primary microscopic repair was not available (Matloub et al, 1994).

Testis

Rupture of the testis is seen with either blunt or penetrating trauma (Aboseif et al, 1993; Altarac, 1994). Physical examination reveals a variable amount of scrotal swelling, hematoma, and tenderness, making the testis and epididymis indistinct. Immediate exploration is indicated if the testis is to be salvaged. The consent form always should include possible orchiectomy. Isotope scan and ultrasonography are helpful in diagnosis of testicular rupture but should not deny or delay surgical exploration. In a series of 16 cases reported by Corrales and associates, five testes that were thought on the basis of ultrasound appearance to be intact were found to be ruptured at exploration; of four thought on the basis of ultrasound appearance to be ruptured, two were intact (Corrales et al, 1993). The combined experience in 41 surgically explored cases from four series reveals the overall accuracy of ultrasonography for detection of traumatic testis rupture as follows: specificity, 75%; sensitivity, 64%; positive predictive value, 77.8%; negative predictive value, 60%.

The injured testis should be irrigated with copious amounts of saline. Extruded and necrotic seminiferous tubules are débrided, and the tunica albuginea is closed with absorbable suture. Failure to close the tunica albuginea re-

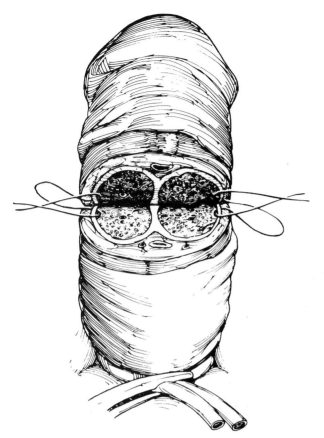

Figure 99–51. Reconstruction of an amputated penis. Complete microscopic vascular reconstruction is preferred. A viable penis sometimes may be obtained by reanastomosis of the corpora and a large dorsal vein if arterial reconstruction of the dorsal arteries is not possible.

sults in continued extrusion of seminiferous tubules. A small drain is placed beneath the tunica vaginalis and brought through a stab in the lower portion of the scrotum. Usually the drain is removed in 24 to 36 hours. Broad-spectrum antibiotic coverage is given for 7 days. The possibility of reimplantation of the amputated testis and cord may be considered in those patients seen within 8 hours of injury. Successful reimplantation of the testis with preserved spermatogenesis on follow-up biopsy has been reported after complete severance of the pedicle (Altarac, 1993).

Scrotum

Loss of the scrotum often occurs when it becomes caught in clothing that has been entangled in farming equipment or machinery. Only a few principles need be remembered. The scrotum may be mobilized a considerable distance in the perineum to replace a large loss of scrotal tissue. The wound must be irrigated and all necrotic and foreign tissue fully débrided. Grossly contaminated wounds are packed with sterile gauze dressings. Cleaner wounds are drained and closed in several layers with absorbable sutures. Scrotum makes a good immediate pedicle flap (Fig. 99–52). The scrotal flaps may be designed to cover exposed testes as advocated by McDougal (1983) (Figure 99–53). Orchiectomy usually is not required owing to loss only of scrotal

skin. If no skin exists to cover the testes as in Figure 99–54, the testes need not be immediately replaced in the thigh but may be treated with daily applications of warm saline or 0.25% acetic acid soaks until scrotal granulations are adequate to permit the application of a mesh or split-thickness skin graft.

Vas Deferens and Epididymis

Techniques for repair of trauma to the vas deferens and epididymis are similar to those used for reanastomosis to restore fertility. The operating microscope or magnifying loupes should be used in all cases. The specific technique of repair (one layer or two) and choice of permanent suture (7–0 to 10–0) depend on the surgeon's preference and experience with microsurgery. A precise, unobstructed, and non-leaking microscopic repair is the goal. Vasoepididymostomy is not recommended in a contaminated field. The vas may be ligated proximally and the epididymis closed, and a delayed elective microscopic vasoepididymostomy to the tail of the epididymis can be performed several months later.

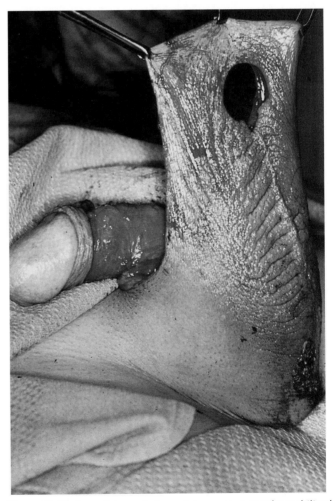

Figure 99–52. A small amount of remaining scrotum may be mobilized as an immediate pedicle flap to cover the entire scrotal area.

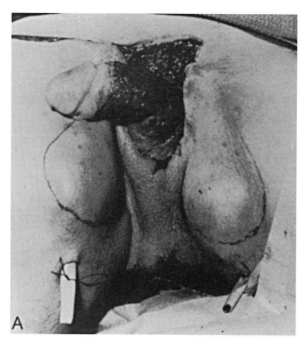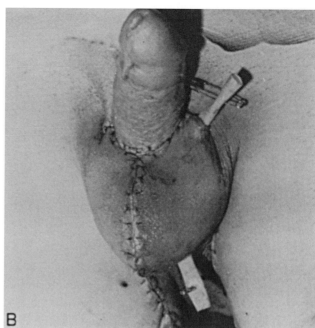

Figure 99–53. *A* and *B,* Scrotal flaps mobilized for immediate testis and penis coverage as suggested by McDougal. (From McDougal WS: J Urol 1983; 129:757–759.)

UROLOGIC TRAUMA IN PREGNANCY

In the evaluation and management of trauma during pregnancy, the physician must consider the well-being of both the mother and the fetus. In general, in emergency circumstances, the health of the mother takes precedence over the health of the fetus. The urologist called to evaluate a pregnant patient for possible urologic trauma should seek early consultation with the obstetrician and share the diagnostic and treatment decisions. Indications for repair of the urinary tract basically are the same as in a nonpregnant patient. The gravid uterus commonly produces relative obstruction of the right ureter producing hydroureteronephrosis during the latter stages of gestation. The right kidney may become predisposed to parenchymal and collecting system injury from trauma as is seen with chronic hydronephrosis.

Ultrasonography may provide evidence for urinary extravasation and urinoma without the use of contrast agents or radiation exposure during the crucial first trimester of pregnancy. Serial ultrasound examinations and repeated physical examination, as the clinical circumstances warrant, are important because of the lesser sensitivity of ultrasound compared with IVP or CT scan in the diagnosis of renal trauma. Major urinary extravasation may be diverted either by cystoscopic insertion of a double-J internal ureteral stent or by percutaneous nephrostomy. Randomized, prospective comparisons of which of these two approaches is least likely to injure the fetus or induce premature labor are not available. Individual urologic and obstetric teams champion one or the other approach.

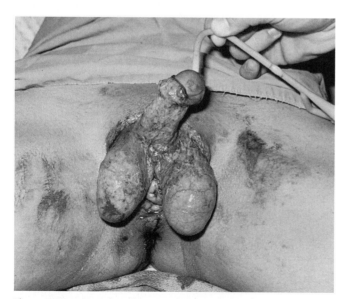

Figure 99–54. Scrotal avulsion. Testis may be covered by rotating flaps as suggested in Figure 99–52 or may be covered with moist 0.25% acetic acid soaks for a few days until split-thickness grafting (0.015 cm) may be done.

REFERENCES

Kidney

Angorn IB: Segmental dearterialization in penetrating renal trauma. Br J Surg 1977; 64:59.

Atala A, Miller FB, Richardson JD, et al: Preliminary vascular control for renal trauma. Surg Gynecol Obstet 1991; 172:386–390.

Baumann L, Greenfield SP, Aker J, et al: Nonoperative management of major blunt renal trauma in children: In-hospital morbidity and long-term followup. J Urol 1992; 148:691–693.

Bernath AS, Schutte H, Fernandez RRD, Addonizio JC: Stab wounds of the kidney: Conservative management in flank penetration. J Urol 1983; 129:468–470.

Bright TC, White K, Peters PC: Significance of hematuria after trauma. J Urol 1978; 120:455–456.

Carlton CE Jr: Injuries of the kidney and ureter. *In* Harrison JH, et al, eds:

Campbell's Urology, Vol. I, 4th ed. Philadelphia, W. B. Saunders, 1978, pp 881–905.

Carlton CE Jr, Scott R Jr, Goldman M: The management of penetrating injuries of the kidney. J Trauma 1968; 8:1071–1083.

Carroll PR, Klosterman PW, McAninch JW: Surgical management of renal trauma: Analysis of risk factors, technique and outcome. J Trauma 1988; 28:1071–1077.

Carroll PR, Klosterman PW, McAninch JW: Early vascular control for renal trauma: A critical review. J Urol 1989; 141:826–829.

Carroll PR, McAninch JW: Staging of renal Trauma. Urol Clin North Am 1989; 16:193–201.

Carroll PR, McAninch HW, Klosterman P, et al: Renovascular trauma: Risk assessment, surgical management, and outcome. J Trauma 1990; 30:547–552.

Carroll PR, McAninch JW, Wong A, et al: Outcome after temporary vascular occlusion for the management of renal trauma. J Urol 1994; 151:1171–1173.

Cass AS: Blunt renal trauma in children. J Trauma 1983; 23:123–127.

Cass AS, Luxenberg M: Management of renal artery injuries from external trauma. J Urol 1987; 138:266–268.

Cass AS, Susset J, Khan A, et al: Renal pedicle injury in the multiple injured patient. J Urol 1979; 122:728–730.

Chandhoke PS, McAninch JW: Detection and significance of microscopic hematuria in patients with blunt renal trauma. J Urol 1988; 140:16–18.

Corriere JN Jr, McAndrew JD, Benson GS: Intraoperative decision-making in renal trauma surgery. J Trauma 1991; 31:1390–1392.

Eastham JA, Wilson TG, Ahlering TE: Urological evaluation and management of renal proximity stab wounds. J Urol 1993; 150:1771–1773.

Eastham JA, Wilson TG, Larsen DW, Ahlering TE: Angiographic embolization of renal stab wounds. J Urol 1992; 148:268–270.

Federle MP, Kaiser JA, McAninch JW, et al: The role of computed tomography in renal trauma. Radiology 1981; 141:455–460.

Guerriero WG, Carlton CE Jr, Scott R Jr, et al: Renal pedicle injuries. J Trauma 1971; 11:53–62.

Hai MA, Pontes JE, Pierce JM Jr: Surgical management of major renal trauma. J Urol 1977; 118:7–9.

Hardeman SW, Husmann DA, Chinn HK, et al: Blunt abdominal trauma and hematuria: Which patients should have radiologic workup. (Abstract.) Urology 1987; 18:66.

Herschorn S, Radomski SB, Shoskes DA, et al: Evaluation and treatment of blunt renal trauma. J Urol 1991; 146:274–277.

Heyns CF, De Klerk DP, De Kock MLS: Stab wounds associated with hematuria—a review of 67 cases. J Urol 1983; 130:228–231.

Heyns CF, De Klerk DP, De Kock MLS: Nonoperative management of renal stab wounds. J Urol 1985; 134:239–242.

Heyns CF, van Vollenhoven P: Increasing role of angiography and segmental artery embolization in the management of renal stab wounds. J Urol 1992; 147:1231–1234.

Husmann DA, Gilling PJ, Perry MO, et al: Major renal lacerations with a devitalized fragment following blunt abdominal trauma: A comparison between nonoperative (expectant) versus surgical management. J Urol 1993; 150:1772–1777.

Husmann DA, Morris JS: Attempted nonoperative management of blunt renal lacerations extending through the corticomedullary junction: The short-term and long-term sequelae. J Urol 1990; 143:682–684.

Maggio AJ Jr, Brosman S: Renal artery trauma. Urology 1978; 11:125–130.

McAninch JW: Renal trauma. (Editorial.) J Urol 1993; 150:1778.

McAninch JW, Carroll PR: Renal trauma: Kidney preservation through improved vascular control—a refined approach. J Trauma 1982; 22:285–290.

McAninch JW, Federle MP: Evaluation of renal injuries with computerized tomography. J Urol 1982; 128:456–460.

Mee SL, McAninch JW, Robinson AL, et al: Radiographic assessment of renal trauma: A 10 year prospective study of patient selection. J Urol 1989; 141:1095–1098.

Moore EE, Shackford SR, Pachter HL, et al: Organ injury scaling: Spleen, liver and kidney. J Trauma 1989; 29:1664–1666.

Nash PA, Bruce JE, McAninch JW: Nephrectomy for traumatic renal injuries. J Urol 1995; 153:609–611.

Nicolaisen GS, McAninch JW, Marshall GA, et al: Renal trauma: Re-evaluation of the indications for radiographic assessment. J Urol 1985; 133:183–187.

Peters PC, Bright TC III: Blunt renal injuries. Urol Clin North Am 1977; 4:17–28.

Sagalowsky AI, McConnell JD, Peters PC: Renal trauma requiring surgery: An analysis of 185 cases. J Trauma 1983; 23:128–131.

Sagalowsky AI, Peters PC, Berman H: A unified approach to renal trauma. In Ehrlich RM, ed: Modern Technics in Surgery. Mount Kisco, NY, Futura Publishing, 1984, Chap. 31, pp 1–11.

Sandler CM, Toombs BD: Computed tomographic evaluation of blunt renal injuries. Radiology 1981; 141:461–466.

Scott RF Jr, Selzman HM: Complications of nephrectomy: Review of 450 patients and a description of a modification of the transperitoneal approach. J Urol 1966; 95:307–312.

Smith EM, Elder JS, Spirnak JP: Major blunt renal trauma in the pediatric population: Is a nonoperative approach indicated? J Urol 1993; 149:546–548.

Teiger CL, Venbrux AC, Quinlan DM, Jeffs RD: Late massive hematuria as a complication of conservative management of blunt renal trauma in children. J Urol 1992; 147:1333–1336.

Thompson IM: Expectant management of blunt renal trauma. Urol Clin North Am 1977; 4:29–32.

Turner WJ Jr, Snyder WH III, Fry WJ: Mortality and renal salvage after renovascular trauma. Am J Surg 1983; 146:848–851.

Ureter

Daly JW, Higgins KA: Injury to the ureter during gynecologic surgical procedures. Surg Gynecol Obstet 1988; 167:19–22.

Orkin LA: Trauma to the Ureter: Pathogenesis and Management. Philadelphia, FA Davis Co, 1964.

Spirnak JP, Hampel N, Resnick MI: Ureteral injuries complicating vascular surgery: Is repair indicated? J Urol 1989; 141:13–14.

Bladder

Carroll PR, McAninch JR: Major bladder trauma: Mechanisms of injury and a unified method of diagnosis and repair. J Urol 1984; 132:254–257.

Corriere JN: Trauma to the lower urinary tract. In Gillenwater J, et al, eds: Adult and Pediatric Urology, 2nd ed. St. Louis, Mosby Year Book, 1991, pp 400–513.

Corriere JN Jr, Sandler CM: Management of the ruptured bladder: 7 years experience with 111 cases. J Trauma 1986; 26:830–833.

McConnell JD, Wilkerson MD, Peters PC: Rupture of the bladder. Urol Clin North Am 1982; 9:293–296.

Parra RO: Laparoscopic repair of intraperitoneal bladder perforation. J Urol 1994; 151:1003–1005.

Peters PC: Intraperitoneal rupture of the bladder. Urol Clin North Am 1989; 16:279–282.

Richardson JR Jr, Leadbetter GW Jr: Non-operative treatment of the ruptured bladder. J Urol 1975; 114:213–216.

Robards VL Jr, Haglund RV, Lubin EN, Leach JR: Treatment of rupture of the bladder. J Urol 1976; 116:178–179.

Urethra

Bandt KE, Khouri RK: Proximal forearm flap. Plast Reconstr Surg 1993; 92:1137–1143.

Baskin LS, McAninch JW: Childhood urethral injuries: Perspectives on outcome and treatment. Br J Urol 1993; 72:241–246.

Boone TB, Wilson WWT, Husmann DA: Postpubertal genitourinary function following posterior urethral disruptions in children. J Urol 1992; 148:1232–1234.

Dixon CM, Hricak H, McAninch JW: Magnetic resonance imaging of traumatic posterior urethral defects and pelvic crush injuries. J Urol 1992; 148:1162–1165.

Herschorn S, Thijssen A, Radomski SB: The value of immediate or early catheterization of the traumatized posterior urethra. J Urol 1992; 148:1428–1431.

Husmann DA, Boone TB, Wilson WT: Management of low velocity gunshot wounds to the anterior urethra: The role of primary repair versus urinary diversion alone. J Urol 1993; 150:70–72.

Marshall FF, Chang R, Gearhart JP: Endoscopic reconstruction of traumatic membranous urethral transection. J Urol 1987; 138:306–309.

Morehouse D, Belitsky P, MacKinnon K: Rupture of the posterior urethra. J Urol 1972; 107:255–258.

Quint HJ, Stanisic TH: Above and below delayed endoscopic treatment of traumatic posterior urethral disruptions. J Urol 1993; 149:484–487.

Spirnak JP, Smith EM, Elder JS: Posterior urethral obliteration treated by endoscopic reconstruction, internal urethrotomy and temporary self-dilation. J Urol 1993; 149:766–768.

Webster GD, Mathes GL, Selli C: Prostatomembranous urethral injuries: A

review of the literature and a rational approach to their management. J Urol 1983; 130:898–902.

External Genitalia

Aboseif S, Gomez R, McAninch J: Genital self mutilation. J Urol 1993; 150:1143–1146.

Altarac S: A case of testicle replantation. J Urol 1993; 150:1507–1508.

Altarac S: Management of 53 cases of testicular trauma. Eur Urol 1994; 25:119–123.

Bhangarada K, Chayaratana T, Pongnumkul C, et al: Surgical management of an epidemic of penile amputations in Siam. Am J Surg 1983; 146:376–382.

Corrales JG, Corbel L, Cipolla B, et al: Accuracy of ultrasound diagnosis after blunt testicular trauma. J Urol 1993; 150:1834–1836.

DeStafani S, Capone M, Carmignani G: Treatment of post-traumatic priapism by means of autologous clot embolization. Eur Urol 1993; 23:506–508.

Devine CJ, Jordan GH, Schlossberg SM: Surgery of the penis and urethra. In Walsh P, et al, eds: Campbell's Urology, 6th ed. Philadelphia, W. B. Saunders, 1992; pp 2957–3032.

Franko ER, Ivatury RR, Schwalb DM: Combined penetrating rectal and genitourinary injuries: A challenge in management. J Trauma 1993; 34:347–353.

Matloub HS, Yousif NJ, Sanger JR: Temporary ectopic implantation of an amputated penis. Plast Reconstr Surg 1994; 93:408–412.

McDougal WS: Scrotal reconstruction using thigh pedicle flaps. J Urol 1983; 129:757–759.

McRoberts JW, Chapman WH, Ansell JS: Primary anastomosis of the traumatically amputated penis: Case report and summary of literature. J Urol 1968; 100:751–754.

Vähäsarja VJ, Serlo W, et al: Treatment of penile incarceration by the string method: 2 case reports. J Urol 1993; 149:372–373.

100
USE OF INTESTINAL SEGMENTS AND URINARY DIVERSION

W. Scott McDougal, M.D.

Bowel is frequently used in reconstructive urologic surgery for ureteral substitutes, bladder augmentation, and bladder replacement. Less commonly, it may be employed as a urethral or vaginal substitute. The stomach, jejunum, ileum, and colon have all been used in these various procedures. The appropriate use of these intestinal segments requires a thorough knowledge of their surgical anatomy, the methods of preparing the intestine for an operative event, the techniques of isolating segments of intestine and reconstituting continuity of the enteric tract, the problems and techniques of anastomosing the urinary tract to the intestine, and the complications that occur with use of the intestine. With this knowledge, reconstruction of the urinary tract may be performed with the proper segment of intestine in the least morbid way. This chapter reviews the technical aspects involved in the use of intestinal segments in urologic surgery that are germane to all types of reconstructive procedures, the difficulties and complications encountered with their use,

and the problems that may arise both acutely and over the long term following their placement in the urinary tract. With these fundamental concepts in mind, the construction of various types of conduit urinary diversions, their advantages, disadvantages, and complications are addressed.

SURGICAL ANATOMY

The segments of bowel with which urologists frequently deal include the ileum, the colon, and the rectum. Less commonly, the jejunum and stomach may be used for reconstructive procedures. A thorough knowledge of the surgical anatomy of these structures is necessary to mobilize and fashion them properly according to the requirements of the often complex reconstructive procedure being performed.

Stomach

The stomach is a vascular organ that receives its blood supply primarily from the celiac axis (Fig. 100–1). **There are three branches of the celiac axis that give rise to the majority of the arterial supply of the stomach:** (1) The **left gastric (coronary) artery** arises directly from the celiac axis and supplies the lesser curvature. (2) The **hepatic artery,** after arising from the celiac axis, gives off the right gastric artery, which also supplies the lesser curve of the stomach and the gastroduodenal artery, which supplies the antrum and duodenum before giving off the right gastroepiploic artery. (3) The **splenic artery** originates from the celiac axis and gives off the vasa brevia, which supply the fundus and cardia, and the left gastroepiploic artery. The right gastroepiploic artery anastomoses with the left gastroepiploic artery, and both supply the greater curve of the stomach. **Using the gastroepiploic vessels, a pedicle of stomach may be mobilized to the pelvis.** The pedicle may consist of the entire antrum pylori or a wedge of the fundus.

The blood supply for these segments is based on either the left or right gastroepiploic artery, depending on the portion of stomach employed. Occasionally the left gastroepiploic artery is atretic at some point in its course and does not provide an adequate blood supply. Under these circumstances, the right gastroepiploic artery must be employed. **When a wedge of fundus is employed, it should not include a significant portion of the antrum and should never extend to the pylorus or all the way to the lesser curve of the stomach.** When based on the left gastroepiploic artery, the short gastric vessels that course from the gastroepiploic artery to the stomach are ligated along the greater curve proximal to the pedicle to the origin of the gastroepiploic artery. The omentum is left attached to the gastroepiploic vessels and helps secure and support them. It may be necessary for proper pedicle mobility to detach the omentum from the colon along the avascular plane located at the point of its attachment to the transverse colon. If an antrectomy is performed, a Billroth I anastomosis reconstitutes gastrointestinal continuity. **The stomach has a thick seromuscular layer, which can easily be separated from the mucosa should a submucosal ureteral reimplantation be necessary.**

Small Bowel

The small bowel is about 22 feet long; however, it may vary from 15 to 30 feet in length. Its largest diameter is in the duodenum, and the lumen becomes smaller in the more distal portions, reaching its smallest diameter in the ileum, approximately 12 inches from the ileocecal valve. **About two fifths of the small bowel is jejunum, whereas the distal three fifths is ileum.** There is no definite demarcation between the two; however, each possesses several unique properties that allow the surgeon to distinguish one from the other intraoperatively. **The ileum, being more distal in location, has a smaller diameter. It has multiple arterial arcades, and the vessels in the arcades are smaller than those in the jejunum. The ileal mesentery is also thicker than the jejunal mesentery. In contrast, the jejunal diameter is larger, the arterial arcades are usually single, and the vessels composing them are larger in diameter.** The arcades anastomose one with another and give off straight vessels, which enter the bowel and form an anastomotic network within the bowel wall. **It has been shown experimentally that up to 15 cm of small bowel can survive lateral to a straight vessel.** Thus, theoretically the mesentery could be cleaned from the small bowel for a length of 15 cm without necrosis of the end. Generally, however, it is unwise to assume that more than 8 cm of small bowel will survive away from a straight vessel. The arcades receive their blood from the superior mesenteric artery. When isolating segments of jejunum or ileum, the mesentery should be transected in such a way that the isolated intestinal segment receives its blood supply from an arcade supplied by a palpable artery of substance that courses through the base of the mesenteric pedicle.

There are **two portions of the small bowel that may lie within the confines of the pelvis** and as such may be exposed to pelvic irradiation and pelvic disease. These two portions are **(1) the last 2 inches of the terminal ileum and (2) 5 feet of small bowel beginning approximately 6 feet from the ligament of Treitz.** The former is often fixed in the pelvis by ligamentous attachments, whereas the mesentery of the latter is the longest of the entire small

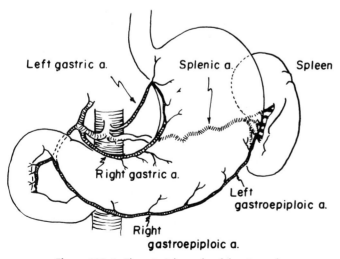

Figure 100–1. The arterial supply of the stomach.

bowel, and, as such, this portion of the small bowel can descend into the pelvis. **In a postirradiated patient, one should try to avoid using these two segments of the small intestine in any reconstructive procedure.**

Colon

The large bowel is divided into the cecum, ascending colon, transverse colon, left colon, sigmoid colon, and rectum. Portions of the large bowel are fixed or retroperitoneal, and other segments lie free within the peritoneal cavity. The cecum, on rare occasion, may lie free within the abdominal cavity and as such may have great mobility. Generally, however, it is fixed in the right lower quadrant. There are two accessory peritoneal bands that bind the cecum and distal ileum to the retroperitoneum and lateral abdominal wall. One band arises from the distal ileum, attaches to the cecum, and is fixed to the retroperitoneum. A second band arises from the cecum and fixes the cecum to the posterior abdominal wall laterally. The remainder of the ascending colon is fixed to the right posterior abdominal wall to the level of the hepatic flexure, at which point the hepatocolic ligament secures this portion of the colon to the liver. The transverse colon lies free within the abdominal cavity and is fixed in the left upper quadrant at the splenic flexure by the phrenocolic ligament. The transverse colon is attached to the stomach by the gastrocolic omentum. The descending colon is fixed to the lateral abdominal wall; however, the sigmoid colon may or may not lie free within the abdominal cavity. The rectosigmoid colon's most cephalad portion is intraperitoneal, and as its distal, more caudad portions are approached, it becomes retroperitoneal and, finally, subperitoneal.

The colon receives its blood supply from the superior mesenteric artery, the inferior mesenteric artery, and the internal iliac arteries (Fig. 100–2). **The major arteries supplying the colon and rectum include the ileocolic, right colic, middle colic, left colic, sigmoid, superior hemorrhoidal, middle hemorrhoidal, and inferior hemorrhoidal arteries.** These arteries anastomose one with the other to form the arc of Drummond and allow for considerable leeway in mobilizing the colon. The middle colic artery arises from the first portion of the superior mesenteric artery and generally ascends the transverse mesocolon to the right of midline. The right colic artery usually arises just below the middle colic artery from the superior mesenteric artery and courses to the right colon. It may arise, however, from the ileocolic or directly from the middle colic artery. If it arises from the ileocolic artery, mobilization of the distal ascending colon is facilitated so that this portion of the colon can be easily brought into the deep pelvis. On occasion, however, it is necessary to sever the right colic artery at its origin to mobilize the distal portion of the ascending colon to the pelvis. This is particularly true if the right colic artery originates from the middle colic artery. The ileocolic artery is the terminal portion of the superior mesenteric artery and supplies the last 6 inches of ileum and ascending colon. The left colic artery arises from the inferior mesenteric artery, and then the inferior mesenteric artery gives off four to six sigmoid branches, the last of which becomes the superior hemorrhoidal artery. This anastomoses with the middle hem-

orrhoidal artery, a branch of the internal iliac artery, which, in turn, anastomoses with the inferior hemorrhoidal artery, the terminal branch of the internal pudendal artery. The middle sacral artery, which originates directly from the aorta, may supply the posterior aspect of the rectum.

Three weak points involving the vascular supply to the colon have been described. Sudeck's critical point, which is located between the junction of the sigmoid and superior hemorrhoidal arteries, was thought to be a particularly tenuous anastomotic area such that if the colon were transected in this region, the anastomosis would heal with difficulty because the blood supply might be compromised. Similarly, the midpoints between the middle colic and right colic arteries and between the middle colic and left colic arteries also have somewhat tenuous anastomotic communications. Although anastomoses in these areas generally heal well, provided that the principles of proper technique are adhered to, it is usually wise to pick an area for the anastomosis to one side of these points.

The ascending colon is mobilized first by transecting the cecal and distal ileal fibrous attachments to the lateral abdominal wall and retroperitoneum described previously and then by detaching it from the lateral abdominal wall along the avascular line of Toldt. This is a bloodless plane, provided that the colonic mesentery is not violated. The transverse colon is mobilized by detaching the gastrocolic omentum along the avascular plane of its attachment to the colon; the hepatocolic ligament, which may have some small vessels coursing through it; and the phrenocolic ligament. The descending colon is mobilized much as the right colon by incising the avascular line of Toldt lateral to the colon. When these attachments are taken down, considerable mobility of the colon is achieved. Further mobility is gained by isolating a pedicle of intestine, which should be based on one of the major arterial vessels described earlier.

SELECTING THE SEGMENT OF INTESTINE

The stomach, jejunum, ileum, and colon have unique properties, each of which gives special advantages and disadvantages. The selection of the proper intestinal segment should be based on the patient's condition, renal function, history of previous abdominal procedures, and type of diversion or substitution required. The stomach has been employed as a replacement for bladder, for augmentation cystoplasty, as a conduit, and for continent diversions (Leong, 1978; Adams et al, 1988; Bihrle et al, 1989). **The advantage of stomach over other intestinal segments for urinary intestinal diversion is that it is less permeable to urinary solutes, it acidifies the urine, it has a net excretion of chloride and protons rather than a net absorption of them, and it produces less mucus.** Urodynamically, it behaves as other intestinal segments. When used in urinary reconstruction, electrolyte imbalance rarely ensues in patients with normal renal function, although a hypochloremic metabolic alkalosis has been described. The incidence of bacteriuria is 25%, much less than the 60% to 80% incidence reported for ileal and colon segments. The acidic urine, which usually has a pH of 5 to 7, does not generally result in an increased incidence of peristomal skin problems.

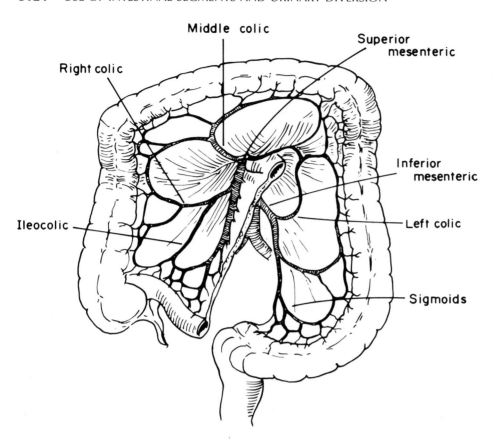

Figure 100–2. The arterial supply to the small bowel and colon.

Generally, serum gastrin levels are normal or minimally elevated depending on what portion of stomach, and how much, is used (Leong, 1978; Adams et al, 1988). Although excluding the antrum from the gastrointestinal tract has not resulted in elevated serum gastrin levels and an ulcer diathesis clinically (Lim et al, 1983), experimentally, antral exclusion results in elevated circulating gastrin levels, which cause major intestinal ulcerative problems in the postoperative period (Tiffany et al, 1986).

There have been no severe ulcerative complications reported thus far in the series that have employed stomach for urinary reconstruction. When the antral portion of stomach is employed, reconstitution is generally by a Billroth I anastomosis. Complications with Billroth I gastroduodenostomy are well documented. Early complications include gastric retention owing to atony of the stomach or edema of the anastomosis; hemorrhage, most commonly originating from the anastomotic site; hiccups secondary to gastric distention; pancreatitis as a consequence of intraoperative injury; and duodenal leakage. Delayed complications include the dumping syndrome, steatorrhea, the small stomach syndrome, increased intestinal transit time, bilious vomiting, afferent loop syndrome, hypoproteinemia, and megaloblastic or iron deficiency anemia. Postoperative bowel obstruction occurs with an incidence of 10% (2 of 21 patients) (Leong, 1978). Gastroduodenal and gastroureteral leaks have also been reported, occasionally resulting in a fatal outcome (Leong, 1978).

The use of stomach for urinary intestinal diversion may be considered when the use of other intestinal segments in a patient with a decreased amount of intestine would result in serious nutritional problems. One advantage of stomach in the patient with severe abdominal adhesions is that, generally, the area of the stomach is adhesion-free and easily mobilized. **Complications specific to its use include the hematuria-dysuria syndrome and uncontrollable metabolic alkalosis in some patients with chronic renal failure.** (See Metabolic Complications.)

The jejunum is usually not employed for reconstruction of the urinary system because its use often results in severe electrolyte imbalance. Generally, diseases that would make the ileum inappropriate to use also make the jejunum inappropriate for use. Rarely, it is the only segment available. Under these circumstances, as distal a segment of jejunum as possible should be employed to minimize the electrolyte problems.

The ileum and colon are used most often for urinary tract reconstruction and have been employed in all types of reconstructive procedures. The ileum is mobile, of small diameter, has a constant blood supply, and serves well for ureteral replacement and the formation of conduits. **Loss of significant portions of the ileum results in nutritional problems because of lack of vitamin B_{12} absorption, diarrhea because of lack of bile salt reabsorption, and fat malabsorption.** On occasion, the mesenteric fat is excessive, making mobility and anastomoses difficult. Also, the mesentery may be so short that it is difficult to mobilize the ileum into the deep pelvis. **Postoperative bowel obstruction occurs in about 10% of patients who have segments isolated from the ileum for urinary tract reconstruction.** One half of the obstructions occur in the early postoperative period (Schwarz and Jeffs, 1975).

The colon requires mobilization from its fixed positions to give it the mobility necessary for use in urinary reconstruction. It has a larger diameter than ileum and is usually easily mobilized into any portion of the abdomen or pelvis. In patients who have received pelvic irradiation, portions of the right, transverse, and descending colon may be used confidently with the knowledge that they have not been exposed to the radiation therapy. Removing segments of colon from the enteric tract results in fewer nutritional problems than removal of segments of ileum, provided that the ileocecal valve is not violated. Should the ileocecal valve be used, diarrhea, excessive bacterial colonization of the ileum with malabsorption, and fluid and bicarbonate loss may occur. **The incidence of postoperative bowel obstruction is 4%—less than that occurring with ileum.** Both ileal and colon segments result in the same type of electrolyte imbalance with similar frequencies. **An antireflux ureterointestinal anastomosis by the submucosal tunnel technique is easier to perform using colon.** In general, ileum and colon are comparable and have few differences, which does not argue strongly for the selection of one over the other except under special circumstances.

BOWEL PREPARATION

Urologic operations in which the bowel is used for genitourinary reconstruction are usually elective, and as such bowel preparation is appropriate. Although the bacterial population in the stomach is relatively low, the remainder of the bowel, including jejunum and ileum, has high bacteria counts and therefore requires mechanical and antibiotic preparation. The need for appropriate bowel preparation is evident from studies that compare bowel anastomoses in unprepared patients with those who have undergone a bowel preparation. **Patients who have intestinal procedures on unprepared bowel have an increased wound infection rate, incidence of intraperitoneal abscesses, and anastomotic dehiscence rate when compared with patients who have had a proper bowel preparation before surgery** (Irvin and Goligher, 1973; Dion et al, 1980). A good mechanical preparation results in collapsed bowel at the time of surgery, which has been shown to reduce the incidence of anastomotic leaks (Christensen and Kronborg, 1981).

In experimental animals, it has been shown that an anastomosis that has vascular compromise at the anastomotic line, which would normally result in perforation, heals if the bowel has been properly prepared with antibiotics. Also, solid feces place strain on the anastomosis in the early phase of healing and result in ischemia with subsequent perforation. **Complications that occur as a result of bacterial contamination are a major cause of morbidity and mortality in patients undergoing urologic procedures.** Infectious complications following radical cystectomy that are a direct result of fecal contamination occur in 18% to 20% of patients who undergo cystectomies and include wound infections, peritonitis, intra-abdominal abscesses, wound dehiscence, anastomotic dehiscence, and systemic sepsis (Bracken et al, 1981).

There are two aspects of bowel preparation: mechanical and antibiotic. Both methods attempt to reduce the complication rate from intestinal surgery. **The mechanical preparation reduces the amount of feces, whereas the antibiotic preparation reduces the bacterial count.** The

bacterial flora in the bowel consists of aerobic organisms, the most common of which are *Escherichia coli* and *Streptococcus faecalis,* and anaerobic organisms, the most common of which are *Bacteroides* species and *Clostridium* species. **The bacterial concentration in the jejunum ranges from 10 to 10^5, in the distal ileum from 10^5 to 10^7, in the ascending colon from 10^6 to 10^8, and in the descending colon from 10^{10} to 10^{12} organisms per gram of fecal content.**

Mechanical Bowel Preparation

A mechanical bowel preparation reduces the total number of bacteria but not their concentration. Thus, the same number of organisms are present per gram of fecal content (Nichols et al, 1972). Therefore, spilling enteric contents during the procedure is less likely to occur with the mechanically prepared bowel because there is less of it to spill; however, once spilled, cubic centimeter for cubic centimeter, the inoculum is the same as if the bowel had not been prepared.

Conventional bowel preparations may exhaust the patient and exacerbate nutritional depletion because they generally require a 3-day preparation period of suboptimal calorie intake (Table 100–1). The use of elemental diets has been advocated to clean the colon of feces while not compromising the nutritional status of the patient. Unfortunately, they have not proven useful because the elemental diets do not empty the colon of feces, and they do not reduce the bacterial flora (Arabi et al, 1978). **In an attempt to reduce the time required for intestinal preparation, to obviate low-calorie intakes, and to contain cost by reducing hospitalization before surgery, whole-gut irrigation has gained popularity.** Originally, whole-gut irrigation was performed by placing a nasogastric tube into the stomach and infusing 9 to 12 L of lactated Ringer's solution or normal saline over a several-hour period. These fluids were subsequently replaced with 10% mannitol, which was equally successful in ridding the bowel of its fecal content; however, the mannitol served as a bacterial nutrient and thereby facilitated microbial growth (Hares and Alexander-Williams, 1982). These solutions have largely been replaced by a polyethylene glycol electrolyte solution. Whole-gut irrigation may be exhausting to the patient and may, in fact, result in a fluid gain, particularly when either saline or mannitol is used. **It is contraindicated in patients with an unstable cardiovascular system, patients with cirrhosis, patients with severe renal disease, patients with congestive heart failure, or those with an obstructed bowel.** Whole-gut irrigation has been found to be no more effective in reducing wound infections and septic complications than conventional preparations (Christensen and Kronborg, 1981), even though there is a reduction of aerobic flora when compared with the conventional preparations (van den Bogaard et al, 1981). **The advantages of the whole-gut irrigation are that it gives the patient dietary freedom, there is a short preparation time, and it eliminates the enema. Its disadvantages are that it may result in patient exhaustion, is rather rigorous, and does result on occasion in fluid overload.**

The use of a polyethylene glycol electrolyte lavage solution (GoLYTELY or the more palatable NuLytely) is an

Table 100–1. MECHANICAL BOWEL PREPARATION

Preoperative Day	Conventional		Whole-Gut Irrigation (Polyethylene Glycol Electrolyte Solutions)	
	Diet	*Cathartic*	*Diet*	*Irrigation*
3	Low residue plus supplements	30–60 ml Fleet Phospho Soda at 10 AM	Regular plus supplements	
2	Clear liquids	30–60 ml Fleet Phospho Soda at 10 AM	Low residue plus supplements	
1	Clear liquids	If rectal effluent is not free of particulate matter 3 L of polyethylene glycol electrolyte solution at 2 PM	Clear liquids	20–30 ml/min (adults) or 25 ml/kg/hour (children) × 5 hours or until rectal effluent clear (not to exceed 10 L in adults)

effective lavage agent in preparing the gut for both elective colon and rectal surgery as well as urologic surgery in which bowel is used. For the adult, 20 to 30 ml/minute or approximately 1 to 1.5 L/hour for 3 hours is given either orally or through a small-caliber nasogastric tube placed into the stomach. If taken by mouth, it is better tolerated if the solution is chilled. The administration of GoLYTELY is stopped when the rectal effluent is clear and there is no particulate matter in it or when 10 L of fluid have been given. This preparation in the adult has been as effective as conventional preparations. The septic complications with its use are approximately 4%. An inadequate preparation occurs in 5% of the patients using this modality (Wolff et al, 1988). For children, even those under the age of 1, GoLYTELY may be used at a rate of 25 ml/kg/hour and given until the rectal effluent is clear and free of particulate matter (Tuggle et al, 1987). Metoclopramide (Reglan) 10 mg is often given simultaneously to control nausea.

The author prefers to begin the mechanical bowel preparation with the patient as an outpatient. Three days before the anticipated date of surgery, the patient is instructed to begin a clear liquid diet. Two days before surgery, 30 to 60 ml of sodium phosphate (Fleet) is taken orally. One day before the surgery, 30 ml of Fleet is taken orally. On the day before surgery, if the rectal effluent is not clear of particulate matter, 3.0 L of polyethylene glycol solution is given orally.

Antibiotic Bowel Preparation

There has been considerable controversy as to whether the addition of antibiotics in elective colon and small bowel surgery reduces mortality and morbidity significantly. The wealth of evidence, however, suggests that **an antimicrobial bowel preparation is advantageous in reducing postoperative complications.** In one study, the septic complication rate was reduced from 68% in the control group to 8% in the antibiotic group (Washington et al, 1974). Most series, however, report a lesser incidence of reduction in wound infection, generally from 35% without antibiotics to 9% with their use (Clarke et al, 1977). Others have suggested that the mortality rate drops from 9% to 3% with the use of antibiotics (Baum et al, 1981). It is clear that the use of antibiotics protects vulnerable bowel in that it may allow the tenuous anastomosis to survive. Other studies, however, have shown that without the use of antibiotics in mechanically prepared

bowel in elective surgery, the septic complication rate is 6%—comparable to those studies using antibiotics (Menaker et al, 1981). In the presence of a bowel obstruction, however, oral antibiotics are of little value because they do little good in sterilizing the bowel. **The disadvantages of antibiotics include a postoperative increase in the incidence of diarrhea; pseudomembranous enterocolitis; a theoretical increased incidence of tumor implantation at the suture line that is not germane to urologic surgery; monilial overgrowth resulting in stomatitis, thrush, and diarrhea; and, with prolonged use, malabsorption of protein, carbohydrate, and fat.** The antibiotics that are most commonly used for bowel preparation include kanamycin, which is the best single agent; neomycin and erythromycin base; and neomycin and metronidazole (Table 100–2). With an appropriate antibiotic preparation, enteric organisms are reduced to 10^2 per gram of feces (Nichols et al, 1972).

The use of perioperative intravenous antibiotics is exceedingly controversial. **Systemic antibiotics must be given before the operative event if they are to be effective.** They appear to be most effective against the anaerobic flora and apparently reduce the complications caused by these organisms (Dion et al, 1980). Perioperative systemic antibiotics when added to the oral regimen reduced the septic complication rate from 15% to 20% to half that rate in several series (Hares and Alexander-Williams, 1982; Gottrup et al, 1985). Other studies, however, have shown no effect of systemic cephalosporin, for example, in reducing septic complications (Wolff et al, 1988). **If perioperative antibiotics are given, they should be effective against anaerobes because it is complications from these organisms against which perioperative antibiotics appear to be particularly effective.**

Diarrhea and Pseudomembranous Enterocolitis

Antibiotic bowel preparations may result in diarrhea and pseudomembranous enterocolitis. The latter is the more severe form of a spectrum of the former. Clinically, this occurs following a bowel preparation in the postoperative period and is heralded by abdominal pain and diarrhea usually in the absence of fever or chills. As the symptoms and infection become more severe, systemic toxicity supervenes. **These patients can develop a toxic megacolon, and if this occurs, the mortality may exceed 15% to 20%.** Historically, pseu-

Table 100–2. ANTIBIOTIC BOWEL PREPARATION

Preoperative Day	Kanamycin	Neomycin plus Erythromycin Base	Neomycin plus Metronidazole
3	1 g kanamycin orally every 1 hour × 4, then 4 times/day	—	—
2	1 g kanamycin orally 4 times/day	—	1 g neomycin 4 times/day plus 750 mg metronidazole 4 times/day
1	1 g kanamycin orally 4 times/day	1 g erythromycin base plus 1 g neomycin at 1 PM, 2 PM, 11 PM	1 g neomycin 4 times/day plus 750 mg metronidazole 4 times/day

domembranous enterocolitis was thought to be due to staphylococcus, but there was, in fact, little evidence to support that organism as the etiologic agent. It is now clear that *Clostridium difficile* **plays a significant role in the majority of cases.** *C. difficile* elaborates at least two toxins that cause diarrhea and enterocolitis. *C. difficile* does not invade the bowel, and it is not normally a significant inhabitant of the fecal flora. It is held in check by other bacteria that inhibit its growth. Thus, antibiotics destroy the bacteria that inhibit the growth of *C. difficile* and thereby allow it to flourish. The toxin produces a diffuse inflammatory response with cream-colored plaque formation, erythema, and edema of the bowel wall. Microscopically the villi appear to be intact, and there is a polymorphonuclear leukocyte infiltrate of the submucosa.

As the disease progresses, large areas of mucosa may slough, and areas of the bowel are denuded of their mucosa. The lesions may involve the colon, in which case it is called pseudomembranous enterocolitis, or the small bowel, in which case it is called pseudomembranous enteritis, or they may involve both. **The diagnosis is suspected by the symptoms or endoscopy and confirmed by culture of the organism or identification of its toxin. Because culture takes a prolonged period of time, it is more expeditious and therefore clinically useful to confirm the diagnosis by identifying the toxin produced by** *C. difficile* through tissue culture techniques. Once diagnosed, **treatment involves the administration of vancomycin or metronidazole and discontinuance of the other antibiotics that the patient is receiving.** Vancomycin or metronidazole is effective in most cases. **Rarely, toxic megacolon supervenes, which requires subtotal colectomy as a lifesaving procedure** (Chang, 1985).

INTESTINAL ANASTOMOSES

Regardless of the type of anastomosis or the methods used to perform it, there are certain fundamental principles that must be observed to minimize morbidity and mortality from intestinal surgery. **In urologic procedures in which gut is used, the most common cause of mortality and morbidity within the immediate postoperative period relates to complications involving the bowel:** either with the enteroenterostomy or with the segment interposed in the urinary tract. Therefore, it cannot be overemphasized that great care must be taken and proper techniques used in handling bowel in urologic procedures. Unfortunately the portion of the procedure that involves mobilization of the intestine and reanastomosis often follows a rather lengthy urologic endeavor and

is performed at a time when the surgical team is not fresh. Therefore, the following principles should be so firmly ingrained in the surgeon that they are performed without the need to recall each one specifically.

The first principle of proper technique for intestinal anastomoses is adequate exposure. The intestine should be mobilized sufficiently so that the anastomosis may be performed without struggling for exposure. If possible, it is preferable to mobilize the intestine sufficiently so that the anastomosis can be performed on the anterior abdominal wall. The area of the anastomosis should be walled off from the rest of the abdominal cavity with Mikulicz pads. This is important so that any inadvertent enteric spills are not distributed throughout the abdominal cavity. The mesentery must be cleared from the bowel segments to be anastomosed for a suitable distance (usually 0.5 cm) from the intestinal clamps at the severed ends so that good serosal apposition may be achieved without interposed mesentery. Sufficient serosa must be exposed so that the seromuscular sutures can be placed directly in the serosa without traversing the mesentery.

The second principle of performing a proper anastomosis is to maintain a good blood supply to the severed ends of the bowel. The blood supply may be compromised by creating an anastomosis under tension, excessive dissection or mobilization of the bowel, excessive use of the electrocautery, and tying the sutures so tight that the intervening tissue is strangulated. A cut margin of bowel that is pink and bleeds freely suggests that the blood supply has not been compromised; however, hemostasis must be ensured before beginning the anastomosis. The site of transection is selected at a point where the blood supply is adequate to both segments. The mesentery should be transilluminated so that the blood supply may be defined before transection of the bowel segment. In urologic surgery, the location of the transection is elective so that an area may be selected in which excellent arcades supply both sections of the transected segment. The area must be selected with an eye to how deep the mesenteric transection must be for proper segment mobility. After locating the appropriate area where the mesentery is to be transected, it is cleaned from the serosa, severed between mosquito clamps, and tied with 4–0 silk sutures.

The third principle involves preventing local spillage of enteric contents. The best way of preventing spills is to operate on bowel properly prepared (i.e., devoid of feces and collapsed). By stripping the enteric contents between the fingers both cephalad and caudad from the proposed transection site and applying a noncrushing occlusive clamp across the bowel, a spill is made even less likely. This clamp should prevent enteric contents from exiting the cut ends of the bowel without interference with the mesenteric blood supply. After applying linen-shod clamps and walling the area off, Allen clamps are applied to the bowel and the bowel transected between the Allen clamps. An anastomotic staple device may be used to transect the bowel at this point in place of Allen clamps (see later). Local spills and local sepsis have an adverse effect on the healing anastomosis, and it is for this reason that noncrushing occlusion clamps, in addition to an adequate bowel preparation, are advisable. If a spill does occur, it should be caught in the Mikulicz pads if the bowel has been properly walled off as described previously. The isolated segment that is to be used in the reconstructive procedure should be irrigated through and through with copious amounts of normal saline. The segment should be walled off. The irrigant is placed in one end of the segment and caught in a kidney basin as it exits the other end. This should be continued until the efflux is clear. This procedure prevents local spills during the ureterointestinal anastomosis and other aspects of reconstruction.

The fourth principle, germane to all intestinal anastomoses, is that **there should be an accurate apposition of serosa to serosa of the two segments of bowel to be anastomosed.** The anastomosis should be watertight and performed without tension. The bowel must be handled gently with the use of noncrushing forceps. The anastomotic line should be inverted and not everted. There is considerable controversy about this issue in that an everted anastomosis has been shown to heal with few complications. It is clear that when marginal conditions occur, an inverted anastomosis is more likely to remain intact than is the everted anastomosis.

The fifth principle is not to tie the sutures so tight that the tissue is strangulated. Obviously the sutures must bring the serosa of the two segments firmly together. Nonabsorbable sutures used for the anastomosis result in a stronger anastomotic line in the early healing phase when compared to reabsorbable sutures, but the difference is minimal and probably not particularly significant.

The final principle involves realignment of the mesentery of the two segments of bowel to be joined. These should be parallel to each other and ensure that, on completion of the anastomosis, there is no twist.

Factors that significantly contribute to anastomotic breakdown include a poor blood supply, local sepsis induced by fecal spillage, drains placed on an intra-abdominal anastomosis, and an anastomosis performed in irradiated bowel. Poor blood supply and local sepsis cause ischemia. Drains placed on the anastomosis increase the likelihood of an anastomotic leak, and an anastomosis performed in irradiated bowel is more likely to result in an anastomotic failure than if performed in nonirradiated tissue. The importance of careful technique and adherence to the aforementioned principles is emphasized by the fact that in one series of urinary intestinal diversion, **75% of the lethal complications that occurred in the postoperative period were related to the bowel. Eighty percent of these patients had received radiation before the intestinal surgery** (Mansson et al, 1979).

Types of Anastomoses

Intestinal anastomoses may be performed using sutures or staples. Properly performed, both have similar complication rates. In selected circumstances, however, one method may have advantages over the other. **In general, sutured anastomoses are preferable for intestinal segments that are exposed to urine** (i.e., suturing intestine to renal pelvis or bladder, closing the proximal end of a conduit [Costello and Johnson, 1984], and forming an intestinal pouch for urine).

Enteroenterostomy by a Two-Layer Suture Anastomosis

A 3–0 silk holding suture is placed on the mesenteric border just beneath the Allen clamps traversing both segments to be anastomosed, and a second suture is placed on the antimesenteric border similarly just beneath the Allen clamps (Fig. 100–3). It is important that the mesentery is cleaned sufficiently so that these sutures are placed in the serosa under direct vision. A row of silk sutures is placed 2 mm apart between the two holding sutures. This is accomplished by rotating the two Allen clamps away from each other, thus apposing the serosal surfaces. Sutures must traverse the muscularis but should not traverse the full thickness of the bowel. After all sutures have been placed, each is tied and the tails of all the sutures cut except those at each end. These are used as holding sutures. The Allen clamps are removed, and hemostasis is achieved, if necessary, with the light application of electrocautery. A 3–0 double-ended chromic intestinal suture is placed in the posterior suture line through all layers and tied to itself. Each end of the suture is then run in a locking fashion away from the midpoint until the mesenteric and antimesenteric borders are approached. As the lateral aspects of the bowel are approached, the suture is converted to a Connell suture (Fig. 100–4), which proceeds onto the anterior bowel wall. The sutures meet anteriorly in the midline and are tied together. The anterior serosa is then apposed with interrupted 3–0 silk sutures. The noncrushing occlusive clamps are removed and the mesentery closed with interrupted 3–0 silk sutures.

Patency of the anastomosis is ensured by palpating the anastomosis with the thumb and forefinger and feeling an annulus of tissue around the fingers. This anastomotic technique is employed when the antrum pylori is removed and

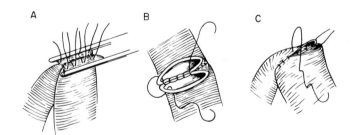

Figure 100–3. Two-layer suture anastomosis. *A*, Two holding sutures of 3–0 silk have been placed at the mesenteric and antimesenteric border, and the posterior wall is approximated with seromuscular sutures of 3–0 silk. *B*, A 3–0 intestinal chromic suture is placed through the full thickness of the bowel posteriorly, tied to itself, and run to the lateral borders with a continuous locking suture. At the lateral borders, it is converted to a Connell suture. *C*, The Connell suture brings the anterior margins together, inverting the suture line. The anastomosis is completed by placing horizontal mattress seromuscular sutures of 3–0 silk over the anterior suture line (not depicted).

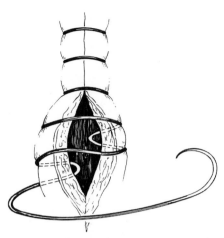

Figure 100–4. Connell suture. The suture traverses the bowel from serosa to mucosa, then from mucosa to serosa on the same side of the anastomosis. The suture is then placed on the opposite side of the anastomosis "outside in/inside out." The sequence is repeated until the two segments are approximated.

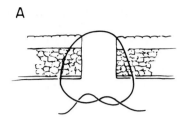

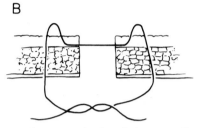

Figure 100–5. *A,* When properly placed, the suture through the intestine should include more serosa than mucosa. *B,* The Gambee stitch: The suture is placed through the full thickness of the bowel, the mucosa is traversed, and then the mirror-image procedure is performed on the segment to be anastomosed.

intestinal continuity is restored by a Billroth I procedure. It is also the most secure of all the anastomoses and should be used when one is forced to do an anastomosis under less than ideal circumstances.

Enteroenterostomy Using a Single-Layer Suture Anastomosis

The mesenteries of the two segments of bowel to be anastomosed are aligned, and a 3–0 silk suture is passed through the seromuscular layers of both segments on the mesenteric side and a second suture similarly placed on the antimesenteric side. The mesenteric suture is tied, and the antimesenteric suture is left untied. The Allen clamps are removed, and hemostasis is achieved with light electrocautery. The critical point of the anastomosis, where most leaks occur, is at the mesenteric border. Leaking generally occurs because the sutures are placed carelessly or the serosa has not been cleaned of mesentery sufficiently so that the sutures are placed through it under direct vision. Because this mesenteric border is the critical area, it is approached first. Two 3–0 silk sutures are placed through the full thickness of the bowel on either side of the mesenteric holding suture. These sutures are placed in such a way as to include more serosa than mucosa, thus causing inversion of the suture line (Fig. 100–5*A*). Some prefer to use a Gambee stitch at this point, which involves placing the suture through the full thickness of the bowel followed by traversing a small segment of mucosa of each segment of bowel before exiting through the full thickness of the bowel of the other segment (Fig. 100–5*B*). The two bowel sutures on the mesenteric border are tied being careful to invert the suture line, thus apposing serosa. Then 3–0 silk sutures are placed 2 mm apart, both on the anterior and on the posterior wall, inverting the suture line, thus apposing the serosa of the two bowel segments to each other. On approaching the antimesenteric holding suture, several sutures are placed before all are tied. A patent anastomosis is confirmed by feeling the annulus with the thumb and forefinger as described previously.

End-to-Side Ileocolic Sutured Anastomosis

The transected end of the colon is closed in the following manner (Fig. 100–6). A 3–0 silk suture is placed beneath the Allen clamp on the mesenteric border and a second suture on the antimesenteric border. These are tied. A 3–0 chromic suture is placed beneath the clamp in a horizontal mattress fashion. Beginning at the mesenteric border, it is tied to itself, and the horizontal mattress suture is placed until the antimesenteric border is reached, at which point the suture is again tied to itself. The clamp is removed, and an over-and-over suture is performed using the same chromic suture throughout the full thickness of the bowel until returning to the point of origin (i.e., the mesenteric border is approached). At this point, the suture is again tied to itself. The suture line is buried by approximating the serosa on each side with interrupted 3–0 silk sutures placed 2 mm apart.

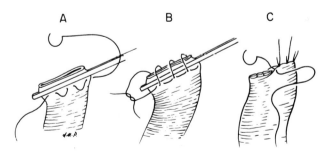

Figure 100–6. Closure of the proximal end of the intestine. *A,* A 3–0 chromic suture is tied to itself at the antimesenteric border and placed beyond the intestinal clamp in a horizontal mattress fashion until the mesenteric border is reached. The suture is then tied to itself at this point. *B,* The intestinal clamp is removed, and an over-and-over suture through the full thickness of the bowel returns the chromic suture to its point of origin, where it is again tied to itself. *C,* Interrupted horizontal mattress seromuscular sutures of 3–0 silk invert the chromic suture line.

The mesenteries are aligned, and the ileal serosa is sutured with interrupted 3–0 silk sutures to the colonic serosa 2 mm below a taenia (Fig. 100–7). The taenia is incised the length of the diameter of the ileum adjacent to it. As described earlier for the two-layer anastomosis, a 3–0 double-ended intestinal chromic suture is placed through all layers of the colon and ileum in the midpoint of the posterior wall and run in a locking fashion laterally to either side of the incision in the taenia. At the lateralmost border, the suture is converted to a Connell suture, and the anterior wall is closed. Seromuscular sutures of 3–0 silk placed from ileum to colon bury the anterior suture line. The mesentery is reapproximated.

Ileocolonic End-to-End Sutured Anastomosis with Discrepant Bowel Sizes

A 3–0 silk suture is placed on the mesenteric border of the ileum and colon (Fig. 100–8). A second 3–0 silk suture is placed on the antimesenteric border of the colon immediately beneath the Allen clamp. The other end of the suture is placed on the antimesenteric border of the ileum at a distance proximal to the Allen clamp, such that the serosal lengths between the two sutures of both ileal and colon segments are equal. Thus, an equal amount of ileal serosa is applied to the length of colonic serosa bordering the severed end of bowel. In the seromuscular layers of ileum and colon, 3–0 silk sutures are placed 2 mm apart, thus apposing the serosa of the ileum to the colon. The Allen clamps are removed. Hemostasis is achieved and the antimesenteric border of the ileum incised to the level of the most proximal suture in the ileum. Thus, the bowel lumens now are of identical size. Using a 3–0 chromic double-ended intestinal suture, the posterior row is run in a locking fashion, laterally converting to a Connell suture, and the anterior row is completed. Seromuscular sutures of 3–0 silk bury the anterior suture line.

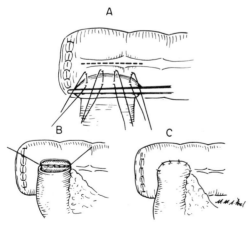

Figure 100–7. End-to-side anastomosis. *A*, The serosa of the ileum is sutured to the serosa of the colon 2 to 3 mm below a taenia. *B*, The taenia is opened for a distance sufficient to accommodate the diameter of the ileum. A 3–0 chromic suture is placed through all layers on the posterior wall, tied to itself, run in a locking fashion to both borders, and converted to a Connell suture laterally, thus completing the inversion anteriorly. *C*, The anterior margin of serosa is reapproximated with interrupted horizontal mattress sutures of 3–0 silk.

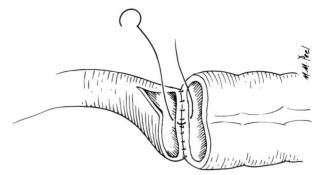

Figure 100–8. Anastomosis of discrepant-sized bowel. A seromuscular suture of 3–0 silk is placed adjacent to each end of the lumen on the mesenteric side. A second 3–0 silk seromuscular suture is placed adjacent to the lumen on the colon and on the antimesenteric border proximal to the cut end of the small bowel at a distance sufficient so that when the antimesenteric border is incised, the lumens are the same size. Interrupted seromuscular sutures of 3–0 silk are then placed at 2-mm intervals between the two holding sutures. The small bowel is opened on its antimesenteric border until the opening in the small bowel is the same size as the opening in the colon. A 3–0 chromic suture is placed through all layers, tied to itself, and run laterally in a running locking fashion. At the borders, it is converted to a Connell suture, thus inverting the anterior margin. The anastomosis is completed with interrupted horizontal mattress 3–0 silk sutures that bring the seromuscular layers together anteriorly. This is similar to the closure depicted in Figure 100–3.

Stapled Anastomoses

The theoretical benefits of a stapled anastomosis are that it provides for a better blood supply to the healing margin, there is reduced tissue manipulation, there is minimal edema with uniformity of suture placement, a wider lumen is created, there is greater ease and less time involved in performing the anastomosis, and the length of postoperative paralytic ileus is reduced. When placed in intestine through which urine traverses, however, stapled anastomoses not infrequently cause stone formation (Bisson et al, 1979; Costello and Johnson, 1984).

Stapled anastomoses evert the suture line. Because staples close in a B and do not crush the tissue, theoretically they prevent ischemia at the suture line. This may be obvious when a staple line is used to transect the bowel and bleeding continues to occur. The bleeding points may be lightly electrocoagulated or tied off with fine absorbable suture. Stapled bowel anastomoses have been shown to be as efficacious as a hand-sewn anastomosis because both have similar complication rates. **They usually require less time to perform when the techniques are properly learned, but for prolonged procedures, they save little, if any, time when the length of time for the whole procedure is taken into account.** In a large prospective, randomized trial in which a two-layer closure was compared to a staple closure, it was found that the complication rate was the same, but the time required to complete the stapled anastomosis was 10 minutes less than that for the hand-sewn anastomosis; when the total operative time was compared between the two, it was the same (Didolkar et al, 1986). **A comparison of complications between sutured and stapled anastomoses reveals a leak and fistula rate of 2.8% for stapled and 3.0% for sutured anastomoses** (Chassin et al, 1978). The clinically significant leak rate, however, is only 0.9% (Fazio et al,

1985). A 4.5% incidence of stapled anastomotic leakage has been reported during ileal conduit construction (Costello and Johnson, 1984).

Thus, the use of staples depends on the preference of the surgeon. Perhaps an area where a stapled anastomosis appears to be superior to a hand-sewn anastomosis is in an esophageal-intestinal anastomosis and a low rectal anastomosis. In these two areas, the circular stapler allows for a more precise anastomosis than is often possible using hand-sewn techniques. Because these are not problems of urologic surgery, staples are used at the discretion of the surgeon. The one area in urology where the author believes the stapling device is superior is in the ileocolonic end-to-side anastomosis. Using the circular stapling device, a widely patent anastomosis can be achieved expeditiously.

There are three staple instruments that are commonly employed in intestinal reconstruction: the linear stapler, the anastomotic stapler, and the circular stapler. The linear stapler places a double row of staggered staples in a straight line. Depending on the cartridge and instrument chosen, various lengths of staple lines and heights of the closed staples may be chosen. The length is selected depending on how long one wishes the staple line to be. **The height of staple is selected according to the tissue to be stapled.** Vascular and pulmonary tissues require staples with a closed height of 1 mm (open height of 2.5 mm). Most intestinal anastomoses are performed with medium staples, which have a closed height of approximately 1.5 mm (open height of 3.5 mm). Occasionally, for thick tissues, large staples are required that have a closed height of 2 mm (open height of 4.8 mm). If there is any doubt in selecting the staple size, the tissue thickness may be measured with a special instrument used for this purpose. In general, **tissues less than 1 mm or greater than 3 mm in thickness are not amenable to the use of staples.**

The anastomotic stapler places two linear double rows of staggered staples. When the knife is advanced, the staple line is divided. The height of the staples is chosen depending on the tissue to be transected.

The circular stapler places two concentric, staggered circular staple rows and cuts the tissue within the circle completely from the surrounding tissue. It may be selected in various diameters and with various heights of staples. The diameter and height are selected according to the tissue to be anastomosed. The diameter to be selected is determined by sizing the diameter of the tissue to be stapled. Special sizers are available for this maneuver. In most intestinal anastomoses in urology, the height of the closed staple is 1.5 to 2.0 mm. The following is a description of various types of stapled anastomoses.

Ileocolonic Anastomosis Using the Circular Stapling Device

The mesenteric borders are cleared for a distance of 1.5 cm from the cut end of both the colon and the ileum (Fig. 100–9). Holding sutures of 3–0 silk are placed on the mesenteric and antimesenteric border of the colon. Two other holding sutures are placed on the medial and lateral walls of the colon, midway between the mesenteric and antimesenteric sutures. A purse-string suture of 2–0 polypropylene (Prolene) is placed around the ileum no more than 2 mm

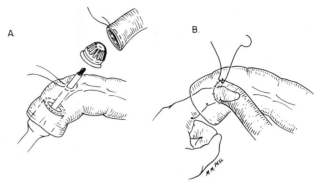

Figure 100–9. Stapled circular anastomosis. *A,* A purse-string suture of 2–0 Prolene is placed around the circumference of the small bowel, and a second purse-string suture 1 cm in diameter is placed on a medial taenia 5 to 6 cm from the open end of the colon. The anvil is removed. A stab wound is made in the center of the purse-string suture in the colon, and the circular stapler is introduced through the end of the colon, with its post thrust through the stab wound. *B,* The anvil is placed on the post and is introduced into the end of the small bowel, the purse-string sutures in the small bowel and colon are tied snugly around the post, and the circular stapler is approximated with a gap of 1.5 to 2 mm, with care taken not to include any mesentery in the gap. The anastomosis is completed by placing interrupted silk sutures around the circumference of the anastomosis.

from the cut end. It is important to take small bites of mucosa to avoid bunching of tissue. Sutures must be placed evenly to avoid a gap. A purse-string instrument is available that can be used for this step, if preferred. The ileal diameter is determined with sizers so that the correct circular stapler diameter instrument may be chosen. A purse-string suture is also placed in a circle, 1 cm in diameter, through which a taenia traverses on the medial aspect of the colon. A stab wound is made in the center of the colonic purse-string suture. The distal anvil of the circular stapler is removed, and the instrument is placed through the open end of the colon with its post passed out the stab wound made in the center of the purse-string on the medial wall of the colon. The purse-string is tied tight. The top anvil is then secured to the post, and the ileum is placed over it. The ileal purse-string is tied.

Care must be taken to align the mesenteries at this point. The instrument is approximated with a staple gap of 1.5 to 2.0 mm. Care must be taken not to catch fat or mesentery in the gap. The instrument is fired and is removed by rotatory movement from the colon. Two doughnuts of tissue should be identified on the instrument, and they should have their complete circumference intact with no gaps. With a finger in the open end of the colon and through the anastomosis, seromuscular sutures of 3–0 silk are placed 3 to 4 mm apart around the circumference of the anastomotic line.

The transected end of the colon may be closed by the suture technique or by the use of staples. If the end is to be closed with sutures, one 3–0 chromic suture is brought out the mesenteric border and another out the antimesenteric border, and both are tied to themselves with the knots on the inside of the bowel. The two sutures are run to each other using a Connell suture until they meet, at which point they are tied to each other. The suture line is inverted by placing a second row of 3–0 silk seromuscular sutures. If staples are preferred, the holding sutures are held up, and a linear stapler is applied across the open end. Excess tissue is trimmed and the stapler removed. By holding the holding sutures up, one is secure in applying the staple line to the serosa and mucosa circumferentially around the bowel. Some invert the staple line with seromuscular sutures of 3–0 silk. This, however, is not necessary. The mesentery between the two segments is now approximated with interrupted 3–0 silk sutures.

End-to-End Stapled Anastomosis: Ileal-Ileal or Ileocolonic Anastomosis

The antimesenteric border of the two bowel segments to be joined is approximated with a 3–0 silk suture 5 to 6 cm from the cut ends of the bowel (Fig. 100–10). A holding suture is placed through both segments of bowel at their cut ends at the midpoint of the antimesenteric borders. Stay sutures are placed at the mesenteric border of each bowel segment, and two other sutures midway between the mesenteric and antimesenteric border on the lateral aspects of the bowel are also placed. The anastomotic stapler is positioned in the lumens of both segments of bowel along the antimes-

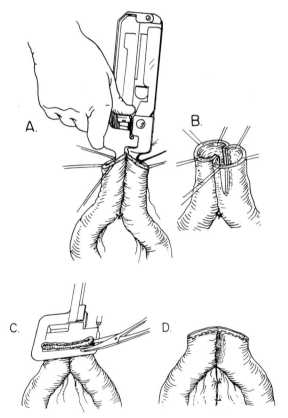

Figure 100–10. Stapled end-to-end anastomosis. *A,* A 3–0 silk suture is placed 5 to 6 cm from the cut ends of the intestine on the antimesenteric borders of both intestinal segments and tied. Holding sutures are placed around the circumference of both intestinal lumens, one suture securing together the antimesenteric borders of both intestinal segments. The linear anastomotic stapler is placed into the lumens, secured and locked in place, and fired, and the knife is advanced. *B,* The appearance of the intestinal anastomosis after firing of the staple device. *C,* The open end of the two intestinal segments is closed with a linear stapler by holding the holding sutures up while applying the linear stapler so that the circumferences of the mucosa and serosa are incorporated in the staple margin. *D,* The anastomosis is completed by closing the mesentery with interrupted 3–0 silk sutures.

enteric border. The antimesenteric holding suture is pulled up adjacent to the stapler. The anastomotic stapler is locked in place, the staples are fired, and the knife is advanced. The staple lines are inspected for bleeders, which if persistent should be suture ligated with an absorbable suture. It is important that several 3–0 silk sutures are placed at the apex of the stapled and cut antimesenteric incision. At this point, slight tension on the anastomotic line can place undue stress on the staple margin and cause a leak. The holding sutures are held up, and a linear stapler is placed across the open end of bowel and fired. Care must be taken so that the staples include the serosa in its entire circumference. Excess bowel tissue is excised flush with the instrument before it is disengaged. The mesentery is then reapproximated.

Postoperative Care

The patient should not be allowed to begin oral alimentation for a minimum of 4 days following surgery. Coordinated small bowel activity begins within hours after the operative event, and stomach activity may return as early as 24 hours postoperatively. Clear liquids may be begun when the paralytic ileus resolves and bowel activity resumes. If clear liquids are tolerated, the diet may be advanced after the patient has a bowel movement. This sequence of events generally takes 4 to 7 days. **If the nutritional condition of the patient is impaired preoperatively, there is a postoperative complication that delays feeding, or the paralytic ileus is still present on the sixth postoperative day, intravenous nutrition that supplies the total caloric requirement (hyperalimentation) should be begun. It is preferable to begin the hyperalimentation the day after surgery if any of these complications are anticipated.** Once started, it is discontinued only when oral intake is sufficient to satisfy the body's caloric requirements. The use of a jejunal feeding tube for the early institution of intestinal feeding has been advocated by some but has not been shown to have any significant advantage over the use of hyperalimentation as outlined here.

The use of nasogastric or gastrostomy decompression during the postoperative period of ileus is somewhat controversial. In a prospective study of elective intestinal anastomoses in which 274 patients had postoperative gastric decompression and 261 patients were given nothing by mouth until bowel activity resumed, **there was no significant difference in major intestinal complications between the two groups; however, those who did not have gastric decompression showed a much greater incidence of abdominal distention, nausea, and vomiting.** It must be understood that only healthy patients with no complications were entered into the study. Sixty percent of the patients initially entered were excluded. Specific exclusion criteria included emergency surgery with peritonitis, extensive fibrous adhesions, enterotomies, previous pelvic irradiation, intra-abdominal infection, pancreatitis, chronic obstruction, prolonged operating time, and difficult endotracheal intubation (Wolff et al, 1988). It is therefore **prudent to decompress all but the most medically fit because vomiting in the postoperative period increases the risk of aspiration and morbidity in the compromised patient.** Moreover, tube decompression allows for the administration of ice chips by mouth before enteric activity resumes, thus enhancing patient comfort. **If the patient has severe pulmonary disease, decompression by placing a gastric tube at the time of surgery facilitates pulmonary toilet and enhances patient comfort. During the period of ileus, the patient should receive a histamine (H_2) blocker and be given an antacid via the stomach tube every 2 hours as necessary to keep the gastric pH above 5.0.** By keeping the gastric contents alkaline in the postoperative period, the incidence of gastric stress ulceration is markedly reduced.

Complications of Intestinal Anastomoses

The complications that occur following anastomoses include leakage of fecal contents, sepsis, wound infections, abdominal abscesses, hemorrhage, anastomotic stenosis, pseudo-obstruction of the colon (Ogilvie's syndrome), and intestinal obstruction. These untoward events increase morbidity and are frequently major contributors to patient mortality. The complication rates for elective colocolonic and ileocolonic anastomoses performed in prepared bowel are intestinal leak, 2%; hemorrhage, 1%; and stenosis or obstruction, 4%. These complications require reoperations in 1% of the patients and result in death in 0.2% of patients (Jex et al, 1987).

Fistulas

Fistulas in the postoperative period are of two types: fecal and urinary. **These generally occur within the first several weeks following the operative event.** They frequently result in sepsis and markedly increase patient morbidity and mortality. Fecal fistulas occur in 4% to 5% of patients (Sullivan et al, 1980; Beckley et al, 1982). **Sepsis is a common complication of these untoward events and carries with it a mortality of 2%** (1 of 47 patients) (Hill and Ransley, 1983).

Sepsis and Other Infectious Complications

Wound infections, pelvic abscesses, and wound dehiscences all may complicate the immediate postoperative period. Although wound dehiscences and pelvic abscesses are rare complications, morbid wound infections occur with an incidence of 5% (3 of 62 patients) (Loening et al, 1982). Many of these complications may be averted by operating on a properly prepared bowel, by walling off the intestine with Mikulicz pads while the anastomosis is being completed, and by irrigating the intestinal segment to be used in the reconstruction until it is free of any residual enteric contents before it is manipulated and its contents are spilled in the abdomen and pelvis.

Bowel Obstruction

The incidence of intestinal obstruction following abdominal procedures for urinary intestinal diversion differs depending on whether the stomach, ileum, or colon is used for the diversion. In patients who have had a segment **of stomach or ileum removed for the diversion, there is a 10% incidence of postoperative bowel obstruction requiring treatment. When the colon is used, the incidence of postoperative obstruction requiring an operation is 5%** (Table 100–3). Half of the bowel obstructions occur in the early postoperative period. In one series, following radical cystectomy and ileal conduit, 15% of the patients had a mild obstruction in the first 6 months that responded to conservative management, whereas 3% required an operation to relieve the obstruction during this period. The occurrence of obstruction following this 6-month period was much less frequent (Sullivan et al, 1980). **Bowel obstruction can be a morbid event, as 21% of patients who develop obstruction following an ileal conduit and require an operation die. The most common cause of the obstruction is adhesions followed by recurrent cancer.** These two causes account for the great majority of the cases. Volvulus and internal hernia account for far fewer cases (Jaffe et al, 1968). Rarely, severe stenosis or obstruction at the anastomotic suture line occurs. The former is a result of edema, poor technique, or performing the anastomosis on ischemic bowel (Fig. 100–11), and the latter of improper technique.

The incidence of postoperative bowel obstruction may be reduced by using nonirradiated bowel, performing the anastomosis on well-vascularized bowel, closing all apertures, reperitonealizing the isolated segment, decompressing the gastrointestinal tract for an adequate period of time, placing omentum over the anastomosis, and reconstituting the pelvic floor following exenterative surgery. The isolated segment is reperitonealized by tacking its antimesenteric border to the lateral abdominal side wall peritoneum. The proximal mesenteric border should be tacked to the posterior parietal peritoneum because failure to obliterate this potential space has resulted in entrapment of bowel, causing a bowel obstruction. The pelvic space left following an anterior exenteration may be closed by placing the sigmoid colon in the area. This effectively prevents small bowel from herniating into the raw pelvis. Omentum may also be mobilized and used to fill any space the sigmoid colon does not fill. In a total exenteration, sufficient sigmoid colon is not available, and often the omentum is not bulky enough to fill the pelvis and thus prevent small bowel from filling the denuded pelvis. This situation is of particular concern in patients who must receive postoperative pelvic irradiation. The bowel may be kept out of the pelvis in these patients by reconstructing the pelvic floor with polyglactin mesh. The mesh is sutured along the posterior pelvic brim to the sacral promontory and presacral fascia and laterally to the adventitia of the iliac vessels. Laterally and anteriorly, it is sewn to the peritoneum two thirds of the distance between the pubis and umbilicus. Omentum is then brought down, placed over the mesh, and sutured in position. This effectively excludes the bowel from the pelvis for 4 to 6 weeks while postoperative irradiation is being administered (Sener et al, 1989).

Hemorrhage

Hemorrhage is a rare complication of intestinal anastomoses. It is much more likely to occur when stomach is used and a Billroth I anastomosis is created. **It is usually due to**

Table 100–3. COMPLICATIONS OF URINARY INTESTINAL DIVERSION*

Complications	Type of Diversion	No. of Patients (Complication/Total No.)	Incidence (%)
Bowel obstruction	Ileal conduit	124/1289	10
	Colon conduit	9/230	4
	Gastric conduit	2/21	10
	Continent diversion	2/250	4
Ureteral intestinal obstruction	Ileal conduit	90/1142	8
	Antireflux colon conduit	25/122	20
	Colon conduit	8/92	9
	Continent diversion	16/461	4
Urine leak	Ileal conduit	23/886	3
	Colon conduit	6/130	5
	Continent diversion		
	Ileum	104/629	17
	Colon	5/123	4
Stomal stenosis/hernia	Ileal conduit	196/806	24
	Colon conduit	45/227	20
	Continent diversion	28/310	9
Renal calculi	Ileal conduit	70/964	7
	Antireflux colon conduit	5/94	5
Pouch calculi	Continent diversion	42/317	13
Acidosis requiring treatment	Ileal conduit	46/296	16
	Antireflux colon conduit	5/94	5
	Gastric conduit	0/21	0
	Continent diversion		
	Ileum	21/263	8
	Colon/colon-Ileum	17/63	27
Pyelonephritis	Ileal conduit	132/1142	12
	Antireflux colon conduit	13/96	13
	Continent diversion	15/296	5
Renal deterioration	Ileal conduit	146/808	18
	Antireflux colon conduit	15/103	15

*Composite from the literature. Follow-up averages 5 years for ileal conduits, 3 years for colon conduits, 2 years for gastric conduits, and 2 years for continent diversions.

Literature reviewed: Adams et al, 1988; Althausen et al, 1978; Beckley et al, 1982; Boyd et al, 1989; Castro and Ram, 1970; Elder et al, 1979; Flanigan et al, 1975; Hagen-Cook and Althausen, 1979; Jaffe et al, 1968; Loening et al, 1982; Malek et al, 1971; Middleton and Hendren, 1976; Pitts and Muecke, 1979; Richie, 1974; Schmidt et al, 1973; Schwarz and Jeffs, 1975; Shapiro et al, 1975; Smith, 1972; Sullivan et al, 1980.

failure to secure bleeding at the time of anastomosis or to anastomotic ulcers that develop on the suture line.

Intestinal Stenosis

Intestinal stenosis occurs at two distinct times: in the immediate postoperative period and over the long term. Intestinal stenosis in the immediate postoperative period is due to technical mishaps or edema. The latter resolves by continuing the intestinal decompression, whereas the former requires a reoperation. Over the long term, it is likely due to ischemia or perienteric infection. Figure 100–11 shows an upper gastrointestinal tract series of a severe intestinal stenosis caused by ischemia. At the time of the ileoileostomy, the suture line was blue. Chronic symptoms of partial small bowel obstruction occurred in the postoperative period.

Pseudo-obstruction

Pseudo-obstruction of the colon, or Ogilvie's syndrome, on rare occasion may complicate the early postoperative period. Its cause is not understood. **It usually occurs within the first 3 days postoperatively in patients with multiple medical illnesses.** The patient complains of severe abdominal pain, and a roentgenogram of the abdomen reveals a dilated cecum. A gentle water-soluble contrast enema eliminates the possibility of a mechanical obstruction. In the

presence of a rising leukocyte count or cecum that is increasing in size and exceeds 12 to 15 cm in diameter, rupture may be imminent. Under these circumstances, an emergency cecostomy should be performed (Clayman et al, 1981). In less acute circumstances, endoscopic decompression may be attempted.

Complications of the Isolated Intestinal Segment

Intestinal Stricture

Strictures of intestinal segments are usually late complications primarily occurring in conduits, although they have been described in ileal ureters as well. **The stricture is thought to be a consequence of lymphoid depletion of the intestine exposed to urine.** The lymphoid depletion contributes to persistent infection, which may result in mid-loop stricture, bacterial seeding of the upper tracts, and renal deterioration (Tapper and Folkman, 1976). Because of the persistent infection and lack of intestinal resistance to the detrimental action of bacteria, submucosal edema with fibrosis and stricture formation occurs. The intestinal segment may also be blocked by encroachment of hypertrophied mesenteric lymph nodes. **Hypertrophied mesenteric lymph nodes, submucosal lymphoid depletion, edema, and fi-**

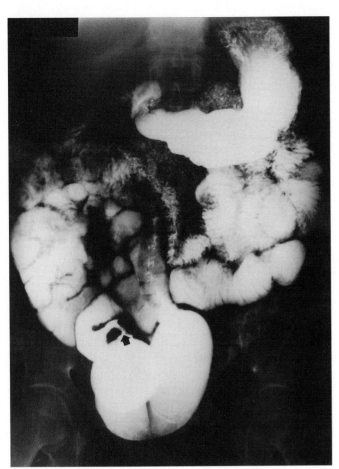

Figure 100–11. Upper gastrointestinal tract series illustrating a small bowel stricture *(arrow)* at the ileoileostomy following ileal conduit urinary diversion. At the time of the initial ileoileostomy, the anastomotic suture line appeared bluish. At subsequent exploration, a bowel lumen of only 2 mm was found. The serosa at the anastomotic site was fibrotic.

brosis are commonly found when intestinal segments that have been chronically exposed to urine are examined pathologically.

Elongation of the Segment

Another complication of the intestinal segment is elongation—occasionally resulting in massive enlargement. When this occurs in conduits or ureteral substitutes, there is usually a distal obstruction. In continent diversions, it may signal failure to catheterize the pouch intermittently frequently enough. If allowed to persist, the increased pressure may result in deterioration of renal function. Enlargement and elongation of the intestine may also result in a volvulus of the segment (Fig. 100–12).

Abdominal Stomas

Two types of stomas may be created on the anterior abdominal wall: those that are flush and those that protrude. The former is preferable for the continent type of diversion in which intermittent catheterization is carried out and over which a small dressing is placed. The latter is preferable

when a collection device is worn. **A properly protruding stoma worn with an appliance results in a lesser incidence of stomal stenosis with epithelial overgrowth and a better appliance fit with fewer peristomal skin problems. There are two types of protruding stomas: the end stoma and the loop end ileostomy. Most complications of stomas are the result of technical errors in their creation.** Therefore, specific technical points must be rigidly adhered to, to minimize such complications.

The site of the stoma should be selected preoperatively. This is done by marking the stomal site with the patient in the sitting position as well as the supine position, care being taken to place it over the rectus muscle at least 5 cm away from the planned incision line. The point chosen should be well away from skin creases, scars, the umbilicus, belt lines, and bony prominences. A site in which radiotherapy has previously injured the area should be avoided. **All stomas should be placed through the belly of the rectus muscle and be located at the peak of the infraumbilical fat roll.** If the stoma is placed lateral to the rectus sheath, a parastomal hernia is likely to occur. The bowel should traverse the abdominal wall perpendicular to the peritoneal lining (i.e., it should come straight out). One should avoid trimming fat or epiploic appendages from around the margin of the stoma, and the appliances should be applied in the operating room.

A circular incision is made at the predetermined site. A

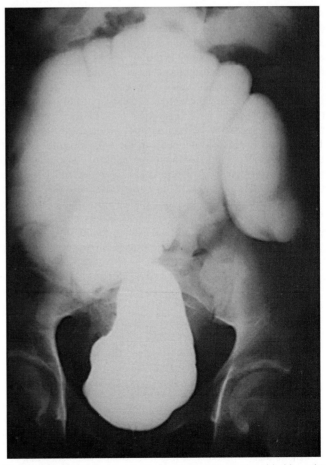

Figure 100–12. Volvulus of an orthotopic right colon bladder. This segment enlarged markedly because of the patient's lack of adherence to a regimen of frequent intermittent catheterization.

perfectly circular opening in the skin may be created by placing the finger hole of a Kelly clamp at the desired point and grasping the skin in the center of the hole with a Kocher clamp. By pulling up on the Kocher and pushing the handle of the Kelly against the abdominal wall, a small button of skin may be removed with a single pass of the knife. This creates a perfectly circular opening in the skin. It should be pointed out, however, that the tendency to remove too much skin is great, resulting in a circular opening that is too large. To avoid this complication, one should not cut the skin flush with the Kelly clamp but rather immediately beneath the Kocher clamp. The subcutaneous tissue is left intact. This is spread, not excising any fat, for the fat falls back adjacent to the bowel and eliminates any dead space. Kocher clamps are placed on the fascia in the incision and pulled medialward so that when the fascia and peritoneum are incised, they are incised directly over the skin line and thus do not result in angulation of the gut when the abdominal incision is closed. The fascia is incised in a cruciate manner, and the rectus muscles are spread. The peritoneum is incised. The opening should accommodate two fingers snugly.

Nipple Stoma: "Rosebud"

A Babcock clamp is placed through the opening, and the bowel is grasped and brought out for a distance of 5 to 6 cm to create a nipple of about 2 to 3 cm in length (Fig. 100–13). Two 3–0 chromic sutures are placed through the seromuscular layer of the bowel and the peritoneum on the anterior abdominal wall. Alternatively the serosa may be sutured to the fascia with two 2–0 chromic sutures. It should be noted that the mesentery is aligned in its normal anatomic direction before suturing the serosa to the peritoneal wall. Usually the ileum is curved concave toward the mesentery. If this is severe, the mesentery may be partially incised 1 cm from the bowel wall (Fig. 100–14). Thus, a portion of mesentery is preserved along the entire length of the bowel. This should straighten the curve in the bowel significantly if not completely. Four 3–0 chromic sutures are placed in quadrants through the full thickness of the bowel edge and through the seromuscular layer of the bowel 3 to 4 cm from the cut edge and then through the subcuticular skin layer. Sutures should not traverse the full thickness of the skin but through the subcuticular and subdermal layers only.

When the sutures are tied, the bowel is everted and forms

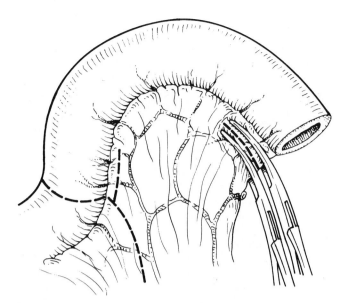

Figure 100–14. The bowel may be straightened if it is tethered by the mesentery by incising the mesentery several centimeters away from the serosa and parallel to the bowel.

a nipple. A more secure nipple may be formed by performing multiple myotomies through the seromuscular layer of the bowel above the skin line before creation of the nipple. The myotomies adhere serosa to serosa and reduce the risk of stomal retraction. This is particularly appropriate for patients who are obese.

Flush Stoma

Quadrant sutures of 3–0 chromic are placed through the full thickness of the bowel and subsequently passed through the subdermal layer of the skin and tied. Several sutures are placed between the quadrant sutures from bowel to subdermal skin. This creates a flush stoma that has a 1-mm raised margin.

Loop End Ileostomy

Obese patients have a thick abdominal wall and often a thick, short ileal mesentery. This makes creation of an end ileal stoma extremely difficult. **The loop end ileostomy obviates some of these problems and is usually easier to perform than the ileal end stoma in the patient who is obese** (Fig. 100–15). To create this type of stoma, the distal end of the ileum is closed as described previously for closing the proximal end of an intestinal segment, and a loop is brought up through the belly of the rectus muscle and onto the anterior abdominal wall. This avoids bringing the mesenteric border onto the abdominal wall and prevents one side of the ileostomy from being involved with mesentery. A slightly larger skin opening is required than for the end stoma. A 3-cm disc of skin is removed. The subcutaneous tissue is spread, the fascia incised, the rectus spread, and the peritoneum incised as described earlier. The opening should admit two fingers comfortably. The loop may be pulled through the opening in the abdominal wall by passing an umbilical tape through a small opening in the mesentery at a distance from the distal end that is sufficient to leave that

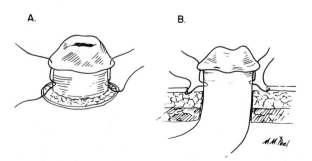

Figure 100–13. *A* and *B,* Nipple stoma. Five to 6 cm of intestine is brought through the abdominal wall. The serosa is scarified, and quadrant sutures of 3–0 chromic are placed through the full thickness of the distal end of the intestine. Each suture is placed in the seromuscular layer 3 cm proximal and then secured to the dermis before it is tied.

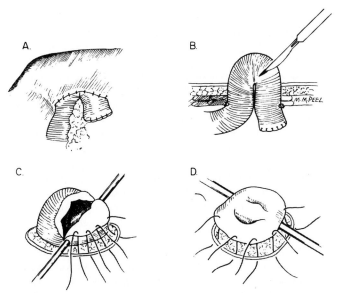

Figure 100–15. Loop end ileostomy. *A,* After the distal end of the loop is closed and the bowel is drawn through the rent in the abdominal wall, the bowel is held in place by a rod passed through the mesentery. The mesentery is realigned, and the peritoneum is sutured to the serosa of the bowel circumferentially. *B,* A transverse incision is made in the bowel four fifths of the loop distance cephalad. *C,* The cephalad portion of the stoma is simply sutured to the dermal layer of skin with interrupted 3–0 chromic sutures. *D,* On the inferior aspect of the incision, sutures of 3–0 chromic are placed through the full thickness of the cut edge and then through the seromuscular layer, then through the dermis. This everts the caudal portion of the stoma.

end in the abdomen when the loop has been pulled through the abdominal wall. By gentle traction on the umbilical tape, the loop is brought onto the abdomen.

The distal portion of the bowel is brought through the opening such that the closed end lies cephalad to the body of the segment. When a sufficient amount of loop protrudes beyond the skin edge, a small rod is placed through the hole in the mesentery at the apex of the loop and holds the bowel on the anterior abdominal wall during suturing. If the rent in the rectus muscle is too large, it may be closed with interrupted 0 chromic sutures from within the abdomen. The serosa is sutured to the peritoneum on the anterior abdominal wall. The bowel wall is opened in a transverse direction at a point four fifths of the distance cephalad to the caudalmost portion of the loop. Using 3–0 chromic sutures, the full thickness of the caudal incision in the bowel is sutured back to itself (serosa) and then to the dermis as in the rosebud technique. The cephalad nonfunctional opening is sutured directly to the dermis. The rod is sutured to the skin and left in place for 7 days.

This type of stoma results in a lesser incidence of stomal stenosis but a higher incidence of parastomal hernias (Emmott et al, 1985). Stomas for the colon may be created in much the same way as end stomas for the ileum. Their suturing, however, is usually more flush than everted.

Complications of Intestinal Stomas

Complications of the abdominal stoma are the single most common problem encountered in the postoperative period after urinary intestinal diversion. **Early complications of abdominal stomas include bowel necrosis, bleeding, dermatitis, parastomal hernia, prolapse, obstruction, stomal retraction, and stomal stenosis.** At some point, virtually every patient has one of these complications. Many of these complications can be reduced by proper construction of the stoma. If periodic visits with the enterostomal therapist are made, products for skin care are appropriately used, nonirritative stomal adhesives are employed, the urine in the collection device is maintained acidic, and properly fitting collection devices are used, most stomal complications can be significantly reduced and many eliminated.

Parastomal skin lesions may be classified as (1) irritative, which are manifested by hypopigmentation, hyperpigmentation, and skin atrophy; (2) erythematous erosive lesions, which appear as macular lesions, scaling of the skin, and loss of the epidermis; and (3) pseudoverrucous, which are wart-like lesions (Borglund et al, 1988).

Stomal stenosis has been reported, on average, in 20% to 24% of patients with ileal conduits and 10% to 20% of patients with colon conduits (see Table 100–3). This incidence has been considerably reduced by better attention to stomal care and better-fitting appliances. Stomal stenosis is less for loop stomas than for end stomas. Parastomal hernias occur rarely (1%–4%) with end stomas but are more likely to occur with loop stomas with reported incidences ranging from 4% to 20%.

Bleeding, stomal stenosis, and dermatitis can be markedly reduced by attention to parastomal skin care and by the use of a properly fitting appliance around a protruding stoma. The other complications are minimized by proper surgical technique.

URETEROINTESTINAL ANASTOMOSES

The ureter may be anastomosed to the colon or small bowel in such a manner as to produce a refluxing or nonrefluxing anastomosis. There is considerable controversy as to whether a nonrefluxing or refluxing anastomosis is desirable in urinary tract reconstruction. Deterioration of the upper tracts for ileal and colon conduits has been reported in 10% to 60% of the patients. In one series, 49% of the upper tracts showed changes after conduit diversion, 16% of which had an increase of the blood urea nitrogen of 10 mg/dl or more (Schwarz and Jeffs, 1975). **Deterioration of the upper tracts is usually a consequence of either infection or stones or less commonly obstruction at the ureteral intestinal anastomosis.** Because bacteriuria occurs in almost all conduits and because the intestine certainly does not inhibit and may, in fact, promote bacterial colonization, many have suggested that a nonrefluxing anastomosis would minimize the incidence of renal deterioration.

The evidence that suggests a nonrefluxing system in urinary intestinal diversions is desirable comes from several observations. **In a group of patients who had nonrefluxing colon conduits constructed, those whose anastomoses remained nonrefluxing had a lesser incidence of renal deterioration than those in whom the antireflux anastomosis failed.** Follow-up for 9 to 20 years revealed that 79% (22 of 28 patients) of the refluxing renal units deteriorated, whereas only 22% (11 of 51 patients) of the nonrefluxing units deteriorated (Elder et al, 1979; Husmann et al, 1989). Others have reported that in continent diversions, the majority of patients who experience reflux show upper tract dilation and deterioration, whereas few show upper tract deterioration when a nonrefluxing anastomosis is present. (Kock et al, 1978). Similar findings have been reported in experimental animals.

If a nonrefluxing ureteral colonic conduit diversion is constructed, only 7% of the renal units show evidence of pyelonephritic scarring after 3 months, whereas if a refluxing anastomosis is constructed, 83% of the renal units show scarring. Half of the conduits in both groups have significant bacteriuria (Richie and Skinner, 1975). **Others have not found the same high incidence of renal deterioration associated with ureteral intestinal reflux.** One group of investigators studying colon conduits noted no difference in the incidence of renal deterioration regardless of whether the colon conduit experienced reflux: 17% (5 of 29) of nonrefluxing renal units showed deterioration compared with 18% (5 of 27) of refluxing units (Hill and Ransley, 1983). In another series, only 3 of 135 renal units with refluxing ureteral intestinal anastomoses that were unobstructed showed evidence of renal deterioration (Shapiro et al, 1975). **It does not appear that conduit pressures are transmitted to the renal pelvis.** The pressure within the renal pelvis in refluxing conduit diversions is not elevated above normal, and it is not dependent on the segment of bowel used (i.e., ileum or colon) (Magnus, 1977; Kamizaki and Cass, 1978; Hayashi et al, 1986). Peristaltic ureteral contractions apparently dampen pressure transmission from intestine to renal pelvis, attesting to the importance of normal ureters. **When bowel is substituted for the ureter, it does not appear that it makes any difference whether there is reflux at the bladder.** The voiding pressure is blunted by the distensible bowel segment. Moreover, there is no difference in ileal and colon conduits between those that experience reflux and those that do not in renal function measured 2 to 5 years postoperatively (Mansson et al, 1984). **Also, the successful creation of an antirefluxing anastomosis does not prevent bacterial colonization of the renal pelvis.** In six of eight patients with nonrefluxing enterocystoplasties and one patient with a nonrefluxing colon conduit in whom the absence of reflux was documented by loopogram, percutaneous renal pelvic aspiration revealed positive cultures (Gonzalez and Reinberg, 1987). **One stated advantage of a refluxing anastomosis in patients who have urothelia that are prone to malignancy is that the upper tracts may be followed by periodically introducing contrast material into the conduit.** From these studies, it appears that reflux associated with impaired ureteral peristalsis in the presence of bacteriuria or obstruction results in renal deterioration, but it has not been established either for conduit or for continent diversions that reflux associated with the normal ureter in the absence of obstruction is detrimental to the adult kidney.

Although many techniques have been described for creating the various types of ureterointestinal anastomoses, certain **basic surgical principles are germane to all the anastomoses** regardless of type. **Only as much ureter as needed should be mobilized** so that there is no redundancy or tension on the anastomosis. **Mobilization should not strip the ureter of its periadventitial tissue** because it is in this tissue that the ureter's blood supply courses. The ureter should be cleaned of its adventitial tissue only for 2 to 3 mm at its distalmost portion where the ureter-to-intestinal mucosa anastomosis is to be performed. **The ureterointestinal anastomosis must be performed with fine absorbable sutures, which are placed so that a watertight mucosa-to-mucosa apposition is created. The bowel should be brought to the ureter and not vice versa** (i.e., the ureter should not be extensively mobilized so that it can be brought into the wound to the bowel lying on the anterior abdominal wall). **At the completion of the anastomosis, the bowel should be fixed to the abdominal cavity, preferably adjacent to the site of the ureterointestinal anastomosis.** If possible, the **anastomosis should be retroperitonealized,** or a pedicle flap of peritoneum should be placed over the anastomosis.

In those diversions in which the intestinal stoma is brought to the abdomen and the proximal end of the bowel fixed to the retroperitoneum, there are two places where the bowel may be conveniently fixed to the retroperitoneum without jeopardizing mesenteric blood supply. The most convenient point of fixation is below the root of the small bowel mesentery at the level of the pelvic brim. The ureterointestinal anastomosis may be retroperitonealized at the level of the pelvic brim, thus fixing the bowel segment to the posterior body wall. In those situations in which the ureters are short, a more cephalad fixation to the posterior peritoneum may be accomplished by placing the proximal end in the right upper quadrant cephalad to the take-off of the right colic artery and immediately below the duodenum. This is a relatively avascular area and places the intestine fairly close to the right and left kidneys, thus reducing the length of ureter required to reach the intestinal segment.

Perhaps one of the most difficult complications of ureterointestinal anastomoses to manage is a **stricture. Strictures are generally caused by ischemia, a urine leak, radiation, or infection.** The incidence of urine leak for all types of ureterointestinal anastomoses is 3% to 5% (see Table 100–3). **This incidence of leak can be reduced to near zero if soft Silastic stents are used.** In one series of ureterointestinal anastomoses done at the same institution, the nonstented group had a 2% anastomotic leak and a 4% stricture rate. When non-Silastic rigid stents were used, there was a 10% incidence of stricture. When a soft Silastic stent was used, however, there were no strictures or leaks (Regan and Barrett, 1985). In a similar series in which colon conduits were created after gynecologic exenterative operations, the nonstented group had an 18% leak rate and an 18% stricture rate, whereas those who had been stented had a 3% leak rate and an 8% stricture rate (Beddoe et al, 1987). Thus, the evidence indicates that modern soft Silastic stents are effective in reducing the leak rate and subsequent stricture formation.

In creating a submucosal tunnel in those procedures in which a nonrefluxing anastomosis is made, it is often helpful to inject saline with a 25-gauge needle submucosally to raise the mucosa away from the seromuscular layer. This makes dissection considerably easier (Menon et al, 1982).

These principles of surgical technique are common to all ureterointestinal anastomoses. Each type of ureterointestinal anastomosis, however, has specific technical points unique to its creation. Techniques involving ureterocolonic anastomoses are discussed first, followed by ureteral small bowel anastomoses.

Ureterocolonic Anastomoses

Combined Technique of Leadbetter and Clarke

This method establishes a nonrefluxing ureterocolonic anastomosis by employing a submucosal tunnel. The technique combines the ureterocolonic anastomosis of Nesbitt, which is a refluxing elliptical anastomosis to the intestine, with the tunneled technique of Coffey (Fig. 100–16) (Leadbetter and Clarke, 1954). The anterior taenia is incised obliquely for 2.5 to 3 cm as close to the mesenteric border as possible. The mucosa is dissected off the muscularis for the entire length of the incision. At the distal end of the incision in the taenia, the mucosa is picked up with a fine Adson forceps, and a small button is excised. The ureter is spatulated for 5 to 7 mm such that an elliptical anastomosis may be created. The ureter is sewn mucosa-to-mucosa with 5–0 PDS either using interrupted sutures with the knots tied on the outside or by a running suture. If the suture line is to be run, it is well to begin the anastomosis at the apex of the ureter. This suture is tied, and the posterior row is run to the distalmost portion of the ureter, which is subsequently tied. A second running suture completes the anterior aspect. The seromuscular layer is then reapproximated loosely over the ureter in such a way as to allow "the ureter [to] lie in the bowel as a hammock without being compressed" (Leadbet-

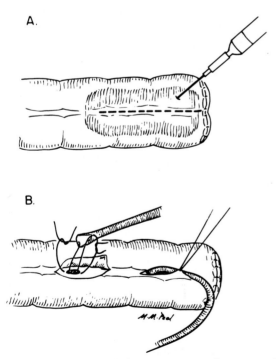

Figure 100–16. Leadbetter-Clarke ureterointestinal anastomosis. *A,* Injection of the submucosal tissues with saline facilitates the dissection. *B,* A linear incision is made in the taenia, the taenia is raised, and the mucosa is identified. A small button of mucosa is removed, and the ureter is spatulated and then sutured to the mucosa with 5–0 PDS. The seromuscular layer is sutured over the ureter, with care taken not to compromise or occlude the ureter.

Table 100–4. COMPLICATIONS OF URETEROINTESTINAL ANASTOMOSES

Procedure	No. of Patients	Stricture (%)	Leakage (%)	Reflux (%)
Colon				
Leadbetter-Clark[1, 2, 3, 4]	127	14	3	4
Strickler[5]	28	14	—	—
Pagano[6]	63	7	—	6
Small Bowel				
Bricker[7, 8]	1809	7	4	—
Wallace-Y[9, 10, 11]	129	3	2	—
Nipple[8]	37	8	—	17
Serosal tunnel[12]	10	10	—	0
LeDuc[13, 14, 15, 16]	82	5	2	13

Literature cited: [1]Hagen-Cook and Althausen, 1979; [2]Leadbetter and Clarke, 1954; [3]Hill and Ransley, 1983; [4]King, 1987; [5]Jacobs and Young, 1980; [6]Pagano et al, 1984; [7]Clark, 1979; [8]Patil et al, 1976; [9]Clark, 1979; [10]Beckley et al, 1982; [11]Wendel et al, 1969; [12]Starr et al, 1975; [13]Hautmann et al, 1988; [14]LeDuc et al, 1987; [15]Klein et al, 1986; [16]Lockhart and Bejany, 1987.

ter and Clarke, 1954). The bowel should be fixed to the peritoneum so that there is no tension on the ureters. The complications reported with this procedure include a leak rate of 2.5%; deterioration of the upper tracts, which varies between 4.3% and 25%; and a stricture rate that varies between 8% and 14% (Table 100–4).

Transcolonic Technique of Goodwin

This method establishes a nonrefluxing ureterocolonic anastomosis by creating a submucosal tunnel (Fig. 100–17). Using this technique, the anastomosis is performed from within the bowel (Goodwin et al, 1953). If it is performed in bowel in continuity with the gastrointestinal tract, a non-

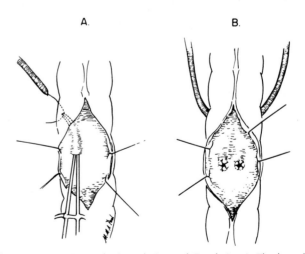

Figure 100–17. Transcolonic technique of Goodwin. *A,* The bowel is opened on its anterior surface; a small rent in the mucosa is made; and, using a mosquito hemostat, the mucosa is raised from the submucosa extending laterally. A 3- to 4-cm tunnel is created before the clamp exits the serosal wall. The ureter is grasped and pulled into the submucosal tunnel. *B,* Both ureters have been drawn into the bowel through their submucosal tunnels before each is spatulated and circumferentially sutured to the mucosa. These sutures should also incorporate a portion of the muscularis for security. Where the ureter enters the colonic sidewall adjacent to the mesentery, the adventitia of the ureter is secured to the colonic serosa with interrupted 5–0 PDS sutures.

crushing occlusive clamp is applied across the bowel cephalad to the desired point of the ureterointestinal anastomosis. This clamp is loosely placed about the bowel and is placed in such a way as not to occlude the arterial supply in the mesentery. A vertical incision is made in the bowel anteriorly, and the desired point of entrance of the ureter into the bowel is identified. A 0.5-cm incision is made in the posterior mucosa, and using a curved hemostat, the mucosa is dissected from the submucosal layer in an oblique fashion coursing from medial to lateral. The hemostat is passed beneath the mucosa for a distance of approximately 3 to 4 cm and then brought through the serosa. A traction suture that has been placed on the ureter is then grasped with the hemostat and the ureter brought into the colon. Both ureters should be brought into the bowel before suturing them to the mucosa. The ureters should lie without tension or angulation. A No. 5 feeding tube is passed through the ureter to be sure that there is no kinking as it passes through the bowel wall. The redundant ureter is excised, and its end is spatulated and sewn with interrupted 5–0 PDS to the mucosa, care being taken to include with the mucosa some muscularis so that the ureter is securely fixed in place. A Silastic stent is placed up both ureters. As the ureters come through the serosa from without the bowel, the adventitia of the ureter is sutured to the serosa of the colon with two 4–0 PDS sutures. The anterior bowel wall is closed in two layers. The reported results with this technique appear to be quite satisfactory; however, specific reliable data on the complication rate are not available.

Strickler Technique

This method establishes a nonrefluxing ureterocolonic anastomosis by creating a submucosal tunnel (Fig. 100–18) (Strickler, 1965; Jacobs and Young, 1980). A 1-cm incision is made on the margin of the taenia. Originally the technique described removal of a 2-mm button of seromuscular tissue. A 2-cm tunnel is formed laterally beneath the seromuscular layer with a hemostat. The seromuscular layer is incised with care being taken not to tent up the mucosa and inadver-

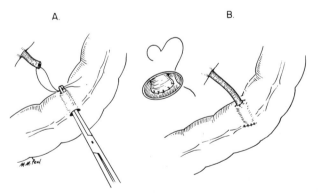

Figure 100–18. Strickler ureterointestinal anastomosis. *A,* A small linear incision is made in the taenia and the submucosa dissected from the mucosa laterally. After a distance of 3 to 4 cm is achieved, a small hole is made in the serosa and the ureter is drawn through. *B,* A button of mucosa is excised and the ureter spatulated and sutured to the mucosa with 5–0 PDS. The rent in the taenia is closed with interrupted sutures, and an adventitial suture at the ureter's entrance point into the colon secures it to the serosa of the colon.

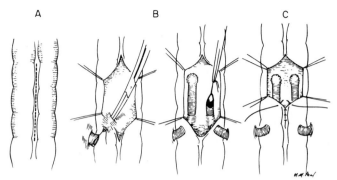

Figure 100–19. Pagano ureterointestinal anastomosis. *A,* A linear incision is made in the taenia between 4 and 5 cm in length. *B,* The submucosa is dissected from the mucosa laterally on both sides to the level of the mesentery. The ureters are drawn into the submucosal tunnel distally and sutured to the mucosa with 5–0 PDS suture proximally. *C,* The serosa is reapproximated, incorporating the mucosa in the midline.

tently incise it. The holding suture in the ureter is grasped and drawn throughout the submucosal tunnel. The ureter is spatulated for 0.5 cm. A button of mucosa is removed, and the full thickness of the ureter is sewn to the mucosa of the bowel with either interrupted or running 5–0 PDS. The serosa is reapproximated over the ureter with 4–0 silk sutures. The serosal suture line is perpendicular to the course of the ureter. Where the ureters enter the serosa, they are also fixed with interrupted 4–0 PDS sutures. A lateral peritoneal flap is placed over the anastomosis. The advantage of this anastomosis is that because the taenia do not need to be aligned, one can form the tunnel according to the normal course of the ureter and avoid angulation. This technique reliably prevents reflux but results in a stricture rate of approximately 14% (see Table 100–4).

Pagano Technique

This method establishes a nonrefluxing ureterointestinal anastomosis by creating a submucosal tunnel (Fig. 100–19) (Pagano, 1980). The taenia is incised for a length of 4 to 5 cm and the seromuscular layer separated from the mucosa on both sides of the taenia laterally as far as the mesenteric border. The ureter is brought in one end (i.e., the distal end) laterally and laid in the 4- to 5-cm tunnel paralleling the mesenteric border. A button of mucosa is excised, and the ureters are spatulated and sutured to the mucosa with either interrupted or running 5–0 PDS. The seromuscular layer is then closed loosely with silk sutures in the midline. Each suture includes the seromuscular layer of the taenia and the mucosa in the midline. This technique has a reported low complication rate. The leakage rate is approximately 3%, the stricture rate is 6%, and the reflux rate is approximately 6% (see Table 100–4) (Pagano et al, 1984).

Cordonnier and Nesbit Technique

These techniques use no tunnel and are direct refluxing anastomoses of the ureter to the colon (Nesbit, 1949; Cordonnier, 1950). They are not desirable for ureterosigmoidostomies, and perhaps their only role lies in creating a refluxing ureterocolonic conduit anastomosis. They are performed in much the same way a Bricker anastomosis would be performed for the small bowel (see later).

Small Bowel Anastomoses

There are a number of ureteral–small bowel anastomoses, which are of two basic types: end-to-side or end-to-end. The end-to-side anastomoses may be constructed in a refluxing or nonrefluxing manner.

Bricker Anastomosis

The Bricker anastomosis is a refluxing end-to-side ureteral small bowel anastomosis that is simple to perform and has a low complication rate (Fig. 100–20) (Bricker, 1950). Although originally described for the small bowel, it may be employed in any suitable intestinal segment. The original description involved suturing the adventitia of the ureter with interrupted silk sutures to the serosa of the bowel. The mucosa and serosa were incised; a small mucosa plug was removed; and using fine reabsorbable chromic sutures, the full thickness of the ureter was sewn to the mucosa of the bowel. The anterior layer of ureteral adventitia was then sewn with interrupted silk sutures to the serosa of the bowel. A less cumbersome method of performing this anastomosis is to excise a small button of seromuscular tissue and mucosa, spatulate the ureter for 0.5 cm, and suture the full thickness of the ureter to the full thickness of the bowel (i.e., mucosa and seromuscular layer to ureteral wall) with either interrupted or running 5–0 PDS. The anastomosis is stented with a soft Silastic catheter. The stricture rate for this anastomosis varies between 4% and 22% (average of 6%) with a leak rate of approximately 3% in the absence of stents (see Table 100–4).

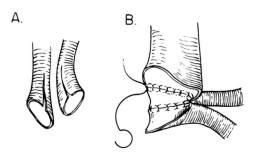
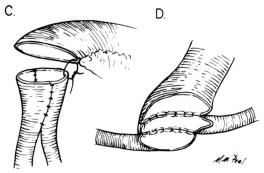

Figure 100–21. Wallace ureterointestinal anastomosis. *A*, Both ureters are spatulated and are laid adjacent to each other. *B*, The apex of one ureter is sutured to the apex of the other ureter with 5–0 PDS. The posterior medial walls of both ureters are then sutured together with interrupted or running 5–0 PDS, the knots tied to the outside. The lateral ureteral walls are then sutured to the intestine. *C*, A Y-type of anastomosis is formed by completing the anterior row of the anterior-lateral ureteral walls of *B* and then suturing the ends of the ureters directly to the intestine. *D*, The head-to-tail anastomosis involves suturing the apex of one ureter to the end of the other. The posterior medial walls are sewn together, then the ends and lateral walls are sewn to the intestine.

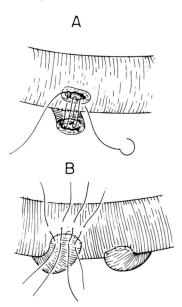

Figure 100–20. Bricker ureterointestinal anastomosis. *A*, The adventitia of the ureter is sutured to the serosa of the bowel. A small full-thickness serosa and mucosal plug is removed. Interrupted 5–0 PDS suture approximates the ureter to the full thickness of the mucosa and serosa. *B*, The anterior layer is completed by interrupted sutures placed through the adventitia of the ureter and the serosa of the small bowel.

Wallace Technique

A frequently employed anastomotic technique is that of Wallace, in which the end of the intestine is sutured to the end of the ureter (Fig. 100–21) (Wallace, 1970; Albert and Persky, 1971). This is a refluxing anastomosis. The intestinal segment employed may be either small bowel or colon. There are three basic types of anastomoses: (1) The end of one ureter is sutured to the end of the other ureter, and this composite anastomosis is sutured to the end of the bowel. (2) A Y anastomosis of the ureters is created, which is sutured to the end of the bowel. (3) A head-to-tail ureteroureteral anastomosis is formed, which is then sutured to the end of the bowel. The ureters are spatulated for 1.5 to 2 cm, and fine 5–0 PDS sutures are used for each anastomosis.

For the first anastomosis, a fine suture is placed at the apex of each ureter with the knot tied to the outside. The posterior medial ureteral walls are sutured together, and the anterior lateral walls are sutured directly to the bowel with interrupted 5–0 PDS. Where the suture line of the end of the ureters comes to the bowel, a horizontal mattress suture is placed to make the anastomosis watertight. If a Y type of anastomosis is desired, after suturing the posterior ureteral walls together as described previously, the anterior walls of the ureters are sutured together, and the end of the composite anastomosis is sutured to the bowel. Again, where the suture lines meet the bowel, a horizontal mattress suture is placed so that the anastomosis is watertight. The head-to-tail anastomosis involves suturing the end of one ureter to the apex of the other. The posterior medial walls of the two ureters are approximated. The anterior lateral walls are sutured to the bowel. The Wallace anastomosis has the lowest complication rate of any of the ureteral intestinal anastomotic techniques. Stricture formation is approximately 3%, deterioration of the upper tracts is about 4%, and leakage is about 2% (see Table 100–4). The Wallace technique is not recommended for patients who have extensive carcinoma in situ or who have a high likelihood of recurrent tumor in the ureter. A recurrence of tumor at the anastomotic line in one ureter would block both ureters causing uremia from bilateral obstruction.

The two small bowel ureterointestinal anastomoses described previously are refluxing in type. The following techniques describe nonrefluxing anastomoses.

Tunneled Small Bowel Anastomosis

This method attempts to establish a nonrefluxing anastomosis by creating a submucosal tunnel (Fig. 100–22) (Starr et al, 1975). Two 0.5-cm incisions are made in the serosa on the antimesenteric border 2.5 cm apart at right angles to the long axis of the bowel. The seromuscular layer is then gently separated from the mucosa with a blunt hemostat. The ureter is pulled through one incision, a button of mucosa removed over the other incision, and the ureter spatulated and sutured to the mucosa with interrupted 5–0 PDS. The serosa is then closed with interrupted 4–0 silk, and the adventitia of the ureter is sutured at its entrance through the serosa of the bowel to the serosa. Good results have been reported, but this technique has not been widely used; therefore, long-term follow-up is not available.

Split-Nipple Technique

This method attempts to establish a nonrefluxing anastomosis by employing a nipple mechanism. It may be applied to either small or large bowel. This technique was described

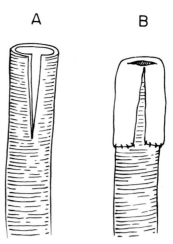

Figure 100–23. *A* and *B*, Split nipple technique. The ureter is spatulated and turned back on itself, and the end of the ureter is secured to the adventitia of the ureter with interrupted 5–0 PDS suture.

by Griffiths and involves forming a nipple in the ureter and implanting it into the small bowel (Fig. 100–23) (Turner-Warwick and Ashken, 1967). A 0.5-cm longitudinal incision in the ureter is made, and the ureteral wall is turned back on itself, creating a nipple at least twice as long as its width. The cuff is stabilized at the corners with sutures. A button of seromuscular and mucosal tissue is removed, and the ureter is then placed into the bowel such that it protrudes through the mucosa. The adventitia just proximal to the point where the ureter has been sewn to itself is sutured to the full thickness of the bowel wall with interrupted 5–0 PDS. The anastomosis is stented. In one series, this type of anastomosis prevented reflux in greater than 50% of the patients, and in other subsequent series, approximately 80% of patients had a nonrefluxing anastomosis with an acceptably low incidence of stenosis (see Table 100–4).

LeDuc Technique

This method establishes a nonrefluxing anastomosis by laying the ureter onto the interior of the bowel wall—eventually resulting in a submucosal tunnel when it is re-epithelialized (Fig. 100–24) (LeDuc et al, 1987). This technique has been used to prevent reflux in the ureteral small intestinal anastomosis. Excellent exposure is required, and therefore the small bowel needs to be opened along its antimesenteric border for a length of approximately 5 cm. The mucosa is incised for a length of 3 cm beginning 2 cm proximal to the cut edge of the bowel. It is important to begin the mucosal tunnel away from the cut edge of the bowel to allow enough distal bowel for closure without jeopardizing the entrance point of the ureter. The ureter is then brought through the serosa at the distalmost portion of the mucosal sulcus, laid in the trough, spatulated, and sutured to the proximal end of the sulcus with interrupted 5–0 PDS using the full thickness of ureteral wall and anchored to the muscularis and mucosal layers of the bowel. The mucosa of the sulcus of the bowel is then sutured to the adventitia of the ureter. The mucosa of the bowel should not be sutured over the ureter but rather to its lateral aspect. The idea is that the mucosa eventually grows over the top of the ureter. Where the ureter enters the

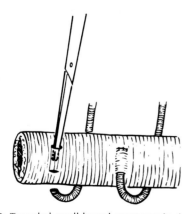

Figure 100–22. Tunneled small bowel anastomosis. A small transverse incision is made in the small bowel, and a second transverse incision 3 cm lateral to it is also made. The submucosal tunnel is created, a button of mucosa removed, and the ureter drawn through the tunnel and sutured directly to the mucosa. The rent in the serosa is closed, and an adventitial ureteral suture is placed and secured to the serosa at the ureter's entrance to the small bowel.

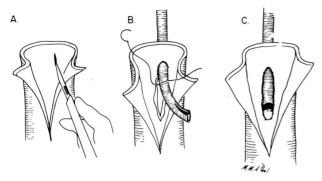

Figure 100–24. LeDuc ureterointestinal anastomosis. *A,* The small bowel is opened for approximately 4 to 5 cm. A longitudinal rent in the mucosa is made and the mucosa raised. *B,* At the distal end of the mucosal rent, a hole is made in the serosa, and the ureter is then drawn through. The entrance of the ureter through the serosa should be at least 2 cm proximal to the cut end of the bowel to allow for sufficient bowel length to close the end. *C,* The ureter is spatulated and sutured to the mucosa and muscular layers. The mucosa is not re-approximated over the top of the ureter but rather sutured to the side of it.

small bowel, its adventitia is sutured to the bowel serosa with 4–0 silk sutures. Stents are placed in the ureter, and their passage must be unimpeded to ensure that there is no angulation. The bowel should be fixed to the body wall near the site of the ureteral implantation so that the ureters do not angulate. The complication rate for this technique is relatively low, although the follow-up is also relatively short. It carries with it an 87% incidence of maintaining an antireflux valve with a 5% incidence of stricture and a 2% incidence of leak (see Table 100–4).

There are several other types of ureteral small intestinal anastomoses mainly involving buried ureter in the small bowel serosa or dissection of mucosa in a funnel-type valve. None of these techniques over the long term have proved to be useful. A slight modification of these techniques, however, does show promise.

Hammock Anastomosis

This type of anastomosis involves conjoining the ureters and implanting them into the small bowel in a nonrefluxing manner. The small bowel is closed at its proximal end, and three 10-cm longitudinal incisions separated by 1 to 2 mm are made through the seromuscular layer to the mucosa. These incisions are cross hatched by multiple incisions. This serves as a hammock. The ureters are conjoined as per the Wallace technique and sutured to the intestinal mucosa. The ureters are buried by closing the intestinal wall over the top of them with seromuscular sutures of 3–0 polyglycolic acid suture (Hirdes et al, 1988). With this technique, there is a 6% incidence of ureteroileal stenosis and approximately a 20% incidence of reflux. Follow-up, however, is relatively short.

Intestinal Antireflux Valves

Another technique of preventing reflux into the ureter involves creation of an antireflux mechanism with bowel distal to the ureterointestinal anastomosis. The ureter is su-

tured by the technique of either Bricker or Wallace (as described earlier) to the end of the bowel, and the bowel is used to create a one-way valve. There are three basic types of antireflux mechanisms commonly employed using the bowel: (1) ileocecal intussusception, (2) ileoileal intussusception, and (3) ileal nipple valve placed into colon.

Intussuscepted Ileocecal Valve

The mesentery is cleaned from the ileum for a length of 8 cm beginning at the cecum and coursing proximal (Fig. 100–25). At least 5 cm of ileum proximal to the detached mesentery must be intact to ensure intestinal viability. Thus, the ileum should not be transected less than 13 cm from the ileocecal junction. A No. 22 catheter is placed through the ileum into the cecum. The ileal serosa is scarified either by multiple cross incisions with a knife or with the electrocautery unit. The 8-cm segment is intussuscepted over the catheter into the cecum. The intussuscepted ileum is secured to the cecal wall with 3–0 silk sutures placed circumferentially 2 mm apart. The valve has a moderate tendency to fail, as the intussusception has a significant chance of reducing. In one series, the antireflux mechanism remained intact in 55% of the patients over the long term (Hensle and Burbige, 1985). The intussusception may be made more secure by employing a modification described by King. The mesentery is cleaned as previously. The cecum is opened along a taenia and the ileum intussuscepted over the catheter under direct vision. Where the intussusception lies adjacent to the cecal wall, mucosa of the intussuscepted ileum and

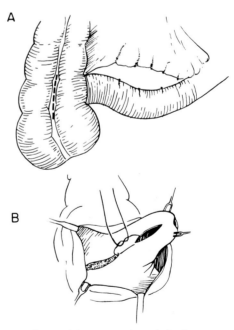

Figure 100–25. Ileocecal intussusception. *A,* An 8-cm segment of ileal mesentery is cleaned from the serosa beginning at the ileocecal junction. At least 5 cm of mesentery remains attached to the proximal ileum. An incision is made along a taenia at the level of the ileocecal valve. *B,* The ileum is intussuscepted over a No. 22 Fr catheter into the cecum under direct vision. The mucosa of the intussuscepted segment is incised, and the mucosa of the cecum adjacent to it is also incised. The muscular coats of both segments are sutured together. The serosa of the ileum is secured to the serosa of the cecum with interrupted 3–0 silk sutures placed circumferentially (not depicted).

the cecal mucosa adjacent to it are incised down to muscle. The muscles are sewn to each other with interrupted 3–0 chromic suture. Long-term follow-up in eight patients reveals maintenance of the antireflux valve in seven using the modified technique (King, 1987; Friedman et al, 1992).

Intussuscepted Ileal Valve

The mesentery is cleaned from an 8-cm segment of ileal serosa (Fig. 100–26). There must be 5 cm of ileal mesentery proximal and distal to the cleared segment to ensure proper blood supply. The ureters are sewn to the proximal end of ileum. The distal end of ileum is opened along its antimesenteric border to within 2 to 3 cm of the cleared mesentery to provide adequate exposure and direct visualization of the intussuscepted segment. A Babcock clamp is placed into the lumen of the bowel, and a portion of bowel wall is grasped by invaginating it into the clamp with a finger. The ileal segment is intussuscepted by pulling on the Babcock clamp with gentle constant traction. If there is resistance, the mesentery is generally too bulky, and it must be defatted carefully before trying again to intussuscept the segment. A 5-cm intussuscepted segment should protrude. Using the gastrointestinal stapler without the knife or the linear stapler, from both of which the distal five to eight staples have been removed, three rows with the former or four rows with the latter are placed in quadrants to secure the intussusception in place. The staple size should be 4.8 mm. The proximal staples are important in securing the intussusception and preventing its reduction, whereas the distal staples are less effective and more prone to be exposed to urine and thus facilitate stone formation. It is for this reason that the distal staples are removed from the staple cartridge before being placed in the stapler and before stapling the intussusception. Using the cautery unit, the mucosa of the intussusception is incised along its length. Adjacent to this incision, another is made in the mucosa of the ileum. The muscularis of both is exposed and sewn together with interrupted 3–0 chromic suture. The distal serosa is then sutured proximally to the

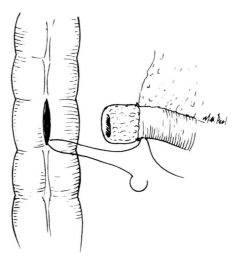

Figure 100–27. Nipple valve. Approximately 8 cm of mesentery is cleaned from the distal end of the ileum, and the serosa is scarified and then turned back on itself to form a nipple of approximately 4 cm in length. The end of the ileum is sutured to itself with interrupted 4–0 PDS suture. A rent is made in the colon through a taenia, and the nipple valve is placed through the rent and secured in place with circumferential interrupted 4–0 PDS sutures placed through the full thickness of the colon and the seromuscular layer of the ileum.

serosa of the intussuscepted segment circumferentially with 3–0 nonreabsorbable sutures. This is meant to secure the intussusception and prevent its reduction with failure of the antireflux mechanism. The valve is successful in preventing reflux 90% of the time (Kock et al, 1982; Skinner et al, 1989).

Nipple Valve

The simplest intestinal antireflux valve to create is the nipple valve using ileum (Fig. 100–27). The mesentery is cleared from the last 8 cm of the cut end of the ileum. The distal 6 cm of serosa is scarified by multiple cross striations and then turned back on itself to form a nipple. The nipple should be at least 4 to 4.5 cm in length. The end of the inverted ileum is then sutured to itself with interrupted 4–0 PDS. An incision on the taenia large enough to accommodate the segment is made. A No. 22 catheter is placed through the segment, and its serosa is sutured to the colon serosa circumferentially with interrupted 3–0 silk sutures placed 2 mm apart. The long-term success rate for this type of valve is unknown but would appear to be less than with the other two methods described previously.

Complications of Ureterointestinal Anastomoses

The complications that occur with ureterointestinal anastomoses include leakage, stricture, reflux in those anastomoses that were performed to prevent reflux, and pyelonephritis. In reviewing the various types of procedures, it appears that of the colonic antirefluxing procedures, the Pagano technique offers the lowest incidence of stricture with an acceptable incidence of reflux. With respect to small bowel antireflux procedures, the LeDuc procedure seems to

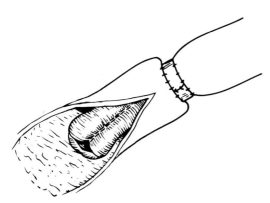

Figure 100–26. Intussuscepted ileal nipple valve. Eight centimeters of ileal mesentery is cleaned from the serosa. The ileum distally is opened within 2 to 3 cm of the rent in the mesentery. Five centimeters of ileum is intussuscepted, and it is secured in place by placing staples in quadrants. The ileal mucosa is incised adjacent to an incision in the intussuscepted segment, and the two muscular coats are sutured together with interrupted 3–0 chromic. The serosa of the intussuscepted segment is sutured circumferentially to the base of the ileum, into which the proximal segment is intussuscepted with interrupted silk suture.

offer the lowest incidence of stricture with the highest success rate in preventing reflux. With respect to stricture formation and leakage, it appears the Wallace technique has the best results. In a comparison of the Bricker, the open technique, the Wallace, and the nipple valve, however, in one series there was no difference in complication rate among any of the procedures. All had an incidence of approximately 29% of some form of obstruction over the long term (Mansson et al, 1979).

Urinary Fistula

Urinary fistulas invariably occur within the first 7 to 10 days postoperatively with an incidence of 3% to 9% (see Table 100–4) (Beckley et al, 1982; Loening et al, 1982). **The incidence of urinary intestinal leak is markedly reduced by the use of soft Silastic stents** (see earlier). A urinary intestinal leak may cause periureteral fibrosis and scarring with subsequent stricture formation.

Stricture

In general, **the antirefluxing techniques have a slightly higher incidence of stricture.** Patients are at risk for ureterointestinal strictures for the life of the anastomosis and must be followed on a scheduled periodic basis. A stricture has been reported to develop 13 years after the procedure (Shapiro et al, 1975). **It is important to note that ureteral strictures also occur away from the ureterointestinal anastomosis. This stricture is most common in the left ureter and is usually found as the ureter crosses over the aorta beneath the inferior mesenteric artery.** It has been suggested that this is due to too-aggressive stripping of adventitia and angulation of the ureter at the inferior mesenteric artery.

Once a stricture has developed, various techniques may be used to rectify the situation. The most successful is re-exploration, removing the stenotic segment and reanastomosing the ureter to the bowel by one of the aforementioned techniques. In a study that compared open surgical correction of ureterointestinal anastomotic strictures with endourologic methods, it was found that the open procedure resulted in approximately 90% success rate, whereas endourologic methods resulted in a 70% early success rate. As follow-up increased, a significant number of strictures treated endourologically failed. The morbidity, of course, with the endourologic procedures was less (Kramolowsky et al, 1988). Open surgical methods may be morbid and difficult procedures. Endourologic procedures employing balloon dilations or incision of the stricture have a lesser morbidity. When several series employing endourologic methods are combined, there is a 50% success rate over the short term. At this juncture, there are no long-term studies that indicate the 50% success will be long-lasting (Kramolowsky et al, 1987).

Pyelonephritis

Acute pyelonephritis occurs both in the early postoperative period and over the long term. Its incidence is approximately 12% in patients diverted with ileal conduits and 9% in those diverted with antirefluxing colon conduits (see Table 100–3). **These complications cause considerable morbidity and, in fact, are associated with significant mortality.** In one series of intestinal segments in the urinary tract, 8 of 178 patients died of sepsis (Schmidt et al, 1973). **That these complications may result in delayed mortality is indicated by the fact that 2 of 115 children and 3 of 127 adults died of septic complications 5 to 14 years after intestinal diversion** (Pitts and Muecke, 1979). **When sepsis is associated with decreasing renal function and uremia, the morbidity and mortality are markedly increased.**

Table 100–4 summarizes the complications and success rates for the various types of anastomoses. The table is derived from composite reports in the literature in which specific anastomoses were reported on and from which the data could be accurately analyzed. Because of these two requirements, it is not possible to comment, for example, on the incidences of reflux or leakage among various anastomotic types inclusively. These complications can be minimized by adhering to the principles of ureterointestinal surgery discussed earlier.

RENAL DETERIORATION

The incidence of renal deterioration after conduit urinary intestinal diversion has varied from 10% to 60%. This variance perhaps is due to the fact that many reports include both renal units that were abnormal as well as those that were normal before diversion. When analyzing abnormal renal units before diversion and documenting progressive disease, it is difficult to be sure whether the urinary diversion caused the progression or whether progression is due to the intrinsic abnormality for which the diversion was created. **When the incidence of renal deterioration is determined by comparing renal units that were normal before diversion and then deteriorated postoperatively, 18% of patients who have ileal conduits show progressive deterioration versus 13% who have nonrefluxing colon conduits** (see Table 100–3). Twenty percent of patients with nonrefluxing continent ileocecal bladders show some evidence of deterioration of the upper tracts when followed over the long term (Benchekroun, 1987). This deterioration leads to a 10% incidence of azotemia in children with ileal conduits (Schwarz and Jeffs, 1975) and a 12% (5 of 41 patients) incidence of renal failure in patients with colon conduits constructed for benign disease (Elder et al, 1979). The incidence of both sepsis and renal failure is greater in patients with ureterosigmoidostomy than those with conduits. Sepsis and renal failure may occur either in the immediate postoperative period or many years later. **The most common cause of death in patients who have had a ureterosigmoidostomy for more than 15 years is acquired renal disease (i.e., sepsis or renal failure).** In this group of patients, approximately 10% to 22% die from these disorders (Zabbo and Kay, 1986), some as late as 4 to 27 years after diversion (Mesrobian et al, 1988). **In patients with ileal conduits, about 6% ultimately die of renal failure** (Richie, 1974).

Renal Function Necessary for Urinary Intestinal Diversion

The amount of renal function required to blunt effectively the reabsorption of urinary solutes by the intestinal segment and prevent serious metabolic side effects depends on the type of urinary intestinal diversion created (i.e., the amount of bowel to be used and the length of time the urine is exposed to the intestinal mucosa). Thus, **a greater degree of renal function is necessary for retentive (continent) diversions than for short conduit diversions.** It is beyond the scope of this chapter to discuss all of the ramifications of renal function, but several points must be understood if patients are to be properly evaluated.

There are five components of renal function: renal blood flow, glomerular filtration, tubule transport, concentration and dilution, and glomerular permeability. Aspects of renal function that must be specifically addressed are glomerular filtration rate, best measured by an inulin clearance, ability of the tubule to acidify as determined by ammonium chloride loading, concentrating ability as determined by water deprivation, and glomerular permeability as reflected by urinary protein concentrations. **In general, patients with normal urinary protein content who have a serum creatinine below 2.0 mg/dl do well with intestine interposed in the urinary tract.** At a level of serum creatinine below 2.0 mg/dl, renal blood flow, glomerular filtration rate, tubule transport, and concentrating and diluting ability are relatively well preserved. **In patients whose serum creatinine exceeds 2.0 mg/dl and who are being considered for retentive diversion or in whom long segments of intestine will be used, a more detailed analysis of renal function is necessary. If the patient is able to achieve a urine pH of 5.8 or less following an ammonium chloride load, a urine osmolality of 600 mOsm/kg or greater in response to water deprivation, has a glomerular filtration rate that exceeds 35 ml/minute, and has minimal protein in the urine, the patient may be considered for a retentive diversion.**

URINARY DIVERSION

This section deals with specific types of conduit urinary diversion. Fundamentally, there are two types of conduits, those using the small bowel, which includes the jejunum or ileum, and those in which a portion of large bowel is used. Conduits made of stomach have been described but are rarely indicated and may carry with them difficult problems of stomal maintenance. Their construction is not discussed here. Each type of conduit has specific indications and advantages, and for each there are specific complications. Some complications, however, are similar among all types. **The indications for a conduit are the need for urinary diversion (1) following a cystectomy; (2) because of a diseased bladder; (3) before transplantation in a patient who has a bladder that cannot adequately receive the transplant ureter; and (4) for dysfunctional bladders that result in persistent bleeding, obstructed ureters, noncompliance with upper tract deterioration, and inadequate storage with total urinary incontinence.**

Preparation

Regardless of whether small or large bowel is used for the conduit, **all patients require both a mechanical and an antibiotic bowel preparation** as outlined earlier. The specific types of ureteral intestinal anastomosis and stomal construction have also been described in previous sections. The complications for the specific types of stoma construction and ureteral intestinal anastomosis are described in previous sections. This section describes features that are unique to the construction of the conduit exclusive of the above-mentioned. The complications sited for each conduit also depend on the length of follow-up and the concomitant procedure performed.

Ileal Conduit

In this procedure, a portion of distal ileum is chosen. **It is the simplest type of conduit diversion to perform and is associated with the fewest number of intraoperative and immediate postoperative complications. It is not advisable to use ileum for a conduit in patients with a short bowel syndrome, in patients with inflammatory small bowel disease, and in those whose ileum has received extensive radiation often as a consequence of prior radiation to a pelvic malignancy.**

Procedure

A segment 10 to 15 cm in length is selected 10 to 15 cm from the ileocecal valve. The cecum and ileal appendage (i.e., that portion of the distal ileum fixed to the retroperitoneum) are mobilized. The ileal mesentery is transilluminated and a major arcade identified to the segment selected. Using a mosquito clamp, the mesentery immediately beneath the bowel is penetrated, and the bowel is encircled with a vessel loop. An area at the base of the mesentery is selected that is to one side of the feeding vessel, and a second vessel loop is placed through the mesentery. At this juncture, the peritoneum overlying both sides of the mesentery is incised from bowel vessel loop to the base of mesentery vessel loop. Using mosquito clamps, the tissue is clamped, severed, and tied with 4–0 silk. A portion of mesentery 2 cm in length is cleaned away from the bowel beneath the mesenteric incision. This procedure is repeated at the other end of the selected segment. The base of the mesentery should be as wide as possible and the mesenteric windows not excessive (generally about 5 cm in length) to prevent ischemia of the segment. Allen clamps are placed across the bowel in an angled fashion such that the antimesenteric portion is shorter than the mesenteric portion. (Some prefer to transect the bowel with staples [i.e., anastomotic stapler]). Thus, a triangular piece of bowel is removed and discarded.

The isolated ileal segment is placed caudad and an ileoileostomy is performed as described earlier (Fig. 100–28). The mesenteric window of the ileoileostomy is closed with interrupted 3–0 silk sutures. The isolated segment is then flushed with copious amounts of saline until the irrigant is clear, at which point the ureters are brought out the retroperitoneum in the right lower quadrant. To accomplish this, the left ureter must be brought over the great vessels and beneath the sigmoid vessels to the rent in the posterior peritoneum. This may be accomplished by mobilizing the cecum cephalad to identify the right ureter. The left ureter may be identified by incising the line of Toldt of the left

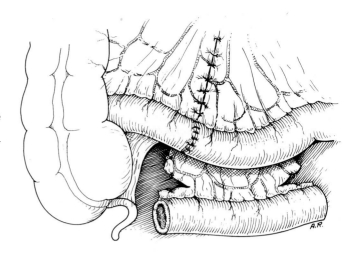

Figure 100–28. The isolated segment of ileum is placed caudal to the ileoileostomy. An incision on the mesentery of the isolated segment 1 cm from the bowel wall straightens the end. This is generally not necessary unless the mesentery is excessively bulky.

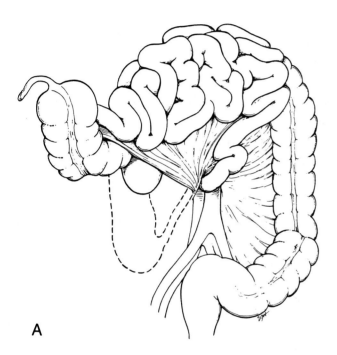

A

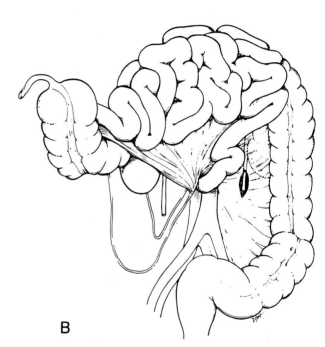

B

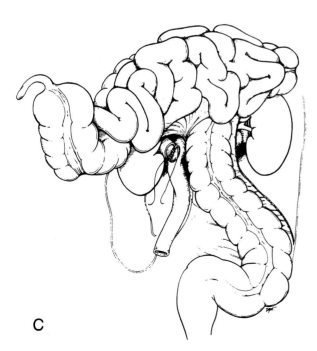

C

Figure 100–29. A, The cecum and root of the mesentery are incised. By blunt dissection, the cecum, ascending colon, and small bowel are mobilized cephalad. B, The right and left ureters are identified. The left ureter is more easily identified by mobilizing the left colon. C, The left colon is mobilized by incising the line of Toldt. This degree of mobilization allows for anastomosing the ileal segment to as proximal a position to the ureter as necessary.

descending colon (Fig. 100–29). This dissection allows for anastomosis of the ileal segment as proximal as is necessary to the ureter. Indeed, the ileum may be anastomosed directly to the renal pelvis on both sides if need be (see Fig. 100–29C). Following a cystectomy, the ureters are identified caudad to the iliac vessels and may be conveniently traced cephalad similarly to the previous description. The ureteral ileal anastomoses are performed as described previously. These anastomoses are stented.

A convenient method of introducing the stent through the loop to the opening in the bowel is illustrated in Figure 100–30. The base of the conduit is fixed to the retroperitoneum in the right lower quadrant by suturing the posterior peritoneum to the conduit, thus effectively retroperitonealizing the ureteral intestinal anastomosis. The stoma is created as described previously. The author prefers to suture the loop segment to the lateral peritoneal wall, thus obviating any chance of herniating small bowel lateral to the conduit. Many, however, prefer to bring the segment directly to the anterior abdominal wall, thus allowing bowel to descend caudad on either side of the loop.

Complications

Early and late postoperative complications are listed in Table 100–5. It is difficult to ascribe clearly these complications solely to creation of the conduit because many are reported in patients undergoing a cystectomy as well. These incidences in Table 100–5 are therefore expected to reflect the high end of the spectrum. **Bleeding may occur from either the stoma or from the conduit itself. Approximately 10% of patients have stomal bleeding. In 4%, it originates from the loop beneath the fascia** (Delgado and Muecke, 1973). Extremely difficult to manage bleeding is due to cirrhosis and varices. In this situation, life-threatening bleeding from the conduit may occur. To stop the bleeding, portal decompression may be required (Chavez et al, 1994). Indeed, this has been successful in several reported cases. **Complications not listed include hypertension, renal failure, decreased renal function, and death.** These complications in large part depend on the concomitant procedure performed, the length of follow-up, and the status of the kidneys before diversion. **Over the long term (≥20 years), 7% of patients have renal failure requiring dialysis, and 60% show deterioration of the upper tracts.** After salvage

cystectomy, **complications are increased so that approximately one third of patients have one of the early complications** (Abratt et al, 1993). Also, the complication rate is increased in patients in whom an intestinal segment is used in those requiring renal transplantation (Nguyen et al, 1990).

One should be cautious in identifying duplex ureters. A failure to identify a second ureter on one side results in intraperitoneal urine leak and can cause excessive morbidity (Evans et al, 1994). The duplex ureters may be dealt with by implanting them separately if they are of sufficient caliber, or they may be spatulated, sewn together, and then implanted into the ileal conduit as a single unit (Fig. 100–31).

Jejunal Conduit

The jejunum has the largest diameter of the small bowel and the longest mesentery. **The jejunum is rarely used for a conduit and should be employed only under circumstances in which there are no other acceptable segments**

Table 100–5. COMPLICATIONS: ILEAL CONDUIT*

	Early	Late
Urine leak	2% (9/356)	
Bowel leak		
Sepsis	3% (7/230)	3% (4/142)
Acute pyelonephritis	3% (21/700)	18% (133/726)
Wound infection	7% (17/230)	2% (4/178)
Wound dehiscence	3% (11/326)	
Gastrointestinal bleed	2% (2/90)	
Abscess	2% (3/168)	
Prolonged ileus	6% (14/230)	
Conduit bleed	2% (3/178)	10% (18/178)
Intestinal obstruction	3% (18/610)	5% (42/878)
Ureteral obstruction	2% (14/610)	6% (56/878)
Parastomal hernia		2% (9/454)
Stomal stenosis		3% (143/486)
Stone formation		7% (59/822)
Excessive conduit length		9% (26/276)
Metabolic acidosis		13% (27/206)
Conduit infarction		2% (2/90)
Volvulus		7% (2/268)
Conduit stenosis		3% (11/320)
Conduit-enteric fistula		<1%

*Incidence as a percent of total number of reported cases from the literature. Numbers in parentheses are number of cases from which percentage is derived.

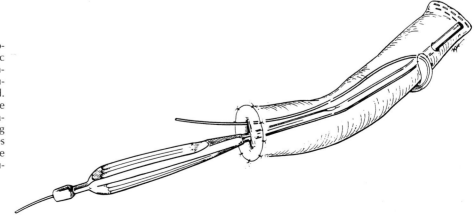

Figure 100–30. The ureteral intestinal anastomoses should be stented with soft Silastic stents. These stents may be conveniently introduced using a Yankauer suction instrument from which the tip has been removed. The suction instrument is introduced via the distal end of the segment to the desired location of the ureteral anastomosis. By cutting down on the instrument, its end protrudes through the bowel at the desired site. The stent is threaded through the suction instrument and the instrument removed.

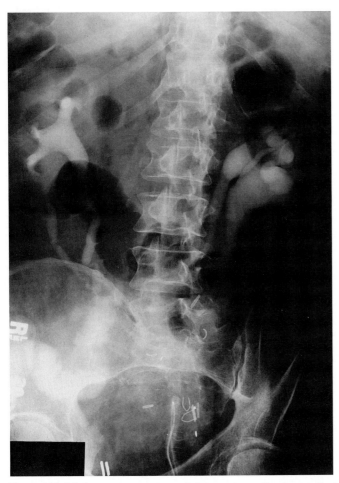

Figure 100–31. Intravenous urogram 6 days postoperative in a patient who had bilateral duplex ureters. The ureters on each side were spatulated, sewn together, and anastomosed to the ileum.

available for use. This might occur in patients who have extensive irradiation that involves the ileum, those with severe adhesions of the ileum and absence of the large bowel, and those who have an absent colon with inflammatory disease of the distal small bowel. **The contraindications to its use are severe bowel nutritional disorders and the presence of another acceptable segment.**

Procedure

The procedure is similar to that for an ileal conduit. A 15- to 20-cm segment of jejunum is isolated as described for the ileal conduit. The portion of jejunum should be chosen as distal as is possible. One should plan for the stoma to be in the upper quadrant, generally the left upper quadrant. The remainder of the technique is as described for the ileal conduit.

Complications

The early and long-term complications are similar to those listed for ileal conduit except that the **electrolyte abnormalities that occur are hyperkalemic, hyponatremic metabolic acidosis** instead of the hyperchloremic metabolic acidosis of ileal diversion (Table 100–6). The treatment of the jejunal

syndrome consists of administering sodium chloride. Thiazides may also be used and are helpful in allaying the hyperkalemia (Hasan et al, 1994).

Colon Conduit

There are three types of colon conduits commonly used: transverse, sigmoid, and ileocecal. Each has specific indications with advantages and disadvantages. **The transverse colon is used when one wants to be sure that the segment of conduit employed has not been irradiated in individuals who have received extensive pelvic irradiation. It is also an excellent segment when an intestinal pyelostomy needs to be performed. The sigmoid conduit is a good choice in patients undergoing a pelvic exenteration who will have a colostomy.** Thus, no bowel anastomosis needs to be made. It also allows for nonrefluxing submucosal reimplantation and provides for an easily placed left-sided stoma when that is desirable. **Contraindications to the use of sigmoid colon include disease of this segment or when the hypogastric arteries have been ligated and the rectum has been left in situ.** The latter circumstance may result in sloughing of the rectum or its mucosa because its blood supply of necessity is interrupted. **It is also unwise to use this segment in individuals with extensive pelvic irradiation** because it likely has been included in the radiation fields.

An ileocecal conduit has the advantage of providing a long segment of ileum when long segments of ureter need replacement as well as the advantage of providing colon for the stoma. It is also used in situations in which free reflux of urine from the conduit to the upper tracts is thought to be undesirable. **Contraindications to the use of transverse, sigmoid, and ileocecal conduits include the presence of inflammatory large bowel disease and severe chronic diarrhea.**

Procedure

Transverse Colon. The segment may be isolated on the right or middle colic arteries—most commonly the latter (Fig. 100–32). The gastrocolic ligament is taken down and the omentum dissected from the portion of colon that is to be isolated. The splenic and hepatic flexures should be mobilized next. The proper length of segment is determined by taking into consideration the desired location of the stoma

Table 100–6. COMPLICATIONS: JEJUNAL CONDUIT*

	Early	Late
Urine leak	14% (3/21)	
Wound dehiscence	5% (1/21)	
Acute pyelonephritis		10% (2/21)
Gastrointestinal bleed	4% (1/27)	
Electrolyte abnormalities		27% (17/62)
Stomal stenosis		7% (2/27)
Bowel obstruction		7% (2/27)
Ureteral stricture		12% (5/41)
Enteric fistula	2% (4/140)	

*Incidence as a percent of total number of reported cases from the literature. Numbers in parentheses are number of cases from which percentage is derived.

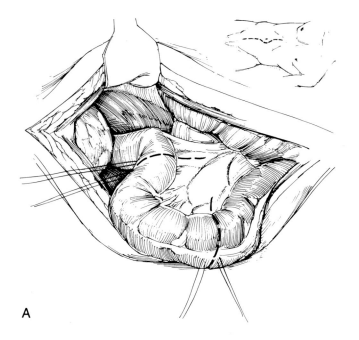

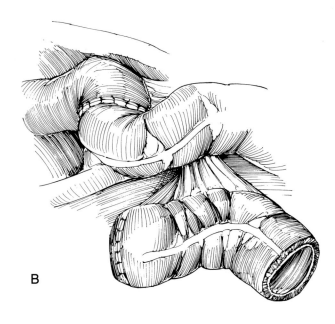

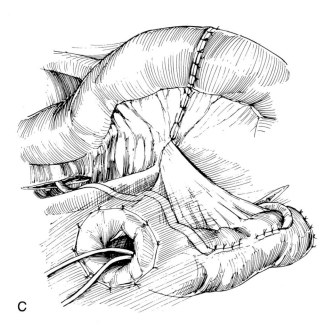

Figure 100–32. *A,* The sigmoid colon is freed of any peritoneal attachments. *B,* The segment is isolated and placed laterally. Bowel continuity is restored and the mesenteric window closed. *C,* The ureters are anastomosed to the colon and stented. (From Hinman F Jr: Atlas of Urologic Surgery. Philadelphia, W. B. Saunders, 1989.)

and the length of available ureters. Generally a length of 15 cm is sufficient. It is important not to isolate a segment that is too short and therefore incapable of reaching the retroperitoneum in such a position that a tension-free uretero-colonic anastomosis may be performed and retroperitone-alized. The segment is isolated between bowel clamps, and a two-layer colocolostomy is performed as outlined earlier. The segment is placed caudad to the anastomosis. If a colopyelostomy is to be performed, the segment should be placed cephalad to the bowel anastomosis. The isolated segment is irrigated with copious amounts of saline until the effluent is clear. The proximal end is closed with a running Connell suture of 3–0 chromic and a second layer of Lembert

sutures of 3–0 silk. This end is anchored to the retroperitoneum close to the midline. The ureterocolic anastomoses are then performed (see earlier). The stoma is usually placed in the right upper quadrant but may be placed anywhere in the abdomen if indicated.

Sigmoid Colon. The sigmoid colon is mobilized by incising its peritoneal attachments and the line of Toldt along the descending colon. The segment is isolated on the sigmoid vessels and placed lateral to the sigmoid colon (Fig. 100–33). The anastomosis of the sigmoid colon and ureterocolic anastomosis are as described for the transverse colon.

Ileocecal Conduit. The ileocecal conduit is based on the terminal branches of the superior mesenteric artery (i.e.,

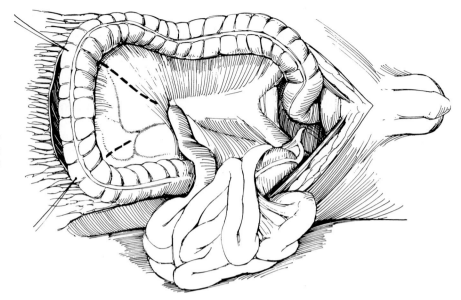

Figure 100–33. Transverse colon conduit may be based on right colic or middle colic arteries (depicted). (From Hinman F Jr: Atlas of Urologic Surgery. Philadelphia, W. B. Saunders, 1989.)

ileocecal artery). The segment is placed caudad, and an ileal ascending colon anastomosis is performed as described previously. The stoma is placed in the right lower quadrant. The ileocecal valve may be reinforced to ensure prevention of reflux. This is described earlier (see Fig. 100–25). For the ureteral intestinal anastomoses, see previously as well.

Complications

Early and late complications following a transverse colon (Beckley et al, 1982; Schmidt et al, 1985; Ravi et al, 1994), sigmoid, or ileocecal conduit are listed in Tables 100–7, 100–8, and 100–9. As is true for the small bowel, complications not listed, including death, renal failure, and renal deterioration, depend on the concomitant procedure performed and the length of follow-up. Interestingly, early reports suggested a lower incidence of renal deterioration with colon conduits; however, more recent series suggest that the incidence of these complications is about the same.

Complications of the ileocecal conduit in one reported series occurred in 21% of patients. (Matsuura et al, 1991). In this series, complications of the ileal conduit were compared with those of the ileocecal conduit, and there appeared to be no difference in the frequency of early and late postoperative complications. Early complications included urinary leakage, bowel obstruction, fecal leakage, acute renal failure, fulminant hepatitis, pneumonia, gastrointestinal bleeding, hemorrhage, perforation of ileum, heart failure, and wound dehiscence. Late complications included stomal prolapse, acute pyelonephritis, bowel obstruction, urinary stones, parastomal hernia, incisional hernia, stomal stenosis, and fecal leakage. There was no difference in the incidence of deterioration of the upper tracts with either form of diversion. Of some note is the fact that at high pressures a large portion of the ileocecal conduits experienced reflux. At low pressures, however, there was minimal to no reflux. Whenever a portion of colon is used for a conduit, chronic diarrhea may be a consequence.

Management Common to All Conduits

All anastomoses are stented with Silastic disposable stents. A convenient method for introducing the stents

Table 100–7. COMPLICATIONS: TRANSVERSE COLON CONDUIT*

	Early	Late
Urine leak	8% (11/137)	8% (2/25)
Acute pyelonephritis		11% (8/75)
Wound infection	5% (5/92)	
Wound dehiscence	7% (8/109)	
Abscess		5% (3/62)
Prolonged ileus	6% (2/30)	
Ureteral stricture	6% (5/84)	17% (37/215)
Bowel obstruction	3% (1/30)	2% (2/109)
Parastomal hernia		4% (5/114)
Stones		11% (11/98)
Enterocutaneous fistula		2% (1/62)
Stomal stenosis		2% (1/62)
Stomal prolapse		11% (6/56)
Metabolic acidosis		12% (3/26)

*Incidence as a percent of total number of reported cases from the literature. Numbers in parentheses are number of cases from which percentage is derived.

Table 100–8. COMPLICATIONS: SIGMOID CONDUIT*

	Early	Late
Urine leak	1% (1/70)	
Wound infection	1% (1/70)	
Wound dehiscence	1% (1/70)	
Acute pyelonephritis		7% (5/70)
Bowel obstruction		6% (4/70)
Ureteral stricture		9% (6/70)
Stones		4% (3/70)
Parastomal hernia		3% (2/70)
Stomal stenosis		3% (2/70)

*Incidence as a percent of total number of reported cases from the literature. Numbers in parentheses are number of cases from which percentage is derived.

Table 100–9. COMPLICATIONS: ILEOCECAL CONDUIT*

	Early	Late
Urine leak	6% (9/147)	
Bowel leak	3% (5/147)	
Gastrointestinal bleed	1% (1/147)	
Wound dehiscence	7% (11/147)	
Acute pyelonephritis		14% (20/147)
Bowel obstruction	3% (5/147)	10% (14/147)
Stomal prolapse		16% (24/147)
Parastomal hernia		5% (7/147)
Stomal stenosis		2% (3/147)
Stones		5% (8/147)
Fecal fistula		2% (3/147)

*Incidence as a percent of total number of reported cases from the literature. Numbers in parentheses are number of cases from which percentage is derived.

through the conduit and into the ureter is illustrated in Figure 100–29. They are removed individually on the fifth and sixth postoperative days; the author routinely obtains an intravenous urogram after their removal. If there is no extravasation, the Jackson-Pratt closed-suction drain is removed. **All conduits are retroperitonealized** with the ureteral intestinal anastomosis being placed in the retroperitoneum. This may be accomplished by suturing the posterior peritoneum to the serosa of the conduit above the ureteral intestinal anastomosis. A drain may then be laid into the retroperitoneum. The author prefers to drain the ureteral intestinal anastomosis with a Jackson-Pratt closed-suction drain laid in the retroperitoneum 3 to 4 cm away from the anastomosis. The peritoneal cavity should not be drained.

All patients are given nothing by mouth until they pass flatus or 4 days postoperatively, whichever is longer. A progressive diet is instituted after confirmation of bowel activity. It has been the author's practice to use nasogastric tube decompression in all patients having a bowel anastomosis. In reported surgical series, it is clear that there are advantages and disadvantages of nasogastric tube decompression after intestinal surgery. Without its use, vomiting is more common. With its use, pulmonary complications are more problematic. For those individuals with severe respiratory disease, consideration should be given to performing a gastrostomy. All patients have compression boots applied as prophylaxis for pulmonary embolus. The author has not employed heparin or warfarin (Coumadin) prophylaxis in this group of patients.

METABOLIC AND NEUROMECHANICAL PROBLEMS OF URINARY INTESTINAL DIVERSION

Problems that occur as a result of interposing intestine in the urinary tract may be conveniently divided into three areas for the purposes of discussion: (1) metabolic, (2) neuromechanical, and (3) technical/surgical. Metabolic complications are the result of altered solute reabsorption by the intestine of the urine that it contains. Neuromechanical aspects involve the configuration of the gut, which affects storage volume and contraction of the intestine, which may lead to difficulties in storage. Finally, technical/surgical complications involve aspects of the procedure that result in

surgical morbidity. The last of these have been discussed following each section on the technical aspects of urinary intestinal diversion. The following is a discussion of metabolic and neuromechanical problems.

Metabolic Complications

Metabolic complications include (1) electrolyte abnormalities, (2) altered sensorium, (3) abnormal drug metabolism, (4) osteomalacia, (5) growth retardation, (6) persistent and recurrent infections, (7) formation of renal and reservoir calculi, (8) problems ensuing from removal of portions of the gut from the intestinal tract, and (9) development of urothelial/intestinal cancer. Many of these complications are a consequence of altered solute absorption across the intestinal segment. **The factors that influence the amount of solute and type of absorption are the segment of bowel used, the surface area of the bowel, the amount of time the urine is exposed to the bowel, the concentration of solutes in the urine, the renal function, and the pH of the fluid.**

Electrolyte Abnormalities

Serum electrolyte complications and the type of electrolyte abnormalities that occur are different depending on the segment of bowel used. If stomach is employed, a hypochloremic metabolic alkalosis may occur. If jejunum is the segment used, hyponatremia, hyperkalemia, and metabolic acidosis occur. If the ileum or colon is used, a hyperchloremic metabolic acidosis ensues. Other electrolyte abnormalities that have been described include hypokalemia, hypomagnesemia, hypocalcemia, hyperammonemia, and elevated blood urea nitrogen and creatinine. Specific abnormalities for each segment of intestine are detailed.

When stomach is used, a hypochloremic, hypokalemic metabolic alkalosis may ensue. This is generally not a significant problem unless the patient has concomitant renal failure, in which case there is a significant impairment of bicarbonate excretion. Under these circumstances, the electrolyte disorder may be difficult to treat. Proton pump blockers (omeprazole) and acidifying the serum may be tried, but often the segment must be taken down and replaced with ileum or colon when this occurs (Gosalbez et al, 1993).

Electrolyte disorders that occur when jejunum is used for urinary intestinal diversion, particularly when proximal jejunum is used, **include hyponatremia, hypochloremia, hyperkalemia, azotemia, and acidosis.** These disorders result from an increased secretion of sodium and chloride with an increased reabsorption of potassium and hydrogen ions. This excessive loss of sodium chloride carries with it water, and thus the patient becomes dehydrated. The dehydration results in hypovolemia, which increases renin secretion and thereby aldosterone production (Golimbu and Morales, 1975). Aldosterone production may also be stimulated by hyperkalemia. The high levels of renin aldosterone facilitate sodium reabsorption by the kidney and potassium loss, which produces a urine low in sodium content and high in potassium. This, when presented to the jejunum, results in a favorable concentration gradient for loss of sodium by the jejunum and increased reabsorption of potassium, thus perpetuating the abnormalities.

These electrolyte abnormalities result in lethargy, nausea, vomiting, dehydration, muscular weakness, and an elevated temperature. If the abnormalities are allowed to persist, the patient may become moribund and finally die. This syndrome may be exacerbated by administering hyperalimentation solutions. The mechanism by which hyperalimentation solutions exacerbate this syndrome in patients with jejunal intestine interposed in the urinary tract is unclear (Bonnheim et al, 1984). The severity of the syndrome depends on the location of the segment of jejunum that is used. The more proximal the segment, the more likely the syndrome is to develop. Its incidence varies from a low of 25% (Klein et al, 1986) to the majority of patients demonstrating significant abnormalities. Treatment for the disorder is rehydration with sodium chloride and correction of the acidosis with sodium bicarbonate. Provided that renal function is normal, the hyperkalemia is corrected by renal secretion. On occasion, a diuretic may be helpful to correct the hyperkalemia. After restoration of normal electrolyte balance, long-term therapy involves oral supplements with sodium chloride. A thiazide diuretic has also been useful in selected cases to control hyperkalemia over the long term (Hasan et al, 1994).

The electrolyte abnormality that occurs with the ileum and colon is hyperchloremic metabolic acidosis. This acidosis occurs to some degree in most patients who have ileum or colon interposed in the urinary tract but is generally of a minor degree. Its clinical significance when it is of a minor degree at this time is unknown. Hyperchloremic acidosis has been reported with a frequency of 68% (19 of 28 patients—10 of the 19 cases were severe enough to require treatment) in patients with ileal conduits (Castro and Ram, 1970). In another study, 70% of patients with ileal conduits followed for 4 years or more had a decreased serum bicarbonate (Malek et al, 1971). Severe electrolyte disturbances occur to a much lesser degree. It has been reported to be a major problem in 18% (8 of 45) of patients with intestinal cystoplasties (Whitmore and Gittes, 1983), in 10% (17 of 178) of patients with ileal conduits (Schmidt et al, 1973), and in 80% (112 of 141) of patients with ureterosigmoidostomies (Ferris and Odel, 1950). In continent diversions involving either ileum and cecum or cecum alone, the majority of patients have an elevated serum chloride and depressed serum bicarbonate (McDougal, 1989; Ashken, 1987). Sixty-five percent of patients with MAINZ pouches require alkali therapy to maintain a normal acid-base balance (Thuroff et al, 1987). Early reports of patients with continent diversions made of ileum have a much lower incidence of electrolyte problems, in the range of 10% to 15% (see Table 100–3) (Allen et al, 1985; Boyd et al, 1989). Symptoms in those in whom the syndrome is severe include easy fatigability, anorexia, weight loss, polydipsia, and lethargy. Those with ureterosigmoidostomies also have an exacerbation of diarrhea.

These electrolyte abnormalities, if significant and allowed to persist, result in major metabolic abnormalities, to be discussed subsequently. In and of themselves, however, they may be lethal to the patient, as severe electrolyte abnormalities have contributed to patient death (Heidler et al, 1979).

The mechanism of hyperchloremic metabolic acidosis is due to the ionized transport of ammonium. Ammonium substitutes for sodium in the Na/H antiport. The exchange of the weak acid NH_4 for a proton is coupled with the exchange of bicarbonate for chloride. Thus, ammonium chloride is absorbed across the lumen into the blood in exchange for carbonic acid (i.e., CO_2 and water). Ammonium may also gain entry to the blood from bowel lumen through potassium channels (McDougal et al, 1995)

The treatment of hyperchloremic metabolic acidosis involves administering alkalizing agents or blockers of chloride transport. Alkalinization with oral sodium bicarbonate is effective in restoring normal acid-base balance. Oral administration of bicarbonate, however, may not be tolerated particularly well because it can produce considerable intestinal gas. Sodium citrate and citric acid solution (Bicitra or Shohl's solution) used together is an effective alternative; however, many patients do not care for the taste. Potassium citrate, sodium citrate, and citric acid solution (Polycitra) may be used instead if excessive sodium administration is a problem because of cardiac or renal disease and if potassium supplementation is desirable or at least not harmful. In those patients in whom persistent hyperchloremic metabolic acidosis occurs and in whom excessive sodium loads are undesirable, chlorpromazine or nicotinic acid may be used to limit the degree of the acidosis. These agents used alone do not correct the acidosis in humans, but they limit its development and thus reduce the need for alkalinizing agents. Chlorpromazine and nicotinic acid inhibit cyclic AMP and thereby impede chloride transport. Chlorpromazine may be given in a dose of 25 mg three times a day. Occasionally, as much as 50 mg three times a day may be necessary, but at such doses, side effects are not uncommon. Chlorpromazine should be used with care in adults because there are many untoward side effects, including tardive dyskinesia. Nicotinic acid may be given in a dose of 400 mg three to four times a day. The drug should not be used in patients with peptic ulcer disease or significant hepatic insufficiency. Side effects that may be observed include exacerbation of liver dysfunction, exacerbation of peptic ulcer disease, headaches, and double vision. Flushing and dermatitis are not uncommon and generally disappear as the patient becomes adapted to the drug.

Hypokalemia and total body depletion of potassium may occur in patients with urinary intestinal diversion. This is more common in patients with ureterosigmoidostomies than it is with patients who have other types of urinary intestinal diversion (Geist and Ansell, 1961). In one study, patients with ureterocolonic diversions had a 30% reduction in total body potassium, whereas those with ileal conduits had, as a group, no significant alteration in total body potassium; individually, however, some had as much as a 14% reduction in total body potassium (Williams et al, 1967). The potassium depletion is probably due to renal potassium wasting as a consequence of renal damage, osmotic diuresis, and gut loss through intestinal secretion. The last-mentioned (probably quantitatively) plays a relatively minor role. Indeed, it has been shown that ileal segments when exposed to high concentrations of potassium in the urine reabsorb some of the potassium, whereas colon is less likely to do so (Koch et al, 1990). Thus, those with ileum interposed in the urinary tract likely blunt the potassium loss by the kidney, whereas those with colon do not, thus explaining why patients with ureterosigmoidostomies and ureterocolonic diversions are more likely to have total body potassium depletion. When the depletion is severe, the patient may develop a flaccid paralysis. In treating these patients, one must remember that if the hypokalemia is associated with severe hyperchloremic metabolic acidosis, treatment must involve both replacement of potassium and correction of the acidosis with bicarbonate. If the acidosis is corrected without attention to potassium replacement, severe hypokalemia may occur, marked flaccid paralysis may develop, and significant morbidity may ensue (Koff, 1975).

Because the bowel transports solutes and because its membrane is not particularly watertight, osmolality generally reequilibrates across the bowel wall. Thus, attempts to deprive a patient of water and determine osmolality as a reflection of renal function are inappropriate because the bowel alters the osmotic content. The bowel also makes the contents more alkaline, and, therefore, it is impossible to determine the ability of the kidney to acidify simply by measuring urinary pH in patients with urinary intestinal diversion. Finally, because urea and creatinine are reabsorbed by both the ileum and the colon, serum concentrations of urea and creatinine do not necessarily accurately reflect renal function (Koch and McDougal, 1985; McDougal and Koch, 1986).

Histologic alterations of the intestine may occur over time when urine is chronically exposed to the mucosa. Villous atrophy and the formation of pseudocrypts may occur, particularly in ileum. These changes are patchy because there is normal ileal mucosa interspersed between these abnormalities. Submucosal inflammatory infiltrates may also be observed. There appear to be fewer changes in the colonic mucosa over the long term. In the colon, a decrease in the size of goblet cells has been described. Over time, some transport processes may be altered, with some solutes less actively transported whereas other processes of solute transport remain active (Philipson et al, 1983). The ability to establish a hyperchloremic metabolic acidosis, however, appears to be retained by most segments of ileum and colon over time.

Altered Sensorium

Alteration of the sensorium may occur as a consequence of magnesium deficiency, drug intoxication, or abnormalities in ammonia metabolism. Patients who develop magnesium deficiency do so either secondary to nutritional depletion or related to magnesium wasting by the kidney in much the same way that calcium wasting occurs (see later). Alterations in the sensorium have also occurred because of diabetic hyperglycemia; however, this is not a consequence of the intestinal diversion. In such patients, reabsorption of urinary glucose can result in hyperglycemia without demonstrable glucosuria (Onwubalili, 1982). Perhaps the more common cause of an altered sensorium is a consequence of altered ammonia metabolism. Ammoniagenic coma in patients with urinary intestinal diversion has been reported in those with cirrhosis (Silberman, 1958), those with altered liver function without underlying chronic liver disease (McDermott, 1957), and those

with normal hepatic function as determined by serum enzymes (Kaufman, 1984; Mounger and Branson, 1972). The syndrome, however, is most commonly associated with decreased liver function and even in those cases in which normal liver function has been reported, the crude methods by which it was assessed in these reports have been unable to confirm the absence of subtle alterations in liver function. The syndrome is most commonly found in patients with ureterosigmoidostomies but has been reported for those with ileal conduits as well (McDermott, 1957).

The treatment of ammoniagenic coma involves draining the urinary intestinal diversion, either with a rectal tube in the case of ureterosigmoidostomy or with a Foley catheter in those with a continent diversion, so that the urine does not remain exposed to the intestine for extended periods of time. Neomycin is administered orally to reduce the ammonia load from the enteric tract, and protein consumption is curtailed, thus limiting the nitrogen load to the patient until serum ammonium levels return to normal. In severe circumstances, arginine glutamate, 50 g in 1000 ml of 5% dextrose in water, may be given intravenously. This complexes the ammonia by providing substrate for the formation of glutamine (Silberman, 1958). Lactulose may be given orally or by rectum (Edwards, 1984) and complexes the ammonia in the gut and prevents its absorption.

Abnormal Drug Absorption

Drug intoxication has been reported in patients with urinary intestinal diversion. Drugs more likely to be a problem are those that are absorbed by the gastrointestinal tract and excreted unchanged by the kidney. Thus, the excreted drug is re-exposed to the intestinal segment, which then reabsorbs it, and toxic serum levels develop. This has been reported for phenytoin (Dilantin) (Savarirayan and Dixey, 1969) and has been seen for certain antibiotics that are excreted unchanged. Although chemotherapy is generally well tolerated by patients with conduits, methotrexate toxicity has been documented in a patient with an ileal conduit (Bowyer and Davies, 1986). In those patients receiving antimetabolites, one must carefully monitor toxic antimetabolites that are excreted in the urine and capable of intestinal absorption lest lethal toxic serum levels develop. Moreover, in patients with continent diversions who are receiving chemotherapy, consideration should be given to draining the pouch during the period of time the toxic drugs are being administered.

Osteomalacia

Osteomalacia or renal rickets occurs when mineralized bone is reduced and the osteoid component becomes excessive. Osteomalacia has been reported in patients with colocystoplasty (Hassain, 1970), ileal ureters (Salahudeen et al, 1984), colon and ileal conduits, and, most commonly, ureterosigmoidostomies (Harrison, 1958; Specht, 1967). The cause of osteomalacia may be multifactorial but commonly involves acidosis. With persistent acidosis, the excess protons are buffered by the bone with release of bone calcium. With its release, it is excreted by the kidney. Support for the theory that chronic acidosis is causative in osteomalacia comes from those patients in whom correction of the acidosis results in remineralization of the bone (Richards et al, 1972; Siklos et al, 1980). It has also been shown, however, that major alterations in serum bicarbonate are not necessary for the development of the syndrome (McDougal et al, 1988; Koch et al, 1988). Moreover, some patients with osteomalacia secondary to urinary intestinal diversion do not have bony demineralization corrected with restoration of normal acid-base balance. **These patients have been found to manifest vitamin D resistance that is independent of the acidosis.** It is likely that this resistance is of renal origin. Resistance can be overcome by supplying 1-alpha-hydroxycholecalciferol, a vitamin D metabolite that is much more potent than vitamin D_2. By providing this substrate in excess amount, remineralization of bone occurs (Perry et al, 1977). Also, it has been shown that reabsorption of urinary solutes may play a role in increasing calcium excretion by the kidney. Sulfate filtered by the kidney inhibits calcium reabsorption and results in both calcium and magnesium loss by the kidney. Thus, if the gut increases its sulfate reabsorption and requires the kidney to increase sulfate excretion, this results in hypercalciuria and hypermagnesuria (McDougal and Koch, 1989). **Osteomalacia in urinary intestinal diversion may be due to persistent acidosis, vitamin D resistance, and excessive calcium loss by the kidney. It appears that the degree to which each of these contributes to the syndrome may vary from patient to patient.**

Patients who develop osteomalacia generally complain of lethargy; joint pain, especially in the weight-bearing joints; and proximal myopathy. Analysis of serum chemistries reveals that the calcium is either low or normal. The alkaline phosphatase is elevated, and the phosphate is low or normal (Harrison, 1958). The treatment as indicated earlier involves correcting the acidosis and providing dietary supplements of calcium. If this does not result in remineralization of the bone, the active form of vitamin D may be administered. If this is not successful, the more active metabolite of vitamin D_3, 1-alpha-hydroxycholecalciferol, should be administered.

Growth and Development

There is considerable evidence to suggest that **urinary intestinal diversion has a detrimental effect on growth and development.** In a study of 93 myelodysplasia patients followed for 17 to 23 years, significant aberrations in growth were noted when morphometric parameters were analyzed. Anthropomorphic measurements in those with urinary intestinal diversion showed a decrease in linear growth in all indices measured, with a statistically significant decrease in biochromial span and in elbow-hand length. (Koch et al, 1992)

Patients with long-term urinary diversions are more prone to fractures and to complications after orthopedic procedures. When myelodysplastic patients with ileal conduits were compared with a similar group of patients on intermittent catheterization, the patients with an ileal conduit had an increased number of fractures as well as malunion and nonunion after orthopedic procedures (Koch et al, 1992). It was found that more patients with urinary intestinal diver-

sion fell below the tenth percentile than did patients who were treated with intermittent catheterization. There was, in fact, no difference in height and weight between the two groups studied (McDougal, 1992; Koch et al, 1992).

There is also experimental evidence for impaired linear growth in urinary intestinal diversion. Rats with unilateral ureterosigmoidostomies when followed over the long term demonstrate significantly decreased femoral bone length when compared to nondiverted controls (Koch and McDougal, 1988). Thus, it appears clear that although obvious alterations in growth and development do not occur, when carefully studied, patients who have urinary intestinal diversions created in childhood and who maintain these diversions for more than 10 years have significant changes in linear growth.

Infection

An increased incidence of bacteriuria, bacteremia, and septic episodes occurs in patients with bowel interposition. A significant number of patients with intestinal cystoplasty develop pyelonephritis, and 13% have septic and major infectious complications (Kuss et al, 1970). The episodes are more frequent following colocystoplasty than ileocystoplasty (Kuss et al, 1970). Acute pyelonephritis occurs in 10% to 17% of patients with colon and ileal conduits (Schmidt et al, 1973; Schwarz and Jeffs, 1975; Hagen-Cook and Althausen, 1979). Approximately 4% (8 of 178) of patients with ileal conduits die of sepsis (Schmidt et al, 1973).

Patients with conduits have a high incidence of bacteriuria. Indeed, **approximately three quarters of ileal conduit urine specimens are infected** (Guinan et al, 1972; Middleton and Hendren, 1976; Elder et al, 1979). It is clear that some patients are merely colonized at the distal end of their conduit because the incidence of positive cultures can be markedly diminished by culturing the proximal portion of the loop by a double-catheter technique (Smith, 1972). Many of these patients, however, show no untoward effects and seem to do quite well with chronic bacteriuria. **Deterioration of the upper tracts is more likely when the culture becomes dominant for *Proteus* or *Pseudomonas*. Thus, patients with relatively pure cultures of *Proteus* or *Pseudomonas* should be treated, whereas those with mixed cultures may generally be observed, provided that they are not symptomatic. Patients with continent diversions also have a significant incidence of bacteriuria and septic episodes** (McDougal, 1986). Indeed, two thirds of patients with Kock continent diversions have positive cultures (Kock, 1987). The reasons for the increased incidence of bacteriuria and sepsis are unclear, but it is likely that the intestine is incapable of inhibiting bacterial proliferation, in contrast to the urothelium. Thus, intestine that normally lives symbiotically with bacteria when interposed in the urinary tract serves as a source for ascending infection and septic complications. Moreover, the intestine may make the urine less bacteriostatic and thereby promote the growth of bacteria.

Stones

One of the consequences of persistent infection is the development of magnesium ammonium phosphate stones.

Indeed, **the great majority of stones formed in patients with urinary intestinal diversions are composed of calcium, magnesium, and ammonium phosphate. Those most prone to develop renal calculi are patients who have hyperchloremic metabolic acidosis, pre-existing pyelonephritis, and urinary tract infection with a urea-splitting organism** (Dretler, 1973). The incidence of renal stones in patients with colon conduits is 3% to 4% (Althausen et al, 1978; Hagen-Cook and Althausen, 1979) and in those with ileal conduits 10 to 12% (Schmidt et al, 1973). In those with continent cecal reservoirs, there is a 20% incidence of calculi within the reservoir (Ashken, 1987). The stones may be due to persistent infection with alkalinization of the urine, persistent hypercalciuria for reasons described previously, and alterations of urinary excretion products by the intestine. A major cause in conduits and pouches of calculus formation is a foreign body, such as staples or nonabsorbable sutures, on which concretions form. In intestinal reservoirs, alterations in bowel mucosa may also serve as a nidus for stone formation.

Short Bowel and Nutritional Problems

Many nutritional problems may occur as the result of a loss of significant intestinal absorptive surface resulting from removing substantial portions of the gut for construction of urinary intestinal diversion. **In patients with a significant loss of ileum, vitamin B_{12} malabsorption has been reported and results in anemia and neurologic abnormalities.** Vitamin B_{12} deficiency has been shown to occur in 10 of 41 patients who received preoperative radiotherapy before radical cystectomy and ileal ureterostomy (Kinn and Lantz, 1984). **Loss of significant portions of ileum also results in malabsorption of bile salts.** Because the ileum is the major site of bile salt reabsorption, the lack of their reabsorption allows them entry into the colon, which causes mucosal irritation and diarrhea. Also, loss of the ileum results in the loss of the "ileal break." The ileal break is a mechanism whereby when lipids come in contact with the ileal mucosa, gut motility is reduced so that increased absorption can occur. With the loss of ileum, the lipid does not result in decreased motility and is presented unmetabolized to the colon, which may result in fatty diarrhea.

Loss of the ileocecal valve may have a number of untoward effects. Because of the loss of the valve, reflux of large concentrations of bacteria into the ileum may occur, which results in small intestinal bacterial overgrowth. This may result in nutritional abnormalities that involve interference with fatty acid reabsorption and bile salt interaction. With the lack of absorption of fats and bile salts, these are presented to the colon and result in diarrhea. Moreover, reflux of bacteria into the small bowel may result in bile salt deficiency. Also, the lack of fat absorption may result in deficiencies of the fat-soluble vitamin A, osteomalacia owing to lack of vitamin D, and complexing calcium with the fats to form soaps and thus lack of its absorption. The ileocecal valve also serves as a break, and an intact valve prolongs transit time of the small bowel and enhances absorption. Thus, its loss may contribute to nutritional abnormalities.

Loss of a significant portion of jejunum may result in malabsorption of fat, calcium, and folic acid; however, significant portions of jejunum are rarely used for urologic reconstructive procedures. Loss of the colon may result in diarrhea because of lack of fluid and electrolyte absorption, loss of bicarbonate because of its increased secretion in the ileum and lack of reabsorption, and dehydration because of the loss of fluids.

Cancer

The incidence of cancer developing in patients with ureterosigmoidostomy varies between 6% and 29% with a mean of 11% (Schipper and Decter, 1981; Stewart et al, 1982; Zabbo and Kay, 1986). There is generally a 10- to 20-year delay before the cancer becomes manifest. **Histologically, the tumors include adenocarcinoma, adenomatous polyps, sarcomas, and transitional cell carcinoma.** Case reports of tumors developing in patients with ileal conduits, colon conduits, and bladder augmentations have been described. Anaplastic carcinomas and adenomatous polyps have been reported in patients with ileal conduits. Adenocarcinoma has developed in patients with colon conduits; patients with bladder augmentations using both ileum and colon have developed adenocarcinoma, undifferentiated carcinoma, sarcomas, and transitional cell carcinomas (Filmer, 1986).

The etiologic mechanism of the development of the carcinoma is not understood. Whether the tumor arises from transitional epithelium or colonic epithelium is unclear. Because most of the tumors are adenocarcinomas, it has been assumed that the tumor arises from the intestinal epithelium. Adenocarcinomas have been shown to arise from transitional cell epithelium exposed to the fecal stream in experimental animals (Aaronson et al, 1989). Furthermore, studies show that the ureters in ureterosigmoidostomy patients have an exceedingly high incidence of dysplasia (Aaronson and Sinclair-Smith, 1984). Moreover, if the transitional epithelium is removed from the enteric tract, patients do not develop adenocarcinomas. **If the urothelium is left in contact with the intestinal mucosa, however, even though the diversion is defunctionalized and the area is not bathed in urine, adenocarcinoma may still develop.** This is illustrated by a case report in which a patient who had a ureterosigmoidostomy that was defunctionalized 9 months after its creation with a conduit developed cancer. The distal ureters at the sigmoid were left in situ. Twenty-two years later, the patient developed a cancer at the site of the ureterointestinal anastomosis (Schipper and Decter, 1981). This suggests that **when ureterointestinal anastomoses are defunctionalized, they should be excised rather than merely ligated and left in situ.** Other evidence including cell staining techniques suggests that the colon is the primary organ of origin (Mundy, 1991, personal communication). Whether the urothelium or intestine is the primary site of origin, it seems likely that tumors can arise from both tissues.

The highest incidence of cancer occurs when the transitional epithelium is juxtaposed to the colonic epithelium and both are bathed by feces (Shands et al, 1989). Nitrosamines, known mutagens, are produced in rats with ureterosigmoidostomy (Cohen et al, 1987), but there appears at least at this juncture no convincing evidence to support a primary role for them in the genesis of the tumor. An abnormal pattern of colonic mucin secretion has been demonstrated in patients with ureterosigmoidostomy, but its significance is unclear (Iannoni et al, 1986). Induction of specific enzymes associated with carcinoma has also been demonstrated. Ornithine decarboxylase, an enzyme that has been found to be elevated in malignant colonic mucosa, is also elevated in experimental animals with vesicosigmoidostomy (Weber et al, 1988). The role epidermal growth factor and other growth factors play is currently being investigated. There is some evidence that these may at least play a role in development if not in induction. At this time, the cause of the genesis of cancer in urinary intestinal diversion is not known. **Because its incidence is significant in patients with ureterosigmoidostomies, they should have routine colonoscopies on a frequent periodic basis.**

NEUROMECHANICAL ASPECTS OF INTESTINAL SEGMENTS

Both small bowel and colon contract to propel luminal contents in an aboral direction. The ability to propel luminal contents is a consequence of muscular activity as well as coordinated nerve activity. Both the small bowel and the colon have an outer longitudinal layer of muscle and an inner circular layer. There is also a muscularis mucosa, which is immediatley beneath the mucosa and may extend into the villi. The outer and inner layers of muscle, however, play the major role in peristalsis. In the colon, the outer longitudinal layer or muscle condenses to form three taeniae coli. The bowel receives its parasympathetic innervation from the vagus. It is also innervated by the sympathetic nervous system. The nerves lie between the circular and longitudinal layers of muscle. The enteral nervous system operates autonomously, and therefore one can denervate the intestine and not affect the coordinated contractions. These contractions are termed *activity fronts* and may be stimulated by feeding, or they may be inhibited by exposing the lumen to various substances (i.e., lipid in the ileum decreases ileal motility). There are two aspects of neuromechanical properties that are particularly germane to urinary intestinal diversion: volume-pressure relationships and motor activity.

Volume-Pressure Considerations

The volume-pressure relationships depend on the configuration of the bowel. If one splits the bowel segment and turns it back on itself, the volume may be doubled if the ends are not closed (Fig. 100–34). In reconstructing intestinal segments for the urinary tract, however, one must close the ends. Thus, the limit of doubling the volume is never quite reached. Indeed, **the greater the ratio of length to diameter, the greater the volume change when the ends are closed. If the ends are closed, when a ratio of 1:3.5, diameter to length is reached, splitting the segment no longer increases the volume. By splitting most segments, one is, in fact, increasing the volume by about 50%. The goal in reconfiguring the bowel is to achieve a spherical storage vessel. This configuration has the most volume for the least surface area.** By increasing the volume, it has been suggested that pressure relationships within

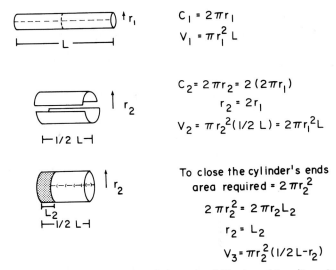

$$C_1 = 2\pi r_1$$
$$V_1 = \pi r_1^2 L$$

$$C_2 = 2\pi r_2 = 2(2\pi r_1)$$
$$r_2 = 2r_1$$
$$V_2 = \pi r_2^2 (1/2\ L) = 2\pi r_1^2 L$$

To close the cylinder's ends area required = $2\pi r_2^2$

$$2\pi r_2^2 = 2\pi r_2 L_2$$
$$r_2 = L_2$$
$$V_3 = \pi r_2^2 (1/2\ L - r_2)$$

Figure 100–34. Effect of "detubularization." The bowel is split on its antimesenteric border and divided in two. By placing the two segments together, the circumference is doubled, thus doubling the volume. Closing the ends of the cylinder requires a reduction in its length equal to the radius of the end. This limits the increase in volume that occurs by reconfiguration.

the confines of the intestine are reduced. This is based on Laplace's law, which states that for a sphere, the tension of its wall is proportional to the product of the radius and pressure. Thus, theoretically, for a given wall tension, the greater the radius, the smaller the generated pressure. This is desirable in an attempt to prevent deterioration of the upper tracts or incontinence. **This relationship (Laplace's law), however, may not be accurately reflected for intestinal segments because they are not perfectly spherical, and the intestinal wall does not conform to Hooke's law but rather demonstrates viscoelastic properties, which tend to distort the relationship between pressure applied at the wall and tension generated in it.** In any event, it does seem desirable to make an attempt to create as spherical a container as possible if one is attempting to create a reservoir.

Over time, the volume capacity of segments increases. This occurs only if they are frequently filled. Their volume decreases with time if they are nonfunctional (Kock et al, 1978). Over time, it can be demonstrated that there is a marked accommodation in volume of pouches created from intestine. For ileal pouches, it has been shown that the capacity increases sevenfold after 1 year (Berglund et al, 1987). As the reservoirs increase in volume, there is a significant increase in smooth muscle thickness of the bowel wall (Philipson et al, 1983).

Motor Activity

It has been suggested that splitting the bowel on its antimesenteric border discoordinates motor activity and thereby creates a lesser intraluminal pressure. Clearly the ideal situation is to provide the patient with a spherical vessel that has few or ineffective contractions of its walls. It can be demonstrated in experimental animals that **by splitting the bowel wall on its antimesenteric border and reconfigur-**

ing it acutely, there is a marked interruption of coordinated activity fronts, which over a period of 3 months return to their normal coordinated state (Concepcion et al, 1988). This has also been demonstrated clinically, as initially after reconfiguring the bowel (detubularization), coordinated activity fronts have been shown to decrease. Over extended periods of time, however, many of the peristaltic waves (activity fronts) reappear and can be readily demonstrated (Fig. 100–35).

The literature is contradictory with respect to the effect of detubularization on segments of ileum and colon used to construct storage vessels for continent diversions. Pressure within the lumen of bowel that has both ends closed may be increased by adding volume or by reducing the size of the bowel through contractions of its wall. Because the bowel wall is freely permeable to water, the higher osmotic content of urine obligates movement of water into the bowel lumen. Most patients with continent diversions excrete 2 to 4 L/day (McDougal, 1986). In evaluating whether motor activity is the primary determinant of intravesical pressure, one must be cognizant of fluid volume changes. Also, as indicated previously, early reports of detubularized segments would be expected to differ from later reports when coordinated activity fronts in these segments return.

These facts are often forgotten, and because pressure measurements are used to infer motor activity rather than directly measuring it as reflected by changes in bowel wall tension, it is not difficult to understand why there are so many contradictions reported in the literature. Detubularization of ileal segments has been reported by some to decrease motor activity at a year compared to immediately postoperatively (Berglund et al, 1987), whereas others have noted increased motor activity at 1 year. Involuntary pressure waves occur in 25% of patients with Kock pouches. Maximum intravesical pressures average 41 cm H_2O in these pouches (Chen et al, 1989). Ileum has also been shown to have less activity fronts per unit period of time than cecum (Berglund et al, 1986). Cecum has been observed to have the same number of activity fronts 1 year postoperatively, but the amplitude of the pressure waves has been observed to decrease over time (Hedlund et al, 1984). Maximum pressures in normal cecum have been shown to range from 18 to 100 cm H_2O (Jakobsen et al, 1987), whereas detubularized cecum has been shown to have pressures that range between 5 and 25 cm H_2O 1 year postoperatively (Hedlund et al, 1984). Others, comparing ileum to cecum, find no difference in pressure generated after a year (Hedlund et al, 1984). The MAINZ pouch, which employs both ileum and cecum, has an average pressure at capacity of 39 cm H_2O with a maximum pressure of 63 cm

H_2O (Thuroff et al, 1987). Thus, **reconfiguring bowel usually increases the volume, but its effect on motor activity and wall tension over the long term is unclear at this time.**

SUMMARY

This chapter has addressed complications both independent of and dependent on the specific type of urinary intestinal diversion. Each unique type of diversion has its own set of individual complications. Moreover, the procedure preceding the urinary intestinal diversion also has a set of complications that must be added to those described previously. It is clear that with current modalities of urinary intestinal diversion, long-term complications significantly contribute to patient mortality and morbidity. Many patients who have intestinal diversion after an extirpative procedure for cancer, however, die of the cancer rather than these long-term complications. Those for whom a urinary intestinal diversion has been created for benign disease and those who are cured of cancer are most likely to experience long-term morbid complications. The knowledge of the frequency of these complications and the correct performance of preoperative preparation, surgical technique, and postoperative care, as outlined in this chapter, should provide the best chance for the least mortality and morbidity in patients undergoing urinary intestinal diversion.

REFERENCES

Aaronson IA, Constantinides CG, Sallie LP, Sinclair-Smith CC: Pathogenesis of adenocarcinoma complicating ureterosigmoidostomy: Experimental observations. Urology 1989; 29:538–543.

Aaronson IA, Sinclair-Smith CC: Dysplasia of ureteric epithelium: A source of adenocarcinoma in ureterosigmoidostomy? Z Kinderchir 1984; 39:364–367.

Abratt RP, Wilson JA, Pontin AR, Barnes RD: Salvage cystectomy after radical irradiation for bladder cancer: Prognostic factors and complications. Br J Urol 1993; 72:756–760.

Adams MC, Mitchell ME, Rink RC: Gastrocystoplasty: An alternative solution to the problem of urological reconstruction in the severely compromised patient. J Urol 1988; 140:1152–1156.

Albert DJ, Persky L: Conjoined end-to-end uretero-intestinal anastomosis. J Urol 1971; 105:201–204.

Allen T, Peters PC, Sagalowsky A: The Camey procedure: Preliminary results in 11 patients. World J Urol 1985; 3:167.

Althausen AF, Hagen-Cook K, Hendren WH III: Nonrefluxing colon conduit: Experience with 70 cases. J Urol 1978; 120:35–39.

Arabi Y, Dimock F, Burdon DW, et al: Influence of bowel preparation and antimicrobials on colonic microflora. Br J Surg 1978; 65:555–559.

Armstrong WM: Cellular mechanisms of ion transport in the small intestine. *In* Johnson LR, ed: Physiology of the Gastrointestinal Tract. New York, Raven Press, 1987, p 1251.

Ashken MH: Urinary cecal reservoir. *In* King LR, Stone AR, Webster GD, eds: Bladder Reconstruction and Continent Urinary Diversion. Chicago, Year Book Medical Publishers, 1987, pp 238–251.

Bartlett JG, Condon RE, Gorback SL, et al: Veterans Administration Cooperative Study on bowel preparation for elective colorectal operations: Impact of oral antibiotic regimen on colonic flora, wound irrigation cultures, and bacteriology or septic complications. Ann Surg 1978; 188:249–254.

Baum ML, Anish DS, Chalmers TC, et al: A survey of clinical trials of antibiotic prophylaxis in colon surgery: Evidence against further use of no-treatment controls. N Engl J Med 1981; 305:795–799.

Beckley S, Wajsman Z, Pontes JE, Murphy G: Transverse colon conduit: A method of urinary diversion after pelvic irradiation. J Urol 1982; 128:464–468.

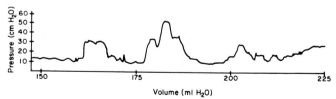

Figure 100–35. Pressure waves recorded 1 year postoperatively from a patient with a continent diversion created from detubularized ileum and right colon. Notice that the coordinated pressure waves are of similar magnitude and frequency to those found in a normal colonic or ileal segment.

Beddoe AM, Boyce JG, Remy JC, et al: Stented versus nonstented transverse colon conduits: A comparative report. Gynecol Oncol 1987; 27:305–313.

Benchekroun A: The ileocecal continent bladder. In King LR, Stone AF, Webster GD, eds: Bladder Reconstruction and Continent Urinary Diversion. Chicago, Year Book Medical Publishers, 1987, pp 224–237.

Berglund B, Kock NG, Myrvold HE: Volume capacity and pressure characteristics of the continent cecal reservoir. Surg Gynecol Obstet 1986; 163:42–48.

Berglund B, Kock NG, Norlen L, Philipson BM: Volume capacity and pressure characteristics of the continent ileal reservoir used for urinary diversion. J Urol 1987; 137:29–34.

Bihrle R, Foster RS, Steidle CP, et al: Creation of a transverse colon-gastric composite reservoir: A new technique. J Urol 1989; 141:1217–1220.

Binder HJ, Sandle GI: Electrolyte absorption and secretion in the mammalian colon. In John LR, ed: Physiology of the Gastrointestinal Tract. New York, Raven Press, 1989, p 1389.

Bisson JM, Vinson RK, Leadbetter GW: Urolithiasis from stapler anastomosis. Am J Surg 1979; 137:280–282.

Bonnheim DC, Petrelli NJ, Steinberg A, Mittelman A: The pathophysiology of the jejunal conduit syndrome and its exacerbation by parenteral hyperalimentation. J Surg Oncol 1984; 26:172–175.

Borglund E, Nordstrom G, Nyman CR: Classification of peristomal skin changes in patients with urostomy. J Am Acad Dermatol 1988; 19:623–628.

Bowyer GW, Davies TW: Methotrexate toxicity associated with an ileal conduit. Br J Urol 1986; 60:592.

Boyd SD, Schiff WM, Skinner DG, et al: Prospective study of metabolic abnormalities in patients with continent Kock pouch urinary diversion. Urology 1989; 33:85–88.

Bracken RB, McDonald MW, Johnson DE: Cystectomy for superficial bladder cancer. Urology 1981; 18:459–463.

Bricker EM: Bladder substitution after pelvic evisceration. Surg Clin North Am 1950; 30:1511–1521.

Camey M, Richard F, Botto H: Bladder replacement by ileocystoplasty. In King LR, Stone AF, Webster GD, eds: Bladder Reconstruction and Continent Urinary Diversion. Chicago, Year Book Medical Publishers, 1987, pp 336–359.

Castro JE, Ram MD: Electrolyte imbalance following ileal urinary diversion. Br J Urol 1970; 42:29–32.

Chang TW: Antibiotic-associated injury to the gut. In Berk JE, ed: Gastroenterology. Philadelphia, WB Saunders, 1985, pp 2585–2590.

Chassin JL, Rifkind KM, Sussman B, et al: The stapled gastrointestinal tract anastomosis: Incidence of postoperative complications compared with the sutured anastomoses. Ann Surg 1978; 188:689–696.

Chavez DR, Snyder PM, Juravsky LI, Heaney JA: Recurrent ileal conduit hemorrhage in an elderly cirrhotic man. J Urol 1994; 152:951–953.

Chen KK, Chang LS, Chen MT: Urodynamic and clinical outcome of Kock pouch continent urinary diversion. J Urol 1989; 141:94–97.

Christensen PB, Kronborg O: Whole-gut irrigation versus enema in elective colorectal surgery: A prospective, randomized study. Dis Colon Rectum 1981; 24:592–595.

Clark PB: End-to-end ureteroileal anastomoses for ileal conduits. Br J Urol 1979; 51:105–109.

Clarke JS, Condon RE, Barlett JG, et al: Preoperative oral antibiotics reduce septic complications of colon operations. Ann Surg 1977; 186:251–259.

Clayman RV, Reddy P, Nivatvongs S: Acute pseudo-obstruction of the colon: A serious consequence of urologic surgery. J Urol 1981; 126:415–417.

Cohen MS, Hilz ME, Davis CP, Anderson MD: Urinary carcinogen (nitrosamine) production in a rat animal model for ureterosigmoidostomy. J Urol 1987; 138:449–452.

Concepcion RS, Koch MO, McDougal WS, Richards WO: Detubularized intestinal segments in urinary tract reconstruction: Why do they work? Abstr Am Urol Assoc 1988; 592.

Cordonnier JJ: Ureterosigmoid anastomosis. J Urol 1950; 63:276–285.

Costello AJ, Johnson DE: Modified autosuture technique for ileal conduit construction in urinary diversion. Aust NZ J Surg 1984; 54:477–482.

Dekleck JN, Lambrechts W, Viljoen I: The bowel as substitute for the bladder. J Urol 1979; 121:22–24.

Delgado GE, Muecke EC: Evaluation of 80 cases of ileal conduits in children: Indications, complications and results. J Urol 1973; 109:210.

Didolkar MS, Reed WP, Elias EG, et al: A prospective randomized study of sutured versus stapled bowel anastomoses in patients with cancer. Cancer 1986; 57:456–460.

Dion YM, Richards GK, Prentis JJ, Hinchey EJ: The influence of oral versus parenteral preoperative metronidazole on sepsis following colon surgery. Ann Surg 1980; 192:221–226.

Dretler SP: The pathogenesis of urinary tract calculi occurring after conduit diversion: I. Clinical study; II. Conduit study; III. Prevention. J Urol 1973; 109:204–209.

Edwards RH: Hyperammonemic encephalopathy related to ureterosigmoidostomy. Arch Neurol 1984; 41:1211–1212.

Elder DD, Moisey CU, Rees RWM: A long-term follow-up of the colonic conduit operation in children. Br J Urol 1979; 51:462–465.

Emmott D, Noble MJ, Mebust WK: A comparison of end versus loop stomas for ileal conduit urinary diversion. J Urol 1985; 133:588–590.

Evans AJ, Manhire AR, Bishop MC: Duplex ureters: A pitfall during ileal conduit urinary diversion. Br J Urol 1994; 73:214–215.

Fall M, Anderstrom C: Funneled ureteroileal anastomosis. J Urol 1982; 128:249–251.

Fazio VW, Jagelman AG, Lavery IC, McGonagle BA: Evaluation of the Proximate-ILS circular stapler: A prospective study. Ann Surg 1985; 201:108–114.

Ferris DO, Odel HM: Electrolyte pattern of blood after ureterosigmoidostomy. JAMA 1950; 142:634–641.

Filmer RB: Malignant tumors arising in bladder augmentations and ileal and colon conduits. Soc Pediatr Urol Newsletter, December 9, 1986.

Flanigan RC, Kursh ED, Persky L: Thirteen year experience with ileal loop diversion in children with myelodysplasia. Am J Surg 1975; 130:535–538.

Friedman RM, Flashner SC, King LR: Effectiveness of a handsewn nipple valve for reflux prevention in bladder reconstruction. J Urol 1992; 147:441–443.

Geist RW, Ansell JS: Total body potassium in patients after ureteroileostomy. Surg Gynecol Obstet 1961; 113:585–590.

Golimbu M, Morales P: Jejunal conduits: Technique and complications. J Urol 1975; 113:787–795.

Gonzalez R, Reinberg Y: Localization of bacteriuria in patients with enterocystoplasty and nonrefluxing conduits. J Urol 1987; 138:1104–1105.

Goodwin WE, Harris AP, Kaufman JJ, Beal JM: Open, transcolonic ureterointestinal anastomosis. Surg Gynecol Obstet 1953; 97:295–330.

Gosalbez R Jr, Woodard, JR, Broecker BH, Warshaw B: Metabolic complications of the use of stomach for urinary reconstruction. J Urol 1993; 150:710–712.

Gottrup F, Diederich P, Sorensen K, et al: Prophylaxis with whole gut irrigation and antimicrobials in colorectal surgery: A prospective randomized double-blind clinical trial. Am J Surg 1985; 149:317–322.

Guinan PD, Moore RH, Neter E, Murphy GP: The bacteriology of ileal conduit urine in man. Surg Gynecol Obstet 1972; 134:78–82.

Hagen-Cook K, Althausen AF: Early observations on 31 adults with nonrefluxing colon conduits. J Urol 1979; 121:13–16.

Hardy BE, Lebowitz RL, Baez A, Colodny AA: Strictures of the ileal loop. J Urol 1977; 117:358–361.

Hares MM, Alexander-Williams J: The effect of bowel preparation on colonic surgery. World J Surg 1982; 6:175–181.

Harrison AR: Clinical and metabolic observations on osteomalacia following ureterosigmoidostomy. Br J Urol 1958; 30:455–461.

Hasan ST, Coorsh J, Tapson JS: Use of bendrofluazide in the management of recurrent jejunal conduit syndrome. Br J Urol 1994; 73:101–102.

Hassain M: The osteomalacia syndrome after colocystoplasty: A cure with sodium bicarbonate alone. Br J Urol 1970; 42:243–245.

Hautmann RE, Egghart G, Frohneberg D, Miller K: The ileal neobladder. J Urol 1988; 139:39–42.

Hayashi T, Ikai K, Kiriyama T, et al: Percutaneous intrapelvic pressure registration in patients with ureterointestinal urinary diversion. Urology 1986; 28:176–178.

Hedlund H, Lindstrom K, Mansson W: Dynamics of a continent caecal reservoir for urinary diversion. Br J Urol 1984; 56:366–372.

Heidler H, Marberger M, Hohenfellner R: The metabolic situation in ureterosigmoidostomy. Eur Urol 1979; 5:39–44.

Hensle TW, Burbige KA: Bladder replacement in children and young adults. J Urol 1985; 133:1004–1010.

Hill JT, Ransley PG: The colonic conduit: A better method of urinary diversion? Br J Urol 1983; 55:629–631.

Hirdes WH, Hoekstra I, Vlietstra HP: Hammock anastomoses: A nonrefluxing ureteroileal anastomosis. J Urol 1988; 139:517–518.

Husmann DA, McLorie GA, Churchill BM: Nonrefluxing colonic conduits: A long-term life-table analysis. J Urol 1989; 142:1201–1203.

Iannoni C, Marcheggiano A, Pallone F, et al: Abnormal patterns of colorectal mucin secretion after urinary diversion of different types: Histochemical and lectin binding studies. Hum Pathol 1986; 17:834–840.

Irvin TT, Goligher JC: Aetiology of disruption of intestinal anastomosis. Br J Surg 1973; 60:461.

Jacobs JA, Young JD Jr: The Strickler technique of ureterosigmoidostomy. J Urol 1980; 124:451–454.

Jaffe BM, Bricker EM, Butcher HR Jr: Surgical complications of ileal segment urinary diversion. Ann Surg 1968; 167:367–376.

Jakobsen H, Steven K, Stigsby B, et al: Pathogenesis of nocturnal urinary incontinence after ileocaecal bladder replacement: Continuous measurement of urethral closure pressure during sleep. Br J Urol 1987; 59:148–152.

Jex RK, van Heerden JA, Wolff BG, et al: Gastrointestinal anastomoses: Factors affecting early complications. Ann Surg 1987; 206:138–141.

Kamizaki H, Cass AS: Conduit and renal pelvic pressure after ileal and colonic urinary diversion in dogs. Invest Urol 1978; 16:27–32.

Kaufman JJ: Ammoniagenic coma following ureterosigmoidostomy. J Urol 1984; 131:743–745.

King LR: Protection of the upper tracts in undiversion. In King LR, Stone AF, Webster GD, eds: Bladder Reconstruction and Continent Urinary Diversion. Chicago, Year Book Medical Publishers, 1987, pp 127–153.

Kinn A, Lantz B: Vitamin B12 deficiency after irradiation for bladder carcinoma. J Urol 1984; 131:888–890.

Klein EA, Montie JE, Montague DK, et al: Jejunal conduit urinary diversion. J Urol 1986; 135:244–246.

Koch MO, Gurevitch E, Hill DE, McDougal WS: Urinary solute transport by intestinal segments: A comparative study of ileum and colon in rats. J Urol 1990; 143:1275–1279.

Koch MO, McDougal WS: Chlorpromazine: Adjuvant therapy for the metabolic derangements created by urinary diversion through intestinal segments. J Urol 1985a; 134:165–169.

Koch MO, McDougal WS: Determination of renal function following urinary diversion through intestinal segments. J Urol 1985b; 133:517–520.

Koch MO, McDougal WS: Nicotinic acid: Treatment for the hyperchloremic metabolic acidosis following urinary diversion through intestinal segments. J Urol 1985c; 134:162–164.

Koch MO, McDougal WS: The pathophysiology of hyperchloremic metabolic acidosis after urinary diversion through intestinal segments. Surgery 1985d; 98:561–570.

Koch MO, McDougal WS, Hall MC, et al: Long-term effects of urinary diversion: A comparison of myelomeningocele patients managed by clean, intermittent catheterization and urinary diversion. J Urol 1992; 147:1343–1347.

Koch MO, McDougal WS: Bone demineralization following ureterosigmoid anastomosis: An experimental study in rats. J Urol 1988; 140:856–859.

Kock NG: The development of the continent ileal reservoir (Kock Pouch), an application in patients requiring urinary diversion. In King LR, Stone AF, Webster GD, eds: Bladder Reconstruction and Continent Urinary Diversion. Chicago, Year Book Medical Publishers, 1987, pp 269–290.

Kock NG, Nilson AE, Nilsson LO, et al: Urinary diversion via a continent ileal reservoir: Clinical results in 12 patients. J Urol 1982; 128:469–475.

Kock NG, Nilson AE, Norlen L, et al: Changes in renal parenchyma and the upper urinary tract following urinary diversion via a continent ileum reservoir: An experimental study in dogs. Scand J Urol Nephrol 1978; 49(suppl):11–22.

Koff SA: Mechanisms of electrolyte imbalance following urointestinal anastomoses. Urology 1975; 5:109–114.

Kramolowsky EV, Clayman RV, Weyman PJ: Endourological management of ureteroileal anastomotic strictures: Is it effective? J Urol 1987; 137:390–394.

Kramolowsky EV, Clayman RV, Weyman PJ: Management of ureterointestinal anastomotic strictures: Comparison of open surgical and endourological repair. J Urol 1988; 139:1195–1198.

Kuss R, Bitker M, Camey M, et al: Indications and early and late results of intestino-cystoplasty: A review of 185 cases. J Urol 1970; 103:53–63.

Leadbetter WF, Clarke BG: Five years' experience with uretero-enterostomy by the "combined" technique. J Urol 1954; 73:67–82.

LeDuc A, Camey M, Teillac P: An original antireflux ureteroileal implantation technique: Long-term follow-up. J Urol 1987; 137:1156–1158.

Leong CH: Use of stomach for bladder replacement and urinary diversion. Ann Roy Coll Surg Engl 1978; 60:283–289.

Lim STK, Lam SK, Lee NW, et al: Effects of gastrocystoplasty on serum gastrin level and gastric acid secretion. Br J Surg 1983; 70:275–277.

Lockhart JL, Bejany D: The antireflux ureteroileal reimplantation in children and adults. J Urol 1986; 135:576–579.

Lockhart JL, Bejany DE: Antireflux ureteroileal reimplantation: An alternative for urinary diversion. J Urol 1987; 137:867–870.

Loening SA, Navarre RJ, Narayana AS, Culp DA: Transverse colon conduit urinary diversion. J Urol 1982; 127:37–39.

Magnus RV: Pressure studies and dynamics of ileal conduits in children. J Urol 1977; 118:406–407.

Malek RS, Burke EC, DeWeerd JH: Ileal conduit urinary diversion in children. J Urol 1971; 105:892–900.

Mansson W: The continent cecal urinary reservoir. In King LR, Stone AR, Webster GD, eds: Bladder Reconstruction and Continent Urinary Diversion. Chicago, Year Book Medical Publishers, 1987, p 209.

Mansson W, Colleen S, Forsberg L, et al: Renal function after urinary diversion: A study of continent caecal reservoir, ileal conduit, and colonic conduit. Scand J Urol Nephrol 1984; 18:307–315.

Mansson W, Colleen S, Stigsson L: Four methods of uretero-intestinal anastomoses in urinary conduit diversion. Scand J Urol Nephrol 1979; 13:191–199.

Matsuura T, Tsujihashi H, Park YC, et al: Assessment of the long-term results of ileocecal conduit urinary diversion. Urol Int 1991;46:154–158.

McDermott WV Jr: Diversion of urine to the intestines as a factor in ammoniagenic coma. N Engl J Med 1957; 256:460–462.

McDougal WS: Bladder reconstruction following cystectomy by uretero-ileo-colourethrostomy. J Urol 1986; 135:698–701.

McDougal WS: Mechanics and neurophysiology of intestinal segments as bowel substitutes. J Urol 1987; 138:1438–1439.

McDougal WS: Metabolic complications of urinary intestinal diversion. J Urol 1992; 147:1199–1208.

McDougal WS, Koch MO: Accurate determination of renal function in patients with intestinal urinary diversion. J Urol 1986; 135:1175–1178.

McDougal WS, Koch MO: Effect of sulfate on calcium and magnesium homeostasis following urinary diversion. Kidney 1989; 35:105–115.

McDougal WS, Koch MO, Flora MD: Ammonium metabolism in urinary intestinal diversion. Abstr Am Assoc GU Surg 1989, p 45.

McDougal WS, Koch MO, Shands C III, Price RR: Bony demineralization following urinary intestinal diversion. J Urol 1988; 140:853–855.

McDougal WS, Stampfer DS, Kirley S, et al: Intestinal ammonium transport by ammonium hydrogen exchange. J Am Coll Surg 1995; 181:241–248.

Menaker GJ, Litvak S, Bendix R, et al: Operations on the colon without preoperative oral antibiotic therapy. Surg Gynecol Obstet 1981; 152:36–38.

Menon M, Yu GW, Jeffs RD: Technique for antirefluxing ureterocolonic anastomosis. J Urol 1982; 127:236–237.

Merricks JW: A continent substitute bladder and urethra. In King LR, Stone AF, Webster GD, eds: Bladder Reconstruction and Continent Urinary Diversion. Chicago, Year Book Medical Publishers, 1987, pp 179–203.

Mesrobian HJ, Kelalis PP, Kramer SA: Long-term follow-up of 103 patients with bladder exstrophy. J Urol 1988; 139:719–722.

Middleton AW Jr, Hendren WH: Ileal conduits in children at the Massachusetts General Hospital from 1955 to 1970. J Urol 1976; 115:591–595.

Mitchell ME, Hensel TW: Total bladder replacement in children. In King LR, Stone AR, Webster GD, eds: Bladder Reconstruction and Continent Urinary Diversion. Chicago, Year Book Medical Publishers, 1987, pp 312–320.

Mounger EJ, Branson AD: Ammonia encephalopathy secondary to ureterosigmoidostomy: A case report. J Urol 1972; 108:411–412.

Mount BM, Susset JG, Campbell J, MacKinnon KJ: Ureteral implantation into ileal conduits. J Urol 1968; 100:605–609.

Nesbit RM: Ureterosigmoid anastomosis by direct elliptical connection: A preliminary report. J Urol 1949; 61:728–734.

Nguyen DH, Reinberg Y, Gonzalez R, et al: Outcome of renal transplantation after urinary diversion and enterocystoplasty: A retrospective controlled study. J Urol 1990; 144:1349–1351.

Nichols RL, Condon RE, Gorback SL, Nyhus LM: Efficacy of preoperative antimicrobial preparation of the bowel. Ann Surg 1972; 176:227–232.

Norlen L, Trasti H: Functional behavior of the continent ileum reservoir for urinary diversion: An experimental and clinical study. Scand J Urol Nephrol 1978; 49(suppl):33–42.

Nurmi M, Puntala P: Antireflux ureteroileal anastomosis in ileal conduit urinary diversion and in ileocystoplasty following cystoprostatectomy. Scand J Urol Nephrol 1988; 22:271–273.

Onwubalili JK: Overt diabetes mellitus without glycosuria in a patient with cutaneous ureteroileostomy. BMJ 1982; 284:1836–1837.

Pagano F: Ureterocolonic anastomoses: Description of a technique. J Urol 1980; 123:355–356.

Pagano F, Cosciani-Cunico S, Dal Bianco M, Zattoni F: Five years of experience with a modified technique of ureterocolonic anastomosis. J Urol 1984; 132:17–18.

Patil U, Glassberg KI, Waterhouse K: Ileal conduit surgery with nippled ureteroileal anastomoses. Urology 1976; 7:594–597.

Perry W, Allen LN, Stamp TCB, Walker PG: Vitamin D resistance in osteomalacia after ureterosigmoidostomy. N Engl J Med 1977; 297:1110–1112.

Philipson BM, Kock NG, Jagenburg R, et al: Functional and structural studies of ileal reservoir used for continent urostomy and ileostomy. Gut 1983; 24:392–398.

Pitts WR Jr, Muecke EC: A 20-year experience with ileal conduits: The fate of the kidneys. J Urol 1979; 122:154–157.

Ravi R, Dewan AK, Pandey KK: Transverse colon conduit urinary diversion in patients treated with very high dose pelvic irradiation. Br J Urol 1994; 73:51–54.

Regan JB, Barrett DM: Stented versus nonstented ureteroileal anastomoses: Is there a difference with regard to leak and stricture? J Urol 1985; 134:1101–1103.

Richards P, Chamerlain MJ, Wrong OM: Treatment of osteomalacia of renal tubular acidosis by sodium bicarbonate alone. Lancet 1972; 2:994–997.

Richie JP: Intestinal loop urinary diversion in children. J Urol 1974; 111:687–689.

Richie JP, Skinner DG: Urinary diversion: The physiological rationale for nonrefluxing colonic conduits. Br J Urol 1975; 47:269–275.

Rowland RG, Mitchell ME, Bihrle R, et al: Indiana continent urinary reservoir. J Urol 1987; 137:1136–1139.

Salahudeen AK, Elliott RW, Ellis HA: Osteomalacia due to ileal replacement of ureters: Report of 2 cases. J Urol 1984; 131:335–337.

Savarirayan F, Dixey GM: Syncope following ureterosigmoidostomy. J Urol 1969; J Urol 101:844–845.

Scher KS, Scott-Conner C, Jones CW, Leach M: A comparison of stapled and sutured anastomoses in colonic operations. Surg Gynecol Obstet 1982; 155:489–493.

Schipper H, Decter A: Carcinoma of the colon arising at ureteral implant sites despite early external diversion: Pathogenetic and clinical implications. Cancer 1981; 47:2062–2065.

Schmidt JD, Bucksbaum HJ, Nachtsheim DA: Long-term follow-up, further experience with and modifications of the transverse colon conduit in urinary tract diversion. Br J Urol 1985; 57:284–288.

Schmidt JD, Hawtrey CE, Flocks RH, Culp DA: Complications, results, and problems of ileal conduit diversions. J Urol 1973; 109:210–216.

Schwarz GR, Jeffs RD: Ileal conduit urinary diversion in children: Computer analysis of follow-up from 2 to 16 years. J Urol 1975; 114:285–288.

Sener SF, Imperato JP, Blum MD, et al: Technique and complications of reconstruction of the pelvic floor with polyglactin mesh. Surg Gynecol Obstet 1989; 168:475–480.

Shands C III, McDougal WS, Wright EP: Prevention of cancer at the urothelial enteric anastomotic site. J Urol 1989; 141:178–181.

Shapiro SR, Lebowitz R, Colodny AH: Fate of 90 children with ileal conduit urinary diversions a decade later: Analysis of complications, pyelography, renal function, and bacteriology. J Urol 1975; 114:289–295.

Siklos P, Davie M, Jung RJ, Chalmers TM: Osteomalacia in ureterosigmoidostomy: Healing by correction of the acidosis. Br J Urol 1980; 52:61–62.

Silberman R: Ammonia intoxication following ureterosigmoidostomy in a patient with liver disease. Lancet 1958; 2:937–939.

Skinner DG, Lieskovsky G, Boyd S: Continent urinary diversion. J Urol 1989; 141:1323–1327.

Smith ED: Follow-up studies on 150 ileal conduits in children. J Pediatr Surg 1972; 7:1–10.

Specht EE: Rickets following ureterosigmoidostomy and chronic hyperchloremia. J Bone Joint Surg 1967; 49:1422–1430.

Starr A, Rose DH, Cooper JF: Antireflux ureteroileal anastomosis in humans. J Urol 1975; 113:170–174.

Stewart M, Macrae FA, Williams CB: Neoplasia and ureterosigmoidostomy: A colonoscopy survey. Br J Surg 1982; 69:414–416.

Stewart WW, Cass AS, Matsen JM: Bacteriuria with intestinal loop urinary diversion in children. J Urol 1979; 122:528–531.

Stone AR, MacDermott JPA: The split-cuff ureteral nipple reimplantation technique: Reliable reflux prevention from bowel segments. J Urol 1989; 142:707–709.

Strickler WL: A modification of the combined uretero-sigmoidostomy. J Urol 1965; 93:370–373.

Sullivan JW, Grabstald H, Whitmore WF Jr: Complications of ureteroileal conduit with radical cystectomy: Review of 336 cases. J Urol 1980; 124:797–801.

Tapper D, Folkman J: Lymphoid depletion in ileal loops: Mechanism and clinical implication. J Pediatr Surg 1976; 11:871–880.

Thuroff JW, Alken P, Hohenfellner R: The MAINZ pouch (Mixed augmentation with ileum 'n' zecum) for bladder augmentation and continent diversion. In King LR, Stone AF, Webster GD, eds: Bladder Reconstruction and Continent Urinary Diversion. Chicago, Year Book Medical Publishers, 1987, p 252.

Tiffany P, Vaughan ED, Marion D, Amberson J: Hypergastrinemia following antral gastrocystoplasty. J Urol 1986; 136:692.

Tuggle DW, Hoelzer DJ, Tunell WP, Smith EI: The safety and cost-effectiveness of polyethylene glycol electrolyte solution bowel preparation in infants and children. J Pediatr Surg 1987; 22:513–515.

Turner-Warwick RT, Ashken MH: The functional results of partial, subtotal, and total cystoplasty with special reference to ureterocaecocystoplasty, selective sphincterotomy and cystocystoplasty. Br J Urol 1967; 39:3–12.

van den Bogaard AEJM, Weidema W, Hazen MJ, Wesdorp RIC: A bacteriological evaluation of three methods of bowel preparation for elective colorectal surgery. Antonie Van Leeuwenhoek 1981; 47:86–88.

Wallace DM: Uretero-ileostomy. Br J Urol 1970; 42:529–534.

Washington JA, Dearing WH, Judd ES, Elveback LR: Effect of preoperative antibiotic regimen in development of infection after intestinal surgery: Prospective, randomized double-blind study. Ann Surg 1974; 180:567–572.

Weber TR, Westfall SH, Steinhardt GF, et al: Malignancy associated with ureterosigmoidostomy: Detection by ornithine decarboxylase. J Pediatr Surg 1988; 23:1091–1094.

Wendel RG, Henning DC, Evans AT: End-to-end ureteroileal anastomosis for iliac conduits: Preliminary report. J Urol 1969; 102:42–43.

Whitmore WF III, Gittes RF: Reconstruction of the urinary tract by cecal and ileocecal cystoplasty: Review of a 15 year experience. J Urol 1983; 129:494–498.

Williams RE, Davenport TJ, Burkinshaw L, Hughes D: Changes in whole body potassium associated with uretero-intestinal anastomoses. Br J Urol 1967; 39:676–680.

Wolff BG, Beart RW Jr, Dozois RR, et al: A new bowel preparation for elective colon and rectal surgery: A prospective, randomized clinical trial. Arch Surg 1988; 123:895–900.

Woods JH, Erickson LW, Condon RE, et al: Postoperative ileus: A colonic problem? Surgery 1978; 84:527–533.

Zabbo A, Kay R: Ureterosigmoidostomy and bladder exstrophy: A long-term follow-up. J Urol 1986; 136:396–398.

101
PRINCIPLES OF CONTINENT RECONSTRUCTION

Howard M. Snyder, III, M.D.

Requirements of Reservoir
Absorption Characteristics

Reservoir Emptying

Continence Mechanisms
Hydraulic Resistance

Nipple Valves
Flap Valves

Complications

The Future

The past two decades have seen striking progress in the development of continent reconstruction of the lower urinary tract in both children and adults. Hendren (1976) was one of the early leaders in promoting the concept of unidiversion and has provided much of the background for current work on continence (Hendren, 1990). The pediatric experience has provided some useful lessons. Spontaneous voiding can often be achieved with quite an abnormal lower urinary tract. To achieve this, however, certain criteria must be satisfied. If the bladder outlet is normal and funnels normally, dropping the pressure gradient between the interior of the bladder and the end of the urethra to a low level, the bladder can empty even if it has a minimal amount of ability to contract. Thus, some patients who have had virtually a complete replacement of the detrusor by an intestinal cystoplasty are still able to empty their bladder satisfactorily, although others inexplicably require clean intermittent catheterization. If there is a normal detrusor with normal neurologic control, one can reconstruct the bladder outlet to provide an adequate resistance to hold urine in the bladder and have some expectation that the detrusor may be able to compensate adequately to produce emptying against this resistance. Unfortunately, there are often instances in which continent reconstruction is desired, but patients have congenital or acquired anomalies of both the outlet and the bladder. This has led to surgical approaches that produce both better reservoir function and a continent outlet. The current success is a reflection of better understanding of the physiologic principles involved in this process. This chapter reviews some of the physiologic principles that are now widely accepted in continent reconstruction.

REQUIREMENTS OF RESERVOIR

The importance of a **low reservoir pressure** cannot be overemphasized. It has been recognized that storage of urine

in the reservoir at pressures of less than 35 to 40 cm H_2O pressure is critical to the avoidance of damage to the upper tracts (McGuire et al, 1981). Although this observation was made initially in the treatment of children with a neurogenic bladder, the principle has now been recognized as valid for adequate reservoir reconstruction at all ages. Physiologic support for this was provided by Thomsen's (1984) work showing that pressures greater than 40 cm H_2O appeared to be capable of altering renal papillary morphology and inducing upper tract damage, even in the absence of infection. Further experience from many centers has supported the importance of avoiding storage pressures greater than 40 cm H_2O (Churchill et al, 1987).

An **adequate capacitance** for the reservoir is also important. More frequent than 4-hourly emptying of the reservoir is often difficult to achieve, and accordingly, one must achieve a reservoir size that permits low-pressure storage of urine with an emptying frequency of four to six times a day. This is an important point to emphasize, particularly in pediatric patients who may have undergone reconstruction following an obstructive uropathy that has left them with a concentrating defect. The total urine volume produced in 24 hours needs to be measured in helping to determine what reservoir size is required to permit a safe storage pressure with a reasonable emptying frequency. A little additional capacitance is always wise. In achieving adequate capacitance using intestinal segments, it is important to emphasize that detubularization of the segment is a gold standard in the use of bowel in continent reconstruction. Although detubularization disrupts the ability of the bowel segment to contract and thus generate pressures in a range that could lead to either incontinence or potentially upper tract abnormality, it also produces a significant increase in the geometric capacity of a tubular intestinal segment, as it is converted into a reconfigured sphere (Hinman, 1988; Koff, 1988).

Absorption Characteristics

In the choice of an intestinal segment to enlarge the bladder, the last two decades have provided adequate clinical experience to permit some broad conclusions to be drawn. The metabolic consequences of intestinal segments have been reviewed (Hall et al, 1991; McDougal, 1992) and are more fully discussed in Chapter 102. All intestinal segments have absorptive and secretory exchanges with urine that influence the choice of segment to be used. The surface area of intestine exposed as well as the dwell time and the metabolic reserve of the patient are important factors. The only bowel segment that is almost never used for reconstruction is the jejunum because its absorptive characteristics leading to hyperchloremia, hyponatremia, and acidosis are manifested so frequently as to make it impractical (Klein et al, 1986). The modern era of use of the stomach to augment the bladder was brought about through the work of Adams and co-workers (1988). The ability of a gastric patch to secrete acid appears to be an advantage in the patient with limited renal reserve who cannot handle the hyperchloremic acidosis that often follows the use of ileum or colon in reconstruction. This has been the clinical experience (Sheldon et al, 1994). A further advantage of the gastric patch has been its availability with little gastrointestinal consequence when other bowel segments have not been available. This has been most commonly seen in patients with cloacal exstrophy who exhibit short gut physiology.

The ileum and colon have had the widest use in creation of an intestinal urinary reservoir (Kass and Koff, 1983; Mitchell and Piser, 1987). Absorptive characteristics are not sufficiently different to make a clinical difference. Success has depended primarily on the size and configuration of the reconstructed reservoir rather than on the origin of the bowel segment employed. Of greatest importance perhaps is a recognition of which segment of intestine the patient can most easily spare (see later). Usually, 25 to 40 cm of bowel is adequate depending on the amount of bladder that can be incorporated into the reconstruction.

With the technique of autoaugmentation (Cartwright and Snow, 1989; Cartwright and Snow, 1994, personal communication), the detrusor is incised to permit the bladder mucosa to herniate outward, increasing capacitance and lowering intrareservoir pressure. The problems seen with this approach have been that results vary considerably, and it is clear that one cannot achieve an adequate reservoir using this technique in a small hypertrophied bladder. The most suitable cases appear to be neurogenic bladders with marginal capacitance, in which the achievement of a 50% or 100% enlargement is adequate. Unfortunately the author has had little success in the exstrophic small bladder. The autoaugmentation procedure has the advantage of avoiding the incorporation of anything other than uroepithelium in the continent reconstruction. This is an advantage from an absorptive standpoint and makes attractive the concept of using a dilated ureter as an alternative source for bladder augmentation (Churchill et al, 1993). The difficulty with this approach is the lack of clinical cases in which there is a sufficiently large ureter that can be spared for this purpose. Perhaps in the future, the most attractive way of augmenting the bladder may result from current ongoing experimental growth of uroepithelium on a matrix template (Atala, 1993;

Kropp, 1995, 1996). In this conceptually attractive approach, one hopes that autologous uroepithelium would line a patch, and in this way one could achieve augmentation while minimizing absorptive complications. It is in the development of alternative sources for augmentation that the greatest potential advances exist for continent reconstruction.

RESERVOIR EMPTYING

Clean intermittent catheterization and the concept that complete low-pressure emptying is more important than sterility in maintaining urinary tract health (Lapides et al, 1972, 1976) have permitted the growth of continent reconstruction as it is known today. The results of surgical efforts to achieve balanced voiding dynamics in the presence of major congenital or acquired anomalies have been poor. Patient compliance with intermittent catheterization, however, is critical, and before undertaking continent reconstruction, one must be certain that a patient will carry out self-catheterization frequently enough to maintain low storage pressures in the reservoir.

One of the consequences of intermittent catheterization is the bacterial colonization of the lower urinary tract (Ehrlich and Brem, 1982). As long as storage pressures are maintained at a low level and emptying is complete, symptomatic episodes of infection appear to be rare both in pediatric and in adult reconstruction (Kass and Koff, 1983; Mansson, 1991). Indeed, the development of symptomatic urinary infection in a patient on a catheterization program should raise questions about the adequacy of the reservoir and appropriate low-pressure storage or the development of urolithiasis. The almost universal presence of bacteriuria in patients with intestine incorporated into the lower urinary tract and the experimental work of Richie and colleagues (1974) have led to emphasis on an antireflux attachment of the upper urinary tract to the reservoir whenever possible.

CONTINENCE MECHANISMS

Hydraulic Resistance

Urinary continence is the result of a complex interaction between bladder outlet resistance and pressure within the bladder or urinary reservoir, as shown in the equation

$$\text{Resistance } \alpha \frac{\text{length, diameter}}{\text{tension in wall}} = \text{normal human bladder outlet}$$

To maintain continence, the bladder outlet resistance must exceed intravesical or intrareservoir pressure, not only at rest but also during changes in posture, coughing, sneezing, or straining. There are several components to this continence mechanism. The intrinsic urethral resistance of the urethra is due to inherent tension in the urethral wall as well as the length and diameter of the urethra (Lapides, 1958; Lapides et al, 1960). The smooth and striated muscular activity of the urethra and the fact that intra-abdominal pressure is transmitted to the proximal urethra also are important. This transmitted pressure increases resistance in the proximal urethra at the time that intra-abdominal pressure produces increased pressure within the bladder or reservoir. With this consideration in mind, it is to be expected that many surgical interventions to treat incontinence narrow, lengthen, or compress the urethra. This type of hydraulic alteration is in essence what underlies the creation of detrusor tubes, the use of the artificial genitourinary sphincter, and the employment of bulk injecting procedures around the urethra, as carried out with collagen or polytef paste. Various suspension procedures lengthen the urethra and reposition it intraabdominally to permit better the transmission of pressure to the urethra. A sling suspension adds a compressive element. The remainder of this section on continence mechanisms focuses on artificial, surgically created continence mechanisms that may be used with a normal bladder, with an augmented one, or in a total intestinal reservoir.

Nipple Valves

The physiologic principle underlying a nipple valve for continence is that filling of the reservoir compresses the nipple, which protrudes into its lumen (Fig. 101–1). This ensures that through hydraulic principles, the resistance to flow through the continence channel exceeds the pressure within the reservoir. This is the principle that underlies the Kock pouch (Kock et al, 1985b; Skinner et al, 1987). This principle was at the heart of a continent reconstruction procedure tried as early as 1950 by Gilchrist and colleagues (1950). Efforts to create a nonrefluxing ileocecal valve continued throughout the 1980s, particularly at the Lahey Clinic (Zinman and Libertino, 1986). Hendren (1980) intussuscepted 4 cm of terminal ileum into the cecum in an effort to create a nipple valve mechanism. Unfortunately, despite all of these efforts, at least one third of patients continued to demonstrate reflux. Gradually, it was realized that the reason for this is that the same intrareservoir pressure that compresses the nipple also has a laterally distracting effect at its base, gradually leading to the effacement of the nipple and thus loss of the continence mechanism. This has led to a

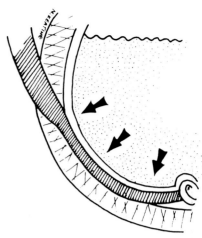

Figure 101–2. Flap valves create continence by having a segment compressed by reservoir filling, as for a reimplanted ureter. The success of this approach lies in a stable, small-diameter, sufficiently long supple segment that is supported on the inner wall of a stable reservoir. Reservoir filling does not cause loss of the continence mechanism, as can occur with a nipple valve.

gradual loss of enthusiasm for the nipple valve principle in continent reconstruction.

Flap Valves

The flap valve principle for a continence mechanism relies on the fact that a segment of the continence channel runs on the inner wall of the reservoir and is fixed in place (Fig. 101–2). As filling of the reservoir occurs, the continence channel is compressed, leading by hydraulic principles to a higher resistance to flow than the pressure produced in the reservoir. This principle is the same as that which underlies the reimplantation of the ureter into the bladder. The secret to success here lies in having a small-diameter, supple structure that has at least a 5:1 length-to-diameter ratio as it is attached to the wall of the reservoir.

Examples of flap valves can be seen in the modified Kock pouch as has been carried out by the group at Columbia (Olsson, 1985) and by Kock himself (Kock et al, 1985a). The ileocecal valve has been intussuscepted and fixed against the wall of the cecum, producing a satisfactory flap valve mechanism in that type of reconstruction as well (Hendren, 1986; Robertson and King, 1986). This same principle has been used with detrusor tubes by Kropp (Kropp and Angwafo, 1986; Belman and Kaplan, 1989) and Salle (Mouriquand, 1995). The most popular type of flap valve mechanism, however, has been the appendix implanted into the bladder or reservoir (Mitrofanoff, 1980). The Mitrofanoff principle describes a small-caliber, supple catheterizable channel implanted with a flap valve mechanism on the inner wall of the reservoir (Duckett and Snyder, 1985, 1986). This concept has been widely used with both appendix and ureter and has been proven to be versatile (Elder, 1992; Sheldon and Gilbert, 1992; Sumfest et al, 1993), thus achieving wide popularity. The stoma in many cases can be cosmetically hidden in the depths of the umbilicus. The small diameter of such a continence channel facilitates catheterization. The most dangerous problem that has been associated with this

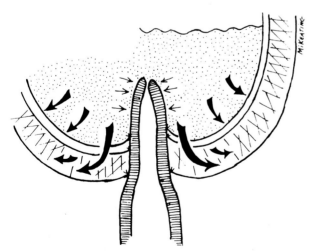

Figure 101–1. Nipple valves produce continence as the protruding nipple is circumferentially compressed by pressure within the reservoir. The same intrareservoir pressure unfortunately has a laterally distractive force on the base of the nipple, often causing eventual shortening of the nipple and thus loss of the continence mechanism.

Table 101–1. POTENTIAL COMPLICATIONS OF CONTINENT RECONSTRUCTION

Chronic bacteriuria
Metabolic alterations
  Acidosis
  Bone demineralization
Disturbances of gastrointestinal function
  Diarrhea
  Anemia (vitamin B_{12} absorption)
Urolithiasis
Reservoir rupture
Malignancy

technique lies in its success. Because the continence channel truly does not give way to high pressure, failure to comply with regular emptying can lead to reservoir or bladder rupture.

COMPLICATIONS

There continue to be multiple potential complications in the continent reconstruction of the urinary tract. These are summarized in Table 101–1 and fully discussed in Chapter 102. There are many problems yet to be solved. One should never discharge these patients from care, as their long-term outcome has not yet been determined.

THE FUTURE

Changes are occurring in medicine now at a more rapid rate than at any time in history. Certainly the field of continent reconstruction will be swept along with current change. In the future, the techniques of molecular biology may permit physicians to carry out genetic manipulation so as to reverse some of the pathologic processes that lead to the need for continent reconstruction. Alternatively the rapid progress that has been made in tissue culture and the recognition of factors important in the stimulus of uroepithelium to multiply may enable researchers to "grow a bladder" on a template (Atala, 1993; Kropp et al, 1995). It is clear that innovative approaches such as this reconstruction will continue to make this field exciting in the twenty-first century.

REFERENCES

Adams MC, Mitchell ME, Rink RC: Gastrocystoplasty: An alternative solution to the problem of urologic reconstruction in the severely compromised patient. J Urol 1988; 140:1152–1156.
Atala A: Implantation in vivo and retrieval of artificial structures consisting of rabbit and human urothelium and human bladder muscle. J Urol 1993; 150:608.
Belman AB, Kaplan GW: Experience with the Kropp anti-incontinence procedure. J Urol 1989; 141:1160–1162.
Cartwright PC, Snow BW: Bladder autoaugmentation: Early clinical experience. J Urol 1989; 142:505–508.
Churchill BM, Aliabadi H, Landon EH, et al: Ureteral bladder augmentation. J Urol 1993; 150:716–720.
Churchill BM, Gilmour RF, Willot P: Urodynamics. Pediatr Clin North Am 1987; 34:1133–1157.
Duckett JW, Snyder HM: Use of the Mitrofanoff principle in urinary reconstruction. World J Urol 1985; 3:191–193.
Duckett JW, Snyder HM: Continent urinary diversion: Variations on the Mitrofanoff principle. J Urol 1986; 135:58–62.
Ehrlich O, Brem AS: A prospective comparison of urinary tract infections in patients treated with either clean intermittent catheterization or urinary diversion. Pediatrics 1982; 70:665.
Elder JS: Continent appendicocolostomy: A variation of the Mitrofanoff principle in pediatric urinary tract reconstruction. J Urol 1992; 148:117–119.
Gilchrist RK, Merricks JW, Hamlin HH, et al: Construction of substitute bladder and urethra. Surg Gynecol Obstet 1950; 90:752.
Hall MC, Koch MO, McDougal WS: Metabolic consequences of urinary diversion through intestinal segment. Urol Clin North Am 1991; 18:725–735.
Hendren WH: Exstrophy of the bladder: Alternative method of management. J Urol 1976; 115:195–202.
Hendren WH: Reoperative ureteral reimplantation: Management of the difficult case. J Pediatr Surg 1980; 15:770.
Hendren WH: Bladder augmentation in children (Abstract 152). AUA Meeting, New York, 1986.
Hendren WH: Urinary tract refunctionalization after long-term diversion. Ann Surg 1990; 212:478–495.
Hinman F Jr: Selection of intestinal segments for bladder substitution: Physical and psychological characteristics. J Urol 1988; 139:522.
Kass EJ, Koff SA: Bladder augmentation in the pediatric neuropathic bladder. J Urol 1983; 129:552–555.
Klein EA, Montie JE, Montague E, et al: Jejunal conduit urinary diversion. J Urol 1986; 135:244.
Kock NG, Norlen LJ, Philipson BM: Management of complications after construction of a continent ileal reservoir for urinary diversion. World J Urol 1985a; 3:152–154.
Kock NG, Norlen L, Philipson BM, et al: The continent ileal reservoir (Koch pouch) for urinary diversion. World J Urol 1985b; 3:146–151.
Koff SA: Guidelines to determine size and shape of intestinal segments used for reconstruction. J Urol 1988; 140:1150.
Kropp KA, Angwafo FF: Urethral lengthening and reimplantation for neurogenic incontinence in children. J Urol 1986; 135:553–536.
Kropp B, Badylak S, Thor KB: Regenerative bladder augmentation: A review of the initial preclinical studies with porcine small intestinal submucosa. In Zderic SA, ed: Muscle, Matrix and Bladder Function. New York, Plenum, 1995, p 229.
Kropp BP, Sawyer BD, Shannon HE, et al: Characterization of small intestinal submucosa regenerated canine detrusor: Assessment of reinnervation, in vitro compliance and contractility. J Urol 1996; 156:599.
Lapides J: Structure and function of the internal vesical sphincter. J Urol 1958; 80:3241–3253.
Lapides J, Ajaemian EP, Stewart BH, et al: Further observation on the kinetics of the urethrovesical sphincter. J Urol 1960; 84:86.
Lapides J, Diokno AC, Gould FR, et al: Further observations on self-catheterization. J Urol 1976; 116:169.
Lapides J, Diokno AC, Silber SJ, et al: Clean intermittent self-catheterization in the treatment of urinary tract disease. J Urol 1972; 107:458.
Mansson W: Continuing experience with the right colon as a continent reservoir for urine. In King L, Stone AR, Webster GD, eds: Bladder Reconstruction and Continent Urinary Diversion, 2nd ed. Chicago, Year Book Medical Publishers, 1991, p 283.
McDougal WS: Metabolic complications of urinary intestinal diversion. J Urol 1992; 147:1199–1208.
McGuire EJ, Woodside JR, Borden TA, et al: Prognostic value of urodynamic testing in myelodysplastic patients. J Urol 1981; 126:205–209.
Mitchell ME, Piser JA: Intestinocystoplasty and total bladder replacement in children and young adults: Followup in 129 cases. J Urol 1987; 138:579–584.
Mitrofanoff P: Cystostomie continente trans-appendiculaire dans le traitement des vessies neurologiques. Chir Pediatr 1980; 21:297–305.
Mouriquand PDE, Sheard R, Phillips N, et al: The Kropp procedure (Pippi Salle procedure): A simplification of the technique of urethral lengthening. Preliminary results in eight patients. Br J Urol 1995; 75:656.
Olsson CA: Cecal reservoirs for continent urinary diversion: Editorial comments: Urinary diversion. World J Urol 1985; 3:197–198.
Richie JP, Skinner DG, Waisman J: The effect of reflux on the development of pyelonephritis in urinary diversion: An experimental study. J Surg Res 1974; 16:256.
Robertson GN, King L: Bladder substitution in children. Urol Clin North Am 1986; 13:333.
Rushton HG, Woodard JR, Parrott TS, et al: Delayed bladder rupture after augmentation enterocystoplasty. J Urol 1988; 140:344.

Sheldon CA, Gilbert A: Use of the appendix for urethral reconstruction in children with congenital anomalies of the bladder. Surgery 1992; 112:805–812.

Sheldon CA, Gilbert A, Lewis AG: Important surgical implications of genitourinary tract anomalies in the management of the imperforate anus. J Urol 1994; 152:196–199.

Skinner DG, Lieskovsky G, Boyd SD: Continuing experience with the continent ileal reservoir (Kock pouch) as an alternative to cutaneous diversion: An update after 250 cases. J Urol 1987; 137:1140–1145.

Sumfest JM, Burns MW, Mitchell ME: The Mitrofanoff principle in urinary reconstruction. J Urol 1993; 150:1875–1878.

Thomsen HS: Pyelorenal backflow. Danish Med Bull 1984; 31:348.

Zinman L, Libertino JA: Right colocystoplasty for bladder replacement. Urol Clin North Am 1986; 13:321.

102
AUGMENTATION CYSTOPLASTY

Richard C. Rink, M.D.
Mark C. Adams, M.D.

Augmentation cystoplasty is now used quite commonly for reconstruction of the dysfunctional bladder when more conservative management fails. The use of bowel for augmentation of the bladder was first described experimentally by Tizzoni and Foggi in 1888 and used in humans by Mickulicz in 1898 (Orr et al, 1958). Since then, much has been learned about the use of bowel. This experience has led to improved results and minimized problems. **Perhaps the most important contribution affecting lower urinary tract reconstruction was the introduction of clean intermittent catheterization (CIC) by Lapides and colleagues** (1972, 1976). It allowed application of augmentation to groups of patients who had not previously been candidates for reconstruction of the urinary tract. Principles learned from experience with intestinocystoplasty have led to the development of techniques for complete bladder replacement, including continent urinary reservoirs and orthotopic neobladders. No intestinal segment is a perfect physiologic substitute for native bladder, and some complications still occur after augmentation cystoplasty. Consequently a great deal of experimental effort is being made to find alternatives to intestinal segments that are accompanied by less morbidity for the patient. At this point, many of these alternatives are still experimental and must be critically compared to intestinal segments that function well for most patients.

This chapter updates the reader on the current state of augmentation cystoplasty. Historical background is included only where it is pertinent to current understanding because it has been well covered in the chapter on this subject in the previous edition (Mitchell et al, 1992).

GENERAL PRINCIPLES OF BLADDER RECONSTRUCTION

Basic Bladder Function

The bladder has two basic functions. The first is urinary storage for an acceptable length of time. For this function, the bladder must act as a large-capacity reservoir and generate little pressure. The sphincter mechanisms prevent leakage by providing outflow pressure greater than vesical pressure. The second function of the urinary bladder is to empty or expel urine. In the normal patient, this is done voluntarily and completely. For emptying, the bladder must generate pressure with a sustained contraction, and the sphincter muscles must synergistically relax to lower outflow resistance. If these two functions are performed well, the patient is continent, the kidneys are protected, and the potential for urinary tract infection is minimized.

Bladder Dysfunction

Bladder dysfunction may be related to a problem with storage, emptying, or both functions. Urinary incontinence is perhaps the most common sign of bladder dysfunction requiring treatment. Urinary frequency, urgency, and the necessity to empty the bladder at unacceptably short intervals in patients able to remain continent may also result from bladder dysfunction, as in those with interstitial cystitis. Upper urinary tract changes, such as hydronephrosis and deterioration of renal function, may also be caused by bladder dysfunction, particularly in the poorly compliant bladder with high outflow resistance. In this setting, there is no relief from high intravesical pressures. Such pressure can give rise to vesicoureteral reflux with its potential for renal scarring. Urinary tract infection may also be a sign of underlying bladder dysfunction.

Problems arise when (1) the bladder does not function as a high-capacity, low-pressure reservoir; (2) the sphincter mechanism does not provide good outflow resistance or does not act in coordination with the bladder; or (3) emptying is poor. These problems may coexist to varying degrees and may be interrelated.

Good urodynamic evaluation is essential to understanding the pathophysiology of bladder dysfunction and deciding which problems predominate and require treatment. Failure to empty the bladder may be approached first by behavioral modification. If adequate spontaneous voiding cannot be achieved in this manner, CIC may be effectively used (Lapides et al, 1972, 1976). Catheterization per urethra is usually well tolerated; however, for occasional patients unable or unwilling to be catheterized per native urethra, construction of a continent abdominal wall stoma is now straightforward. This allows easy catheterization that is well tolerated (Mitrofanoff, 1980; Keating et al, 1993).

Inadequate outflow resistance owing to a poorly functioning sphincter mechanism is most commonly a problem in pediatric patients. Increasing urethral outflow resistance to adequate levels may be a difficult challenge. Alpha-adrenergic agonists produce smooth muscle contraction of the bladder neck and proximal urethra; beta-adrenergic antagonists may potentiate these alpha-adrenergic effects. Such medications may produce some clinical improvement but rarely result in adequate resistance when impairment is significant. This is particularly true in patients with neurogenic dysfunction, in whom urethral resistance tends to be fixed. Surgical techniques to improve outflow resistance are numerous, and a discussion of such procedures is beyond the scope of this chapter. It is imperative, however, that a compliant reservoir is present or will be created when undertaking a procedure to increase outflow resistance to protect the kidneys (Rink and Mitchell, 1990). McGuire and associates have documented that sustained bladder pressure over 40 cm H_2O puts the upper tracts at risk (McGuire et al, 1981).

Indications for Augmentation Cystoplasty

Augmentation cystoplasty is an attempt to improve the function of the urinary bladder as a compliant storage vessel. The goals of bladder augmentation are to improve bladder capacity while decreasing bladder pressure. Bladder augmentation does not, in itself, increase outflow resistance, and it does not improve bladder emptying. In fact, spontaneous emptying may be more difficult. When a patient with bladder dysfunction is proven to have a noncompliant bladder, treatment should be undertaken. Bladder augmentation is reserved for patients who fail more conservative therapy. Efforts should first be made to improve bladder compliance using anticholinergic or antispasmodic medications. The possibility of improvement on such medications often relates to the underlying cause of the noncompliant bladder. Patients with neurogenic bladder dysfunction often respond well to anticholinergic medications and may be managed frequently with a combination of medications and intermittent catheterization (Rink and Mitchell, 1984). Patients with bladder dysfunction caused by tuberculosis or irradiation seldom respond to the same treatment. Nonetheless, attempts should be made to treat all patients with medication before augmentation cystoplasty. Direct bladder stimulation (Kaplan, 1994) and nerve root stimulation (Schmidt et al, 1990) may provide effective treatment for some of these patients in the future, although experience is quite limited with these techniques at this time.

Failure of medical management warrants a surgical approach. Augmentation cystoplasty has generally been the first choice, but this procedure to increase bladder compliance may be achieved at a cost to the patient. The potential complications and problems related to bladder augmentation are discussed in this chapter. The surgeon and patient considering such a procedure must understand that bladder augmentation results in decreased efficiency of bladder emptying by spontaneous voiding to some degree (Gleason et al, 1972). Each patient must understand and accept the possibility of long-term, even permanent, CIC as a necessity for bladder emptying.

PATIENT SELECTION: ANATOMIC AND PHYSIOLOGIC CONSIDERATIONS

Many anatomic and physiologic variables must be considered before enterocystoplasty to ensure an optimal result.

Proper preoperative evaluation requires an understanding of not only the pathophysiology of the urinary tract but also the psychosocial situation and commitment of the patient. Physiologic considerations include not only the bladder and sphincter but also the entire urinary tract.

Renal Function

Renal function should be considered in any patient undergoing bladder augmentation. Consequently, each patient should have determinations of serum electrolytes, blood urea nitrogen (BUN), and serum creatinine. For patients with elevation of the serum creatinine or significant hydronephrosis, a 24-hour urine collection both for creatinine clearance and for urine volume should be obtained. **Demos (1962) and Koch and McDougal (1985) have demonstrated that urinary solutes, particularly chloride, are absorbed from urine in contact with the mucosa of small and large bowel.** For patients with normal renal function, the kidneys are able to handle the resorbed load of chloride and acid without difficulty. Patients with decreased renal function, however, may develop significant metabolic acidosis secondary to such resorption, particularly if any acidosis existed preoperatively (Mitchell and Piser, 1987). The first renal function to deteriorate after obstruction or infection is usually concentrating ability. These patients may generate an enormous volume of urine in 24 hours. **The bladder volume achieved through augmentation must be adequate to handle the patient's urinary output for an acceptable period of time (usually 4 hours).** Patients with renal failure or other medical problems may conversely develop oliguria. Low urinary output may also affect the augmented bladder because there is greater potential for collection and inspissation of mucus. There is also less urine for dilution and buffering of gastric secretions if stomach is considered for augmentation.

Other Organ Systems

The function of other organ systems may also affect the risk of augmentation cystoplasty. Liver function tests and arterial blood gas studies may be appropriate for some patients. Resorption of ammonia by large or small intestine in contact with urine may be dangerous for patients with hepatic failure (McDougal, 1992). Some medications excreted in the urine may be resorbed by bowel mucosa (Savauagen and Dixey, 1969).

Ureteral Dynamics

Each patient should have upper tract imaging before augmentation cystoplasty. **If hydronephrosis is present, obstruction and vesicoureteral reflux should be sought with a functional study and voiding cystogram.** Reflux should be excluded in any pediatric patient with bladder dysfunction. **If these problems exist, they should be corrected at the time of bladder augmentation.** Particular attention should be given to chronically scarred, dilated ureters, which

may be incapable of peristalsis. Such ureters may drain poorly when reimplanted, even when good bladder compliance is achieved.

Bladder and Sphincter Dynamics

Proper assessment of bladder and urethral dynamics is critical to achieve an optimal result and may be obtained only with good urodynamic evaluation. The cystometrogram should define a bladder of small capacity or poor compliance (or both). Compliance may be underestimated if the bladder is filled too quickly; carbon dioxide is used as an infusant; or the study is done soon after an infection, which may irritate the bladder. Joseph (1992) has shown that measured detrusor pressure can be affected by varying the fill rate. Bauer (1994) has suggested that the cystometrogram be performed with a fill rate of no greater than 10% of the predicted bladder volume per minute.

The most difficult bladders to assess in terms of compliance are those previously diverted or those with low urethral resistance (Mitchell et al, 1992). Both may demonstrate a small capacity, and even if a flat tonus limb exists up to capacity, it can be hard to predict how such a bladder will stretch. Urodynamics done with the bladder outlet occluded with a Foley balloon may be helpful in those patients with low outlet resistance. Repeated bladder cycling is also beneficial, and information regarding the bladder's ability to stretch may be determined in as little time as a day with repeated cycling (McGuire, personal communication, 1993). Urethral and bladder neck function are ideally interpreted without a catheter through the urethra; however, this is difficult to do from a practical standpoint. The smallest catheter possible should be used through the urethra when evaluating outflow resistance, so as to avoid an obstruction to leakage, which may cause overestimation of urethral resistance. Measurement of the urethral pressure profile may help to define outflow resistance; however, McGuire and associates have found leak point pressure to be the most simple technique to define and use (McGuire et al, 1981). The accurate point and pressure of leakage is most difficult to define in patients with a small, noncompliant bladder in whom the rate of change of bladder pressure may be rapid. The bladder filling rate should be as slow as possible in such cases. **For most patients, a leak point pressure of approximately 40 cm H_2O is necessary for reliable continence.** If the leak point pressure is considerably lower than 40 cm H_2O, surgical techniques for increasing outflow resistance are usually necessary to achieve reliable continence.

Bladder Emptying

The patient's ability to empty the bladder before augmentation should also be assessed urodynamically. Useful parameters related to bladder emptying include synergistic relaxation of the external sphincter on electromyography, urinary flow rate, and measurements of postvoid residual urine. Neurologically normal patients who are able to empty the bladder well are much more likely to be able to continue to empty adequately after bladder augmentation than are patients who have neurogenic dysfunction or who are unable to empty well preoperatively. **No test ensures that a patient will be able to void spontaneously and empty well after a bladder augmentation under any circumstances.** Therefore, all patients must be prepared to perform CIC after augmentation cystoplasty. The native urethra should be examined for the ease of catheterization. Ideally, the patient learns CIC and practices it preoperatively until the patient and surgeon are comfortable that catheterization can and will be done reliably. Physical and psychosocial limitations of the patient must be considered in regard to the ability to self-catheterize and perform self-care. **Failure to catheterize and empty reliably after augmentation may result in upper tract deterioration, urinary tract infection, or bladder perforation despite a technically perfect operation.**

PATIENT PREPARATION

Bowel Preparation

Even by today's standards, augmentation cystoplasty remains a significant operative procedure, and the patient should be well prepared. Each patient should undergo preoperative bowel preparation to minimize the potential risk of the surgery. Two days of a clear liquid diet before bowel preparation aid in effective clearing of solid stool. The patient should then undergo full mechanical bowel preparation on the day before surgery. Historically, such bowel preparations have been done in the hospital. Increasingly, however, some are being done on an outpatient basis. Augmentation cystoplasty is often part of a major reconstructive effort requiring many hours of operative time with large fluid shifts. It is critical that the patient be well hydrated at the time of surgery. Consequently, there should be a low threshold for the use of intravenous fluids preoperatively. The use of oral antibiotics in bowel preparation, once dogma, is now a matter of personal preference. Special attention must be paid to the bowel preparation of patients with neurogenic dysfunction. Most of these patients have neuropathic bowel dysfunction as well, which is often manifest by chronic constipation. Good bowel preparation is challenging in such patients.

Antiembolism stockings or lower extremity sequential compression devices are used in adults or younger patients on oral contraceptives. Most surgeons use parenteral antibiotics perioperatively for prophylaxis. Theoretically, gastric contents are sterile, and such antibiotics, or a routine bowel preparation, are not necessary before gastrocystoplasty. Nonetheless, it is safest to follow such guidelines for all patients because intraoperative considerations may preclude the use of stomach and necessitate ileocystoplasty or colocystoplasty.

Urine Culture

All patients should have a urine culture performed at least several days before augmentation cystoplasty to rule out infection. It is a mistake to open the bladder and spill infected urine intraperitoneally when it can be avoided, particularly in those patients with a ventriculoperitoneal shunt. Any patient with a positive preoperative culture should undergo treatment for the infection and have a second culture to document sterile urine.

Cystoscopy

Preoperative cystoscopy may be helpful for evaluating the native bladder, outflow, or the ureteral orifices, particularly in pediatric patients. In that setting, endoscopy should be performed immediately before augmentation under the same anesthetic. In adult patients with interstitial cystitis or irritative bladder symptoms requiring augmentation cystoplasty, cystoscopy should be performed well before augmentation to rule out urothelial carcinoma in situ with certainty. Bladder biopsy and cytologic examination of the urine may be helpful in excluding tumor. Consideration for performance of colonoscopy or a barium enema should be given in older patients when bladder augmentation with a colonic segment is planned, particularly in the presence of any gastrointestinal symptoms.

SURGICAL TECHNIQUE

Regardless of the bowel segment to be selected, the initial approach to the patient for augmentation cystoplasty is the same. Cystoscopy should be performed preoperatively to avoid any unsuspected anatomic abnormalities that may affect the surgery or postoperative care. If there are other bladder procedures to be performed, such as ureteral reimplantation, the bladder is left full. If only augmentation is to be performed, the bladder is emptied after endoscopy to allow easy access into the peritoneal cavity.

As a general rule, a midline incision is performed for intestinocystoplasty, although these procedures can be done through a lower abdominal transverse incision if there has been no previous abdominal surgery. For gastrocystoplasty, the incision needs to extend from the pubis to the xiphoid. Associated procedures on the bladder, such as bladder neck reconstruction or ureteral reimplantation, should be performed before opening the peritoneal cavity to limit third space fluid loss. After completion of the procedures on the native bladder, the peritoneum is opened.

Management of Native Bladder

There have been differing opinions about the management of the native bladder. In the past, many have recommended excision of the "diseased" bladder. This has meant excision of the entire supratrigonal bladder. A cuff of bladder is left surrounding the trigone for anastomosis to the intestinal segment. **More recently, however, most have believed that native bladder can be preserved as long as the bladder is widely open to prevent a narrow-mouthed anastomosis, which could result in the augmentation segment behaving as a diverticulum** (Fig. 102–1). A sagittal incision to bivalve the bladder is generally recommended, which allows a technically easier anastomosis and leaves the native bladder to add to the overall capacity. The incision is carried from a point several centimeters cephalad to the bladder neck anteriorly to a position just above the trigone posteriorly. A

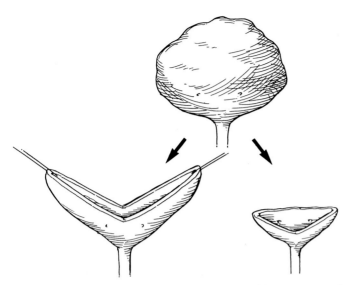

Figure 102–1. The native bladder can be managed by supratrigonal excision of the diseased bladder or by opening the bladder in the sagittal plane.

greater surface area can be provided, if need be, by opening the bladder in a stellate fashion, which simply requires a second transverse incision into the two bladder halves.

Management of Intestinal Segments

Hinman (1988) and Koff (1988) have demonstrated well the advantages of opening the bowel segment on its antimesenteric border, which allows detubularization and reconfiguration of that intestinal segment. **Reconfiguration into a spherical shape provides multiple advantages, including maximizing the volume achieved for any given surface area of bowel, blunting of bowel contractions, and improving overall compliance.** Furthermore, a shorter intestinal segment can be used to achieve the same capacity than if left in the tubular form. Detubularization and reconfiguration should always be performed during augmentation cystoplasty. The authors and others have produced graphs to determine intraoperatively the length of bowel segment necessary to achieve a desired volume, but these are cumbersome (Rink and Mitchell, 1990). Depending on the volume to be achieved, 20 to 40 cm of ileum or approximately 20 cm of colon are used for cystoplasty. Unless otherwise contraindicated, one should err by making the bladder too large rather than too small.

Ileocystoplasty

Technique

Goodwin and colleagues have demonstrated multiple ways of anastomosing the ileum to the native bladder (Goodwin et al, 1959). At this time, all surgeons believe that ileum should be detubularized and reconfigured to achieve the most spherical shape possible.

A segment of ileum at least 15 to 20 cm proximal to the ileocecal valve is selected. This segment needs to be 20

to 40 cm in length depending on patient size, native bladder capacity, and desired capacity. **The segment should have an adequate mesentery to reach the native bladder easily.** After selecting the bowel segment, the mesentery is cleared from the bowel at each end for a short distance to create a window at each end. The bowel is divided at these ends, and a two-layer hand-sewn ileoileostomy or stapled anastomosis is performed. The ileal segment for augmentation is irrigated clear with 0.25% neomycin solution and is then opened on its antimesenteric border (Fig. 102–2A). **The ileum is then folded in a U shape most commonly, although it can be folded further with longer segments into an S or W configuration.** The ileum is anastomosed to itself with running absorbable suture (Fig. 102–2B). If not previously opened, the bladder is next incised in the sagittal plane extending near the bladder neck anteriorly and near the trigone posteriorly. The anastomosis of the ileum to the native bladder is technically easiest when started posteriorly and may be done in a one-layer or two-layer fashion (an inner layer of running interlocking 3–0 chromic and an outer layer of running 3–0 Vicryl suture) (Fig. 102–2C). A suprapubic tube is brought out through the native bladder and secured. The anterior layer of the anastomosis is then completed. Permanent suture should never be used for any cystoplasty to avoid a nidus for stone formation. The mesenteric window at the bowel anastomosis is closed. A drain is placed near the bladder and brought out of the pelvis through a separate stab incision. The wound is irrigated, and the abdomen is closed in layers.

Vesicoureteral Reflux

As a general rule, if vesicoureteral reflux exists, the authors recommend reimplantation of the ureter into the native bladder. If that is not possible, implantation into a bowel segment is necessary. Ileum is not the authors' choice for any tunneling procedure. **With short ureters, however, a tail of ileum can be useful to reach the foreshortened ureters. This requires creation of an ileal nipple valve to prevent reflux** as in the Kock or the hemi-Kock pouch. This type of reconstruction may require up to 60 cm of small intestine.

Cecocystoplasty, Ileocecocystoplasty

Technique

Use of the cecum for bladder augmentation dates back to Couvelaire's description in 1950. Numerous reports about simple cecocystoplasty have appeared in the literature since then. In the 1990s, simple cecocystoplasty is an uncommon operative procedure and is not discussed because it has largely been replaced by various forms of ileocecocystoplasty. In this procedure, the cecum is opened, reconfigured, and used to augment the bladder alone, leaving a segment of ileum to reach the ureters or create a continent abdominal stoma. Conversely, the ileal segment can be opened as well and used as a patch on the cecal segment before augmentation cystoplasty. There have been many descriptions of varying techniques of ileocecocystoplasty, but all start with mobilization of the cecum and right colon

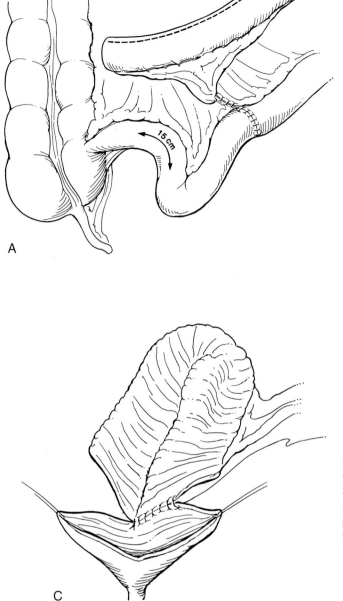

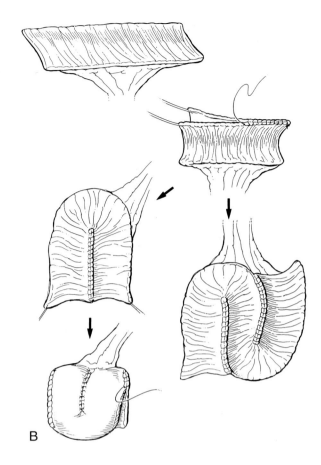

Figure 102–2. *A,* Ileocystoplasty. A 20- to 40-cm segment of ileum at least 15 cm from the ileocecal valve is removed and opened on its antimesenteric border. Ileoileostomy reconstitutes the bowel. *B,* The opened ileal segment should be reconfigured. This can be done in a U, S, or W configuration. It can be further folded as a cup patch. *C,* The reconfigured ileal segment is anastomosed to the native bladder.

by incising the peritoneum along the white line of Toldt to the hepatic flexure. Approximately 15 to 30 cm of the terminal ileum is used in this procedure. The length of ileal segment used depends on the technique employed. As with all intestinocystoplasties, before division of the bowel segment, it must be first demonstrated that it will easily reach the bladder (Fig. 102–3A).

The isolated ileocecal segment is irrigated clear with 0.25% neomycin solution and then opened on its antimesenteric border through its entirety, including the ileocecal valve. In the standard ileocecal augmentation, the ileal and cecal segments are of equivalent length such that the borders of the open segments can be anastomosed and then folded on themselves to form a cup for cystoplasty (Fig. 102–3B). This anastomosis of the reconfigured segments is done in either a one-layer or two-layer closure. The opening should

be left large enough to provide a wide anastomosis to the bivalved bladder. **If more volume is necessary, the ileal segment used can be significantly longer, allowing it to be folded before anastomosis to the cecum.** The MAINZ ileocecocystoplasty uses an ileal segment twice the length of the cecal segment. The opened edge of the cecal portion is anastomosed to the first portion of the ileal segment. The first and second portions of the ileal segment are then anastomosed together. This compound ileocecal patch is then anastomosed to the bladder (Fig. 102–4). The mesenteric window is closed, and a suprapubic tube is placed through the native bladder wall and secured to the abdominal wall.

Appendix

Continent urinary reservoirs, many of which are based on use of the appendix, currently enjoy a great deal of popular-

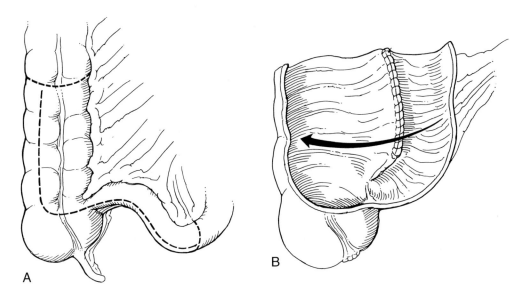

Figure 102–3. *A,* Ileocecocystoplasty. An ileocecal segment is selected. The length of segment chosen depends on the technique employed. After removal, it is opened on the antimesenteric border *(dashed lines). B,* The opened ileal and cecal segments are anastomosed to form a cup in the standard ileocecal cystoplasty.

ity. The appendix may be tunneled into the cecal segment or native bladder, or its junction with the cecum can be reinforced to provide a continence mechanism. The appendix may be brought to the abdominal wall as a catheterizable stoma. If the appendix is not to be used, an appendectomy is performed. After identification of the appropriate ileocecal segment, the bowel is divided, and an ileocolostomy is performed.

Ileocecal Valve

The ileocecal segment has found a great deal of use in the adult population undergoing reconstruction. It has been used much less frequently in children because the majority undergo augmentation for neurovesical dysfunction. Removal of the ileocecal valve in these children can result in intractable diarrhea (Gonzalez and Cabral, 1987; King, 1987). There are advantages to the use of the ileocecal segment. Antireflux tunnels can easily be performed into the cecum, and the ileum can be used to create a continent or antireflux nipple. Again for the short ureter, a tail of ileum can be left intact to reach the ureters. Cain and Husmann (1994) have proposed using the ileocecal segment as in the Indiana pouch for augmentation with the plicated ileal segment to the abdominal wall as a catheterizable stoma.

Sigmoid Cystoplasty

Technique

The use of the sigmoid colon for augmentation cystoplasty continues to be quite common. It was first reported in 1912 by Lemoine (Chargi et al, 1967). **Because of the strong unit contractions of the sigmoid, it is imperative to detubularize and reconfigure the segment to provide maximal compliance and disruption of contractions.** A sigmoid segment is selected and removed from the gastrointestinal tract, and a colocolostomy is performed (Fig. 102–5*A*). The sigmoid segment for augmentation is opened on its antimesenteric border. Sigmoid is generally reconfigured in one of two ways.

Fifteen to 20 cm of sigmoid colon is identified and mobilized by incising along the white line of Toldt. The mesentery is transilluminated to identify a vascular arcade for the use of the proposed segment. After identification of this vasculature, one must be certain again that this bowel segment can reach the bladder easily without tension. If so, the bowel segment is divided between bowel clamps, and a colocolostomy is performed. This colonic segment can be brought on either side of the reanastomosed bowel to reach the bladder successfully. The opened bowel segment is irrigated clear with 0.25% neomycin solution. The rest of the abdominal cavity is packed to prevent contamination from the opened sigmoid segment. Detubularization and reconfiguring is done at this time in a fashion determined by the surgeon's preference. The bowel-to-bowel reconfiguration is done in either a single-layer or a two-layer closure. This sigmoid flap is anastomosed to the bivalved bladder in a manner similar to that described previously for ileocystoplasty. Again a large-bore suprapubic tube is brought out through the native bladder and secured to the bladder and then the abdominal wall. Drains are placed as previously noted.

Reconfiguration of Sigmoid

Mitchell (1986) has popularized closing the two ends of the sigmoid segment and then opening the segment longitudinally opposite its blood supply. This segment easily fits on the bivalved bladder. The bowel segment fits in either the sagittal or the coronal plane (Fig. 102–5*B*). Sidi and colleagues have folded this in a U shape to provide a reconfigured patch similar to that described for ileocystoplasty (Sidi et al, 1987) (Fig. 102–5*C*). The basic procedures, however, are the same regardless of which type of reconfiguration is performed.

Gastrocystoplasty

Technique Using Antrum

Two basic techniques exist for the use of stomach in bladder augmentation. Leong and Ong (1972) first de-

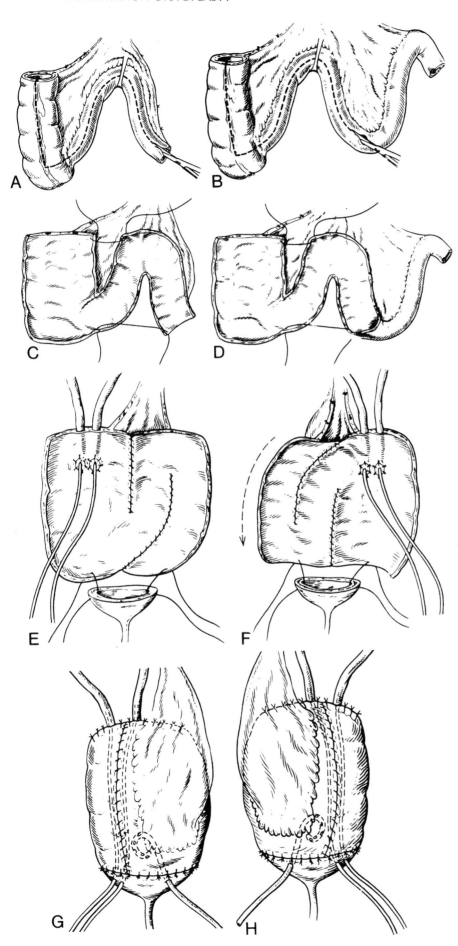

Figure 102–4. The MAINZ ileocecocystoplasty. The ileal segment is twice the length of the cecal segment (A and B). It is opened on the antimesenteric border (C and D). The ureters can be reimplanted into the opened cecal segment if necessary (E and F). The ileocecal segment is anastomosed to the native bladder (G and H). (From Thuroff JW, et al: *In* King LR, et al, eds: Bladder Reconstruction and Continent Urinary Diversion. Chicago, Year Book Medical Publishers, 1987.)

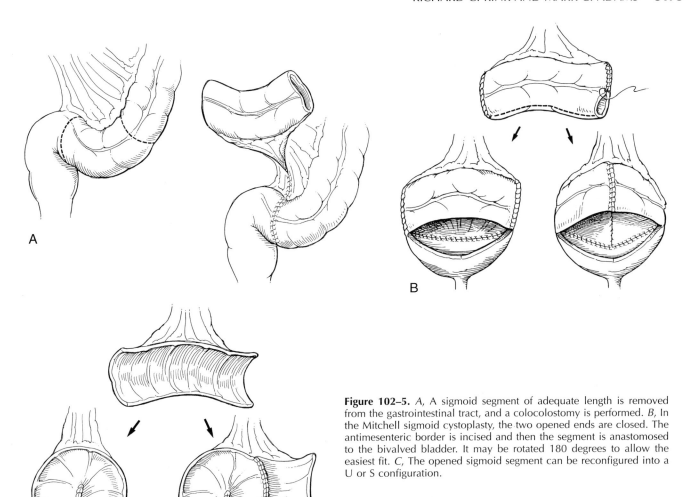

Figure 102–5. *A,* A sigmoid segment of adequate length is removed from the gastrointestinal tract, and a colocolostomy is performed. *B,* In the Mitchell sigmoid cystoplasty, the two opened ends are closed. The antimesenteric border is incised and then the segment is anastomosed to the bivalved bladder. It may be rotated 180 degrees to allow the easiest fit. *C,* The opened sigmoid segment can be reconfigured into a U or S configuration.

scribed the use of the entire gastric antrum with a small rim of body for bladder replacement. With this technique, the left gastroepiploic artery is always used as a vascular pedicle. If the right gastroepiploic artery is dominant and the left vessel ends high on the greater curvature, a strip of body along the greater curvature from the left gastroepiploic artery to the antrum is maintained for blood supply (Leong, 1988). Continuity of the gastrointestinal tract is restored by a Billroth I gastroduodenostomy.

Technique Using Body

Alternatively a gastric wedge based along the midportion of the greater curvature may be used (Adams et al, 1988) (Fig. 102–6A). **The gastric segment used in this technique is made up mainly of body and consequently has a higher concentration of acid-producing cells. The right or left gastroepiploic artery may be used as a vascular pedicle to this segment.** The right artery is more commonly dominant and thus more commonly used. The wedge-shaped segment of stomach includes both the anterior and the posterior wall of the stomach. **The segment used may be 10 to 20 cm in length along the greater curvature depending**

on patient age and size and the needed volume (Fig. 102–6B). **The incision into the stomach is stopped just short of the lesser curvature to avoid injury to the branches of the vagus nerve controlling gastric emptying.** Branches of the left gastric artery are suture ligated in situ just cephalad to the apex. This is done before incision to avoid significant bleeding. Parallel atraumatic bowel clamps are placed on each side of the gastric incisions to avoid excessive bleeding or spillage of gastric contents. Alternatively the stomach may be incised using a GIA stapling device that places a double row of staples on each side of the incision (Mitchell et al, 1992). The staple lines, however, must be excised in their entirety. The native stomach is closed in two layers using permanent sutures on the outer seromuscular layer.

Branches of the gastroepiploic artery to the antrum on the right or to the high corpus on the left are divided to provide mobilization of the isolated segment and pedicle. The pedicle must not be free floating within the peritoneum. The gastric segment and pedicle may be passed through windows in the transverse mesocolon and mesentery of the distal ileum and carefully secured to the posterior peritoneum. Despite careful consideration for an adequate pedicle length, the gastric

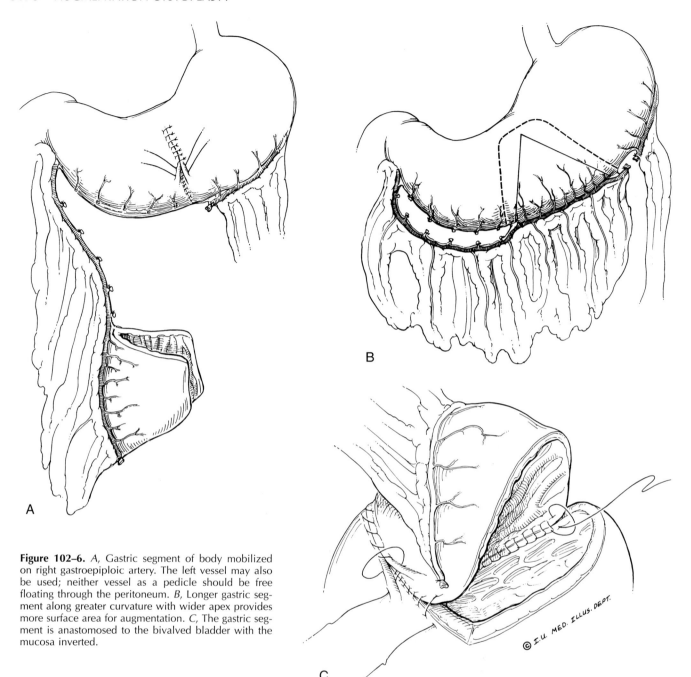

Figure 102–6. *A*, Gastric segment of body mobilized on right gastroepiploic artery. The left vessel may also be used; neither vessel as a pedicle should be free floating through the peritoneum. *B*, Longer gastric segment along greater curvature with wider apex provides more surface area for augmentation. *C*, The gastric segment is anastomosed to the bivalved bladder with the mucosa inverted.

segment initially does not reach the bladder without tension on occasion. Either gastroepiploic artery may be mobilized closer to its origin for further length. The first few branches from the gastroepiploic artery to the isolated gastric segment may also be divided to provide further mobilization. Because of the rich submucosal arterial plexus in the stomach, devascularization does not result. Rarely, it may be necessary to approximate some of the isolated gastric segment to itself in one corner. The gastric segment should be approximated to the native bladder using two layers of absorbable sutures, taking care to invert the mucosa (Fig. 102–6C).

Raz and colleagues and Lockhart and associates have described the use of a much longer, more narrow segment of stomach based along the greater curvature (Lockhart et al, 1993; Raz et al, 1993). Use of this segment, which includes

both body and antrum, somewhat narrows the lumen of the stomach along its entire length except at the fundus and pylorus. Raz and colleagues have isolated the segment using a GIA stapler so that the native stomach is never opened (Raz et al, 1993). The segment used in both of these series is similar to that first described by Sinaiko (1956), the first surgeon to use stomach for bladder replacement. **Postoperative bladder and gastric drainage is no different than that described previously for intestinocystoplasty.**

POSTOPERATIVE MANAGEMENT
Early Management

Care of patients following augmentation cystoplasty is similar regardless of the gastrointestinal segment used. **All** patients are maintained on nasogastric decompression until bowel function recovers, including patients following gastrocystoplasty. Attention to fluid and electrolyte management is important because third space losses may be significant after extensive reconstructive surgery. Continuous drainage of the bladder is achieved by suprapubic cystostomy. Mucus production from small or large bowel segments may be excessive and can potentially occlude the drainage catheter. **The suprapubic tube should be irrigated at least three times daily and whenever drainage is slowed by mucus.** A cystogram is usually performed before patient discharge, although suprapubic drainage is continued until approximately 3 weeks after augmentation cystoplasty. All patients are then started on CIC every 2 to 3 hours during the day and one to two times at night. The suprapubic tube is removed after catheterization is successfully underway and well tolerated. The time between catheterizations is gradually stretched out over several weeks but should not exceed 4 to 5 hours during the day. Patients without neurologic impairment may eventually attempt to void spontaneously. All must check postvoid residual volumes and continue catheterizations if the residuals are significant.

Late Management

Routine radiographic surveillance of the upper urinary tract is indicated at 6 weeks, 6 months, and 1 year following augmentation cystoplasty. Likewise, serum electrolytes, BUN, and creatinine levels along with urine cultures are performed at 3-month intervals during the first year following surgery. Evaluation by ultrasonography and serum chemistries is then appropriate once a year. Eventually, yearly endoscopy for tumor surveillance should be performed.

RESULTS AND COMPLICATIONS OF CYSTOPLASTY

The effect of augmentation cystoplasty on the patient should be considered in two main categories. One must first consider the effect of removing a relatively small segment of the gastrointestinal tract for use in the lower urinary tract. **Any more than rare development of gastrointestinal problems would be prohibitive,** even if results were perfect from the standpoint of the urinary bladder. Second, the effect of augmentation cystoplasty on the urinary bladder must be reviewed. The primary goal of augmentation is to construct a compliant urinary reservoir; therefore, **the primary consideration after augmentation is the compliance that is achieved. Any other effect on the urinary bladder is a side effect or complication that exists because bowel is not a perfect physiologic substitute for native bladder.**

Gastrointestinal Effects

Bowel Obstruction

Postoperative bowel obstruction is uncommon after augmentation cystoplasty. Obstruction has occurred in approximately 3% of patients after augmentation (Gear-

hart et al, 1986; King, 1987; Mitchell and Piser, 1987; Hollensbe et al, 1992; Rink et al, 1995). The rate of obstruction is equivalent to or better than that noted after conduit diversion or continent urinary diversion (McDougal, 1992). Delicate handling of tissues, closure of mesenteric windows, and elimination of sites of internal herniation help to avoid obstructions. The incidence of bowel obstruction is low regardless of the gastrointestinal segment used and should not influence the choice of a particular segment for enterocystoplasty.

Diarrhea

Reports of chronic diarrhea after bladder augmentation alone have been rare. Diarrhea can occur after removal of large segments of ileum from the gastrointestinal tract, although the segments typically used for augmentation rarely are problematic unless other problems coexist. Likewise, resection of a typical colonic segment for augmentation only rarely results in a change in bowel function and is probably less of a risk than the use of ileum. **Removal of the ileocecal valve from the gastrointestinal tract is most likely to cause diarrhea.** King (1987) has noted that 10% of children with neurogenic dysfunction have significant diarrhea after ileocecal valve resection. Patients with neurogenic impairment depend on controlled constipation for fecal continence.

Removal of the ileocecal valve from the gastrointestinal tract may significantly decrease bowel transit time. Loss can also allow bacterial backflow into the ileum, in which the organisms may interfere with fat and vitamin B_{12} metabolism.

Vitamin B_{12} Deficiency

Ileum is the sole site of vitamin B_{12} absorption. **Removal of the distal ileum from the gastrointestinal tract may therefore result in vitamin B_{12} deficiency and megaloblastic anemia. Certainly the terminal 15 to 18 cm of ileum should not be used for augmentation, although problems may arise even if that segment is preserved.** Thirty-five percent of patients followed over 5 years after a Kock pouch were found to be deficient in vitamin B_{12} in one series (Akerlund et al, 1989). In general, the length of ileum used for augmentation is less than one half of that used for a Kock pouch, so that vitamin B_{12} deficiency seems unlikely following routine bladder augmentation with ileum. Canning and associates evaluated 26 patients after bladder augmentation or replacement and found no patient with either fat malabsorption or vitamin B_{12} deficiency (Canning et al, 1989). Only three patients, however, were followed longer than 3 years, and longer observation is necessary because existing body vitamin B_{12} stores may last considerably longer (Rowland, 1991). Eventually, determinations of vitamin B_{12} levels or injections of the vitamin may be appropriate after ileocystoplasty.

Bladder Compliance After Augmentation

Compliance

One lesson learned from past clinical experience with augmentation cystoplasty has been the value of detubularization and reconfiguration of the bowel segment (Hinman, 1988; Koff, 1988). **Bowel in its native, tubular form continues to demonstrate peristalsis or mass contraction. The tubular form also does not maximize the volume achieved for the surface area of bowel used.** Although many patients who underwent augmentation cystoplasty with a tubular segment of bowel have done well, there have also been failures caused by continued pressure rises in the bladder. Some surgeons have concluded that ileum is superior to other segments in terms of compliance after augmentation (Goldwasser and Webster, 1986; Rink and McLaughlin, 1994); however, good results have been achieved with all bowel in most cases, and it is more important to use a bowel segment well than to choose a particular bowel segment.

Lytton and Green (1989) demonstrated mass contractions generating pressure of 60 to 110 cm H_2O in right colon reservoirs, despite detubularization. Such pressures approach those observed in native cecum (Jakobsen et al, 1987). Hedlund and co-workers, however, reported pressures in detubularized cecum of only 25 cm H_2O 1 year postoperatively (Hedlund et al, 1984). Patching a cecal segment with ileum may be a more effective means of decreasing mass contractions than simple reconfiguration (Thuroff et al, 1987). Sidi and associates demonstrated peak bladder pressures of 41 cm H_2O following cup-patch sigmoid cystoplasty in the first postoperative year; these improved with time (Sidi et al, 1986). A comparison of enterocystoplasty using detubularized ileum and detubularized colon demonstrated contractions greater than 15 cm H_2O in 42% of patients after ileocystoplasty versus 60% of those with colocystoplasties (Goldwasser et al, 1987). Significant contractions, defined as those greater than 40 cm H_2O at a volume less than 200 ml, were not noted in any of the ileal augmentations but persisted in 10% of cecal augmentations. In continent urinary diversions, ileal reservoirs have been noted to have lower basal pressures and less motor activity (Berglund et al, 1987).

Uninhibited Contractions

Rhythmic contractions after augmentation have also been noted following gastrocystoplasty. In virtually all cases following gastrocystoplasty, as with other intestinal segments, an adequate bladder volume is achieved with a flat tonus limb (Adams et al, 1988; Atala et al, 1993; Gosalbez et al, 1993a). Rhythmic sinusoidal contractions, however, have been noted in all three series in up to 62% of patients. The segment of stomach initially described for augmentation was much smaller in surface area when compared to segments of ileum or colon commonly used for augmentation. Since observing these contractions, Adams and colleagues have used a slightly larger gastric segment that is longer along the greater curvature and noted improved urodynamics following augmentation, with less prominent contractions (Adams et al, 1995).

For most patients, these differences in pressure contractions noted urodynamically are of theoretical interest only and have not affected the clinical result. Contractions that begin at low amplitude later in filling and progress in amplitude only near capacity may be of no clinical significance at all. In the authors' series of patients (Hollensbe et al, 1992; Rink et al, 1995), 11 of 234 patients demonstrated contractions of clinical significance after augmentation cystoplasty.

The contractions appeared to result in persistent incontinence, delayed perforation, or vesicoureteral reflux. The segments used for primary augmentation in those 11 patients include sigmoid colon in 5 patients, stomach in 4 patients, ileum in 2 patients, and cecum in 1 patient. A secondary patch augmentation has improved the clinical status and urodynamic findings in eight of nine patients.

Metabolic Complications

Chloride Absorption and Acidosis

The development of hyperchloremic metabolic acidosis related to the storage of urine in intestinal segments was first recognized in 1950 after ureterosigmoidostomy (Ferris and Odel, 1950). The metabolic derangements were marked by patient fatigue, weakness, anorexia, and polydipsia. **Koch and McDougal (1985) nicely demonstrated the mechanisms by which acid was resorbed from urine by intestinal segments.** Resorption in the form of ammonium basically results in chronic acid loading, although in patients with normal renal function, the kidneys are generally able to handle the resorbed load of chloride and acid without frank acidosis. **Mitchell and Piser (1987) noted that essentially every patient after augmentation with an intestinal segment had an increase in serum chloride and a decrease in serum bicarbonate level, although acidosis was rare if the patient's renal function was normal.** Such trends of increased serum chloride and decreased serum bicarbonate have been noted with ileal conduits (Malek et al, 1971) and continent urinary reservoirs as well (Allen et al, 1985; McDougal, 1986; Ashken, 1987; Thuroff et al, 1987; Boyd et al, 1989). More severe electrolyte disturbances requiring treatment despite normal renal function have been reported (Schmidt et al, 1973; Whitmore and Gittes, 1983). Such derangements may be debilitating to the patient if not recognized, and patient death has been reported (Heidler et al, 1979). **Hall and colleagues have noted that there is an increase in the urinary acid load with wasting of bony buffers even in the absence of frank acidosis** (Hall et al, 1991). Such wasting may result in bone demineralization, which could potentially cause retarded growth in children after augmentation cystoplasty. Patients with acidosis should receive bicarbonate therapy. Whether all patients with intestine in the lower urinary tract might benefit from supplemental bicarbonate is controversial. In severe cases, chloride transport can be blocked with chlorpromazine and nicotinic acid.

Although jejunum is rarely used for bladder reconstruction, storage of urine in this segment results in a unique metabolic pattern. Hyponatremic, hypochloremic, and hyperkalemic acidosis can result and are often associated with significant hypovolemia.

Chloride Secretion

Gastric mucosa acts as a barrier to chloride and acid resorption after its incorporation in the bladder and, in fact, secretes hydrochloric acid (Piser et al, 1987). This difference was the primary factor in the initial consideration of stomach for use in the urinary tract. The secretory nature of the gastric segment was shown to be beneficial in azotemic dogs during acid loading (Piser et al, 1987; Kennedy et al, 1988). **Serum chloride does decrease and serum bicarbonate does increase slightly after gastrocystoplasty whether using antrum or corpus in patients with normal and impaired renal function** (Adams et al, 1988; Ganesan et al, 1991). In a series of 21 patients with renal insufficiency, serum bicarbonate improved in all patients except one after gastrocystoplasty, and many patients requiring oral bicarbonate therapy before augmentation did not do so after gastrocystoplasty (Ganesan et al, 1991). Similar results have been noted in a smaller group of patients with renal failure (Sheldon and Gilbert, 1991).

Alkalosis

The secretory nature of gastric mucosa, however, may at times be detrimental to the patient and results in two unique complications of gastrocystoplasty. The authors have noted severe episodes of hypokalemic, hypochloremic metabolic alkalosis after an acute gastrointestinal illness in 5 of 37 patients following gastrocystoplasty (Hollensbe et al, 1992). These episodes were severe enough to require hospitalization in all cases and have been recurrent in two patients. Three of these five patients had significant renal insufficiency and would not have been candidates for augmentation with other segments. Ganesan and associates noted similar episodes of alkalosis in 5 of 21 patients with renal insufficiency after gastrocystoplasty (Ganesan et al, 1991). **Apparently, those patients with the primary indication for the use of stomach may be the ones at greatest risk for this complication.** It has been proposed that the alkalosis results from ongoing chloride loss from the gastric segment in the bladder in the face of decreased oral intake. McDougal (1992) suggested that decreased ability to excrete bicarbonate from an impaired kidney may be primarily responsible for the problem. Gosalbez and associates, however, demonstrated persistently increased fractional excretion of chloride despite profound hypochloremia, suggesting that inappropriate gastric secretion may be a primary problem (Gosalbez et al, 1993b). One patient in that series eventually required resection of three quarters of the gastric segment because of recurrent problems. All patients with stomach in the urinary tract should be made aware of this potential derangement.

Hematuria and Dysuria Syndrome

The secretory nature of gastric mucosa may result in another unique problem, the hematuria and dysuria syndrome. Nguyen and co-workers have characterized this syndrome well (Nguyen et al, 1993). **All patients after gastrocystoplasty, particularly those with normal sensation, have occasional hematuria or dysuria with voiding or catheterization beyond that which is expected with other intestinal segments. All patients should be warned of this potential problem, although in most patients these symptoms are intermittent, are mild, and do not require treatment.** In Nguyen and co-workers' experience, 36% of patients have developed signs or symptoms of the hematuria and dysuria syndrome (Nguyen et al, 1993). Fourteen percent of patients have required medications, 9% on a regular basis. Nguyen and co-workers believe that patients who are

incontinent or have decreased renal function are at increased risk for these symptoms. In the authors' experience, 35% of patients have required medications at least on an intermittent basis, and 8% of patients have required long-term medications for the problem (Hollensbe et al, 1992; Rink et al, 1995). It is the authors' experience, and that of Nguyen and colleagues, that the symptoms of the hematuria and dysuria do respond well to H_2 blockers and hydrogen ion pump blockers. Bladder irrigation with baking soda may also be effective. **It has been demonstrated that urinary pH may decrease remarkably after meals following gastrocystoplasty** (Bogaert et al, 1995). The signs and symptoms of the hematuria and dysuria syndrome are most likely secondary to acid irritation. Such problems are less frequent but can occur after antral cystoplasty (Ngan et al, 1993).

Leong first noted glanular excoriation after gastrocystoplasty in one patient with voiding symptoms (Ngan et al, 1993). The authors have noted similar meatal irritation in two patients after gastrocystoplasty; both have had significant dysuria. Nguyen and associates have noted skin excoriation in 8 of 57 patients after gastrocystoplasty; all 8 patients had some element of urinary incontinence (Nguyen et al, 1993). **It is imperative to achieve urinary continence in patients undergoing gastrocystoplasty because urinary leakage not only may result in the exposure of the skin to gastric secretions but also may result in gastric secretions that are poorly diluted and buffered by less urine in the bladder.** Such dilution and buffering is important because Reinberg and co-workers have noted a perforation of a gastric segment in a defunctionalized bladder after gastrocystoplasty (Reinberg et al, 1992). They evaluated the influence of urine on gastrocystoplasties in dogs (Castro-Diaz et al, 1992). In their experience, all dogs developed marked inflammation of the gastric segment and native bladder after creation of a dry gastrocystoplasty, and three of nine dogs developed ulceration and perforation. Use of H_2 blockers resulted in some protection for these animals; however, such a clinical situation in humans should certainly be avoided. The authors have not noted any ulceration of a gastric segment or native bladder at cystoscopy in any patient with or without the hematuria and dysuria syndrome.

Tumor Formation

Another well-recognized complication of ureterosigmoidostomy has been the development of tumors at the ureterocolonic anastomotic site. In Husmann and Spence's (1990) review of reported tumors after ureterosigmoidostomy, the latency period for development of such tumors averaged 26 years and ranged from 3 to 53 years. Adenocarcinomas were the prominent tumors that developed, but benign polyps and other types of carcinoma were also noted. It has been estimated that the risk for developing such tumors increases 7000-fold over age-matched controls after ureterosigmoidostomy (Eraklus and Folkman, 1978). The exact etiology of such tumors is unknown; however, N-nitrosocompounds thought to originate from the admixture of urine and feces may be carcinogenic. These compounds have been noted in the urine of patients with conduit diversions and augmentation (Treiger and Marshall, 1991). Husmann and Spence (1990) have suggested that these compounds are more likely enhancing agents rather than a lone cause for tumor development. It has also been proposed that inflammatory reaction at the anastomotic site may induce growth factor production, which, in turn, increases cellular proliferation and nitrosamine or oxygen free radical production. **Filmer and Spencer (1990) identified 14 patients with tumor formation in an augmented bladder.** Nine of these tumors occurred in patients after ileocystoplasty and five after colocystoplasty. **Experimental work in the rat has demonstrated hyperplastic growth in the augmented bladder using all intestinal segments, with no segment showing any particular increased risk** (Klee et al, 1990; Buson et al, 1993; Spencer et al, 1993; Little et al, 1994). The applicability of such findings to humans is uncertain. The long latency noted for tumor development after ureterosigmoidostomy suggests that short-term follow-up looking for tumors after augmentation cystoplasty is not adequate. **Patients undergoing augmentation cystoplasty should be made aware of this potential risk. Yearly surveillance of the augmented bladder with endoscopy should eventually be performed.**

Mucus

Gastrointestinal segments continue to produce mucus after placement in the urinary tract. Mucus can potentially impede bladder drainage by spontaneous voiding or CIC, particularly in pediatric patients in whom the use of small-caliber catheters is necessary. Mucus may also serve as a nidus for infection or stone formation when it remains in the bladder for a long period of time. Mucus production increases with urinary tract infections, particularly after colocystoplasty. Kulb and associates have shown experimentally in dogs that colonic segments produce more mucus than ileum and that stomach produces the least amount of mucus (Kulb et al, 1986). This has been noted clinically by the authors as well. Most patients do not require any bladder irrigations for mucus after gastrocystoplasty. Villous atrophy in the ileum has been noted with long-term storage of urine. It has been suggested that such atrophy may result in decreased mucus production (Gearhart, 1987), although Murray and colleagues were unable to demonstrate any decrease in mucus production with time in ileal or cecal segments (Murray et al, 1987). Hendren and Hendren (1990) noted a decrease in mucus production from colonic segments following colocystoplasty over time; however, amounts were not quantitated, and this has not been the authors' experience (Rink et al, 1995). Glandular atrophy in colonic mucosa has not been noted histologically (Mansson et al, 1984). **Routine use of daily bladder irrigations to prevent mucus buildup often prevents complications related to mucus from any intestinal segment.**

Urinary Tract Infections

Bacteriuria is quite common following intestinocystoplasty (Gearhart et al, 1986; Hendren and Hendren, 1990; King, 1991). More recent experience with bowel neobladders has demonstrated that patients who are able to void well and empty a bowel bladder spontaneously generally maintain sterile urine. The major difference in the groups of patients is the requirement of CIC in most to empty after bladder augmentation because of their underlying problem. **It appears that the use of CIC is a prominent factor in the development of bacteriuria in these patients.** Bacteriuria has been noted even when patients are maintained on daily antibiotics in the face of catheterizations (Gearhart et al, 1986). In Hirst's (1991) experience, persistent or recurrent bacteriuria occurred in 50% of patients augmented with sigmoid colon versus 25% of those following ileocystoplasty. Hollensbe and co-workers noted asymptomatic bacteriuria much more commonly in patients requiring CIC (Hollensbe et al, 1992). Symptomatic episodes of cystitis occurred in 23% of their patients after ileocystoplasty, compared to 17% of patients after sigmoid cystoplasty, 13% after cecocystoplasty, and 8% after gastrocystoplasty. Febrile urinary tract infections occurred in 13% of those 231 patients after augmentation. The same trend among different bowel segments was noted for these febrile infections. There was no statistically significant difference, however, among the various enteric segments. **The incidence of pyelonephritis is quite similar to that noted for conduit diversion, whether refluxing or not** (McDougal, 1992).

Not every episode of asymptomatic bacteriuria needs treatment in patients requiring CIC. **Certainly, bacteriuria should be treated if symptoms such as incontinence, suprapubic pain, hematuria, foul-smelling urine, or remarkably increased mucus production result. Bacteriuria requires treatment if the urine culture demonstrates growth of a urea-splitting organism that may predispose to stone formation.** To help avoid infection, patients requiring CIC must perform it on a regular basis and work to empty the bladder completely. This includes periodic irrigation of mucus, which can occlude the catheter and result in residual urine. Special care must be taken by patients catheterizing through a continent abdominal wall stoma, who may have more difficulty completely emptying the bladder but who can empty well with effort (Ludlow et al, 1995). Although catheterization is not a sterile technique, proper clean technique should be stressed.

Calculi

Bladder calculi have been noted with increasing frequency in series of patients following augmentation cystoplasty. Hendren and Hendren (1990) and Hirst (1991) noted bladder calculi in 18% of patients after augmentation. Blythe and associates noted calculus formation in 30% of 87 patients, with those patients catheterizing through an abdominal wall stoma having the highest risk (Blythe et al, 1992). Such patients may have a more difficult time emptying the bladder because the catheter is not as dependent. Palmer and co-workers noted urolithiasis in 52% of patients, whereas the authors have noted only an 8% rate of bladder stone formation in 231 patients following enterocystoplasty (Palmer et al, 1993; Rink et al, 1995). The reason for these remarkable differences is not clear. **The overwhelming majority of stones in this patient population are struvite in composition, and bacteriuria is an important risk factor.** Any infection with a urea-splitting organism should be treated aggressively. Care must be taken to make sure that all patients requiring CIC, particularly those who have already formed stones, make every effort to empty the bladder completely with each catheterization. The association of urinary stasis with stone formation is well established. Routine bladder irrigations to avoid buildup of inspissated mucus may remove a nidus for stone formation. Stones have been noted after the use of all intestinal segments with no significant difference noted between segments except that no struvite stone has been noted after gastrocystoplasty (Hirst, 1991; Hollensbe et al, 1992; Blythe et al, 1992; Palmer et al, 1993). A single uric acid stone has been noted in a bladder after gastrocystoplasty (Garzotto and Walker, 1995). Clearly, foreign bodies serve as a nidus for stone formation, and the use of permanent suture or staples should be avoided during enterocystoplasty.

Delayed Spontaneous Bladder Perforation

Incidence

Perhaps the most disturbing complication of augmentation cystoplasty is delayed bladder perforation. This problem has been noted with increasing frequency in all gastrointestinal segments (Elder et al, 1988; Rink et al, 1988; Rushton et al, 1988; Sheiner and Kaplan, 1988; Rosen and Light, 1991; Hollensbe et al, 1992). Early postoperative leaks from the bowel-to-bladder anastomosis after augmentation cystoplasty are rare and represent a technical error or problem with early healing (Hollensbe et al, 1992). **Delayed perforations more commonly occur within a bowel segment and represent a problem with long-term storage of urine within bowel.** There may be no particular increased risk of one intestinal segment over another. At Riley Children's Hospital, perforations were noted in 22 of 264 patients undergoing augmentation cystoplasty (Rink et al, 1992). Multivariant analysis of the patients noted that the use of sigmoid colon was the only significant increased risk in that series. Several other large series of patients with sigmoid cystoplasty have noted a low incidence of delayed perforation (Sidi et al, 1987; Hendren and Hendren, 1990). At the Boston Children's Hospital, the incidence of perforation has been highest in ileum (9.3%) following augmentation; perforations have occurred after 4.3% of ileocecal cystoplasties, 4.2% of sigmoid augmentations, and 2.9% of gastrocystoplasties (Bauer et al, 1992).

Presentation and Diagnosis

Patients presenting with spontaneous perforation are generally quite ill with abdominal pain, distention, and fever. Sepsis has not been uncommon. Nausea and vomiting, decreased urine output, and shoulder pain from diaphragmatic irritation have all been noted frequently. **Patients with neurogenic dysfunction often have impaired lower abdominal sensation and present later in the course of the illness.** Patients with perforation after gastrocystoplasty often present promptly owing to acid irritation of the peritoneum. **A high index of suspicion for the diagnosis is necessary. Series have demonstrated that contrast cystography is diagnostic in most cases** (Braverman and Lebowitz, 1991; Rosen and Light, 1991; Bauer et al, 1992). Braverman and Lebowitz (1991) noted that the technique of cystography is important. Earlier reports of perforations noted a significant false-negative rate on cystography (Rushton et al, 1988; Sheiner and Kaplan, 1988) and suggested that ultrasonography and computed tomography improve diagnostic accuracy. They recommended that one of those studies be done in any child suspected to have a perforation if the initial cystogram is negative.

Etiology

The etiology of delayed perforations within a bowel segment is unknown. Several early reports suggested that perforation might be secondary to traumatic catheterization (Elder et al, 1988; Rushton et al, 1988). Perforation of a bladder not previously augmented has been recognized after catheterization (Reisman and Preminger, 1989), although it seems unlikely that catheterization trauma is the lone cause in most patients. The location of perforations has been variable among patients and even in a single patient with multiple perforations. Rosen and Light (1991) have reported perforations in three patients after augmentation who did not catheterize at all. Trauma to the bowel because of fixed adhesions resulting in shearing forces with emptying and filling of the bladder has also been suggested as an etiology (Elder et al, 1988). Chronic urinary tract infection with transmural infection of the bowel wall has also been proposed as an etiology in some patients. **Crane and associates reviewed histologic sections of bowel segments adjacent to areas of perforation and noted necrosis, vascular congestion, hemorrhage, and hemosiderin deposition compatible with chronic bowel wall ischemia** (Crane et al, 1991). **Chronic overdistention of the bladder might result in such ischemia.** Experimentally, Essig and co-workers noted decreased perfusion in dog bowel used for augmentation with high intravesical pressure (Essig et al, 1991). These changes were noted most prominently at the antimesenteric border of the bowel. It does appear that chronic ischemia may play a significant role in at least some bladder perforations.

Anderson and Rickwood (1991) reported three perforations occurring in bladders with significant hyperreflexia after augmentation. **They suggested that high outflow resistance might maintain pressure generated in the bladder rather than allowing urinary leakage and venting of the pressure.** Persistent hyperreflexia after augmentation has been noted in several other patients after perforation (Bauer et al, 1992; Rink et al, 1992). Hyperreflexia alone is not a common cause because spontaneous bladder perforation was essentially never recognized in the era before bowel detubularization and reconfiguration, when persistent hyperreflexia was more common after augmentation cystoplasty. **Once bowel is reconfigured, however, it may be more prone to ischemia if high pressure does persist.** The majority of patients suffering perforations have had myelodysplasia. The role of neurogenic dysfunction in the etiology of perforations is unclear. No matter what the etiology, there is likely some field effect on the entire bowel segment. Once a patient has suffered a spontaneous perforation, the chance of a recurrence is significant (Hollensbe et al, 1992). Consideration must eventually be given to removal and replacement of a segment after recurrent perforation.

Treatment

The standard of treatment for documented spontaneous perforation of the augmented bladder has been surgical repair, as it is for an intraperitoneal leak of the bladder following trauma. Slaton and Kropp (1994) reported a series of conservative management for suspected perforations. Their use of catheter drainage, antibiotics, and serial abdominal examinations was successful in 87% of cases, although only 2 of their 13 patients with suspected ruptures had x-ray documentation of perforation. Such management is a consideration in a stable patient with sterile urine; however, the surgeon should certainly have a low threshold for surgical exploration and repair. The majority of perforations have occurred in myelomeningocele patients who generally present late in the course of the disease owing to impaired sensation. Sepsis is not uncommon at presentation, and death of the patient may result from a delay in diagnosis or treatment.

ALTERNATIVES TO GASTROINTESTINOCYSTOPLASTY

Theoretical Considerations

Because of the significant number of complications and side effects related to removal of a gastrointestinal segment or its incorporation into the urinary tract, many surgeons have searched for alternative ways to achieve a large-capacity, highly compliant reservoir. These efforts have covered the spectrum from synthetic materials and autologous grafts to augment the bladder, some of which act as a biodegradable scaffold for regeneration, to creation of a bladder diverticulum (autoaugmentation) and to various forms of neural stimulation. **Some of these alternatives appear to hold great promise, but none have stood the test of time for true comparison to intestinocystoplasty.**

An ideal tissue for increasing capacity and improving compliance would have transitional epithelium so as to be relatively impermeable and avoid electrolyte changes and be free of mucus production or increased tumor potential. Avoidance of violation of the peritoneal cavity would also decrease morbidity. A native urinary tract tissue could meet such criteria. Two alternative procedures are ureterocystoplasty and autoaugmentation. With ureterocystoplasty, there is good muscle backing of transitional epithelium, whereas collagen backs the transitional mucosa of an autoaugmentation.

Ureterocystoplasty

Results

It has been noted now for some time that in patients with posterior urethral valves, unilateral reflux may behave as a "pop-off" valve to lower intravesical pressures and protect the contralateral upper tract (Hoover and

Duckett, 1982; Rittendberg et al, 1988; Kaefer et al, 1994). In many of these patients, the refluxing ureter is massively dilated, draining a poorly functioning or nonfunctioning kidney. **It is a logical extension to use this ureteral tissue to augment the bladder.** Early reports suggested this could be technically achieved after nephrectomy by bivalving the bladder through the ureterovesical junction and laying in the opened ureter (Mitchell et al, 1992; Bellinger, 1993). Later reports have modified and improved this procedure by noting that with meticulous surgical technique, the vascularity to the entire renal pelvis could be preserved, allowing more tissue for ureterocystoplasty (Churchill et al, 1993; Landau et al, 1994; McKenna and Bauer, 1995; Reinberg et al, 1995). Furthermore, as with intestinocystoplasty, folding this ureter into a more spherical configuration, which is now standard technique, maximizes the volume that can be stored. In the massively dilated ureter draining a functioning kidney, the distal ureter alone may be used for augmentation with the proximal ureter either reimplanted into the bladder or anastomosed to the contralateral ureter (transureteroureterostomy) (Bellinger, 1993). More than 50 patients have been reported after bladder augmentation using ureter, some with follow-up as long as 5 years (Mitchell et al, 1992; Bellinger, 1993, 1995; Churchill et al, 1993; Wolf and Turzan, 1993; Dewan et al, 1994a; Hitchcock et al, 1994; Landau et al, 1994; Lindgren and Flom, 1995; Reinberg et al, 1995). The upper tracts have remained stable or improved in all patients. Complications have been uncommon, with only a rare early extravasation of urine being noted (Churchill et al, 1993). Landau and colleagues reported a comparison of age-matched and diagnosis-matched children having ureterocystoplasty or ileocystoplasty (Landau et al, 1994). **The total mean bladder capacity was 417 ml in the ureterocystoplasty group and 381 ml in the ileocystoplasty group. Bladder volumes at 30 cm H_2O were 413 ml and 380 ml after ureterocystoplasty and ileocystoplasty, respectively.** Ureter seemingly provided both volume and compliance. There was one failure from a compliance standpoint in a child in whom the distal ureter did not provide enough volume. The main disadvantage to ureterocystoplasty is that the patient population with a nonfunctioning kidney draining into a megaureter is limited. McKenna and Bauer (1995) have now reported the use of a normal-size ureter with success. Atala and colleagues presented an experimental technique to dilate slowly a normal ureter for later use (Atala et al, 1994). For clinical use, this research model needs modification.

This procedure using a megaureter has been universally successful in the authors' hands (Rink, 1995). There are no electrolyte or mucus problems created by the procedure because the lining is urothelial. One patient with severe renal insufficiency has developed to renal failure as expected but has had successful renal transplantation into the ureterally augmented bladder. The ultimate success using normal size ureters for augmentation requires further study.

Technique

Generally, ureterocystoplasty is performed through a midline, intraperitoneal incision after bowel preparation. This provides access to the intestine should mobilization of the ureter for augmentation prove unsuccessful. **Bellinger**

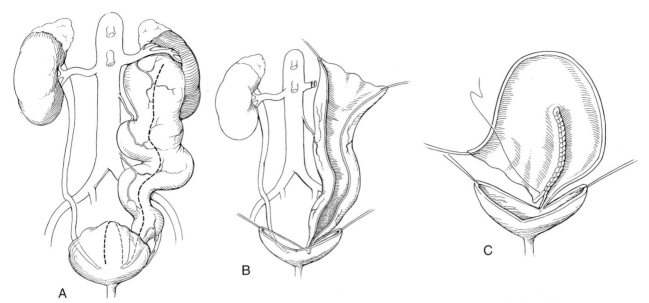

Figure 102–7. *A,* After nephrectomy, the bladder is bivalved, with the posterior aspect of the incision carried off the midline to enter the ureteral orifice. The ureter is not detached from the bladder. *B,* The ureter is opened opposite its main blood supply. *C,* The ureter is reconfigured into a U similar to intestinocystoplasty.

(1993), Dewan and colleagues (1994a), and Reinberg and colleagues (1995), however, have shown that this can be done through two incisions, remaining extraperitoneal (flank or posterior lumbotomy for nephrectomy and Pfannenstiel for the augmentation). In both situations, the technique is the same. A standard nephrectomy is performed with great care to preserve the renal pelvic and upper ureteral blood supply. All tissue is swept from the peritoneum toward the ureter during ureteral mobilization with care to protect the ureteral blood supply, which arises medially in the proximal ureter. As the ureter enters the true pelvis, the blood supply arises posterolaterally. After mobilization of the ureter into the pelvis, the bladder is opened in the sagittal plane. Posteriorly, this incision is carried off-center directly into the ureteral orifice of the ureter used for augmentation. This bivalves the bladder. The ureter is *not* detached from the bladder but is then opened longitudinally along its entire length, taking care to avoid its main blood supply (Fig. 102–7*A* and *B*). The ureter is folded upon itself and the ureter-to-ureter (Fig. 102–7*C*) and ureter-to-bladder anastomosis is performed with running-interlocking absorbable suture. A suprapubic tube is left indwelling through the native bladder and remains indwelling for 3 weeks, at which time ICC is started.

Autoaugmentation

Techniques and Results

Cartwright and Snow (1989a, 1989b) reported an ingenious way to improve bladder compliance and capacity using native urothelial tissue in an effort to avoid the complications of gastric or intestinocystoplasty. In their procedure, known as *autoaugmentation,* they excise the detrusor muscle over the dome of the bladder, leaving the mucosa intact to protrude as a wide-mouthed diverticulum. Initially a midline bladder muscle-only incision is made (Fig. 102–8*A*). Aided

by having the bladder filled with saline, the muscle is excised laterally in each direction from the bulging mucosa (Fig. 102–8*B*). The lateral edges of the detrusor muscle are secured to the psoas muscle bilaterally to prevent collapse of the diverticulum (Fig. 102–8*C*). Their early experience noted compliance to be improved in four of five patients, with capacity increasing in three of five (Cartwright and Snow, 1989a).

This procedure has since been modified by a number of surgeons, each providing a different name for the procedure depending on whether the detrusor muscle is simply incised to allow the mucosa to bulge or excised to create the diverticulum. In an effort to determine if incision or excision provided superior results, Johnson and co-workers performed 16 vesicomyotomies and 16 vesicomyectomies in rabbits after previously having reduced the bladder capacity (Johnson et al, 1994). Functional bladder capacity in these animals increased by 43.5%, and leak point pressure decreased by an average of 48%, but there was no statistical difference between the two groups. Armed with these findings in animals, they performed vesicomyotomy (incision) in 12 patients with neurogenic bladders and demonstrated a mean increase in capacity of 40% and a mean decrease in leak point pressure of 33% (Stothers et al, 1994). They again believed that detrusor excision offered no advantage over incision in humans. All patients demonstrated some increase in capacity (15%–70%), and no patient in early follow-up clinically deteriorated, requiring enterocystoplasty.

Detrusorectomy, leaving a small cap of muscle at the dome through which a suprapubic tube is placed, has been reported by Landa and Moorhead (1994). **They have been concerned that although these procedures usually improve compliance, increase in volume is "modest at best." The same findings have been noted by Cartwright and Snow** (personal communication, 1995). In a report of 12 detrusorectomies, 5 patients were considered to have excellent results, 2 were considered to have acceptable re-

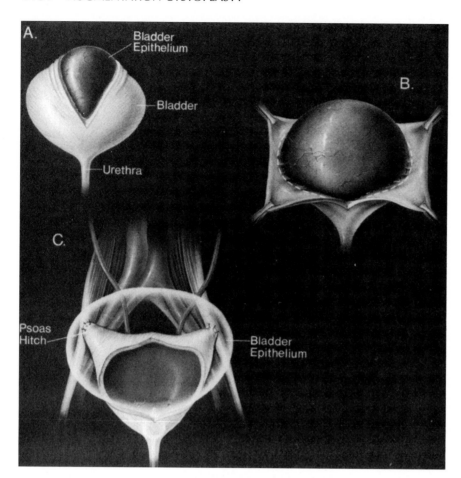

Figure 102–8. Autoaugmentation. *A,* Detrusor incised. *B,* Detrusor stripped and excised from mucosa. *C,* Bulging mucosa with bladder filling. (From Cartwright PC, Snow BW: J Urol 1989; 142:505.)

sults, and 1 was lost to follow-up (Landa and Moorhead, 1994). There were four failures (one increasing hydronephrosis, two persistent incontinence, one worsening renal insufficiency), of which three have so far undergone gastrocystoplasty or ileocystoplasty. Reoperative enterocystoplasty was not hampered by the prior detrusorectomy. The urothelial diverticulum at the time of augmentation cystoplasty was noted to be thick and fibrous, similar to a leather bag.

There are obvious advantages to autoaugmentation and its variants. Native urothelial tissue is used, which avoids mucus production and electrolyte changes and limits tumor potential. This is an extraperitoneal procedure, which shortens operative time and avoids the risks of intestinal surgery and adhesions. It is compatible with CIC and does not seem to complicate subsequent intestinocystoplasty should failure occur.

Complications from these procedures are generally uncommon and of little clinical significance. Perforation, a major concern after intestinocystoplasty, has not been reported. Inadvertent opening of the mucosa during the procedure can make the procedure more difficult and may promote prolonged postoperative extravasation. Such leakage has stopped with bladder drainage (Landa and Moorhead, 1994; Stothers et al, 1994). If concomitant ureteral reimplantation or bladder neck surgery is necessary, it is recommended that it be done first and the bladder then closed before detrusorectomy (Stothers et al, 1994).

Ehrlich and Gershman (1993) performed a laparoscopic seromyotomy (incision) in a patient with clinical success,

although postoperative urodynamics could not be obtained. A laparoscopic approach limits incision size and perhaps shortens postoperative hospitalization; however, it has the disadvantage of being an intraperitoneal procedure with no way to secure the detrusor open.

Concerns

The main disadvantage is a limited increase in capacity such that an adequate preoperative volume may be the most important predictor of success (Landa and Moorhead, 1994). Landa and Moorhead (1994) have noted that if the maximum capacity and the volume of urine held at 40 cm H_2O are similar, the patient may be better served by intestinocystoplasty. It is of note that many patients have demonstrated clinical improvement after these procedures without a significant change in the urodynamics. The exact reasons for the improvement are unknown. In Hinman's (1989) experience, only rarely do these procedures provide adequate compliance and capacity. Furthermore, many times after detrusorectomy, the bladder has not seemed to expand at the time of the operative procedure, and it was elected to proceed with enterocystoplasty at that time (Landa and Moorhead, 1994). These patients are not included in the failure rate. Lastly, there is concern that any increase in capacity obtained may not last long-term (Dewan et al, 1994b; Gonzalez, personal communication, 1994). In the rabbit, the surface area of the autoaugmentation site was noted to decrease approximately 50% at 12 weeks. Progressive thickening of the site was also noted because of fibrous infiltrate (Johnson et al, 1994).

Seromuscular Enterocystoplasty

With concerns about fibrosis of the diverticulum in autoaugmentation and its variants, some surgeons have elected to combine that procedure with demucosalized enteric segments. The use of demucosalized bowel segments is not new. Shoemaker and colleagues reported their use in bladder reconstruction in the mid-1950s but chose the serosal side of the bowel to face the bladder lumen (Shoemaker and Marucci, 1955; Shoemaker et al, 1957). Urothelium soon replaced the serosa. Gonzalez's group repeated these efforts at reversed seromuscular augmentation cystoplasty in rats with good results, but contracture of the patch occurred when attempted in canines (De Badiola et al, 1991; Long et al, 1992).

The authors and others have used bowel for augmentation in dogs with the demucosalized surface toward the lumen but have met problems with patch contracture (Salle et al, 1990). It had been noted that the demucosalized segment reepithelializes with urothelium in the rat and dog (Oesch, 1988; Salle et al, 1990).

A combination of autoaugmentation and detrusorectomy covered with a demucosalized enteric segment has now been attempted in an effort to achieve the best of both procedures while eliminating the negative aspects of each. Dewan and Byard (1993) reported the use of demuco-

salized stomach covering an autoaugmentation in sheep. Their early clinical results in five patients (Dewan and Stefanek, 1994) found improved bladder function in all, but two remained incontinent. Another patient has been reoperated on for a *double bladder*. This technique has now been reported in 11 other humans by several groups (Horowitz and Mitchell, 1993; Horowitz et al, 1994; Robinson et al, 1994). Their patients reportedly are dry on CIC. In those studied with urodynamics, compliance has improved, and capacity has increased. They noted no significant complications.

Buson and co-workers reported the use of reconfigured, demucosalized sigmoid colon placed over the urothelium after detrusorectomy in the dog and called this an SCLU (seromuscular colocystoplasty lined with urothelium) procedure (Buson et al, 1994) (Fig. 102–9). They noted that if the intestinal submucosa was removed with the mucosa, the sigmoid patch contracted, but fibrosis did not occur when the submucosa was preserved.

This SCLU procedure has since been reported in 16 patients using 25 cm of sigmoid colon, with postoperative capacity increasing an average of 2.4-fold (139–335 ml) in 14 of the 16 patients (Gonzalez et al, 1994). End filling pressures decreased from an average of 51.6 to 27.7 cm H_2O. Two patients failed and required ileocystoplasty, and their urodynamic data were excluded. Two other patients developed an hourglass deformity. Ten patients have had biopsies of the bladder; in one, urothelium with islands of colonic mucosa was noted. In two others, only colonic mucosa was demonstrated. Histologic studies using the gastric

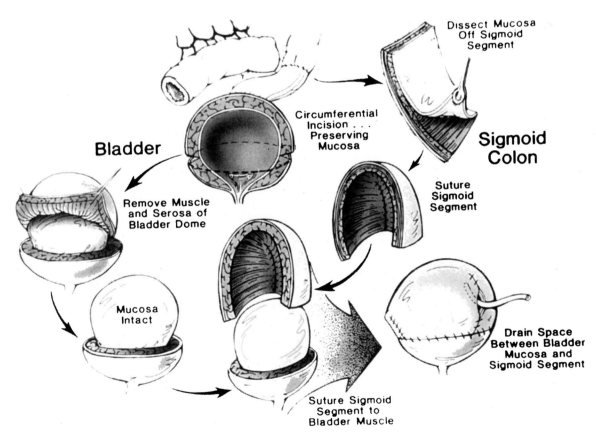

Figure 102–9. Seromuscular enterocystoplasty using sigmoid colon. (Reprinted by permission of the publisher from Buson H, Manivel JC, Dayanc M, et al: Seromuscular colocystoplasty lined with urothelium: Experimental study. Urology 1994; 44:745. Copyright 1994 by Elsevier Science Inc.)

segments have not been reported. It appears that the removal of *all* mucosa is important when using sigmoid to prevent mucoceles or overgrowth of intestinal mucosa (Gonzalez et al, 1994; Lutz and Frey, 1994).

These procedures are associated with more blood loss and longer operative time and are technically more demanding than simple augmentation or autoaugmentation (Gonzalez et al, 1994; Horowitz et al, 1994), particularly those using stomach. Although these seromuscular, urothelial-lined augmentations are theoretically attractive, the results reported have short-term follow-up at this time. The long-term effects on the urothelium by the seromuscular segment or vice versa are unknown.

Bladder Regeneration

The use of alloplastic materials for bladder substitution has had only limited success since research efforts began in the mid-1950s. Gleeson and Griffith (1992) have reviewed the history of such efforts. They noted that polyvinyl sponge, ethylene glycol, nylon velour, tetron membrane, silicone rubber, and polypropylene have all been used as a bladder patch. Several substances such as acrylic mold, polyethylene, gelatin sponge, and paper have been used to provide a scaffold for bladder regeneration. Although multiple problems arose, including infection, hydronephrosis, fistula, peritonitis, bladder contracture, stone formation, and extrusion, it was clear from these early efforts that there was potential for bladder regeneration. Further work using biodegradable, collagen-rich tissues to function as a scaffold for bladder regeneration has also been reported. Kelami (1971) used lyophilized dura, Fishman and colleagues (1987) tried placental membranes, and Kambic and associates (1992) reported experience with biodegradable pericardial implants. More encouraging results were noted in these studies. The bladder appears to have a natural ability to repair and remodel itself, particularly if provided with a suitable scaffold. More recent work has focused on the potential use of native bladder for augmentation. Kropp and colleagues have continued to search for the best tissue to act as the best scaffold for bladder regeneration (Kropp et al, 1995). Their work using pig small intestine submucosa (Kropp et al, 1995) to augment the rat bladder is encouraging. The small intestine submucosa patch was remodeled and replaced by all three layers of the normal bladder. Further studies are ongoing to determine if small intestine submucosa is a viable alternative to bladder augmentation.

Atala and co-workers approached this problem by harvesting bladder cells for later expansion in culture (Atala et al, 1992, 1993b; Cilento et al, 1994). Their work has now advanced to the point that they believe there is a possibility to expand these cells in tissue culture in a quantity sufficient for bladder reconstruction (Atala et al, 1994).

Although the above-noted research using native bladder to regenerate in vivo or in vitro for use in reconstruction is exciting, it is preliminary. Clinical applicability in the human for use in bladder replacement requires a great deal more study. Because of the above-noted complications with other forms of augmentation cystoplasty, this type of research is encouraged.

CONCLUSIONS

Since the initial work of Tizzoni and Foggi, extraordinary advances have been made in the use of bowel in urinary tract reconstruction. Bladder augmentation is used for patients with bladder dysfunction related to a noncompliant storage vesical. **Enterocystoplasty results in good bladder compliance in virtually all cases when medical management fails.** The cornerstone of preoperative evaluation before bladder augmentation is good urodynamic testing to understand fully bladder and urethral dynamics. Such an understanding aids in optimizing results while minimizing complications. Attention to detail and careful surgical technique are also imperative. Unfortunately, no bowel segment is a physiologic substitute for native bladder; side effects and complications still may occur after augmentation cystoplasty with any intestinal segment.

It is obvious from the previous discussion that there is no one single bowel segment that is perfect for augmentation in all patients. All gastrointestinal segments have been used and continue to be used with good results. Unremitting medical problems or complications requiring surgical intervention are relatively rare after augmentation cystoplasty. No one bowel segment has a clear advantage over others when all such problems are considered. Patient diagnosis, anatomy, physiology, and physical or mental capabilities may suggest that one bowel segment is preferable for a particular patient. Each surgeon interested in augmentation cystoplasty should be familiar with the advantages and disadvantages of each gastrointestinal segment in different settings.

In many routine cases, any gastrointestinal segment may be chosen for cystoplasty, based purely on the personal preference and familiarity of the surgeon. The authors believe that no one bowel segment is the best choice in all patients and that optimal results and the most efficient uses of bowel are achieved when the bowel segment is chosen based on the needs of the particular patient and that segment is then used correctly.

Because side effects of augmentation cystoplasty persist and are significant for some patients, efforts continue to find suitable alternatives to the use of intestinal segments in bladder reconstruction. Continued experience and longer follow-up are necessary to compare critically any of these alternatives to augmentation cystoplasty. Transurethral electrical bladder stimulation may increase bladder growth in some patients with neurogenic bladder dysfunction (Kaplan, 1994) but is unlikely to change a noncompliant bladder to a compliant one and significantly change the outcome of most patients now requiring augmentation cystoplasty. Autoaugmentation may function well for rare patients with a noncompliant bladder of relatively large capacity. It should not be expected to increase dramatically the bladder capacity of patients starting with a small capacity. Concerns about the persistence of improvements in bladder function that do occur after autoaugmentation have arisen, secondary to the fibrotic process that surrounds the exposed mucosa. Such concerns have led to experimental techniques to provide seromuscular intestinal backing to an intact transitional cell diverticulum. Although reported clinical experience with this technique, whether the demucosalized gastrointestinal segment is stomach or colon, has produced good results for some patients, follow-up is short, and some problems have occurred. Use of native ureteral tissue to augment the bladder seems ideal, and results thus far have been encouraging. Widespread use is presently limited by the absence of a dilated ureter. Continued effort with these and other techniques to find a suitable alternative to intestinal segments is certainly warranted.

No matter which gastrointestinal segment is used to augment the bladder or whether or not a good alternative is available in the future, one factor will continue to determine the long-term outcome more than any other. Proper preoperative evaluation and good surgical technique remain important, but the patient's outcome depends most on that person's commitment to achieving the desired results. The importance of proper patient selection and education cannot be overlooked.

REFERENCES

Adams MC, Bihrle R, Rink RC: The use of stomach in urologic reconstruction. AUA Update Series 1995; 27:218–223.

Adams MC, Mitchell ME, Rink RC: Gastrocystoplasty: An alternative solution to the problem of urological reconstruction in the severely compromised patient. J Urol 1988; 140:1152–1156.

Akerlund S, Lelin K, Kock NG, et al: Renal function and upper tract configuration following urinary diversion to a continent ileal reservoir (Kock pouch): A prospective 5 to 11 year follow up after reservoir construction. J Urol 1989; 142:964.

Allen T, Peters PC, Sagalowsky A: The Camey procedure: Preliminary results in 11 patients. World J Urol 1985; 3:167.

Anderson PAM, Rickwood AMK: Detrusor hyper-reflexia as a factor in spontaneous perforation of augmentation cystoplasty for neuropathic bladder. Br J Urol 1991; 67:210–212.

Ashken MH: Urinary cecal reservoir. In King LR, Stone AR, Webster GD, eds: Bladder Reconstruction and Continent Urinary Diversion. Chicago, Year Book Medical Publishers, 1987, pp 238–251.

Atala A, Bauer SB, Hendren WH, et al: The effect of gastric augmentation on bladder function. J Urol 1993a; 149:1099.

Atala A, Freeman MR, Vacanti JP, et al: Implantation in vivo and retrieval of urothelial structures consisting of rabbit and human bladder muscle. J Urol 1993b; 150:608.

Atala A, Lailas NG, Cilento BG, Retik AB: Progressive ureteral dilation for subsequent ureterocystoplasty. Presented at the Section on Urology Meeting, American Academy of Pediatrics, Dallas, 1994.

Atala A, Vacanti JP, Peters CA, et al: Formation of urothelial structures in vivo from disassociated cells attached to biodegradable polymer scaffolds. J Urol 1992; 148:658.

Bauer SB: An approach to neurogenic bladder. Prob Urol 1994; 8:441–459.

Bauer SB, Hendren WH, Kozakewich H, et al: Perforation of the augmented bladder. J Urol 1992; 148:699.

Bellinger MF: Ureterocystoplasty: A unique method for vesical augmentation in children. J Urol 1993; 149:811–813.

Bellinger MF: Uretcrocystoplasty. Curr Surg Tech Urol 1995; 8:2–7.

Berglund B, Kock NG, Norlen L, Philipson BM: Volume capacity and pressure characteristics of the continent ileal reservoir used for urinary diversion. J Urol 1987; 137:29.

Blythe B, Ewalt DH, Duckett JW, Snyder HM: Lithogenic properties of enterocystoplasty. J Urol 1992; 148:575.

Bogaert GA, Mevorach RA, Kim J, et al: The physiology of gastrocystoplasty: Once a stomach, always a stomach. J Urol 1995; 153:1977.

Boyd SD, Schiff WM, Skinner DG, et al: Prospective study of metabolic abnormalities in patients with continent Kock pouch urinary diversion. Urology 1989; 33:85–88.

Braverman RM, Lebowitz RL: Perforation of the augmented urinary bladder in nine children and adolescents: Importance of cystography. AJR 1991; 157:1059.

Buson H, Castro-Diaz D, Manivel JC, et al: The development of tumors in experimental gastroenterocystoplasty. J Urol 1993; 150:730.

Buson H, Manivel JC, Dayanc M, et al: Seromuscular colocystoplasty lined with urothelium: Experimental study. Urology 1994; 44:743–748.

Cain MP, Husmann DA: Cecal bladder augmentation with a tapered catheterizable stoma: A modification of the Indiana pouch. Presented at the Urology Section Meeting, American Academy of Pediatrics, Dallas, 1994.

Canning DA, Perman JA, Jeffs RD, Gearhart JP: Nutritional consequences of bowel segments in the lower urinary tract. J Urol 1989; 142:509.

Cartwright PC, Snow BW: Bladder autoaugmentation: Early clinical experience. J Urol 1989a; 142:505.

Cartwright PC, Snow BW: Bladder augmentation: Partial detrusor excision to augment the bladder without use of bowel. J Urol 1989b; 142:1050.

Castro-Diaz D, Froemming C, Manivel JC, et al: The influence of urinary diversion on experimental gastrocystoplasty. J Urol 1992; 148:571–574.

Chargi A, Charbonneau J, Gauthier G: Colocystoplasty for bladder enlargement and bladder substitution: A study of late results in 31 cases. J Urol 1967; 97:849.

Churchill BM, Aliabadi H, Landau EH, et al: Ureteral bladder augmentation. J Urol 1993; 150:716–720.

Cilento BG, Freeman MR, Scheneck FX: Phenotypic and cytogenetic characterization of human bladder urothelia expanded in vitro. J Urol 1994; 152:665–670.

Couvelaire R: La "Petite Vessle" des tuberculeux genitourinaires. Essai de classification place et variantes des cysto-intestinoplasties. J Urol 1950; 56:381.

Crane JM, Scherz HS, Billman GF, Kaplan GW: Ischemic necrosis: A hypothesis to explain the pathogenesis of spontaneously ruptured enterocystoplasty. J Urol 1991; 146:141–144.

De Badiola F, Manivel JC, Gonzalez R: Seromuscular enterocystoplasty in rats. J Urol 1991; 146:559–562.

Demos MP: Radioactive electrolyte absorption studies of small bowel, comparison of different segments for use in urinary diversion. J Urol 1962; 88:638.

Dewan PA, Byard R: Autoaugmentation gastrocystoplasty in a sheep model. Br J Urol 1993; 72:56–59.

Dewan PA, Nicholls EA, Goh DW: Ureterocystoplasty: An extraperitoneal urothelial bladder augmentation technique. Eur Urol 1994a; 26:85–89.

Dewan PA, Stefanek W: Autoaugmentation gastrocystoplasty: Early clinical results. Br J Urol 1994; 74:460–464.

Dewan PA, Stefanek W, Lorenz C, Byard RW: Autoaugmentation omentoplasty in a sheep model. Urology 1994b; 43:888–891.

Ehrlich RM, Gershman A: Laparoscopic seromyotomy (autoaugmentation) for non-neurogenic neurogenic bladder in a child: Initial case report. Urology 1993; 42:175–178.

Elder JS, Snyder HM, Hulbert WC, Duckett JW: Perforation of the augmented bladder in patients undergoing clean intermittent catheterization. J Urol 1988; 140:1159.

Eraklus AJ, Folkman MJ: Adenocarcinoma at the site of ureterosigmoidostomies for exstrophy of the bladder. J Pediatr Surg 1978; 13:730.

Essig KA, Sheldon CA, Brandt MT, et al: Elevated intravesical pressure causes arterial hypoperfusion in canine colocystoplasty: A fluorometric assessment. J Urol 1991; 146:551–553.

Ferris DO, Odel MH: Electrolyte pattern of blood after ureterosigmoidostomy. JAMA 1950; 142:634.

Filmer RB, Spencer JR: Malignancies in bladder augmentations and intestinal conduits. J Urol 1990;143:671.

Fishman IJ, Flores FN, Scott FB, et al: Use of fresh placental membranes for bladder reconstruction. J Urol 1987; 138:1291–1294.

Franco I, Storrs B, Firlit CF, et al: Selective sacral rhizotomy in children with high pressure neurogenic bladders: Preliminary results. J Urol 1992; 148:648–650.

Ganesan GS, Mitchell ME, Adams MC, et al: Use of stomach for reconstruction of the lower urinary tract in patients with compromised renal function. Presented at the Urology Section Meeting, American Academy of Pediatrics, New Orleans, 1991.

Garzotto MG, Walker RD: Uric acid stone and gastric bladder augmentation. J Urol 1995; 153:1976.

Gearhart JP: Mucus secretions in augmented bladder. Dialog Pediatr Urol 1987; 10:6.

Gearhart JP, Albertsen PC, Marshall FF, et al: Pediatric applications of augmentation cystoplasty: The Johns Hopkins experience. J Urol 1986; 136:430.

Gleason DM, Gittes RF, Bottaccini MR, Byen JC: Energy balance of voiding after cecal cystoplasty. J Urol 1972; 108:259–264.

Gleeson MJ, Griffith DP: The use of alloplastic biomaterials in bladder substitution. J Urol 1992; 148:1377–1382.

Goldwasser B, Barrett DM, Webster GD, et al: Cystometric properties of ileum and right colon after bladder augmentation, substitution or replacement. J Urol 1987; 138:1007.

Goldwasser B, Webster GD: Augmentation and substitution enterocystoplasty. J Urol 1986; 135:215.

Gonzalez R, Buson H, Reid C, Reinberg Y: Seromuscular colocystoplasty lined with urothelium: Experience with 16 patients. Urology 1994; 45:124–129.

Gonzalez R, Cabral BHP: Rectal continence after enterocystoplasty. Dialog Pediatr Urol 1987; 10:3–4.

Goodwin WE, Winter CC, Barker WF: Cup-patch technique of ileocystoplasty for bladder enlargement or partial substitution. Surg Gynecol Obstet 1959;108:240.

Gosalbez R Jr, Woodard JR, Broecker BH, et al: The use of stomach in pediatric urinary reconstruction. J Urol 1993a; 150:438.

Gosalbez R Jr, Woodard JR, Broecker BH, et al: Metabolic complications of the use of stomach for urinary reconstruction. J Urol 1993b; 150:710–712.

Hall MC, Koch MO, McDougal WS: Metabolic consequences of urinary diversion through intestinal segments. Urol Clin North Am 1991; 18:725.

Hedlund H, Lindstrom K, Mansson W: Dynamics of a continent cecal reservoir for urinary diversion. Br J Urol 1984; 56:366–372.

Heidler H, Marberger M, Hohenfellner R: The metabolic situation in ureterosigmoidostomy. Eur Urol 1979; 5:39–44.

Hendren WH, Hendren RB: Bladder augmentation: Experience with 129 children and young adults. J Urol 1990; 144:445.

Hinman F Jr: Selection of intestinal segments for bladder substitution: Physical and physiological characteristics. J Urol 1988; 139:519.

Hinman F Jr: Bladder augmentation. In Hinman FJ, ed: Atlas of Urologic Surgery. Philadelphia, W.B. Saunders, 1989, p 534.

Hirst G: Ileal and colonic cystoplasties. Prob Urol 1991; 5:223.

Hitchcock RJI, Duffy PG, Malone PS: Ureterocystoplasty: The 'bladder' augmentation of choice. Br J Urol 1994; 73:575–579.

Hollensbe DW, Adams MC, Rink RC, et al: Comparison of different gastrointestinal segments for bladder augmentation. Presented at the American Urological Association Meeting, Washington, D.C., 1992.

Hoover DL, Duckett JW: Posterior urethral valves, unilateral reflux and renal dysplasia: A syndrome. J Urol 1982; 128:994.

Horowitz M, Mitchell ME: DAWG procedure (demucosalized augmentation with gastric segment). Presented at Genitourinary Reconstructive Surgeon's Meeting, San Francisco, 1993.

Horowitz M, Mitchell ME, Nguyen DH: The DAWG procedure: Gastrocystoplasty made better. J Urol 1994; 151:503A.

Husmann DA, Spence HM: Current status of tumor of the bowel following ureterosigmoidostomy: A review. J Urol 1990; 144:607.

Jakobsen H, Steven K, Stigsby B, et al: Pathogenesis of nocturnal urinary incontinence after ileocaecal bladder replacement: Continuous measurement of urethral closure pressure during sleep. Br J Urol 1987; 59:148–152.

Johnson HW, Nigro MK, Stothers L, et al: Laboratory variables of autoaugmentation in an animal model. Urology 1994; 44:260–263.

Joseph DB: The effect of medium-fill and slow-fill saline cystometry on detrusor pressure in infants and children with myelodysplasia. J Urol 1992; 147:444–446.

Kaefer M, Keating MA, Adams MC, Rink RC: Posterior urethral valves, pressure pop-offs and bladder function. Presented at Section on Urology, American Academy of Pediatrics, Dallas, 1994.

Kambic H, Kay R, Chen JF, et al: Biodegradable pericardial implants for bladder augmentation: A 2.5 year study in dogs. J Urol 1992; 148:539–543.

Kaplan WE: Alternative to enterocystoplasty: II. Bladder stimulation. Prob Urol 1994; 8:410–415.

Keating MA, Rink RC, Adams MC: Appendicovesicostomy: A useful adjunct to continent reconstruction of the bladder. J Urol 1993; 149:1091–1094.

Kelami A: Lyophilized human dura as a bladder wall substitute: Experimental and clinical results. J Urol 1971; 105:518–522.

Kennedy HA, Adams MC, Mitchell ME, et al: Chronic renal failure in bladder augmentation: Stomach versus sigmoid in the canine model. J Urol 1988; 140:1138–1140.

King LR: Protection of the upper tracts in children. In King LR, Stone AR, Webster GD, eds: Bladder Reconstruction and Continent Urinary Diversion. Chicago, Year Book Medical Publishers, 1987, p 127.

King LR: Cystoplasty in children. In King LR, Stone AR, Webster GD, eds: Bladder Reconstruction and Continent Urinary Diversion, 2nd ed. St. Louis, Mosby Year Book, 1991, pp 115–125.

Klee LW, Hoover DM, Mitchell ME, Rink RC: Long term effects of gastrocystoplasty in rats. J Urol 1990; 144:1283.

Koch MO, McDougal WS: The pathophysiology of hyperchloremic metabolic acidosis after urinary diversion through intestinal segments. Surgery 1985; 98:561.

Koff SA: Guidelines to determine the size and shape of intestinal segments used for reconstruction. J Urol 1988; 140:1150.

Kropp BP, Eppley BL, Prevel CD, et al: Experimental assessment of small intestine submucosa as a bladder wall substitute. Urology 1995; 46:396–400.

Kulb TB, Rink RC, Mitchell ME: Gastrocystoplasty in azotemic canines. Presented at the American Urological Association, North Central Section Meeting, Palm Springs, Florida, 1986.

Landa HM, Moorhead JD: Detrusorectomy. Prob Pediatr Urol 1994; 8:404–409.

Landau EH, Jayanthi VR, Khoury AE, et al: Bladder augmentation: Ureterocystoplasty versus ileocystoplasty. J Urol 1994; 152:716–719.

Lapides J, Diokno AC, Gould FR, et al: Further observations on self-catheterization. J Urol 1976; 116:169.

Lapides J, Diokno AC, Silber SJ, Lowe BS: Clean intermittent self-catheterization in the treatment of urinary tract disease. J Urol 1972; 107:458.

Leong CH: The use of gastrocystoplasty. Dialog Pediatr Urol 1988; 11:3–5.

Leong CH, Ong GB: Gastrocystoplasty in dogs. Aust N Z J Surg 1972; 41:272–279.

Lindgren BW, Flom LS: Augmentation ureterocystoplasty. Dialog Pediatr Urol 1995; 18:3–5.

Little JS, Klee LW, Hoover DM, Rink RC: Long term histopathologic changes observed in rats subjected to augmentation cystoplasty. J Urol 1994; 152:720–724.

Lockhart JL, Lotenfoe RR, Davies R, et al: An alternative continent urinary reservoir for patients with short bowel, acidosis or radiation. Presented at the American Urological Association Meeting, San Antonio, 1993.

Long R, Buson H, Manivel JC, Gonzalez R: Seromuscular enterocystoplasty in dogs. J Urol 1992; 147:430a.

Ludlow J, McLaughlin KP, Rink RC, et al: Do appendicovesicostomies empty effectively? Presented at the North Central Section—AUA, Minneapolis, 1995.

Lutz N, Frey P: Evaluation of modified enterocystoplasties using a pediculated detubularized and demucosed sigmoid patch in the mini-pig. Presented at the Section on Urology Meeting, American Academy of Pediatrics, Dallas, 1994.

Lytton B, Green DF: Urodynamic studies in patients undergoing bladder replacement surgery. J Urol 1989; 141:1984.

Malek RS, Burke EC, DeWeerd JH: Ileal conduit urinary diversion in children. J Urol 1971; 105:892–900.

Mansson W, Colleen S, Sundin T: The continent cecal reservoir for urine. Scand J Urol Nephrol 1984; 85(suppl.):8.

McDougal WS: Bladder reconstruction following cystectomy by uretero-ileo-colourethrostomy. J Urol 1986; 135:698–701.

McDougal WS: Metabolic complications of urinary intestinal diversion. J Urol 1992a; 147:1199–1208.

McDougal WS: Use of intestinal segments in the urinary tract: Basic principles. In Walsh PC, Retik AB, Stamey TA, Vaughan ED Jr, eds: Campbell's Urology, 6th ed. Philadelphia, W.B. Saunders, 1992b, pp 2595–2629.

McGuire EJ, Woodside JR, Borden TA, Weiss RM: Prognostic value of urodynamic testing in myelodysplastic patients. J Urol 1981; 126:205–209.

McKenna PH, Bauer SB: Bladder augmentation with ureter. Dialog Pediatr Urol 1995; 18:4.

Mitchell ME: Use of bowel in undiversion. Urol Clin North Am 1986; 13:349.

Mitchell ME, Piser JA: Intestinocystoplasty and total bladder replacement in children and young adults: Follow-up in 129 cases. J Urol 1987; 138:579–584.

Mitchell ME, Rink RC: Urinary diversion and undiversion. Urol Clin North Am 1985; 12:111.

Mitchell ME, Rink RC, Adams MC: Augmentation cystoplasty, implantation of artificial urinary sphincter in men and women, and reconstruction of the dysfunction urinary tract. In Walsh PC, Retik AB, Stamey TA, Vaughn ED Jr, eds: Campbell's Urology, 6th ed. Philadelphia, W.B. Saunders, 1992, pp 2630–2653.

Mitrofanoff P: Cystostomie continente trans-appendiculaire dans le traitement des vessies neurolgiques. Chir Pediatr 1980; 21:297.

Murray K, Nurse D, Mundy AR: Secreto-motor function of intestinal segments used in lower urinary tract reconstruction. Br J Urol 1987; 60:532.

Ngan JHK, Lau JLT, Lim STK, et al: Long-term results of antral gastrocystoplasty. J Urol 1993; 149:731–734.

Nguyen DH, Bain MA, Salmonson KL, et al: The syndrome of dysuria and hematuria in pediatric urinary reconstruction with stomach. J Urol 1993; 150:707–709.

Oesch I: Neourothelium in bladder augmentation: An experimental rat model. Eur Urol 1988; 14:328.

Orr LM, Thomley MW, Campbell MF: Ileocystoplasty for bladder enlargement. J Urol 1958; 79:250.

Palmer LS, Franco I, Kogan SJ, et al: Urolithiasis in children following augmentation cystoplasty. J Urol 1993; 150:726.

Piser JA, Mitchell ME, Kulb TB, et al: Gastrocystoplasty and colocystoplasty in canines: The metabolic consequences of acute saline and acid loading. J Urol 1987; 138:1009–1012.

Raz S, Ehrlich RM, Babiarz JW, et al: Gastrocystoplasty without opening the stomach. J Urol 1993; 150:713–715.

Reinberg Y, Allen RC, Vaughn M, McKenna PH: Nephrectomy combined with lower abdominal extraperitoneal ureteral bladder augmentation in the treatment of children with the vesicoureteral reflux dysplasia syndrome. J Urol 1995; 153:777–779.

Reinberg Y, Manivel JC, Froemming C, et al: Perforation of the gastric segment of an augmented bladder secondary to peptic ulcer disease. J Urol 1992; 148:369–371.

Reisman EM, Preminger GM: Bladder perforation secondary to clean intermittent catheterization. J Urol 1989; 142:1316–1317.

Rink RC: Choice of materials for bladder augmentation. Curr Opin Urol 1995; 9:300–305.

Rink RC, Hollensbe D, Adams MC: Complications of augmentation in children and comparison of gastrointestinal segments. AUA Update Series 1995; 14:122–128.

Rink RC, Hollensbe DW, Adams MC, et al: Is sigmoid enterocystoplasty at greatest risk for perforation? Observation and etiology in 22 bladder perforations in 264 patients. Presented at the International Meeting on Continent Urinary Reconstruction, Lund, Sweden, 1992.

Rink RC, McLaughlin KP: Indications for enterocystoplasty and choice of bowel segment. Prob Urol 1994; 8:389–403.

Rink RC, Mitchell ME: Surgical correction of urinary incontinence. J Pediatr Surg 1984; 19:637.

Rink RC, Mitchell ME: Role of enterocystoplasty in reconstructing the neurogenic bladder. In Gonzales ET, Roth D, eds: Common Problems in Pediatric Urology. St. Louis, Mosby Year Book, 1990, pp 192–204.

Rink RC, Woodbury PW, Mitchell ME: Bladder perforation following enterocystoplasty (Abstract). J Urol 1988; 139:234a.

Rittendberg MH, Hulbert WC, Synder HM III, Duckett JW: Protective factors in posterior urethral valves. J Urol 1988; 140:993.

Robinson RG, Delahunt B, Pringle KC: Autoaugmentation gastrocystoplasty. J Urol 1994; 151:500a.

Rosen MA, Light JK: Spontaneous bladder rupture following augmentation enterocystoplasty. J Urol 1991; 146:1232–1234.

Rowland RG: Intestine for bladder augmentation and substitution. In King LR, Stone AR, Webster GD, eds: Bladder Reconstruction and Continent Urinary Diversion. St. Louis, Mosby Year Book, 1991, pp 22–28.

Rushton HG, Woodard JR, Parrott TS, et al: Delayed bladder rupture after augmentation enterocystoplasty. J Urol 1988; 140:344.

Salle JL, Fraga JC, Lucib A, et al: Seromuscular enterocystoplasty in dogs. J Urol 1990; 144:454–456.

Savauagen F, Dixey GM: Syncope following ureterosigmoidostomy. J Urol 1969; 101:844.

Schmidt JD, Hawtrey CE, Flocks RH, Culp DA: Complications, results, and problems of ileal conduit diversions. J Urol 1973; 109:210–216.

Schmidt RA, Kogan BA, Tanaglo EA: Neuroprosthesis in the management of incontinence of myelomeningocele patients. J Urol 1990; 143:779.

Schneidau T, Franco I, Zebold K, et al: Selective sacral rhizotomy for the management of neurogenic bladders in spina bifida patients: Long-term follow up. J Urol 1995; 154:766–768.

Sheiner JR, Kaplan GW: Spontaneous bladder rupture following enterocystoplasty. J Urol 1988; 140:1157.

Sheldon CA, Gilbert A: Gastrocystoplasty allows safe pretransplant urinary reconstruction without acidosis. Presented at the American Urological Association Meeting, Toronto, 1991.

Shoemaker WC, Bower R, Long DM: A new technique for bladder reconstruction. Surg Gynecol Obstet 1957 ;105:645–650.

Shoemaker WC, Marucci HD: The experimental use of seromuscular grafts in bladder reconstruction: Preliminary report. J Urol 1955; 73:314–321.

Sidi AA, Aliabadi H, Gonzalez R: Enterocystoplasty in the management and reconstruction of the pediatric neurogenic bladder. J Pediatr Surg 1987; 22:153.

Sidi AA, Reinberg Y, Gonzalez R: Influence of intestinal segment and configuration on the outcome of augmentation enterocystoplasty. J Urol 1986; 136:1201.

Sinaiko ES: Artificial bladder from segment of stomach and study effect of urine on gastric secretion. Surg Gynecol Obstet 1956; 102:433–438.

Slaton JW, Kropp KA: Conservative management of suspected bladder rupture after augmentation enterocystoplasty. J Urol 1994; 152:713–715.

Spencer JR, Steckel J, May M, et al: Histological and bacteriological findings in long-term ileocystoplasty and colocystoplasty in the rat. J Urol 1993; 150:1321.

Steiner MS, Morton RA: Nutritional and gastrointestinal complications of the use of bowel segments in the lower urinary tract. Urol Clin North Am 1991; 18:743.

Stothers L, Johnson H, Arnold W, et al: Bladder autoaugmentation by vesicomyotomy in pediatric neurogenic bladder. Urology 1994; 44:110–113.

Thuroff JW, Alken P, Hohenfellner R: The MAINZ pouch (mixed augmentation with ileum 'n' zecum) for bladder augmentation and continent diversion. In King LR, Stone AR, Webster GD, eds: Bladder Reconstruction and Continent Urinary Diversion. Chicago, Year Book Medical Publishers, 1987, p 252.

Tizzoni G, Foggi A: Die Wiederherstellung der Harnblase. Zentralbl Chir 1888; 15:921.

Treiger BFG, Marshall FF: Carcinogenesis and the use of intestinal segments in the urinary tract. Urol Clin North Am 1991; 18:737.

Whitmore WF III, Gittes RF: Reconstruction of the urinary tract by cecal and ileocecal cystoplasty: Review of a 15-year experience. J Urol 1983; 129:494–498.

Wolf JS, Turzan C: Augmentation ureterocystoplasty. J Urol 1993; 149:1095–1098.

103
CONTINENT URINARY DIVERSION

Mitchell C. Benson, M.D.
Carl A. Olsson, M.D.

This chapter reviews all forms of continent urinary diversion used in the adult patient population. The principles and techniques of bowel surgery as well as complications resulting therefrom are covered elsewhere in this text. Similarly, techniques of ureterointestinal anastomosis and complications resulting from these anastomoses are reviewed in another chapter. These features are not repeated except when essential to the appropriate description of the operative procedures reviewed here.

Continent diversion has become widely accepted by both urologists and patients. Orthotopic urethral anastomotic procedures and continent catheterizable stomal reservoirs are standing the test of time, and both procedures should be considered for all appropriate patients. The chapter on urinary diversion in the previous edition attempted to cover all published procedures regardless of the popularity or success rate of the operation. This chapter focuses more on those procedures the authors believe to be associated with the highest success rates. All operations that have been reported in substantial numbers of patients, however, are mentioned.

Despite the considerable enthusiasm for continent urinary diversion operations, procedures that require the use of external urinary collecting appliances remain the most common. Although continent urinary diversion is certainly appropriate in selected patients, some of the procedures are technically more challenging and have potentially higher complication rates than those operations that use collecting devices. The operating time associated with these more complex procedures has been significantly reduced, however, by the wide-

spread use of absorbable and metal staples in the construction of the reservoirs and limbs. The techniques used to create reservoirs and neobladders using absorbable and metal staples are discussed in detail later.

PATIENT SELECTION

Because the ability to self-catheterize or to care for a neobladder is essential to the patient undergoing continent diversion, **the patient must be assessed for the ability to care for himself or herself.** An enterostomal therapist in consultation with the patient and the urologist is extremely helpful in this regard. Certain categories of patients may not be able to comprehend the regimens that must be followed after continent urinary diversion, or they may lack the motor skills to perform self-care. Patients with severe multiple sclerosis, quadriplegic patients, frail patients, and mentally impaired patients require the care of members of the family or visiting nurse attendance; the authors view such patients as poor candidates for any form of continent diversion. These patients may also require assistance with external appliances, but such assistance is much less burdensome on the patient and society. Usually a collecting appliance can simply be emptied when full; nighttime bedside drainage equipment can be attached to the collecting appliance so that long periods of uninterrupted sleep may be experienced. Continent catheterizable diversion and neobladder care require round-the-clock attention and may limit patient and family options when determining nursing home placement.

PATIENT PREPARATION

The authors prepare all patients undergoing anticipated continent urinary diversion for the possibility that a traditional ileal conduit might be performed. Although it is rare to abandon a continent diversion owing to unanticipated problems, this remains a possible outcome. Therefore, before the operation, the site for an external stoma should be selected with extreme care. In general, the location must be free from fat creases in both standing and sitting positions, and it should not be close to prior abdominal scars that might interfere with proper adherence of an external appliance. Here again, the aid of an enterostomal therapist is extremely helpful. In general, the stoma should be brought through the right (or left) lower quadrant of the abdomen on a line extending between the umbilicus and the anterosuperior iliac spine. The stoma should be as far lateral from the midline as possible but should always be selected so as to require the bowel segment comprising the stoma to traverse the rectus muscle. Failure to adhere to this latter feature promotes the incidence of parastomal hernias. The selected site for the stoma should be marked with an X scratched on the anterior abdominal wall. Marking the stoma site with ink should be avoided because the ink may be washed away during the antiseptic preparation of the skin.

The surgeon undertaking continent urinary diversion should be familiar with more than one type of continent diversion procedure. At times, unanticipated anatomic variations may be encountered that do not allow for the intended bowel segment to be used. In these circumstances, it is prudent that the surgeon be able to elect an alternative form of continent diversion from that originally intended.

Renal and hepatic function must be reviewed carefully in the patient selected for continent diversion. The reabsorption and recirculation of urinary constituents and other metabolites require that liver function be normal and that serum creatinine levels be in the normal range or certainly below the level of 1.8 mg/dl. In cases in which renal function is borderline, creatinine clearance should be measured. A minimal level of creatinine clearance of 60 ml/minute should be documented before the patient is deemed an appropriate candidate for continent diversion. In patients with bilateral hydronephrosis, in whom renal functional improvement might be anticipated on relief of the ureteral obstruction, the urologist may veer from these serum creatinine and creatinine clearance standards. The authors' prejudice in such cases is to drain the upper tract (by percutaneous nephrostomy(ies), if needed) with re-evaluation of renal function thereafter, before opting for a continent diversion.

Procedures that require the use of a large intestinal segment should always be preceded by a radiologic or colonoscopic assessment of the entire large intestine. Sigmoidoscopy only for a sigmoid colon procedure is insufficient because more proximal disease may leave the patient with a short colon syndrome. No evaluation guarantees the durability of the entire colon, but the authors believe that one should do all one can to ensure the health of the bowel

to be used. The authors do not routinely perform colon evaluation if small intestine is used.

Healthy patients undergoing radical cystectomy can be admitted to the hospital on the day of surgery. A polyethylene glycol–electrolyte solution (GoLYTELY) 1-gallon bowel preparation is administered after a liquid dinner on the night before surgery. The patient is instructed to drink copious amounts of water, and at 8 PM and 10 PM, the patient is administered oral metronidazole 500 mg. The patient receives cefoxitin 1 g intravenously 1 hour before the skin incision.

SURGICAL CYSTECTOMY PROCEDURE

All operations described require a midline incision, skirting the umbilicus to the side opposite the selected stoma site. As an alternative, a paramedian incision may be used opposite the preselected stoma location. The incision for a right colon pouch usually extends from the pubis to the xyphoid. For a neobladder constructed from ileum or sigmoid, the incision need extend only a few fingerbreadths above the umbilicus.

After abdominal exploration, urinary diversion operations proceed by the isolation, transection, and transposition of the ureters to an appropriate place for subsequent diversion. The right retroperitoneum is opened over the iliac artery to expose the right ureter. In the typical circumstance of bowel diversion, the ureter may be transected at the level of the iliac artery or slightly below this level. The sigmoid colon is then freed from its lateral peritoneal attachments by incising along the line of Toldt. After the colon is medially reflected, the left ureter can be identified and dissected somewhat more distally than the right. A wide tunnel is created by blunt finger dissection ventral to the aorta and common iliac arteries beneath the inferior mesenteric artery. This affords left ureteral access to the previously exposed right retroperitoneum. In cases of uroepithelial malignancy, a small portion of the distalmost ureter on each side should be sent for frozen section analysis for possible urothelial neoplasm. The left ureter is directed to the right retroperitoneum through the tunnel beneath the inferior mesenteric artery. In carrying out sigmoid colon conduit diversion, the procedures are reversed, with longer segments of right ureter transected and directed to the left retroperitoneum. In the case of some neobladder operations, the ureters must be left sufficiently long to reach the pouch when situated deep in the pelvis. In these cases, the ureters remain on their respective sides of the sigmoid colon and rectum. A unique property of the hemi-Kock and the Studer neobladders is their ability to be fashioned in a manner that compensates for short ureteral length.

All sutures used in the urinary tract should be absorbable. An individual surgeon's preference dictates the caliber of suture material used as well as whether simple chromic catgut or synthetic absorbable materials should be used. **In general, when carrying out bowel surgery for those urinary diversions requiring bowel, the authors prefer a stapled bowel segment division as well as stapled reconstruction of bowel continuity. The authors believe that this shortens operative time greatly and affords safe**

bowel anastomoses. Suturing techniques are not necessary except to take one or two silk Lembert sutures at the apex of side-to-side stapled bowel anastomoses. End-to-end stapled reconstruction requires reinforcing sutures. To avoid stone formation on the stapled butts of conduits, the simple expedient of oversewing the stapled end of the conduit with absorbable material or the single application of an absorbable staple proximal to the metal stapled margin isolates the metal staple line from urinary contact.

In constructing a nonappendiceal continent urinary diversion stoma, a skin button matching the diameter of the structure to be used in the diversion is circumcised. Cutaneous tissues are separated down to the level of the anterior rectus fascia, and a similar diameter circle is excised from this fascia or the fascia is opened in cruciate fashion. In carrying out this maneuver, the surgeon should take care that the fascia and skin are properly aligned, so that angulation does not occur. Rectus muscle fibers are separated bluntly, and an instrument is passed through to the posterior peritoneum (and fascia). A similar-size circle of posterior fascia and peritoneum is removed, or these tissues are incised, again taking care to ensure proper alignment of all layers of the abdominal wall. For appendiceal stomas, the authors prefer to perform a Y-shaped cutaneous incision, which allows for a Y-V-plasty incision between the appendiceal limb and the skin (Fig. 103–1). It has been the authors' experience that this decreases the likelihood of subsequent stomal stenosis.

The authors prefer to use diverting stents in all cases of urinary diversion, regardless of whether standard diversion or continent diversion is selected. The authors also prefer to use stents that drain urine externally, ensuring that urine is safely diverted beyond any anastomotic site during the early healing interval. Finally, the authors prefer to use stents that can be replaced if needed. Therefore, any number of long end-hole, single-J type of ureteral diverting stent is preferred. The proximal end of the J stent should be patent to allow replacement of the stent, if necessary, by means of guide wire exchange. The end hole also allows for the passage of a straight wire through the stent before removal. This maneuver decreases the likelihood of anastomotic trauma at the time of stent removal and allows for the observation of drainage with the stent out.

The authors advocate the use of closed-suction drains in all cases of urinary diversion in which anastomotic leaks may be experienced. Soft silicone rubber suction drains are preferred because they have less potential for tissue damage or migration into pouches. These are usually brought through a stab wound in the left lower quadrant, traverse the pelvis, and are brought to the area of the ureteral anastomosis.

Abdominal closure is performed according to the surgeon's preference. The authors believe that a single-layer closure, using No. 2 nylon, Surgilene, or Prolene taken through all layers of fascia and muscle, provides a rapid, secure abdominal closure in the majority of patients. In obese patients, patients with tissues of poor quality, or nutritionally depleted patients, through-and-through stay sutures are also used. Subcutaneous sutures are placed to close dead space, and skin is closed with staples. Ureteral stents are always brought through separate abdominal stab wounds,

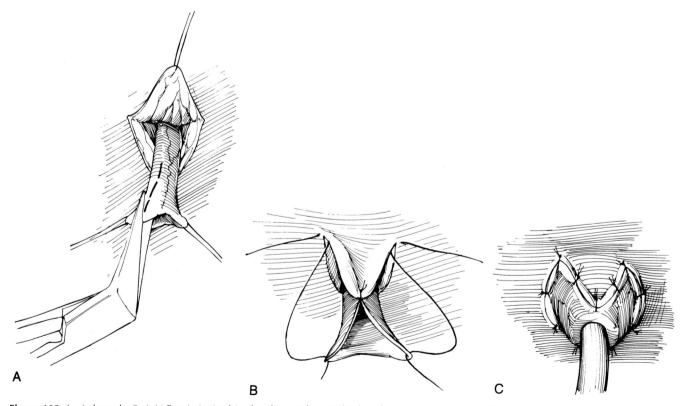

Figure 103–1. *A* through *C*, A V-flap is incised in the skin, and a similar length incision is made on the adjacent appendiceal surface. This is similar to the technique used to mature a cutaneous ureterostomy. For an appendiceal stoma, no eversion is required. (From Hinman F Jr: Atlas of Urologic Surgery. Philadelphia, W. B. Saunders, 1989.)

sutured to the anterior abdominal wall, and directed into separate drainage bags to monitor urine output. The authors ascertain that there is adequate drainage of the reservoir for safety against pouch rupture, should the ureteral stents become dislodged. Therefore, in the case of limited pouch access such as with an appendiceal stoma, a Malecot tube is always placed directly into the reservoir and secured to the skin. When a suprapubic tube is used, the reservoir is sutured to the abdominal wall to prevent urine leakage into the peritoneal cavity after tube removal.

POSTOPERATIVE CARE AND COMMENTS

Paralytic ileus is nearly always experienced after all forms of urinary diversion procedures. Therefore, gastric decompression is always achieved by means of either nasogastric intubation or the provision of a gastrostomy at the time of the operation. Gastric decompression is maintained for 24 to 48 hours. Nasogastric tubes suffice in the majority of patients. Certain patients, however, may best be managed by formal gastrostomy decompression. These include individuals in whom multiple prior abdominal procedures have been performed and prolonged ileus may be anticipated. In addition, patients with chronic pulmonary disease may benefit from the improved pulmonary toilet that can be achieved in the absence of a nasogastric tube. If formal gastrostomy is carried out, this is achieved by means of puncturing the anterior wall of the stomach and inserting a Malecot catheter. A purse-string suture is taken to ensure against gastric content leakage. A small stab wound is made in the left upper quadrant through which the Malecot catheter can be directed. The stomach wall is sutured around the margins of the tube exit site to the posterior fascia to prevent intraperitoneal leakage of gastric contents after tube removal. When gastrostomy tubes are used, they may be clamped on resolution of the ileus. If gastric residuals are small, they can be simply removed and the tube site heals quickly. If the duration of paralytic ileus is projected to be in excess of 4 to 5 days, intravenous hyperalimentation is initiated on the second postoperative day. If the patient is nutritionally depleted to begin with, hyperalimentation has been suggested to be of value if initiated during the preoperative interval (Hensle, 1983; Askanazi et al, 1985).

Ureteral stents are generally removed 1 week after surgery. Before removal, pouch x-ray studies are performed to ensure that the pouch is intact. Similarly, at the time of removal, radiologic contrast studies are carried out to ensure against ureteral anastomotic leakage or obstruction. The authors inject each stent with contrast material, looking first for extravasation. If none is seen, guide wires are advanced to each kidney and left in place, and the stents are removed over the wires. Subsequent films are obtained to document good drainage. If there is any question of extravasation, stents can be advanced over the wires, positioned fluoroscopically, and left in situ for re-evaluation after additional healing has taken place.

CONTINENT URINARY DIVERSION

Continent urinary diversion can be divided into three major categories. First, ureterosigmoidostomy and its varia-

tions, such as ileocecal sigmoidostomy, rectal bladder, and sigmoid hemi-Kock operation with proximal colonic intussusception, are discussed. These techniques allow for excretion of urine by means of evacuation. Orthotopic voiding pouches, which were first used almost exclusively in the male patient but are now being offered to female patients with an intact sphincteric apparatus, are then discussed. Finally discussed is the large category of continent diversions requiring clean intermittent catheterization for emptying urine at intervals from the constructed pouch.

The past 15 years have seen an acceleration of interest in the continent diversion of the upper urinary tract. The concept of refashioning bowel so that it serves as a urinary reservoir rather than a conduit has become universally accepted. This concept is based on original pioneering observations by Goodwin and others in the development of the cystoplasty augmentation procedure (Goodwin et al, 1958). The destruction of peristaltic integrity and refashioning of bowel has led to the development of many innovative urinary reservoirs constructed from bowel, using antireflux procedures to avoid upper tract urinary sepsis and additional surgical techniques to achieve urinary continence.

Because there are more than 40 variants of continent urinary diversion used worldwide, a complete review of all operative techniques is beyond the scope of this chapter. Many of the procedures, however, are simple modifications of parent procedures; this chapter addresses each parent operation as well as major modifications in detail. The fact that there are as many continent urinary diversion procedures described reveals that the "best" continent diversion has yet to be devised. There is to date no unanimity of opinion to indicate that one continent diversion is superior to another, but it is becoming apparent that certain procedures are associated with lower early and late complication rates. Remaining points of controversy include which bowel segment is most appropriate for fashioning into a urinary reservoir, the best techniques to use for achieving urinary continence, and the best technique for prevention of reflux of urine into the upper urinary tract.

It should be emphasized that all continent diversions allow for substantial reabsorption of urinary constituents. This places an increased workload on the kidneys. No patient with substantial renal impairment should be considered for these procedures. As mentioned, the authors require that the preoperative serum creatinine level be less than 1.8 mg/dl. Patients with a serum creatinine above 1.8 are more likely to experience significant acid-base disturbances and may experience a more rapid deterioration in renal function.

The long-term sequelae of conduit urinary diversion are well understood and, unfortunately, involve a considerable degree of damage to renal units. It has been suggested that the absence of reflux to the upper urinary tract (in catheterizing pouches) and the relative absence of bacteriuria in orthotopic voiding pouches (as well as the absence of reflux in most) may greatly reduce the long-term impact of the newer continent diversion procedures on renal function. It should be cautioned, however, that long-term data have yet to be achieved in these newer operations.

Many studies have suggested an improved psychosocial adjustment of the patient undergoing continent urinary and fecal diversion compared with those patients with diversions requiring collecting appliances (Gerber, 1980; McLeod and

Fazio, 1984; Boyd et al, 1987; Salter, 1992a, 1992b; Bjerre et al, 1995). Although this is indeed true and is best exemplified by the individual with a conduit who desires conversion to a continent procedure, it is also true that many individuals seem to adjust well to wearing appliances. The sense of body image is a remarkably personal and subjective parameter that is variable from patient to patient. For this reason, the authors believe that each patient facing urinary diversion should be interviewed separately by the urologist and the enterostomal therapist so that the patient becomes aware of the impact of wearing a urinary appliance as well as the price of opting for an alternative form of urinary diversion.

The process of patient counseling that the authors employ always refers to conduit urinary diversion as the gold standard against which the newer operations must be compared. The patient is well advised that long-term data are not yet available for continent diversion procedures and that continent diversion, in general, is associated with a longer hospital stay, higher complication rate, and greater potential for need of reoperative surgery, all other considerations being equal. An extensive review from the authors' institution, however, has demonstrated no statistically significant difference in reoperations, mortality, or hospital stay in patients undergoing continent diversion versus conduit diversion by the same three surgeons over a 3-year period (Benson et al, 1992). Analysis of the two patient groups showed that, in general, those selected for continent diversion were 12 years younger and four times less likely to have significant intercurrent illness. What this review indicates is that, **with proper patient selection, continent diversion operations can be conducted at the same cost to society and to the patient as conduit diversions.**

Rectal Bladder Urinary Diversion

Various innovative surgical techniques have been advocated for separating the fecal and urinary streams while still employing ureterosigmoidostomy principles. These operations can generally be discussed together as rectal bladder urinary diversions. In each of these operations, ureters are transplanted to the rectal stump, and the proximal sigmoid colon is managed by terminal sigmoid colostomy or, more commonly, by bringing the sigmoid to the perineum, using the anal sphincter in an effort to achieve both bowel and urinary control.

Although these operations continue to be popular abroad, they have never been well accepted in the United States for a variety of reasons. The principal reason is the calamitous complication of combined urinary and fecal incontinence, presumably occurring as a consequence of damage to the anal sphincter mechanism during the dissection processes (Culp, 1984).

If the urologist selects one of these procedures, the preoperative evaluation should include all of the caveats of ureterosigmoidostomy. Dilated ureters are not acceptable. The patient with prior extensive pelvic irradiation is not a candidate. Existing renal insufficiency disqualifies a patient from candidacy. Anal sphincteric tone must be judged competent before electing these operations, and finally colonoscopy must be carried out before the procedure to ensure against pre-existing colorectal disease as well as after the procedure

to guard against the potential development of colonic cancer after surgery. The procedures that separated the fecal and urinary streams but brought both out through the rectal sphincter are not described here. Those wishing a detailed description of these procedures can find this in the previous edition. In this chapter, the technique of ureterosigmoidostomy and the more modern surgical procedures that use the intact anal sphincter for urinary and fecal continence are described.

Ureterosigmoidostomy

Ureterosigmoidostomy can be regarded as the original continent urinary diversion; reports of this procedure can be found in the medical literature dating back to the 1870s (Smith, 1879). The operation has vacillated in its appeal to the urologic surgeon because of the considerable complications associated with transplantation of the ureters directly to the intact fecal stream. Complications, including hyperchloremic acidosis, hypokalemia with nephropathy, pyelonephritis, and development of colonic malignancy, have already been reviewed elsewhere.

Nevertheless, some authors believe that despite its pitfalls, ureterosigmoidostomy continues to offer a form of continent urinary diversion that is rather simple in comparison to the newer operative techniques devised for creating urinary reservoirs by means of complex refashioning of bowel segments.

The selection of the patient for continent diversion by ureterosigmoidostomy is most important. Because the potentially adverse long-term sequelae of this operation are so severe, most urologists use the procedure only for patients of advanced age. The operation is not suitable for the patient with neurogenic bladder because there may be associated bowel or anal sphincter dysfunction in such patients. Patients with dilated ureters are not candidates for ureterosigmoidostomy owing to the development of either obstruction or reflux. Patients with already established renal impairment are poor candidates for ureterosigmoidostomy or any continent diversion. The patient who has undergone extensive pelvic irradiation is not a good candidate for ureterosigmoidostomy, owing to the condition of the irradiated bowel as well as the irradiated distal ureters (Ambrose, 1983; Spirnak and Caldamone, 1986). Finally, patients with hepatic dysfunction should not undergo ureterosigmoidostomy (or perhaps any continent diversion) because of the possibility of ammonia intoxication (Silberman, 1958).

Preoperative evaluation of the patient selected for ureterosigmoidostomy should include studies for bowel disease that might contraindicate the operation. The presence of diverticulitis or colon polyps may be investigated by means of barium studies of the large bowel or colonoscopy. By no means should any patient undergo ureterosigmoidostomy without having an adequate test of anal sphincter integrity preoperatively. Incontinence of the mixture of stool and urine is a calamitous complication that can be avoided by a simple assessment. Various tests have been proposed to assess sphincter integrity; the most useful are those that require the patient to retain an enema solution of solid and liquid material for a specified time in the upright and ambulating position without soilage. A thin mixture of oatmeal and water serves well in this regard (Spirnak and Caldamone, 1986).

The authors have the patient retain 400 to 500 ml for 1 hour in the upright position.

PROCEDURE

Immediately before surgery, a multiperforate No. 28 Fr rectal tube is advanced through the anus and sutured in place to the perianal skin. This tube should be advanced sufficiently far so that it can be easily reached at the time of surgery.

A longitudinal incision in the posterior peritoneum overlying the right ureter is made, so that the distalmost ureter can be retrieved (Fig. 103–2A). The surgeon should keep in mind that a submucosal tunnel requires additional ureteral length. The white line of Toldt is incised along its course deep into the pelvis and the sigmoid colon reflected medially. The left ureter is identified and similarly transected at a low level (Fig. 103–2B)

Because the authors believe that all urinary diversion procedures should be protected by means of indwelling ureteral stents bilaterally, the open colotomy approach is preferred for ureterosigmoidostomy (Fig. 103–2C). These stents can be directed to the outside through the lumen of the rectal tube (Fig. 103–2D). The open colotomy approach affords greater ease in achieving this maneuver, although intubation of the ureters and direction of the stent through the rectal tube can be accomplished somewhat awkwardly using the Leadbetter technique of implantation.

The various techniques of ureterocolostomy have already been described in a previous chapter. If the open colon technique is used, an anterior colotomy is made in the region of appropriate taenia selection for the ureteral transplantation sites. After completing ureteral anastomosis and intubation, the colon can be closed with a simple two-layer technique (Fig. 103–2E). The inner layer should be closed with a running suture of absorbable material taken through all layers of intestine, whereas the outer layer is closed with seromuscular nonabsorbable material.

At the surgeon's preference, an attempt at retroperitonealizing the ureterocolonic anastomoses may be made. On the right side, this is somewhat easier to achieve because the peritoneal incision can simply be closed. On the left side, the colon can be rotated toward the left so that the lateral peritoneal incision used to expose the ureter can be sutured in place to the anterior sigmoid wall (Fig. 103–2F).

POSTOPERATIVE CARE AND COMMENTS

The ureteral stents are placed within the lumen of a urinary drainage device, which can then be directly fitted to the rectal tube. The total diversion of urine in this operation serves the additional function of decreasing postoperative concern for electrolyte disturbances.

Radiologic studies of the stents are carried out on the sixth or seventh postoperative day. Before conducting the stent studies, a Gastrografin enema may be given through the rectal tube itself to ensure that the region of ureterocolonic anastomoses is intact. Follow-up films are taken to ensure prompt drainage of the upper urinary tracts into the rectosigmoid region. The rectal tube may be removed at this point, but it is usually advisable to have it reinserted for evening drainage over the forthcoming week. The patient can be

instructed in this function so that he or she can be discharged from the hospital early. The patient is instructed to empty the colon at intervals of no more than every 2 hours, particularly in the early postoperative period.

When the rectal tube is removed, the patient must be closely monitored for the development of hyperchloremic acidosis. This occurs in the majority of instances, and it is wise to initiate a bicarbonate replacement program at the outset. Because hypokalemia is also a feature of ureterosigmoidostomy, replacement of base along with potassium may be achieved with potassium citrate medication. Routine nightly insertion of a rectal tube is advocated in the long-term care of the patient. Many patients, however, reject this practice as uncomfortable and unappealing. Nighttime urinary drainage must be mandated in any patient who cannot maintain electrolyte homeostasis with oral medication.

Obviously, all patients have exposure of the urinary tract to fecal flora. Most authors advocate long-term antibacterial agent administration in all patients (Duckett and Gazak, 1983; Spirnak and Caldamone, 1986). Ureteral strictures require reoperative surgery and are experienced in 26% to 35% of cases over time (Williams et al, 1969; Duckett and Gazak, 1983).

Because of the definite concern for the occurrence of rectal cancer some 5 to 50 years (average 21 years) after ureterosigmoidostomy (Ambrose, 1983), it is suggested that patients with long-term ureterosigmoidostomy be subjected to annual colonic investigation by means of colonoscopy (Filmer and Spencer, 1990). Barium enemas are relatively contraindicated because reflux of this material into the kidneys (if the antireflux procedure fails) can result in dire consequences (Williams, 1984). A further suggestion that might be used in monitoring for colon carcinoma is monitoring for blood in the stool and attempted cytologic examination of a mixed urine and feces specimen (Filmer and Spencer, 1990).

Augmented Valved Rectum

Kock developed this technique to be used in certain Third World countries where stoma appliances were not readily available (Kock et al, 1988). This operation is similar to standard ureterosigmoidostomy except that a proximal intussusception of the sigmoid colon confines the urine to a smaller surface area, thus minimizing the problems of electrolyte imbalance. Additionally the rectum is patched with ileum to improve the urodynamic properties of the rectum as a urinary reservoir. Preoperative evaluation is similar to that used in ureterosigmoidostomy. The large bowel must be studied for pre-existing disease, and anal sphincteric integrity must be tested before surgery.

PROCEDURE

Immediately before surgery, a multiperforate No. 28 Fr rectal tube is advanced through the anus and sutured in place to the perianal skin. This tube should be advanced sufficiently far so that it can be easily reached at the time of surgery.

The left colon and sigmoid are freed from their attachments to the line of Toldt. The anterior wall of the rectum is opened from the rectosigmoid junction inferiorly for a

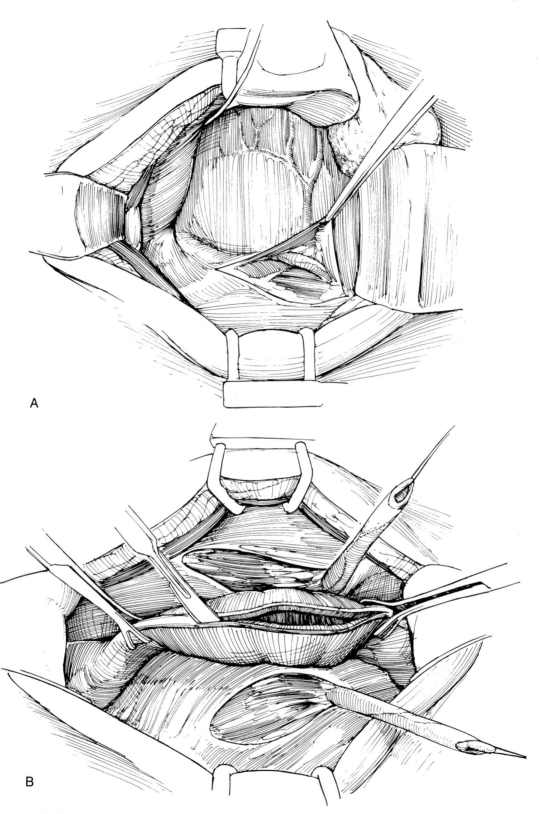

Figure 103–2. *A*, A longitudinal incision is made in the posterior peritoneum overlying the right ureter. *B*, The sigmoid colon reflected medially and the left ureter identified and transected.

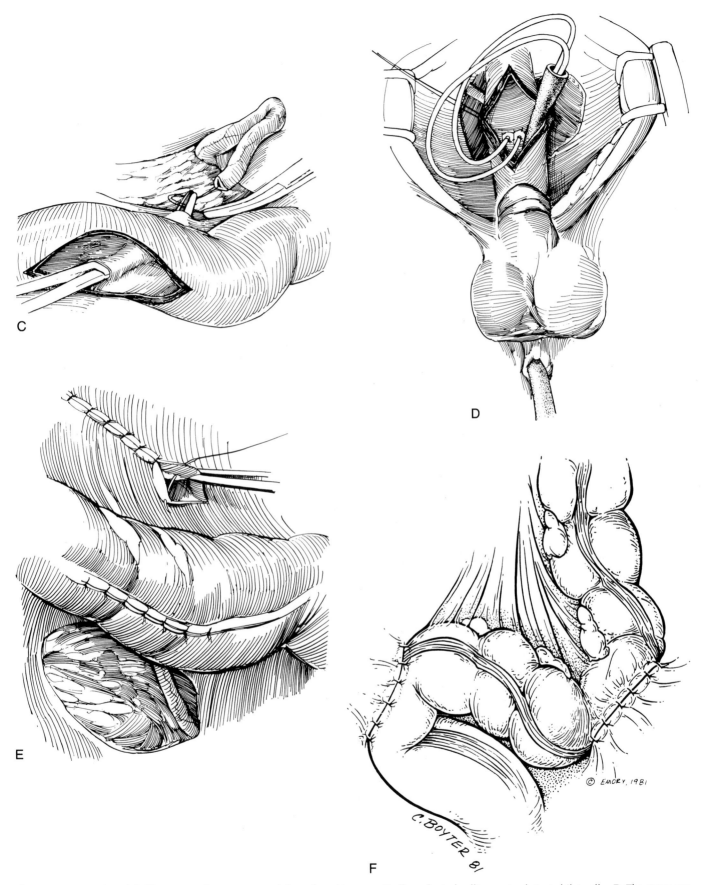

Figure 103–2 *Continued C,* The open colotomy approach is preferred because it allows for indwelling ureteral stents bilaterally. *D,* The stents are directed to the outside through the lumen of the rectal tube. *E,* The colon is closed with a simple two-layer technique. The retroperitoneal windows are closed with a running suture. *F,* The ureteral colonic anastomoses are retroperitonealized if possible. (From Hinman F Jr: Atlas of Urologic Surgery. Philadelphia, W. B. Saunders, 1989.)

distance of 10 cm. A 6- to 8-cm portion of distal sigmoid is cleared of its mesenteric attachments and appendices epiploacae by means of electrocautery. A Babcock clamp is directed into the sigmoid lumen through the rectal opening and the full thickness of sigmoid grasped. This is pulled down into the rectum as an intussusceptum, which is then stapled with four applications of the TA-55 stapler (Fig. 103–3A). The distal four to five staples are removed from the staple cartridge before firing to ensure that no staples reside at the tip of the nipple valve. If the stabilizing pin is used to ensure proper alignment of the staples and anvil, resulting pinholes are closed with figure-of-eight absorbable sutures. The opposing faces of the nipple valve and rectum are cauterized to denude the mucosa, and a fifth staple line is placed from the outside to fix the intussusceptum to the rectal wall. This is performed by sliding the anvil of the stapling device between the leaves of the intussusceptum, from the outside of the bowel.

The ureters are then anastomosed to the rectum by leading them down between the leaves of the intussuscipiens to buttonholes created bluntly at the summit of the nipple valve. The ureters are sewn to the buttonholes with absorbable sutures. The nipple valve is further stabilized by attaching the rectum to the intussuscepted sigmoid with interrupted seromuscular sutures.

A 20-cm segment of ileum is isolated and ileoileostomy employed to reconstitute the bowel. After closing the mesenteric trap, the ileal segment is opened on its antimesenteric border and folded in the shape of an upside-down U whose adjacent borders are sutured together with absorbable material. This broad ileal plate is used to close the rectal incision by patch graft technique (Fig. 103–3B).

POSTOPERATIVE CARE AND COMMENTS

There are no substantial differences in the postoperative care of these patients compared with those undergoing standard ureterosigmoidostomy. The patched rectal pouch has been studied urodynamically by Kock and associates and found to expand in volume from 200 ml perioperatively to 700 ml at 6 months postoperatively (Kock et al, 1988). Basal pressures increased gradually to only 30 cm H_2O at capacity. All patients reported excellent daytime and nighttime control.

Because of the limited surface area bathed by urine, no metabolic disturbances were reported, and no patient required sodium bicarbonate or potassium citrate therapy. No episodes of large bowel obstruction were reported despite the presence of a sigmoid intussusception. Reoperation for bowel obstruction was reported in 1 of 19 patients.

Hemi-Kock Procedure with Valved Rectum

In their description of the augmented valved rectum procedure, Kock and associates described the use of a foreshortened hemi-Kock pouch to be used as a rectal patch when the ureters were too dilated to bring down between the leaves of the intussuscepted sigmoid (Kock et al, 1988). Skinner and colleagues then modified this procedure by using an entire hemi-Kock segment to augment the rectum after sigmoid intussusception (Skinner et al, 1989).

The surgery consists of the construction of a hemi-Kock pouch employing doubly folded, marsupialized ileum and a proximal intussusception to prevent pouch-ureteral reflux. This hemi-Kock pouch is then anastomosed to the rectum, and contact of urine with the proximal colon is avoided by the intussusception of the sigmoid colon proximal to the anastomotic site. Because the competence of the intussuscepted ileocecal valve is approximately the same as that of the ileal intussusception achieved with the hemi-Kock operation, this latter feature of confining the urinary absorption area to a smaller portion of bowel remains the most compelling reason for conducting this complicated surgery in comparison to simple ileocecal sigmoidostomy.

Many of the same caveats are applicable to this procedure as in other colonic diversions. Anal sphincteric integrity must be intact before selecting this operation; the patient must have reasonable renal function to undergo this form of urinary diversion. Finally, the large bowel should be ascertained to be free of disease before surgery as evidenced by colonoscopy or barium studies. In contrast to direct ureterocolonic anastomotic procedures, however, dilated ureters may be accommodated by this operation.

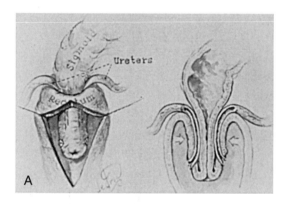

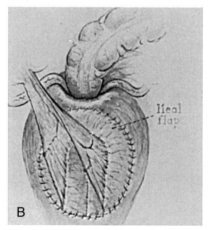

Figure 103–3. *A,* The anterior wall of the rectum is opened from the rectosigmoid junction inferiorly for a distance of 10 cm. A 6- to 8-cm portion of distal sigmoid is cleared of its mesenteric attachments and directed into the sigmoid lumen through the rectal opening and secured with a TA-55 stapler. The ureters are anastomosed to the rectum. *B,* A 20-cm segment of ileum is opened on its antimesenteric border and folded in the shape of an upside-down U. This ileal plate is used to close the rectal incision. (From Kock NG, Ghoneim MA, Lycke KG, Mahran MR: J Urol 1988; 140:1375–1379.)

PROCEDURE

After abdominal incision, the ureters are transected and led to the right retroperitoneum in the fashion as described for ileal conduit diversion. A 55-cm segment of ileum is selected, preserving the distal 10 to 20 cm of ileum. The distal ileal resection margin should be selected at the avascular plane of Treves, which separates the portion of ileum supplied by the ileocolic artery from that segment dependent on more proximal vascular supply. At the proximal ileal resection margin, a small triangular wedge of mesentery is resected along with approximately 5 cm of ileum to achieve appropriate hemi-Kock mobility while preserving adequate blood supply (Skinner et al, 1987a).

The lower 40 cm of ileum is then marsupialized along its antimesenteric border, using electrocautery, and the opened ileum is fashioned in the shape of a U (Fig. 103–4A). The posterior plate is formed by sewing together the medial limbs of the U with multiple running sutures of absorbable material (Fig. 103–4B). Once the posterior plate has been created, an intussusception of the proximal limb is required. Beginning approximately 3 cm from the end of the plate, the intact ileal limb is freed from its mesenteric attachments by means of electrocautery over a distance of 6 to 8 cm. Freeing the mesenteric attachments from the middle portions of the intussuscipiens prevents the potential of mesenteric tension disrupting the intussusception. A Babcock clamp is directed inside the intact proximal ileal limb, and, grasping full thickness of ileum, intussusception is carried out, creating at least a 5-cm intussuscipiens. This is stapled in two or three quadrants with the TA stapling device from which four or five inner staples have been removed (Fig. 103–4C). This simple maneuver avoids the deposition of staples at the distal aspect of the nipple valve (Skinner et al, 1984). More proximal staples are usually well covered by mucosa and not in contact with urine to serve as a nidus for stone formation. A fourth stapled line is taken in an additional quadrant to attach the intussuscipiens to the sidewall of the reservoir (Fig. 103–4D). This can be achieved in one of two fashions (see Kock pouch). Again, pinholes from the stabilizing pin of the stapling device must be oversewn. After the proximal intussusception is completed, ureteroileal anastomoses can be carried out as in ileal conduit urinary diversion and ureteral stents placed from the renal pelves through the proximal limb. The caudal margin of the posterior plate may then be brought cephalad to close one half of the pouch (Fig. 103–4E). This closure is accomplished with running absorbable sutures that are interrupted frequently at distances of 8 to 10 cm. The remaining inferior portion of the pouch is left patent for anastomosis to the rectum.

A 10-cm linear enterotomy is made on the anterior rectal surface, after freeing the entire sigmoid colon from the line of Toldt. A 6- to 8-cm segment of distal sigmoid colon is freed from its mesenteric blood supply, and sigmoid intussusceptions performed as in the augmented valved rectum procedure.

When this has been completed, the rectal enterotomy receives the inferior hemi-Kock pouch margin, and anastomosis of these two structures is carried out by interval running absorbable suture technique (Fig. 103–4F). Just before closing the entire anastomosis, the ureteral stents are directed to a rectal tube previously placed at the initiation of the procedure.

POSTOPERATIVE CARE AND COMMENTS

Postoperative management and complications associated with this operation are similar to those that might be experienced after the augmented valved rectum. The hemi-Kock procedure with valved rectum has one theoretical advantage over the valved rectum operation itself. Because transitional ureteral epithelium is not in contact with colonic epithelium, there might be less opportunity for development of colonic malignancy. This procedure has the potential for all the complications associated with the afferent limb of the Kock pouch (see Kock pouch). As in the augmented valved rectum, there is potentially less of a tendency toward hyperchloremic acidosis with this procedure because the ability of urine to contact larger portions of colonic epithelium is impeded by the proximal colonic intussusception. Nevertheless, attention should be paid to electrolyte levels after removal of stents and rectal tubes.

Simoneau and Skinner (1995) reported on the results of this procedure in 15 patients operated on between 1987 and 1991. Four patients had a prior bladder exstrophy and were converted to an ileoanal reservoir, and 11 patients underwent the procedure as a form of primary diversion after cystectomy. At the time of this report, 10 patients were still alive and evaluable. Early postoperative complications occurred in three patients (20%) and included a colocutaneous fistula in two patients, urine leak in one patient, and a deep venous thrombosis in one patient. Late complications included partial small bowel obstruction in four patients (two requiring surgery), urinary retention requiring surgery in two patients, and metabolic acidosis in five patients. Two of the 11 patients undergoing primary construction never achieved continence; both were over 68 years old. Simoneau and Skinner summarized their experience by concluding that the operation is best suited for the younger exstrophy patient and that it is essential to avoid colonic redundancy distal to the reservoir.

Sigma Rectum Pouch, MAINZ II

A variation of ureterosigmoidostomy was described by Fisch and Hohenfellner in 1991. This operation, which they termed the sigma rectum or the MAINZ II pouch, creates a low-pressure rectosigmoid reservoir of increased capacity. They viewed the simplicity and reproducibility of the operation as one if its major advantages.

Preoperative evaluation included radiologic imaging of the colon to rule out diverticulosis or polyps. Patients are given a 300-ml water enema, which they are asked to hold for 2 to 3 hours. Additionally an anal sphincter profile is performed to evaluate the integrity of the rectal sphincter (Fisch et al, 1992a).

PROCEDURE

At the rectosigmoid junction, the sigmoid colon is opened proximally through a taenial line for a distance of 10 to 12 cm. Stay sutures are placed at the midportion of the taenial incision, and the sigmoid colon is folded on itself in a U (Fig. 103–5A). The medial plate is closed in two layers using running sutures of 4–0 polyglycolic acid. The ureters are then implanted into 4- to 5-cm submucosal tunnels. These are intubated with No. 8 Fr ureteral stents that are led out

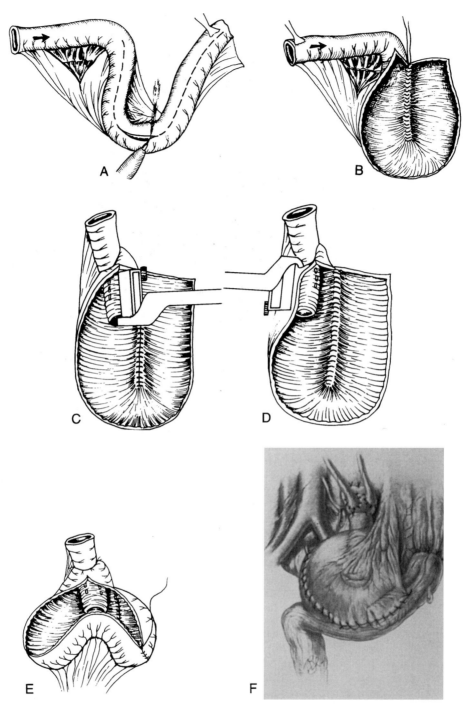

Figure 103–4. *A,* A 55-cm segment of ileum is selected, preserving the distal 10 to 20 cm of ileum. The lower 40 cm of ileum is marsupialized along its antimesenteric border. *B,* The posterior plate is formed by sewing together the medial limbs of the U with running sutures. *C,* A 5-cm intussusception is secured in two or three quadrants with the TA stapling device. *D,* An additional staple line is taken to attach the intussuscipiens to the side wall of the reservoir. *E,* The caudal margin of the posterior plate may be brought cephalad to close one half of the pouch. The inferior portion of the pouch is left patent for anastomosis to the rectum. *F,* A 10-cm linear enterotomy is made on the anterior rectal surface. A 6- to 8-cm segment of distal sigmoid colon is freed from its mesenteric blood supply and sigmoid intussusception performed as in the augmented valved rectum procedure. The rectal enterotomy receives the inferior hemi-Kock pouch margin. (*A–E* from Ghoneim MA, Kock NG, Kycke G, Shehab El-Din AB: J Urol 1987; 138:1150–1154. *F* from Skinner DG, Lieskovsky G, Boyd S: J Urol 1989; 141:1323–1327.)

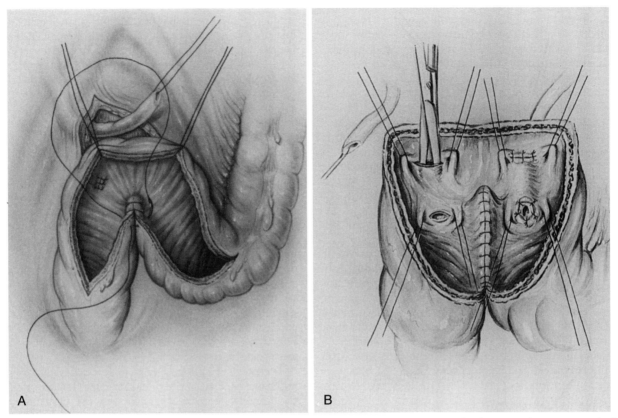

Figure 103–5. *A,* The rectosigmoid junction is identified and the bowel opened along an antimesenteric border taenia for 6 cm in each direction (12-cm incision). The segment is folded on itself and the posterior plate closed in two layers. *B,* The ureters are reimplanted into the posterior plate using a Goodwin technique and the reservoir closed in two layers. (From Fisch M, Wammack R, Hohenfellner R: The sigma-rectum pouch [MAINZ pouch II]. *In* Hohenfellner R, Wammack R, eds: Continent Urinary Diversion. Edinburgh, Churchill Livingstone, 1992, pp 165, 166.)

with a previously placed rectal tube (Fig. 103–5*B*). To prevent dislocation of the pouch and ureteral kinking, the posterior plate is secured to the area of the sacral promontory with two full-thickness interrupted absorbable sutures, which are placed after the ureteral implantation. The anterior wall of the pouch is then closed in two layers with interrupted sutures of 4–0 polyglycolic acid.

POSTOPERATIVE CARE AND COMMENTS

The rectal tube is removed on the third to fifth postoperative day, and the ureteral stents are removed around the eighth day. On the 15th postoperative day, the MAINZ group performs an intravenous pyelogram to assess the upper tracts and the sigma rectum pouch construction. Pouchography is performed on the 17th postoperative day. **The authors prefer to close the reservoir with a heavier suture using 3–0 polyglycolic acid for the mucosa and 2–0 polyglycolic acid for the bowel wall.** Although leakage is not reported as a significant problem, the use of 4–0 polyglycolic acid would cause the authors some concern.

The results of the MAINZ II pouch were presented by Fisch and co-workers (1995). Between 1990 and 1993, 73 patients (59 adults and 14 children) underwent the MAINZ II pouch procedure. Early complications were encountered in 5 of 73 patients (6.8%). These included single examples of a dislodged ureteral stent, pneumonia, pulmonary embolism, wound dehiscence, and ileus necessitating operative inter-

vention. Eight (10.9%) late complications required operative intervention. Ureteral stenosis occurred in five patients (6.8%), nephrolithiasis was treated with extracorporeal shock-wave lithotripsy in one patient, rupture of the anterior suture line required temporary colostomy in one patient, and one patient experienced perianal bleeding after chemotherapy that required endoscopic coagulation. Six patients presented with pyelonephritis (8.2%) and were treated with antibiotics. Daytime continence was reported at 94.5%, and nighttime continence was 98.6%. Oral alkalinization to prevent metabolic acidosis was used in 49 of 73 patients (67.1%). Two patients who refused any oral medication developed metabolic acidosis. The MAINZ group concluded that the overall complication rate was low and comparable to other techniques of continent urinary diversion. The high incidence of need for alkalinization is not dissimilar to standard ureterosigmoidostomy, however, so there is no apparent comparative advantage to this operation. In fact, the only difference between this operation and standard ureterosigmoidostomy is the partial reconfiguration of the rectosigmoid junction. It is possible that the reduced intracolonic pressures that may result from the partial reconfiguration decrease the incidence of upper tract problems, but this remains to be demonstrated.

Orthotopic Voiding Diversions

A variety of operative procedures were developed for the provision of a urinary pouch of low pressure and high capacity that accommodates the collection of urine and allows the male patient to initiate voiding by pelvic floor relaxation and Valsalva maneuver after cystoprostatectomy. More recently, these same principles have been successfully applied to selected female patients whose distal two thirds of urethra can be preserved (Colleselli et al, 1994; Stein et al, 1994). All of these operations were initially popularized by the singular work of Camey, whose Camey I operation using an intact ileal segment was a pioneer step in this form of urinary diversion (Camey and LeDuc, 1979). Because the concepts of bowel refashioning and interruption of peristaltic integrity are now well accepted, however, the only operations described in this section are those procedures that incorporate reconfigured intestinal segments.

All orthotopic neobladder operations share similar features. First, continence depends on the preservation of the external sphincteric apparatus in the both the male and the female. The preserved male sphincter results in a daytime continence rate in orthotopic voiding operations well in excess of 95%, and early results suggest that female daytime continence may exceed the 95% level seen in the male. The high level of male continence may result from the improved identification of the prostatic apex described in the nerve-sparing prostatectomy. This anatomic dissection results in better identification and preservation of the sphincteric apparatus (Walsh et al, 1983; Schlegel and Walsh, 1987).

Nocturnal enuresis is common to all orthotopic voiding procedures. The reason for enuresis in these operations, as contrasted with radical prostatectomy (in which enuresis is rare), is secondary to at least two phenomena. First, in radical prostatectomy, the native bladder and its reflexes remain intact. During bladder filling, a spinal reflex arc ensures the continued recruitment of external sphincteric contraction. Because the bladder has been removed in the patient undergoing orthotopic voiding diversion, this reflex is ablated, and external sphincteric recruitment does not occur except under voluntary conscious control (Jakobsen et al, 1987). **Interestingly, the authors have observed the acquisition of a *wake reflex* in many of their younger patients** (Benson et al, 1996). **The acquisition of this reflex, which is seen in both men and women, is a testimony to the tremendous ability of the human cerebrum to adapt to change.** Second, after neobladder construction, there is a significant reabsorption and recirculation of urinary constituents and other metabolites that result in the production of an increased urine volume. For this reason, it is important to ascertain that serum creatinine levels are in the normal range or certainly below the level of 1.8 mg/dl.

The incidence and degree of enuresis varies from series to series and appears independent of the type of bowel used to construct the voiding pouch. Nevertheless, most series suggest that at least some patients are bothered by nocturnal wetting (Melchior et al, 1988; Thuroff et al, 1988; Kock et al, 1989; Schreiter and Noll, 1989; Studer et al, 1989; Wenderoth et al, 1990; Benson et al, 1996). Means of managing this wetting vary as well. In the usual patient, the simple technique of waking two or three times per night results in a dry sleep period. If this does not suffice, the patient can undergo various sphincter operations, as suggested by others (Skinner et al, 1989; Lange P, personal communication, 1991). Finally, male patients who may not wish to undergo

sphincter placement may be suitably managed by condom catheter drainage or the simple wearing of a penile incontinence clamp during sleeping hours. In female patients, enuresis appears to be a lesser problem for reasons that remain unclear. Perhaps it is related to the hypercontinence (urinary retention requiring clean intermittent catheterization) that is sometimes encountered in the female patient.

The additional feature shared by all of the orthotopic voiding procedures when they are used for treatment of bladder cancer is the risk of urethral cancer recurrence. In the male bladder cancer patient, the incidence of anterior urethral recurrence is approximately 4% to 5% overall (Cordonnier and Spjut, 1961). This is obviously too low a percentage to warrant routine urethrectomy in all patients. The risk of urethral transitional cell carcinoma is slightly higher in patients with diffuse carcinoma in situ of the bladder and may approach 35% or more in those patients who have transitional cell cancer of the prostatic urethra (Schellhammer and Whitmore, 1976; Raz et al, 1978; Stockle et al, 1990). **Although the risk of urethral recurrence may be slightly higher in those patients with diffuse bladder carcinoma in situ, the authors do not consider this an indication for urethrectomy unless the process involves the prostatic urethra.**

The incidence of delayed female urethral recurrence has not been as well studied because the female urethra has traditionally been incorporated into the cystectomy specimen. The frequency of incidental female urethral involvement coexisting with bladder cancer has been reported. A study by DePaepe and colleagues identified urethral involvement in 8 of 22 (36%) unselected female cystectomy specimens (DePaepe et al, 1990). An extensive study by Stein and co-workers reviewed the incidence of urethral cancer in 65 female cystectomy specimens; 56 of these patients underwent cystectomy for transitional cell cancer (Stein et al, 1994). Of the 56, 16 (28%) had histologic evidence of atypia, carcinoma in situ, or frank tumor at the bladder neck, and 7 of the 16 also had urethral atypia or carcinoma. None of the 40 patients in whom the bladder neck was uninvolved had a urethral abnormality. Stein and co-workers concluded that in the absence of bladder neck involvement, the female urethra could be safely retained.

One other concern in the woman being selected for orthotopic neobladder diversion is the involvement of the anterior vaginal wall. Anterior vaginal wall involvement was identified in 4 of 67 cystectomy specimens (Stein et al, 1994). All four of these patients had bladder neck involvement, and two had urethral involvement. **Therefore, it appears safe to conclude that in the absence of bladder neck involvement, the female urethra can be preserved and that either the vaginal wall can be left in place or a narrow strip can be resected without compromising the margins of the cystectomy.**

If urethrectomy is required, the patient is not a candidate for continent voiding diversion. To ensure the proper selection of patients for this operation, the authors perform prostatic urethral biopsy in all men being considered and biopsy of the bladder neck of women. The authors agree with others and have not routinely disqualified patients with in situ carcinoma from continent voiding diversion (Hickey et al, 1986). The authors advocate formal transurethral resection of the prostatic urethra in these instances, mandating that all of the transitional epithelium in the prostate is free of disease before suggesting that an orthotopic voiding procedure is safe. **Finally, it should be emphasized that only long-term experience will clarify the exclusion criteria appropriately, and these have not yet been developed.**

One feature regarding metachronous urethral recurrence in the patient undergoing orthotopic voiding diversion is that monitoring for potential of urethral recurrence is greatly simplified. In the patient with an alternative form of urinary diversion in whom the urethra remains after cystoprostatectomy for urothelial cancer, urethral washings are required at intervals to monitor for malignant change in the urethral remnant. In patients undergoing continent voiding diversion, simple voided urine may be used in this respect for cytologic examination.

Whatever the risk of urethral recurrence or enuresis, continent voiding diversion appears to be the most popular among all candidates (male and female) undergoing cystectomy. Patients can be restored to micturition that is nearly normal, and if the nerve-sparing technique is used, the male patient may have preservation of sexual function as well (Marshall et al, 1990). Female patients not requiring total vaginectomy can likewise maintain sexual function. The removal of only a 1- to 2-cm strip of anterior vagina has not resulted in a compromise of vaginal capacity, nor has it resulted in any compromise to appropriate excision of all cancer in orthotopic female diversion.

All patients, male and female, should be advised of the possible need for clean intermittent catheterization. A rare male patient is unable to void by Valsalva maneuver (Marshall et al, 1990). In women, the incidence of urinary retention requiring clean intermittent catheterization may be as high as 50% (Hautmann et al, 1995). Furthermore, there have been reports of greatly distended pouches occurring with the passage of time after continent voiding diversion (Camey et al, 1987; Keetch et al, 1992). Such patients are necessarily assigned to permanent clean intermittent catheterization to achieve urinary emptying. In an effort to obviate the silent development of this complication, the authors advise patients to self-catheterize at least monthly to measure postvoid residual volume. The authors further insist that all patients without enuresis and men employing nighttime penile clamps wake at least once nightly to void.

If a patient does develop an invasive urethral recurrence after cystectomy and neobladder, it is necessary to remove the reservoir and urethra and convert the patient to a conduit. The Studer neobladder is perhaps the most amenable to this conversion by virtue of its 15- to 20-cm isoperistaltic proximal ileal limb. The hemi-Kock is also more amenable to conversion than a reservoir in which the ureters are implanted into the wall of the pouch. For superficial urethral papillary recurrence, local resection may in some instances suffice (Benson and Miller, 1995). Such a patient must be monitored closely.

The literature is replete with opinion relative to the bowel segment that is best to employ in orthotopic voiding diversion. Most procedures use the small bowel in whole or in part, and there does appear to be somewhat less contractility in the reformed small bowel compared to large bowel. Furthermore, there is evidence that mucosal atrophy, with resultant decrease in reabsorption of urinary constituents, is more dependable in small bowel than in large bowel (Norlen and

Trasti, 1978). It is clear, however, that continent voiding diversion procedures employing large bowel in part (MAINZ pouch) or in whole (sigmoid pouch) appear to work equally well in all regards. Similar degrees of daytime and nocturnal incontinence are reported; similar freedom from metabolic complications has been experienced (Reddy, 1987; Thuroff et al, 1988).

Common to the operative and postoperative care of all voiding pouches is the management of tubes and drains. Long single-J end-hole stents are used to drain the kidneys externally. A Foley catheter can be used transurethrally, and if there is a small urethral capacity (as in most men), it may be preferable to direct the stents through a stab wound, usually in the right lower quadrant. A suprapubic tube is optional; if used, it can be led out with the ureteral stents. Pouch integrity should always be tested intraoperatively by saline insufflation. A suction drain is placed through another stab wound in the left lower quadrant. This is directed toward the ureteral anastomoses and traverses across the membranous urethral pouch anastomosis as well. If stents or a suprapubic tube are led through the bowel wall, the bowel puncture sites are secured with purse-string sutures to diminish urinary leakage after stent removal. Similarly the pouch can be sutured to the anterior abdominal wall at the stab wound site to prevent urine leakage into the peritoneal cavity.

Postoperatively the urethral catheter or suprapubic tube must be irrigated at 4- to 6-hour intervals to ensure that tubes remain clear of mucus plugs. As soon as practical, the patient can be taught to carry out this process alone. Before the stents are removed, a radiographic pouch study is performed. The authors routinely carry this out at about 7 days postoperatively. If the pouch shows no leakage of contrast material, the stents are removed, again with radiologic control (as previously described) to ensure that the ureteral anastomoses are intact and that the kidneys drain promptly. If a suprapubic tube has been used, it may be removed at this time as well, along with the suction drains, so that the patient may then be discharged with only a urethral catheter to care for.

The patient is taught to irrigate the urethral catheter at home, on a 4- to 6-hourly program, with additional irrigation anytime suprapubic pressure or discomfort occurs. By 14 days, the patient returns to the office for removal of the urethral catheter and institution of a voiding trial. The authors have patients catheterize once daily for irrigation of mucus debris during the subsequent 2 weeks. If there is only a small amount of mucus remaining after voiding, catheterizing intervals can be lengthened to weekly and then monthly. In the early postoperative period, pouch capacities may be quite small (as little as 100 ml), especially in the case of small intestinal neobladders. To afford restful sleep to the patient overnight during the first 6 weeks after surgery, the patient inserts a Foley catheter at bedtime. No attempt is made to address management of nighttime voiding or enuresis until daytime control is well established and the voided volumes are at least 200 ml.

Orthotopic Diversion: Surgical Techniques

Orthotopic diversion to the male urethra mimics the operative techniques used in radical prostatectomy. One major difference is the dissection of the prostatic apex. In patients undergoing radical prostatectomy, great care must be exercised in the apical dissection to ensure a negative surgical margin. In patients undergoing orthotopic diversion, the prostate apex is still excised, but if some apical capsular tissue is inadvertently left, the ramifications are less significant. The authors are aggressive in dissecting the urethral stump into the prostate before urethral transection. This is accomplished by using a peanut dissector to reflect the apex of the prostate proximally by about 0.6 to 1.0 cm. In all instances, these patients have had undetectable postoperative serum prostate-specific antigen determinations, even when a hypersensitive assay was employed.

In women, the technique of radical cystectomy must be modified if an orthotopic diversion to the urethra is anticipated (Stein et al, 1994). The cystectomy proceeds antegrade to the level of the vaginal apex. At the vaginal apex, a plane can be established between the bladder and the vagina if there is no tumor involvement of the bladder base and trigone. **If tumor does involve any aspect of the floor, the authors still remove an anterior strip (1–2 cm) of vagina with the bladder specimen.** The procedure continues antegrade to the level of the bladder neck. Distal to the bladder neck, it is important not to interfere with the lateral neurovascular supply to the urethra. The authors have accomplished this portion of the procedure by placing a Satinsky vascular clamp across the urethra, with its proximal side at the level of the bladder neck. The Foley catheter is then deflated and the clamp secured as the catheter is removed. This prevents spillage of bladder contents as the urethra is transected. This maneuver also results in resection of a portion of the proximal urethra, which is important if hypercontinence (urinary retention) is to be avoided. On removal of the specimen, the distal bladder neck–urethral margin is sent for frozen section. Anastomosis of the reservoir to the urethral stump can then be performed in the usual manner.

A final caveat in the fashioning of a continent voiding diversion is the mobility of the bowel segment employed. After cystectomy, and before division of the bowel segment, a Babcock clamp should be placed on the selected bowel, directing it toward the urethral stump to ensure that the bowel segment comfortably reaches the anastomotic region. In obese patients with fatty mesentery, there may be some degree of tension, which can usually be obviated by adjusting the degree of hyperextension of the operating room table. Whenever there is any anastomotic tension at all, the authors keep the patient in a semi-Fowler's position for the first 2 postoperative days.

Camey II Operation

The Camey II operation is a modification of the original technique developed by Camey that accommodates the principle of refashioning bowel so that peristaltic integrity is abrogated (Camey, 1990). A length of ileum measuring 65 cm is selected for its ability to reach the region of the membranous urethral anastomosis without tension (Fig. 103–6A). This point is marked, and the ileal segment is isolated from the bowel (Fig. 103–6B). After ileoileostomy has been used to restore bowel integrity and the mesenteric trap is closed, the ileum is opened along its antimesenteric border

throughout its entire length, with the exception of the region previously marked for ileourethral anastomosis. At this point, the spatulation curves toward the mesenteric border (Fig. 103–6C). The totally spatulated ileum is then folded over itself in the form of a transverse U with the medial borders of the U sutured to one another with running absorbable suture material (Fig. 103–6D). A fingertip opening is made in the ileal wall at the site selected for ileourethral anastomosis, and the entire broad, wide plate of ileum is advanced into the pelvis for ileourethral and ureteral anastomosis. Eight urethral sutures, previously placed from inside to outside the urethra, are completed by taking full thickness of ileum at the posterior margin of the ileourethral anastomosis. As the ileum is advanced into the pelvis, these sutures are tied so that the knots lie within the lumen of the anastomosis.

Ureteral anastomoses are carried out by the LeDuc technique (LeDuc et al, 1987), already described in Chapter 100. The remaining ileum is then closed by folding the plate so as to complete the pouch construction (Fig. 103–6E). At these points, the ileal plate is sutured to the pelvic fascia to reduce tension on the anastomoses. Here again, closure is achieved with running sutures of absorbable material (Fig. 103–6F).

POSTOPERATIVE CARE AND COMMENTS

Daytime continence rates of 96% are reported by Camey (1990). There is time lag to the development of total daytime continence. Sphincter exercises are used uniformly for this and can be initiated preoperatively among most patients. More than 75% of men have achieved nocturnal continence as a consequence of the simple expedient of voiding at two or three planned awakenings.

Baseline pouch pressures of 10 cm H_2O have been reported, and minimal contractility averaging 32 cm H_2O has been observed during pouch fillings. Full pouch pressures averaged 30 cm H_2O, and mean pouch capacity was 434 ml. In an unselected series of 57 patients, Camey describes the need for reoperation in 10 (17%). None of the complications requiring reoperation were related to the urinary pouch construction (Camey, 1990). In 1995, Lugagne and colleagues reported on the fate of the upper tracts in patients undergoing both the Camey I (nondetubularized) and the Camey II operations (Lugagne et al, 1995). For both operations, LeDuc ureteral anastomoses were performed. They found no statistical differences in upper tract preservation between the two groups. Among 232 renal units evaluable at 2 years or more, 11.2% demonstrated obstruction; 3.8% required reimplantation and 2.1% nephrectomy. **This rate of upper tract obstruction is higher than that seen in neobladders that do not rely on the LeDuc ureteral anastomosis technique.**

There are no substantial differences in postoperative care of these patients with voiding pouches and other procedures other than the sphincteric exercises and ensuring that the patient recognizes the sense of pelvic fullness associated with the need to void.

Vesica Ileale Pouch

A technique of ileal bladder replacement similar to the Camey II procedure was developed by the group in Padova,

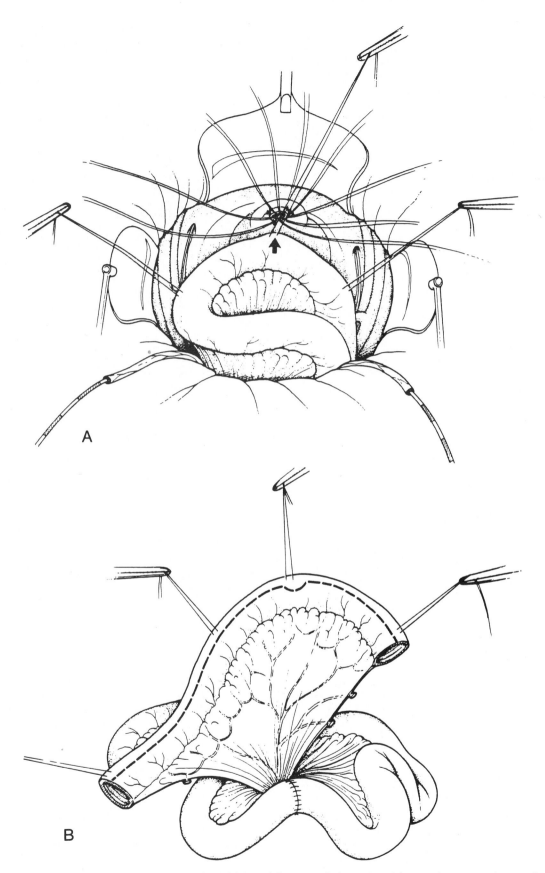

A

B

Figure 103–6. *A*, A length of ileum measuring 65 cm is selected for its ability to reach the region of the membranous urethra. *B*, The ileal segment is isolated and opened along its antimesenteric border throughout its length.

Illustration continued on following page

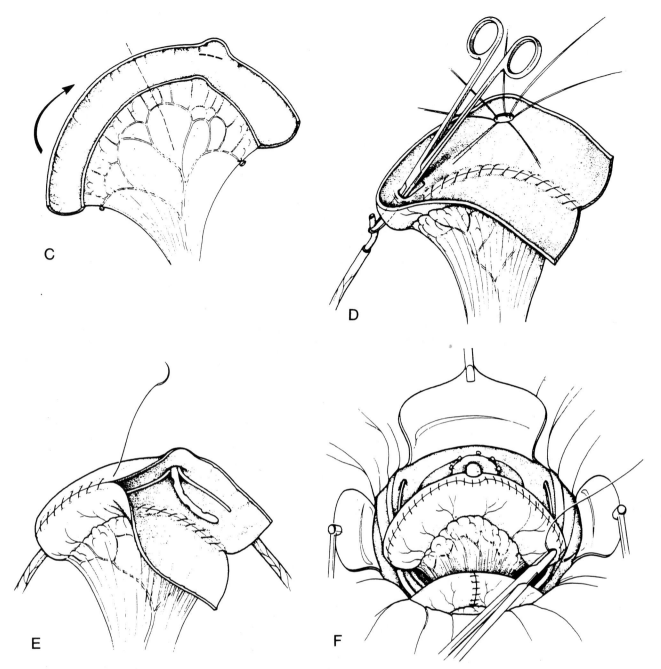

Figure 103–6 *Continued C,* In the region of the ileourethral anastomosis, the incision is spatulated to curve toward the mesenteric border. *D,* The ileum is then folded in the form of a transverse U with the medial borders of the U sutured to one another. A fingertip opening is made in the ileal wall at the site selected for ileourethral anastomosis. The ureters are reimplanted by the LeDuc technique. Eight urethral sutures are tied so that the knots lie within the lumen of the anastomosis. *E,* The ileum is closed by folding the plate so as to complete the pouch construction. *F,* The ileum is sutured to the pelvic fascia to reduce tension on the anastomoses. (From Camey M: Curr Surg Tech Urol 1990; 3:1–8.)

Italy (Pagano et al, 1990). This was called the vesica ileale Padovana (VIP) pouch. The operation is similar to the Camey II in many regards. An approximately 60-cm length of ileum is employed, and ileourethral anastomosis is carried out in a similar fashion. LeDuc ureteral implants are similarly performed. The only difference is in the way the spatulated bowel is refashioned. In the VIP pouch, the spatulated ileum is rolled on itself, as in a jelly roll, to produce the posterior plate, which is then closed anteriorly (Fig. 103–7).

POSTOPERATIVE CARE AND MANAGEMENT

There are no substantial differences in the postoperative care of these patients as compared with patients undergoing Camey II orthotopic diversion. The Padova group reported a 90% daytime continence rate that increased to 100% if patients with "very rare leakage during straining" were considered dry (Pagano et al, 1992). Nighttime continence was defined as dry for 6 hours; 80% of patients fulfilled that definition. An additional 12% were dry with two to three

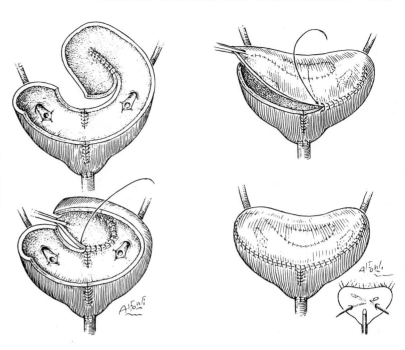

Figure 103–7. A 60-cm length of ileum is employed, and ileourethral anastomosis is carried out. LeDuc ureteral implants are performed. The spatulated bowel is refashioned in a jelly roll to produce the posterior plate, which is then closed anteriorly. (From Pagano F, Artibani W, Ligato P, et al: Eur Urol 1990; 17:149–154.)

planned awakenings, but 7% continued to experience enuresis. Ultimate bladder capacities ranged from 400 to 650 ml; basal pouch pressures of 3 to 5 cm H_2O and capacity pressures of 10 to 30 cm H_2O were reported.

In 61 patients, early complications included one postoperative death secondary to pulmonary embolism and two anastomotic leaks with spontaneous closure. Long-term complications related to the neobladder were reported in 41 patients and included three (7%) ureteroileal stenoses, five (12%) urethroileal stenoses, and two (5%) urethral stenoses. All complications were treated endoscopically. No metabolic complications were reported. The incidence of ureteral anastomotic obstruction is lower than that usually encountered with LeDuc reimplants and may be related to a shorter follow-up interval in the Pagano (1992) report.

S-Bladder

Schreiter and Noll (1989, 1991) described a technique of total spatulation of an isolated 75-cm segment of terminal ileum that is refashioned into a broad plate by means of S or incomplete W configuration (Fig. 103–8). Here again, LeDuc ureteral anastomosis was performed. Results were reported in 52 patients, 46 men and 6 women. Full daytime continence was reported in 49 (94%), and 44 (85%) were reported to be continent day and night. To achieve this result, 16 patients were treated with an artificial sphincter, but in fairness to the authors of this study, 11 of the 16 had cystectomy performed for neurogenic bladders, and these 11 were preoperatively known to have urethral incompetence. An overall complication rate of 13.5% was reported.

Ileal Neobladder

This operation, devised at the University of Ulm in Germany, is an additional extension of the Camey principle incorporating Goodwin cup cystoplasty principles (Hautmann et al, 1988; Wenderoth et al, 1990). It has become a popular neobladder and has been used worldwide (Fair, 1991).

PROCEDURE

A segment of ileum 70 cm in length is chosen while preserving the distal 15 cm of terminal ileum (Fig. 103–9A). The distal resection margin is at the junction of ileocolic and superior mesenteric blood supplies. After reconstituting the bowel and closing the mesenteric trap, the isolated ileum is spatulated at its antimesenteric border except for the area selected for ileourethral anastomosis, where the incision is made at the anterior mesenteric border creating a U-shaped flap (as in the Camey II operation), which serves as the new bladder neck. The bowel is arranged in an M or W configuration, and the four limbs are sutured one to another with running absorbable suture material to form a broad ileal plate (Fig. 103–9B).

A button of tissue is removed from the previously selected ileourethral anastomotic site. This button is approximately

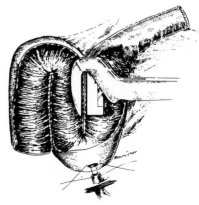

Figure 103–8. The ileum is reconfigured in an S or W shape. (From Schreiter F, Noll F: J Urol 1989; 142:1197–1200.)

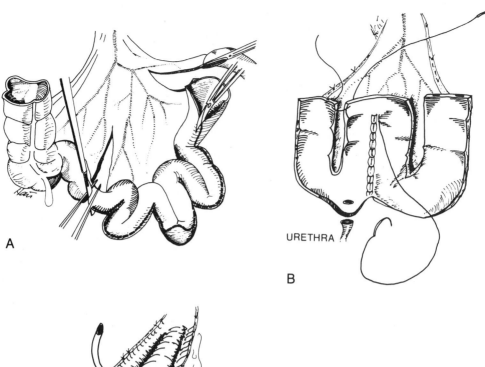

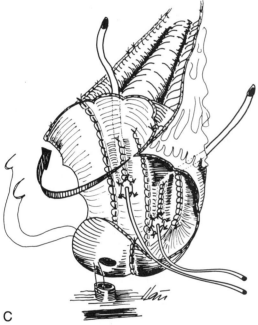

Figure 103–9. *A*, A segment of ileum 70 cm in length is chosen while preserving the distal 15 cm. *B*, The isolated ileum is spatulated at its antimesenteric border except for the area selected for ileourethral anastomosis. The segment is arranged in an M or W configuration, and the four limbs are sutured one to another with running absorbable suture material. *C*, A button of tissue is removed from the selected ileourethral anastomotic site. Six separate absorbable sutures are placed from the inside of the ileal plate to the urethra, with the ends brought back into the ileourethral aperture. LeDuc ureteral implants are performed, and the plate itself is closed into a pouch. (From Wenderoth UK, Bachor R, Egghart G, et al: J Urol 1990; 143:492–497.)

the size of a fingertip. Six separate absorbable sutures are placed from the inside of the ileal plate to the urethra, with the ends brought back into the ileourethral aperture. A Foley catheter is placed through the urethra into the ileal aperture, and all six sutures are tied on the inside of the pouch while traction on the catheter directs the ileal plate to the urethral stump. LeDuc ureteral implants are then carried out in the posterior margin of the ileal plate, and then the plate itself is closed into a pouch (Fig. 103–9*C*).

POSTOPERATIVE CARE AND COMMENTS

The Ulm group recommends that ureteral stent studies be carried out at 12 days and that urethral catheter drainage be maintained for 3 weeks. This prolonged period of ureteral and urethral catheter drainage may be necessary because these authors do not attempt to create a watertight closure.

The Ulm group believes that the neobladder will close and that the efforts necessary to ensure that the neobladder is watertight given the long suture lines are unnecessary. **It has always been the authors' practice to create a watertight reservoir or neobladder.**

Bladder capacities averaging 755 ml were reported with the mean intravesical pressure at capacity of 26 cm H_2O; one-half capacity intravesical pressures were 10 cm H_2O. In a report of 229 patients undergoing cystectomy for invasive bladder cancer, the Ulm group reported a perioperative mortality of 2.4% and a 10.5% incidence of early reoperation (Steiner et al, 1994). Bowel obstruction occurred in 3.8%. Late complications included urethroileal stricture (6.7%) and ureteroileal stenosis (3.3%). Despite a strict definition of continence (patients dry but waking at night to void were considered incontinent), 77% of patients were totally continent day and night, and an additional 12% of patients experienced only occasional enuresis or had mild stress urinary incontinence in the daytime. Only 2 of 229 patients had grade 3 incontinence with 2-year follow-up.

The ileal neobladder has been adopted by numerous surgeons who have achieved excellent results (Fair, 1991). A major concern is the relatively high incidence of early reoperations reported by Steiner and colleagues (1994). With regard to urinary continence, however, the operation is unsurpassed.

Orthotopic Hemi-Kock Pouch

This operation was designed by Ghoneim and associates to accommodate the male patient facing cystectomy (Ghoneim et al, 1987). In this operation, prevention against ureteral reflux depends on the construction of a nipple valve. As previously described, nipple valve construction usually requires the use of staples to stabilize the intussusception of the bowel. Thus, this form of voiding pouch has some potential for the development of urinary calculi within the pouch, a feature not shared by the other orthotopic voiding operations.

PROCEDURE

The operative procedure is carried out precisely as has been previously described for orthotopic hemi-Kock with sigmoid intussusception. The sole difference is that the closure of the inferior portion of the pouch leaves a smaller aperture patent to be used for the urethral anastomosis. Alternatively the entire pouch may be closed and a buttonhole opening used (Fig. 103–10). The authors fashion this opening such that it accept a No. 24 Fr catheter without resistance. Ileourethral anastomosis is carried out in the usual fashion, employing four to eight interrupted absorbable sutures, previously placed in the urethral stump.

Some authors advocate the use of double-J stents whose lower portion resides within the pouch after traversing the nipple valve. The authors use open-end, single-J stents brought out through the reservoir (previously described in surgical cystectomy procedure) to divert the urine from the entire pouch.

POSTOPERATIVE CARE AND COMMENTS

The postoperative management of this voiding pouch is the same as the others. The only specific complication of this procedure relative to the others is the potential for the

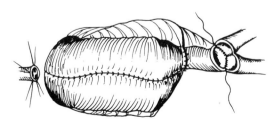

Figure 103–10. The operative procedure is carried out precisely as has been previously described (see Fig. 103–4). The closure of the inferior portion of the pouch leaves a small aperture patent to be used for the urethral anastomosis. (From Ghoneim MA, Kock NG, Kycke G, Shehab El-Din AB: J Urol 1987; 138:1150–1154.)

development of stones on any exposed staples in the urinary tract. If stones are found at a small enough size, they can usually be managed cystoscopically by forceps extraction (along with the offending staple). If somewhat larger stones are found, electrohydraulic or ultrasound lithotripsy units may be used to fracture the stone and the fragments and staple removed by a combination of forceps and irrigating techniques.

Ghoneim and associates reported 100% daytime continence (Ghoneim et al, 1987). Nocturnal control or only mild urinary spotting was seen in 12 of the first 16 patients studied. At 3 months, pouch capacity was 300 ml on average and expanded to 750 ml by 11 months. Urodynamic evaluation showed pressures below 20 cm H_2O until reservoir capacity was reached. In a later article reporting results in 34 evaluable patients (Kock et al, 1989), 30 patients (88%) were continent day and night. One patient required reoperation early for bowel obstruction, and nearly half the patients required surgery to correct a slipped antireflux valve.

The largest clinical experience with orthotopic hemi-Kock ileal reservoirs has been amassed by Elmajian and colleagues (1995). They reported on 266 patients operated on between May 1986 and June 1993. Fifty-two early complications were experienced by 47 of 266 patients (7.7%); 19 were related to the neobladder, and 33 were unrelated. There was no perioperative mortality. With a median follow-up of 2.9 years, 40 late complications were experienced by 35 of 266 patients (13.2%); 26 were related to the neobladder, and 14 were unrelated. Neobladder-related complications included nine patients (3.4%) with reservoir calculi; six patients with afferent nipple stenoses (2.3%); five patients with ureteroileal stenosis (1.9%); two patients with a prolapsed afferent nipple (0.8%); and one patient each (0.4%) with reflux, Kock-cutaneous fistula, diarrhea, and metabolic acidosis. Of interest is that 18 of 26 of the late neobladder-related complications were directly or indirectly attributable to the Kock neobladder operation and might not have been experienced if an alternative procedure had been employed by these authors. Nevertheless, the overall short-term and long-term complication rates reported by these authors are commendable.

Continence was evaluable in 156 of 202 patients still alive and responding to the survey. Of patients, 99 (64.7%) reported good and 34 (22.2%) reported satisfactory daytime continence. Good nighttime continence was reported by 69 patients (44.2%), and an additional 65 (41.7%) reported satisfactory nocturnal continence.

Low-Pressure Bladder Substitute

A variation of the orthotopic hemi-Kock procedure is the pouch described by Studer and co-workers (1988). This procedure is much simpler in its construction because it avoids the need for an intussuscepted proximal limb. It has now been used by the authors for more than 6 years in men and for 1 year in women with excellent results (Benson et al, 1994, 1996). A report by Rogers and Scardino (1995) also confirmed the reliability and simplicity of Studer's procedure.

PROCEDURE

An ileal segment measuring 60 to 65 cm in length is isolated, leaving the distal 25 cm of ileum intact. After reconstituting the bowel and closing the mesenteric trap, the ileum is rotated 180 degrees on its mesentery so that its proximal end reaches the right retroperitoneum (Fig. 103–11A). Studer described the oversewing of both ileal ends with absorbable material (may be managed by application of absorbable staples). The authors oversew only the proximal end and open the distal segment to its terminus and include it in the reservoir to maximize pouch volume. The distal 40 to 45 cm is opened along the antimesenteric border and folded in the configuration of a U, facing the patient's right side. The posterior plate is completed by joining the limbs of the U with running absorbable sutures. Standard ureteroileal (refluxing) anastomoses are carried out at the apex of the intact limb of ileum (Fig. 103–11B). Anastomosis of the posterior plate of ileum to the urethra is carried out with six previously placed urethral sutures. The left side of the ileal plate is brought to the patient's right, and the plate is closed in a cup cystoplasty configuration with running absorbable suture material (Fig. 103–11C). Ureteral stents are brought through a separate abdominal incision, and suction drainage is achieved. Studer (1989) described the use of a suprapubic tube, but the authors have performed this operation with only urethral drainage.

POSTOPERATIVE CARE AND COMMENTS

Studer and colleagues reported 10-year results in 100 consecutive patients using the ileal low-pressure bladder substitute (Studer et al, 1995). Eleven patients experienced early complications, including pulmonary embolism (three patients); severe sepsis (three patients, two fatal); fascial dehiscence (two patients); and cerebrovascular accident, myocardial infarction, and femoral artery thrombosis (one patient each). None of the early complications were directly attributable to the neobladder. Late complications requiring rehospitalization or reoperation were experienced by 18 patients. Six patients were hospitalized for treatment of metabolic disturbances, four patients developed inguinal or abdominal wall hernias, and two patients developed deep venous thrombosis. There were two cases each of ureteral stenosis and urethral stricture. One patient developed intestinal obstruction and one developed pouch necrosis at delayed times from surgery.

The median immediate postoperative neobladder capacity in Studer and colleagues' series was 120 ml after catheter removal (Studer et al, 1995). Median functional capacity was 300 ml at 3 months, 450 ml at 6 months, and 500 ml at 12 months. After 3 months, basal pressure was 20 cm H_2O and at capacity varied from 20 to 35 cm H_2O (Studer et al, 1995). Daytime continence was 92% at 1 year; 80% of patients reported good nighttime continence after 2 years. Studer and colleagues reported that 45% of patients required sodium bicarbonate replacement in the early postoperative period. Only three patients were reported to require permanent bicarbonate replacement.

The concept of using the intact 20-cm proximal ileal limb for prevention of deleterious effects of reflux is novel. Indeed, the maintenance of the peristaltic integrity of the proximal limb serves to dampen the effects of any but the most overfilled reservoir, according to Studer's radiographic studies and the authors' experience. Because patients with voiding pouches can often maintain a sterile urine, more definitive techniques to avoid reflux into the upper urinary tract may not be important. The authors' experience in more than 30 patients supports all of Studer's conclusions (Benson et al, 1996). The authors have found excellent preservation

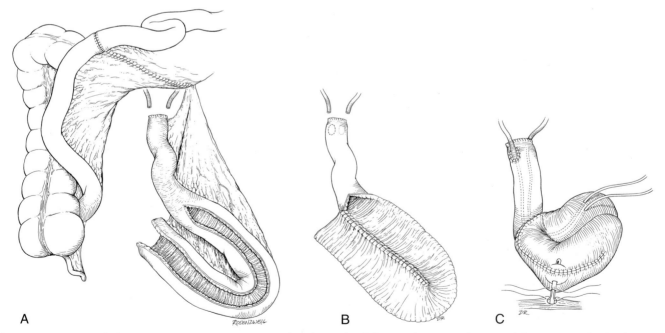

Figure 103–11. *A,* An ileal segment measuring 60 to 65 cm in length is isolated, leaving the proximal 25 cm of ileum intact. The distal 40 to 45 cm is opened along the antimesenteric border and folded in the configuration of a U. *B,* The posterior plate is completed by joining the limbs of the U with running absorbable sutures. Standard ureteroileal (refluxing) anastomoses are performed. Stents are brought out through separate stab wounds. *C,* Anastomosis of the posterior plate of ileum to the urethra is carried out with six urethral sutures. The left side of the ileal plate is brought to the patient's right, and the plate is closed in a cup cystoplasty configuration.

of the upper tracts and urinary continence, day and night, equivalent to other neobladder operations. The ileal ureter allows for a simple end-to-side ureteroileal anastomosis. This procedure avoids many of the pitfalls of the hemi-Kock operation because many of the complications reported are related to the nipple valve construction.

Ileocolonic Orthotopic Diversions

Orthotopic MAINZ Pouch

The MAINZ pouch is actually two separate operations, sharing the common principle of employing the cecum and two limbs of distal ileum to create a broad intestinal plate, which can then be closed in a spherical fashion (Thuroff et al, 1985, 1987). One variation of the MAINZ pouch is a catheterized version (described later). The MAINZ pouch variant that allows for orthotopic voiding is described here.

PROCEDURE

A segment of bowel, including 10 to 15 cm of cecum as well as 20 to 30 cm of distal ileum, is isolated from the bowel, and an ileo–ascending colostomy is used to re-establish intestinal continuity (Fig. 103–12A). After closing the mesenteric trap, the entire bowel segment is marsupialized along its antimesenteric border, sacrificing the ileocecal valve (Fig. 103–12B). The bowel is then fashioned in the shape of an incomplete W, with the first limb of the W represented by cecum and the middle two limbs of the W

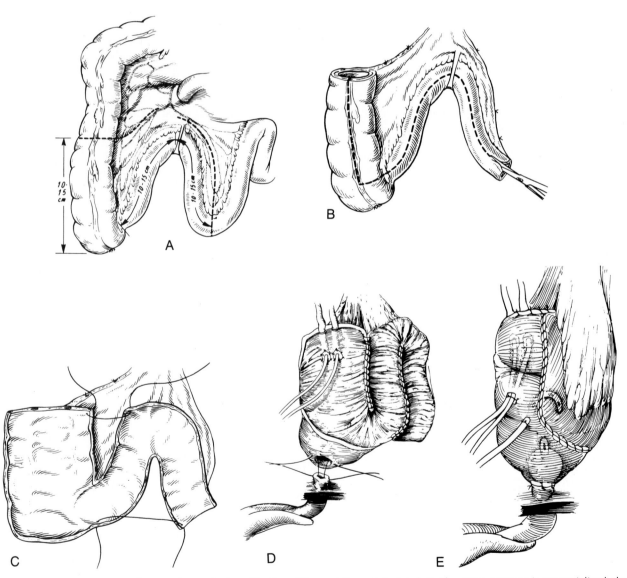

Figure 103–12. *A,* Ten to 15 cm of cecum in continuity with 20 to 30 cm of ileum is isolated. *B,* The entire segment is marsupialized along its antimesenteric border. *C,* A broad posterior plate is created by suturing the apposing margins of the three limbs of the incomplete W. *D,* At the apex of the cecal portion of the posterior plate, tunneled ureterocolonic anastomoses are performed. Appendectomy is routinely performed, and a buttonhole incision made at the base of the cecal portion of the reservoir serves as the site for urethrointestinal anastomosis. *E,* The ileal portions of the faceplate are brought anteriorly and to the right side to close the pouch. (From Thuroff JW, Alken P, Hohenfellner R: The MAINZ pouch [mixed augmentation with ileum 'n' zecum] for bladder augmentation and continent diversion. *In* King LR, Stone AR, Webster GD, eds: Bladder Reconstruction and Continent Urinary Diversion. Chicago, Year Book Medical Publishers, 1987.)

represented by marsupialized ileum. A broad posterior plate of one-third cecum and two-thirds ileum is created by suturing together the apposing margins of the three limbs of the incomplete W with running absorbable material (Fig. 103–12C).

At the apex of the cecal portion of the posterior plate, tunneled ureterocolonic anastomoses can be carried out. Long ureteral stents are placed into the renal pelves bilaterally. These are led out through the urethra or a separate suprapubic site, depending on the capacity of the urethra.

Appendectomy is routinely performed, and a buttonhole incision is made at the base of the cecal portion of the reservoir (Fig. 103–12D). Urethrointestinal anastomosis is carried out as previously described, using gentle traction on a Foley catheter balloon to reduce tension on the sutures until the anastomosis is complete. The ileal portions of the faceplate are then brought anteriorly and to the right side to close the pouch (Fig. 103–12E). This is accomplished with running sutures of absorbable material.

POSTOPERATIVE CARE AND COMMENTS

The postoperative care of the orthotopic MAINZ pouch is identical to other voiding diversions. Mean pouch capacities of 510 ml are reported. Pressures recorded range from 33 cm H_2O at 50% capacity to 41 cm H_2O at 100% capacity. In a report of 27 patients, daytime continence was reported in 100% (Fisch et al, 1992b). Nocturnal continence was reported in 24 of 27 (89%) patients, provided that they woke two to three times to void.

Fisch and colleagues did not report on complications for patients undergoing orthotopic MAINZ neobladder procedures as a separate population (Fisch et al, 1992b). The

reservoir is large and fills at low pressure. Therefore, the late complication risks include ureteral stenosis, metabolic disorders secondary to the loss of the terminal ileum, and diarrhea. Complications of the MAINZ pouch are discussed later.

Ileocolonic Pouch (Le Bag)

A modification of the MAINZ pouch that uses a single segment of ileum along with cecum was described by Light and Scardino (1986). This procedure is slightly simpler because it avoids one of the ileal folds.

PROCEDURE

A 20-cm segment of ascending colon and cecum is isolated along with an equal length of distal ileum. After reconstituting bowel integrity and closing the mesenteric trap, the entire mesenteric border of the large and small bowel segments is split to create two flat sheets, which are then sewn to one another posteriorly. Light and Scardino (1986) believe that metal stapling techniques can be used in this regard (Fig. 103–13A). When the first variant of this operation was described, the most proximal few centimeters of ileum were left intact, and the pouch was rotated 180 degrees cephalad to caudad so that the intact ileal stump could be used for ileourethral anastomosis (Fig. 103–13B). With increasing experience, suggesting that the intact ileal segment was peristaltic and promoted urinary wetting, the technique was modified to spatulate the entire bowel (Light and Marks, 1990). The urethra is anastomosed end-to-side to the cecum in the modern variant, and ureterocolonic anastomoses are

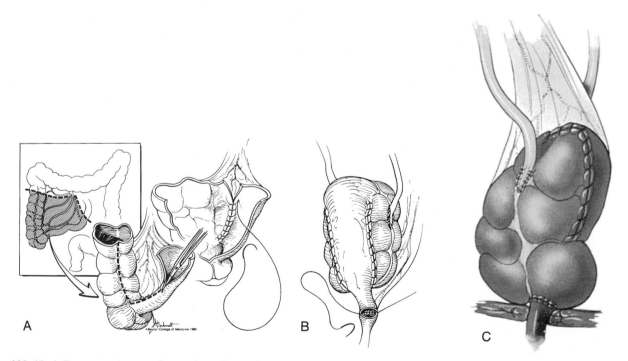

Figure 103–13. *A*, Twenty centimeters of ascending colon and cecum is isolated along with an equal length of distal ileum. The entire antimesenteric border of the large and small bowel segments is split to create two flat sheets, which are then sewn to one another posteriorly. *B*, The first variant of this operation left intact the proximal ileum. *C*, The entire bowel segment is spatulated. (*A* and *B* from Light JK, Scardino PT: Urol Clin North Am 1986; 13:261–270. *C* from Light JK, Marks JL: Br J Urol 1990; 65:467–472.)

carried out according to the surgeon's preference (Fig. 103–13C).

POSTOPERATIVE CARE AND COMMENTS

No alterations in postoperative care are necessary. Pouch capacities varied from 400 to 700 ml, and cystometry 6 weeks after surgery showed low-pressure contractions. End pressures of 20 to 58 cm H_2O were reported. The initial reports of this procedure were based on only 11 patients (Light and Scardino, 1986). Since the initial description, there have been two subsequent reports of this procedure (Vara et al, 1992; Kolettis et al, 1995). Vara and associates described their results in 17 patients. They reported minor modifications to the procedure and noted an overall daytime and nighttime continence rate of 94%. More recently, Kolettis and associates reported on their experience with Le Bag in 35 patients, the last 19 of whom had the pouch constructed with absorbable staples. They reported an overall complication rate of 31% (17% early and 14% late). In this series, three patients (8.6%) required reoperation for ureteral

obstruction. The daytime continence rate was reported to be 92%. At night, the authors stated that 74% of patients either were completely dry or experienced only mild incontinence. Most patients were reported to experience some degree of hyperchloremic acidosis, which in some required electrolyte replacement. The authors correlated the severity of the acidosis directly with pouch length.

Right Colon Pouch

Two groups have reported using the right colon exclusively. Goldwasser and Benson (1986) described a technique of replacing bladder using a partly detubularized right colon. This procedure was later modified to incorporate a fully detubularized right colon (Mansson and Colleen, 1990; Goldwasser, 1995).

PROCEDURE

The entire right colon is isolated on a pedicle fed by the ileocolic and right colic arteries (Fig. 103–14A). Ileocolonic

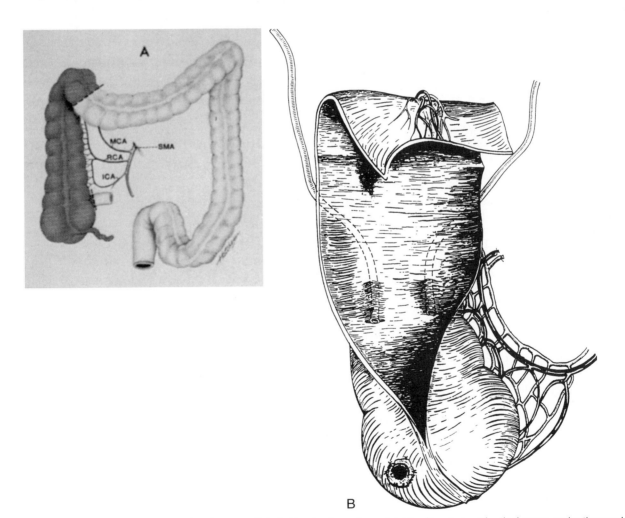

Figure 103–14. *A*, The entire right colon is isolated on a pedicle fed by the ileocolic and right colic arteries. The ileal stump at the ileocecal valve is closed by a running suture of absorbable material, and the colon segment is opened along the anterior taenia, leaving the proximal 2 to 3 inches of cecum intact. Appendectomy is performed, and ureters are implanted by standard antireflux technique. Urethrocecal anastomosis is performed over a ureteral catheter. *B*, The entire colon is spatulated. (*A* from Goldwasser B, Barrett DM, Benson RC Jr: Complete bladder replacement using the detubularized right colon. *In* King LR, Stone AR, Webster GD, eds: Bladder Reconstruction and Continent Urinary Diversion. Chicago, Year Book Medical Publishers, 1987. *B* from Mansson W, Colleen S: Scand J Urol Nephrol 1990; 24:53–56.)

anastomosis is used to restore bowel continuity, and the mesenteric trap is closed. The ileal stump at the ileocecal valve is closed by a running suture of absorbable material, and the colon segment is opened along the anterior taenia leaving the proximal 2 to 3 inches of cecum intact. Appendectomy is performed, and ureters are implanted by standard antireflux technique. The spatulated upper colon is closed in a Heinecke-Mikulicz fashion, using multiple running absorbable sutures (Fig. 103–14B). Urethrocecal anastomosis is performed over a ureteral catheter.

POSTOPERATIVE CARE AND COMMENTS

Although the use of a pouch constructed solely of right colon has some theoretical attractiveness (e.g., preservation of the terminal ileum for enterohepatic circulation and vitamin B_{12} absorption), most surgeons have opted for the use of a combined terminal ileum and right colon pouch. As a result, there have been too few procedures reported to allow for an extensive evaluation of day and night continence. Mansson and Colleen (1990) reported that all patients were continent in the daytime. Nocturnal continence was not reported. Pouch capacities varied from 320 to 600 ml. Measuring at high-level pouch filling, low basal pressures were recorded (11–22 cm H_2O).

Sigmoid Pouch

The use of the sigmoid colon for creation of a voiding reservoir was initially popularized in the United States at the University of Minnesota and was promulgated in Egypt. Originally employing a nonreconfigured U-shaped portion of colon (similar to the Camey I operation), the Minnesota group soon abandoned that technique because of high-pressure contractions in the unreconfigured pouch. A partially detubularized segment was then reported that improved the urodynamic characteristics of the pouch (Reddy, 1987). Later a fully reconfigured sigmoid was employed (Lange P, personal communication, 1990). The group at Al-Azhar University in Cairo has also reported on a series of totally reconfigured sigmoid pouches (Khakaf I, personal communication, 1991). In 1994, DaPozzo and co-workers reported on their 6-year experience with a fully detubularized sigmoid colon neobladder.

The use of the sigmoid colon as a continent voiding pouch offers a few potential advantages as well as disadvantages. With regard to the latter, the sigmoid colon is often affected by diverticulosis, malignancy, or both. For this reason, it might not be a suitable bowel segment to use for longer-term urinary diversion. The facility with which the sigmoid colon can be brought to the membranous urethral region and the simplicity with which it can be reconfigured by the Heinecke-Mikulicz maneuver, however, afford distinct advantages over other bowel segments. Furthermore, the loss of the sigmoid colon has little if any impact on the nutritional status or bowel habits of the patient.

PROCEDURE

As described by Reddy (1987), a portion of sigmoid and descending colon measuring 35 cm is isolated and folded in the shape of a U with the curve of the U oriented to the pelvis (Fig. 103–15A). The medial taenia of the U is incised down to a point a few centimeters cephalad to the site of the urethral anastomosis (Fig. 103–15B). Medial limbs of the U are sutured together with running absorbable suture material (Fig. 103–15C). Tunneled ureteral implantation is carried out with stents brought through separate stab wounds. A small button of tissue is removed from the inferiormost portion of the pouch, and urethral anastomosis is carried out with previously placed urethral stump sutures (Fig. 103–15D). Foley catheter drainage is achieved transurethrally. The pouch is closed with running absorbable suture material by rotating each side medially to meet one another. The pouch is, therefore, only partially detubularized, with its inferior aspect (shaped like the bottom half of a doughnut) intact.

A more advantageous form of bowel reconfiguration involves the total reconfiguration of the sigmoid segment. This has been reported by Khakaf and DaPozzo and co-workers and used by the authors with considerable success (Khakaf I, personal communication, 1991; DaPozzo et al, 1994). In this instance, the entire sigmoid colon is opened on its antimesenteric border and reconfigured by either a Heinecke-Mikulicz procedure or classic Goodwin cup principles. The remaining portions of the operative procedure are identical.

POSTOPERATIVE CARE AND COMMENTS

In the single case study reported by Reddy (1987), the partially detubularized sigmoid resulted in a capacity of 760 ml and pressures less than 20 cm H_2O until capacity was reached. The Cairo group reported excellent urodynamic characteristics with total bowel reconfiguration in a large series (Khakaf I, personal communication, 1991). In 24 patients, DaPozzo and co-workers reported daytime continence rates of 95% but nocturnal continence in only 43% (DaPozzo et al, 1994). The surgical complication rate was said to be minimal.

Continent Catheterizing Pouches

Numerous operative techniques have been developed for continent diversion in which urine is emptied at intervals by patient self-catheterization, conducted in a clean fashion. The majority of these operations are described, although certain pioneering procedures such as those of Gilchrist and colleagues (1950), Ashken (1987), Mansson and Colleen (1984, 1987), Benchekroun (1987), and others are not described because intact bowel was used. This is not to discredit the pioneers in the field but simply to allow the chapter to focus on those pouches that incorporate modern principles attempting to achieve a spherical configuration and disruption of peristaltic integrity.

A few initial comments about self-catheterizing pouches are appropriate. First, it is mandatory that patients undergoing these procedures have sufficient hand-eye coordination to perform clean intermittent catheterization. Quadriplegic patients and some individuals with multiple sclerosis or other neurologic disorders may not be candidates for this operation. Furthermore, patients with any degree of dementia that would interfere with their understanding of the catheterizing process are not appropriate candidates. The location of

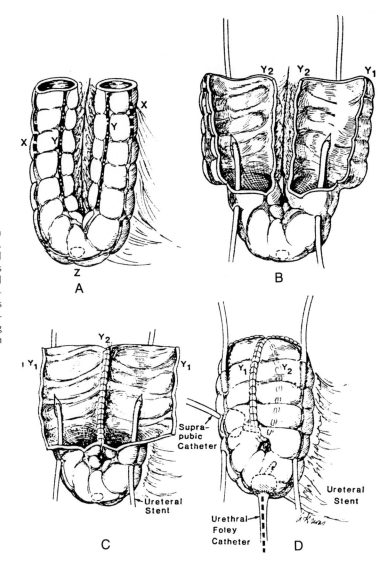

Figure 103–15. *A*, A portion of sigmoid and descending colon measuring 35 cm is isolated and folded in the shape of a U. *B*, The curve of the U is oriented to the pelvis, and the medial taenia of the U is incised down to a point a few centimeters cephalad to the site of the urethral anastomosis. *C*, The medial limbs of the U are sutured together, and tunneled ureteral implantation is performed (Y_2 to Y_2). *D*, A button of tissue is removed from the inferiormost portion of the pouch, and urethral anastomosis is performed. The pouch is closed by rotating each side of the pouch medially and suturing Y_1 to Y_1. (From Reddy PK: Urology 1987; 29:625–628.)

the catheterizing portal differs according to individual authors' preference. The two favored sites for stomal location are at the umbilicus and in the lower quadrant of the abdomen, through the rectus bulge and below the "bikini" line. This location is often preferred because it affords both men and women the opportunity to conceal the stoma. The umbilicus is a preferred location for the individual confined to a wheelchair. This location makes it far easier for the paraplegic individual to catheterize without the need for chair transfer and disrobing. The umbilical stoma location is actually preferred by some authors, even in those patients who are not wheelchair confined. In individuals with a recessed umbilicus, the umbilical location of a stoma is barely perceptible from a normal umbilical dimple. Generally, the stoma site is covered with a gauze or square Band-Aid to avoid mucous soiling of clothing.

Patients undergoing continent urinary diversion to an umbilical location should be advised to wear a medical alert bracelet that informs the examiner of the umbilical stoma. The authors consulted on a "Jane Doe" patient who in the past had undergone an umbilical continent bladder augmentation with closure of her bladder neck secondary to a neurogenic bladder. She presented to the emergency department unconscious, and the emergency department staff were unable to catheterize her via her retained, blind-ending urethra. The initial diagnosis was bladder neck contracture. Inspection of her abdomen eventually led to the correct diagnosis, and her reservoir was catheterized. One can imagine other circumstances in which a delay in understanding prior surgery could have grave consequences.

Orthotopic location of a catheterizing portal has been carried out in certain patients. Particularly in women, the construction of a neourethra to the introitus is attractive, provided that there is no substantial difficulty in the catheterizing process. Because it can be so difficult to direct a catheter through the "chimney" of an intussuscepted nipple valve, particularly if there is a long portion of bowel leading to the chimney, those continent diversions employing nipple valves are not particularly adaptable to orthotopic location, although they have been performed with success in a small number of patients (Olsson, 1987). In contrast, however, the imbricated and tapered ileal segment leading to an Indiana pouch is relatively easier to catheterize and can be used for orthotopic catheterizing diversion (Rowland et al, 1987). It may be difficult, however, to obtain sufficient mesenteric length in some patients. The appendix has been used as a neourethra, and in this instance, mesenteric length should be less of a problem (Hubner and Pfluger, 1995).

The relative surgical complexity required in the construction of various of the catheterizing pouches should be mentioned. Perhaps the single most demanding technical feature of each pouch is the construction of the continence mechanism. Furthermore, the integrity or failure of this mechanism ensures the success or failure of the diversion.

Four general techniques have been employed to create a dependable, catheterizable continence zone. For right colon pouches, appendiceal techniques or ileocecal valve plication are adaptable. Appendiceal tunneling techniques are the simplest of all to perform in that they use established surgical techniques that are already in the urologic armamentarium. In these procedures, the in situ or transposed appendix is tunneled into the cecal taenia in a fashion similar to ureterocolonic anastomosis. Appendiceal continence mechanisms have been criticized for three general reasons. First, the appendix may be unavailable in some patients owing to prior appendectomy. Second, the appendiceal stump may be too short to reach the anterior abdominal wall or umbilicus while still maintaining sufficient length for tunneling. This criticism has been addressed by an operative variation described by Burns and Mitchell (1990), in which the appendiceal stump can be lengthened by the inclusion of a tubular portion of proximal cecum (Fig. 103–16). Finally, appendiceal continence mechanisms share the feature of allowing for only small-diameter catheters to be used for intermittent catheterization. The large amount of mucus produced by an intestinal reservoir is more easily emptied or irrigated by using a catheter of No. 20 to 22 Fr size rather than the typical catheter that would be admitted through an appendiceal stump (No. 14–16 Fr).

The second major type of continence mechanism used in right colon pouches is the tapered or imbricated terminal ileum and ileocecal valve. The technology is rather simple, with imbrication or plication of the ileocecal valve region along with tapering of the more proximal ileum in the fashion of a neourethra (Rowland et al, 1985; Lockhart, 1987; Bejany and Politano, 1988). These techniques afford a reliable continence mechanism.

One feature of right colon pouches that has been criticized is the loss of the ileocecal valve. Although this does result in frequent bowel movements for some patients, at least in the short-term, the majority experience bowel regularity either through intestinal adaptation or with the use of pharmacologic therapy. Some patients, however, have developed striking diarrhea or steatorrhea after the loss of the ileocecal valve. This may be particularly true in the pediatric patient in whom there is neurogenic bowel dysfunction (the myelomeningocele patient) (Mitchell ME, personal communication, 1991).

The third surgical principle used in constructing the continence mechanism is the use of the intussuscepted nipple valve. The creation of these nipple valves is by far the most technologically demanding of all the continence mechanisms. **Before the surgeon achieves reproducible and dependable results, a significant learning curve must be overcome. For this reason, nipple valve construction should probably not be chosen by the surgeon who occasionally performs construction of continent pouches.** Furthermore, it should be noted that the past decade has seen the introduction of numerous modifications of the original technique of Kock for construction of a stable nipple valve. The singular reason for all of these modifications is the disappointing long-term stability of the nipple valve in some patients.

One of the major advances in nipple valve construction has been the removal of mesenteric attachments from the middle 6 to 8 cm of bowel to be used for nipple valve construction (Hendren, 1980). This reduces the tethering effect of the mesentery that otherwise induces eversion and effacement of the intussusception. The second major advance has been the attachment of the nipple valve to the reservoir wall itself. This has been achieved by two or three different stapling techniques as well as by a suturing technique described by Hendren and King (Hendren, 1976; Skinner et al, 1984; King, 1987). Nevertheless, nipple valve failure can be anticipated in 10% to 15% of cases despite the best, experienced surgeons.

A final feature of stapled nipple valves is the potential for stone formation on exposed staples. This has been greatly

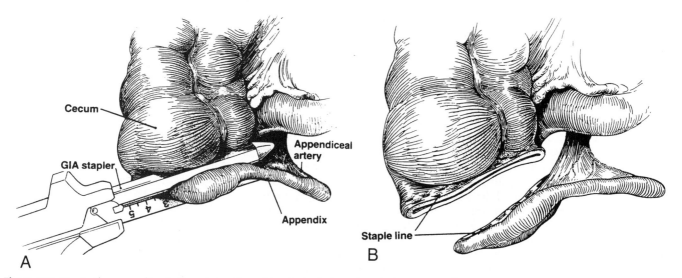

Figure 103–16. *A,* The appendiceal stump is lengthened by the inclusion of a tubular portion of proximal cecum by the application of the GIA stapler to the terminal cecum. *B,* The added length is demonstrated. (From Burns MW, Mitchell ME: Contemp Urol 1990; May:10–12.)

lessened by the omission of staples at the tip of the intussuscepted nipple valve as suggested by Skinner and associates (1984). More proximal staples, however, occasionally erode into the pouch and serve as a nidus for stone formation. These stones are usually manageable endoscopically with forceps extraction of the stone and staple or electrohydraulic or ultrasonic disintegration of the stone with subsequent forceps staple extraction. Although exposed staples may serve as a nidus for stone formation, continent urinary diversion results in more urinary excretion of calcium, magnesium, and phosphate as compared to ileal conduit diversion (Terai et al, 1995). Thus, all patients undergoing continent diversion are at an increased risk for the formation of reservoir stones.

The fourth major technique of continence mechanism construction is the provision of a hydraulic valve as in the Benchekroun nipple (Benchekroun, 1987). In this procedure, a small bowel segment is isolated, and a reversed intussusception is carried out, apposing the mucosal surfaces of the small bowel. Tacking sutures are taken to a portion of the circumference of the intussusception to stabilize the nipple valve while allowing urine to flow freely between the leaves of apposed ileal mucosa. As the pouch fills, hydraulic pressure closes the leaves, ensuring continence. Although the authors have no personal experience with these types of hydraulic valves, clinical reports of their use have suggested long-term success. Stomal stenosis, especially in children, and nipple destabilization in general remain concerns (Sanda et al, 1995).

General Methodology

During construction of the pouch, intraoperative testing for pouch integrity is always performed. The continence mechanism is also tested for ease of catheterization as well as continence after the pouch construction has been completed. The pouch is filled with saline, the continence mechanism catheter is removed, and the pouch can be compressed slightly to look for points of leakage as well as to test the continence mechanism for its ability to contain urine. **Thereafter the continence mechanism is catheterized to ensure ease of catheter passage. This is an extremely important maneuver because the inability to catheterize is a serious complication that often results in the need for reoperation.**

Postoperatively, in all catheterizing pouches, certain principles must be adhered to. The larger-bore catheter used for drainage of the pouch should be irrigated at frequent intervals to ensure against mucus obstruction. This can be performed at 4-hour intervals by simple irrigation with 45 to 50 ml of saline. Less frequent intervals of irrigation can be employed when the urine is totally diverted from the kidneys by means of long indwelling stents. As soon as possible, the patient is instructed in conducting his or her own irrigation program. This is performed to familiarize the patient with the catheterization process, to reduce the work burden on the nursing staff, and to allow for earlier discharge.

On the seventh postoperative day a contrast study is performed to ensure pouch integrity. Thereafter, ureteral stents may be removed, again with radiologic control. When it has been ascertained that the ureteral anastomoses and pouch are intact, the suction drain is removed. The suprapubic tube (if

employed) can also be removed at this time, or it can be left in place until the patient is confident of the catheterization technique. The patient is taught to irrigate the tube traversing the continence mechanism at 4-hour intervals and instructed to irrigate whenever any episode of intra-abdominal pressure or discomfort is experienced. Once these procedures are mastered and the patient is tolerating a regular diet, the patient can be discharged. This usually occurs between hospital days 8 and 10.

Instruction in clean self-catheterization and care for the continence mechanism stoma can begin 1 week after discharge in an outpatient setting. The authors are impressed by the value of and rely heavily on the enterostomal therapist's patient instructions not only during these office visits, but also throughout the preoperative and postoperative period. The numerous insecurities and questions posed by patients are always best resolved by an individual with extensive experience in addressing seemingly minor, but from the patient's standpoint truly important, everyday issues.

Following is a summary of common patient questions and everyday solutions:

> *"What kind of catheter do I use?"* For nipple valves, a straight ended No. 22 to 24 Fr tube; for ileocecal plication, a No. 20 to 22 Fr coudé-tip catheter; and for appendiceal sphincters, a No. 14 to 16 Fr coudé-tip catheter.
>
> *"How do I carry my catheter?"* In a Zip-Lock bag that can be placed in a woman's purse or a man's coat pocket.
>
> *"How do I clean the stoma before catheterizing in a public facility?"* With a benzalkonium chloride wipe, which can be purchased in individual foil-wrapped packets.
>
> *"How do I lubricate the catheter?"* By tearing off the end of an individual-use foil pack of water-soluble lubricant and inserting the tip of the catheter into the pack.
>
> *"What do I do with the stoma after catheterizing?"* Cover it with a Band-Aid.
>
> *"How do I clean my catheter after draining my pouch?"* By rinsing ordinary tap water through the inside channel and over the outside surface before replacing it in its Zip-Lock bag.

In the case of gastric or Kock pouches, pouch capacity is initially low (150 ml). Therefore, the frequency of catheterization has to be significantly different in these individuals compared with those with right colon pouches, in whom initial comfortable capacities well in excess of 300 ml are experienced. To ensure restful sleeping hours, smaller-capacity pouches may best be managed by indwelling catheterization during sleeping hours. The patient is instructed in irrigation of mucus debris on a two- to three-times-daily basis initially, with increasing intervals as mucus production decreases with time.

General Care

Because all patients with catheterized pouches have chronic bacteriuria, the problem of antibiotic management should be discussed. Most authors suggest that bacteriuria in the absence of symptoms does not warrant antibiotic treatment (Skinner et al, 1987b). The construction of an effective antireflux mechanism in all of these pouches may ensure against clinical episodes of pyelonephritis, in contrast to patients diverted by means of free refluxing conduits. Obviously, if clinical pyelonephritis does occur, antibiotic treatment should be instituted.

A condition has been described that is manifested by pain in the region of the pouch along with increased pouch contractility (*pouchitis*). It should be mentioned that this latter condition, although infrequent, may result in temporary failure of the continence mechanism because of the hypercontractility of the bowel segment employed for construction of the pouch. The patient typically presents with a history of sudden explosive discharge of urine through the continence mechanism (rather than dribbling incontinence) along with discomfort in the region of the pouch. Appropriate antibiotic therapy usually results in resolution of these symptoms. In the authors' experience, short courses of antibiotics are not usually successful when treating pouch infections. Perhaps this is due to the larger amount of foreign material (mucus and sediment) within intestinal pouches as opposed to the bladder. Intestinal crypts may also serve as bacterial sanctuaries. Therefore, whenever a pouch infection is treated, a minimal course of antibiotic therapy is 10 days. Pyelonephritis may, of course, require longer courses of therapy.

Urinary retention is an infrequent but serious occurrence in catheterizable pouches. It is most commonly seen with pouches with a nipple valve as the continence mechanism. In these circumstances, if the chimney of the nipple valve is not near the abdominal surface, the catheter can be directed into folds of bowel rather than into the nipple valve proper such that urinary retention results. **Pouch urinary retention represents a true emergency, and the patient must seek immediate attention so that catheterization and drainage by experienced personnel can be achieved promptly.** Sometimes the use of a coudé-tip catheter is helpful in this regard. Rarely a flexible cystoscope is necessary. After the immediate problem has been resolved by emptying the pouch, a catheter should be left indwelling for 2 to 3 days to allow the edema and trauma to the catheterization portal to resolve. Subsequently the patient should be observed for ability to catheterize successfully on a number of occasions. The appropriate angle of entry can be taught to the patient until he or she is comfortable with the use of the new catheter. In fact, the authors prefer to use coudé-tip catheters with non-nipple valve pouches routinely.

Intraperitoneal rupture of catheterizable pouches has been reported (Kristiansen et al, 1991; Thompson and Kursh, 1992; Watanabe et al, 1994). In general, these episodes are more common in the neurologic patient in whom sensation of pouch fullness may be less distinct (Hensle TW, personal communication, 1991; Mitchell ME, personal communication, 1991). Often, there is associated mild abdominal trauma, such as a fall, that is antecedent to the rupture. In general, these patients require immediate pouch decompression and radiologic pouch studies. If the amount of urinary extravasation is small and the patient does not have a surgical abdomen, catheter drainage and antibiotic administration may suffice in treating intraperitoneal rupture of a pouch. The authors have successfully employed this nonoperative approach on patients with a ruptured right colon pouch. For patients with large defects, surgical exploration and pouch repair is required.

Continent Ileal Reservoir (Kock Pouch)

This operation was first reported for use in urinary diversion by Kock and associates in 1982. This report was singularly responsible for the reawakened interest in continent diversion procedures. An outgrowth of the Kock procedure for continent ileostomy (Kock, 1971), the Kock pouch combined reasonably dependable techniques for securing continence of urine and preventing reflux to the upper urinary tract (nipple valves) along with carefully refashioned bowel that provided a low-pressure urinary reservoir. Skinner and co-workers have carefully studied and improved the technique over the years, while amassing a prodigious experience with the operation and its variants (Skinner et al, 1989; Skinner, 1992). Their operative description is followed closely in this chapter.

PROCEDURE

Seventy to 80 cm of small bowel is isolated from a point at the avascular plane of Treves cephalad. If the patient has a pre-existing ileal conduit and is undergoing conversion to a Kock pouch, the previous small bowel anastomosis should be resected and the length of ileum measured cephalad from this point. A 5-cm segment of proximal ileum and mesentery is sacrificed to provide added mobility of the isolated segment.

The middle portion of the ileum is folded in the shape of a U with each limb of the U measuring 20 to 22 cm in length (Fig. 103–17A). The medial borders of the U may be sutured to one another on the serosal surface before opening the bowel, or the bowel may be opened along its antimesenteric border, extending into each ileal terminus for a few centimeters before closing the posterior wall of the ileal plate with running absorbable material (Fig. 103–17B and C). A 10-cm length of ileum is selected on both the afferent and the efferent ileal terminus for creating the intussuscepted nipple valves. The middle 6 to 8 cm of the 10-cm segment is denuded of mesentery by electrocoagulation. An Allis or Babcock clamp is advanced into the ileal terminus, grasping the full thickness of the intussusceptum and inverting the ileum into the pouch (Fig. 103–17D).

Using the TA-55 stapler, three rows of 4.8-mm staples are applied to the intussuscepted nipple valve (Fig. 103–17E). The distal six staples from each cartridge are removed before staple application to ensure that the tip of the valve is free of the staples. Most authors suggest that the pin of the stapling instrument should always be kept in place so that staple misalignment does not occur. This results in a pinhole puncture site at the base of the nipple valve, and this pinhole should be oversewn with absorbable suture material to prevent fistula formation after staple application is complete. The nipple valve is then fixed by one of two stapling techniques to the back wall of the reservoir (Skinner et al, 1984). A small buttonhole may be made in the back wall of the ileal plate so that the anvil of the stapler can be passed through the buttonhole and advanced into the nipple valve before application of the fourth row of staples (Fig. 103–17F). If this is carried out, the buttonhole is oversewn

Text continued on page 3223

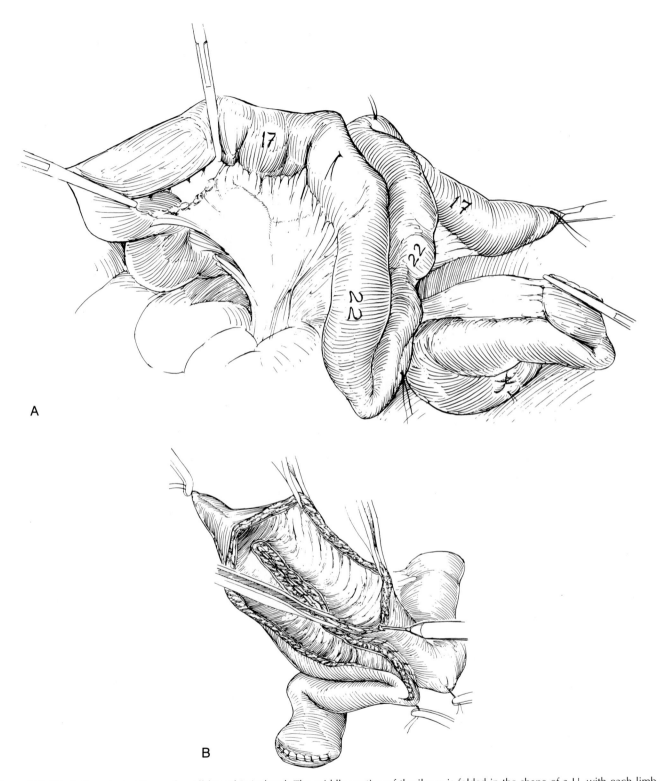

Figure 103–17. *A*, Seventy to 80 cm of small bowel is isolated. The middle portion of the ileum is folded in the shape of a U, with each limb of the U measuring 20 to 22 cm in length. *B*, The medial borders of the U may be sutured on the serosal surface before opening the bowel.

Illustration continued on following page

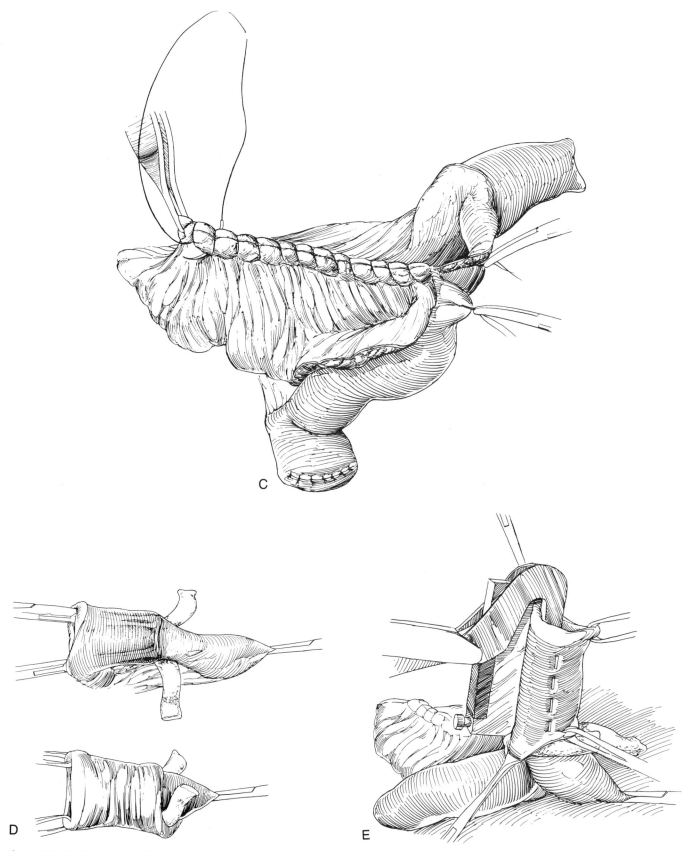

Figure 103–17 *Continued C*, The bowel being opened along its antimesenteric border before closing the posterior wall of the ileal plate. *D*, An Allis or Babcock clamp is advanced into the ileal terminus, the full thickness of the intussuscipiens is grasped, and it is prolapsed into the pouch. *E*, Three rows of 4.8-mm staples are applied to the intussuscepted nipple valve using the TA-55 stapler.

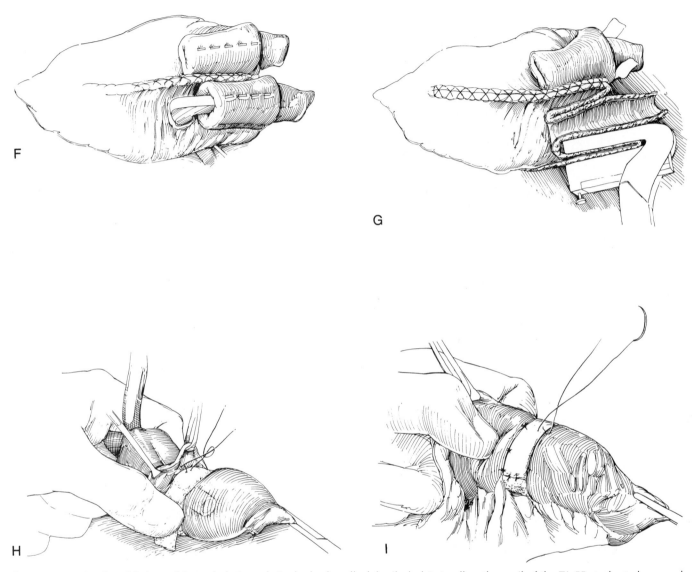

Figure 103–17 *Continued F,* A small buttonhole is made in the back wall of the ileal plate to allow the anvil of the TA-55 stapler to be passed through and advanced into the nipple valve. A fourth row of staples is applied. *G,* The anvil of the stapler can be directed between the two leaves of the intussuscipiens and the fourth row of staples applied in this manner. *H,* A 2.5-cm-wide strip of absorbable mesh is placed through additional windows of Deaver at the base of each nipple valve. The mesh strips are fashioned into collars. *I,* The collars are sewn to the base of the pouch as well as to the ileal terminus with seromuscular sutures.

Illustration continued on following page

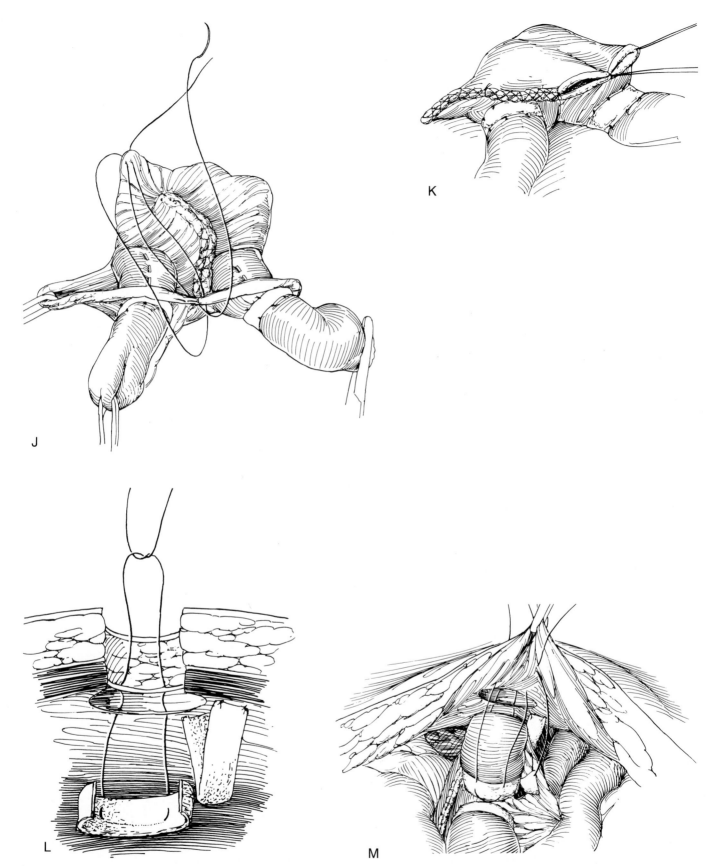

Figure 103–17 *Continued J* and *K,* The posterior plate is closed to create the pouch by folding the ileum in a cup cystoplasty fashion. *L* and *M,* A button of skin is removed with small plugs of anterior and posterior fasciae. If a collar has been employed, separate heavy absorbable sutures are taken from anterior fascia in a horizontal mattress fashion to the cuff so as to anchor the cuff to the anterior fascia. (From Hinman F Jr: Atlas of Urologic Surgery. Philadelphia, W. B. Saunders, 1989.)

afterward with absorbable material. Alternatively the anvil of the stapler can be directed between the two leaves of the intussuscipiens and the fourth row of staples used to fix the inner leaf of the nipple valve to the pouch wall (Fig. 103–17G). Again, pinhole puncture sites are oversewn.

Some authors, including Skinner and colleagues (1989), have suggested the use of absorbable mesh collars to anchor the base of the nipple valve subsequently. If collars are used, 2.5-cm-wide strips of absorbable mesh are placed through additional windows of Deaver at the base of each nipple valve. The mesh strips are fashioned into collars and sewn both to the base of the pouch and to the ileal terminus with seromuscular sutures of absorbable material (Fig. 103–17H and I). The posterior plate is then closed to create the pouch by folding the ileum in a cup cystoplasty fashion (Fig. 103–17J and K). The closure is completed by running absorbable suture material. The pouch can then be inverted on its own mesentery to achieve proper anterior-posterior alignment of the ileal termini. The proximal terminus is prepared for ureteroileal anastomosis, which can be conducted according to the surgeon's preference. The use of a Yankauer suction tip is useful to traverse the two nipple valves and direct long ureteral stents from the renal pelves out through the distal valve. The distal ileal terminus is directed to the previously selected stoma site. A small button of skin is removed with small plugs of anterior and posterior fasciae. The distal terminus is led out between bluntly separated bundles of the rectus muscle. If a collar has been employed, separate heavy absorbable sutures are taken from the anterior fascia in a horizontal mattress fashion to the cuff to anchor the cuff to the anterior fascia (Fig. 103–17L and M). This ensures a short chimney. Alternatively the base of the pouch may be fixed to the posterior fascia or peritoneal margins with interrupted heavy absorbable sutures.

The presence of a bulky mesentery at the cephalad extent of the stoma is an invitation to parastomal herniation. To avoid this problem, the authors "defat" the mesentery before it is led through the stoma site or remove some of the mesentery from the ileal terminus. Alternatively, Skinner and co-workers have suggested the use of a Marlex sling, which is passed through the window of Deaver used for the collar and sutured to each side of the stoma site to prevent parastomal herniation (Fig. 103–17L and M) (Skinner et al, 1984).

Excess ileum is transected at the skin level, and a flush stoma is created by suturing the ileum to the skin with interrupted absorbable material. A No. 30 Fr Medina catheter is advocated by Skinner for postoperative drainage. The authors use a No. 24 Fr multiperforate rubber tube, which is sutured to the anterior abdominal wall along with ureteral stents.

POSTOPERATIVE CARE AND COMMENTS

General comments have already been made about postoperative care of all catheterizable pouches. Specific to the Kock pouch is the small initial pouch capacity. Skinner and colleagues have advised leaving the Medina tube in place for 3 weeks, and Kock and associates have suggested that the patient clamp the tube until a point of discomfort before releasing after the second week (Kock et al, 1982; Skinner et al, 1989). If double-J stents have been left in the pouch,

the pouch is examined endoscopically with a cystoscope on tube removal and stents are removed. Patients are trained in intermittent catheterization, and catheterization intervals are increased by 1 hour weekly.

Average pouch capacities exceeding 500 ml are achieved by 3 to 6 months. Overall the Kock pouch affords average capacities of 700 ml or more, and urodynamic evaluations suggest pouch pressures averaging 4 to 8 cm H_2O in the long term (at two-thirds' pouch capacity) (Chen et al, 1989).

Management of the complications of stone formation has already been discussed. Managing a failed nipple valve is considerably more complicated. Three general reasons for failure can be cited. Pinhole fistulas at the base of the nipple are a consequence of setting the aligning pin of the staple instrument. Such fistulas can be simply oversewn during formal re-exploration. Nipple valve prolapse may occur, in which case bowel can be intussuscepted once more, restapled, and fixed to the reservoir wall with suture or stapling techniques. Shortening of the nipple length beneath the 2.5 and 3 cm necessary for urinary continence probably occurs as a consequence of ischemia. Repair of this necessitates the isolation of 15 cm of ileum, which is used to create a new nipple valve (Lieskovsky et al, 1987). One end of this ileum is fashioned into a new stoma, whereas the other is spatulated and sewn onto the established pouch.

It should be emphasized that nipple valve failure of one sort or another may occur at any time after surgery. Even in the most experienced of hands, a failure rate of 15% or higher is experienced. With an individual surgeon's initial experience in constructing nipple valves, the failure rate is higher still. Excluding the original patients in Kock's own series in which a reoperation rate exceeding 80% was noted (Berglund et al, 1987), other authors have reported the need for repeat surgery in approximately one third of patients (DeKernion et al, 1985; Waters et al, 1987).

MAINZ Pouch

The catheterizable MAINZ pouch has undergone considerable modification over the years (Thuroff et al, 1985; Stein et al, 1995). Problems with the nipple valve represented the primary reason for modifications to be carried out. The operative technique has now been modified to use the intact ileocecal valve as a means of further stabilizing the intussusception (Thuroff et al, 1988). This procedure is described here without further reference to earlier prototypes.

PROCEDURE

The catheterizable MAINZ pouch varies somewhat from the orthotopic voiding MAINZ pouch. First, a longer segment of bowel is used. A 10- to 15-cm portion of cecum and ascending colon is isolated along with two separate equal-sized limbs of distal ileum and an additional portion of ileum measuring 20 cm (Fig. 103–18A). The entire colon and distal segments of ileum are spatulated, taking care to preserve the ileocecal valve. These three bowel segments are folded in the form of an incomplete W, and their posterior aspects are sutured to one another to form a broad posterior plate (Fig. 103–18B). A portion of the intact proximal ileal terminus is freed of its mesentery for a distance of 6 to 8

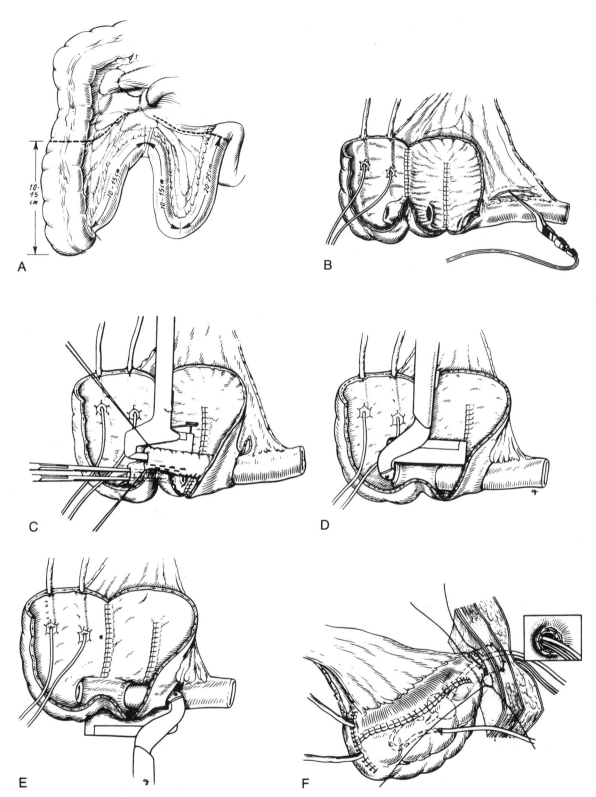

Figure 103–18. *A*, A 10- to 15-cm portion of cecum and ascending colon is isolated along with two separate equal sized limbs of distal ileum and an additional portion of ileum measuring 20 cm. *B*, A portion of the intact proximal ileal terminus is freed of its mesentery for a distance of 6 to 8 cm. *C*, The intact ileum is intussuscepted and two rows of staples are taken on the intussuscipiens itself. *D*, The intussuscipiens is led through the intact ileocecal valve, and a third row of staples is taken to stabilize the nipple valve to the ileocecal valve. *E*, A fourth row of staples is taken inferiorly, securing the inner leaf of the intussusception to the ileal wall. *F*, A button of skin is removed from the depth of the umbilical funnel and the ileal terminus is directed through this buttonhole. Excess ileal length is resected, and ileum is sutured at the depth of the umbilical funnel. (*A* from Thuroff JW, Alken P, Hohenfellner R: The MAINZ pouch (mixed augmentation with ileum 'n' zecum) for bladder augmentation and continent division. *In* King LR, Stone AR, Webster GD, eds: Bladder Reconstruction and Continent Urinary Diversion. Chicago, Year Book Medical Publishers, 1987, p 252. *B–F* from Thüroff JW, Alken P, Riedmiller H, et al: J Urol 1988; 140:283–288.)

cm, and intussusception of the segment is achieved. Two rows of staples are applied on the intussusceptum itself (Fig. 103–18C). Thereafter the intussusceptum is led through the intact ileocecal valve, and a third row of staples is applied to stabilize the nipple valve to the ileocecal valve (Fig. 103–18D). Finally, a fourth row of staples is applied inferiorly, securing the inner leaf of the intussusceptum to the ileal wall (Fig. 103–18E).

Ureterocolonic anastomoses are created at the apex of the reservoir, which is then folded on itself in a side-to-side fashion to complete the pouch construction. The entire pouch is rotated cephalad so as to bring the ileal terminus to the region of the umbilicus. A small button of skin is removed from the depth of the umbilical funnel, and the ileal terminus is directed through this buttonhole (Fig. 103–18F). The pouch is secured to the posterior fascia with interrupted absorbable sutures, and the ileal terminus is sewn similarly to anterior fascia. Excess ileal length is resected, and ileum is sutured at the depth of the umbilical funnel with interrupted absorbable sutures.

POSTOPERATIVE CARE AND COMMENTS

No specific differences in postoperative care or complications associated with the MAINZ pouch need be addressed. Initial pouch capacities are higher than in the Kock pouch. Final mean capacity averaging greater than 600 ml has been reported. Pouch pressures are 23 cm H_2O at half capacity and 31 cm H_2O when the pouch is full. Contraction waves, beginning at 50% pouch fullness, can be recorded at an amplitude of 12 cm H_2O. Thus, this pouch seems to produce a reasonably low-pressure urinary reservoir, although the pressures are not as low as that achieved with the use of small bowel alone.

The 10-year experience with the MAINZ pouch and the variations created by its developers has been presented (Stein et al, 1995). Between 1983 and July 1994, 374 patients underwent a MAINZ I operation. In 116, the appendix was used as the continence mechanism, 248 patients had the invaginated ileum used as the continent stoma, and 10 underwent a modified nipple technique (appendiceal continence mechanisms are described later). The early complication rate was 6.7%. Early complications included mechanical ileus requiring open revision in seven patients (1.9%), pouch leakage requiring revision in seven patients (1.9%), wound dehiscence in three patients (0.8%), and fatal pulmonary emboli in two patients (0.5%).

The late complication rate was 25% and predominantly attributable to the pouch. Incontinence owing to nipple prolapse occurred in 26 patients (7%) and was directly related to the continence mechanism. No patient (0 of 116) with an appendiceal continence mechanism was incontinent. Therefore, the incontinence rate among patients with nipple valves was actually 26 of 258 (10.1%). The developers of this procedure were innovative in their attempts to bring the incontinence rate down to an acceptable level. To this end, they tried alloplastic stoma (4 of 4 incontinent), sutured intussusception (8 of 8 incontinent), stapled intussusception (5 of 22 [23%] incontinent), and stapled ileocecal intussusception (10 of 204 [4.9%] incontinent). The stapled ileocecal intussusception described previously is the current recommendation. Other late complications include ureteral stenosis

in 30 patients (8%). Stomal stenosis occurred in 29 patients with an ileal nipple (11.7%) and in 17 patients with an appendiceal stoma (14.7%).

Calculus formation in the pouch occurred in 30 patients (8%). These 30 patients underwent 37 percutaneous and 4 open procedures. Despite the loss of the terminal ileum, the authors have not seen a significant drop in serum vitamin B_{12} levels, and no patient has developed macrocytic anemia or neurologic symptoms. Twenty-five percent of patients are on oral alkalinization to avoid metabolic acidosis.

The overall complication rate for this procedure since its inception has been high (31%). Stein and co-workers have pointed out, however, that 50% of the complications were manageable with percutaneous techniques (Stein et al, 1995). Additionally, since 1988 the incontinence rate has been only 3.2%, and no patient with an appendiceal continence mechanism has been incontinent.

The authors share Stein and co-workers' enthusiasm for the use of the appendix as a continence mechanism. In the authors' experience, it has also been a reliable technique that is easy to perform. In constructing right colon pouches employing appendiceal sphincter technology, the authors use the entire right colon inclusive of the hepatic flexure to form the reservoir, thereby preserving more terminal ileum. This has the theoretical advantage of fewer metabolic complications, but Thüroff and colleagues (1988) have not experienced significant metabolic problems.

With the introduction of the appendiceal continence mechanism greatly increasing the acceptance of their procedure, Thüroff and colleagues have two new techniques for construction of a Mitrofanoff (appendiceal) type of tube for use in patients whose appendix is either unsuitable or absent (Lampel et al, 1995a, 1995b). Both techniques use a small-caliber conduit fashioned from the large intestine in the region of the cecum. One technique uses a full-thickness tube lined by mucosa (Fig. 103–19) and the other a seromuscular tube lined by serosa (Fig. 103–20). With short follow-up, both techniques appear to be successful, although the full-thickness tube was associated with a lower complication rate and a higher success rate in a limited number of patients (Lampel et al, 1995b). Other groups have used tapered ileum to create a tunneled access into the right colon (Fig. 103–21) (Woodhouse and MacNeily, 1994; Hampel et al, 1995). Using tapered ileum for this purpose has the advantage of a blood supply independent of the reservoir and no length restrictions while having the disadvantage of further limiting intestinal absorptive surface.

Right Colon Pouches with Intussuscepted Terminal Ileum

Additional pouches using nipple valve technology for the continence mechanism include those right colon pouches in which intussusception of the terminal ileum and ileocecal valve is employed. As such, they are variations on the continent cecal reservoir initially described by Mansson (1987) employing an intact cecal segment. These three pouches are the UCLA pouch (Raz S, personal communication, 1991), the Duke pouch (Webster and King, 1987), and Le Bag (Light and Scardino, 1986). These operations differ from one another by only a few features, predominantly

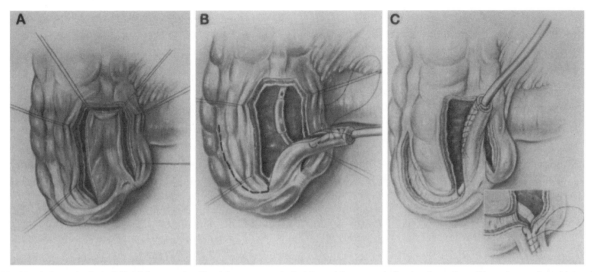

Figure 103–19. *A* through *C*, A full-thickness tube lined by mucosa is fashioned for tunneled reimplantation. (From Lampel A, Hohenfellner M, Schultz-Lampel D, Thuroff JW: J Urol 1995; 153:308–315.)

related to the technique employed for stabilizing the nipple valve.

PROCEDURES

The UCLA pouch is created by isolating the entire right colon along with 15 cm of distal ileum (Fig. 103–22*A*). The entire colon segment is incised along the anterior taenia (Fig. 103–22*B*). (The authors prefer to incise along the antimesenteric border, preserving all possible taenial sites for ureteral reimplantation.)

Measuring from the tip of the projected intussusception, 6 to 8 cm of ileum is cleared of mesenteric attachment, and the ileum is intussuscepted through the ileocecal valve into the cecum. Staples are used to stabilize the nipple valve. Two rows of staples are placed using the bladeless GIA device. The anvil of the device is then directed between the leaves of the intussuscipiens so that the inner leaf of the nipple valve can be stapled to the anterior and inferior walls of the marsupialized cecal pouch (Fig. 103–22*C*). Further anchoring of the nipple to the sidewall of the pouch is achieved by multiple runs of continuous absorbable suture material sewing the nipple to the pouch (Fig. 103–22*D*). An absorbable mesh collar is advocated at the base of the nipple valve.

Ureterocolonic anastomosis is carried out by typical tunneling technique, and the pouch is closed by folding the colon in a Heinecke-Mikulicz configuration using multiple running absorbable sutures (Fig. 103–22*E*). The stoma construction proceeds as in the Kock pouch.

The Duke pouch consists of the isolation of a similar segment of distal ileum and cecum with ascending colon. The cecum and ascending colon are detubularized by incising the antimesenteric border (Fig. 103–23*A*). Ureterocolonic anastomoses are carried out in the usual tunneled fashion.

A length of 6 to 8 cm of mesentery is freed from the middle portion of the planned intussusception. The ileum is intussuscepted through the ileocecal valve (Fig. 103–23*B*). Stabilization of the intussusception is carried out by suture technique rather than stapling technique. A broad patch of

mucosa is excised from the posterior cecal plate. One entire thickness of the intussuscipiens is incised so as to reveal the serosa of the inner leaf of the intussuscipiens. Seromuscular sutures taken in this structure are placed into the muscularis of the back wall of the cecum, and mucosal sutures connect the edge of the outer leaf to the edge of the cecal denudation (Fig. 103–23*C*). The pouch is then closed by serial applications of running absorbable sutures taken to close an angled Heinecke-Mikulicz configuration into the form of a pouch (Fig. 103–23*D* and *E*).

This pouch has the advantage of requiring no staples in its construction. The authors have found that the stabilization achieved by this suturing technique is as dependable as affixing the nipple valve to the sidewall using staples. In fact, the authors prefer to combine the two techniques using both staple fixation and suture fixation (by this variant of the Hendren [1976] concept) to the reservoir sidewall.

A final adaptation using an ileocecal bowel segment and an intussuscepted nipple valve is the variation of Le Bag previously described in the section on orthotopic voiding diversions. In this variation, a somewhat longer length of distal ileum is taken and remains intact for construction of the nipple valve in the usual fashion, after removing mesentery from the midportion of the intussuscipiens. The nipple valve is stapled to itself in three quadrants, and the fourth-quadrant staple line attaches the nipple valve to the posterior reservoir wall. The completely marsupialized colon and ileum are sewn to one another with running absorbable suture material (Fig. 103–24). In the catheterizing Le Bag pouch, there is believed to be no need for further nipple valve stabilization by means of absorbable mesh collars. The stoma is brought flush to the umbilical funnel so that the reservoir wall lies immediately beneath the skin level.

POSTOPERATIVE CARE AND COMMENTS

There are no substantive differences in the management of these patients compared with those patients undergoing MAINZ pouch diversion. The UCLA group has not reported its urodynamic data. Pouch capacities have varied between

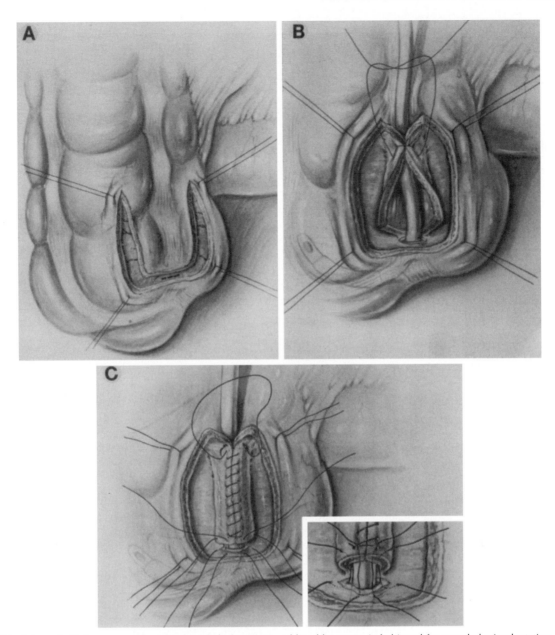

Figure 103–20. *A* through *C*, A seromuscular tube denuded of mucosa and lined by serosa is fashioned for tunneled reimplantation. (From Lampel A, Hohenfellner M, Schultz-Lampel D, Thuroff JW: J Urol 1995; 153:308–315.)

600 and 700 ml. Thirty of 34 patients were dry night and day, and only one operation for a fistula at the base of a nipple valve was required. One additional reoperation is planned. The outcome of the Duke and Le Bag pouches is unknown as of this writing. There have been no further published reports on these variations since the previous edition of this text.

Indiana Pouch

The concept of using the buttressed ileocecal valve as a dependable continence mechanism that can withstand the trauma of intermittent catheterization was first reported from Indiana University by Rowland and colleagues (1987). This operation, involving partial spatulation of the cecal segment and attachment of an ileal patch, represented major contribu-

tions to the original ileocecal reservoir described by Gilchrist and co-workers (1950), in which the intact bowel reservoir was employed, and no attempt was made to strengthen the ileocecal valve. Originally, strengthening the ileocecal valve consisted of a double row of imbricating sutures taken to the entire ileal segment (Rowland et al, 1985, 1987). It soon became apparent that this was necessary only in the region of the ileocecal valve. *Neourethral* pressure profiles showed that the continence zone was confined to the region of the reconfigured ileocecal valve (Bejany and Politano, 1988). The remaining neourethra could be tapered and brought through an abdominal or perineal stoma. At Indiana as well as other institutions, it became clear that marsupializing only a portion of the ascending colon segment left sufficient peristaltic integrity in the cecal region to generate pressures sufficiently high to overcome the continence mechanism in

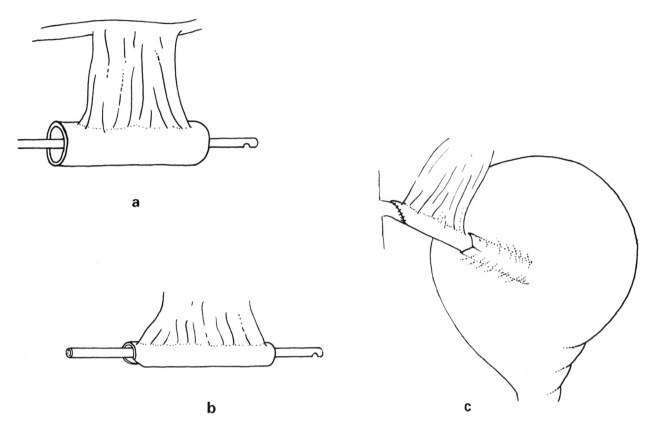

a

b

c

Figure 103–21. *A* through *C*, Woodhouse tapered ileum. (From Woodhouse CR, MacNeily AE: Br J Urol 1994; 74:447–453.)

some patients. A number of groups contributed to the concept of using the entire right colon or more, marsupializing the entire structure, and refashioning it in a Heinecke-Mikulicz configuration (Lockhart, 1987; Bejany and Politano, 1988; Benson et al, 1988; Rowland RG, personal communication, 1988). These variations have been named the Florida pouch (Lockhart, 1987) and the University of Miami pouch (Bejany and Politano, 1988). They represent relatively minor variations on the theme of the Indiana pouch.

PROCEDURE

The Indiana pouch, in its present form, involves isolating a segment of terminal ileum approximately 10 cm in length along with the entire right colon to the junction of the right and middle colic artery blood supplies (Fig. 103–25*A*). After bowel continuity is re-established, appendectomy is performed, and the appendiceal fat pad obscuring the inferior margin of the ileocecal junction is removed by cautery (Fig. 103–25*B*). The entire right colon is opened along its antimesenteric border, and ureteral-taenial implants are fashioned (Fig. 103–25*C*). The ileocecal junction is buttressed according to different techniques depending on the author. Interrupted Lembert sutures are taken over a short distance (3–4 cm) in two rows for the double imbrication of the ileocecal valve as described at Indiana (Fig. 103–25*D*). Nonabsorbable material is used for this, and the second row of sutures should attempt to bring the opposite mesenteric edges of ileum together, usually over a No. 12 to 14 Fr catheter. These two rows of sutures should be placed approximately 8 mm from one another, and the initial suture in each row may be taken in a purse-string fashion around the

cecal margin as well. Alternatively, the University of Miami group suggest that purse-string sutures be taken in the ileum in the same region (Bejany and Politano, 1988). Finally, the Tampa group suggest that apposing Lembert sutures be taken on each side of the terminal ileum (Fig. 103–25*E*). The remaining ileum can be tapered over the catheter and excess ileum removed by stapling technique (Fig. 103–25*F*).

It is important to carry out the imbrication while the cecal reservoir is still open (Rowland RG, personal communication, 1988). In this fashion, one can easily observe the gradual closure of the ileocecal valve. The pouch is then closed in a Heinecke-Mikulicz configuration with running absorbable suture material. Ureteral stents and a suprapubic tube are taken through a stab wound in the pouch and led through the right lower abdominal quadrant. The pouch is rotated so as to bring the ileal neourethra as close as possible to the selected stoma site. A fingerbreadth-width skin button is transected along with a similar button from the anterior and posterior fascia. The ileal neourethra is advanced between bundles of the rectus muscle through the stoma, and excess ileum is transected. The ileal edges are sewn to skin with interrupted sutures to create a flush stoma.

In addition to the differences in the technique of ileocecal valve imbrication, both the University of Miami and the Florida pouch differ in the amount of colon used. The entire ascending colon and the right third or half of the transverse colon are isolated along with 10 to 12 cm of ileum. The entire upper extremity of the large bowel is mobilized laterally in the fashion of an inverted U (Fig. 103–26*A*). The medial limbs of the U are sutured to one another after the bowel is spatulated (Fig. 103–26*B*). The bowel plate is then closed side-to-side (Fig. 103–26*C*). This inverted U closure,

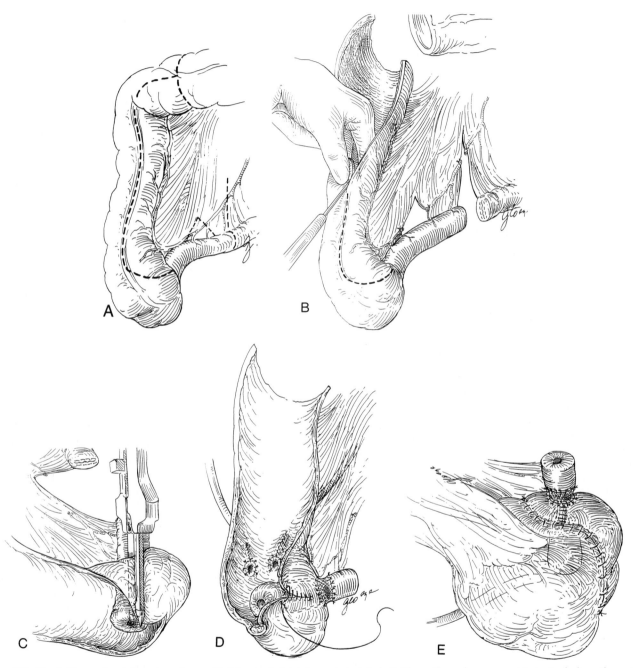

Figure 103–22. *A*, The entire right colon along with 15 cm of distal ileum is isolated. *B*, The entire colon segment is incised along the anterior taenia. Six to 8 cm of ileum is cleared of mesenteric attachments. *C*, The ileum is intussuscepted through the ileocecal valve, and staples are used to stabilize the nipple valve. *D*, The nipple is also anchored to the sidewall of the pouch with continuous absorbable sutures. An absorbable mesh collar is placed at the base of the nipple valve. *E*, The pouch is closed by folding the colon in a Heinecke-Mikulicz configuration. (Courtesy of S. Raz.)

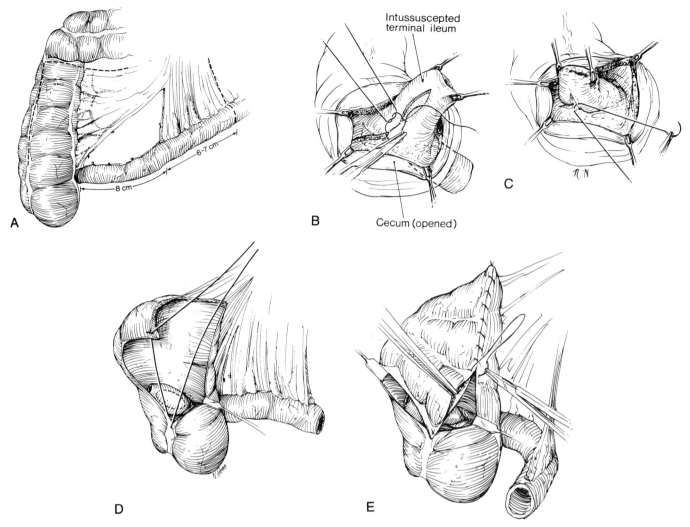

Figure 103–23. *A,* Fifteen-centimeter segments of distal ileum and cecum with ascending colon are isolated. *B,* The ileum is intussuscepted through the ileocecal valve and stabilized with sutures. A patch of mucosa is excised from the posterior cecal plate, and one entire thickness of the intussuscipiens is incised so as to reveal the serosa of the inner leaf of the intussuscipiens. Seromuscular sutures taken in this structure are placed into the muscularis of the back wall of the cecum. *C,* Mucosal sutures connect the edge of the outer leaf to the mucosal edge of the cecal denudation. *D* and *E,* The pouch is closed with running sutures in a Heinecke-Mikulicz configuration. (*A, D,* and *E* from Webster GD, King LR: Further commentary: Cecal bladder. *In* King LR, Stone AR, Webster GD, eds: Bladder Reconstruction and Continent Urinary Diversion. Chicago, Year Book Medical Publishers, 1987, pp 206–208. *B* and *C* from Robertson CM, King LL: Urol Clin North Am 1986; 13:333–344.)

however, is exactly the same as a Heinecke-Mikulicz reconfiguration.

Modifications to the Indiana reservoir allow for more rapid construction and a lower complication rate (Rowland, 1996). The modifications incorporate the use of metal staples to create the efferent limb and absorbable staples to fashion the reservoir. The concept of using a metal GIA stapler to fashion the efferent limb was first introduced by Bejany and Politano (1988). Carroll and Presti (1992) reported on the urodynamic features of the stapled and plicated terminal ileum and found that the stapled limb performed equally well and was easier to construct. The use of absorbable staples to create this and other types of reservoirs is described later.

POSTOPERATIVE CARE AND COMMENTS

The postoperative care of the patient with an Indiana pouch or its variants is not substantially different from that in patients with other right colon catheterizable diversions.

Rowland (1996) recommended discharging the patient with the suprapubic tube in place until readmission to the hospital 3 weeks later for tube removal and instruction in self-catheterization. In the current medical climate, which places a premium on outpatient procedures, tube removal and catheterization instruction are now ambulatory procedures at most institutions.

Average pouch capacities 400 to 500 ml have been reported by the Indiana group (Rowland et al, 1987). Combining the partially and totally spatulated bowel procedures, this group reported a reoperation rate of 26%. Overall continence rates of 93% were achieved (Scheidler et al, 1989). Elegant urodynamic studies were conducted in Indiana pouch variants by Carroll and associates (1989). They found only 86% of patients totally continent in a small series. Their pouch capacities, however, exceeded 650 ml. Peak contractions of 47 cm H$_2$O were recorded at capacity.

The last 81 patients operated on by Rowland underwent construction of a stapled efferent limb, and in the last 20,

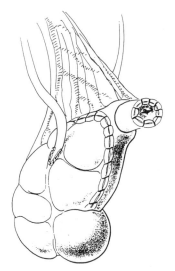

Figure 103–24. A completely marsupialized colon and ileum are sewn to one another with running absorbable suture material.

the reservoir was created with absorbable staples (Rowland, 1996). The results in this group of patients were extremely favorable. Early pouch-related complications occurred in only three patients (3.7%). Two patients experienced a pouch leak, which was managed conservatively, and one patient required open revision of the efferent limb owing to difficulty with catheterization. Early complications not directly attributable to the pouch occurred in seven patients (8.6%).

Transient small bowel obstruction was the most common complication occurring in four patients (4.9%). One patient developed a superficial wound infection, and one patient developed an abdominal abscess requiring surgery (1.2%). Late complications related to the reservoir occurred in 23 patients (28.4%). Incontinence occurred in six patients (7.4%). The incontinence was secondary to high pouch pressures in five patients and secondary to failure of the efferent limb in one patient. One of the former patients and the latter patient underwent reoperation. Three patients (3.7%) developed stomal stenosis, and three had parastomal hernias; all six underwent surgery. Pouch stones occurred in three patients; one underwent open removal, and two had endoscopic extraction. Acute pyelonephritis was seen in four patients (4.9%). The most common late complication not related to the pouch was small bowel obstruction; this was seen in six patients and was managed conservatively in five. The early reoperation rate was 2.5% and the late reoperation rate 14.8%. At 1 year, day and nighttime dry intervals of 4 hours or greater were achieved in 98% of patients. Eighty-four percent of patients stated they slept through the night without the need to awake for catheterization.

The Florida pouch procedure has been performed in more than 190 patients (Helal et al, 1993). In 165 patients involving 326 ureters, no attempt was made to create a tunneled reimplantation. This approach was adopted owing to the high incidence of ureteral obstruction encountered in the first 30 ureters that were tunneled into a Florida pouch (4 of 30 [13.3%]). In the latter 165 patients, primary obstruction developed in 16 of 326 ureters (4.9%), and patients were

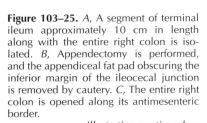

Figure 103–25. *A,* A segment of terminal ileum approximately 10 cm in length along with the entire right colon is isolated. *B,* Appendectomy is performed, and the appendiceal fat pad obscuring the inferior margin of the ileocecal junction is removed by cautery. *C,* The entire right colon is opened along its antimesenteric border.

Illustration continued on following page

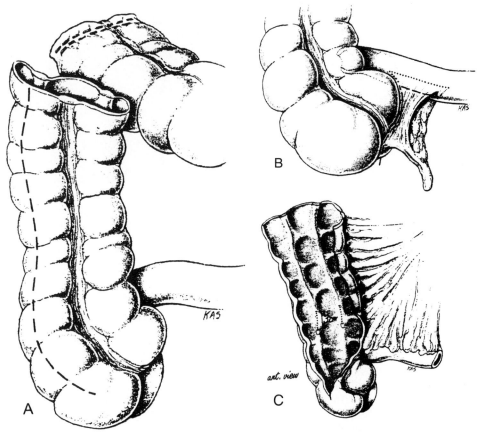

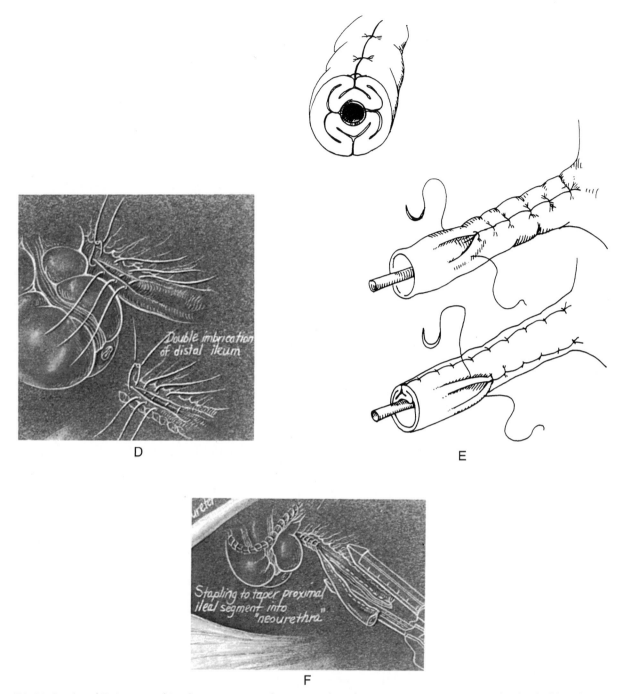

Figure 103–25 *Continued D,* Interrupted Lembert sutures are taken over a short distance (3–4 cm) in two rows for the double imbrication of the ileocecal valve as described at Indiana. *E,* Application of opposing Lembert sutures on each side of the terminal ileum. *F,* Excess ileum can be tapered by stapling technique. (*A–C* from Benson MC, Sawczulk IS, Hensle TW, et al: Curr Surg Tech Urol 1988; 1:1–8. *D* and *F* from Olsson CA: Contemp Urol 1989; Aug/Sept:62–68; *E* courtesy of J. Lockhart.)

treated by percutaneous balloon dilation, nephrectomy, or observation. Although no attempt is made to create an antirefluxing anastomosis, only 7.1% of the ureters implanted demonstrated reflux. All are being followed conservatively, and no renal deterioration has been demonstrated. In the initial 100 patients, a 7.2% reoperation rate was reported (Lockhart, 1987). Although hyperchloremia was noted in 70% of patients, only four patients (including those who had pre-existing renal disease) required treatment. Reservoir capacities ranged from 400 to 1200 ml, and maximal reser-

voir pressures at capacity ranged from 18 to 55 cm H_2O (Lockhart, 1987). The reason why these authors experienced such a high incidence of ureteral obstruction with both nontunneled and tunneled ureteral colonic anastomoses is not clear. It is also surprising that only 23 of 326 ureters anastomosed end-to-side refluxed.

The University of Miami group have reported on their results in 75 patients. Early complications occurred in 19 patients (25%). Sixteen patients experienced late complications (21%). The success rate of the ureterocolonic anasto-

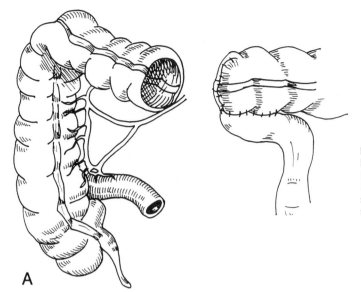

A

Figure 103–26. *A,* The entire ascending colon and the right third or half of the transverse colon are isolated along with 10 to 12 cm of ileum. *B,* The entire upper extremity of the large bowel is mobilized laterally in the fashion of an inverted U. The medial limbs of the U are sutured after the bowel is spatulated. *C,* The bowel plate is then closed side-to-side. (Courtesy of J. Lockhart.)

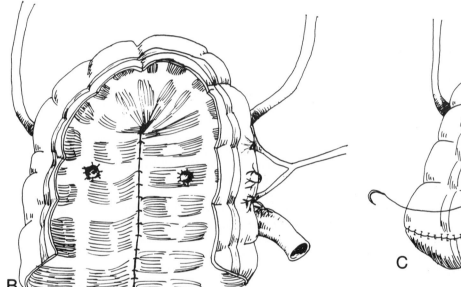

B

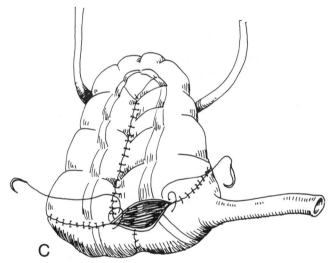

C

mosis was 90%. Total continence occurred in 98.6%. Average pouch capacities were 750 ml or higher. End filling pressures of 20 cm H_2O were reported. No patient required alkali therapy.

Penn Pouch

The Penn pouch was the first continent diversion employing the Mitrofanoff principle, in which the appendix served as the continence mechanism. As mentioned earlier, this operation enjoys the singular feature of affording a catheterizable continent diversion that can be performed using techniques already in the urologic armamentarium.

PROCEDURE

Two techniques of appendiceal continence mechanisms have been reported. Mitrofanoff reported excising the appen-

dix with a button of cecum and reversing it on itself before tunneled reimplant (Duckett and Snyder, 1986). Alternatively, Riedmiller and co-workers have left the appendix attached to the cecum and buried it into the adjacent taenia by rolling it back onto itself (Riedmiller et al, 1990). A wide tunnel is created in the taenia extending 5 to 6 cm from the base of the appendix (Fig. 103–27). Windows are created in the mesoappendix between blood vessels. The appendix is folded cephalad into the tunnel, and seromuscular sutures are placed through the mesoappendix windows to complete the tunneling. The tip of the appendix is amputated and brought to the selected stoma site.

As described by Duckett and Snyder (1986), an ileocecal pouch is created by isolating a segment of cecum up to the junction of the ileocolic and middle colic blood supplies along with a similar length of terminal ileum. These two structures are marsupialized on the antimesenteric borders and sutured to one another in the form of a neotubularized

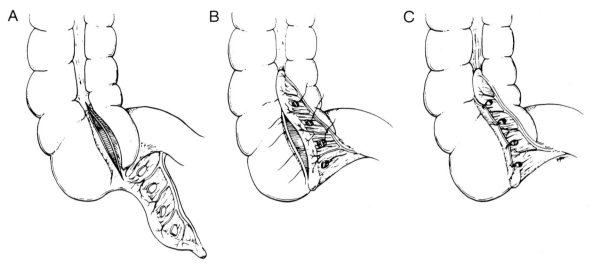

Figure 103–27. *A* through *C,* The appendix is left attached to the cecum and buried into the adjacent cecal taenia by rolling it back onto itself. A wide tunnel is created that extends 5 to 6 cm from the base of the appendix. Windows are created in the mesoappendix between blood vessels. The appendix is folded cephalad into the tunnel, and seromuscular sutures are placed through the mesoappendix.

pouch. The superior margin of the pouch is sutured in a transverse fashion (all sutures being of absorbable material). A button of cecum surrounding the origin of the appendix is circumcised and the resulting cecal aperture closed with running absorbable suture. The mesentery of the appendix is dissected carefully from the base of the cecum, preserving its blood supply. The appendix is then reversed on itself, so that the cecal button can reach the anterior abdominal wall and the tail of the appendix can be directed to the taenia of the colon (Fig. 103–28). The appendiceal tip is obliquely transected and may be spatulated. A tunneled appendiceal-taenial implantation is carried out. If additional appendiceal length is required, the variation proposed by Burns and Mitchell (1990), creating a tube of the base of the cecum, may be employed (see Fig. 103–16*A* and *B*). Instead of simply removing the appendix with a button of cecum before preparing it for tunneling, the entire base of the cecum leading to the appendix can be resected in continuity with the appendix by the application of the GIA stapler. The authors have found that spatulating the distal tip of the

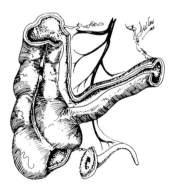

Figure 103–28. A segment of cecum up to the junction of the ileocolic and middle colic blood supplies along with a similar length of terminal ileum is isolated and marsupialized on the antimesenteric borders. A button of cecum surrounding the origin of the appendix is circumcised. The mesentery of the appendix is dissected carefully from the base of the cecum, preserving its blood supply. (From Duckett JW, Snyder HM III: Semin Urol 1987; 5:55–62.)

appendix until a catheter at least No. 12 to 14 Fr in size can be passed is helpful.

POSTOPERATIVE CARE AND COMMENTS

Although not shown in Duckett's surgical drawings (see Fig. 103–28), the authors suggest that a large-bore suprapubic tube be used to drain the pouch in the early postoperative interval. The size of the catheter admitted by the appendiceal stump is insufficient to allow for the passage of ureteral stents along with the No. 12 to 14 Fr catheter. In addition, safe irrigation of mucus debris is best managed by a larger-bore catheter.

Many groups have used the Mitrofanoff principle owing to the simplicity and reliability of the continence mechanism (Burger et al, 1992; Bissada, 1993; Sumfest et al, 1993; Woodhouse and MacNeily, 1994; Hampel et al, 1995). Woodhouse and MacNeily (1994) reported on a series of 100 patients operated on from 1985 through 1993. They employed the seven different catheterizable Mitrofanoff principle tubes into six different types of reservoirs. Although they found the Mitrofanoff principle to be versatile and associated with a high success rate (91% continence rate), the reoperation rate for tube complications was 33%. Sumfest and associates affirmed the use of the appendix as the Mitrofanoff segment of choice (Sumfest et al, 1993). They reported a continence rate of 96%. In their hands, late complications included difficulty with catheterization in 10.6% and stomal stenosis in 19.1%. Urodynamic properties and pouch capacities are a function of the reservoir constructed. Most often, the appendix is used in situ (Burger et al, 1992), and the right colon either alone or with associated terminal ileum (MAINZ) serves as the reservoir. The authors have used the in situ appendix with a detubularized right colon reservoir and the native ileocecal valve as an antireflux mechanism (ureters implanted end-to-side into terminal ileum). In the authors' hands, this has resulted in an excellent success rate with no upper tract problems. The adequacy of the ileocecal valve as an antireflux mechanism was also reported by Alcini and colleagues (1994). In their series, however, the reservoir was not always detubularized, and, as expected, upper tract complications ensued because of high reservoir pressures.

Benchekroun Hydraulic Ileal Valve

Benchekroun (1987) described the concept of creating an ileal hydraulic valve that would sit atop an ileal or ileocecal reservoir. The premise was that, as the reservoir filled, the pressure within the valve would also increase, thereby creating continence. This procedure continues to be employed by Benchekroun (1992) and has been reported on by Leonard and Quinlan (1991) but has been abandoned by others owing to poor long-term results (Sanda et al, 1995).

PROCEDURE

The Benchekroun hydraulic valve can be fashioned in continuity with either the ileum or the ileocecal segment, or it can be transplanted to the top of any other bowel segment. Twelve to 14 cm of ileum is isolated on its mesentery. A reverse intussusception is then performed such that serosa covers the entire segment, and the mucosa apposes mucosa (Fig. 103–29*A*). The ends of the invagination are then fixed to each other with interrupted full-thickness absorbable sutures. This leaves the mucosa-to-mucosa internal surface open to fill with urine as pouch pressures increase. The outside ileal wall is then anastomosed to the reservoir with full-thickness sutures, leaving a mucosally lined channel, which coapts the internal serosally lined channel as pouch pressures increase (Fig. 103–29*B*). If the terminal ileum is used in pouch construction, the catheterizing element can be formed in situ by internally intussuscepting the more proximal ileum and circumferentially securing the two leaves from within the cecum.

POSTOPERATIVE CARE AND COMMENTS

Benchekroun (1992) has the largest experience with this technique. He has used the hydraulic valve to create more than 210 continent urostomies. In his 1992 report, the hydraulic valve was placed atop 184 ileocecal reservoirs (8 detubularized), 15 ileal reservoirs, 3 sigmoid reservoirs, 1

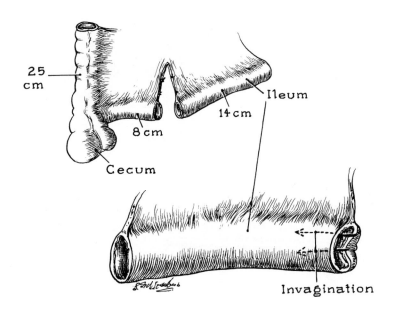

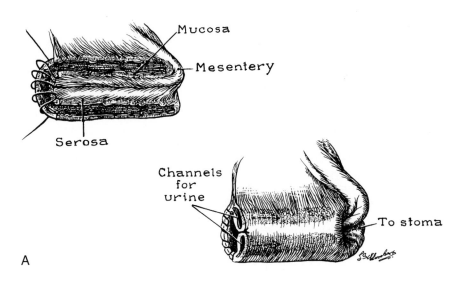

Figure 103–29. *A,* The ileal segment is invaginated and secured by interrupted sutures. Open channels are left for urine to access the valve mechanism.

Illustration continued on following page

A

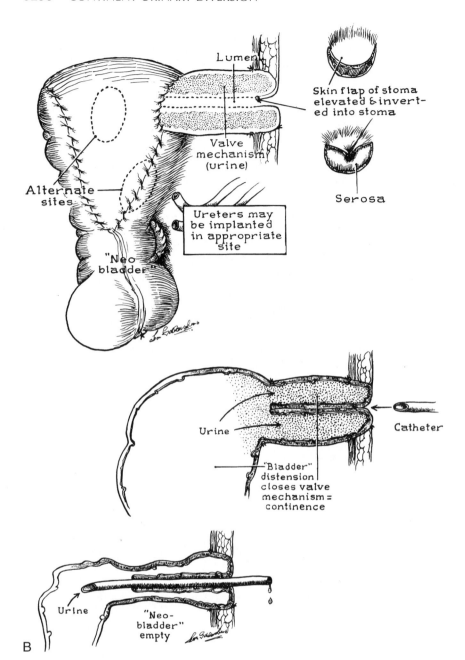

Figure 103–29 *Continued B*, The valve can be attached to a separate reservoir or can be created in situ using terminal ileum. (From Leonard MP, Quinlan DM: Urol Clin North Am 1991; 18:717–724.)

rectum, 1 transverse colon, and 6 bladders. Continence was immediately achieved in 155 of 210 patients (73.8%). The continence rate is reported to rise to 91.5% after valve repair.

Leonard and Quinlan (1991) labeled the Benchekroun hydraulic ileal valve their continence mechanism of choice. This conclusion was based on a need for surgical revision in only 5 of 15 patients, whereas their revision rate among patients undergoing a plicated terminal ileum was 58%. This 58% failure rate for the Indiana mechanism is higher than that experienced in other published series.

The Benchekroun hydraulic ileal valve was used extensively on the pediatric service at Johns Hopkins Hospital from 1989 to 1991 (Leonard et al, 1990). Although initial results were promising, only a 13% surgical revision rate at 18 months, long-term data (at least 40 months) are not as favorable (Sanda et al, 1995). At 5 years, the surgical revi-

sion rate was 91%. The common late complications requiring major revisions included stomal stenosis in 73% and devagination in 36%. Although the authors report that stomal stenosis was occasionally managed by superficial revision with skin flaps and grafts, most required complete replacement of the valve mechanism. Repair was successfully achieved by converting the hydraulic valve into a Mitrofanoff implanted tube.

The Benchekroun hydraulic ileal valve may be the one diversion in which reservoir detubularization actually impairs the continence rate because the valve mechanism is dependent on pouch pressure for continence. Without elevated pouch pressure, there is no forceful apposition of the serosal leaves of the valve, and as a result, one might expect low-volume, low-pressure or high-volume, low-pressure incontinence. Furthermore, the initial success rate (before open surgical revision) of 75% is lower than that seen with other continence mechanisms. The authors have no personal experience with this procedure.

Gastric Pouches

Pioneering animal experimentation demonstrated the feasibility of employing stomach as a bladder patch or urinary reservoir (Sinaiko, 1956; Rudick et al, 1977). The use of the stomach to create a urinary reservoir has theoretical and real advantages (Adams et al, 1988). First, electrolyte reabsorption would be greatly diminished by using this bowel segment in the reservoir. This potentially makes the stomach the selected reservoir for individuals with pre-existing metabolic acidosis or renal insufficiency. Hyperchloremic acidosis would not be an anticipated problem; in fact, in addition to presenting a barrier against the absorption of chloride and ammonium, the gastric mucosa secretes chloride ions (Piser et al, 1987). Furthermore, in patients in whom shortening of the bowel may be expected to lead to degrees of malabsorption, the use of stomach is an attractive alternative. Finally, when the entire lower bowel has been irradiated, stomach may provide healthy nonirradiated tissue to use in performing continent diversion. Given these theoretical advantages, a number of groups have initiated trials with gastric pouches, particularly in the pediatric population (Adams et al, 1988).

PROCEDURE

A wedge-shaped segment of stomach whose greatest width is 7 to 10 cm is fashioned from the greater curvature. Care is taken not to extend the wedge through to the lesser curvature to preserve vagal innervation and normal gastric emptying. The left gastroepiploic artery is preferentially used as the blood supply for the isolated gastric wedge, dividing the short gastric vessels from the more proximal artery up to the gastric fundus. Alternatively, if there is a problem with the left artery, the right gastroepiploic vessel may be employed, dividing the short gastrics to the level of the pylorus (Fig. 103–30A and B). The stomach is then closed according to the surgeon's preference. Neither gastroduodenostomy nor gastrojejunostomy is mandatory, unless the antrum of the stomach has been used. The isolated wedge is refashioned into nearly a sphere by folding it back on itself and suturing the edges together with running absorbable material. Before pouch closure, one ureter is tunneled into the reservoir according to the surgeon's preferred antireflux technique. Contralaterally, proximal transureteroureterostomy is performed. The contralateral distal ureter is used to create the continence mechanism. The distal ureter is tunneled into the reservoir in a fashion similar to an appendiceal implant. The free portion of the ureter can then be brought to the skin or to the introitus (or urethral stump in men) to serve as a catheterization portal (Fig. 103–30C).

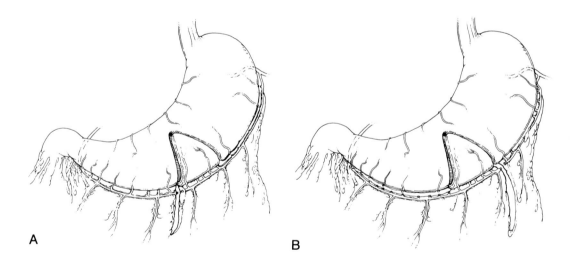

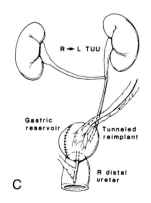

Figure 103–30. *A* and *B*, A wedge-shaped segment of stomach whose greatest width is 7 to 10 cm is fashioned from the greater curvature. The left gastroepiploic artery is preferentially used as the blood supply for the isolated gastric wedge, by dividing the short gastric vessels up to the gastric fundus. Alternatively, if there is a problem with the left artery, the right gastroepiploic vessel may be employed. *C,* The isolated wedge is refashioned into nearly a sphere by folding it back on itself and suturing the edges together with running absorbable material. One ureter is tunneled into the reservoir. A proximal transureteroureterostomy is performed. The ipsilateral distal ureter is tunneled into the reservoir with its distal extent brought to the introitus to serve as a catheterization portal. (From Adams MC, Mitchell ME, Rink RC: J Urol 1988; 140:1152–1156.)

Adams and colleagues reported mean pouch capacities of 245 ml and end filling pressures averaging 35 cm H_2O in a small patient sample (Adams et al, 1988). Combining their experience of gastric continent diversion and gastrocystoplasty, they reported minimal mucus production; only 3 of 13 patients required any irrigations, and the majority maintained a sterile urine. Urine pH values have ranged from 4 to 7, but no introital ulceration from acid urine was reported. Three patients had minor elevations of serum gastrin, and none of the continent divisions required reoperation. Leong (1978) has used similar concepts in gastric pouch construction and has alluded to the creation of a voiding pouch created from stomach as well.

The construction of reservoirs entirely from stomach has not seen widespread acceptance. Rather, there has been greater use of stomach segments either for bladder augmentation or as a portion of a reservoir (composite) either alone or with an in situ catheterizable tube fashioned from a portion of the stomach (Gosalbez et al, 1994; Carr and Mitchell, 1996).

Gosalbez and co-workers reported on 15 patients who received a gastric tube as part of a composite gastric patch (Gosalbez et al, 1994). Complications associated with the gastric patch and in situ tube included one each of early traumatic perforation of the tube, distal tube stenosis, and mucosal redundancy. Two of these patients required reoperation. Peristomal skin irritation from acid secretion occurred in two patients but was not considered severe. This is a more frequent complication in other reports and has resulted in skin breakdown in some instances.

Over a 10-year period from January 1985 to June 1995, Carr and Mitchell (1996) reported on the use of stomach in 12 patients. Seven had urinary reservoirs totally constructed from stomach, and five had composite reservoirs. They reported continence in all patients but that the continence mechanisms have often required revision. Average bladder capacity was 309 ml, and average compliance was 12.9 ml/cm H_2O. When stomach is used as a bladder augment or as a portion of a neobladder, a dysuria and hematuria syndrome has been reported (Nguyen et al, 1993).

The use of stomach has particular appeal in the pediatric population, in which the stomach's unique acid-base properties can be used not only to reconstruct, but also to help correct the metabolic problems that are often associated with the need for pediatric urinary reconstruction (Carr and Mitchell, 1996). Although experience with stomach remains small, its various unique intrinsic properties as a reservoir suggest that its use will continue in selected clinical situations.

VARIATIONS IN OPERATIVE TECHNIQUE

Conduit Conversion to a Continent Reservoir

The major indication for conversion of a functioning conduit to a continent urinary reservoir is the patient's desire for improved quality of life. Pow-Sang and associates reported on conversion in 20 patients (Pow-Sang et al, 1992). Fifteen were converted from an ileal conduit and one each from a cecal conduit, ureterosigmoidostomy, cutaneous ureterostomy, sigmoid conduit, and suprapubic tube. In 14 of 20, the conduit was discarded or used only as a patch to a colonic reservoir. It was observed that renal units that were obstructed preoperatively were associated with a 71% failure rate. Metabolic acidosis was seen in 15 of 20 (75%) but was believed to be mild. Pouch-related complications are in general a function of the reconstruction selected and need not be higher in this setting. Patient selection is important in determining appropriate candidates for conversion.

The authors prefer to use the conduit in some form whenever possible. This strategy was supported in a report on two patients by Oesterling and Gearhart (1990). The use of an existing bowel segment has the potential to diminish metabolic sequelae and may result in a lower complication rate. The form of continent reconstruction chosen depends on intraoperative findings, and no one procedure is more amenable then another. Before undertaking conversion, the patient should be fully evaluated for disease recurrence, renal functional status, urinary anatomy, hydronephrosis, intestinal length, and intestinal health.

Absorbable Stapling Techniques in Continent Urinary Diversion

The principle of bowel detubularization to increase reservoir capacity and diminish the effects of peristalsis is a fundamental principle of all contemporary continent urinary diversions. The process of detubularization and refashioning of the spatulated bowel segment approximates at least 1 hour of operating time and is by far the most time-consuming and tedious aspect of pouch construction. The employment of devices applying absorbable staples (absorbable staplers) has substantially reduced the time required to fashion bowel reservoirs.

Bonney and Robinson (1990) first demonstrated the potential use of absorbable staplers to substitute for conventional suturing of bowel reservoirs. These authors used a bulky absorbable stapler (Polysorb staples in a TA Premium 55 stapler, U.S. Surgical Corp., Norwalk, CT) to construct an S-pouch configuration in a canine ileal urinary pouch model. Although the same stapler was used in humans by Cummings KB (personal communication, 1995), its clinical use was never widely adopted because the bulky staple configuration destroyed a significant portion of the bowel diameter, particularly when applied to the small intestine. The fact that up to 20 costly staple cartridges were required to complete the closure of a bowel reservoir further reduced the potential benefits of absorbable pouch construction.

A 75-mm GIA instrument (PolyGIA, U.S. Surgical Corp.) incorporating substantially smaller absorbable staples was made available for clinical use in 1992. The stapler delivers four rows of polyglactic acid and polyglycolic acid blend copolymer (absorbable) staples that divide the bowel between the second and third rows. Thus, each staple line of the pouch has a double staggered stapled closure. This device has enabled both refashioning and closure of bowel pouches to be performed with fewer staple applications and is strong and watertight. Finally, the width of bowel sacrificed with the new instrument is appreciably less than with the older staple device. Several investigators have subsequently used the new absorbable GIA stapler to construct catheterizable pouches and neobladders (Olsson et al, 1993; Montie et al, 1994, 1995; Olsson and Kirsch, 1995).

Surgical Techniques

Right Colon Pouch

In 1993, the authors described a technique using absorbable GIA staplers to detubularize fully and refashion large

bowel (Olsson et al, 1993). The technique of colon pouch construction described here incorporates the principles of bowel detubularization and refashioning using absorbable staplers in a simple one-step process.

The right colon and 10 cm of terminal ileum are mobilized by incising the peritoneum along the white line of Toldt and along the base of the mesentery and isolated using metal GIA staplers (Fig. 103–31A). After bowel continuity is restored with standard metal GIA and TA staplers, the distal staple line of the right colon is excised, and the bowel lumen is irrigated to remove residual enteric contents. Using electrocautery, a small opening (2 cm) is created on the antimesenteric border of the cecum to fit the absorbable

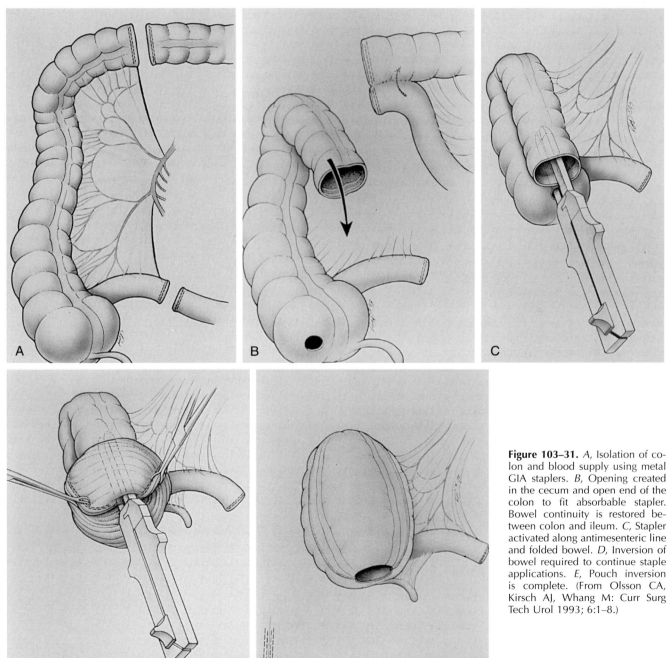

Figure 103–31. *A,* Isolation of colon and blood supply using metal GIA staplers. *B,* Opening created in the cecum and open end of the colon to fit absorbable stapler. Bowel continuity is restored between colon and ileum. *C,* Stapler activated along antimesenteric line and folded bowel. *D,* Inversion of bowel required to continue staple applications. *E,* Pouch inversion is complete. (From Olsson CA, Kirsch AJ, Whang M: Curr Surg Tech Urol 1993; 6:1–8.)

stapler. The distal open end of the colon is aligned with the cecostomy by folding the right colon on itself as depicted in Figure 103–31*B*. The limbs of the absorbable GIA stapler are inserted into the distal open end and into the cecostomy, and the stapler is fired along the antimesenteric line of the apposed folded bowel (Fig. 103–31*C*). It is necessary to evert the bowel to continue subsequent staple applications. This may be achieved by placing Babcock clamps on each side of the distal staple line (Fig. 103–31*D*). A small incision at the junction of each staple line is made to prevent overlap of the absorbable staple rows and allow for the next staple application. Because of this incision, there is often a short unstapled area at the junction between each application of the stapler; a simple figure-of-eight of 2–0 absorbable suture is applied to each of these points. The last staple application traverses the apex of the fold of bowel. In adults, three applications of the stapling device have been required to construct the right colon pouch, whereas in children, two to three staplers suffice. The appearance of the nearly completed pouch is illustrated in Figure 103–31*E*.

Once the generic right pouch has been fashioned, several options exist for ureteral anastomosis and formation of a sphincter mechanism. These maneuvers may be approached through the coalesced distal colon opening and cecostomy, which accesses the pouch interior (see Fig. 103–31*E*). Likewise, this opening permits appropriate stent placement or inspection of a buttressed ileocecal valve. If an appendiceal sphincter mechanism is desired and a short appendiceal stump exists, it may be lengthened by resecting the entire base of the cecum in continuity with the appendix by the application of the absorbable GIA stapler (see Fig. 103–16*A* and *B*). An additional cecostomy can be fashioned for placement of a suprapubic tube or for leading long ureteral stents through a lower abdominal stab wound. Once construction of a continence mechanism and ureteral anastomoses have been performed, the opening can be closed with a running 2–0 absorbable suture or the application of an absorbable TA stapler of appropriate length.

Continent diversion procedures commonly employ the right colon or the cecum and terminal ileum. The array of right colon pouches that can be facilitated by this technique include all of the reservoirs described earlier. Reservoirs using terminal ileum and cecum such as the Penn pouch and the MAINZ pouch can also be fashioned in this manner.

Stapled Sigmoid Neobladder

The same stapling maneuvers can be applied to create an orthotopic neobladder constructed from the sigmoid colon (Olsson and Kirsch, 1995). A portion of the sigmoid and descending colon measuring approximately 35 cm is mobilized by incising the peritoneum along the white line of Toldt. Once mesenteric windows have been created, the segment of colon is isolated using metal GIA staplers (Fig. 103–32*A*). Restoration of bowel continuity is achieved with GIA, TA, or EEA staple devices.

Each of the metal stapled ends of the isolated colon is excised, and the bowel lumen is irrigated. The isolated sigmoid is folded on itself in a U configuration, aligning both open ends (Fig. 103–32*B*). The absorbable GIA stapler is inserted into the open bowel ends and fired along the antimesenteric line of the folded bowel (Fig. 103–32*C*).

Following the procedure for bowel eversion described earlier completes the reservoir. Again, usually two or three applications of the stapler are required to complete the pouch, cutting each staple line tip to avoid staple overlap.

After bowel reinversion, ureteral implants into the tinea can be carried out, using the residual colon opening to facilitate stent passage. These stents and a suprapubic tube are led through a separate stab wound in the pouch and brought through a lower abdominal wall stab incision. Anastomosis is performed between a separate enterotomy at the lower portion of the pouch and the urethra, using six to eight separately placed absorbable sutures, tied after insertion of a Foley catheter. The catheter is inflated to allow traction to facilitate suture tying. The superior colon opening can then be closed with a running suture of absorbable material (Fig. 103–32*D*) or the single application of absorbable TA staples. A suction drainage tube in the vicinity of the urethral and ureteral anastomoses is brought through a stab wound in the left lower quadrant.

W-Stapled Ileal Neobladder

Montie and co-workers used the absorbable GIA stapler to construct ileal neobladders in patients undergoing cystoprostatectomy (Montie et al, 1994). A segment of ileum measuring 50 cm is divided with a standard metal GIA stapler 20 cm from the ileocecal valve. The terminal ends of each limb of the isolated ileal segment are closed with an absorbable TA-55 stapler, and the metal staple line is resected. The bowel is aligned in a W configuration, and an enterotomy is made 10 cm from each end (Fig. 103–33*A*). To facilitate closure of the enterotomy with a TA instrument (see Fig. 103–33*A*, inset), the enterotomy must be made midway between the mesentery and antimesenteric border. The absorbable GIA device is inserted through the enterotomy and is activated. This maneuver adjoins the two adjacent bowel segments. The enterotomy may be closed with the absorbable TA-55 instrument or running absorbable suture, completing the distal segment of the W. The middle and proximal segments are constructed similarly (Fig. 103–33*B*). Montie stressed that the segments of the W must be offset to avoid staple lines that overlap each other. Exceeding a 3- to 6-cm overlap may result in bowel ischemia.

In creating W-configuration pouches, three applications of the absorbable GIA device are used. Because of its dependent nature, the distal segment of the W is most suitable for ileal-urethral anastomosis. Anastomosis between an enterotomy (1 cm) made along the anterior surface of the pouch and the urethra completes the neobladder procedure.

Stapled Ileal Neobladder with Additional ("Chimney") Afferent Limb

Vates and Cummings (Vates TS, Cummings KB, personal communication, 1995) have described an adaptation of the W-stapled ileal neobladder incorporating an additional limb of ileum to receive the ureters, thereby mimicking the Studer (Studer et al, 1988) neobladder. In this procedure, a 60-cm ileal segment is configured as a W for the reservoir with an additional afferent limb (twice the length of the other limbs) to receive the ureters. Enterotomies are made sequentially from right to left. The absorbable GIA stapler is fired be-

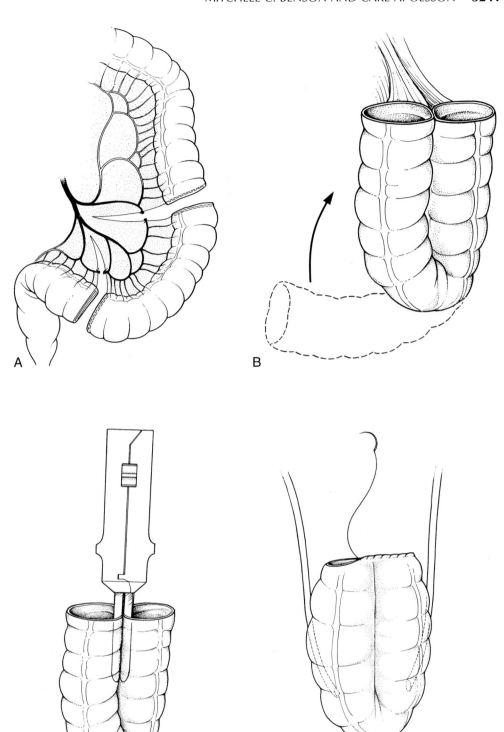

Figure 103–32. *A,* Isolation of colon and blood supply using metal GIA staplers. *B,* Sigmoid bowel folded in U shape. *C,* Stapler fired along antimesenteric border of folded sigmoid. *D,* Oversewing of superior open end completes pouch construction. (From Olsson CA, Kirsch AJ, Whang M: Curr Surg Tech Urol 1993; 6:1–8.)

tween the limbs, care being taken to displace the mesentery posteriorly (Fig. 103–34*A*). The enterotomies in the first two limbs of the pouch are closed with a running absorbable suture, whereas the remaining two enterotomies are temporarily left open to facilitate ureteral stent placement. Four applications of the stapler are required to complete reservoir construction. The cutaway view of the pouch (Fig. 103–34*B*) illustrates the fully stapled and detubularized bowel seg-

ments. The pouch is then anastomosed to the urethra using several interrupted absorbable sutures.

Postoperative Care and Comments

The rapid construction of bowel reservoirs for continent diversion using the absorbable stapler has several advantages

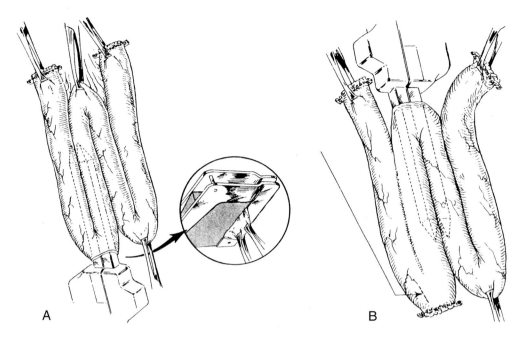

Figure 103–33. *A,* Following closure of butt ends of the reservoir with TA-55 stapler, an enterotomy is made in the dependent portion of first limb of W. Absorbable stapler is inserted through the enterotomy and fired, creating a common lumen between two adjacent limbs. *Arrow* indicates closeup of closure of enterotomy with TA-55 stapler. *B,* In middle limb of W, stapler is placed through the enterotomy at the apex, and again a common lumen is created. Staple lines are not directly opposing for their entire distance to avoid ischemia between adjacent staple lines. *Arrow* indicates site of enterotomy where urethroileal anastomosis will be performed. (From Pontes JE: Genitourinary Oncologic Pelvic Surgery. New York, John Wiley & Sons, 1993. Copyright 1993 John Wiley & Sons. Reprinted by permission of Wiley-Liss, Inc., a subsidiary of John Wiley & Sons, Inc.)

compared to conventional suturing. Because neither bowel spatulation nor reservoir refashioning is required by these modified techniques, there is considerable time saved in pouch construction. The time spent to create the generic pouch (between the point at which the bowel segment is mobilized and the point before ureteral anastomosis or construction of a sphincter mechanism) approximates only 15 to 20 minutes with practice. This represents a saving of approximately 1 hour of operating time per case as well as reduction of overall blood loss.

In the first 15 adult patients to undergo the authors' absorbable stapling technique in right colon pouch construction, with at least 2 years' follow-up, there have been no complications attributed to absorbable staples. Similar results have been reported by Rowland (1996). In the pediatric population, the authors have applied the absorbable stapler to

continent urinary diversion as well as bladder augmentation (Hensle et al, 1995). In the first 18 children followed for up to 3 years, there have been no instances of pouch perforation or inadequate pouch capacity, and to date, only one of the patients developed a reservoir calculus.

Montie and colleagues used absorbable staplers to create W-stapled ileal neobladders in 25 patients (Montie et al, 1994). Ileal pouch construction was performed in approximately 20 minutes, and functional aspects were comparable to bowel reservoirs constructed by conventional suturing. Urodynamic evaluation at 6 months, however, documented a small-capacity reservoir requiring augmentation enterocystoplasty in 3 of 25 patients (12%). Montie and colleagues attributed this complication to either the size of the staples or reservoir fibrosis secondary to foreign body reaction. It is conceivable that a similar situation would arise when

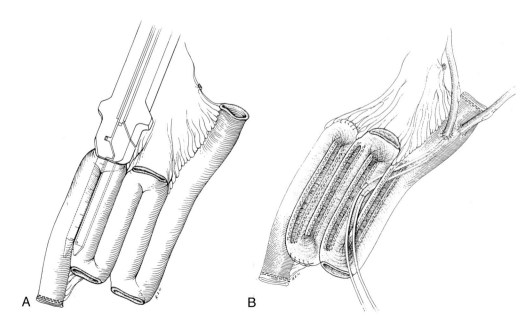

Figure 103–34. *A,* Modified W configuration with additional afferent limb ("chimney"). *B,* Cut-away view of stapled and detubularized pouch. (Courtesy of Kenneth Cummings, M.D.)

constructing the more extensive modified (Studer) W-stapled ileal neobladder described by Vates and Cummings (Vates TS, Cummings KB, personal communication, 1995), although they reported that this has not constituted a problem clinically.

The authors have used the absorbable stapler to construct both large and small bowel reservoirs. In the authors' experience, colonic pouches appear better suited for construction with the absorbable stapler because of their relatively larger lumen. As opposed to small bowel, there is no problem with overlap of staple lines and subsequent risk of bowel ischemia in using colonic segments. The introduction of stapling devices delivering still smaller staples may prevent the problems presently seen when ileal pouches are constructed with current technology.

REFERENCES

Adams MC, Mitchell ME, Rink RC: Gastrocystoplasty: An alternative solution to the problem of urological reconstruction in the severely compromised patient. J Urol 1988; 140:1152–1156.

Alcini E, Racioppi M, D'Addessi A, et al: Refluxes in orthotopic neobladders: Can the ileocecal sphincter be considered an adequate antireflux mechanism. Urology 1994; 44:38–45.

Althausen AF, Hagen-Cook K, Hendren WH III: Non-refluxing colon conduit: Experience with 70 cases. J Urol 1978; 120:35–39.

Ambrose SS: Ureterosigmoidostomy. In Glenn JF, ed: Urologic Surgery. Philadelphia, J.B. Lippincott, 1983, pp 511–520.

Ashken MH: Urinary cecal reservoir. In King LR, Stone AR, Webster GD, eds: Bladder Reconstruction and Continent Diversion. Chicago, Year Book Medical Publishers, 1987, pp 238–251.

Askanazi J, Hensle TW, Starker P, et al: Effect of immediate postoperative nutritional support on length of hospitalization. J Urol 1985; 134:1032–1036.

Bejany DE, Politano VA: Stapled and nonstapled tapered distal ileum for construction of a continent colonic urinary reservoir. J Urol 1988; 140:491–494.

Benchekroun A: The ileocecal continent bladder. In King LR, Stone AR, Webster GD, eds: Bladder Reconstruction and Continent Urinary Diversion. Chicago, Year Book Medical Publishers, 1987, pp 224–237.

Benchekroun A: Hydraulic valve for continence and antireflux: A 17 year experience of 210 cases. Scand J Urol Nephrol 1992; 142(suppl):70–72.

Benson MC, Miller M: The management of superficial urethral recurrence following cystectomy and neobladder by transurethral resection. J Urol 1996; 156:1768.

Benson MC, Sawczuk IS, Hensle TW, et al: Modified Indiana University continent diversion. Curr Surg Tech Urol 1988; 1:1–8.

Benson MC, Seaman EK, Olsson CA: The ileal ureter neobladder is associated with a high success and a low complication rate. J Urol 1996; 155:1585–1588.

Benson MC, Seaman E, Tannenbaum S, Olsson CA: The ileal ureter neobladder (Studer) is associated with a high success and a low complication rate. J Urol 1994; 151:60a.

Benson MC, Slawin KM, Wechsler MH, Olsson CA: Analysis of continent versus standard urinary diversion. Br J Urol 1992; 69:156–162.

Berglund B, Kock NG, Norlen L, Philipson BM: Volume capacity and pressure characteristics of the continent ileal reservoir used for urinary diversion. J Urol 1987; 137:29–34.

Bissada NK: Characteristics of the in-situ appendix as a continent catheterization stoma for continent urinary diversion in adults. J Urol 1993; 150:151–152.

Bjerre BD, Johansen C, Steven K: Health-related quality of life after cystectomy: Bladder substitution compared with ileal conduit diversion. A questionnaire survey. Br J Urol 1995; 75:200–205.

Bonney WW, Robinson RA: Absorbable staples in continent ileal urinary pouch. Urology 1990; 3:57–62.

Boyd SD, Feinberg SM, Skinner DG, et al: Quality of life survey of urinary diversion patients: Comparison of ileal conduits versus continent Kock ileal reservoirs. J Urol 1987; 138:1386–1389.

Burger R, Wammack R, Fisch M, et al: The appendix as a continence mechanism. Eur Urol 1992; 22:255–262.

Burns MW, Mitchell ME: Tips on constructing the Mitrofanoff appendiceal stoma. Contemp Urol 1990; May:10–12.

Camey M: Detubularized U-shaped cystoplasty (Camey 2). Curr Surg Tech Urol 1990; 3:1–8.

Camey M, LeDuc: L'enterocystoplastie avec cystoprostatectomie totale pour cancer de la vessie. Ann Urol 1979; 13:114.

Camey M, Richard F, Botto H: Bladder replacement by ileocystoplasty. In King LR, Stone AR, Webster GD, eds: Bladder Reconstruction and Continent Urinary Diversion. Chicago, Year Book Medical Publishers, 1987, pp 336–359.

Carr MC, Mitchell ME: Continent gastric pouch. World J Urol. 1996; 14:112–116.

Carroll PR, Presti JC Jr: Comparison of plicated and stapled continent ileocecal stoma. Urology 1992; 40:107–109.

Carroll PR, Presti JC Jr, McAninch JW, Tanagho EA: Functional characteristics of the continent ileocecal urinary reservoir: Mechanisms of urinary continence. J Urol 1989; 142:1032–1036.

Chen KK, Chang LS, Chen MT: Urodynamic and clinical outcome of Kock pouch continent urinary diversion. J Urol 1989; 141:94–97.

Colleselli K, Strasser H, Mirriggl B, et al: Hemi-Kock to the female urethra: Anatomical approach to the continence mechanism of the female urethra. J Urol 1994; 151(part 2):500A.

Cordonnier JJ, Spjut HJ: Urethral occurrence of bladder carcinoma following cystectomy. Trans Am Assoc Genitourin Surg 1961; 53:13.

Culp DA: Commentary: Heitz-Boyer-Havelacque procedure: Not the procedure of choice. In Whitehead ED, Leiter E, eds: Current Operative Urology, 2nd ed. Philadelphia, Harper & Row, 1984, pp 782–783.

DaPozzo LF, Colombo R, Pompa P, et al: Detubularized sigmoid colon for bladder replacement after radical cystectomy. J Urol 1994; 152:1409–1412.

DeKernion JB, Den Besten L, Kaufman J, Ehrlich R: The Kock pouch as a urinary reservoir: Pitfalls and perspectives. Am J Surg 1985; 150:83.

DePaepe ME, Andre R, Mahadevia P: Urethral involvement in female patients with bladder cancer: A study of 22 cystectomy specimens. Cancer 1990; 65:1237–1241.

Duckett JW, Gazak JM: Complications of ureterosigmoidostomy. Urol Clin North Am 1983; 10:473–481.

Duckett JW, Snyder HM III: Use of the Mitrofanoff principle in urinary reconstruction. Urol Clin North Am 1986; 13:271–274.

Duckett JW, Snyder HM III: The Mitrofanoff principle in continent urinary reservoirs. Semin Urol 1987; 5:55–62.

Elmajian DA, Esrig D, Freeman JA, et al: Orthotopic lower urinary tract reconstruction utilizing the Kock ileal reservoir: Updated experience in 266 patients. J Urol 1995; 153(part 2):241a.

Fair WR: The ileal neobladder. Urol Clin North Am 1991; 18:555–559.

Filmer RB, Spencer JR: Malignancies in bladder augmentations and intestinal conduits. J Urol 1990; 143:671–678.

Fisch M, Hohenfellner R: Der sigma rectum pouch: Eine modifikation der harnleiterdarn implantation. Aktuelle Urologie Operative Techniken, vol 22, 1991.

Fisch M, Klinkowski U, Wammack R, Hohenfellner R: The sigma-rectum pouch (MAINZ pouch II): Critical analysis after 3 years of clinical experience. J Urol 1995; 153:61a.

Fisch M, Wammack R, Hohenfellner R: The sigma-rectum pouch (MAINZ pouch II). In Hohenfellner R, Wammack R, eds: Continent Urinary Diversion. Edinburgh, Churchill Livingstone, 1992a, pp 163–182.

Fisch M, Wammack R, Hohenfellner R: Seven years experience with the MAINZ Pouch procedure. Archivos Españoles de Urologia 1992b; 45:175–185.

Gerber A: Improved quality of life following a Kock continent ileostomy. West J Med 1980; 133:95.

Ghoneim MA, Kock NG, Kycke G, Shehab El-Din AB: An appliance-free, sphincter-controlled bladder substitute: The urethral Kock pouch. J Urol 1987; 138:1150–1154.

Gilchrist RK, Merricks JW, Hamlin HH, Rieger IT: Construction of a substitute bladder and urethra. Surg Gynecol Obstet 1950; 90:752–760.

Goldwasser B: The colonic orthotopic bladder. Urology 1995; 45:190–192.

Goldwasser B, Barrett DM, Benson RC Jr: Complete bladder replacement using the detubularized right colon. In King LR, Stone AR, Webster GD, eds: Bladder Reconstruction and Continent Urinary Diversion. Chicago, Year Book Medical Publishers, 1987, pp 360–366.

Goldwasser B, Benson RC Jr: Continent urinary diversion. Mayo Clin Proc 1986; 61:615–621.

Goodwin WE, Turner RD, Winter CC: Results of ileocystoplasty. J Urol 1958; 80:461–466.

Gosalbez R, Padron OF, Singla AK, et al: The gastric augment single pedicle tube catheterizable stoma: A useful adjunct to reconstruction of the urinary tract. J Urol 1994; 152:2005–2007.

Hampel N, Hasan ST, Marshall C, Neal DE: Continent urinary diversion using the Mitrofanoff principle. Br J Urol 1995; 74:454–459.

Hautmann RE, Egghart G, Frohneberg D, Miller K: The ileal neobladder. J Urol l988; 139:39–42.

Hautmann RE, Paiss T, Kleinschmidt K, DePetriconi R: The ileal neobladder in the female: Why it works or not. J Urol 1995; 153(part 2):58a.

Helal M, Pow-Sang J, Sanford E, et al: Direct (non-tunneled) uretrocolonic reimplantation in association with continent reservoirs. J Urol 1993; 150:835–837.

Hendren WH: Urinary diversion and undiversion in children. Surg Clin North Am 1976; 56:425.

Hendren WH: Reoperative ureteral reimplantation: Management of the difficult case. J Pediatr Surg 1980; 15:770–786.

Hensle TW: Nutritional support of the surgical patient. Urol Clin North Am 1983; 10:109.

Hensle TW, Kirsch AJ, Olsson CA: Bowel reservoirs created with absorbable staples in a pediatric population. Presented at the annual meeting of the American Academy of Pediatrics, San Francisco, 1995.

Hickey DP, Soloway MS, Murphy WM: Selective urethrectomy following cystoprostatectomy for bladder cancer. J Urol 1986; 136:828–833.

Hubner WA, Pfluger H: Functional replacement of bladder and urethra after cystectomy for bladder cancer in a female patient. J Urol 1995; 153(part 2):1043–1046.

Jakobsen H, Steven K, Stigsby B, et al: Pathogenesis of nocturnal urinary incontinence after ileocaecal bladder replacement: Continuous measurement of urethral closure pressure during sleep. Br J Urol 1987; 59:148–152.

Keetch DW, Klutke CG, Catalona WJ: Late decompensation of neobladder. J Urol 1992; 148:806.

King LR: Protection of the upper tracts in undiversion. In King LR, Stone AR, Webster GD, eds: Bladder Reconstruction and Continent Urinary Diversion. Chicago, Year Book Medical Publishers, l987, pp 127–153.

Kirsch AJ, Hensle TW, Olsson CA: Rapid right colon pouch construction with absorbable stapler: Initial clinical experience. Urology 1994; 43:228–231.

Kirsch AJ, Hensle TW, Olsson CA: Absorbable stapling techniques in bowel reservoirs. Atlas Urol Clin North Am 1995; 3:69–80.

Kock NG: Ileostomy without external appliance: A survey of 25 patients provided with intestinal reservoir. Ann Surg 1971; 173:545.

Kock NG, Ghoneim MA, Lycke KG, Mahran MR: Urinary diversion to the augmented and valved rectum: Preliminary results with a novel surgical procedure. J Urol 1988; 140:1375–1379.

Kock NG, Ghoneim MA, Lycke KG, Mahran MR: Replacement of the bladder by the urethral Kock pouch: Functional results, urodynamics and radiological features. J Urol 1989; 141:1111–1116.

Kock NG, Nilson AE, Nilsson LO, et al: Urinary diversion via a continent ileal reservoir: Clinical results in 12 patients. J Urol 1982; 128:469.

Kolettis PN, Klein EA, Novick AC: The LeBag continent urinary diversion: The Cleveland Clinic experience. J Urol 1995; 153:303A.

Kramolowsky EV, Clayman RV, Weyman PJ: Endourological management of ureteroileal anastomotic strictures: Is it effective? J Urol 1987; 137:390–394.

Kramolowsky EV, Clayman RV, Weyman PJ: Management of ureterointestinal anastomotic strictures: Comparison of open surgical and endourological repair. J Urol 1988; 139:1195–1198.

Kristiansen P, Mansson W, Tyger J: Perforation of continent caecal reservoir for urine twice in one patient. Scand J Urol Nephrol 1991; 25:279–281.

Lampel A, Hohenfellner M, Schultz D, Thuroff JW: Submucosal seromuscular tube and submucosal bowel flap tube: Two new stoma techniques for MAINZ pouch continent cutaneous urinary diversion. J Urol 1995a; 153:305A.

Lampel A, Hohenfellner M, Schultz-Lampel D, Thuroff JW: In situ tunneled bowel flap tubes: 2 new techniques of a continent outlet for MAINZ pouch cutaneous diversion. J Urol 1995b; 153:308–315.

LeDuc A, Camey M, Teillac P: An original antireflux ureteroileal implantation technique: Long term follow-up. J Urol 1987; 137:1156–1158.

Leonard MP, Gearhart JP, Jeffs RD: Continent urinary reservoirs in pediatric urological practice. J Urol 1990; 144:330–334.

Leonard MP, Quinlan DM: The Benchekroun ileal valve. Urol Clin North Am 1991; 18:717–724.

Leong CH: Use of stomach for bladder replacement and urinary diversion. Ann R Coll Surg Eng 1978; 60:283–289.

Lieskovsky G, Boyd SD, Skinner DG: Management of late complications of the Kock pouch form of urinary diversion. J Urol 1987; 137:1146.

Light JK, Marks JL: Total bladder replacement in the male and female using the ileocolonic segment (Le Bag). Br J Urol 1990; 65:467–472.

Light JK, Scardino PT: Radical cystectomy with preservation of sexual and urinary function: Use of the ileocolonic pouch ("Le Bag"). Urol Clin North Am 1986; 13:261–270.

Lockhart JL: Remodeled right colon: An alternative urinary reservoir. J Urol 1987; 138:730–734.

Lugagne PM, Herve JM, Barre P, et al: Long term evolution of upper urinary tract after cystoprostatectomy with neo-ileal-bladder. J Urol 1995; 153(part 2):52a.

Mansson W: The continent cecal urinary reservoir. In King LR, Stone AR, Webster GD, eds: Bladder Reconstruction and Continent Urinary Diversion. Chicago, Year Book Medical Publishers, 1987, p 209.

Mansson W, Colleen S: Experience with a detubularized right colonic segment for bladder replacement. Scand J Urol Nephrol 1990; 24:53–56.

Mansson W, Colleen S, Forsberg L, et al: Renal function after urinary diversion: A study of continent caecal reservoir, ileal conduit, and colonic conduit. Scand J Urol Nephrol 1984; 18:307–315.

Marshall FF: Creation of an ileocolic bladder after cystectomy. J Urol 1988; 139:1264–1268.

Marshall FF, Mostwin JC, Radebaugh LC, et al: Ileocolic neobladder post cystectomy: Continence and potency. J Urol 1991; 145:502–504.

McLeod RS, Fazio VW: Quality of life with the continent ileostomy. World J Surg 1984; 8:90.

Melchior H, Spehr C, Knop-Wagemann I, et al: The continent ileal bladder for urinary tract reconstruction after cystectomy: A survey of 44 patients. J Urol 1988; 139:714–718.

Montie JE, Pontes JE, Parulkar BG, Selby T: W-stapled ileal neobladder formed entirely with absorbable staples. J Urol 1994; 151:1188–1192.

Montie JE, Pontes JE, Powell IJ: Orthotopic ileal neobladder after cystectomy: Comparison of hand-sewn vs. absorbable staples for reservoir formation. J Urol 1995; 153:305a.

Nguyen DH, Bain MA, Salmonson KL, et al: The syndrome of dysuria and hematuria in pediatric urinary reconstruction with stomach. J Urol 1993; 150:707–709.

Norlen L, Trasti H: Functional behavior of the continent ileum reservoir for urinary diversion: An experimental and clinical study. Scand J Urol Nephrol 1978; 49(suppl):33–42.

Oesterling JE, Gearhart JP: Utilization of ileal conduit in construction of continent urinary reservoir. Urology 1990; 36:15–19.

Olsson CA: Continent urinary diversion. J Urol 1984; 132:1157–1158.

Olsson CA: Kock continent ileal reservoir for urinary diversion. In King LR, Stone AR, Webster GD, eds: Bladder Reconstruction and Continent Urinary Diversion. Chicago, Year Book Medical Publishers, 1987, pp 291–310.

Olsson CA, Kirsch AJ: Stapled sigmoid neobladder. Curr Surg Tech Urol 1995; 8:1–8.

Olsson CA, Kirsch AJ, Whang M: Rapid construction of right colon pouch. Curr Surg Tech Urol 1993; 6:1–8.

Pagano F, Artibani W, Ligato P, et al: Vesica ileale Padovana: A technique for total bladder replacement. Eur Urol 1990; 17:149–154.

Pagano F, Artibani W, Villi G, et al: The vesica ileale Padovana. In Wammack R, Hohenfellner R, eds: Continent Urinary Diversion. Edinburgh, Churchill Livingstone, 1992, pp 117–125.

Piser JA, Mitchell ME, Kulb TB, et al: Gastrocystoplasty and colocystoplasty in canines: The metabolic consequences of acute saline and acid loading. J Urol 1987; 138:1009.

Pow-Sang JM, Helal M, Figueroa E, et al: Conversion from external appliance wearing or internal urinary diversion to a continent urinary reservoir (Florida Pouch I, II): Surgical technique, indications and complications. J Urol 1992; 147:356–360.

Raz S, McLorie G, Johnson S, Skinner DG: Management of the urethra in patients undergoing radical cystectomy for bladder carcinoma. J Urol 1978; 120:298.

Reddy PK: Detubularized sigmoid reservoir for bladder replacement after cystoprostatectomy. Urology 1987; 29:625–628.

Riedmiller H, Steinbach F, Thuroff J, Hohenfellner R: Continent appendix stoma: A modification of the MAINZ pouch technique. Presented at the E.A.U. Congress, Amsterdam, 1990.

Rogers E, Scardino PT: A simple ileal substitute bladder after radical cystectomy: Experience with a modification of the Studer Pouch. J Urol 1995; 153:1432–1438.

Rowland RG: Editorial comment. Urology 1994; 43:231.

Rowland RG: Present experience with the Indiana pouch. World J Urol 1996; 14:92–98.

Rowland RG, Mitchell ME, Bihrle R: The cecoileal continent urinary reservoir. World J Urol 1985; 3:185–190.

Rowland RG, Mitchell ME, Bihrle R, et al: Indiana continent urinary reservoir. J Urol 1987; 137:1136–1139.

Rudick J, Schonholz S, Weber HN: The gastric bladder: A continent reservoir for urinary diversion. Surgery 1977; 82:1.

Salter MJ: What are the differences in body image between patients with a conventional stoma compared with those who have had a conventional stoma followed by a continent pouch. J Adv Nursing 1992a; 17:841–848.

Salter MJ: Aspects of sexuality for patients with stomas and continent pouches. J Adv Nursing 1992b; 19:126–130.

Sanda MG, Jeffs RD, Gearhart JP: Evolution of outcomes with the ileal hydraulic valve continent diversion: Re-evaluation of the Benchekroun catheterizable stoma. World J Urol 1996; 14:108–111.

Scheidler DM, Klee LW, Rowland RG, et al: Update on the Indiana continent urinary reservoir. J Urol 1989; 141:302A.

Schellhammer PF, Whitmore WF Jr: Transitional cell carcinoma of the urethra in men having cystectomy for bladder cancer. J Urol 1976; 115:56.

Schlegel PN, Walsh PC: Neuroanatomical approach to radical cystoprosta-tectomy with preservation of sexual function. J Urol 1987; 138:1402.

Schreiter F, Noll F: Kock pouch and S bladder: 2 different ways of lower urinary tract reconstruction. J Urol 1989; 142:1197–1200.

Schreiter F, Noll F: The S bladder, an ideal bladder substitution. Acta Urol Belg 1991; 59:251–264.

Silberman R: Ammonia intoxication following ureterosigmoidostomy in a patient with liver disease. Lancet 1958; 2:937–939.

Simoneau AR, Skinner DG: Ileo-anal reservoir. J Urol 1995; 153:305A.

Sinaiko E: Artificial bladder segment of stomach and study of effect of urine on gastric secretion. Surg Gynecol Obstet 1956; 102:433.

Skinner DG: The Kock pouch for continent urinary reconstruction focusing on the afferent segment and the reservoir. Scand J Urol Nephrol 1992; 142:77–78.

Skinner DG, Boyd S, Lieskovsky G: Clinical experience with the Kock continent ileal reservoir for urinary diversion. J Urol 1984; 132:1101–1107.

Skinner DG, Lieskovsky G, Boyd S: Continuing experience with the conti-nent ileal reservoir (Kock Pouch) as an alternative to cutaneous urinary diversion: An update after 250 cases. J Urol 1987a; 141:1140–1145.

Skinner DG, Lieskovsky G, Boyd S: Continent urinary diversion. J Urol 1989; 141:1323–1327.

Skinner DG, Lieskovsky G, Skinner E, Boyd S: Urinary diversion. Curr Prob Surg 1987b; 24:401–471.

Smith T: An account of an unsuccessful attempt to treat extroversion of the bladder by a new operation. St Barth Hosp Rep 1879; 15:29–35.

Spirnak JP, Caldamone AA: Ureterosigmoidostomy. Urol Clin North Am 1986; 13:285–294.

Stein JP, Stenzl A, Esrig D, et al: Lower urinary tract reconstruction in women following cystectomy using the Kock ileal reservoir with bilateral ureteroileal urethrostomy: Initial clinical experience. J Urol 1994; 152:1404–1408.

Stein R, Matani Y, Doi Y, et al: Continent urinary diversion using the MAINZ pouch I technique—ten years later. J Urol 1995; 153:251a.

Steiner U, Miller K, Hautmann R: Functional results and complications of the ileal neobladder in over 200 patients. Urologe-Ausgabe A 1994; 33:53–57.

Stockle M, Gokcebay E, Riedmiller H, Hohenfellner R: Urethral tumor recurrences after radical cystoprostatectomy: The case for primary cysto-prostatourethrectomy? J Urol 1990; 143:41.

Studer U, Ackermann D, Casanova GA, Zingg EJ: A newer form of bladder substitute based on historical perspectives. Semin Urol 1988; 6:57–65.

Studer U, Ackermann D, Casanova GA, Zingg EJ: Three years' experience with an ileal low pressure bladder substitute. Br J Urol 1989; 63:43–52.

Studer U, Danuser H, Hochreiter W, et al: Ten years' experience with an ileal low pressure bladder substitute with an afferent tubular isoperistaltic segment. World J Urol 1996; 14:29–39.

Sumfest JM, Burns MW, Mitchell ME: The Mitrofanoff principle in urinary reconstruction. J Urol 1993; 150:1875–1878.

Terai A, Arai Y, Kawakita M, et al: Effect of urinary intestinal diversion on urinary risk factors for urolithiasis. J Urol 1995; 153:37–41.

Thompson ST, Kursh ED: Delayed spontaneous rupture of an ileocolonic neobladder. J Urol 1992; 148:1890–1891.

Thüroff JW, Alken P, Hohenfellner R: The MAINZ pouch (mixed augmen-tation with ileum 'n zecum) for bladder augmentation and continent diversion. In King LR, Stone AR, Webster GD, eds: Bladder Reconstruc-tion and Continent Urinary Diversion. Chicago, Year Book Medical Publishers, 1987, p 252.

Thüroff JW, Alken P, Riedmiller H, et al: The MAINZ pouch (mixed augmentation ileum 'n zecum) for bladder augmentation and continent diversion. World J Urol 1985; 3:179–184.

Thüroff JW, Alken P, Riedmiller H, et al: 100 cases of MAINZ pouch: Continuing experience and evolution. J Urol 1988; 140:283–288.

Vara AR, Shanberg AM, Sawyer DE, et al: Modification of LeBag ileoco-lonic pouch with improved results: Review of 17 cases. Urology 1992; 40:221–226.

Walsh PC, Lepor H, Eggleston JC: Radical prostatectomy with preservation of sexual function: Anatomical and pathological considerations. Prostate 1983; 4:473.

Watanabe K, Kato H, Misawa K, Ogawa A: Spontaneous perforation of an ileal neobladder. Br J Urol 1994; 73:460–461.

Waters WB, Vaughan DJ, Harris RG, Brady SM: The Kock pouch: Initial experience and complications. J Urol 1987; 137:1151.

Webster GD, King LR: Further commentary: Cecal bladder. In King LR, Stone AR, Webster GD, eds: Bladder Reconstruction and Continent Urinary Diversion. Chicago, Year Book Medical Publishers, 1987, pp 206–208.

Wenderoth UK, Bachor R, Egghart G, et al: The ileal neobladder: Experi-ence and results of more than 100 consecutive cases. J Urol 1990; 143:492–497.

Williams DF: Commentary: The value of ureterosigmoidostomy. In Whitehead ED, Leiter E, eds: Current Operative Urology, 2nd ed. Phila-delphia, Harper & Row, 1984, pp 742–744.

Williams DF, Burkholder GV, Goodwin WE: Ureterosigmoidostomy: A 15-year experience. J Urol 1969; 101:168–170.

Woodhouse CR, MacNeily AE: The Mitrofanoff principle: Expanding upon a versatile technique. Br J Urol 1994; 74:447–453.

104

URINARY UNDIVERSION: REFUNCTIONALIZATION OF THE PREVIOUSLY DIVERTED URINARY TRACT

W. Hardy Hendren, M.D.

General Considerations
  Renal Function
  Psychologic Factors
  Anesthesia
  Assessment of Bladder Function

Surgical Principles
  Wide Transabdominal Exposure
  Psoas Hitch

Transureteroureterostomy or
  Transureteropyelostomy
  Bladder Augmentation

Selected Cases

Results and Complications

Conclusion

Diversion of the urinary tract by a variety of means was used widely in treating certain urologic problems in infants and children (Johnston, 1963; Retik et al, 1967; Perlmutter and Patil, 1972; Zinman and Libertino, 1975; Hendren, 1976; Mitchell, 1981a, 1981b; Mitchell and Rink, 1987; Mor et al, 1992). A good example is the child with myelomeningocele and neuropathic bladder. In the 1950s, many children were maintained on long-term urethral or suprapubic catheter drainage to make them dry and relieve pressure on the upper tracts if there was hydronephrosis. This treatment provided a poor quality of life because of recurrent infection, stones, and the complications from inlying tubes.

The ileal loop urinary diversion was considered to be a major advance (Bricker, 1950). In time, however, it was clear that the ileal loop urinary diversion also had many complications, including recurring infection because of reflux, stones, and stricture of the stoma or the bowel segment itself (Smith, 1972; Richie et al, 1974; Shapiro et al, 1975; Middleton and Hendren, 1976; Pitts and Muecke, 1979). This diversion also required living with a bag on the abdomen to collect urine.

Today the majority of children with a neuropathic bladder can be managed by either intermittent catheterization, popularized by Lapides and co-workers (1976), or various reconstructive operations, depending on the state of continence, whether vesicoureteral reflux is apparent, the size and in-

nervation of the bladder, and other factors. Intermittent catheterization has made it possible to reverse prior urinary diversion in myelodysplastic bladders (Perlmutter, 1980).

Progress has been made in managing various obstructive uropathies, such as in boys with urethral valves (Hendren, 1970, 1971, 1974a; Bauer et al, 1974; Duckett, 1974; Campaiola et al, 1985; Glassberg, 1985; Mitchell and Close, 1995), in children with ureteroceles (Hendren and Mitchell, 1979; Smith et al, 1994; Coplen and Duckett, 1995), and in children with major malformations such as epispadias and exstrophy of the bladder (Jeffs, 1986). Many advances have allowed the repair of these problems instead of resorting to urinary diversions, which in the past provided an "easy way out" for the surgeon but not a good long-term solution for the patient.

Continent urinary diversion (Gilchrist et al, 1950; Mitrofanoff, 1980; Kock et al, 1982; Skinner et al, 1984; King et al, 1987a, 1987b; Thuroff et al, 1988; Sheldon and Gilbert, 1992; Sumfest et al, 1993), which entails construction of an internal reservoir or pouch of bowel for storage of urine that can be intermittently catheterized by the patient, has come into use in the past several years, similar to the ileal loop in the 1950s and 1960s. **The author hopes that the continent diversion does not become overused, to the extent that it is selected instead of appropriate reconstructive surgery for those complex problems that can be repaired.**

Table 104–1. URINARY UNDIVERSION: 216 CASES, 1969–1995*

74	Ileal loop (14 pyeloileal)	144	Permanent diversions
18	Colon conduit (3 had been ileal loops)	72	Temporary diversions
		87	Females
41	Loop ureterostomy or pyelostomy	129	Males
18	End ureterostomy	54	Patients had one kidney (3 had a transplant)
54	Cystostomy or vesicostomy		
8	Nephrostomy	1	Patient anephric (later transplanted)
2	Ureterosigmoidostomies		
1	Continent diversion		

*13 diversions by the author; 203 had been performed elsewhere.

This chapter summarizes a 26-year experience in reconstructing the previously diverted urinary tract of 216 patients. Table 104–1 shows the types of urinary diversions present in these patients. Many reasons were given for the original diversions, such as complex anatomy, thought to be unsalvageable except by diversions; failed ureteral reimplantation surgery; urinary incontinence; and hydronephrosis, thought to be too severe to be corrected. In most such cases today, diversions can be avoided (Hendren, 1978a, 1980a; Sheldon, 1995). The majority of the patients had diversions originally planned as permanent measures. Others had undergone diversions as temporary measures, such as loop ureterostomy, nephrostomy, and vesicostomy. In many instances, however, the "temporary" diversion had been present for many years.

Fifty-four of the patients had only one kidney: in three of those 54 patients, the kidney was a transplanted one. One of those three had been transplanted into an ileal loop, and the other two were transplanted into bladders that had a vesicostomy. Another patient had no kidneys at all, having been on hemodialysis after two failed transplants. He also had the same poor, noncompliant bladder that had initially led to renal deterioration. The lower urinary tract was reconstructed and augmented, and a third transplant was performed successfully with a living related donor, his mother.

Figure 104–1 shows the ages of the patients. Any patient with a urinary diversion, regardless of age, should be thought of as a possible candidate for undiversion. Indeed, a series of undiversions in adults has been reported (Goldstein and Hensle, 1981).

Figure 104–2 shows the duration of urinary diversion. The longest was an ileal loop, which had been done 35 years previously, when the patient was only 3 years old. Thus, a long duration of a urinary diversion is not a contraindication to eventual repair.

GENERAL CONSIDERATIONS

When considering an individual patient for possible refunctionalization of the diverted urinary tract, a number of factors must be weighed. Every patient differs in some respect from all of the others that one may have treated. It is important to examine why the patient's urinary tract was previously diverted. The most common causes encountered include severe obstructive uropathy from urethral valves, the prune-belly syndrome, failed ureteral reimplantation, failed megaureter repair, failed surgery for urinary incontinence, stricture of the urethra, and myelodysplasia causing neurogenic bladder.

If the patient was originally incontinent, obviously, undiversion requires not only joining the upper tract to the bladder, but also correcting the problem. Correction may involve revising the bladder outlet, creating a urethra (Hendren, 1980b), increasing the size and compliance of the bladder, or all of these. Bladder augmentation can be done by a variety of techniques.

Renal Function

Many patients with diverted urinary tracts have reduced renal function. About a third of those for whom the author has performed undiversions had such severe upper tract damage at the outset that it could be predicted that trans-

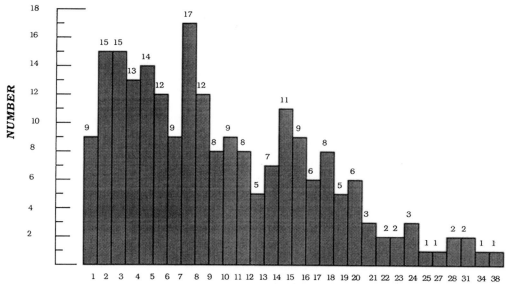

Figure 104–1. Age in 216 patients with undiversions.

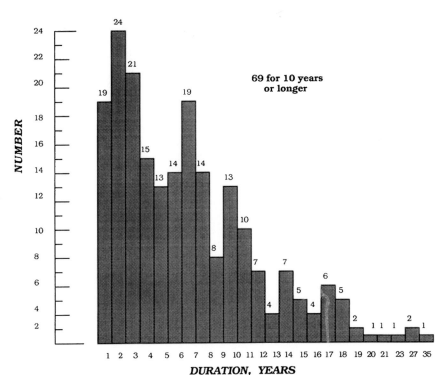

Figure 104–2. Duration of diversion in 216 patients with undiversions.

plantation would be necessary in the future. To date, 29 of the patients have undergone renal transplantations (3 antedated reconstruction). Approximately 43 others from the group will likely need transplantations as they grow older, judging from their present creatinine clearance rates and the state of their upper tracts. It is common to see a steady rise in serum creatinine as young patients grow, especially at adolescence when the body mass increases to a size greater than poor kidneys can support.

In patients with borderline renal function, undiversion has invariably improved the quality of life between the time of reconstruction and the time when dialysis or transplantation was needed. Many patients with diversions have chronic bacilluria. It is often possible to maintain a sterile urinary tract after undiversion. When transplantation is necessary in these patients, it is much better done into a functioning lower urinary tract than into a urinary diversion that imposes additional possible complications (Sheldon et al, 1994).

If bowel is to be used in the urinary tract, one should anticipate solute resorption through the bowel surface (Ferris and Odel, 1950; Koch and McDougal, 1985). The patients so treated must be followed closely. All patients with diminished renal function are managed collaboratively with a nephrologist. This collaborative monitoring is of great help in maintaining metabolic homeostasis when there is declining renal function. This practice has provided a smooth transition to dialysis and transplantation for patients who have reached that stage.

Psychologic Factors

A patient with a long-term urinary diversion has grown accustomed to it as a way of life. If undiversion should require temporary or permanent intermittent self-catheteriza-

tion postoperatively to empty the bladder, such as in neuropathic bladder, the patient must be fully prepared to cooperate and to do this. Failure to comply with this regimen is one of the factors that can lead to spontaneous rupture of the bladder, if augmentation cystoplasty has been performed (Elder et al, 1981; Rushton et al, 1988; Sheiner and Kaplan, 1988).

Anesthesia

Undiversion operations are long and complicated—seldom do they last less than 5 to 6 hours. The most difficult one the author has performed lasted 20 hours. The child had undergone 13 prior operations. Undiversion required repair of ureters, bladder neck, urethra, and vagina and simultaneous repositioning of a previously pulled-through rectum. Obviously, expert anesthesia management is mandatory. Constant monitoring of acid-base balance and blood gases should be in effect along with replacement of blood and fluids. These patients cannot withstand inadequate fluid replacement, which can cause renal tubular necrosis. Fluid replacement for ordinary intra-abdominal pediatric surgical operations is in the range of 5 ml/kg body weight per hour.

In the author's experience, these patients generally require four to five times that volume (i.e., 20–25 ml/kg/hour) to maintain a satisfactory urinary output intraoperatively. These amounts are reduced appropriately for older adult patients. Wide retroperitoneal dissection and exposure of the intestines create enormous fluid losses and *third spacing*.

If only parameters of blood pressure and hematocrit are followed to estimate fluid requirements, replacement falls behind. The author routinely measures urinary output intraoperatively as a guide for the anesthesiologist. Even when the urinary tract has been taken apart, by securing a catheter within each ureter while working, a timed output can be obtained for each kidney, draining the end of the catheter into a small receptacle in the operative field. This gives a good guide to speeding up or slowing down fluid administration during these long cases. Invariably the anesthesiologist who has not had experience with long and complex cases falls behind in replacement of fluid and blood. Renal shutdown from inadequate volume replacement is a preventable complication, and its importance cannot be overemphasized. Many patients with renal failure and inability to concentrate urine have an obligatory high output. Preoperatively, they are not placed on an ordinary NPO (nothing by mouth) after midnight regimen. They are maintained on intravenous fluid therapy from the time oral intake is stopped, to be adequately hydrated when entering the operating room.

Nitrous oxide should be avoided in these long cases. It diffuses into the gut and creates distention, which makes intraoperative exposure and later wound closure significantly more difficult. Nitrous oxide should be avoided not only during these cases, but also during the induction of anesthesia. The author has opened many bellies containing bowel filled with gas, which required milking the gas up to the stomach to evacuate it. This is a poor way to start a major operation. Continuous epidural analgesia has proven helpful in the last several years, reducing the amount of anesthesia required intraoperatively and providing pain relief postoperatively. This analgesia gives reduced sensation to the legs and feet. Safeguards must be taken against compression of the lower extremities by tightly fitting bandages, which can cause pressure sores. Pneumatic boots to provide venous milking of the legs intraoperatively are used in all patients in their teens or older.

Assessment of Bladder Function

Urodynamic evaluation of the lower urinary tract is an important tool in modern-day urology and can help in some cases (Bauer et al, 1980). Nevertheless, it has not been the keystone for predicting how a long defunctionalized bladder will function when urine flow is re-established. Cystography demonstrates bladder size and sensation as well as the presence of diverticula, urethral valves, and reflux into ureteral stumps. Cystoscopy can provide additional information. Usually the long-diverted bladder is small and has a smooth lining, which bleeds readily when filled with irrigating solution under pressure. It is important not to overfill the bladder, which can cause it to rupture, a complication the author has encountered on four occasions when attempting to stretch a bladder preoperatively under anesthesia.

Preoperative "bladder cycling" can help (Kogan et al, 1976; Kogan and Levitt, 1977). A small Silastic catheter is introduced during cystoscopy. The patient is taught to fill the bladder with saline to test continence, ability to empty, and stretch. Some bladder capacities increase rapidly in just a week or two from a small initial capacity of 2 or 3 ounces to a normal or near-normal capacity—others do not. The latter finding may signify the need for augmentation during undiversion. The length of time spent doing bladder cycling may vary from a few days to several months, depending on the findings, the degree of cooperation of the patient, and other factors. Optimally the patient should fill the bladder by rapid drip from a reservoir bottle about 3 to 4 feet above the level of the bladder. This is done as many times during the day as possible. The irrigating fluid is tap water to which 2 teaspoons of salt per quart are added (boiled to sterilize it and cooled before use). A few milliliters of 0.5% neomycin or other antibiotic solution is added to this solution to reduce the likelihood of contamination and infection.

Occasionally the catheter passes through the bladder neck into the urethra so that irrigation does not fill the bladder. In this instance, it can be pulled back an appropriate distance to remedy the problem. If the patient's original problem was urinary incontinence, it is of no avail to attempt cycling the bladder. Similarly, if it is a tiny scarred bladder that leaks after a few milliliters are introduced into it, cycling proves fruitless. In point of fact, the author cycles bladders today preoperatively much less often than 15 years ago. This change is in part from being more willing to augment the bladder when it is too small and in part, perhaps, from having a selectively poorer group of patients on whom to do undiversions compared with earlier patients.

When urethral valves are encountered at cystoscopy in a patient whose bladder is diverted, they can be destroyed by fulguration if bladder cycling is to commence immediately. Conversely, urethral valves should never be fulgurated in a "dry urethra" that remains dry postoperatively. In several cases, the author has seen that fulguration leads to impermeable strictures (Crooks, 1982), creating a need for an additional reconstructive operation.

SURGICAL PRINCIPLES

The bowel is cleansed thoroughly preoperatively. Clear liquids are taken by mouth for 2 days preoperatively. Gastrointestinal lavage takes place the night before using GoLYTELY. This polyethylene glycol-electrolyte gastrointestinal lavage solution is a powder that is diluted with tap water and administered orally. It passes rapidly through the gastrointestinal tract, cleaning it well. An adult patient drinks 4 L of this solution, taking one 8-ounce glass by mouth every 10 minutes until the entire 4 L is consumed. By the time the fourth or fifth glass is swallowed, the first begins passing by rectum, washing out the gastrointestinal tract effectively. A reduced amount is given to children. Pediatric patients are usually given the solution by tube because most will not voluntarily drink a large volume of fluid. It has a slightly salty taste. Rapid administration is essential for it to be effective. The author believes that a GoLYTELY bowel preparation may dehydrate the patient somewhat, an added point to bear in mind, especially in the patient with high-output renal failure as mentioned earlier. Preoperative and intraoperative broad-spectrum antibiotic administration is given in these cases.

Wide Transabdominal Exposure

Wide transabdominal exposure is essential. Although some patients have had previous urologic surgery through a transverse lower abdominal incision, a long midline incision is preferred, usually from the pubis to the xiphoid. This incision gives access to all levels of the urinary tract. A large ring retractor is desirable. To expose the kidneys and ureters, the right and left colons are mobilized and reflected medially. When the ureter is mobilized, all of its periureteral tissue should be kept with it, skeletonizing the other structures in the retroperitoneum, not the ureter (Fig. 104–3). The gonadal vessels should be maintained with the ureter for collateral blood supply. The author has done this many times without loss of a testis or an ovary. Similarly the kidney can be mobilized and moved downward and medially to facilitate obtaining sufficient length for a foreshortened ureter, whether it is to be joined to the bladder or to the contralateral renal pelvis or ureter.

Psoas Hitch

Psoas hitch is a most helpful adjunct (Fig. 104–4). It can compensate for some shortness of the ureter, which must be implanted without tension. It can also allow a super-long tunnel to be obtained, which is necessary if reflux is to be prevented when reimplanting a bowel segment or a slightly dilated and scarred ureter. Obtaining a ratio of tunnel length to ureter diameter of 5:1 may mandate having a tunnel 5 to 10 cm long. Fixation to the psoas muscle allows that. It anchors the ureteral hiatus, and when the bladder fills, no angulation and obstruction of the ureter occur. The hitch is done with monofilament nonabsorbable sutures (Prolene), taking care not to enter the bladder lumen. Note that the reimplant is performed before the bladder psoas hitch.

Transureteroureterostomy or Transureteropyelostomy

Transureteroureterostomy or transureteropyelostomy is another extremely useful adjunct in these cases (Fig. 104–5)

(Hodges et al, 1963; Hendren and Hensle, 1980). It is rarely feasible to join two ureters to the bladder in reoperative cases. Most often, the better ureter is implanted, draining the other across into it. This maneuver must be done without tension. It is important to avoid angulation of a ureter beneath a mesenteric vessel, especially the inferior mesenteric artery. When mobilizing a ureter to be swung over to the opposite side, the same principle should be employed as shown in Figure 104–3 (i.e., mobilizing it with all of its periureteral tissue and the gonadal vessels) so that its blood supply is well maintained.

The contralateral ureter to receive it is not mobilized and is not brought over to meet the end of the ureter to be drained into it. Each ureter is routinely drained by a soft, No. 5 Fr plastic catheter, passed through the abdominal wall, the sidewall of the bladder, and up the common ureter, threading one to each kidney before the anastomosis is completed. These catheters provide individual drainage of each kidney and are also useful to determine differential function. A contrast study is performed 10 to 12 days postoperatively to exclude a leak. (None has been encountered in >170 transureteroureterostomies.) The catheters are removed one at a time, a day apart.

Bladder Augmentation

Bladder augmentation is an indispensable part of the urologic armamentarium (Courvelaire, 1950; Goodwin et al, 1958, 1959; Smith et al, 1977; Turner-Warwick, 1979; Mitchell, 1981a; Kass and Koff, 1983; Linder et al, 1983; Whitmore and Gittes, 1983; Stephenson and Mundy, 1985; Goldwasser and Webster, 1986; Mitchell et al, 1986; Mitchell and Piser, 1987; Sidi et al, 1986, 1987; Churchill et al, 1993). In 82 of 216 undiversion cases, augmentation was needed. Although bladder augmentation was at one time

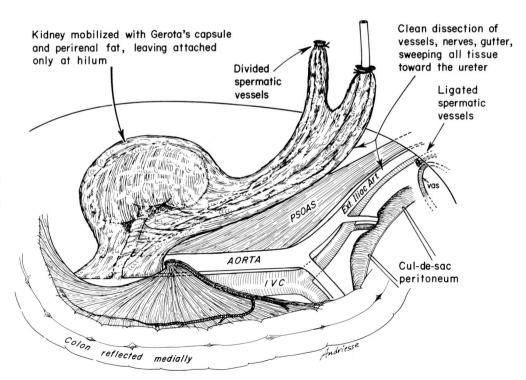

Figure 104–3. Technique for mobilizing the kidney and ureter to gain additional length by wide dissection of structures, while preserving periureteral tissue for blood supply, including gonadal vessels. IVC, inferior vena cava; vas, vas deferens.

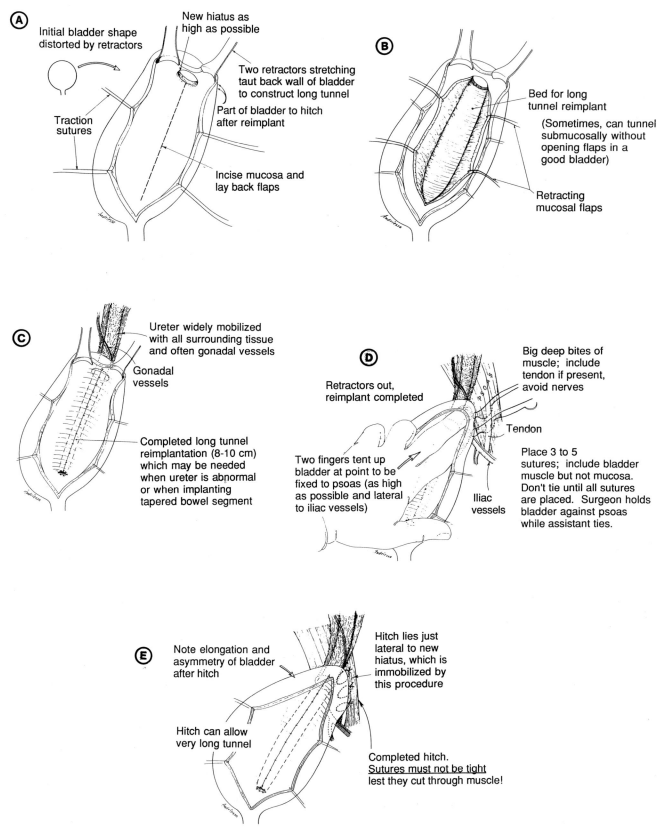

Figure 104–4. *A* to *E,* Technique for psoas hitch, which allows the creation of a long reimplantation tunnel and prevents angulation of the ureter or tapered bowel segment when the bladder fills. Monofilament nonabsorbable suture material is used to fix the bladder to psoas muscle. Care must be taken to avoid entering the bladder, which might cause stone formation on a suture.

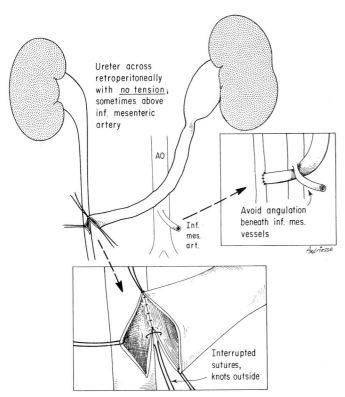

Figure 104–5. Technique for transureteroureterostomy (AO, aorta; inf. mes. art., inferior mesenteric artery).

used principally in adult patients with bladder tuberculosis, interstitial cystitis, and carcinoma, in later years it has become a mainstay of urologic reconstructive surgery in all ages. The author's experience with augmentation includes 201 cases with a wide variety of indications, but the need in all was to enlarge the capacity of the bladder (Hendren and Hendren, 1990) or make a continent catheterizable reservoir. The segments used were cecum in 73 cases, sigmoid in 40, small intestine in 43, stomach in 61, left colon in 2, and right colon in 3; 21 patients had two augmentation operations. Experience has shown that whatever segment is added to the bladder, it should be *detubularized* so that the bowel cannot exert peristaltic waves, which may exceed in amplitude the resistance of the bladder neck and cause incontinence.

In some patients, the surgeon may have a wide choice of bowel segment to use. In others, this may be restricted, such as with cloacal exstrophy, in which there is little or no colon. The small bowel may be short, making gastrocystoplasty the only reasonable choice. The stomach has some outstanding advantages as a means for augmentation (Leong, 1978; Adams et al, 1988; Kennedy et al, 1988; Sheldon et al, 1995). Stomach is metabolically better than bowel or colon regarding chloride absorption and base loss, which occur in segments of small bowel and colon. The small bowel segments tend to lose bicarbonate and potassium and to a lesser extent sodium, while reabsorbing chloride. Gastric mucosa secretes chloride ion and is, therefore, better in patients with poor renal function who cannot tolerate an increase in solute resorption, which can aggravate acidosis. Furthermore, the urine is more often sterile after gastrocystoplasty because it is less alkaline. Bladder pain and hematuria can accompany use of gastrocystoplasty. It can be treated with hydrogen ion

blockade with ranitidine or bladder washout using dilute sodium bicarbonate solution. Oral vitamin C can be helpful also. Bladder stones rarely occur in gastrocystoplasty but are common after use of colon or small intestine. If a patient with a gastric augment develops gastroenteritis with vomiting or diarrhea or both, electrolyte depletion can occur quickly because of the chloride loss through the augment. Therefore, close observation and intravenous supplementation may be needed.

In regard to ureteral drainage in patients undergoing bladder augmentations, the author prefers to place one or both ureters into the bladder if that is possible. Frequently the ureters are too short, however, or the bladder is too scarred to accomplish even one good ureteral reimplantation. Therefore, it may be necessary to implant the ureter into the augmentation. A good ureter (not too wide, not too scarred, and of adequate length) can be implanted with a tunnel in the colon, cecum, or stomach. The author prefers the technique in which the ureter is tunneled beneath the mucosa from inside the bowel (Goodwin et al, 1953). If the ureters are too short or dilated to reimplant, they can be joined to the terminal ileum of a cecal cystoplasty, making an antireflux nipple of the intussuscepted terminal ileum (Fig. 104–6). An antireflux nipple does not stand the test of time, unless it is sewn to the adjacent wall of the cecum to prevent its popping out of the cecum and allowing reflux. When there is no ureter, an inadequate terminal ileum, or a failed antireflux nipple, the technique shown in Figure 104–7 can be employed to drain the upper tracts into the cecum to prevent reflux.

When small bowel or sigmoid is chosen to augment the bladder, it is opened longitudinally, sewing the edges to one another to produce a cup-like dome to join to the bladder. A simple patch of bowel is used less often.

Although stomach provides an excellent source of tissue for increasing the size of the bladder, the author believes it is technically more difficult and hazardous because of the long vascular pedicle required to bring the middle third of the stomach down to the pelvis. In sigmoid colon, the mesentery is adjacent to the bladder. Little danger exists of compromising the vascular pedicle. Similarly the ileal mesentery or ileocecal mesentery seldom presents a problem in reaching the pelvis without tension. When stomach is to be used, the right gastroepiploic pedicle is best, although alternative techniques have been described (Leong, 1978).

The many small branches running from the right gastroepiploic artery to the greater curvature of the gastric antrum are divided in a meticulous manner. The length of this mobilization depends on the distance to which the stomach must be brought. Resecting the middle third of the stomach, while maintaining intact the lesser curvature, yields a large diamond-shaped patch with excellent blood supply. This patch is brought through the transverse mesocolon, usually to the right of the middle colic vessels. A generous tunnel is then made beneath the small bowel mesentery, emerging at the terminal ileum to bring the patch and its pedicle to the bladder. The part of stomach most distant from the pedicle is sewn to the lowest part of the bladder opening, lastly closing the upper part of the opening near the vascular pedicle. It is important to avoid tension on the vascular pedicle.

In any type of augmentation, the bladder is doubly drained, using one catheter through the urethra and the other

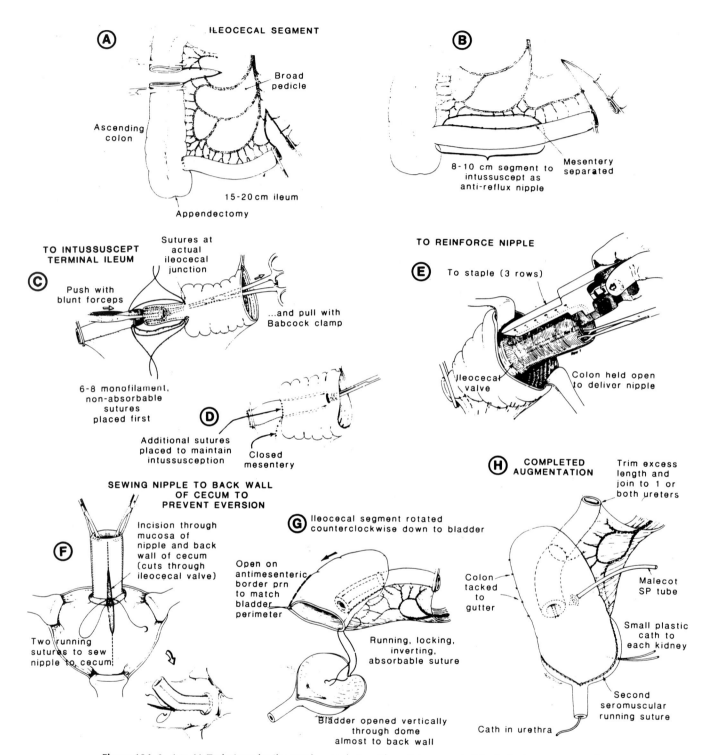

ILEOCECAL SEGMENT

(A) Broad pedicle

Ascending colon

15-20 cm ileum

Appendectomy

(B) 8-10 cm segment to intussuscept as anti-reflux nipple

Mesentery separated

TO INTUSSUSCEPT TERMINAL ILEUM

(C) Push with blunt forceps

Sutures at actual ileocecal junction

...and pull with Babcock clamp

6-8 monofilament, non-absorbable sutures placed first

(D) Additional sutures placed to maintain intussusception

Closed mesentery

TO REINFORCE NIPPLE

(E) To staple (3 rows)

Ileocecal valve

Colon held open to deliver nipple

SEWING NIPPLE TO BACK WALL OF CECUM TO PREVENT EVERSION

(F) Incision through mucosa of nipple and back wall of cecum (cuts through ileocecal valve)

Two running sutures to sew nipple to cecum

(G) Ileocecal segment rotated counterclockwise down to bladder

Open on antimesenteric border prn to match bladder perimeter

Running, locking, inverting, absorbable suture

Bladder opened vertically through dome almost to back wall

(H) **COMPLETED AUGMENTATION**

Trim excess length and join to 1 or both ureters

Colon tacked to gutter

Malecot SP tube

Small plastic cath to each kidney

Second seromuscular running suture

Cath in urethra

Figure 104–6. *A* to *H*, Technique for ileocecal cystoplasty with an intussuscepted ileal nipple to prevent reflux.

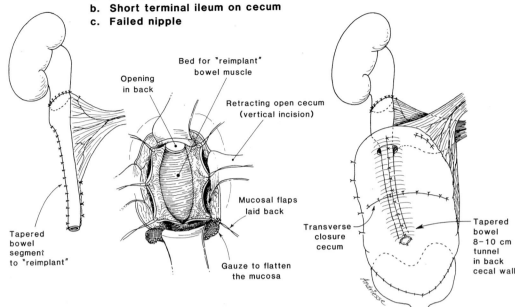

CECAL AUGMENTATION:
Preventing reflux when:
a. No ureter
b. Short terminal ileum on cecum
c. Failed nipple

Figure 104–7. "Ureter" created from a tapered small bowel.

as a suprapubic tube through the augmentation and out the abdominal wall. The suprapubic tube remains postoperatively until the patient can void or self-catheterize. It can take a great deal of time and patience to teach a patient to catheterize, especially when an extensive narrowing of the urethra and bladder neck has been performed, such as in patients with myelodysplasia or exstrophy-epispadias. Catheterization is not attempted until 2 weeks postoperatively. It often requires endoscopy under anesthesia to locate the passage and to dilate it to make catheterization possible. If the passage is not easily visualized because of postoperative edema and the presence of sutures in the reconstructed bladder outlet, a ureteral catheter is passed upward, following it with the endoscope, just as one might negotiate a urethral stricture.

Blind dilatation is not safe because it risks making a false passage. Catheterization can be done with a straight catheter, a coudé-tipped catheter, or a catheterizing sound, depending on what is simplist in a given patient. The suprapubic tube is never removed until it is evident that the bladder can be emptied by either voiding or catheterization. Emptying should be done on a regular schedule, about every 4 hours, to avoid overfilling an augmentation. In boys whose urethra will accept only small catheters, saline irrigation and syringe aspiration may be necessary. Mucus can block a small catheter. Production of mucus seems to decrease in time when colon or small bowel is used. Mucus is less of a problem when stomach augments the bladder.

A cardinal principle in reconstructing previously diverted urinary tracts is to lay out all of the anatomic structures at the operating table, listing the various options available and choosing the one that has the greatest likelihood of success. In the author's experience, failure is much more likely when the surgeon attempts to get by with a minor procedure, with the aim of avoiding a major one. Generally, most of the more extensive procedures succeed if they are well conceived

and skillfully executed. The patient cannot tolerate a major complication, such as leakage from an anastomosis under tension, ureteral obstruction, or devascularization of a part of the urinary tract.

SELECTED CASES

The following cases, and others that have been described previously, illustrate some of the technical details to be encountered in undiversion surgery (Hendren, 1973, 1974b, 1987, 1990). Because the ileal loop is the most common type of previous diversion extant, it is emphasized here. The same principles apply, however, with undiversions in patients with long-standing diversions by vesicostomy, end ureterostomy, loop ureterostomy, pyelostomy, or nephrostomy.

The principal options available in reconstruction of the urinary tract in patients with ileal loop diversions are shown in Figure 104–8. Autotransplantation is indicated only rarely. Whenever the bowel loop can be discarded, using one or both ureters to drain the upper tracts into the bladder is preferred. Often this is not possible, however.

Case 1 (Figs. 104–9 and 104–10)

An 11-year-old boy was referred in 1974 with an ileal loop done at age 3 years. His original pathologic condition was urethral valves with hydronephrosis, infection, and stones. Prior surgery included suprapubic cystostomy at age 3 months, bilateral pyelolithotomies at age 2 years, urinary diversion at age 3 years, and later a second left pyelolithotomy. The ileal loop was tapered and reimplanted with a long tunnel to prevent reflux. The patient is now 32 years old, more than 21 years after undiversion. He is well and free from urinary infection or stones. Originally a scrawny youngster, with a bag on his abdomen and chronic urinary infection, he is now a

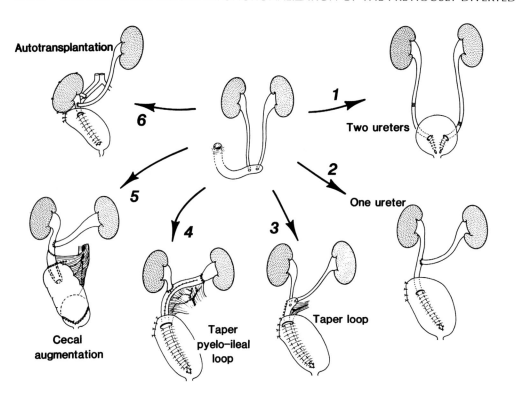

Figure 104–8. Principal options available for undiversion of an ileal loop.

robust adult (6 feet, 3.5 inches tall). Creatinine clearance is 48 L/m²/body surface area (BSA) per day (i.e., about 50% of normal).

Comment. In tapering an ileal loop that is to serve as a substitute ureter, several important points must be respected. Mobilization of the ileal loop from the abdominal wall should be done with great care because it may be necessary to use the full length of the bowel segment. In dissecting free the intra-abdominal part of the loop,

catheters through the loop and up the ureters can prove helpful. This dissection can be facilitated by gently distending the system with saline with a ligature occluding the end of the loop around the catheters. It is often necessary to incise the mesentery to straighten the loop, taking care not to devascularize the bowel.

The strip of bowel to be removed on its antimesenteric border should be marked with a skin pencil to ensure accuracy, resecting

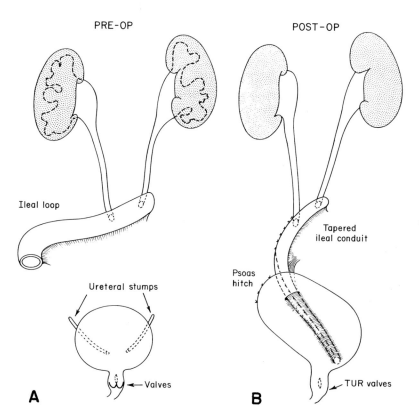

Figure 104–9. Case 1. Before *(A)* and after *(B)* reconstruction. TUR, transurethral.

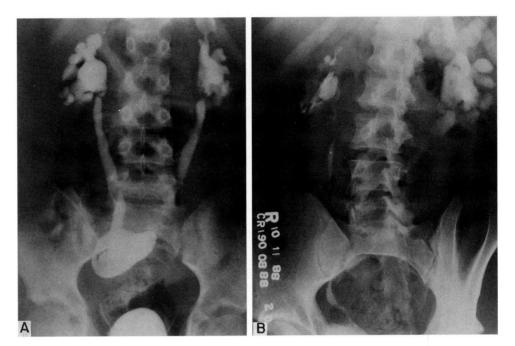

Figure 104–10. Case 1 roentgenograms. *A,* Preoperative simultaneous loopogram and cystogram. Note the small bladder and short unusable ureteral stumps. *B,* Intravenous pyelogram 14 years after undiversion. Bladder size was normal.

not more than one third of the circumference of the bowel. A two-layer inverting closure with catgut sutures requires several additional millimeters of bowel circumference. The first layer is running, inverting sutures. The second layer is interrupted sutures. It is important to create a nonrefluxing anastomosis of the tapered bowel to the bladder.

Because the bowel loop, even when tapered, is 1 to 1.5 cm in diameter, the tunnel must be long (5–10 cm). Obviously, this length is possible only in a favorable bladder of good size. It is fruitless to attempt reimplantation of a tapered small bowel segment into a small, scarred, contracted bladder. The optimal method for making a long tunnel is shown in Figure 104–4.

Mucosal flaps are dissected sharply to prepare a bed for the tapered bowel. The tapered bowel is tacked to the muscle of the back wall of the bladder, with its suture line lying posteriorly, not adjacent to the mucosa to be closed over it, to avert fistula formation. Psoas hitch is essential to immobilize the hiatus through which the tapered bowel segment enters the bladder wall. This practice prevents angulation when the bladder fills.

In tapering 29 ileal loops and reimplanting them into the bladder, 20 attempts were completely successful, as in this patient. Nine patients required reoperation because of reflux. In six patients, it was possible to make a longer tunnel, which stopped the reflux. The bladders were basically good—in which a longer tunnel could be made. Three were poor bladders, indicating that it had been an error in judgment to attempt implantation of a tapered loop in the first place. Ileocecal cystoplasty solved the problem in these small, noncompliant bladders. Avoiding the pitfalls learned from experience, which have been mentioned previously, should lead to a high success rate when implanting a tapered bowel segment is necessary.

Patients with intestine in the urinary tract notice mucus in their urine. Occasionally a blob of mucus temporarily obstructs the urethra in a male during micturition. The amount of mucus and the patient's awareness of it seem to diminish in time. Late stricture is a well-known complication of ileal loop urinary diversions. Late stricture of a tapered bowel segment has been noted in three cases as well as in two other cases that were referred, with untapered bowel serving as ureter (Hendren and McLorie, 1983). This problem underscores the need to maintain long-term, continuing surveillance of all patients with bowel in the urinary tract, especially when it has been used as a substitute ureter. When bowel has been used as a ureter, a straight endoscope is easily introduced from

below. In two cases in which narrowing occurred later from a mucosal web, it was incised with a cutting electrode, dilated, and injected with triamcinolone diacetate to help prevent future scar formation. This late stricture phenomenon may result from lymphocyte depletion of the bowel wall that is bathed by urine.

Case 2 (Figs. 104–11 and 104–12)

A 15-year-old boy with the prune-belly syndrome was referred in 1973 for possible undiversion. Bilateral nephrostomies had been done at birth. Later an ileal loop was done, but it had never drained. The left ureter was obstructed by the left colic artery; the right kidney was blocked by ureteropelvic junction obstruction. An extensive reconstruction was performed, converting the conduit to a pyeloileal conduit to correct obstruction of both ureters. The conduit was then tapered and implanted with a long tunnel to prevent reflux. Creatinine clearance at that time was 30 L/m^2/BSA. The patient's clinical status was excellent during the next 9 years.

At age 25 years, after treatment of a duodenal ulcer with cimetidine, the serum creatinine rose to 12 mg/dl. Dialysis was begun, and he received a kidney transplant from his brother. Now, at age 37 years, and 12 years after transplantation, the patient is in good general health and works full-time as a stockbroker.

Comment. There were 14 patients with pyeloileal conduits among the 74 patients with ileal loops for undiversion. It is well recognized that patients with pyeloileal loops have the greatest degree of long-term deterioration when the loop drains into a bag on the abdominal wall. Thus, these patients in particular can benefit from eliminating the bags and diverting the drainage into the bladder, provided that it is done in a manner that averts reflux. Bladder cycling was not used in 1975, but the bladder, which had been defunctional since birth, increased in size and functioned well nevertheless. Nephritis is a rare complication of cimetidine therapy. Evidently, this tipped a precarious balance with his renal function, which had been stable for several years. Considering the bad state of his kidneys at birth, this patient represents a striking example of how careful metabolic management by an excellent nephrologist prevented the need for renal transplantation until age 25 years.

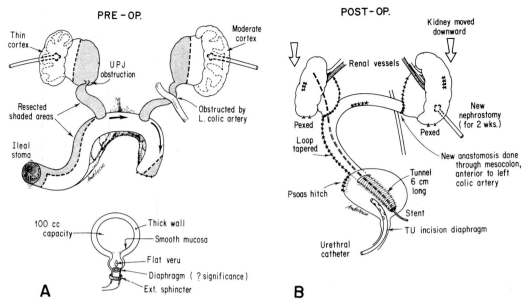

Figure 104–11. Case 2. Before *(A)* and after *(B)* reconstruction. UPJ, ureteropelvic junction; TU, transurethral.

Case 3 (Figs. 104–13 and 104–14)

A 16-year-old boy was referred in 1982 with an ileal loop performed 8 years previously, after failed ureteral reimplantation surgery elsewhere two times. Hydrostatic stretching preoperatively increased the bladder size from about 50 to 250 ml. The boy was able to retain saline instilled into the bladder, and he could void it at will. At operation, both previously reimplanted lower ureters were too short to be useful. The strictured ileal loop also was unusable. Because the two kidneys and upper ureters were nearly normal, and this was a favorable bladder in which reimplantation of a ureter would be relatively simple, autotransplantation of the right kidney was done, draining the left kidney by transureteropyelostomy. The patient convalesced uneventfully after this lengthy operation. He is now age 29 years, works full-time as a mechanic, has a child, and is free from urologic problems.

Comment. Autotransplantation is an operation that can be con-

sidered in selected cases. The author has considered it the best choice in only two patients to date. Both had strictured ileal loops, raising the possibility that a bowel segment to be employed as a ureter might become strictured. Both had two good kidneys, lending a margin of safety in case the transplanted kidney should sustain a serious complication, although that is a low risk. It is vital to consider all possible methods in each case. Generally the best choice becomes clear when all factors are taken into account: renal function, length of the ureters, state of the bladder, and so on.

Case 4 (Figs. 104–15 and 104–16)

A 15-year-old girl was referred in 1982 with an ileal loop that had been present for 10 years. The underlying problem was a neurogenic bladder secondary to sacral agenesis. Y-V-plasty had been performed to the bladder neck at age 2 years for inability to

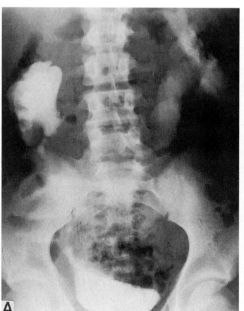

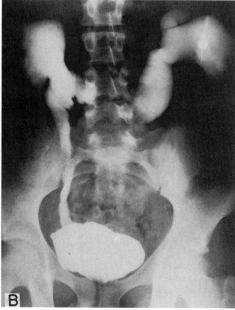

Figure 104–12. Case 2. Antegrade perfusion pyelography 8 years postoperatively. *A,* Bladder on drainage. *B,* Bladder being allowed to fill during the study. Note the needle in the left kidney.

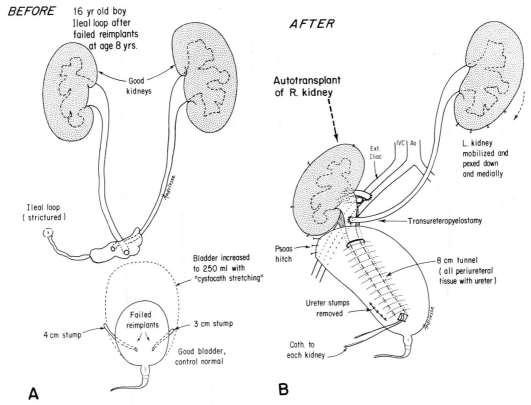

Figure 104–13. Case 3. Before *(A)* and after *(B)* reconstruction.

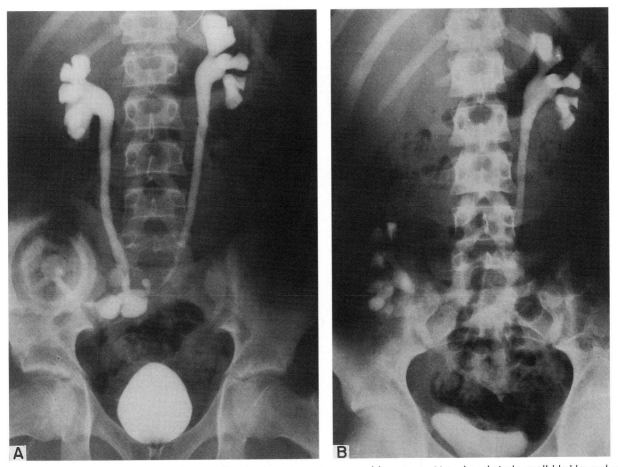

Figure 104–14. Case 3 roentgenograms. *A,* Preoperative simultaneous cystogram and loopogram. Note the relatively small bladder and severely strictured ileal loop. *B,* Intravenous pyelogram 1 year postoperatively. Note the autotransplanted right kidney in the right lower quadrant.

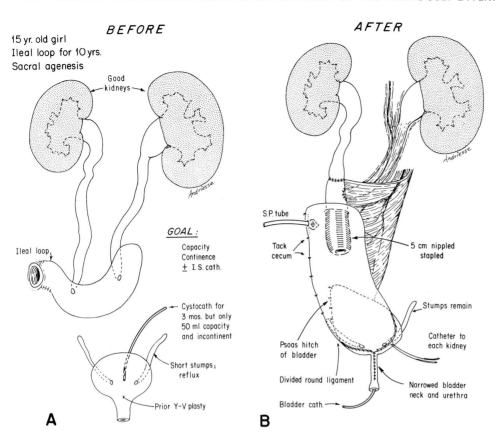

BEFORE

15 yr. old girl
Ileal loop for 10 yrs.
Sacral agenesis

Good kidneys

Ileal loop

GOAL:

Capacity
Continence
± I.S. cath.

Cystocath for
3 mos. but only
50 ml capacity
and incontinent

Short stumps;
reflux

Prior Y-V plasty

A

AFTER

S.P. tube

Tack cecum

5 cm nippled stapled

Psoas hitch
of bladder

Stumps remain

Catheter to
each kidney

Divided round ligament

Narrowed bladder
neck and urethra

Bladder cath.

B

Figure 104–15. Case 4. Before *(A)* and after *(B)* reconstruction.

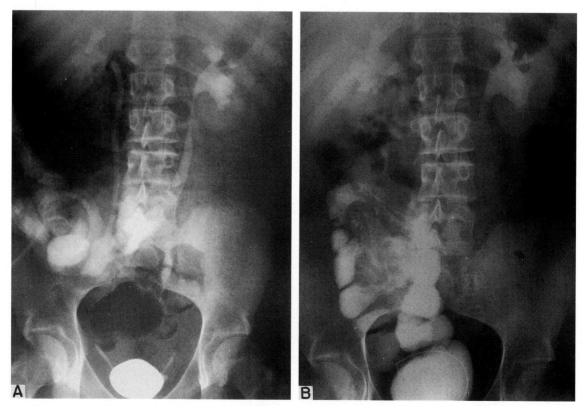

A

B

Figure 104–16. Case 4 roentgenograms. *A*, Simultaneous loopogram and cystogram preoperatively. Note the small bladder and sacral agenesis. *B*, Intravenous pyelogram 9 months postoperatively. Note the cecal augmentation of the small bladder and the filling defect in the cecum, which is intussuscepted terminal ileum. Note the staples in the nipple.

empty the bladder. Ileal loop was elected later because she was incontinent. Hydrostatic "cycling" of the bladder showed that there was a small capacity and complete incontinence. It could be predicted, therefore, that undiversion would require increasing outlet resistance as well as augmenting the bladder to provide a low-pressure reservoir of good size.

The patient's neurologic deficit showed that she must be prepared to do intermittent self-catheterization. Undiversion consisted of narrowing the bladder neck and urethra to increase outlet resistance and augmenting the bladder with cecum. The ureters were not satisfactory for reimplantation into the bladder or into the cecal wall. An antireflux mechanism was constructed by intussuscepting the terminal ileum to make a nipple, stapling the nipple, and sewing it to the back wall of the cecum. The right ureter was joined end-to-end and the left ureter end-to-side into the terminal ileum.

Postoperative urodynamic study showed urethral resistance of 85 cm H$_2$O, with a functional urethral length of 3.5 cm. The bladder capacity was 400 ml. The cecum did not exhibit uninhibited contraction waves. Now age 28 years, she has done well during the 14 years since undiversion. She empties the bladder without difficulty by self-catheterization, using a metal hollow sound. She is dry and free from urinary infection, and her kidneys have remained stable.

Comment. If an ileocecal nipple is made for prevention of reflux, it must be sewn to the back wall of the cecum or the nipple will pop out of the cecum and allow reflux (Friedman et al, 1992). A report has been made in which ileocecal augmentation was performed in a patient with myelodysplasia, which resulted in diarrhea and required putting the ileocecal valve back into the gastrointestinal tract (Gonzalez et al, 1986). Many patients with spina bifida and neurogenic bladder have alternating constipation and overflow diarrhea. Therefore, it may be better to retain the ileocecal valve in that group of patients if another method of augmentation and reflux prevention can be done. Loss of the ileocecal valve alters bile salt resorption in the terminal ileum, which can cause diarrhea from excessive bile in the colon. Oral

cholestyramine, which binds bile salts, can be helpful for these patients.

The author has found staples more reliable than simple sutures in approximating the walls of an intussuscepted nipple. Whenever staples are used, endoscopy should be performed several months later. Most become covered by mucosa. If some are still exposed, stones form on them. They can be plucked out easily using alligator forceps, through a panendoscope. If they are not removed, the stones can become large and difficult to remove. In the author's opinion, staples should never be used in the urinary tract in a location that is not easily accessible with a straight endoscope and an alligator forceps.

Artificial sphincters are used today in some medical centers to create continence in patients with these problems (Scott et al, 1974; Mitchell and Rink, 1983; Light and Engelmann, 1985; Gonzalez et al, 1989; Bosco et al, 1991). In the author's opinion, however, increasing outlet resistance and resorting to intermittent catheterization may prove safer and more satisfactory in the long-term for most patients. There is still a substantial long-term failure rate with prosthetic devices. Narrowing the bladder neck does not "burn any bridges." If sphincter technology advances in the future to a point at which there is no failure from erosion or mechanical malfunction, it would be relatively simple to open the previously narrowed bladder neck by endoscopic resection, creating incontinence, and subsequently implanting an artificial sphincter to control it.

Case 5 (Figs. 104–17 and 104–18)

A 3-year-old boy was referred in 1977 with bilateral loop cutaneous ureterostomies, suprapubic cystostomy, and complete stricture of the membranous urethra. Imperforate anus had been treated by colostomy when he was a newborn. Subsequent urinary tract evaluation at 6 months disclosed urethral valves and hydronephrosis. Cutaneous vesicostomy was performed, but the bladder pro-

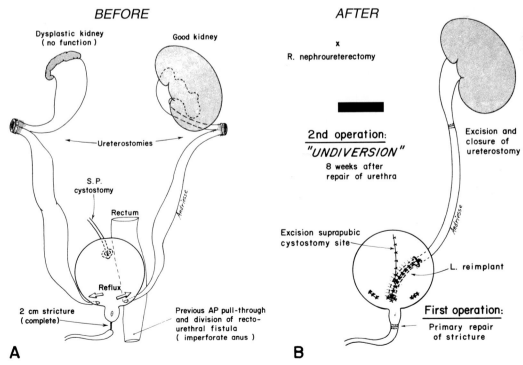

Figure 104–17. Case 5. Before *(A)* and after *(B)* reconstruction.

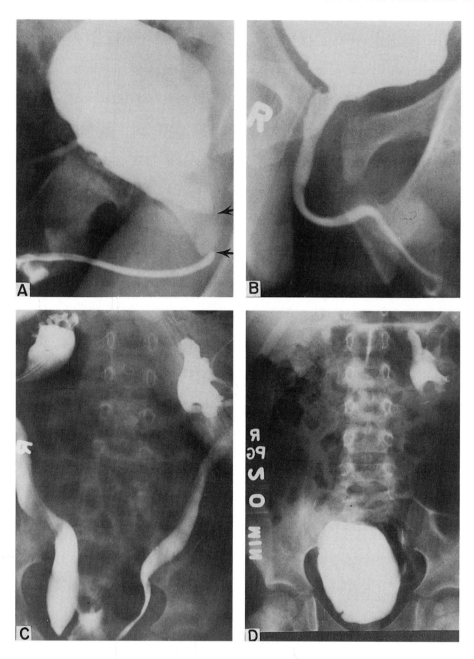

Figure 104–18. Case 5 roentgenograms. A, Preoperative cystourethrogram showing long stricture (arrows). B, Cystourethrogram after repair of stricture by excision and anastomosis. C, Preoperative ureterograms via the bilateral cutaneous loop ureterostomies; the right kidney was nonfunctional. D, Intravenous pyelogram 1 year after undiversion. Note the normal bladder and normal left ureter.

lapsed, causing increasing hydronephrosis. Bilateral skin ureterostomies were performed. Later the valves were resected, and a rectal pull-through was done. The vesicostomy was closed and converted into a suprapubic cystostomy. Pyocystis was treated by antibiotic irrigation. Ileal loop urinary diversion was recommended but was declined by the parents, who then sought further advice.

Hydrostatic testing of the bladder showed good function despite previous diversion and pyocystis. At the first operation, the urethral stricture was resected and continuity was re-established by primary anastomosis. Undiversion was accomplished 8 weeks later. This included removing the nonfunctional right kidney, closing the left ureterostomy, reimplanting the left ureter, and excising the suprapubic cystostomy site. Today, 18 years later, the patient is age 22 years, is 6 feet, 1 inch tall, and weighs 190 pounds. He has normal urinary control and normal bowel control. Recent blood chemical values disclosed blood urea nitrogen (BUN), 13 mg/dl; creatinine, 1.5 mg/dl; and creatinine clearance, 60 L/m²/BSA, which is about 60% of normal. This clinical picture likely bodes well for the future because he has already attained full adult growth.

Comment. This case illustrates several points. First, cutaneous vesicostomy was a simple procedure to perform, but it set the stage for a series of major complications. It failed to drain the bladder adequately because of prolapse, following which ureterostomies were performed. It would have been better to resect the valves in the first place, probably followed by left ureteral reimplantation and right nephroureterectomy. Second, it is probable that complete stricture of the membranous urethra was caused by endoscopic resection of valves when there was a "dry urethra" (i.e., supravesical diversion of the urine).

Rectal pull-through with division of the rectourethral fistula may also have contributed to that complication, however. Ileal loop diversion was suggested elsewhere as being the best alternative, "since reconstruction would be difficult and might be fraught with some uncertainties."

In the author's experience, however, worse results come from a lesser procedure, as compared with a major reconstructive procedure that is well planned and skillfully performed. In performing reconstructive surgery in the patient who has undergone loop ureterostomy, the author has found that it is best to do the entire reconstruction at one procedure—repair the obstructive problem and close the ureterostomies simultaneously (Hendren, 1978b).

Case 6 (Figs. 104–19 and 104–20)

A 17-year-old girl was referred in 1987 for urinary tract reconstruction. During infancy, she had closure of a meningocele and ventricular peritoneal shunt for hydrocephalus. At age 2 years, an ileal loop was performed for urinary incontinence of the myelodysplastic bladder. During the next 15 years, there were many episodes of infection. Progressive dilatation of the upper tract and multiple strictures of the ileal loop were noted. Bladder cycling was not performed because the bladder was completely incontinent when filled with saline.

At operation, the urethra was lengthened and narrowed to increase outlet resistance. It was possible to reimplant the left ureter, with a psoas hitch, draining the right ureter by transureteroureterostomy. A 30-cm-long segment of sigmoid colon was detubularized and reconfigured to augment the bladder. She tolerated this 16-hour operation well. Now 8 years later and age 25, the patient is well and free from urinary infection, being maintained on prophylactic medication. Unexpectedly, she is able to void by abdominal effort and Credé's maneuver, which she does every 3 to 4 hours to empty the bladder. She has been instructed, however, to catheterize at least twice daily in the morning and evening to make certain that the bladder is being emptied completely. Urodynamic study postoperatively showed the bladder capacity to be 550 ml with little rise in pressure during filling. At capacity, there were contrac-

tion waves from 10 to 30 cm H_2O, but they caused no leakage. Resistance at the repaired bladder neck measured 60 cm H_2O.

Comment. This patient was an ideal candidate for undiversion, being an intelligent and highly motivated teenager who was anxious to get rid of the bag on her abdomen and end the recurrent episodes of infection. She and one other female are the only ones of the 21 neurogenic bladder cases in this series who have been able to void most of the urine without self-catheterization. It is, nevertheless, important to check the residual at least twice daily, to avert overdistention and possible spontaneous perforation of the bowel segment in a patient with myelodysplasia and diminished sensation. Urinary diversion was a common operation for this type of patient in the past. There are, therefore, many like this patient who could undergo undiversion today. Her long-term outlook will be greatly improved not only from the standpoint of stopping recurrent infection from reflux, but also from the standpoint of her greatly improved social status. The upper urinary tract is now much more delicate in appearance than it was originally with hydronephrosis (see Fig. 104–20).

Case 7 (Fig. 104–21)

A 19-year-old man was referred in 1986 for urologic reconstruction. Urinary infection had occurred, and study showed a large bladder with massive reflux. At age 9 years, ureteral reimplantation and 50% cystectomy were performed. He continued to have severe infection with deteriorating upper tracts, and so ileal loop was performed at age 14 years.

Magnetic resonance imaging of the lumbosacral spine was performed to rule out a spinal cord malformation because the etiology

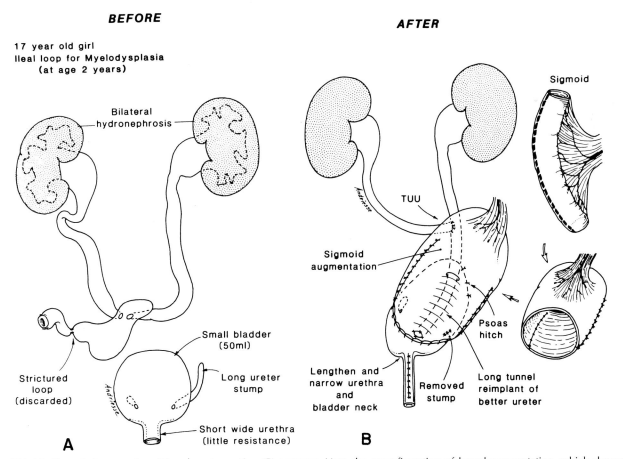

Figure 104–19. Case 6. Preoperative *(A)* and postoperative *(B)* anatomy. Note the reconfiguration of bowel augmentation, which dampens its peristalsis and increases its volume. TUU, transureteroureterostomy.

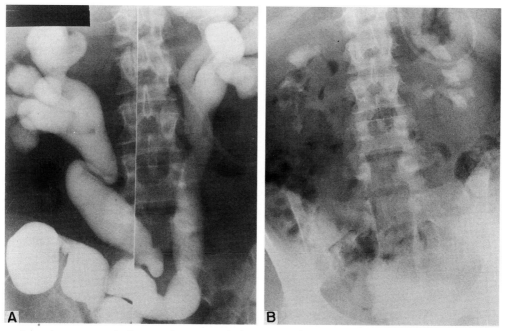

Figure 104–20. Case 6 roentgenograms. *A*, Preoperative retrograde loopogram showing multiple strictures of ileal loop, massive reflux, and hydronephrosis. The patient had long-term recurring urinary infections. *B*, Postoperative intravenous pyelogram that showed relatively delicate upper tracts that are draining well into the bladder augmented with sigmoid. Cystogram showed no reflux. Unexpectedly, this patient does not require intermittent catheterization to empty the bladder.

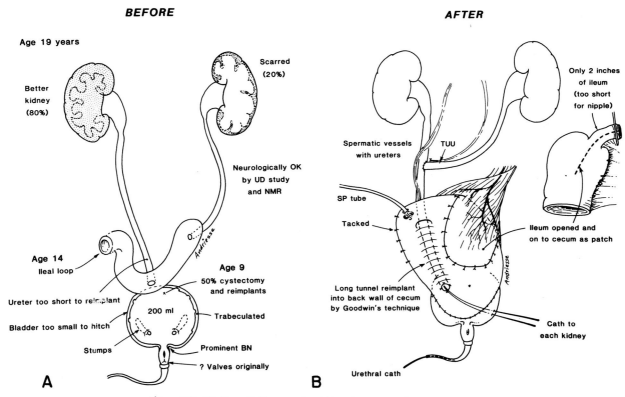

Figure 104–21. Case 7. Preoperative *(A)* and postoperative *(B)* anatomy.

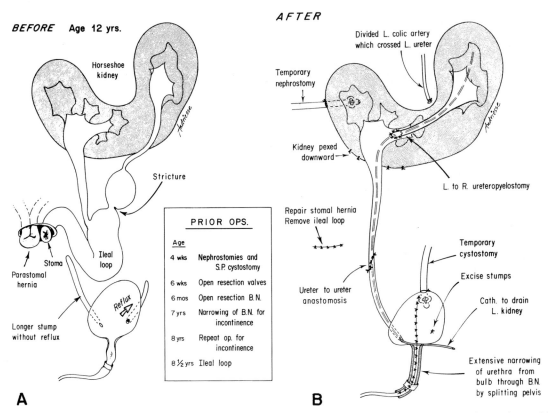

Figure 104-22. Case 8. Preoperative *(A)* and postoperative *(B)* anatomy. The symphysis pubis was split to narrow the urethra and bladder neck.

of his bladder problem was not clear. The study results were normal. Bladder cycling was not attempted because much of the bladder had been surgically removed. The bladder was augmented with cecum. The right ureter was implanted, employing a submucosal tunnel in the back wall of the cecum. The terminal ileum was too short to make a nipple to prevent reflux, but that did not matter because the right ureter was satisfactory for a tunneled reimplantation, which is the preferred method. The terminal ileum was opened and placed on the anterior wall of the cecum to render it incapable of producing strong peristaltic waves. Transureteroureterostomy was performed.

The patient's preoperative urodynamic study showed normal urethral sphincter function. As expected, he proved able to empty the bladder without difficulty postoperatively and is clinically well. BUN measures 20 mg/dl, and the serum creatinine level 1.3 mg/dl (normal is 0.5–0.8 mg/dl). Creatinine clearance measures 54 $L/m^2/$ BSA. The patient's postoperative status has been good except for one episode of epididymitis and traumatic small bowel perforation in an industrial accident.

Comment. Early detection of urinary infection and technically successful ureteral reimplantation would have almost certainly prevented the severe scarring with which this patient presented, in which little function remained in the left kidney. Enlargement of the bladder is common with massive reflux. That enlargement would probably have disappeared with technically successful antireflux surgery. Thus, partial cystectomy was probably not necessary at age 9 years, and it made necessary augmentation of the bladder as part of the reconstructive surgery.

Case 8 (Figs. 104–22 and 104–23)

A 12-year-old boy was referred in 1975 with a strictured ileal loop and a parastomal hernia. Previous surgery had included neph-

rostomies and suprapubic cystostomy at age 1 month, resection of urethral valves at age 6 weeks, resection of the bladder neck at age 6 months, two operations for urinary incontinence, and an ileal loop at age 8.5 years. There was a good right ureteral stump without reflux. The right ureter of his horseshoe kidney was joined to it, and the left side of the horseshoe was drained by left-to-right ureteropyelostomy.

By splitting the pubic symphysis for exposure, the urethra and bladder neck were narrowed extensively to provide more outlet resistance. The bladder increased gradually in size. Urinary wetting occurred initially, but it disappeared during the next 2 years. Now 20 years later and age 32, the patient works full-time and is in good general health. He has psychologic problems, however, secondary to multiple hospitalizations as a young child.

Comment. Endoscopic resection of the urethral valves during infancy would have likely sufficed in this patient who first had tube diversion and then open resection of valves, which left him incontinent, followed by failed surgery for incontinence, and finally an ileal loop for permanent urinary diversion. Modern fiberoptic infant panendoscopes have greatly changed the treatment of urethral valves during infancy. The author has found that splitting the symphysis pubis has proved key in achieving urinary continence in some patients who require narrowing of the urethra and bladder neck to increase outlet resistance (Peters and Hendren, 1990). A high-pressure, small-volume, noncompliant "valve bladder" develops in some boys with urethral valves. Augmentation is needed to prevent back pressure on their upper tracts.

Case 9 (Figs. 104–24, 104–25, 104–26, and 104–27)

A 9-year-old boy was referred in 1976 with a strictured ileal loop and hydronephrosis and a small, scarred bladder following

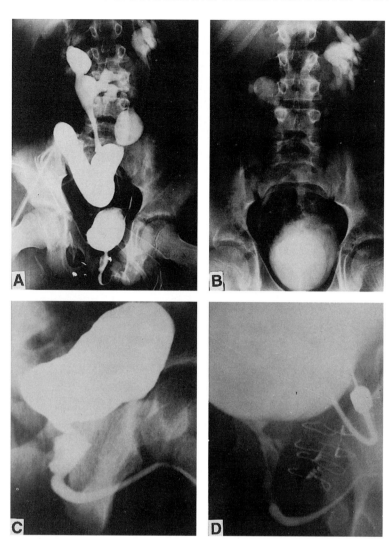

Figure 104–23. Case 8 roentgenograms. *A,* Preoperative loopogram and cystogram. *B,* Postoperative intravenous pyelogram. It has remained stable for 20 years. *C,* Preoperative cystogram of defunctionalized bladder. Note the wide prostatic urethra, despite two previous attempts to narrow bladder outlet. *D,* Postoperative cystogram (note the needle in the bladder) showing a narrowed prostatic urethra and a higher bladder neck. The patient is now continent. Splitting the symphysis pubis was key in this repair.

chemotherapy and radiation therapy for sarcoma of the prostate 4 years earlier. A nonrefluxing colon conduit was constructed because this is far better than the ileal loop that allows reflux (Kelalis, 1974; Hendren, 1975; Richie and Skinner, 1975; Skinner et al, 1975; Althausen et al, 1982). The bladder was extremely fibrotic, and so it was decided to defer undiversion. Meanwhile, drainage was converted to a nonrefluxing colon conduit (see Fig. 104–24). Five years later, total obstruction of the membranous urethra and secondary pyocystis developed. The stricture was repaired (see Fig. 104–25). The bladder was still small, but the bladder neck was no longer densely fibrotic as it had been 5 years earlier. After the stricture repair, the patient could hold saline instilled into the bladder.

Undiversion was performed by adding the cecum to the bladder and joining the nonrefluxing colon conduit to it (see Fig. 104–26). The patient voided by abdominal straining and he was continent. His upper tracts remained stable. At age 27, a large bladder stone developed. Its transvesical removal would have been simple. A transurethral lithotripsy procedure was attempted elsewhere, however, proving to be traumatic and creating a severe restricturing of the urethra, which had been satisfactory for 11 years. At age 28, he developed Hodgkin's disease. When treatment for that is completed, another stricture repair will be performed. Meanwhile the bladder is drained by vesicostomy.

Comment. This patient is one of 17 patients who had a nonrefluxing colon conduit made with the plan to consider undiversion later. He demonstrates how radiation therapy and chemotherapy

can cure some genitourinary rhabdomyosarcomas but result in a badly scarred urinary tract, which requires major reconstructive surgery. He was continent despite stricture resection at the site of the membranous urethra because the bladder neck is intact. The finding of a bladder stone a decade later illustrates that these patients can never be discharged from medical supervision. A simple open cystolithotomy would have been a far superior way to deal with the bladder stone than a long, traumatic endoscopic procedure through a previously radiated and repaired urethra.

Case 10 (Figs. 104–28, 104–29, and 104–30)

A 3-year-old girl was referred in 1988 for reconstructive surgery. Born with severe bilateral obstructive megaureters and hydronephrosis, bilateral end ureterostomies had been performed at age 1 month. The ureterostomies did not drain well. Therefore, bilateral loop cutaneous ureterostomies were performed at age 1 year. Hydronephrosis improved. The ureterostomies were later closed, but severe hydronephrosis recurred.

Preoperative assessment showed the bladder volume to be only 10 ml. When contrast material was introduced through the end ureterostomy stomas, the ureters drained well, but contrast material remained in the kidneys, indicating functional ureteropelvic junction obstruction on both sides. At operation, the better ureter was reimplanted with as long a tunnel as possible in her tiny bladder, together with psoas hitch. Transureteroureterostomy

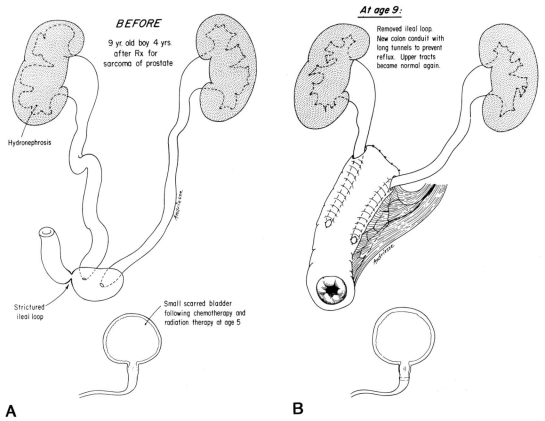

BEFORE

9 yr. old boy 4 yrs.
after Rx for
sarcoma of prostate

Hydronephrosis

Strictured
ileal loop

Small scarred bladder
following chemotherapy and
radiation therapy at age 5

At age 9:

Removed ileal loop.
New colon conduit with
long tunnels to prevent
reflux. Upper tracts
became normal again.

A

B

Figure 104–24. Case 9. Preoperative anatomy *(A)* and anatomy following nonrefluxing colon conduit *(B)*. Upper tracts then showed dramatic improvement on follow-up roentgenogram.

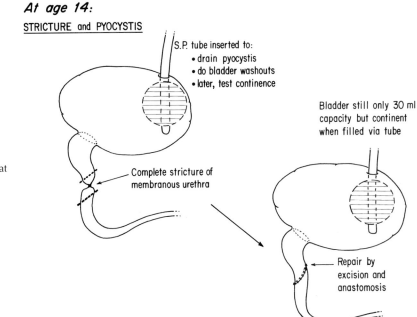

At age 14:

STRICTURE and PYOCYSTIS

S.P. tube inserted to:
• drain pyocystis
• do bladder washouts
• later, test continence

Bladder still only 30 ml
capacity but continent
when filled via tube

Complete stricture of
membranous urethra

Repair by
excision and
anastomosis

Figure 104–25. Case 9. Urethral stricture and its repair at age 14 years, when pyocystis developed.

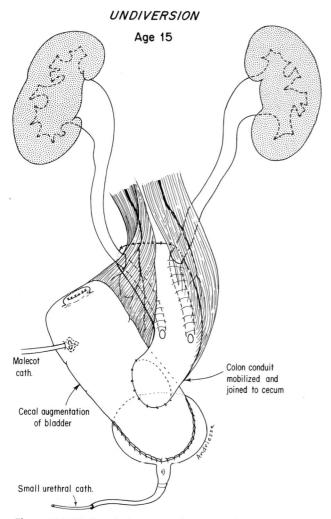

UNDIVERSION

Age 15

Malecot cath.

Cecal augmentation of bladder

Small urethral cath.

Colon conduit mobilized and joined to cecum

Figure 104–26. Case 9. Anatomy using composite augmentations.

drained the opposite ureter. Both upper ureters were obstructed from angulation at the site of the ureterostomy closures. Therefore, bilateral dismembered pyeloplasties were performed, maintaining ureteral blood supply in the surrounding periureteral tissues.

The bladder was augmented with stomach, based on the right gastroepiploic artery. The patient tolerated this 13-hour operation well. Bladder emptying was performed initially by intermittent catheterization by her mother. The child gradually learned to void to completion, and catheterization was stopped.

Postoperative evaluation showed reflux. Subureteric injection of Teflon paste beneath the ureteral orifice stopped the reflux (O'Donnell and Puri, 1980; Puri and O'Donnell, 1987). Now 7 years later and age 10, the patient voids normally, is dry, and is free from urinary infection.

Blood chemical values are remarkably normal considering the degree of hydronephrosis originally present: BUN, 10 mg/dl; serum creatinine, 0.3 mg/dl; and creatinine clearance, 121 L/m²/BSA. Postoperative urodynamic study showed bladder capacity to be 275 ml, with no uninhibited contractions, and normal sphincter function.

Comment. The stomach for bladder augmentation has some outstanding advantages over small bowel and colon. It is metabolically superior regarding chloride absorption and base loss that are seen with segments of small bowel and especially colon. Those segments tend to lose bicarbonate and potassium and, to a lesser extent, sodium while resorbing chloride.

If potassium loss is replaced as potassium chloride, bicarbonate

loss can be accelerated, aggravating acidosis. In comparison, gastric mucosa secretes chloride ion and is, therefore, preferred in patients with poor renal function who cannot tolerate increased solute resorption and resulting acidosis.

The urine is more often sterile after operation because it is not so alkaline in pH. Ureters can be tunneled and implanted without difficulty into gastric wall. Stomach is durable, yet quite compliant.

The stomach may be the only reasonable means for reconstructing certain cases of cloacal exstrophy, with little or no colon and possibly a short small bowel. The stomach's metabolic superiority probably makes it the augmentation of choice in patients with poor renal function. These patients do not have excess mucus in the urine, which is an added advantage because mucus provides a nidus for stones. Because gastrocystoplasty has been used only recently in children, as compared with intestine and colon, long-term observations are needed. Cutaneous ureterostomy was a common type of temporary diversion in infants several years ago. It can cause many complications, however, as shown in this case.

Case 11 (Fig. 104–31)

A 16-year-old girl was referred in 1995 with an ileal loop and the hope of getting rid of the external appliance. Cystostomy had been performed for rhabdomyosarcoma of the bladder at age 1 year. Right renal function was poor, although loopogram showed reflux and no obstruction. Left renal function was good, although there was mild left obstruction. There was midvaginal stenosis.

The patient preferred a catheterizable stoma in the lower abdomen and not at the site of her former urethra. Therefore, a continent diversion was performed as shown in Figure 104–31. The patient is dry and catheterizes easily.

Comment. Although reconstruction with no stoma is the ultimate goal, there are some patients such as this and such as wheelchair-bound myelodysplasia patients for whom a catheterizable stoma on the abdomen of appendix or tapered bowel is a good alternative. Ten of the 216 patients in this series, all within the last 5 years, underwent this type of undiversion to discard a bag appliance on the abdominal wall.

RESULTS AND COMPLICATIONS

No early postoperative deaths occurred, indicating that these global reconstructions can be performed with safety if meticulous attention is paid to avoid ureteral obstruction, anastomotic leakage, and so on. Nine late deaths (1–14 years after operation) were recorded, the causes for which were trauma (two), septicemia during hemodialysis (one), massive stroke (one), varicella infection after renal transplantation (one), acute leukemia (one), anaphylactic reaction during intravenous pyelogram examination (one), failure to take prescribed immunosuppressive drugs (one), and heart attack at age 26 years in a young woman undiverted 9 years previously (one). She had surgery for coarctation of the aorta as a child.

Renal transplantation was performed, to date, in 29 patients. These included three patients who had undergone transplantation before undiversion and one patient who was anephric at the time of bladder reconstruction. Approximately 43 more of the 216 patients will probably require renal transplantation within the coming decade, judging from their original and current renal function values. Renal function did not fail in any patient soon after undiversion from an obstruction or other complication. In most patients, the

Figure 104–27. Case 9 roentgenograms. *A,* Preoperative loopogram. Note the severe ileal loop stricture and dilated upper tracts. The patient was having recurrent urinary infections. *B,* Postoperative intravenous pyelogram showing excellent upper tracts, which have remained stable.

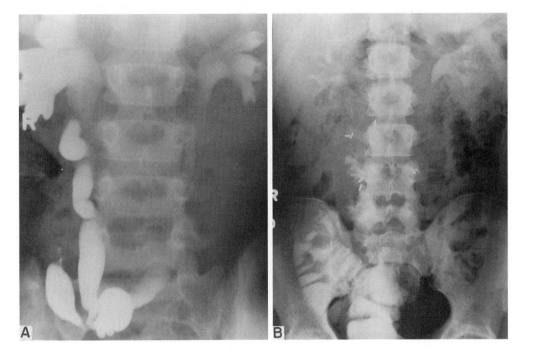

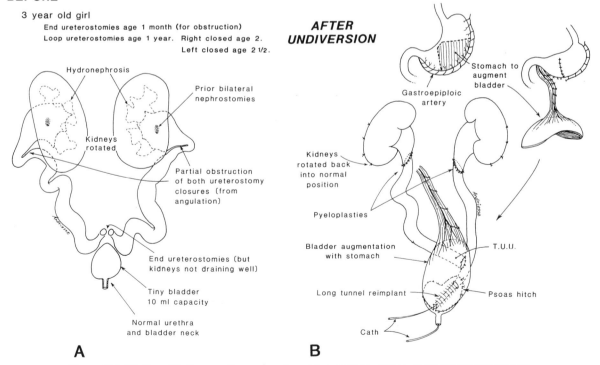

BEFORE

3 year old girl

End ureterostomies age 1 month (for obstruction)
Loop ureterostomies age 1 year. Right closed age 2.
Left closed age 2 1/2.

AFTER UNDIVERSION

Hydronephrosis

Prior bilateral nephrostomies

Kidneys rotated

Partial obstruction of both ureterostomy closures (from angulation)

End ureterostomies (but kidneys not draining well)

Tiny bladder 10 ml capacity

Normal urethra and bladder neck

Stomach to augment bladder

Gastroepiploic artery

Kidneys rotated back into normal position

Pyeloplasties

Bladder augmentation with stomach

Long tunnel reimplant

Cath

T.U.U.

Psoas hitch

A

B

Figure 104–28. Case 10. Preoperative and postoperative anatomy. T.U.U., transureteroureterostomy.

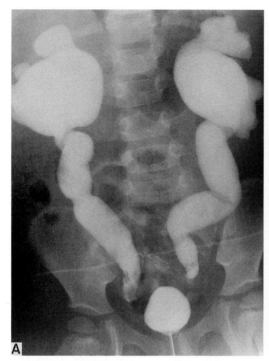

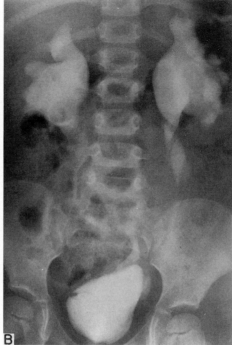

Figure 104–29. Case 10 roentgenograms. *A,* Preoperative simultaneous retrograde ureterograms and cystogram. The ureters emptied quickly, but contrast material remained in the renal pelvis on both sides, each being partially obstructed from angulation at closure of former ureterostomies. Note the small bladder. *B,* Intravenous pyelography 1 year later. The upper tracts are draining well, with less hydronephrosis.

expected decline in creatinine clearance, which occurs with growth and increase in body weight, resulted in relative renal insufficiency. For example, the author's third undiversion patient was reconstructed at age 6 years in 1969. Creatinine clearance was then only 24 L/m^2/BSA, about 20% of normal. Renal transplantation was performed 20 years later at age 26 years in 1989.

Some 23 patients required reoperation for persisting reflux. Sites of reflux included the ureter (nine), bowel ureter (six), and an ileocecal nipple (eight). Longer tunnels were made for the ureters. Longer tunnels were made in three of the bowel ureters, and three were converted to ileocecal conduits. The nipples were revised by sewing them to the cecal wall or substituting a tapered and tunneled bowel segment. Two patients had perforations of bladder augmentations, one from a karate kick and the other from a spontaneous event. This is a known risk of bladder augmentation. Both perforations were successfully closed surgically.

Ten patients required reoperation for partial obstruction. The partial obstructions in seven were in a ureter. Late stricture of a bowel ureter occurred in three, each localized. An endoscope can be passed up a bowel ureter (1) to incise a web, (2) to inject a steroid solution, or (3) to dilate. Urinary tract stones developed in 14 patients and required removal. Most of the stones had a staple nidus. When staples have been used, the author always performs a cystoscopy several months later to remove any staples not covered by mucosa. Otherwise, staples can form stones on the nipple or drop off into the bladder and grow larger, which occurred in two patients who did not return soon for follow-up examination.

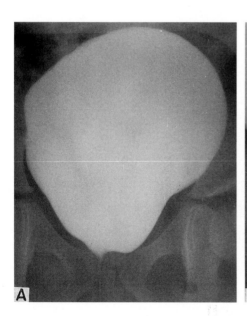

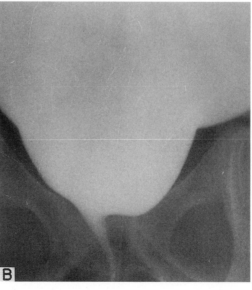

Figure 104–30. Case 10 roentgenograms. *A,* Bladder filled to 275 ml. Most of the bladder wall is gastric augmentation. *B,* Voiding film showing a normal bladder neck and urethra. The patient empties the bladder completely by abdominal effort, while voluntarily opening the bladder neck and sphincter.

BEFORE

16 year old girl
Cystectomy and diversion at
age 1 year for sarcoma

AFTER

Continent diversion

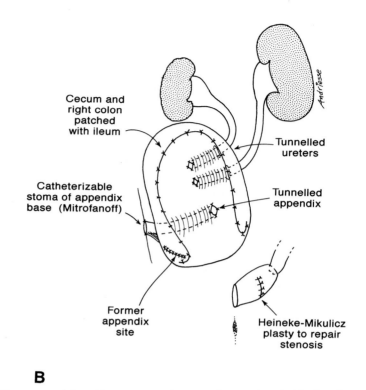

A

Good kidney
89% of renal function

Poor kidney
11%

Right
reflux

Left
obstruction

Ileal
loop

Cystectomy ———x

Rectum
normal

Vaginal
stenosis

Cecum and
right colon
patched
with ileum

Tunnelled
ureters

Catheterizable
stoma of appendix
base (Mitrofanoff)

Tunnelled
appendix

Former
appendix
site

Heineke-Mikulicz
plasty to repair
stenosis

B

Figure 104–31. Case 11. Preoperative *(A)* and postoperative *(B)* anatomy of Case 11, reconstructed as a continent catheterizable diversion.

Three patients had postoperative leaks, and each closed spontaneously. Two patients had pigment gallstones on follow-up, presumably from a large intraoperative transfusion requirement during undiversion. Cholecystectomy was done in each of these patients. One patient had a traumatic urethral vaginal fistula that required closure. Thirteen patients required a secondary operation for persistent wetting.

One patient had an artificial sphincter (Rosen type) placed. It worked well but later eroded the urethra and was removed. Many successes have been reported with the use of artificial sphincters; however, the author prefers to avoid them, opting to narrow the outlet surgically and catheterize to empty, if necessary.

CONCLUSION

Urinary undiversion should be considered for patients who have undergone diversion in the past. Reconstructions of this magnitude require meticulous attention to all technical surgical details. Many of these patients have poor renal function. This is not a contraindication to undiversion, however, because restoration of bladder function gives a much better quality of life. Furthermore, it is ultimately better to transplant a kidney into a bladder than into a cutaneous diversion. Undiversion may reduce urinary infection and prolong the time before transplantation is needed.

REFERENCES

Adams MC, Mitchell ME, Rink RC: Gastrocystoplasty: An alternative solution to the problem of urological reconstruction in the severely compromised patient. J Urol 1988; 140:1152–1156.

Althausen AF, Hagen-Cook K, Hendren WH: Non-refluxing colon conduit: Experience with 70 cases. J Urol 1982; 120:35–39.

Bauer SB, Colodny AH, Hallet M, et al: Urinary undiversion in myelodysplasia criteria for selection and predictive value of urodynamics. J Urol 1980; 124:89–93.

Bauer SB, Dieppa RA, Labib KK, Retik AB: The bladder in boys with posterior urethral valves, a urodynamic assessment. J Urol 1974; 121:769–773.

Bosco PJ, Bauer SB, Colodny AH, et al: The long-term results of artificial sphincters in children. J Urol 1991; 146:396–399.

Bricker EM: Bladder substitution after pelvic evisceration. Surg Clin North Am 1950; 30:1511–1521.

Campaiola JM, Perlmutter AD, Steinhardt GF: Noncompliant bladder resulting from posterior urethral valves. J Urol 1985; 134:708–710.

Churchill BN, Aliabadi H, Landau EH, et al: Ureteral bladder augmentation. J Urol 1993; 150:716–720.

Coplen DE, Duckett JW: Modern approach to ureteroceles. J Urol 1995; 153:166–171.

Courvelaire R: La "petite vessie" des tuberculeaux genitourinaires. Essai de classification place et variantes des cysto-intestino-plasties. J Urol Paris 1950; 56:381–434.

Crooks KK: Urethral strictures following transurethral resection of posterior urethral valves. J Urol 1982; 127:1153–1154.

Duckett JW Jr: Current management of posterior urethral valves. Urol Clin North Am 1974; 1:471–483.

Elder JS, Snyder HM, Hulbert WC, Duckett JW: Perforation of the augmented bladder in patients undergoing clean intermittent catheterization. J Urol 1981; 140:1159–1162.

Ferris DO, Odel HM: Electrolyte pattern of the blood after bilateral uretero-sigmoidostomy. JAMA 1950; 142:634–641.

Friedman RM, Flashner SC, King LR: Effectiveness of handsewn nipple valve for reflux prevention in bladder reconstruction. J Urol 1992; 147:441–443.

Gilchrist RK, Merricks JW, Hamlin HH, et al: Construction of a substitute bladder and urethra. Surg Gynecol Obstet 1950; 90:752–760.

Glassberg KI: Current issues regarding posterior urethral valves. Urol Clin North Am 1985; 12:175–185.

Goldstein HR, Hensle TW: Urinary undiversion in adults. J Urol 1981; 128:143–150.

Goldwasser B, Webster GD: Augmentation and substitution enterocystoplasty. J Urol 1986; 135:215–224.

Gonzalez R, Koleilat N, Austin C, et al: The artificial sphincter AS800 in congenital urinary incontinence. J Urol 1989; 142:512–515.

Gonzalez R, Sidi A, Zhang G: Urinary undiversion: Indications, technique and results in 50 cases. J Urol 1986; 136:13–16.

Goodwin WE, Harris AP, Kaufman JJ, Beal JM: Open transcolonic uretero-intestinal anastomosis: A new approach. Surg Gynecol Obstet 1953; 97:295–300.

Goodwin WE, Turner RD, Winter CC: Results of ileocystoplasty. J Urol 1958; 80:461–466.

Goodwin WE, Winter CC, Barker WF: "Cup-patch" technique of ileocystoplasty for bladder enlargement of partial substitution. Surg Gynecol Obstet 1959; 108:240–244.

Hendren WH: A new approach to infants with severe obstructive uropathy: Early complete reconstruction. J Pediatr Surg 1970; 5:184–199.

Hendren WH: Posterior urethral valves in boys: A broad clinical spectrum. J Urol 1971; 106:298–307.

Hendren WH: Reconstruction of previously diverted urinary tracts in children. J Pediatr Surg 1973; 8:135–150.

Hendren WH: Urethral valves: Diagnosis and endoscopic resection. Eaton Film Library, 1974a.

Hendren WH: Urinary tract refunctionalization after prior diversion in children. Ann Surg 1974b; 180:494–510.

Hendren WH: Non-refluxing colon conduit for temporary or permanent urinary diversion in children. J Pediatr Surg 1975; 10:381–398.

Hendren WH: Urinary diversion and undiversion in children. Surg Clin North Am 1976; 56:425–449.

Hendren WH: Some alternatives to urinary diversion in children. J Urol 1978a; 119:652–660.

Hendren WH: Complications of ureterostomy. J Urol 1978b; 120:269–281.

Hendren WH: Reoperative ureteral reimplantation: Management of the difficult case. J Pediatr Surg 1980a; 15:770–786.

Hendren WH: Construction of female urethra from vaginal wall and a perineal flap. J Urol 1980b; 123:657–664.

Hendren WH: Techniques for urinary undiversion. *In* King LR, Stone AR, Webster GD, eds: Reconstruction and Continent Urinary Diversion. Chicago, Year Book Medical Publishers, 1987, p 101.

Hendren WH: Urinary tract refunctionalization after long-term diversion: A 20 year experience with 177 patients. Ann Surg 1990; 212:478–495.

Hendren WH, Hendren RB: Bladder augmentation: Experience with 129 cases in children and young adults. J Urol 1990; 144:445–453.

Hendren WH, Hensle TW: Transureteroureterostomy: Experience with 75 cases. J Urol 1980; 123:826–833.

Hendren WH, McLorie GA: Late stricture of intestinal ureter. J Urol 1983; 129:584–590.

Hendren WH, Mitchell ME: Surgical correction of ureteroceles. J Urol 1979; 121:590–597.

Hodges CV, Moore RJ, Lehman TH, Behnam AM: Clinical experiences with transureteroureterostomy. J Urol 1963; 90:552–562.

Jeffs R: Exstrophy of the urinary bladder. *In* Welch KJ, Randolph JG, Ravitch MM, et al, eds: Pediatric Surgery. Chicago, Year Book Medical Publishers, 1986, pp 1212–1241.

Johnston JH: Temporary cutaneous ureterostomy in the management of advanced congenital urinary obstruction. Arch Dis Child 1963; 38:161–166.

Kass EJ, Koff SA: Bladder augmentation in the pediatric neuropathic bladder. J Urol 1983; 129:552–555.

Kelalis P: Urinary diversion in children by sigmoid conduits: Its advantages and limitations. J Urol 1974; 112:666–672.

Kennedy HA, Adams MC, Mitchell ME, et al: Chronic renal failure and bladder augmentation: Stomach versus sigmoid colon in the canine model. J Urol 1988; 140:1138–1140.

King LR, Stone AR, Webster GD, eds: Bladder Reconstruction and Continent Urinary Diversion. Chicago, Year Book Medical Publishers, 1987a.

King LR, Webster GD, Bertram RA: Experience with bladder reconstruction in children. J Urol 1987b; 138:1002–1006.

Koch MO, McDougal WS: The pathophysiology of hyperchloremic metabolic acidosis after urinary diversion through intestinal segments. Surgery 1985; 98:561–570.

Kock NG, Nilson AE, Nilsson LO, et al: Urinary diversion via a continent ileal reservoir: Clinical results in 12 patients. J Urol 1982; 128:469–475.

Kogan SJ, Kim K, Levitt SB: Preoperative evaluation of bladder function prior to renal transplantation or urinary tract reconstruction in children: Description of a method. J Pediatr Surg 1976; 11:1007–1008.

Kogan SJ, Levitt SB: Bladder evaluation in pediatric patients before undiversion in previously diverted urinary tracts. J Urol 1977; 118:443–446.

Lapides J, Diokno AC, Gould FR, Low BS: Further observations on self-catheterization. J Urol 1976; 116:169–171.

Leong CH: Use of the stomach for bladder replacement and urinary diversion. Ann R Coll Surg Engl 1978; 60:283–289.

Light JK, Engelmann UH: Reconstruction of the lower urinary tract: Observations on bowel dynamics and the artificial urinary sphincter. J Urol 1985; 133:594–597.

Linder A, Leach GE, Raz S: Augmentation cystoplasty in the treatment of neurogenic bladder dysfunction. J Urol 1983; 129:491–493.

Middleton AW Jr, Hendren WH: Ileal conduits in children at the Massachusetts General Hospital from 1955 to 1970. J Urol 1976; 115:591–595.

Mitchell ME: The role of bladder augmentation in undiversion. J Pediatr Surg 1981a; 16:790–798.

Mitchell ME: Urinary tract diversion and undiversion in the pediatric age group. Surg Clin North Am 1981b; 61:1147–1164.

Mitchell ME, Close CE: Early primary valve ablation for posterior urethral valves. Semin Pediatr Surg 1995; 5:66–71.

Mitchell ME, Kulf TB, Backes DJ: Intestinocystoplasty in combination with clean intermittent catheterization in the management of vesical dysfunction. J Urol 1986; 136:288–291.

Mitchell ME, Piser JA: Intestinocystoplasty and total bladder replacement in children and young adults: Follow-up in 129 cases. J Urol 1987; 138:579–584.

Mitchell ME, Rink RC: Experience with the artificial urinary sphincter in children and young adults. J Pediatr Surg 1983; 18:700–706.

Mitchell ME, Rink RC: Pediatric urinary diversion and undiversion. Pediatr Clin North Am 1987; 34:1319–1332.

Mitrofanoff P: Cystostomie continente trans-appendiculaire dans le traitement des vessies neurologiques. Chir Pediatr 1980; 21:297–305.

Mor Y, Ramon J, Raviv G, et al: Low loop cutaneous ureterostomy and subsequent reconstruction: 20 years of experience. J Urol 1992; 147:1595–1598.

O'Donnell B, Puri P: Technical refinements in endoscopic correction of vesicoureteral reflux. J Urol 1980; 40:1101–1102.

Perlmutter AD: Experiences with urinary undiversion in children with neurogenic bladder. J Urol 1980; 123:402–406.

Perlmutter AD, Patil J: Loop cutaneous ureterostomy in infants and young children: Late results in 32 cases. J Urol 1972; 107:655–659.

Peters CA, Hendren WH: Splitting the pubis for exposure in difficult reconstructions for incontinence. Urol Clin North Am 1990; 17:37–45.

Pitts WR Jr, Muecke EC: A 20 year experience with ileal conduits: The fate of the kidneys. J Urol 1979; 122:154–157.

Puri P, O'Donnell B: Endoscopic correction of grades IV and V primary vesicoureteric reflux: Six to 30 month follow-up in 42 ureters. J Pediatr Surg 1987; 22:1087–1091.

Retik AB, Perlmutter AD, Gross RE: Cutaneous ureteroileostomy in children. N Engl J Med 1967; 277:217–222.

Richie JP, Skinner DG: Urinary diversion: The physiological rationale for non-refluxing colonic conduits. Br J Urol 1975; 47:269–275.

Richie JP, Skinner DG, Waisman J: The effect of reflux on the development of pyelonephritis in urinary diversion: An experimental study. J Surg Res 1974; 16:256–261.

Rushton HG, Woodward JR, Parrot TS, et al: Delayed bladder rupture after augmentation enterocystoplasty. J Urol 1988; 140:344–346.

Scott FB, Bradley WE, Tumm GW: Treatment of urinary incontinence by an implantable prosthetic urinary sphincter. J Urol 1974; 112:75–80.

Shapiro SR, Lebowitz R, Colodny AH: Fate of 90 children with ileal conduit urinary diversion a decade later: Analysis of complications, pyelography, renal function and bacteriology. J Urol 1975; 114:89–95.

Sheiner JR, Kaplan GW: Spontaneous bladder rupture following enterocystoplasty. J Urol 1988; 140:1157–1158.

Sheldon CA: Urinary reconstruction (rather than diversion) for continence in difficult pediatric urologic disorders. Semin Pediatr Surg 1995; 5:8–15.

Sheldon CA, Gilbert A: Use of appendix for uretheral reconstruction in children with congenital abnormalities of the bladder. Surgery 1992; 112:805–812.

Sheldon CA, Gilbert A, Wacksman J, et al: Gastrocystoplasty: Technical and metabolic characteristics of the most versatile childhood bladder augmentation modality. J Pediatr Surg 1995; 30:283–288.

Sheldon CA, Gonzalez R, Burns MW, et al: Renal transplantation into the dysfunctional bladder: The role of adjunctive bladder reconstruction. J Urol 1994; 152:972–975.

Sidi AA, Aliabadi H, Gonzalez R: Enterocystoplasty in the management and reconstruction of the pediatric neurogenic bladder. J Pediatr Surg 1987; 22:153–157.

Sidi AA, Reinberg Y, Gonzalez R: Influence of intestinal segment and configuration on the outcome of augmentation enterocystoplasty. J Urol 1986; 136:1201–1204.

Skinner DG, Boyd SD, Lieskovsky G: Clinical experience with the Kock continent ileal reservoir for urinary diversion. J Urol 1984; 132:1101–1107.

Skinner DG, Gottesman JE, Richie JP: The isolated sigmoid segment: Its value in temporary urinary diversion and reconstruction. J Urol 1975; 113:614–618.

Smith C, Gonsalbez TS, Parrott JR, et al: Transurethral puncture of ectopic ureteroceles in neonates and infants. J Urol 1994; 152:2110–2112.

Smith ED: Follow-up studies on 150 ileal conduits in children. J Pediatr Surg 1972; 7:1–10.

Smith RB, VanCangh P, Skinner DG, et al: Augmentation enterocystoplasty: A critical review. J Urol 1977; 118:35–39.

Stephenson TP, Mundy AR: Treatment of the neuropathic bladder by enterocystoplasty and selective sphincterotomy or sphincter ablation and replacement. Br J Urol 1985; 57:27–31.

Sumfest JM, Burns MW, Mitchell ME: Mitrofanoff principle in urinary reconstruction. J Urol 1993; 150:1875–1878.

Thuroff JW, Alken P, Riedmiller H, et al: 100 cases of Mainz pouch; Continuing experience and evolution. J Urol 1988; 140:283–288.

Turner-Warwick R: Cystoplasty. Urol Clin North Am 1979; 6:259–264.

Whitmore WF III, Gittes RF: Reconstruction of the urinary tract by cecal and ileocecal cystoplasty: Review of a 15-year experience. J Urol 1983; 129:494–498.

Zinman L, Libertino JA: Ileocecal conduit for temporary and permanent diversion. J Urol 1975; 113:317–323.

105
SURGERY OF THE BLADDER

Fray F. Marshall, M.D.

SURGICAL APPROACHES

The bladder is approached surgically through incisions below the umbilicus. Incisions are typically vertical or transverse. Vertical incisions include a midline incision or a paramedian incision. Transverse incisions include the Pfannenstiel or Cherney incision. The Pfannenstiel incision is a transverse incision made 1 to 2 cm above the pubis. The anterior rectus fascia is divided transversely, and upper and lower fascia flaps are dissected off the rectus muscle. The rectus muscles are then divided in the midline. The Cherney incision is made somewhat higher and is also transverse but divides the rectus sheath and rectus muscles transversely. The Pfannenstiel incision may be more cosmetic, but the vertical midline incision is easier to perform and can be extended superiorly if necessary. Small midline incisions such as the *mini-lap* can be used for small operations on the bladder or for pelvic lymphadenectomy (Steiner and Marshall, 1993). These small incisions are facilitated by the use of small ring retractors or other fixed retractors that provide superficial and deep retraction through a small incision.

The urinary bladder has a rich blood supply so that it usually heals well and can be mobilized extensively. As a result, hemostasis is important because the compliance of the bladder can allow bleeding as there is little tamponade. Absorbable sutures are always used because of the possibility of calculus formation and infection with any permanent suture.

This chapter includes detailed descriptions of radical cystectomy in the male as well as urethrectomy. There are major differences in cystectomy between the two sexes, and radical cystectomy in the female represents an anterior exenteration when performed for bladder carcinoma. Simple cystectomy with a retrograde approach is covered as well as partial cystectomy. Surgery for benign disease includes vesical diverticulectomy and repair of vesical fistulas. Lastly, Y-V-plasty of the bladder neck for bladder neck contracture and a suprapubic cystostomy are also described.

RADICAL CYSTECTOMY IN THE MALE

Radical cystectomy is typically performed for invasive carcinoma of the bladder. The first cystectomy was performed in the late 1800s, but in 1926 Young and Davis indicated that a high mortality rate and poor success made cystectomy unjustifiable. In 1939, a mortality rate of 34.5% was reported in Hinman's large series of 250 cystectomies (Hinman, 1939). **Improvements in surgical and anesthetic techniques as well as perioperative care reduced the mortality rate to 1% to 3% in most contemporary series** (Bracken et al, 1981; Hendry, 1986).

Preoperative radiation therapy was proposed in the 1970s as additional treatment to improve survival. Subsequent evaluation, however, has not demonstrated any significant advantage for the use of this treatment (Thrasher and Crawford, 1993). As combination chemotherapy trials have demonstrated increased efficacy in the treatment of transitional cell carcinoma of the bladder, the precise place of neoadjuvant or adjuvant chemotherapy remains to be determined (Thrasher and Crawford, 1993). For localized or regional transitional cell carcinoma of the bladder, radical cystectomy remains an effective treatment. In the future, surgery will likely be used in association with other treatment modalities.

Indications

Radical cystectomy is performed for muscle-invasive transitional cell carcinoma of the bladder and for some patients with recurrent transitional cell carcinoma in situ that does not respond to topical chemotherapy. Occasionally, it may be a palliative procedure when the morbidity of the disease from bleeding or frequency is severe. In this situation, urinary diversion and adjunctive chemotherapy can be helpful.

Preoperative Evaluation and Management

The preoperative evaluation is most important, both medically and urologically. Any medical problems that may affect surgery necessitate a careful medical evaluation for treatment of any other significant medical diseases. It is also recommended that the patients stop taking aspirin, lose weight if necessary, stop smoking, and take vitamins.

Urologically the patient is staged with a transurethral resection of the bladder tumor and multiple bladder and urethral biopsies. If any transitional cell carcinoma is found in the prostate or prostatic urethra, a urethrectomy should be considered as well.

Radiologic evaluation includes computed tomographic (CT) evaluation of the pelvis and abdomen. If there appears to be a sizable bladder tumor, it is preferable to obtain this study before transurethral resection because staging is more accurate. CT scan of the chest is also recommended. Liver function tests are obtained. A bone scan is sometimes recommended, although if the alkaline phosphatase is normal and there are no symptoms, bony metastatic disease is not likely. Barium enema or colonoscopy or both are recommended for those patients who have possible gastrointestinal

disease or if a continent urinary diversion is being considered. If adenocarcinoma is found on biopsy, an extravesical site such as colon should also be considered. Primary vesical adenocarcinoma can also occur in the dome and may represent a urachal carcinoma. It is also often recommended that the patient donate 2 to 3 units of blood and take ferrous gluconate 300 mg three times a day.

The risk of deep venous thrombosis and possible pulmonary emboli always exists. Some have recommended warfarin (Coumadin) or subcutaneous heparin perioperatively, but there has been an associated increased risk of postoperative lymphocele as well as the potential for serious bleeding complications. Perioperative external compression boots, aggressive early ambulation, and avoidance of sitting may reduce the risk of deep venous thrombosis. Patients who have had a previous pulmonary embolus or have a significant history of previous phlebitis are considered high risk and typically receive anticoagulation postoperatively.

Bowel preparation is exceedingly important, particularly if continent diversion with an extensive length of bowel or large bowel is used. Clear liquids are recommended for the 2 days before surgery. Polyethylene glycol-electrolyte solution (GoLYTELY) is given on the day before surgery, and oral antibiotics containing both neomycin and erythromycin base, 1 g each, are administered in three doses on the day before surgery. **Although many patients are now brought into the hospital the day of surgery, it remains important to have an adequate bowel preparation, especially for continent diversions employing large bowel.** In some older patients, dehydration can also become a serious issue. For those reasons, an admission the night before surgery may still be indicated in some patients.

More than a decade ago, all patients who underwent radical cystoprostatectomy were impotent postoperatively. It is now possible to preserve the neurovascular bundles for a radical cystoprostatectomy in much the same fashion as has been described for radical prostatectomy (Schlegel et al, 1987; Marshall, 1991). With preservation of the neurovascular bundles and a continent urinary diversion with a urethral anastomosis, it is now possible to have a patient who is potent and can void with complete control.

Operative Technique

The patient is positioned with the table split, which opens the area between the umbilicus and the pubis. A No. 22 Fr urethral catheter with a 30-ml balloon is placed into the bladder, and at least 50 ml of sterile water is instilled into the balloon.

A midline lower abdominal incision is made to the umbilicus. If additional length is required, it is extended usually around the left side of the umbilicus. If patients have had a previous partial cystectomy or suprapubic tube, this tract is generally excised with the incision. The space of Retzius is developed. The peritoneal cavity is entered and is systematically explored for any possible metastatic disease. The position of the nasogastric tube is verified, and any other obvious abnormalities are duly noted. The urachus is identified and ligated below the umbilicus. The peritoneum is incised along each side of the bladder. The vasa deferentia are identified lateral to the bladder and are ligated and divided. Usually the descending colon has a few adhesions that need to be dissected free on the left side. A moist pack and an additional moist towel are then placed with the ends in each colonic gutter so that the bowel can be isolated from the pelvis and remains in the upper abdomen away from the operative field. **A self-retaining retractor such as a Wilkinson ring, Omni-Tract retractor, or Buchwalter retractor helps with exposure.** A blade is placed on each side of the abdomen so that the ascending and descending colon as well as the small bowel contents remain packed in the upper abdomen.

A bilateral pelvic lymphadenectomy is performed (Figs. 105–1 and 105–2). The dissection is initiated below the genitofemoral nerve residing on the psoas muscle. The entire external iliac artery and vein are dissected, with the dissection extending from the bifurcation of the common iliac artery superiorly to the lateral fascia of the rectum medially. The node dissections are initiated by incising the adventitia overlying the external iliac artery and vein. The lymphatic package is then dissected free of the iliac vessels and extends

into the obturator fossa (Fig. 105–3). The bladder is retracted medially by a Harrington blade. Care should be taken to avoid tearing an accessory obturator vein, which is present frequently. The obturator nerve is visualized. The node of Cloquet is mobilized at the junction of the femoral canal, and a clip is applied to the lymphatic package in this area before dividing lymphatics (Fig. 105–4). The nodes are then dissected from the hypogastric artery and vein.

At the time of the dissection of the hypogastric vessels, the obliterated umbilical and superior vesical arteries are divided. Branches of the hypogastric artery are divided, but the hypogastric artery is not ligated to avoid potential compromise of blood flow to the internal pudendal artery and possible vasculogenic impotence (Fig. 105–5).

After division of the vessels, the ureters are then identified and divided close to the bladder. **The margins of the ureter are then sent to pathology for frozen section.** Occasionally, carcinoma in situ can necessitate multiple resections of the ureter. The retrovesical cul-de-sac is exposed, and the

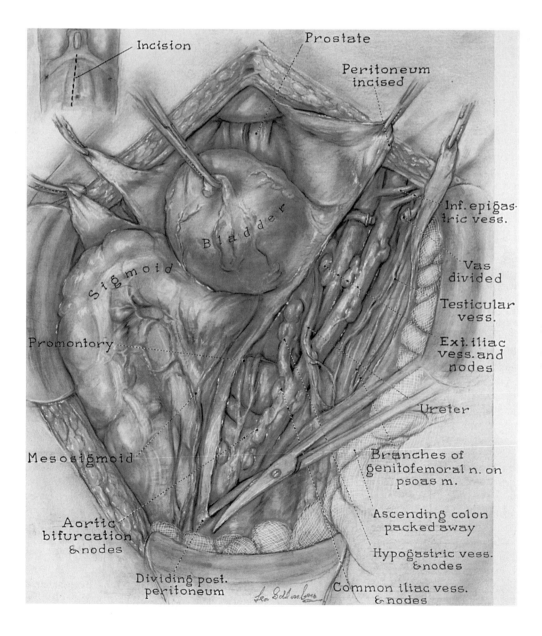

Figure 105–1. Exposure of the right iliac vessels and pelvic lymph nodes after incision of the peritoneal reflection. (From Walsh PC, Schlegel PN: Radical cystectomy. *In* Marshall FF, ed: Operative Urology. Philadelphia, W. B. Saunders, 1991.)

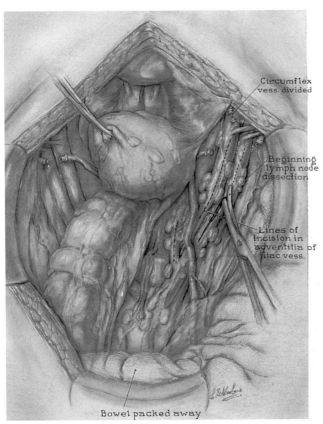

Figure 105–2. Position of incisions along iliac vessels performed at the commencement of the right pelvic and iliac lymph node dissections. (From Walsh PC, Schlegel PN: Radical cystectomy. *In* Marshall FF, ed: Operative Urology. Philadelphia, W. B. Saunders, 1991.)

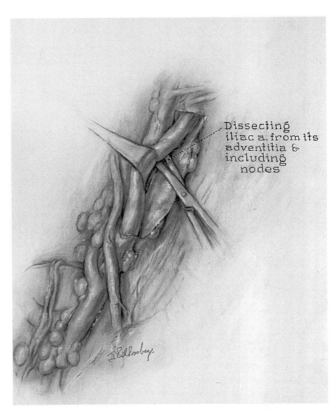

Figure 105–3. Dissection of the right external iliac lymph nodes away from the isolated external iliac artery. (From Walsh PC, Schlegel PN: Radical cystectomy. *In* Marshall FF, ed: Operative Urology. Philadelphia, W. B. Saunders, 1991.)

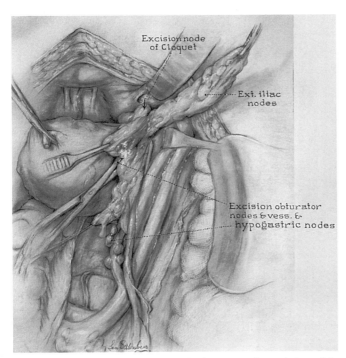

Figure 105–4. Right pelvic lymph node dissection after isolation of the external iliac vessels and excision of the node of Cloquet from the femoral canal. (From Walsh PC, Schlegel PN: Radical cystectomy. *In* Marshall FF, ed: Operative Urology. Philadelphia, W. B. Saunders, 1991.)

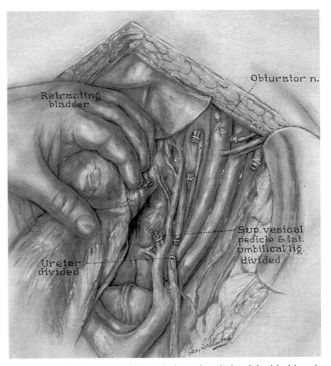

Figure 105–5. Dissection of the right lateral pedicle of the bladder after division of the right ureter, superior vesicle pedicle, and lateral umbilical ligament (umbilical artery). (From Walsh PC, Schlegel PN: Radical cystectomy. *In* Marshall FF, ed: Operative Urology. Philadelphia, W. B. Saunders, 1991.)

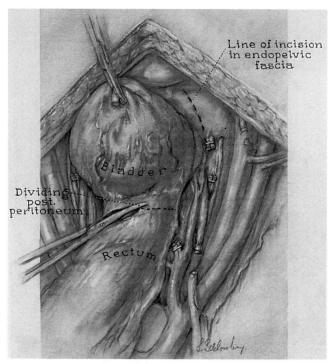

Figure 105–6. Incision of the posterior peritoneum in the rectovesical cul-de-sac. The site of incision of the endopelvic fascia lateral to the prostate is also demonstrated. (From Walsh PC, Schlegel PN: Radical cystectomy. *In* Marshall FF, ed: Operative Urology. Philadelphia, W. B. Saunders, 1991.)

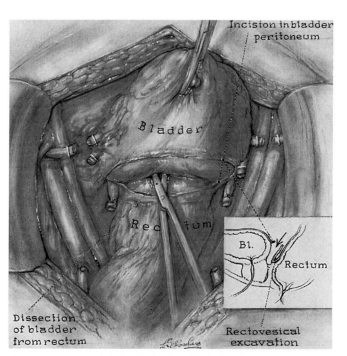

Figure 105–7. Initial dissection of the bladder specimen off the rectum and site of entry into the rectovesical cul-de-sac. (From Walsh PC, Schlegel PN: Radical cystectomy. *In* Marshall FF, ed: Operative Urology. Philadelphia, W. B. Saunders, 1991.)

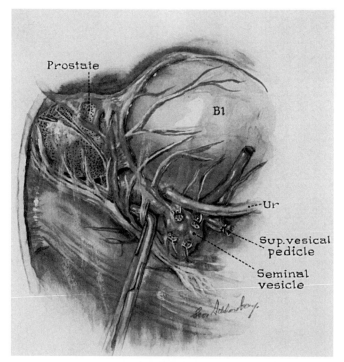

Figure 105–8. Schematic illustration of division of the left posterior pedicle to the bladder containing branches of the inferior vesicle artery and vein. Note the preservation of the autonomic innervation to the corpora cavernosa posterior to the seminal vesicle. (From Walsh PC, Schlegel PN: Radical cystectomy. *In* Marshall FF, ed: Operative Urology. Philadelphia, W. B. Saunders, 1991.)

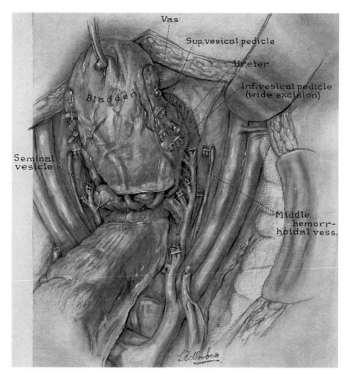

Figure 105–9. The bladder specimen, after wide excision of the right posterior pedicle of the bladder with sacrifice of the right neurovascular bundle, is demonstrated. (From Walsh PC, Schlegel PN: Radical cystectomy. *In* Marshall FF, ed: Operative Urology. Philadelphia, W. B. Saunders, 1991.)

posterior peritoneum is incised (Fig. 105–6). A plane between the bladder and rectum is then developed (Fig. 105–7). Usually, this dissection can proceed under direct vision, and the bladder and prostate can be separated from the rectum. The seminal vesicles can then be visualized posteriorly. Unless the tumor is quite large, it is not common to find transitional cell carcinoma extending through the prostate into the area of the neurovascular bundle in invasive bladder cancer. If there is any question, wide excision of the neurovascular bundle on that side is indicated. It is sometimes difficult in an obese male to continue the dissection in an antegrade manner (Figs. 105–8 and 105–9), although this can be done in a slender man.

At this time, a retrograde dissection is initiated similar to a radical prostatectomy. The endopelvic fascia is divided, and the puboprostatic ligaments are divided. The dorsal vein complex is divided and oversewn. The urethra is then divided. If a urethrectomy is to be performed, the urethra is dissected under the symphysis so that the perineal dissection is facilitated. **If a continent urinary diversion is being considered, frozen section verification of the prostatic urethra and the apex of the prostate is performed to verify there is no carcinoma in the urethra.** The external striated urethral sphincter is divided (Fig. 105–10). The neurovascular bundle is dissected off the prostate, the remainder of the pedicles are ligated and divided, and the specimen is removed. It is wise to pass a heavy ligature around the urethra and tie it at the level of the apex of the prostate to prevent leakage of urine after division of the urethra. If a urethrectomy is to be performed, it may be reasonable to divide the striated muscle of the urethra and mobilize the posterior lateral neurovascular bundles off the urethra distally.

Once the specimen has been removed, the appearance of the pelvis should include the rectum, urethral stump, and dorsal vein complex. If one neurovascular bundle has been excised, the other remains (see Fig. 105–10B).

Postoperative Management and Complications

The overall complication rate after radical cystectomy and urinary diversion may be as high as 25% to 35%. Atelectasis and respiratory complications are common and require aggressive attention in almost all patients. Early mobilization is important not only for respiratory problems, but also for prevention of deep venous thrombosis. Wound infections may occur especially in an obese population. Intraoperative wound irrigation remains important as well as hemostasis. Extensive use of the cautery also predisposes to infection.

Gastrointestinal complications can occur with rectal injury, intestinal obstruction, or fistula. If a rectal injury occurs, it can be repaired primarily, provided that the tissue appears healthy and it is not irradiated. If there is previous radiation, a colostomy is indicated.

Impotence is another recognized complication, but potency can be maintained in the majority of patients with careful dissection of the neurovascular bundle (Schlegel and Walsh, 1987). It is usually feasible to preserve the neurovascular bundles during a cystectomy because the transitional cell carcinoma does not frequently extend beyond

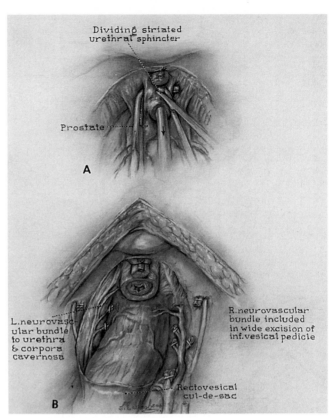

Figure 105–10. *A,* The prostate is being retracted superiorly using gentle traction on the urethral catheter. The attachment of the striated urethral sphincter to the prostate is isolated with a right-angle clamp and divided sharply. *B,* The pelvic fossa after removal of the radical cystectomy specimen. The neurovascular structures on the left side have been preserved. Wide excision of the right posterior pedicle including the neurovascular bundle has been performed, with preservation of only the middle hemorrhoidal vessels and internal pudendal vessels. (From Walsh PC, Schlegel PN: Radical cystectomy. *In* Marshall FF, ed: Operative Urology. Philadelphia, W. B. Saunders, 1991.)

the prostate. Age is an important prognostic factor; older patients, especially over 70 years, frequently become impotent. Younger patients (<60 years) do better. The author's experience has been favorable in this younger population without massive tumor (Marshall et al, 1991). It is possible to cure a patient with invasive bladder cancer and still maintain continence and sexual function.

URETHRECTOMY

Indications

The indications for urethrectomy include carcinomatous involvement of the urethra, typically the prostatic urethra. The prognosis is even more serious when the transitional cell carcinoma involves the prostatic stroma. If there is even a solitary tumor at the bladder neck or multifocal disease, urethrectomy may be required in only 4% of patients, but if there is involvement of the prostate, urethrectomy may be required in 17% to 30% of patients (Levinson et al, 1990). If the urethra is followed closely with urethral washings, even patients with multifocal tumors or carcinoma in situ may be candidates for orthotopic urinary diversion.

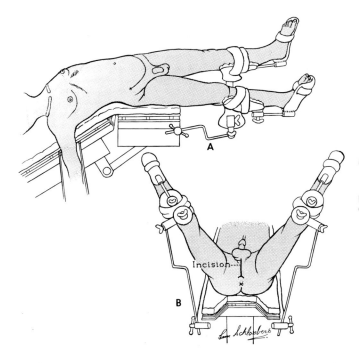

Figure 105–11. *A,* Patient position for radical cystoprostatectomy. Umbilicus is placed over break of table, and table is fully flexed and tilted into Trendelenburg's position, until legs are parallel to floor. *B,* Patient position for urethrectomy. Leg braces are elevated until hips are flexed 60 degrees and knees are fully extended.

Figure 105–12. *A,* Urethra is ligated with 1–0 silk suture to prevent spillage of urine around catheter. NVB, neurovascular bundle; Pros, prostate. *B,* Mobilization of membranous urethra from urogenital diaphragm with Kitner dissector. *C,* Further mobilization of membranous urethra. *D,* Lateral view shows membranous urethra (Ur) fully mobilized with neurovascular bundles displaced posterolaterally. *E,* Urethra is transected, and catheter is drawn cephalad into wound. Neurovascular bundles are seen intact, lateral to the urethra.

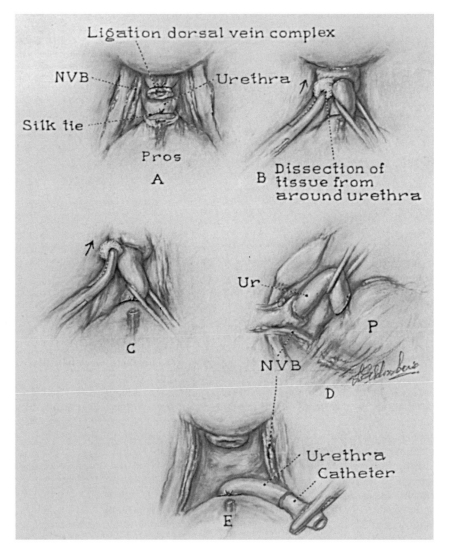

The cavernous nerves course along the bladder and prostate, then posterolaterally to the membranous urethra as they go through the urogenital diaphragm (Schlegel and Walsh, 1987). The most likely cause of impotence appears to be neurovascular injury when the urethra is mobilized in the area of the membranous urethra. With careful dissection, it may be possible to preserve potency in a few patients through a retropubic approach (Brendler et al, 1990). The easiest time to dissect this membranous urethra is during a cystoprostatectomy because the subsequent perineal dissection is greatly facilitated.

Operative Technique

The patient is placed supine on the operating table with the table flexed at the level of the umbilicus and is tilted into Trendelenburg's position until the patient's legs are parallel with the floor (Fig. 105–11).

If a concomitant radical cystoprostatectomy is being performed, the initial dissection involves division of the dorsal vein in the penis and suturing with a 3–0 absorbable suture. The ligature is passed around the urethra and ligated to prevent spillage of potential tumor cells from the bladder (Fig. 105–12A). With a Kitner dissector, the urethra can be dissected from the urogenital diaphragm (Fig. 105–12B). The neurovascular bundles can then be dissected away from the membranous urethra gently (Fig. 105–12C and D). The urethra can then be dissected into the urogenital diaphragm and then ultimately transected (Fig. 105–12E). This dissection facilitates preservation of the neurovascular bundle as well as the subsequent perineal dissection. The remainder of the cystoprostatectomy is then performed, and the specimen is removed.

Frozen section analysis of the membranous urethra is obtained at the operation. Depending on the course of the cystoprostatectomy, a simultaneous urethrectomy can be performed, especially if the frozen section findings are positive. Some surgeons prefer to wait several weeks to avoid excessive mobilization of the cavernous nerves.

The urethrectomy from the perineal approach is most easily performed in the exaggerated lithotomy position by raising the leg braces until the hips are flexed 60 degrees (see Fig. 105–11B). It is somewhat more difficult to perform this procedure in a lower lithotomy position, but it can be done and depends partly on body habitus.

A No. 26 Fr Van Buren sound can be passed through the urethra to the level of the urogenital diaphragm. A vertical incision is made, or additional exposure can be obtained with an inverted Y incision extending from the base of the scrotum toward the anus (see Fig. 105–12B). After the initial incision has been made through the subcutaneous tissue, a ring retractor such as a Turner-Warwick ring retractor or a Brantley-Scott retractor can be helpful with this surgery. The bulbocavernosus muscle is divided in the midline to the central perineal tendon. The urethra can then be dissected usually fairly easily, with the larger sound in place. After initial dissection of the urethra, a Penrose drain can be placed around the urethra and facilitates retraction (Fig. 105–13). A larger catheter can also be placed in the urethra to the level of the urogenital diaphragm and allows easy movement of the urethra during dissection. The urethra is

then dissected anteriorly toward the glans penis by sharply incising Buck's fascia, and the urethra can then be dissected from each adjacent corpora cavernosa (Fig. 105–14).

The penis can be easily everted, and the urethral dissection can be continued to the glans penis. Although a T-shaped incision can be made on the ventral surface of the corona of the glans and the glans split, transitional cell epithelium does not typically extend to the meatus, so it is not always necessary to split the glans to complete the dissection. This dissection can be carried into the glans, and the urethra is divided from the inside. If there is significant bleeding, a tourniquet around the base of the penis can reduce bleeding.

Once the urethra is divided distally, it then becomes easier to dissect the bulbar urethra. The urethra can be dissected anteriorly under the symphysis (Fig. 105–15). **Care must be taken to identify and expose the bulbar urethral arteries in a posterior lateral position because inadvertent avulsion or cutting of these vessels often prompts some difficult bleeding in a deep wound** (Fig. 105–16). The bulbar urethral artery should be clipped or tied (see Fig. 105–16). Extensive fulguration in this area may cause injury to the internal pudendal arteries. These arteries provide blood supply to the corpora cavernosa (see Fig. 105–16C). The perineal dissection is then completed and again is facilitated because there has been significant dissection through or into the urogenital diaphragm from the previous retropubic approach (Fig. 105–17).

The dissection is easier if the perineal dissection is done at the time of radical cystoprostatectomy. Later, it may be more difficult, and there may be considerably more fibrosis, which can make the deeper perineal dissection more difficult.

After the urethra has been removed, good hemostasis is required. A small drain, typically a Jackson-Pratt drain, is placed in the bed of the urethra and brought out through a stab wound lateral to the incision. The bulbocavernosus muscles are reapproximated with absorbable suture. An additional subcutaneous layer can be closed, and a subcuticular skin closure is performed with a 4–0 absorbable suture so that no sutures need subsequent removal (Fig. 105–18). A T-binder is usually used as a dressing because it is difficult to dress this area.

Postoperative Management and Complications

Most significant drainage usually stops after 1 to 2 days and the drains can be removed. Typically, extensive irrigation with antibiotic solution is given during the procedure, but postoperative antibiotics are not given routinely. Ambulation is encouraged the day after surgery, and usually the patient tolerates the perineal operation well. If a concomitant cystectomy has been performed, management relates primarily to the cystectomy.

RADICAL CYSTECTOMY IN THE FEMALE (ANTERIOR EXENTERATION)

Indications

Radical cystectomy in the female patient is a different operation compared to a radical cystoprostatectomy. Typi-

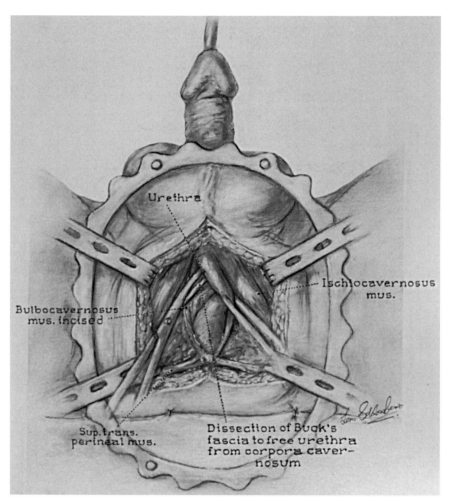

Figure 105–13. Turner-Warwick ring retractor positioned and bulbocavernosus muscle incised to expose bulbar urethra.

Figure 105–14. Incision in Buck's fascia to liberate urethra from corpora cavernosa.

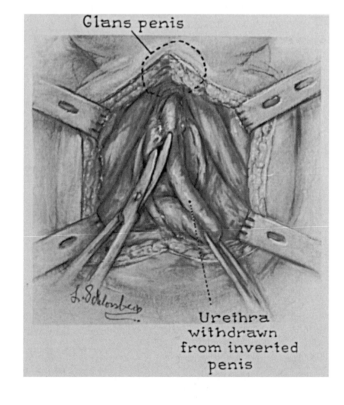

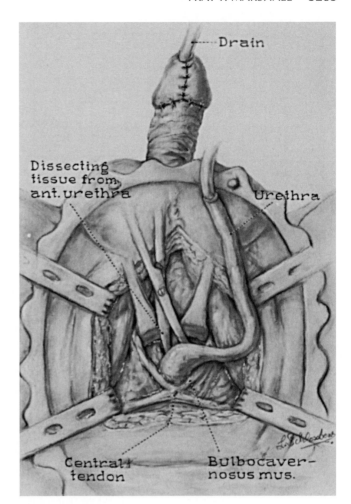

Figure 105–15. Initial dissection of tissue anterior to bulbar urethra to facilitate subsequent exposure and control of posterolateral bulbar urethral arteries.

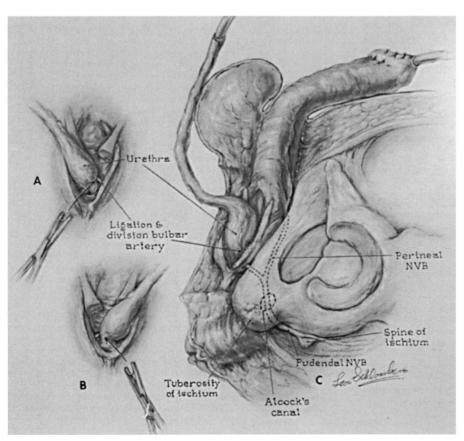

Figure 105–16. *A* and *B,* Ligation of the bulbar urethral arteries with hemoclips. *C,* Lateral view shows the relationship between the internal pudendal and bulbar arteries and the ischium and inferior ramus of the pubis. The bulbar arteries should not be fulgurated to prevent injury to the internal pudendal arteries, from which they arise and which provide arterial supply to corpora cavernosa. NVB, neurovascular bundle.

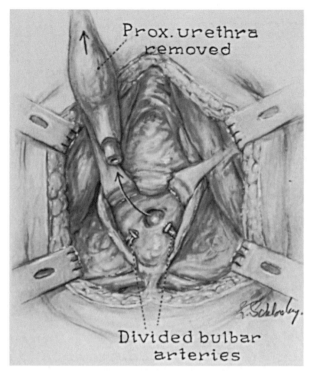

Figure 105–17. Completed urethrectomy. Dissection of bulbar urethra is completed without difficulty because the membranous urethra has previously been mobilized through the pelvis.

cally, this operation is performed for invasive transitional cell carcinoma. Although this operation has been described with a vaginal approach (Marshall and Schnittman, 1947; San Felippo and Kessler, 1978), an anterior approach is typically preferred (Marshall and Treiger, 1991). **In the patient undergoing a cystectomy for invasive cancer, the anterior approach allows a simultaneous pelvic lymphadenectomy, cystectomy, urethrectomy, hysterectomy, salpingo-oophorectomy, and partial vaginectomy.** Removal of these adjacent organs helps provide for local tumor control even if there is extensive invasive disease. In addition, it allows for accurate staging of the tumor. In some instances, adjuvant chemotherapy may be recommended in high-risk patients, particularly ones with positive nodes. In the past, often both ovaries and much of the vagina were excised so that there was no potential for sexual activity in these patients. In younger patients undergoing an anterior exenteration, it is possible to leave one ovary and reconstruct the vagina. Sexual function can then be maintained in the female. Recurrence rates of 15% to 28% have been reported in the area of the vagina (Chin et al, 1985) so that a strip of anterior vaginal wall is typically removed with the specimen. In the present age of more accurate diagnosis with CT scan, the incidence of invasion of the vagina is probably considerably lower, and as a result, vaginal reconstruction can be considered more often. The urethra is typically removed because in one study, 8 of 22 patients (36%) with transitional cell carcinoma of the bladder had urethral involvement (Paepe et al, 1990). More recent studies (Stein et al, 1994) indicate that with careful evaluation it may be possible to preserve the urethra and achieve orthotopic functional reconstruction of the urinary tract with a neoblad-

der to the urethra in women. An initial pelvic lymph node dissection is performed, and if there are grossly positive nodes, sometimes an exenteration might not be performed. If there is minimal nodal involvement, adjunctive chemotherapy and cystectomy remain an option.

Preoperative Evaluation

Transitional cell carcinoma typically occurs in an older population, often with a positive smoking history. For these reasons, all patients deserve a careful medical evaluation before the operation to ascertain their anesthetic risk. Metastatic evaluation is performed with CT evaluation of the chest, abdomen, and pelvis. A concomitant cystoscopic and pelvic examination usually helps determine the gross extent of tumor, especially if there is tumor extending toward the pelvic sidewall. The usual laboratory evaluation with hematologic and chemistry studies is performed, including liver function tests. If the patient has a smaller lesion, a normal alkaline phosphatase, and no other symptoms, a bone scan is not always obtained.

An extensive bowel preparation is given with GoLYTELY. Erythromycin and neomycin are given orally, and intravenous fluids are given the night before, particularly in older patients who might become dehydrated. If a continent diversion is considered, a bowel preparation becomes even more crucial. Although insurance companies may argue against admission the day before surgery, it is sometimes in the patient's best interest to be admitted to the hospital and have

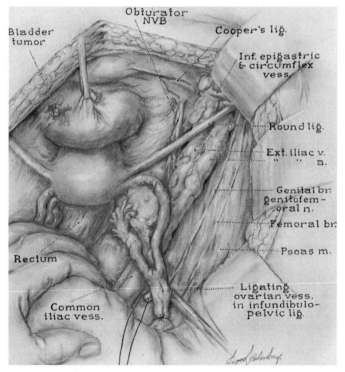

Figure 105–18. General exposure after initial division of the umbilical ligaments and peritoneum. The sigmoid colon has also been dissected free. A moist towel has been placed up each colic gutter to provide exposure. Initial ligation and division of the ovarian vessels is performed. (From Marshall FF, Treiger BFG: Urol Clin North Am 1991; 18:765–775.)

an adequate bowel preparation, appropriate hydration, and preoperative antibiotics. The author has had experience with suboptimal bowel preparations, even with careful instruction as an outpatient. The marking of a potential stoma site for an ileal conduit is also important, although in some patients the author has used the umbilicus as a stoma. Certainly the umbilicus is cosmetic and easier to catheterize than the orthotopic position, particularly in some obese females.

Surgical Technique

Stirrups or leg braces have been used frequently in the past for positioning of female patients undergoing an anterior exenteration because of the necessity of a vaginal dissection. **The author has seen problems related to peroneal nerve palsy or anterior compartment syndrome in the leg and as a result have used the split-leg fluoroscopy table.** The patient's legs can be placed together during the initial part of the dissection, but with the vaginal dissection the legs can be abducted and elevated. Although this position may not provide as good exposure as the formal lithotomy position, it is feasible to perform this operation in this manner, and the author has experienced no problems with the lower extremities since using this approach.

The patient is placed on the table with the bend in the table at the level of the umbilicus. The table is then flexed to provide better exposure of the pelvis. The patient is then widely prepared and draped, and the vagina is prepared carefully. A Foley catheter is inserted. A midline incision is then made to the left of the umbilicus. It may not be necessary to extend the incision above the umbilicus unless mobilization of the colonic hepatic flexure is required for continent urinary diversion. The retroperitoneal space is entered, and the peritoneum is mobilized off the transversalis fascia. The median and lateral umbilical ligaments are ligated and divided, and any adhesions in the peritoneal cavity are dissected. Frequently, it is necessary to dissect the sigmoid colon out of the left lower quadrant. The peritoneal contents are then inspected carefully, including palpation of the liver and the retroperitoneum along the great vessels. Any retroperitoneal lymphadenopathy is noted or biopsied.

The peritoneum lateral to the bladder is divided, and the dissection is carried down to the round ligament, which is ligated and divided. The ovarian vessels can then be identified, ligated, and divided, and this maneuver allows the peritoneal contents to be packed away from the pelvis and the primary operative field (see Fig. 105–18). A moist pack and rolled towel combined with a ring retractor or Omni-Tract retractor provide excellent superficial and deep exposure. It is easier to operate in the female pelvis because exposure is easier with its broader expanse compared to the male pelvis.

Pelvic Lymphadenectomy

The pelvic lymphadenectomy is commenced above and lateral to the external iliac vessels. The genitofemoral nerve is seen coursing on the psoas muscle (Fig. 105–19), and the dissection is initiated in this area. A nodal package over the external iliac artery and vein is then divided. Usually, this

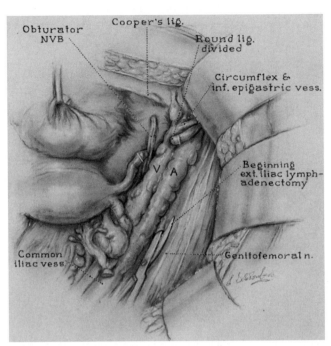

Figure 105–19. Pelvic lymphadenectomy. The dissection is initiated lateral to the external iliac artery. The genitofemoral nerve is avoided. (From Marshall FF, Treiger BFG: Urol Clin North Am 1991; 18:765–775.)

dissection is commenced at the junction of the hypogastric artery and external iliac artery. A superior dissection to the bifurcation of the aorta is not performed. The dissection can then be carried down the pelvic sidewall behind the vessels to the level of the obturator vessels. This maneuver often facilitates the overall dissection. The lymphatic package is then mobilized, and it coalesces in the angle between Cooper's ligament and the inferior aspect of the iliac vein (Fig. 105–20). It is important to place a clip in this area. A Gil-Vernet retractor provides excellent elevation of the external iliac artery and vein. Usually the lymphatic package can be mobilized off the obturator neurovascular bundle (Fig. 105–21), particularly if the entire package has been freed posteriorly. A clip can then be placed on the lymphatic package at its point of division along the hypogastric vessels (see Fig. 105–21B). Dissecting from lateral to medial facilitates the dissection. If one tries to dissect anteriorly, small perforating vessels are avulsed more often.

Pelvic Dissection

In conjunction with the pelvic lymphadenectomy, dissection is usually carried down the hypogastric artery. Each branch of the hypogastric artery to the pelvic viscera is individually dissected, ligated, and divided, usually with 2–0 absorbable ties (Fig. 105–22). These vascular branches usually include the superior vesical, middle or inferior vesicals, and vascular branches (see Fig. 105–22). Large suture ligatures with Kelly clamps are avoided.

At this point, the dissection is carried down to the ureteral insertion into the bladder. Each ureter is carefully dissected and divided. **A frozen section is always obtained of the distal ureter.** If carcinoma in situ is present, additional

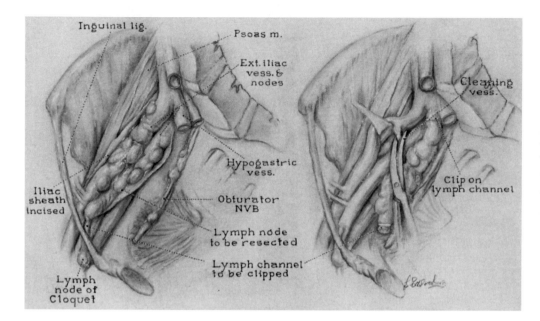

Figure 105–20. The lymphatic tissue is dissected from the iliac artery and vein. A clip is placed on the coalescence of the lymphatic package in the angle between the iliac vein and Cooper's ligament. (From Marshall FF, Treiger BFG: Urol Clin North Am 1991; 18:765–775.)

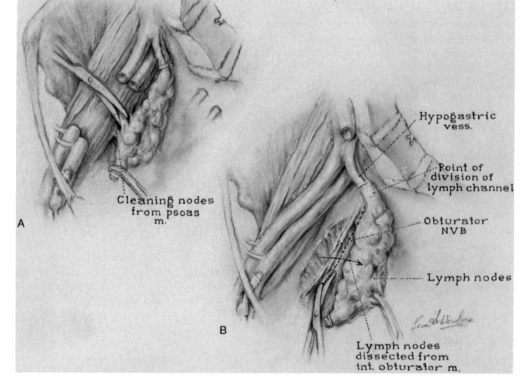

Figure 105–21. Pelvic lymphadenectomy. *A*, The lymphatic package is dissected from underneath the iliac vessels. *B*, The package is rotated medially. The obturator neurovascular bundle can easily be dissected superiorly, where the lymphatics are again clipped. (From Marshall FF, Treiger BFG: Urol Clin North Am 1991; 18:765–775.)

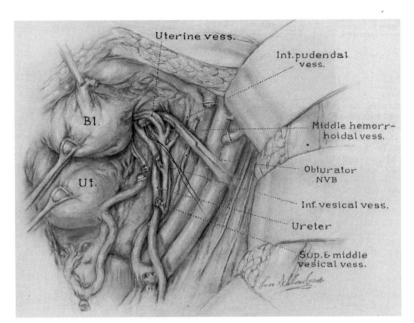

Figure 105–22. Dissection of the hypogastric artery. Superior and inferior divisions of the vesical artery are ligated with individual ties. (From Marshall FF, Treiger BFG: Urol Clin North Am 1991; 18:765–775.)

resection of the ureter is necessary. The ureter is divided at 6 o'clock and is spatulated, and a feeding tube is sutured in place so that the ureter is not manipulated extensively with any instruments (Fig. 105–23). This allows easy mobilization of the ureter as needed for subsequent urinary diversion.

Traction can then be placed on the uterus, or sometimes a Babcock clamp can be placed on each fallopian tube and the uterus elevated and at the same time traction can be placed on the rectosigmoid. This maneuver provides good exposure for an incision in the cul-de-sac. The vaginal wall can then be mobilized off the rectosigmoid (Fig. 105–24). **Placement of a sponge stick within the vagina can greatly aid in identification of the cervix in the posterior vagina.** With mobilization of the vagina posteriorly, the cervix can usually

be easily palpated, and an incision can be made into the vagina below the cervix. Often to identify the vagina more carefully, a small portion of the cardinal ligament is ligated and divided laterally (Fig. 105–25). The vessels to the vagina run in this thick ligament.

The cautery is usually used to incise the vagina under the cervix (Fig. 105–26). Because the vagina is quite vascular, stay sutures are placed in the thick vaginal wall to help provide hemostasis and traction. Previous external mobilization of the vagina allows preservation of it for subsequent vaginal reconstruction. It is easy to excise large segments of the vagina inadvertently. If the tumor is not large, vaginal construction can be considered. Additional cardinal ligament can be ligated and divided, and typically a small portion of

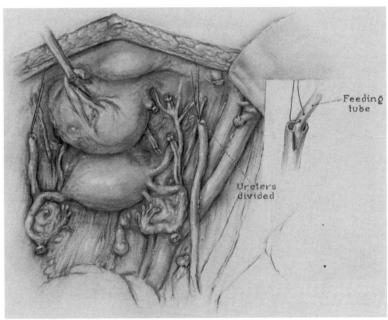

Figure 105–23. The ureters are divided. After frozen section is obtained, a feeding tube is sutured in place after the ureter is spatulated. This maneuver allows easy atraumatic manipulation of the ureter. (From Marshall FF, Treiger BFG: Urol Clin North Am 1991; 18:765–775.)

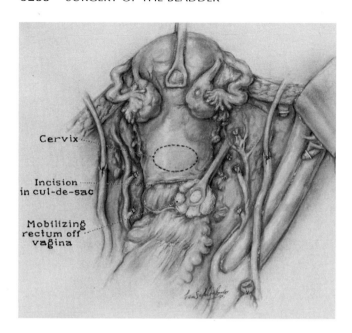

Figure 105–24. Dissection of the cul-de-sac. Traction is maintained superiorly on both the uterus and the rectosigmoid to allow easy identification of the cul-de-sac and palpation of the cervix. (From Marshall FF, Treiger BFG: Urol Clin North Am 1991; 18:765–775.)

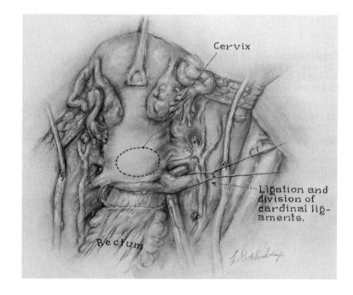

Figure 105–25. The vasculature within the cardinal ligament is ligated and divided to allow exposure of the vagina after the vagina has been mobilized off the rectosigmoid. (From Marshall FF, Treiger BFG: Urol Clin North Am 1991; 18:765–775.)

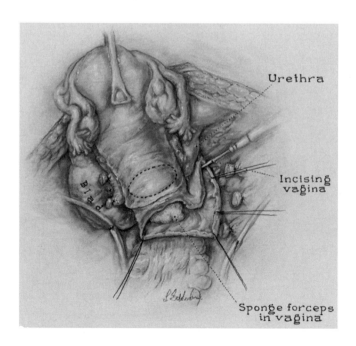

Figure 105–26. A sponge stick is placed in the vagina, and the cautery is used to incise the vagina directly. Stay sutures facilitate the dissection and improve hemostasis. (From Marshall FF, Treiger BFG: Urol Clin North Am 1991; 18:765–775.)

the anterior vaginal wall remains with the cystectomy specimen. Additional sutures are placed for hemostasis as required.

Anterior Dissection

Once the posterior dissection is essentially complete, the anterior dissection is started and is similar to that in the male in many respects. The endopelvic fascia is divided (Fig. 105–27). The pubourethral suspensory ligaments are divided, and they are analogous to the puboprostatic ligaments in the male. The urethra and bladder drop inferiorly. The dorsal vein of the clitoris is identified and oversewn in a manner similar to the dorsal vein in the penis (see Fig. 105–27). The urethra can then be dissected under the dorsal vein complex. Ultimately the only remaining attachments of the specimen are the urethral meatus and a small portion of the vagina. **Some of the urethra can be maintained, and continent diversion has been performed to the urethra in the female** (Stein et al, 1994).

Vaginal Dissection and Completion of Operation

At this point in the operation, the ovaries, fallopian tubes, uterus, anterior vagina, and cervix are attached only by a small portion of the anterior vagina and urethra (Fig. 105–28). The remaining vagina can be incised.

At this time, the patient's legs are spread and elevated. A Guelpi retractor can be placed to spread the labia, and the urethral meatus can be incised circumferentially. Usually,

there is a minimal amount of resection required to free the meatus. The dissection is carried along the urethra, and the entire specimen can then be removed (Fig. 105–29).

If the patient is sexually active and the tumor is not large, the vagina can be reconstructed. The vaginal flap can be closed in either a posterior-anterior or vertical plane, depending on the amount of vagina present. Usually a povidone-iodine (Betadine) pack is left in place.

Later, vaginal reconstruction can be accomplished by skin grafts, various muscle flaps, and bowel segments. Colonic segments appear to be preferable to small bowel segments. It is preferable to defer vaginal reconstruction, if necessary, to a later date when there is no tumor recurrence or chemotherapy. The patient and the surgeon can then decide if an elective additional surgery is indicated.

Hemovac or suction drains are placed, and then the urinary diversion is performed. Typically the author has closed the midline incision with either a heavy nylon or heavy monofilament absorbable suture.

Postoperative Management and Complications

The Betadine pack is usually removed 36 to 48 hours after the operation. Hemovac drains are removed after the urinary tract is verified to be intact radiographically. The urinary diversion often dictates much of the postoperative management. If women have a continent urinary diversion, they are often sent home with drainage tubes and suprapubic tubes for 1 month and are asked to return for tube removal and catheterization instructions.

The usual postoperative complications can occur, includ-

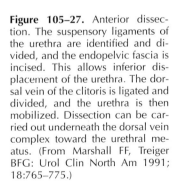

Figure 105–27. Anterior dissection. The suspensory ligaments of the urethra are identified and divided, and the endopelvic fascia is incised. This allows inferior displacement of the urethra. The dorsal vein of the clitoris is ligated and divided, and the urethra is then mobilized. Dissection can be carried out underneath the dorsal vein complex toward the urethral meatus. (From Marshall FF, Treiger BFG: Urol Clin North Am 1991; 18:765–775.)

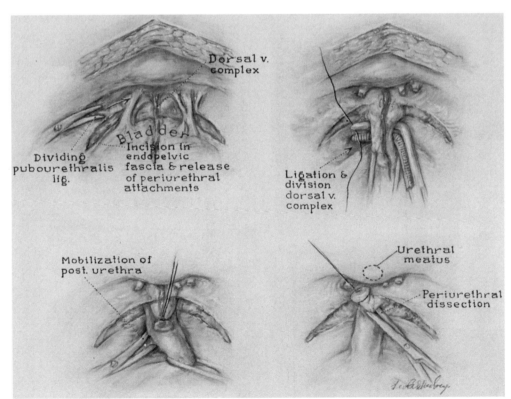

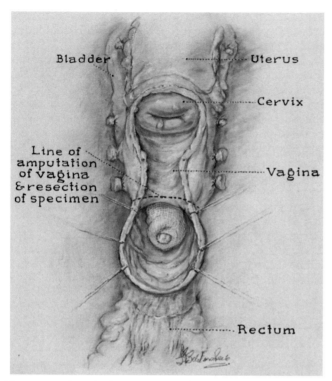

Figure 105–28. Only the vaginal wall and urethra remain. The vagina is amputated. (From Marshall FF, Treiger BFG: Urol Clin North Am 1991; 18:765–775.)

ing pulmonary, venous, or wound problems. Because of potential contamination with a vaginal dissection, extensive intraoperative irrigation with antibiotic solution is performed. Attempts are made to avoid all the usual problems of phlebitis, atelectasis, or infection. It is still possible to preserve sexual function postcystectomy in the woman (Schover and von Eschenbach, 1985).

Summary

Radical cystectomy in the female or anterior exenteration can be performed with a disciplined anatomic approach. The

pelvic lymphadenectomy provides for staging, and excision of the uterus and adjacent organs reduces the potential for pelvic recurrence. In certain patients, vaginal reconstruction and continent urinary diversion can provide for continued sexual function and urinary continence if there is no neoplastic involvement of the urethra or the immediate bladder neck (Coloby et al, 1994).

SIMPLE CYSTECTOMY

Indications

Simple cystectomy is not performed commonly. It is more typically performed for benign conditions rather than malignancy. It is defined as removal of the bladder but maintaining of the urethra in women or the prostate and seminal vesicles in men. **Various conditions may warrant simple cystectomy, including pyocystis in patients with neurogenic bladders,** particularly if they have already had some form of permanent urinary diversion. **There may be other rare indications, such as interstitial cystitis or fistulas in which the bladder is nonfunctional.** Other problems may relate to radiation cystitis or the effects of chemotherapy, particularly cyclophosphamide (Cytoxan) cystitis with severe hematuria, frequency, and dysuria.

Surgical Technique

The technique of antegrade simple cystectomy can be similar to that described for radical cystectomy earlier. This retrograde approach may be attractive, especially if there has already been a urinary diversion performed. The bladder is distended after a catheter has been placed to allow somewhat easier dissection. The veins on the surface of the prostate at 12 o'clock coursing over the prostate to the bladder can be ligated and divided. The cautery is used to divide the bladder neck (Fig. 105–30). If necessary, individual bleeding points can be sutured or ligated (Fig. 105–31). The bladder neck is divided entirely, and the ureteral orifices are visualized. The

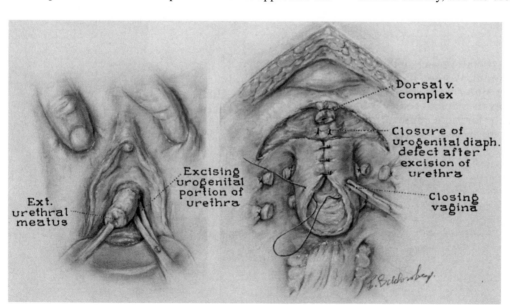

Figure 105–29. The vaginal dissection completes the operation with a circumscribed incision around the urethral meatus. The specimen can then be removed. The vagina is reconstructed. (From Marshall FF, Treiger BFG: Urol Clin North Am 1991; 18:765–775.)

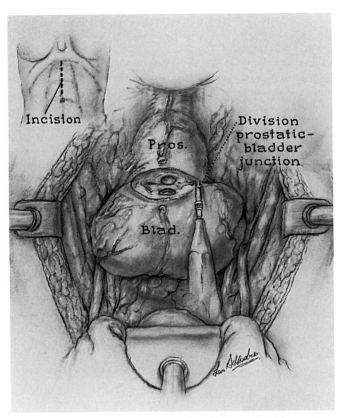

Figure 105–30. The cautery is used to divide the bladder neck.

incision is extended through the bladder neck to the area of the seminal vesicles.

The dissection is then carried along the seminal vesicles, and the bladder is immobilized off the ampulla of the vas and seminal vesicles (see Fig. 105–31). The prostate itself is oversewn. Some additional tissue may be resected so that it can be closed in two layers with running absorbable suture (see Fig. 105–31). Allis clamps can be placed on the bladder and the dissection continued along the rectum (Fig. 105–32). Often, this plane can be continued to the peritoneal reflection. The peritoneum is dissected off the superior aspect of the bladder.

The remaining superior middle vesical branches are individually ligated and divided (Fig. 105–33), and the specimen is then removed.

Alternatively the antegrade approach can involve initial dissection of the bladder with it slightly inflated, which can facilitate the dissection. The dissection can be initially carried down the hypogastric vessels with ligation of the superior vesical and middle vesical arteries. The peritoneum can be dissected off the dome, and the plane behind the bladder to the level of the prostate can be dissected bluntly. Seminal vesicles and ampulla of the vas can sometimes be identified if the patient is not too obese.

The remainder of the vesical pedicles can be ligated and divided, and the cautery can be used to divide the bladder

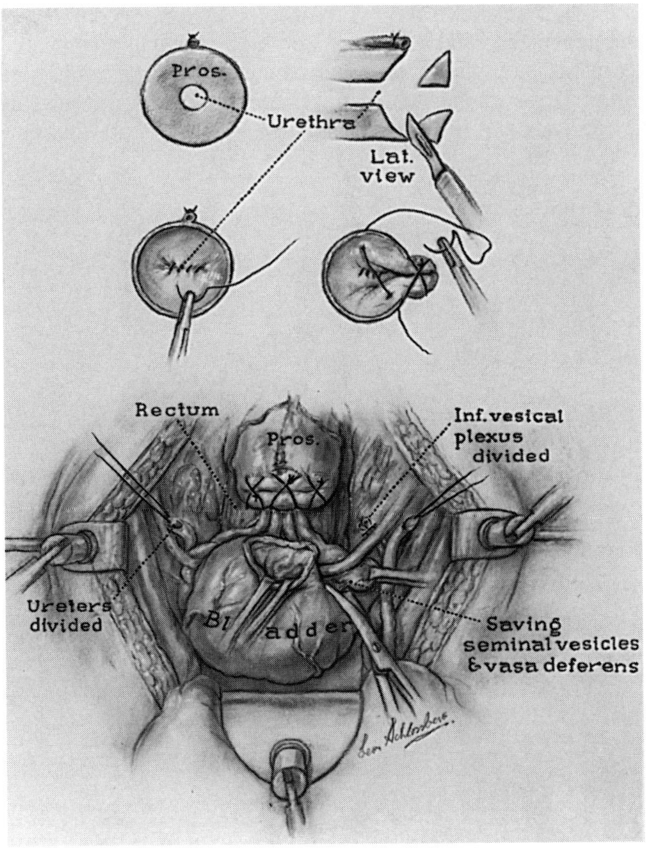

Figure 105–31. The bladder neck is divided, and the prostate is incised so that it can be closed in two layers.

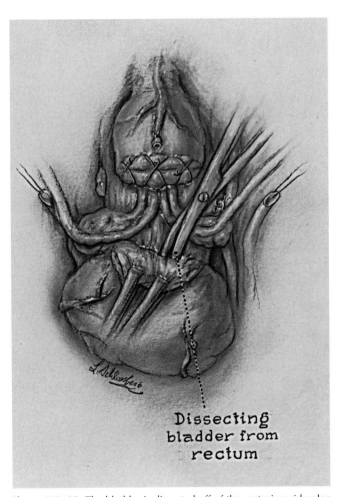

Figure 105–32. The bladder is dissected off of the rectosigmoid colon.

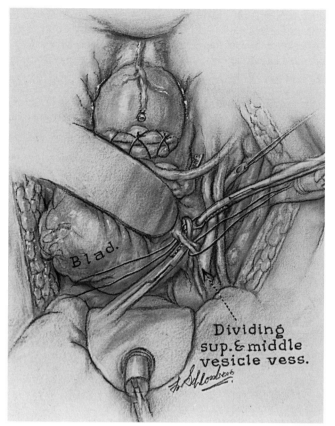

Figure 105–33. The superior and middle vesical branches are individually ligated and divided.

neck. The prostate is oversewn as previously indicated. The wound is irrigated, and typically a drain is left for several days.

Postoperative Management and Complications

The complications of simple cystectomy relate in part to the reasons for the cystectomy. Complications may be related to tumor if the cystectomy is only for palliation, or there can be problems with rectal injury or infection if there has been fistula formation, radiation, or previous infection.

PARTIAL CYSTECTOMY

Indications

Partial cystectomy has been performed since the 1800s but became more popular in the 1950s when it was thought that many bladder cancer patients would be candidates for this operation. Transurethral resection, however, made it possible initially to resect most tumors, and many patients were found to have widespread transitional cell carcinoma, which precluded resection of a portion of the bladder. As many as half of the patients undergoing partial cystectomy developed recurrent bladder tumor (Lindahl et al, 1984).

Although performed relatively infrequently, there still

is a place for partial cystectomy in an appropriate candidate. **If there is a transitional cell carcinoma located toward the dome of the bladder away from the bladder neck and trigone, a partial cystectomy may be indicated if there is no evidence of tumor anywhere else on random biopsy specimens.** If there is a tumor within a diverticulum, a partial cystectomy may be indicated. **Another indication is a urachal adenocarcinoma that occurs in the dome** and may extend up the urachus toward the umbilicus (Burnett et al, 1991). A partial cystectomy is not indicated when there are multiple tumors at many sites within the bladder, in the presence of carcinoma in situ, or with tumors involving the bladder neck or posterior urethra. Although some have suggested that tumors can be excised with a partial cystectomy in the area of the trigone with ureteral reimplants (Brannan et al, 1978; Kaneti, 1986), it is probably not a good idea to consider this kind of resection frequently.

Before surgery, cystoscopy and multiple biopsy specimens can determine whether there is widespread flat carcinoma in situ. Bimanual examination may help determine the extent of the tumor. A CT scan should be performed to rule out any metastatic disease in the pelvis, abdomen, or chest. After this careful evaluation, a partial cystectomy can then be considered.

Surgical Technique

The patient is placed flat on the table with the umbilicus over the break in the table, and the table is bent to open the pelvis. Typically a vertical midline incision is made extending from above the symphysis to below the umbilicus. The retroperitoneal space is entered. Urachal adenocarcinoma can be treated with a partial cystectomy (Burnett et al, 1991). The urachus and obliterated umbilical arteries are resected up to the umbilicus, and this resection is then

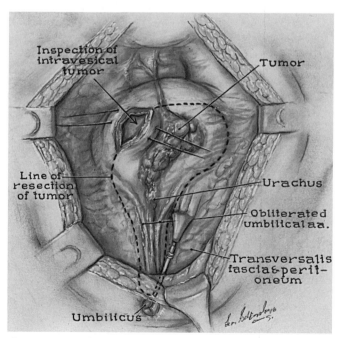

Figure 105–34. The urachus and obliterated umbilical vessels are included en bloc with the partial cystectomy specimen.

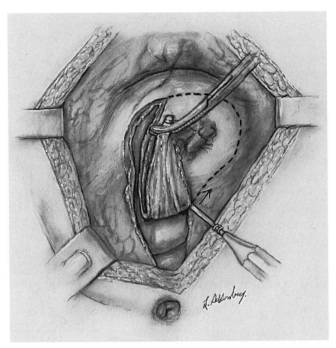

Figure 105–35. A 1- to 2-cm margin is included around the gross tumor.

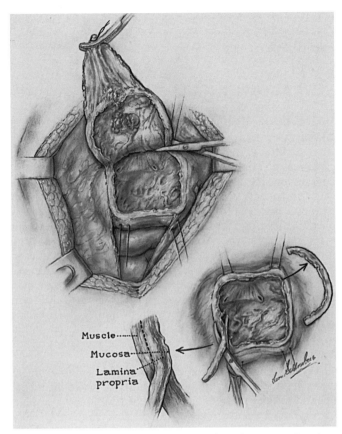

Figure 105–36. A wide margin is excised, and an extensive, long segment of remaining bladder is excised for frozen microscopic pathologic evaluation.

extended down toward the bladder (Fig. 105–34). The peritoneum is dissected off the bladder laterally, but a portion of the peritoneum may be taken if there is any adherence in the area of the tumor. The bladder should be carefully mobilized so that there is abundant bladder wall available beyond any palpable tumor. Sometimes the initial dissection is facilitated by filling the bladder so that one can dissect around the sides of the bladder more easily. The lateral wall of the bladder is dissected. Then the urine is removed through the previously placed catheter, and a small vesicostomy is made so that the tumor can be carefully inspected. All of the other tissue in the pelvis is packed off so that there will not be any obvious spillage (see Fig. 105–34). Cautery is then used to dissect around the tumor mass with at least a 1- to 2-cm margin of tissue in apparent normal bladder (Fig. 105–35).

Stay sutures are placed, which often facilitate the dissection. Cautery or scissors can be used to excise remaining bladder wall with an apparent wide margin of normal tissue (Fig. 105–36). On completion of resection of the specimen, a frozen section margin is obtained, with a portion of the lateral aspects of the bladder wall excised all the way down on each side. Each side is sent separately (see Fig. 105–36). Assuming the frozen sections are negative and no other lesions are seen, the bladder is then closed in two layers, first a running mucosal and submucosal suture usually with chromic suture. An additional second layer of running suture is also performed (Fig. 105–37). A catheter is left in the bladder, and the bladder is inflated to be sure there is no leak.

A drain is brought out through a separate stab wound lateral to the incision. The fascia is usually closed with a No. 1 polydioxanone (PDS) suture. Typically a urethral catheter rather than a suprapubic tube is left as drainage.

Postoperative Management and Complications

Tumor recurrence is frequent in a partial cystectomy patient and has occurred in from one third to three quarters of patients (Kaneti, 1986). Other immediate problems include prolonged urinary drainage, but usually this resolves if the bladder is closed properly and drained satisfactorily. Good technique reduces wound infection or development of a hernia.

Patients who have undergone partial cystectomy should have cystoscopy and urinary cytologic examination every 3 months for at least 2 years. Regular CT scans of the pelvis and abdomen are recommended, par-

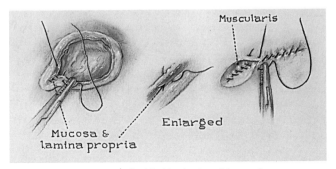

Figure 105–37. The bladder is closed in two layers.

ticularly in the first several years of follow-up. In well-selected patients, partial cystectomy can yield favorable results (Brannan et al, 1978) with a survival rate of 58%.

VESICAL DIVERTICULECTOMY

Indications and Preoperative Management

Vesical diverticula result from herniation of bladder mucosa through the muscular wall. Typically, vesical diverticula occur in patients with obstructive lower urinary tract problems and are found frequently in older men. Primary congenital diverticula are less common. **Most vesical diverticula occur anterolateral to the ureteral orifice because this is a weak point within the bladder.** The presence of a diverticulum is not a specific indication for surgery. Persistent infection, stone formation, or ureteral obstruction may be specific indications for surgery (Fox et al, 1962; McLean and Kelalis, 1968). Tumors occurring within a diverticulum are worrisome and often associated with a worse prognosis because of the poor detrusor wall around the diverticulum (Melekos et al, 1987).

An intravenous pyelogram should be obtained to evaluate the upper tracts and determine anatomically where the diverticulum resides. A voiding cystourethrogram may also help the assessment of the bladder and the diverticulum. Cystoscopy is important to be certain there is no tumor or other important feature that may be unrecognized.

Surgical Technique

Bladder diverticulectomy can be performed in three ways: intravesically, extravesically, or transurethrally. Complete destructionly transurethrally may be difficult.

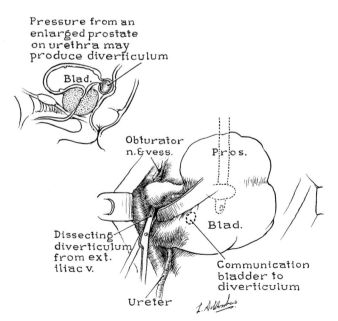

Figure 105–38. Initial dissection of the diverticulum along the pelvic side wall also identifies the vasculature.

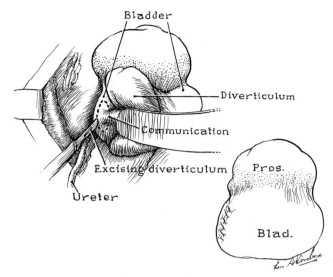

Figure 105–39. The mouth of the diverticulum is identified, and the ureter is identified. The bladder is closed in two layers.

With a larger diverticulum, an extravesical or intravesical approach may be most feasible. An intravesical approach was originally described by Young in 1906. The mucosal lining can sometimes be removed without excising the entire pseudocapsule. Some of these diverticula can be difficult to dissect and may be adherent to vessels, rectum, or other vital structures.

The extravesical approach may require dissection from the iliac vessels (Fig. 105–38). After dissection along the pelvic sidewall, the bladder diverticulum and its smaller mouth can be identified, and then the diverticulum can be excised. Ligation and division of multiple vesical vascular branches may be required to facilitate this dissection. The bladder is then oversewn in two layers (Fig. 105–39). Typically the mucosa is oversewn with running absorbable suture, and then the muscularis is closed in a second layer.

At times, it may be easier to open the bladder and identify the opening of the diverticulum. It is typically adjacent to the ureteral orifice, so catheterization of the ureter may be helpful. To avoid injury to the ureter during the dissection, the bladder can then be opened into the ostium of the diverticulum. Then either the diverticulum can be dissected in its entirety, or the mucosa can be dissected depending on the extent of the diverticulum.

Ultimately the bladder can then be closed, and a drain is typically left in this area to ensure adequate drainage if there is a small urine leak. This repair has been summarized by Brendler (1991).

Postoperative Management and Complications

Postoperative urinary drainage is exceedingly important following open diverticulectomy. If there is any question about the ureter, a reimplant may be performed, and radiographic verification of the ureter should be obtained postoperatively.

VESICAL FISTULAS

Vesicovaginal Fistula

Vesicovaginal fistulas are covered in part in Chapter 37. Outside the United States and in many parts of the world, vesicovaginal fistulas are often related to trauma during labor and delivery. **In the United States, vesicovaginal fistula is more likely to be iatrogenic, particularly following gynecologic procedures, especially hysterectomy.** A fistula can occur between the vagina and the bladder or ureter (Selzman et al, 1995) (Fig. 105–40).

Preoperative Management

Complete urologic evaluation is important, including an intravenous pyelogram, cystoscopy, and vaginoscopy. Fluoroscopy may be helpful in identifying a ureteral fistula with a retrograde pyelogram. If urinary leakage is not clear, methylene blue can be instilled into the bladder with a pack in the vagina.

Surgical Technique

The approaches can be vaginal or abdominal. For a small fistula, a vaginal approach may be reasonable. The fistula can be excised circumferentially. The wound is then closed with multiple layers with the closure first of the bladder wall. An interposition of a Martius flap may be helpful from the labia (Martius, 1928). The vagina can then be closed in multiple layers with an attempt to avoid overlapping suture lines.

A transabdominal approach can be performed for larger, more complicated fistulas. This retroperitoneal approach is usually employed with a midline vertical incision or a Pfannenstiel incision. The bladder is opened, and the fistula can

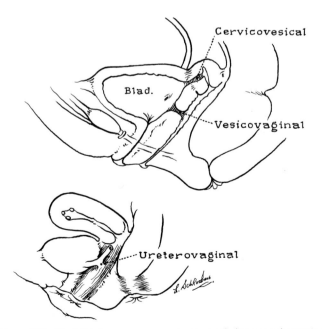

Figure 105–40. A fistula can occur most commonly between the vagina and the bladder or ureter.

be identified, usually close to the trigone. The bladder can be dissected or divided down to this fistula tract. The fistula tract can be excised, and then the bladder and vagina can be closed separately and omentum can be placed to improve the repair (Turner-Warwick, 1976).

Postoperative Management and Complications

Antibiotic therapy is usually maintained, and catheters and drains are left in place. A cystogram is typically obtained before a voiding trial to be sure there is no leak, and then a voiding trial is initiated.

Vesicoenteric Fistula

A fistula connection between bladder and bowel is usually caused by bowel disease. **Vesicoenteric fistulas are most commonly associated with diverticulitis in about half of patients** (Kirsh et al, 1991). **Crohn's disease** (Billips and Marshall, 1989), **carcinoma of the colon, or other pelvic malignancies can also produce fistulas.** Although barium enema has been advocated as an excellent method of diagnosing this condition, cystoscopy and a cystogram have been perhaps more effective in making this diagnosis (Kirsh et al, 1991). CT can also be highly effective in diagnosing a fistula. Small amounts of gas can be seen in the bladder or fistula tract, and associated lesions can also be diagnosed. As one might expect, a fistula on the left side of the dome of the bladder suggests diverticulitis. On the right side, it might be more likely to be associated with Crohn's disease.

Spontaneous closure of vesicoenteric fistula is unusual. Malignancies, diverticulitis, and Crohn's disease (Fig. 105–41) all require different treatment. Surgical repair is typically directed at the primary bowel process, and the bladder is a secondary feature. **Ordinarily a segment of bowel is resected** after appropriate bowel preparation and antibiotic coverage. Sometimes a staged repair and colostomy may be necessary. Usually a portion of the bladder wall is resected and closed in multiple layers. Omentum used as interposition can be helpful. A Foley catheter is usually left in place for 8 to 10 days, and a cystogram is done before removal.

Y-V-PLASTY OF THE BLADDER NECK

Indications

The primary indication for a Y-V-plasty of the bladder neck is a bladder neck contracture. Frequently, this occurs after suprapubic prostatectomy or transurethral resection of the prostate. More commonly, transurethral incision of a bladder neck contracture suffices, and an open bladder neck plasty is not necessary. If there has been extensive scarring and transurethral incisions have failed, an open revision may be required.

Surgical Technique

A small suprapubic incision is made through the bladder neck and through the scarred area. This full-thickness inci-

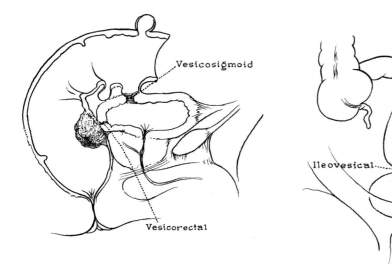

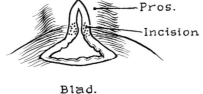

Figure 105–41. Colovesical fistulas commonly occur from carcinoma or diverticulitis on the left side. On the right side, inflammatory bowel is more common.

sion then allows advancement of more pliable detrusor musculature through the bladder neck into the prostatic urethra (Fig. 105–42). A large Foley catheter is left in place for at least 7 days and then is removed.

SUPRAPUBIC CYSTOSTOMY

Although there are many percutaneous methods of performing a suprapubic cystostomy, open placement is sometimes performed in conjunction with prostatectomy, vesicolithotomy, or vesicodiverticulectomy. **It is important to create a direct tract so that the suprapubic tube is not angled** (Fig. 105–43). The bladder can be tacked to the

transversalis fascia. This straight tract allows easy changing of the suprapubic tube at a later date if the catheter is to be left in place for a longer period of time. Absorbable sutures are used.

ACKNOWLEDGMENTS

The author would specifically like to recognize the significant previous contributions of Peter Schlegel and Patrick Walsh for their chapter on Radical Cystectomy (in the male) that appeared in *Operative Urology* (Marshall FF, editor; Philadelphia, W. B. Saunders, 1991) and Charles Brendler for his chapter on Urethrectomy that appeared in *Campbell's Urology*, 6th edition.

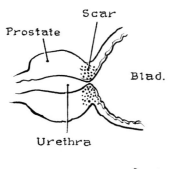

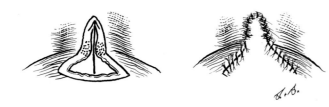

Figure 105–42. An incision through the entire scarred contracted bladder neck allows placement of supple detrusor musculature in this space.

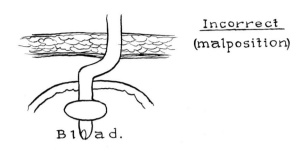

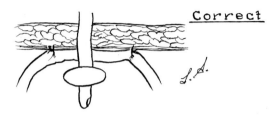

Figure 105–43. A straight, short tract is best for placement of a suprapubic tube.

REFERENCES

Radical Cystectomy in the Male

Bracken RB, McDonad MW, Johnson DE: Complications of single stage radical cystectomy and ileal conduit. Urology 1981; 27:141–146.

Brendler CB, Steinberg GD, Marshall FF, et al: Local recurrence and survival following nerve-sparing cystoprostatectomy. J Urol 1990; 144:1137–1140.

Hendry WF: Morbidity and mortality of radical cystectomy (1971–78 and 1978–85). J R Soc Med 1986; 79:395–400.

Hinman F: The technique and late results of ureterointestinal implantation and cystectomy for cancer of the bladder. Int Soc Urol Rep 1939; 7:464–524.

Marshall FF, Mostwin JL, Radebaugh LC, et al: Ileocolic neobladder postcystectomy: Continence and potency. J Urol 1991; 145:502–504.

Schlegel PN, Walsh PC: Neuroanatomical approach to radical cystoprostatectomy with preservation of sexual function. J Urol 1987; 138:1402–1406.

Steiner MS, Marshall FF: Mini-laparotomy staging pelvic lymphadenectomy (minilap): Alternative to standard and laparoscopic pelvic lymphadenectomy. Urology 1993; 41:201–206.

Thrasher JB, Crawford ED: Current management of invasive and metastatic transitional cell carcinoma of the bladder. J Urol 1993; 149:957–972.

Young HH, Davis DM: Young's Practice of Urology, Vol 12. Philadelphia, W. B. Saunders, 1926.

Urethrectomy

Brendler CB, Schlegel PN, Walsh PC: Urethrectomy with preservation of potency. J Urol 1990; 144:270–273.

Levinson AK, Johnson DE, Wishnow KI: Indications for urethrectomy in an era of continent urinary diversion. J Urol 1990; 144:73–75.

Schlegel PN, Walsh PC: Neuroanatomical approach to radical cystoprostatectomy with preservation of sexual function. J Urol 1987; 138:1402–1406.

Radical Cystectomy in the Female

Chin JL, Wolf RM, Huben RP, Pantes JE: Vaginal recurrence after cystectomy for bladder cancer. J Urol 1985; 134:58–61.

Coloby PJ, Kakizoe T, Tobisu K, Sakamoto M: Urethral involvement in female bladder cancer patients: Mapping of 47 consecutive cysto-urethrectomy specimens. J Urol 1994; 152:1438–1442.

Marshall FF, Treiger BFG: Radical cystectomy (anterior exenteration) in the female patient. Urol Clin North Am 1991; 18:765–775.

Marshall VF, Schnittman M: Vaginal cystectomy. J Urol 1947; 57:848–857.

Paepe ME, Rubin A, Mahaderia P: Urethral involvement in female patients with bladder cancer. Cancer 1990; 65:1237.

San Felippo CJ, Kessler R: Vaginal cystectomy. Urology 1978; 12:542–544.

Schover LR, von Eschenbach AC: Sexual function and female radical cystectomy: A case series. J Urol 1985; 134:465.

Stein JP, Stenzl A, Essrig D, et al: Lower urinary tract reconstruction following cystectomy in women using the Kock ileal reservoir with bilateral ureteroileal urethrostomy: Initial clinical experience. J Urol 1994; 152:1404–1408.

Partial Cystectomy

Brannan W, Ochsner MG, Fuselier HA Jr, Landry GR: Partial cystectomy in the treatment of transitional cell carcinoma of the bladder. J Urol 1978; 119:213.

Burnett AL, Epstein JI, Marshall FF: Adenocarcinoma of the urinary bladder: Classification and management. Urology 1991; 37:315–321.

Kaneti J: Partial cystectomy in the management of bladder carcinoma. Eur Urol 1986; 12:249.

Lindahl F, Jorgensen P, Egvad K: Partial cystectomy for transitional cell carcinoma of the bladder. Scand J Urol Nephrol 1984; 18:125.

Vesical Diverticulectomy

Brendler CB: Vesical diverticulectomy. In Marshall FF, ed: Operative Urology. Philadelphia, W. B. Saunders, 1991, pp 119–123.

Fox M, Power RF, Bruce AW: Diverticulum of the bladder-presentation and evaluation of treatment of 115 cases. Br J Urol 1962; 34:286.

McLean P, Kelalis PP: Bladder diverticulum in the male. Br J Urol 1968; 40:321.

Melekos MD, Asbach HW, Barbalis GA: Vesical diverticula: Etiology, diagnosis, tumor genesis, and treatment. Urology 1987; 30:453–457.

Young HH: The operative treatment of vesical diverticulum with report of four cases. Johns Hopkins Hosp Rep 1906; 13:411.

Fistulas

Billups KL, Marshall FF: Urologic complications. In Bayless T, ed: Current Management of Inflammatory Bowel Disease. Philadelphia, B. C. Decker, 1989, pp 187–191.

Kirsh GM, Hampel N, Schack JM, Resnick MI: Diagnosis and management of vesicoenteric fistulas. Surg Gynecol Obstet 1991; 173:91–97.

Martius H: The repair of vesicovaginal fistulae with interposition pedicle graft of labial tissue. Zentrabl Gynakol 1928; 52:480.

Selzman AA, Spirnak JP, Kursh ED: The changing management of uretero-vaginal fistulas. J Urol 1995; 153:626–628.

Turner-Warwick R: The use of omental pedicle graft in urinary tract reconstruction. J Urol 1976; 116:341.

106
SURGERY OF THE SEMINAL VESICLES

Richard D. Williams, M.D.
Jay I. Sandlow, M.D.

The seminal vesicles were first described by Fallopius in 1561 (Brewster, 1985) as paired male organs. **Primary pathology within the seminal vesicles is rare, but secondary lesions are more common.** In the past, insufficient imaging methods led to infrequent definition of either primary or secondary seminal vesicle pathology. **The use of ultrasonography, computed tomography (CT), and magnetic resonance imaging (MRI) has improved diagnostic visibility and facilitated the diagnosis and treatment of seminal vesicle pathology.** Surgical intervention is rarely needed but may be required with congenital cysts with infection or obstruction causing infertility; ureteral ectopy into a seminal vesicle with resultant obstruction or dysplasia of the ipsilateral kidney; and primary tumors, either benign or malignant. Surgical access to the seminal vesicles is mostly by way of routes familiar to the urologic surgeon, but surgery on the seminal vesicles alone (without adjacent organ removal) is a unique challenge.

EMBRYOLOGY

Normal Development

An understanding of the normal embryologic development of the seminal vesicles is necessary for the diagnosis and treatment of diseases involving these structures. **The seminal vesicle, a strictly male organ (no female homologue), develops as a dorsolateral bulbous swelling of the distal mesonephric duct at approximately 12 fetal weeks** (Arey, 1965; Brewster, 1985). Initially the cloaca is subdivided by downward growth of the urorectal septum into the posterior anal canal and the anterior urogenital sinus (Fig. 106–1A). The division is completed around the seventh week. The mesonephric duct (wolffian duct) is thus included in an area termed the *vesicourethral canal* within the urogenital sinus. The ureter is a bud initiating from the mesonephric duct at 4 weeks that eventually attains a separate opening into the bladder by absorption and cranial migration (Fig. 106–1B). The mesonephric duct becomes the vas deferens, which normally drains into the urethra at the ejaculatory duct where it is surrounded by the prostatic glands. **Separate symmetric buds extend from the distal mesonephric duct just proximal to the ejaculatory duct at approximately 12 weeks to form the seminal vesicles** (Fig. 106–1C).

Embryologic Abnormalities

Developmental anomalies form by alteration of this orderly process. If the ureteral bud arises too far cranially on

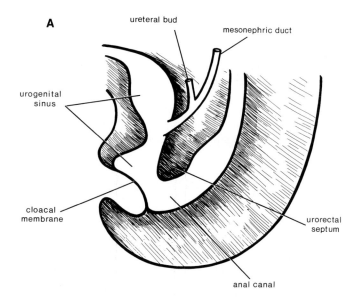

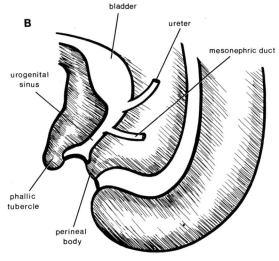

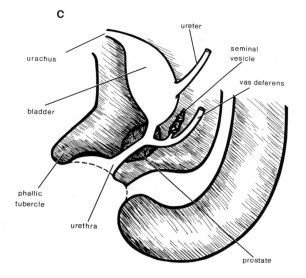

Figure 106–1. Intrauterine (fetal) development of the seminal vesicles. *A,* Fifth week. *B,* Eighth week. *C,* Thirteenth week. (Redrawn from Langman J: Medical Embryology, 4th ed. Baltimore, Williams & Wilkins, 1981, pp 242–243.)

the mesonephric duct, it is absorbed late. This results in failure to meet the metanephric blastema, thus leading to renal dysplasia or agenesis as well as causing the ureter to enter ectopically anywhere along the vas deferens or posterior urethra (MacDonald, 1986; Tanagho, 1976). **Gordon and Kessler (1972) have shown that 50% of ectopic ureters in males enter the posterior urethra, whereas 30% join the seminal vesicle. The remainder enter the vas deferens or the ejaculatory ducts.** Because formation of the seminal vesicles occurs at week 12 of embryogenesis, an alteration in ureteral bud development from the mesonephric duct may have an impact on formation of the seminal vesicles. There is an association between absence of the seminal vesicle and ipsilateral renal anomalies (see later).

PHYSIOLOGY

The physiologic role of the seminal vesicle is not entirely known; however, the secreted fluid is important in the motility and metabolism of ejaculated sperm. **The secretions from the seminal vesicle contribute approximately 50% to 80% of the ejaculate volume, with an average volume of 2.5 ml and a pH in the neutral-to-alkaline range** (Mawhinney, 1992). Seminal vesicle secretions contain primarily carbohydrates such as fructose, a necessary component for sperm motility, and prostaglandins E, A, B, and F as well as a coagulation factor (Tauber et al, 1975, 1976).

ANATOMY

General Description

The normal adult seminal vesicle is 5 to 10 cm in length and 3 to 5 cm in diameter. The volume capacity of the seminal vesicle averages 13 ml. The right gland is slightly larger than the left in one third of men, but the size of both decreases with advancing age (Redman, 1987). There are three major anatomic types, but the most common contains one central canal with minimal tortuosity and only a few side branches (Aboul-Azm, 1979). The major canal of the seminal vesicle empties into the ejaculatory duct (2.2 cm average length) at the terminal portion of the vas deferens within the prostate.

Vasculature and Innervation

The blood supply to the seminal vesicle is from the vesiculodeferential artery, a branch of the umbilical artery (Braithwaite, 1952). Occasionally the inferior vesicle artery provides a communicating vessel. **Venous drainage is from the vesiculodeferential veins and the inferior vesical plexus.** The seminal vesicles are innervated by the pelvic nerve and the hypogastric nerve. The hypogastric nerve sends both adrenergic and cholinergic fibers to the seminal vesicles (Mawhinney, 1992). Lymphatic drainage is by way of the internal iliac nodes.

PHYSICAL EXAMINATION AND LABORATORY TESTING

Previously, physical diagnosis and vasography were the only diagnostic tools available for studying the seminal vesicle. Transrectal ultrasound (TRUS), CT, and MRI have each added substantially to examination and diagnosis of pathologic conditions of the seminal vesicle (Fig. 106–2).

The normal seminal vesicle and adjacent ducts are not palpable in the normal male. On rectal examination, the area directly craniad to the base of the prostate where the seminal vesicles reside is soft and nondescript. The seminal vesicles lie anterior to the surrounding relatively thick and inelastic two layers of Denonvilliers' fascia, but no anatomic detail of the vesicles or ducts is usually appreciated by palpation even if the glands are asymmetric. The area immediately above the prostate on rectal examination may be enlarged and relatively compressible in the presence of a seminal vesicle cyst or solid and firm if there is a seminal vesicle tumor. These lesions may compress the bladder base anteriorly instead and, thus, not be readily palpable. Secondary involvement of the seminal vesicle from the prostate or bladder is palpated as hard areas above the prostate but may not be absolutely definable on physical examination.

Laboratory examination of seminal vesicle fluid requires obtaining a semen sample and testing directly for exclusively seminal vesicle excretions, such as fructose, and indirectly by measuring the volume and observing liquefaction of the semen sample. **A low semen volume and lack of both fructose and liquefaction imply either absent seminal vesicles or ejaculatory duct obstruction.** Although the terminal portion of the ejaculate originates from the seminal vesicles, split ejaculate bacterial cultures are more likely

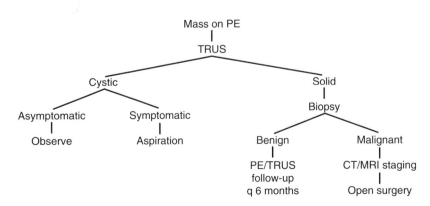

Figure 106–2. Algorithm for work-up of seminal vesicle mass on physical examination. PE, physical examination; TRUS, transrectal ultrasound; CT, computed tomography; MRI, magnetic resonance imaging.

contaminated by multiple other sites along the lower urinary tract and, thus, are not useful for localizing the site of infection (Stamey, 1980). TRUS-guided perineal aspiration cultures and abscess drainage have been successful, however (Lee et al, 1986).

Ultrasound

Ultrasound, by either the transabdominal or transrectal (preferred) route, **has become one of the most accurate methods of evaluating the seminal vesicle.** The advent of probes with high resolution at short focal lengths has allowed rapid, noninvasive, inexpensive, and accurate seminal vesical examination in an outpatient setting.

The normal seminal vesicle on TRUS is an elongated, flat, paired structure between the rectum and bladder just superior to the prostate (Fig. 106–3). The seminal vesicle appears predominantly symmetric and is smooth with apparent saccularity. The center of the seminal vesicle is echopenic with occasional areas of increased echogenicity relating to luminal folds within the vesicle itself (Carter et al, 1989). The ampulla of the vas can usually be seen, particularly near the prostate, as a tortuous tube on sagittal scans. The ejaculatory duct may also be seen within the substance of the prostate, but the lumen is not usually visible. The verumontanum is characteristically seen as a more densely echoic structure in the midline at the termination of the ejaculatory ducts. **Although sagittal images are best for examining the length of seminal vesicles and adjacent ductular anatomy, transaxial scans are best for detecting symmetry and volume.** TRUS of the seminal vesicles does not require any special preparation, although a half-full bladder allows easier differentiation of the vesicles and adjacent structures.

Abnormal findings on TRUS include seminal vesicle aplasia, atrophy, or cyst formation. Aplasia and atrophy are commonly associated with infertility in up to 2.5% of infertile men (Carter et al, 1989). Cysts, although quite rare, may be congenital and associated with an ipsilateral ectopic ureter or an agenetic kidney (or both) or acquired as a result of obstruction following transurethral prostatectomy. In one study, however, 5% of men screened for prostate cancer were found to have asymptomatic cystic dilation of the seminal vesicles (Wessels et al, 1992). The majority of patients with a seminal vesicle cyst are asymptomatic; however, they may present with urinary tract symptoms, including dysuria, painful ejaculation, hematospermia, or recurrent epididymitis. Ultrasound reveals these cystic lesions to be anechoic masses within the substance of the seminal vesicle or larger anechoic saccular lesions, which might rise out of the pelvis and displace the bladder and other pelvic structures (Steers and Corriere, 1986). Ultrasonography can be used to guide needle placement for drainage or contrast studies to delineate the lesion more fully (Shabsigh et al, 1989). Ultrasound has also been used to attempt to differentiate inflammatory conditions of the seminal vesicle; however, other than calcifications with chronic bilharziasis, the TRUS findings in patients with chronic prostatourethritis, prostatodynia, and other conditions are relatively nonspecific (Littrup et al, 1988).

Sonographic findings of a tumor within the seminal vesicle depend on whether the tumor is primary or secondary. Primary tumors are usually unilateral, whereas secondary tumors more likely involve both seminal vesicles and may be difficult to distinguish as to their origin (i.e., from the rectum, bladder, or prostate). The TRUS image of a solid tumor is isoechoic with respect to the prostate but relatively hyperechoic with respect to the normal seminal vesicle. **There are no image characteristics indicative of benign versus malignant or primary versus secondary tumors** except that primary tumors are commonly unilateral and tend not to be contiguous with the prostate, whereas prostate cancer invading the seminal vesicle may be at the base of both seminal vesicles and contiguous with the prostate tumor. Ultrasound-guided transrectal or perineal aspiration cy-

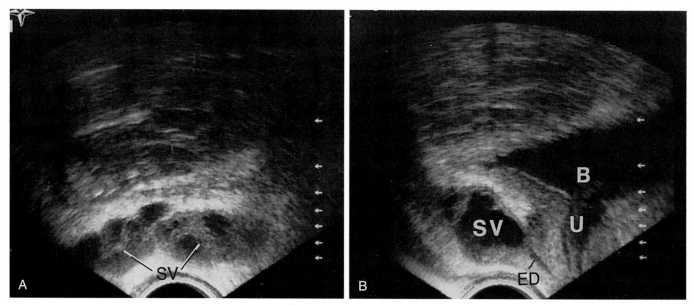

Figure 106–3. Transrectal ultrasound of normal seminal vesicles. *A,* Transverse view. *B,* Sagittal view. B, bladder; SV, seminal vesicle; U, urethra; ED, ejaculatory duct.

tologies or core biopsies can be useful to diagnose pathologically a seminal vesicle neoplasm.

Computed Tomography

CT is a considerable improvement over conventional radiography for evaluation of the pelvis. Evaluation of seminal vesicle pathology by CT, however, has not been systematically studied. Silverman and colleagues reviewed a group of 50 patients with normal seminal vesicles by CT and determined that the mean length was 3.1 cm, width 1.5 cm, and overall area 3.6 cm (Silverman et al, 1985). The volume tended to decrease with age, and the shape varied from ovoid (70%) to tubular (20%) to rounded (10%). The seminal vesicles were symmetric in 67% of those studied. **The seminal vesicles themselves are medium contrast structures (similar to muscle) routinely seen directly below the bladder.** The surrounding Denonvilliers' fascia is not discernible on CT. Goldstein and Schlossberg (1988) studied CT in patients who had absent vasa deferentia and found that not all had absent seminal vesicles, concluding that CT was accurate for detection of the presence of seminal vesicles. **CT has been used to detect congenital anomalies, and perhaps this may be its best use in seminal vesicle diagnosis** (Fig. 106–4). Cystic structures have CT attenuation numbers (Hounsfield units) from 0 to 10 similar to most clear fluid–filled structures, although the density may be higher secondary to debris, pus, or hemorrhage.

Tumors within the seminal vesicle are readily seen on CT as an enlarged vesicle with a higher CT attenuation number in the area of the tumor mass than in normal seminal vesicle and with a normal bladder and prostate (Fig. 106–5). The lesion may be cystic, however, as a result of tumor necrosis (King et al, 1989). **CT cannot distinguish between benign and malignant tumors and cannot routinely distinguish between primary and secondary tumors,** although tissue planes are usually obliterated by secondary tumors invading from prostate or rectum (Sussman et al, 1986). Inflammatory masses in the seminal vesicles, such as tuberculosis or old bacterial abscesses, can be calcified (Patel and Wilbur, 1987; Schwartz et al, 1988; Birnbaum et al, 1990) and thus distinguished from tumors,

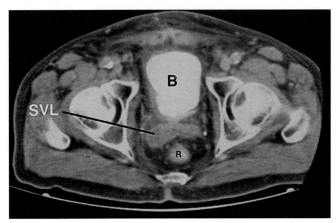

Figure 106–5. Computed tomography scan of seminal vesicle lymphoma (SVL). B, bladder; R, rectum.

although a history of infection and related symptoms can usually be elicited. A long-term history of diabetes mellitus has also been associated with seminal vesicle calcification (King et al, 1989).

Magnetic Resonance Imaging

Although MRI is not, in general, more sensitive than CT or ultrasound for diagnosis, the anatomic relationships are more clearly seen, multiplanar imaging is readily available, and the minimal amount of fat in the pelvis and **the characteristics of the magnetic resonance phenomenon (T1-weighted and T2-weighted image) allow for more definitive diagnosis of cystic lesions and more accurate staging of solid neoplasms in the pelvis.** In the normal situation, the anatomic relationships of the seminal vesicles are similar to those shown on CT except that on **T1-weighted images, seminal vesicles are of low signal intensity that increases substantially on T2-weighted images** (Fig. 106–6). This is thought to be secondary to the secretions present in the ductular lumen of the seminal vesicle. The surrounding Denonvilliers' fascia is of low intensity on both T1-weighted and T2-weighted images. In general, the T2-weighted images have lower signal intensity than fat in prepubertal children, similar to or higher than that of fat in adults, and similar to or lower than that of fat in patients older than 70 years of age. Endocrine and radiation therapy influence the size and intensity of the seminal vesicles (Secaf et al, 1991). Seminal vesicle cysts are similar to cysts in other locations in that the T1-weighted image is low intensity but the T2-weighted image is that of a unilocular smooth wall with a uniform high intensity and well-defined margin (Genevois et al, 1990; Hihara et al, 1993). Hemorrhagic cysts have a high intensity signal on both T1-weighted and T2-weighted images (Sue et al, 1989). Seminal vesiculitis shows a decreased signal intensity on T1-weighted image, whereas the T2-weighted image intensity is higher than that of both fat and the normal seminal vesicle.

MRI of seminal vesicle tumors shows a heterogeneous mass with a medium intensity on T1-weighted image and a heterogeneous intensity on T2-weighted image. There has been no systematic MRI study of seminal vesicle tumors,

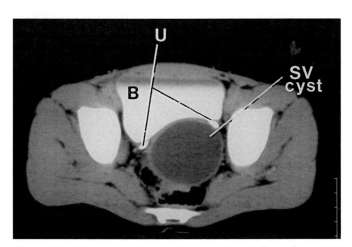

Figure 106–4. Computed tomography scan of seminal vesicle cyst (SV cyst). U, ureters; B, bladder.

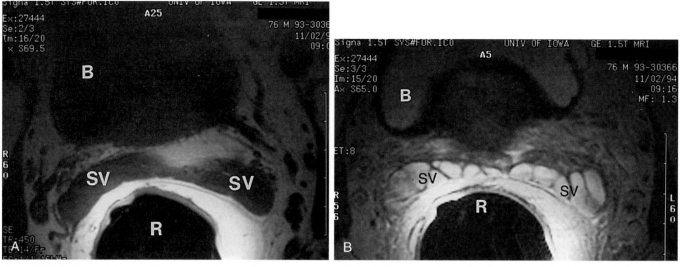

Figure 106–6. Transaxial magnetic resonance image of normal seminal vesicles (SV) using endorectal coil. *A*, T1-weighted image. *B*, T2-weighted image. B, bladder; R, rectum.

and it cannot distinguish between benign and malignant solid masses within the seminal vesicle.

Patients with a suspected seminal vesicle abnormality or mass felt on rectal examination should first have a TRUS (see Fig. 106–2). If the mass is solid and noncystic, a transperineal or TRUS-guided biopsy is a reasonable next step. If tumor is confirmed, a CT scan should be done next for staging purposes; MRI is necessary only to confirm the hemorrhagic nature of the mass or to stage more definitively the extent of the mass to contiguous organs within the pelvis. Definitive treatment for most seminal vesicle lesions, however, can be appropriately determined without MRI.

Vasography

Vasography, accomplished by either transurethral contrast injection at the seminal colliculus or surgical exposure of the scrotal vas and contrast injection, **was the preferred means to image the seminal vesicles until only recently** (Fig. 106–7). Transurethral routes of injection were often unsuccessful because of the time, special equipment, and expertise required. Antegrade injection through the surgically exposed vas is highly successful, particularly in evaluating duct obstruction in azoospermic individuals or those with prior surgical trauma (Al-Omari et al, 1985). **Vasogra-**

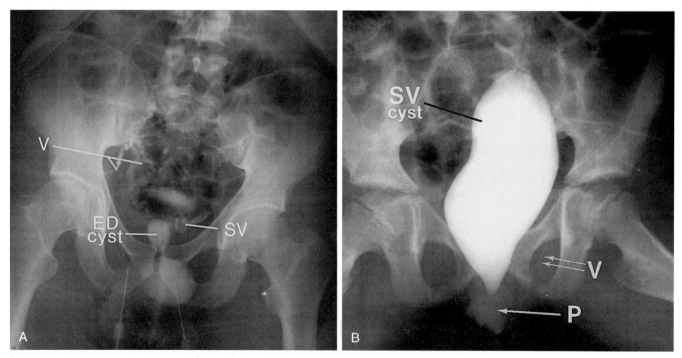

Figure 106–7. Vasograms in patients with ejaculatory duct/seminal vesicle cysts. *A*, Bilateral vasogram in a patient with right ejaculatory duct obstruction. *B*, Vasogram showing seminal vesicle cyst in patient from Figure 106–4. V, vas deferens; SV, seminal vesicle; ED, ejaculatory duct; P, prostate.

phy does not, however, provide accurate demonstration of the pathology of the seminal vesicles in patients with vesiculitis, cysts, or tumors (Dunnick et al, 1982; King et al, 1989). Direct transrectal needle seminal vesiculography has also been reported as a method for diagnosis or drug delivery but is not recommended for routine cases (Meyer et al, 1979; Fuse et al, 1988).

PATHOLOGY

Congenital Lesions

Agenesis of the Seminal Vesicles

Unilateral agenesis of the seminal vesicles is not uncommon, with an incidence of 0.6% to 1.0%. It may be associated with unilateral absence of the vas deferens as well as ipsilateral renal anomalies (Fig. 106–8). This is thought to result from an embryologic insult before the separation of the ureteral bud from the mesonephric duct, which typically occurs at 7 weeks' gestation. It is believed that if the insult occurs after 7 weeks' gestation, the seminal vesicle anomaly may not be associated with renal agenesis (Hall and Oates, 1993). The frequency of associated renal anomalies varies, but in one series, 79% of patients with absence of a seminal vesicle or vas deferens had ipsilateral renal agenesis, 12% had ipsilateral renal abnormalities, and only 9% had normal kidneys bilaterally (Donohue and Fauver, 1989).

Bilateral absence of the seminal vesicles is frequently found in association with bilateral congenital absence of the vas deferens. This is commonly associated with cystic fibrosis. Sixty percent to 80% of men with bilateral absence of the vas or seminal vesicles are carriers for the genetic mutation associated with cystic fibrosis (Anguiano et al, 1994; Chillon et al, 1995). Conversely, 80% to 95% of men with cystic fibrosis have bilateral absence of the vas deferens or seminal vesicles (Holsclaw et al, 1971; Boat et al, 1989). **Lack of a vas deferens does not necessarily imply an absent seminal vesicle, however, unless the ipsilateral**

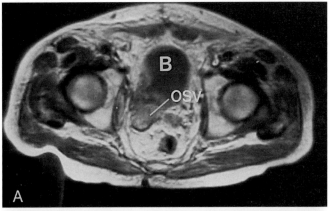
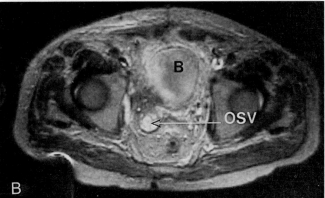

Figure 106–9. Magnetic resonance image (MRI) of an obstructed right seminal vesicle (OSV) as a result of invasive bladder cancer (B, bladder). *A*, Transaxial T1-weighted MRI. *B*, Transaxial T2-weighted MRI.

ureter is also not present (Goldstein and Schlossberg, 1988). Seminal vesicle agenesis requires no treatment.

Obstruction of the Seminal Vesicles

Although absence of the seminal vesicle(s) may be asymptomatic, obstruction is frequently associated with symptoms. Unilateral obstruction may be due to entrance of an ectopic ureter, leading to infection of the obstructed organ. The kidney associated with the ectopic ureter is frequently dysplastic. Obstruction may also be due to local invasion of bladder or prostate cancer (Fig. 106–9). Bilateral obstruction (Fig. 106–10) is frequently associated with infertility (Donohue and Fauver, 1989; Hall and Oates, 1993).

Infection

Vesiculitis

Infection of the seminal vesicles is an uncommon problem today in the United States. In less developed countries, tuberculosis and schistosomiasis remain common causes of seminal vesicle masses, abscesses, and calcification. Chronic bacterial vesiculitis is rare and difficult to diagnose; however, transrectal or perineal needle aspiration for diagnosis or treatment of abscesses has been successful. **Bacterial infections are commonly due to colonic flora and are thought to be secondary to bacterial prostatitis.** In the distant past,

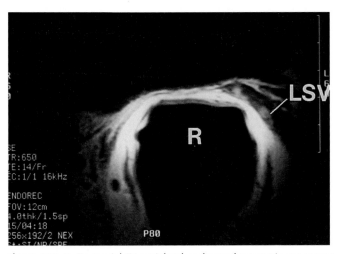

Figure 106–8. Transaxial T1-weighted endorectal magnetic resonance image of absent right seminal vesicle. R, rectum; LSV, left seminal vesicle.

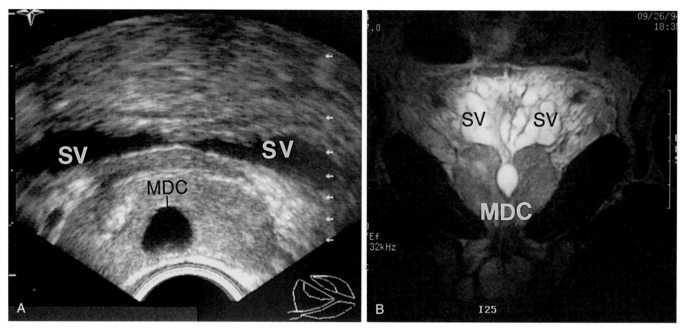

Figure 106–10. *A,* Transrectal ultrasound of patient with seminal vesicle obstruction because of müllerian duct cyst. *B,* T2-weighted magnetic resonance image of same patient. SV, seminal vesicle; MDC, müllerian duct cyst.

bilateral seminal vesiculectomy was used as treatment for infections of the seminal vesicle, but today, selected systemic antibiotics are usually curative, obviating surgery (Gutierrez et al, 1994). Occasionally, chronic bacterial seminal vesiculitis may require surgical removal to eliminate symptoms and prevent recurrent septicemia. Any of the surgical approaches described subsequently are appropriate (Indudhara et al, 1991).

Abscess

Abscesses of the seminal vesicles usually have an unknown etiology, although predisposing factors include diabetes mellitus, a chronic indwelling catheter, and endoscopic manipulation. Signs and symptoms vary but are typically related to inflammation. Conservative drainage via a percutaneous route is occasionally successful, but **most abscesses of the seminal vesicles require open drainage** (Gutierrez et al, 1994; Kore et al, 1994). Imaging of the abscess is best accomplished with MRI because of the high fluid content of the seminal vesicles. In contrast to the normal hypointense T1-weighted image, inflammation results in a less intense image. The normally hyperintense signal found on T2-weighted image is increased further with inflammation. The use of systemic gadolinium diethylenetriamine penta-acetic acid (DTPA) offers better enhancement and visualization (Chandra et al, 1991; Doringer et al, 1991).

Calculi

Stones within the seminal vesicles are usually related to obstruction, infection, or both (Li, 1991; Wilkinson, 1993). Patients usually present with either pain or infection related to the stone, although hematospermia or infertility can be the presenting complaint. **Treatment requires removal of the stone,** usually through an open vesiculectomy.

Adjuvant treatment with antibiotics may be necessary, particularly in cases of systemic infection.

Masses

Most masses within the seminal vesicles are not neoplastic. Tumors of the seminal vesicles are extremely rare. Benign primary tumors are the most common, including papillary adenoma, cystadenoma, fibroma, and leiomyoma (Mostofi and Price, 1973; Lundhus et al, 1984; Narayana, 1985; Mazur et al, 1987; Bullock, 1988). **Simple cysts of the seminal vesicle** are not uncommonly seen and **may be associated with other genitourinary anomalies,** such as ipsilateral renal agenesis or malformation (Lynch and Flannigan, 1992; Sheih et al, 1993).

Seminal Vesicle Cysts

Cysts of the seminal vesicles may be either congenital or acquired (King et al, 1991) **and are believed to be due to obstruction of the ejaculatory duct** (Heaney et al, 1987; Conn et al, 1992). Numerous authors have reported an **association between seminal vesicle cysts and other abnormalities, including renal agenesis** (Kimchi and Wiesenfeld, 1963; Roehrborn et al, 1986), **infertility** (Nazli et al, 1994), **hematospermia** (Mayersak and Viviano, 1992; Wang et al, 1993), **and genitourinary infection** (Beeby, 1974; Roehrborn et al, 1986; Lynch and Flannigan, 1992).

Others have reported an association between seminal vesicle cysts and adult polycystic kidney disease (Alpern et al, 1991; Hihara et al, 1993). In contrast to the typical benign cysts, some believe that the pathogenesis of these cysts associated with polycystic kidney disease is due to a general defect in the basement membrane of multiple organs, including the seminal vesicles. These authors recommend that all patients with cysts of the seminal vesicles undergo imaging of the kidneys to rule out polycystic kidney disease (Alpern et al, 1991).

Unless these cystic lesions are symptomatic, treatment is not usually necessary (Surya et al, 1988). If the lesion causes symptoms, percutaneous transperineal drainage of the cysts with TRUS guidance can be successful (Kirkali et al, 1991; Wang et al, 1993); if not, open surgical excision may be necessary. If an ectopic ureter is present, a nephroureterectomy, including removal of the seminal vesicle, should be curative.

Benign Tumors

PAPILLARY ADENOMA AND CYSTADENOMA

Papillary adenoma and cystadenoma may mimic simple seminal vesicle cysts in their presentation and imaging. These benign tumors generally occur in middle-aged men and involve one side, with only one case of bilateral involvement reported (Mazur et al, 1987). Some believe that they originate from embryologic remnants (Tock et al, 1991; Mazzucchelli et al, 1992; Ranschaert et al, 1992). Open surgical removal is the treatment of choice because preoperative diagnosis is rarely made.

AMYLOID OF THE SEMINAL VESICLES

Subepithelial deposits of amyloid in the seminal vesicles have been reported in 4% to 17% of male autopsies, with an incidence up to 20% in men older than 76 years of age (Pitkanen et al, 1983; Ramchandani et al, 1993). Because of the increased incidence in the older population, it is frequently present concomitant with other conditions, such as bladder or prostate cancer. Therefore, it is possible to misinterpret enlargement of the seminal vesicles from senile amyloidosis as carcinomatous invasion. MRI of the pelvis usually can distinguish tumor invasion, although not with complete accuracy (Kaji et al, 1992). In contrast to senile amyloidosis, the systemic form of amyloidosis may involve multiple organ systems with amyloid deposits seen in the blood vessels and muscle cells as opposed to the subepithelium (Coyne and Kealy, 1993). If asymptomatic, no treatment is necessary.

Malignant Tumors

The diagnosis of seminal vesical neoplasms can be difficult because they often do not cause symptoms until late in their course. General symptoms that may occur include urinary retention, dysuria, hematuria, or hematospermia. A mass is often palpable above the prostate and is usually nontender. TRUS is usually the next step in diagnosis and may be accompanied by needle aspiration or biopsy for diagnosis. CT or MRI is then appropriate to stage the patient. Because prostate cancer may be mistaken for primary seminal vesicle cancer, serum prostate-specific antigen (PSA) and prostatic acid phosphatase (PAP) as well as tissue immunohistochemical stains for both enzymes should, if positive, help to define the prostate as the site of primary malignancy.

The main difficulty encountered with seminal vesicle neoplasms is determining that they are, in fact, primary

within the seminal vesicles. Indeed, it is more common for carcinoma in situ of the bladder, adenocarcinoma of the prostate, lymphoma, or rectal carcinoma to involve the seminal vesicle secondarily (Mostofi and Price, 1973; Jakse et al, 1987; Ro et al, 1987).

To date, few primary tumors of the seminal vesicles have been reported. This is due in part to the paucity of symptoms and lack of detection on physical examination for the small benign tumors and, until recently, the lack of diagnostic imaging capable of accurately depicting the seminal vesicles. It is surprising that a tumor arising from an analogue similar to that of the prostate and responding to similar hormonal influences has so few recognized pathologic conditions. Perhaps the extremely low proliferative activity of seminal vesicle epithelium accounts for this in part (Meyer et al, 1982).

ADENOCARCINOMA

Characteristics of a primary seminal vesicle adenocarcinoma include the following: (1) the tumor commonly occurs in patients over the age of 50; (2) when discovered, the tumor usually extends locally into prostate, bladder, or rectum; (3) prostatic or ureteral obstruction is common; (4) pathology reveals a mucin-producing papillary or anaplastic carcinoma that may also contain lipofuscin in a patient with no other pelvic primary tumor; (5) serum markers for prostate cancer (PSA and PAP) are normal; and (6) serum carcinoembryonic antigen (CEA) may be elevated (Mostofi and Price, 1973; Benson et al, 1984; Tanaka et al, 1987; Chinoy and Kulkarni, 1993). A report of a CA^{125}-producing adenocarcinoma suggested that the tumor may have originated from the müllerian-wolffian duct system (Ohmori et al, 1994).

SARCOMA

Sarcomas of the seminal vesicles have been reported by various authors and are extremely rare. They are usually diagnosed late in the course of the disease. There are no distinguishing features except for biopsy findings (Benson et al, 1984; Chiou et al, 1985; Schned et al, 1986; Tanaka et al, 1987; Davis et al, 1988; Kawahara et al, 1988). These include leiomyosarcoma (Amirkhan et al, 1994), angiosarcoma (Lamont et al, 1991), and a müllerian adenosarcoma-like tumor (Laurila et al, 1992). These all display aggressive behavior. Treatment is similar to that for carcinomas, with radical extirpation yielding varying results.

Other Pathology

Other pathology includes hydatid cysts (Kuyumcuoglu et al, 1991; Whyman and Morris, 1991) and **carcinoid** (Soyer et al, 1991). Other primary malignant tumors of the seminal vesicles that have been reported include **cystosarcoma phyllodes** (Fain et al, 1993) and **primary seminoma** (Adachi et al, 1991). Hydatid disease affecting the seminal vesicles can cause hematospermia, infertility, infection, or pain. Carcinoid of the seminal vesicle appears homogeneous, with intense enhancement, on CT. On MRI, hypointense images are demonstrated on both T1-weighted and T2-

weighted images, with T2-weighted images demonstrating heterogeneity (Soyer et al, 1991).

TREATMENT

If a solid lesion identified in the seminal vesicle shows no evidence of local spread and is benign on biopsy, treatment depends on symptoms. If the patient is asymptomatic, close follow-up consisting of repeat rectal examination and TRUS to determine subsequent growth of the tumor is reasonable, although it may be difficult to be certain the tumor is not malignant. If the mass enlarges or the patient has symptoms referable to the mass, simple seminal vesiculectomy is advisable. This may be accomplished through one of several routes described later.

If the mass is quite large and solid and has questionable margins or the biopsy shows malignant columnar or poorly differentiated carcinoma cells, the treatment of choice is quite different. **Because fewer than ten cases of primary tumors of the seminal vesicles have been treated at any one institution, it is difficult to define optimum treatment with any degree of certainty. Radical excision,** which usually includes a cystoprostatectomy with pelvic lymphadenectomy, **is the treatment of choice unless the tumor is extremely small.** This recommendation is based on the extensive nature of the majority of the cancers when detected. The excision may include the rectum (total pelvic exenteration) if the tumor is thought to be invading the surrounding structures. Adjuvant therapy has no proven efficacy, although the only long-term survivors in the literature had radical surgery with subsequent pelvic radiation therapy or androgen deprivation therapy. No chemotherapeutic regimen is known to be efficacious.

Surgical Approaches

The surgical approaches to the seminal vesicle have varied considerably since the first seminal vesicle was removed by Ullmann in 1889 (De Assis, 1952). Descriptions of large series (up to 700 by one surgeon) of seminal vesiculectomies have been described—most for tuberculosis or suspected inflammation. **Today, seminal vesiculectomy is rarely necessary.** The most useful open surgical methods include transperineal, similar to a radical perineal prostatectomy; transvesical, by incising through the posterior bladder wall; paravesical; retrovesical; or transcoccygeal. The choice of surgical approach depends partly on the characteristics of the lesion to be treated but probably more on the experience and expertise of the surgeon. For the most part, **congenital lesions require an abdominal approach so that the ipsilateral kidney can be dealt with concomitantly,** if necessary. Benign or small malignancies could be approached perineally; however, the risk of impotence is high even if a nerve-sparing approach is attempted. Larger benign tumors or cysts are best handled by an anterior abdominal approach, although a transcoccygeal method may be as useful. Patients with a malignancy require radical extirpation, which commonly includes a cystoprostatoseminal-vesiculectomy and pelvic lymphadenectomy. This operation is no different from

a routine procedure for bladder cancer and, thus, is not described here.

Indications

The majority of surgeries on seminal vesicles currently are done in conjunction with radical surgical treatment of pelvic neoplasms, such as bladder, prostate, or urethral cancer and occasionally for treatment of rectal cancer. The indications and surgical principles entailed for treatment of these conditions are discussed in other chapters in this book.

Treatment of conditions of the seminal vesicles alone are limited to (1) transperineal and transvesical aspiration of seminal vesicle cysts or abscesses, (2) transurethral unroofing of seminal vesicle cysts or abscesses, (3) laparoscopic dissection, and (4) open resection of one or both seminal vesicles.

Preoperative Preparation

Preoperative preparation for open seminal vesicle surgery depends on the extent of the pathology and the planned incision. The transperineal, transcoccygeal, and transvesical approaches should be prefaced by a complete bowel preparation. The authors use a mechanical preparation with GoLYTELY orally the evening before surgery followed by the standard antibiotic regimen including oral neomycin/erythromycin. This is in anticipation of the uncommon, but not unlikely, possibility of a rectal laceration. A prophylactic systemic antibiotic of choice is administered perioperatively (i.e., immediately before surgery and for 36 hours after). Some method of attempted prevention of phlebothrombosis in the legs, such as intermittent compression stockings during and immediately after surgery, is advisable. The blood loss expected from seminal vesicle surgery depends on the surgical approach used. One to 2 units should be prepared for perineal and transcoccygeal approaches and 2 to 3 units for an anterior approach. Autologous blood can be obtained because these operations are rarely emergencies.

Endoscopic Treatment

Transurethral Resection

If the cyst or abscess is adjacent to the prostate (not in the mid or distal end of the seminal vesicle), **it may be possible to unroof the cavity with a deep transurethral resection** into the prostatic substance just distal to the bladder neck at the 5-o'clock or 7-o'clock position (Frye and Loughlin, 1988; Honnens de Lichtenberg and Hvidt, 1989). Vasal urinary reflux, with resultant postvoid dribbling and possible infection, however, is a potential complication (Goluboff et al, 1995). One group reported the treatment of a seminal vesicle cyst through aspiration via a No. 6.9 Fr ureteroscope (Razvi and Denstedt, 1994).

Laparoscopic Approach

The majority of laparoscopic surgery performed on seminal vesicles has been in conjunction with radical perineal prostatectomies. The laparoscopic approach allows for greater visualization, particularly of the vasculature and the tip of the seminal vesicle. Drawbacks include the need for a transperitoneal approach and the increase in operative time (Kavoussi et al, 1993). Excision of a benign symptomatic seminal vesicle cyst has been accomplished laparoscopically (Carmignani et al, 1995).

Medical and Radiologic Treatment

Small seminal vesicle cysts obstructing ejaculatory ducts or causing local symptoms should undergo initial transperineal or TRUS-guided aspiration. If this is not successful because the cyst reaccumulates, consideration could be given to reaspiration with injection of a sclerosing solution such as tetracycline. Similarly an abscess in the seminal vesicle could be aspirated for culture and drained perhaps even with a short-term indwelling catheter by way of a transperineal or transvesical percutaneous route using TRUS or CT guidance (Frye and Loughlin, 1988; Shabsigh et al, 1989; Gutierrez et al, 1994). Direct irrigation of the cavity and subsequent antibiotic injection may be curative (Fuse et al, 1988; Fox et al, 1988).

Open Surgical Techniques

Patients with chronic seminal vesiculitis or a small benign tumor of the seminal vesicle can have a seminal vesiculectomy by way of the perineal route similar to a radical perineal prostatectomy. **Large benign tumors or cysts require removal through either an anterior incision or a transcoccygeal approach** because the perineal route limits the ability to reach more than a few centimeters craniad to the bladder neck or to remove large masses physically through the relatively small opening.

Patients with an ectopic ureter into a seminal vesicle cyst require an anterior approach so that the kidney, ureter, and seminal vesicle can be removed in toto. We prefer a midline incision so that the kidney and ureter can be approached transperitoneally, after mobilizing the colon. The ureter can then be followed and dissected from the bladder in a paravesical approach similar to performing a nephroureterectomy for urothelial cancer.

Transperineal Approach

The transperineal approach follows the standard positioning and incision described for a radical perineal prostatectomy. To find the seminal vesicles above the prostate, the rectal wall needs to be dissected free and released higher on the base of the prostate and seminal vesicles than is usually necessary for initiation of the radical prostatectomy. The incision in Denonvilliers' fascia is then made either transversely, just above the level of the base of the seminal vesicles on the prostate (Fig. 106–11), or vertically, if attempting to save the neurovascular bundles responsible for potency (Weldon and Tavel, 1988). In this latter case, Denonvilliers' fascia is carefully dissected laterally away from the underlying seminal vesicle and ampulla of the vas so as not to tear the longitudinal tissue carrying the neurovascular bundle. The dissection at the base of the

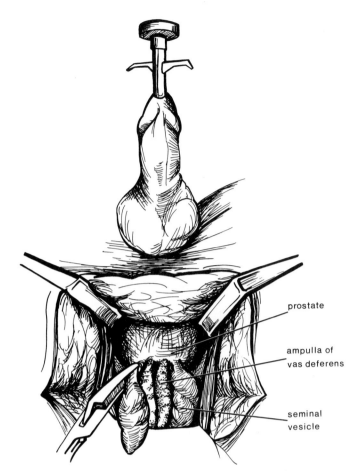

Figure 106–11. Transperineal approach to seminal vesiculectomy. (Redrawn from Hinman F Jr: Atlas of Urologic Surgery. Philadelphia, W. B. Saunders Company, 1989, p 381.)

seminal vesicle may be enhanced by posterior traction on a Lowsley tractor placed through the urethra into the bladder, thus elevating the prostate and putting tension on Denonvilliers' fascia. The two ampullae of the vasa deferentia should easily be dissected directly above the prostate and just under Denonvilliers' fascia. They are somewhat friable but can be clipped with metal clips (not placed too tightly) if necessary. **In the case of a simple seminal vesicle cyst or small adenoma, the vas can be spared,** and the dissection then proceeds to the vesicle of concern. **If the reason for surgery is cancer or recurrent infection, a wider resection including the ampulla of the vas may be advisable.** If the diagnosis is benign, the dissection can begin directly on the seminal vesicle. There is usually an easily dissected plane that can be found between the seminal vesicle, surrounding retroperitoneal tissue, and Denonvilliers' fascia. After dissecting around the seminal vesicle at the base of the prostate, it is usually possible to pass a right-angle clamp around the seminal vesicle and use an absorbable 2–0 suture to ligate the stump of the seminal vesicle directly on the prostate. A second tie or clip on the distal seminal vesicle keeps the secretions from obscuring the field after the vesicle is cut across, which is the next step. Although some surgeons may prefer to attempt to dissect out the seminal vesicle completely before ligating its entry into the prostate, this makes the operation more difficult and lengthy as well as serving no useful purpose when the seminal vesicle is being removed for a benign condition. Once the seminal vesicle has been ligated and cut across at the base, an Allis clamp can be used on the cut edge to put countertraction on the seminal vesicle so that spreading dissection with Metzenbaum scissors can free the seminal vesicle from the surrounding tissue. The vascular pedicle is usually encountered within 1 cm of the distal tip, and after it is ligated with metal clips and cut across, the organ can be removed. The wound is then closed in layers exactly as outlined for a radical perineal prostatectomy. A Penrose drain is left in the bed of the seminal vesicle and removed within 24 hours if no drainage is noted.

The perineal approach is extremely well tolerated by patients, affording them minimal blood loss, early ambulation, and minimal postoperative pain. Because there is no urethral anastomosis, patients may be ready for discharge in 24 to 48 hours. Intraoperative complications primarily entail inadvertent rectal wall laceration, although it is possible to lacerate the trigone area of the bladder or the ipsilateral ureter during deep dissection of the distal tip of the seminal vesicle. If an adequate bowel preparation has been given preoperatively and no gross fecal contamination is seen, a two-layer closure of the rectum using a running mucosal layer of 3–0 absorbable suture and a submucosal layer of interrupted 4–0 silk is usually sufficient. Anal dilatation before awakening the patient may be useful. A large laceration or fecal contamination should cause consideration of a temporary colostomy, although such a measure has not been necessary in the authors' experience. If a bladder injury is noted, it should be closed in two layers with absorbable suture as in any bladder incision and a urethral catheter left indwelling for 7 to 10 days postoperatively. If a ureteral injury occurs, an attempt to place a self-retaining (double-J) catheter should be made and the ureter then repaired with absorbable suture. If the ureter cannot be catheterized, flexible cystoscopy and retrograde placement of a ureteral stent should be performed on the table with the stent left in place for 10 to 14 days postoperatively.

Transvesical Approach

The transvesical approach to the seminal vesicle has been described by numerous authors (Walker and Bowles, 1968; Politano et al, 1975). A midline extraperitoneal suprapubic incision is made up to the umbilicus, and the rectus muscles are separated on the midline. The space of Retzius is opened by downward displacement of the transversalis fascia on the pubis, and an Omni retractor is placed to expose the anterior bladder wall. The bladder is opened longitudinally approximately 7 to 10 cm, ending 2 to 3 cm away from the bladder neck. Moist 4 × 8 sponges are placed on the bladder wall laterally and at the dome of the bladder, and specialized blades are placed to put the open bladder on stretch. Although it is not absolutely necessary, it is preferable to place long No. 8 feeding tubes in the ureters at this point for definition of the orifices and to help with identification of the subtrigonal ureters to prevent their injury later during the dissection. Using a bovie cutting stylet, a vertical incision is made through the trigone on the posterior midline approximately 5 cm in length (Fig. 106–12A). Alternatively a transverse incision just above the

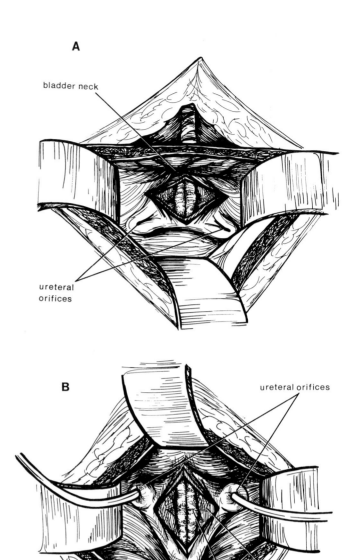

Figure 106–12. Transvesical approach to seminal vesiculectomy. *A,* Transverse incision 2 cm superior to the bladder neck below the ureteral orifices. *B,* Vertical incision between the ureteral orifices. (Redrawn from Hinman F Jr: Atlas of Urologic Surgery. Philadelphia, W. B. Saunders Company, 1989, p 382.)

bladder neck could be used but is not preferred (Fig. 106–12B). The vertical incision is deepened through the bladder muscle, and directly beneath the bladder neck the ampullae of the vasa should be recognized. They can be dissected by scissors down to their entrance into the prostate and then either ligated and divided or left intact depending on the pathology, as described in the perineal approach. Just lateral to the ampullae on the prostate base, the seminal vesicles should be identified and the plane surrounding them entered easily unless there has been prior inflammatory disease. The seminal vesicles should be encircled and dissected completely free. Metal clips should be placed on the vascular pedicle and a 2–0 chromic tie on the distal end at the prostate. A clip is placed across the proximal end to prevent seminal vesicle contents from obscuring the field, and then the vesicle is transected and removed. If there is a moderate-sized cyst, the dissection is more involved but usually is made simple because the perivesical plane is usually more pronounced. The plane may be difficult to establish if there was prior vesiculitis, and in this instance the ureteral catheters are a welcome safeguard—care must be taken not to dissect completely through Denonvilliers' fascia posteriorly and into the rectum. The posterior bladder incision is then closed with a running 2–0 absorbable suture in the muscle layer followed by a running 4–0 absorbable suture in the mucosal layer. The ureteral stents and 4 × 8 sponges are removed, a No. 20 Fr urethral catheter is placed, and the anterior bladder wall is closed as was the posterior wall. Suprapubic tube placement is an option but is not necessary. A suction drain is placed through a separate stab incision and positioned in the prevesical space away from the suture line. The drain is left for 2 to 3 days and then removed when the drainage has proved not to be urine and is less than 50 ml/day. The urethral catheter is removed in 5 to 7 days. Early ambulation is the rule, and the patient is usually discharged within 3 to 5 days after surgery.

This approach is more prone to blood loss and ureteral injury than the perineal approach, but a rectal laceration is much less likely. These complications are handled as described previously.

Paravesical Incision

The paravesical incision is used in children or when there is a large unilateral cyst that lies lateral to and above the bladder and when nephroureterectomy is required. A midline or Pfannenstiel extraperitoneal suprapubic incision is made. The bladder is finger dissected away from the lateral pelvic sidewall on the affected side. The vas deferens is identified, placed on tension, and dissected down toward the base of the bladder. If the seminal vesicle mass is distended, it should be visible rather quickly as the vas comes close to the bladder posteriorly. Placing a catheter in the bladder and emptying it usually allows the plane between the bladder and the cyst to be readily identified. The plane is incised with scissors and the seminal vesicle cyst carefully dissected away sharply. When the tip of the cyst is clearly identified, a 1–0 chromic suture is placed into it to provide traction, making further dissection easier. As the dissection proceeds, it must be remembered that the ureter crosses the vas and must be identified to prevent its injury. In addition, the superior vesicle artery and perhaps the inferior vesicle artery may be sacrificed to gain access to the base of the seminal vesicle. This causes no harm and should be done without major concern. As the dissection proceeds, the bladder is progressively rolled over medially, and the mass is dissected away from the bladder laterally. The plane is easily maintained with sharp dissection. Any vessels feeding the seminal vesicles should be suture ligated or metal clipped. **As the prostate is approached, caution must be used to stay directly on the mass so as not to injure the neurovascular bundle lying just lateral to the seminal vesicle.** At the prostate base, the neck of the seminal vesicle is encircled

and ligated with a 2–0 absorbable suture. A clamp is placed across just distal to the tie, and the seminal vesicle is severed. There may be no need to clip the vas. A suction drain is placed in the bed of the seminal vesicle and brought out through a separate stab incision. The wound is then closed in layers. Postoperative care is as previously described except that with this approach, the drain can be removed within 24 hours if there is no drainage, and the urethral catheter can be removed within 24 hours. The patient may be discharged within 2 to 3 days. Complications include ureteral injury and excessive blood loss. If the principles outlined previously are followed, these are unlikely events.

Retrovesical Approach

The retrovesical approach should be considered in patients requiring bilateral excision of small seminal vesicle cysts or benign masses (De Assis, 1952). A midline suprapubic incision is made into the peritoneal space. A catheter is placed, and the urine is evacuated. The reflection of the peritoneum over the rectum at the posterior bladder wall is incised transversely, being careful not to incise into the rectum (Fig. 106–13A). The bladder is peeled back from the rectum progressively with sharp dissection until the ampullae of the vasa and tips of the seminal vesicles come into view (Fig. 106–13B). The seminal vesicles are dissected down to the base of the prostate much as described in the transvesical approach, and the neck of the seminal vesicle is ligated and divided bilaterally. The ampullae are usually not taken unless necessary. A suction drain is left in the area posterior to the bladder and brought out as before. Postoperative care is per the description for a paravesical resection. Complications include rectal injury, bladder laceration, and hemorrhage. In this situation, a rectal injury would be within the peritoneum well above the levator ani muscles. Following a two-layer closure as before, strong consideration should be given to placement of omentum over the closure between the bladder base and the rectum as well as a temporary colostomy.

Transcoccygeal Approach

The transcoccygeal approach may not be familiar to most urologic surgeons and is unlikely to be a common choice because of the fear of rectal injury and impotence. **In individuals in whom the perineal or supine position may be difficult to maintain or who have had multiple suprapubic or perineal surgeries, the transcoccygeal approach may be useful.** The patient is placed on the table ventral side down (prone) and in a relative jackknife position (Kreager and Jordan, 1965). The incision is made in an L shape from midway on the sacrum (10 cm from the tip of the coccyx) and angled at the tip of the coccyx down the gluteal cleft within 3 cm of the anus (Fig. 106–14A). The incision is carried down to the lateral side of the coccyx, which is dissected free from the underlying rectum and eventually totally removed (Fig. 106–14B). The gluteus maximus muscle layers are moved aside and the rectosigmoid encountered and dissected carefully from the underside of the sacrum. With careful dissection, the lateral wall of the rectum on the side of the lesion is dissected medially from the levator ani muscle and surrounding tissue until the prostate is encountered (Fig. 106–14C). It is possible that the

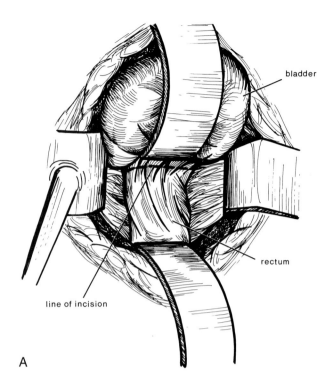

A

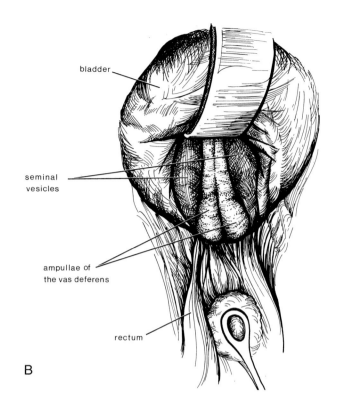

B

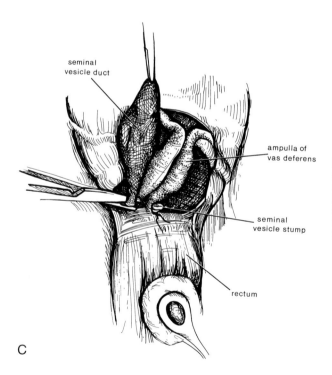

C

Figure 106–13. Retrovesical approach to seminal vesiculectomy. *A,* Incision line between base of bladder and peritoneal reflection over the rectum. *B,* Caudal dissection reveals the ampullae of the vas deferens on the midline and seminal vesicles immediately lateral to them. *C,* The duct of the seminal vesicle is ligated and transected. (Redrawn from Hinman F Jr: Atlas of Urologic Surgery. Philadelphia, W. B. Saunders Company, 1989, pp 379–380.)

neurovascular bundle will be recognized from this approach; if the dissection is unilateral, injury may be of little consequence. Once the prostate is palpated, dissection of the tissue directly superior to the base on the midline should reveal the ampulla of the vas and lateral to it the seminal vesicle (Fig. 106–14*D*). If difficulty dissecting the rectum away from the prostate is encountered, a finger in the anus via an O'Connor sheath allows the correct plane to be determined. Dissection and removal of the seminal vesicles should follow

the principles outlined previously. A Penrose drain should be left in the area exiting through a separate stab incision at closure. The rectum should be carefully scrutinized for injury and, if found, closed in two layers as previously described. The wound is closed in layers as well. Postoperative care is not different from that previously described except that, similar to the perineal approach, patients should have a rapid, easy recovery. The drain should be removed within 2 to 3 days if there is no drainage.

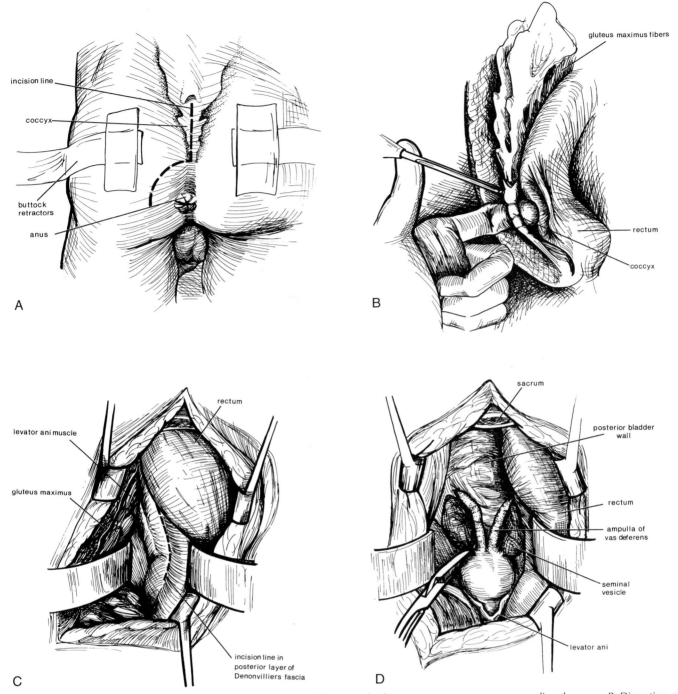

Figure 106–14. Transcoccygeal seminal vesiculectomy. *A,* Incision line over the lower sacrum on coccyx surrounding the anus. *B,* Dissection of the coccyx. *C,* Incising Denonvilliers' fascia after the rectum has been displaced. *D,* Exposure of the prostate and seminal vesicles. (Redrawn from Hinman F Jr: Atlas of Urologic Surgery. Philadelphia, W. B. Saunders Company, 1989, pp 385–388.)

CONCLUSION

The seminal vesicles are difficult organs to access, but they fortunately have a small number of primary pathologic conditions. Today there are few reasons to operate solely on the seminal vesicles, but when the indications are appropriate, the approach and surgical principles are not particularly different from other pelvic conditions more frequently encountered by the urologic surgeon.

REFERENCES

Aboul-Azm TE: Anatomy of the human seminal vesicles and ejaculatory ducts. Arch Androl 1979; 3:287.

Adachi Y, Rokujyo M, Kojima H, Nagashima K: Primary seminoma of the seminal vesicle: Report of a case. J Urol 1991; 146:857.

Al-Omari H, Girgis SM, Hanna AZ: Diagnostic value of vaso-seminal-vesiculography. Arch Androl 1985; 15:187.

Alpern MB, Dorfman RE, Gross BH, et al: Seminal vesicle cysts: Association with adult polycystic kidney disease. Radiology 1991; 180:79.

Amirkhan RH, Molberg KH, Wiley EL, et al: Primary leiomyosarcoma of the seminal vesicle. Urology 1994; 44:132.

Anguiano A, Oates RD, Amos JA, et al: Congenital bilateral absence of the vas deferens: A primarily genital form of cystic fibrosis. JAMA 1994; 267:1794.

Arey LB: The urinary system. *In* Developmental Anatomy. Philadelphia, W. B. Saunders, 1965, p 313.

Beeby DI: Seminal vesicle cyst associated with ipsilateral renal agenesis: Case report and review of literature. J Urol 1974; 112:120.

Benson RC Jr, Clark WR, Farrow GM: Carcinoma of the seminal vesicle. J Urol 1984; 132:483.

Birnbaum BA, Friedman JP, Lubat E, et al: Extrarenal genitourinary tuberculosis: CT appearance of calcified pipe-stem ureter and seminal vesicle abscess. J Comput Assist Tomogr 1990; 14:653.

Boat TF, Welsh MJ, Beaudet AL: Cystic fibrosis. *In* Scriver CR, Beaudet AL, Sly WS, Valle D, eds: The Metabolic Basis of Inherited Disease, Vol 2, 6th ed. New York, McGraw-Hill, 1989, p 2649.

Braithwaite JL: The arterial supply of the male urinary bladder. Br J Urol 1952; 24:64.

Brewster SF: The development and differentiation of human seminal vesicles. J Anat 1985; 143:45.

Bullock KN: Cystadenoma of the seminal vesicle. J R Soc Med 1988; 81:294.

Carmignani G, Gallucci M, Puppo P, et al: Video laparoscopic excision of a seminal cyst associated with ipsilateral renal agenesis. J Urol 1995; 153:437.

Carter SStC, Shinohara K, Lipshultz LI: Transrectal ultrasonography in disorders of the seminal vesicles and ejaculatory ducts. Urol Clin North Am 1989; 16:773.

Chandra I, Doringer E, Sarica K, et al: Bilateral seminal vesicle abscesses. Eur Urol 1991; 20:164.

Chillon M, Casals T, Mercier B, et al: Mutations in the cystic fibrosis gene in patients with congenital absence of the vas deferens. N Engl J Med 1995; 332:1475.

Chinoy RF, Kulkarni JN: Primary papillary adenocarcinoma of the seminal vesicle. Ind J Cancer 1993; 30:82.

Chiou RK, Limas C, Lange PH: Hemangiosarcoma of the seminal vesicle: Case report and literature review. J Urol 1985; 134:371.

Conn IG, Peeling WB, Clements R: Complete resolution of a large seminal vesicle cyst—evidence for an obstructive aetiology. Br J Urol 1992; 69:636.

Coyne JD, Kealy WF: Seminal vesicle amyloidosis: Morphological, histochemical and immunohistochemical observations. Histopathology 1993; 22:173.

Davis NS, Merguerian PA, DiMarco PL, et al: Primary adenocarcinoma of seminal vesicle presenting as bladder tumor. Urology 1988; 32:466.

De Assis JS: Seminal vesiculectomy. J Urol 1952; 68:747.

Donohue RE, Fauver HE: Unilateral absence of the vas deferens: A useful clinical sign. JAMA 1989; 261:1180.

Doringer E, Chandra I, Sarica K, et al: MRI of bilateral seminal vesicle abscesses. Eur J Radiol 1991; 12:60.

Dunnick NR, Ford K, Osborne D, et al: Seminal vesiculography: Limited value in vesiculitis. Urology 1982; 20:454.

Fain JS, Cosnow I, King BF, et al: Cystosarcoma phyllodes of the seminal vesicle. Cancer 1993; 71:2055.

Fox CW Jr, Vaccaro JA, Kiesling VJ Jr, Belville WD: Seminal vesicle abscess: The use of computerized coaxial tomography for diagnosis and therapy. J Urol 1988; 139:384.

Frye K, Loughlin K: Successful transurethral drainage of bilateral seminal vesicle abscesses. J Urol 1988; 139:1323.

Fuse H, Sumiya H, Ishii H, et al: Treatment of hemospermia caused by dilated seminal vesicles by direct drug injection guided by ultrasonography. J Urol 1988; 140:991.

Genevois PA, Van Sinoy ML, Sintzoff SA Jr, et al: Cysts of the prostate and seminal vesicles: MR imaging findings in 11 cases. AJR 1990; 155:1021.

Goldstein M, Schlossberg S: Men with congenital absence of the vas deferens often have seminal vesicles. J Urol 1988; 140:85.

Goluboff ET, Kaplan SA, Fisch H: Seminal vesicle urinary reflux as a complication of transurethral resection of the ejaculatory ducts. J Urol 1995; 153:1234.

Gordon HL, Kessler R: Ectopic ureter entering the seminal vesicle associated with renal dysplasia. J Urol 1972; 108:389.

Gutierrez R, Carrere W, Llopis J, et al: Seminal vesicle abscess: Two case reports and a review of the literature. Urol Int 1994; 52:45.

Hall S, Oates RD: Unilateral absence of the scrotal vas deferens associated with contralateral mesonephric duct anomalies resulting in infertility: Laboratory, physical and radiographic findings, and therapeutic alternatives. J Urol 1993; 150:1161.

Heaney JA, Pfister RC, Meares EM Jr: Giant cyst of the seminal vesicle with renal agenesis. Am J Radiol 1987; 149:139.

Hihara T, Ohnishi H, Muraishi O, et al: MR imaging of seminal vesicle cysts associated with adult polycystic kidney disease. Radiat Med 1993; 11:24.

Holsclaw DS, Perlmutter AD, Jockin H, Shwachman H: Genital abnormalities in male patients with cystic fibrosis. J Urol 1971; 106:568.

Honnens de Lichtenberg M, Hvidt V: Transurethral, transprostatic incision of a seminal vesicle cyst. Scand J Urol Nephrol 1989; 23:303.

Indudhara R, Das K, Sharma M, Vaidyanathan S: Seminal vesiculitis due to *Mycobacterium gastri* leading to male infertility. Urol Int 1991; 46:99.

Jakse G, Putz A, Hofstadter F: Carcinoma in situ of the bladder extending into the seminal vesicles. J Urol 1987; 137:44.

Kaji Y, Sugimura K, Nagaoka S, Ishida T: Amyloid deposition in seminal vesicles mimicking tumor invasion from bladder cancer: MR findings. J Comput Assist Tomogr 1992; 16:989.

Kavoussi LR, Schuessler WW, Vancaillie TG, Clayman RV: Laparoscopic approach to the seminal vesicles. J Urol 1993; 150:417.

Kawahara M, Matsuhashi M, Tajima M, et al: Primary carcinoma of seminal vesicle. Urology 1988; 32:269.

Kimchi D, Wiesenfeld A: Cyst of seminal vesicle associated with ipsilateral renal agenesis: Case report. J Urol 1963; 89:906.

King BF, Hattery RR, Lieber MM, et al: Seminal vesicle imaging. Radiographics 1989; 9:653.

King BF, Hattery RR, Lieber MM, et al: Congenital cystic disease of the seminal vesicle. Radiology 1991; 178:207.

Kirkali Z, Yigitbasi O, Diren B, et al: Cysts of the prostate, seminal vesicles, and diverticulum of the ejaculatory ducts. Eur Urol 1991; 20:77.

Kore RN, McLoughlin J, Kabala J, Sibley GN: Seminal vesicle abscess. Br J Urol 1994; 73:331.

Kreager JA, Jordan WP: Transcoccygeal approach to the seminal vesicle. Am Surg 1965; 31:126.

Kuyumcuoglu U, Erol D, Germiyanoglu C, Baltaci L: Hydatid cyst of the seminal vesicle. Int Urol Nephrol 1991; 23:479.

Lamont JS, Hesketh PJ, de las Morenas A, Babayan RK: Primary angiosarcoma of the seminal vesicle. J Urol 1991; 146:165.

Laurila P, Leivo I, Makisalo H, et al: Müllerian adenosarcoma-like tumor of the seminal vesicle. Arch Pathol Lab Med 1992; 116:1072.

Lee SB, Lee F, Solomon MH, et al: Seminal vesicle abscess: Diagnosis by transrectal ultrasound. J Clin Ultrasound 1986; 14:546.

Li YK: Diagnosis and management of large seminal vesicle stones. Br J Urol 1991; 68:322.

Littrup PJ, Lee F, McLeary RD, et al: Transrectal US of the seminal vesicles and ejaculatory ducts: Clinical correlation. Radiology 1988; 168:625.

Lundhus E, Bundgaard N, Sorensen FB: Cystadenoma of the seminal vesicle. Scand J Urol Nephrol 1984; 18:341.

Lynch MJ, Flannigan GM: Seminal vesicle cyst, renal agenesis, and epididymitis in a 50-year-old patient. Br J Urol 1992; 69:98.

MacDonald GR: The ectopic ureter in men. J Urol 1986; 135:1269.

Mawhinney MG: Male accessory sex organs and androgen action. *In* Lipshultz LI, Howards SS, eds: Infertility of the Male, 2nd ed. New York, Churchill Livingstone, 1992, p 124.

Mayersak JS, Viviano CJ: Unilateral seminal vesicle cyst presenting as hematospermia: Diagnosis established by transrectal prostatic ultrasound. Wisc Med J 1992; 11:629.

Mazur MT, Myers JL, Maddox WA: Cystic epithelial-stromal tumor of the seminal vesicle. Am J Surg Pathol 1987; 11:210.

Mazzucchelli L, Studer UE, Zimmermann A: Cystadenoma of the seminal vesicle: Case report and literature review. J Urol 1992; 147:1621.

Meyer JJ, Hartig PR, Koos GW, McKinley CR: Transrectal seminal vesiculography. J Urol 1979; 121:129.

Meyer JS, Sufrin G, Martin SA: Proliferative activity of benign human prostate, prostatic adenocarcinoma and seminal vesicle evaluated by thymidine labeling. J Urol 1982; 128:1353.

Mostofi FK, Price EB: Tumors of the seminal vesicle. *In* Mostofi FK, Price EB, eds: Tumors of the Male Genital System. Washington, D.C., Armed Forces Institute of Pathology, 1973, p 259.

Narayana A: Tumors of the epididymis, seminal vesicles, and vas deferens (spermatic cord). *In* Culp DA, Loening SA, eds: Genitourinary Oncology. Philadelphia, Lea & Febiger, 1985, p 385.

Nazli O, Apaydin E, Killi R, et al: Seminal vesicle cyst, renal agenesis, and infertility in a 32-year-old man. Br J Urol 1994; 73:467.

Ohmori T, Okada K, Tabei R, et al: CA^{125}-producing adenocarcinoma of the seminal vesicle. Pathol Int 1994; 44:333.

Patel PS, Wilbur AC: Cystic seminal vesiculitis: CT demonstration. J Comput Assist Tomogr 1987; 11:103.

Pitkanen P, Westermark P, Cornwell GG III, Murdoch W: Amyloid of the seminal vesicles: A distinctive and common localized form of senile amyloidosis. Am J Pathol 1983; 110:64.

Politano VA, Lankford RW, Susaeta R: A transvesical approach to total seminal vesiculectomy: A case report. J Urol 1975; 113:385.

Ramchandani P, Schnall MD, LiVolsi VA, et al: Senile amyloidosis of the seminal vesicles mimicking metastatic spread of prostatic carcinoma on MR images. AJR 1993; 161:99.

Ranschaert ER, Van Mulders P, Usewils R, et al: An unusual low-abdominal tumor: Cystadenoma of the seminal vesicle. J Belg Radiol 1992; 75:105.

Razvi HA, Denstedt JD: Endourologic management of seminal vesicle cyst. J Endourol 1994; 8:429.

Redman JF: Anatomy of the genitourinary system. *In* Gillenwater JY, Grayhack JT, Howards SS, Duckett JW, eds: Adult and Pediatric Urology. Chicago, Year Book Medical Publishers, 1987, p 45.

Ro JY, Ayala AG, Naggar A, Wishnow KI: Seminal vesicle involvement by in situ and invasive transitional cell carcinoma of the bladder. Am J Surg Pathol 1987; 11:951.

Roehrborn CG, Schneider HJ, Rugendorff EW, Hamann W: Embryological and diagnostic aspects of seminal vesicle cysts associated with upper urinary tract malformation. J Urol 1986; 135:1029.

Schned AR, Ledbetter JS, Selikowitz SM: Primary leiomyosarcoma of the seminal vesicle. Cancer 1986; 57:2202.

Schwartz ML, Kenney PJ, Bueschen AJ: Computed tomographic diagnosis of ectopic ureter with seminal vesicle cyst. Urology 1988; 31:55.

Secaf E, Nuruddin RN, Hricak H, et al: MR imaging of the seminal vesicles. AJR 1991; 156:989.

Shabsigh R, Lerner S, Fishman IJ, Kadmon D: The role of transrectal ultrasonography in the diagnosis and management of prostatic and seminal vesicle cysts. J Urol 1989; 141:1206.

Sheih CP, Liao YJ, Li YW, Yang LY: Seminal vesicle cyst associated with ipsilateral renal malformation and hemivertebra: Report of 2 cases. J Urol 1993; 150:1214.

Silverman PM, Dunnick NR, Ford KK: Computed tomography of the normal seminal vesicles. Comput Radiol 1985; 9:379.

Soyer P, Rougier P, Gad M, Roche A: Primary carcinoid tumor of the seminal vesicles: CT and MR findings. J Belg Radiol 1991; 74:117.

Stamey TA: Urinary infections in males. *In* Stamey TA, ed: Pathogenesis and Treatment of Urinary Tract Infections. Baltimore, Williams & Wilkins, 1980, p 417.

Steers WD, Corriere JN Jr: Case profile: Seminal vesicle cyst. Urology 1986; 27:177.

Sue DE, Chicola C, Brant-Zawadzki MN, et al: MR imaging in seminal vesiculitis. J Comput Assist Tomogr 1989; 13:662.

Surya BV, Washecka R, Glasser J, Johanson KE: Cysts of the seminal vesicles: Diagnosis and management. Br J Urol 1988; 62:491.

Sussman SK, Dunnick NR, Silverman PM, Cohan RH: Case report: Carcinoma of the seminal vesicle: CT appearance. J Comput Assist Tomogr 1986; 10:519.

Tanagho EA: Embryological basis for lower ureteral anomalies: A hypothesis. Urology 1976; 7:451.

Tanaka T, Takeuchi T, Oguchi K, et al: Primary adenocarcinoma of the seminal vesicle. Hum Pathol 1987; 18:200.

Tauber PF, Zaneveld LJD, Propping D, et al: Components of human split ejaculate. J Reprod Fertil 1975; 43:249.

Tauber PF, Zaneveld LJD, Propping D, et al: Components of human split ejaculate: II. Enzymes and proteinase inhibitors. J Reprod Fertil 1976; 46:165.

Tock EP, Hoe J, Foo KT: Haemorrhagic papillary cystadenoma of the seminal vesicle mimicking giant seminal vesicle cyst: MRI appearances. Ann Acad Med Sing 1991; 20:792.

Walker WC, Bowles WT: Transvesical seminal vesiculectomy in treatment of congenital obstruction of seminal vesicles: Case report. J Urol 1968; 90:324.

Wang TM, Chuang CK, Lai MK: Seminal vesicle cyst: An unusual cause of hematospermia—a case report. Chang Keng I Hsueh 1993; 16:275.

Weldon VE, Tavel FR: Potency-sparing radical perineal prostatectomy: Anatomy, surgical technique and initial results. J Urol 1988; 140:559.

Wessels EC, Ohori M, Grantmyre JE, et al: The prevalence of cystic dilatation of the ejaculatory ducts detected by transrectal ultrasound (TRUS) in a self-referred (screening) group of men. J Urol 1992; 147:456A.

Whyman MR, Morris DL: Retrovesical hydatid causing haemospermia. Br J Urol 1991; 68:100.

Wilkinson AG: Case report: Calculus in the seminal vesicle. Pediatr Radiol 1993; 23:327.

107

SURGERY OF THE PENIS AND URETHRA

Gerald H. Jordan, M.D.
Steven M. Schlossberg, M.D.
Charles J. Devine, M.D.

Improvements in microsurgery and tissue transfer techniques have greatly expanded the repertoire of the urologic surgeon and the genitourinary reconstructive surgeon in particular. As a result, urologists are now able to reconstruct congenital and acquired genitourinary abnormalities with greater facility. Microvascular and microneurosurgical techniques have made it possible to create a phallus that allows a patient to stand to void and enjoy erotic sensibility, and because the flap has both erotic and protective sensibility, the patient can eventually have prosthetic implantation that allows a relatively acceptable sexual life. This chapter discusses the techniques involved in genitourinary reconstructive surgery.

PRINCIPLES OF RECONSTRUCTIVE SURGERY

Many of the techniques involved in reconstructive surgery require transfer of skin. The physical properties of skin vary among individuals as well as among areas on the same patient. Anatomic variables such as color, texture, thickness, extensibility, innate skin tension, and blood supply can be used in various situations.

The outermost layer of the skin (average thickness of 0.8–1.0 mm) is the epidermis. Composed of keratinocytes that differentiate and die, rising to the surface as a cornified external membrane, this layer of stratified squamous epithelium has a high metabolic rate and cell turnover rate. The epidermal layer also contains the skin appendages, which in some areas extend deep into the dermis.

The layer lying immediately beneath the epidermis is the dermis. The dermal layer beneath the epidermis containing the skin appendages is known as the periadnexal dermis, and the layer beneath the epidermis that is free of skin appendages is referred to as the papillary dermis. Other terms used to describe the dermal layers include the adventitial dermis, a collective term referring to the superficial layer of the dermis, and the reticular dermis, or the deep layer.

The dermal layer accounts for most of the physical characteristics of the skin, which are a reflection of the relationship between collagen, elastin, and the mucopolysaccharide matrix. These characteristics are attributed mostly to the deep layer, or the reticular dermis, and the inclusion or lack of reticular dermis thus accounts for the physical characteristics of a graft.

The blood supply to the skin is provided by two plexuses. The superficial (intradermal) plexus lies approximately at the interface of the adventitial dermis and the papillary projections of the epidermis and is characterized by numerous small vessels. The subdermal plexus lies at the interface between the reticular dermis and subcuticular adipose tissue and is composed of less numerous, but larger, vessels. The nature of these plexuses accounts for the fastidiousness of each skin graft's *take* characteristics.

Grafts

Graft **is a term that implies transfer of tissue from a donor site to a recipient site without an intact blood supply.** Neovascularization, or the development of a new blood supply to the graft tissue, allows for the process of graft take. Graft take occurs in two phases: **imbibition** and **inosculation.** The initial phase, **imbibition,** lasts 48 hours. During this phase, the pale graft exists below core body temperature and survives by imbibing nutrients from the adjacent graft bed, causing the graft to increase in weight. Imbibition has been viewed as a latent phase during which the graft is held in suspended animation. Although this is an oversimplified view, no graft can live long in this phase, and progress into the second phase must occur rapidly for graft take to be successful.

The second phase of graft take, **inosculation,** is characterized by anastomoses of the exposed vessels of the host bed, with the vessels exposed on the undersurface of the graft. Angiogenesis appears to be initiated by anoxic metabolism, mediated by lactate. These growth factors induce capillary sprouting from the host bed and penetration for anastomosis to the vessels of the graft. During this phase, lasting an additional 48 hours, the graft develops true vascularity, assumes body temperature, and re-establishes lymphatic drainage that carries off the imbibed fluid.

Four conditions are necessary to ensure success during the 96-hour process of neovascularization: a well-vascularized graft bed, rapid onset of imbibition, immobilization of the graft at the host site, and rapid onset of inosculation. Because of its poor vascularity, scar tissue is not an optimal host bed. Also, collections, such as hematomas, seromas, or purulence, separate the vessels of the undersurface of the graft from the underlying host bed, leading to failure of take. After a graft has been harvested, it should be kept wrapped in saline-soaked sponges to avoid desiccation of the surface because desiccation can inhibit imbibition and the release of vascular growth factors. Grafts must be fixed securely to the graft host bed. The authors also routinely use prophylactic broad-spectrum antibiotics.

A **full-thickness skin graft** is composed of the full thickness of the skin, with the dermal surface of the graft trimmed of the underlying fat or subcutaneous tissues to expose the vessels of the subdermal plexus (Fig. 107–1A). The combination of the thickness associated with the full-thickness skin graft and its sparsely distributed vessels makes it a graft that is slowly revascularized and thus fastidious with regard to conditions of take. Because the entire dermis is included, however, the full-thickness skin graft carries with it the innate physical characteristics of the skin.

In contrast, a **split-thickness skin graft** contains the epidermis and a portion of the dermis. It can be harvested at various thicknesses, with a graft that is 0.0016 to 0.0018 inch thick considered to be a medium split-thickness skin graft and a graft harvested at greater than 0.002 to 0.0022 inch considered to be a thick split-thickness skin graft. Little of the reticular dermis is included, and these grafts tend to be brittle, with a marked tendency to contract in unsupported tissues. More plentifully distributed vessels of the intradermal plexus are exposed on the undersurface of a split-thickness skin graft, however, and this factor combined with a decreased total volume of the graft (owing to its reduced thickness) allows more rapid inosculation. In addition, lymphatics, primarily distributed in the reticular dermis, are not carried in the split-thickness skin graft. Rapid inosculation and the lack of lymphatics make split-thickness skin grafts

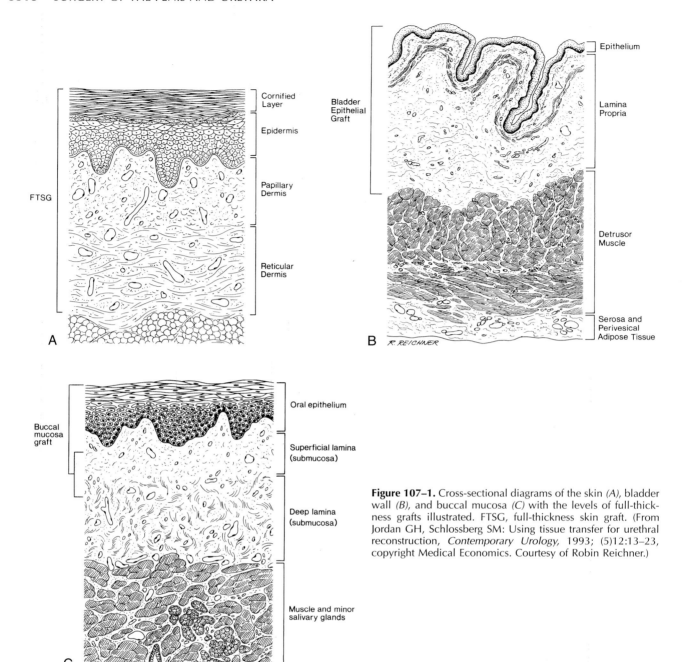

Figure 107–1. Cross-sectional diagrams of the skin *(A)*, bladder wall *(B)*, and buccal mucosa *(C)* with the levels of full-thickness grafts illustrated. FTSG, full-thickness skin graft. (From Jordan GH, Schlossberg SM: Using tissue transfer for urethral reconstruction, *Contemporary Urology,* 1993; (5)12:13–23, copyright Medical Economics. Courtesy of Robin Reichner.)

useful for acute trauma and for coverage after excision of lymphedematous tissue.

A **meshed graft is a special application of a split-thickness skin graft** in which many slits are cut in the sheet graft. The slits allow for graft bed collections to escape and provide a much greater interface between the graft and host bed. Cut with a meshing dermatome, a template design is used to create a specific expansion ratio (1.5:1 is most useful for genital reconstruction). Meshed grafts are advantageous for less than optimal host beds and when the potential exists for the development of collections beneath the graft. Although the meshed graft can be expanded when it is used in coverage situations, in genitourinary reconstructive surgery, it is usually not expanded.

A **dermal graft** is taken from the dermis at the junction of the epidermis and superficial papillary dermis, and the subcutaneous or adipose tissue is removed from the deep surface. The graft is therefore composed almost entirely of reticular dermis, with only a small portion of the adventitial dermis included. Because the dermal graft carries the entire reticular dermis and its collagen elastin mucopolysaccharide network, it has little tendency to contract and maintains good extensibility at maturation. Furthermore, because the intradermal plexus is exposed on the superficial surface and the subdermal plexus is exposed on the deep surface, it is believed that inosculation can occur on both surfaces, resulting in an extremely reliable graft.

A dermal graft can be harvested freehand. The area of the proposed graft may be de-epithelialized using either a large scalpel blade and magnification or a dermatome. The use of a dermatome often creates a square defect that is difficult to close. The graft excision is oriented along Langer's lines to allow for closure of the dermal graft donor site with an acceptable scar. The authors close the graft donor site per primam.

Flaps

A flap is tissue that has been excised and transferred from a donor site, either with its own blood supply intact or with the blood supply re-established by way of microvascular techniques at the recipient site. Whereas graft take is dependent on the two-phase process of imbibition and inosculation, flap survival is dependent on venous runoff and the arterial supply.

Flaps can consist of any of several tissues. Although the most commonly recognized are skin flaps, flap reconstructions can also consist of muscle, omentum, or intestinal tissue. Terms seen in the literature such as free graft and pedicle graft are misleading. The term free graft is redundant, and by definition, a graft has no pedicle, making a pedicle graft actually a flap. The appropriate reconstructive surgical terms are grafts and flaps.

Flaps can be **classified according to both vascularity and elevation technique** (Fig. 107–2). When using a vascular classification, the term **random flap** represents a flap that is dependent on the subdermal and intradermal plexuses for survival. Characterized by random vascularity, these flaps lack identifiable arteries and veins in the base and do not have a predictable cuticular vascular territory. Random flaps are generally taken from areas that are vascularized by way of either the musculocutaneous or the fasciocutaneous system (defined later).

A second flap defined under the vascular classification is an **axial flap.** An axial flap is planned so that a large artery and vein are contained in the base of the flap. The survival of the axial flap is therefore dictated by the cutaneous vascular territory supplied by this major vessel. The cutaneous vascular territory of an axial flap is predictable and well defined and does not demonstrate marked differences among individuals. In addition, an axial flap is not limited by length-to-width ratios. The survival of the entire flap unit is instead related to the length of the direct artery in the pedicle, plus the additional distal skin that is carried via the intradermal and subdermal plexuses.

A number of terms are used to subclassify axial flaps. A **direct cuticular flap** is one in which the flap is supplied by a cutaneous artery and vein that are mobilized with the subcuticular portion of the flap base. A classic example of a direct cuticular flap is the groin flap.

A second subclassification of axial flaps is the **musculocutaneous flap** (Fig. 107–3A). These flaps are composed of muscle, subcutaneous fat, and the overlying skin island or paddle. With the flap elevated as a unit based on the vascular supply or the pedicle in the muscle, the vascularity to the skin is carried via perforating vessels that emanate from the muscle, penetrating the fascia and the subcutaneous tissue to connect with the dermal plexuses of the skin. Musculocutaneous flaps are often bulky, a characteristic that may be viewed as either an advantage or a hindrance, depending on the application.

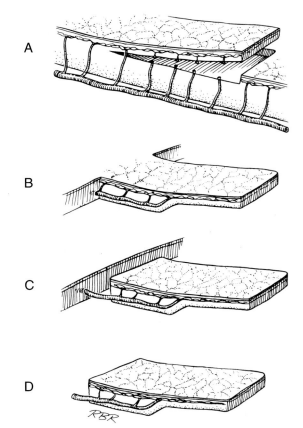

Figure 107–2. *A*, Random flap. The arterial connections have been interrupted, and flap survival depends on the intradermal and subdermal plexuses. *B*, Axial flap. Large vessels enter the base of the flap. Survival depends on them and on the random distal vascularity. *C*, Island flap. The vascular pedicle is intact; the skin has been divided. These axial vessels are unsupported. *D*, Microvascular free transfer flap. The skin and vascular connections are interrupted at the base of the flap. Vascular continuity is reconstituted in the recipient area by a microsurgical anastomosis. (From Jordan GH, Schlossberg SM, McCraw JB: AUA Update Series, Lesson 10, Vol 7, 1988.)

A final subclassification of axial flaps is the **fasciocutaneous flap** (Fig. 107–3B). A fasciocutaneous flap is one with identifiable axial vessels that are deep to the fascia, with perforator vessels penetrating within the fascial septa to fan out and form subfascial and superfascial plexuses. These plexuses then connect to the subcuticular tissue and overlying skin with perforator vessels. Examples of fasciocutaneous flaps include the dartos fascial flap (with its overlying penile skin) as well as all the other local flaps that have revolutionized genital reconstruction.

Terms used to classify flaps according to elevation techniques include **peninsula flap, island flap, and microvascular free transfer flap.** A **peninsula flap** is one that is elevated such that the base of the flap leaves the continuity of the skin, subcuticular tissues, and vascular pedicle intact. Peninsula flaps can be either random or axial.

An **island flap** is one in which the arteriovenous pedicle is preserved while the subcuticular and cuticular connections at the flap base are interrupted. All island flaps are, by definition, axial flaps. A **true island flap connotes dangling vessels.** True island flaps are seldom used, however, because they are somewhat difficult to transfer. The term island flap should be separated from the terms skin paddle and skin

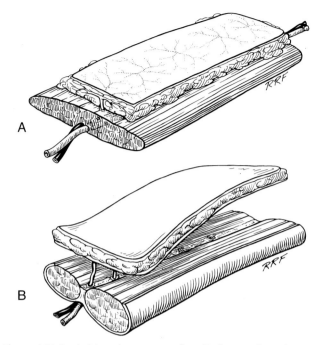

Figure 107–3. *A,* Musculocutaneous flap. Perforators from the artery to a muscle vascularize the skin and overlying subcutaneous fat via musculocutaneous perforators. They may be transferred as free flaps but are usually transferred locally, left attached to the fasciolar pedicle. *B,* Fasciocutaneous flap. Perforating blood vessels from rich plexuses on the superficial and deep aspects of the fascia connect to perforator vessels that communicate with the microvasculature. In genital reconstruction, these flaps are based on the dartos fascia of the penis or as free flaps from the forearm. (From Jordan GH, Schlossberg SM, McCraw JB: AUA Update Series, Lesson 10, Vol 7, 1988.)

island. The skin that is carried with a fascial or muscle flap is termed the skin paddle or island. It is helpful to the surgeon to view these flaps as if the muscle or fascia is the flap, and the overlying adipose and skin are passengers situated on the muscle.

A **microvascular free transfer flap** is one in which the arteriovenous pedicle in the flap is interrupted and, when the flap is transferred, reconnected to the recipient vessels as a means of re-establishing vascularity of the flap. As with the island flap, all free flaps are axial flaps.

The usefulness of these flaps and grafts is illustrated in the discussion of surgical techniques. Because an understanding of anatomy is of utmost importance to reconstructive surgery, however, the anatomic relationships of the male genitourinary structures in the penis and male perineum precede the discussion of reconstructive surgical techniques.

ANATOMY OF THE PENIS AND MALE PERINEUM

The penile shaft (Fig. 107–4) is made up of three erectile bodies, the two corpora cavernosa and the corpus spongiosum containing the urethra with their enveloping fascial layers, nerves, and vessels, all covered by skin. All of these structures continue into the perineum. The corpora cavernosa make up the bulk of the penis. They contain erectile tissue within a dense elastic sheath of connective tissue called the tunica albuginea. The corpora cavernosa are not separate

structures but constitute a single space with free communication through a midline septum, composed of multiple strands of elastic tissue similar to that making up the tunica albuginea. The septum becomes more complete toward the base of the penis, but the corpora truly become independent only as they split to form the crus attached to the inferior ramus of the pubis and ischium.

The erectile tissue containing arteries, nerves, muscle fibers, and venous sinuses lined with flat endothelial cells fills the space of the corpora, making its cut surface look like that of a sponge. This tissue is separated from the tunica albuginea by a thin layer of areolar connective tissue, which was described by Smith (1966). The paired cavernosal arteries run near the center of the corpora. Blood inflow through these arteries returns through the erectile space of the corpus and numerous anastomotic channels.

An artificial erection, produced by placing a tourniquet on the base of the penis and injecting a saline solution into one side of the corpora cavernosa, fills both sides, the corpus spongiosum, the glans penis, and the superficial and deep veins of the penis. With normally functioning erectile vasculature, however, contrast material injected into one corpus cavernosum, after having established a pharmacologically evoked erection, fills only the two corpora because the other anastomotic channels have been occluded by the neuroendocrine processes of erection.

The third erectile body, the corpus spongiosum, lies in the ventral groove between the two corpora cavernosa. The tunica albuginea of the corpus spongiosum is thinner than the tunica of the corpora cavernosa, and there is less erectile tissue. Another thin layer of tunica encloses the urethra, which traverses the length of the penis within the corpus spongiosum. At its distal end, the corpus spongiosum expands to form the glans penis, a broad cap of erectile tissue covering the tips of the corpora cavernosa. The urethral meatus is slit-like, lying slightly on the ventral aspect of the tip of the glans, with its long axis oriented vertically. The edge of the glans overhangs the penile shaft, forming a rim called the corona, with the sulcus just proximal. A fold of skin, the frenulum, is attached at the most ventral point, just

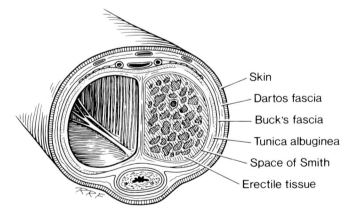

Figure 107–4. Transverse section of the penis at the junction of its middle and distal thirds. The septum is correctly illustrated as strands that interweave with the tunica albuginea both ventrally and dorsally. (From Jordan GH: Peyronie's disease and its management. *In* Krane RJ, Siroky MB, Fitzpatrick J, eds: Clinical Urology. Philadelphia, J. B. Lippincott, 1994, pp 1282–1297.)

proximal to the meatus, where the corona forms a distally pointing V.

At its base, the penis is supported by two ligaments, composed primarily of elastic fibers, that are continuous with the fascia of the penis. Posterior to this attachment, the right and left corpora cavernosa diverge, and the corpus spongiosum broadens between the two crura to form the bulbospongiosus (bulb).

Figure 107–5 illustrates the relationship of the erectile bodies and the urethra to the structures in the perineum. For the discussion of reconstruction, it is convenient to depart from the common usage of the terms anterior and posterior urethra and subdivide the urethra into five separate areas. The portions of the urethra are numbered in Figure 107–5: (1) The fossa navicularis is the portion of the urethra that is contained within the spongy erectile tissue of the glans penis and terminates at the junction of the urethral epithelium with the skin of the glans. This portion of the urethra is lined with stratified squamous epithelium. (2) The penile or pendulous urethra lies distal to the investment of the ischiocavernosus musculature but is also invested by the corpus spongiosum and maintains a constant lumen size roughly centered in the corpus spongiosum. The pendulous urethra is lined with simple squamous epithelium. (3) The bulbous urethra is covered by the midlying fusion of the ischiocavernosus musculature and is invested by the bulbospongiosus and corpus spongiosum. It becomes larger and lies closer to the dorsal aspect of the spongy tissue, exiting from its dorsal surface before the posterior attachment of the bulbospongiosus to the perineal body. The bulbous urethra is lined distally with squamous epithelium, which gradually changes to the transitional epithelium found in the membranous urethra as it swings upward (Devine and Horton, 1977). (4) The membranous urethra is the portion that traverses the perineal pouch and is surrounded by the external urethral sphincter. This segment of the urethra is unattached to fixed structures, has the distinction of being the only portion of the urethra that is not invested by another structure, and is lined with a delicate transitional epithelium. (5) The prostatic urethra is the portion of the urethra that is proximal to the verumontanum and surrounded by the prostatic glandular tissue. Its epithelium is continuous with that of the trigone and bladder.

A submucosal layer is noted throughout the length of the urethra, with an outer sphincter composed of an active muscular layer in the prostatic and membranous portions. Numerous glands of Littre open into the urethra along its dorsal surface. At times, these form small diverticula called lacunae of Morgagni. Often, there is a larger lacuna magna in the dorsal wall of the fossa navicularis. The ducts of Cowper's glands open into the urethra in the bulb and travel to the glands located in the urogenital diaphragm (the perineal membrane) adjacent to the membranous urethra.

In the penis, the erectile bodies are surrounded by Buck's fascia, dartos fascia, and skin. Buck's fascia is the tough, elastic layer immediately adjacent to the tunica albuginea. On the superior aspect of the corpora cavernosa, the deep dorsal vein, paired dorsal arteries, and multiple branches of the dorsal nerves lying on the tunica albuginea are attached to the inner surface of the fascia. In the midline groove on the underside of the corpora cavernosa, Buck's fascia splits to surround the corpus spongiosum. Consolidations of the fascia, lateral to the corpus spongiosum, attach it to the tunica albuginea of the corpora cavernosa. Attached distally to the undersurface of the glans penis at the corona, Buck's fascia extends into the perineum, enclosing each crus of the corpora cavernosa and the bulb of the corpus spongiosum and firmly fixing these structures to the pubis, ischium, and the inferior fascia of the perineal membrane.

Distally, the skin of the penis is confluent with the glabrous skin covering the glans. At the corona, it is folded on itself to form the foreskin (prepuce) that overlies the glans. The dartos fascia, a layer of areolar tissue remarkable for its lack of fat, separates these two layers of skin and continues into the perineum, where it fuses with the layers of the superficial perineal (Colles') fascia. In the penis, the dartos fascia is loosely attached to the skin and the deeper layer of Buck's fascia and contains the superficial arteries, veins, and nerves of the penis.

Blood is supplied to the skin of the penis by the left and right superficial external pudendal vessels (Fig. 107–6) that arise from the first portion of the femoral artery, cross the upper medial portion of the femoral triangle, and divide into two main branches, running dorsolaterally and ventrolaterally in the shaft of the penis with a collateralization across

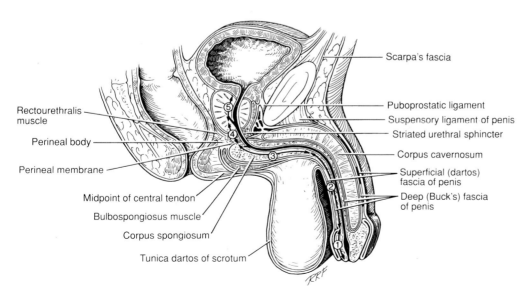

Rectourethralis muscle

Perineal body

Perineal membrane

Midpoint of central tendon

Bulbospongiosus muscle

Corpus spongiosum

Tunica dartos of scrotum

Scarpa's fascia

Puboprostatic ligament

Suspensory ligament of penis

Striated urethral sphincter

Corpus cavernosum

Superficial (dartos) fascia of penis

Deep (Buck's) fascia of penis

Figure 107–5. Diagram of the sagittal section of the penis and perineum illustrating the fascial layers. The divisions of the urethra are enumerated. (From Devine CJ Jr, Angermeier KW: AUA Update Series, Part 1, Lesson 2, Vol 8, 1994.)

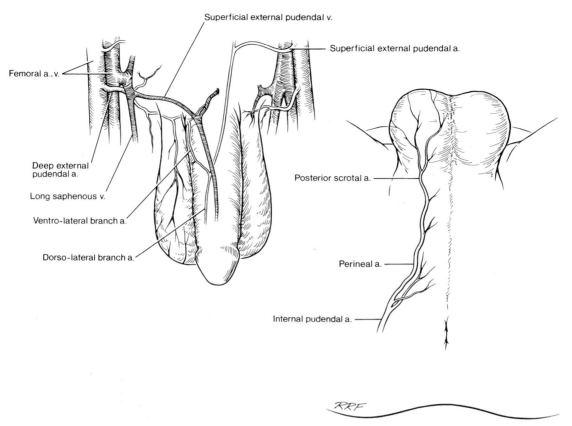

Figure 107–6. Vasculature to the genital skin. *On the left,* the superficial external pudendal vessels arborize to become the fascial blood supply contained in the dartos fascia of the penis. The scrotal artery is a terminal branch of the deep internal pudendal artery. This artery is thought to arborize in the tunica dartos of the scrotum and Colles' fascia of the perineum.

the midline. At intervals, they give off fine branches to the skin, forming a rich subdermal vascular plexus that can sustain the skin after its underlying dartos fascia has been mobilized. The arteries are accompanied by venous tributaries that are more prominent and easily seen than the arteries. Because of its remarkable thinness and mobility and the character of its vascular supply, the skin covering the penis is an ideal substitute in urethral reconstruction. A flap of skin may be elevated, and the fascia containing its blood supply can be mobilized, to create a subcutaneous pedicle allowing distal islands of preputial or penile skin to be transferred to virtually any part of the urethra.

Venous Drainage

The penis is drained by three venous systems: superficial, intermediate, and deep (Fig. 107–7) (Aboseif et al, 1989). The superficial veins contained in the dartos fascia on the dorsolateral aspects of the penis unite at its base to form a single superficial dorsal vein. The superficial dorsal vein usually drains into the left saphenous vein (rarely into the right) and occasionally forms two trunks that drain into both. Veins from more superficial tissue may drain into the external superficial pudendal veins.

The **intermediate system** contains the deep dorsal and circumflex veins, lying within and beneath Buck's fascia. Emissary veins begin within the erectile space of the penis and, following a perpendicular or oblique course through the

tunica albuginea, emerge from the lateral and dorsal surfaces of the corpora cavernosa to empty into the circumflex veins or the deep dorsal vein. The circumflex veins are channels present in the distal two thirds of the penile shaft. They arise from the corpus spongiosum and receive emissary veins as they travel around the lateral aspect of the corpora, passing beneath the dorsal arteries and nerves to empty into the deep dorsal vein. They communicate with one another and those of the opposite side to form 3 to 12 common venous channels, usually accompanied by branches of the dorsal nerve and artery. The circumflex veins also become confluent ventrally, forming periurethral veins on each side. These become important in the treatment of impotence caused by veno-occlusive incompetence. Additionally, venae comitantes travel with the dorsal arteries and their branches.

The deep dorsal vein is formed by five to eight small veins emerging from the glans penis to form the retrocoronal plexus, which drains into the deep dorsal vein lying in the midline groove between the corporal bodies. In a number of patients, the authors have found a connection between the superficial and deep dorsal veins. In the shaft of the penis, the deep dorsal vein often consists of two, and sometimes three, tributaries that anastomose with each other. The vein gathers blood from the emissary and circumflex veins, and passing beneath the pubis at the level of the suspensory ligament, it leaves the shaft of the penis at the crus and drains into the periprostatic plexus.

The **deep drainage system** consists of the crural and cavernosal veins. The crural veins arise in the midline, in

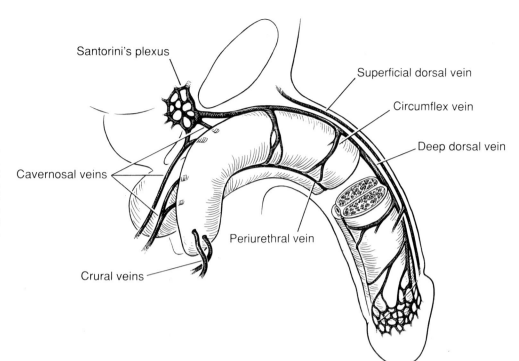

Figure 107–7. Deep venous drainage of the penis. (From Horton CE, Stecker JF, Jordan GH: Management of erectile dysfunction, genital reconstruction following trauma and transsexualism. *In* McCarthy JG, May JW Jr, Littler JW, eds: Plastic Surgery, Vol 6. Philadelphia, W. B. Saunders, 1990, pp 4213–4245.)

the space between the crura. Normally, they are small and almost indiscernible, joining the deep dorsal vein or the periprostatic plexus. If the deep dorsal vein has been ligated or obliterated following trauma, striking development of these veins can be noted as the intracrural space is entered during the perineal dissection for urethral repair. Emissary veins in the proximal third of the crura, near their attachment to the ischial tuberosities, join to form several thin-walled trunks on the dorsomedial surface of each corpus cavernosum. Some pass medially, joining the dorsal or crural veins, or extend proximally, entering the periprostatic plexus. Most consolidate into one or two cavernosal veins on each side. Running in the penile hilum, deep and medial to the cavernosal arteries and nerves, they join to form a large venous channel that drains into the internal pudendal vein. Three or four small cavernosal veins emerge from the dorsolateral surface of each crus and course laterally between the bulbospongiosus and the crus of the penis for 2 to 3 cm, before draining into the internal pudendal veins. These usually insignificant vessels become larger and can be noted more readily in patients with veno-occlusive erectile dysfunction. The internal pudendal veins (usually two) run together with the internal pudendal artery and nerve in Alcock's canal to empty into the internal iliac vein.

Arterial System

The **blood supply to the deep structures of the penis is derived from the common penile artery,** which is a continuation of the internal pudendal artery after it gives off its perineal branch (Fig. 107–8). From that point, the artery travels along the medial margin of the inferior pubic ramus. As it nears the urethral bulb, the artery divides into its three terminal branches as follows:

1. The bulbourethral artery is a short artery of large caliber that pierces Buck's fascia to enter the bulbospongiosus.

2. The dorsal artery generally travels along the dorsum of the penis between the deep dorsal vein medially and the dorsal nerves laterally, with a coiled rather than a straight configuration. The artery uncoils as the penis elongates with erection, allowing flow to be maintained. Along its course, it gives off three to ten circumflex branches that accompany the circumflex veins around the lateral surface of the corpora. Its terminal branches supply the glans penis. Occasionally a branch penetrates the tunica and in some individuals may help supply the erectile tissue. Proximally the circumflex arteries are also a part of the blood supply of the urethra.

3. The cavernosal artery, usually a single artery, arises on

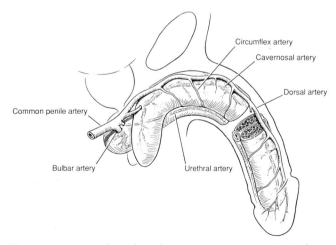

Figure 107–8. Arterial supply to the penis. (From Horton CE, Stecker JF, Jordan GH: Management of erectile dysfunction, genital reconstruction following trauma and transsexualism. *In* McCarthy JG, May JW Jr, Littler JW, eds: Plastic Surgery, Vol 6. Philadelphia, W. B. Saunders, 1990, pp 4213–4245.)

each side as the terminal branch of the penile artery. It enters the corpus cavernosum at the hilum and runs the length of the penile shaft, giving off the many helicine arteries that constitute the arterial portion of the erectile apparatus. The arteries frequently branch before entering the corporal body. Sometimes a branch enters the opposite corpus, and occasionally a single artery branches in the penile shaft to supply both sides. The authors have seen some of these variations during duplex ultrasound evaluation of the penis following a pharmacologically induced erection.

Lymphatics

Lymph drainage from the glans penis collects in large trunks in the area of the frenulum. The lymph vessels circle to the dorsal aspect of the corona, where they unite with those from the other side. The vessels traverse the penis beneath Buck's fascia, terminating mostly in the deep inguinal lymph nodes of the femoral triangle. Some drainage is to the presymphyseal lymph nodes and by way of these to the lateral lymph nodes of the external iliac group.

Nerve Supply

The nerves of the penis are derived from the pudendal and cavernosal nerves. The pudendal nerves supply somatic motor and sensory innervation to the penis. The cavernosal nerves and a combination of the parasympathetic and visceral afferent fibers constitute the autonomic nerves of the penis. These provide the nerve supply to the erectile apparatus.

The pudendal nerves enter the perineum with the internal pudendal vessels through the lesser sciatic notch at the posterior border of the ischiorectal fossa. They run in the fibrofascial pudendal canal of Alcock to the edge of the urogenital diaphragm (Fig. 107–9A). Each dorsal nerve of the penis arises in Alcock's canal as the first branch of the pudendal nerve. Traveling ventral to the main pudendal trunk above the internal obturator and under the levator ani, the dorsal nerves perforate the transverse perinei muscles to attain the dorsum of the penis and continue distally along the respective dorsolateral penile surface lateral to the dorsal artery. On the shaft, their fascicles fan out to supply proprioceptive and sensory nerve terminals in the tunica of the corpora cavernosa and sensory terminals in the skin. These nerves terminate in the glans penis.

The autonomic innervation of the pelvic organs and external genitalia arises from the pelvic plexus. The plexus is formed by preganglionic parasympathetic visceral efferent and afferent fibers arising from the sacral center (S2–S4) and sympathetic preganglionic afferent and visceral afferent fibers from the thoracolumbar center (T11–L2). Beyond the prostate, the parasympathetic nerves enter the cavernosal nerves and run adjacent to and through the wall of the membranous urethra. As they pierce the urogenital diaphragm, these nerves pass close to and supply Cowper's gland before entering the corpora cavernosa—where they are readily identified in the hilum of the penis, dorsomedial to the cavernosal arteries.

Perineum

The perineum is the diamond-shaped outlet bounded anteriorly by the pubic arch and the arcuate ligaments of the pubis, posteriorly by the tip of the coccyx, and laterally by the inferior rami of the pubis and ischium. **A transverse line between the ischial tuberosities divides the perineum into an anterior triangle** containing the external urogenital organs and a **posterior anal triangle** (Fig. 107–9B).

Colles' Fascia

In the anterior triangle, Colles' fascia (see Fig. 107–9A) attaches at its posterior margin to the perineal body, at the posteroinferior margin of the perineal membrane or urogenital diaphragm. The fascia curves below the superficial transverse perinei muscles and projects forward as two layers attached laterally to the ischium and the inferior ramus of the pelvis. The loose superficial layer is fatty and is continuous with the more substantial dartos fascia of the scrotum. In the scrotum, the dartos fascia layer contains muscle fibers that cause the rugous appearance of the scrotum. The fascia also projects (but without muscle fibers) into the midline, to form the septum between the two halves of the scrotum. The median raphe in the skin delineates the separation of the two halves of the scrotum and is continued anteriorly as a dark-colored streak in the ventral midline of the penis and posteriorly as the median raphe of the perineum terminating at the anus.

The deep membranous layer of Colles' fascia is a more substantial layer and forms a roof over the scrotal cavity separating it from the superficial perineal pouch. At the anterior aspect of the scrotum, Colles' fascia joins with the dartos fascia of the scrotum, and a fold of this fascia projects backward beneath the fibers of the bulbospongiosus muscle. At the base of the penis, it is continuous with the dartos fascia of the penis. Thickenings of the fascia at this level form the two suspensory ligaments of the penis. First, the outer fundiform ligament, which is continuous with the lower end of the linea alba, splits into laminae that surround the body of the penis and unite beneath it. Second, the inner triangular-shaped suspensory ligament is attached to the anterior aspect of the symphysis pubis and blends with the dartos fascia of the penis below it.

Anteriorly, Colles' fascia fuses and becomes continuous with the membranous layer of the subcutaneous connective tissue of the anterior abdominal wall (Scarpa's fascia). Laterally, Colles' fascia fuses to the pubic arch and with the fascia lata. Posteriorly, Colles' fascia sweeps beneath the transverse perinei muscles, fusing with the posterior aspect of the perineal membrane. The space beneath the continuous plane formed by these fascial attachments is the superficial perineal pouch, in which infections or extravasations of urine and collections of blood following trauma to the urethra may be confined.

Superficial Perineal Space

In males, the superficial perineal space contains the continuation of the corpora cavernosa, the proximal part of the

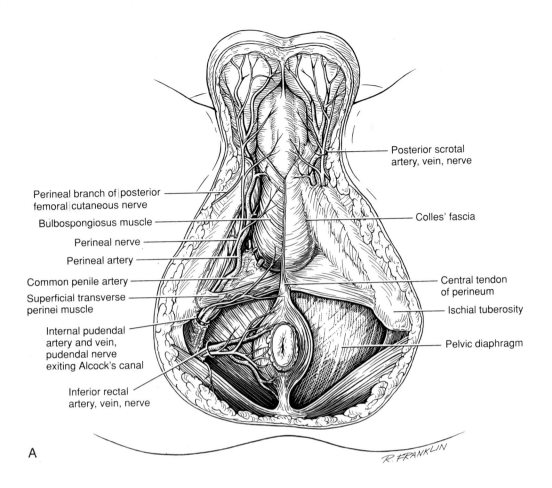

Perineal branch of posterior femoral cutaneous nerve

Bulbospongiosus muscle

Perineal nerve

Perineal artery

Common penile artery

Superficial transverse perinei muscle

Internal pudendal artery and vein, pudendal nerve exiting Alcock's canal

Inferior rectal artery, vein, nerve

Posterior scrotal artery, vein, nerve

Colles' fascia

Central tendon of perineum

Ischial tuberosity

Pelvic diaphragm

A

R. FRANKLIN

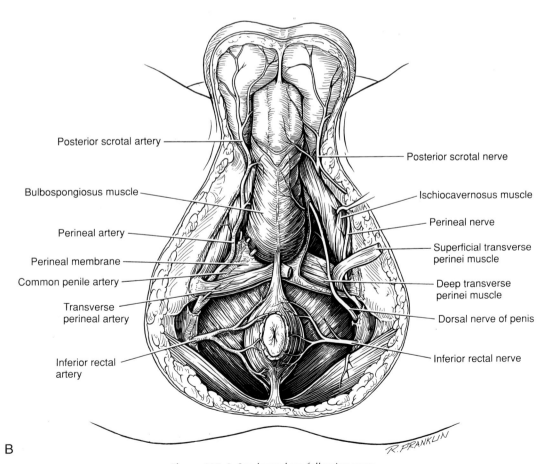

Posterior scrotal artery

Bulbospongiosus muscle

Perineal artery

Perineal membrane

Common penile artery

Transverse perineal artery

Inferior rectal artery

Posterior scrotal nerve

Ischiocavernosus muscle

Perineal nerve

Superficial transverse perinei muscle

Deep transverse perinei muscle

Dorsal nerve of penis

Inferior rectal nerve

B

R. FRANKLIN

Figure 107–9 *See legend on following page*

Illustration continued on following page

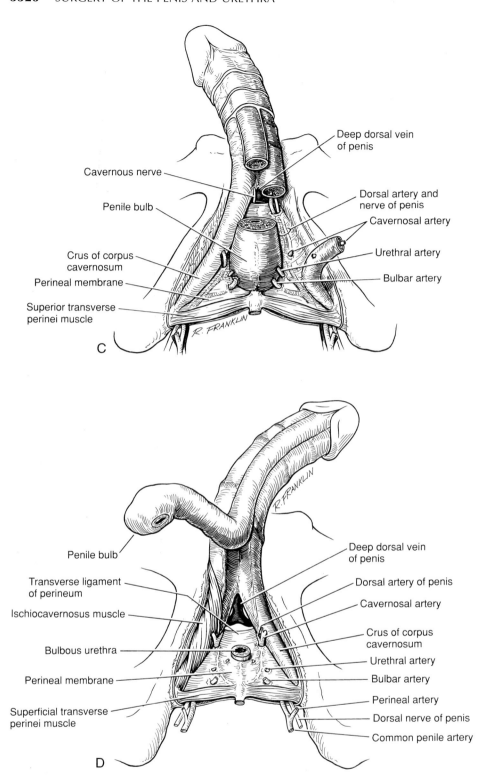

Figure 107–9. "Peel-away" diagrams of the anatomy of the perineum. *A,* The skin and subcuticular tissues have been removed. *B,* In the anterior perineal triangle, Colles' fascia has been removed. In the posterior anal triangle, the pelvic diaphragm has been removed. Note the division of the superficial transverse perinei muscle exposing the deep transverse perinei muscle. *C,* Anterior perineal triangle has been dissected to expose the erectile bodies. *D,* The corpus spongiosum has been divided at the departure of the urethra from the penile bulb. The intracrural space is exposed. (From Devine CJ Jr, Angermeier KW: AUA Update Series, Part 1, Lesson 2, Vol 8, 1994.)

corpus spongiosum and urethra, the muscles associated with them, and the branches of the internal pudendal vessels and pudendal nerves (see Fig. 107–9B).

The ischiocavernosus muscles cover the crura of the corpora cavernosa. They attach to the inner surfaces of the ischium and ischial tuberosities on each side and insert at the midline into Buck's fascia, surrounding the crura at their junction below the arcuate ligament of the penis. The

bulbospongiosus muscles are located in the midline of the perineum. They are attached to the perineal body posteriorly and to each other in the midline as they encompass the bulbospongiosus and crura of the corpora cavernosa at the base of the penis. These muscles are confluent with the ischiocavernosus muscles laterally and at their insertion into Buck's fascia, covering the dorsal vessels and nerves at the base of the penis.

Central Perineal Tendon (Perineal Body)

Lying just anterior to the anus, as a part of the plane separating the anterior and posterior perineal triangles, the perineal body is formed by the interconnection of eight muscles of the perineum (see Fig. 107–9A and B). The perineal body receives fibers from the anterior portion of the anal sphincter and is the central point of insertion of the superficial transverse perinei muscles that arise at the ischial tuberosities. The bulbospongiosus muscle is fixed to the perineal body by its posteriormost fibers. The deep transverse perinei muscles and fibers from the anterior portions of the levator ani muscles attach to the deep aspect of the perineal body.

Deep Perineal Space

The urogenital diaphragm constitutes the deep perineal space (Fig. 107–9C and D). It is contained within two layers of fascia and incompletely covers the outlet of the pelvis anterior to the deep layer of the perineal body. The deep layer of fascia is an indistinct structure—the continuation of the endopelvic obturator fascia. The superficial fascia attaches laterally to the ischial rami and the inferior ramus of the pubis. This fascia blends with the deep layer behind the perineal body and anteriorly, where it terminates with a thickened edge—the transverse perineal ligament. A space between this ligament and the arcuate ligament of the pubis accommodates the deep dorsal vein of the penis.

The deep perineal pouch (see Fig. 107–9D; Fig. 107–10) contains the deep transversus perinei muscles, the external sphincter of the urethra, the bulbourethral (Cowper's) glands, and the blood vessels and nerves associated with the structures within it. The sphincter urethra muscle fibers arise from the medial surface of the inferior pubic rami and pass medially toward the urethra, where they meet the fibers from the opposite side. In males, the muscle encircles the membranous urethra to function as the somatic sphincter of the urethra.

URETHRAL HEMANGIOMA

Although the lesion of a urethral hemangioma is rare, it is usually persistent and offers a challenge to the surgeon in those cases in which excision is deemed necessary. Patients typically present with hematuria or a bloody urethral discharge and occasionally with obstructive symptoms. The lesions may be either single or multiple, and the urethral meatus is a common location. Although diagnosis is often made at cystoscopy, which readily visualizes the dilated blood vessels, the lesion often extends beyond the point at which it is seen with cystoscopy.

Because all reported cases of urethral hemangioma have been benign, management depends on the size and location of the lesion. Asymptomatic lesions do not require treatment and should be observed because hemangiomas can regress spontaneously. Symptomatic lesions that require treatment must be completely excised to prevent recurrence.

Although electrofulguration has been reported as a possible treatment for urethral hemangioma, it should be used only to control an acute episode. For smaller lesions, laser treatment has been successful and produces less scarring. Lasers that are used for this purpose include argon, potassium titanyl phosphate (KTP) 532, and the neodymium:yttrium-aluminum-garnet (Nd:YAG) laser. The preferred treatment for larger lesions is open excision and urethral reconstruction. In addition, good initial success has been reported using polidocanol injected into the hemangioma transurethrally, as a sclerosing agent for extensive urethral hemangiomas.

REITER'S SYNDROME

Reiter's syndrome is characterized by a classic triad of arthritis, conjunctivitis, and urethritis. In addition, some pa-

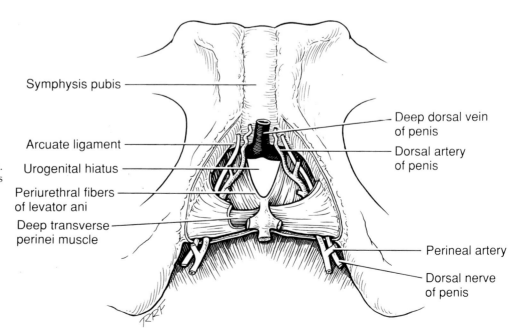

Figure 107–10. Infrapubic space. The urethra has been dissected, as has been the perineal diaphragm.

Symphysis pubis

Arcuate ligament

Urogenital hiatus

Periurethral fibers of levator ani

Deep transverse perinei muscle

Deep dorsal vein of penis

Dorsal artery of penis

Perineal artery

Dorsal nerve of penis

tients experience an episode of diarrhea before developing arthritis. In most cases, however, the classic triad is not present, and patients present only with arthritis, affecting the knees, ankles, and feet in an asymmetric distribution. The history of urethritis is then obtained on detailed questioning.

Urethral involvement is usually mild, self-limiting, and a minor portion of the disease. In approximately 10% to 20% of patients, a glanular lesion is present. Referred to as circinate balanitis, this lesion is diagnostic of Reiter's syndrome and typically appears as a shallow, painless ulcer with gray borders. Occasionally the lesion appears as small, red macules, 1 to 2 mm in diameter. When the urethritis is mild and self-limiting, no treatment is necessary.

In rare cases, urethritis occurs with severe inflammation with necrosis of the mucosa, producing uncompromising stricture disease. The authors have not been successful in excision and replacement of the urethra in these cases. Alternatively, the authors create a perineal urethrostomy and excise the entire distal urethra. This approach may decrease the rheumatic manifestations associated with Reiter's syndrome.

BALANITIS XEROTICA OBLITERANS

Balanitis xerotica obliterans (BXO) is the term used to describe genital lichen sclerosus in the male. Histologically, it is characterized by hyperkeratosis, homogenization of the collagen in the papillary dermis in association with stromal edema, and a lymphocytic infiltrate.

The most common cause of meatal stenosis, BXO appears as a whitish plaque that may involve the prepuce, glans penis, urethral meatus, and fossa navicularis. In severe, long-standing cases, the inflammation often involves the skin of the penile shaft. In uncircumcised men, the prepuce becomes edematous and thickened and often may be adherent to the glans (Bainbridge et al, 1971). Diagnosis is made through biopsy.

Although previously believed to be rare, BXO is commonly found at the time of circumcisions performed beyond the neonatal period (Rickwood et al, 1980; Ledwig and Weigrand, 1989; Meuli et al, 1994). If only the foreskin is involved, circumcision is curative. More commonly, however, the glans and meatus are also involved. A combination of topical steroids and antibiotics may help to stabilize the inflammation around the meatus. Conservative therapy may be warranted in patients whose meatus can easily be maintained at No. 14 to 16 Fr. In these cases, intermittent catheterization with lubrication of the catheter or meatal dilator with 0.1% triamcinolone may be adequate treatment. This nonsurgical approach to treatment is used in older patients who are not good surgical candidates for other medical reasons or all older patients and younger patients who have demonstrated stable disease.

In young patients with severe meatal stenosis, surgery is indicated. Because patients with long-standing BXO and meatal stenosis often have urethral stricture disease, these patients should have a retrograde urethrogram before initiation of therapy. The etiology of stricture disease associated with BXO is unclear. Possible causes include iatrogenic stricture resulting from repeated instrumentation and pressure voiding associated with meatal stenosis causing secondary intravasation of urine into the glands of Littre (Fig. 107–11). In cases of early BXO with only meatal fossa stenosis, prompt reconstruction using penile island flaps has been extremely successful and seems to avoid the sequelae of panurethral stricture disease. Long-standing cases with long lengths of urethral stricture are amenable to techniques of reconstruction but can be quite challenging.

The authors have also seen patients present with the clinical picture of a buried penis. This occurs when the skin of the penile shaft has been lost because of severe inflammation and the penis is trapped in the penopubic and scrotal skin. These patients are often profoundly overweight, they have often had prior surgical procedures, and their management is complex and ultimately determined by their desire and need for functional reconstruction. In some patients with severe urethral stricture disease, the authors have completely reconstructed the urethra, and in others they have simply performed a perineal urethrostomy. Younger patients have requested mobilization and release of the penis with place-

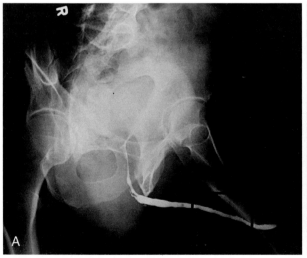
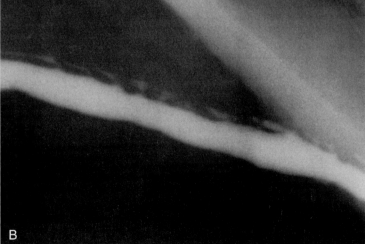

Figure 107–11. *A,* Urethrogram in a patient with urethral stricture disease secondary to balanitis xerotica obliterans. *B,* Intravasation of contrast material, during voiding, into the dilated glands of Littre. (From Jordan GH: Reconstruction for strictures of the fossa navicularis. *In* McAninch J, ed: Topics in Clinical Urology: New Techniques in Reconstructive Urology. New York, Igaku-Shoin, 1996, p 10.)

ment of a split-thickness skin graft. Because the inflammation involves the glans penis (which is not removed), however, the secondary inflammation may also involve the skin graft. Therefore, lifelong monitoring of these patients for the secondary effects of inflammation is necessary. In addition, several reports have appeared suggesting the development of squamous cell carcinoma in patients with a long history of BXO (Dore et al, 1990; Pride and Tyler, 1993).

URETHROCUTANEOUS FISTULA

A fistula is a tract lined with epithelium, leading from the urethra to the skin. The size of a urethral stricture may vary from a pinpoint to quite large. A urethral fistula may be the result of a complication of urethral surgery, or it may develop secondary to periurethral infection associated with inflammatory strictures or treatment of a urethral growth (condyloma or papillary tumor). Treatment of a urethral fistula must be directed not only toward the defect but also at the underlying process that led to its development and therefore varies depending on the cause of the fistula.

After urethral surgery, a fistula may develop as either an immediate or a delayed complication. An early fistula is the result of poor local healing secondary to hematoma, infection, or tension on the tissues. In addition, breakdown of the urethral and overlying skin closures might occur. Occasionally, with aggressive local care and continued urinary diversion, the fistula closes spontaneously.

If a fistula is noted after removal of a urethral stent for a voiding trial, urinary diversion is reinstituted. Before reinsertion of a urethral stent in the management of such an acute fistula, cystoscopy may be helpful to determine if meatal stenosis or other complicating factors are present. If these measures fail, repair of the fistula should be delayed for 6 months to allow for complete resolution of the inflammation.

The authors use several methods to close fistulas. Endoscopic and radiographic evaluation of the urethra should be performed before the repair. If the fistula is small and closure of the hole does not decrease the lumen of the urethra, a button of skin is removed from around the fistula, and its edges are cut even with the urethra (Fig. 107–12). The urethra is closed with 6–0 or 7–0 polydioxanone sutures (PDS), inverting the mucosal edge, and the authors test the repair to ensure that it is watertight. A second layer of tissue is closed over the sutures, and a widely mobilized flap of skin is placed over the repair so that the suture lines are not apposed. The authors leave a small silicone stent tube in the urethra for 10 to 14 days to reduce pressure during voiding. The operating microscope can be useful for the closure of small fistulas. Use of the microscope allows for the use of 8–0 polyglycolic acid suture.

If the fistula is so large that simple closure compromises the lumen of the urethra, a trap-door flap of penile skin is left attached to one edge of the fistula, and the other edges are incised even with the urethral mucosa (Fig. 107–13). The flap is trimmed to fit exactly and sewn in place with interrupted 7–0 PDS to invert the mucosa. The authors leave

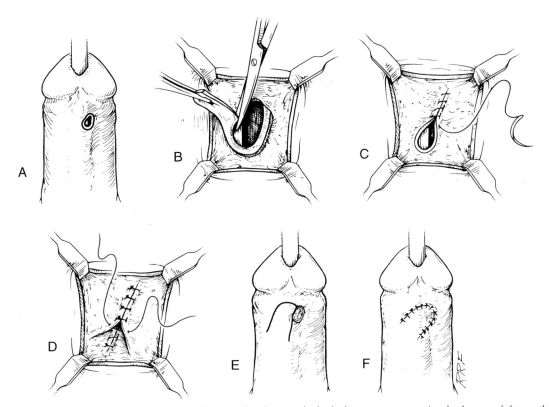

Figure 107–12. *A,* An incision is marked surrounding a fistula—the closure of which does not compromise the lumen of the urethra. *B,* The skin is dissected peripherally, and the fistula tract is excised. *C,* A running extraepithelial 6–0 polydioxanone suture secures a watertight closure. *D,* A second layer of sutures buries the urethral closure. *E,* A skin flap is designed to cover the repair without overlapping suture lines. *F,* The closure is complete—a Bioclusive dressing is applied. The patient voids through a silicone stent for 2 weeks. (From Jordan GH, Schlossberg SM, McCraw JB: AUA Update Series, Lesson 10, Vol 7, 1988.)

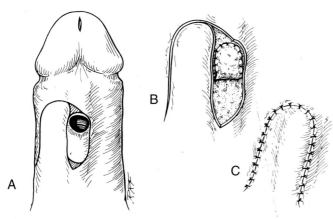

Figure 107–13. A, A trapdoor flap is outlined to fill the defect when simple closure would compromise the urethral lumen. B, The flap has been mobilized and sewn into the fistula defect. C, A skin flap is transposed to cover the repair to avoid overlapping suture lines. A Bioclusive dressing is applied. (From Jordan GH, Schlossberg SM, McCraw JB: AUA Update Series, Lesson 10, Vol 7, 1988.)

a urethral stent in place for 10 to 14 days and occasionally divert the urine for several days with a feeding tube passed through it.

Fistulas associated with inflammatory strictures occur as periurethral tracts and develop secondary to high-pressure voiding of infected urine. As multiple tracts develop, this problem becomes what is known as a "watering-pot perineum." Repair requires suprapubic drainage, and treatment of the infection requires incision and drainage of any abscesses present. The authors widely excise the fistula tracts and associated inflammatory tissue and wait 4 to 6 months before repairing the underlying stricture. In cases in which tissue is available, a flap urethroplasty is the authors' first choice; however, a staged meshed graft procedure (see further discussion) is also an excellent choice.

Treatment of a fistula occurring after electrocautery or laser destruction of a urethral lesion follows the principles outlined previously. If the original lesion was a papillary tumor or condyloma, however, it is imperative to determine if there has been any seeding of the tract that must be excised at the time of repair.

URETHRAL DIVERTICULUM

A diverticulum is an epithelium-lined pouch. These can result from a distention of a segment of the urethra or can consist of an outpouching attached to the urethra by a narrow ostium. In males, a congenital urethral diverticulum may result from incomplete development of the urethra, with a defect in only the ventral wall and subsequent distention of this segment by the hydraulic force of the voiding stream. Furthermore, the downstream lip of the defect may serve as a valvular obstruction, increasing the pressure in the lumen and the rate at which the diverticulum enlarges. Injuries of the urethra may also cause defects (fistula or diverticulum), and these are often associated with urethral strictures.

A congenital diverticulum in the prostatic urethra may be a large remnant of the müllerian duct associated with intersex. It often occurs in proximal hypospadias, however,

and represents an enlarged utricle (Fig. 107–14A) (Devine et al, 1980a). These diverticula may not be demonstrated with voiding urethrography but are demonstrated with cystoscopy or retrograde urethrography. The tip of a urethral catheter tends to catch in this opening, necessitating the use of a catheter guide. Other than requiring caution during evaluation, they do not usually cause problems or require treatment.

Occasionally, however, a large diverticulum holds urine postvoiding and leads to dribbling, recurrent infection, or obstruction (Fig. 107–14B). A surgical approach to small lesions can be through a suprapubic incision, possibly opening the bladder to go through the center of the trigone. Large diverticula, however, can be approached transsacrally, using the Peña approach (Peña and Devries, 1982). Although this is a complex procedure, it seems to be associated with much less morbidity than an abdominal or a perineal approach. The authors excise the diverticulum after exposing and dissecting its communication with the urethra. After ensuring that there is no distal obstruction to interfere with healing, the authors close the urethra.

Diverticula of the female urethra may result from dilation of the periurethral glands or may follow maternal birth trauma. In some cases, it is believed that the diverticulum arises secondary to obstruction of the periureteral glands with subsequent microabscess formation (infected or sterile). The diverticulum then forms as the microabscess decompresses into the urethral lumen. Urethral dribbling after voiding may be an early finding. Diverticula can cause severe pain when they become infected and distended with pus. Diagnosis is made by palpation of a mass and expression of urine or infected material from the urethra. Most cases require radiographic confirmation before surgery. Sometimes a diverticulum fills on a voiding urethrogram; however, its delineation may require a special catheter that occludes the bladder neck and external meatus with balloons, while an opening between them allows the urethra to fill with contrast material. Ultrasound can document the presence of a fluid-filled structure and can aid in defining the extent of the diverticulum, especially if it extends anteriorly around the urethra. Cancer occurs extremely rarely in a diverticulum.

Repair of a urethral diverticulum can be accomplished by excising the diverticulum and closing its neck through a vertical or U-shaped vaginal incision or by simply opening the sac to allow drainage. A catheter in the urethra and, if possible, a Fogarty balloon placed in the sac aid in the dissection. The urethra may be opened back to the neck of the diverticulum and a urethroplasty accomplished after excision of the diverticulum. Spence and Duckett (1970) and O'Conor and Kropp (1969) have shown that it is possible to marsupialize a distal urethral diverticulum by incising the urethra and the wall of the diverticulum, allowing the tract to granulate. The authors' experience with this procedure has not been good, however, and they select it for only the smallest and most distal lesions. Patients have noted considerable tenderness in these opened urethras.

PARAPHIMOSIS, BALANITIS, AND PHIMOSIS

Paraphimosis, or painful swelling of the foreskin distal to a phimotic ring, may occur if the foreskin has been retracted

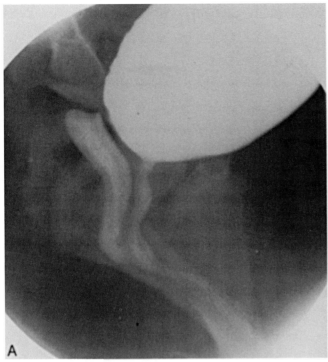

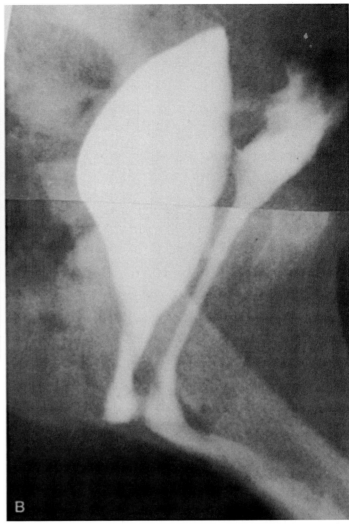

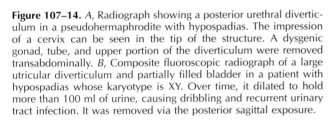

Figure 107–14. *A,* Radiograph showing a posterior urethral diverticulum in a pseudohermaphrodite with hypospadias. The impression of a cervix can be seen in the tip of the structure. A dysgenic gonad, tube, and upper portion of the diverticulum were removed transabdominally. *B,* Composite fluoroscopic radiograph of a large utricular diverticulum and partially filled bladder in a patient with hypospadias whose karyotype is XY. Over time, it dilated to hold more than 100 ml of urine, causing dribbling and recurrent urinary tract infection. It was removed via the posterior sagittal exposure.

for a prolonged period of time. Swelling may be sufficient to prevent its subsequent replacement over the glans. To reduce paraphimosis, gentle, steady pressure must be applied to the foreskin to decrease the swelling. Especially with a child, this is best accomplished in a quiet room by a parent squeezing it in the hand. Elastic wrap may be helpful in some cases. When the swelling has been reduced, the surgeon can push against the glans with the thumbs, pulling on the foreskin with the fingers. Because paraphimosis tends to recur, a circumcision should be carried out as an elective procedure at a later date. An occasional patient presents with acute paraphimosis that has been present for many hours or days. This is typically seen in an adolescent who is reluctant to reveal the problem to his parents. In these cases, reduction may be impossible and should be dealt with by emergency dorsal slit or circumcision.

Balanitis, or inflammation of the glans, can occur as a result of poor hygiene from failure to retract and clean under the foreskin. The subsequent swelling makes cleaning more difficult, but the inflammation usually responds to local care and antibiotic ointment. Occasionally an oral antibiotic may be necessary.

Phimosis, or the inability to retract the foreskin, can result from repeated episodes of balanitis. In older patients, bala-

nitis may be a presenting sign of diabetes. In these cases, circumcision may be warranted.

URETHRAL MEATAL STENOSIS

A small urethral meatus in the newborn is probably not called to a urologist's attention unless the stenosis is associated with other congenital deformities (e.g., hypospadias) or causes voiding difficulties or urinary tract infection (Allen and Summers, 1974). If the urethral meatus of a boy appears exceptionally narrow and there are associated symptoms, a meatotomy should be considered. To make this decision, voiding should be observed to note that the meatus opens as a full, forceful stream is passed. If the stream is narrow and excessively forceful, stenosis is probably present. The occluding skin is generally a thin layer that can be seen to pouch out, with the meatus opening in its center as the child voids.

A **ventral urethral meatotomy** can at times be accomplished using local anesthesia (Fig. 107–15). It is important to insert the needle into the skinfold from the underside, so that the tip of the needle can be observed and controlled. If insertion is done from the outside, the needle passes through

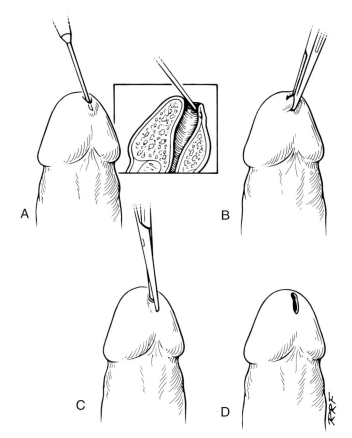

Figure 107–15. Ventral meatotomy. This procedure is useful for children with meatal stenosis secondary to ammoniacal meatitis. *A,* If performed under local anesthesia, a needle can be introduced into the obstructing diaphragm tissue from the inside. *B,* The ventral diaphragm is crushed using a small hemostat. *C,* The crushed tissue is incised. *D,* The appearance of the meatus following ventral meatotomy. The child's parent is instructed to use a meatal dilator, thus separating the crushed edges during healing.

both layers of the fold, and a wheal cannot be raised because of leakage of the anesthetic solution. After the meatotomy, the edges of the cut seal together, unless they are kept open. The tip of a pediatric meatal dilator is the best instrument for this purpose. The child's parents are instructed to separate the edges gently with the tip of the tube, three times a day, for 7 to 10 days. The surgeon should observe the parents as they use the ointment for lubrication and the wedge-shaped tip for gentle dilation.

Meatal stenosis occurs in adults following inflammation, specific or nonspecific urethral infection, and trauma (especially in association with indwelling catheters or urethral instrumentation). It may also be the result of the failure of a previous hypospadias repair. To perform a ventral meatotomy in a normally developed penis in adolescents and adults, it is often necessary to place sutures to approximate the urethral mucosal edges to control bleeding. This step usually requires three sutures: one at the apex and one on each side. The authors find a dilator made by Cook (Cook Urological, Spencer, IN) to be helpful in keeping the meatus open. In some cases, it may be necessary to perform a dorsal rather than a ventral meatotomy. This can be accomplished as a **Y-V-plasty,** after the excision of any scarred ridge of neourethra (Fig. 107–16).

CIRCUMCISION

Controversy continues as to whether neonatal circumcision should or should not be performed (Poland, 1990; Schoen, 1990). Much attention has been focused on this issue, but despite this most male infants in the United States are circumcised. Ritual circumcision will continue; however, in ritual circumcision, it is not necessary to remove the skin but only to draw blood. It is important not to circumcise any boy with a penile abnormality (e.g., hypospadias) that may require the foreskin for repair.

Most circumcisions performed just after birth are done with the Gomco clamp or one of the plastic disposable devices made for this purpose. Caution should be used to free the foreskin from the glans completely and to apply appropriate tension when pulling the foreskin into the clamp, to prevent either a too generous or an inadequate circumcision.

The most common complication is bleeding as a result of inadequate control with vascular compression. Application of an epinephrine-soaked sponge may help in controlling a minimal ooze. Infection can also occur and responds to local care. Any resulting skin separation should be repaired after the inflammation resolves. Sometimes too much skin is removed, or the urethra is included in the clamp, resulting in a fistula. If the entire penis is "scalped," it is best managed with a split-thickness skin graft or with reapplication of the excised skin after preparing it as a graft. In complicated cases, burying the penis in the scrotum and repairing it at a later date may be the best option. Monopolar electrocautery should be avoided in a neonatal circumcision because penile loss from the field distribution of the current can occur.

At present, the consensus is that a newborn who has lost his penis as a result of such a mishap should be gender reassigned (Oesterling et al, 1987; Gearhart and Rock, 1989). The authors' experience with phallic construction now includes a number of children and youths, and some of these older patients had been converted to female after a circumcision accident, and as they passed through puberty they realized that this sexual assignment was wrong. **The authors believe that with the present knowledge of reconstructive techniques, the matter should receive more thought because most of these boys could undergo reconstruction in such a manner as to preserve reproductive function.**

In adults, circumcision can be done using local anesthesia, by blocking the dorsal nerves at the base of the penis and circumferentially infiltrating the superficial layers of the

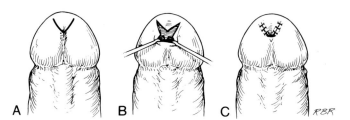

Figure 107–16. The procedure for dorsal Y-V meatotomy. *A,* Skin incisions are outlined by the dotted line. The V-shaped flap of glans is incised and elevated. *B,* An incision is made on the dorsal surface of the urethra. *C,* The flap of glans has been advanced into the urethra. (From Jordan GH: Reconstruction of the meatus/fossa navicularis using flap techniques. *In* Schreiter F, ed: Plastic Reconstructive Surgery in Urology. Stuttgart, Germany, Georg Thieme Publishers. In press.)

penile base. The authors favor a sleeve circumcision in men and older boys (Fig. 107–17). With the foreskin in its retracted position, a marking pen outlines an incision approximately 1 cm proximal to the corona. This mark should go straight across the base of the frenulum. This incision is made and carried through the dartos fascia down to the superficial lamina of Buck's fascia. The foreskin is reduced, and a second incision is marked, following the outlines of the corona and the V of the frenulum on the ventral side. The frenulum usually retracts into a V. In some cases, the frenulum can be lengthened by closing the edges of the V in a longitudinal orientation for a short length (frenuloplasty) (see Fig. 107–17D). If frenuloplasty is done, the proximal incision does not need to follow the V of the retracted frenulum in that the ventral skin is straight. The authors make the skin incision and fulgurate bleeding vessels with bipolar cautery, as the incision is deepened and the skin edge mobilized. In older boys, the vessels are more substantial

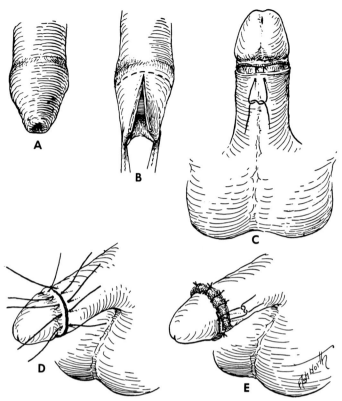

Figure 107–18. Circumcision in a patient with phimosis. *A,* Phimosis to be corrected by circumcision. *B,* Incision in the dorsal aspect of the foreskin, which has been drawn over the glans. Broken line indicates point of incision for removal of foreskin. *C,* Suture in frenulum. *D,* Closure. Note that the sutures have been left long. *E,* Sutures are tied around a strip of Xeroform gauze.

and not easily sealed by compression, no matter how vigorous. Thus, circumcision clamps are often ineffective and are not recommended even though larger sizes are available. After the sleeve of prepuce has been removed, hemostasis is obtained, and the skin edges are reapproximated.

In smaller boys, this sleeve procedure may be considered tedious and difficult by some. If this is the case, after marking the skin, a dorsal slit is made through both layers of the prepuce back to the level of the corona (Fig. 107–18). Following the marks, the two layers of the prepuce are incised. Bleeders are controlled, and the skin edges are reapproximated.

Complications should be uncommon. Most patients develop some hyperesthesia of the glans, which resolves. A hematoma is probably the most common immediate complication. Some patients notice minor cosmetic imperfections that are functionally insignificant. One of the most distressing problems seen by the authors, however, is a patient who complains that the surgeon has removed too much skin. To avoid this occurrence, a circumcision should be done precisely, and, whatever the procedure to be carried out, the incisions should first be marked with the skin lying undistorted on the shaft.

FAILED HYPOSPADIAS REPAIR

When treating a patient in whom hypospadias repair has failed, it is important to obtain all available records to help

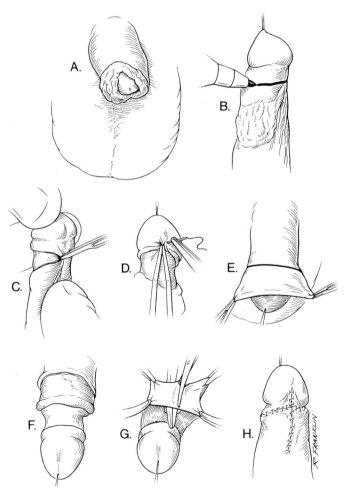

Figure 107–17. Technique of sleeve circumcision. *A,* Appearance of the penis. The redundant penile or preputial skin is reduced over the glans. *B,* The skin is retracted, and the distal incision is marked. *C,* The incision is created and carried sharply down to Buck's fascia. *D,* Frenuloplasty is performed. *E,* The proximal incision is marked. *F,* The incision is carried down deeply into the dartos fascia. *G,* The sleeve of tissue is divided in the midline, and the redundant tissue is excised. *H,* Appearance of the ventrum of the penis after closure. Notice in this child there was circumferential redundancy of the penile skin, and hence a wedge incision of the ventrum has been performed to improve the closure.

determine what may have contributed to the complication. A hypospadias repair may fail as a result of an inadequate correction of chordee or an inadequate urethra, with a stricture, fistula, or diverticulum (Winslow et al, 1986). Many times, from the records, it becomes readily apparent that not all aspects of the hypospadias deformity (Fig. 107–19) (i.e., ventrally displaced meatus, ventral chordee, and some expression of ventral tissue fusion inadequacy) were addressed in the previous repairs. Adults with urethral strictures are often seen who have had hypospadias surgery as a child. Depending on the age of the patient and the preference of the treating urologist, a variety of different techniques may have been used to repair the original hypospadias. Some of these patients have persistent chordee and a subcoronal meatus. Adults have also been seen who have had long-standing evidence for urethral fistula. In addition, some patients may have clinical findings not related to hypospadias that should have been recognized previously, especially when hypospadias is an aspect of intersex. In years past, problems associated with previous failures have been caused by errors in design, technique, or postoperative care (Devine et al, 1978). With more modern techniques available and with most hypospadias treated by surgeons with considerable experience, failures are seen with postoperative infections or other factors that have an adverse impact on wound healing. Complex hypospadias repair failures are being encountered with much less frequency, and most that are encountered are patients that had their last procedures more than 10 years ago.

Evaluation of a failed hypospadias repair includes retrograde urethrogram, voiding cystourethrogram, and cystoscopy. In an older patient, a reliable preoperative assessment of residual chordee can be made based on history and photographs taken at home. In younger patients, complete evaluation of more complex situations using anesthesia may be necessary.

In the adult patient, a detailed discussion must occur about the positive and negative aspects of the various approaches. Patients who were initially operated on before the late 1970s likely underwent either a graft or some form of repair using almost exclusively ventral tissue. Some of these patients still have the remnants of a dorsal hood or enough dorsal skin to perform a dorsal transverse penile skin island flap reconstruction.

The authors believe that **surgical correction of complex cases requires an aggressive attitude** (Secrest et al, 1993). All residual dysgenetic and scarred tissue causing chordee must be excised and the penis straightened, employing various techniques as necessary. All of the fibrotic tissue around the neourethra must be excised. If the urethra is inadequate, it too must be excised. The most difficult cases clearly present a challenge to the reconstructive surgeon. The techniques for release of chordee and repair of urethral strictures are discussed later. In particular, the authors have found the dorsal transverse penile skin island flap repair, the buccal epithelial onlay graft procedure, and the staged meshed split-thickness skin graft technique especially useful for this group of complicated re-do hypospadias patients.

RESIDUAL GENITAL ABNORMALITY IN PATIENTS WITH REPAIRED EXSTROPHY

Residual genital defects in men who have had exstrophy repaired as a child can cause functional, esthetic, and psychologic problems. The emotional effects of these problems are compounded in men who have undergone urinary diversion and who must wear stomal appliances. Except in the most severe forms of bladder exstrophy or cloacal exstrophy when the penis or two halves of the bifid penis are truly inadequate, successful reconstruction is possible. Even then, if normal testes are present, the success of newer techniques of phallic construction (see subsequent discussion) should lend support to consideration of the option of raising the child as a boy, preserving his reproductive potential through puberty. In these difficult cases, the authors believe that the parents must be presented with both options: gender reassignment versus prepubertal phalloplasty. Remarkable progress has been made in the treatment of difficult cases (Johnston, 1975; Hendren, 1979; Jeffs, 1979; Snyder, 1990). Many patients, however, need further genital surgery as they experience the hypertrophic growth spurt of the penis associated with puberty. The goals of reconstructive surgery in male patients with exstrophy or epispadias are to produce a dangling penis with erectile bodies of satisfactory length and shape to allow sexual function and to construct a urethra that serves as a conduit for the passage of urine and ejaculate.

Many patients who have undergone surgery as children do not present for correction of inadequacies of the external genitalia until after they have completed puberty and realize that the situation has not improved and likely will not improve. The authors employ a systematic approach to accomplishing the reconstruction necessary to correct the anatomic defects in these patients (Winslow et al, 1988). Surgery is undertaken in a sequential fashion beginning with the simplest procedure that can achieve the desired functional result.

SURGICAL TECHNIQUE
Release and Lengthening of the Penis

The **W flap incision** (Fig. 107–20) allows mobilization of superiorly based random flaps of skin lateral to the base of

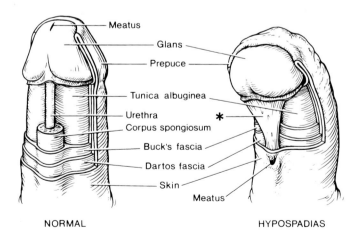

Figure 107–19. Anatomy of the normal penis and one with hypospadias. The fan-shaped band of fibrous tissue marked with an asterisk is the tissue that contributes to chordee. (From Devine CJ Jr, Horton CE: Bent penis. Semin Urol 1987; 5:252.)

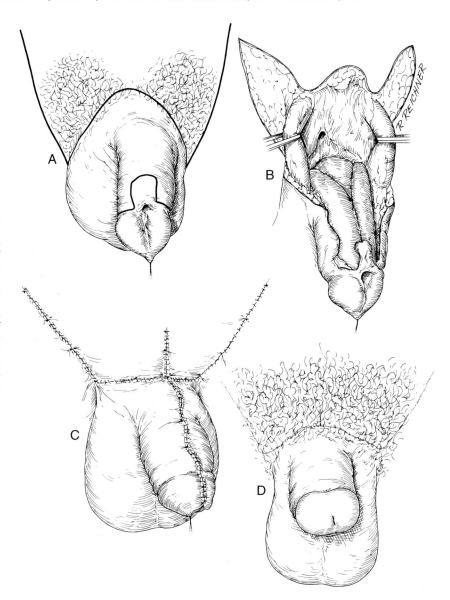

Figure 107–20. *A*, Development of the superiorly based W flap for exposure of the penile shaft and correction of the abnormal distribution of the pubic hair. *B*, The flap is developed, and the structures of the cord are immobilized and retracted laterally. A midline incision in the skin exposes the penile shaft. *C*, At completion of the repair, the penile skin is closed, and transposition of the limbs of the W to the midline has placed the pubic hair above the base of the penis. *D*, After healing, the growth of hair hides the scars of the incision. (From Winslow BH, Horton CE, Gilbert DA, Devine CJ Jr: Epispadias and exstrophy of the bladder. *In* Mustarde JC, Jackson IT, eds: Plastic Surgery in Infancy and Childhood, 3rd ed. New York, Churchill Livingstone, 1988, p 527.)

the penis, affording optimal exposure of the infrapubic region. The penis can then be mobilized by meticulous dissection. When the penis dangles, the authors proceed using one of a number of possible techniques designed to correct intrinsic chordee until an artificial erection confirms that the penis is straight. If necessary, the urethra can be constructed using graft or flap techniques or in many cases can be transposed to the ventrum as in the **Cantwell-Ransley procedure** (Gearhart et al, 1992). All of the midline abdominal and penopubic scar tissue is excised and the attached skin released, while preserving the vascularity in the layer deep to the skin.

Care must be taken while mobilizing these flaps in patients who have had inguinal herniorrhaphies, not an unusual situation in exstrophy patients. The presence of herniorrhaphy scars is not a contraindication to the use of the W flap. The flap must be more cautiously elevated, preserving all of the remaining blood supply to the tip. A dorsal midline incision in the penile skin may be extended distally to meet a circumcising incision proximal to the coronal margin of the epispadiac glans to expose the shaft of the penis. If one antici-

pates using a Cantwell-Ransley type of technique, a paired incision along the lateral margins of the urethra may be preferable.

With the W flap, closure of the incision reconstructs the bifid escutcheon. Likewise, some reconstruction of the lower abdominal wall is accomplished. The bifid escutcheon is brought medially and superiorly into a more normal location by transposition of the tips of the W flap to the midline (see Fig. 107–20*C* and *D*). The incisions are closed with subcutaneous polyglactin 910 (Vicryl) sutures and subcuticular long-acting absorbable monofilament sutures.

With the incisions created, a sound is placed in the native urethra or neourethra of a patient who has had previous urethral reconstruction; this helps to identify these structures and avoid injury to them. Because of the inguinal anomalies associated with exstrophy, the spermatic cord structures may be unusually superficial (see Fig. 107–20*B*). On each side, they should be identified as the tips of the W flap are elevated. They can be mobilized and retracted laterally with Penrose drains. The dorsal penile branches of the pudendal vessels and nerves stand on to the dorsal surface laterally at the base of each corporal body and must be preserved during any dissection on the shaft of the penis.

After the W flaps are elevated and retracted, the authors evaluate the corporal bodies. Relative shortening, dorsal chordee, and sometimes torsion of the penis may be caused by one or more of the following factors:

1. Inelastic fibrous bands of scar tissue that attach the penis to the bone or fascia in the anterior part of the ring of the pelvis.
2. Shortness of a dorsally placed native urethra or shortness and possible scarring of a previously constructed neourethra.
3. Inelasticity of abnormal attachments of the deeper dartos and Buck's fascial layers.
4. Dysgenetic development or inelasticity of the dorsal aspect of the tunica albuginea of the paired corpora cavernosa.

The skin of the penis is elevated to dissect any restricting tissue from the shaft. If the epispadiac urethra or neourethra prevents release of the penis during this mobilization, the authors transect the urethra distally and mobilize the proximal portion, releasing the vascular spongy tissue of the corpus spongiosum. This tissue lies deep to the urethra in the midline, between the divergent proximal ends of the corporal bodies. Bleeding from the thin-walled venous spaces of the corpus spongiosum may be troublesome if entered. The dissection is continued releasing the proximal portions of the erectile bodies from their attachment to the widespread inferior pubic rami and excising dysgenetic or scar tissue encountered during the dissection. The authors have not routinely completely detached the corpora as has been described (Kelley and Eraklis, 1971) for fear of devascularization of the corporal bodies.

When at any point in this dissection the penis has been released so that it dangles, the authors move to the next step to straighten the penile shaft. The divergent corporal bodies cause the base of the penis to be wide; however, sewing the corporal bodies together to narrow the base of the penis would also shorten the penile shaft. If urethral reconstruction is not undertaken at this time, the proximal urethra can and should be released and passed between the corporal bodies to open on the underside of the penis.

Correction of Chordee

After release of the penis, the authors assess the degree of chordee by artificial erection. Because the **corpora in exstrophy and epispadias do not communicate,** an artificial erection requires the use of two needles and syringes. If the artificial erection demonstrates that the penis is straight, further dissection is not required. This is seldom the case, however, because the penis usually is not straight. The location, direction, and degree of curvature are identified, and the authors then proceed with its correction. After each step of the sequence, shaft straightness is reassessed with another artifical erection. When the penis is straight, the authors may proceed with urethral reconstruction followed by penile shaft skin coverage.

The **first step in correction of chordee involves the resection of all dysgenetic restrictive bands** from the dor-

sal surface of the corporal bodies, carefully preserving the dorsolateral vessels and nerves. **If chordee persists** after this dissection, the problems are related to dysgenetic development of the corporal bodies themselves. There are **three treatment options possible,** depending on the extent and location of the chordee:

1. Excision of ellipses of the tunica albuginea from the convex (i.e., ventral) aspect of the corporal bodies and approximation of the cut edges (Fig. 107–21A). This technique tends to shorten what is already a short penis but is useful for the patient who has a well-functioning urethra that should be preserved (Horton and Devine, 1973; Vorstman and Devine, 1987).
2. Koff and Eakins (1984) described inward corporal rotation to correct chordee (Fig. 107–21B). After mobilizing the ventral aspects of the corporal bodies, several deep midline PDS are placed to rotate the corporal bodies inward, attaching them in the midline. If artificial erection now shows the penis to be straight, the tunica of each corporal body is incised and joined by suturing the respective edges together to ensure persistence of the rotation.
3. Most commonly, the authors lengthen the dorsal aspect of the corpora by insertions with dermal graft inlay (Fig. 107–22). During artificial erection, the dorsal aspect of each

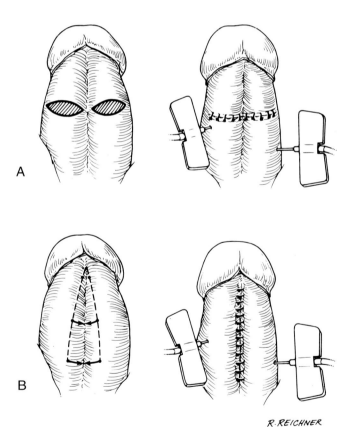

R. REICHNER

Figure 107–21. *A,* Nesbit-type ellipses are excised from the ventral aspect of the two erectile bodies. Closure of these can straighten the chordee. *B,* Koff's procedure. The corporal bodies are rotated to the midline and tacked in place. If this maneuver corrects the chordee, a longitudinal incision is made in the tunica, and the rotation is fixed with absorbable monofilament sutures. (From Winslow BH, Horton CE, Gilbert DA, Devine CJ Jr: Epispadias and exstrophy of the bladder. *In* Mustarde JC, Jackson IT, eds: Plastic Surgery in Infancy and Childhood, 3rd ed. New York, Churchill Livingstone, 1988, p 527.)

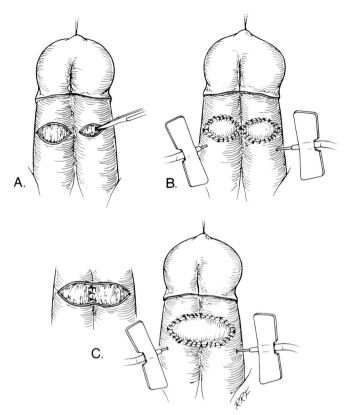

Figure 107–22. Correction of chordee with dermal graft. *A,* Transverse incisions are made in the dorsal aspect of the corporal bodies. *B,* A lenticular dermal graft is placed in each of these defects, or, *C,* the medial ends of the incision are sewn together with absorbable mono-filament sutures, and the conjoined defect is closed with a simple dermal graft. (From Winslow BH, Horton CE, Gilbert DA, Devine CJ Jr: Epispadias and exstrophy of the bladder. *In* Mustarde JC, Jackson IT, eds: Plastic Surgery in Infancy and Childhood, 3rd ed. New York, Churchill Livingstone, 1988, p 527.)

of the corporal bodies is marked at the point of maximum concavity. Incisions at these marks extend from the medial midline of the corporal bodies to the lateral midline, thus allowing the tunica to elongate, leaving the vascular erectile tissue exposed. To preserve the increased length, the defects are patched with dermal graft inlays. Lenticular grafts (see Fig. 107–22B) can be used, each individually placed in the defects in the corpora. In most cases, the medial aspects of the incisions are approximated, and then the merged defect is covered with a single dermal graft (see Fig. 107–22C). Details concerning the harvest and inlay of dermal grafts are covered later in the section dealing with Peyronie's disease.

Urethral Construction

At this point, the shaft of the penis should be straight and free to dangle. In each case, the complexity of the procedures required and of those necessary to create a urethra determines whether completion of the reconstruction is to be staged or accomplished at the time of the current surgery. Graft-graft interfaces must be avoided because of the potential for interference with take in the area where the grafts are coapted. If a dermal graft has been used to straighten the penis and it appears that a graft is necessary for urethral

reconstruction, it is advisable to proceed with urethral construction at another stage. The authors would not construct the urethra with a tubed graft at this stage unless it could be placed in the ventral groove between the corpora without overlapping the dorsally placed dermal grafts. It is preferable to complete urethral construction in one stage, and this may be possible using one of the following techniques: (1) A tubed graft can be brought to the ventral aspect of the penis by passing it between the corporal bodies at their base, keeping it well away from the dermal grafts, and (2) a flap of ventral penile skin can be used, which can be tubed to form a urethra and brought between the corpora to rest on the dermal graft or left on the ventral surface. If transposed dorsally, the dartos fascia probably enhances the vascular bed for the dermal grafts (Duckett, 1981).

For patients with epispadias and for patients with exstrophy who still have sufficient penile skin, the skin from the ventrum of the penis is preferable for urethral construction. Redundancy of the penile skin is usually not present, and thus urethral construction might require a tube graft. As with all urethral reconstruction, the graft options include penile or preputial skin, bladder epithelium, or buccal mucosa (see Fig. 107–1). In reality, it is not advisable to diminish the closed exstrophy bladder compliance and volume by harvesting a bladder epithelial graft. Likewise, usually, penile skin is at a premium, leaving (as of this writing) the buccal mucosa graft as the most likely option for graft urethral construction. In some patients presenting for secondary exstrophy reconstruction, the midline abdominal skin is not scarred, and the tumble-tube technique described by Snyder (1990) may be helpful.

If a patient has undergone previous urinary diversion, construction of a urethra may not be necessary, and coverage of the penis completes the procedure. In these patients, however, if they have a remnant of their bladder neck, a sinus must be created to allow the escape of prostatic secretions, ejaculate, or both. Failure to create such a sinus tract allows these fluids to collect in what becomes rather sizable suprapubic cysts. The sinus may be placed in the abdominal wall above the base of the penis, or if there is a posterior urethral remnant that can be formed into a tube, it can be brought out between the corpora to open in the skin below the penis.

Repair of the Escutcheon in Exstrophy

In exstrophy, as part of the midline abnormality, as already mentioned, the hair-bearing skin of the escutcheon is located lateral to the penis and scrotum (see Fig. 107–20A). Usually, there is no umbilicus as the cord enters from the upper edge of the exstrophic bladder patch. When present, the umbilicus is usually caudally displaced and prone to hernia formation. In some centers, the umbilical stump is dissected from the "dome" of the bladder patch and transposed through the abdominal wall to the normal anatomic location. As they mature, these children then have a true umbilicus. The lower abdominal wall exhibits diastasis recti, and the lower midline area is often quite scarred. The W flaps nicely transpose the skin, making the escutcheon appear more anatomically correct, but, more important, there is a contouring of the suprapubic area. Often a large amount of dead space is created by the elevation of these flaps. The interface between the flaps must be drained using small suction drains. In some cases, it is helpful to fill the space at the base of the penis with a vertical inferior rectus abdominis muscle flap.

Skin Coverage

If possible, coverage of the penile shaft is accomplished with flaps of penile skin. These tissues provide proper sensation and have correct pigmentation. In many multiply operated patients, however, skin coverage can be a problem because the remaining genital skin is scarred and insufficient to cover the length of the straightened penis. If well vascularized, the penile shaft can be covered with a skin graft. If a dermal graft was employed to correct chordee or if a tubed graft was employed to create a neourethra in a patient in whom there is insufficient penile skin, the authors would not choose a skin graft to cover the penile shaft. Local flaps must be developed to cover the penis; the authors have used the groin flap in the past (Devine and Horton, 1979). Revision of the penile skin coverage can be done in 6 months. Often the skin of the penis and the graft or flap has become so elastic that at the time of scar revision, one is able to excise completely the redundancy of the tissue and close the penile skin primarily.

Umbilicoplasty

As mentioned, the technique of transposing the umbilicus to an anatomically correct position during primary exstrophy closure avoids the need for umbilicoplasty. If a child does not have an umbilicus, it can be a disturbing defect, particularly when the child is young. Thus, for children, reconstruction of the umbilicus is important. The umbilicus can be

constructed by elevating a small, superiorly based semicircular flap in the midline at the level of the iliac crests. After removing the subcutaneous fat and exposing the fascia of the abdominal wall, the flap is sutured to the fascia with absorbable monofilament suture. The remaining defect at the lower edge of this wound is covered by a graft of full-thickness or split-thickness skin (Fig. 107–23A through C). If the graft is taken from the area of the genitalia, it creates a color contrast and further emphasizes the umbilicus. Another method of umbilicoplasty merely creates a contour defect, which is grafted with a thin split-thickness skin graft (Fig. 107–23D and E).

Penetrating Trauma of the Penis

Penetrating injuries of the penis can involve the urethra, the corporal bodies, or both. The authors' choice in managing the acute injury is exploration and attempted immediate anatomic repair. In some cases placement of a suprapubic tube is necessary should extensive urethral reconstruction be required. Later, reconstruction is directed at the urethral stricture if it occurs or curvature of the penis, which may occur secondary to damage of the corporal bodies. Fistulas that result from penetrating trauma to the penis are usually treatable by primary closure with imposition of superficial tissue layers between the urethra and the skin. Large fistulas may require more complex tissue transfer and in many ways become urethral reconstruction as if for stricture. The principles are discussed elsewhere.

Amputation of the Penis

Amputation is the ultimate penile injury. If the patient presents acutely with the amputated distal part of the penis,

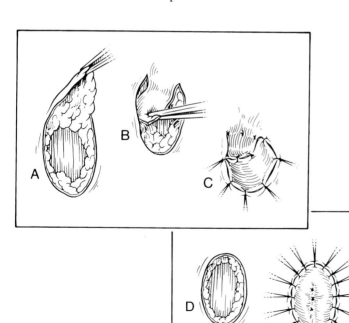

Figure 107–23. Techniques of umbilicoplasty. *A,* Rostrally based semicircular flap is elevated. *B,* The defect is defatted. The flap is tacked to the fascia. *C,* Split-thickness graft is used to cover the defect. *D,* A defect is created down to the level of the fascia. *E,* A split-thickness skin graft is taken from an area of different pigmentation and tacked to the defect.

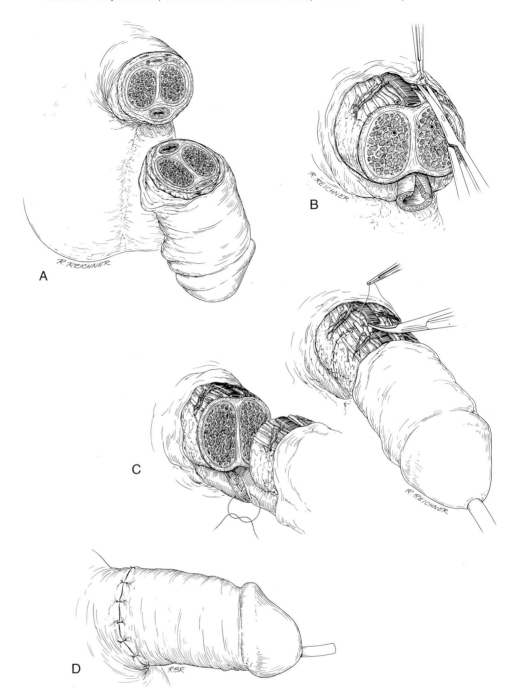

Figure 107–24. Technique of microscopic replantation following amputation of the penis. *A,* The typical appearance of a penile amputation injury. *B,* The urethra, corpora cavernosa, and dorsal neurovascular structures are exposed and minimally debrided. *C,* A two-layer spatulated urethral anastomosis is completed. Microvascular coaptation of the dorsal vein, deep dorsal artery, and dorsal nerves is accomplished. *D,* Coverage is accomplished using the native skin. If the patient is circumcised, the sleeve of skin between the amputation injury and the old circumcision scar should not be discarded. Should chronic edema develop, revision can be accomplished at a later date. *Note:* Diversion is via suprapubic cystostomy tube. The urethral reconstruction is stented. (From Jordan GH, Gilbert DA: Management of amputation injuries of the male genitalia. Urol Clin North Am 1989; 16:359–367.)

microvascular reimplantation is the favored approach (Fig. 107–24). If there is no microvascular surgeon at the center where the patient presents, the patient should be transferred. The penis should be cleaned, wrapped in a sponge soaked in sterile saline, and placed in a sterile Ziploc bag. This is kept in ice water, and reimplantation can be accomplished as long as 18 hours after amputation. Often the amputation is self-inflicted, usually during an acute mental crisis. This should not preclude reimplantation unless the patient adamantly refuses such treatment. Even then, with court order or the agreement of two or more surgeons, reimplantation can be undertaken. The patient's condition or other circumstances may prevent his transfer for microvascular reimplantation. If so, reimplantation by the technique described by McRoberts (1968) should be carried out. His series and other series showed that a high degree of success can be expected following reimplantation without microvascular reanastomosis.

If the patient presents with the distal part having been disposed of or otherwise unavailable, the wound should be closed. Often the penis has been stretched out during the amputation, and an excess of skin has been removed leaving a length of intact but denuded shaft structures proximal to the amputation wound. The authors close the corporal bodies with 4–0 or 5–0 PDS, spatulate the urethral meatus to the tunica, and immediately cover the penile shaft with a split-thickness skin graft. Others bury the shaft beneath the skin of the scrotum. In some of these patients, primary grafting of the stump allows a functional penis. Most, however, require phallic/penile reconstruction.

A number of sophisticated techniques for reconstruction of the traumatized penis are available. The radial forearm flap has become the mainstay of penile reconstructive procedures (see subsequent discussion). The initial stage of reconstruction of the amputated penis consists of mobilizing the penile and urethral stumps.

Degloving Injuries of the Penis

Degloving injuries occur when the skin of the penis or scrotum is trapped and stripped from the deeper structures, exposing the uninjured corpora and the testicles. The tear is deep to the elastic dartos fascia. Bleeding is usually not a problem because there are not many large vessels in this space. The appearance of the bare testicles and penile shaft, however, is impressive.

After defining the extent of the damage, **most degloving injuries can be managed acutely with immediate reconstruction by application of split-thickness skin grafts.** The shaft is covered with a sheet graft of split-thickness skin. The testicles are sutured together in the midline, placed surgically in their anatomically correct position, and covered with a meshed split-thickness skin graft. After take of this graft, the meshing gives the appearance of rugations. With time, the effect of gravity on the testicles causes the reconstructed scrotum to become pendulous and sometimes even redundant. In this repair, split-thickness skin grafts are more successful than full-thickness skin grafts because the host bed is less than optimal after a degloving injury. Although split-thickness grafts cannot be employed for single-stage urethroplasty because of contraction, contraction has not been a problem with such grafts applied to the penile shaft or testicles. Adequate shaft sensation is achieved by way of the structures deep to the graft.

Some surgeons bury the shaft of the penis in a subcutaneous tunnel on the abdomen and bury the testicles in subcutaneous thigh pouches. McDougal (1983) has described a technique to mobilize the buried testicles with the overlying thigh skin, combining scrotal reconstruction with testicular replacement (Fig. 107–25). In patients so managed, this is a good way of transposing the testicles and overlying tissues to an anatomically correct location. When the authors have managed patients who have been previously managed acutely with placement of testicles and penis in subcutaneous tunnels, the authors have mobilized the testicles and the penile shaft from their tunnels and immediately applied grafts of split-thickness skin, as already discussed.

Genital Burns

The ability to reconstruct the damage caused by genital burns often depends on how well the normal structures have been maintained after the acute injury. Careful débridement is the rule in acute management of genital burns. Corporal tissue cannot be replaced with transferred tissue. The physiologic functions of genital tissues cannot be accurately duplicated. The unique vascularity of genital tissue

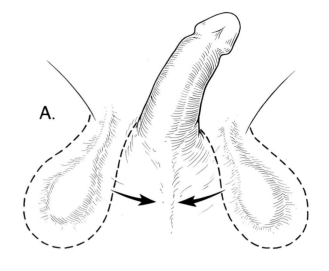

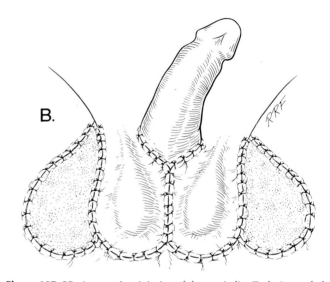

Figure 107–25. Amputation injuries of the genitalia. Technique of elevation and transposition of testicles from thigh pouches. *A,* Testicles in thigh pouches with a random, superiorly based flap outlined. *B,* Flaps and testicles are transposed to the correct anatomic area, and the lateral defects are covered with a skin graft. (Redrawn from McDougal WS: Scrotal reconstruction using thigh pedicle flaps. J Urol 1983; 129:757–759.)

allows for less aggressive rather than more aggressive débridement.

Devastating urethral injuries occur with many burns. Reconstruction of the urethra depends on the nature of the injuries. When the urethra has been nearly obliterated, there usually is not sufficient, uninvolved, nonhirsute local genital tissue that could be transferred for urethral reconstruction. Vascularized tissue must be imported to support reconstruction of the urethra with a graft. In many patients, the penis becomes incarcerated in contracted scar tissue after healing of the acute injury. Successful transposition of a gracilis musculocutaneous flap introduces compliant vascular tissue and skin into the area, allowing release of the penile shaft. Subsequently the penile shaft can be covered with a split-thickness skin graft. In some patients, the genital scarring is so severe that microvascular transfer of a free flap is necessary to replace the penile shaft.

For many patients, reconstruction requires a number of stages. In several patients, the urethra has been obliterated from the entry of the membranous urethra into the bulbospongiosus to the tip of the penis. A perineal urethrostomy has been required while transfer of vascular tissues to the area of the perineum and penis was accomplished. When these tissues are in place, subsequent reconstruction of the urethra can be undertaken with meshed split-thickness skin grafts, bladder epithelial grafts, or buccal mucosa grafts. For coverage, the posterior thigh flap offers excellent bulky, sensate tissues.

Radiation Trauma

Radiation trauma to the penis occurs in two patient subsets: (1) patients in whom radiation has been used therapeutically for a lesion on the penis and (2) those in whom radiation to the pelvis has caused chronic lymphedema. **Therapeutic radiation can produce chronic suppurative gangrene.** These lesions **are not amenable to reconstruction** and are best managed by partial penectomy and later reconstruction. Also, the authors have treated several patients who developed tissue atrophy and further fibrosis after radiation therapy for Peyronie's disease. Delivered at near tumoricidal doses, this radiation made dermal graft repair much more difficult.

In patients with lymphedema the penis can readily be reconstructed. Lymphedema of the penis involves the tissues of the dartos fascia and the dermis layer of the skin. In the penis, the lymphedematous tissue can be excised by removing the dartos fascia and skin, dissecting in the layer superficial to Buck's fascia. In the scrotum, Colle's fascia (the tunica dartos) and the skin of the scrotum must be removed. When the lymphedematous tissue has been excised, the testicles are free, and, as in a degloving injury, they must be fixed in the midline in an anatomically correct position. Often, scrotal skin peripheral to the edema is normal and can be advanced to cover the testicles. The shaft of the penis should be covered with a split-thickness skin graft. If the scrotum cannot be closed, a meshed split-thickness skin graft is used to cover the testicles. Grafts provide optimal reconstruction in these patients.

In contrast to the full-thickness skin graft, split-thickness skin carries little of the reticular dermis and hence few of the lymphatic channels. Reaccumulation of lymphedema can occur within a full-thickness skin graft. Local skin flaps should be avoided because they seldom give good cosmetic results, and often they reaccumulate lymphedema once they have been transposed to the area of the genitalia. As previously noted, grafts do not develop sensation. Good sensation usually develops, however, derived from the deep structures. The glans almost never accumulates disabling edema, and the sensation of the glans remains intact because the lymphedematous tissue has been excised in the plane superficial to Buck's fascia, sparing the dorsal nerves of the penis.

The authors have managed one patient who had organic impotence in addition to chronic lymphedema. He wanted the lymphedematous tissue excised but also desired that a prosthesis be implanted. With lymphedema involving all of the genital tissues, he was not considered to be a good candidate for a hydraulic device. An articulated prosthesis was selected. After excision of the lymphedematous tissue, the articulated device was placed in the penis by way of subcoronal corporotomies, which were meticulously closed. The remaining subcuticular tissue of the glans was superimposed over these closures, and a split-thickness skin graft was placed on the shaft of the penis. The patient had an excellent cosmetic and functional result. The authors believe that placement of a prosthesis at the same time as the graft carried a diminished possibility of morbidity compared with placement of a prosthesis beneath the graft at a later stage.

Direct radiation to the penis can cause urethral injury. It is unusual for the urethra to be injured without damage to adjacent structures. Often, because of the vascularity of the corpus spongiosum, minimal débridement can be accomplished leaving the patient with a fistula that can be reconstructed at a later date. The success of such reconstruction depends on the damage that the radiation has done to the adjacent structures.

URETHRAL STRICTURE DISEASE

The term urethral stricture generally refers to anterior urethral disease, or a scar in the spongy erectile tissue of the corpus spongiosum (spongiofibrosis) (Fig. 107–26). The corpus spongiosum underlies the urethral epithelium, and, in some cases, the scarring process extends through the tissues of the corpus spongiosum and into adjacent tissues. Contraction of this scar reduces the urethral lumen. For example, if a normal urethra measures No. 30 Fr, its diameter is 10 mm and the area of the lumen is approximately 78 mm^2. If scarring has resulted in a urethra that measures No. 15 Fr, the lumen is only 55 mm^2, or 25% reduced. It is therefore evident that scar contraction caused by anterior urethral stricture disease can be associated with marked voiding symptoms.

In contrast, posterior urethral strictures are not included in the common definition of urethral stricture. Posterior urethral stricture is an obliterative process in the posterior urethra that has resulted in fibrosis and is generally the effect of distraction in that area caused by either trauma or radical prostatectomy.

Urethral Anatomy

Although urethral anatomy was described in the previous section on anatomy, it is useful to re-emphasize key anatomic points. The urethra is eccentrically placed in relation to the corpus spongiosum in the bulbous urethra and is much closer to the dorsum of the penile structures (Fig. 107–27). As one moves distally, the pendulous or penile urethra becomes more centrally placed within the corpus spongiosum.

The genital skin has a dual (proximal and distal) and bilateral blood supply, forming a fasciocutaneous system (see Fig. 107–6). The corpus spongiosum receives blood from the common penile artery, the terminal branch of the internal pudendal artery (see Fig. 107–8). The corpus spongiosum also has a dual blood supply, with both a proximal

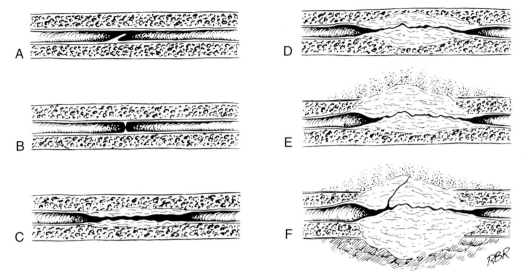

Figure 107–26. The anatomy of anterior urethral strictures. *A,* Mucosal fold. *B,* Iris constriction. *C,* Full-thickness involvement with minimal fibrosis in the spongy tissue. *D,* Full-thickness spongiofibrosis. *E,* Inflammation and fibrosis involving tissues outside the corpus spongiosum. *F,* Complex stricture complicated by a fistula. This can proceed to the formation of an abscess, or the fistula may open to the skin or the rectum. (From Jordan GJ: Management of anterior urethral stricture disease. *In* Webster GD, ed: Problems in Urology. Philadelphia, J. B. Lippincott, 1987, p 199.)

Figure 107–27. Diagrammatic cross sections of the anterior urethra. *A,* The bulbous urethra is eccentrically placed in the corpus spongiosum. Proximally, the corpora cavernosa have split into individual crura, with the urethra lying against the triangular ligament. *B,* In the shaft of the penis, the urethra lies more centrally placed, and the corpora cavernosa are intimately fused, separated only by septal fibers. *C,* At the coronal margin, the urethra remains relatively centrally placed, and the corpora cavernosa are fused, again separated by septal fibers. The spongy tissue of the corpus spongiosum has become incorporated as the deep tissues of the glans. *D,* The fossa navicularis widens somewhat in caliber and is totally surrounded by the spongy erectile tissue of the glans penis. (From Jordan GH, Schlossberg SM: Complications of interventional techniques for urethral stricture disease: direct visual internal urethrotomy, stents and laser intervention. Courtesy of Culley C. Carson, III, MD, from the book Topics in Clinical Urology: Complications of Interventional Techniques. Igaku-Shoin Medical Publishers, New York, NY, 1996, pp 86–94.)

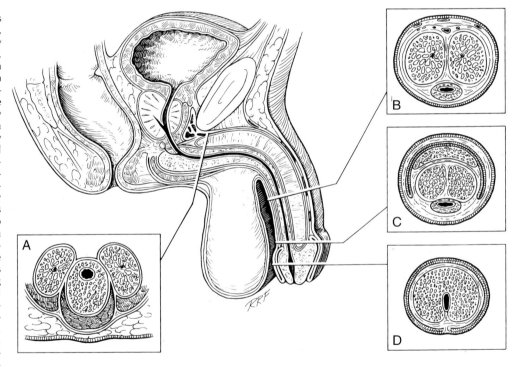

blood supply and a retrograde blood supply by way of the dorsal arteries as they arborize in the glans penis.

Etiology

Any **process that injures the urethral epithelium** or the underlying corpus spongiosum to the point that **healing results in a scar** can cause an anterior urethral stricture. Today, urethral strictures are generally the result of trauma (usually straddle trauma). This trauma to the urethra often goes unrecognized until the patient presents with voiding symptoms resulting from the obstruction of the stricture or scar. Unfortunately, iatrogenic trauma to the urethra still exists, but with the development of small endoscopes and the limitation of indications for cystoscopy in boys, fewer iatrogenic strictures are seen today than in the past. Finally, posterior urethral distraction injuries, traumatic by definition, result in strictures that are associated with extensive periurethral fibrosis.

Inflammatory strictures were the most commonly seen in the past and are less common now. Gonorrhea accounted for the bulk of inflammatory strictures in the past; however, with the advent of prompt, effective antibiotic treatment, gonococcal urethritis now progresses less often to gonococcal urethral strictures. The place of chlamydia and *Ureaplasma urealyticum* (i.e., nonspecific urethritis) in the development of anterior urethral strictures is not clear. To date, no clear association between nonspecific urethritis and the development of anterior urethral stricture has been established.

There is, however, a definite association between the development of an inflammatory stricture and BXO. BXO usually begins with inflammation of the glans and inevitably causes meatal stenosis, if not a true stricture of the fossa navicularis. The cause of this distal penile skin and urethral inflammation is not known. As discussed, there is some evidence to suggest that the progression of the stricture eventually to involve the entire anterior urethra may be due to high-pressure voiding that causes intravasation of urine into the glands of Littre, inflammation of these glands, and, perhaps, microabscesses and deep spongiofibrosis (see Fig. 107–11).

A congenital stricture is an entity that is difficult to understand. If a stricture is found at a natural place in embryologic development where a fusion of structures occurs (i.e., the posterior and anterior urethra), a congenital stricture might be a reasonable assumption. The term congenital stricture, however, is used by some to define a stricture for which there is no identifiable etiology. The authors propose, however, that it is reasonable to define a stricture as congenital only if it is not an inflammatory stricture; it is a short-length stricture; and it is not associated with a history of, or potential for, urethral trauma. This then limits congenital stricture to those strictures of the anterior urethra found in infants before their attempting erect ambulation. So defined, congenital strictures are clearly the rarest cause encountered.

Diagnosis and Evaluation

Patients who have urethral strictures most often present with obstructive voiding symptoms or urinary tract infections, such as prostatitis or epididymitis. Some patients also present with urinary retention. On close inquiry, however, many of these patients are found to have tolerated notable voiding symptoms for a long time before progressing to complete obstruction.

When a patient cannot void, an attempt is made to pass a urethral catheter. If the catheter does not pass, the nature of the obstruction is determined by way of dynamic retrograde urethrography. Although most patients are managed with acute dilation, there are many instances in which this is not the best course for the patient. When there is doubt, the authors place a suprapubic cystostomy catheter to treat the acute situation and allow time for an appropriate treatment plan to be devised. The practice of blind passage of filiforms and blind dilation, without knowledge of the anatomy of the urethral stricture, is condemned. Although detailed imaging is not always available, flexible endoscopy is almost universally available in the United States. At the least, the stricture can be visualized and a guide wire passed under direct vision through the lumen.

To devise an appropriate treatment plan, it is important to determine the location, length, depth, and density of the stricture (spongiofibrosis). The length and location of the stricture can be determined using radiographs, urethroscopy, and ultrasound. **The depth and density** of the scar in the spongy tissue can be deduced from the physical examination, the appearance of the urethra in contrast studies, the amount of elasticity noted on urethroscopy, and the depth and density of fibrosis as evidenced by ultrasound evaluation of the urethra.

Contrast studies of the urethra are best carried out by or under the direct supervision of the surgeon responsible for treatment of the patient. In 1979, McCallum described the use of dynamic radiographic studies and emphasized the need for these studies to be dynamic as opposed to static (Fig. 107–28). At the authors' center, imaging includes dynamic studies that are accomplished during retrograde injection of contrast material and while the patient is voiding. Even with gentle technique, extravasation during retrograde urethrography is possible in patients in whom the urethra is markedly inflamed (Fig. 107–29). For this reason, contrast studies should be carried out with contrast material that is suitable for intravenous injection and used either directly from the bottle or diluted according to the manufacturer's guidelines. Contrast materials that have been thickened with lubricating jelly can be a source of problems and offer little with regard to enhancement of radiographic studies. Real-time ultrasound evaluation of the urethra after it has been filled with a lubricating jelly has been described by McAninch and colleagues (1988). Finally, during contrast urethrography, more than one projection may be necessary to visualize the stricture (Fig. 107–30).

Endoscopic examination may be necessary after the contrast studies. Use of the flexible cystoscope has simplified this evaluation, and when local anesthesia is used, there is little discomfort associated with it. The scope can be passed to the stricture, and many times it is not necessary to pass it beyond that level. In addition, it is not always necessary to dilate the stricture at the time of the initial endoscopic evaluation. Pediatric endoscopic equipment has proven to be extremely valuable for examining the urethra proximal to a

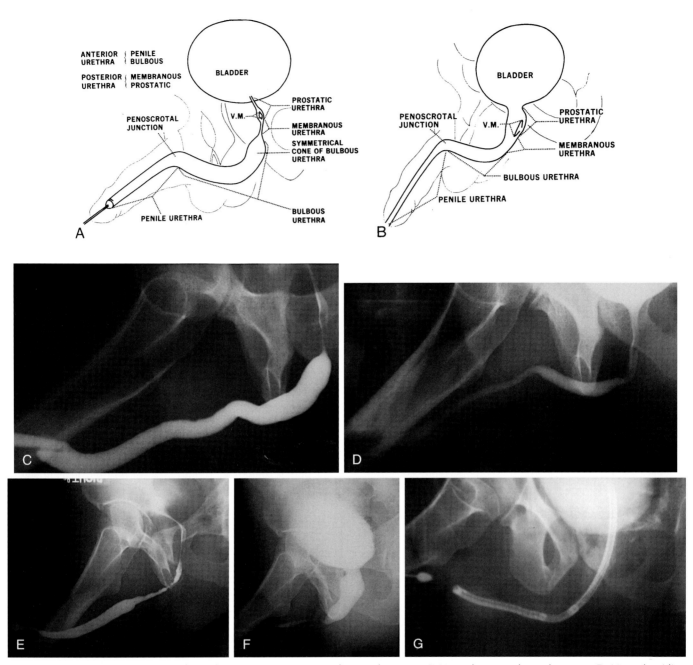

Figure 107–28. *A,* Dynamic retrograde urethrogram. *B,* Dynamic voiding urethrogram. *C,* Normal retrograde urethrogram. *D,* Normal voiding urethrogram. *E,* Retrograde urethrogram showing area of meatal stricture and area of proximal bulbous urethral stricture. *F,* Voiding urethrogram in same patient as *E.* Notice the distal stricture is obscured because of the severity of the functional implications of the proximal stricture. *G,* Technique of simultaneous endoscopy and bougienage illustrating the usefulness of this technique for the estimation of length in totally obliterating defects. (*A* and *B* from McCallum RW: The adult male urethra: normal anatomy, pathology, and method of urethrography. Radiol Clin North Am 1979; 17:227.)

narrow-caliber area without the need to dilate the most narrow area.

It is imperative, however, to evaluate completely the urethra proximal and distal to the stricture with endoscopy and bougienage during surgery, to ensure that all of the involved urethra is included in the reconstruction. Although hydraulic pressure generated by voiding may keep segments proximal to the stricture patent, unless the segments are included in the repair, they contract after obstruction of the narrow-caliber segment is relieved with reconstruction, causing a new stricture. For this reason, areas of

the urethra that are proximal to a narrow-caliber segment of the stricture must be treated with suspicion. If the lumen does not appear to demonstrate evidence of diminished compliance, the authors presume that area to be uninvolved in active stricture disease. Coning down of the urethra, however, suggests its involvement in the scar.

In some patients, the urethra proximal to a narrow area may be confusing with regards to its potential for continued constriction after reconstruction. In select patients, the authors place a suprapubic tube to defunctionalize the urethra. After 6 to 8 weeks, if there is going to be constriction of an

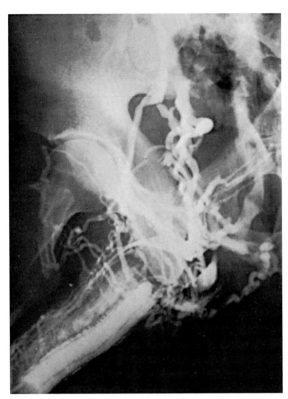

Figure 107–29. Venogram of the penis, pelvis, and inferior vena cava following gentle retrograde urethrogram. (From Horton CE, Devine PC: Strictures of the male urethra. *In* Converse JM, ed: Reconstructive Plastic Surgery. Philadelphia, W. B. Saunders, 1977.)

area that was hydrodilated with voiding, the tendency for that constriction to occur should become apparent.

Treatment

Although the treatment of urethral stricture disease dates back to the foundations of urology, significant progress, made over the last 30 years, allows for many of the most complex strictures to be reliably reconstructed in one stage. In the past, a concept known as the reconstructive ladder was used as a treatment guideline for urethral strictures. That concept was based on the principle that the simplest procedure was always attempted first, and sometimes repeated after failure, before moving on to more complex approaches. This approach is considered archaic in modern urethral reconstruction.

A good understanding by both the patient and the physician regarding the goal of treatment is mandatory before the treatment choice is made. To this end, treatment options should be discussed with the patient, with care taken to emphasize the anticipated outcome with regards to cure. Some patients may prefer stricture management and choose to have periodic dilations in the office, at home, or in the hospital rather than undergo technically detailed open surgery. Others may have cure as a goal and choose surgical management, which today has a success rate of greater than 90% to 95% for most strictures.

Dilation

Urethral dilation is the oldest and simplest treatment for urethral stricture disease, and for the patient with an epithelial stricture without spongiofibrosis, it is curative. The goal of this treatment, a concept that is frequently forgotten, is to stretch the scar without producing more scarring. If bleeding occurs during dilation, the stricture has been torn rather than stretched, further injuring the involved area.

The least traumatic method to stretch the urethra is to use soft techniques over multiple treatment sessions. The authors believe that the safest method of urethral dilation currently available involves use of a urethral balloon dilating catheter. These catheters may be passed over a guide wire attached to a filiform tip or may come with an integral coudé tip.

Internal Urethrotomy

Internal urethrotomy refers to any procedure that opens the stricture by incising or ablating it transurethrally. The urethrotomy procedure involves incising healthy tissue to allow the scar to expand (release of scar contracture) and the lumen to heal enlarged (Fig. 107–31). The goal is for

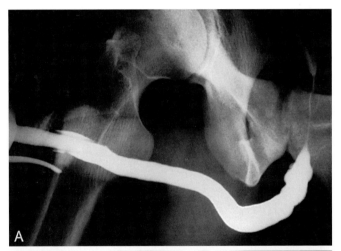

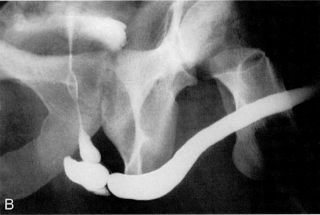

Figure 107–30. *A,* A right posterior oblique dynamic retrograde urethrogram does not define the situation. Contrast material flows past an irregular area in the posterior bulb and through the tonic external sphincter outlining the verumontanum. *B,* A left posterior oblique dynamic retrograde urethrogram shows the stricture in the same patient with intervening diverticulum.

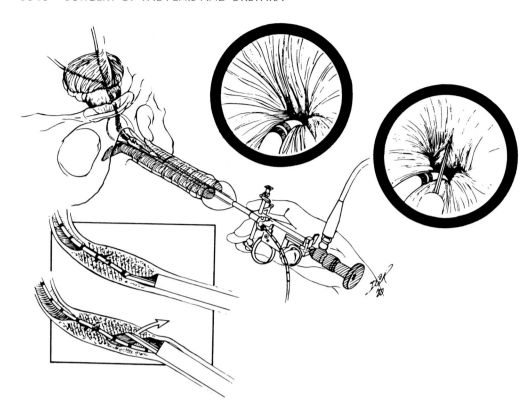

Figure 107–31. Internal urethrotomy under vision with a cold knife. A ureteral catheter is passed through the stricture, and the cold knife is advanced under vision into the stricture guided by this catheter. As the proximal end of the urethrotome is depressed, the stricture is incised. In short strictures, only one cut may be necessary, but in longer ones the ureteral catheter allows the blade to be advanced farther and the incision to be elongated. The urethra is incised until a No. 24 Fr silicone catheter can be passed with ease in an adult or an appropriately smaller one in a child. (From Devine CJ Jr, Devine PC: Operations for urethral stricture. *In* Stewart BH, ed: Operative Urology. Baltimore, Williams & Wilkins, 1982, pp 243–270.)

the resultant larger luminal caliber to be maintained after healing.

With epithelial apposition, wound healing occurs by primary intention. Internal urethrotomy does not provide an epithelial approximation but rather aims to separate the scarred epithelium, so that the healing occurs by secondary intention. In healing by secondary intention, epithelialization progresses from the wound edges and slows. In an effort to aid epithelialization, nature invokes the forces of wound contraction, not to be confused with scar contraction. Wound contraction closes the wound defect and limits the size of the area that requires epithelialization, hastening the healing of the surface defect. In the case of internal urethrotomy, however, wound contraction merely tries to reapproximate the edges of the scar. If epithelialization progresses completely before wound contraction significantly narrows the lumen, the internal urethrotomy is a success. If wound contraction significantly narrows the lumen before completion of epithelialization, stricture can recur.

Many surgeons have learned to perform internal urethrotomy by making a single incision at the 12 o'clock position. This location might be questioned, however, based on the location of the urethra within the corpus spongiosum (see Fig. 107–27). On examination of a cross-section of the corpus spongiosum, it can be seen that the thinnest portion of the anterior aspect is from 10 o'clock to 2 o'clock. The distance between the anterior wall of the corpus spongiosum and the corpora cavernosa is somewhat displaced in the bulbous urethra, and a single 12 o'clock cut could rapidly penetrate the corpus spongiosum and extend through the triangular ligament; although it may not enter the corpora cavernosa, a deep cut could enter the intracrural space. A deep incision in the more distal aspects of the anterior urethra certainly enters the corpora cavernosa, and these incisions have been associated with the creation of erectile

dysfunction believed to be due to local cavernosal veno-occlusive dysfunction. Vigorous incisions at 10 o'clock and 2 o'clock in the bulbous urethra risk the same problem. It should be kept in mind that if deep spongiofibrosis is present, stricture cure is impossible by way of internal urethrotomy, and therefore these deep incisions are counterproductive.

The most common complication of internal urethrotomy is recurrence of stricture. Less commonly noted complications of internal urethrotomy include bleeding (almost always associated with erections immediately following the procedure) and extravasation of irrigation fluid into the perispongiosal tissues. These complications are rare today, however, because of the less frequent use of aggressive internal urethrotomy as a treatment modality for urethral strictures.

A major problem with assessing the success rates of internal urethrotomy is that the nature of the strictures that have been treated with internal urethrotomy has been poorly reported. In addition, the literature is not clear about the goal of internal urethrotomy. For many, an internal urethrotomy is successful if it offers temporary relief. Therefore, in many cases, internal urethrotomy has been reported as successful despite the fact that it has been associated with eventual stricture recurrence. A report by McAninch and colleagues (1988), using actuarial techniques, shows the curative success rate of internal urethrotomy to be approximately 20%. A similar **evaluation by Pansadoro and Emiliozzi (1996)** shows the curative success rate of direct visual internal urethrotomy to be approximately 35%. His analysis also shows that there is virtually **no increase in success rate with a second internal urethrotomy.**

Because of this dismal success rate, several techniques have been employed to oppose the process of wound contraction and prevent stricture recurrence. One method is to leave an indwelling Foley catheter for as long as 6 weeks after urethrotomy, hoping that the urethra will mold around the catheter as it heals. Studies have shown, however, that the failure rate of long-term catheterization after internal urethrotomy is similar to that seen with 3 to 7 days of catheterization, and even 6 weeks is not sufficient time to oppose the forces of wound contraction.

Another technique used to oppose the forces of wound contraction after internal urethrotomy is home self-catheterization or urethral obturation. After internal urethrotomy, patients generally have an indwelling catheter placed for a period of 3 to 5 days. When the catheter is removed, the patient is begun on a urethral obturation regimen. Most regimens require more frequent catheterizations early in the recovery period, with a tapering schedule over the next 3 to 6 months. Anecdotally, many researchers have reported an improved cure rate using self-catheterization in combination with internal urethrotomy. In the authors' experience, however, the stricture inevitably recurs when the patient stops self-dilation, regardless of how long it has been used.

Urethral stents (removable or permanently implantable) are another modality used in opposing the forces of wound contraction after internal urethrotomy or dilation. Removable urethral stents are designed to prevent the process of epithelialization from incorporating the stent into the urethral wall and are left in place for as long as 6 months to a year before they are removed. The greatest experience with these removable stents comes from Israel, and centers there report good success in small series.

The majority of experience with permanently implantable stents comes from Europe and the United Kingdom. Milroy (1993) has reported a success rate of 84% using the permanently implantable Urolume. The Urolume, made of an alloy, is designed to be incorporated into the wall of the urethra and corpus spongiosum (Fig. 107–32). Available data show that the stent is best employed for relatively short-length strictures of the bulbous urethra associated with minimal spongiofibrosis. **These are the strictures, however, that are most successfully reconstructed with open techniques that offer better long-term success rates.**

Permanently implantable stents are associated with some unique complications. The stents must be placed only in the bulbous urethra; when placed beyond the area of the scrotal urethra, placement has been associated with pain on sitting and intercourse. Some patients complain of perineal pain, particularly with vigorous activity, even following implantation of the stent in the deep bulbous urethra. In addition, longer bulbous strictures require the use of two stents that are placed overlapping. These stents can migrate away from each other, leaving a gap between them where recurrence of stricture is inevitable. When this occurs, the stricture recurrence is excised, and a third stent is placed to span the gap.

There are also specific contraindications to the use of the Urolume. Patients who have undergone prior substitution urethral reconstruction, particularly in whom skin has been incorporated into the urethra, have been shown to be poor candidates for implantation with the Urolume stent because contact of the stent with the skin is associated with a virulent hypertrophic reaction. These patients experience postvoid dribbling, and, in some cases, the hypertrophic reaction can be so severe that functional recurrence of the stricture recurs. Another subset of patients shown to be poor candidates for the use of the Urolume are those in whom deep spongio-

fibrosis exists. Patients who fall into this category have had urethral distraction injuries and straddle injuries associated with deep fibrosis. As of this writing, the Urolume is nearing Food and Drug Administration approval and will soon be released in the United States. Many view the Urolume as a panacea. There appears, however, to be a great deal of opportunity for misuse of the device, and its use should therefore be approached with the utmost caution. Some centers in Europe now advocate the use of the Urolume only in patients who are over 50 years old or who have significant medical problems that make the option of lengthy open urethral reconstruction less appealing.

Lasers

Types of lasers used for the treatment of urethral stricture disease include carbon dioxide, argon, KTP, Nd:YAG, holmium:YAG, and excimer lasers. Figure 107–33 shows the laser wavelengths compared with those of hemoglobin and water.

The ideal laser for use in treatment of urethral stricture disease is one that totally vaporizes the tissue, exhibits negligible peripheral tissue destruction, is not absorbed by water, and is easily propagated along a fiber. Although the carbon dioxide laser appears to be ideally suited, it must be used with a gas cystoscope, which carries the potential threat of a carbon dioxide embolus.

For both the argon and Nd:YAG lasers, the predominant mode of action is thermal necrosis, which leads to a significant potential for peripheral tissue injury rather than vaporization. The Nd:YAG laser has also been used with a bare fiber in the contact mode. A bare fiber carries with it a risk of forward scatter. When used in the contact mode, the YAG energy is transferred to a sapphire tip. Advocates of the use of a contact laser suggest that it obliterates the scar via vaporization; however, results of using these fibers are no better than those using direct cold knife visual internal urethrotomy.

A KTP laser is essentially an Nd:YAG laser that has passed through a KTP crystal, resulting in a reduced depth of penetration. A urethrotomy performed using a KTP laser is accomplished by passing the fiber over the scar tissue to make urethrotomy cuts. The holmium:YAG laser has similar properties to the KTP laser and, similar to the KTP laser, provides both direct contact cutting and vaporization with minimal forward scatter.

The excimer laser is a true vaporizing laser that has little forward scatter or peripheral tissue necrosis associated with it. Little experience has been reported with the use of this laser, but future investigation is clearly warranted. **To date, the results of laser urethrotomy are less than promising.** With the advent of new lasers and experience with them, however, future data may show better results.

OPEN RECONSTRUCTION

Excision and Reanastomosis

It has now been demonstrated with certainty that the **most dependable technique of anterior urethral reconstruction is the complete excision of the area of fibrosis, with a**

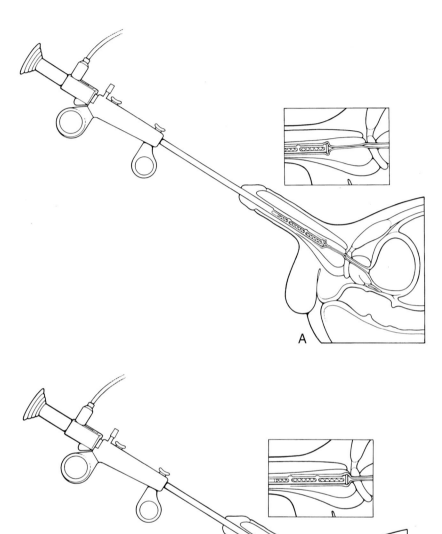

Figure 107–32. Technique of placement of a permanently implanted urethral stent (Urolume) for proximal bulbous urethral stricture. *A*, Urethral stricture has been dilated or incised. The delivery tool with stent is advanced to the area of stricture. *B*, The delivery tool is advanced to just distal to the external urethral sphincter.

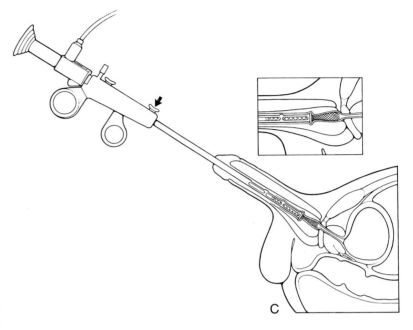

C

Figure 107–32 *Continued C,* The stent is advanced but not deployed from the delivery tool. The correct position with relation to the external sphincter is visualized directly. *D,* The stent, after being correctly placed, is deployed from the delivery tool.

Illustration continued on following page

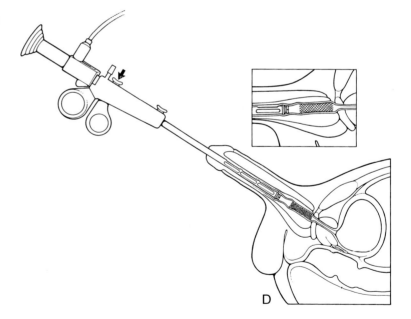

D

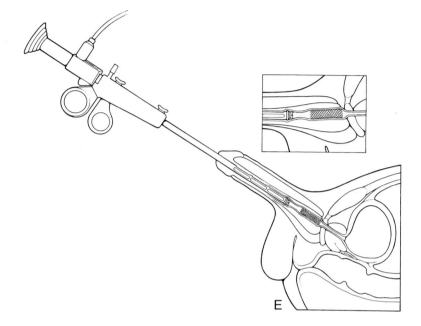

Figure 107–32 *Continued E*, The delivery tool is removed, leaving the stent positioned across the area of stricture. (Courtesy of American Medical Systems, Inc., Minnetonka, MN.)

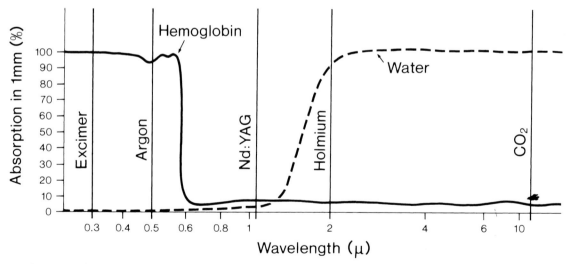

Figure 107–33. Absorption of hemoglobin and water as a function of medical lasers that have been used for the treatment of strictures. (From Jordan GH, Schlossberg SM: Complications of interventional techniques for urethral stricture disease: Direct visual internal urethrotomy, stents and laser intervention. Courtesy of Culley C. Carson, III, MD, from the book Topics in Clinical Urology: Complications of Interventional Techniques. Igaku-Shoin Medical Publishers, New York, NY, 1996, pp 86–94.)

primary reanastomosis of the normal ends of the anterior urethra (Fig. 107–34). The best results are achieved when the following technical points are observed: (1) the area of fibrosis is totally excised; (2) the urethral anastomosis is widely spatulated, creating a large ovoid anastomosis (see Fig. 107–34*B*); and (3) the anastomosis is tension-free.

The success of this procedure relies on vigorous mobilization of the corpus spongiosum. With vigorous mobilization, development of the intracrural space, and detachment of the bulbospongiosus from the perineal body, significant lengths of stricture can be excised and reanastomosed (see Fig. 107–34*A*). Strictures of 1 to 2 cm are generally easily excised with reanastomosis. In some cases, strictures as long as 3 to 4 cm can be totally excised, and a primary reanastomosis of the anterior urethra can be performed. At the authors' center, all cases of urethral reconstruction are diverted with a suprapubic catheter. The urethral repair is stented with a soft silicone small urethral catheter. When the length of stricture precludes total excision of fibrosis with primary anastomosis, tissue transfer is required.

Reconstruction with Tissue Transfer

Four grafts that have been used for urethral reconstruction are the full-thickness skin graft (see Fig. 107–1*A*), **the split-thickness skin graft, the bladder epithelial graft** (see Fig. 107–1*B*), **and the buccal mucosal graft** (see Fig. 107–1*C*). Similar to that of the skin, the microvascularity of the bladder epithelium consists of two plexuses: a deep laminar plexus and a superficial laminar plexus. Also the contraction characteristics of a bladder epithelial graft appear to be similar to those of a full-thickness skin graft (approximately 10%–15%). There have been reports that bladder epithelial grafts form diverticula. The authors believe, however, that proper tailoring yields a graft that is no more prone to diverticula formation than the other grafts discussed.

Differing from the layered distribution found in the skin and bladder, the microvasculature of the lamina propria of the buccal mucosa exhibits a fairly uniform distribution. The uniform microvasculature of the buccal mucosal graft allows it to be harvested at various levels in the lamina, with the vascular take characteristics relatively unaffected. In addition, despite the level of graft harvest, the contraction characteristics appear to be similar to those of a full-thickness skin graft. Split-thickness skin in unsupported tissues contracts significantly and thus is not appropriate for use in single-stage reconstruction.

If graft transfer is contemplated, **nonhirsute full-thickness grafts are preferred for repair of urethral stricture disease.** Grafts have been shown to be most successfully employed in the area of the bulbous urethra, where the urethra is invested by the musculature of the ischiocavernosal muscle group. The graft can be applied to the ventrum of the urethra; however, a ventral urethrotomy is advantageous only if one contemplates the use of the spongioplasty maneuver (Fig. 107–35*A*). The use of the spongioplasty procedure requires that the corpus spongiosum adjacent to the area of the stricture be relatively normal and free of fibrosis. The authors prefer the use of a lateral urethrostomy (Fig. 107–35*B*). Placing the urethrostomy there allows one to expose the urethra while cutting through the corpus spongiosum where it is relatively thinner, thus limiting bleeding and maximizing exposure. Additionally, the graft can be sutured to the underlying muscle bed, improving, it is hoped, graft bed immobilization and approximation. In circumstances in which **nonhirsute genital skin is not available, bladder epithelium or buccal mucosal grafts are good options. Another option is the two-staged application of a mesh split-thickness skin graft** (Fig. 107–36). In the first stage, a medium-thickness skin graft is placed over the dartos fascia. If it is placed immediately onto the tunica albuginea or corpora cavernosa, contraction makes second-stage tubularization difficult. At a later date, second-stage

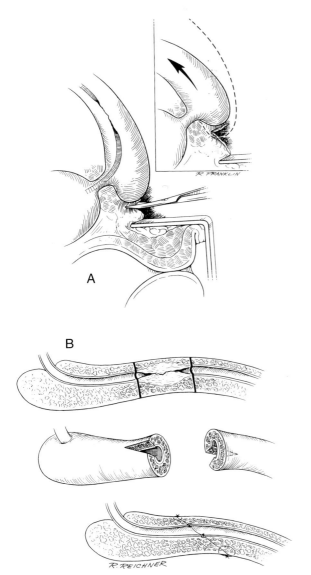

Figure 107–34. Techniques for excision and primary reanastomosis of anterior urethral stricture. *A*, The bulbospongiosus is released from its attachment to the perineal bodies. The arteries to the bulb are not divided. This technique allows the urethra to be mobilized distally. This technique combined with development of the intracrural space can shorten the path of the urethra by approximately 1 to 1.5 cm. *B*, Technique of a primary spatulated anastomosis following excision of an anterior urethral stricture. (*B* From Jordan GH: Principles of plastic surgery. *In* Droller MJ, ed: Surgical Management of Urologic Disease: An Anatomic Approach. Chicago, Mosby Year Book, 1992, p 824.)

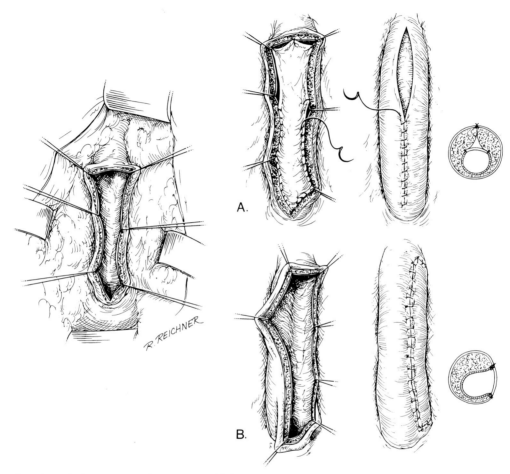

Figure 107–35. Patch graft. With the patient in the exaggerated lithotomy position, exposure of the urethra in the bulb is achieved. The spongy tissue of the bulb and the epithelium of the urethral stricture have been opened for placement of a full-thickness graft patch to repair the stricture. The spongy tissue can be seen between the epithelium of the urethra and the tunica of the bulb, which are approximated by the stay sutures. If there is excessive bleeding, a running 5–0 or 6–0 chromic suture closes this gap. *A,* The skin graft has been fitted to the urethral epithelium. The erectile tissue is mobilized so that it covers the graft as the tunica of the bulb is closed. *B,* Because of fibrosis in the spongy tissue, the urethrotomy has been placed laterally. With this amount of spongiofibrosis, the authors often fill the defect with a flap. In this instance, the graft is inset to both layers—the epithelium and the tunica. The bulbospongiosus muscle serves as the host bed. (From Devine CJ Jr, Jordan GH: Surgery of anterior urethral strictures. *In* Marshall FF, ed: Operative Urology. Philadelphia, W. B. Saunders, 1991, p 316.)

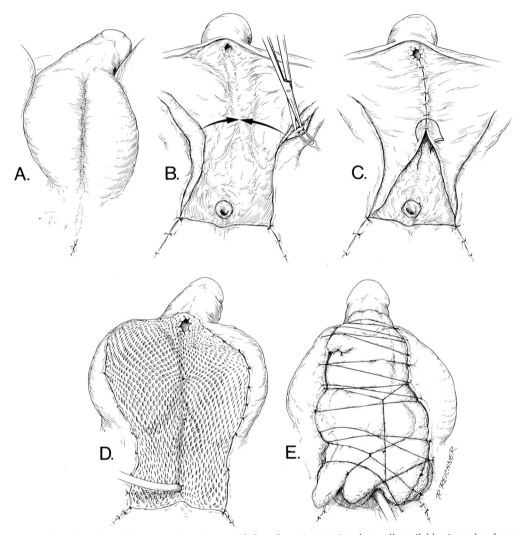

Figure 107–36. Mesh graft urethroplasty, first stage, in patients with lengthy strictures in whom all available tissue has been expended. *A,* The strictured urethra is excised completely or only a dorsal strip of epithelium is left. *B* and *C,* The dartos fascia is mobilized and brought in to cover tunica albuginea and the scar in the defect with vascularized tissue. *D,* A split-thickness skin graft is harvested from the buttocks or inner surface of the thigh, meshed on the Padgett dermatome with a carrier using a 1:5:1 ratio, and placed in the site of the excised urethra as an open-faced graft, without expanding the mesh. If a roof strip is left, the epithelium of the urethra is sewn to the graft. *E,* The graft is covered with Xeroform gauze, and a thick bolster of Dacron batting is secured in place with tie-over sutures. A Foley catheter is left in the proximal urethra. (From Devine CJ Jr, Jordan GH: AUA Update Series, Lesson 26, Vol 9, 1990.)

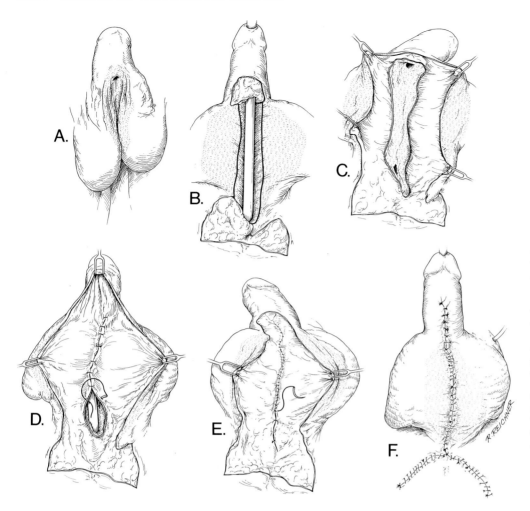

Figure 107–37. Meshed graft urethroplasty, second stage. *A,* In 3 to 6 months, the new epithelial surface is smooth and elastic. At 1 year, the patient is brought back to the operating room. The proximal and distal portions of the urethra are evaluated with an à-boule bougie and cystoscopy. *B,* A catheter is passed through the penile urethra and into the bladder. A 3-cm-wide strip is marked to form the new urethra, outlining flaps at each end to tailor the junction of the tube to the existing urethra. *C,* The strip is not undermined, but dissection is carried out laterally to mobilize the remaining skin graft and scrotal skin. *D,* Interrupted sutures are placed to approximate the epithelial edges, tying the knots in the lumen. *E,* A running subepithelial monofilament absorbable suture is placed to roll the edges in and to make the suture line watertight. *F,* The skin is closed, leaving suction drains. The urine is diverted with a suprapubic tube. (From Devine CJ Jr, Jordan GH: AUA Update Series, Lesson 26, Vol 9, 1990.)

surgery is performed to tubularize the graft (Fig. 107–37). Although Schreiter and Noll (1989), who first described the procedure, often proceed to the second stage within 3 months, the authors wait 12 months between the first-stage and second-stage surgeries. This procedure has been found useful for select cases in both the United States and Europe. In the United States, its use has been confined to only the most difficult cases, however, with single-stage reconstruction still applied to the vast majority of cases.

A number of applications of **genital skin islands, mobilized in either the dartos fascia of the penis or the tunica dartos of the scrotum,** have been proposed for repair of urethral stricture disease. In the past, these were considered to be separate procedures. The authors suggest that all of

Figure 107–38. A dorsal transverse island (Duckett) of penile skin applied to a stricture of the urethra. The flap has been elevated on the dartos fascia, and a lateral incision has been made into the urethra. The flap is secured in place *(right).* (From Jordan GH: Management of anterior urethral stricture disease. *In* Webster GD, ed: Problems in Urology. Philadelphia, J. B. Lippincott, 1987, p 217.)

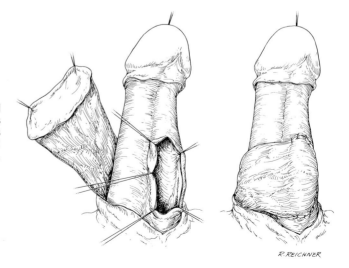

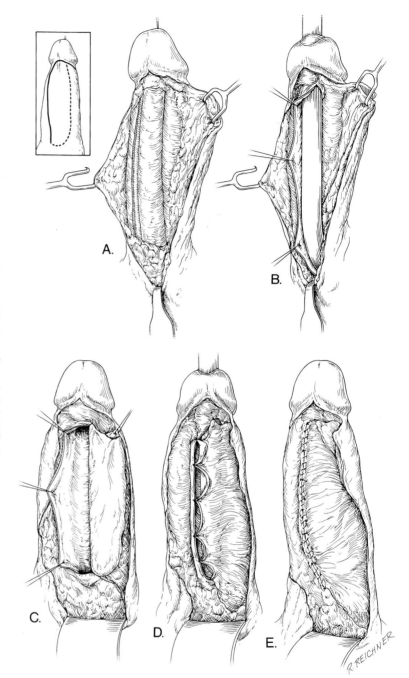

Figure 107–39. Urethral longitudinal skin island (Orandi flap). The incisions to be made to mobilize the flap are demonstrated in the *inset*. The heavy line is the primary incision made full thickness through the dartos fascia and superficial Buck's fascia lateral to the corpus spongiosum. *A,* Dissection elevates the dartos fascial flap well past the corpus spongiosum in the midline. *B,* A lateral urethrotomy placed to face the flap has opened the entire length of the stricture. *C,* The skin paddle of the flap has been developed by making the incision outlined by the dotted line (see *inset*) and undermining the skin lateral to it. The medial edge of the flap has been fixed to the edge of the urethrotomy. *D,* The flap is inverted into the defect. *E,* A watertight subepithelial suture line has been completed with a running absorbable monofilament suture. The skin is closed with subcutaneous sutures and interrupted cutaneous sutures. (From Jordan GH: Management of anterior urethral stricture disease. *In* Webster GD, ed: Problems in Urology. Philadelphia, J. B. Lippincott, 1987, p 214.)

these procedures are different applications of a single concept, proposed by the microinjection studies of Quartey (1983). Skin islands, as mentioned, can be viewed as passengers on fascial flaps, and the design of flaps for urethral reconstruction can be paralleled to the design of flaps for reconstruction in general.

There are **three important considerations for the use of flaps in urethral reconstruction:** (1) the nature of the flap tissue, (2) the vasculature of the flap, and (3) the mechanics of flap transfer. The skin must be nonhirsute for urethral reconstruction. In addition, it is most convenient to use the areas of redundant nonhirsute genital skin.

If the redundancy is dorsal, the skin island can be oriented transversely and mobilized on the dorsal dartos fascia after

the techniques described by Duckett (1981) and Standoli (1982) (Fig. 107–38). If there is redundancy of the ventral skin, the skin island can be mobilized as a ventral longitudinal island. These islands can be either vigorously mobilized on a laterally oriented dartos fascial flap for transposition to the perineum or less vigorously mobilized and transposed and inverted into a pendulous urethral stricture defect (Figs. 107–39 and 107–40). Ventral islands can be oriented transversely (Fig. 107–41) as well as longitudinally. Longer skin islands can be mobilized by orienting the island both ventrally and transversely at the distal extent. This "hockey stick" orientation allows for islands as long as 7 to 9 cm (Fig. 107–42).

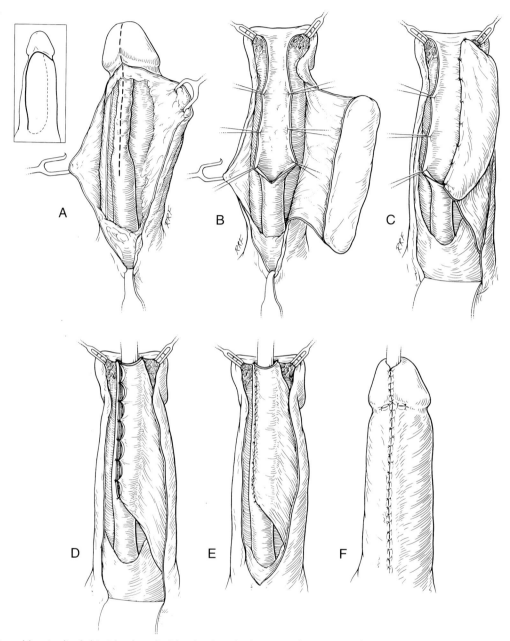

Figure 107–40. Ventral longitudinal skin island applied for distal urethral stricture disease extending to the meatus. In this case, the flap is elevated more aggressively on the dartos fascia, allowing for inversion of the skin island into the defect with advancement to the meatus. *A,* The corpus spongiosum is exposed. *B,* Urethrostomy is performed; the skin island is elevated on the dartos fascia. *C,* The skin island inlay is being accomplished. *D,* The flap is inverted with the contralateral suture line tacked. *E,* The skin island onlay is complete. *F,* The appearance of the ventrum of the closed penis. (From Jordan GH: Reconstruction of the meatus/fossa navicularis using flap techniques. *In* Schreiter F, ed: Plastic Reconstructive Surgery in Urology. Stuttgart, Germany, Georg Thieme Publishers. In press.)

scrotum (Fig. 107–44). The fascial flap must be based laterally and when so oriented has been shown to be extremely reliable. Because the tunica dartos has a significant muscular component, the skin island must be carefully tailored. If these skin islands are correctly tailored at the outset, they are not attended with diverticular development as some have thought in the past. The authors have used these flaps in more than 60 patients with excellent results and good long-term follow-up (as of this writing >7 years).

These procedures using skin islands oriented on the penile dartos fascia have also been useful for reconstruction of the fossa navicularis (Figs. 107–45 and 107–46). In the past, meatal stenosis and strictures of the fossa navicularis were managed with repeated dilations or sequential meatotomies. Because these meatotomies were seldom successful in the long-term, techniques were developed that allowed for the spatulation of random penile skin flaps into the meatotomy defects (see Fig. 107–45A–C). These procedures functionally improved the results; however, the cosmetic appearance of the penis was less than optimal. With the use of skin islands elevated on the dartos fascia, excellent functional as well as cosmetic results became the norm (see Figs. 107–45D and 107–46A–D). Again the design of these islands must take into consideration the location of hair on the shaft of the penis as well as considerations of the mechanics of flap transfer (i.e., transposition versus advancement). In addition, full-thickness skin has been used to reconstruct the fossa navicularis (see Fig. 107–45E), but skin grafts are not believed appropriate for reconstruction in cases of BXO, when they can be avoided.

The literature has made it clear that onlay procedures are attended with a higher success rate than tubularized grafts or tubularized skin islands. Tubularized grafts and skin islands should therefore be avoided, if possible. In instances in which tubularized segments cannot be avoided, the length of these segments can be limited by combining aggressive mobilization and excision.

A flap procedure that can be used as an alternative to the split-thickness skin grafts when nonhirsute skin is unavailable is the epilated midline genital skin island. Like the split-thickness skin graft, this procedure must be viewed as a staged procedure, with the epilations being the initial stage(s). Epilation can be accomplished using either a narrow gauge needle and monopolar cautery or epilation needles and machines. The interval between the epilations must be 6 to 8 weeks, and urethral reconstruction cannot be accomplished until 10 to 12 weeks after the last epilation. The actual stricture repair involves elevation of the midline skin island, based on both the dartos fascia of the penis and the tunica dartos of the scrotum. As with nonhirsute scrotal skin islands in general, the importance of meticulous tailoring of the scrotal portion of the island cannot be overemphasized.

Mundy (1994) analyzed a large series of urethral reconstruction. His data show that when follow-up is limited to a year, the success rate using tissue transfer clusters is about 95%. With longer follow-up, however, there is a deterioration over time. Rosen and colleagues' actuarial regression analysis suggested a similar phenomenon. With excision and primary anastomosis, the success seen at 1 year seems to be durable, however, and does not appear to deteriorate with time (Rosen et al, 1994).

Text continued on page 3362

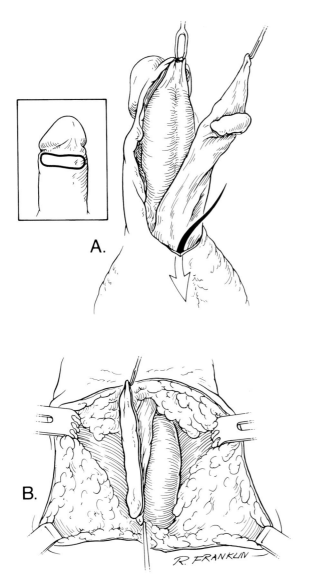

Figure 107–41. A ventral transverse skin island is elevated on the penile dartos fascia, inverted to the area of the perineum where flap onlay is accomplished. *A*, The skin island is elevated on the dartos fascia. *B*, The appearance of the flap transposed to the area of the perineum for onlay in a proximal bulbous urethral stricture.

Where there is general redundancy to the penile skin, the islands can be oriented circumferentially (Fig. 107–43). These circular skin islands are mobilized on the entire penile dartos fascia, and the mechanics of transposition suggest that they are most efficient when they are ventrally based, with the pedicle split dorsally. In some cases, circular skin islands as long as 15 cm can be obtained.

Many times, it is beneficial to combine excision of the stricture with a skin island onlay (see Fig. 107–43). The authors have found that **narrow-caliber, nearly (or totally) obliterating segments are difficult to deal with.** These segments can often be completely excised, a roof strip anastomosis of the urethra performed, and the remaining urethrotomy defect filled with a skin island onlay. In some patients, there are relatively large nonhirsute areas of the scrotal skin that can be elevated on the tunica dartos of the

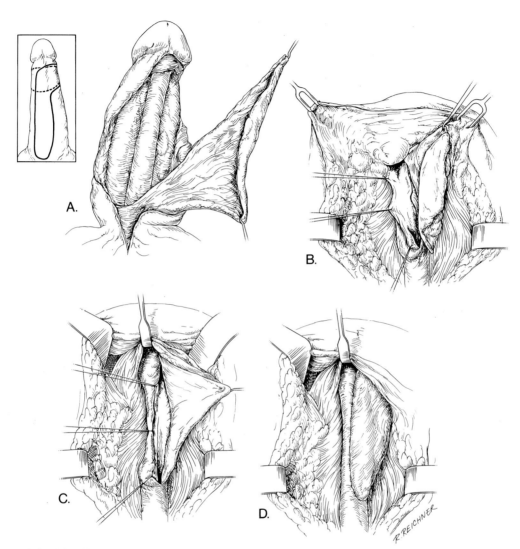

Figure 107–42. Ventral skin island for long bulbous stricture. The skin paddle of the flap is developed on the ventral midline of the penis and can be extended around the penile shaft at its distal end. *A,* The paddle of the flap has been incised and its pedicle elevated. This pedicle includes Buck's and dartos fascia denuding the tunica of the corpus spongiosum and the corpora cavernosa. The pedicle (the dartos fascia bilaterally) is based on the superficial external pudendal vessels and the internal pudendal vessels in the scrotum. Development of this pedicle allows the flap to be moved to any area of the urethra. *B,* The flap has been passed through a tunnel beneath the scrotum created by dissecting along the corpus spongiosum. A laterally placed urethrostomy has opened the urethral stricture. *C,* The deep edge of the flap is secured employing the suture techniques previously described. *D,* Anastomosis of the flap has been completed. The pedicle can be seen extending beneath the scrotum. (From Jordan GH, McCraw JB: AUA Update Series, Lesson 11, Vol 7, 1988.)

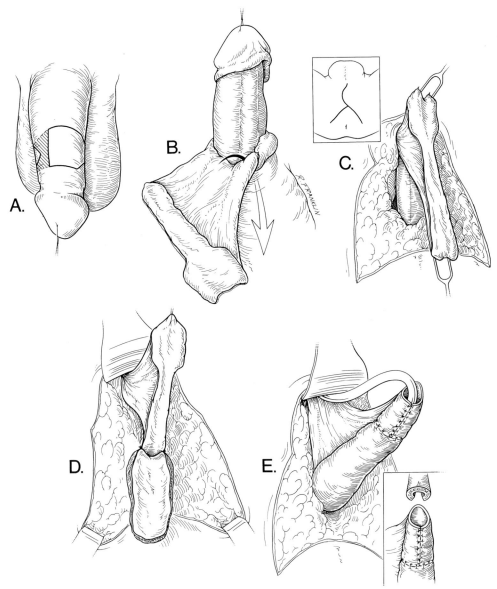

Figure 107–43. Circular skin island combined with excision of stricture with reanastomosis. *A*, The skin island is marked on the skin of the penis. *B*, The skin island is elevated on the complete penile dartos fascia. *C*, Lambda-shaped perineal incision has been accomplished. The flap is transposed to the perineum. *D*, The corpus spongiosum has been divided through an area of total obliteration of the anterior urethra. The area of obliteration has been excised. The patient's proximal bulbous urethra is detected and spatulated dorsally. The patient, proximal to the area of total obliteration, had severe stenosis to the level of the departure of the urethra from the bulbospongiosus. The skin island onlay is accomplished on the dorsal aspect of the urethra. *E*, Appearance after the skin island onlay has been accomplished. Notice the distal tubularized section, which is then anastomosed to the distal anterior urethra with a spatulated anastomosis. (From Jordan GH, Schlossberg SM: Using tissue transfer for urethral reconstruction, *Contemporary Urology*, 1993; (5)12: 13–23, copyright Medical Economics. Courtesy of Robin Reichner.)

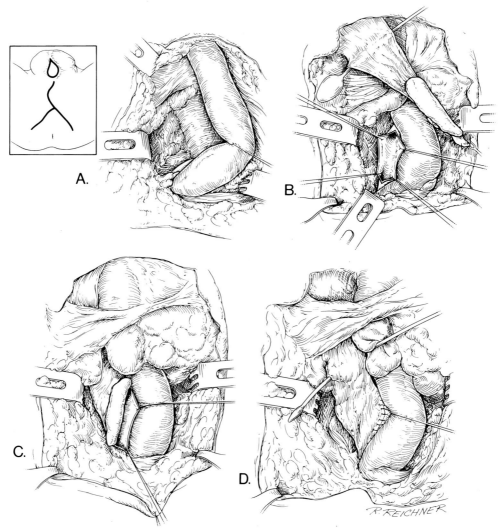

Figure 107–44. Hairless scrotal island flap. *A,* In the *inset,* the incisions are planned so that a hairless area of skin in the midline of the scrotum can be transferred on the tunica dartos of the scrotum to repair a stricture in the bulbomembranous portion of the urethra. With the patient in the exaggerated lithotomy position, the lambda incision is made in the perineum. The right lateral aspect of the bulb is mobilized, isolating the membranous portion of the urethra as it departs. *B,* The skin paddle has been elevated; the bougie lies beneath the pedicle of the fascial flap. *C,* The flap has been anastomosed to the deep edge of the incision in the lateral aspect of the urethra. *D,* The superficial edge of the skin island has been sewn into place, and the closure is watertight. A probe lies behind the transposed fascial flap. (From Jordan GJ: Management of anterior urethral stricture disease. *In* Webster GD, ed: Problems in Urology. Philadelphia, J. B. Lippincott, 1987, p 199.)

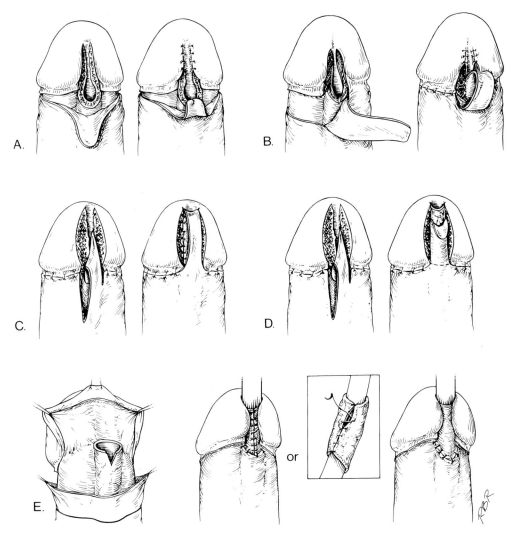

Figure 107–45. Collage of techniques for reconstruction of the fossa navicularis and meatus. *A,* Technique after Blandy, in which a random penile skin island is advanced into a meatotomy defect. *B,* Technique after Cohney, in which a transversely oriented random flap is advanced into the meatotomy defect. *C,* Technique after Brannen, in which a midline random flap is advanced into the meatotomy defect. This technique was an attempt to improve the cosmetic result of prior procedures. *D,* Technique after DeSy, in which a ventral longitudinal skin island is advanced into the meatotomy defect. The skin island is created by de-epithelializing a portion of the longitudinal flap. *E,* Technique after Devine, in which the fossa navicularis is resurfaced. The entire stenotic fossa navicularis is excised. A full-thickness skin graft is tubularized to replace the fossa navicularis and restore the meatus. As described by Devine, the suture line was ventral. The skin graft suture line, however, can be placed dorsally. (From Jordan GJ: Management of anterior urethral stricture disease. *In* Webster GD, ed: Problems in Urology. Philadelphia, J. B. Lippincott, 1987, p 199.)

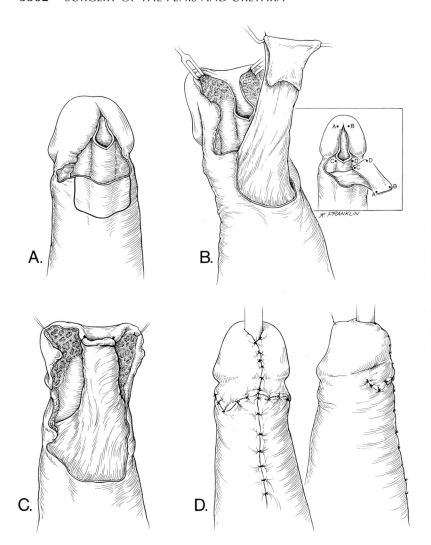

A.

B.

C.

D.

Figure 107–46. Technique of reconstruction of the fossa navicularis after Jordan. *A,* The ventral corpus spongiosum is exposed, and the urethra is opened ventrally through the area of stenosis. A transverse ventral skin island is outlined on the distal penile skin. *B,* The skin island is elevated on the ventral dartos fascia. *C,* The skin island is transposed and inverted into the meatotomy defect (see *inset*). *D,* Appearance of the penis closed after the procedure. (From Jordan GH: Reconstruction of the meatus/fossa navicularis using flap techniques. *In* Schreiter F, ed: Plastic Reconstructive Surgery in Urology. Stuttgart, Germany, Georg Thieme Publishers. In press.)

DISTRACTION INJURIES OF THE URETHRA

Urethral distraction injuries are the result of blunt pelvic trauma and accompany abut 10% of pelvic fracture injuries. Although it is possible to disrupt the urethra totally with a straddle injury, these injuries most commonly involve only the bulbous urethra. The ensuing fibrosis can be associated with complete obliteration of the urethra.

Distraction injuries of the membranous urethra have been compared to plucking an apple (prostate) off its stem (the membranous urethra). This analogy implies that the injury most frequently occurs at the apex of the prostate. Experience shows that this is not the case, however, and the **most frequent point of distraction is at the departure of the membranous urethra from the bulbospongiosus.** The distraction can involve all, or any portion, of the membranous urethra between the departure of the bulbospongiosus and the apex of the prostate. In the **postpubescent male, the injury seldom involves the prostatic urethra. In the prepubescent male,** in whom **the prostatic urethra is more fragile,** the injury can extend into that area.

Many injuries appear not to distract totally the entire circumference of the urethra. Instead, a strip of epithelium is left intact. In these patients, the placement of an aligning catheter may allow the urethra to heal virtually unscarred or with an easily managed stricture. Because of flexible endoscopy equipment, placement of an aligning catheter is relatively straightforward (Fig. 107–47). The difference between partial and complete distraction cannot be readily ascertained acutely. Thus, if the patient's general condition allows, placement of an aligning catheter in the first days immediately after distraction is strongly advocated. If distraction is complete, the catheter then serves to align the obliterated urethral ends, and reconstruction is facilitated.

Evaluation

As with the repair of any stricture, it is **important to define the precise anatomy of the distraction defect before undertaking treatment:** depth, density, length, and location. In posterior urethral distraction defects, the depth and density of fibrosis are predictable. Although location of the distraction injury has been demonstrated to be an important factor in continence after reconstruction, this information should be a factor only in patient counseling before the reconstruction and not in the treatment approach. The

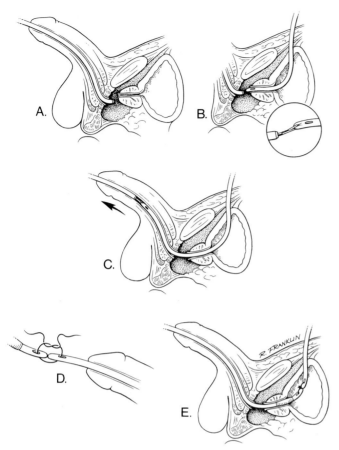

Figure 107–47. Technique of placement of an aligning catheter following urethral distraction defect. *A,* Urethroscopy is performed with the flexible cystopanendoscope. *B,* A cystotomy has been created, and a catheter is advanced in antegrade fashion through the bladder neck. The catheter is visualized and grasped. *C,* The catheter is withdrawn through the urethra. *D,* The aligning catheter is sutured to the catheter from above. *E,* The aligning catheter is placed and can be secured either with inflation of the balloon or to a Prolene loop stitch to the abdominal wall. *Note:* The catheters are placed for alignment only. Traction is not placed on the catheter.

length of the defect is an important consideration and must be determined as precisely as possible.

Contrast studies are a first-line tool for the evaluation of distraction defects. A cystogram outlines the bladder and provides information about rostral displacement of the proximal urethra. Lack of contrast in the posterior urethra gives some information about the integrity of the bladder neck.

When the patient is successfully relaxing to void and the cystogram outlines the posterior urethra, simultaneous retrograde urethrograms nicely outline the length of the distraction defect. This situation is the exception rather than the rule, however, and retrograde urethrograms are most useful for determining whether the anterior urethra is normal. If the anterior urethra is normal, in the authors' experience, a successful anastomotic repair is assured.

In cases in which the proximal urethra is not visualized on simultaneous cystogram with urethrogram, endoscopy through the suprapubic tract in combination with retrograde urethrogram can be used to outline the defect. After assessing the endoscopic appearance of the bladder neck, the flexible endoscope can be advanced through the bladder neck and into the posterior urethra to the level of the obstruction. Simultaneous retrograde urethrogram then outlines the anterior urethra, with the space not visualized representing the distraction defect.

Magnetic resonance imaging has also been advocated by some for the evaluation of patients with distraction injuries. The authors have had little experience with this modality for that purpose.

Repair

The timetable for reconstruction of distraction defects is determined by the type and extent of associated injuries. If possible, it is desirable to proceed within 4 to 6 months after trauma. Orthopedic injuries of the lower extremities, however, often necessitate delay in proceeding with urethral reconstruction.

In the majority of cases, distraction injuries are not long, and the resultant obliteration is amenable to a technically straightforward mobilization of the corpus spongiosum with a primary anastomotic technique. The classic reconstruction consists of a spatulated anastomosis of the proximal anterior urethra to the apical prostatic urethra. Experience has demonstrated, however, that anastomosis of the proximal anterior urethra to any segment of the posterior urethra (apical, prostatic, or below) can be successfully accomplished using a widely spatulated anastomosis in which optimal epithelial apposition is achieved. About 10% of distraction injuries are associated with more complex injuries and can be associated with fistulas (most commonly urethrorectal fistulas). Reconstruction of these injuries is technically more demanding.

Several series support the concept that **most distraction injuries,** even the most difficult cases, **can be managed by way of the perineal approach.** In fact, the use of a transpubic or an abdominal perineal approach, as pioneered by Waterhouse and co-workers, is not necessary for the reconstruction of a distraction injury (Waterhouse et al, 1973).

Alternatively the above-and-below approach does have merit for cases in which concomitant surgery is planned in the region of the bladder neck. The authors have found that the competence of the bladder neck is difficult to assess accurately before the re-establishment of urethral continuity. In the past, great reliance was placed on whether the bladder neck was closed or open on cystogram. Now, contrast material can opacify the prostatic urethra in cases in which the bladder neck is more than adequately competent for purposes of continence. Similarly, confidence has been placed in the appearance of the bladder neck on endoscopic examination through the suprapubic tube. Again, even in cases in which an obvious scar is noted to involve the bladder neck, follow-up of these patients after the urethral reconstruction establishes continuity of the urethra has found many patients with more than adequate continence. Still other patients are believed to have incontinence owing to scar incarceration of the bladder neck, created by the extensive fibrosis left behind by resolution of the hematoma. In the authors' experience, however, this is an infrequent occurrence, and the appearance of the bladder neck by any modality available is not predictive of continence. Therefore, the authors re-establish the continuity of the urethra and, in cases in which there are concerns about continence, forewarn the patient before the urethral reconstruction. If these patients find that they experience less than adequate continence postoperatively, the problem is addressed in a subsequent procedure.

At the time of reconstruction, before positioning the patient into lithotomy position, endoscopy is performed through the meatus and again through the suprapubic tube sinus. Endoscopy on the table is designed to ensure that there is no concomitant vesicolithiasis. This endoscopy is performed with a rigid scope that is manipulated through the suprapubic tube sinus and the bladder neck and positioned against the area of total obliteration. On gentle manipulation of the scope, if the impulse of the scope tip is felt on the patient's perineum, the impulse will be palpable during reconstruction at the time the perineum is opened, and an instrument is manipulated through the bladder neck. If the impulse is not palpable perineally at this time, it may not be palpable during dissection. In those cases, the authors create a temporary vesicostomy, allowing the surgeon to identify palpably the bladder neck before passing the curved Hagrove staff into the posterior urethra. This maneuver has eliminated the occurrence of false passages of the Hagrove staff, the tip of which can be seen in Figure 107–51H, and also has eliminated the occurrence of misanastomosis of the anterior urethra to sites other than the apical proximal urethra.

The authors use the exaggerated lithotomy position for the perineal approach (Fig. 107–48). This position is safe and provides optimal exposure to the area of the membra-

nous and apical prostatic urethra. The authors prefer a custom Skytron table, modified to allow for the exaggerated lithotomy position, or a Stille-Scandia table, designed to place patients in the lithotomy position. The legs are carefully positioned in the Allen or Guardian style stirrups. Care is taken to avoid pressure on the lateral aspects of the lower extremities and calf muscles (Fig. 107–49). The patient's hips are elevated into position by raising the buttocks portion of the operating table. The boots are positioned to avoid stretch injuries of the common peroneal nerves (Fig. 107–50).

After correctly positioning the patient, the perineal approach to reconstruction begins with an incision and dissection anterior to the transverse perinei musculature (anterior perineal triangle). This is in contrast to the approach posterior to the transverse perinei musculature (posterior anal triangle), useful for perineal prostatectomy. The authors use a lambda-shaped incision (Fig. 107–51) that is carried sharply down to the midline fusion of the ischiocavernosus musculature, then beneath the scrotum, to expose the uninvested portion of the corpus spongiosum. The authors then place a self-retaining ring retractor.

The fusion of the ischiocavernosus musculature is divided, and the musculature is cleanly dissected from the corpus spongiosum and bulbospongiosus. The corpus spongiosum is detached from the ligament overlying the intracrural space and corpora cavernosa, the bulbospongiosus is detached from the perineal body, and the dissection is carried further down to the infrapubic space. Posterior detachment of the bulbospongiosus is carried anteriorly, and the dissection is eventually carried through the area of fibrosis.

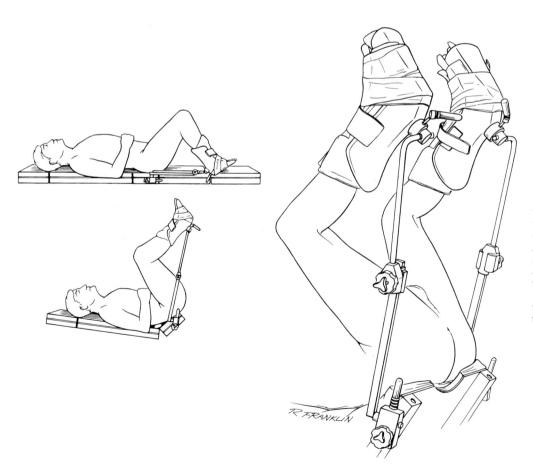

Figure 107–48. Patient placed in an exaggerated lithotomy position. Note that hips have been rotated into position by elevating the buttocks portion of a specially modified table. Note that the legs are suspended from boot-style stirrups. Also note that the legs are suspended with as little flexion of hips and knees as allowed by design of the stirrups. (From Angermeier KW, Jordan GH: Complications of the exaggerated lithotomy position: a review of 177 cases. J Urol 1994; 151:866–868.)

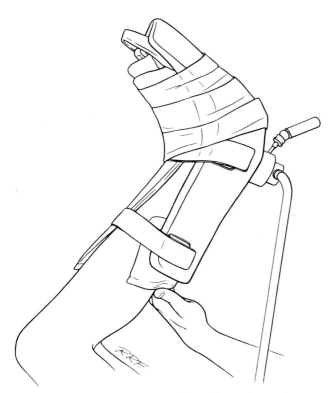

Figure 107–49. Positioning of feet and lower legs in boot-style stirrups. Note that there is absolutely no pressure on calves and that feet hang in stirrups. (From Angermeier KW, Jordan GH: Complications of the exaggerated lithotomy position: a review of 177 cases. J Urol 1994; 151:866–868.)

In some cases, the proximal blood supply is encountered and must be controlled. The authors have found that these arteries are easily controlled with a sharp-tipped hemostat and monopolar cautery. Suture ligature should be avoided in the case of the circumflex cavernosal arteries because of their proximity to the nerves as they are coursing into the corpora cavernosa.

The authors then incise the triangular ligament and vigorously develop the intracrural space down to the pubis (Fig. 107–52). If the dorsal vein is encountered, it is ligated and divided. It is important to make sure that the arteries were not rolled into the intracrural space when the tissues were dislocated during trauma. It is not uncommon to see the penetration of the cavernosal arteries or the dorsal arteries rolled into this space. If there is doubt about the nature of the vessels encountered, the Doppler should be used. When the pubis is exposed, the periosteal elevator can be gently introduced onto the retropubic surface, releasing and allowing for the descent of the tissues from beneath the pubis.

The authors then introduce a Hagrove staff into the suprapubic sinus and through the bladder neck, to the distal limits of the posterior urethra (see Fig. 107–51H). The impulse is palpated, and the fibrosis is resected until normal tissue planes are encountered. The tissue is submitted for histology. The tip of the Hagrove staff is eventually concealed only by the normal urethral epithelium, at which point the authors open the epithelium and control it with either a skin hook or a stitch. The authors then perform endoscopy to ensure that the urethrotomy is at the distal

limits of the posterior urethra. If a tension-free anastomosis is not possible, the authors mobilize the corpus spongiosum beneath the scrotum from its attachment to the corpora cavernosa. Aggressive mobilization of the corpus spongiosum is the last maneuver undertaken because it is believed to have possible ill effects on the retrograde blood supply, which in the patient with pelvic fracture may be tenuous. Meticulous detachment of the investment of Buck's fascia from the corpus spongiosum increases the compliance of the corpus and limits the need for aggressive mobilization.

It is important to try to avoid the creation of chordee during the repair of a distraction injury. To prevent chordee, the detachment cannot be carried beyond the area of the penopubic attachment. It is warranted in some cases, however, to counsel patients preoperatively that they may have chordee after aggressive mobilization that results in a primary anastomotic repair. Primary anastomotic repairs carry success rates in the high 90% range. If a technique of tissue transfer is needed, the long-term cure rates may eventually be in only the mid-80% range. The vast majority of these patients are young, and successful reconstruction is of paramount importance. If chordee results, it is most often mild; not disabling sexually; and, in the authors' and other surgeons' minds, probably a fair trade for optimizing the urethral reconstruction.

The proximal urethrotomy is spatulated so that it accepts

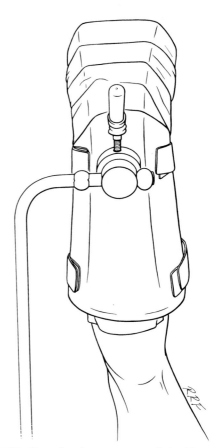

Figure 107–50. Note that legs are suspended without any internal rotation of feet in stirrups. This position is believed to lessen potential for neurapraxia injuries associated with prolonged positioning. (From Angermeier KW, Jordan GH: Complications of the exaggerated lithotomy position: a review of 177 cases. J Urol 1994; 151:866–868.)

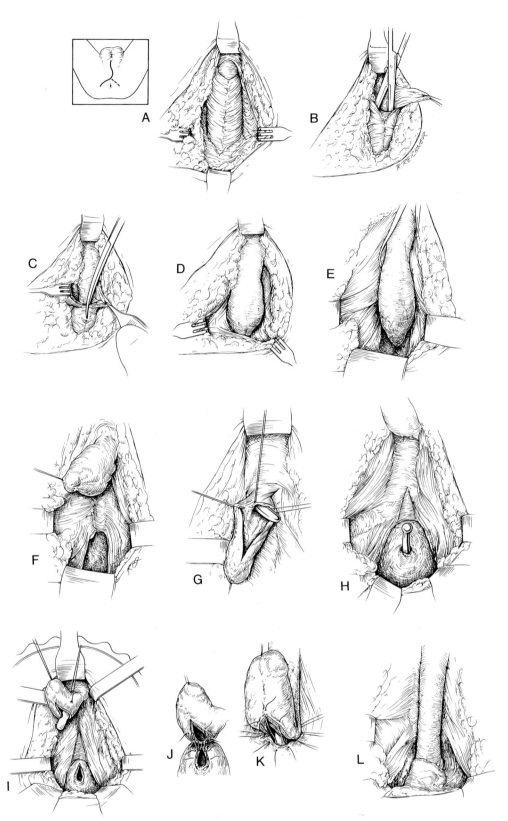

Figure 107–51. Perineal repair of membranous urethral stricture. A lambda incision extends from the midline of the scrotum to the ischial tuberosities. *A*, Colles' fascia has been opened to expose the bulbospongiosus muscles and the tunica of the corpus spongiosum distal to the edge of the muscles. *B*, The scissors are introduced to develop the space between the muscle and the bulb of the urethra. *C*, An incision is made in the midline with the scissors exposing the length of the bulb. *D*, The ischial cavernosus muscle is retracted to expose the full length of the bulb. *E*, The self-retaining retractor is placed to expose the inferior fascia of the genitourinary diaphragm. The bulb of the corpus spongiosum (bulbospongiosus) can now be mobilized to gain access to the strictured area of the urethra. *F*, The strictured urethra is incised, freeing the bulb. *G*, The urethra is opened, to create an adequate lumen. *H*, The Hagrove staff has been passed through the suprapubic cystostomy. Resection of the scar has allowed it to pass into the perineum. *I*, The scar tissue has been removed from the anterior aspect of the prostatic urethra, and the urethra has been opened for the anastomosis. *J*, Sutures have been placed to approximate the epithelial edges of the proximal and distal segments of the urethra. *K*, The catheter has been passed, the anterior sutures have been tied, and the posterior sutures are about to be tied. *L*, Anastomosis is completed, with the reinforcing sutures between the tunica of the corpus spongiosum and corpora cavernosa in place.

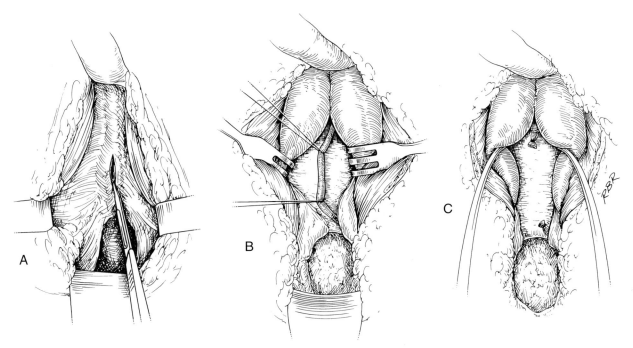

Figure 107–52. Division of the triangular ligament and development of the intracrural space. *A,* When the prostatic urethra is displaced and the arc that the urethra must traverse needs to be shortened, length can be shortened by incising the triangular ligament. *B,* Incision and mobilization of the perichondrium and periosteum of the symphysis pubis allow placement of retractors without trauma to the erectile bodies. Lateral displacement of the crura exposes the dorsal vein of the penis, which after careful identification can be ligated and divided. *C,* Completion of the dissection affords additional exposure for resection of the fibrosis that surrounds the prostate and the proximal end of the disrupted urethra. (From Jordan GH: Reconstruction of the meatus/fossa navicularis using flap techniques. *In* Schreiter F, ed: Plastic Reconstructive Surgery in Urology. Stuttgart, Germany, Georg Thieme Publishers. In press.)

at least a No. 32 Fr bougie á-boule, and 10 to 12 anastomotic sutures are placed and tagged to allow identification of their position in the proximal anastomosis. The authors use a combination of 3–0 Monocryl sutures and 3–0 PDS for this purpose. Special needles are not required for the placement of these sutures. A Heaney needle driver and a Ravich needle driver can be useful in difficult cases. A lighted sucker is also beneficial at this point of the procedure.

After spatulation of the proximal urethrotomy and placement of the sutures, the authors spatulate the proximal portion of the anterior urethra (see Fig. 107–51*I*). The spatulation is continued until the urethrotomy accepts a No. 32 Fr bougie á-boule, and the anastomotic sutures are placed in their respective locations. Before seating the anastomosis, the authors introduce a soft silicone Silastic-ribbed urethral stenting catheter through the anastomosis under direct vision (see Fig. 107–51*K*). The wound is then copiously irrigated to reduce the clot around the area of the anastomosis, and the anastomosis is seated.

Next, the authors reattach the corpus spongiosum to the corpora cavernosa and the bulbospongiosus to the perineal body. The authors then place a small suction drain deep to the closure of the ischiocavernosus musculature and Colles' fascia and a second one superficial to that closure and beneath the subcutaneous closure.

In those cases in which the proximal urethra is significantly distracted in a rostral direction, the surgeon must be prepared to perform infrapubectomy (Fig. 107–53) or corporal rerouting. The performance of the infrapubectomy, along with the development of the intracrural space, allows for exposure of the apical prostatic urethra. In cases in which the prostatic urethra remains rostrally displaced, the impulse

of the sound or instrument placed through the cystostomy tract into the bladder neck is often not readily apparent. In these situations, it is comforting to be able to palpate the bladder neck and the properly placed sound before embarking on a dissection beneath the pubis. In addition, if the rostral distraction is significant, the path of the anterior urethra over the hilum of the penis into the infrapubectomy often does not allow for a tension-free anastomosis, and the infrapubectomy can be continued beneath one side of the corpora cavernosa, allowing for rerouting of the corpus spongiosum (Fig. 107–54).

Postoperative Management

The authors use a soft silicone Silastic stenting catheter. Urine is diverted by way of the suprapubic cystostomy, and the urethral catheter is plugged and serves as a stent only. After the reconstruction, patients are initially kept at bed rest and then ambulated and discharged with the suprapubic catheter and stenting urethral catheter in place. They are also discharged on oxybutynin and a suppressive antibiotic. The drains are removed as drainage allows.

A voiding trial with contrast material is performed between 21 and 28 days postoperatively. Patients are directed to stop taking oxybutynin 24 hours before the voiding trial. In anastomoses that are technically straightforward, the trial is performed at 21 days, and in those cases with more rostral distraction of the proximal urethra, the trial is delayed for 3 to 5 days longer. The trial involves removing the urethral catheter, filling the patient's bladder with contrast material, and instructing him to void. The voiding film is examined

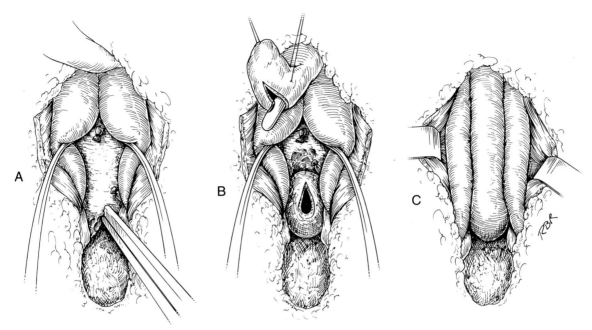

Figure 107–53. Infrapubectomy. *A,* If the prostate is elevated behind the symphysis pubis, the inferior aspect of the symphysis is resected using a Kerrison rongeur. *B* and *C,* As much of the bone can be removed as necessary to afford a simple approximation of the ends of the urethra.

to ensure that there is no evidence of extravasation and that the reanastomosis appears widely patent. A urine culture is also obtained, and the suprapubic catheter is plugged. The patient is allowed to void per urethra for 5 to 7 days, and the suprapubic catheter is then removed.

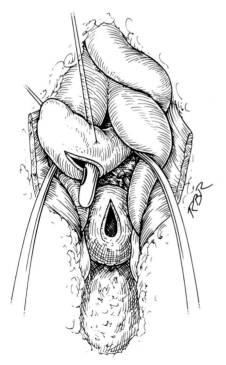

Figure 107–54. Resection of the pubis and rerouting of the urethra over a crus. When the prostate is markedly displaced, it may be necessary to expand the infrapubectomy. Sometimes, despite the crura's having been separated to the full extent possible, the two ends of the urethra do not meet when brought directly through the crus. It is necessary to bring the urethra lateral to one of the crura to make up this length.

Patients remain on the suppressive antibiotic until they are tube-free and a culture and sensitivity have been obtained. At that time, they are placed on a short regimen of culture-specific antibiotic.

At approximately 6 months and again at 1 year postoperatively, the patients are evaluated with a flexible endoscope. At that time, the authors consider the reconstruction to be mature, and it should be widely patent. In the absence of the reappearance of symptoms, no further routine follow-up is done.

The authors have almost completely replaced postoperative retrograde studies with the use of the flexible endoscope. The authors have not found flow studies to be valuable in following these patients and have found in many cases (anterior urethral reconstruction) that retrograde urethrography was more confusing than helpful.

Using the techniques discussed, or similar techniques, curative rates for reconstruction of posterior urethral distraction injuries is in the high 90% range. **Failures are not, in large centers, due to technical problems** (i.e., anastomotic restenosis). In general, failures **are indicative of ischemia of the proximal corpus spongiosum** with ensuing stenosis of the mobilized corpus spongiosum. This occurs because with mobilization, the corpus spongiosum, in essence, becomes a flap with the vascular pedicle being the retrograde vascularity from the arborization of the dorsal arteries through the glans.

The authors have studied this phenomenon in trauma patients and believe they can **predict the patients at risk for this ischemic atrophic phenomenon.** Initially, the authors studied with pudendal angiography all trauma patients who seemed to be at risk for bilateral deep internal pudendal artery injury at the time of trauma. These are patients who have evidence of injury to the dorsal penile nerves, patients who were failures of reconstruction referred from other centers, patients with lateral impact pelvic fractures, and patients whose pelvic fractures were of the "windswept" variety. The authors found that many patients had evidence of either unilateral or bilateral pudendal artery lesions but that most had evidence of vascular reconstitution. Patients with an intact pudendal artery on one side often were potent and were reliably cured with reconstruction. Patients with only reconstituted vessels, either unilateral or bilateral, never were potent but were reliably reconstructed. These patients were optimal candidates for corporal arterial revascularization to improve potency. Because the authors noted this relationship to potency, they began looking at patients with duplex Doppler ultrasonography. The authors found that patients with normal pudendal arteries, either unilateral or bilateral, demonstrated normal arterial parameters on duplex evaluation. Those with only reconstituted arteries, either bilateral or unilateral, never had normal arterial parameters on duplex Doppler ultrasonography.

The authors proceed to pudendal angiography only in those patients with abnormal arterial parameters on ultrasonography, with the patients whose ultrasonography was normal predictably doing well with reconstruction. The data also show that patients do well with reconstruction if they have at least one side that is reconstituted, and the only patients at risk for ischemic stenosis are those with bilateral complete obstruction of the internal pudendal vessels. In such patients, the authors perform corporal arterial revascularization to augment the vascularity and with that accomplished then proceed to urethral reconstruction.

Summary

Using the maneuvers outlined previously, **the authors have found that virtually all distraction injuries can be reconstructed by way of a perineal approach using an anastomotic technique.** Although the above-and-below approach is used in cases in which concomitant bladder neck surgery is performed, the inability to identify those patients accurately has led the authors to perform bladder neck surgery at a second setting. The authors have therefore abandoned a transpubic approach as applied to posterior urethral distraction injuries.

Although the authors favor primary reconstruction of posterior urethral distraction injuries, others choose to manage these injuries endoscopically. The endoscopic management of urethral distraction defects is not a simple procedure and must be undertaken by a skilled and experienced surgeon. Many of these procedures can be categorized as a "cut for light" procedure. Although some surgeons report success, the majority of "cut for light" procedures are not done with sufficient precision to allow for adequate realignment of the urethra. The authors have seen many disasters that have resulted from these procedures and in most cases condemn the use of these modalities.

In 1989, Marshall described his method of using stereotactic techniques for endoscopic alignment of the ends of the urethra (Marshall, 1989). He emphasized the length of time it takes to obtain precise alignment before undertaking the endoscopic portion of the procedure. In his procedure, he passes a wire through the aligned ends of the urethra, minimally dilating the channel and widening it with transurethral resection. The scar is stabilized by a period of self-catheter-

ization. Marshall has limited the applications of this procedure and does not advocate it as a primary modality. Patients whose medical condition, age, or concomitant orthopedic injury prevents them from being placed in the exaggerated lithotomy position or reconstructed by way of a transpubic approach may be managed with this technique.

VESICOURETHRAL DISTRACTION DEFECTS

Enthusiastic use of radical prostatectomy has unfortunately led to a large experience with patients who have had total obliteration of their vesicourethral anastomosis. In some patients, there is distraction of the vesicourethral anastomosis, with either a totally obliterating distraction defect or severe anastomotic stenosis. Additionally, with the proposal that bladder tube interposition might enhance continence, a new entity, the stenotic or obliterated vesicourethral anastomosis owing to ischemia of the bladder tube, is now encountered.

As with other defects, it is important to determine the length of the defect accurately. This can be accomplished using simultaneous cystogram with retrograde urethrogram or simultaneous retrograde urethrogram and antegrade endoscopy through the suprapubic tube (Fig. 107–55).

The authors place patients in a low lithotomy position and use an abdominoperineal combined approach. The authors create a lower midline incision, exposing the bladder and dissecting it from the lateral sidewall and further mobilizing the anterior portion of the bladder from beneath the pubis as aggressively as can be safely undertaken from above. The authors then open the peritoneum and develop the retrovesical space, again taking care to complete the dissection as safely as can be accomplished from above.

A second surgeon then begins the perineal dissection, using a curvilinear perineal incision similar to that used for a radical perineal prostatectomy. The authors dissect posterior to the transverse perinei musculature (posterior anal

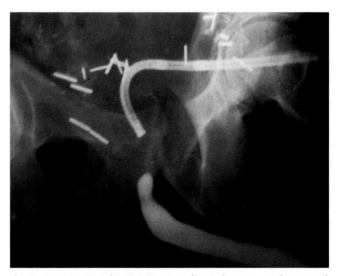

Figure 107–55. Simultaneous retrograde urethrogram and antegrade endoscopy through suprapubic tube in a patient after radical prostatectomy with vesicourethral distraction.

triangle) and carefully carry the dissection up the anterior rectal wall to the area where fibrosis from the prior radical prostatectomy dissection is encountered. At this point the impulse of the perineal surgeon's digits can usually be felt adjacent and lateral to the area of fibrosis and distraction. In addition, the abdominal surgeon places his or her finger at the limits of the retrovesical dissection from above, to provide further palpable landmarks and ensure a safe dissection anterior to the rectal wall and posterior to the bladder and trigone. The authors carry this dissection to join the abdominal dissection, completely dropping the rectal wall off the area of fibrosis associated with the distraction defect. The authors then place drains between the rectum and the distraction defect, encircling the area of fibrosis.

This dissection beneath the pubis is made easier by the excision of an ellipse of the rim of the superior pubic ramus. Total pubectomy is not required. The partial pubectomy can be performed using the reciprocating attachment of the Aesculap surgical drilling device, improving the exposure for dissection and resection of the distraction fibrosis and making placement of the sutures technically straightforward.

At this point, the authors open the bladder, determine its caudad extent, and place a sound per urethra to the caudad area of obliteration. The authors are then able to resect the well-defined area of fibrosis completely. The urethral stump is exposed and opened, and the site of the neobladder neck is identified and opened. The authors marsupialize the bladder epithelium as described by Walsh (1985), place anastomotic sutures in the urethral stump, and pass a stenting catheter.

Before seating the vesicourethral anastomosis, the omentum is mobilized and placed between the posterior wall of the anastomosis and the anterior rectal wall. The authors then seat the anastomosis and wrap the omentum around the area of anastomosis, tacking it into place. The lateral vesical spaces are drained with closed-suction drains, and a suprapubic tube is left in place when closing the vesicostomy.

Postoperative care is the same as for a radical prostatectomy. The patients are discharged when their drainage and ambulation allows and their diet has been resumed. The authors evaluate the patients at 6 weeks postoperatively with the stenting urethral catheter removed and the bladder filled via the suprapubic tube. In most of these cases, the stenting urethral catheter, although a Foley catheter, does not have the balloon inflated. It is positioned and held in place by way of a monofilament suture looped to an abdominal wall button. In cases in which there may be tension on the anastomosis, it can be performed in association with Vest sutures (Vest, 1940).

The authors have successfully reconstructed by way of open anastomosis all but one of six patients. Four of the six procedures have resulted in continence that the patients deem adequate for their lifestyle, whereas one patient who is incontinent has been managed with placement of an artificial sphincter.

CURVATURES OF THE PENIS

Normal elasticity and compliance of all tissue layers of the penis are critical for erectile function, tumescence, and rigidity. Tissues must expand in all dimensions as the penis engorges with blood, and eventually the tissues of the tunica albuginea and the septal fibers of the corpora cavernosa are stretched to the limits of their compliance, and tumescence is converted to rigidity. **In the normal penis, the tissues are symmetrically elastic,** and the erection is straight. **In curvature of the penis, there is relative asymmetry of one aspect of the erect penis.** In some cases, this arises from diminished compliance of one aspect of the tunica albuginea or outright foreshortening of one aspect of the erectile bodies.

In proper usage, the term chordee means curvature. In common usage, chordee has been used as if it refers to the tissues causing the curvature. This misuse of the term is seen in the phrase "the chordee was resected." Correct usage of this term would be "the correction of chordee can be accomplished by resecting the inelastic tissues that are causing the chordee."

Curvatures of the penis can be congenital or acquired. Some confusion also exists regarding the common usage of the term congenital curvature of the penis. The terms congenital curvature of the penis and chordee without hypospadias have often been used interchangeably. The authors reserve chordee without hypospadias for those patients in whom the meatus is properly located on the tip of the glans penis, yet a ventral curvature is associated with abnormalities of the ventral fascial tissues or corpus spongiosum. It has long been recognized that hypospadias is a condition that is associated in some males with either smallness of the penis or a micropenis. Although a small penis is not diagnostic of hypospadias, it is highly unusual for a patient with hypospadias to have an exceptionally large erect penis. In contrast, other congenital curvatures of the penis (ventral, lateral, or dorsal) are inevitably associated with the finding of a large erect penis.

The term acquired curvature implies that the patient was born, traversed puberty, and existed during some years of adulthood with a penis that was perfectly straight and then, as a result of trauma to the penis, developed curvature as an adult. In that the trauma that results in acquired curvature is virtually always associated with intercourse, the occurrence of acquired curvature is nil before the onset of puberty. The authors have seen some patients in whom there was a history of trauma during vigorous masturbation, but these patients are the exception. As with congenital curvatures of the penis, the acquired curvatures may be dorsal, lateral, ventral, or complex.

Congenital Curvatures of the Penis

The urethra begins as an epithelial groove in the midline of the ventral surface of the developing penis. As the groove extends, it deepens, with the edges eventually meeting to fuse into a tube. Fusion begins proximally and progresses distally. During normal development, the fusion of the urethral tube eventually reaches the tip of the glans penis. Proliferating mesenchyme surrounds the tube, separating it from the skin, and differentiates to form the corpus spongiosum, Buck's fascia, dartos fascia, and the overlying ventral skin of the penis. **Fetal development of the penis is regulated by testosterone, produced by the fetal testis, that is converted by 5α-reductase to dihydrotestosterone.** Dihydrotestosterone acts directly on cells with androgen receptors and all layers of the male external genitalia. This embryologic process explains the development of the anterior urethra that is unique to males.

Maturation of these tissues into normal structures depends on the same growth factors that control the formation of the urethra. Even though urethral development has progressed normally, mesenchymal tissue development in the penis may be deficient or abnormal and result in dysgenic and inelastic fascial layers. El-Galley and associates have shown that, at least in hypospadias, there is a deficiency of epidermal growth factors in the ventral penile skin (El-Galley et al, 1997). Research is currently underway to investigate the levels of these growth factors in the deeper tissues.

In some patients, there is an intimate association between congenital curvature and the hypospadias anomaly (see Fig. 107–19). Ventral curvature of the penis is most frequently associated with hypospadias in which the mesenchyme distal to the meatus ceases proper differentiation, becoming a fan-shaped layer of dysgenic fascia. The apex of this inelastic tissue surrounds the urethral meatus and inserts into the undersurface of the glans penis. In most cases of hypospadias, the defect represents a panventral anomaly of the penile tissues. In classic hypospadias, there is nonfusion of the ventral glans, and the preputial skin is distributed dorsally. As with many, if not all, congenital anomalies, however, there is a spectrum of penetrance, and the hypospadias anomaly can represent a spectrum from a perineal location of the meatus, with total malfusion of the ventral tissues involving the scrotum and the shaft of the penis, to a normally located urethral meatus, fused preputial skin, and apparently properly fused ventral penile skin but with persistent abnormalities of the fascial layers or corpus spongiosum. In proximal hypospadias, for example, there is inappropriate development of all of the ventral penile tissues, superficial to the tunica albuginea of the corpora cavernosa. Buck's fascia is abnormal or not present, the dartos fascia is abnormal or not present, and the ventral skin is abnormal. It appears that the anomaly in hypospadias is due to premature cessation of the production of testosterone or to delayed production of testosterone between fetal weeks 8 and 12, during the critical phases of genital development (Devine et al, 1980a).

In 1973, Devine and Horton proposed **a typing of the various congenital curvatures** (Fig. 107–56). In type I congenital curvature, the urethral meatus is at the tip of the glans. None of the surrounding layers is normally formed, and the epithelial urethra is associated with malfusion of the corpus spongiosum and all of the tissues superficial to the urethra. Skin coverage of the epithelial tube is present. In type II, a dysgenic band of fibrous tissue believed to be derived from the mesenchyme, which would have produced Buck's fascia and the dartos fascia, lies beneath and lateral to the urethra. The urethra is contained within a normally developed and fused corpus spongiosum.

In type III, the urethra, corpus spongiosum, and Buck's fascia are all normally developed and ventrally fused. There is an area of inelastic tissue in the dartos layer of the penis that causes a relatively sharp bend. Abnormal development of the dartos fascia is frequently associated with complex curvatures. With extensive involvement, the inelastic dartos can be sufficient to restrain the penis and conceal the penile shaft. In many of these cases, there also appears to be abnormal prominence of the mons fat pad. These stigmata

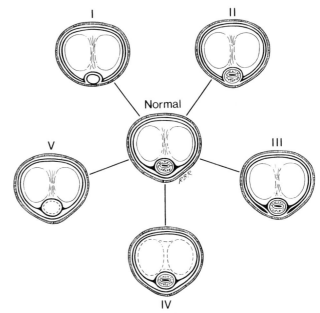

Figure 107–56. Cross section of the penis displaying the forms of congenital curvatures of the penis. The normal penis is in the center. *Class I*: Epithelial urethra beneath the skin. Dysgenic tissue beneath it represents undeveloped corpus spongiosum, Buck's fascia, and dartos fascia. *Class II*: Normal urethra and spongiosum but abnormal Buck's and dartos fascia. *Class III*: Abnormal dartos fascia only. *Class IV*: Normal urethra and fascial layers with abnormal corpocavernosal development. *Class V*: Congenital short urethra (rare). (From Devine CJ Jr, Horton CE: Bent penis. Semin Urol 1987; 5:252.)

are believed to be associated with an abnormality in the proper progression of virilization during fetal development.

In type IV, although the urethra, corpus spongiosum, and fascial layers are normally developed, there is relative shortness or inelasticity of one aspect of the tunica albuginea of the corpora cavernosa. Experience has shown that most patients whose congenital curvature is type IV seem to demonstrate evidence of a hypercompliance of the tunica albuginea. In these patients, the flaccid penis is normal in size and not necessarily impressively large, whereas the erect penis is large. The tunica albuginea of the corpora is required to expand through a wide range, and if there is asymmetry in the compliance of the tunica, curvature occurs. It is not uncommon for patients with type IV curvature to have noticed curvature before puberty but to have noticed an increase in the curvature as they traverse puberty, owing to the penile hypertrophic growth spurt that occurs during this time.

Type V congenital curvature is also known as the congenital short urethra. This implies that there has been correct fusion of all elements of the penis (i.e., tunica albuginea, urethral epithelium, corpus spongiosum, Buck's fascia, dartos fascia, and the ventral skin). During erection, however, the correctly fused urethra and corpus spongiosum are not long or compliant enough to match the compliance of the other ventral tissue layers.

If type V congenital curvature exists at all, it occurs so rarely that when it is encountered one should doubt the finding. Although in the past discussion of the condition centered on the best location to "cut the urethra" during the repair, in the rare occasions when this condition is encountered, the authors believe that it should be diagnosed and treated only by the most experienced surgeons. In general, if the urethral meatus has developed to the tip of the glans and the urethra is of adequate caliber, the urethra should not be divided to correct ventral curvature of the penis. Although there may be extremely rare exceptions to this bold statement, if those exceptions are encountered, their existence should still be questioned.

Congenital curvatures types I, II, and III all represent forms of hypospadias anomaly, and the authors refer to them collectively under the term chordee without hypospadias. This term implies that although the meatus is not improperly placed, curvature is present because of inappropriate fetal development of the ventral penile structures. The authors refer to type IV anomaly as congenital curvature of the penis. If a patient has findings of hypercompliance of the corpora cavernosa and a ventral curvature, the patient is diagnosed as having congenital ventral curvature of the penis; if the hypercompliance causes a lateral curvature, it is referred to as congenital lateral curvature of the penis (left or right). Although, as mentioned, the type V anomaly is so rarely encountered that it deserves its own diagnosis, the authors believe its correction is best discussed with types I, II, and III, under the category of chordee without hypospadias.

Chordee Without Hypospadias in Young Men

Patients with chordee without hypospadias usually present with either ventral curvature or ventral curvature associated with torsion (complex curvature). These young men do not typically have a greater than average stretched penile length (13.1 cm; Schonfeld and Beebe, 1942) (or 12.4 cm; Wessels et al, 1996) and have noted curvature throughout life. If prepubescent, they have obvious curvature with erection, and if postpubescent, they may offer a history of increasing curvature as they pass through puberty.

In many cases, there are abnormalities of the ventral penile skin. These might consist of either an element of hooded preputial skin or a high insertion of the penoscrotal junction. Although the patients have fusion of the preputial skin, there is also often a wrinkled appearance dorsally, which is a form of the classic hooded preputial skin. In addition, in most cases, the tissues on the ventrum of the penis, deep to the corpus spongiosum, seem inelastic as the patient's penis is examined on stretch. This palpable inelasticity on the ventral aspect of the penis consists of dysgenic fibrous tissue, which can replace the Buck's and dartos fascia layers, and, in some cases, consists of an element of inelasticity of the tunica itself.

During surgical exploration, Devine and Pepe (unpublished data, 1991) obtained tissue from these patients for evaluation of 5α-reductase. These data suggested a deficiency of that enzyme in the ventral dysgenic tissue. Although the values were inconclusive at the time, the study was discontinued (Devine and Pepe, 1991). As mentioned, Galloway (1995) also looked at tissues in males with hypospadias for epidermal growth factor deficiency and found a correlation. To the authors' knowledge, however, a growth factor analysis has not been undertaken in patients with true chordee without hypospadias or in patients with congenital curvature of the penis.

An important part of the preoperative evaluation is submission of Polaroid photographs taken by the patient of the erect penis, documenting the curvature. The Polaroid photographs are especially helpful in differentiating the patients with chordee without hypospadias from those with congenital curvatures of the penis. In patients who have chordee without hypospadias, the photograph reveals an erect penis commensurate with the size of the detumesced penis, whereas in the congenital curvature patient, the erect penis is noticeably large.

Because of their congenital anomaly, these patients often become relatively reclusive and have poor self-images and genital images. For a successful surgical outcome, it is important to address the psychologic aspects of the condition as an integral part of the treatment. Many of the authors' patients are also evaluated preoperatively by a sex therapy colleague.

Corrective surgery for chordee without hypospadias is highly successful, and in almost all cases, an effective correction can be accomplished with a single operation (Devine et al, 1991). In some cases, the penis has been straightened by excising all the dysgenic tissues from the ventral side of the penis and widely mobilizing the corpus spongiosum from the glans penis into the perineum.

Even in patients with obvious abnormalities of the corpus spongiosum (i.e., poor ventral fusion or frank bifid corpus spongiosum), wide mobilization usually reveals that it is not the corpus spongiosum that remains as the ventral limiting factor. In many patients, the penis remains curved owing to the inelasticity of the ventral aspect of the corpora cavernosa themselves. Furthermore, as mentioned, in occasional patients, the corpus spongiosum becomes atretic distally on the shaft, and the urethra itself is only an epithelium-lined tube. In these patients, however, wide mobilization of the epithelial distal portion and proximal corpus spongiosum usually does not reveal that the corpus spongiosum or the epithelial tube is limiting the ventral erection. If the epithelial urethra has served as an adequate conduit (i.e., it is not stenotic), the morbidity of urethral division and subsequent need for urethral reconstruction must be considered before undertaking such a procedure. With the evolution of hypospadias repairs accomplished by wide mobilization of the corpus spongiosum and epithelial and corpus spongiosal elements distal to the meatus, allowing for onlay procedures, the greater morbidity of urethral division must be strongly considered, and the authors believe that the morbidity can usually be avoided.

In children, after mobilization and excision of the dysgenic fibrous tissues, if there is residual chordee, it can usually be corrected by making a longitudinal incision, with a sharp blade, in the ventral midline of the corpora cavernosa, while maintaining an artificial erection. The incision can often be extended between the corporal bodies without entering the erectile tissue for a significant distance, allowing the edges of the ventral tunica to move laterally. The penis noticeably straightens with erection.

If this maneuver is not sufficient, the dorsal neurovascular structures can be mobilized in concert with Buck's fascia, and a small ellipse or ellipses of dorsal tunica albuginea can be excised and closed with watertight plicating sutures. Caution is important, however, when the dorsal neurovascular structures are mobilized because with poor development of the ventral structures, which occurs in some patients, the arborization of the dorsal arteries provides the dominant vascularity to the glans.

Surgical Approaches to Congenital Curvatures of the Penis

Patients with congenital curvature of the penis can have ventral, lateral (which is most often to the left), or, unusually, dorsal curvature. Polaroid photographs of the erect penis demonstrate a smooth curvature that generally involves the entire pendulous portion of the penile shaft.

Patients usually present as otherwise healthy young men between the ages of 18 and 30. Many have noticed curvature before passing through puberty but have presumed it to be normal. With puberty, however, they discover that the curvature is not normal, they become sexually active and discover that the curvature impedes their efforts, or they notice increasing curvature as they pass through puberty, which, in their minds, clearly would preclude sexual intercourse. Occasionally a patient waits until after age 30 to deal with the anomaly; less often, a younger adolescent presents who has a relationship such that he can discuss his genitalia with his parents.

The authors' surgical approach to patients with a congenital ventral curvature is illustrated in Figure 107–57. Most of the authors' patients have been circumcised, and new pat-

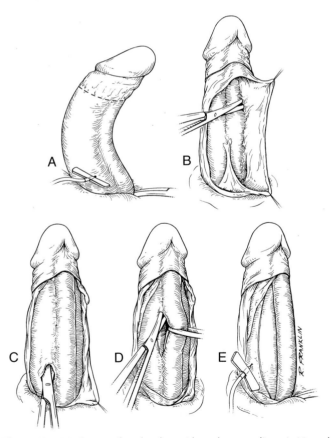

Figure 107–57. Surgery for chordee without hypospadias. *A,* Ventral curvature demonstrated with artificial erection. *B,* Dysgenic dartos fascia is elevated and will be excised. *C,* The dysgenic layer of Buck's fascia is undermined by spreading the scissors. *D,* The inelastic fascia is excised as the corpus spongiosum and urethra are mobilized. *E,* Artificial erection demonstrates correction of the curvature.

terns of venous and lymph drainage of the skin have been established by that procedure. In circumcised patients, the authors make an incision through the circumcision scar, which, in many cases, is displaced well down on the penile shaft. Even with relatively significant displacement of the circumcision scar on the shaft of the penis, however, the reincision should be through the circumcision scar. The penis is degloved by dissecting the layer immediately superficial to the superficial lamina of Buck's fascia.

An artificial erection is performed using normal saline. A high-pressure pump is useful for this purpose. The authors do not routinely recommend a tourniquet device because constricting devices can conceal the proximal limits of the curvature. This is most significant in cases with ventral curvature, which frequently extends proximally. Occasionally, some element of perineal pressure is initially required, but these are patients with normal erectile function, and their veno-occlusive function is normal. Also, the authors do not use pharmacologic agents to induce erection, although some centers favor this approach.

The artificial erection demonstrates the character of the curvature and the location of maximal deflection. In patients with ventral curvature, there may be some thickening of the dartos and Buck's fascia, and in those patients, the fibrous tissue is mobilized and completely excised. The corpus spongiosum is detached from the corpora cavernosa and mobilized from the glans to the penoscrotal junction.

After excising these tissues, the artificial erection is repeated; occasionally, the curvature is completely straightened. Most patients, however, suffer from a differential elasticity between the dorsal and ventral aspects of the corporal bodies, and although the curvature may have been lessened, it persists unless further procedures are done to straighten the penis.

In the adult patient with persistent curvature, there are two options for surgical correction: (1) to lengthen the ventral aspect of the penis by making transverse incisions in the ventral tunica and placing an autologous tissue graft (the authors favor the dermal graft) or (2) to shorten the dorsal aspect of the penis by elevating the neurovascular bundle, excising an ellipse or ellipses from the dorsum of the tunica albuginea, and closing the defects in watertight fashion (Fig. 107–58) (Nesbit procedure) (Nesbit, 1965). Because the length of the erect penis is usually not a problem in these cases of congenital curvature, the authors generally choose the second option. The recovery period is much shorter, and the variabilities of graft take do not have to be considered. Additionally, when using a dermal graft, there is always the possibility, although uncommon, of the development of graft-induced veno-occlusive dysfunction. It is therefore preferable to shorten the longer dorsal aspect of the penis in patients with congenital curvature. If the patient falls into the category of chordee without hypospadias, and shortness of the penis is an issue, the authors use incisions with grafts to correct the curvature (Devine and Horton, 1975).

After the decision to proceed with excisions of ellipses of dorsal tunica has been made, Buck's fascia can be elevated, in concert with the dorsal neurovascular structures, by beginning just lateral to the corpus spongiosum and carrying the dissection dorsally across the midline. Alternatively the tunica can be exposed by excising the deep dorsal vein of the penis and opening the inner lamina of Buck's fascia, elevat-

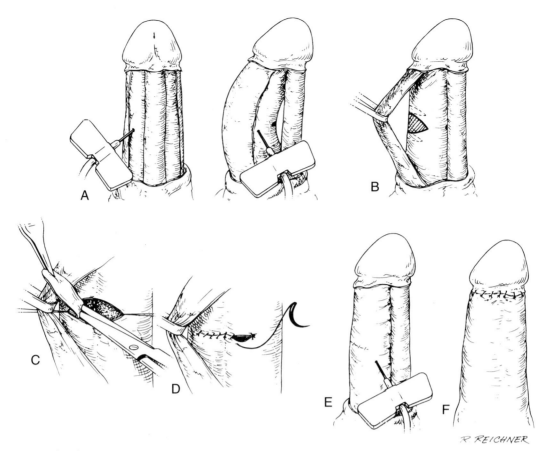

R. REICHNER

Figure 107–58. Surgery for chordee without hypospadias. *A*, A circumcision incision has been made, and the urethra has been mobilized by resecting the dartos and Buck's fascia. The needle is in place for an artificial erection. The erection shows continuing chordee. The elastic urethra is not the cause of this curvature. The point of maximum concavity has been marked. *B*, An ellipse of tissue is outlined opposite the point of maximum concavity. As an alternative, two smaller ellipses are shown. *C*, Excision of the ellipse of tunica. Note the tips of the septal strands in the midline. *D*, Closure of the edges of the incision. *E*, Artifical erection revealing a straight penis. When the bend is more complex, ellipses must be excised in other locations. *F*, The skin is closed. (From Devine CJ Jr, Horton CE: Bent penis. Semin Urol 1987; 5:4.)

ing the neurovascular structures by dissecting from the dorsal midline laterally around to the corpus spongiosum and from the coronal margin to the penopubic junction, thus limiting the effects of stretching the dorsal structures with exposure of the dorsum of the penis.

An artificial erection is performed to plan the proposed ellipse excisions. The authors use several small ellipses rather than try to correct the curvature with one large ellipse. The first ellipse is usually positioned at the point of maximum convexity. The edges of the planned ellipse are then apposed using polypropylene (Prolene) suture. The artificial erection is repeated to assess the effects of that excision. If there is good straightening in that area of the shaft, the incisions are again well marked, the plicating sutures are removed, and the ellipses of tunica are created using a sharp scalpel blade. By dissecting in the space of Smith and removing only an ellipse of tunica, the ellipse can be carefully excised to avoid damage to the underlying erectile tissue. The edges of the ellipse are reapproximated with a combination of interrupted 4–0 PDS and a watertight running 5–0 PDS.

After closure, the authors repeat the artificial erection to assess the results of the first ellipse and determine the need for other excisions. A final artificial erection demonstrates the penis to be perfectly straight. In cases of ventral curva-

ture or cases in which complex curvatures are associated with an element of ventral curvature, a minimal degree of dorsal curvature is acceptable. In most of these cases, as the sutures dissolve, the penis either remains minimally dorsiflexed or becomes perfectly straight.

Buck's fascia is closed. Two small suction drains are placed superficial to Buck's fascia but deep to the dartos fascia. The authors then replace the skin sleeve, with its edges apposed with interrupted small Vicryl or Monocryl sutures, placing a small Foley catheter in all patients. The catheter is removed on the first postoperative day. The two small suction drains are also removed at 24 to 36 hours, but not both at the same time. Depending on edema, patients are discharged from the hospital on the second or third postoperative day.

Congenital lateral curvature of the penis is often associated with some complexity of curvature, and patients frequently notice lateral curvature associated with a ventral or, less commonly, a dorsal curvature. Some patients present with only lateral curvature, however, with the right side larger than the left and curvature to the left.

In some cases, the repair of the lateral curvature can be approached through a small incision at the point of maximal curvature (Fig. 107–59). If this incision is possible, after induction of anesthesia, an artificial erection is performed.

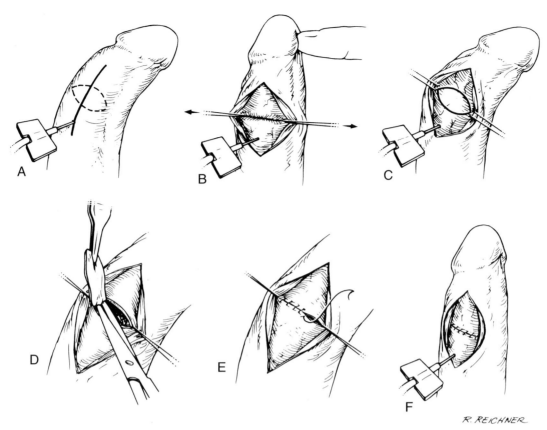

R. REICHNER

Figure 107–59. Congenital lateral curvature. *A,* An artificial erection reveals the curvature. The incision to gain access to the potential ellipse of tissue is marked. *B,* The tunica albuginea has been exposed by mobilizing Buck's fascia, and Prolene sutures have been placed at the dorsal and ventral tips of the potential ellipse. While maintaining the artificial erection, tension is established on the two sutures as the penile shaft is straightened. The fold produced in the tunica is marked. *C,* When the penis is relaxed, this mark defines the ellipse of tunica to be removed. *D,* The tunica is excised. *E,* The edges are approximated. *F,* The penis is straight. Buck's fascia and the skin are closed.

The point of maximum concavity is marked, and a small incision is created contralaterally at the site of maximal convexity. After opening the dartos fascia and Buck's fascia, some minimal mobilization of the dorsal neurovascular bundle is required. Prolene sutures are placed, and an artificial erection is again performed. The size of the ellipse is assessed, excised, and closed as discussed previously.

As mentioned, however, cases of lateral curvature are associated with complex curvatures. In these patients, correction of the curvature is similar to that described for patients with ventral curvature, using a circumcising incision with the skin reflected. In contrast to ventral curvature, however, with lateral curvature, the entire dorsal neurovascular bundle does not need to be reflected, and therefore it is seldom required or considered beneficial to excise the deep dorsal vein when approaching the dorsum of the penis. The postoperative care is the same as described for a ventral curvature.

For the uncommon patient with a congenital dorsal curvature of the penis, the repair is best accomplished by partially mobilizing the corpus spongiosum to allow small ellipses to be positioned lateral to the midline on the ventrum of the penis, using the technique described previously. Again, postoperative care is as described of a ventral the curvature.

Although described as a method of plication for the curvature associated with Peyronie's disease, the procedure described by Yachia (1993) is useful also the correction of congenital curvatures (Fig. 107–60). This procedure essen-

tially creates longitudinal incisions in the tunica albuginea that are closed transversely. Thus, the "long side" is plicated without the need for excision; however, the plication is durable in that the tunica is opened and closed resulting in a scar rather than relying only on the strength of sutures as was originally described by Nesbit (1965). With this technique, closure is done with absorbable monofilament suture.

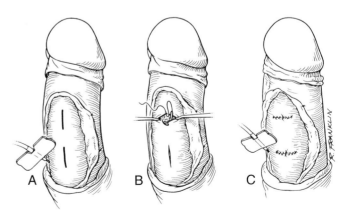

Figure 107–60. Technique after Yachia for correction of curvature, in this case, a patient with congenital lateral curvature. *A,* Buck's fascia is reflected exposing the lateral tunica albuginea. *B,* Longitudinal incisions are created at the area of maximal curvature as demonstrated by artificial erection. *C,* The longitudinal closures are closed transversely, with artificial erection demonstrating good straightening of the penis.

Acquired Curvatures of the Penis

Acquired curvature of the penis inevitably follows trauma to the penis. Many are associated with the findings of Peyronie's disease, believed to be associated with trauma to the penis during intercourse. Patients who have had vigorous internal urethrotomy occasionally develop significant curvature. In these patients, the incision has extended outside of the urethra and corpus spongiosum to involve the tunica of the corporal bodies, causing scarring that is significant enough to be associated with curvature.

Acquired Curvatures of the Penis That Are Not Peyronie's Disease

When a young man presents with an acquired curvature of the penis, one must always consider the possibility of Peyronie's disease. In many of these patients, close questioning reveals a history of minimal lateral curvature of the penis and a clear memory of a lateral buckling injury occurring during intercourse. In some cases, the patient remembers hearing a "snap" and noticing immediate detumescence and significant ecchymosis of the penis. These patients often are referred with a diagnosis of **fractured penis.** Owing to the noticeable events associated with fracture of the penis, most patients now present acutely, and reconstruction can be accomplished at that time.

Occasionally, however, a patient or his primary care physician ignores the stigmata of the trauma, and the patient presents with a noticeable lateral scar that causes both indentation of the lateral aspect of the penis and, in some cases, curvature. Patients who had pre-existing lateral curvature may actually notice that their penis has been straightened by the trauma, but they are disturbed by the indentation caused by the scar. In others, the small linear scar causes a significant lateral curvature.

Another group of patients present after having noticed a similar buckling trauma to the penis but not associated detumescence or ecchymosis. These patients report noticing that their erections were quite painful for a period of time after the trauma and then the development of a nodule in the lateral aspect of the penis. Eventually, they present with a lateral linear scar that has led to curvature and indentation at the site. The authors refer to this injury as a **subclinical fracture of the penis.**

The pathology of a subclinical fracture of the penis is believed to be due to disruption of the outer longitudinal layer of the tunica albuginea during the buckling trauma. The inner, circular layer is not disrupted, however, and maintains the blood-tight continuity of the corpus cavernosum. In some patients, it may be that both layers of the tunica albuginea are disrupted, but the closely applied Buck's fascia remains intact, thus precluding the usual findings of fracture of the penis.

These patients always have normal erectile function, and there is no association with concomitant global cavernosal veno-occlusive dysfunction. In addition, these injuries are not associated with shortening of the penis. Indeed, the lack of erectile dysfunction and penile shortening distinguishes these patients from patients with Peyronie's disease. If a detailed history leads one to suspect blighted erectile func-

tion, an evaluation of erectile function should be accomplished before proceeding with surgery. At the authors' institution, they begin with a nocturnal penile tumescence study with sleep monitoring. These studies are performed in a sleep laboratory, but a Rigi-scan can also be used. If the sleep tumescence study is abnormal, the patient should be assessed with more detailed studies (duplex ultrasound plus cavernosography or dynamic infusion pharmacocavernosography and cavernosometry).

Although foreshortening of the penis is neither a characteristic of the injury itself nor the resulting scar in either of these injuries, these patients are not thought to be best treated by approaching the opposite aspect of the scar and excising an ellipse of the tunica. This results in bilateral scars, which cause bilateral indentations of the penis, and although the penis has been straightened by the correction, most patients are upset by the cosmetic and functional result of a near circumferential indentation of the penis. Instead, the authors excise the scar as is done in Peyronie's disease and place a dermal graft to replace the corporotomy defect created by the scar excision. Because these scars are on the lateral aspect of the penis, minimal mobilization of Buck's fascia, associated dorsal neurovascular structures, and the corpus spongiosum is required at the site. The surgical correction described has been extremely effective, with all curvatures treated at the authors' institution successfully corrected with a single operation.

PEYRONIE'S DISEASE

Although described by others before, Peyronie's disease was named for Francois de la Peyronie, who discussed the condition in his paper of 1743. **Peyronie's disease is characterized by a lesion in the tunica albuginea of the corpora cavernosa.** During erection, this lesion causes functional shortening and curvature of the involved aspect of the corporal body. The lesion has commonly been called a plaque.

Not a rare condition, Peyronie's disease is seen in about 1% of white men. Although the disease has been reported in younger patients, there is a clear predominance between the ages of 45 and 60 years. Few of the authors' patients have been black, and the majority of those patients who were black have had diabetes mellitus and an element of erectile dysfunction diagnosed before the onset of Peyronie's disease. To date, the authors have not treated any Orientals for Peyronie's disease.

Peyronie's disease is also called plastic induration of the penis and penile fibromatosis. In this case, the term fibromatosis describes the scarring processes of the tunica albuginea of the corpora cavernosa. This is in contradistinction to the term penile fibrosis, which commonly has been applied to a fibrotic process involving the intracorporeal erectile tissue. In addition, other physiologically important elastic tissues can be involved by processes similar to Peyronie's disease, such as scarring of the palmar fascia, termed Dupuytren's contracture; contracture of the plantar fascia, termed Lederhose's disease; and a scar of the eardrum, termed tympanosclerosis. Approximately 30% of the authors' patients have associated Dupuytren's contracture. A familial association is noted in patients with these conditions, but no association with the B7 group of HLA antigens has been found (Leffell, 1997).

Pathophysiology

Although the cause of Peyronie's disease is not completely understood, laboratory work has illuminated some possible causative factors. In 1966, Smith described its pathology and thought that the lesion resulted from perivascular inflammation in the space he described as lying between the tunica albuginea and the erectile tissue. The space between the tunica albuginea and the underlying spongy erectile tissue has since been referred to as Smith's space. Histology does show inflammation present in this space, but it is also present in and beneath Buck's fascia, where it overlies the lesion. Smith (1969) was never able to define the cause of the inflammation; however, most of the nonsurgical treatments for Peyronie's disease since that time have been aimed at controlling this inflammation. The authors believe the inflammation to be a result of the underlying processes in the tunica. There are no reports with good supporting evidence showing that patients have done better on the many anti-inflammatory medical regimens other than those in small series of patients reported by Williams and Thomas (1970) with no treatment at all. **The plaque is a scar and not the result of inflammatory or autoimmune processes that have been identified to date.**

Although Peyronie's plaques may extend laterally to involve adjacent aspects of the tunica albuginea, **all plaques the authors have seen have been located in the dorsal or ventral midline and are associated with the attachment of the strands of the midline septum.** Tissue sections from plaque, stained using a technique that defines elastic fibers, collagen, and fibrin, exhibit characteristically disordered collagen and abnormal deposition of elastic fibers. Both biochemical and immunologic criteria have identified extravascular material in these sections as fibrin. Although there is excessive deposition of collagen in the plaques, plaque cells do not show excessive collagen production in tissue culture. They do show strongly reduced production of elastin (Somers et al, 1982).

Evidence indicates that the inciting event in Peyronie's disease is trauma. Several investigators, including DeSanctis and Furey (1967), Godec and Van Beek (1983), Hinman (1983), and McRoberts (1969), have associated the development of Peyronie's disease with trauma in susceptible individuals occurring during sexual intercourse. The authors agree with these investigators and believe that they can define the process by which this occurs. A number of patients also present after trauma that has occurred during a period of diversion following a prostatic transurethral resection. The authors believe that the buckling mechanism still applies to these patients, but with the buckling force being the result of a nocturnal erection with a large-caliber catheter, rather than during vigorous intercourse.

Although buckling does appear to be an important factor, trauma to the tissues of the tunica albuginea from other forces appears to lead in some cases to the same result. For example, the authors have seen patients who have been involved in motor vehicle and industrial accidents that resulted in direct trauma to the penis and led to the development of scars identical to those of Peyronie's disease. Finally, there continue to be reports of patients who develop Peyronie's disease and are adamant that they have not had any trauma to the penis owing to intercourse or any other source. Some patients, in fact, seemingly develop Peyronie's disease after a radical prostatectomy and an ensuing long period of abstinence from sexual activity. Interestingly, these patients complain of curvature with erection, yet they deny being sexually active. The precise dynamics of this population are not yet explained.

Peyronie's disease is also associated with the development of erectile dysfunction in most patients. It appears that in most cases, however, the erectile dysfunction precedes the development of Peyronie's disease. With destabilization of the axial erectile rigidity mechanism, which may be caused by minimal erectile dysfunction, the potential exists for either chronic or acute buckling, which is discussed later.

As mentioned, the tunica albuginea is a laminated structure throughout most of its circumference (see Fig. 107–4). The fibers of the outer lamina run lengthwise, and the fibers of the inner lamina are circular in orientation. The bilaminar orientation is present both dorsally and laterally; however, there does appear to be some attenuation of the longitudinal fibers in the ventral midline, where the tunica albuginea may be monolaminar. The fibers of the septal strands fan out and are interwoven with the strands of the inner layer of the tunica albuginea, which are circumferentially oriented. Normally the tissues of the corpora are symmetrically elastic, and the penis remains relatively straight as it fills with blood and becomes erect. As they stretch, the tissues of the tunica become thinner, and without an inner supporting fiber structure, the penis would have little rigidity. An intercavernosal fiber framework contributes to this characteristic, with the strands of the septum affording most of the ventral-dorsal, axial rigidity of the erect penis.

When the sheath of the tunica and the septal fibers have been stretched to the limit of their distensibility, the configuration of the septum forms an inflated "I beam," resisting dorsal and ventral bending forces (Fig. 107–61). The pressures accumulated in the corpora cavernosa are hydraulic pressures, exerted at right angles to the layer that contains

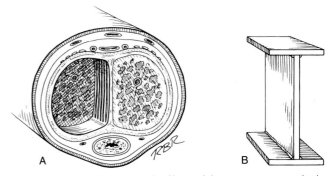

Figure 107–61. *A,* The penis. The fibers of the septum are attached to the inner surface of the tunica albuginea of the corpora cavernosa along the dorsal and ventral midlines. Plaques of Peyronie's disease occur in the tunica albuginea at the site of attachment of the septal strands. *B,* An I-beam illustrates the configuration of the septum that is responsible for the ultimate rigidity of the penile erection. This function leads to the occurrence of Peyronie's disease. (From Devine CJ, Jordan GH, Somers KD: AUA Today, 1989; 2:1–3.)

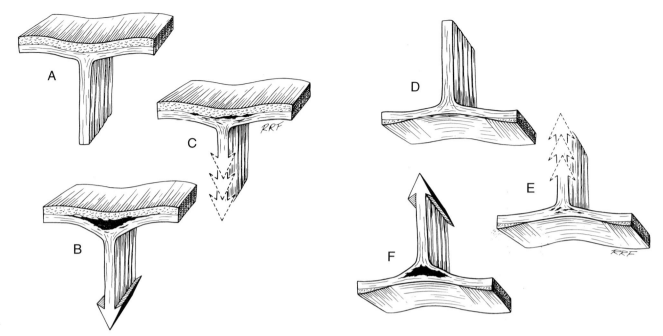

Figure 107–62. Demonstration of the mechanism of injury during buckling injuries to the penis. *A,* Fibers of the septal strands dorsally fan out and are interwoven with the inner circular lamina fibers of the tunica albuginea. The outer lamina consists of longitudinal fibers. *B,* The acute form of Peyronie's disease—bending the erect penis out of column—produces tension on the strands of the septum, delaminating the layers of the tunica albuginea. Bleeding occurs, and the space fills with clots. The scar generated by the response of the tissue to this process becomes the Peyronie's disease plaque. *C,* In the chronic form of Peyronie's disease, less turgid erections allow flexion of the penis during intercourse, producing elastic tissue fatigue, further reducing elasticity of the tissue and leading to multiple smaller ruptures of the fibers of the tunica with smaller collections of blood producing multiple scars. *D,* The situation on the ventrum of the penis, where the bilaminar arrangement of the tunica albuginea becomes thinned, with the midline being monolaminar. The fibers of the septal strands fan out and are interwoven with the inner circular layer. There is no outer circular layer. *E,* In the chronic form of Peyronie's disease, less turgid erections allow for buckling of the penis as per *C. F,* In the acute form of Peyronie's disease, buckling of the erect penis out of column produces tension of the strands of the septum, causing the septal fibers to tear. The scar forms as per *B.*

them. Functionally the dorsum of the tunica albuginea has vectors pushing that "plate" dorsally, and as the ventral plate pushes ventrally, both dorsal and ventral vectors of force stretch the midline septal strands. When the penis flexes in the dorsoventral aspect, the stress on the system (compression on the concave side and tension on the convex side) is focused at the connection of the septal strands with the tunica, where plaques of Peyronie's disease occur as scars in the tunica albuginea (Fig. 107–62). The buckling thus causes either delamination of layers of the tunica where the septal fibers implant with intravasation of blood into the intralaminar space or shearing of the septal fibers where they are interwoven with the inner circular lamina of the tunica albuginea. Trauma combined with intravasation of blood leads to inflammation, induration, and eventual scarring in the susceptible patient (Somers and Dawson, in press, 1997).

The process by which a buckling injury to the penis leads to Peyronie's disease begins with diminution of the modulus of elasticity of the aging tissues of the tunica albuginea. The rapidity of the loss of elasticity may be genetically determined, accounting for a familial association that the authors have noted. Furthermore, it does not appear that the trauma has to be severe to initiate the process, and tension generated at the attachment of the stressed septal strands, by an acute bending of the outer column of the turgid penis, can be sufficient to delaminate the fibers of the tunica. This tear disrupts many small vessels, with bleeding and formation of a clot within the tunica or snapping of the septal fibers.

As the clot resolves, fibrin remains in the injured tissue.

Retained fibrin then activates fibroblasts (causing cellular proliferation), enhances vascular permeability, and generates chemotactic factors for inflammatory cells (histiocytes). Although this is a normal part of the healing process, the tunica is hypovascular, and the fibrin is not removed during the phase of remodeling that takes place in all tissues during healing. Because this original stimulus is not cleared, or perhaps because of repeated trauma leading to further fibrin deposition, the lesion does not appear to resolve, inflammation persists, collagen is trapped, and the pathologic fibrosis ensues.* The course of this active process, during which the body attempts to remodel the scar, takes approximately 1 to 1.5 years (Devine, 1997; Devine et al, 1997).

Not all patients who have a buckling injury of the penis develop a scar in the tunica albuginea, however. In most patients, after trauma to the penis, a stage of induration and inflammation occurs that involves the tissues of the tunica albuginea as well as the peritunical spaces and tissues. There is evidence in surgical patients showing that the inflammation, although not directly involving Buck's fascia, clearly involves the space between the tunica and Buck's fascia. In many patients, that stage of induration and inflammation resolves with what appears to be complete resolution of Peyronie's disease. In fact, what has occurred is that in these

*Research from Somers KD: Cell Biology and Immunology of Peyronie's Disease. NIH Grant No. 1546055378A2. Other participants are listed in the references (VandeBerg et al, 1981, 1982; Somers et al, 1982, 1987, 1989; Schmidt et al, 1987; Devine et al, 1988; Somers and Dawson, 1997).

patients, the injury has healed without the resultant virulent scarring reaction that is characteristic of the Peyronie's disease patient. Patients predisposed to elastic tissue fibromatosis secondary to trauma, however, appear to develop the scarring reaction that is characteristic of Peyronie's disease.

As stated earlier, Peyronie's disease is a disease of middle age and is seen less frequently in younger and older men. Young men accumulate intracorporeal pressures sufficient to resist the deforming force and limit flexion during intercourse. Despite the turgor of the erection or the vigor of intercourse, if a bend occurs, the elasticity of youthful tissues allows the structures to stretch with the stress and spring back. As men age, however, their tissue becomes less elastic, the rigidity diminishes, and if the force of intercourse persists, it can cause the penis to bend, generating a tear, as described previously. Many patients retain a vivid memory of an acute episode, perhaps a week to a month before the onset of the disease. With many older men, intercourse is often less vigorous, and even despite diminished elasticity and rigidity, there is less likelihood of such trauma.

The predilection for the Peyronie's couple to engage in frequent, and often vigorous, intercourse is well recognized. Frequently, men with Peyronie's disease have intercourse three to four times a week, if not on a daily basis, well into middle age. In addition, positions that are traumatic to the penis are often frequently employed by these couples. In the authors' patient population, at least half of the patients have intercourse with the female partner on top at least 50% of the time, and many describe that position as preferred. Many couples also describe a pattern of achieving anterior vaginal wall stimulation by forcing the penis into the woman's pubis during thrusting. Peyronie's is a disease of aging tissues in the patient with a youthful libido.

The two presentations of Peyronie's disease represent two subsets of patients. In many patients, the onset of Peyronie's disease is insidious. These men have lost much of the turgor of erection. Tension on the septal strands is decreased during active and vigorous sexual performance, allowing the attachments to the tunica to "work back and forth" generating tissue fatigue. This factor further reduces the elasticity of the attachments of the septal strands and leads to multiple small tears, with either vascularized disruptions or outright disruption of the strands. These patients notice pain or a painful lump in the penis, followed by minimal curvature that may slowly progress. In contrast, about half of the authors' patients notice that the condition appears suddenly, with little or no further progression. Patients notice a curvature, appearing almost overnight, and the curvature does not progress or improve from the time it was first noted.

Evaluation

The history and physical examination usually provide a diagnosis. Associations with medications and concurrent diseases seem to be happenstance, although the association of diabetes with erectile dysfunction may clearly put the predisposed man at risk for buckling and trauma. Pain during erection has been considered pathognomonic of Peyronie's disease; however, pain with erection can occur following other trauma to the penis that runs a different course than Peyronie's disease (as described earlier). Only approximately

one third to one half of the authors' patient population describe having had painful erections (Snow and Devine, 1981).

The physical examination should include Polaroid photographs, helpful in demonstrating the distortion of the penis, palpation of the penis to locate the plaque, and radiography to identify calcification within the plaque. Whenever possible, the authors initially evaluate the patient with his sex partner. It is important to reassure them that the lesion is not a tumor or cancer. It is also important to reassure the couple that the condition can be treated, and it does not represent an end to sexual interactions. Many of these couples have been previously told by physicians that there is no treatment or cure for Peyronie's disease, and although this is semantically correct, Peyronie's patients are treatable if resumption or continuation of sexual activity is the goal of therapy.

It is also important for the treating physicians to recognize that Peyronie's disease is an evolving one and that in some patients it can apparently resolve or improve to the degree that surgical treatment is unnecessary. Thus, **most Peyronie's disease patients require a waiting period between their first presentation and the decision to undertake definitive treatment.**

Sexual intercourse is of major importance to these couples and may cause a great deal of distress during the waiting period. Therefore, it is essential to make the patient feel as if something is being done for him and his disease during this time. Administering medication allows the time to pass more quickly and the patient to feel that "something is being done."

The authors treat with vitamin E 400 mg twice a day. Vitamin E is inexpensive, has no side effects, and may be effective because it anecdotally appears to improve some patients. Vitamin E is a scavenger of free radicals.

The beneficial effects of para-aminobenzoic acid (PABA) have been reported in anecdotal series with small numbers of patients. PABA may be effective; however, it is effective only at a recommended dosage of 12 g/day (24 500-mg tablets or 6 2-g packets). The medication is very expensive, and the recommended dose can be accompanied by significant gastrointestinal side effects.

The authors have occasionally used the nonspecific antihistamine terfenadine (Seldane) in young patients in whom painful erections are reported as problematic. The rationale of its use results from the theory that the inflammation characteristic of the early phase of Peyronie's disease may be histamine-mediated. Terfenadine has been associated with a number of side effects, so recently we have switched to using fexofenadine (Allegra) for a 3-month course of 60 mg twice a day. Again, although there are no conclusive pharmacologic studies validating the use of terfenadine or fexofenadine in Peyronie's disease, anecdotal reports support its effectiveness.

The benefit of colchicine in Peyronie's disease is also anecdotal. The authors initially use colchicine 0.6 mg twice daily for a period of 2 to 3 weeks. The patient's collective blood count is then checked for evidence of bone marrow suppression, and if none is found, he is continued on colchicine 0.6 mg three times daily to complete a 3- to 4-month course of therapy. Young men who are treated with colchicine should be warned before starting therapy about the potentially negative effects on their sperm count. Many patients cannot tolerate colchicine because of its gastrointestinal side effects. Tamoxifen has been used in Europe. Again, its effectiveness is reported anecdotally only.

The injection of pharmacologic agents directly into plaques is also advocated by some physicians. Steroids are used at some centers. At the authors' center, however, a number of patients were seen referred after they noted a deterioration of their condition following the injection of steroids. Many of these patients had reached what was reported to be a relatively stable stage in Peyronie's disease before the injection of steroids; afterwards the trauma of the injection appears to have led to further inflammation, induration, or curvature.

Levine and co-workers have injected calcium channel blockers into Peyronie's plaques (Levine et al, 1994). Although Levine's method has not been shown to alleviate the curvature, in patients who have areas of constriction, it appears to lead to some diminution in the scarring process and resulting fibrosis.

Gelbard and colleagues have investigated the use of collagenase in Peyronie's plaques (Gelbard et al, 1985). In an initial double-blind study, Gelbard and colleagues included relatively small numbers and did not demonstrate dramatic improvements in the patients studied. A planned double-blind study that is larger may define better the use of collagenase for Peyronie's disease plaque injections.

Radiation therapy appears to have a place in the management of Peyronie's disease only as a means of reducing inflammation. The authors use radiation extremely sparingly, administering it with the beta beam of the linear accelerator. It has been used exclusively in patients who have had an especially protracted, painful early disease course. Occasional studies of the use of dimethyl sulfoxide, ultrasound therapy, and iontophoresis with steroids all suffer from a lack of validation with regard to effectiveness.

In many patients, Peyronie's disease appears to develop with a concomitant background of erectile dysfunction. **When the physician is confident that the disease has reached a mature stage, disabling curvature of the penis and the presence of disabling erectile dysfunction are indications for surgical correction of Peyronie's disease. At this point, the authors believe that a preoperative evaluation of the surgical candidate's erectile function is necessary.** In some patients, the history suggests that severe erectile dysfunction may actually be the disabling factor, and defining that dysfunction may allow for its treatment in advance of the surgery to straighten the penis. Some patients may find that improvement in erectile function using modalities such as intracavernosal injection or vacuum erection devices reveals that the curvature itself is not disabling, and a return to sexual activity can be achieved without the need for surgery.

The authors currently use duplex Doppler evaluation with pharmacologically induced erection to define erectile function initially. If this study reveals evidence of veno-occlusive abnormality, the authors proceed to **dynamic infusion pharmacocavernosometry and cavernosography.** The authors have found these studies to be useful in defining which patients respond well to corrective surgery. **Caution should be used, however, not to over-rely on vascular testing.** For some patients, sympathetic tone persists despite the injection of vasoactive material, inaccurately indicating veno-occlusive dysfunction. Therefore, if pharmacoerectile

testing does not match the patient's report of erectile function, the results of these studies must be validated with nocturnal penile tumescence testing.

Finally, the patient's goals should be defined before undertaking surgical correction of Peyronie's disease. Although most patients would like to have their penis as it was before their affliction with Peyronie's disease, it must be understood that this is impossible. Therefore, it must be **explained to the patient that, at best, surgery can create a penis that is adequately straightened such that any residual curvature does not impede sexual intercourse and erectile function can be preserved at preoperative levels. Any greater goal than this is unobtainable,** and the patient must be counseled so that he has realistic expectations in approaching surgery.

In addition to being counseled by the authors, all patients are screened by a sex therapist, who often discovers problem areas that must be dealt with before surgery. The sex therapist also ensures that the patient and his sex partner have appropriate expectations of surgical outcomes and recovery.

Surgical Correction

A number of surgical procedures have been used for the straightening of the deformity of Peyronie's disease. Pryor and Fitzpatrick (1979) described excision and plication of the aspect of the corporal bodies opposite the Peyronie's lesion. This procedure counteracted the effects of the inelastic lesion by shortening the opposite compliant aspect of the corpora cavernosa.

Lue (1989) performed a correction in a series of patients in whom he omitted the excision of the tunica albuginea and merely plicated the opposite aspect of the corpora cavernosa. Although this technique has not yielded durable results in patients with congenital curvatures, in the Peyronie's patients, in whom accumulated intracavernosal pressures are probably less, he has reported good early results. Although the techniques of both Pryor and Fitzpatrick (1979) and Lue (1989) are valid in some patients, many patients are concerned by the shortening of the penis as a result of Peyronie's disease, and surgery that offers the suggestion of further shortening of the penis may be unacceptable to them. The procedure described by Yachia (1993) (discussed earlier under the correction of congenital curvatures) represents another plication technique that can be effectively used for curvatures associated with Peyronie's disease.

Poutasse (1973) described an unsuccessful procedure for straightening of the Peyronie's disease deformity. He created incisions in the Peyronie's plaque, and Buck's fascia was reapproximated over the incision. With time, however, the incision rescarred and the deformity was recreated. This procedure is mentioned, therefore, only to decry its use.

Gelbard (personal communication, 1989) also described a surgical technique that involved incising the Peyronie's plaque. He reported a series of patients in whom incisions were made in the Peyronie's plaque, and a graft of temporalis fascia was used to fill the defect. His technique was based on the theory that by creating a number of incisions and filling them with compliant material, a smoother curvature would result. He has reported good results with this procedure.

Das and Amar (1982) described a procedure in which the

Peyronie's plaque is excised, and the corporotomy defects are filled with tunica vaginalis graft. Das believed that the tunica vaginalis was an easy donor site for the urologist, and he believed that it gave the same results as the dermal graft. The authors' experience has been that tunica vaginalis is a suitable substitute for dermis in select patients with well-defined, small lesions. In patients in whom the corporotomy defect is large, however, the authors have not been pleased with the use of tunica vaginalis.

Lockhart (personal communication, 1991) has employed a procedure in which the Peyronie's plaque is excised, and the corporotomy defect is closed using tunica vaginalis as a flap based on the dartos, fascial, and cremasteric pedicle. He found that his results were better with the improved vascularity of the tunica vaginalis, transposed as a paddle on a flap.

Stefanovic and associates reported an experimental animal series in which a corporotomy defect was replaced with temporalis fascia transferred to the area of the penis as a microvascular free transfer flap (Stefanovic et al, 1994). To date, this procedure has not been reported in humans.

Lue (1989) has also described a procedure using incisions but patching the corporotomy defects with a vein graft. He initially thought that the excised deep dorsal vein provided an adequate donor site for vein grafts. With time, however, Lue found that the donor site offered inadequate amounts of donor tissue, and he now harvests saphenous vein to create vein graft patches. Lue believes that the intracorporal space represents a large vessel, and therefore a patch of vessel wall represents a physiologic procedure. He reported good results with this procedure in a relatively small series.

Hellstrom (1994) discussed his use of Silastic sheeting used as a graft to patch the corporotomy defect. He reports good results. The authors' experience is that nonautologous grafts (e.g., Silastic, Gore-Tex, Dacron), in the absence of concomitant prosthetic replantation, inevitably yield poor results (Devine et al, 1995).

Devine and Horton (1974) described a procedure for correction of deformity of Peyronie's disease in which the plaque is excised and replaced with a dermal graft. The authors use this procedure or a modification. The authors now also have a relatively large series of patients who have been treated by creating incisions through the Peyronie's plaque and patching the corporotomy defects with dermis. With the exception of patients with severely calcified plaques, in recent years the authors have preferentially used the technique of incisions with dermal grafting. Early results indicate that the technique of plaque incision is at least as successful as the technique of plaque excision; however, it has not yet been determined whether there is a difference between the techniques with regards to preservation of erectile function or limitation of the occurrence of graft-induced veno-occlusive dysfunction.

The initial incision depends on the location of the lesion (Figs. 107–63 and 107–64). Ventral plaques can be approached through a midline incision on the ventral aspect of the penis, and dorsal plaques are most effectively approached using a circumcision incision. In the patient who has been previously circumcised, the incision should be placed through the original circumcision incision. In many patients, the circumcision scar may be displaced far down the shaft of the penis. The authors have not encountered any problems, however, with reapproaching the penis through the circumcision incision even when this is the case.

For both dorsal and ventral plaques, the shaft of the penis is degloved to its base. This maneuver gives good exposure for midshaft and distal lesions. For proximal plaques or in patients who have relatively redundant foreskin, a second incision is created on the scrotum, lateral to the base of the penis (Fig. 107–65). After degloving the shaft of the penis, it is delivered into the scrotal incision, laying the shaft skin aside and covering it with a warm sponge. This protects the penile skin from trauma until the end of the procedure, when it is returned to the shaft.

The dorsal neurovascular bundle is elevated in concert with Buck's fascia. This can be accomplished by several techniques. Incisions can be made just lateral to the corpus spongiosum, with Buck's fascia and the dorsal neurovascular bundle dissected off the lateral and dorsal aspects of the corpora cavernosa. Alternatively, the authors currently approach dorsal plaques by dissecting sharply through the bed of the deep dorsal vein and perform a modified vein dissection. The authors initially used this approach to investigate the potential effect of a modified vein dissection with regard to limitation of graft-induced veno-occlusive dysfunction. Although the beneficial effects with regard to limitation of graft-induced veno-occlusive dysfunction are yet to be determined, approaching the dorsal plaque through the bed of the dorsal vein appears to be a superior approach technically.

In the past, if preoperative testing suggested veno-occlusive dysfunction, the authors proceeded with a formal vein dissection, ligation, and excision. More recent experience has shown, however, that vein dissection does not offer durable results in Peyronie's disease patients, and it is currently thought that patients who demonstrate severe veno-occlusive dysfunction are better treated by using a surgical approach to straightening the penis and prosthetic implantation for their erectile dysfunction.

After dorsal or ventral exposure of the tunica, the inelasticity of the plaque is evident, and its extent can be delineated by feeling the surface of the tunica albuginea. An artificial erection also aids in defining the curvature. Incisions can then be planned either across or to excise the plaque. Using Prolene, the authors place stay sutures in the midline, both proximally and distally to the plaque, and mark the planned incisions. Depending on the technique selected, the authors then excise (see Figs. 107–63 and 107–64) or incise (Figs. 107–66 and 107–67) the plaque. If an excisional technique is employed, lateral incisions in the tunica are used to convert the corporotomy defect from ovoid to stellate (see Figs. 107–63 and 107–64). This serves to release the tightness of the defect's edges and to increase the areas of the corporotomy defect by approximately 1.5 to 2 times the size of the plaque that was excised. The authors do not favor the use of a tourniquet either for the control of bleeding or for induction of an artificial erection because tourniquets can conceal proximal curvatures.

Once the plaque has been excised or incisions created, the authors measure the defect, stretching the penis to ensure accurate coverage. The dermal graft is then outlined on the donor site (Fig. 107–68). The authors use the skin of the abdomen just above the iliac crest, lateral to the hair line. The graft site is de-epithelialized, either freehand or using a

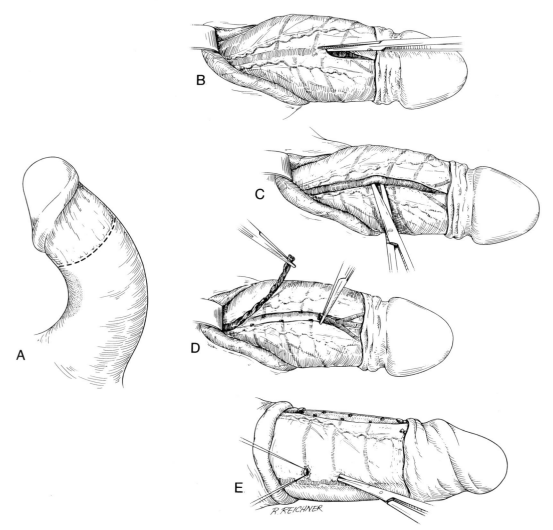

Figure 107–63. *A,* An erection demonstrates the dorsal curvature of the penis caused by the inelastic scar tissue in a dorsal plaque of Peyronie's disease. The incision to be made in the scar of the previous circumcision has been marked. *B,* The skin has been degloved to the base of the penis by dissecting in the layer immediately superficial to Buck's fascia. An incision in the dorsal midline of Buck's fascia exposes the deep dorsal vein. The coiled dorsal arteries and the circumflex veins are demonstrated. *C,* The deep dorsal vein is mobilized. *D,* After dividing the deep dorsal vein, it is dissected proximally, dividing the emissary veins and ligating. *E,* The circumflex veins are isolated and are oversewn.

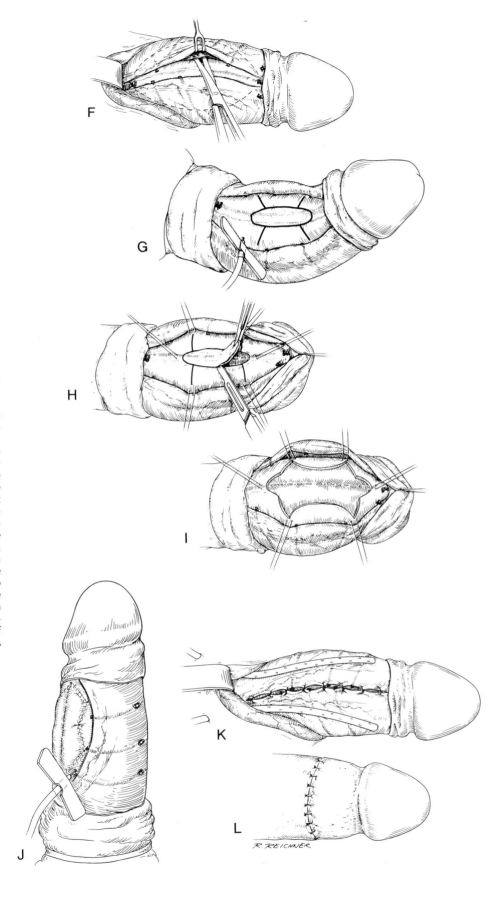

Figure 107–63 *Continued F*, Buck's fascia is elevated from the Peyronie's plaque. The area of dissection is outlined by the dashed line in the diagram, continued far enough proximally, distally, and laterally to allow excision of the plaque without distraction stretching the nerves in Buck's fascia. *G*, An artificial erection demonstrates the curvature caused by the inelastic plaque, which has been outlined on the tunica. Stellate releasing incisions have been marked. *H*, Prolene sutures have been placed distal and proximal to the plaque and at the tip of each of the releasing incisions. An incision has been made outlining the plaque, and the plaque is excised. The strands of the septum have been incised and are seen in the midline of the defect. *I*, The plaque has been excised. This defect must now be filled with a dermal graft. To determine the size of the patch, the defect in the tunica is measured while stretching it first longitudinally, then laterally. *J*, The dermal graft has been obtained and inlaid in the defect. An artificial erection shows the penis to be straight. If there is a leak in a suture line, it is oversewn. *K*, Buck's fascia is loosely reapproximated in the midline with interrupted sutures. One or two small suction drains are left in the space superficial to Buck's fascia. *L*, The skin closure is completed. A Bioclusive dressing is applied. A light pressure wrap of Kling dressing is left on 3 to 4 hours. A No. 14 Fr urethral catheter is placed.

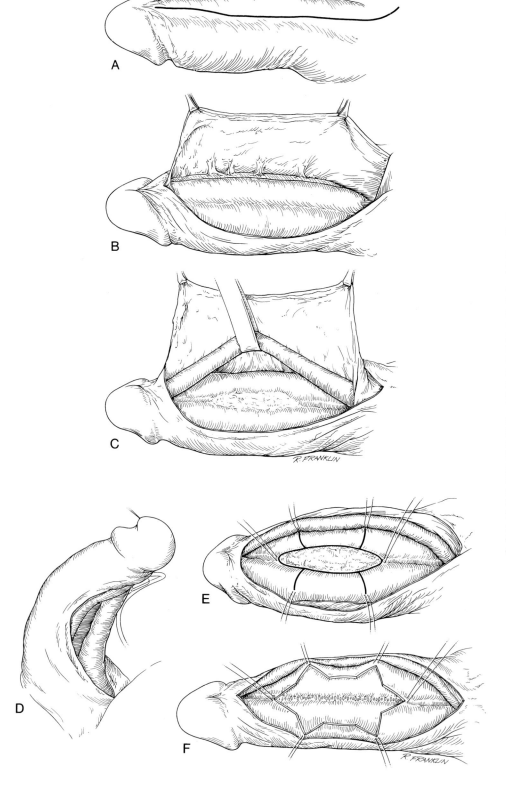

Figure 107–64. Exposure of a ventral plaque of Peyronie's disease. *A,* A midline incision marked on the ventral aspect of the penis is continued into the scrotum for a more proximal plaque. This can also be extended distally by combining it with an incision in the old circumcision scar. *B,* The skin is elevated with the full thickness of the dartos fascia elevated to expose the corpus spongiosum. *C,* The corpus spongiosum is mobilized by incising Buck's fascia on each side. The connections of the circumflex veins with the veins running lateral to the corpus spongiosum are ligated during this dissection. The inelastic plaque of Peyronie's disease is seen on the ventrum of the corporal bodies. *D,* An artificial erection demonstrating the extent of the curvature. *E,* The incision to excise the plaque and the releasing incisions have been marked. Stay sutures of Prolene are placed at the ends of the plaque and the releasing incisions. *F,* Resection of the plaque is complete. The defect is ready for the dermal graft. Note the ends of strands of the septum in the midline of this space.

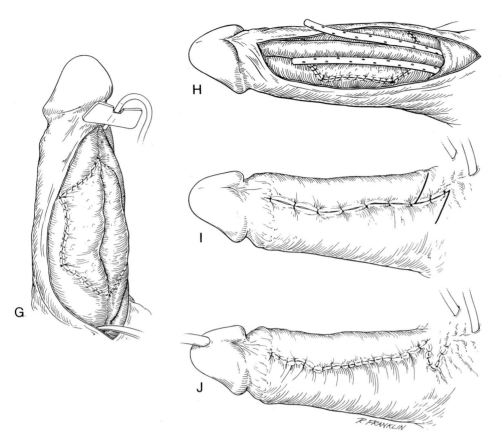

Figure 107–64 *Continued G*, A dermal graft has been obtained and placed in the defect. An artificial erection shows the penis to be straight. Note that the expansion of the graft is restrained by its attachment to the strands of the septum in the midline. *H*, The corpus spongiosum is reattached to the ventral tunica albuginea. The suction drains are placed on the ventrum superficial to Buck's fascia. *I*, The skin is approximated and a Z-plasty has been marked where the incision crosses the penoscrotal junction. *J*, Closure is complete; Bioclusive dressing is applied, and a No. 14 Fr catheter is placed.

dermatome. The epidermis is discarded, and the dermal graft is harvested and meticulously defatted. The donor site is closed per primam with subcuticular sutures, using either a pullout or the newer absorbable long-acting monofilament suture.

The authors carefully tailor the graft to measure approximately 30% larger in all dimensions than the corporotomy defect and place it into either the incisional or the excisional defect (Figs. 107–63, 107–64, 107–66, 107–67, and 107–69). After completing the closure using PDS, the authors perform another artificial erection to demonstrate that the penis is straight and the suture lines are watertight. If there are leaks, they are oversewn. If the penis is not straight during surgery, it will not be straight postoperatively. If curvature persists, therefore, further modifications by way of incisions and grafting are necessary.

After completion of the dermal graft inlays, the penis is anatomically closed. Buck's fascia is reapposed using PDS, and small suction drains are placed superficial to Buck's fascia but deep to the dartos layer. The authors then coapt the skin incisions using either chromic or small Vicryl sutures. If a ventral midline incision was created that crosses the penoscrotal junction, a Z-plasty should be used to prevent penoscrotal tethering.

The penis is dressed with a Bioclusive plastic dressing, loosely applied and extending from the base of the penis to the level of the midglans. A mildly compressive Kling dressing is placed over the Bioclusive dressing to limit edema and allow better collapse of the surgical spaces around the suction drains. The Kling dressing is left in place for a period of 4 hours, during which the glans is checked every

30 minutes. The authors place a No. 14 Fr Foley catheter until the patient ambulates and remove the suction drains at 24 to 48 hours. Erections are suppressed with diazepam and amyl nitrate, and patients are discharged on the second or third postoperative day.

Dermal grafts mature in the same manner as other grafts: first nourished by imbibition of tissue fluids, while inosculation occurs from adjacent blood vessels. Remodeling takes place during the late phase of maturation, with the graft tending first to contract and then become compliant. In the first 3 months, the graft may contract enough to recreate some of the curvature, but as the graft softens, straightening occurs. Patients should be forewarned of this sequence of events to avoid undue anxiety.

After the first 2 weeks, the authors encourage patients to have erections but discourage them from intercourse. During this time, it is desirable for the penis to be manipulated so that the skin does not adhere to the deeper layers of the penis. Additionally, erections stretch the graft and aid in the maturation phases of graft take.

Although there is a place for prosthetic implantation in the treatment of erectile dysfunction associated with Peyronie's disease, in the authors' experience, most patients do not require prosthetic placement. Patients who demonstrate poor erectile function before contemplation of surgery, however, are properly treated with placement of a prosthesis and an associated procedure to straighten the penis.

For this purpose, the authors have used incisions with dermal grafting and placement of a prosthesis. Others have elected incisions with Gore-Tex or Dacron grafting. Montague and associates (1993) have treated a number of patients

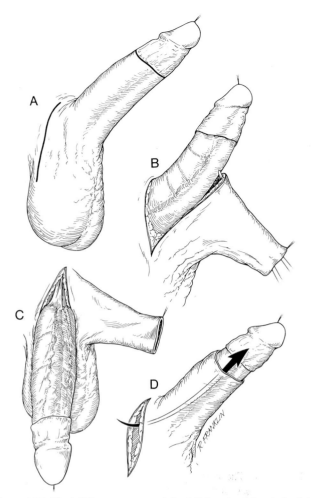

Figure 107–65. *A,* When exposure of the full length of the shaft of the penis is necessary, two incisions are marked: one in the scar of the previous circumcision and the other lateral to the base of the penis and carried down into the scrotum. *B,* The two incisions are completed, and the shaft of the penis is freed by a degloving dissection. The shaft of the penis is delivered into the scrotal incision. *C,* Retraction of the penis exposes the full length of the shaft and with minimal dissection the suspensory ligaments can be visualized. With further dissection, complete resection of the dorsal vein can be accomplished. *D,* At the conclusion of the surgical procedure, the shaft of the penis is replaced within the relatively untraumatized sleeve of skin. (From Devine CJ Jr, Horton CE: Bent penis. Semin Urol 1987; 5:252.)

with implantation of the AMS-700 CX prosthesis. After the placement of the prosthesis, Montague's technique involves remodeling the penis by stressing the plaque manually, which in some cases yields a cracking sensation of the plaque. Montague and associates have not encountered any associated morbidity with this technique of plaque remodeling and have been successful in a large number of cases in straightening the penis with implantation of the prosthesis and manual manipulation of the plaque.

TOTAL PENILE RECONSTRUCTION

The principal techniques for penile reconstruction were originally developed to treat trauma patients, and in many cases these patients were victims of war injuries. In 1936, Borgoraz reported a series of cases describing a technique

for phallic construction in war-injured patients, and in 1944, Frumkin followed with a series from Russia. Aware of the work in Russia, in 1948, Gilles and Harrison reported a series of patients in whom they had accomplished penile reconstruction while stationed at a major hospital in the outskirts of London during World War II. In their series, there were a number of patients with complete absence of the penis.

Initially, all procedures for phallic construction involved delayed formation and transfer of tubed abdominal flaps. These tubes were produced from random flaps of skin and because of their size were based on a tenuous blood supply. To allow new vascular patterns to become established in the transferred tissue, they were formed in stages, with a delay between the stages. In the tube-within-a-tube design, the inner tube allowed for placement of a baculum during intercourse, and the outer tube provided skin coverage. Patients voided through a proximal urethrostomy. (A baculum is a rod-like device that is inserted temporarily in the urethra or, in the case of a phallis, in a pocket, thus supplying rigidity for intercourse. In the 17th and 18th centuries they were constructed of wood or glass and later they were made of rubber or plastic.) This continued to be the state-of-the-art phallic construction and penile reconstruction until 1972, when Orticochea described total reconstruction of the penis using the gracilis musculocutaneous flap.

In 1978, Puckett and Montie reported a series in which they constructed the penis using a tubed groin flap. In early cases in this series, the flap was transferred in delayed fashion to the area of the penile stump. Later in the series, a microvascular free transfer technique was employed.

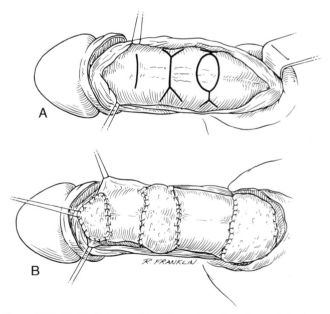

Figure 107–66. Technique of incisions through a Peyronie's plaque with dermal grafting. *A,* The dorsum of the penis has been exposed. The dorsal neurovascular bundle is reflected from the dorsum by removing the dorsal vein of the penis and reflecting the Buck's fascia in concert with the neurovascular structures. Artificial erection has identified the point of maximal curvature. At that point, a partial excision of the plaque is performed. The remaining incisions are marked. *B,* The dermal graft has been harvested, and the graft inlay into the corporotomy defect is completed. Artificial erection demonstrates good straightening of the penis.

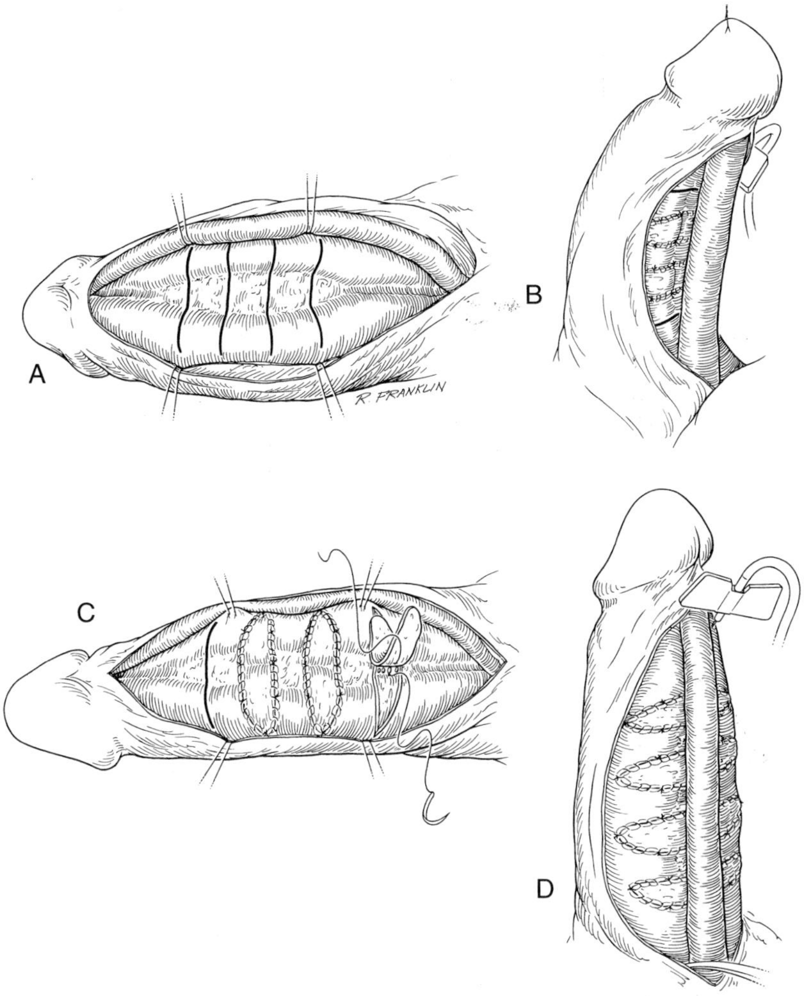

Figure 107–67. Technique of incision with dermal grafting for a ventral Peyronie's plaque. *A,* The skin has been opened in the ventral midline; the dartos fascia has been opened in the ventral midline, and the corpus spongiosum is dissected and detached from the area of plaque on the ventrum of the penis. Incisions are planned across the area of the plaque. Artificial erection demonstrates the area of maximal curvature. *B,* Two incisions with dermal graft inlay have been performed. Some residual curvature remains with artificial erection. *C,* The third incision has been created, and dermal graft inlay is being accomplished. Notice that the dermal graft is sutured to the midline septal fibers. *D,* Four incisions with dermal graft inlay have been performed. Artificial erection now demonstrates the penis to be straight.

In 1984, Chang and Hwang popularized the forearm flap, based on the radial artery, for phallic reconstruction (Fig. 107–70). Biemer (1988) reported a modification of the forearm flap, which was also based on the radial artery; and in 1990, Farrow and associates reported their "cricket bat modification" of the radial forearm flap. **Today, forearm flaps are the most commonly employed method for total phallic construction and penile reconstruction.**

The forearm flap is usually elevated from the nondominant forearm. Preoperatively, patients are carefully screened for arterial insufficiency, using the Allen test. This test involves compressing the radial and ulnar arteries in the wrist while the patient makes a fist to express blood from his hand. As he opens his hand, the fingers are pale, but if palmar circulation is normal and the artery is patent, the fingers turn pink when one of the arteries is released. The test is then repeated, releasing the other artery. If, based on either the Allen test or the patient history, there is any doubt concerning the integrity of the radial and ulnar arteries or the palmar arch, upper extremity angiography is performed.

As described, the forearm flap is a fasciocutaneous flap vascularized by the radial artery; however, the ulnar artery also vascularizes the forearm fascia and most of the forearm skin. The radial artery arises as a continuation of the brachial artery and proximally lies beneath the belly of the brachioradialis muscle, becoming more superficial at the wrist. The ulnar artery is also a continuation of the brachial artery and vascularizes a similar area of skin and underlying adipose tissue. The vascularity of the overlying skin is achieved by way of the underlying (antebrachial) fascia, which is the superficial fascia investing the musculature of the forearm.

The forearm flap can be elevated and transferred on the superficial fascia. The lateral and medial antebrachial cutaneous nerves appear proximally beneath the fascia. The cephalic, basilic, and medial antebrachial veins are also included in the flap and constitute a portion of the venous drainage. In some patients, the vena comitans is the dominant venous drainage system. At the time of flap transfer, it is imperative to assess both the vena comitans and the superficial veins, to determine which is the dominant system in the individual patient.

The various modifications of the forearm flap do not represent changes in the technique of flap elevation but rather modifications in the design of the skin island and the relative position of the urethral paddle in relation to the skin that eventually becomes shaft coverage. Each of these modifications has advantages in different situations.

In the forearm flap as described by Chang and Hwang (1984) (see Fig. 107–70A), the shaft coverage is accomplished using the radial aspect of the skin paddle. A deepithelialized strip is created, and a second skin island, on the ulnar aspect of the skin paddle, is tubed to form the

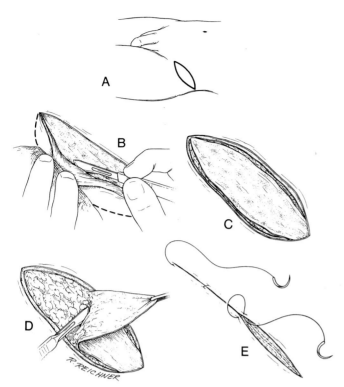

Figure 107–68. Technique of harvest of the dermal graft. *A,* The area of nonhirsute skin immediately superior to the iliac crest is identified. The dermal graft is marked, designed to be approximately 30% larger in all dimensions than the corporotomy defect. *B,* The dermal graft is meticulously de-epithelialized. *C,* After de-epithelialization is accomplished, the incision is carried into the subcuticular adipose tissue. *D,* The graft is harvested with meticulous defatting of the deep aspect. *E,* The dermal graft donor site is closed per primam.

urethra. The urethral tube is then rolled within the tube of skin to form a tube-within-a-tube design. In the white population, this flap has demonstrated a tendency to lead to ischemic stenosis of the lateral paddle, where the urethra is constructed.

In the cricket bat modification (see Fig. 107–70*B*), the urethral tube extends distally, closely overlying either the radial or the ulnar artery. The authors have experience with elevation of the cricket bat modification on each of these arteries. Proximal to the urethral strip, a broader portion of the skin paddle provides coverage of the shaft. The urethral portion is tubed and transposed by inverting it into the center of the shaft portion of the skin paddle. The advantage of this modification lies in centering the urethral portion over the respective artery, in contrast to the Chinese design, in which the ulnar aspect is far distal from the radial artery, with the potential for ischemic stenosis or loss of that portion. The cricket bat modification has been useful in trauma patients, particularly in those who have a significant stump of erectile bodies and urethra left after the injury.

Biemer's modification (see Fig. 107–70*C*) also centers the urethral portion of the flap over the artery. As described by Biemer (1988), the flap is elevated on the radial artery and includes a vascularized piece of the radial bone intended to provide rigidity to the new penis. The inclusion of cartilage and bone has not been universally successful, however, and rigidity in these flaps is obtainable by the use of either an externally applied or internally implanted prosthesis. If the

bone is not elevated, the Biemer flap design can be elevated on either the radial or the ulnar artery. At the authors' center, the flap is most often elevated on the ulnar artery, without including the bone, in a modification of the Biemer design.

Modifications of the Biemer design also include the glans construction technique that was originally described by Puckett and Montic (1978). In the original Biemer design, a central strip becomes the urethra, and lateral to that strip two de-epithelialized portions and two lateral islands (lateral aspects of that skin paddle) are fused dorsally and ventrally to cover the shaft. With the Puckett modification (Puckett et al, 1982), a large island is left distal and flared back over the tip of the tubed flaps, creating the illusion of a glans penis. The Biemer design, especially when it is combined with Puckett's design for glanular construction, offers superior cosmetic results.

There are several disadvantages to the use of a forearm flap for phallic construction. The **major disadvantage of forearm flaps,** which yield **an unsightly scar,** is the obvious donor site deformity. The authors have reconstructed the donor site using full-thickness skin grafts taken from the area of the inguinal crease, and the cosmetic result is far superior to that obtained when the donor site is reconstructed using split-thickness skin grafts (even thick split-thickness

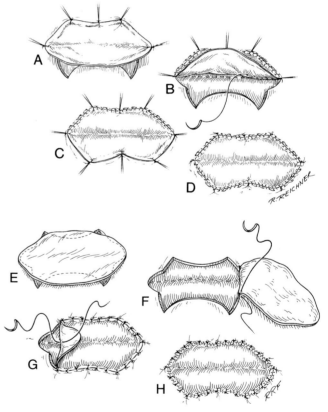

Figure 107–69. Techniques of dermal graft inlay following plaque excision. *A,* Stellate plaque excisional defect with the dermal graft loosely placed. *B,* The dermal graft is meticulously tailored, and one aspect of the suture line is complete. The midline of the dermal graft inlay is sutured to the midline septal fibers. *C,* The contralateral aspect is tacked. *D,* The suture line is complete. *E,* Alternatively, the dermal graft is shown overlying the corporotomy defect. *F,* The dermal graft inlay is begun at one end. The graft is tacked laterally and attached to the midline septal fibers. *G,* The tacking of the graft and tailoring are almost complete. *H,* The watertight suture line is complete.

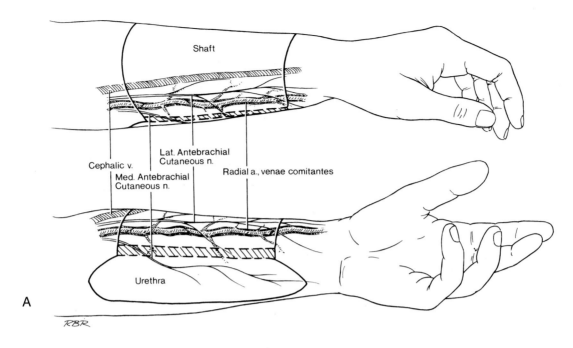

Cephalic v.

Lat. Antebrachial
Cutaneous n.

Med. Antebrachial
Cutaneous n.

Radial a., venae comitantes

Shaft

Urethra

A

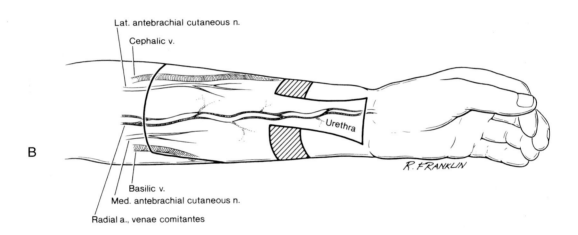

Lat. antebrachial cutaneous n.

Cephalic v.

Urethra

B

Basilic v.
Med. antebrachial cutaneous n.

Radial a., venae comitantes

R. FRANKLIN

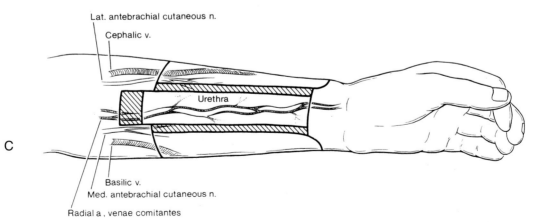

Lat. antebrachial cutaneous n.

Cephalic v.

Urethra

C

Basilic v.
Med. antebrachial cutaneous n.

Radial a., venae comitantes

Figure 107–70. Variations of the forearm flap for phallic construction. *A,* The Chang V "Chinese" flap based on the radial artery. Notice the skin island has two separate paddles. An ulnar urethral paddle is separated from the shaft coverage paddle by a de-epithelialized strip. *B,* The cricket bat modification of the radial forearm flap proposed by Farrow and Boyd. The urethral portion extends centered over the artery. The shaft coverage portion is on the proximal forearm. The de-epithelialized areas (cross-hatched) add bulk to the glans. The urethral portion is flipped into the middle of the flap and tubularized. *C,* Modification of the forearm flap as proposed by Biemer. The urethral paddle is a midline strip separated by the two lateral paddles by de-epithelialized strips. The lateral paddles are tubularized, with the urethral paddle tubularized in the center.

skin). A second disadvantage lies in the possibility of cold intolerance developing in the hand of the donor side. Early in their experience with the forearm flap, the authors reconstructed the radial artery using an interposition vein graft. The authors have since abandoned this procedure in the majority of their series and have not seen cold intolerance in patients. Another disadvantage occurs in both male and virilized transgender patients when the forearm skin is hirsute because the hair can be problematic if it is included in the portion of the flap used for urethral construction.

For patients who only need vascularized tissue to cover the shaft of the penis, the authors have used the upper lateral arm flap (Fig. 107–71). This is a fasciocutaneous flap, and its cutaneous vascular territory is centered on the radial collateral artery. The skin of the lateral upper arm is thin, with little subcutaneous adiposity. To mark the location of the lateral intramuscular septum and the course of the superior radial collateral artery, the authors draw a line joining the insertion of the deltoid with the lateral epicondyle. The authors begin the dissection posteriorly, elevating the superficial fascia until the posterior lateral portion of the intramuscular septum has been identified. A potential disadvantage of this flap lies in the fact that the entire venous drainage is dependent on the vena comitans, and although superficial veins do traverse the flap, none of them seem to provide significant venous drainage. Although this is disquieting, thus far, the authors have found the flap to be completely reliable, with no losses owing to venous insufficiency.

This flap has also been used for total phallic construction. For this purpose, the flap is expanded using a tissue expander and elevated across the elbow, and the distal flap is elevated on the recurrent radial artery (Shenaq and Saleh, 1992). As with the forearm flap, the donor site from an upper lateral arm flap can be quite disfiguring. Because the scar is on the upper arm, however, it is more easily concealed beneath a shirtsleeve than a scar in the forearm.

All of the flaps described allow for microneurosurgical coaptation of the flap's cutaneous nerves with recipient nerves. With total phallic construction, the cutaneous nerves can be attached either to the dorsal nerves of the penis or, in the transsexual patient, to the dorsal nerves of the clitoris. These nerves are believed to provide the best restoration of erogenous cutaneous sensibility. In situations in which these nerves are not available, the nerves can be coapted to the pudendal nerve, which in most patients requires an interposition graft. The authors have also coapted the flap's cutaneous nerves to the ilioinguinal nerves, which provide sensation to the inner aspect of the thigh and the lateral aspect of the scrotum, and achieved a reasonable degree of erogenous sensibility.

In most patients, the recipient vasculature for flap transfer is the deep inferior epigastric vessels. These vessels are medial branches of the iliac system and lie on the dorsal aspect of the rectus muscle. The artery usually remains deep to the muscle, although in some patients, an early penetration of the artery into the muscle can be observed. The artery classically bifurcates at the level of the umbilicus and is generally accompanied by two or more venae comitantes. These vessels have been elevated by several methods, and Lund and Winfield (1995) described their elevation for penile revascularization using laparoscopic techniques. When the deep inferior epigastric vessels are used, it is often necessary to include a saphenous vein for further venous runoff.

In some patients, these vessels are not available, and the recipient vessels are created by connecting a saphenous interposition graft to the superficial femoral artery. Using this technique, the authors mobilize the saphenous vein well down the upper aspect of the thigh and then attach the vein to the femoral artery, creating a temporary arteriovenous fistula. The fistula is divided, with the saphenous vein becoming the venous runoff and the interposition graft provid-

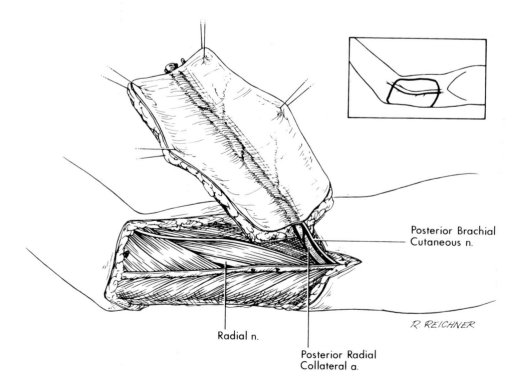

Posterior Brachial Cutaneous n.

Radial n.

Posterior Radial Collateral a.

R. REICHNER

Figure 107–71. Upper lateral arm flap. This fasciocutaneous flap based on the posterior radial collateral artery, one of the first branches of the axillary artery located in the interosseous septum in the upper forearm, is elevated with the superficial fascia of the upper arm. The cutaneous vascular territory is centered roughly on a line between the groove of the deltoid and the lateral epicondyle of the elbow. In elevating the vessels, care must be taken not to injure the radial nerve, which runs proximate to the posterior radial collateral artery. (From Jordan GH, Schlossberg SM, McCraw JB: AUA Update Series, Lesson 10, Vol 7, 1988.)

ing the arterial in-flow. The authors find this system of recipient vessels less desirable than the deep inferior epigastric vessels.

In the latter part of their series, **the authors included the routine transfer of gracilis muscle to cover the area of the urethral anastomosis,** increasing the vascularity to that area and significantly altering the incidence of anastomotic fistula and stricture formation. The authors have also elevated a bipedicled flap from the base of the penile shaft, transposing it beneath the phallic flap (Fig. 107–72). This flap provides increased bulk and a modicum of scrotal construction, and when combined with the gracilis muscle, its thickness provides excellent coverage for the juncture of the flap with the base of the neoscrotum.

During the phallic construction procedure, urine is diverted by way of a suprapubic cystostomy tube, and the urethra is stented with a No. 14 Fr soft silicone Silastic catheter. A voiding study is usually performed between the third and fourth postoperative week.

As already mentioned, rigidity for intercourse in the patient with phallic construction is usually achieved by either an externally applied or a permanently implanted prosthesis. **Prosthetic implantation is never undertaken until a year after phallic construction because protective sensibility must be demonstrated in the flap.** When the flap is transferred, it is, by definition, rendered insensate. At about 3 to 4 months after reconstruction, however, as nerve regeneration occurs, sensation becomes noticeable. In addition, before undertaking prosthetic implantation, the urethra must be patent and proven to be durable.

At their center, the authors now have a large series of patients with internally implanted devices. The authors have implanted both hydraulic and articulated prostheses encased in Gore-Tex neocorpora. These devices are anchored to the ischial tuberosity and the pubis by anchoring the neocorpora to these bony structures. In most patients, two cylinders or rods are implanted. Early in their series, the authors had problems with hematoma and seroma formation and subsequent infection. Since modifying the antibiotic regimen and including the routine use of suction drains with the implant procedure, however, the authors have enjoyed excellent success with implantation.

The authors also have implanted testicular prostheses in a number of patients. In patients in whom a hydraulic device has been used, the authors have implanted the pump in one neohemiscrotum and a testicular prosthesis in the opposite one.

RECONSTRUCTION FOLLOWING TRAUMA

In many ways, the problems of trauma patients are more challenging to solve than those of patients who require total phallic construction. The authors have treated a large number of patients who have had devastating injuries to the penis following complicated prosthetic surgery or surgery to correct penile curvatures of Peyronie's disease.

Acutely, urine must be diverted, necrotic tissue must be carefully débrided, and any foreign bodies that may have been implanted must be removed. Vigorous acute wound management stabilizes the wounds and allows active granulation to progress. In all trauma patients, an attempt should be made to save as much of the penile structure as possible.

Primary reconstruction can be undertaken approximately 3 to 6 weeks after trauma, although in some patients, the authors have elected to wait 4 to 6 months, depending on the situation. In cases in which significant adjacent tissue loss has occurred, the adjacent areas must be well reconstructed before proceeding with either phallic construction or penile reconstruction.

It is imperative that in the trauma patient, well-vascularized tissues are eventually transposed to the adjacent areas, and reconstruction of these areas can be accomplished with a number of flaps. For groin reconstruction, the tensor fascia lata flap has been useful. The rectus femoris flap, characteristically long and large, can be transposed to the area of the lower abdomen and has been an extremely useful flap for inguinal and lower abdominal reconstruction. The gracilis muscle is an excellent flap for reconstruction of the perineum and the groin. Alternatively the posterior thigh flap can be used for reconstruction of the groin and perineum and, in some cases, transposed to the lowermost portion of the lower abdomen.

Variations of the flap designs described previously for

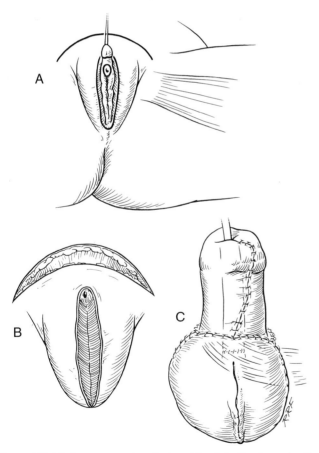

Figure 107–72. In transsexual patients, a bipedicle flap is used with a gracilis muscle flap. *A,* Transsexual patient after urethral lengthening procedure. Notice the gracilis muscle marked on the left thigh. *B,* A bipedicle flap is elevated from the site of the proposed location for the phallic flap. The flap is transposed ventral to the phallic flap. *C,* The transposed bipedicle flap is sutured in place. Note the mobilized gracilis flap surrounding the area of the urethral anastomosis to the elongated native urethra.

complete phallic construction have successfully been applied in select patients for penile reconstruction. An example is seen in one patient who suffered an injury to the penis with a shotgun blast. The blast injured a large portion of the patient's right corpus cavernosum, and the majority of the penile skin was either destroyed or used for urethral reconstruction. In this patient, a forearm flap based on the Chinese design was elevated. Because the urethral reconstruction was accomplished using a penile skin island, however, the ulnar portion of the flap was not needed for that purpose. Therefore, the ulnar portion was de-epithelialized and tubularized to form bulk and a new right corporal body. This patient is now sexually active, and the bulk of the tube's dermal section gives adequate support to the penis for intercourse.

Another patient required only distal urethral construction and glans reconstruction. For this patient, the authors based a flap on the Biemer design to create a glans. The proximal portions of the flap were de-epithelialized, allowing for fixation of the neoglans on the tips of the corporal bodies, and an excellent functional and cosmetic result was achieved for this patient.

FEMALE-TO-MALE TRANSSEXUALISM

Female-to-male transsexual patients present a unique challenge, and **no patient should be considered for definitive reassignment surgery without having undergone complex screening and evaluation by a team consisting of mental health professionals as well as surgeons who are skilled in undertaking transgender surgery. It is imperative that an ongoing, stable, therapeutic relationship be established between the patient and a mental health professional at the time of definitive general reassignment surgery.** At the authors' institution, the Harry Benjamin (Ramsey, 1996) criteria are strictly adhered to, and surgery is accomplished by a team of urologists, plastic surgeons, and gynecologists.

In most patients, the first stage of female-to-male transsexual surgery consists of bilateral salpingo-oophorectomy, hysterectomy, vaginectomy, and urethral lengthening with colpocleisis. Even in the virginal patient, surgeons at the authors' institution have become skilled at accomplishing a hysterectomy and bilateral salpingo-oophorectomy via transvaginal surgery. The authors perform a vaginectomy at the same operation, leaving the anterior vaginal wall to be transposed as a random flap to lengthen the female urethra and allow for colpocleisis (Fig. 107–73). Lengthening of the female urethra brings the base of the native urethra up to what will be the base of the phallic flap and, along with the transfer of gracilis muscle, has significantly altered surgical results with regard to urethral anastomotic fistula and stricture. Urine is diverted with a suprapubic tube, and a voiding trial is performed in approximately 21 days. Patients are generally in the hospital for 2 to 3 days and return to surgery 3 to 4 months later for phallic construction.

For phallic construction in the transgender patient, as already discussed, a bipedicled flap of skin is elevated from the area where the phallic structure is to be implanted and transposed to the undersurface of the neopenis (see Fig. 107–72). The patient is generally in the hospital for a period of 10 to 14 days after total phallic construction, and a

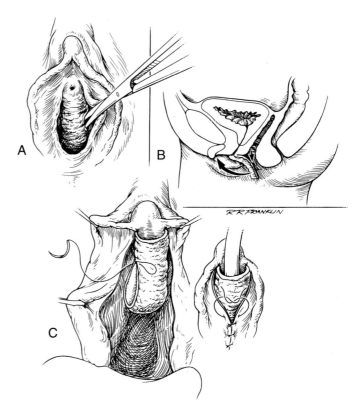

Figure 107–73. Technique of vaginectomy with colpocleisis and urethral lengthening. *A,* Vaginectomy has been performed leaving an anterior vaginal flap. The flap is mobilized. *B,* The flap is then flipped to be sutured to the urethral strip extending on the ventrum of the clitoris. *C,* The urethral lengthening procedure is completed by suturing the lateral aspect of the flap. The vaginectomy defect is collapsed using concentric sutures. The urethral meatus is thus brought out to the ventrum of the glans clitoris.

voiding trial with contrast material is accomplished at about 28 days postoperatively. After a year, when erogenous sensibility is demonstrated and the urethra is proven to be durable, prosthetic implantation is considered.

REFERENCES

Aboseif SR, Breza J, Lue TF, Tanagho E: Penile venous drainage in erectile dysfunction: Anatomical, radiological and functional considerations. Br J Urol 1989; 64:183–190.

Allen JS, Summers JL: Meatal stenosis in children. J Urol 1974; 112:526.

Bainbridge DR, Whitaker RH, Shepheard BGF: Balanitis xerotica obliterans and urinary obstruction. Br J Urol 1971; 43:487.

Biemer E: Penile construction by the radial arm flap. Clin Plast Surg 1988; 15:425.

Borgoraz NA: Plastic restoration of the penis. Sovet Khir No 1936; 8:303–307.

Chang TS, Hwang WJ: Forearm flap in one-stage reconstruction of the penis. Plast Reconstr Surg 1984; 74:251.

Das S, Amar AD: Peyronie's disease: Excision of the plaque and grafting with tunica vaginalis. Urol Clin North Am 1982; 9:1.

DeSanctis PN, Furey GA: Steroid injection therapy for Peyronie's disease: A 10-year summary and review of 38 cases. J Urol 1967; 97:114.

Devine CJ: Introduction to the International Conference on Peyronie's disease: Advances in basic and clinical research. J Urol 1997; 157:272–275.

Devine CJ Jr, Blackley SK, Horton CE, Gilbert DA: The surgical treatment of chordee without hypospadias in post adolescent men. J Urol 1991; 146:325–329.

Devine CJ Jr, Franz JP, Horton CE: Evaluation and treatment of patients with failed hypospadias repair. J Urol 1978; 119:223–226.

Devine CJ Jr, Gonzales-Serva L, Stecker JF Jr, Devine PC: Utrical configuration in hypospadias and intersex. J Urol 1980a; 123:407.

Devine CJ Jr, Horton CE: Chordee without hypospadias. J Urol 1973; 110:264–271.

Devine CJ Jr, Horton CE: The surgical treatment of Peyronie's disease with a dermal graft. J Urol 1974; 111:44.

Devine CJ Jr, Horton CE: Use of dermal graft to correct chordee. J Urol 1975; 113:56.

Devine CJ Jr, Horton CE: Penile reconstruction of epispadias associated with exstrophy. The Eaton Collection, Penn Com, Inc., Ridgefield, CT. (16 mm. color and sound, 925) 1979.

Devine CJ Jr, Horton CE, Scarff JE: Epispadias. Urol Clin North Am 1980b; 7:465–476.

Devine CJ Jr, Jordan GH, Schlossberg SM: Peyronie's disease. In Cohen MS, Reskick MI, eds: Reoperative Urology. Boston, Little Brown and Co., 1995, pp 221–233.

Devine CJ Jr, Somers KD, Jordan GH, Schlossberg SM: Proposal: Trauma as the cause of the Peyronie's lesion. J Urol 1997; 185:290.

Devine CJ Jr, Somers KD, Wright GL Jr, et al: A working model for the genesis of Peyronie's disease derived from its pathobiology (Abstract 495). J Urol 1988; 139:286A.

Devine PC, Horton CE: Strictures of the male urethra. In Converse JM, ed: Reconstructive Plastic Surgery, Vol 7, 2nd ed. Philadelphia, W. B. Saunders, 1977, pp 3883–3895.

Dore B, Irani J, Aubert J: Carcinoma of the penis in lichen sclerosus atrophicus. Eur Urol 1990; 18:153–155.

Duckett JW: The island flap technique for hypospadias repair. Urol Clin North Am 1981; 8:503.

El-Galley RES, Smith E, Cohen C, et al: Epidermal growth factor (ECG) and EGF receptor in hypospadias. Br J Urol 1997; 79:116–119, 1997.

Farrow GA, Boyd JB, Semple JL: Total reconstruction of the penis employing the "cricket bat flap" single stage forearm free graft. AUA Today 1990; 3:7.

Frumkin AP: Reconstruction of male genitalia. Am Rev Sov Med 1944; 2:14–21.

Galloway NT: Hypospadias: Difficult surgery on incompetent tissues. Presented at S.E. Section AUA, Orlando, FL, April, 1995.

Gearhart JP, Leonard MP, Burgers JK, Jeffs RD: The Cantwell-Ransley technique for repair of epispadias. J Urol 1992; 148:851–854.

Gearhart JP, Rock JA: Total ablation of the penis after circumcision and electrocautery: A method of management and long-term followup. J Urol 1989; 42:799.

Gelbard MK, Linder A, Kaufman JJ: The use of collagenase in the treatment of Peyronie's disease. J Urol 1985; 134:280.

Gilles HD, Harrison RH: Congenital absence of the penis. Br J Plast Surg 1948; 1:8–28.

Godec CJ, Van Beek AL: Peyronie's disease is curable—is it also preventable? Urology 1983; 21:257.

Hellstrom WJG: The use of prosthetic materials in the surgical management of Peyronie's disease. Int J Impotence Res 1994; 6(Suppl):32.

Hendren WH: Penile lengthening after previous repair of epispadias. J Urol 1979; 121:527.

Hinman F Jr: Peyronie's disease: Etiological considerations. Prog Reprod Biol Med 1983; 9:5–12.

Horton CE, Devine CJ Jr: Peyronie's disease. Plast Reconstr Surg 1973; 52:503.

Jeffs RD: Exstrophy. In Harrison JH, Gittes RF, Perlmutter A, et al, eds: Campbell's Urology, 4th ed. Philadelphia, W. B. Saunders, 1979.

Johnston JH: The genital aspects of exstrophy. J Urol 1975; 113:701.

Jordan CH: Peyronie's disease and its management. In Krane RJ, Siroky MB, Fitzpatrick J, eds: Clinical Urology. Philadelphia, J. B. Lippincott, 1994, pp 1282–1297.

Jordan GH, Schlossberg SM: Complications of interventional techniques for urethral stricture disease: Direct visual internal urethrotomy, stents and laser intervention. In Carson CC III, ed: Topics in Clinical Urology: Complications of Interventional Techniques. New York, Igaku-Shoin, 1996, pp 86–94.

Jordan GH, Schlossberg SM, McCraw JB: Tissue transfer techniques for genitourinary reconstructive surgery. AUA Update Series, Lessons 9, 10, 11, 12, Vol 7, 1988.

Kelley JH, Eraklis AJ: A procedure for lengthening the phallus in boys with exstrophy of the bladder. J Pediatr Surg 1971; 6:645.

Koff SA, Eakins M: Treatment of penile chordee using corporal rotation. J Urol 1984; 131:931.

Ledwig P, Weigrand D: Late circumcision and lichen sclerosus et atrophicus of the penis. J Am Acad Dermatol 1989; 20:211–214.

Leffell MS: Is there an immunogenetic basis for Peyronie's disease. J Urol 1997; 157:295–297.

Levine LA, Merrick PF, Lee RC: Intralesional verapamil injection for the treatment of Peyronie's disease. J Urol 1994; 151:1522–1524.

Lue TF: Penile venous surgery. Urol Clin North Am 1989; 16:607–611.

Lund GO, Winfield HN, Donovan JF: Laparoscopically assisted penile revascularization for vasculogenic impotence. J Urol 1995; 153:1923–1926.

Marshall F: Endoscopic reconstruction of traumatic urethral transections. Urol Clin North Am 1989; 16:313–318.

McAninch JW, Laing FC, Jeffrey RB Jr: Sonourethrography in the evaluation of urethral strictures: a preliminary report. J Urol 1988; 139:294.

McCallum RW: The adult male urethra: normal anatomy, pathology, and method of urethrography. Radiol Clin North Am 1979; 17:227.

McDougal WS: Scrotal reconstruction using thigh pedicle flaps. J Urol 1983; 129:757–759.

McRoberts JW: Peyronie's disease. Surg Gynecol Obstet 1969; 12:1291.

McRoberts JW, Chapman WH, Ansell JS: Primary anastomosis of the traumatically amputated penis: case report and summary of the literature. J Urol 1968; 100:751.

Meuli M, Briner, J, Hanimann B, Sacher P: Lichen sclerosus et atrophicus causing phimosis in boys: A prospective study with 5-year follow-up after complete circumcision. J Urol 1994; 152:967–989.

Milroy E: Treatment of sphincter strictures using permanent UroLume stent. J Urol 1993; 150:1729–1733.

Montague DK, Lakin MM: Erectile prosthesis in Peyronie's disease. Presented at the International Conference on Peyronie's Disease, Bethesda, 1993.

Mundy AR: A comparison of urethral reconstruction techniques. Presented at Genitourinary Reconstructive Surgeons Meeting, London, 1994.

Nesbit RM: Congenital curvature of the phallus: A report of three cases with description of corrective operation. J Urol 1965; 93:230.

O'Conor VJ Jr, Kropp KA: Surgery of the female urethra. In Glen JF, Boyce WH, eds: Urologic Surgery. New York, Harper & Row, 1969, p 572.

Oesterling JE, Gearhart JP, Jeffs RD: A unified approach to early reconstructive surgery of the child with ambiguous genitalia. J Urol 1987; 138:107.

Orticochea M: Musculo-cutaneous flap method: Immediate and heroic substitute for the method of delay. Br J Plast Surg 1972; 25:106.

Pansadoro V, Emiliozzi P: Internal urethrotomy in the management of anterior urethral strictures: Long-term follow-up. J Urol 1996; 156:78–79.

Peña A, Devries PA: Posterior sagittal anorectoplasty: Important technical considerations and new applications. J Pediatr Surg 1982; 17:796–811.

Peyronie F de la: Sur quelques ostacles qui s'opposent a l'ejaculation naturelle de la semence. Memoires de l'Academie de Chirurgie 1743; 1:318.

Poland RL: The question of routine neonatal circumcision: Sounding board. N Engl J Med 1990; 322:1312–1315.

Poutasse EF: Peyronie's disease. In Horton CE, ed: Plastic and Reconstructive Surgery of the Genital Area. Boston, Little, Brown, 1973, pp 621–625.

Pride FM III, Tyler W: Penile squamous cell carcinoma arising from balanitis xerotica obliterans. J Am Acad Dermatol 1993; 29:469–473.

Pryor JP, Fitzpatrick JM: A new approach to the correction of the penile deformity in Peyronie's disease. J Urol 1979; 122:622.

Puckett CL, Montie JE: Construction of male genitalia in the transsexual using a tubed groin flap for the penis and a hydraulic inflation device. Plast Reconstr Surg 1978; 61:523.

Puckett CL, Reinisch JF, Montie JE: Free flap phalloplasty. J Urol 1982; 128:294.

Quartey JKM: One-stage penile/preputial cutaneous island flap urethroplasty for urethral stricture. J Urol 1983; 129:284.

Ramsey G: Transsexuals: Candid Answers to Private Questions. Freedom, CA, The Crossing Press, 1996. In press.

Rickwood AM, Hamalatha V, Batcup G, Spitz L: Phimosis in boys. J Urol 1980; 52:147–150.

Rosen MA, Nash PA, Bruce JE, McAninch JW: The accurial success rate of surgical treatment of urethral strictures. J Urol 1994; 151:360A.

Schmidt KH, Somers KD, Devine CJ Jr, et al: Development of an in vivo model of Peyronie's disease in the nude mouse (Abstract 147). J Urol 1987; 137:140A.

Schoen EJ: The status of circumcision of newborns: Sounding board. N Engl J Med 1990; 322:1309–1311.

Schonfeld WA, Beebe GW: Normal growth and variation in the male genitalia from birth to maturity. Am J Dis Child 1942; 64:759.

Schreiter F, Noll F: Mesh graft urethroplasty using split thickness skin graft or foreskin. J Urol 1989; 142:1223–1226.

Secrest CL, Jordan GH, Winslow BH, et al: Repair of the complications of hypospadias surgery. J Urol 1993; 150:1138–1142.

Shenaq SM, Saleh M: Extended upper lateral arm flaps for phallic reconstruction. Presented at the Eleventh Congress of the International Microsurgical Society, Rhodes, Greece June 24–27, 1992.

Smith BH: Peyronie's disease. Am J Clin Pathol 1966; 45:670.

Smith BH: Subclinical Peyronie's disease. Am J Clin Pathol 1969; 52:385.

Snow R, Devine CJ Jr: The conservative management of Peyronie's disease. Unpublished data, 1981.

Snyder H: The surgery of bladder exstrophy and epispadias. In Frank JD, Johnston JH, eds: Operative Paediatric Urology. London, Churchill Livingstone, 1990, pp 153–185.

Sommers KD, Dawson DM: Fibrin deposition in Peyronie's disease plaque. J Urol, 1997, in press.

Somers KD, Dawson DM, Wright GL Jr, et al: Cell culture of Peyronie's disease plaque and normal penile tissue. J Urol 1982; 127:585.

Somers KD, Sismour EN, Wright GL Jr, et al: Isolation and characterization of collagen in Peyronie's disease. J Urol 1989; 141:629.

Somers KD, Winters BA, Dawson DM, et al: Chromosome abnormalities in Peyronie's disease. J Urol 1987; 137:672.

Spence HM, Duckett JW Jr: Diverticulum of the female urethra: Clinical aspects and presentation of a simple operative technique for cure. J Urol 1970; 104:432.

Standoli L: One stage repair of hypospadias: Preputial island flap technique. Ann Plast Surg 1982; 9:81–88.

Stefanovic KB, Clark SA, Buncke HJ: Microsurgical vascularized free temporoparietal fascia transfer for Peyronie's disease: An experimental study. J Reconstr Microsurg 1994; 10:39–45.

VandeBerg JS, Devine CJ Jr, Horton CE, et al: Peyronie's disease: An electron microscopic study. J Urol 1981; 126:33.

VandeBerg JS, Devine CJ Jr, Horton CE, et al: Mechanisms of calcification in Peyronie's disease. J Urol 1982; 127:52.

Vest SA: Radical perineal prostatectomy, modification of closure. Surg Gynecol Obstet 1940; 70:935–937.

Vorstman B, Devine CJ Jr: Penile torsion, curvature and Peyronie's disease. In Pryor J, Lipshultz LI, eds: Andrology. London, Butterworths, 1987, pp 69–91.

Walsh PC: Radical prostatectomy with preservation of sexual function: Pathological findings in the first 100 cases. J Urol 1985; 134:1146–1148.

Waterhouse K, Abrahams HG, Hackett RE, Peng BK: The transpubic approach to the lower urinary tract. J Urol 1973; 109:486.

Wessels H, Lue TF, McAninch JW: Penile length in the flaccid and erect states: Guidelines for penile augmentation. J Urol 1996; 156:995–997.

Williams J, Thomas G: The natural history of Peyronie's disease. J Urol 1970; 103:75.

Winslow BH, Horton CE, Gilbert DA, Devine CJ Jr: Epispadias and exstrophy of the bladder. In Mustarde JC, Jackson IT, eds: Plastic Surgery in Infancy and Childhood, 3rd ed. New York, Churchill Livingstone, 1988, pp 511–527.

Winslow BH, Vorstman B, Devine CJ Jr: Complications of hypospadias surgery. In Marshall FF, ed: Urologic Complications, Medical and Surgical, Adult and Pediatric. Chicago, Year Book Medical Publishers, 1986, pp 411–426.

Yachia D: Corporal plication for surgical correction of Peyronie's disease. J Urol 1993; 149:869.

108

SURGERY OF PENILE AND URETHRAL CARCINOMA

Harry W. Herr, M.D.

Cancer of the penis and urethra is uncommon. Surgery is the primary treatment for both penile and urethral neoplasms. This chapter describes surgical techniques commonly used for cancer of the penis and provides an overview of urethral cancer in men and women.

SURGERY OF PENILE CANCER

Carcinoma arising from the prepuce, glans, or shaft of the penis often remains localized for prolonged periods. **When metastasis occurs, it usually follows a stepwise pattern—first to the inguinal (groin) nodes and second to the pelvic lymph nodes.** A favorable natural history permits surgical cure of most localized penile cancers and many with inguinal metastases.

Primary Tumor

Histologic Diagnosis

Histologic verification of penile cancer is the essential first step to staging and the formulation of a treatment plan. Tumors of the penis lend themselves to convenient excisional, incisional, or needle biopsy. Adjacent normal tissue should be included to evaluate invasion, a critical differential point with regard to planning definitive surgery.

Partial Penectomy

Successful local control by partial penectomy depends on division of the penis 2 cm proximal to the gross tumor extent (Fig. 108–1). After the lesion is excluded by a towel or surgical glove secured along the proposed line of amputation, a tourniquet is applied at the base of the penis. The skin is incised circumferentially, and the cavernous bodies are divided sharply to the urethra. The dorsal vessels are ligated, and the urethra is dissected proximally and distally to attain a 1-cm distal redundancy. The urethra is divided without sacrifice of the tumor margin, and the corpora are secured with interrupted sutures opposing the margins of Buck's fascia. The tourniquet is removed, and additional hemostasis is obtained as necessary. The urethra is spatulated on both its dorsal and ventral surfaces. A skin-urethra anastomosis is performed using 3–0 or 4–0 chromic or Dexon absorbable suture material. The redundant skin is approximated dorsally to complete the closure (Fig. 108–2). A small urinary catheter is placed, and a light dressing is applied. Both may be removed the following day.

Modified Partial Penectomy

When the penile stump after partial penectomy is too short for directing the urinary stream, further length can be obtained by releasing the corpora from the suspensory ligament, dividing the ischiocavernosus muscle, and partially separating the crura from the undersurface of the pubic rami. The scrotum is incised along the raphe, and skin flaps are

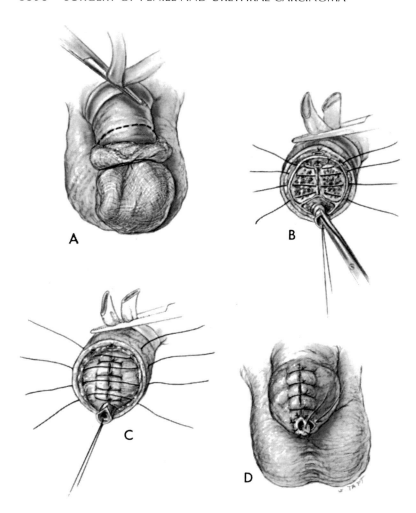

Figure 108–1. Partial penectomy. *A* and *B*, After exclusion of the lesion from the field, the corpora are divided with a 2-cm gross margin. *C*, The dorsal vessels are ligated, the cut margins of the tunica albuginea approximated, and the urethra spatulated. *D*, Simple skin closure and urethral meatus formation complete the procedure.

fashioned for penile coverage. The testes are secured in subcutaneous pouches, and the scrotum is reconstructed cephalad to the transposed phallus.

Total Penectomy

The urethra is transposed to the perineum if the size of the primary lesion precludes a partial penectomy (Fig. 108–3). After appropriate draping of the primary lesion, an elliptic incision is made around the base of the penis. Dissection along the corpora is performed with division of the suspensory ligament and dorsal vessels. The urethra is dissected sharply from the corpora to the bulbar region. This dissection is aided by distal division of the urethra and ventral traction. The corpora are further dissected from their attachments to the inferior pubic rami, divided, and ligated with chromic sutures.

A 1-cm ellipse of skin is removed from the region of the perineal body, and a tunnel is created bluntly in the perineal subcutaneous tissue. The urethra is grasped and transposed through the perineum without angulation. Spatulation of the urethra and skin-to-urethra anastomosis are performed. The primary incision is closed superiorly, with drainage transversely to elevate the scrotum away from the new meatus. A urethral catheter is placed, and the wound is dressed.

Groin Metastasis

When nodal disease (N+) has been proven by biopsy, surgical dissection of the ileoinguinal lymph nodes should follow.

Anatomic Considerations

The inguinal lymph nodes are divided into superficial and deep groups, which are anatomically separated by the deep fascia of the thigh—the fascia lata. The superficial group of nodes is composed of 4 to 25 glands (average of 8), which are situated in the deep membranous layer of the superficial fascia of the thigh—Camper's fascia. The superficial group drains to the two or three deep inguinal nodes that lie along the femoral vessels within the femoral sheath. The node of Cloquet is the most cephalad of this deep group and is situated within the femoral canal (medial to the femoral vein). The external iliac lymph nodes receive drainage from the deep inguinal, obturator, and hypogastric groups. In turn, drainage progresses to the common iliac and para-aortic nodes.

The blood supply to the skin of the inguinal region derives from branches of the common femoral artery—the superficial external pudendal, the superficial circumflex iliac, and the superficial epigastric arteries. Complete inguinal dissec-

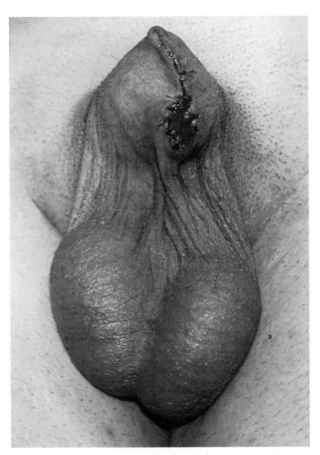

Figure 108–2. Completed partial penectomy.

involved by metastatic penile cancer. When the superior medial superficial inguinal lymph node is negative, all other groin nodes are negative at dissection; when only one node is positive, it is the sentinel; and when multiple nodes are positive, the sentinel node is always involved as well. Patients with a negative sentinel node biopsy finding can avoid a more extensive dissection with a relatively good prognosis. Patients with a positive sentinel node biopsy finding still need a radical groin dissection. If the sentinel node only is involved, 5-year survival increases overall from 50% to 70%. This concept needs further clinical confirmation, however, because patients with negative sentinel node biopsy findings have developed extensive regional metastases (Perinetti et al, 1980).

The location of the saphenofemoral junction is estimated to be at a point two fingerbreadths lateral and inferior to the pubic tubercle. A transverse incision through this point exposes the fossa ovalis and the greater saphenous vein with its medial tributaries—the superficial epigastric and the external pudendal veins (Fig. 108–4). Within the space bounded by these branches, the tissue is excised and submitted for microscopic examination. The superomedial area may contain several nodes, and all should be removed to ensure complete sampling. With histologic confirmation of metastatic involvement, complete dissection is indicated.

The surgeon should anticipate the direction of the preferred incision for groin dissection so that the biopsy incision may be included with the specimen if the results should dictate a complete ilioinguinal lymphadenectomy.

Radical Ilioinguinal Node Dissection

A 6-week interval after treatment of the penile lesion allows for reduction of any inflammatory component of the regional adenopathy and minimizes the incidence of wound suppuration. Preliminary preparations for regional node dissection include mechanical preparation of the bowel, wearing of elastic support wraps or stockings for the legs, and administration of preoperative antibiotics.

The patient is positioned with the involved thigh slightly abducted and externally rotated. The flexed knee is supported as necessary. A urethral catheter is placed, and the scrotum is positioned or sutured out of the operative field. A fungating tumor is excluded from the field by suturing a laparotomy sponge to the skin around the lesion before the routine skin preparation.

Various incisional approaches to the regional nodes in carcinoma of the penis have been described (Fig. 108–5). For cases that require bilateral dissection, **an oblique or elliptic incision below and parallel to the inguinal ligament is commonly used for excision of the superficial and deep inguinal nodes.** Addition of a lower midline extraperitoneal incision allows access to the pelvic nodal component and is recommended for bilateral management. Such an approach is preferred because these incisions, coupled with thick skin flaps, virtually eliminate problems of skin necrosis (Whitmore and Vagaiwala, 1984).

A double incisional unilateral approach has been promoted with reported decreased wound morbidity (Fraley and Hutchens, 1972). The inability to excise conveniently a previous biopsy scar or areas of cutaneous involvement is a limitation

tion necessitates ligation of these branches. Viability of the skin flaps raised during the dissection depends on anastomotic vessels in the superficial fatty layer of Camper's fascia that course parallel to the natural skin lines. **Because lymphatic drainage of the penis to the groin runs beneath Camper's fascia, this layer can be preserved and left attached to the overlying skin in fashioning the superior and inferior skin flaps. This technique prevents serious skin slough, especially if an oblique incision with removal of an ellipse of skin overlying adherent nodes is employed.** Such incision least disrupts the collateral circulation and best preserves vascular integrity to the reapproximated skin margins. The femoral nerve lies deep to the fascia iliacas and supplies motor function to the pectineus, quadriceps femoris, and sartorius muscles. In addition, this nerve provides cutaneous sensation to the anterior thigh and should be preserved. Some of the sensory branches, however, are commonly sacrificed in the regional node dissection.

The femoral triangle, the area that contains the pertinent lymphatic groups, is bounded by the inguinal ligaments superiorly, the sartorius laterally, and the adductor longus medially. The floor of the triangle is composed of the pectineus medially and the iliopsoas laterally.

Sentinel Node Biopsy

A sentinel node concept has been proposed by Cabanas (1977). This involves a limited dissection of the primary "landing" site of regional nodes most likely to be first

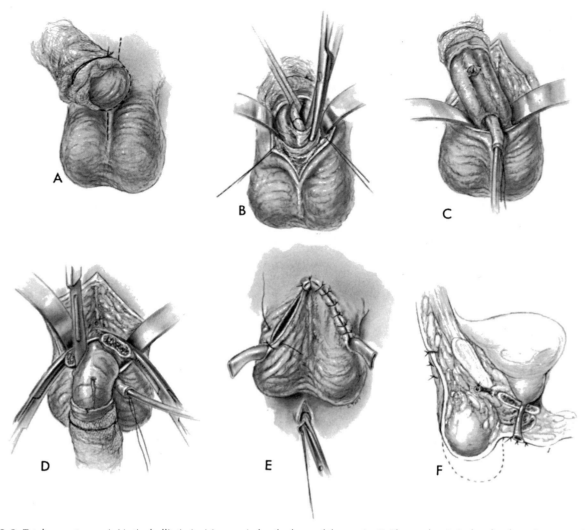

Figure 108–3. Total penectomy. *A,* Vertical elliptic incision encircles the base of the penis. *B,* The urethra is isolated at least 2 cm proximal to the gross lesion. *C,* The suspensory ligament has been divided. The urethra is transected and dissected from the corpora. *D,* The dorsal vessels are ligated, and the crura are transected with the stumps ligated. *E,* A button of perineal skin is excised, and the urethra is transposed and spatulated to form the perineal urethrostomy. *F,* Horizontal closure of the primary incision with drainage serves to elevate the scrotum away from the urinary stream.

of the double incision technique. The single oblique incision is recommended for cases that require unilateral dissection.

The inguinofemoral dissection is performed through a separate elliptic incision centered on the saphenofemoral junction at the base of the femoral triangle. The dimensions are determined by the patient's size and subcutaneous fat distribution and by the features of the inguinal adenopathy. The incision is planned to encompass a liberal soft tissue margin peripheral to metastatic lymph nodes and, simultaneously, to remove the skin at greatest risk of devitalization from dissection.

The elliptic incision extends from the anterior superior iliac spine toward the pubic tubercle, parallel to the inguinal ligament and usually about 4 to 6 cm. The incision is beveled outward, while it is deepened through the subcutaneous tissue, so that a pyramidal wedge of skin and subcutaneous fat truncated by the skin surface results. The base of this pyramid rests on the external oblique aponeurosis superiorly, the sartorius muscle laterally, and the adductor muscles medially.

The encompassed fat and areolar tissue are dissected from the external oblique aponeurosis and the spermatic cord to the inferior border of the inguinal ligament. This maneuver usually begins 4 to 5 cm above the level of the inguinal ligament. The inferior angle of the inguinofemoral exposure is at the apex of the femoral triangle, during which dissection of the long saphenous vein is identified and divided. Dissection is deepened through the fascia overlying the sartorius muscle laterally and adductor muscle medially. At the apex of the femoral triangle, the femoral artery and vein are identified and dissection continued superiorly along the femoral vessels. The saphenous vein is divided at the saphenofemoral junction and the dissection continued superiorly until continuity with the pelvic dissection is attained at the femoral canal (Fig. 108–6). The anterior and lateral aspects of the femoral vessels are dissected, but the femoral vessels are not skeletonized, and the femoral nerve is not necessarily seen as it runs beneath the iliac fascia.

After dissection of the femoral triangle, the sartorius muscle is mobilized from its origin at the anterior superior iliac spine and either transposed or rolled medially to cover the femoral vessels (Fig. 108–7). Its origin is sutured to the inguinal ligament superiorly, and its margins are sutured to the muscles of the thigh immediately adjacent to the femoral vessels. The femoral canal is closed by suturing the shelving edge of Poupart's ligament to Cooper's ligament, being careful not to compromise the lumen of the external iliac vein or injure the inferior epigastric vessels in the process.

Primary closure of the inguinofemoral dissection, despite the skin excision, is usually possible with no or minimal further mobilization of the excision margins. When circumstances demand a particularly large area of inguinal soft tissue sacrifice, primary closure using scrotal skin rotation flaps may suffice. With extensive defects, coverage by a myocutaneous flap is preferred.

Pelvic lymphadenectomy is best accomplished through the lower midline extraperitoneal approach familiar to most urologic surgeons and is not reviewed here. For unilateral dissection, however, there are three basic routes to this region through the recommended single oblique inguinal incision described by Spratt and co-workers (1965). The inguinal ligament can be divided vertically over the vessels or at the anterior superior iliac spine. Another approach is incision of the external oblique fascia and, reflecting the spermatic cord cephalad, division of the inguinal floor from

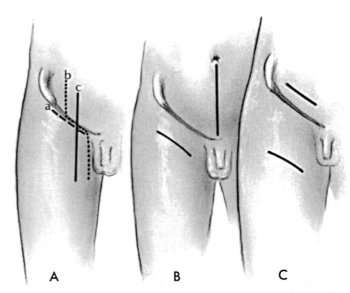

Figure 108–5. *A,* Single incisional approaches include (a) oblique, (b) S-shaped, and (c) vertical techniques. *B,* Double incisional techniques may combine a lower midline with an inguinal incision. *C,* Alternatively an oblique abdominal incision may provide unilateral access to the pelvic nodes.

the internal ring to the pubic tubercle, with ligation of the inferior epigastric vessels. This maneuver permits wide pelvic and retroperitoneal access. The preferred approach is incision in the anterior abdominal musculature 4 to 5 cm above and parallel to the inguinal ligament with medial mobilization of the peritoneum. This approach widely exposes the iliac region for nodal dissection (Fig. 108–8). The pelvic lymphadenectomy includes the distal common iliac,

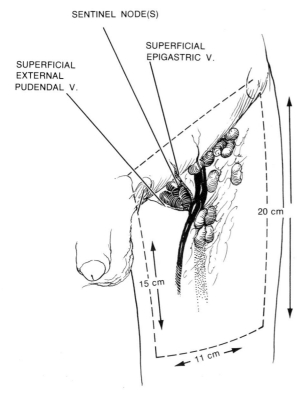

Figure 108–4. Sentinel node biopsy. An incision is centered on a point two fingerbreadths lateral and inferior to the pubic tubercle. The saphenous vein and its medial tributaries are isolated at the fossa ovalis. All fibroadipose node–bearing tissue is removed from this region and submitted for pathologic study. Also depicted are the topography and dimensions of the quadrangle within which all inguinal nodal tissue is predictably situated. This area can be marked after positioning and draping to avoid excessive dissection and excessive compromise of collateral blood supply to the skin flaps. (From Spaulding J: *In* Javadpour N, ed: Principles and Management of Urologic Cancer. Baltimore, Williams & Wilkins, 1979.)

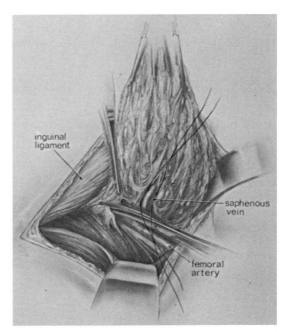

Figure 108–6. The flaps having been dissected, the entire circumference of this area is divided, and the ascending lymphatics are ligated. The tissue is mobilized from lateral to medial with exposition and skeletonization of the femoral vessels. Branches and tributaries are sacrificed, including the greater saphenous vein, which is double-ligated at its junction with the common femoral vein.

external iliac, and obturator groups of nodes. No further therapeutic benefit is gained from proximal iliac or para-aortic dissection.

The specimen is delivered from the pelvis en bloc through the femoral canal and should be carefully labeled. Alternatively the inguinal and pelvic components are submitted separately, so that the extent of regional disease can be accurately determined.

Closed-suction catheters are introduced into the area of dissection from a point peripheral to the skin flaps to obliterate dead space and prevent seroma formation. The catheters eliminate the need for compressive dressings over skin flaps. The catheters are removed after 5 to 7 days, when the aspirate volume is negligible and good flap adherence is evident. The skin is closed with fine absorbable sutures without tension. Scrotal flaps may be fashioned to cover some residual groin skin defects. This technique or other rotational or myocutaneous flaps are preferable to primary closure under tension.

Efforts should be made to minimize lymph flow during the initial postoperative period. Thigh-length elastic wraps or stockings should be worn. The foot of the bed is elevated slightly. Because the patient should be at bed rest for at least 5 days, postoperative anticoagulation has been recommended (Skinner et al, 1972), but prophylactic low-dose heparin therapy (Sogani et al, 1981) may increase postoperative complications (e.g., prolonged lymphatic drainage, infection, and lymphocele).

A low-residue diet is introduced to minimize fecal contamination. The urinary catheter may be removed on the first or second postoperative day. When primary healing appears well established, ambulation can be resumed. Prophylactic application of fitted elastic stockings and limb elevation reduce the incidence and severity of lymphedema after groin dissection.

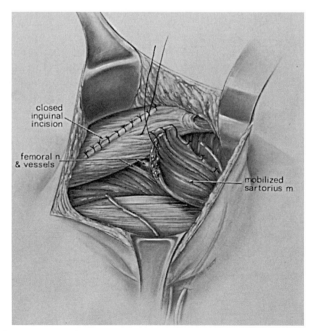

Figure 108–7. Closure of the wound includes repair of the access to the retroperitoneum, transposition of the sartorius muscle, placement of closed-suction catheter drainage, and approximation of the skin edges without tension.

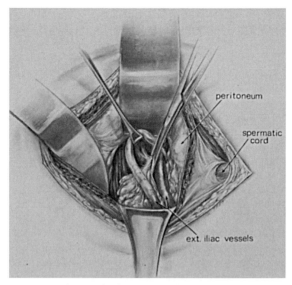

Figure 108–8. When only the ipsilateral pelvic component is to be addressed, access is readily gained to the retroperitoneum through an abdominal incision 4 to 5 cm above and parallel to the inguinal ligament. Nodal tissue is dissected from the iliac vessels, specifically including the external iliac and obturator groups.

Modified Groin Lymphadenectomy

For patients with clinically negative nodes or with equivocally or minimally enlarged nodes, a modified (limited) therapeutic lymphadenectomy has been proposed (Catalona, 1988). This procedure is a compromise between the sentinel lymph node biopsy, which may not be therapeutic for patients with more than one positive node, and the standard extended inguinal lymphadenectomy, which may not be absolutely necessary in patients with minimal regional metastases.

The modified groin dissection (Fig. 108–9) differs from the standard dissection in that (1) the skin incision is shorter; (2) the node dissection is limited, excluding regions lateral to the femoral artery and caudad to the fossa ovalis; (3) the saphenous veins are preserved; and (4) the transposition of the sartorius muscles is eliminated. The dissection is designed to remove completely the superficial inguinal lymph nodes, situated at the anterior and medial aspects of the saphenofemoral junction and the deep inguinal nodes, which are clustered around the femoral vessels situated deep to the fascia lata.

The patient is positioned in a manner similar to that for radical ilioinguinal lymphadenectomy. The skin is opened with a 10-cm incision placed 1.5 cm below the groin crease, deepened to the level of Scarpa's fascia. The superior flap is developed deep to Scarpa's fascia for a distance of about 8 cm. A funiculus of adipose and lymphatic tissue, coursing from the base of the penis to the superficial inguinal lymph nodes, is divided. The spermatic cord is identified and reflected medially. All fibrofatty tissue below this structure is reflected caudad as a "package" that contains the superficial inguinal nodes.

The inferior flap is now developed for a distance of 6 cm below the incision. The saphenous vein is seen in the center of the field, emerging from the package of lymph node–

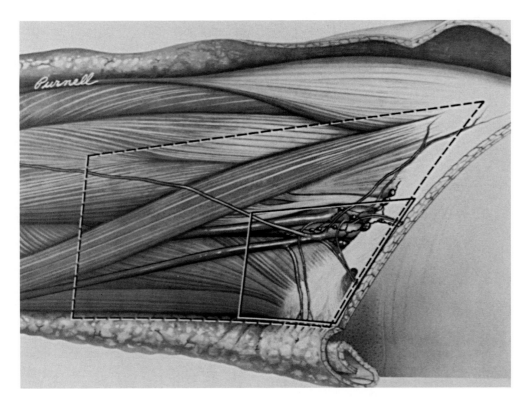

Figure 108–9. Boundaries of the standard ilioinguinal lymph node dissection and the modified (limited) groin dissection.

bearing tissue. This tissue is dissected of the fascia lata and the fossa ovalis in the lateral-to-medial fashion. The saphenous vein is carefully preserved. The superficial inguinal lymph nodes are then dissected laterally and off the saphenofemoral junction and surrounding surfaces (Fig. 108–10). As the dissection proceeds, the numerous lymphatic channels encountered are isolated and ligated.

The deep inguinal nodes, clustered around the femoral vessels, are dissected superiorly to the level of the inguinal ligament and excised (Fig. 108–11). At the end of the procedure, the saphenofemoral junction is intact. The medial margin of the dissection is the adductor longis muscle, the lateral margin is the femoral artery, the superior margin is the spermatic cord, and the inferior margin is the fossa ovalis. The incision is closed with skin staples. Suction catheters are placed inferiorly to drain the skin flaps.

MALE URETHRAL CANCER

General Considerations

Carcinoma of the male urethra is rare. Approximately 600 cases have been reported. Most patients are older than 50 years of age, although urethral carcinoma has been reported in boys as young as 13 years of age and in men in their nineties. Significant etiologic factors have not been identified, but chronic inflammation appears to play a role because many patients have prior sexually transmitted disease, urethritis, or urethral stricture. The incidence of urethral stricture in men with carcinoma of the urethra ranges from 24% to 76%. **The most frequent site of stricture is the bulbomembranous urethra, which is also the most frequent portion of the urethra to be involved with tumor.** No racial predisposition has been noted.

The lesion is often insidious at onset with symptoms attributed to benign stricture disease rather than to malignancy. Men most often present with a palpable urethral mass or obstructive symptoms. Urethral stricture or bleeding, perineal pain, or onset of a urethral fistula in an elderly man should suggest the possibility of urethral carcinoma.

Pathology

Tumors of the male urethra can be categorized according to the location and histology of the cells lining the urethra (Mostafi et al, 1992). Cancers occur in the bulbomembranous urethra in 60%, penile urethra in 30%, and prostatic urethra in about 10%. Histologically, 80% of male urethral cancers are squamous cell carcinoma, 15% are transitional cell carcinoma, and 5% are adenocarcinoma and undifferentiated tumors.

Male urethral carcinoma spreads by direct extension to adjacent structures and usually involves the vascular spaces of the corpus spongiosum and the periurethral tissues. Carcinoma of the bulbomembranous urethra extends to the urogenital diaphragm, prostate, perineum, and scrotal skin. Hematogenous spread is uncommon except in advanced disease. Metastasis occurs by lymphatic embolization to regional lymph nodes. The lymphatics from the anterior urethra drain into the superficial and deep inguinal lymph nodes and occasionally to the external iliac lymph nodes. The lymphatics from the posterior urethra drain into the external iliac, obturator, and hypogastric lymph nodes. Tumors of the posterior urethra most commonly spread to the pelvic lymph nodes, although exceptions occur. Palpable inguinal lymph nodes occur in about 20% of cases and almost always represent metastatic disease.

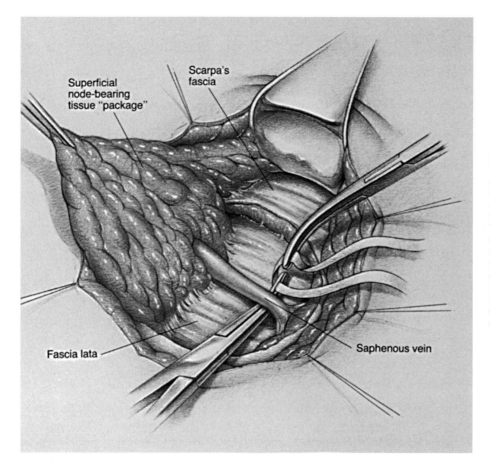

Figure 108–10. Development of the inferior flap has been extended deep to Scarpa's fascia for a distance of approximately 6 cm below the incision. The saphenous vein is seen in the center of the field, emerging from the "package" of lymph node–bearing tissue. This tissue is dissected off the fascia lata and the fossa ovalis in a lateral-to-medial fashion. (From Catalona WJ: Urologic Surgery: Modified Groin Lymphadenopathy for Carcinoma of the Penis. deKernion JB, conferee. Drawings by William B. Westwood. Courtesy of LTI Medica and Bristol-Myers Company. Copyright 1988 by Learning Technology Incorporated.)

Evaluation and Staging

The TNM staging classification is based on depth of invasion of the primary tumor and the presence or absence of regional lymph node involvement and distant metastasis (Table 108–1) (Beahrs et al, 1992). Examinations under anesthesia consisting of inspection, palpation of the external genitalia and perineum, and bimanual palpation aid in evaluating the extent of local involvement by tumor. Cystourethroscopy and transurethral or needle biopsy are also performed. Cytologic studies of voided urine may be helpful for diagnosing some patients. Local soft tissue, lymph node involvement, and bone extension are best evaluated by a computed tomography scan of the abdomen and pelvis or magnetic resonance imaging scan.

Treatment

The primary mode of therapy for carcinoma of the male urethra is surgical excision, and its extent depends on the location and stage of the tumor. In general, anterior urethral carcinoma is more amenable to surgical control, and the prognosis is better than posterior urethral carcinoma. Although some instances of tumor control by irradiation have been reported, in general radiation has been reserved for patients with early-stage lesions of the anterior urethra who refuse surgery. Radiation therapy has the advantage of preserving the penis but may result in urethral stricture and chronic edema and does not prevent new tumor occurrence.

Combination chemotherapy has achieved encouraging results in patients with metastatic urothelial cancer and is now increasingly being employed with irradiation and definitive surgery in patients with locally advanced urethral carcinoma.

Carcinoma of the Distal Urethra

Carcinoma of the penile urethra may be treated by transurethral resection, local excision, partial amputation, or radical amputation with or without emasculation. For superficial, papillary, or in situ tumor, transurethral resection and fulguration is sufficient. For tumor infiltrating the corpus and localized to the distal half of the penis, a partial amputation with a 2-cm margin proximal to visible or palpable tumor is an accepted and generally successful treatment. If infiltrating tumor is located in the proximal penile urethra or involves the entire urethra, total penectomy is indicated. Ilioinguinal node dissection is indicated if the inguinal nodes are palpable. There is no benefit from prophylactic groin dissection.

Carcinoma of the Bulbomembranous Urethra

Early lesions of the bulbomembranous urethra have been treated successfully by transurethral resection or by resection of the involved urethral segment with end-to-end anastomosis, but cases appropriate for limited resection are rare. Poor survival figures have been recorded for all forms of treatment, but it appears that radical excision offers the best

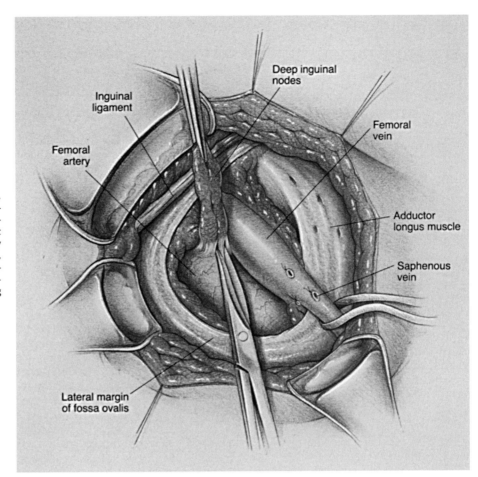

Figure 108–11. The deep inguinal nodes, clustered around the femoral vessels, are dissected out superiorly to the level of the inguinal ligament. (From Catalona WJ: Urologic Surgery: Modified Groin Lymphadenopathy for Carcinoma of the Penis. deKernion JB, conferee. Drawings by William B. Westwood. Courtesy of LTI Medica and Bristol-Myers Company. Copyright 1988 by Learning Technology Incorporated.)

opportunity for long-term disease control and the lowest incidence of local recurrence.

Radical cystoprostatectomy, pelvic lymphadenectomy, and total penectomy are usually required. Extending the operation to include in-continuity resection of the pubic rami and adjacent urogenital diaphragm may improve the margin of resection and local control (Bracken, 1982; Klein et al, 1983; Mackenzie and Whitmore, 1968; Shuttleworth and Lloyd-Davies, 1969).

With the patient in a low lithotomy position to allow perineal access, the standard abdominal mobilization of the bladder is completed except for preservation of the endopelvic fascia and the anterior pubic attachments. In the male, an inverted U-shaped perineal incision is initiated, based just medial to the ischial tuberosities, with the apex in the midperineum. The ischiorectal fossae are developed as in perineal prostatectomy, and a tunnel is bluntly dissected just anterior to the rectum, extending from one fossa to the other. The inferior skin flap is mobilized by sharply dividing the intervening subcutaneous tissue and rectourethralis muscle.

The superior flap is mobilized by sharply incising the subcutaneous tissue to the superficial Colles' fascia. The dissection is continued bilaterally to the adductor musculature at the inferior pubic rami. Anteriorly the dissection is carried along the phallus to the penoscrotal junction. Wider exposure, if necessary, results from dividing the scrotum in the midline. Bulky tumors may necessitate sacrifice of portions of the scrotum or perineal skin. The testicles may still be preserved and placed in thigh pouches.

To complete the pubic arch resection, the adductor musculature is sharply divided bilaterally from the length of the inferior pubic ramus along the medial margin of the obturator foramen. A Gigli saw is passed along the inferior ramus just posterior to the origins of the transverse perineal muscles. An inferiorly beveled transection is made bilaterally. The bevel is important to simplify perineal delivery of the specimen. The entire symphysis is resected for bulky urethral lesions involving the presymphyseal tissues and is accomplished by division of the superior rami at their junction with the symphysis. The Gigli saw is introduced, and laterally beveled ostomies are completed.

For most lesions, the bulk of the symphysis can be preserved with resection of the subsymphyseal arch. This procedure is preferred, when possible, to preserve stability of the pelvic girdle. The Gigli saw is passed through the obturator foramina to incise the symphysis transversely, joining the foramina with an upward beveled osteotomy (Fig. 108–12). The specimen is delivered en bloc (Fig. 108–13). After hemostasis is secure, the omentum is mobilized to cover the bowel. Myocutaneous flaps can be fashioned to close large perineal defects (Larson and Bracken, 1982).

Carcinoma of the Prostatic Urethra

Carcinoma arising from the prostatic urethra is rare. Tumors may be transitional or adenocarcinoma, and the diagnosis is based on a solitary tumor in the prostatic urethra

Table 108–1. TNM CLASSIFICATION OF CARCINOMA OF THE URETHRA

Primary Tumor (T) (Male and Female)

TX	Primary tumor cannot be assessed
T0	No evidence of primary tumor
Ta	Noninvasive papillary, polypoid, or verrucous carcinoma
Tis	Carcinoma in situ
T1	Tumor invades subepithelial connective tissue
T2	Tumor invades the corpus spongiosum or the prostate, or the periurethral muscle
T3	Tumor invades the corpus cavernosum or beyond the prostatic capsule, or the anterior vagina or bladder neck
T4	Tumor invades other adjacent organs

Regional Lymph Nodes (N)

NX	Regional lymph nodes cannot be assessed
N0	No regional lymph node metastasis
N1	Metastasis in a single lymph node, ≤2 cm in greatest dimension
N2	Metastasis in a single lymph node, >2 cm but <5 cm in greatest dimension; or multiple lymph nodes, none >5 cm in greatest dimension
N3	Metastasis in a lymph node >5 cm in greatest dimension

Distant Metastasis (M)

MX	Presence of distant metastasis cannot be assessed
M0	No distant metastasis
M1	Distant metastasis

From Beahrs O, Henson D, Hutter R, Kennedy BJ: Manual for Staging of Cancer. Philadelphia, J. B. Lippincott, 1992.

without associated coexisting or pre-existing urothelial tumors within the bladder or bladder neck.

There are no characteristic symptoms of this lesion. Patients generally present with hematuria or obstructive urinary symptoms. Prostatic induration on rectal examination represents advanced disease. The serum prostate-specific antigen and acid phosphatase values are normal. Diagnosis depends on transurethral biopsy of the prostate.

Superficial lesions of the prostatic urethra are managed successfully by transurethral resection in the majority of patients (Bretton and Herr, 1989). In the majority of instances, the tumor involves the bulk of the prostate and

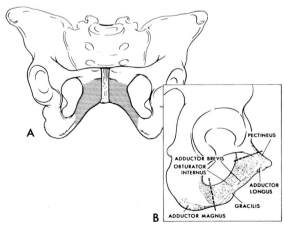

Figure 108–12. *A,* The shaded area is resected. *B,* Muscle groups encountered in resection of the pubis. (From Klein FA, et al: CANCER 1983; 51:1241. Copyright © 1983, American Cancer Society. Reprinted by permission of Wiley-Liss, Inc., a subsidiary of John Wiley & Sons, Inc.)

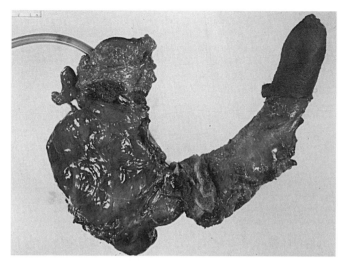

Figure 108–13. Extended resection of posterior urethral cancer in a man.

often extends into the base of the bladder. In this situation, cystoprostatectomy and total urethrectomy is the treatment of choice, although the overall 5-year survival of patients with infiltrating cancers is less than 20%.

There are anecdotal reports of successful treatment of primary adenocarcinoma of the prostatic urethral stroma with combination chemotherapy plus radiotherapy or extensive transurethral resection of the prostate or radical prostatectomy. Although these cases are few, this multimodal approach has the advantage of retaining the patient's bladder. It remains to be seen whether a combination approach can better control the primary tumor and offer survival advantages over surgery alone (Table 108–2).

Radiation Therapy

Radiotherapy has been used as a palliative measure, as an adjunct to surgical excision, and as a primary therapy. The long-term results of radiotherapy are mixed because only a few reports are available for patients treated with this modality (Raghavaiah, 1978).

MANAGEMENT OF THE RETAINED URETHRA AFTER CYSTECTOMY

General Considerations

The potentially multifocal nature of transitional cell carcinoma places the entire urothelium at risk in the patient

Table 108–2. FIVE-YEAR SURVIVAL IN CARCINOMA OF THE MALE URETHRA

Site	Treatment	No. Patients	No. Survival
Fossa navicularis	Partial penectomy	12	11 (92%)
Penile	Partial or total penectomy	100	34 (34%)
Bulbomembranous	Total penectomy, urethrectomy, cystoprostatectomy	64	10 (16%)
Prostatic			
Superficial	Transurethral resection	45	39 (87%)
Invasive	Cystoprostatectomy, urethrectomy	78	29 (37%)

Data from Ray et al, 1977; Zeidman et al, 1992; Grigsby and Herr, 1995.

with bladder cancer. The prostatic and penile urethra is uncommonly involved at the time of cystectomy. Therefore, the entire urethra from the membranous portion to the meatus is generally not removed with the specimen. Because this urothelium remains at risk, close follow-up with urethral washings for cytology, flow cytometry (if available), and biopsy (if necessary) is required at 3- to 4-month intervals for at least 5 years. It is important to maintain a high index of suspicion if incontinuity urethrectomy is not performed at the time of cystectomy. The incidence of subsequent severe epithelial atypia or frank in situ urethral carcinoma is estimated at 12.5% in male patients in whom urethrectomy was not performed prophylactically during total cystectomy for bladder cancer (Schellhammer and Whitmore, 1976).

Urethrectomy is indicated as an isolated procedure after cystectomy if the findings determined from urethral washings become positive for malignant cells or if a bloody urethral discharge develops. Secondary urethrectomy may be a less adequate operation than primary urethrectomy because the perineal scarring and proximity of the small bowel to the urogenital diaphragm after radical cystectomy render complete excision of the membranous portion of the urethra more difficult and less certain.

Operative Technique

A modified lithotomy position is employed for urethrectomy, with hips and knees gently flexed and the lower limbs adducted in foot stirrups.

A 5-cm midline or an inverted U–shaped perineal incision

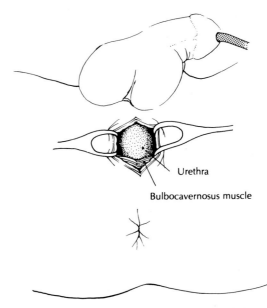

Figure 108–15. The bulbocavernous muscle is retracted, demonstrating the underlying urethral bulb. (Copyright Royal Victoria Hospital. From Herr HW: Urethrectomy. *In* Glenn JF, ed: Urologic Surgery, 3rd ed. Philadelphia, J. B. Lippincott, 1983. Courtesy of Balfour M. Mount.)

may be used (Fig. 108–14). **The perineal incision affords simpler access to the urethral arteries and greater exposure of the urethral bulb and urogenital diaphragm.** The subcutaneous tissue and bipenniform bulbocavernosus muscle are divided in the midline and retracted to expose the corpus spongiosum (Fig. 108–15), which is isolated. A small tape is passed around the urethra, and traction is applied to facilitate sharp dissection of the urethra distally, thus separating the corpus spongiosum from the adjacent corpora cavernosa (Fig. 108–16).

As dissection proceeds, the penis becomes inverted as the

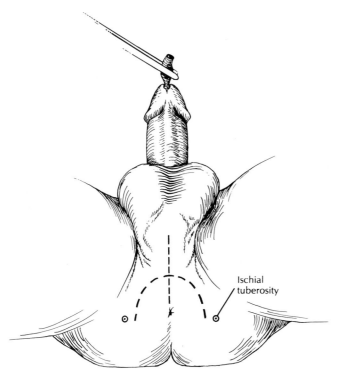

Figure 108–14. A midline or inverted U–shaped perineal incision between the ischial tuberosities or a combination thereof is used to expose the urethral bulb. (From Herr HW: Urethrectomy. *In* Glenn JF, ed: Urologic Surgery, 3rd ed. Philadelphia, J. B. Lippincott, 1983. Courtesy of Balfour M. Mount.)

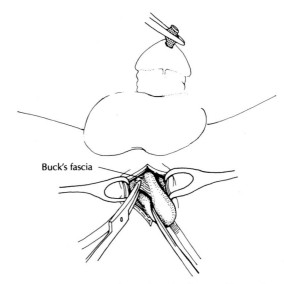

Figure 108–16. Sharp dissection of Buck's fascia with traction on the urethra separates the corpus spongiosum from the corpora cavernosa. (Copyright Royal Victoria Hospital. From Herr HW: Urethrectomy. *In* Glenn JF, ed: Urologic Surgery, 3rd ed. Philadelphia, J. B. Lippincott, 1983.)

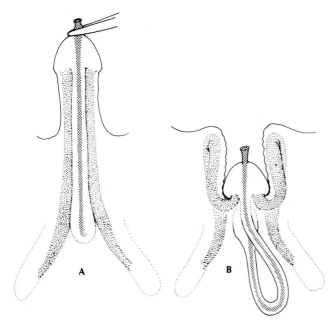

Figure 108–17. Catheterized pendulous urethra *(A)* before dissection and *(B)* with penis inverted at completion of distal dissection to glans penis. (Copyright Royal Victoria Hospital. From Herr HW: Urethrectomy. *In* Glenn JF, ed: Urologic Surgery, 3rd ed. Philadelphia, J. B. Lippincott, 1983. Courtesy of Balfour M. Mount.)

corpora cavernosa become bowed and the glans recedes into the phallus as it follows the line of traction on the urethra (Fig. 108–17). **In this manner, the penis is turned inside-out onto the perineum, and dissection is completed to the base of the glans (Fig. 108–18).** To excise the meatus and glandular urethra, the penis is replaced in its anatomic position, and an incision is made around the meatus and extended on each side down the ventral aspect of the glans (Fig. 108–19). The distal urethra is then freed from its investments within the glans penis employing sharp dissection. The isolated pendulous urethra may now be delivered onto the perineum, and the filleted glans penis is reapproximated to minimize blood loss.

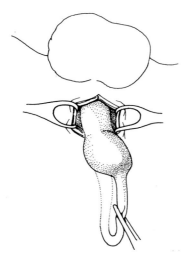

Figure 108–18. Completion of distal dissection to the undersurface of the glans penis. (Copyright Royal Victoria Hospital. From Herr HW: Urethrectomy. *In* Glenn JF, ed: Urologic Surgery, 3rd ed. Philadelphia, J. B. Lippincott, 1983. Courtesy of Balfour M. Mount.)

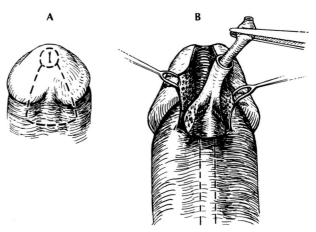

Figure 108–19. *A* and *B,* Incision used for dissection of the urethral meatus and the glandular urethra. Note that the penis has been placed in its normal anatomic position. (From Herr HW: Urethrectomy. *In* Glenn JF, ed: Urologic Surgery, 3rd ed. Philadelphia, J. B. Lippincott, 1983. Courtesy of Balfour M. Mount.)

Proximal sharp dissection of the urethral bulb is completed to the level of the perineal membrane and inferior fascia of the urogenital diaphragm. Further sharp and blunt dissection is used to enlarge the urethral hiatus and to free the urethra above the level of the urogenital diaphragm, all or a portion of which may be included with the specimen.

The urethral branches of the internal pudendal arteries are isolated, ligated, and divided as they enter the bulb at 4 o'clock and 8 o'clock, just inferior to the perineal membrane (Fig. 108–20). Care must be exercised in completing the proximal dissection in view of the possible postcystectomy adherence of intestine to the superior surface of the urogenital diaphragm. All that remains of the membranous urethra proximally is an ill-defined fibrotic band. Frozen-section analysis of this region adds some assurance that a negative proximal margin has been attained.

Closure of the bulbocavernosus muscle, subcutaneous tissue, and skin with interrupted absorbable sutures completes the procedure. A light pressure dressing is applied. A small Penrose drain exiting near the frenulum is used to drain the urethral bed. Defects created in the corpora cavernosa during sharp dissection of the urethra require suture ligature to control bleeding before closure. The patient is ambulated on the first postoperative day, and the Penrose drain is removed.

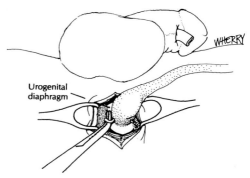

Figure 108–20. Isolation and division of the artery to the urethral bulb, with a drain in the bed of the corpus spongiosum. (Copyright Royal Victoria Hospital. From Herr HW: Urethrectomy. *In* Glenn JF, ed: Urologic Surgery, 3rd ed. Philadelphia, J. B. Lippincott, 1983. Courtesy of Balfour M. Mount.)

The urethrectomy is completed in less than 1 hour. Superficial hematoma, edema along the penile shaft, and infection are uncommon complications.

FEMALE URETHRAL CANCER

General Considerations

Urethral carcinoma is much more common in women than in men. The majority of patients are older than 50 years of age, and the disease is more prevalent among whites. The cause of urethral carcinoma has not been established with certainty, although there appears to be a relation between chronic irritation, urinary tract infection, and malignancy. Proliferate lesions, such as caruncles, papillomas, adenomas, and polyps, have been associated with subsequent malignancy. Leukoplakia of the urethra is considered a premalignant lesion.

Most patients present with urinary frequency, hesitancy, obstruction, and a palpable urethral mass or induration. Tumors may present as a papillary growth within the urethra and later become a soft fungating mass that bleeds easily. Ulcerative lesions produce a foul-smelling discharge. The tumor may present first as a submucosal mass in the anterior wall of the vagina. Spread from the primary lesion is by local extension and infiltration with subsequent involvement of the bladder neck, vagina, or vulva. It may be difficult on initial physical examination to differentiate malignant tumors of the urethra from those of the vulva or vagina.

The anterior urethra and labia drain to the superficial and then deep inguinal nodes, while the posterior urethra drains to the external iliac, hypogastric, and obturator lymph nodes. These boundaries are not distinct and anatomic cross-overs are possible. Clinically palpable inguinal nodes are found in one third of patients and represent neoplasm in more than 90%. Pelvic node involvement occurs in 20%, and an additional 15% of patients develop metastatic disease during follow-up. Metastasis outside the pelvis at the time of initial presentation is uncommon.

Tumor histology is a reflection of the site of origin within the urethra, with squamous cell carcinoma being the predominant tumor type and usually presenting in the proximal two thirds of the urethra. In general, carcinomas of the anterior urethra are low grade and less extensive. Carcinomas of the proximal or entire urethra are high grade and locally advanced. Squamous cell carcinoma accounts for 60%, transitional cell carcinoma 20%, adenocarcinoma 10%, undifferentiated tumor and sarcomas about 8%, and melanoma 2%. Histologic characteristics do not appear to affect the prognosis significantly, and different histologic types are treated in a similar fashion.

Evaluation and Staging

A pelvic examination under anesthesia combined with urethroscopy, cystoscopy, and biopsies is required. Radiographic evaluation consists of a chest x-ray, computed tomography scan of abdomen and pelvis, and, in symptomatic patients, a barium enema and bone scan.

The TNM staging system for female urethral cancer is presented in Table 108–1. Although incorporation of the TNM staging system is desirable, the practical fact is that staging, treatment, and prognosis are simplified by dividing tumors into anterior versus posterior or entire urethra.

Treatment

The most significant prognostic factor for local control and survival is the anatomic location and extent of the tumor. For example, a meatal tumor if diagnosed early is associated with an excellent 5-year survival. The treatment is based primarily on the tumor stage at the time of presentation.

Most urethral cancers in women are locally advanced when detected and involve the proximal one third or entire urethra. Such lesions clearly do worse than localized, low-grade, anterior urethral lesions. The poor prognosis is due to advanced stage (high tumor volume), adjacent organ involvement, inability to obtain a clear surgical margin owing to soft tissue infiltration, nodal disease, morbidity of extensive treatment, and inadequate systemic therapy for metastatic disease. Single-modality therapy often fails for advanced disease and is successful only in selected cases.

Surgery

Local excision is often sufficient for carcinoma of the distal urethra. Such tumors are superficial and well localized. The incidence of lymph node metastasis is low. Local excision controls the primary tumor, and urinary continence is maintained.

For tumors involving the proximal urethra or with extension beyond the urethra into adjacent structures, more aggressive therapy is required, both for local control and palliation. When surgery is considered, extensive resection is necessary, including total urethrectomy, cystectomy with pelvic lymph node dissection, and removal of most, if not all, of the vagina. En bloc resection of the inferior aspect of the pubic symphysis, similar to extensive dissection in males, and adjacent urogenital diaphragms may improve local control. Inguinal lymph node dissection is usually not performed in the absence of palpable disease in the groin. Even extensive surgery fails, however, owing to soft tissue infiltration by tumor beyond the confines of the bladder neck, urethra, and vagina. Local recurrence after surgery alone is common.

Radiation Therapy

Radiation alone, as with surgical excision, is often sufficient to control small lesions in the distal urethra. Radiation of small lesions can be accomplished with brachytherapy with iridium 192 implant. Interstitial or intracavitary irradiation delivering a 50- to 65-Gy tumor dose has been demonstrated to be sufficient to control small distal urethral lesions.

Tumors of the proximal urethra, bladder neck invasion, or involvement of the entire urethra requires combined external irradiation and brachytherapy. The pelvis is treated with 50 Gy by combined whole-pelvis and split-field technique, and the pelvic sidewall dosage can be boosted to 60 Gy in the presence of lymphadenopathy. The primary tumor site is boosted with one or two interstitial implants to bring the total tumor dose to 70 to 80 Gy depending on tumor size. The overall control rate for proximal urethral tumors in women is no more than 20%. Complications from radiation include bowel obstruction, fistula formation, urethral stricture, and incontinence. Table 108–3 shows results of treatment of female urethral cancer.

Combined Modality Therapy

Although the number of cases of advanced female urethral carcinoma is small, it is obvious that either extensive surgery alone or high-dose irradiation alone produces an unacceptably high morbidity rate and low tumor control rate. Several studies have recommended combined-modality approaches of preoperative irradiation and chemotherapy (M-VAC, or combined mitomycin-C and 5-fluorouracil) followed by radical cystourethrectomy. Long-term results from combined treatment policy are unavailable. The combined modality regimen to achieve local control and survival with the least morbidity is currently under investigation.

Specific Surgical Techniques

Local Excision

Circumferential local excision of the distal urethra and adjacent portions of the anterior vaginal wall can be accomplished for small, exophytic, and well-differentiated lesions of the external meatus or distal third of the urethra. Spatulation of the urethra and approximation to the subjacent vagina and labia provide a patent meatus and preserve urinary continence.

For entire or proximal urethral invasive lesions, cystourethrectomy (anterior exenteration), including a wide margin of vagina and in some cases the entire vagina, is required. For bulky female urethral lesions or local recurrences, an extended excision may be necessary. The perineal incision is similar to but wider than that for standard transvaginal anterior pelvic exenterations. The labia majora are retracted, and the introital incision is initiated anterior to the clitoris. The incision continues inferiorly to include the labia minora to the lower midvagina, where it joins the vaginotomies initiated from the pelvis. Dissecting anteriorly, the symphysis is cleared, whereas lateral dissection exposes the fascia overlying the origins of the adductors along the inferior pubic rami. If resection of the pubic arch or its subsym-

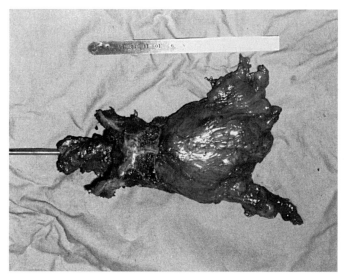

Figure 108–21. Extended resection of urethral cancer in a woman.

physeal portion is required, this is accomplished in a manner similar to that described for the male (Fig. 108–21).

Regional Metastasis

The significant morbidity associated with groin dissection and the observation that cancer of the female urethra often metastasizes systemically without regional node involvement caution against the indiscriminate, routine, or prophylactic employment of lymphadenectomy in a patient with no clinically suspected regional lymphatic spread. Groin dissection is reserved for the patient who presents initially with histologically confirmed regional lymph nodes without distant metastases or one who subsequently demonstrates lymph node involvement. Groin dissections in the female are performed in a fashion identical to that in the male for penile cancer. For transitional carcinomas metastatic to the inguinal or pelvic lymph nodes, chemotherapy is expected to play a greater role in combination with surgery.

REFERENCES

Airhart RA, DeKernion JB, Guillermo EO: Tensor fascia lata myocutaneous flap for coverage of skin defect after radical groin dissection for metastatic penile carcinoma. J Urol 1982; 128:599.

Arconti JS, Goodwin WE: Use of scrotal skin to cover wound defects in the groin and pubic area. J Urol 1956; 75:292.

Beahrs O, Henson D, Hutter R, Kennedy B: Manual for Staging of Cancer. Philadelphia, J.B. Lippincott, 1992.

Bracken RB: Exenterative surgery for posterior urethral cancer. Urology 1982; 19:248.

Bracken RB, Grabstald H: Primary carcinoma of the urethra. J Urol 1976; 116:188.

Bretton PR, Herr HW: Intravesical BCG therapy for in situ transitional cell carcinoma involving the prostatic urethra. J Urol 1989; 141:853–856.

Cabanas RM: An approach for the treatment of penile carcinoma. Cancer 1977; 39:456.

Catalona WJ: Modified inguinal lymphadenectomy for carcinoma of the penis with preservation of saphenous vein: Technique and preliminary results. J Urol 1988; 140:306–310.

Dinney CP, Johnson PE, Swanson DA, et al: Therapy and prognosis for male urethra carcinoma. AUA Update 1994; 43:506.

Foens CS, Hussey JHJ, Staples JJ, et al: A comparison of the roles of

Table 108–3. FIVE-YEAR SURVIVAL IN FEMALE URETHRAL CANCER

Stage	Treatment	No. Patients	No. Survival
Early	Radiotherapy	140	94 (67%)
	Surgery	24	20 (83%)
	Radiotherapy plus surgery	5	4 (80%)
Advanced	Radiotherapy	157	54 (34%)
	Radiotherapy plus surgery	39	21 (54%)

Data from Narayan and Konety, 1992; Grigsby and Herr, 1995.

surgery and radiation therapy in the management of carcinoma of the female urethra. Int J Radiat Oncol Biol Phys 1991; 21:961–968.

Fraley EE, Hutchens HC: Radical ilioinguinal node dissection—skin bridge technique. J Urol 1972; 108:279.

Grabstald H: Tumors of the urethra in men and women. Cancer 1973; 32:1236.

Grabstald H, Whitmore WF: Cancer of the female urethra. JAMA 1966; 197:835.

Grigsby PW, Corn BW: Localized urethral tumors in women: Indications for conservative versus exenterative therapies. J Urol 1992; 147:1516–1520.

Grigsby PW, Herr HW: Urethral tumors. Vogelzang N, Cardino PTS, Shipley WU, Coffey DS, eds: Comprehensive Textbook of Genitourinary Oncology. Baltimore, Williams and Wilkins, 1996, pp 1117–1123.

Hahn P, Krepart G, Malaker K: Carcinoma of the female urethra: Manitoba experience, 1958–1987. Urology 1991; 37:106–109.

Johnson DE, et al: Rotational skin flaps to cover defect in groin. Urology 1975; 6:461.

Johnson DE, O'Connell JR: Primary carcinoma of female urethra. Urology 1983; 21:42.

Kaplan GW, et al: Carcinoma of the male urethra. J Urol 1967; 98:365.

Klein FA, Herr HW, Whitmore WF, et al: Inferior pubic rami resection with en bloc radical excision for invasive proximal urethral carcinoma. Cancer 1983; 51:1238.

Konnak JW: Conservative management of low-grade neoplasms of the male urethra: A preliminary report. J Urol 1980; 123:175.

Larson DL, Bracken RB: Use of gracilis musculocutaneous flap in urologic cancer surgery. Urology 1982; 14:148.

Levine RL: Urethral cancer. Cancer 1980; 45:1965.

Mackenzie AR, Whitmore WF: Resection of pubic rami for urologic cancer. J Urol 1968; 100:546.

Mayer R, Fowler JE Jr, Clayton M: Localized urethral cancer in women. Cancer 1987; 60:1548–1551.

Mostafi FK, Davis CJ, Sesterhenn IA: Carcinoma of the male and female urethra. Urol Clin North Am 1992; 19:347–358.

Mullen EM, Anderson EE, Paulson DF: Carcinoma of the male urethra. J Urol 1974; 112:610.

Narayan P, Konety B: Surgical treatment of female urethral carcinoma. Urol Clin North Am 1992; 19:373–382.

Perinetti E, Catalona WJ: Unreliability of sentinel lymph node biopsy for staging penile carcinoma. J Urol 1980; 124:734.

Prempree T, et al: Radiation therapy in primary carcinoma of the female urethra. Cancer 1984; 54:729.

Raghavaiah NV: Radiotherapy in the treatment of carcinoma of the male urethra. Cancer 1978; 41:1313.

Ray B, Grabstald H: Experience with primary carcinoma of the male urethra. J Urol 1977; 117:591.

Sailer SL, Shipley WU, Wang CC: Carcinoma of the female urethra: A review of results with radiation therapy. J Urol 1988; 140:1–5.

Schellhammer PF, Whitmore WF Jr: Transitional cell carcinoma of the urethra in men having cystectomy for bladder cancer. J Urol 1976; 115:56.

Scher HI, Herr HW, Yagoda A, et al: Neoadjuvant M-VAC (methotrexate, vinblastine, doxorubicin, and cisplatin) for extravesical urinary tract tumors. J Urol 1988; 139:475–477.

Shuttleworth KED, Lloyd-Davies RW: Radical resection for tumors involving the posterior urethra. Br J Urol 1969; 41:739.

Skinner DG: Management of extensive localized neoplasms of the lower abdominal wall. Urology 1974; 3:34.

Skinner DG, et al: The surgical management of squamous cell carcinoma of the penis. J Urol 1972; 107:273.

Sogani PC, Hindsley P, Whitmore WF: Lymphocele after pelvic lymphadenectomy for urologic cancer. Urology 1981; 17:39.

Spratt JS, et al: Anatomy and Surgical Technique of Groin Dissection. St. Louis, C. V. Mosby, 1965.

Whitmore WF Jr, Vagaiwala MR: A technique of ilioinguinal lymph node dissection for carcinoma of the penis. Surg Gynecol Obstet 1984; 159:573.

Zeidman EJ, Desmond P, Thompson I: Surgical treatment of carcinoma of the male urethra. Urol Clin North Am 1992; 19:3569.

109
SURGERY OF TESTICULAR NEOPLASMS

Eila C. Skinner, M.D.
Donald G. Skinner, M.D.

Primary Testis Cancer
    Diagnosis
    Radical Orchiectomy
    Management of Scrotal Tumor Contamination
    Delayed Orchiectomy in Advanced Disease
    Pathology

Staging

Surgery for Low-Stage Germ Cell Tumors
    Role of Surgery in Pure Seminoma
    Retroperitoneal Lymph Node Dissection Versus
        Observation for Clinical Stage I Disease
    Fertility in Low-Stage Testicular Cancer
    Rationale for a Limited Retroperitoneal Lymph
        Node Dissection
    Prospective Nerve-Sparing Retroperitoneal
        Dissection
    Intraoperative Nerve Stimulation
    Management of Stage II Disease

Surgical Technique of Retroperitoneal Lymph Node Dissection
    Choice of Surgical Approach
    Preoperative Preparation
    Technique of Thoracoabdominal Node Dissection
    Prospective Nerve-Sparing Technique
    Complications
    Technique of Transabdominal Node Dissection

Surgery for Advanced-Stage Disease
    Timing of Retroperitoneal Dissection in Stage III
        Disease
    Management of Residual Mass in Advanced
        Seminoma
    Technique of Retroperitoneal Node Dissection for
        Advanced Disease

Testicular cancer continues to be the most curable solid tumor in men. The modern approach to this disease exemplifies the successful integration of multimodal therapies and requires active cooperation between the surgeon, oncologist, and radiation therapist. Despite the tremendous effectiveness of platinum-based chemotherapy regimens, surgery continues to remain a cornerstone in the treatment of testicular cancer.

PRIMARY TESTIS CANCER

Diagnosis

Testis cancer primarily occurs in men between 17 and 40 years of age, and most patients present with a painless, hard lump in the testis. Many patients have dull or even severe acute pain in the testis, however, and others complain primarily of symptoms caused by metastatic disease (back pain, gastrointestinal symptoms, hemoptysis, a neck mass, or gynecomastia). Patients often give a history of a recent scrotal trauma, which most likely simply drew the patient's attention to the abnormal testis, rather than actually causing the tumor. **Delays in diagnosis as a result of physician error continue to be fairly common.**

Scrotal ultrasound is the definitive diagnostic test for testicular tumors. It is greater than 90% sensitive and specific in identifying a solid mass within the parenchyma of the testis (Benson, 1988) and is especially helpful in the face of an equivocal examination or an obscuring hydrocele. If the ultrasound is inconclusive, however, inguinal exploration and biopsy may be required.

Blood for serum beta human chorionic gonadotropin (beta hCG) and alpha-fetoprotein (AFP) should be drawn before orchiectomy. These tests cannot be used for screening because most seminomas and a third of nonseminomas have normal serum marker levels. Preorchiectomy markers are critical in staging, however, and helpful in treatment planning and follow-up.

If the ultrasound study is highly suggestive of testis tumor, and especially if tumor markers are elevated, it is preferable to perform a staging computed tomography (CT) scan of the abdomen and pelvis **before** orchiectomy. There have been case reports of patients who bled into the retroperitoneum after orchiectomy leading to misinterpretation of the subsequent CT scan as showing metastatic disease (Bochner et al, 1995). A day or two delay in orchiectomy to obtain the scan is preferable to the risk of overtreatment.

Percutaneous needle or core biopsies of the testis should be avoided. An exception might be a young leukemia patient with probable leukemic involvement of the testes because orchiectomy is not always required in that setting.

Radical Orchiectomy

The first surgical step in treatment of any testis tumor is radical inguinal orchiectomy. **The inguinal approach avoids interruption of the scrotal lymphatics, which would risk changing the metastatic pathway of the tumor, and allows complete removal of the spermatic cord up to the internal ring.**

The technique is straightforward. A transverse oblique inguinal incision is made approximately 4 to 6 cm in length, beginning 2 cm lateral and superior to the pubic tubercle. The external oblique fascia is identified and divided from the external ring superiorly in line with its fibers (Fig.

109–1). The ilioinguinal nerve is identified and retracted to one side, and the spermatic cord is gently mobilized up to the internal ring. A noncrushing clamp across the cord is placed at this point to avoid any potential tumor spread by way of the veins or lymphatics during mobilization of the testis. Alternatively, if the diagnosis is certain, the cord can simply be ligated and divided before manipulating the testis.

The testis is mobilized from the scrotum into the wound using blunt dissection (Fig. 109–2). If the tumor is large, it may be necessary to extend the incision toward the scrotum to allow delivery of the testis. If diagnostic biopsy is planned, the wound should be carefully draped off before opening the tunica vaginalis, and a wedge biopsy sample may be taken from the parenchyma of the testis. To complete the orchiectomy, the cord is mobilized at least 1 to 2 cm inside the internal inguinal ring and suture ligated with a large permanent suture to allow easy identification of the stump should a retroperitoneal lymph node dissection be required later.

The wound and scrotum are irrigated, and a testis prosthesis may be placed at this point if so desired. The internal ring is obliterated with a No. 1 polyglycolic acid (PGA) suture, and the external oblique fascia closed with a running 3–0 PGA suture. The skin may be closed with skin clips or a subcuticular suture.

This procedure can usually be done as an outpatient, and complications are rare. The most serious complication is bleeding. Several units of blood can collect surreptitiously

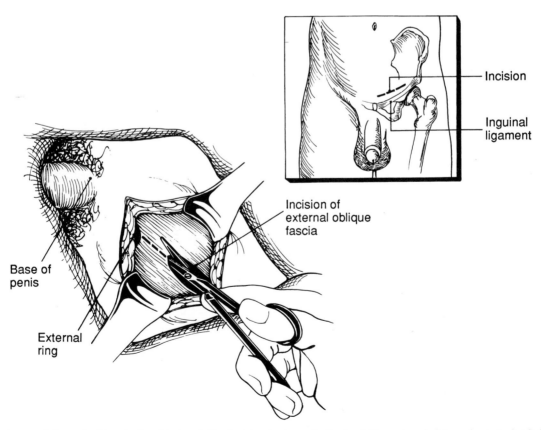

Figure 109–1. Approach for radical inguinal orchiectomy. The incision is shown in the *inset*. The external oblique fascia is divided in line with its fibers down to the external inguinal ring. (Adapted from Gottesman JE: *In* Crawford ED, ed: Current Genitourinary Cancer Surgery. Philadelphia, Lea & Febiger, 1990, p 319.)

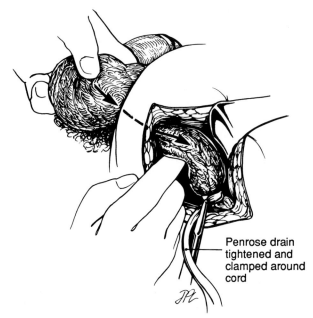

Figure 109–2. After the cord has been controlled with a tightened Penrose drain or rubber-shod clamp, the testicle is mobilized out of the scrotum using blunt dissection. (Adapted from Gottesman JE: *In* Crawford ED, ed: Current Genitourinary Cancer Surgery. Philadelphia, Lea & Febiger, 1990, p 319.)

in the retroperitoneum before the complication is recognized. A large hematoma can be misinterpreted on CT scan as representing metastatic tumor, resulting in serious overtreatment of the patient (Bochner et al, 1995). Therefore, the ligated cord should be inspected carefully before allowing it to retract into the retroperitoneum. Other complications, such as wound infection or seroma formation, are seen only occasionally (Moul et al, 1989).

Management of Scrotal Tumor Contamination

The possible diagnosis of testicular cancer should always be considered before performing any scrotal surgery in a man between 17 and 40 years old. Errors clearly occur, however, and as many as 14% of testis cancer patients referred to one treatment center had undergone transscrotal orchiectomy or biopsy (Boileau and Steers, 1984). It was previously believed that scrotal surgery markedly increased the risk of local recurrence and inguinal node metastasis (Markland et al, 1973). Further evidence now suggests that this risk has been overestimated and that a formal hemiscrotectomy or prophylactic inguinal node dissection is rarely indicated in these cases (Boileau and Steers, 1984; Giguere et al, 1988; Capelouto et al, 1995). A meta-analysis of all evaluable reported series (1182 total cases, 206 with scrotal violation) found that the risk of local recurrence increased from 0.4% to 2.9% with scrotal violation, but there was no difference in the distant recurrence or survival rates. They also could not demonstrate any advantage to adjuvant treatment regimens, although the numbers in each group were small (Capelouto et al, 1995). Giguere and colleagues (1988) demonstrated a markedly increased local recurrence rate in

patients with gross tumor contamination of the scrotum (e.g., open biopsy) who did not have subsequent hemiscrotectomy. Based on these data, the following management is currently recommended:

1. In stage A pure seminoma, prophylactic retroperitoneal radiation should be extended to include the ipsilateral hemiscrotum and inguinal nodes. This may increase the risk of subsequent azoospermia (Amelar et al, 1971), which must be discussed with the patient.

2. In stage A nonseminoma, the previous scrotal scar should be widely excised at the time of retroperitoneal lymph node dissection, along with any remaining spermatic cord stump. If a lymph node dissection is not planned, these structures should be excised as a separate procedure. In the case of gross contamination, a formal hemiscrotectomy should be performed.

3. In advanced disease treated with full-dose platinum chemotherapy, no further treatment of the scrotum is necessary. The inguinal nodes should be carefully examined at each follow-up visit.

Delayed Orchiectomy in Advanced Disease

A young man may present with an obvious advanced nonseminomatous germ cell tumor in whom there is no doubt about the diagnosis, for example, a testicular mass, elevated AFP, and multiple pulmonary metastases. In this setting, it may be in his best interest to begin chemotherapy immediately without performing an orchiectomy. A similar situation may arise in a patient whose tissue diagnosis has been established through needle biopsy of a metastatic lesion.

It is important that eventual inguinal orchiectomy be carried out in these patients, even if a complete response from chemotherapy is achieved. There have been several reports of viable tumor identified within a retained testis following full-dose platinum combination chemotherapy (Fowler and Whitmore; 1981; Calvo et al, 1983; Simmonds et al, 1995). This suggests that the testis may act as a "privileged site" that is protected from the chemotherapy effects.

The delayed orchiectomy can be performed at the time of retroperitoneal lymph node dissection (RPLND) by pulling the spermatic cord and testis up through the inguinal canal from above. The gubernacular attachments must be carefully coagulated as they are divided to prevent scrotal hematoma, and the inguinal ring should be formally closed afterward.

If a patient does not require node dissection, the orchiectomy should be performed through a standard inguinal technique shortly after completing chemotherapy. If both testes remained normal throughout the course of treatment, by both palpation and ultrasound, this suggests an extragonadal primary tumor. In that case, the testes may be left in place and closely monitored at follow-up visits. If the retroperitoneal disease localizes to one side, however, the authors' policy is to remove the testis on that side at the time of lymphadenectomy. This occasionally reveals a small scar or tiny focus of tumor in a palpably normal testis.

Pathology

Germ cell tumors of the testis are categorized as either pure seminoma or pure or mixed nonseminomatous tumors. A detailed discussion of testis cancer pathology is presented in Chapter 78. Only a few comments are made here relevant to the surgical plan.

Because testicular cancer is relatively rare, not all pathologists are adept at dealing with this disease. Errors in primary diagnosis are fairly common, for example, mistaking anaplastic seminoma for embryonal cell carcinoma. Often, important prognostic factors in the pathologic evaluation are not reported. **If there is any question, tissue should be sent for a second opinion to a center with expertise in testicular cancer pathology.**

Seminoma

It is of central importance that the diagnosis of pure seminoma be made only after step sectioning of the testis. The differentiation between various subtypes of seminoma is not thought to be of prognostic significance (Wetlaufer, 1984).

Most seminomas do not cause an elevation of serum tumor markers. **AFP is produced *only* by embryonal or yolk sac elements, so by definition if the AFP is elevated in a seminoma, there must be occult nonseminomatous elements present.** Beta hCG, however, may be elevated in up to 40% of pure seminomas (Javadpour, 1978; Fossa and Fossa, 1989). This protein is believed to originate from syncytiotrophoblastic giant cells that may be identified in seminomas. Some reports have suggested a worse prognosis for patients with an elevated beta hCG (Maier and Sulak, 1973), but others have failed to confirm this relationship (Schwartz et al, 1984).

High levels of beta hCG (>200 mIU/ml) almost certainly reflect occult metastatic nonseminomatous elements, but lower levels do not exclude them. The authors have seen one patient with a moderate elevation (47 mIU/ml) who was found to have a 4-cm focus of embryonal cell carcinoma in the retroperitoneum (Pritchett et al, 1985). Because of this concern, the authors recommend that a patient with pure seminoma and a beta hCG greater than 20 mIU/ml or a lower elevation in the absence of identifiable syncytiotrophoblastic giant cells on pathology be treated as having a nonseminoma tumor.

Nonseminoma

Several aspects of the pathologic evaluation of the primary nonseminomatous testis tumor have been identified as having an impact on prognosis, including the extent of the primary tumor, the presence of lymphovascular invasion, and the relative amount of embryonal histology.

The prognostic significance of T stage has been established in both patients undergoing retroperitoneal lymphadenectomy (Fung et al, 1988) and in those on surveillance protocols that did not exclude higher-stage tumors (Freedman et al, 1987). Patients with T2 and above primary stage with negative metastatic work-up have a twofold increase in the incidence of positive nodes at retroperitoneal lymphade-

nectomy compared with patients with T1 tumors (38% versus 18%).

Lymphovascular invasion is perhaps even more powerful in predicting the presence of metastatic disease. In surveillance protocols, the risk of relapse has been reported in an average of 52% of patients with lymphovascular invasion (Freedman et al, 1987; Dunphy et al, 1988), compared to 10% to 15% in those without this finding.

Beyond these prognostic variables, nonseminomatous testis cancers are essentially all treated the same, regardless of the specific histology types. **Importantly, pure mature teratoma is considered a malignant histology in the adult testis and must be treated appropriately.**

Non–Germ Cell Tumors

Non–germ cell malignancies make up less than 10% of all testicular tumors and are discussed in detail in Chapter 78. These tumors include gonadal stroma tumors (Leydig's and Sertoli cell tumors), gonadoblastomas, and sarcomas of the cord or testis. The initial approach to all of these tumors is inguinal orchiectomy, which establishes the pathologic diagnosis. RPLND is generally recommended for these tumors, although there are a few exceptions. The surgical techniques are identical to those used for germ cell tumors.

Lymphomas also occur in the testis and account for the majority of tumors in men over age 50. Testicular lymphoma most often occurs in patients with the established diagnosis of lymphoma. In these cases, the diagnosis may be established by ultrasound. Rarely a lymphoma may present with a testis mass as the chief complaint at initial diagnosis. These patients often have occult disseminated disease, but as many as half of patients with testicular lymphoma appear initially to have disease limited to the testis (Turner et al, 1981; Moller et al, 1994). **Orchiectomy is recommended, but RPLND is *not* indicated in lymphoma of the testis. The cornerstone of treatment is systemic chemotherapy, even in patients whose disease is apparently confined to the testicle.** The prognosis generally is good.

STAGING

The spread of testicular germ cell tumors occurs along predictable routes in the majority of patients, primarily following the lymphatic drainage of the testis. The initial staging work-up should include preorchiectomy and postorchiectomy tumor markers, a CT scan of the abdomen and pelvis, and chest film. Bone scan, CT of the chest, and magnetic resonance imaging (MRI) of the brain are reserved for patients with established extraretroperitoneal disease. Routine CT scan of the chest has been shown to be unnecessary in low-stage disease and may show significant false-positive findings, which result in many additional costly tests that do not change the ultimate treatment outcome (Fernandez et al, 1994).

Bipedal lymphangiography (LAG) is rarely used in the United States, although it continues to be popular in some areas. The study is difficult to perform and interpret and uncomfortable for the patient. Many studies have failed to show any additional advantage of LAG over conventional CT scan (Ehrlichman et al, 1981; Wishnow et al, 1989a).

Table 109–1. STAGING SYSTEMS FOR GERM CELL TUMORS

Skinner/Walter Reed

A/I	Confined to testis
B/II	Retroperitoneum only
B1/IIa	<6 positive nodes, all <2 cm
B2/IIb	>6 nodes, or any node >2 cm
B3/IIc	bulky disease, >5 cm
C/III	Disease beyond retroperitoneum

UICC (TNM) System

T1	Confined to testis	N0	No nodes
T2	Beyond tunica albuginea	N1	1 ipsilateral node <2 cm
T3	Rete testis, epididymis	N2	Multiple nodes or one >2 cm
T4a	Invasion of cord	N3	Nodes >5 cm
T4b	Scrotal wall		

Some centers continue to require LAG before enrollment in a surveillance protocol for nonseminomas, and some radiation therapists use LAG in treatment planning for low-stage seminoma.

MRI has added little to the accuracy of staging of retroperitoneal nodes. The technology is evolving, and the use of enhancing materials may improve on this in the future. Currently, MRI does not seem to have any advantage over conventional CT scan in staging retroperitoneal lymph nodes, and the cost is considerably higher.

All currently available staging techniques are accurate in detecting retroperitoneal nodes greater than 2 cm in size. No technique short of surgery, however, is able to identify microscopic metastases. By the same token, false-positive results consistently occur in 20% to 25% of cases with a mass less than 5 cm in diameter and may result in unnecessary overtreatment (Donohue et al, 1995).

There are several staging systems in common use in the United States and around the world. They are all similar in that they divide patients into those with tumor confined to the testicle (stage A or I), those with retroperitoneal metastasis (stage B or II), and those with tumor beyond the retroperitoneum (stage C or III). Three of the different systems are compared in Table 109–1. The TNM system adds significant additional prognostic information about the extent of the primary tumor.

Stage C or III includes patients with widely different prognoses depending on the site and extent of disease. This has stimulated several centers to modify the staging systems to reflect these differences, but none of these modifications has been widely accepted.

SURGERY FOR LOW-STAGE GERM CELL TUMORS

Role of Surgery in Pure Seminoma

In general, surgery beyond orchiectomy has a relatively minor role in the treatment of pure testicular seminoma. Prophylactic retroperitoneal irradiation remains the standard of care for stage A patients, reducing the risk of recurrence from 10% to 20% down to below 3% and nearly eliminating the risk of retroperitoneal recurrence. Several groups have explored surveillance protocols for these patients, but follow-up is problematic because of the absence of effective tumor

markers, and late recurrences beyond 5 years are common (Duchesne et al, 1990; Horwich et al, 1992; van der Maase et al, 1993). Low-dose retroperitoneal irradiation carries little or no long-term risk and seems well worth the investment.

Retroperitoneal Lymph Node Dissection Versus Observation for Clinical Stage I Disease

The development of effective chemotherapy for advanced testicular cancer caused some investigators to question the role of RPLND in early-stage disease. Approximately 70% to 75% of patients with clinical stage I (N0) nonseminoma have pathologically negative nodes and presumably gain no benefit from the dissection. At the same time, a full bilateral dissection in the past carried an almost certain side effect of anejaculation and resultant infertility. Therefore, protocols were designed at several medical centers that called for careful observation of clinical stage I patients, with chemotherapy and possible node dissection reserved for those who demonstrated progression.

Results are now available from many different protocols, including several large cohorts of patients (Pizzocaro et al, 1985; Gelderman et al, 1987; Freedman et al, 1987; Dunphy et al, 1988; Sturgeon et al, 1992; Nicolai and Pizzocaro, 1995). The following conclusions can be drawn from these studies:

1. Consistently 25% to 35% of patients develop metastatic disease on observation protocols that include all stage I patients.

2. Overall survival is 98%, similar to primary RPLND series.

3. Fifty percent to 75% of cancers that recur do so in the retroperitoneum, with the rest recurring in the lung or elsewhere. This points out the central importance of routine CT scan of the abdomen in surveillance protocols.

4. Numerous cases of late failures have been documented, even beyond 5 years, emphasizing the need for long-term follow-up (Nicolai and Pizzocaro, 1995).

A typical surveillance regimen is shown in Table 109–2. It is an intensive program, requiring considerable resources and a compliant patient. Because of the rapid growth rate of testicular cancer, patients who miss one or more visits are at high risk of developing bulky disease that may be resistant to subsequent treatment efforts.

Several studies have identified patients at lowest risk for

Table 109–2. SURVEILLANCE PROTOCOL FOR STAGE I NONSEMINOMA

Year 1	CXR, markers (AFP, β HCG), examination every month CT abdomen and pelvis every 3 months
Year 2	CXR, markers, examination every 2 months CT abdomen and pelvis every 4 months
Years 3–5	CXR, markers, examination every 3 months CT abdomen and pelvis every 6 months
Years 6 +	CXR, markers, examination every 6 months CT abdomen and pelvis every year

CXR, Chest x-ray; CT; computed tomography.

relapse and therefore most suited to an observation protocol. The pathology of the primary testis tumor, if carefully evaluated, can give important prognostic information. **Pathologic factors contributing to a higher risk of relapse include**

1. **Higher T stage (T2 or T3 tumors).**
2. **Lymphovascular invasion.**
3. **Greater proportion of embryonal cell histology.**

Wishnow and co-workers found no recurrences in 30 patients with none of these pathologic findings and preorchiectomy AFP less than 80 ng/dl (Wishnow et al, 1989b). That compared to 46% recurrence rate in patients who had one or more of these findings. Similarly, Freiha and Torti (1989) found only three relapses in 23 patients with T1 tumors without lymphovascular invasion. Thus, offering surveillance only to selected patients may improve the results with this approach.

Quality of life aspects of the surveillance protocols are more difficult to quantify. The development of modified nerve-sparing node dissection techniques has greatly reduced the risk of anejaculation after this surgery (see later), so the issue of fertility is no longer the driving force behind the decision. A program with initial node dissection with adjuvant chemotherapy for IIB disease is completed within 4 months. At that point, the patient knows his risk of recurrence is less than 10%, and he can go on with his life with less frequent follow-up visits and without the need for subsequent CT scans. By comparison, patients in the surveillance protocol must contend with the fact that up to one third or more of them will need chemotherapy and perhaps a delayed node dissection, sometimes months to years later. This makes it difficult to plan for work, school, marriage, and other activities.

Compliance with follow-up visits is central to the success of surveillance protocols. Young and colleagues found that patients on surveillance tended to miss a significant number of follow-up appointments and tended to downplay their risk of relapse or the seriousness of their disease (Young et al, 1991).

Differences in costs to the health care system have not been formally analyzed to date. Lowe (1993) estimated that a surveillance program would cost an average of 25% less than a program with primary RPLND. He estimated a 1-week average hospital stay for surgery, with 20% of patients requiring an additional week or two for postoperative complications. This is clearly a significant overestimate (Baniel et al, 1994). Aass and colleagues, however, also found that estimated costs were less with an observation approach in the Norwegian system (Aass et al, 1990).

Clearly the winners in the surveillance protocol are the patients who remain free of disease with no further treatment beyond orchiectomy. Many patients may be willing to take that gamble, which should be offered only in a setting with a well-defined protocol for patient follow-up. For most patients, however, the authors believe that a limited node dissection is the best initial therapy.

Fertility in Low-Stage Testicular Cancer

Patients with testis cancer have long been recognized as having impaired fertility compared with other men, for reasons not well understood. When measured before orchiectomy, up to 50% of men with testis cancer have a poor semen analysis (Lange et al, 1984).

When node dissection was performed routinely on every patient with low-stage nonseminomatous tumor, it was impossible to measure directly the effect of the surgery on fertility. Instead, investigators performed fairly complex statistical estimates to try to understand this issue (Lange et al, 1987). Now this question can be answered by observing fertility in men treated with either orchiectomy alone or orchiectomy with a successful nerve-sparing node dissection. Foster and colleagues (1994) reported on 51 men who had semen analysis after orchiectomy. They found that 75% of the men had normal semen analysis after orchiectomy but before node dissection. It is not certain, however, that the 25% who were in the subfertile range would remain so in the long-term. In a larger sample who responded to a questionnaire, 76% of 66 men who attempted to achieve a pregnancy after a nerve-sparing node dissection were successful. Bar-Charma and colleagues reported that 16 of 19 men (84%) treated with orchiectomy alone who had tried to father children had been successful (Bar-Charma et al, 1992). **Thus, it appears that at least three fourths of men with low-stage nonseminomatous testis cancer can expect to be fertile, making attempts to preserve ejaculation reasonable.**

Treatment is also available for patients who have anejaculation following RPLND. Initial therapy should consist of sympathomimetics given for short periods around ovulation. Regimens used include imipramine (25 mg three times a day), phenylpropanolamine (75 mg four times a day), and pseudoephedrine (90–120 mg four times a day). If these regimens fail to produce an ejaculate, postorgasm urine should be checked for presence of sperm, which could be washed and used for insemination (Presti et al, 1993). Finally, electroejaculation is nearly always successful in obtaining semen from patients who have undergone this surgery (Ohl et al, 1991). Advances in techniques for assisted reproduction make the prospect for future fertility for men with poor sperm counts in this group even better.

Future fertility must also be considered when assessing the impact of alternative treatments for low-stage testis cancer. Four cycles of platinum-based chemotherapy predictably result in transient azoospermia for all patients. Only 50% to 75% of these patients eventually recover sperm production, a process that may take 2 to 4 years (Drasga et al, 1983; Hansen et al, 1990). The impact of shorter courses of chemotherapy is unknown. A surveillance protocol is estimated to *increase* the percentage of patients who require chemotherapy from 15% to 20% up to 30% to 35% when compared with primary lymphadenectomy series. Others have recommended primary chemotherapy for all high-risk patients in clinical stage I (Sternberg, 1993; Studer et al, 1993). Fertility results have not been directly reported from any of these alternative approaches to date and need to be examined.

Rationale for a Limited Retroperitoneal Lymph Node Dissection

Historically the standard RPLND included a full bilateral dissection from above the renal hila to below the aortic bifurcation. Anejaculation was nearly guaranteed, especially because the sympathetic ganglia were often routinely sacrificed. Many investigators sought to limit the extent of dissection based on elegant studies by Donohue and co-workers mapping the extent of positive nodes in patients with only microscopic disease (stage IIA) (Fig. 109–3) (Donohue et al, 1982; Lange et al, 1984; Richie, 1990). **By sparing the area overlying the aorta below the inferior mesenteric artery (IMA) where the confluence of the postganglionic sympathetic fibers is located, ejaculation is preserved in 80% to 90% of cases.** The extent of such a dissection is shown in Figure 109–4. This approach allows the surgeon to use a straightforward template approach, removing all of the fibroareolar tissue in the area and ensuring a complete dissection.

The authors reported results using this approach in 47 patients (Doerr et al, 1993). Preservation of ejaculation occurred in 81% of the patients and was more common with right-sided dissections (88%) than left (62%). There were no retroperitoneal recurrences, and overall survival was 100%. Richie (1990) used a similar template and was able to preserve ejaculation in 75 of 85 patients (88%), with an additional 5 patients able to ejaculate with the aid of imipramine. He also reported no retroperitoneal recurrences.

It is important to include the interaortocaval area in **both right-sided and left-sided dissections.** The mapping studies have shown that this is an area of extensive crossover, especially with right-sided tumors crossing to the area around the aorta. Pizzocaro and Fossa and their colleagues described truly unilateral dissections for left-sided tumors, which would be predicted to miss approximately 20% of microscopically positive nodes (see Fig. 109–3) (Fossa et al, 1985; Pizzocaro et al, 1985).

The limited dissection has clearly passed the test of time. Retroperitoneal recurrences have been either absent or extremely rare in all reports, indicating that this dissection is adequate for patients with grossly negative nodes.

Prospective Nerve-Sparing Retroperitoneal Dissection

A better understanding of the anatomy of the sympathetic nerves in the retroperitoneum was derived from cadaver studies by Colleselli and associates (1990). Jewett and Donohue and their colleagues separately reported their early experience attempting to dissect out the branches of the sympathetic chain that course over the anterior aorta (Fig. 109–5) (Jewett et al, 1988; Donohue et al, 1990, 1993).

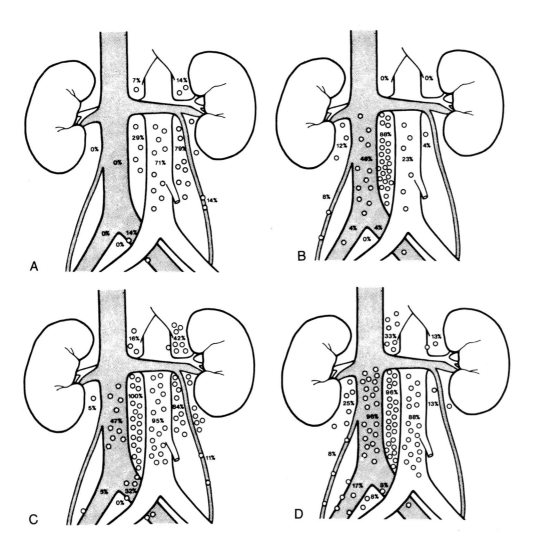

Figure 109–3. Distribution of positive nodes in patients with various pathologic stages of disease. *A*, Left-sided stage IIA. *B*, Right-sided stage IIA. *C*, Left-sided stage IIB. *D*, Right-sided stage IIB. (From Donohue JP, Zachary JM, Maynard BR: J Urol 1982; 128:315. © by Williams & Wilkins, 1982.)

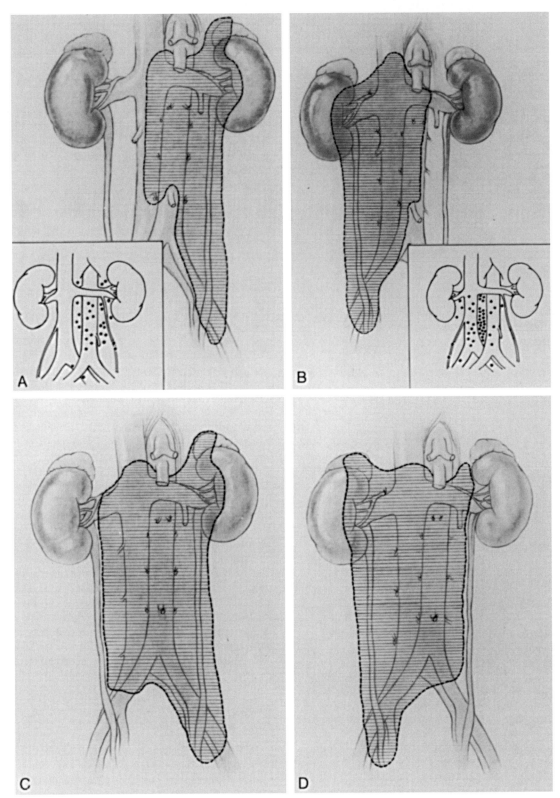

Figure 109–4. Adopted limits of dissection for retroperitoneal lymphadenectomy. *Insets in A and B* show distribution of positive nodes in patients with microscopic disease, stage IIA. *A,* Limited left-sided dissection. *B,* Limited right-sided dissection. *C,* Full bilateral left-sided dissection. *D,* Full bilateral right-sided dissection. (From Wise PG, Scardino PT: *In* Skinner DG, Lieskovsky G, eds: Diagnosis and Management of Genitourinary Cancer. Philadelphia, W. B. Saunders Company, 1988, p 779.)

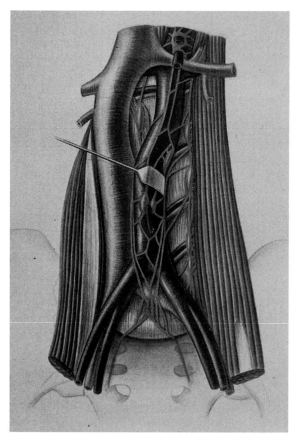

Figure 109–5. Branches of the lumbar sympathetic nerves, coursing over the anterior aorta. Note that the branches interconnect both above and below the root of the inferior mesenteric artery. The branches arise from the sympathetic ganglia, which course just lateral to the lumbar segmental vessels. (Adapted from Colleselli K, Poisel S, Schachtner W, Bartch G: J Urol 1990; 144:293–298.)

Ejaculation was maintained in virtually 100% of patients in the hands of these experienced surgeons.

The initial concern about such an approach was the question of the completeness of the dissection. Donohue and co-workers initially recommended against ligation of the lumbar artery branches off the aorta, making it difficult to clear the tissue completely posterior to the aorta. They found no instance, however, of retroperitoneal recurrence in 61 patients with negative nodes or in 13 of 14 patients with microscopically positive nodes (stage IIA) and no decrease in overall survival (Donohue et al, 1990). In the authors' experience, the lumbar vessels can indeed be ligated after dissecting out the nerve branches, without compromising the preservation of ejaculation. This facilitates a complete, careful dissection.

There have been isolated reports of using this technique in cases with grossly positive nodes. Although it may be technically feasible, great care must be taken not to compromise the extent of dissection or increase the risk of a local recurrence. Such cases need to be followed carefully with regular CT scan postoperatively, which is not necessary if a full bilateral node dissection has been performed. This surgery is technically difficult and is perhaps best left in the hands of surgeons with considerable experience with standard RPLND.

Intraoperative Nerve Stimulation

Some surgeons have attempted to refine the approach to nerve sparing using intraoperative electrical stimulation of the nerves. Intraoperative stimulation of the nerves can cause ejaculation, but repeated stimulation may not be useful because of a limited volume of available ejaculate (Dieckmann et al, 1992). Weidner and colleagues reported that the effect of stimulation could be measured by recording the increase in intravesical pressure that results from sympathetic stimulation (Weidner et al, 1994). With excellent results reported in the absence of electrical stimulation, it is not clear what additional benefit is obtained by such cumbersome techniques in stage I patients. It may improve the outcome, however, with selective preservation of one or more nerve branches in patients with more bulky lymphadenopathy. At this time, such techniques remain in the realm of research investigation.

Management of Stage II Disease

Extension to Full Bilateral Dissection

Approximately 10% of patients with negative CT scan and markers are found to have grossly positive nodes at retroperitoneal lymphadenectomy (Fung et al, 1988). Because the limited node dissection has been shown to be adequate for stage IIA (microscopic) disease, the authors do not routinely perform frozen section analysis of normal-appearing nodes at the time of surgery. When enlarged or indurated nodes are encountered, the decision must be made whether or not to extend the limits of dissection. The authors are influenced by the location of the positive nodes, which can be confirmed by frozen section in questionable cases. If the positive nodes are near the origin of the IMA, it is necessary to extend the dissection over the lower aorta and down the contralateral common iliac artery. Retrograde lymphatic spread can occur when these nodes are blocked by tumor. In such cases, loss of ejaculation is likely. When the positive nodes are located only superiorly, the authors still attempt to preserve the lower aorta. The dissection should be extended to the contralateral ureter, with full mobilization of the aorta and vena cava. The main sympathetic ganglia can still be preserved unless the disease is adherent to the psoas adjacent to the vertebral bodies. Bilateral suprahilar dissections are performed routinely in the presence of high grossly positive nodes.

Primary Surgery Versus Chemotherapy for Clinical Stage IIA or IIB

Patients are classified as clinical stage IIA or IIB when they have persistently elevated tumor markers after orchiectomy or minimal to moderate retroperitoneal adenopathy on CT scan. Currently, two approaches can be taken for these patients: (1) primary chemotherapy followed by node dissection for residual disease or (2) primary node dissection with or without adjuvant chemotherapy. The results in terms of survival are similar, but there are various advantages and disadvantages of each approach (Logothetis et al, 1987; Vugrin and Whitmore, 1985).

Patients treated with primary surgery have the advantage of more accurate staging. **Up to 23% of patients with apparent lymphadenopathy on CT scan are overstaged, especially with nodes less than 2 cm in size** (Donohue et al, 1995). These patients may not require chemotherapy at all. With small-volume disease, the surgery may be easier, especially with nerve sparing, and there is significantly lower morbidity before exposure to bleomycin. In addition, RPLND effectively eliminates the retroperitoneum as a site for future relapse, simplifying follow-up. Finally, patients who have teratomatous elements in the primary tumor have a high risk of late progression in the retroperitoneum and are best treated with node dissection, even after chemotherapy (Logothetis et al, 1982).

Up to 75% of patients with clinical stage IIA and IIB disease, especially those with pure embryonal cell carcinoma, achieve a complete remission with primary chemotherapy and may not require a node dissection (Logothetis et al, 1987). **In the authors' experience, the CT scan tends to underestimate the extent of disease more often than overestimating it. Clearly the surgeon must avoid the situation of an incomplete resection, tumor spill, or surgical injury as a result of encountering more disease than expected.** With significant disease, the lymph node dissection is safer following chemotherapy because of the fibrous capsule that forms around the tumor. The ability to preserve ejaculation may also occasionally be enhanced by the reduction in tumor volume that can result from chemotherapy.

The decision to approach a particular patient with primary surgery or chemotherapy ultimately depends on the relative weight of these advantages as well as the skill and experience of the surgeon. **The authors currently recommend primary lymph node dissection for patients with questionable disease or a mass less than 2 to 3 cm on CT scan, especially with teratomatous elements in the primary tumor. For those with multiple nodes or a mass greater than 5 cm on CT scan, the authors begin with chemotherapy. Intermediate-sized tumors are approached on a case-by-case basis.**

Adjuvant Chemotherapy for Pathologic Stage IIA and IIB After Node Dissection

The risk of tumor recurrence after node dissection alone is estimated to be 8% to 20% for microscopic disease stage IIA and 50% to 60% for stage IIB. These relapse rates have been markedly reduced in several series using a variety of different adjuvant chemotherapy regimens (Skinner, 1976; Scardino, 1980; Williams et al, 1987). Most reported series using platinum-based combinations have shown rare recurrences in patients who received adjuvant treatment. Such a program requires treatment of many patients who would have been otherwise cured by surgery alone, and the results must be compared with those obtained by simply treating the recurrences when they develop.

A multicenter trial was completed in 1984, with 195 IIA and IIB patients randomized to observation or chemotherapy with two courses of platinum, vinblastin, and bleomycin (PVB) or cis-platin, vinblastine, actinomycin D, bleomycin, and cyclophosphamide (VAB-4) following RPLND. The relapse rate in the observation group was approximately 50%,

with only one relapse in the adjuvant treatment group (in a patient who had undergone unilateral node dissection). There were three cancer-related deaths in the observation group and one in the treatment group, but the difference was not statistically significant. Richie and Kantoff (1991) subsequently reported that only 3 of 39 IIA patients followed without adjuvant treatment had a recurrence, 2 in the lung and 1 in the retrocrural region, and all 3 were salvaged with chemotherapy.

Other issues must be discussed in relation to this question. In many ways, they parallel those raised by the observation protocols for patients with stage I disease. The most important issue is compliance with follow-up in this population group. In the randomized study cited previously, the mean number of visits per year was 9 (of 12 planned), and 25% of the patients made 6 or fewer visits (Williams et al, 1987). If a patient is judged as being at high risk of noncompliance, perhaps adjuvant treatment is the safer route.

Second, the treatment of a documented recurrence requires three or four cycles of standard PVB or PEB (platinum, VP-16, bleomycin), which has significant potential toxicity. Besides the acute risk of treatment-related sepsis, long-term side effects occur frequently, including peripheral neuropathy, Raynaud's phenomenon, renal insufficiency, and azoospermia in up to 50% (Vogelsang et al, 1981; Roth et al, 1988; Osanto et al, 1992). Adjuvant chemotherapy programs generally include only one or two cycles of chemotherapy, with much less attendant toxicity (Williams et al, 1987; Weiss et al, 1988). The philosophical question is whether to expose all of the patients to the lower toxicity to avoid the greater toxicity for 50% or 60%.

We continue to recommend adjuvant chemotherapy for all patients with stage IIB disease, using four weekly cycles of bleomycin, vincristine (Oncovin), platinum, and VP-16 (BOP-VP16) or two monthly cycles of standard PEB. Patients with stage IIA are offered the alternatives of adjuvant treatment or observation alone.

SURGICAL TECHNIQUE OF RETROPERITONEAL LYMPH NODE DISSECTION

Choice of Surgical Approach

Multiple surgical approaches to the retroperitoneum have been described. The two most popular currently are the transabdominal and the thoracoabdominal incisions. A laparoscopic approach has also been used in a few centers (Stone et al, 1993; Gerber et al, 1994). Each type of approach has its specific advantages.

The thoracoabdominal incision provides superb exposure to the upper retroperitoneum, with the renal hilum essentially in the middle of the operative field. This approach is crucial in the patient with advanced disease who may have a large retroperitoneal mass and requires a thorough suprahilar dissection. In patients with less disease, this approach can be performed entirely extraperitoneally, reducing postoperative ileus and the risk of late small bowel obstruction.

The transabdominal approach, however, offers faster opening and closing and is more familiar to most surgeons. Exposure to the suprahilar area can be achieved

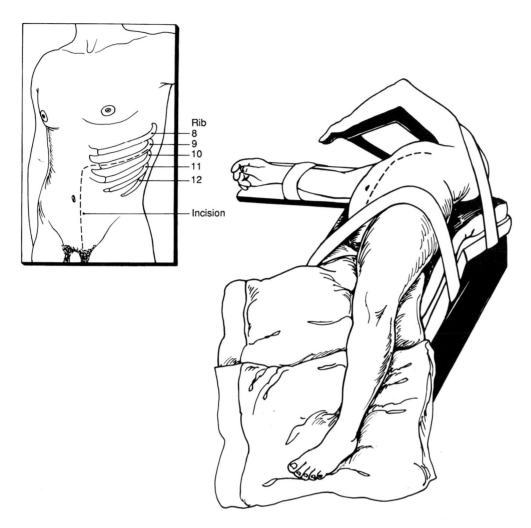

Figure 109–6. Thoracoabdominal position. Patient is positioned at the edge of the table, with the break just above the iliac crest. The contralateral leg is flexed 30 degrees at the hip and 90 degrees at the knee, and the ipsilateral leg lies over the top with a pillow in between. The ipsilateral arm is supported on an "airplane," and the table is fully flexed. The incision is shown in the *inset*.

but requires mobilization of the pancreas and spleen. The chest is not entered, which decreases the potential pulmonary complications and decreases postoperative pain. Mobilization of the bowel may result in a longer ileus, however, and puts the patient at risk for a later small bowel obstruction.

The laparoscopic approach is still new but appears to offer the advantages of a much more rapid postoperative recovery, perhaps at the cost of longer operating time and a potentially less thorough dissection. The learning curve has generally been steep for laparoscopic procedures. No long-term data have yet been reported on effectiveness in terms of avoiding later retroperitoneal recurrence (Stone et al, 1993; Gerber et al, 1994).

The overall incidence of major complications in patients with low-stage disease is 3% to 4% in most series regardless of surgical approach, with less than 0.1% operative mortality. Ultimately the training of the individual surgeon is probably the most important determinant in the type of incision chosen.

Preoperative Preparation

The preoperative evaluation is routine and should include serum tumor markers (AFP and beta hCG). A bowel prepara-

tion is not routinely used in low-stage disease but is crucial in the patient with a significant retroperitoneal mass after chemotherapy. Overnight intravenous hydration is ideal, but most patients are now admitted the morning of surgery to reduce cost.

Technique of Thoracoabdominal Node Dissection

The technique of a full left-sided dissection is described in detail, with specific comments about the right-sided and more limited dissections. A demonstration of the technique is also available on film (Skinner and Lieskovsky, 1984).

The patient is positioned as in Figure 109–6. He is placed supine near the ipsilateral edge of the table, with the break in the table located just above the iliac crest. The ipsilateral arm is rotated over the head onto an adjustable "airplane" arm rest. The lower leg is flexed 30 degrees at the hips and 90 degrees at the knee, and the upper leg is placed straight on a pillow. Sheet rolls are placed on either side to support the patient. All pressure points are carefully padded, with special attention to the inferior leg. The table is flexed completely, and the patient is secured in place using wide adhesive tape.

An incision is made over the bed of the eighth or ninth rib from the midaxillary line to the midepigastrium (see Fig. 109–6). It is then carried inferiorly as a paramedian incision, 1 cm lateral to the umbilicus. The rib is resected subperiostially, and the anterior rectus fascia is divided. The body of the ipsilateral rectus muscle is divided superiorly and retracted laterally, and the transversus abdominis is split in line with the incision.

The pleural cavity is entered through the posterior periosteum of the rib. Blunt Mayo scissors are passed behind the costochondral junction anterior to the peritoneum, and the cartilage is divided (Fig. 109–7). This maneuver allows the plane to be developed between the abdominal wall muscles and fascia and the peritoneal cavity using blunt and sharp dissection. The dissection begins laterally and continues medially, where the peritoneum may be quite adherent along the lateral rectus sheath. A small peritoneotomy is not uncommon, but an attempt should be made to complete the extraperitoneal dissection for the length of the incision. The posterior rectus fascia is freed from the peritoneum to its terminus at the arcuate line and is divided longitudinally.

Using the left hand with gentle downward and medial traction on the spleen (or liver on the right), the attachments between the peritoneum and the underside of the diaphragm are separated all the way back to the central tendon of the diaphragm. This allows complete mobilization of the peritoneal envelope medially (Fig. 109–8). This maneuver is best achieved by gently pushing off the muscular fibers of

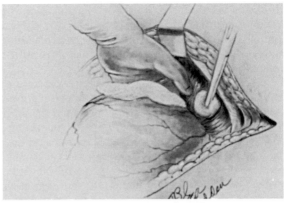

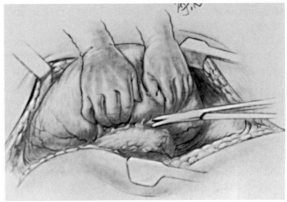

Figure 109–8. The attachments between the diaphragm and peritoneal envelope are divided back to the central tendon of the diaphragm. The peritoneum and Gerota's fascia together are mobilized off the posterior abdominal wall muscles. The avascular plane between the posterior peritoneum and the anterior leaf of Gerota's fascia is then identified and developed across the midline to the vena cava. The inferior mesenteric artery can be divided, if necessary. (From Wise PG, Scardino PT: *In* Skinner DG, Lieskovsky G, eds: Diagnosis and Management of Genitourinary Cancer. Philadelphia, W. B. Saunders Company, 1988, p 779.)

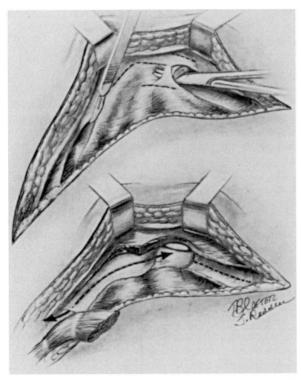

Figure 109–7. A subperiosteal rib resection has been completed. The anterior rectus fascia is divided in the abdominal portion of the wound. Scissors are passed behind the costochondral junction anterior to the peritoneum, allowing the surgeon to develop the plane between the peritoneum and the transversalis fascia bluntly. (From Wise PG, Scardino PT: *In* Skinner DG, Lieskovsky G, eds: Diagnosis and Management of Genitourinary Cancer. Philadelphia, W. B. Saunders Company, 1988, p 779.)

the diaphragm as they attach to the peritoneum using the open tips of blunt Mayo scissors. The diaphragm is then divided for a few centimeters from the costochondral junction posteriorly. A Finochietto retractor is placed with the protruding costal cartilage fixed in the holes in the retractor blades. Palpation of the lung is carried out to detect any unexpected nodules, which may be resected at the end of the procedure.

The peritoneum and Gerota's fascia are then bluntly swept off the back muscles over to the side of the aorta. Incision into the fascia of the psoas muscle facilitates this move. The next step is mobilization of the posterior peritoneum off the anterior surface of Gerota's fascia. Beginning superiorly at the top of the kidney, one can usually identify the plane between the two layers, remembering that the peritoneal envelope curves posteriorly around Gerota's fascia. A thin fascial layer surrounds both the peritoneum and Gerota's fascia and must be sharply incised. The loose fibroareolar tissue in the avascular plane is then encountered, which then can be bluntly developed over to the anterior aorta and vena cava (see Fig. 109–8). Only three structures penetrate through Gerota's fascia: the celiac artery, superior mesenteric artery (SMA) and IMA. If a full bilateral dissection is planned for a left-sided tumor, we routinely divide the IMA, which allows access to the opposite common iliac vessels. This should be avoided in elderly patients who may have compromised collateral blood supply to the left colon. In a limited or nerve-sparing dissection, the IMA is usually left intact.

The node dissection begins with identification of the root of the SMA, which is a key landmark in the retroperitoneum. The left renal vein is mobilized inferiorly, and the origin of the SMA is skeletonized, clipping the small lacteals that run alongside the vessel to prevent chylous leak. The left crus of the diaphragm is identified, and the tissue overlying it is clipped and divided (Fig. 109–9). This usually includes the left celiac plexus, which is often mistaken for indurated nodes.

The dissection continues laterally, dividing the superior attachments of Gerota's fascia to the diaphragm. The adrenal gland may be left intact or may be removed with Gerota's fascia if there is disease in the hilum of the kidney. On the left side, the adrenal vein is routinely divided, as is the inferior adrenal artery, which usually arises directly from the aorta. There is generally sufficient blood supply, however, arising from the phrenic branches. If the adrenal is to be preserved, the dissection should proceed across Gerota's fascia between the adrenal and the kidney.

The dissection then proceeds over the top of the left renal vein to the anterior vena cava and inferiorly down the center of the vena cava (Fig. 109–10). The gonadal and ascending lumbar veins draining into the left renal vein are ligated. The ipsilateral lumbar veins below the renal vein are care-

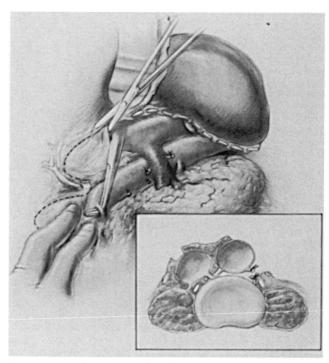

Figure 109–10. The tissue overlying the aorta is split down to the origin of the inferior mesenteric artery, and the ipsilateral lumbar arteries are ligated and divided. Care must be taken to identify and protect any accessory renal arteries that may be present. The tissue over the inferior vena cava is then split in the midline, clipping the lateral limits of the dissection. *Inset* shows the great vessels in cross section, demonstrating the "split-and-roll" technique. (From Wise PG, Scardino PT: *In* Skinner DG, Lieskovsky G, eds: Diagnosis and Management of Genitourinary Cancer. Philadelphia, W. B. Saunders Company, 1988, p 779.)

fully ligated with fine suture. In a bilateral dissection, the authors continue the dissection over to the right ureter, and the lumbar veins are divided bilaterally. In either case, the right gonadal vein is generally ligated, and the dissection continues inferiorly over the vena cava to the lower limits at the level of the IMA.

Attention is then turned to the anterior aorta. The tissue over the top of the aorta is split down to the origin of the IMA. In a limited dissection, the authors stop here, taking care not to disturb the aorta below the IMA (Fig. 109–11). In a full dissection, the IMA is again doubly ligated at its origin and the tissue split down to the bifurcation. The aorta is then further skeletonized. The left renal artery is identified and carefully skeletonized toward the hilum. Before this dissection, the patient is given 12.5 to 25 g mannitol intravenously to maintain renal perfusion and decrease the risk of arterial spasm. The contralateral renal artery is also dissected out, taking care to identify any accessory branches. The contralateral suprahilar area is generally not dissected in low-stage disease, so the contralateral renal artery represents the upper limit of dissection in these cases. The tissue behind the right renal artery overlying the crus of the diaphragm should be carefully clipped because it often contains the cisterna chyli.

The gonadal arteries are ligated at the aorta, as are the paired lumbar arteries between the renal arteries and the IMA (Fig. 109–12). The authors believe that division of the lumbar arteries is necessary in both the limited and the full

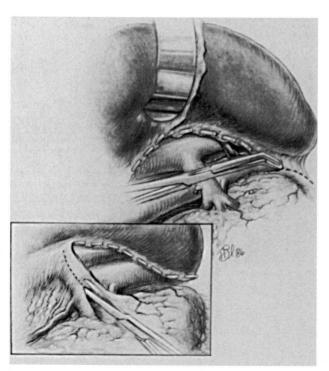

Figure 109–9. The root of the superior mesenteric artery (SMA) is identified just medial to the junction of the inferior mesenteric vein and splenic vein. The lacteals running parallel to the SMA are clipped distally, and the root of the SMA is cleaned. The tissue over the left renal vein is divided anteriorly, and the left renal artery is identified. (From Wise PG, Scardino PT: *In* Skinner DG, Lieskovsky G, eds: Diagnosis and Management of Genitourinary Cancer. Philadelphia, W. B. Saunders Company, 1988, p 779.)

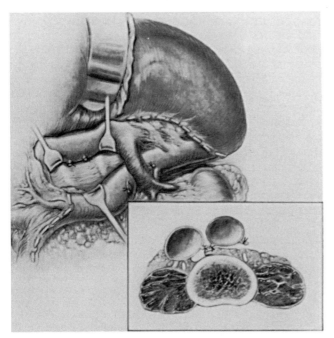

Figure 109–11. The opposite renal artery has been identified, and the tissue overlying the right crus of the diaphragm has been swept inferiorly. Gerota's fascia surrounding the left kidney has been split along the back of the kidney and swept inferiorly with the specimen. *Inset* shows a cross section of the great vessels with the lumbar vessels ligated. (From Wise PG, Scardino PT: *In* Skinner DG, Lieskovsky G, eds: Diagnosis and Management of Genitourinary Cancer. Philadelphia, W. B. Saunders Company, 1988, p 779.)

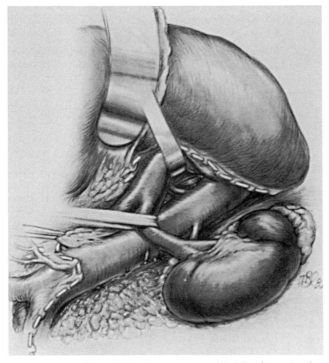

Figure 109–12. The right lumbar arteries and left lumbar veins have been ligated, completely freeing the aorta off the posterior abdominal wall. The interaortocaval tissue is then swept under the aorta to the left side. (From Wise PG, Scardino PT: *In* Skinner DG, Lieskovsky G, eds: Diagnosis and Management of Genitourinary Cancer. Philadelphia, W. B. Saunders Company, 1988, p 779.)

dissections to allow adequate access to the nodal tissue behind the aorta and between the vena cava and aorta. These arteries generally arise in three evenly spaced pairs posteriorly. The ligatures should be carefully placed because a dislodged tie results in troublesome bleeding with a risk of damaging the sympathetic chain during attempts to control it.

At this point, Gerota's fascia is divided over the lateral kidney, allowing half to pass posteriorly and half anteriorly. It is further taken off the hilum, allowing careful dissection of the branches of the renal artery and vein. The ureter is dissected out and mobilized away from the gonadal vein complex (Fig. 109–13). It is easily inadvertently injured and must be carefully protected during the inferior dissection.

In a full bilateral dissection, the authors continue over the bifurcation, dissecting out the common iliac artery and vein and the tissue overlying the sacral promontory. The median sacral artery is ligated posteriorly. In a limited dissection (shown in the figures), the authors continue down the center of the left common iliac artery to avoid injury to the contralateral sympathetic fibers.

The stump of the spermatic cord is then dissected out of the internal iliac ring, taking care not to injure the ureter or the peritoneum. Every effort should be made to identify and

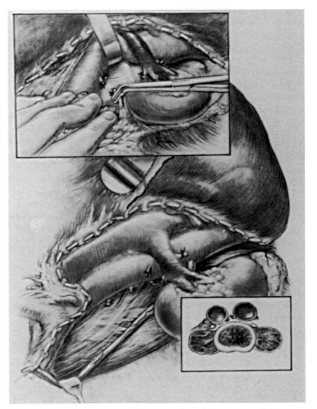

Figure 109–13. The ureter is skeletonized, and the stump of the spermatic cord is removed from the internal inguinal ring. As the specimen is dissected off the anterior spinous ligament, the lumbar vessels are again clipped with hemoclips as they dive into the foramina. The sympathetic chain, not shown here, can usually be clearly identified in the groove between the vertebral body and the psoas muscle and should be protected. Note that the dissection does not disturb any tissue anterior to the aorta below the origin of the inferior mesenteric artery. (From Wise PG, Scardino PT: *In* Skinner DG, Lieskovsky G, eds: Diagnosis and Management of Genitourinary Cancer. Philadelphia, W. B. Saunders Company, 1988, p 779.)

remove the suture that was placed on the end of the cord at the time of orchiectomy.

All of the tissue anterior to the great vessels has now been divided, and the limits of dissection clipped. The "split-and-roll" technique is then used to sweep the posterior lymphatic tissue to the ipsilateral side (Fig. 109–14). The authors begin by elevating the vena cava slightly and clipping and dividing the tissue beneath the cava. This forms the lateral posterior limit of dissection. The aorta can be completely elevated and the tissue swept behind the aorta to the ipsilateral side, sharply dividing the attachments to the anterior vertebral ligaments.

In a limited dissection, the sympathetic chains bilaterally should be identified and protected while sweeping the posterior tissue laterally. They can be found most easily just above the common iliac artery, coursing in the groove between the psoas muscle and the sacrospinalis muscles. Each ligated lumbar artery and vein is encountered a second time as it enters the lumbar foramen and should carefully be clipped again at that level. When the tissue has been swept off the psoas muscles, it can then be removed as an en bloc specimen.

Meticulous hemostasis is crucial, and the authors reinforce the ligatures on the lumbar branches off the aorta with small hemoclips for added security. A small chest tube is routinely placed and generally removed the following morning. The diaphragm is closed with two layers of running No. 0 PGA suture. The abdomen and chest are closed in a single layer of interrupted No. 1 nylon or other permanent suture in a single layer. In the medial portion of the chest incision, the diaphragm should be included in this suture layer to avoid serous leakage into the pleural cavity.

Postoperative care is routine. Intravenous fluid requirements may be high for the first 24 to 48 hours because of third spacing into the retroperitoneum. Postoperative ileus is minimized by the retroperitoneal approach, and most patients are discharged in 3 to 6 days.

Prospective Nerve-Sparing Technique

This technique, as described by Donohue and colleagues (1990) and Jewett (1988), can be used in either a thoracoabdominal or transabdominal procedure and is appropriate in any patient with clinically negative lymph nodes. Setting up of the surgical field is identical to that described previously for a template approach, with the peritoneal envelope mobilized off Gerota's fascia over to the great vessels.

Before beginning the dissection, the first step is to identify the postganglionic nerve fibers coursing in the retroperitoneal fat overlying the anterior aorta from the sympathetic chains bilaterally. These fibers are quite variable and tend to intertwine, as shown in Figure 109–5. Identification of these fibers is relatively easy in a thin individual but may be challenging in someone with significant retroperitoneal fat. Note that the right-sided fibers arise from behind the vena cava and pass anteriorly between the cava and the aorta.

The sympathetic chains can be identified just above the common iliac arteries. As each branch is identified, it is carefully dissected free from the surrounding fat and tagged with a fine vessel loop. The loop can be used to move the fibers back and forth as the lymphatic tissue is dissected out from behind them. The most important fibers to preserve are those arising from the L3 and L4 ganglia, which generally coalesce around the root of the IMA. It is often possible, however, to preserve three or four separate fibers on each side.

Once the nerve fibers have been identified, the authors complete the dissection much in the same way as described previously, simply working around the sympathetics as the tissue is clipped and divided. The lumbar arteries and veins are carefully divided because the nerve fibers are often close by these structures.

Dissecting the nerve fibers clearly adds significant time to the procedure and makes the surgery a bit more tedious. It

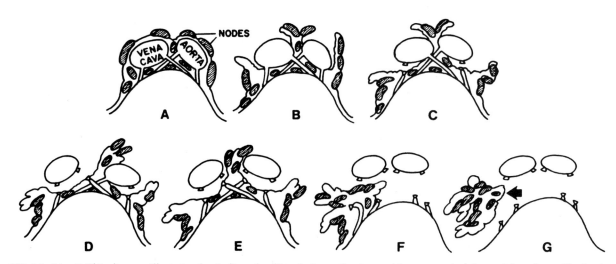

Figure 109–14. *A* to *G*, This diagram illustrates the "split-and-roll" technique allowing en bloc removal of the nodal package. The lumbar vessels must be divided twice, first at the wall of the great vessels and again as they enter the foramina alongside the vertebral bodies. The sympathetic ganglia run in the lateral grooves between the great vessels and psoas muscles, just lateral to the lumbar vessels as they enter the foramina. (From Donohue JP: Urol Clin North Am 1977; 4:509.)

appears, however, to increase significantly the probability of preservation of antegrade ejaculation, especially in left-sided dissection.

Complications

Complications directly caused by the thoracoabdominal approach consist of primarily pulmonary problems. Atelectasis is common but easily managed. Intercostal anesthetic blocks may help the patient who is splinting because of incisional pain. Occasional patients have a high chest tube output or reaccumulate pleural fluid after the chest tube has been removed. This represents leak of retroperitoneal serous fluid into the chest through the diaphragm. If the chest tube is still in, it should be placed on water seal only, which avoids drawing fluid into the chest. If the chest tube is out and the patient is symptomatic, any pleural fluid accumulation may be tapped percutaneously, which generally resolves the problem quickly.

The other problems are common to any retroperitoneal node dissection. The most common intraoperative complication is an inadvertent injury to one of the major vascular structures. Aortic injuries can usually be repaired primarily with 4–0 or 3–0 cardiovascular silk or Prolene, but if difficulty arises or if there is a large defect, a patch graft should be used. Vena cava injuries can essentially always be oversewn, taking care not to narrow the lumen more than 50%. Damage to the main renal artery can also occur and should be repaired if possible. Primary repair may risk subsequent stenosis and hypertension or loss of the unit, and patch or interposition graft material may give a better result. If a small polar artery is ligated or injured, it is best left alone because repairs are rarely successful. All of Gerota's fascia should be stripped from the involved kidney to reduce the chance of hypertension from a collateral vessel (Skinner et al, 1982). Bleeding from an avulsed lumbar vessel should be controlled with an Allis clamp until the area has been completely dissected out and the injury can be clipped or oversewn. Bleeding from deep in the lumbar foramina is controlled with a deep figure-of-eight suture, incorporating some of the periosteum of the vertebral body.

Ureteral injury during dissection is best repaired by ureteroneocystotomy whenever possible. A midureteral or proximal ureteral injury is problematic because of the extensive mobilization of the ureter required during the dissection, with elimination of the collateral blood supply from the gonadal vessels. Ureteroureterostomy can be attempted but should always be stented because of a significant risk of late anastomotic leak or stenosis. Other alternatives include placement of a nephrostomy tube with delayed repair or autotransplantation of the kidney into the pelvis. Nephrectomy may also be considered in the presence of a normal contralateral kidney.

Concern about compromise to the vascular supply to the spinal cord resulting from ligation of the lumbar arteries is unwarranted. The anterior spinal artery syndrome, which has been reported rarely in patients undergoing abdominal aortic aneurysm repair, has not been seen in the authors' experience (Skinner et al, 1982).

Postoperative lymphocele probably occurs more often than reported but is not generally a clinically significant problem. If a symptomatic lymphocele occurs, it is managed first by simple aspiration, then by resection of the wall if it recurs.

Perioperative mortality from this dissection in a patient who has not received chemotherapy should be extremely rare or nonexistent. The one long-term complication is anejaculation, which is discussed in detail subsequently.

Technique of Transabdominal Node Dissection

This surgical approach has been described in detail (Donohue, 1977; Donohue et al, 1988) and continues to be popular because of its familiarity to most surgeons. Once the retroperitoneum has been exposed, the technique and limits of dissection are essentially identical to those detailed earlier. Comments here focus on setting up the surgical exposure, which is identical for right-sided and left-sided tumors.

The incision is made in the midline, from the symphysis pubis to the xiphoid. It is carried down through the subcutaneous tissues, and the linea alba and peritoneum are opened. The abdomen is explored for any unexpected pathology. A self-retaining retractor is placed.

The posterior peritoneum is divided along the root of the small bowel mesentery from the ligament of Treitz to the cecum. Superiorly the inferior mesenteric vein is routinely divided between ligatures to facilitate mobilization of the left colon mesentery (Fig. 109–15). For a limited dissection, the right colon is not mobilized. For a bilateral dissection,

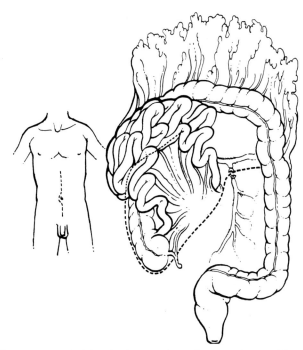

Figure 109–15. Incisions in the posterior peritoneum that provide exposure to the retroperitoneum. In a limited dissection, the incision extends only down to the area of the cecum. In a full dissection, the right colon is completely mobilized, and the small bowel and ascending colon are placed in a plastic bag on the chest. (From Donohue JP: Urol Clin North Am 1977; 4:509.)

the incision in the posterior peritoneum is continued around the cecum and up to the foramen of Winslow. The right colon is mobilized off Gerota's fascia, and the colon and small bowel are placed in a Lahey bag on the chest. The IMA can also be divided at its origin off the aorta to facilitate mobilization of the sigmoid mesentery.

Suprahilar Dissection

In stage IIB disease, the suprahilar areas should be dissected bilaterally. To accomplish this, the head and body of the pancreas are elevated off Gerota's fascia and retracted under two deep Harrington retractors, protected with laparotomy pads. The inferior mesenteric vein must be ligated and divided near its confluence with the splenic vein to accomplish this. The origin of the SMA is identified and skeletonized, clipping the lymphatics around it. The renal arteries are identified bilaterally and dissected a few centimeters toward the renal hilum. The tissue above the renal arteries overlying the crura of the diaphragm, including the celiac ganglia, is clipped in its upper limit and swept inferiorly. The upper limit of dissection over the inferior vena cava is just below the first hepatic vein. On the right, the cisterna chyli is identified overlying the right crus and is clipped. Then the right adrenal vein is carefully ligated and divided. The tissue is dissected off the medial edge of the adrenal gland and off the crus of the diaphragm and removed. On the left, the adrenal vein and small arterial branch off the aorta are individually ligated and divided. Again the tissue is dissected off the medial edge of the adrenal and crus and removed separately. Alternatively the tissue may be passed behind the renal artery and removed en bloc with the infrahilar dissection (Fig. 109–16).

Infrahilar Dissection

Below the renal vessels, the dissection is essentially identical to that described earlier for the retroperitoneal approach. The limits of the inferior dissection are those shown in Figure 109–4, and the "split-and-roll" technique is used to dissect the nodal tissue from around the great vessels and off the posterior abdominal wall muscles (Fig. 109–17).

Postoperative care is routine, although a nasogastric tube may be necessary for several days until the postoperative ileus resolves.

Complications

The main postoperative complication associated with this surgical approach that is not seen in the thoracoabdominal approach is a 3% to 6% incidence of small bowel obstruction, which may require a second surgery (Baniel et al, 1994). Other complications are identical to those discussed previously. Complications that extend the hospital stay more than 2 days occurred in less than 10% of patients in one large series (Baniel et al, 1994).

SURGERY FOR ADVANCED-STAGE DISEASE

Timing of Retroperitoneal Dissection in Stage III Disease

There is general agreement that all patients with advanced testicular cancer, stage IIC (palpable retroperitoneal disease or a mass >10 cm) or stage III (disease beyond the retroperi-

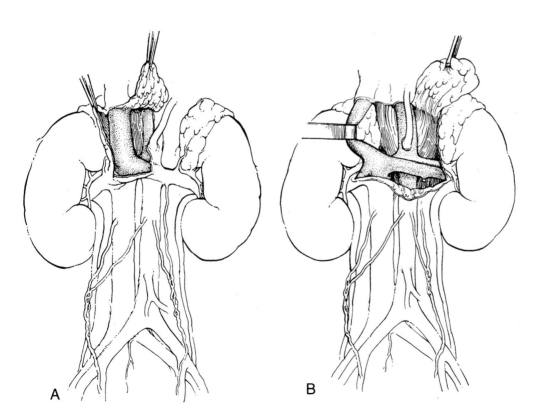

Figure 109–16. Right *(A)* and left *(B)* suprahilar dissections extending 4 to 6 cm above the renal arteries, exposing the crura of the diaphragm. (From Donohue JP: Urol Clin North Am 1977; 4:509.)

A   B

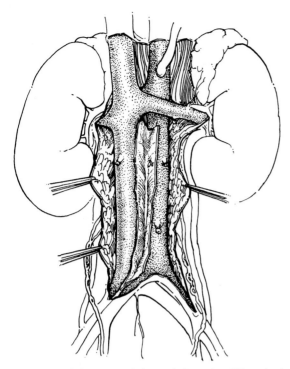

Figure 109–17. Infrahilar transabdominal dissection. When the lumbar arteries and veins have been divided, the great vessels are elevated and the nodal package is swept off the anterior vertebral ligament and posterior abdominal wall muscles. In a limited dissection, the division of the tissue overlying the aorta would extend only down to the origin of the inferior mesenteric artery. (From Donohue JP: Urol Clin North Am 1977; 4:509.)

toneal lymphatics) should be treated primarily with full-dose, platinum-based chemotherapy. The specifics of the chemotherapy are beyond the scope of this chapter. The patient must be treated until the serum markers normalize, or a minimum of four cycles of the standard PEB regimen. Repeat CT scan of the abdomen and chest is then performed.

If the patient has any evidence of residual retroperitoneal disease on CT scan or if the primary tumor contained teratomatous elements, he is scheduled for a node dissection 4 to 6 weeks after the last chemotherapy treatment.

In the authors' experience, it is rare for a patient with a significant pretreatment mass to achieve a radiographic complete response (Carter et al, 1987). The patient with minimal to moderate retroperitoneal disease and lung metastases, however, especially with pure embryonal cell carcinoma, may have a normal CT scan after chemotherapy (Dexeus et al, 1989). In the Indiana University experience, 70% to 80% of all patients with stages IIC and III nonseminoma have been managed without retroperitoneal dissection (Donohue et al, 1987). Some investigators have suggested that patients with small residual masses or greater than 90% reduction in the size of the mass could also be managed with observation alone (Donohue et al, 1987; Toner et al, 1990). Herr and colleagues, however, found that 8 of 43 patients who fit these criteria had either malignancy or teratoma on retroperitoneal dissection (Herr et al, 1991). This included several patients who had no teratoma in the primary tumor. They concluded that all patients with a prechemotherapy mass greater than 3 cm should undergo surgical resection.

Mature teratoma in the retroperitoneum is not effectively eradicated by chemotherapy and has a tendency for persistent growth over many years (Logothetis et al, 1982). Although the metastatic potential of such growth is controversial, there is no doubt that it can cause significant, life-threatening problems owing to renal obstruction, mediastinal compression, and possible malignant degeneration. **Therefore, all patients with teratoma in the primary tumor are best served by retroperitoneal dissection shortly after completing chemotherapy, regardless of the CT scan findings.**

Patients with residual disease outside the retroperitoneum require resection of that disease in addition to retroperitoneal dissection. The order of these surgeries is decided on an individual basis. Neck dissection and thoracotomy for pulmonary disease are generally well tolerated with a short postoperative recovery time. These are often best performed initially, allowing the patient to proceed with retroperitoneal dissection soon after the other surgeries. In addition, if the patient is found to have residual viable cancer in the neck or lungs, he is best referred for salvage chemotherapy before retroperitoneal dissection.

A large retroperitoneal mass should probably be dealt with first because of the risk of progressive involvement of surrounding structures. Ipsilateral pulmonary disease can certainly be resected at the same time as the retroperitoneal dissection if a high thoracoabdominal incision is used. Interestingly, Gerl and colleagues (1994) found that 15 of 38 patients undergoing multiple surgical resections had dissimilar histology in the two locations, with 3 showing less favorable histology in the smaller mass. They underlined the importance of proceeding with retroperitoneal dissection even if initial pulmonary resection shows only fibrosis.

Patients with rising tumor markers are rarely cured with surgery alone. They should be treated with salvage chemotherapy before resection of any residual masses, perhaps with consideration for autologous bone marrow transplantation. Occasionally, surgery is indicated as a last attempt to achieve a cure in a patient who has failed all chemotherapy, but the results are disappointing.

The histology of the residual mass in postchemotherapy dissections is fibrosis or scar tissue in 27% to 58%, mature teratoma in 22% to 38%, and viable carcinoma in 12% to 35% (Vugrin et al, 1981; Donohue and Rowland, 1984; Stoter et al, 1984; Loehrer et al, 1986; Carter et al, 1987). **Patients with residual malignant elements should receive additional chemotherapy, with an expected long-term cure rate of 70% compared to less than 50% without it** (Skinner, 1976; Donohue et al, 1994). If such patients have already received salvage chemotherapy, however, continued chemotherapy does not appear to have any additional benefit (Donohue et al, 1994).

Patients with pathologic findings of mature teratoma in the retroperitoneal dissection are generally followed without additional treatment. They may be at somewhat higher risk of late recurrence than those with fibrosis only, and these recurrences may be in the form of mature or immature teratoma or frank carcinoma (Loehrer et al, 1986). With a meticulous retroperitoneal dissection, these recurrences should be outside the area of dissection. Therefore, careful follow-up is mandatory for at least 5 years in these patients.

Occasionally the histology of the residual mass may demonstrate sarcomatous elements, such as embryonal rhabdomyosarcoma or angiosarcoma. This finding occurred in 11 of 269 patients at Indiana University over 6 years. Often the non–germ cell elements were present in the primary tumor as well and perhaps were unmasked by the disappearance of the metastatic germ cell elements with chemotherapy. Alternatively, this histology may represent true degeneration of metastatic teratomatous elements. Regardless of the etiology, the presence of these sarcomatous elements carries a poor prognosis, and the optimum therapy is unknown (Loehrer et al, 1986).

Management of Residual Mass in Advanced Seminoma

Similar to nonseminomatous disease, advanced seminoma is best treated with platinum-based chemotherapy (Peckham et al, 1985; Loehrer et al, 1987). The management of residual tumor after chemotherapy remains controversial. Viable tumor cells are discovered in the residual mass in 0% to 43% of patients, depending in part on the size of the mass (Motzer et al, 1988; Schultz et al, 1989). **Completing a thorough RPLND is often difficult or impossible in these cases, owing to a thick sheet of fibrous reactive tissue that encases the great vessels.** Many workers recommend an excision of the mass alone, rather than a full node dissection (Motzer et al, 1988).

All series have relatively small numbers, and it has not been proven that resection of residual masses translates to a survival advantage in these cases. If residual viable tumor is identified, however, those patients should receive further chemotherapy or radiation therapy. Routine consolidation radiation therapy of residual masses does not appear to prevent relapse and can significantly limit the tolerance of further chemotherapy (Peckham et al, 1985).

The authors' current policy is to resect surgically any residual retroperitoneal mass greater than 3 cm after chemotherapy. Masses less than 3 cm are observed with CT scan every 3 to 4 months the first year and every 6 to 12 months for at least 5 years.

Technique of Retroperitoneal Node Dissection for Advanced Disease

Preoperative Preparation

Patients who have been exposed to chemotherapy require special attention to prepare them for such extensive surgery. The white blood cell and platelet counts must be at normal levels before surgery. Patients who have received bleomycin should have pulmonary function assessed. **The anesthesiologist must be advised about the need to maintain a low inspired oxygen level and low crystalloid replacement throughout the perioperative period** (Viljoen et al, 1988). In addition, patients may have other problems, such as renal insufficiency or anemia, which should be addressed.

The authors do a routine mechanical bowel preparation on these patients, with full antibiotic preparation on those suspected to have small or large bowel involvement by tumor. In selected cases, other consultants are involved, such

as the vascular surgeon if replacement of the abdominal aorta or an external iliac vessel is anticipated.

Surgical Technique

RPLND following chemotherapy is one of the most difficult surgeries undertaken by urologists. The CT scan often underestimates the extent of disease, and there is nearly always extensive fibrosis around the great vessels and renal hilum, making dissection tedious and risky. This surgery should not be attempted by the occasional surgeon and requires training in vascular techniques.

Patients with a significant retroperitoneal mass are best approached through a thoracoabdominal incision. Suprahilar dissections are necessary, often extending high into the retrocrural space, and the exposure to this area is clearly superior through a high (sixth to eighth rib) thoracoabdominal incision. In patients with minimal retroperitoneal disease, the dissection may be completed entirely retroperitoneally, as described previously. With a significant mass, however, the authors routinely open the peritoneal cavity.

The patient positioning and initial steps of the exposure are identical to those described previously for low-stage disease. It is helpful to separate the peritoneal envelope from the diaphragm back to the central tendon before opening the peritoneum because this facilitates mobilization of the liver or spleen and pancreas. The peritoneum is then opened, and the right colon and root of the small bowel mesentery are mobilized off the retroperitoneum (Fig. 109–18). The bowel is placed in a Lahey bag on the chest. It is not uncommon to find invasion of the duodenum by the mass,

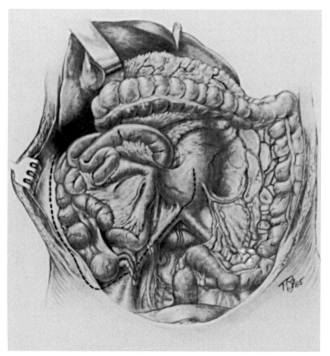

Figure 109–18. Exposure of the retroperitoneum via a thoracoabdominal, transperitoneal approach for advanced disease following chemotherapy. The posterior peritoneum is incised from the ligament of Treitz down along the root of the small bowel mesentery, around the cecum, and up the right colic gutter. This maneuver allows all of the small bowel and ascending colon to be placed into a plastic bag on the chest.

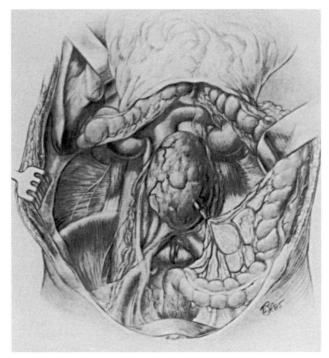

Figure 109–19. The inferior mesenteric artery, which often is encased in the mass, is divided. The left colon is mobilized off Gerota's fascia. The sigmoid mesentery may be adherent to the mass and can be resected, provided that the marginal artery remains intact.

which may require partial duodenal resection. The posterior peritoneum is divided lateral to the left colon, and the sigmoid mesentery is mobilized off Gerota's fascia. The IMA is divided if tumor extends to the inferior aorta. The sigmoid mesentery may also be invaded by tumor, and the mesenteric vessels may be divided, provided that the marginal artery and veins are left intact (Fig. 109–19).

The SMA must be identified early and its root dissected, clipping the small lymphatic channels running along its surface. The renal vein is mobilized, and both the right and the left renal arteries are dissected. If this area is encased by tumor, normal areas of the vena cava and aorta should be mobilized above and below the tumor before beginning the dissection to obtain vascular control.

The "split-and-roll" technique is used throughout the dissection. The tumor mass is divided over the vena cava and aorta, finding the plane between the fibrous capsule of the tumor and the wall of the great vessels. If dissection proceeds too superficially (e.g., within the tumor capsule), tumor spill is likely, and an incomplete resection results. Too-deep dissection on the aorta results in a thinned-out wall, which may result in a delayed rupture. The gonadal vessels are ligated bilaterally, as are all lumbar arteries and veins below the renal vessels. The latter may be difficult if a large amount of retroaortic disease is present.

The ureters should be dissected early, before approaching the renal arteries. If one ureter is completely encased or directly invaded by tumor, that kidney may best be sacrificed rather than risking an incomplete dissection. Once the ureters are free, the renal arteries bilaterally are dissected from the aorta to the renal hilum. Often, multiple arteries make this dissection difficult. If a polar artery is injured or divided,

care should be taken to strip off Gerota's fascia completely from that kidney to reduce the risk of late hypertension.

Specialized vascular techniques may be required during the dissection, including suture repair; vascular patch graft; or complete replacement of the aorta, renal, or iliac vessels (Kelly et al, 1995). The vena cava may require repair or formal resection. The vena cava can safely be ligated below the renal veins if tumor extends into it in the form of a tumor thrombus or directly invades the wall. The patient may develop significant edema of the lower extremities, but this gradually resolves.

Superiorly the tissue overlying the crura of the diaphragm is resected and swept inferiorly with the main nodal package. If there is any question of retrocrural disease, the crus should be divided alongside the vertebral body. The retrocrural tissue is dissected as far superiorly as possible. The lumbar vessels should not be ligated if possible because there is some risk of devascularization of the spine. On the right, the thoracic duct should be carefully clipped, and the hemiazygous vein may be ligated if necessary. The crus should be repaired after removing the nodal tissue.

When the great vessels have been fully mobilized, the tumor is dissected off the posterior body wall. The lumbar arteries and veins are again clipped as they dive into the foramina. Tongues of tumor may extend down into the foramina alongside the lumbar vessels and should be teased out if possible. The anterior psoas fascia should be removed with the tumor, and some of the muscle itself may need to come with the tumor. This may result in significant bleeding that is difficult to control.

In the case of a large mass, generally no attempt is made to preserve the sympathetic trunks. Some authors, however, have advocated a modified template for dissection even in postchemotherapy patients (Wood et al, 1992). The key is patient selection. If the prechemotherapy mass was centered around the IMA (as shown in Fig. 109–19), the dissection must be carried down over the lower aorta and presacral area, to the level of the bifurcation of the common iliac arteries, and anejaculation is inevitable. If all the disease was up around the renal vessels, a modified approach to the lower limits of dissection may be reasonable. In that setting, even postganglionic sympathetic fibers can occasionally be dissected inferiorly. **Most importantly, metastatic testicular cancer is a curable disease when treated appropriately, and any risk of leaving tumor behind in the hopes of preserving ejaculation is not acceptable in this setting.** One should remember that fertility is already compromised in many of these patients because of effects of the chemotherapy (see previous discussion).

Complications

Major intraoperative and postoperative complications are more common in patients with large-volume retroperitoneal disease (Donohue and Rowland, 1981; Skinner et al, 1982; Baniel et al, 1995). Vascular complications, discussed in detail previously, are common but should not pose a problem if the surgeon is prepared. Complete replacement of the infrarenal aorta has been accomplished in selected patients, with excellent results (Kelly et al, 1995).

Major postoperative complications occurred in 9 of 52

patients (17%) with stage IIC or II disease in the authors' series (Skinner et al, 1982) and 125 of 603 patients (20.7%) in the Indiana University experience (Baniel et al, 1995). The perioperative mortality in both series was under 1%. The most devastating complication is fatal adult respiratory distress syndrome associated with bleomycin toxicity. Gold-finger and Schweizer (1979) associated this risk with increased inspired oxygen and overhydration. This risk must be kept in mind constantly and requires the cooperation of the anesthesiologist, surgeon, and intensivists to avoid problems. The authors generally ventilate the patients with room air during surgery, never raising inspired FIO_2 to exceed 25% to 30%. The authors also use a colloid-to-crystalloid ratio of 2:1 during the perioperative period and carefully avoid overhydration.

Many other major complications have been reported, including other pulmonary complications, hemorrhage, thrombophlebitis, small bowel obstruction, wound infection or dehiscence, and pancreatitis. Pneumonia and wound infections accounted for nearly half of all of the complications seen (Baniel et al, 1995).

Despite the magnitude of this surgery, patients tolerate the procedure remarkably well, and there have been few long-term complications other than anejaculation. The efficacy of the procedure is attested to by the fact that retroperitoneal recurrences are exceedingly rare after a complete node dissection, even with advanced disease.

REFERENCES

Aass N, Fossa SD, Ous S, et al: Is routine primary retroperitoneal lymph node dissection still justified in patients with low stage non-seminomatous testicular cancer? Br J Urol 1990; 65:385–390.

Ahlering TA, Skinner DG: Vena caval resection in bulky metastatic germ cell tumors. J Urol 1989; 142:1497–1499.

Amelar RD, Dubin L, Hotchkiss RS: Restoration of fertility following unilateral orchiectomy and radiation therapy for testicular tumors. J Urol 1971; 106:714–718.

Baniel J, Foster RS, Rowland RG, et al: Complications of primary retroperitoneal lymph node dissection. J Urol 1994; 152:424–427.

Baniel J, Foster RS, Rowland RG, et al: Complications of post-chemotherapy retroperitoneal lymph node dissection. J Urol 1995; 153:976–980.

Bar-Charma N, Herr HW, Sogani PC, Whitmore WF Jr: The fertility of males with stage I nonseminomatous germ-cell tumor of the testis managed with surveillance alone (Abstract). J Urol 1992; 147:337A.

Bennett CJ, Seager SWJ, McGuire E: Electroejaculation for recovery of semen after retroperitoneal lymph node dissection: Case report. J Urol 1987; 137:513–515.

Benson CJ: The role of ultrasound in diagnosis and staging of testicular cancer. Semin Urol 1988; 6:189–202.

Bochner BH, Lerner SP, Kawachi M, et al: Post radical orchiectomy hemorrhage: Should an alteration in staging strategy for testicular cancer be considered? Urology 1995; 46:408–411.

Boileau MA, Steers WD: Testis tumors: The clinical significance of the tumor-contaminated scrotum. J Urol 1984; 132:51–54.

Calvo F, Hodson N, Barrett A, Peckham MJ: Chemotherapy of primary (in situ) testicular tumors: Response in advanced metastatic disease. Br J Urol 1983; 55:560–563.

Capelouto CC, Clark PE, Ransil BJ, Loughlin KR: A review of scrotal violation in testicular cancer: Is adjuvant local therapy necessary? J Urol 1995; 153:981–985.

Carter GE, Lieskovsky G, Skinner DG, Daniels JR: Reassessment of the role of adjunctive surgical therapy in the treatment of advanced germ cell tumors. J Urol 1987; 138:1397–1401.

Colleselli K, Poisel S, Schachtner W, Bartch G: Nerve-preserving bilateral retroperitoneal lymphadenectomy: Anatomical study and operative approach. J Urol 1990; 144:293–298.

Dexeus FH, Shirkhoda A, Logothetis CJ, et al: Clinical and radiological correlation of retroperitoneal metastasis from nonseminomatous testicular cancer treated with chemotherapy. Eur J Can Clin Oncol 1989; 23:35–43.

Dieckmann KP, Huland H, Gross AJ: A test for the identification of relevant sympathetic nerve fibers during nerve sparing retroperitoneal lymphadenectomy. J Urol 1992; 148:1450–1452.

Doerr A, Skinner EC, Skinner DG: Preservation of ejaculation through a modified retroperitoneal lymph node dissection in low stage testis cancer. J Urol 1993; 149:1472–1474.

Donohue JP: Retroperitoneal lymphadenectomy: The anterior approach including bilateral suprarenal-hilar dissection. Urol Clin North Am 1977; 4:509–521.

Donohue JP, Foster RS, Rowland RG, et al: Nerve-sparing retroperitoneal lymphadenectomy with preservation of ejaculation. J Urol 1990; 144:287–292.

Donohue JP, Fox EP, Williams SD, et al: Persistent cancer in postchemotherapy retroperitoneal lymph-node dissection: Outcome analysis. World J Urol 1994; 12:190–195.

Donohue JP, Rowland RG: Complications of retroperitoneal lymph node dissection. J Urol 1981; 125:338–340.

Donohue JP, Rowland RG: The role of surgery in advanced testicular cancer. Cancer 1984; 54:2716–2721.

Donohue JP, Rowland RG, Bihrle RG: Transabdominal retroperitoneal lymph node dissection. In Skinner DG, Lieskovsky G, eds: Diagnosis and Management of Genitourinary Cancer. Philadelphia, W. B. Saunders, 1988, pp 802–916.

Donohue JP, Rowland RG, Kopechky K, et al: Correlation of computerized tomographic changes and histologic findings in 80 patients having radical retroperitoneal lymph node dissection after chemotherapy for testis cancer. J Urol 1987; 137:1170–1175.

Donohue JP, Thornhill JA, Foster RS, et al: Retroperitoneal lymphadenectomy for clinical stage A testis cancer (1965 to 1989): Modifications of technique and impact on ejaculation. J Urol 1993; 149:237–243.

Donohue JP, Thornhill JA, Foster RS, et al: The role of retroperitoneal lymphadenectomy in clinical stage B testis cancer: The Indiana University experience (1965–1989). J Urol 1995; 153:85–89.

Donohue JP, Zachary JM, Maynard BR: Distribution of nodal metastases in nonseminomatous testis cancer. J Urol 1982; 128:315–320.

Drasga RE, Einhorn LH, Williams SD, et al: Fertility after chemotherapy for testicular cancer. J Clin Oncol 1983; 1:179–183.

Duchesne GM, Horwich A, Dearnaley DP, et al: Orchidectomy alone for stage I seminoma of the testis. Cancer 1990; 65:1115–1118.

Dunphy CH, Ayala AG, Swanson DA, et al: Clinical stage I nonseminomatous and mixed germ cell tumors of the testis: A clinicopathologic study of 93 patients on a surveillance protocol after orchiectomy alone. Cancer 1988; 62:1202–1206.

Ehrlichman RJ, Kaugman SL, Siegelman SS, et al: Computerized tomography and lymphangiography in staging testis tumors. J Urol 1981; 126:179–181.

Fernandez EB, Colon E, McLeod DG, Moul JW: Efficacy of radiographic chest imaging in patients with testicular cancer. Urology 1994; 44:243–248.

Fossa A, Fossa SD: Serum lactate dehydrogenase and human choriogonadotrophin in seminoma. Br J Urol 1989; 63:408–415.

Fossa SD, Ous S, Abyholm T, Loeb M: Post-treatment fertility in patients with testicular cancer: I. Influence of retroperitoneal lymph node dissection on ejaculatory potential. Br J Urol 1985; 57:204–209.

Fossa SD, Qvist H, Steinwig AL, et al: Is postchemotherapy retroperitoneal surgery necessary in patients with nonseminomatous testicular cancer and minimal residual tumor mass? J Clin Oncol 1992; 10:569–573.

Foster RS, McNulty A, Rubin LR, et al: The fertility of patients with clinical stage I testis cancer managed by nerve sparing retroperitoneal lymph node dissection. J Urol 1994; 152:1139–1143.

Fowler JE, Whitmore WF Jr: Intratesticular germ cell tumors: Observations on the effect of chemotherapy. J Urol 1981; 126:412–414.

Freedman LS, Jones WG, Peckham MJ, et al: Histopathology in the prediction of relapse of patients with stage I testicular teratoma treated by orchiectomy alone. Lancet 1987; 2:295–297.

Freiha F, Torti F: Orchiectomy only for clinical stage I non-seminomatous germ cell testis tumors: Comparison with pathologic stage I disease. Urology 1989; 34:347–348.

Fung CY, Kalish LA, Brodsky GL, et al: Stage I nonseminomatous germ cell testicular tumor: Prediction of metastatic potential by primary histopathology. J Clin Oncol 1988; 6:1467–1473.

Gelderman WAH, Koops HS, Sleijfer DT, et al: Orchidectomy alone in stage I nonseminomatous testicular germ cell tumors. Cancer 1987; 59:578–580.

Gerber GS, Bissada NK, Hulbert JC, et al: Laparoscopic retroperitoneal lymphadenectomy: Multi-institutional analysis. J Urol 1994; 152:1188–1191.

Gerl A, Clemm C, Schmeller N, et al: Sequential resection of residual abdominal and thoracic masses after chemotherapy for metastatic nonseminomatous germ cell tumours. Br J Cancer 1994; 70:960–965.

Giguere JK, Stablein DM, Spaulding JT, et al: The clinical significance of unconventional orchiectomy approaches in testicular cancer: A report from the testicular cancer intergroup study. J Urol 1988; 139:1225–1228.

Goldfinger PL, Schweizer O: The hazards of anesthesia and surgery in bleomycin treated patients. Semin Oncol 1979; 6:121–124.

Hansen SW, Berthelsen JG, von der Maase H: Long-term fertility and Leydig cell function in patients treated for germ cell cancer with cisplatin, vinblastine, and bleomycin versus surveillance. J Clin Oncol 1990; 8:1695–1698.

Herr HW, Toner GC, Geller NL, Bosl GJ: Patient selection for retroperitoneal lymph node dissection after chemotherapy for nonseminomatous germ cell tumors. Eur Urol 1991; 19:1–5.

Horwich A, Alsanjari N, Ahern R, et al: Surveillance following orchidectomy for stage I testicular seminoma. Br J Cancer 1992; 65:775–778.

Javadpour N: Biological tumor markers in the management of testicular and bladder cancer. Urology 1978; 12:177–183.

Jewett MAS, Kong Y-S, Goldberg SD, et al: Retroperitoneal lymphadenectomy for testis tumor with nerve sparing for ejaculation. J Urol 1988; 139:1220–1224.

Jewett MA, Wesley JT: Early and late complications of retroperitoneal lymphadenectomy in testis cancer. Can J Surg 1991; 34:368–373.

Kelly R, Skinner DG, Yellin AE, Weaver FA: En bloc aortic resection for bulky metastatic germ cell tumors. J Urol 1995; 153:1849–1851.

Lange PH, Chang WY, Fraley EE: Fertility issues in the therapy of nonseminomatous testicular tumors. Urol Clin North Am 1987; 24:731–747.

Lange PH, Narayan P, Fraley EE: Fertility issues following therapy for testicular cancer. Semin Urol 1984; 2:264–274.

Lieskovsky G, Weinberg AC, Skinner DG: Surgical management of early-stage nonseminomatous germ cell tumors of the testis. Semin Urol 1984; 2:208–216.

Loehrer PJ Sr, Birch R, Williams SD, et al: Chemotherapy of metastatic seminoma: The Southeastern Cancer Study Group experience. J Clin Oncol 1987; 5:1212–1220.

Loehrer PJ Sr, Hui S, Clark S, et al: Teratoma following cisplatin-based combination chemotherapy for nonseminomatous germ cell tumors: A clinico-pathological correlation. J Urol 1986; 135:1183–1189.

Logothetis CJ, Samuels ML, Trindade A, Johnson DE: The growing teratoma syndrome. Cancer 1982; 50:1629–1635.

Logothetis CJ, Swanson DA, Dexeus F, et al: Primary chemotherapy for clinical stage II nonseminomatous germ-cell tumor of the testis: A follow-up of 50 patients. J Clin Oncol 1987; 5:906–911.

Lowe BA: Surveillance versus nerve-sparing retroperitoneal lymph node dissection in stage I nonseminomatous germ-cell tumors. Urol Clin North Am 1993; 20:75–83.

Maier JG, Sulak NH: Radiation therapy in malignant testis tumors: Carcinoma. Cancer 1973; 32:1217–1226.

Markland C, Kedia K, Fraley EE: Inadequate orchiectomy for patients with testicular tumors. JAMA 1973; 224:1025–1026.

Moller MB, d'Amore F, Christensen BE: Testicular lymphoma: A population-based study of incidence, clinicopathological correlation and prognosis: The Danish Lymphoma Study Group. Eur J Cancer 1994; 30A:1760–1764.

Motzer RJ, Bosl GJ, Geller NJ, et al: Advanced seminoma: The role of chemotherapy and adjunctive surgery. Ann Intern Med 1988; 108:513–518.

Motzer RJ, Geller NL, Tan CC, et al: Salvage chemotherapy for patients with germ cell tumors: The Memorial Sloan Kettering Cancer Center experience (1979–1989). Cancer 1991; 67:1305–1310.

Moul JW, Robertson JE, George SL, et al: Complications of therapy for testicular cancer. J Urol 1989; 142:1491–1496.

Nicolai N, Pizzocaro G: Ten year follow-up of a surveillance study in clinical stage I non-seminomatous germ cell tumors of the testis (NSGCTT) (Abstract). J Urol 1995; 153:245A.

Ohl DA, Denil J, Bennett CJ, et al: Electroejaculation following retroperitoneal lymphadenectomy. J Urol 1991; 145:980–983.

Osanto S, Bukman A, Van Hoek F, et al: Long-term effects of chemotherapy in patients with testicular cancer. J Clin Oncol 1992; 10:574–579.

Peckham MJ, Horwich A, Hendry WF: Advanced seminoma: Treatment with cis-platinum-based combination chemotherapy or carboplatin (JM8). Br J Cancer 1985; 52:7–13.

Pizzocaro G, Salvioni R, Zanoni F: Unilateral lymphadenectomy in intraoperative stage I nonseminomatous germinal testis cancer. J Urol 1985; 134:485–489.

Presti JC, Herr HW, Carroll PR: Fertility and testis cancer. Urol Clin North Am 1993; 20:173–179.

Pritchett TR, Skinner DG, Selser SF, Kern WH: Seminoma with elevated human chorionic gonadotrophin: The case for retroperitoneal lymph node dissection. Urology 1985; 25:344–346.

Richie JP: Clinical stage I testicular cancer: The role of modified retroperitoneal lymphadenectomy. J Urol 1990; 144:1160–1163.

Richie JP, Kantoff PW: Is adjuvant chemotherapy necessary for patients with stage B testicular cancer? J Clin Oncol 1991; 9:1393–1396.

Roth BJ, Greist A, Kubilis PS, et al: Cisplatin-based chemotherapy for disseminated germ cell tumors: Long-term follow-up. J Clin Oncol 1988; 6:1239–1247.

Sagalowsky AI, Ewalt DH, Molberg K, Peters PC: Predictors of residual mass histology after chemotherapy for advanced testis cancer. Urology 1990; 35:537–542.

Scardino PT: Adjuvant chemotherapy is of value following retroperitoneal lymph node dissection for nonseminomatous testicular tumors. Urol Clin North Am 1980; 7:735–745.

Schultz SM, Einhorn LH, Conces DJ Jr, et al: Management of postchemotherapy residual mass in patients with advanced seminoma: Indiana University experience. J Clin Oncol 1989; 7:1497–1503.

Schwartz DA, Johnson DE, Hussey DH: Should an elevated human chorionic gonadotrophin titer alter therapy for seminoma? J Urol 1984; 131:63–65.

Sheinfeld J, Bajorin D: Management of the postchemotherapy residual mass. Urol Clin North Am 1993; 20:133–143.

Simmonds PD, Mead GM, Lee AH, et al: Orchectomy after chemotherapy in patients with metastatic testicular cancer: Is it indicated? Cancer 1995; 75:1018–1024.

Siracusano S, Sau G, Aiello I, et al: The skin response in evaluation of the sympathetic chains after retroperitoneal lymphadenectomy: Preliminary report. Scand J Urol Nephrol 1994; 28:405–407.

Skinner DG: Non-seminomatous testis tumors: A plan of management based on 96 patients to improve survival in all stages by combined therapeutic modalities. J Urol 1976; 115:65–69.

Skinner DG, Lieskovsky G: The thoracoabdominal approach for management of nonseminomatous germ cell tumors of the testis (Movie). Norwich, New York, Norwich Eaton, Inc., 1984.

Skinner DG, Melamud A, Lieskovsky G: Complications of thoracoabdominal retroperitoneal lymph node dissection. J Urol 1982; 127:1107–1110.

Sternberg C: Role of primary chemotherapy in stage I and low-volume stage II nonseminomatous germ-cell testis tumors. Urol Clin North Am 1993; 20:93–109.

Stone NN, Schlussel RN, Waterhouse RL, Unver P: Laparoscopic retroperitoneal lymph node dissection in stage A nonseminomatous testis cancer. Urology 1993; 42:610–614.

Stoter G, Vendrick CP, Struyvenberg A, et al: Five-year survival of patients with disseminated nonseminomatous testicular cancer treated with cisplatin, vinblastine, and bleomycin. Cancer 1984; 54:1521–1524.

Studer UE, Fey MF, Calderoni A, et al: Adjuvant chemotherapy after orchiectomy in high-risk patients with clinical stage I non-seminomatous testicular cancer. Eur Urol 1993; 23:444–449.

Sturgeon JF, Jewett MA, Alison RE, et al: Surveillance after orchidectomy for patients with clinical stage I nonseminomatous testis tumors. J Clin Oncol 1992; 10:564–568.

Swanson DA, von Eschenbah AC, Babaian RJ, Dinney CP: The advantage of retroperitoneal lymph node dissection instead of initial chemotherapy for clinical stage II nonseminomatous germ cell testicular tumors (Abstract). J Urol 1995; 153:244A.

Toner GC, Panicek DM, Heeland RT, et al: Adjunctive surgery after chemotherapy for nonseminomatous germ cell tumors: Recommendations for patient selection. J Clin Oncol 1990; 8:1683–1694.

Turner RR, Colby TV, MacKintosh FR: Testicular lymphomas: A clinico-pathologic study of 35 cases. Cancer 1981; 48:2095–2102.

van der Maase H, Specht L, Jacobsen GK, et al: Surveillance following orchidectomy for stage I seminoma of the testis. Eur J Cancer 1993; 29A:1931–1934.

Viljoen JF, Thangathurai D: Anesthetic management in radical surgery for urologic malignancies. *In* Skinner DG, Lieskovsky G, eds: Diagnosis and Management of Genitourinary Cancer. Philadelphia, W. B. Saunders, 1988, pp 595–600.

Vogelsang NJ, Bosl GJ, Johnson K, Kennedy BJ: Raynaud's phenomenon: A common toxicity after combination chemotherapy for testicular cancer. Ann Intern Med 1981; 95:288–292.

Vugrin D, Whitmore WF Jr: The role of chemotherapy and surgery in the treatment of retroperitoneal metastases in advanced nonseminomatous testis cancer. Cancer 1985; 55:1874–1878.

Vugrin D, Whitmore WF Jr, Sogani PC, et al: Combination chemotherapy and surgery in the treatment of advanced germ-cell tumors. Cancer 1981; 47:2228–2231.

Weidner W, Zoller G, Sauerwein D, et al: A modified technique for nerve-sparing retroperitoneal lymph node dissection in stage II nonseminomatous germ cell tumors using intraoperative measurement of bladder neck pressure alterations following sympathetic nerve fiber electrostimulation. Eur Urol 1994; 26:67–70.

Weiss RB, Stablein DM, Muggia FM, et al: Toxicity comparisons between 2 chemotherapy regimens as adjuvant or salvage treatment in nonseminomatous testicular cancer. Cancer 1988; 62:18–23.

Wetlaufer JN: The management of advanced seminoma. Semin Urol 1984; 2:257–263.

Williams SD, Stablein DM, Einhorn LH, et al: Immediate adjuvant chemotherapy versus observation with treatment at relapse in pathological stage II testicular cancer. N Engl J Med 1987; 317:1433–1438.

Wishnow KI, Johnson DE, Tenney DM: Are lymphangiograms necessary before placing patients with nonseminomatous testicular tumors on surveillance? J Urol 1989a; 41:1133–1135.

Wishnow KI, Johnson DE, Tenney DM, et al: Identifying patients with low-risk clinical stage I nonseminomatous testicular tumors who should be treated by surveillance. Urology 1989b; 34:339–343.

Wood DP Jr, Herr HW, Heller G, et al: Distribution of retroperitoneal metastases after chemotherapy in patients with nonseminomatous germ cell tumors. J Urol 1992; 148:1812–1816.

Young BJ, Bultz BD, Russell JA, Trew MS: Compliance with follow-up of patients treated for non-seminomatous testicular cancer. Br J Cancer 1991; 64:606–608.

INDEX

Note: Page numbers in *italics* refer to illustrations; page numbers followed by t refer to tables.

Berry aneurysm, in autosomal dominant polycystic kidney disease, 1771
Beta-inhibin, 1393t, 1395
Betamethasone, biologic activity of, 2940t
Beta-microseminoprotein, 1393t, 1395
Bethanechol chloride (Duvoid, Urecholine), bladder effects of, 882, 883, 883t, 884
    complications of, 991
    in geriatric incontinence, 956
    in neuropathic voiding dysfunction, 990–991
    ureteral effects of, 850
Bethanechol test, during cystometry, 936
Bezoar, fungal, Candida in, 781, 781, 784, 784, 786, 2836–2837, 2837t
    percutaneous removal of, 2836–2837, 2837t
Bias, in clinical trials, 1459–1460
Bicarbonate, in acute renal failure, 325
    renal reabsorption of, 2673, 2673
        chloride levels and, 300
        in neonate, 1657, 1659
    serum, after augmentation cystoplasty, 3178
    urinary, in renal tubular acidosis, 2686–2687
Bicarbonate buffer system, 297–298
Biceps femoris musculocutaneous unit, in inguinal reconstruction, 2478
Bicornuate uterus, 2121t
Bile salts, malabsorption of, after urinary intestinal diversion, 3156
Bilharcil (metrifonate), in schistosomiasis, 747
Bilharzial bladder cancer syndrome, 750, 752–754
Bilharzioma, 757
Bilirubin, urinary, 152–153
Biltricide (praziquantel), in schistosomiasis, 747
Biofeedback, cystometric, in urinary incontinence, 1033
    in neuropathic voiding dysfunction, 972, 982–983
    in pelvic floor exercises, 1032–1033
Bioglass, in endoscopic vesicoureteral reflux, 1894
Bioplastique, for periurethral injection therapy, 1111
Biopsy, bladder, in diverticulum tumor, 2358
    in interstitial cystitis, 643
    in tuberculosis, 823
    in penile squamous cell carcinoma, 2460
    needle, in prostate cancer, 2498, 2500–2501, 2519
    percutaneous, 253–255, 255
    percutaneous, 253–255, 255
    of urothelial lesion, 248
    renal, 2808–2809
    testicular, 1332–1334, 1333, 1334
        in children, 2199
        in hypogonadotropic hypogonadism, 1305
        in male infertility, 1303–1305, 1304
    transrectal ultrasonography–guided, 2509, 2510. See also Transrectal ultrasonography (TRUS)–guided biopsy.
Biothesiometry, in erectile dysfunction evaluation, 1188
Bismuth sclerotherapy, for renal cysts, 1793–1794
Bisphosphonates, in hypercalcemia, 2680–2681
Bladder, 107–110. See also at Cysto-; Vesical; Vesico-.
    acetylcholine effect on, 883t, 894
    adenocarcinoma of, 2344–2345
        in children, 2244–2245
        in exstrophy, 1969–1970
    adenosine triphosphate effects on, 883t, 885–886, 885t
    adrenergic receptors of, 884–885, 885t, 918
    afferent fibers of, 900–903, 901, 902
    agenesis of, 1982–1983

Bladder (Continued)
    anatomy of, 96, 98, 99, 106, 107, 872–874, 872
        for percutaneous interventions, 241
    angiosarcoma of, 2383
    angiotensin II effect on, 887
    antibodies to, in interstitial cystitis, 641
    arginine vasopressin effect on, 887
    arteries of, 110
    atropine effect on, 881
    atropine resistance of, 972
    augmentation of. See Cystoplasty, augmentation.
    autonomous, alpha-adrenergic blocker treatment of, 976–977, 995
    baclofen effect on, 893, 894
    bethanechol effect on, 882, 883, 883t, 884
    biomechanics of, 878–879, 878, 879
    biopsy of, in bladder cancer, 1523, 1523, 2358
        in diverticulum tumor, 2358
        in interstitial cystitis, 643
        in tuberculosis, 823
    bombesin effect on, 883t, 887
    bradykinin effect on, 883t
    calcifications of, in schistosomiasis, 740, 740, 741, 746, 746
    calcitonin gene-related peptide effect on, 887
    calculi of, 2715–2716, 2716
        after augmentation cystoplasty, 3180–3181
        after renal transplantation, 526
        endemic, 2720
        in benign prostatic hyperplasia, 1441
        treatment of, 1525–1527
            lithotripsy in, 1526–1527, 2742
            vesicolithopaxy in, 1525–1526, 1526
    cancer of. See Bladder cancer.
    Candida infection of, 780–781, 781
    capacity of, 934
    carcinoma in situ of, 2339–2340, 2340, 2349, 2365. See also Bladder cancer.
    carcinosarcoma of, 2382
    cells of, for regeneration repair, 3186
    CGRP effect on, 883t
    cholecystokinin effect on, 884, 894
    chondrosarcoma of, 2383
    choriocarcinoma of, 2383
    collagen of, 877–878
    compliance of, 934–935
        after augmentation cystoplasty, 3177–3178
        cystometric evaluation of, 934, 935–936, 935, 936
        embryology of, 1577–1578, 1578
        low, definition of, 1011
            etiology of, 1016, 1016t
            treatment of, 1024–1026, 1025t
    congenital megacystis of, 1605, 1605, 1983–1984
    corticotropin-releasing hormone effects on, 894
    decompression of, postoperative, 970
    denervation of, in neuropathic voiding dysfunction, 981–982
    detrusor muscle of, 107–109, 108. See also Detrusor muscle.
    development of, 1568t, 1572, 1575–1578, 1577, 1578, 1940, 1942, 1943
    diverticulum of, congenital, 1983
        intravenous urography in, 182
        treatment of, 3294, 3294
        tumor in, 2347
            biopsy of, 2358
        ultrasonography of, 206, 207
        vesicoureteral reflux with, 1876, 1877, 1878
        voiding cystourethrography in, 190, 192, 193
    dopamine effect on, 883t, 892–893

Bladder (Continued)
    duplication of, 1983, 1983
    during pregnancy, 597
    dysplasia of, in schistosomiasis, 752
    electric stimulation of, in neuropathic voiding dysfunction, 992
    emptying of, 917–920, 919, 926t, 1007–1010, 1008–1011, 3168
        abnormalities of, 919, 925, 1008–1009, 1008, 1009. See also Enuresis; Incontinence; Voiding dysfunction.
        before augmentation cystoplasty, 3169–3170
    biomechanics of, 878–879, 879
    in benign prostatic hyperplasia, 1458–1459
    in infant, 2055–2056
    initiation of, 919
    neuropharmacology of, 890–895, 891, 892
    pain with, in children, 1624
    physiology of, 1007–1008, 1008
    pressure-flow studies of, 939–944, 940–944
    reflex of, 895–899, 896–899, 919, 1007–1008, 1008
        inhibition of, 1029–1030, 1030
        manual initiation of, 989–990
        neurologic interruption of, 1008–1010, 1009–1011
        voluntary control of, 1008, 1009
    timed, in voiding dysfunction, 972
    urethral pressure studies of, 936, 945–947, 947
    uroflowmetric evaluation of, 937–939, 937t, 938, 939
    voluntary initiation of, 919
    endothelin effect on, 883t, 888
    enkephalin effect on, 883t, 884, 887, 893–894, 895
    enlargement of, acetylcholinesterase staining in, 881
        in myelodysplasia-related neurogenic bladder, 2030
    epithelial permeability barrier of, in interstitial cystitis, 639–640
    epithelium of, 871–872, 2337–2338
        atypical hyperplasia of, 2338
        carcinoma in situ of, 2339–2340, 2340
        dysplasia of, 2338–2339, 2339
        eosinophilic liquefaction of, 2338
        hyperplasia of, 2338
        leukoplakia of, 2339
        metaplasia of, 2338
        von Brunn's nests of, 2338
    estrogen effects on, 889
    estrogen receptors of, 889
    examination of, 139–140, 140
    excision of. See Cystectomy.
    exstrophy of. See Bladder exstrophy.
    fetal, aspiration of, 1611
        drainage of, 1611–1613, 1612
        functional reserve of, 1611
        ultrasonography of, 1603
    filling of, 917, 918–919, 926t
        abnormalities of, 919. See also Voiding dysfunction.
    biomechanics of, 878, 878
    in children, 2021–2022
    urethral pressure during, 919
    fistula of, computed tomography of, 223
        excision of, 3295, 3296
    function of, 917–918, 3168. See also Enuresis; Incontinence; Voiding dysfunction.
    galanin effect on, 883t, 887
    gamma-aminobutyric acid effects on, 888, 893–894
    glutamate effects on, 891, 891, 892
    glycine effects on, 892, 893

Bladder *(Continued)*
  granular cell myoblastoma of, 2383
  histamine effect on, 883t
  histology of, 872
  hormone effects on, 888–889
  hydrodistention of, in interstitial cystitis, 645–646
  hypertonic, small capacity, 2041–2042, *2041, 2042*
  hypoplasia of, 1983
  imaging of. See *Cystography.*
  in acquired immunodeficiency syndrome, 697t
  in cloacal exstrophy, 1976
  in prune-belly syndrome, 1919, *1920*
  in spinal shock, 960
  incisional approaches to, 3274
  infection of. See *Cystitis.*
  innervation of, 110, 879–880, *879,* 1029
    acetylcholine release in, 881–883, *881–884,* 883t, 893
    adenosine triphosphate release in, *881,* 885–886, 885t
    afferent, 900–903, *901, 902*
    calcitonin gene-related peptide release in, 887
    dopamine effect on, 892–893
    endothelin release in, 888
    enkephalin release in, 893–894, *895*
    galanin release in, 887
    gamma-aminobutyric acid release in, 888, 893–894
    glutamate effects on, 891, *891, 892*
    glycine effect on, *892,* 893
    hormone impact on, 888–889
    neurokinin A release in, 886–887
    neurokinin B release in, 886–887
    neuropeptide Y release in, *884,* 886, *886*
    nitric oxide synthesis in, 887
    norepinephrine release in, 883–885, *884,* 893
    opiate release in, 893–894, *895*
    parasympathetic, 879–880, *879*
    prostaglandin release in, 888
    serotonin release in, 888, 891–892, *892*
    somatostatin release in, 887
    substance P release in, 886–887
    sympathetic, *879,* 880, 918
    tachykinin release in, 886–887
    vasoactive intestinal polypeptide release in, *881,* 886
  intraoperative injury to, during laparoscopy, 2905
    during vaginal surgery, 1091
  intravesical pressure of, 875, 875t, 918, 941–942, *941, 942*
    cystometric evaluation of, 933–937, *934–936*
    urine transport and, 854
  inverted papilloma of, 2338, *2339*
  involuntary contraction of, 920
  ion transport by, 871
  irrigation of, after augmentation cystoplasty, 3180
  leiomyosarcoma of, 2244, 2383
  leukoplakia of, 2339
  liposarcoma of, 2383
  lymphatic drainage of, *103,* 110
  lymphohemangioma of, 2245
  lymphoma of, 2383
  malacoplakia of, 581
  malignant melanoma of, 2383
  mast cells of, 637–638, *637*
  megacystis of, 1605, *1605,* 1983–1984
  mesonephric adenocarcinoma of, 2339
  muscarinic receptors of, 881–882, *881, 882*
  nephrogenic adenoma of, 2339

Bladder *(Continued)*
  neurofibroma of, 2245, 2382
  neurogenic. See *Voiding dysfunction, neuropathic.*
  neurokinin A effect on, 883t, 886–887
  neuromedin-U effect on, 887
  neuropeptide Y effect on, 883t, *884,* 886, *886*
  nitric oxide effect on, 883t, 887–888
  nonepithelial tumors of, 2382–2383
  norepinephrine effect on, 883–885, 883t, *884,* 893
  of infant, 2056
  opiate effects on, 887, 893–894, *895*
  osteosarcoma of, 2383
  overdistention of, in neuropathic voiding dysfunction treatment, 979
  pain in, in children, 1624
    in patient history, 132–133
    mechanisms of, 902–903
  painful disease of. See *Cystitis.*
  palpation of, in neurourologic evaluation, 930
  paralytic, motor, 923
  pear-shaped, 419, 419t
  Penicillium citrinum infection of, 796
  perforation of, after augmentation cystoplasty, 3179, 3181–3182
  peripheral denervation of, in neuropathic voiding dysfunction, 981–982
  phenol infiltration of, in neuropathic voiding dysfunction, 982
  pheochromocytoma of, 2382–2383
  pine cone appearance of, 192
  plasmacytoma of, 2383
  polyposis of, schistosomal, 749–751, *750*
  postcystourethropexy instability of, 1101
  postoperative appearance of, on voiding cystourethrography, 192
  postoperative spindle cell nodule of, 2339
  postvoid residual urine in, in benign prostatic hyperplasia, 1446–1447, 1458–1459
    in geriatric incontinence, 1051
    in prune-belly syndrome, 1919
    intraindividual variation in, 1446
  preservation of, in augmentation cystoplasty, 3170–3171, *3171*
  progesterone effects on, 889
  prolapse of, 2136, *2136*
  prostaglandin effect on, 883t, 888
  pseudosarcoma of, 2339
  reconstruction of. See *Cystoplasty.*
  regeneration of, 3168
  rhabdomyosarcoma of, 2383
  rupture of. See also *Bladder, trauma to.*
    cystography in, 181, 188
    in neonate, 1638, 1640
    with umbilical arterial catheterization, 1643
  sarcoma of, 2383
  schistosomiasis of, 749–756
    carcinoma and, *750,* 752–754
    fibrosis in, 751, *751*
    histologic grade of, 749, 749t
    polyposis and, 749–751, *750*
    squamous metaplasia in, *750, 752, 753*
    ulcers in, *750,* 751
    urothelial hyperplasia in, 751, *752*
  sensation in, 935
  serotonin effects on, 883t, 888, 891–892, *892*
  small cell carcinoma of, 2381–2382
  smooth muscle of, 874–878, 874t, 875t. See also *Detrusor muscle.*
    calcium channels of, 876
    contractile proteins of, 875–876, *875*
    energetics of, 877
    gap junctions of, 875
    potassium channels of, 876–877
    stretch-activated channels of, 877

Bladder *(Continued)*
  somatostatin effect on, *884,* 887
  spasm of, after hypospadias repair, 2113
  spinning top deformity of, 2041, *2041,* 2136, 2137, *2137*
  squamous cell carcinoma of, 2343–2344
    etiology of, 2343
    histology of, 2343, *2344*
    in exstrophy, 1970
    treatment of, 2343–2344
  squamous metaplasia of, in schistosomiasis, *750, 752, 753*
  storage function of, 917, 3168
    abnormalities of, 919, 925. See also *Enuresis; Incontinence; Voiding dysfunction.*
    cystometric evaluation of, 933–937, *934–936*
    evaluation of, 933–937, *934–936*
    reflexes of, 899–900
  stress relaxation of, 918
  structure of, 107–109, *108*
  substance P effects on, 883t, 886–887, 894
  suprapubic aspiration of, 546–547, *547,* 1693
  thimble, in tuberculosis, 822, *822*
  training of, in enuresis, 2063–2064
    in neuropathic voiding dysfunction, 972
    in urinary incontinence, 1035–1036
  transection of, in neuropathic voiding dysfunction, 982
  transitional cell carcinoma of, 2329–2383. See also *Bladder cancer.*
  transvaginal partial denervation of, in neuropathic voiding dysfunction, 982
  trauma to, 3104–3108
    anatomic considerations in, 3104
    classification of, 3105–3106
    cystography in, 181, 188, 3104–3105
    extraperitoneal, 3105–3106, *3107,* 3108
    intraperitoneal, 3106, *3107,* 3108
    mechanisms of, 3105–3106, *3107*
    patient history in, 3104
    pelvic rupture with, 3105–3106, *3107*
    physical examination in, 3104
    radiologic evaluation of, 3104–3105
    treatment of, 3106, 3108
    urinalysis in, 3104
  trigone of, 109–110, *109*
    anatomy of, 872, *872*
    development of, 1571, 1573–1575, *1574–1576*
    in vesicoureteral reflux, 859–860
  tuberculosis of, 815, *816*
  ulcers of, in schistosomiasis, *750,* 751
  ultrasonography of, 206, *206, 207*
    in pediatric urinary tract infection, *1697,* 1698–1699
  ureteral jets in, color Doppler imaging of, 201
  vasoactive intestinal polypeptide effects on, *881, 884,* 886, 894
  veins of, 110
  viscoelasticity of, 918
  yolk sac tumor of, 2383
Bladder cancer, 2329–2383
  N-acetyltransferase 2 in, 2335
  after augmentation cystoplasty, 3179–3180
  age and, 2331
  4-aminobiphenyl in, 2335
  analgesic abuse in, 2336
  angiogenic factors in, 2346
  artificial sweeteners in, 2336
  autopsy in, 2331
  biopsy of, 1523, *1523,* 2358
  bone scan in, 2360
  cell growth in, 2261
  chest radiography in, 2360
  cigarette smoking in, 2334–2336

Breast, cancer of, hypercalcemia in, 2678–2679, 2680
  intratumor pressure of, 2273t
  metastases from, 2276
  NM23 gene in, 2276
  transgenic animal development of, 2276
  development of, 2148
Breast milk, antituberculosis drugs in, 829–830
Breast-feeding, pediatric urinary tract infection and, 1690–1691
Bredinim (mizoribine), immunosuppressive activity of, 496t, 497
  structure of, 495
Brequinar sodium, immunosuppressive activity of, 496t, 498
  structure of, 495
Brief Male Sexual Function Inventory for Urology, 1183
Bristol nomogram, for uroflowmetry, 939
BRL 38227, ureteral effect of, 864
Broad ligaments, 1065–1066
  development of, 1595
Brödel's line, 239
Bromocriptine, in erectile dysfunction, 1201
  in hyperprolactinemia, 1244
Bronchopulmonary dysplasia, furosemide for, nephrolithiasis with, 1643
Bropiramine, in bladder cancer, 2367
Brugia, lymphatic obstruction by, 761–762
Brugia malayi, 757, 759, 760
Brugia timori, 757, 759
Brush biopsy, percutaneous, 253–254, 255
BSD-300 device, in benign prostatic hyperplasia, 1493
Buccal mucosal graft, in hypospadias repair, 2110, 2111
Buck's fascia, 120, 120, 3321, 3321
Buffer systems, bicarbonate, 297–298
  in acid-base balance, 298, 298, 301
  phosphate, 299
Bulbocavernosus reflex, in erectile dysfunction, 1188
  in voiding dysfunction, 929, 1022
Bulbospongiosus muscles, 119
Bulbourethral artery, 3323, 3323
Bulbourethral glands, 96, 114, 1384
  development of, 1586, 1587
Bulla, 718
Bullous pemphigoid, of male genitalia, 722
Bumetanide, in geriatric incontinence etiology, 1046t
  in neuropathic voiding dysfunction, 986
Burch retropubic colposuspension, 1098–1099, 1099
  enterocele after, 1081–1082
  laparoscopic, 1100
Burkitt's lymphoma, testicular tumor and, 2248
Burns, genital, 3340–3341
Buschke-Löwenstein tumor, 712, 725, 2457
Buspirone, sexual function effects of, 1167
Butyrates, in prostate cancer treatment, 2656
Bypass graft(s), aortorenal, 476–479, 477–479
  gastroduodenal–to–renal artery, 480–482, 481, 482
  hepatic–to–renal artery saphenous vein, 480–482, 481, 482
  iliac–to–renal artery, 482, 483
  splenorenal, 479–480, 480
  superior mesenteric–to–renal artery saphenous vein, 482, 482

C3, of seminal plasma, 1395–1396
Cachexia, in physical examination, 139
E-Cadherin, in prostate cancer, 1410, 2491

E-Cadherin (Continued)
  in prostate gland growth, 1409–1410
  in transitional cell bladder cancer, 2346
N-Cadherin, 1409
P-Cadherin, 1409
Cadmium, prostate cancer and, 2494
  renal cell carcinoma and, 2293
Caffeine, male infertility and, 1289, 1315
Calcification(s), bladder, in schistosomiasis, 740, 740, 741, 746, 746
  computed tomography of, 215–216
  in medullary sponge kidney, 173, 173
  in renal artery aneurysm, 1734
  in renal cysts, 1791
  in renal osteogenic sarcoma, 2318
  in schistosomiasis, 746, 746
  in tuberculosis, 813–814, 814, 820, 821–822, 821, 822
  retroperitoneal, recurrent hematoma and, 411, 411
  scrotal, in filariasis, 762, 763
  ureteric, in tuberculosis, 820
Calcineurin, in antiallograft response, 493
Calcitonin, in hypercalcemia, 2681
Calcitonin gene–related peptide, bladder effect of, 887
  in erectile dysfunction, 1204, 1206
  ureteral effect of, 851–852
Calcium. See also Hypercalcemia.
  citrate complexation of, 2673–2674, 2684
  dietary, absorption of, 2670–2671, 2671
    after urinary intestinal diversion, 3156
    in urinary lithiasis treatment, 2708–2709, 2709, 2733
    urinary lithiasis and, 2665
  extracellular, 283
  in action potential, 841
  in acute tubular necrosis, 319–320
  in ureteral peristalsis, 843–845, 844
  metabolism of, 2670–2672, 2671
  renal excretion of, 281, 283–285, 2674–2677, 2675, 2676, 2677t
    neonatal, 1661
  renal reabsorption of, distal tubule in, 283, 283
    diuretics and, 284–285
    extracellular fluid volume in, 284, 284t
    loop of Henle in, 283, 283
    parathyroid hormone in, 283–284, 284, 284t
    pH and, 283
    proximal tubule in, 283, 283
    vitamin D in, 284
  renal transport of, 283–285, 284t
  serum, in chronic renal failure, 335
  urinary, 2674–2677, 2675, 2676, 2677t. See also Hypercalciuria.
Calcium antagonists, in neuropathic voiding dysfunction, 975
Calcium channel, of smooth muscle, 876
Calcium channel blockers, after ureteral obstruction release, 379
  in acute renal failure, 322
  in geriatric incontinence, 1054, 1054t
  in geriatric incontinence etiology, 1046t, 1047
  in Peyronie's disease, 3380
  ureteral effect of, 864
Calcium oxalate calculi, 2674–2677, 2675, 2676, 2677t. See also Urinary lithiasis, calcium oxalate.
Calcium oxalate crystals, in urinary sediment, 155, 155
Calcium phosphate calculi, 2686, 2701
  renal tubular acidosis and, 2686, 2687
Calcium-calmodulin complex, in ureteral peristalsis, 844, 844
Calcium-creatinine ratio, in children, 1672–1673

Calcium-creatinine ratio (Continued)
  in neonate, 1661
Calcium-specific binding proteins, 44, 44t
Calculus(i). See also Urinary lithiasis.
  ammonium acid urate, 2698
  calcium oxalate, 2668, 2674–2677, 2675, 2676, 2677t. See also Urinary lithiasis, calcium oxalate.
  calcium phosphate, 2686, 2701
    renal tubular acidosis and, 2686, 2687
  chemical analysis of, 2703–2704, 2703t
  composition of, 2664t
  culture of, 552, 552
  cystine, 2695–2696, 2701
  dihydroxyadenine, 2696–2697
  in children, 1673, 2718–2720, 2719t, 2827, 2829, 2829t
  in medullary sponge kidney, 1795
  in pregnancy, 2720–2721
  in urinary tract infection, 552, 552
  in very-low-birth-weight infant, 2718
  matrix, 2697
  of calyceal diverticulum, 2839, 3030–3031, 3033
  of kidneys. See Urinary lithiasis, renal.
  of prostate, 616–617, 623, 2716–2717, 2717
  of seminal vesicles, 3306
  of ureters. See Urinary lithiasis, ureteral.
  of urethra, 2717–2718
  of urethral diverticulum, 1146
  preputial, 2718
  radiography of, 2699–2702, 2701, 2702, 3017
  silicate, 2697
  spurious, 2698
  staghorn, 2692–2695, 2693, 2694t, 2701. See also Urinary lithiasis, staghorn.
  struvite (magnesium ammonium phosphate), 2691–2695, 2692t, 2693, 2694t. See also Urinary lithiasis, struvite (magnesium ammonium phosphate).
  triamterene, 2697
  ureteral function with, 860–861
  uric acid, 2688–2690, 2689, 2690, 2701
  xanthine, 2697
Calmodulin, in ureteral peristalsis, 844, 844
Calpain, in acute tubular necrosis, 319–320
Calymmatobacterium granulomatis, 664t, 676–677
Calyx(calyces), 71, 73
  abscess of, misdiagnosis of, 2801, 2802
    percutaneous drainage of, 2801, 2802
  absence of, 84
  anatomy of, 79, 82, 83, 84–85, 2758–2759
    for percutaneous interventions, 239–240
  anomalous, 1738, 1739
  clubbing of, in reflux nephropathy, 1763
    in renal hypodysplasia, 1763
  congenital anomalies of, 1734–1738
  cystic dilatation of, 1735, 1736
  development of, ureteric bud branching in, 1550–1551, 1552–1553
  diverticulum of, 1734–1735, 1735, 1800–1801, 1801, 1802
    calculi in, 3030–3031, 3033
      extracorporeal shockwave lithotripsy for, 2839
      ureteroscopy for, 2839
    endosurgical treatment of, 248–249, 249, 2837–2839, 2838, 2839t
    vs. hydrocalyx, 2840
  elongation of, 85
  enlargement of, 84
    nonobstructive, 1736–1737, 1736, 1737
  extrarenal, 1738, 1738
  in horseshoe kidney, 1726
  in tuberculosis, 820, 821–822, 821

Computed tomography (CT) *(Continued)*
 in testicular cancer, 2420–2421, 3411, 3419
 in transitional cell carcinoma, *223*
 in tuberculosis, 823
 in upper tract urothelial tumors, 2389–2390
 in ureteral obstruction, 348, 388
 in ureteral tumors, 2389–2390
 in urinary lithiasis, 215, *217,* 2700
 in urinary tract infection, 553, 1699
 in urothelial tumors, 217, *220*
 in Wilms' tumor, 2221
 in xanthogranulomatous pyelonephritis, 220,
   580, *580*
 of adrenal gland, *235*
 of seminal vesicles, 3303, *3303*
 spiral, in renovascular hypertension, 436, *436*
Concealed penis, 2122–2123, *2123*
Concussion, voiding dysfunction after, 956
Conditioning therapy, for enuresis, 2064
Condom catheter, in geriatric incontinence,
   1054, 1055
Condyloma acuminatum, 664t, 677–678, 678t
 diagnosis of, 2455
 giant, 2457
 in acquired immunodeficiency syndrome, 699
 in bladder cancer, 2336–2337
 of penis, *713,* 2455–2456, 2467
 vs. Buschke-Lowenstein tumor, 2457
Congenital adrenal hyperplasia, 2150, *2150,*
   2919
 ambiguous genitalia in, 1641, *1642,* 2155–
   2156, 2155t. See also *Ambiguous genitalia; Intersexuality.*
 clitoromegaly in, *2159*
 male infertility and, 1296, 1309–1310
 testicular hyperplastic nodules in, 2247
 urogenital sinus defect in, 2158, *2160,* 2161–
   2162, *2161–2166*
Congenital urologic abnormalities. See *Children;
   Fetus; Neonate* and specific disorders.
Congestive heart failure, hyponatremia in, 293
Conjoint tendon, 94
Connell suture, 3128, *3128, 3129*
Connexin 43, in erection, 1166
Conn's syndrome. See *Hyperaldosteronism.*
Conray (iothalamic acid), 171
Constipation, in prune-belly syndrome, 1922
 pediatric urinary tract infection and, 1686
 urinary incontinence and, 2043
Contact dermatitis, of male genitalia, 721–722
Continence, urinary. See also *Enuresis;
   Incontinence; Voiding dysfunction.*
 abdominal pressure and, 919–920
 mechanisms of, 3163–3164
 neuropharmacology of, *892*
 reflexes of, 899–900
Continuous arteriovenous hemofiltration, in
   neonate, 1647–1648
Continuous incontinence, 1019, 1020t. See also
   Incontinence.
Contraception, vasectomy for, 1338–1344. See
   also *Vasectomy.*
Contraceptives, oral, rifampicin effects on, 829
Contrast media, extravasation of, 172
 for diagnostic uroradiology, 170–172
 high-osmolality, 171, 172
 low-osmolality, 171, 172
 reactions to, 171–172, 268, 318, 2800
Cooper's (pectineal) ligament, 89, *95*
Cordotomy, micturition reflex pathways after,
   897, *897*
Cornelia de Lange syndrome, 1620t
Corpus cavernosum (corpora cavernosa), 118,
   118, 119, 1158–1159, 3320
 alpha-adrenoceptors of, 1164
 biopsy of, in erectile dysfunction, 1198–1199

Corpus cavernosum (corpora cavernosa)
   (Continued)
 electromyography of, 1162
 in erectile dysfunction, 1189, *1190*
 in erection, 1159–1161, *(1161)*
 injection of, in erectile dysfunction evaluation,
   1191–1192
 muscarinic receptors of, 1164
 papaverine injection of, priapism with, 1173
 transverse section of, *3320*
 tunical covering of, 1158, *1158*
Corpus spongiosum, 118–119, *118,* 120, *120,*
   1159, 3320–3321
 development of, 1581
 hypoplasia of, in chordee, 2098–2099
 in erection, 1161–1162
 transverse section of, *3320*
Cortical collecting duct, HCO_3^- reabsorption by,
   299
 potassium transport by, *273, 278, 278*
 sodium reabsorption by, *273, 274*
 urine concentration/dilution by, *290*
Cortical microcystic disease, 1778
Corticosteroids, immunosuppressive activity of,
   496, 496t
 in immune-mediated male infertility, 1316–
   1317
Corticotropin-releasing hormone (CRH), bladder
   effects of, 894
 in ACTH secretion, 2920–2921
 in gonadotropin-releasing hormone regulation,
   1241, 1242
Cortisol, adrenal production of, 2919, *2920*
 C18 methyloxygenation metabolites of, in primary hyperaldosteronism, *2942, 2942,*
   2946
 hypersecretion of. See *Cushing's syndrome.*
 metabolism of, 2922
 plasma, in primary hyperaldosteronism, 2945
 urinary, in Cushing's syndrome, 2926–2927,
   2928
Cortisone, biologic activity of, 2940t
Corynebacterium minutissimum, 726
Corynebacterium parvum, in renal cell
   carcinoma, 2312
Corynebacterium tenuis, 726
Costovertebral ligament, 54–55
Co-trimoxazole, in urinary tract infection
   prevention, 594t
Cotton swab test, in urethral hypermobility,
   1022, 1051
Coudé catheter, for urethral catheterization, 160,
   160, 161
Coumarin, in renal cell carcinoma, 2313
Council catheter, for percutaneous nephrostomy,
   2797–2798, *2799*
 for urethral catheterization, 161, *162*
Countercurrent multiplier principle, 288–289,
   289
Cowper's glands, *96,* 114, 1384
 development of, 1586, *1587*
Cowper's syringocele, 1586
Creatinine, drug effects on, 316
 during pregnancy, 597, 597t
 in benign prostatic hyperplasia, 1443
 in children, 1701–1702, 1702t
 in fetus, 1565, *1566*
 in neurourologic evaluation, 931
 production of, 316
Creatinine clearance, calculation of, 271, 1658
 in children, 1672
 in diuretic renography, 345, *345*
 in glomerular filtration rate assessment, 271
 in neonate, 1658, *1658*
 in neurourologic evaluation, 931
Credé maneuver, in neuropathic voiding
   dysfunction, 989

Cremasteric artery, 1256
Cremasteric muscle, 122
Cremasteric reflex, in cryptorchidism, 2174
CRH. See *Corticotropin-releasing hormone
   (CRH).*
Crick, Francis, 5
Crohn's disease, hypomagnesuria in, 2685
 interstitial cystitis and, 634
 male genitalia in, 723
 ureteral obstruction in, 400–402, *402*
Cromakalim, in neuropathic voiding dysfunction,
   976
 ureteral effect of, 864
Cromolyn sodium, intravesical, in interstitial
   cystitis, 649
Crural veins, 3322–3323, *3323*
Crust, 718
Cryoprobe, in urethral syndrome, 655
Cryotherapy, in prostate cancer, 2617–2623. See
   also *Prostate cancer, treatment of,
   cryotherapy in.*
Cryptococcosis, 788–790
 adrenal, 789
 diagnosis of, 788–789
 epidemiology of, 788
 genital, 790
 predisposition to, 788
 prostatic, 789–790, *790*
 renal, 789
 treatment of, 799t
Cryptococcus neoformans, 788–790, *790*
Cryptorchidism, 1623, 2172–2183, 2193–2199
 abdominal, 2176–2177, 2194
   microvascular autotransplantation for,
     2196–2197
   tumors in, 2249
   two-step vasal pedicle orchiopexy for,
     2198–2199, *2198*
 angiography in, 2178
 bilateral, 2174
   neoplasia and, 2179
 canalicular, 2176–2177
 classification of, 2176–2177, *2177,* 2178t
 complications of, 2179–2181, *2179*
 diagnosis of, laparoscopic, 2887–2890
   indications for, 2887–2888
   results of, 2889–2890, *2891*
   technique of, 2888–2889, *2888–2890*
   ultrasonography in, 211, *212,* 2890
 diethylstilbestrol and, 2181
 ectopic, 2176–2177, *2177*
 endocrine aspects of, 2175–2176, *2176*
 femoral, *2194*
 gonadotropin releasing hormone for, 2182–
   2183
 hernia with, 2180
 herniography in, 2178
 histology of, 2178–2179
 human chorionic gonadotropin for, 2181–
   2183, *2182*
 hypospadias and, 2095–2096
 hypothalamic-pituitary-testicular axis in,
   2175–2176, *2176*
 imaging of, 211, *212,* 2178, 2890
 in cystic fibrosis, 2181
 in genetic syndromes, 2175, 2181
 in prune-belly syndrome, 1920, 1933–1935,
   1934
 in testicular feminization syndrome, 2184
 incidence of, 2173–2174, 2174t
 infertility with, 1312–1313, 2180–2181
 inguinal, *2194*
 microvascular autotransplantation for, 2196–
   2197
 neoplasia and, 2179–2180, *2179, 2180,* 2249,
   2415–2416

Fibroplasia (*Continued*)
  medial, of renal artery, 426t, 427–428, *428*
  perimedial (subadventitial), of renal artery,
    426t, 428, *429*
Fibrosarcoma, renal, 2318–2319, *2318*
Fibrosis, in urinary tract obstruction, 349–350,
    349
  retroperitoneal, 403–410. See also *Retroperitoneal fibrosis.*
Filarial fever, 762–763
Filariasis, 757–766
  amicrofilaremic, 765
  amyloidosis in, 770
  asymptomatic microfilaremia in, 763
  chyluria in, 764
  clinical manifestation of, 763–765, *763*
  diagnosis of, 765
  elephantiasis in, 762–763, *763, 764*
  epidemiology of, 759
  fever in, 763–764
  funiculoepididymitis in, 764
  hydrocele in, 762, *762,* 764
  immune response in, 763–764
  inflammation of, 761
  late period of, 761–763, *762, 763*
  lymphatic obstruction in, 761–763
  occult, 760, 764–765
  of epididymis, *759,* 761, *761,* 762, 764
  orchitis in, 764
  pathogenesis of, 760–762, *760, 761*
  pathology of, *758,* 759–760, *759*
  prepatent period of, 760
  prevention of, 766
  prognosis for, 766
  progression of, 760–763, *760, 761*
  scrotal calcifications in, 762, *763*
  scrotal edema in, 764
  treatment of, 765–766
  tropical pulmonary eosinophilia in, 764–765
Filiforms, for urethral dilation, 163–164, *164*
Fimbriae, bacterial, in urinary tract infection,
    541–543, *541, 543, 544*
Finasteride (Proscar), in benign prostatic
    hyperplasia, 1468–1470, *1468,* 1469t,
    1471–1472, 1471t
  in geriatric incontinence, 1055
  in prostate cancer prevention, 2495
  prostate-specific antigen levels with, 2521
Fish oil, post-transplantation, 499
Fistula(s). See also *Urethrovaginal fistula;
    Vesicovaginal fistula.*
  after intestinal anastomoses, 3133
  after ureterointestinal anastomoses, 3145
  arteriovenous, renal, 462, *463, 464,* 1734
    post-traumatic, 451
    with percutaneous nephrostomy, 249
  fecal, after radical perineal prostatectomy,
    2603
  pancreatic, after radical nephrectomy, 3006–
    3007
  postoperative, intravenous urography in, *182*
  urethral, 2128–2129, *2128*
    treatment of, 3329–3330, *3329, 3330*
  urethrocutaneous, after circumcision, 1633
    after hypospadias repair, 2115
    after urethral reconstruction, 1967–1968
    treatment of, 3329–3330, *3329, 3330*
  urinary, after partial nephrectomy, 3015, 3016
    in pelvic malignancy, 2863–2864, *2864*
    incontinence in, 135
  vesicocutaneous, percutaneous treatment of,
    2863–2864, *2864,* 2865t
  vesicoenteric, cystography in, *190*
    excision of, 3295, *3296*
Fixed drug reaction, of male genitalia, *714,*
    719–720

FK506 (tacrolimus), immunosuppressive effects
    of, 495–496, *495, 496*t
  in renal transplantation, 521–524, 523t, 524t
  structure of, *495*
Flank incision, for renal surgery, 2979–2982,
    2979–2982
Flank pain, in urinary tract infection, 549
Flap(s), 3319–3320, *3319, 3320*
  axial, 3319
  cuticular, direct, 3319
  fasciocutaneous, 3319, *3321*
  for penile reconstruction, 3387–3391, *3389–
    3391*
  forearm, for penile reconstruction, 3387–3390,
    3389
  gracilis muscle, in penile reconstruction, 3391,
    3391
  in urethral reconstruction, 3354–3357, *3354–
    3362*
  island, 3319–3320
  microvascular, 3320
  musculocutaneous, 3319, *3321*
  peninsula, 3319–3320
  random, 3319, *3319*
  upper arm, for penile reconstruction, 3390–
    3391, *3390*
Flap valves, in continent reconstruction,
    3164–3165, *3164*
Flavoxate hydrochloride (Urispas), in geriatric
    incontinence, 1053, 1054t
  in neuropathic voiding dysfunction, 974
Florida pouch, 3228, 3231–3233, *3233*
Flow cytometry, cross-match by, 500
  in bladder cancer, 2352–2353
  in upper tract urothelial tumors, 2388
  of cell cycle, 2261–2262, 2261t
  of testicular cells, 2199
Fluconazole, 799–800, 799t, 800t
  adverse effects of, 799–800
  in candidal infection, 785–786, *785*
  resistance to, 800
Flucytosine, 798, 799t, 800t
  adverse effects of, 798
  in candidal infection, 785, 798
  pharmacology of, 798
  resistance to, 798
Fluid(s), after renal transplantation, 519–521
  body, 286–288
    osmolality of, 286–288, 287t, *288*
  in cystine calculi treatment, 2696
  in uric acid calculi treatment, 2690
  in urinary lithiasis treatment, 2707–2708
Fluid volume, extracellular, in renal calcium
    reabsorption, 284
  renal urate excretion and, 286
Fluorescent image analysis, in bladder cancer,
    2353
Fluorescent treponemal antibody absorption
    (FTA-ABS) test, 676
Fluoroquinolones, contraindications to, 557t
  in urinary tract infection, 556t, 557t, 558–559
  in urinary tract infection prevention, 592–593
  seminal plasma concentration of, 1397
  side effects of, 557t
Fluoroscopy, for percutaneous nephrostomy,
    2790, *2790*
  for shock-wave lithotripsy, 2737, 2737t, 2744
  for urodynamic testing, 944–945, *945*
5-Fluorouracil, in condyloma acuminatum, 2456
  in penile carcinoma, 2475
  in prostate cancer, 2650t, 2651t, 2652t, 2654t
  in renal cell carcinoma, 2312
Flush stoma, for urinary intestinal diversion,
    3136
Flutamide, in benign prostatic hyperplasia, 1470
  in prostate cancer, 2636, 2636t, 2637–2638,
    2637

Focal proliferative glomerulonephritis, in chronic
    renal failure, 329
Focal segmental glomerulosclerosis, in children,
    1678
  in chronic renal failure, 329
  in persistent asymptomatic proteinuria, 1677
Foley Y-V plasty, for congenital ureteropelvic
    junction obstruction, 3045–3046, *3046*
Foley-type catheter, for urethral catheterization,
    160, *160,* 161
Folic acid, malabsorption of, after urinary
    intestinal diversion, 3156
Follicle-stimulating hormone (FSH), 1239, *1240*
  age-related changes in, 1248, *1248*
  deficiency of, in male infertility, 1309
  gonadal hormone feedback regulation of,
    1244–1246, *1245*
  in children, 1247–1248, *1247*
  in isolated hypogonadotropic hypogonadism,
    1309
  in male infertility, 1296, 1296t, 1298–1299,
    1299
  in spermatogenesis, 1246–1247, 1266–1268
  inhibin regulation of, 1245
  secretion of, 1243
Folliculitis, of male genitalia, 726
Force-length relations, of muscle, 847–848, *848*
Force-velocity relations, of smooth muscle, 848,
    849
Fordyce, angiokeratoma of, *710*
Foreign body, penile, 2454
  renal, *249*
Foreskin. See also *Circumcision.*
  development of, 1582–1583, *1583*
  manual retraction of, 2121
  physiologic phimosis of, 2121
Formalin, intravesical, in bladder cancer, 2381
Formin, in renal agenesis, 1554
Forward motility protein, of epididymal fluid,
    1276
Fournier's gangrene, 91, 603–605, *708,* 727
Fowler-Stephens orchiopexy, 2196, 2197–2198,
    2894, *2894*
  in prune-belly syndrome, 1933
Fracture, after urinary intestinal diversion, 3155
  metastasis-associated, 2613
  pelvic, bladder rupture and, 3105–3106, *3107*
    pudendal artery injury in, 3368–3369
    urethral distraction injury with, 3362–3369,
      3363–3368
  penile, 3376
Fraser syndrome, 1620t
Fructose, in semen analysis, 1295
  of seminal plasma, 1390–1391
FSH. See *Follicle-stimulating hormone (FSH).*
Fumagillin, in cancer therapy, 2277, *2277*
Fungus(i), 779–801. See also specific organisms.
  bezoar of, *Candida* in, 781, *781,* 784, *784,*
    786, 2836–2837, 2837t
    percutaneous removal of, 2836–2837, 2837t
  in prostatitis, 627
Funiculoepididymitis, filarial, 764
Furosemide (Lasix), bronchopulmonary dysplasia
    treatment with, nephrolithiasis with, 1643
  in geriatric incontinence etiology, 1046t
Furosemide (Lasix) washout renogram. See
    Renography, diuretic.
Furunculosis, of male genitalia, 726–727
Fusarium, 794
Fusobacterium, in urinary tract infection, 540

G proteins, in signal transduction, 42–43, *43*
G syndrome, 1620t
Gal 4 protein, 34–35, *35*

Incontinence *(Continued)*
transcutaneous, 1035
estrogens in, 1026–1027
musculotropic relaxing agents in, 1026
pelvic floor exercises in, 1030–1033
biofeedback in, 1032–1033
history of, 1031–1032
outcome of, 1032
patient assessment for, 1031, *1032*
periurethral injection therapy in, 1109–1119. See also *Periurethral injection therapy.*
tricyclic antidepressants in, 1026
urethrolysis in, 1025
unconscious, 1019, 1020t
urge, 136, 1018–1019, 1020t
in depression, 892
in neurourologic evaluation, 931
stress incontinence with, 1028
Valsalva leak point pressure in, 1024
Inderal. See *Propranolol (Inderal).*
Indiana pouch, for urinary continent diversion, 3227–3228, 3230–3233, *3231–3233*
in bladder cancer treatment, 2376
in myelodysplasia-related neurogenic bladder, 2031
Indinavir, in acquired immunodeficiency syndrome, 704–705
Indium 111–labeled leukocyte imaging, in urinary tract infection, 553
Indomethacin, fetal effects of, 1663
in renal colic, 378
maternal use of, 1663
neonatal effects of, 1663
ureteral effect of, 863
Infant. See also *Children; Fetus; Neonate.*
acid-base regulation in, 1657
amino acid excretion in, 1661
aminoaciduria in, 1661
bladder neck in, 107
bladder of, 2056
calcium excretion in, 1661
captopril effects in, 1662
congenital nephrosis in, 1777–1778
creatinine clearance in, 1658, *1658*
cryptorchidism in, 2172–2183. See also *Cryptorchidism.*
fractional tubular phosphorus reabsorption in, 1661
glomerular filtration rate in, 1601, 1601t, 1657
angiotensin-converting enzyme inhibitor effect on, 1662
evaluation of, 1657–1659, *1658*
glucose excretion in, 1661
glucose transport in, 1657
glucosuria in, 1661
gonadotropin levels in, 1247, *1247*
hydrocele in, 2184
indomethacin effects in, 1663
inguinal hernia in, 2183–2184
kidneys of, 68. See also *Kidney(s), development of.*
evaluation of, 1657–1661, *1658, 1659*
hormonal regulation of, 1661–1663
reduced mass of, 1665
laparoscopic nephrectomy in, 2898–2900, *2899*
micturition in, 2055–2056
multicystic kidney in, 1782–1786. See also *Multicystic kidney disease.*
nonsteroidal anti-inflammatory drug administration to, 1663
oliguria in, 1657, 1659
phosphorus excretion in, 1661
polyuria in, 1657, 1660–1661
premature, anesthesia for, 1630

Infant *(Continued)*
maternal bacteriuria and, 598–599
renal function in, 1657
renal blood flow in, 1657, 1665
renal tubular acidosis in, 1659–1660, *1659*
renin in, 1664
sodium excretion in, 1657, 1659
testicular torsion in, 2185
tubular function in, 1659–1661, *1659*
urinary acidification in, 1659–1660, *1659*
urinary concentration in, 1660–1661
urinary tract infection in, 1681–1702. See also *Urinary tract infection, pediatric.*
urine production of, first, 1657
Infection, 533–605. See also *Urinary tract infection.*
after artificial genitourinary sphincter placement, 1131
after hypospadias repair, 2114
after intestinal anastomoses, 3133
after partial nephrectomy, 3016
after radical nephrectomy, 3008
after retropubic prostatectomy, 1536
after ureterointestinal anastomoses, 3145
after urinary intestinal diversion, 3155
circumcision and, 1633
enteric, 679
epididymal, 1353–1354
geriatric incontinence and, 1045
male infertility and, 1302–1303
opportunistic, in acquired immunodeficiency syndrome, 696, 697t, *698*
renal, chronic renal failure and, 332–333
renal transplantation and, 507–508
retroperitoneal, ureteral obstruction and, 410–411, *411*
small capacity hypertonic bladder and, 2041
urinary tract obstruction and, 343–344
with bacille Calmette-Guérin bladder cancer therapy, 2366
Infection calculi, 2691–2695, 2692t, *2693,* 2694t. See also *Struvite calculi.*
Inferior vena cava. See *Vena cava, inferior.*
Infertility, female, 1289–1290
sexually transmitted disease in, 670
male, 1287–1322
absent ejaculation in, 1297–1298, *1298*
acrosome reaction study in, 1306–1307
alcohol ingestion and, 1315
androgen abnormalities and, 1309–1310, 1312
antisperm antibodies in, 1301–1302
assisted reproductive techniques for, 1320–1332
asthenospermia in, 1299–1300, *1300*
azoospermia in, 1297t, 1298–1299, *1299,* 1305, *1305*
bilateral anorchia and, 1312
caffeine ingestion and, 1315
chemotherapy and, 1314–1315
chromosomal abnormalities and, 1311–1312
cigarette smoking and, 1315
clomiphene citrate treatment in, 1318
cocaine use and, 1315
congenital adrenal hyperplasia and, 1296, 1309–1310
cryptorchidism and, 1312–1313, 2180–2181
diethylstilbestrol exposure and, 1315
differential diagnosis of, 1296–1301, 1297t, *1298–1301*
ejaculatory duct obstruction in, 1318–1319, 1358–1359, *1359*
ejaculatory problems and, 1319–1320
end-stage testes in, 1304
epididymal obstruction in, 1354–1358, *1355–1358*

Infertility *(Continued)*
epididymectomy and, 1353
estrogen excess and, 1310
etiology of, 1308–1320
post-testicular, 1318–1320
pretesticular, 1308–1310
testicular, 1310–1318
FSH deficiency and, 1309
genetic abnormalities in, 1310–1312
genital examination in, 1290–1291, 1290t
germinal aplasia in, 1304
glucocorticoid excess and, 1310
gonadotoxic agents and, 1314
gonadotropin-releasing hormone treatment in, 1318
hemizona assay in, 1307
hormonal evaluation in, 1296, 1296t
human chorionic gonadotropin treatment in, 1318
hypogonadotropic hypogonadism and, 1308–1309
hypospermatogenesis in, 1304, *1304*
idiopathic, 1317–1318, 1317t
immune-mediated, 1316–1317
in Kallmann's syndrome, 1308–1309
in Klinefelter's syndrome, 1311
in myotonic dystrophy, 1314
in Noonan's syndrome, 1312
in Prader-Willi syndrome, 1309
in Sertoli cell–only syndrome, 1314
in vanishing testes syndrome, 1312
in vitro fertilization for, 1320–1321
in XX male, 1311–1312
in XYY syndrome, 1311
infection and, 1302–1303
intracytoplasmic sperm injection for, 1332, 1363–1364, *1364*
intrauterine insemination for, 1320
low-volume ejaculate in, 1297–1298, *1298*
luteinizing hormone deficiency and, 1309
marijuana use and, 1315
maturation arrest in, 1304, *1304*
mesterolone treatment in, 1318
micromanipulation for, 1321–1322
multiple defects in, 1300–1301, *1301*
oligospermia in, 1299
orchitis and, 1316
patient history in, 1288–1289, 1288t
percutaneous fine needle aspiration cytology in, 1305
physical examination in, 1290–1291, 1290t
pituitary disease and, 1308
prolactin excess and, 1310
prostatitis and, 628
pyospermia in, 1302–1303
radiation exposure and, 1315
retrograde ejaculation and, 1319–1320
semen analysis in, 1291–1296
computer-aided, 1292–1293
fructose measurements in, 1295
normal values in, 1295–1296
physical characteristics in, 1291–1292
sample collection for, 1291
sperm concentration in, 1292
sperm morphology in, 1293, *1294,* 1295
sperm motility in, 1293
seminal vesiculography in, 1338
sperm penetration assay in, 1307
sperm retrieval for, 1359–1363, *1361, 1362*
sperm–cervical mucus interaction assays in, 1306
tamoxifen treatment in, 1318
teratospermia in, 1300
testicular biopsy in, 1303–1305, *1304,* 1332–1334, *1333, 1334*
testolactone treatment in, 1318

Laparoscopy *(Continued)*
　renal function with, 2903–2904
　trocar configuration for, 2880–2881, *2880–2882*
　trocar placement for, 2878–2879, *2878, 2879*
　　secondary, 2880
　ureteral injury during, 399–400, *401*
Lapides classification, of voiding dysfunction, 922–923, 922t
Laplace's equation, 854, 878, *878*
Large bowel, 3123, *3123.* See also *Colon.*
Laser(s), 2467
　argon, 2467
　balloon, in benign prostatic hyperplasia, 1490
　CO_2, 2467
　diode, in benign prostatic hyperplasia, 1490
　holmium-YAG, in benign prostatic hyperplasia, 1490
　in bladder cancer, 2361
　in condyloma acuminatum, 2456, 2467
　in genital hemangioma, 2132
　in hypospadias repair, 2113
　in interstitial cystitis, 650
　in penile carcinoma in situ, 2467–2468
　in penile squamous cell carcinoma, 2467, 2468
　in premalignant penile lesions, 2467–2468
　in ureteral surgery, 3065–3066
　in urethral hemangioma, 3327
　in urethral stricture, 3347, *3350*
　KTP, 2467
　Nd:YAG, 2467
　　in benign prostatic hyperplasia, 1482–1490. See also *Benign prostatic hyperplasia (BPH), treatment of, laser therapy in.*
　　interstitial, in benign prostatic hyperplasia, 1488–1490
Laser lithotripsy, in ureteral calculi treatment, 2777, 2779, 2824
Laser welding, for hypospadias repair, 2113
Lasix (furosemide), bronchopulmonary dysplasia treatment with, nephrolithiasis with, 1643
　in geriatric incontinence etiology, 1046t
Laurence-Moon-Bardet-Biedl syndrome, 1620t
　male infertility in, 1309
　micropenis in, 2125
　renal cysts in, 1776
Lazy bladder syndrome, 2044–2045, *2045*
Leak point pressure, before augmentation cystoplasty, 3169
　in urinary incontinence, 1024–1025
Leflunomide (HWA 486), *495*
　immunosuppressive activity of, 496t, 498
Leiomyoma, testicular, 2442
Leiomyosarcoma, of bladder, 2244, 2383
　of kidney, 2318
　of prostate gland, 2504
　of spermatic cord, 2446–2447
　paratesticular, 2446–2447
Leiotonin, in smooth muscle contraction, 844
Lentigo, of penis, *709*
Lentiviruses, 687–688, *687.* See also *Human immunodeficiency virus (HIV).*
Leprosy, nephropathy in, 769–770
Lesch-Nyhan syndrome, uric acid levels in, 2690
　xanthine calculi in, 2697
Leucine aminopeptidase, of seminal plasma, 1395
Leucine zipper, *13,* 14
Leukemia, hyperuricosuria in, 2690
　L1210 model of, 2270
　of penis, 2479
　of testis, 2199, 2444
　renal tumors and, 2231
Leukocyte esterase, urinary, 153
Leukocyte esterase test, in neurourologic evaluation, 930

Leukocyte esterase test *(Continued)*
　in pediatric urinary tract infection, 1693
Leukocytes, in prostatitis, 617
　in semen specimen, 1293, 1302–1303
　in urinary sediment, 154, *154*
　in urinary tract infection, 548
Leukoplakia, of penis, 2455
Leukotriene(s), in renal hemodynamics, 268
　in unilateral ureteral obstruction, 358
Leukotriene A_4, synthesis of, *352,* 353–354
Leukotriene C_4, in renal hemodynamics, 268
Leukotriene D_4, in renal hemodynamics, 268
Levator ani muscle, *97*
　denervation of, 117
　innervation of, 104, *104*
　of female pelvis, 117, 1060, *1060–1063,* 1065
　tendinous arch of, 94, *97, 98, 99*
Levator fascia, 1061, *1061–1063,* 2568, *2568*
Levator plate, 95, *97,* 116, *116,* 117
Levsin (Levsinex, hyoscyamine sulfate), in neuropathic voiding dysfunction, 973
Lewis blood group, in urinary tract infection, 545
Lewisˣ antigen, in bladder cancer prognosis, 2349
　in bladder cancer screening, 2356
Leydig cell, 1257, *1258, 1259*
　androgen production by, 1257–1258, *1259, 1260,* 1397–1399, *1399,* 2628
　in hypergonadotropic hypogonadism, 1249
　luteinizing hormone response of, 1247
　prepubertal, 2174
Leydig cell tumors, 2247, 2439–2440
　vs. hyperplastic nodules, 2247
LH. See *Luteinizing hormone (LH).*
LHRH (luteinizing hormone–releasing hormone), in prostate cancer treatment, 2633t, 2634–2636, *2635*
　prostate gland effects of, 1397, *1398*
Libido, in patient history, 136
Lice, 678–679
Lichen nitidus, 719
Lichen planus, *708,* 719
Lichen sclerosis, 720
Lichen sclerosis et atrophicus, *716,* 720, 729, 2454–2455
　after hypospadias repair, 2094
　treatment of, 3328–3329, *3328*
Lichen simplex chronicus, *715*
Lichenoid reaction, 719
Lich-Grégoir antireflux procedure, 1888–1889, *1889,* 2900–2902, *2901*
Lidocaine, in interstitial cystitis, 649
Lienorenal ligament, 73
Lifestyle, in erectile dysfunction evaluation, 1199
Li-Fraumeni syndrome, TP53 gene mutation in, 2265
Limiting dilution assay, of tumor stem cells, 2270–2271, *2270*
Lindane, in scabies, 678
Linea alba, 91, *92, 93*
Linsidomine, in erectile dysfunction, 1204–1205
Lioresal (baclofen), bladder effect of, 893, *894*
　in neuropathic voiding dysfunction, 978, 997–998
Lipids, inositol, in signal transduction, 43–44, *44*
　of seminal plasma, 1392
Lipoma, in urogenital sinus development, 1588
　renal, 2291–2292
Lipomatosis, pelvic, cystitis glandularis in, 418, 419
　diagnosis of, 418–419, *418, 419*
　ureteral obstruction and, 417–419, *418, 419*
Lipomeningocele, 2031–2034. See also *Myelodysplasia.*

Lipomeningocele *(Continued)*
　diagnosis of, 2031–2033, *2032*
　pathogenesis of, 2033–2034, *2033*
　ultrasonography in, 2034, *2034*
　urodynamic testing in, 2033, *2033*
Lipomyelomeningocele, 2022
Lipopolysaccharide, in septic shock, 584–585, *585*
Liposarcoma, of bladder, 2383
　of kidney, 2318
　of spermatic cord, 2447
Lipoxins, in renal hemodynamics, 268
　synthesis of, 354
5-Lipoxygenase inhibitor (MK886), in bilateral ureteral obstruction, 369, *370*
Lisinopril, in geriatric incontinence etiology, 1046t, 1047
Lithiasis, urinary. See *Urinary lithiasis.*
Lithium, in syndrome of inappropriate antidiuretic hormone secretion, 294
Lithotomy position, for radical perineal prostatectomy, 2590, 2591, *2591*
Lithotripsy. See *Shock-wave lithotripsy (SWL).*
Lithotriptors, 2749, 2749t
　electrohydraulic, 2746–2748, 2746t, *2747, 2748*
　electromagnetic, 2746t, 2748–2749
　piezoelectric, 2746t, 2749
Littre, glands of, 1384
Liver. See also *Hepatic; Hepatitis; Hepato-.*
　anatomy of, for percutaneous interventions, 240
　antituberculosis drug toxicity to, 828–829
　cirrhosis of, benign prostatic hyperplasia and, 1432–1433
　disease of, in polycystic kidney disease, 1767, 1771
　injury to, with percutaneous nephrostomy, 250
　　with shock-wave lithotripsy, 2739
　metastatic cancer of, 2227, 2233, *2234*
　　intratumor pressure of, 2273t
　neuroblastoma metastases to, 2233, *2234*
　schistosomiasis of, 757
　transplantation of, in hyperoxaluria, 2682
　Wilms' tumor metastases to, 2227
Loop (Bradley) classification, of voiding dysfunction, 922
Loop end ileostomy, in urinary diversion, 3136–3137, *3137*
Loop of Henle, 79, *81.* See also *Nephron(s).*
　calcium reabsorption by, 283
　potassium reabsorption by, 277–278
　sodium reabsorption by, 272–273, *273*
　urine concentration/dilution by, 289–290, *289*
Loopography, 194–195
Losartan, 432
Losoxantrone, in prostate cancer, 2651t
Low back pain, in abdominal aortic aneurysm, 390
Lower motor neurons, lesions of, voiding dysfunction after, 921, 921t
LSD (lysergic acid diethylamide), in retroperitoneal fibrosis, 404
Lumbar arteries, 58, 100
Lumbar lordosis, 89, *90*
Lumbar plexus, *61*
Lumbar veins, *56,* 58
　intraoperative hemorrhage from, during radical nephrectomy, 3000–3001, *3001, 3002*
Lumbocostal ligament, posterior, 53
Lumbodorsal fascia, 49, 54, *54*
　anterior layer of, 49, *53*
　middle layer of, 49, *53*
　posterior layer of, 49, *52, 53*
Lumbodorsal incision, 54, *54*
Lumbodorsal ligament, 54–55

Meckel's syndrome, 1620t
  renal cysts in, 1779t
Meconium hydrocele, 2133
Meconium peritonitis, 2132
Medial fibroplasia, of renal artery, 426t,
  427–428, *428*. See also *Renovascular
  hypertension.*
Medial preoptic area, in erection, 1162, 1163,
  1168
Median raphe, cyst of, 728, 2132
Mediastinum, germ cell tumor of, 2438–2439
Medications. See also *specific drugs.*
  erectile effects of, 1167, 1171, 1173, 1173t
  in patient history, 138
  in urinary lithiasis evaluation, 2704
Medstone STS lithotriptor, 2746t, 2747
Medullary collecting duct, 274
  inner, 274
  outer, 274
  potassium secretion by, 278–279
  sodium reabsorption by, 274
  urine concentration/dilution by, 290
Medullary sponge kidney, 1794–1796, *1794*
  clinical features of, 1794–1795
  diagnosis of, 1795
  histopathology of, 1795
  hypercalcemia in, 1795
  intravenous urography of, 173, *173*
  plain film radiography of, 173, *173*
  prognosis for, 1796
  treatment of, 1795–1796
  urinary stones in, 1795
Megacalyces, *84*
Megacalycosis, 1736–1737, *1736*
  megaureter with, 1737, *1737*
Megacystis, 1983–1984
  prenatal diagnosis of, 1605, *1605*
Megalourethra, 2087, *2088*
  glans canalization in, 1583
  in prune-belly syndrome, 1920, *1921*, 1929,
    1933
  prenatal diagnosis of, 1605–1606, *1607*
Megameatus intact prepuce, 2095, 2103–2104,
  2105. See also *Hypospadias.*
Megaureter, 1829–1830, 1897–1910
  augmentation cystoplasty with, 3182–3183,
    3183
  classification of, 1829t
  definition of, 1898, *1898*
  diuretic renography in, 1901, *1903*
  evaluation of, 1901–1902, *1902, 1903*
  intravenous urography in, 1901
  megacalycosis with, 1737, *1737*
  nonrefluxing, nonobstructive, primary, 1900–
    1901, *1901, 1902,* 1903
    secondary, 1900
    pathogenesis of, 1830
  obstructive, primary, 1829, 1829t, 1899–1900,
    1899, 1900, 1903
    secondary, 1900, 1903
  pathology of, 1829–1830
  pathophysiology of, 1898–1901, *1898–1902*
  postnatal follow-up of, *1615*
  prenatal diagnosis of, 1605, *1605*
  refluxing, primary, 1898, 1902–1903
    secondary, 1898, 1903
  renal hypodysplasia and, 1762–1763, *1762*
  treatment of, 1830, 1902–1903
    surgical, 1904, 1906, *1906–1910*
  ultrasonography in, 1901, *1902, 1903*
  Whitaker's perfusion test in, 1902
Megavitamins, in bladder cancer, 2368
Megestrol acetate, in prostate cancer, 2638
Meglumine, 171
Melanoma, intratumor pressure of, 2273t
  NM23 gene in, 2276

Melanoma *(Continued)*
  of bladder, 2383
  of male genitalia, 725, 2478
Melanosis, penile, 728
Melatonin, gonadotropin secretion and,
  1240–1241
Membranous nephropathy, in children, 1678
Menarche, in blind girls, 1241
Mendel, Gregor, 3
Meningocele, 2022. See also *Myelodysplasia.*
Menkes syndrome, 1620t
Menstrual cycle, epithelial cell–bacterial
  adherence and, 546, *546*
Mental status examination, in voiding
  dysfunction, 929
2-Mercaptoethanesulfonic acid (mesna), in
  nonseminomatous germ cell neoplasm,
  2437, 2437t
  with cyclophosphamide administration, 2337
α-Mercaptopropionylglycine, in cystine calculi
  treatment, 2696
Mersilene (Dacron), for pubovaginal sling, 1105
Mesenchymal inductive mediators, in prostate
  gland growth, 1415
Mesenteric artery, 55, 57
Mesenteric vein, 58
Mesna (2-mercaptoethanesulfonic acid), in
  nonseminomatous germ cell neoplasm,
  2437, 2437t
  with cyclophosphamide administration, 2337
Mesoblastic nephroma, congenital, 1637–1638
Mesonephric (wolffian) duct, development of,
  1550, *1550, 1551,* 1589–1590, *1589*
Mesonephros, 1550, *1550, 1551,* 1655, *1656*
Mesothelioma, paratesticular, 2445
  testicular, 2442, 2443
Mesterolone, in idiopathic male infertility, 1317t,
  1318
Metabolic acidosis, 302–305
  aldosterone insufficiency in, 304
  anion gap, 302, 302t, 303t
  compensatory response to, 299t
  glomerular filtration rate in, 304–305
  hyperchloremic, 302–305, *303,* 303t
  in chronic renal failure, 335
  neonatal, 1659–1660, *1659*
  renal citrate metabolism and, 2674
  renal tubular, 303–304, *303*
  treatment of, 305
  urinary pH in, 145–146
Metal intoxication, in chronic renal failure, 331
Metal sounds, for urethral dilation, 162, *163*
Metalloproteinase inhibitors, in prostate cancer,
  2655
Metanephros, 1655–1656, *1656*
Metapyrone stimulation test, in Cushing's
  syndrome, 2928
Metastasis, 2273–2276, *2274.* See also *specific
  cancers.*
  mechanical theory of, 2274–2275
  radionuclide imaging of, 225, *226*
  seed and soil theory of, 2274–2275, *2275*
  suppression of, genes for, 2275–2276
Methacholine (Mecholyl), ureteral effects of, 850
Methantheline (Banthine), in neuropathic voiding
  dysfunction, 973
  ureteral effects of, 850
Methenamine hippurate, in urinary tract infection
  prevention, 594t
Methenamine mandelate, during pregnancy, 600
  in urinary tract infection prevention, 594t
Methotrexate, in penile carcinoma, 2475, 2476
  toxicity of, after urinary intestinal diversion,
  3154
Methoxyflurane anesthesia, in hyperoxaluria,
  2682

5-Methyl cytosine, 6, *7*
Methyl methacrylate, in retroperitoneal fibrosis,
  409, *409*
Methyldopa (Aldomet), erectile dysfunction
  with, 1171
  in retroperitoneal fibrosis, 404
Methylhistamine, in interstitial cystitis, 638t
Methylprednisolone, in septic shock, 588t
Methysergide (Sansert), in retroperitoneal
  fibrosis, 404
Metoclopramide (Reglan), in neuropathic
  voiding dysfunction, 991
Metrifonate (Bilharcil), in schistosomiasis, 747
Metronidazole, in bowel preparation, 3126,
  3127t
Metyrapone, in Cushing's syndrome, 2930
Metyrosine, in pheochromocytoma, 2956
Meyers-Kouvenaar syndrome, 760, 764–765
Micaceous growth, of penis, 2454
Michaelis-Gutmann bodies, in malacoplakia, 581
Miconazole, 798, 799t, 800t
  in candidal infection, 785
Microcoleus, restriction enzyme of, 18t
Microexplosive generator, in shock-wave
  lithotripsy, 2737
$β_2$-Microglobulin, in uremic syndrome, 335
Micropenis, 2121t, 2123–2124, *2124,* 2169,
  2169
  in pseudohermaphroditism, 2151
  prenatal diagnosis of, 1606
  vs. hypospadias, 2096
Micturition, 917–920, 919t, 926t, 1007–1010,
  1008–1011
  abnormalities of. See also *Enuresis; Inconti-
    nence; Voiding dysfunction.*
  biomechanics of, 878–879, *879*
  in benign prostatic hyperplasia, 1458–1459
  in infant, 2055–2056
  initiation of, 919
  neuropharmacology of, 890–895, *891, 892*
  pain with, 1624
  pathophysiology of, 903–906, *905,* 1008–
    1009, *1008, 1009*
  physiology of, 1007–1008, *1008*
  pressure-flow studies of, 939–944, *940–944*
  reflexes of, 895–899, *896–899,* 1007–1010,
    1008–1011
  urethral pressure studies of, *936,* 945–947,
    947
  uroflowmetric evaluation of, 937–939, 937t,
    938, 939
  voluntary initiation of, 919
Micturition diary, in incontinence evaluation,
  1020, *1021*
Micturition reflex, 895–899, *896–899,* 919,
  1007–1008, *1008*
  inhibition of, 1029–1030, *1030*
  manual initiation of, 989–990
  neurologic interruption of, 1008–1010, *1009–
    1011*
  voluntary control of, 1008, *1009*
Midbrain, 1240
Mifepristone, in Cushing's syndrome, 2930
Migraine, methysergide for, retroperitoneal
  fibrosis and, 404
Milk, urinary lithiasis and, 2665
Milk-alkali syndrome, 2680
Minerals, metabolism of, 2670–2674, *2671–2673*
Minimal change disease (nil disease), 328–329,
  1678
Minipress. See *Prazosin hydrochloride
  (Minipress).*
Minisatellite deoxyribonucleic acid, 19
Minnesota Multiphasic Personality Inventory, in
  erectile dysfunction evaluation, 1187
Minoxidil, in erectile dysfunction, 1202

Polycythemia, in Wilms' tumor, 2220
Polyethylene glycol (GoLYTELY), for bowel preparation, 3125–3126, 3126t
for urinary diversion preparation, 3250
Polyhydramnios, 1603
Polymerase, in DNA transcription, 10, *11,* 12
Polymerase chain reaction, 22–23, *22*
in prostate cancer, 2532–2533
Polyomavirus, in acute hemorrhagic cystitis, 1700
Polypropylene, for pubovaginal sling, 1105
Polyps, urethral, prostatic, 2089
Polystyrene sodium sulfonate (Kayexalate), in neonatal renal tubular acidosis, 1660
Polytetrafluoroethylene (polytef), periurethral injection of, 1110, 1116, 1118. See also *Periurethral injection therapy.*
in neuropathic voiding dysfunction, 985
in urinary incontinence, 1028
Polyuria, 134. See also *Hypernatremia.*
after ureteral obstruction release, 375–376, *376*
definition of, 376
differential diagnosis of, *378*
etiology of, 377t
evaluation of, 296, *297*
hypernatremia in, 295
neonatal, 1657, 1660–1661
nocturnal, enuresis and, 2058–2059
Polyvinyl alcohol (Ivalon), in endoscopic vesicoureteral reflux treatment, 1894
POMC (proopiomelanocortin), in ACTH production, 2920, *2920*
Pontine micturition center, 896–899, *896–899,* 1008, *1030*
Pontine-sacral reflex interaction, in myelodysplasia, 2026, *2028*
Porcine dermis, for pubovaginal sling, 1105
Post-coital test, in male infertility, 1306
Posterior urethral valves, 2069–2085
ascites in, 1638, 2073, *2074*
classification of, 2069–2072, *2070*
clinical presentation of, 2072–2074
glomerular filtration in, 2075–2076
hydronephrosis and, 1605, *1606,* 2076–2077, *2077, 2078*
pathophysiology of, 2074–2079
prenatal identification of, 1605, *1606,* 2083–2085, 2084t
prognosis for, 2085
pulmonary hypoplasia and, 2073–2074, 2084
renal dysplasia and, 2075–2076, 2085
renal hypodysplasia and, 1764, *1764*
renal tubular function and, 2076
treatment of, 2076, 2079–2083
diet in, 2076
endoscopic valve ablation in, 2080
high-loop ureterostomy in, 2080–2081, *2081*
prenatal, 2083–2085, 2084t
renal transplantation in, 2085
valve ablation in, 2079–2080, *2080*
vesicostomy in, 2081–2082, *2082–2083*
type I, 2069–2072, *2070, 2071*
valve ablation in, 2079–2080, *2080*
type II, *2070,* 2072
type III, *2070,* 2072, *2072, 2073*
type IV, 2072
ultrasonography in, 2074, *2075*
urinary incontinence and, 2077–2079
urodynamic studies in, 2077
vesical dysfunction and, 2077–2079
vesicoureteral reflux and, 1862, 2077
wind-sock membrane in, 2072, *2073*
Postpartum ovarian vein thrombophlebitis, 393
Posture, lumbar lordosis of, 89, *90*

Posture test, in primary hyperaldosteronism, 2945, *2945*
Postvoid dribble, 1019–1020, 1020t. See also *Incontinence.*
Postvoid residual urine, in benign prostatic hyperplasia, 1446–1447, 1458–1459
in geriatric incontinence, 1051
in prune-belly syndrome, 1919
intraindividual variation in, 1446
Potassium, deficiency of, after urinary intestinal diversion, 3153–3154
dietary, potassium excretion and, 279
disorders of, 280–281, 281t, *282*
extracellular, 276–277, *277*
in acid-base balance, 300
in aldosterone secretion, 2921, *2921*
in primary hyperaldosteronism, 2940, 2944, *2944, 2945*
in resting membrane potential, 840–841, *840*
intracellular shift of, 277
renal excretion of, 276–281
acid-base balance and, 279–280
after bilateral ureteral obstruction release, 373
after unilateral ureteral obstruction, 363–364
aldosterone in, 279
cortical collecting tubule in, 278, *278*
distal tubule in, 278
diuretics and, 279, *280*
flow rate in, 279
glomerular filtration in, 277
loop of Henle in, 277–278
luminal sodium supply in, 279
magnesium balance and, 280
medullary collecting tubule in, 278–279
potassium intake and, 279
proximal tubule in, 277, *278*
Potassium bicarbonate, in renal tubular acidosis, 2688
Potassium binding resins, in acute renal failure, 325
Potassium channel, of smooth muscle, 876–877
Potassium channel openers, in neuropathic voiding dysfunction, 975–976
ureteral effect of, 864
Potassium citrate, in renal tubular acidosis, 2688
in urinary lithiasis, 2712–2713
Potter facies, in bilateral renal agenesis, 1710, *1710*
Potter's syndrome, 1563
Pouches. See also *Urinary diversion, continent (intestinal).*
Florida, 3228, 3231–3233, *3233*
gastric, 3237–3238, *3237*
hemi-Kock, 3209, *3209*
ileocolonic, 3212–3213, *3212*
Indiana, 3227–3228, 3230–3233, *3231–3233*
Kock (continent ileal reservoir), 3218–3223, *3219–3222*
low-pressure, 3209–3211, *3210*
MAINZ, 3211–3212, *3211,* 3223–3225, *3224, 3226–3228*
Penn, 3233–3235, *3234*
right colon, 3213–3214, *3213*
absorbable staple technique with, 3239–3240, *3239*
with intussuscepted terminal ileum, 3225–3227, *3229–3231*
sigmoid, 3214, *3215*
UCLA, 3225–3227, *3229–3231*
vesica ileale, 3204, 3206–3207, *3207*
Pouchitis, with catheterizing pouch, 3218
Povidone-iodine wash, in urinary tract infection prevention, 594t
Prader-Willi syndrome, 1620t

Prader-Willi syndrome *(Continued)*
cryptorchidism in, 2181
male infertility in, 1309
micropenis in, 2125
Praziquantel (Biltricide), in schistosomiasis, 747
Prazosin hydrochloride (Minipress), erectile dysfunction with, 1171
in geriatric incontinence etiology, 1046t, 1047
in neuropathic voiding dysfunction, 977, 995
in pheochromocytoma, 2956
prophylactic, for postoperative urinary retention, 970
pRB, in cell cycle regulation, 2263–2264, *2264*
Precalyceal canalicular ectasia, 1794–1796, *1794*
Precipitancy, in geriatric incontinence, 1049
Precipitant leakage, in geriatric incontinence, 1049
Prednisolone, biologic activity of, 2940t
in tuberculosis, 827
Prednisone, biologic activity of, 2940t
in immune-mediated male infertility, 1316–1317
in prostate cancer, 2653t
in renal transplantation, 522, 523t
Pregnancy, after renal transplantation, 527–528
antimicrobial toxicity during, 599–600
antituberculosis drugs during, 829
bacteriuria during, 597–598, 1691–1692
bladder changes in, 597
Cushing's syndrome during, 2931, *2931*
cystitis during, 559t
ectopic, in ureteral obstruction, 396
sexually transmitted disease in, 670
glomerular filtration rate in, 597, *597*
hydroureter in, *596,* 597, 861–862
in bladder exstrophy, 1970–1971
myelodysplasia and, 2031
ovarian vein syndrome in, 392–393
pheochromocytoma in, 2949–2950
pubovaginal slings and, 1107
pyelonephritis during, 598, 1878–1879
treatment of, 560, 560t
renal artery aneurysm during, 453
renal enlargement in, 596–597
renal insufficiency and, 600–601
renal scarring during, 1879
schistosomiasis during, 749
serum creatinine in, 597, 597t
shock-wave lithotripsy contraindication in, 2739
trauma during, 3118
ureteral obstruction during, 395–396, *395*
ureteroscopy in, 2767–2768
urinary calculi in, 2720–2721
urinary tract infection during, 596–601, 1691–1692
anemia with, 599
complications of, 598–599
diagnosis of, 599
natural history of, 598
treatment of, 599–601
vesicoureteral reflux with, 1878–1879
without sperm, 1364
Pregnenolone, cholesterol conversion to, *2919*
Premature infant. See also *Neonate.*
anesthesia for, 1630
undescended testes in, 2173–2174, 2174t
Preprostatic plexus, 122, *122*
Preprostatic sphincter, 107–109, *108*
Prepuce, development of, 1584, 2095, *2095*
Preputial calculi, 2718
Preputial transverse island flap and glans channel, for hypospadias repair, 2105–2109, *2107, 2108*
Pressure-flow micturition studies, 939–944, *940,* *941*

Pseudohermaphroditism (*Continued*)
  male, 2151, 2155t, 2156
    laparoscopic diagnosis of, 2805–2806,
      2806t
    neovagina construction in, 2162, 2166–
      2168, *2166–2168*
    urethral diverticulum in, *3331*
    vs. hypospadias, 2096
Pseudohyponatremia, 292
Pseudomonas, after urinary intestinal diversion,
  3155
Pseudomonas aeruginosa, bezoar of, 2837t
Pseudomonas exotoxin, in bladder cancer,
  2367–2368
  in cancer therapy, 2278
Pseudomonas oxalitcus, in oxalate metabolism,
  2672
Pseudo–prune-belly syndrome, 1924
Pseudosarcoma, of bladder, 2339
Pseudotumor, of kidneys, 1738, *1739*
  of penis, 2454
Pseudovaginal-perineal-scrotal hypospadias, 2096
Psoas hitch, 3070–3071, *3071, 3072*
  in urinary undiversion, 3251, *3252, 3256*
  in vesicoureteral reflux, 1892, *1893*
  suture placement in, 103
Psoas muscle, *50–51*, 54, *55*
  abscess of, ureteral obstruction and, 410–411,
    411
Psoriasis, of male genitalia, *707*, 718–719
Psychologic disorders, in geriatric incontinence,
  1047
Psychologic interview, in erectile dysfunction
  evaluation, 1187
Psychologic non-neuropathic bladder,
  2045–2047, *2046*, 2047t, *2048*
Psychometry, in erectile dysfunction, 1187
Psychophysiologic testing, in erectile
  dysfunction, 1186–1187
Psychosexual history, in erectile dysfunction,
  1183, 1187
Psychosexual therapy, in erectile dysfunction,
  1200, 1200t
Psychotherapy, in erectile dysfunction, 1200
PTH. See *Parathyroid hormone (PTH)*.
Puberty, melatonin levels and, 1241
Pubes, 91
  congenital nonunion of, 91
Pubic hair, digital manipulation of, in
  neuropathic voiding dysfunction, 989–990
Pubic tubercles, 89, *90*
Pubocervical fascia, 1063
Pubococcygeus muscle, 94, *97*, 1060
Puboprostatic ligament, 98, 114, *116, 121*
Puborectalis muscle, *97*
Pubourethral ligament, *98, 99, 116*, 117, 1062
Pubovaginal sling, 1103–1107
  abdominal approach to, 1106, *1106*
  care after, 1107
  history of, 1103–1104
  in geriatric incontinence, 1055
  in neuropathic voiding dysfunction, 985
  in stress incontinence, 1027, 1028
  indications for, 1103–1105
  intermittent catheterization after, 1105
  materials for, 1105
  pregnancy and, 1107
  preoperative antimicrobials for, 1106
  preoperative preparation for, 1105–1106
  technique of, 1106–1107, *1106, 1107*
  thromboembolic prophylaxis with, 1106
  vaginal approach to, 1106–1107, *1106, 1107*
Pubovesical ligament, 98
Pubovisceral hiatus, 94–95
Pubovisceral muscle, 117
Pudendal artery, 119, *119*, 1159, *1160*, 2566,
  3321–3322, *3322*

Pudendal artery (*Continued*)
  accessory, 120, *121*
  internal, 100
  trauma to, 3368–3369
Pudendal nerve, *61*, 104, 114, 119, *119*, 2569,
  3324, *3325*
  interruption of, in neuropathic voiding dysfunc-
    tion, 999–1000
  stimulation of, detrusor inhibition and, 929–
    1030, *1031*
Pudendal vein, 119
Puerperal septic pelvic vein thrombophlebitis,
  393
Pulmonary disease, erectile dysfunction with,
  1172
Pulmonary edema, in renovascular hypertension,
  434
Pulmonary embolism, gas, during laparoscopy,
  2905
  in postpartum ovarian vein thrombophlebitis,
    393
  in radical prostatectomy, 2554–2555
Purine, dietary, in hyperuricosuria, 2683, 2684
  in urinary lithiasis treatment, 2732
  urinary lithiasis and, 2665
Pustule, 718
P21/WAF1 gene, 2266, *2266*
Pyelography, antegrade, 243, *243*
  in tuberculosis, 822
  in upper tract urothelial tumors, 2389
  intravenous. See *Urography, intravenous*.
  retrograde, 167–169, 177, 179, 181, *188*
    complications of, 179
    contraindications to, 179, 181
    contrast extravasation with, 179
    in preureteral vena cava, *1851*
    in retroperitoneal fibrosis, 406, *407*
    in tuberculosis, 822
    in upper tract urothelial tumors, 2389
    in ureterocele, *1832*
    in ureteropelvic junction obstruction, *188*
    in urinary lithiasis, 2702
    in Wilms' tumor, 2221
    indications for, 167
    patient preparation for, 167
    technique of, 167–168, *168*, 179
    ureteral stents in, 168–169, *168*
Pyelolithotomy, coagulum, 3028, 3028t, 3030,
  3030, 3030t
  extended, 3028, *3029*
  laparoscopic, 2887
  standard, 3024–3025, *3027*, 3028
Pyelolysis, 2844
Pyelonephritis, 568–573
  acute, 568–570. See also *Urinary tract infec-
    tion*.
    angiography in, 569
    bacteriology of, 568–569
    clinical presentation of, 568
    computed tomography in, 217, 220, *221*,
      569
    definition of, 534
    during pregnancy, 598, 599
    in acute renal failure, 319
    intravenous urography in, 177, 569
    laboratory findings in, 568
    pathology of, 569
    radiographic findings in, 569
    treatment of, 560, 560t, 569–570, *570*
      in women, 560, 560t
    ultrasonography in, 204, 569
    vs. perinephric abscess, 578–579
  after ureterointestinal anastomoses, 3145
  after urinary intestinal diversion, 3155
  bacterial ascent in, 540
  Candida in, 782

Pyelonephritis (*Continued*)
  chronic, 570–573
    clinical presentation of, 572
    definition of, 534
    immune system in, 570–571
    in chronic renal failure, 331
    intravenous urography in, 572
    laboratory findings in, 572
    pathogenesis of, 570–571
    pathology of, 572
    radiologic findings in, 572
    reflux nephropathy in, 571
    sequelae of, 572–573
    voiding cystourethrography in, 572
  cryptococcal, 789
  during pregnancy, 1691–1692, 1878–1879
  emphysematous, 573–574
    clinical presentation of, 573
    in diabetes mellitus, 568, 573–574, *573*
    management of, 573–574
    radiologic findings in, 573, *573*
  Escherichia coli in, 1873–1874
  immunoglobulin response in, 551
  in Ask-Upmark kidney development, 1762
  in pediatric urinary tract infection, 1683–1684
  radionuclide imaging in, 227–229, *228, 229*
  renal failure and, 1875–1876
  schistosomiasis with, 756
  ultrasonography in, 203, 204, 569, 915
  ureteral peristalsis in, 860
  vesicoureteral reflux in, 1872–1874, *1874*
  xanthogranulomatous, 579–581
    bacteriology of, 580
    clinical presentation of, 579–580
    pathogenesis of, 579
    pathology of, 579
    radiologic findings in, 220, 580, *580*
    treatment of, 580–581
Pyeloplasty, 3041–3048
  Culp-DeWeerd, 3046, *3047*
  dismembered, 3044–3045, *3044, 3045*
  failure of, 3048–3049
  Foley Y-V, 3045–3046, *3046*
  history of, 3043–3044
  laparoscopic, 2887
    in children, 2900
    in infant, 2897
  principles of, 3041–3043, *3043*
  Scardino-Prince, 3046–3048, *3047*
Pyelostomy, cutaneous, in prune-belly syndrome,
  1927
Pyelotomy, slash, after ureteropelvic junction
  obstruction repair, 3043
Pyeloureterography, antegrade, in retroperitoneal
  fibrosis, 406
Pygeum africanum, in benign prostatic
  hyperplasia, 1472
Pyloric stenosis, hypertrophic, in autosomal
  dominant polycystic kidney disease,
  1771–1772
  ureteropelvic junction obstruction in, 1567
Pyocalyx, misdiagnosis of, 2801, *2802*
  percutaneous drainage of, 2801, *2802*
Pyoderma gangrenosum, of male genitalia, *716*,
  723
Pyonephrosis, 576, *576*
  percutaneous drainage of, 2801
  with percutaneous nephrostomy, 246
Pyospermia, in infertility, 1300, *1300*
Pyrazinamide, hepatotoxicity of, 829
  hypersensitivity reactions to, 829t
  in tuberculosis, 825
  side effects of, 829
Pyridium test, of vaginal drainage, 1136
Pyridoxine, in hyperoxaluria, 2681–2682
Pyrotech, in benign prostatic hyperplasia,
  1481–1482

Pyuria, 145
  definition of, 534
  in urinary tract infection, 547–548

Q-tip test, of urethral hypermobility, 1022, 1051
Quinolones, in urinary tract infection, 555t

Race, prostate cancer and, 2493, *2493*
Radiation, protection from, 241–242
Radiation pneumonitis, in prostate cancer, 2614
Radiation sensitizers, in bladder cancer
    treatment, 2372
Radiation therapy, basic fibroblast growth factor
    prophylaxis in, 2273
  in bladder cancer, 2361–2362, 2371–2373,
    2381
  in bladder cancer etiology, 2337
  in female urethral cancer, 3407–3408
  in male urethral cancer, 3404
  in metastasis-related spinal cord compression,
    2613
  in neuroblastoma, 2239
  in penile cancer, 2464–2467, 2466t, 2475,
    2476
  in Peyronie's disease, 3380
  in prostate cancer, 2560, 2605–2616. See also
    *Prostate cancer, treatment of, radiation
    therapy in.*
  in renal cell carcinoma, 2309, 2312
  in rhabdomyosarcoma, 2243–2244
  in upper tract urothelial tumors, 2394
  in Wilms' tumor, 2225, 2227, 2228–2229
  male infertility and, 1315
  penile injury during, 3341
  salvage cystectomy with, in bladder cancer,
    2372–2373
  systemic, in prostate cancer, 2614–2616,
    2614t, 2615t
  ureteral obstruction and, 409–410
  urethral injury during, 3341
  vesicovaginal fistula and, 1141
Radiculitis, 139
Radioimmunoassay, in urinary tract infection,
    551
Radiology. See *Uroradiology.*
Radionuclide imaging, 224–229, *226–229*
  adrenal masses on, 236
  in bladder cancer, 2360
  in epididymitis, 229, *230*
  in erectile dysfunction, 1196
  in extrinsic ureteral obstruction, 388
  in neurourologic evaluation, 931
  in prostate cancer, 2530–2531
  in pyelonephritis, 226, 227–229, *228, 229*
  in renal infection, 227–229, *228, 229*
  in renal transplantation, 225–226, 227, *228*
  in renovascular hypertension, 226–227
  in scrotal evaluation, 229, *230*
  in skeletal metastases, 225, *226*
  in testicular torsion, 229, *230*
  in urinary tract infection, 553–554
  in vesicoureteral reflux, 229, *229*, 1869–1870,
    1870
Radionuclide therapy, in prostate cancer,
    2614–2616, 2614t, 2615t
Randolph abdominoplasty, in prune-belly
    syndrome, 1936–1937
Rapamycin (sirolimus), *495*
  immunosuppressive activity of, 496–497, 496t
Ras oncogene, in prostate cancer, 2491
Rathke's plicae, 1570, *1571*
Raz needle bladder neck suspension, in stress
    urinary incontinence, 1069–1071, *1070*

Raz vaginal wall sling, in stress urinary
    incontinence, 1072–1075, *1072, 1073*
Rb gene, 1416
  in bladder cancer, 2333, 2351
  in prostate cancer, 2491
  in tumor suppressor gene replacement therapy,
    2267–2268
  mutation in, 2264–2265
Rb protein, inhibition of, 2264–2265
Receptor(s), alpha-adrenergic, of prostate gland,
    1388
  of ureter, 850–851
  beta-adrenergic, of ureter, 850–851
  androgen, embryologic development of, 1407
    gene for, 1406–1408, *1407*
    of prostate gland, 1406–1408, *1407*
    variable response to, 1408
  cholinergic, of bladder, 881–882, *881, 882*
    of corpus cavernosa, 1164
    of prostate gland, 1388
    of ureter, 849–850
  estrogen, in urogenital sinus development,
    1587
    of bladder, 889
    of prostate gland, 1405–1406, 1434
  for angiotensin I, 432
  for angiotensin II, 354, *430*, 432
  for atrial natriuretic peptide, 268, 355
  for endothelin, 267–268, *267*, 356
  for platelet activating factor, 356
  for prostanoids, 353
  for thromboxane A₂, 353
  for vasopressin, 268
  opiate, 893
Rectal artery, 100, *119*
Rectal bladder urinary diversion, 3194–3201,
    3196–3198, 3200, 3201
Rectal nerve, *119*
Rectal prolapse, in bladder exstrophy, 1945
Rectal veins, 119
Rectocele, 1075v
  treatment of, 1080–1081, *1081*
Rectogenital septum (Denonvilliers' fascia), 91,
    95
Rectourethralis muscle, 106, *118*
Rectouterine pouch (of Douglas), 98, 104, *106,
    107*
Rectovaginal septum, 116, *116*
Rectovesical pouch, 104
Rectum, anatomy of, 91, 104–106, *104, 106, 116*
  in cloacal malformations, 1993, *1995*
  cancer of, after ureterosigmoidostomy, 3195
  digital stimulation of, in neuropathic voiding
    dysfunction, 989–990
  examination of, in female, 142
    in male, 141–142
    in male infertility, 1291
    in neurourologic evaluation, 930
    in urinary incontinence, 1022
  injury to, during radical perineal prostatec-
    tomy, 2603
  malformation of, prenatal diagnosis of, 1606,
    1610
  schistosomiasis of, 756
  valved, augmented, for continent urinary diver-
    sion, 3195, 3198, *3198*
    hemi-Kock procedure with, for continent uri-
    nary diversion, 3198–3199, *3200*
Rectus abdominis muscle, 92, 93
  hematoma of, ureteral obstruction and, 411
Rectus abdominis musculocutaneous flap, in
    inguinal reconstruction, 2477, *2478*
Rectus fascia, for pubovaginal sling, 1105
Rectus sheath, 91, 92
  anterior, 91, *93*
  cross section of, *93*

Rectus sheath (*Continued*)
  posterior, 91, 93, *93*
Red blood cells, dysmorphic, 1671, *1671, 1672*
  in hematuria, 147, 1671, *1671, 1672*, 1673,
    1675–1677
  eumorphic, 1671
  in hematuria, 1671, 1673
  in urine, 154, *154*, 1670–1671, *1671, 1672.*
    See also *Hematuria.*
  oxalate exchange of, 2683
5α-Reductase, deficiency of, in male
    pseudohermaphroditism, 2151
  in benign prostatic hyperplasia, 1434
  in DHT production, 1404–1405, *1404*, 1404t
  isozymes of, 1404–1405, 1404t
5α-Reductase inhibitor, in geriatric incontinence,
    1055
Reflectance analysis, infrared, of urinary calculi,
    2704
Reflex sympathetic dystrophy, in interstitial
    cystitis, 640
Reflux, after transurethral ejaculatory duct
    resection, 1359
  prenatal diagnosis of, 1605, *1605*
  vesicoureteral, 1859–1897. See also *Vesicoure-
    teral reflux.*
Reflux nephropathy, 571, 1678
  in children, 1871–1876, 1871t, *1872–1875.*
    See also *Vesicoureteral reflux.*
  in chronic renal failure, 331
Regitine. See *Phentolamine methylate (Regitine).*
Reglan (metoclopramide), in neuropathic voiding
    dysfunction, 991
Reifenstein syndrome (type I pseudo-
    hermaphroditism), *vs.* hypospadias, 2096
Reiter's syndrome, 712, 719, 3327–3328
Renal artery(ies), 55, *56*, 74–76, 75–77, 238–239
  accessory, 1731, *1733*
    in congenital ureteropelvic junction obstruc-
    tion, 1743
  accidental ligation of, *225*
  aneurysm of, 452–453, *453*, 461–462
    acquired, 1733
    classification of, 1733
    congenital, 1731, 1733–1734
    dissecting, 461, *462*
    during pregnancy, 453
    extracorporeal shock-wave lithotripsy and,
    2745
    fusiform, 461, *462*
    intrarenal, 462, *463*
    resection of, 452, 453, *453*
    rupture of, 452, 453
    saccular, 461, *461*
    treatment of, 452, 453, *453*, 462
      autotransplantation in, 482–484, *483–486*
  anterior branches of, *74*, 75, *75*
  atheromatous plaque of, 427, *427*
  atherosclerosis of, *426*, 426t, 427, *427*. See
    also *Renovascular hypertension.*
  aortorenal bypass graft for, 476–479, *477–
    479*
  chronic renal failure and, 332
  endarterectomy for, 473–476, *474, 475*
  nonsignificant, 425–426, *425*
  percutaneous atherectomy for, 488
  percutaneous transluminal angioplasty for,
    487–488, *488*
  renal autotransplantation in, 482–484, *484–
    486*
  renal stent for, 488, *488*
  splenorenal bypass graft for, 479–480, *480*
  branches of, 1731, *1731*, 1732t
  cholesterol embolism of, 449, 449t
  congenital anomalies of, 1730–1734, *1731,
    1732*, 1732t, *1733*

Seminal plasma *(Continued)*
  prostate-specific protein–94 of, 1395
  prostatic acid phosphatase of, 1394–1395
  proteolytic enzymes of, 1396
  spermidine of, 1391
  spermine of, 1391
  transferrin of, 1396
  zinc of, 1392–1393
  Zn-α2-glycoprotein of, 1395
Seminal vesicle(s), abscess of, 3306
    transurethral resection in, 3308
  adenocarcinoma of, 3307
  agenesis of, 3305
  amyloid of, 3307
  anatomy of, *96, 103, 106, 112,* 114, 1385–
    1386, 3301
  aplasia of, ultrasonography of, 3302
  atrophy of, ultrasonography of, 3302
  calculi of, 2717, 3306
  clusterin in, 357
  computed tomography of, 3303, *3303*
  congenital cystic dilatation of, ultrasonography
    of, *210*
  cystadenoma of, 3307
  cysts of, 3302–3311
    computed tomography of, 3303, *3303*
    treatment of, 3307–3311
      paravesical approach in, 3311
      percutaneous drainage in, 3307
      retrovesical approach in, 3311, *3312*
      transperineal approach in, 3309–3310,
        3309
      transurethral resection in, 3308
      ultrasound-guided aspiration in, 3309
    ultrasonography of, 3302
    ureteral drainage to, 1574–1575
    vasography of, 3304–3305, *3304*
  development of, 1586, 3299–3301, *3300*
  developmental anomalies of, 3299, 3301
  epithelium of, 1385–1386
  fructose formation in, 1390–1391
  hydatid cysts of, 3307–3308
  infection of, 628, 3305–3306
  innervation of, 3301
  laparoscopic approach to, 2887
  layers of, 1386
  lymphoma of, 3303, *3303*
  magnetic resonance imaging of, *234,* 3303–
    3304, *3304*
  masses of, 3306–3307
  normal, *207, 209*
  obstruction of, 3305, *3305*
  papillary adenoma of, 3307
  physical examination of, 3301–3305, *3301*
  physiology of, 3301
  prostaglandins of, 1392
  radiography of, 1338
  sarcoma of, 3307
  schistosomiasis of, 749
  secretory proteins of, 1396
  species variation in, 1385
  surgical approaches to, 3308–3312
    laparoscopic, 3308–3309
    open, 3309–3312, *3309, 3310, 3312, 3313*
    paravesical, 3311
    retrovesical, 3311, *3312*
    transcoccygeal, 3311–3312, *3313*
    transperineal, 3309–3310, *3309*
    transvesical, 3310–3311, *3310*
  tumors of, 3307–3308
    computed tomography of, 3303, *3303*
    magnetic resonance imaging of, 3303–3304
    treatment of, 3308
      transperineal approach in, 3309–3310,
        3309
    ultrasonography of, 3302–3303

Seminal vesicle(s) *(Continued)*
  ultrasonography of, *207, 209,* 3302–3303,
    3302
  vasculature of, 3301
  vasography of, 3304–3305, *3304*
  weight of, 1384
Seminiferous tubules, 123, *124,* 1258–1262
  blood-testis barrier of, 1261–1262, *1262*
  epithelium of, 1263–1266
  gonocytes of, 1264–1265
  peritubular structures of, 1259, *1260*
  Sertoli cell of, 1259–1261, *1261*
  structure of, 1255, *1255, 1256*
Seminogelin, 1396
Seminoma, 2247, 2413t, 2424–2428. See also
  Testis (testes), seminoma of.
  retroperitoneal, 2438–2439
Senior-Loken syndrome, 1775
Sensory examination, in voiding dysfunction,
  929, *930*
Sepsis, 583–587, 583t. See also *Septic shock.*
  after intestinal anastomoses, 3133
  after percutaneous nephrostolithotomy, 2816–
    2817
  after percutaneous nephrostomy, 249
  after ureterointestinal anastomoses, 3145
  after urinary intestinal diversion, 3155
Septic shock, 583–587, 583t
  bacterial cell-wall components in, 584
  bacteriology of, 586, 586t
  clinical presentation of, 585–586
  cytokines in, 584–585, *585*
  endotoxin antibodies in, 584
  management of, 586–587, 587t
  pathophysiology of, 584–585, *584*
  treatment of, *585,* 588
Seromuscular enterocystoplasty, 3185–3186,
  3185
Seromyotomy, laparoscopic, for
  autoaugmentation cystoplasty, 3184
Serotonergic drugs, in erectile dysfunction, 1202
Serotonin, bladder effects of, 883t, 888, 891–892
  in gonadotropin-releasing hormone regulation,
    1241, 1242
  in retroperitoneal fibrosis, 404
  in sexual function, 1166, 1167
  of prostate gland, 1387
Serratia, in sepsis, 586, 586t
Sertoli cell(s), 1259–1261, *1261*
  estrogen effects on, 1261
  germ cell associations of, 1262–1263, *1263*
  P-Mod-S factor effects on, 1259
  secretory products of, 1259–1261
  tight junctions of, 1261–1262, *1262*
Sertoli cell tumors, 2248, 2440–2441
Sertoli cell–only syndrome, male infertility and,
  1314
  testicular biopsy in, 1304, *1304*
Sex accessory tissues. See *Bulbourethral glands;*
  Prostate gland; Seminal vesicle(s).
Sex assignment, by fetal ultrasonography, 1603
Sex cord–mesenchyme tumors, 2439–2441
Sex reversal syndrome, male infertility in,
  1311–1312
Sex therapy, in erectile dysfunction, 1200
Sex workers, human immunodeficiency virus in,
  695
Sexual abuse, examination for, *1626,* 1627
Sexual function. See also *Erectile dysfunction;*
  Erection.
  after radical prostatectomy, 2577, 2586–2587
  in Peyronie's disease, 3377, 3379
  myelodysplasia and, 2031
Sexual infantilism, 2153, *2153*
Sexual stimulation testing, in erectile
  dysfunction, 1186–1187

Sexually transmitted diseases, 663–680, 664t.
  See also specific diseases.
  contact tracing in, 665
  in acquired immunodeficiency syndrome, 696,
    698
  in urethral syndrome, 653, 654
  incidence of, 664–665
  patient history in, 663–664
  treatment of, in women, 670
Sézary syndrome, 725
Sheath of Waldeyer, 109–110, *109*
Shigella, 664t
Shock, septic, 583–587. See also *Septic shock.*
Shock-wave lithotripsy (SWL), 2735–2749
  abdominal aortic aneurysm and, 2745
  administration of, 2744
  after renal transplantation, 526
  bioeffects of, 2739
  bleeding with, 2743
  cardiac pacemakers and, 2745–2746
  care after, 2745
  cavitation component of, 2738–2739, *2738*
  coagulopathy and, 2739
  complications of, 2742–2743
  compressive component of, 2738, *2738*
  contraindications to, 2721, 2739–2740, 2815
  cost-effectiveness of, 2815
  Direx Tripter X-1 lithotriptor for, 2748
  Dornier HM-3 lithotriptor for, 2746, *2746,*
    2746t
  Dornier HM-4 lithotriptor for, 2746, 2746t
  Dornier MPL-5000 lithotriptor for, 2747, *2748*
  Dornier MPL-9000 lithotriptor for, 2747
  DP-1 lithotriptor for, 2748
  EDAP LT lithotriptor for, 2749
  electrohydraulic generator in, 2736, *2736,*
    2736t
  electromagnetic generator in, 2736–2737,
    2736t, *2737*
  electromagnetic lithotriptors for, 2748–2749
  failure of, 2813
  fluoroscopy for, 2737, 2737t, 2744
  gastrointestinal effects of, 2739, 2743
  hypertension and, 2739–2740, 2743
  in bladder calculi, 2742
  in calyceal calculi, 2740–2741
  in calyceal diverticula calculi, 2741
  in children, 2745
  in distal ureteral calculi, 2742
  in horseshoe kidneys, 2745, 2827, 2828t
  in midureteral calculi, 2741–2742
  in misdiagnosed pyocalyx, 2801, *2802*
  in pelvic kidneys, 2745
  in proximal ureteral calculi, 2741
  in renal insufficiency, 2826–2827
  in renal pelvic calculi, 2741
  in staghorn calculi, 2741
  in struvite calculi, 563–564, 2693, 2694t
  in ureteral calculi, 2741–2742, *2763,* 2776–
    2777, *2781,* 2823, 2824, 2825
    vs. transurethral ureteroscopy, 2761–2762,
      2762, 2763
  indications for, 2810, 2813
  laser, in bladder calculi treatment, 1526
    in ureteral calculi treatment, 2777, 2779,
      2824
  lithotriptors for, 2746–2748, 2746t, *2747,*
    2748, 2749, 2749t
  mechanisms of, 2738–2739, *2738*
  Medstone STS lithotriptor for, 2746t, 2747
  microexplosive generator in, 2737
  mortality rate with, 2743
  Northgate SD-3 lithotriptor for, 2748
  obesity and, 2746
  ovarian effects of, 2740
  pain after, 2745

Shock-wave lithotripsy (SWL) (Continued)
  patient positioning for, 2744
  patient preparation for, 2743–2744, 2743t
  percutaneous nephrostomy with, 246–247, 248
  piezoelectric generator in, 2736t, 2737, 2737
  piezoelectric lithotriptor for, 2749
  pneumatic, in ureteral calculi treatment, 2780,
    2824–2825, 2826
  pregnancy and, 2739
  pulmonary effects of, 2739
  radiography for, 2737, 2737t
  renal artery aneurysm and, 2745
  renal effects of, 2739
  results of, 2810, 2813, 2814t, 2815
  Richard Wolf Piezolith lithotriptor for, 2749
  shock wave generation in, 2736–2737, 2736t
  Siemens Lithostar lithotriptor for, 2748–2749
  spalling process of, 2738, 2738
  steinstrasse after, 2742
  stone size and, 2740
  stone type and, 2740, 2740t
  Storz Modulith lithotriptor for, 2749
  Technomed Sonolith 3000 lithotriptor for,
    2746t, 2747–2748
  tensile component of, 2738, 2738
  Therasonics Lithotripsy System for, 2749
  ultrasonography for, 2737–2738, 2737t, 2744
  urinary tract infection and, 2740
  urinary tract obstruction and, 2740
Shorr regimen, in urinary lithiasis, 2733
Short gut syndrome, in cloacal exstrophy, 1973
Short Marital Adjustment Test, in erectile
  dysfunction evaluation, 1187
Shy-Drager syndrome, voiding dysfunction in,
  955t, 957–958
  vs. Parkinson's disease, 958
Sialic acid, of epididymal fluid, 1276
Sialidase, in urinary lithiasis, 2670
Sickle-cell anemia, chronic renal failure in, 332
  priapism in, 1172–1173, 1208
Sickle-cell nephropathy, 1676
Siemens Lithostar lithotriptor, 2748–2749
Sigma rectum pouch, for continent urinary
  diversion, 3199, 3201, 3201
Sigmoid colon, for vaginal replacement,
  2167–2168, 2167, 2168
Sigmoid cystoplasty, 3173, 3175
Sigmoid neobladder, absorbable staple technique
  with, 3240, 3241
Sigmoid pouch, for orthotopic voiding
  diversions, 3214, 3215
Signal transduction, 42–44
  calcium-specific binding proteins in, 44, 44t
  diacylglycerol in, 43–44, 44
  in antiallograft response, 493–494, 494t
  inositol lipids in, 43–44, 44
  nuclear hormone receptors in, 44
Sildenafil (phosphodiesterase inhibitor), in
  erection enhancement, 1167
Silicate calculi, 2697
Silicone, in endoscopic vesicoureteral reflux
  treatment, 1894
Silicone balloon, in endoscopic vesicoureteral
  reflux treatment, 1894–1895, 1895
Silicone polymers, for periurethral injection
  therapy, 1111, 1116
Silver nitrate, intravesical, in interstitial cystitis,
  648
Sinequan (doxepin), in geriatric incontinence,
  1054, 1054t
  in neuropathic voiding dysfunction, 978
Single potential analysis of cavernous electrical
  activity, in erectile dysfunction evaluation,
  1189
Single-photon emission computerized
  tomography, in vesicoureteral reflux,
  1869–1870, 1870

Sinus, urachal, external, 1986, 1986
Sipple's syndrome, 2950–2951
Siroky nomogram, for uroflowmetry, 938
Sirolimus (rapamycin), immunosuppressive
  activity of, 496–497, 496t
  structure of, 495
Sjögren's syndrome, interstitial cystitis and, 635
Skeletal radiography, in prostate cancer, 2530
Skene's glands, 117
Skin, blood supply to, 3317
  candidal infection of, 780, 780
  grafts of, 3317–3319, 3318
  Histoplasma lesions of, 793
  layers of, 3317
  parastomal, lesions of, 3137
  radiation injury to, 241–242
  schistosomiasis of, 757
  sympathetic response of, in erectile dysfunc-
    tion evaluation, 1189
Skin diseases, of external genitalia, 717–730.
  See also specific diseases.
Skin graft, split-thickness, for neovagina
  construction, 2162, 2166–2167, 2166
Skin tag, 729
Sleep, enuresis and, 2057–2058, 2058t. See also
  Enuresis, nocturnal.
  imipramine effects on, 2063
  vasopressin secretion and, 2058
Sling procedure. See Pubovaginal sling.
SLT 7 laser fiber, in benign prostatic
  hyperplasia, 1488
Small bowel, 3122–3123. See also Urinary
  diversion, continent (intestinal).
  blood supply to, 3124
  obstruction of, in transabdominal lymph node
    dissection, 3426
Small bowel anastomoses, Bricker technique of,
  3139t, 3141, 3141
  Hammock technique of, 3143
  LeDuc technique of, 3139t, 3142–3143, 3143
  split-nipple technique of, 3139t, 3142, 3142
  tunneled, 3142, 3142
  Wallace technique of, 3139t, 3141–3142, 3141
Small capacity hypertonic bladder, 2041–2042,
  2041, 2042
Small-cell carcinoma, of bladder, 2381–2382
  of prostate gland, 2503, 2503
Smith-Lemli-Opitz syndrome, 1620t
Smoking, in patient history, 138
Smooth muscle, 874–878, 874t, 875
  actin of, 875–876, 875
  anatomy of, 839–840
  calcium channels of, 876
  contractile activity of, 843–847, 844–847
  electrical activity of, 840–843, 840–843, 877
  energetics of, 877
  force-length relations of, 847–848, 848
  force-velocity relations of, 848, 849
  gap junctions of, 875
  hysteresis of, 848, 848
  mechanical properties of, 847–849, 848, 849
  myosin of, 875–876, 875
  potassium channels of, 876–877
  pressure-length-diameter relations of, 848–
    849, 849
  stress relaxation of, 848, 848
  stretch-activated channels of, 877
Snake venom, converting enzyme inhibiting
  action of, 433, 438
Snap gauge, in erectile dysfunction, 1185–1186
Sodium, angiotensin II effect on, 432
  dietary, in renal hypercalciuria, 2676
    in renin secretion, 432
    in urinary lithiasis treatment, 2709
  disorders of metabolism of. See Hyperna-
    tremia; Hyponatremia.

Sodium (Continued)
  in action potential, 841
  in resting membrane potential, 840, 841
  luminal concentration of, in renal potassium
    excretion, 279
  plasma osmolality and, 287, 287t
  renal excretion of, angiotensin II in, 275, 432
    fetal, 1656
    in acute renal failure, 323–324
    neonatal, 1657, 1659
  renal reabsorption of, 272–274
    at cortical collecting duct, 273, 273, 274
    at loop of Henle, 272–273, 272, 273
    at medullary collecting tubule, 274
    at proximal tubule, 270, 272
    in primary hyperaldosteronism, 2940
  urinary, fetal, 1657
    neonatal, 1659
Sodium acid urate, in calcium oxalate calculi
  formation, 2683
Sodium bicarbonate, in uric acid calculi
  treatment, 2690
Sodium cellulose phosphate, in urinary lithiasis
  treatment, 2712
Sodium nitroprusside, in erectile dysfunction,
  1205
Sodium pentosan polysulfate, in interstitial
  cystitis, 647
Sodium polystyrene sulfonate (Kayexalate), in
  acute renal failure, 325
Sodium potassium citrate, in urinary lithiasis
  treatment, 2712–2713
Sodium wasting nephropathy, after ureteral
  obstruction release, 376
Sodium-loading tests, in primary
  hyperaldosteronism, 2945–2946
Somatostatin, bladder effect of, 884, 887
Sonoblate Probe, in benign prostatic hyperplasia,
  1480–1482, 1480, 1481
Southern blotting, 15–18, 17
SPACE (single potential analysis of cavernous
  electrical activity), in erectile dysfunction
  evaluation, 1189
Space of Retzius, 99, 107
Spasticity, baclofen treatment of, 997–998
Specific gravity, urinary, in neurourologic
  evaluation, 931
Spectroscopy, infrared, of urinary calculi,
  2703–2704
Sperm. See Spermatozoon (spermatozoa).
Sperm granuloma, 1344
  with vasectomy, 1343–1344
  with vasography, 1338
Sperm motility–inhibiting factor, of epididymal
  fluid, 1276
Sperm penetration assay, in male infertility, 1307
Sperm survival factor, of epididymal fluid, 1276
Spermatic artery, 50–51, 57, 1256
Spermatic cord, 123
  examination of, 141
  leiomyosarcoma of, 2446–2447
  liposarcoma of, 2447
  mesenchymal tumors of, 2445–2447
  rhabdomyosarcoma of, 2446
Spermatic fascia, 122, 123, 123
Spermatic veins, balloon occlusion of, for
  varicocele, 1370
Spermatocele, alloplastic, 1363
  autogenous, 1362–1363, 1362
  resection of, 1354
Spermatocelectomy, 1354
Spermatocytes, blood-testis barrier migration by,
  1261–1262, 1262
  primary, 1264, 1264, 1265, 1266
  secondary, 1264, 1264, 1266
  Sertoli cell associations with, 1262–1263,
    1263

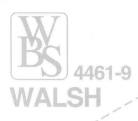

WBS 4461-9

WALSH

ISBN 0-7216-4464-3

90038

9 780721 644646